DeLee & Drez's

Orthopaedic
Sports Medicine

DeLee & Drez's
Orthopaedic Sports Medicine

PRINCIPLES AND PRACTICE

Volume Two

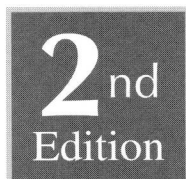

Jesse C. DeLee, MD
Clinical Professor of Orthopaedics
Director, University of Texas
Health Sciences Center at San Antonio
Sports Medicine Fellowship Program
San Antonio, Texas

David Drez Jr., MD
Clinical Professor of Orthopaedics
Head, Louisiana State University Knee and
Sports Medicine Fellowship Program
Lake Charles, Louisiana

Associate Editor:
Mark D. Miller, MD
Associate Professor of Orthopaedic Surgery
Co-Director, Division of Sports Medicine
University of Virginia
Charlottesville, Virginia

SAUNDERS
An Imprint of Elsevier

SAUNDERS
An Imprint of Elsevier
The Curtis Center
Independence Square West
Philadelphia, PA 19106

Notice

Orthopaedic sports medicine is an ever-changing field. Standard safety precautions must be followed, but as new research and clinical experience broaden our knowledge, changes in treatment and drug therapy may become necessary or appropriate. Readers are advised to check the most current product information provided by the manufacturer of each drug to be administered to verify the recommended dose, the method and duration of administration, and contraindications. It is the responsibility of the treating physician, relying on experience and knowledge of the patient, to determine dosages and the best treatment for each individual patient. Neither the Publisher nor the editor assumes any liability for any injury and/ or damage to persons or property arising from this publication.

The Publisher

First Edition 1994.

Mayo Foundation retains copyright of illustrations to the following chapters: 23A, 23B, 23F1, 23G1, 23H, 23I1, and 23J.

Library of Congress Cataloging-in-Publication Data

DeLee & Drez's orthopaedic sports medicine; principles and practice/[edited by] Jesse C. DeLee, David Drez, Jr. ; associate editor, Mark D. Miller.—2nd ed.
    p. ; cm.
  Includes bibliographical references and index.
  ISBN-13: 978-0-7216-8845-9 (set)   ISBN-10: 0-7216-8845-4 (set)
    1. Sports injuries. 2. Orthopedic emergencies. 3. Sports medicine. I. Title:
Orthopaedic sports medicine. II. DeLee, Jesse. III. Drez, David. IV. Miller, Mark D.
  [DNLM: 1. Athletic Injuries. 2. Orthopedics. 3. Sports Medicine. QT 260 D346 2002]
  RD97 .D455 2002
  617.1'027—dc21   2001032001

set ISBN-13: 978-0-7216-8845-9
set ISBN-10: 0-7216-8845-4
VOL.1: Part No. 9997635175
VOL.2: Part No. 9997635183

Editor-in-Chief: Andrew Stevenson
Acquisitions Editor: Richard Lampert
Developmental Editors: Melissa Dudlick, Hilarie Surrena
Project Manager: Linda Van Pelt
Book Designer: Andrew Johnson

MC/MVY
Printed in the United States of America.

Last digit is the print number: 9 8 7 6 5 4

We dedicate these volumes
to our wives,
Anne and Judy,
to our families who support us,
and to all our teachers
past and present.
J.D., D.D.

To my children,
each an outstanding athlete
in their own right,
with a promise that I will become
a better fan.
M.M.

CONTRIBUTORS

Karim Abdollahi, MD
Instructor of Orthopaedics, Department of Orthopaedic Surgery, Loma Linda University School of Medicine; Orthopaedic Surgeon, Loma Linda University Medical Center, Loma Linda, California
Thoracic Outlet Syndrome

P. David Adelson, MD, FACS, FAAP
Associate Professor of Neurosurgery, University of Pittsburgh School of Medicine; Director, Pediatric Neurotrauma, and Associate Director, Trauma and Trauma Research, Children's Hospital of Pittsburgh, Pittsburgh, Pennsylvania
Pediatric Sports-Related Head Injuries

John P. Albright, MD
Professor, Department of Orthopaedic Surgery, University of Iowa College of Medicine; Director, Sports Medicine Services, University of Iowa Hospitals & Clinics, Iowa City, Iowa
The Use of Knee Braces in Sports Medicine

David B. Allen, MD
Professor of Pediatrics, University of Wisconsin Medical School; Director of Endocrinology and Residency Training, University of Wisconsin Children's Hospital, Madison, Wisconsin
Diabetes Mellitus

Louis C. Almekinders, MD
Professor, Department of Orthopaedics, University of North Carolina at Chapel Hill School of Medicine, Chapel Hill, North Carolina
Muscle and Tendon

John L. Andary, MD, MBA
Idaho Falls, Idaho; Formerly Sports Medicine Fellow, Department of Orthopaedics, Jacksonville Memorial Hospital, Miami, Florida
Thermal Modification of Connective Tissue: Basic Science Considerations

Robert Anderson, BS
President, Stretching Inc., Palmer Lake, Colorado
Stretching

James R. Andrews, MD
Clinical Professor of Orthopaedics and Sports Medicine, University of Virginia School of Medicine, Charlottesville, Virginia; Clinical Professor, Department of Surgery, Division of Orthopaedic Surgery, University of Alabama School of Medicine, Birmingham; Medical Director, American Sports Medicine Institute; Orthopaedic Surgeon, Alabama Sports Medicine and Orthopaedic Center, Birmingham, Alabama
Throwing Injuries in the Adult

Jack T. Andrish, MD
Orthopaedic Surgeon, Cleveland Clinic Foundation, Cleveland, Ohio
The Leg

Christopher C. Annunziata, MD
Clinical Instructor, Department of Orthopaedics, Georgetown University School of Medicine, Washington, District of Columbia
Posterior Cruciate Ligament Injuries in the Adult; Posterior Cruciate Ligament Injuries in the Child

John Antoniou, MD, PhD, FRCSC
Assistant Professor, Mc Gill University, Faculty of Medicine; Orthopaedic Surgeon, Jewish General Hospital, Montreal, Quebec, Canada
Arthroscopic Knot Tying

Col. (ret.) Robert A. Arciero, MD
Associate Professor, Department of Orthopaedic Surgery, University of Connecticut School of Medicine, Farmington, Connecticut
Sports Medicine Terminology; Patellar Fractures in the Adult; Knee Extensor Mechanism Injuries in Athletes

Steven P. Arnoczky, DVM
Wade O. Brinker Professor of Veterinary Surgery, College of Veterinary Medicine, Department of Small Animal Clinical Sciences, Michigan State University, East Lansing, Michigan
Thermal Modification of Connective Tissue: Basic Science Considerations

Bernard R. Bach Jr., MD
Professor, Department of Orthopaedic Surgery, and Director, Sports Medicine Section, Rush Medical College of Rush University; Staff, Rush-Presbyterian-St. Luke's Medical Center, Chicago, Illinois
Anterior Cruciate Ligament Reconstruction in the Adult

Marianne Backer, MD
Orthopaedic Surgeon and Senior Registrar, Bispebjeg Hospital and University Hospital of Copenhagen, Copenhagen, Denmark
Glenohumeral Instability in Adults

F. Alan Barber, MD, FACS
Plano Orthopedic and Sports Medicine Center, Plano, Texas
Suture Anchors

Sue D. Barber-Westin, BS
Director, Clinical Studies, Cincinnati Sportsmedicine Research and Education Foundation, Cincinnati, Ohio
High Tibial Osteotomy in the Anterior Cruciate Ligament–Deficient Knee with Varus Angulation

Carl J. Basamania, MD
Assistant Professor, Division of Orthopaedic Surgery, Duke University Medical Center; Chief, Orthopaedic Surgery, Durham Veterans Administration Hospital, Durham, North Carolina
Clavicle Fracture in Adult Athletes; Clavicle Injuries in the Pediatric and Adolescent Athlete

James B. Bennett, MD
Clinical Professor, Department of Orthopedic Surgery, University of Texas–Houston Medical School; Chief of Staff, Texas Orthopedic Hospital, Houston, Texas
Soft Tissue Injury and Fractures of the Arm in the Adult; Neurovascular Injury of the Arm

Thomas M. Best, MD, PhD
Assistant Professor of Family Medicine and Orthopedic Surgery, University of Wisconsin Medical School, Madison, Wisconsin
Muscle and Tendon

Bruce D. Beynnon, MS, PhD
Professor of Orthopaedics and Rehabilitation, University of Vermont College of Medicine, Burlington, Vermont
Biomechanics; Relevant Biomechanics of the Knee

Tim Bollom, MD
Chief Resident, Department of Orthopaedics and Rehabilitation, University of Florida Health Science Center, Gainesville, Florida
Biodegradable Materials

Christine M. Bonci, MS, ATC
Co-Director, Division of Athletic Training/Sports Medicine, Intercollegiate Athletics, University of Texas at Austin, Austin, Texas
Functional Training Progressions for the Prevention of Anterior Cruciate Ligament Injuries in Female Athletes

Leslie Bonci, MPH, RD
Adjunct Assistant Professor, Department of Orthopaedics, University of Pittsburgh School of Medicine; Director, Sports Nutrition, University of Pittsburgh Medical Center, Pittsburgh, Pennsylvania
Nutrition for Sports

R. Luke Bordelon, MD
Clinical Professor, Louisiana State University School of Medicine in New Orleans; Attending, Children's Hospital, New Orleans; Director, Foot Clinic, Doctor's Hospital of Opelousis, Opelousis, Louisiana
Heel Pain

Andrew H. Borom, MD
Tallahassee Orthopedic Clinic, Tallahasse, Florida
Sports Shoes and Orthoses

LTC Craig R. Bottoni, MD
Clinical Instructor in Surgery, Department of Surgery, Uniformed Services University of the Health Sciences F. Edward Hébert School of Medicine, Bethesda, Maryland; Chief, Sports Medicine, Orthopaedic Surgery Service, Tripler Army Medical Center, Honolulu, Hawaii
Patellar Fractures in the Adult; Knee Extensor Mechanism Injuries in Athletes

James P. Bradley, MD
Clinical Associate Professor, Department of Orthopedic Surgery, University of Pittsburgh School of Medicine; Staff Orthopedic Surgeon, UPMC–St. Margaret; Orthopedic Team Physician, Pittsburgh Steelers, Pittsburgh, Pennsylvania
Elbow Injuries in Children and Adolescents; Osteochondritis Dissecans of the Humeral Capitellum, Pediatric Elbow Fractures and Dislocations, Pediatric Elbow Dislocations

Brad E. Brautigan, MD
Team Physician, Muskingum College, Orthopaedic Associates of Zanesville, Zanesville, Ohio
Allograft Tissues

Mark R. Brinker, MD
Clinical Professor of Orthopaedic Surgery, Tulane University School of Medicine, New Orleans, Louisiana; Clinical Professor of Orthopaedic Surgery, Texas Tech University Health Sciences Center School of Medicine, Lubbock, Texas; Director of Acute and Reconstructive Trauma and Co-Director, The Center for Problem Fractures and Limb Restoration, Texas Orthopedic Hospital; Fondren Orthopedic Group LLP, Houston, Texas
Bone

James W. Brodsky, MD
Clinical Professor of Orthopaedic Surgery, University of Texas Southwestern Medical Center at Dallas Southwestern Medical School; Director, Foot and Ankle Surgery Fellowship, Baylor University Medical Center Dallas, Texas
Stress Fractures of the Foot and Ankle

Andrew W. Brown, MD
Assistant Professor of Clinical Orthopaedic Surgery, University of Arizona College of Medicine Tucson, Arizona
The Use of Knee Braces in Sports Medicine

Treg D. Brown, MD
Assistant Professor of Orthopaedics, Tulane University
School of Medicine; Division of Sports Medicine &
Shoulder Reconstruction, Tulane Institute of Sports
Medicine; Active Staff, Tulane University Hospital &
Clinics, New Orleans, Louisiana
Adult thigh; Pediatric thigh

James F. Bruce Jr., MD, FAAOS
Orthopedic Clinic of West Georgia, LaGrange, Georgia
The Wrist in the Adult

Michael E. Brunet, MD
Professor of Orthopaedic Surgery, Tulane University
School of Medicine; Section Chief, Division of Sports
Medicine, Tulane Institute of Sports Medicine; Active
Staff, Tulane University Hospital & Clinics, New Orleans,
Louisiana
Adult Thigh; Pediatric Thigh

Joseph A. Buckwalter, MD
Professor and Head, Department of Orthopaedics,
University of Iowa College of Medicine; Department of
Orthopaedic Surgery, University of Iowa Hospitals and
Clinics, Iowa City, Iowa
*Ligaments; Effects of Medications in Sports Injuries at the
Tissue Level; Anticular Cartilage; Meniscus*

Edmund R. Burke, PhD
Professor, Biology Department, University of Colorado at
Colorado Springs, Colorado Springs, Colorado
Stretching

Kenneth P. Butters, MD
Clinical Senior Instructor Department of Orthopaedics and
Rehabilitation, Oregon Health Sciences University School
of Medicine, Portland; Upper Extremity Orthopedist,
Sacred Heart Hospital, Eugene, Oregon
*Nerve Lesions of the Shoulder; Olecranon Bursitis;
Osteochondroses of the Elbow*

David M. Caborn, MD
Professor of Orthopaedic Surgery, University of
Louisville, Louisville, Kentucky
Allograft Tissues

S. Terry Canale, MD
Professor and Chairman, Department of Orthopaedic
Surgery, University of Tennessee, Memphis, College of
Medicine; Chief-of-Staff Emeritus, Campbell Clinic,
Memphis, Tennessee
*Osteochondroses and Related Problems of the Foot and
Ankle*

Robert C. Cantu, MA, MD, FACS, FACSM
Clinical Instructor, Neurosurgery/Pediatrics, Boston
University School of Medicine, Boston; Chief,
Neurosurgery Service, and Director, Service Sports
Medicine, Emerson Hospital, Concord, Massachusetts;
Medical Director, National Center for Catastrophic Sports
Injury Research, University of North Carolina at Chapel
Hill, Chapel Hill, North Carolina
Head Injuries in Adults

Mark M. Casillas, MD
Clinical Assistant Professor, Department of Orthopaedics,
University of Texas Medical School at San Antonio, San
Antonio, Texas
Ligament Injuries of the Foot and Ankle in Adult Athletes

Frank M. Chang, MD
Associate Professor, Department of Orthopaedic Surgery
and Department of Pediatrics, University of Colorado
School of Medicine; Director, Orthopaedic Surgery, and
Co–Medical Director, Center for Gait and Motion
Analysis, The Children's Hospital, Denver, Colorado
The Disabled Pediatric Athlete

John D. Childs, MPT, MBA, OCS, CSCS
Doctoral Student, Department of Physical Therapy,
University of Pittsburgh School of Health and
Rehabilitation Sciences, Pittsburgh, Pennsylvania
The Language of Exercise and Rehabilitation

Chang-Hyuk Choi, MD
Assistant Professor, Department of Orthopaedic Surgery,
Hanyang University Medical School, Hanyang University
Hospital, Seoul, Korea
Injuries of the Proximal Humerus in Adults

Thomas O. Clanton, MD
Professor and Chairman, Department of Orthopaedics,
University of Texas–Houston Medical School, Houston,
Texas
*Etiology of Injury to the Foot and Ankle; Sports Shoes and
Orthoses*

Henry D. Clarke, MD
Attending Orthopaedic Surgeon, Insall-Scott Kelly
Institute for Orthopaedics and Sports Medicine, Beth
Israel Medical Center, New York, New York
Knee Replacement in the Recreational Athlete

Robert O. Cone III, MD
Radiologist, South Texas Radiology, San Antonio, Texas
Imaging Sports-Related Injuries of the Knee

Kathryn M. Coughlin, MS
Biomedical Engineer, University of Vermont, Burlington
Vermont
Relevant Biomechanics of the Knee

Michael J. Coughlin, MD
Clinical Professor, Division of Orthopaedic Surgery and
Rehabilitation, Oregon Health Sciences University,
Portland, Oregon
Conditions of the Forefoot

Frances Cuomo, MD
Assistant Professor, Department of Orthopaedic Surgery,
New York University School of Medicine; Chief,
Shoulder and Elbow Service, New York University
Hospital for Joint Diseases, New York, New York
Injuries of the Proximal Humerus in Adults

Ralph J. Curtis Jr., MD
Clinical Assistant Professor, Department of Orthopedics, University of Texas Medical School at San Antonio, San Antonio, Texas
Anatomy, Biomechanics, and Kinesiology of the Child's Shoulder; Glenohumeral Instabilities in the Child

Samuel D. D'Agata, MD
Team Orthopedic Surgeon, Gettysburg College, Gettysburg; Director of Sports Medicine, Rehabilitation Center, and Chairman, Department of Surgery, Hanover Hospital, Hanover, Private Practice, Hanover, Pennsylvania
Factors Predisposing to Knee Injury

Michael J. D'Amato, MD
Sports Medicine Fellow, Rush Medical College of Rush University; Staff, Rush-Presbyterian-St. Luke's Medical Center, Chicago, Illinois
Anterior Cruciate Ligament Reconstruction in the Adult

Allen Deutsch, MD
Clinical Assistant Professor, Department of Orthopaedic Surgery, Baylor University College of Medicine; Kelsey Seybold Clinic, Houston, Texas
Glenoid and Scapula Fractures in Adults and Children; Fractures of the Coracoid in Adults and Children

Lee H. Diehl, MD
Fellow, Sports Medicine, Section of Orthopaedic Surgery and Rehabilitation Medicine, University of Chicago, Chicago, Illinois
Acute Dislocation of the Patella in the Adult

Keith Duerler, MS, PT
Physical Therapist, Lexington Sports Medicine Center, Lexington, Kentucky
Electrical Stimulation; Application of Heat

Jeffrey R. Dugas, MD
Clinical Instructor and Attending Orthopaedic Surgeon, American Sports Medicine Institute, Birmingham, Alabama
Throwing Injuries in the Adult

James S. Dunnick, MD, FACC
Department of Medicine, Division of Cardiology, Louisiana State University School of Medicine–Lake Charles Campus; Medical Director, Nuclear Cardiology, CHF Clinic, and Cardiac Rehabilitation, Lake Charles Memorial Heart and Vascular Center, Lake Charles, Louisiana
Athletes and Sudden Cardiac Death

Craig J. Edson, MS, PT/ATC
Physical Therapist, Geisinger Medical Center, Danville, Pennsylvania
The Multiple Ligament–injured Knee

William P. Elsass, MD
Chief, Pediatric Behavioral Medicine, Ramstein AFB, Germany
Psychological Aspects of Sports in Children and Adolescents

Frank J. Eismont, MD
Professor and Vice Chairman, Department of Orthopedics, University of Miami, Jackson Memorial Hospital, Miami, Florida
Thoracolumbar Spine in the Adult

Mark A. Erickson, MD
Assistant Professor, Department of Orthopaedics, University of Colorado Children's Hospital, Denver, Colorado
Medial Ligament Injuries in Children; Lateral and Posterior Injuries of the Knee in Children

Gregory C. Fanelli, MD
Chief, Arthroscopic Surgery and Orthopaedic Sports Medicine, Geisinger Clinic Medical Center, Danville, Pennsylvania
The Multiple Ligament–injured Knee

Daniel D. Feldmann, MD
Resident in Orthopaedic Surgery, Geisinger Medical Center, Danville, Pennsylvania
The Multiple Ligament–injured Knee

Gerald A. M. Finerman, MD
Professor and Chairman, Department of Orthopaedic Surgery, University of California Los Angeles, UCLA School of Medicine, Los Angeles, California
Physeal Injuries in Young Athletes; Hip and Pelvis: Adult

Peter J. Fowler, MD, FRCSC
Professor, Orthopaedic Surgery, University of Western Ontario Faculty of Medicine; Medical Director, Fowler Kennedy Sports Medicine Clinic, London, Ontario, Canada
Anterior Cruciate Ligament Injuries in the Child

Freddie H. Fu, MD, DSc
Chairman, Department of Orthopaedic Surgery, University of Pittsburgh Medical Center, Pittsburgh, Pennsylvania
Meniscal Injuries in the Adult

John P. Fulkerson, MD
Clinical Professor of Orthopaedic Surgery, University of Connecticut School of Medicine; Orthopaedic Surgeon, Orthopaedic Associates of Hartford, Farmington, Connecticut
Anterior Knee Pain and Patellar Subluxation in the Adult

Chris Fults-Ganey, MD, PhD
Radiologist, Wilford Hall Medical Center, San Antonio, Texas
Imaging of Sports-Related Injuries

Dina H. Galvin, MD
Orthopedic Hand Surgeon, Jordan Hospital, Plymouth, Massachusetts
Hand Injuries in Children

Ralph Garretson, MD
Staff, Rush-Presbyterian-St. Luke's Medical Center,
Chicago, Illinois
*Injuries to the Acromioclavicular Joint in Adults and
Children; Sternum and Rib Fractures in Adults and Children*

William E. Garrett Jr., MD, PhD
Frank C. Wilson Professor and Chair, Department of
Orthopaedics, University of North Carolina at Chapel Hill
School of Medicine, Chapel Hill, North Carolina
*Muscle and Tendon; Acute Dislocation of the Patella in the
Adult*

Christian Gerber, MD
Professor and Chairman, Department of Orthopaedic
Surgery, University of Zurich Faculty of Medicine,
Zurich, Switzerland
Suture Materials

J. Robert Giffin, MD, FRCSC
Assistant Professor, Orthopaedic Surgery, University of
Western Ontario Faculty of Medicine; Fowler Kennedy
Sports Medicine Clinic, London, Ontario, Canada
*Meniscal Injuries in the Adult; Posterior Cruciate Ligament
Injuries in the Adult; Posterior Cruciate Ligament Injuries in
the Child*

Martin J. Gillespie, MD
Assistant Professor, Department of Orthopaedics,
University of Texas Medical School at San Antonio,
Chief, Sports Medicine and Arthroscopy, University
Hospital, and Veterans Affairs Hospital, and Audie
Murphy Memorial Hospital, San Antonio, Texas
The Effects of Medications in Sports Injuries

James S. Gilley, MD
Assistant Professor of Radiology, University of Texas
Medical School at San Antonio; Medical Director, South
Texas Radiology Imaging Centers, San Antonio, Texas
Imaging of Sports Injuries of the Foot and Ankle

John E. Glorioso, Jr., MD
Director, Primary Care Sports Medicine, Department of
Family Practice, and Emergency Medical Services, Tripler
Army Medical Center, Honolulu, Hawaii
Viral Disease

David M. Gloystein, BS
Medical Student, University of Texas Medical School at
San Antonio, San Antonio, Texas
The Effects of Medications in Sports Injuries

Jorge E. Gómez, MS, MD
Associate Professor and Director, Program in Pediatric
Sports Medicine and Fitness, Department of Pediatrics,
University of Texas Medical School at San Antonio;
Medical Team Physician, University of Texas at San
Antonio, San Antonio, Texas
Paired Organ Loss

**Frank A. Gottschalk, MD, FRCSEd,
FCS(SA)Orth**
Professor, Department of Orthopaedic Surgery, University
of Texas Southwestern Medical Center at Dallas
Southwestern Medical School; Attending, Zale Lipshy
University Hospital and Parkland Memorial Hospital,
Dallas, Texas
The Orthopaedically Disabled Athlete

Thomas J. Graham, MD
Chief, Curtis National Hand Center, Union Memorial
Hospital, Baltimore, Maryland
Athletic Injuries of the Adult Hand

William A. Grana, MD, MPH
Professor and Head, Department of Orthopaedic Surgery,
University of Arizona College of Medicine, Tucson,
Arizona
Application of Cold

Gary A. Green, MD
Clinical Associate Professor, Department of Family
Medicine, Division of Sports Medicine, University of
California, Los Angeles, UCLA School of Medicine, Los
Angeles; Team Physician, Pepperdine University, Malibu,
California; Team Physician, U.S. Soccer
Recreational Drug Use in Athletes

Donald E. Greydanus, MD FAAP, FSAM
Professor, Department of Pediatrics and Human
Development, Michigan State University College of
Human Medicine, Kalamazoo, Michigan
*Sports and the Neurodevelopment of the Child and
Adolescent*

Letha Y. Griffin, MD, PhD
Adjunct Professor, Department of Kinesiology and Health,
and Team Physician, Georgia State University, Atlanta,
Georgia
The Female Athlete

George W. Gross, MD
Professor of Radiology, University of Maryland School of
Medicine; Director of Pediatric Radiology, University of
Maryland Medical Center, Baltimore, Maryland
Differences between the Immature and the Mature Skeleton

Dan Guttmann, MD
Clinical Instructor, Department of Orthopaedic Surgery,
University of New Mexico School of Medicine,
Albuquerque; Director, Upper Extremity Surgery, Taos
Orthopaedic Institute, Taos, New Mexico
Injuries of the Proximal Humerus in Adults

Bettina M. Gyr, MD
Fellow, Pediatric Orthopaedic Surgery, Primary Children's
Medical Center and Shriner's Hospital for Children, Salt
Lake City, Utah
Strength Training in Children and Adolescents

Christopher D. Harner, MD
Blue Cross of Western Pennsylvania Professor, University of Pittsburgh School of Medicine Medical Director, UPMCS–Center for Sports Medicine, Pittsburgh, Pennsylvania
Posterior Cruciate Ligament Injuries in the Adult; Posterior Cruciate Ligament Injuries in the Child

Douglas T. Harryman II, MD*
Associate Professor, Department of Orthopaedics, University of Washington School of Medicine, Seattle, Washington
Arthroscopic Knot Tying

Richard J. Hawkins, MD, FRCSC(c)
Clinical Professor, Department of Orthopaedic Surgery, University of Colorado School of Medicine, Denver; Orthopaedic Consultant, Steadman Hawkins Clinic, Vail, Colorado
Rotator Cuff and Impringement Lesions in Adult and Adolescent Athletes

Morley A. Herbert, PhD
Manager, Biomedical and Surgical Research, Medical City Dallas Hospital, Dallas, Texas
Suture Anchors

M. Alan Hinton, MD
Clinical Assistant Professor and Assistant Director for Sports Medicine, Department of Orthopaedics, Louisiana State University School of Medicine, Louisiana State University at New Orleans; Lake Charles Memorial Hospital and Christus St. Patrick Hospital, Lake Charles, Louisiana
Heat Intolerance

Edward G. Hixson, MD
Adirondack Surgical Group, Saranac Lake, New York
Cold Injury; Altitude Stress

Stephen M. Howell, MD
Adjunct Associate Professor of Mechanical Engineering and Adjunct Associate Professor of Biomedical Engineering, University of California, Davis, California
Construction and Fixation of a Tendon Anterior Cruciate Ligament Graft

L. M. Hull, MS, PhD
Professor of Mechanical Engineering and Professor of Biomedical Engineering, University of California, Davis; Scientific Staff, Shriners Hospital, Sacramento, California
Construction and Fixation of a Tendon Anterior Cruciate Ligament Graft

David M. Hunter, MD
Assistant Professor, Department of Orthopaedic Surgery, University of California, Los Angeles, UCLA School of Medicine, Los Angeles, California
Hip and Pelvis: Adult

Jon Hyman, MD
Peachtree Orthopaedic Clinic, Atlanta, Georgia
Patellofemoral Tendinopathy

Peter A. Indelicato, MD
Professor and Chief, Orthopaedics and Rehabilitation, University of Florida, Gainesville, Florida
Medial Ligament Injuries in the Adult

James J. Irrgang, PhD, PF, ATC
Assistant Professor and Vice Chairman for Clinical Services, Department of Physical Therapy, University of Pittsburgh School of Health and Rehabilitation Sciences; Vice President of QI and Outcomes and Director of Sports and Orthopaedic Physical Therapy, Centers for Rehab Services, Pittsburgh, Pennsylvania
The Language of Exercise and Rehabilitation

Nizar N. Jarjour, MD
Associate Professor of Medicine, Section of Pulmonary and Critical Care, Department of Medicine, University of Wisconsin Medical School, Madison, Wisconsin
Exercise-Induced Asthma

Darren L. Johnson, MD
Associate Professor and Chairman, Department of Surgery, University of Kentucky School of Medicine; Lexington, Kentucky
Research Design and Statistics in Sports Medicine; Allograft Tissues

Robert J. Johnson, MD
Professor, Department of Orthopaedics and Rehabilitation, University of Vermont College of Medicine, Director, Sports Medicine Center, Fletcher Allen Health Care, Burlington, Vermont
Relevant Biomechanics of the Knee

Ron M. Johnson, PT, MPT, ATC, CSCS
Physical Therapist and HealthSouth National Clinical Education Instructor, HealthSouth Sports Medicine, Houston, Texas
Open and Closed Chain Exercises (Non–Weight-Bearing and Weight-Bearing Exercises); Exercise Modalities: Cycle Ergometry, StairMaster, Elliptical Fitness Trainer, Slideboard, Elastic Resistance

James S. Keene, MD
Professor of Orthopedic Surgery, Department of Orthopedic Surgery and Rehabilitation Medicine, University of Wisconsin Medical School, Madison, Wisconsin
Tendon Injuries of the Foot and Ankle

W. Ben Kibler, MD
Associate Clinical Professor, University of Kentucky College of Medicine; Medical Director, Lexington Sports Medicine Center, Lexington, Kentucky
Electrical Stimulation; Application of Heat

Donald T. Kirkendall, PhD
Department of Orthopaedics, University of North Carolina at Chapel Hill School of Medicine, Chapel Hill, North Carolina
Muscle and Tendon

Scott H. Kitchel, MD
Athletic Medicine Staff, University of Oregon, Eugene, Oregon
Thoracolumbar Spine in the Adult

John J. Klimkiewicz, MD
Assistant Professor of Orthopaedic Surgery and Sports Medicine, Georgetown University School of Medicine; Georgetown University Hospital—MEDSTAR Health; Head Team Physician, Georgetown University Hoyas, Washington, District of Columbia
Pediatric Elbow Fractures and Dislocations; Pediatric Elbow Dislocations

Mininder Kocher, MD, MPH
Instructor of Orthopaedic Surgery, Harvard Medical School; Program in Clinical Effectiveness, Harvard School of Public Health; Attending Orthopaedic Surgeon, Department of Orthopaedic Surgery, Children's Hospital, Boston, Massachusetts
Hip and Pelvic Injuries in the Young Athlete

DeAnn M. Koehler, MS, ATC, CSCS, CFT
Assistant Athletic Trainer, Intercollegiate Athletics, University of Texas at Austin, Austin, Texas
Functional Training Progressions for the Prevention of Anterior Cruciate Ligament Injuries in Female Athletes

Jon D. Koman, MD
Orthopaedic Specialty Center, Baltimore, Maryland
The Wrist in the Adult

John O. Krause, MD
Clinical Assistant Professor of Surgery, University of Texas Medical School at San Antonio, San Antonio, Texas; Assistant Professor of Surgery, Uniformed Services University of the Health Sciences F. Edward Hébert School of Medicine, Bethesda, Maryland; Chief, Orthopedic Foot and Ankle Service, Wilford Hall Medical Center, Lackland AFB, Texas
Stress Fractures of the Foot and Ankle

Sumant G. Krishnan, MD
Assistant Clinical Professor, Department of Orthopaedic Surgery, University of Texas Southwestern Medical Center at Dallas Southwestern Medical School; Staff, Shoulder Service, W.B. Carrell Memorial Clinic, Dallas, Texas
Rotator Cuff and Impingement Lesions in Adult and Adolescent Athletes

John E. Kuhn, MD
Associate Professor, Department of Orthopaedic Surgery, Division of Sports Medicine and Shoulder Surgery, University of Michigan Medical School; Team Physician, University of Michigan, and Team Physician, USA Hockey National Team Development Program, Ann Arbor, Michigan
Scapulothoracic Crepitus and Bursitis in Athletes

Frank A. Kulling, EdD
Associate Professor, School of Applied Health and Educational Psychology, Oklahoma State University, Stillwater, Oklahoma
Exercise Physiology

Roger V. Larson, MD
Associate Professor, Department of Orthopaedics and Sports Medicine, University of Washington School of Medicine, Seattle, Washington
Lateral and Posterolateral Instability of the Knee in Adults

William C. Lauerman, MD
Associate Professor of Orthopaedic Surgery, Georgetown University School of Medicine; Chief, Division of Spine Surgery, Department of Orthopaedic Surgery, Georgetown University Hospital, Washington, District of Columbia
Sports Injuries to the Thoracolumbar Spine in Children and Adolescents

Kenneth M. Leclerc, MD, FACC
Director, Cardiac Rehabilitation Unit and Staff Cardiologist, Brooke Army Medical Center, San Antonio, Texas
Hypertension and Other Cardiac Disease in Athletes

Robert F. Lemanske Jr., MD
Professor of Pediatrics and Medicine, University of Wisconsin School of Medicine; Head, Division of Pediatric Allergy, Immunology, and Rheumatology, University of Wisconsin Medical School, Madison, Wisconsin
Exercise-Induced Asthma

Scott M. Lephart, PhD ATC
Associate Professor of Orthopaedic Surgery and Associate Professor of Health and Rehabilitation Sciences, University of Pittsburgh School of Medicine; Director, Neuromuscular Research Laboratory, University of Pittsburgh Medical Center, Pittsburgh, Pennsylvania
Role of Proprioception in Functional Joint Stability

Thomas N. Lindenfeld, MD
Volunteer Instructor, Department of Orthopaedic Surgery, University of Cincinnati College of Medicine; Associate Director, Cincinnati Sportsmedicine and Orthopaedic Center, Cincinnati, Ohio
Complex Regional Pain Syndromes Including Reflex Sympathetic Dystrophy and Causalgia

Russell C. Linton, MD
Attending, Baptist Memorial Hospital–Golden Triangle,
Columbus, Mississippi
Medial Ligament Injuries in the Adult

Jeffrey L. Lovallo, MD
Assistant Clinical Professor, Department of Orthopaedics,
Georgetown University School of Medicine, Washington,
District of Columbia; Staff, Anderson Orthopedic Clinic,
Arlington, Virginia
Wrist Injuries in the Child; Hand Injuries in Children

Lisa D. Lowe, MEd ATC, CSCS, USAW, CFT
Strength and Conditioning Specialist, Intercollegiate
Athletics, University of Texas at Austin, Austin, TX
*Functional Training Progressions for the Prevention of
Anterior Cruciate Ligament Injuries in Female Athletes*

Walter R. Lowe, MD
Clinical Associate Professor, Department of Orthopaedics,
Baylor University College of Medicine; Baylor Sports
Medicine Institute; Team Physician, Houston Rockets,
Houston, Texas
Superior Labral Injuries

Christopher C. Madden, MD
Private Practice, Longs Peak Sports and Family Medicine
and Longs Peak Family Practice, Longmont; Team
Physician, Niwut High School, Niwut, Colorado
*The Team Physician: The Preparticipation Examination and
On-Field Emergencies*

Mark W. Maffet, MD
Clinical Assistant Professor, Department of Orthopedics,
Baylor University College of Medicine; Baylor Sports
Medicine Institute; Team Physician, Houston Comets,
Houston Texas
Superior Labral Injuries

David Maish, MD
Resident in Orthopaedic Surgery, Geisinger Medical
Center, Danville, Pennsylvania
The Multiple Ligament–injured Knee

Roger A. Mann, MD
Associate Clinical Professor, Department of Orthopaedic
Surgery, University of California at San Francisco School
of Medicine, San Francisco; Director, Foot Fellowship
Program, Oakland, California
*Biomechanics of the Foot and Ankle Linkage; Entrapment
Neuropathies of the Foot*

Carl G. Mattacola, PhD, ATC
Assistant Professor and Director, Division of Athletic
Training, College of Allied Health Professions, University
of Kentucky, Lexington, Kentucky
Research Design and Statistics in Sports Medicine

Augustus D. Mazzocca, MD
Assistant Professor, Department of Orthopaedic Surgery,
University of Connecticut School of Medicine,
Farmington, Connecticut
*Injuries to the Acromioclavicular Joint in Adults and
Children; Sternum and Rib Fractures in Adults and Children*

Frank C. McCue III, MD
Professor of Orthopaedic Surgery and Plastic Surgery of
the Hand, Department of Orthopaedic Surgery; Division
Head, Division of Sports Medicine, University of Virginia
Medical Center, Charlottesville, Virginia
The Wrist in the Adult

Edward R. McDevitt, MD
Assistant Clinical Professor of Surgery, Uniformed
Services University of the Health Sciences F. Edward
Hébert School of Medicine, Bethesda; Orthopaedic Staff,
Anne Arundel Medical Center, Annapolis, and North
Arundel Medical Center, Glen Burnie, Maryland
Ergogenic Drugs in Sports

Patrick J. McMahon, MD
Assistant Professor, Department of Orthopaedic Surgery,
University of Pittsburgh School of Medicine; Assistant
Team Physician, Football, Shoulder and Elbow Surgery,
University of Pittsburgh, Pittsburgh, Pennsylvania
Functional Anatomy and Biomechanics of the Adult Shoulder

Thomas L. Mehlhoff, MD
Team Physician, Houston Astros; Staff, Texas Orthopedic
Hospital, Houston, Texas
*Soft Tissue Injuries and Fractures of the Arm in the Adult;
Neurovascular Injury of the Arm*

Sacheen H. Mehta, MD
Sportsmedicine Fellow, Cincinnati Sportsmedicine and
Orthopaedic Center, Cincinnati, Ohio
*Complex Regional Pain Syndromes Including Reflex
Sympathetic Dystrophy and Causalgia*

Keith Meister, MD
Associate Professor and Team Physician, Department of
Orthopedics, University of Florida, College of Medicine,
Orthopaedic Surgeon, Shands Hospital, Gainesville,
Florida
Biodegradable Materials

Morris B. Mellion, MD
Adjunct Associate Professor, Department of Family
Practice and Orthopaedic Surgery, University of Nebraska
College of Medicine, Adjunct Professor, School of
Health, Physical Education, and Recreation, University of
Nebraska at Omaha; Team Physician Emeritus, University
of Nebraska at Omaha, Omaha, Nebraska
*The Team Physician: The Preparticipation Examination and
On-Field Emergencies*

Mark D. Miller, MD
Associate Professor of Orthopaedic Surgery and Co-
Director, Division of Sports Medicine, University of
Virginia School of Medicine, Charlottesville, Virginia;
Associate Professor, Department of Surgery, Uniformed
Services University of the Health Sciences F. Edward
Hébert School of Medicine, Bethesda, Maryland
Basic Arthroscopic Principles

Michael B. Millis, MD
Associate Professor of Orthopaedic Surgery, Harvard
Medical School; Director, Adolescent and Young Adult
Hip Unit, Children's Hospital, Boston, Massachusetts
Hip and Pelvic Injuries in the Young Athlete

Bernard F. Morrey, MD
Professor of Orthopedics, Mayo Medical School; Emeritus
Chairman, Department of Orthopedics, Mayo Clinic,
Mayo Foundation, Rochester, Minnesota
*Biomechanics of the Elbow and Forearm; Tendinopathies
about the Elbow; Osteochondritis Dissecans of the Elbow
and Forearm in the Adult; Fractures of the Elbow in Adults;
Heterotopic Bone about the Elbow; Elbow Dislocation in the
Adult Athlete; Entrapment Neuropathies about the Elbow*

Col. Charles T. Morton, MD, USAF, MC
Clinical Assistant Professor, University of Texas Medical
School at San Antonio, San Antonio, Texas; Clinical
Assistant Professor, Uniformed Services University of the
Health Sciences F. Edward He(c)bert School of Medicine,
Bethesda, Maryland; Chief, Developmental Pediatrics
Service, San Antonio Military Pediatric Center, Lackland
AFB, Texas
The Child Athlete with Chronic Disease

Van C. Mow, PhD
Chairman, Department of Biomedical Engineering,
Columbia University, New York; Director, Orthopaedic
Research Laboratory, New York Presbyterian Hospital,
New York, New York
Articular Cartilage; Meniscus

Kenneth J. Mroczek, MD
Assistant Professor of Orthopaedic Surgery, New York
University School of Medicine; Attending Surgeon,
Department of Orthopaedic Surgery, Hospital for Joint
Diseases Orthopaedic Institute, New York, New York
Factors Predisposing to Knee Injury

Daniel J. Mullen, MD
Curtis National Hand Center, Union Memorial Hospital,
Baltimore, Maryland
Athletic Injuries of the Adult Hand

Joseph B. Myers, PhD, ATC
Assistant Professor of Kinesiology, Louisiana State
University, Baton Rouge, Louisiana
Role of Proprioception in Functional Joint Stability

Blaise A. Nemeth, MD
Chief Resident, Department of Pediatrics, University of
Wisconsin Hospital and Clinics, Madison, Wisconsin
Diabetes Mellitus

David C. Neuschwander, MD
Clinical Instructor, Department of Orthopaedic Surgery,
University of Pittsburgh School of Medicine, Pittsburgh;
Orthopedic Associates of Pittsburgh, Monroeville,
Pennsylvania
Peripatellar Pathology

John E. Novotny, MS, PhD
Professor of Mechanical Engineering, University of
Delaware, Newark, Delaware
Biomechanics

Frank R. Noyes, MD
Volunteer Professor, Department of Orthopaedic Surgery,
University of Cincinnati College of Medicine; Chairman,
Cincinnati Sportsmedicine and Orthopaedic Center,
Cincinnati Sportsmedicine Research and Education
Foundation, Cincinnati, Ohio
*High Tibial Osteotomy in the Anterior Cruciate
Ligament–Deficient Knee with Varus Angulation*

Stephen L. Nuccion, MD
Resident, Department of Orthopaedic Surgery, UCLA
Medical Center, Los Angeles, California
Hip and Pelvis: Adult

James P. O'Leary, MD
Sports Medicine Consultant, University of South Carolina,
Columbia, South Carolina
Meniscal Injuries in the Adult

Russell M. Paine, PT
Rehab. Consultant Houston Rockets, Houston Astros, and
NASA; Clinical Director, HealthSouth Sports Medicine,
Houston, Texas
*Open and Closed Chain Exercises (Non–Weight-Bearing and
Weight-Bearing Exercises); Exercise Modalities: Cycle
Ergometry, StairMaster, Elliptical Fitness Trainer,
Slideboard, Elastic Resistance*

William D. Parham, PhD, ABPP
Associate Director of Clinical Services, Student
Psychological Services, and Consultant, Department of
Intercollegiate Athletics, University of California, Los
Angeles; Consulting Psychologist, Department of Health
Psychology, Children's Hospital of Orange County,
Orange, California
Sports Psychology and Injured Athletes

Dilip R. Patel, MD, FAAP, FAACPDM
Professor, Department of Pediatrics and Human
Development, Michigan State University College of
Human Medicine, East Lansing, Michigan; Kalamazoo
Center for Medical Studies, Kalamazoo, Michigan
*Sports and the Neurodevelopment of the Child and
Adolescent*

Robert A. Pedowitz, MD, PhD
Associate Professor and Chief, Sports Medicine,
Department of Orthopaedics, University of California, San
Diego, School of Medicine, San Diego, California
Use and Abuse of the Pneumatic Tourniquet

Russell S. Petrie, MD
Team Physician, Vanguard University, Costa Mesa; Staff
Orthopedic Surgeon, Hoag Memorial Hospital, Newport
Beach, California.
*Elbow Injuries in Children and Adolescents; Osteochondritis
Dissecans of the Humeral Capitellum*

Marilyn M. Pink, PhD, PT
Director of Biomechanics Laboratory, Centinela Hospital
Medical Center, Inglewood, California
Functional Anatomy and Biomechanics of the Adult Shoulder

Peter D. Pizzutillo, MD
Professor, Department of Orthopaedic Surgery and
Department of Pediatrics, MCP Hahnemann School of
Medicine; Director, Orthopedic Surgery, St. Christopher's
Hospital for Children, Philadelphia, Pennsylvania
The Cervical Spine in the Child

Helen D. Pratt, PhD, DABPS
Professor, Department of Pediatrics and Human
Development Michigan State University College of
Human Medicine, Kalamazoo, Michigan
*Sports and the Neurodevelopment of the Child and
Adolescent*

William D. Regan, MD
Assistant Professor of Orthopaedic Surgery, University of
British Columbia Faculty of Medicine, Vancouver, British
Columbia, Canada
*Tendinopathies about the Elbow; Entrapment Neuropathies
about the Elbow*

Bruce Reider, MD
Professor, Department of Surgery, Section of Orthopaedic
Surgery and Rehabilitation Medicine, University of
Chicago Division of the Biological Sciences Pritzker
School of Medicine; Director of Sports Medicine,
University of Chicago Hospitals, Chicago, Illinois; Editor,
American Journal of Sports Medicine
Factors Predisposing to Knee Injury

Bryan L. Riemann, PhD, ATC
Assistant Professor of Athletic Training, Graduate
Athletic Training Program, Georgia Southern University,
Statesboro, Georgia
Role of Proprioception in Functional Joint Stability

Rudy Robbe, MD
Resident, University Hospital, Lexington, Kentucky
Allograft Tissues

Charles A. Rockwood Jr., MD
Professor and Chairman Emeritus, Department of
Orthopaedics, University of Texas Medical School at San
Antonio; Chief, Shoulder Service, University Hospital of
University of Texas HSC, San Antonio, Texas
Injuries to the Sternoclavicular Joint in the Adult and Child

Scott A. Rodeo, MD
Instructor of Orthopaedic Surgery, Weill Medical College
of Cornell University; Assistant Scientist, Department of
Research, The Hospital for Special Surgery, New York,
New York
Patellofemoral Tendinopathy

Anthony A. Romeo, MD
Associate Professor, Department of Orthopaedic Surgery,
Rush Medical College; Director, Shoulder Service, Rush-
Presbyterian-St. Luke's Medical Center, Chicago, Illinois
*Injuries to the Acromioclavicular Joint in Adults and
Children; Sternum and Rib Fractures in Adults and Children*

Richard Rozencwaig, MD
Clinical Instructor of Surgery, Nova Southeastern
University, Fort Lauderdale; Orthopaedic Surgeon,
Orthopaedic Care and Sports Medicine Center, Aventura,
Florida
Arthroscopic Knot Tying

Timothy G. Sanders, MD
Assistant Clinical Professor, Department of Radiology,
University of Texas Medical School at San Antonio;
Chairman, Department of Radiology, Wilford Hall
Medical Center, San Antonio, Texas
*Imaging of Sports-Related Injuries, Imaging of the
Glenohumeral Joint*

Jeffrey R. Sawyer, MD
Associate Professor of Orthopaedics, Rush Medical
College of Rush University; Pediatric Orthopedic, and
Spinal Deformity, Rush-Presbyterian-St. Luke's Medical
Center, Chicago, Illinois
*Pediatric Elbow Fractures and Dislocations; Pediatric
Elbow Dislocations*

Robert C. Schenck Jr., MD
Professor and Division Chief, Sports Medicine Section,
Department of Orthopaedics and Rehabilitation,
University of New Mexico School of Medicine; Staff,
University Hospital, Albuquerque; New Mexico
The Effects of Medications in Sports Injuries

Gregory A. Schmale, MD
Assistant Professor, Department of Orthopaedic Surgery,
Children's Hospital and Regional Medical Center of
Washington, Seattle, Washington
*Medial Ligament Injuries in Children; Lateral and Posterior
Injuries of the Knee in Children*

Alberto G. Schneeberger, MD
Assistant Professor, Department of Orthopaedic Surgery,
University of Zurich Faculty of Medicine, Zurich,
Switzerland
Suture Materials

W. Norman Scott, MD
Clinical Professor of Orthopaedics Surgery Albert
Einstein Medical College of Yeshiva University, Bronx;
Chairman, Department of Orthopaedic Surgery, and
Director, Insall-Scott Kelly Institute for Orthopaedics and
Sports Medicine, Beth Israel Medical Center, New York,
New York
Knee Replacement in the Recreational Athlete

Robert Sellards, MD
Assistant Professor, Department of Orthopaedic Surgery, Louisiana State University School of Medicine, Baton Rouge, Louisiana
Injuries to the Acromioclavicular Joint in Adults and Children

Benjamin S. Shaffer, MD
Clinical Assistant Professor of Orthopaedic Surgery, Georgetown University School of Medicine; Team Physician, Washington Capitals, Washington, District of Columbia
Sports Injuries to the Thoracolumbar Spine in Children and Adolescents

Matthew S. Shapiro, MD
Orthopaedic Surgeon, Orthopedic Healthcare Northwest, Inc., Eugene, Oregon
Olecranon Bursitis; Osteochondroses of the Elbow

Barry P. Simmons, MD
Associate Professor of Orthopedic Surgery, Harvard Medical School; Chief, Hand and Upper Extremity Service, and Senior Orthopedic Surgeon, Brigham and Women's Hospital, Boston, Massachusetts
Wrist Injuries in the Child; Hand Injuries in Children

Richard Simon, MD
Orthopaedic Surgeon, Orthopaedic Center of South Florida, Plantation, Florida
High Tibial Osteotomy in the Anterior Cruciate Ligament–Deficient Knee with Varus Angulation

Kenneth M. Singer, MD
Clinical Associate Professor in Orthopaedic Surgery, Oregon Health Sciences University School of Medicine, Portland; Adjunct Assistant Professor, Department of Health and Movement Science, University of Oregon–Eugene, Eugene, Oregon
Nerve Lesions of the Shoulder; Olecranon Bursitis; Osteochondroses of the Elbow

Douglas K. Smith, MD
Musculoskeletal Radiologist, South Texas Radiology Group, Southwest Texas Methodist Hospital, San Antonio, Texas
Imaging of Sports Injuries of the Foot and Ankle

Carl L. Stanitski, MD
Professor of Orthopaedic Surgery, Medical University of South Carolina, Charleston, South Carolina
Overuse Injuries in the Skeletally Immature Athlete; Meniscal Injuries in the Skeletally Immature Patient; Patellar Instability in the Skeletally Immature Patient; Acute Tibial Tubercle Avulsion Fractures in the Skeletally Immature Patient; Patellofemoral Mechanism; Articular Cartilage Lesions and Osteochondritis Dissecans of the Knee in the Adult; Articular Cartilage Lesions and Osteochondritis Dissecans of the Knee in the Skeletally Immature Patient

Keith L. Stanley, MD
East Oklahoma Orthopaedic Center, Tulsa, Oklahoma
Preparticipation Evaluation of the Young Athlete

Enrico J. Stazzone, MD
Assistant Professor, Division of Pediatric Orthopaedics, Carrie Tingley Hospital, Albuquerque, New Mexico
Physeal Injuries in Young Athletes

Kevin L. Stevenson, MD
Chief Resident, Department of Neurological Surgery, University of Pittsburgh Medical Center, Pittsburgh, Pennsylvania
Pediatric Sports-Related Head Injuries

J. Andy Sullivan, MD
Professor and Don H. O'Donoghue Chair, Department of Orthopaedics, University of Oklahoma College of Medicine, Children's Hospital of Oklahoma, Oklahoma City, Oklahoma
Ligament Injuries of the Foot/Ankle in the Pediatric Athlete

Dean C. Taylor, MD
Clinical Assistant Professor of Surgery, Uniformed Services University of the Health Sciences F. Edward He(c)bert School of Medicine, Bethesda, Maryland; Director, U.S. Army Joint and Soft Tissue Trauma Fellowship, Keller Army Hospital, West Point, New York
Sports Medicine Terminology; Patellar Fractures in the Adult; Knee Extensor Mechanism Injuries in Athletes

Peter C. Theut, MD
Orthopaedic Surgeon, Orthopaedic Associates of Grand Rapids, Grand Rapids, Michigan
Anterior Knee Pain and Patellar Subluxation in the Adult

James E. Tibone, MD
Professor, Department of Orthopaedics, University of Southern California School of Medicine; Associate, Kerlan-Jobe Orthopaedic Clinic, Los Angeles, California
Functional Anatomy and Biomechanics of the Adult Shoulder

Edwin M. Tingstad, MD
Clinical Instructor, Department of Orthopaedics and Sports Medicine, University of Washington School of Medicine, Seattle, Washington
Lateral and Posterolateral Instability of the Knee in Adults

Joseph S. Torg, MD
Professor of Orthopaedics, Temple University School of Medicine, Philadelphia, Pennsylvania
Cervical Spine Injuries in the Adult

Thomas C. Turturro, PT, OCS
Department of Physical Therapy, University of Texas Health Sciences Center, San Antonio, Texas
Continuous Passive Motion

Marc W. Urquhart, MD
Clinical Faculty, Liberty Orthopaedics, Springfield, New Jersey; St. Barnabas Sports Medicine Institute, Livingston, New Jersey
Meniscal Injuries in the Adult

C. Thomas Vangsness Jr., MD
Professor of Orthopaedic Surgery, Department of Orthopaedic Surgery, University of Southern California, Los Angeles, California
Articular Cartilage Lesions and Osteochondritis Dissecans of the Knee in the Adult

W. Michael Walsh, MD
Clinical Associate Professor of Orthopaedic Surgery, Department of Orthopaedic Surgery and Rehabilitation, University of Nebraska, College of Medicine; Adjunct Graduate Associate Professor, School of Health, Physical Education, and Recreation, and Team Orthopaedic Surgeon, University of Nebraska at Omaha, Omaha, Nebraska
The Team Physician: The Preparticipation Examination and On-Field Emergencies; Recurrent Dislocation of the Knee in the Adult

Keith L. Wapner, MD
Clinical Professor of Orthopaedic Surgery, University of Pennsylvania School of Medicine; Professor of Orthopaedic Surgery, MCP Hahnemann School of Medicine, Director, Foot and Ankle Orthopaedic Fellowship Program, Pennsylvania Hospital, Philadelphia, Pennsylvania
Heel Pain

Russell F. Warren, MD
Professor of Surgery (Orthopaedics) and Chairman, Division of Orthopaedic Surgery, Weill Medical College of Cornell University; Surgeon-in-Chief, Department of Orthopaedic Surgery, The Hospital for Special Surgery, New York, New York
Glenohumeral Instability in Adults

Daniel C. Wascher, MD
Associate Professor and Chief, Division of Sports Medicine, Department of Orthopaedics and Rehabilitation, University of New Mexico Health Science Center, Albuquerque, New Mexico
Physeal Injuries in Young Athletes

Thomas Wickiewicz, MD
Professor of Clinical Orthopaedic Surgery, Weill Medical College of Cornell University; Attending Orthopaedic Surgeon, The Hospital for Special Surgery, New York, New York
Patellofemoral Tendinopathy

John H. Wilckens, MD
Clinical Assistant Professor of Surgery, Uniformed Services University of Health Sciences F. Edward He(c)bert School of Medicine, Bethesda; Orthopaedic Surgeon and Head Team Physician, U.S. Naval Academy, Annapolis, Maryland
Viral Disease

Kaye E. Wilkins, DVM, MD
Professor, Department of Orthopedics and Department of Pediatrics, University of Texas Medical School at San Antonio, San Antonio, Texas
Fractures of the Proximal Humerus in the Child; Fractures and Soft Tissue Injuries of the Arm in the Child

Gerald R. Williams Jr., MD
Associate Professor, University of Pennsylvania School of Medicine; Chief, Shoulder and Elbow Surgery, University of Pennsylvania Health System, and Chairman, Orthopaedic Surgery, Presbyterian Medical Center, Philadelphia, Pennsylvania
Glenoid and Scapula Fractures in Adults and Children; Fractures of the Coracoid in Adults and Children

Ilaina M. Wingler, MA
Staff Psychologist and Chief, Substance Abuse, MacDill AFB, Florida
Psychological Aspects of Sports in Children and Adolescents

Michael A. Wirth, MD
Associate Professor, Department of Orthopaedics, University of Texas Medical School at San Antonio; Chief, Orthopaedic Shoulder Service, Audie Murphy Veterans Hospital, San Antonio, Texas
Injuries to the Sternoclavicular Joint in the Adult and Child

Edmund G. Witkowski, MD
Private Practice, Suncoast Orthopaedic Surgery and Sports Medicine, Venice, Florida
Clavicle Injuries in the Pediatric and Adolescent Athlete

Savio L.-Y. Woo, PhD, DSc
A. B. Ferguson Professor, Department of Orthopaedic Surgery, University of Pittsburgh School of Medicine, and Professor of Bioengineering, Professor of Mechanical Engineering, and Professor of Rehabilitation Science and Technology, University of Pittsburgh; Vice Chairman for Research, Department of Orthopaedic Surgery, and Director, Musculoskeletal Research Center, University of Pittsburgh Medical Center, Pittsburgh, Pennsylvania
Ligaments; Effects of Medications in Sports Injuries at the Tissue Level

Robert M. Wood, MD, FRCS
Orthopedic Surgeon, Sports Medicine North, Lynnfield, and North Shore Medical Center, Salem, Massachusetts
Etiology of Injury to the Foot and Ankle

Virchel E. Wood, MD
Professor, Department of Orthopaedic Surgery, Loma Linda University School of Medicine; Consulting Chief, Hand Surgery Service, Loma Linda University Medical Center, Loma Linda, California
Thoracic Outlet Syndrome

Richard J. Wyzykowski, MD
John Muir Medical Center, Walnut Creek, California
Wrist Injuries in the Child

Kazunori Yasuda, MD, PhD
Professor and Chairman, Department of Medical Bioengineering and Sports Medicine, Hokkaido University School of Medicine, Sapporo, Japan
Construction and Fixation of a Tendon Anterior Cruciate Ligament Graft

Mary L. Zupanc, MD
Associate Professor, Department of Pediatrics, Columbia University College of Physicians and Surgeons, New York; Director, Pediatric Epilepsy Program, Children's Hospital of New York City, New York, New York
Sports and Epilepsy

PREFACE

One might ask, "Why publish a book on sports medicine when the subspecialty simply treats athletes with orthopaedic injuries?" There is no question the orthopaedic sports medicine specialist must be soundly schooled in orthopaedic knowledge; however, the athletes often present special considerations that are not part of the everyday practice of orthopaedics. The intense desire and determination of the athlete to return to sports are not commonly encountered in the day-to-day practice of orthopaedics. The various stress syndromes of the musculoskeletal system that occur secondary to training and athletic competition and the specialized rehabilitation techniques also present special problems not seen in other orthopaedic patients.

The contributors to this two-volume treatise on orthopaedic sports medicine are leaders in their subspecialty. They have shared with us their experience and perspectives by addressing specific problems of the athlete in their areas of expertise. Each contributor gives an excellent review of the particular topic and completes the contribution with preferred treatment.

The early chapters address certain nonorthopaedic conditions that the orthopaedic sports medicine specialist must address when caring for the athlete. Nutrition, heat illness, biomechanics, and sports psychology are areas that must be part of the orthopaedic sports medicine physician's data base.

In the later chapters, contributors discuss diagnosis and various methods of treatment and present their chosen method of treatment of specific athletic injuries. When to return an athlete to activity is an important responsibility the orthopaedic sports medicine specialist must assume. Each contributor has addressed this issue for his or her particular anatomic area.

It is our hope that this work will prove useful to our fellow orthopaedic surgeons. If so, it will be a tribute to the contributors who have shared with us their expertise. We are indebted to them for their time and effort.

We also offer our sincere appreciation to Marti Daigle and to the staff at Elsevier Science for their patience and untiring efforts in bringing these volumes to publication.

JESSE C. DeLEE, M.D., DAVID DREZ, JR., M.D.,
MARK D. MILLER, M.D.

CONTENTS

CHAPTER TWENTY-FOUR

Wrist and Hand

Section A

Wrist

1. THE WRIST IN THE ADULT

Frank C. McCue III, MD ■ James F. Bruce Jr., MD ■ Jon D. Koman, MD

For many years, the wrist joint has been an enigma. Even today, our understanding of problems concerning the wrist remains incomplete. Questions persist in regard to basic function and the effect of trauma and disease on that function. Methods of treatment in many cases have been derived from trial and error rather than from a basic understanding of this unique collection of joints. The long-term effect of some treatment modalities has not been fully determined.

The wrist is a complex structure with multiple parts, and an infinite combination of positions and motions is possible. Understanding these complexities requires a thorough knowledge of the anatomy and the kinematics of the normal wrist. The effect of trauma and disease on the wrist must be appreciated to deliver optimal care to the injured athlete.

It is beyond the scope of this chapter to include an exhaustive review of all the contributors to our understanding of the wrist. Reference is made in each section to those pioneers whose work was pertinent. It is enough to say that great strides have been made that now permit us to diagnose and treat disorders of this complex articulation more accurately.

Biomechanics

Anatomy

Osseous Anatomy

Eight bones make up the carpus. Some authors consider the pisiform a sesamoid rather than one of the carpal bones. The other seven carpal bones are aligned in two transverse rows, with the scaphoid bridging the proximal and distal carpal row (Fig. 24A1–1).

The carpal bones each have multiple articulations. The carpus as a unit basically functions as two articulations: (1) the radiocarpal joint between the distal radius and the proximal carpal row, and (2) the midcarpal joint between the proximal and distal carpal rows. The carpometacarpal articulation is relatively fixed and does not contribute significantly to carpal motion.

There are no tendon insertions on the seven carpal bones except the flexor carpi ulnaris, which inserts on the pisiform. Motion of the wrist therefore results from a complex combination of indirect forces exerted by muscle units attaching proximal or distal to the carpus and from the complex osseous and ligamentous orientation.

Ligamentous Anatomy

There are two excellent studies of the ligamentous anatomy of the wrist, one by Taleisnik[131] and one by Mayfield and associates.[96] Although there are some minor discrepancies between the two studies, they agree in general. The major points have been summarized well by Green[60] as follows:

1. The major ligaments of the wrist are intracapsular and are covered by the wrist capsule.

2. The volar ligaments are much more substantial than the dorsal ligaments (Fig. 24A1–2).

3. The prime stabilizer of the proximal pole of the scaphoid is the volar radioscapholunate ligament.

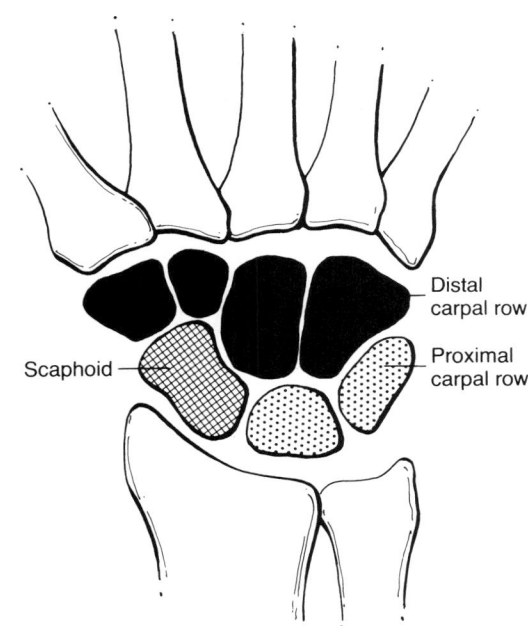

Figure 24A1–1. The carpal bones are aligned in two transverse rows, with the scaphoid bridging the proximal and distal carpal rows. (Illustration by Elizabeth Roselius, © 1988. Reprinted with permission from Green DP: Operative Hand Surgery, 2nd ed. New York, Churchill Livingstone, 1988.)

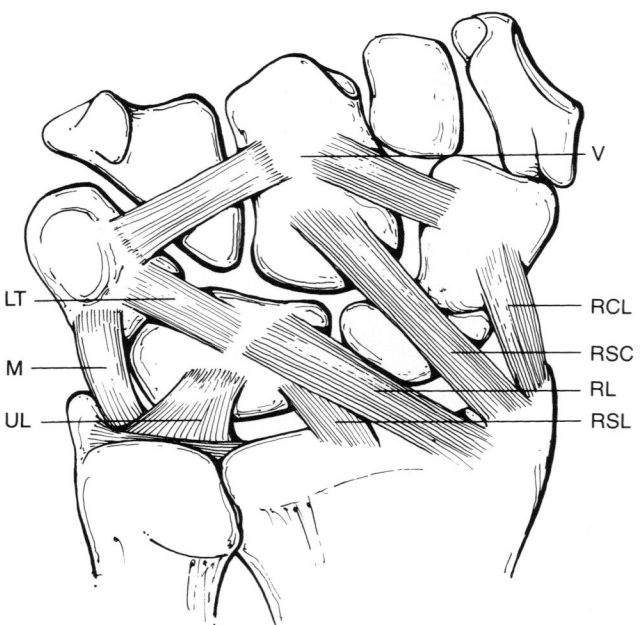

Figure 24A1–2. The volar carpal ligaments from Taleisnik. LT, lunotri-quetral ligament; M, ulnocarpal meniscus homologue; RCL, radial collat-eral ligament; RL, radiolunate ligament; RSC, radioscaphocapitate liga-ment; RSL, radioscapholunate ligament; UL, ulnolunate ligament; V, deltoid ligament. (Illustration by Elizabeth Roselius, © 1985. Reprinted with permission from Taleisnik J: The Wrist, New York, Churchill Living-stone, 1985.)

4. The collateral ligaments do not exist as static stabiliz-ers of the wrist.

Vascular Anatomy

The wrist has an excellent vascular supply with multiple anastomoses between the radial, the ulnar, and the anterior interosseous arteries.[133] These vessels supply three pairs of transverse arches, which are located volarly and dorsally (Fig. 24A1–3).[50] Despite their excellent collateral blood supply, there is an increased incidence of avascular necrosis in the scaphoid, the lunate, and the capitate.[117] It has been found that each of these bones is dependent on a single external vessel or group of vessels for its blood supply.[108] The proximal poles of both the scaphoid and the capitate are supplied by intraosseous vessels coursing retrograde from the waist (Fig. 24A1–4).[49] These bones are therefore more susceptible to vascular disruption and avascular ne-crosis subsequent to trauma.

Function

Biomechanical Concepts

Our understanding of the biomechanics of the wrist has evolved greatly since Navarro described carpal mechanics in 1921.[102] Several different models have been developed to help explain the complex pattern of motion that exists in the wrist. Lambrinudi[54] proposed the link mechanism of the wrist joint: The distal radius, the proximal carpal row, and the distal carpal row function as links in a chain that is stable in tension but inherently unstable in compression. The scaphoid bridges the proximal and distal carpal rows, provides stability, and helps control motion (Fig. 24A1–5). Taleisnik[132] modified Navarro's columnar column concept to explain patterns of carpal instability (Fig. 24A1–6). The scaphoid is the mobile lateral column, the triquetrum is the rotary medial column, and the lunate and the entire distal carpal row function as a flexion-extension column. We-ber[140] proposed a slightly different concept, dividing the carpus into two longitudinal columns (Fig. 24A1–7). The radial side of the carpus functions as a force-bearing col-umn, whereas the ulnar aspect of the carpus acts to control

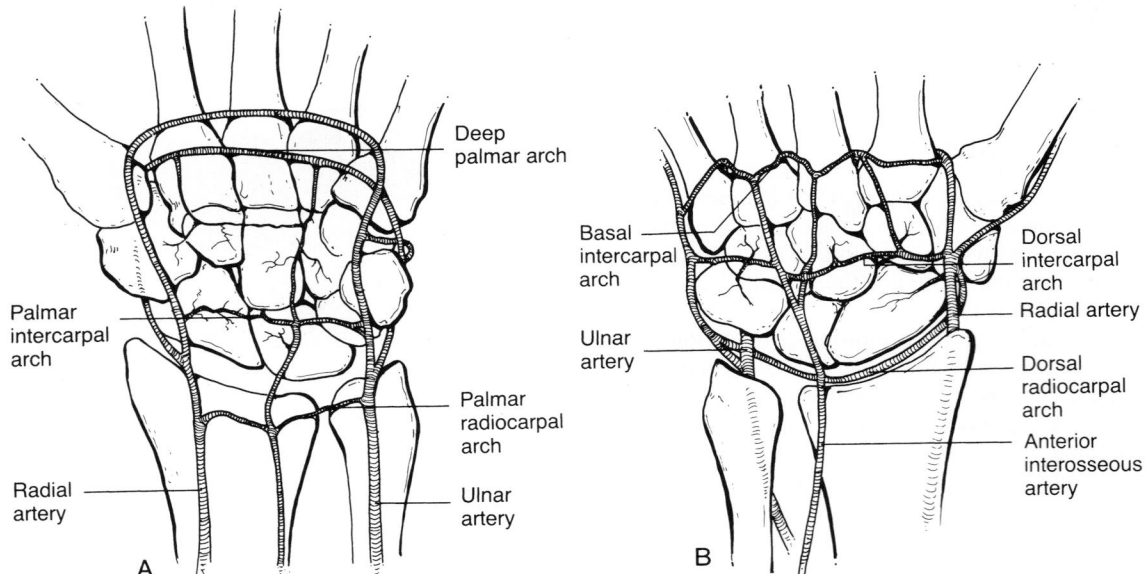

Figure 24A1–3. The arterial supply of the wrist. Anastomoses from the radial ulnar and anterior interosseous arteries form three transverse arches. *A,* The arterial supply of the palmar aspect of the wrist. *B,* The arterial supply of the dorsal aspect of the wrist.

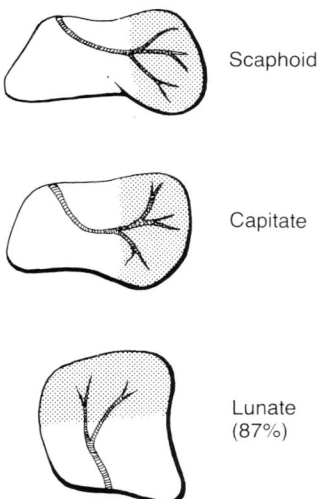

Figure 24A1–4. The scaphoid, the capitate, and occasionally the lunate are each dependent on a single intraosseous vessel for their blood supply. (Redrawn from Gelberman RH, Gross MS: The vascularity of the wrist. Clin Orthop 202:42, 1986.)

the position of the lunate relative to the capitate. Lichtman[87] has proposed an oval ring concept (Fig. 24A1–8). The carpus is viewed as two mobile links that allow reciprocal motion between the proximal and distal carpal rows. The mobile links are at the scaphotrapezial joint and the triquetrohamate joint. Although these models differ in their concepts of wrist mechanics, each serves to explain carpal motion and helps increase our understanding of carpal injury patterns.

Patterns of Injury

Mayfield[96] has demonstrated the perilunate pattern of injury to the wrist (Fig. 24A1–9). With increased force,

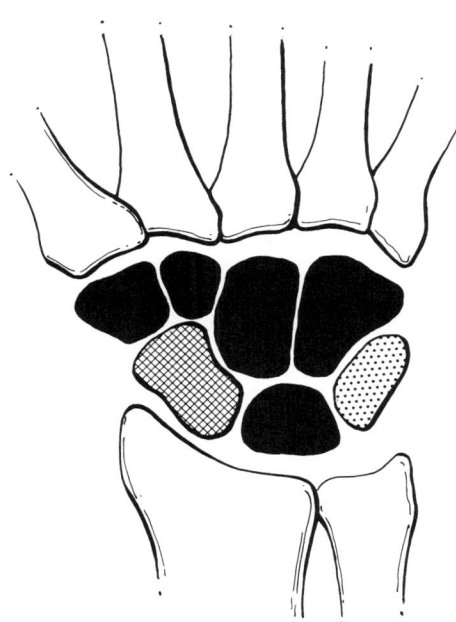

Figure 24A1–6. The columnar column concept of Taleisnik. (Redrawn from Lichtman DM, Schneider JR, Swafford AR, Mack GR: Ulnar midcarpal instability—clinical and laboratory analysis. J Hand Surg 6:522, 1981.)

there is a progression of ligamentous injury from the scapholunate joint continuing around the lunate until all ligamentous support is disrupted. Stage I corresponds to a scapholunate dissociation, whereas stage IV results in a lunate or a perilunate dislocation. Various fracture patterns can accompany the ligamentous injury. Varying the position of the hand can change the pattern of injury.[142] With pro-

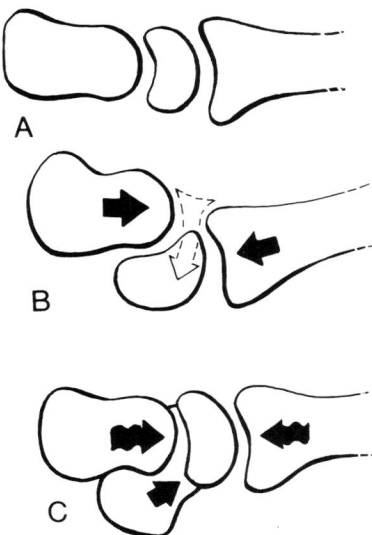

Figure 24A1–5. *A–C,* The link mechanism of Lambrinudi, which is inherently unstable in compression. The scaphoid bridges the proximal and distal carpal rows, providing stability in compression. (Redrawn from Gilford WW, Baltar RH, Lambrinudi C: The mechanics of the wrist joint. Guy's Hosp Rep 92:52–59, 1943.)

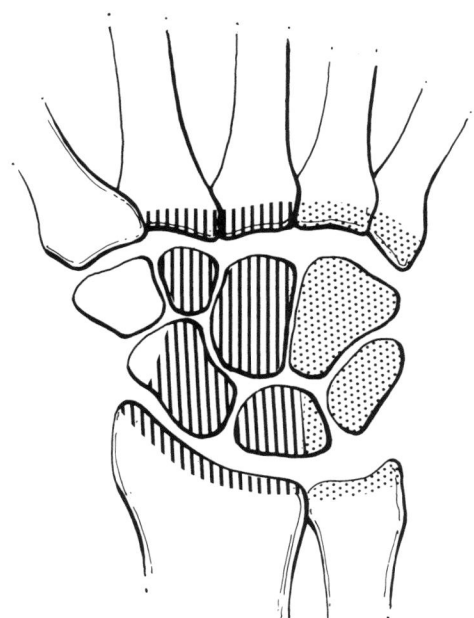

Figure 24A1–7. The longitudinal column concept of Weber. (Redrawn from Weber ER: Concepts governing the rotational shift of the intercalated segment of the carpus. Orthop Clin North Am 15:196, 1984.)

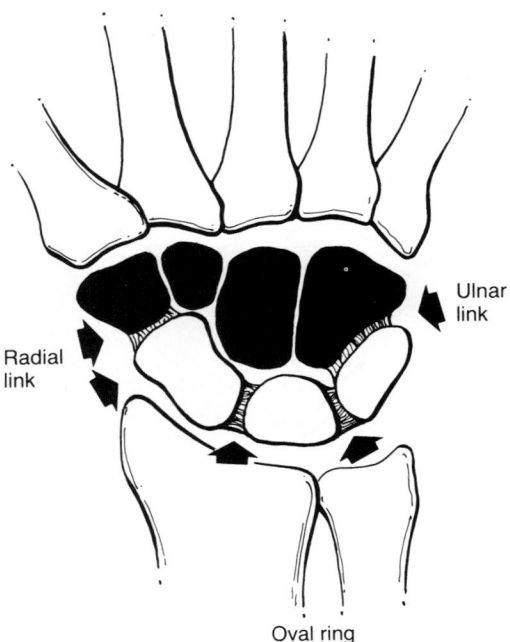

Figure 24A1–8. The oval ring concept of Lichtman. (Redrawn from Lichtman DM, Schneider JR, Swafford AR, Mack GR: Ulnar midcarpal instability—clinical and laboratory analysis. J Hand Surg 6:522, 1981.)

gressive radial deviation, the path of injury moves from a lesser arc about the lunate to a greater arc in a more peripheral course through the carpus.

Kinematics

Flexion and extension of the wrist occur through both the radiocarpal joint and the midcarpal joint,[146] although

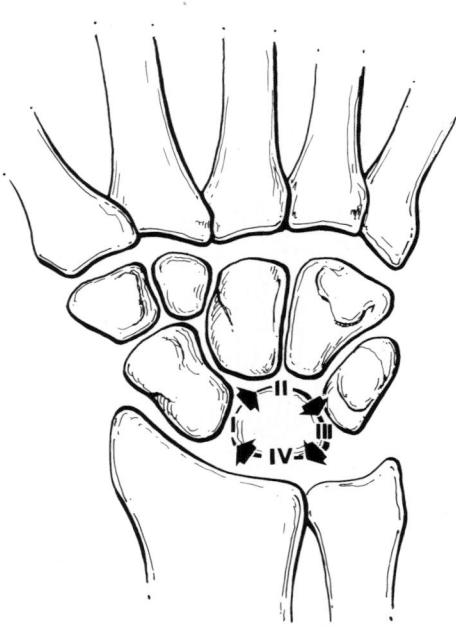

Figure 24A1–9. The perilunate pattern of injury from Mayfield. (Redrawn from Mayfield JK: Mechanism of carpal injuries. Clin Orthop 149: 50, 1980.)

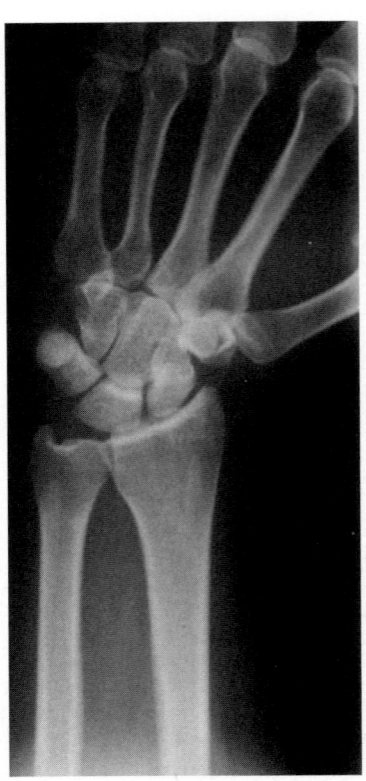

Figure 24A1–10. In radial deviation, the scaphoid appears shortened owing to its more vertical alignment, and the triquetrum has moved to a proximal position on the hamate.

the relative contribution of each joint has been disputed. The radiocarpal joint participates more prominently in dorsiflexion, whereas the midcarpal joint is the major contributor to palmar flexion. Ulnar and radial deviation involve more complex intercarpal motion. In radial deviation, the scaphoid palmar-flexes and becomes more vertical relative to the long axis of the forearm. This in effect shortens the radial column of the wrist. As the wrist moves into ulnar deviation, the scaphoid orients in a more longitudinal position, which lengthens the radial column (Fig. 24A1–10). This has the effect of locking the midcarpal joint, preventing further flexion or extension from occurring through the midcarpal joint. On the ulnar side of the wrist, the helicoid triquetrohamate joint allows the triquetrum to move proximally and distally relative to its position on the hamate (Fig. 24A1–11). This allows a similar shortening and lengthening of the ulnar column in ulnar and radial deviation, respectively. The position of the lunate is influenced by the scaphoid and the triquetrum; this results in dorsiflexion of the lunate in ulnar deviation and palmar flexion in radial deviation. Understanding these relationships is important in evaluating radiographs and appreciating patterns of ligamentous instability.

Radiography of the Wrist

Although a thorough history and physical examination are critical in diagnosis of injuries to the carpus, radiogra-

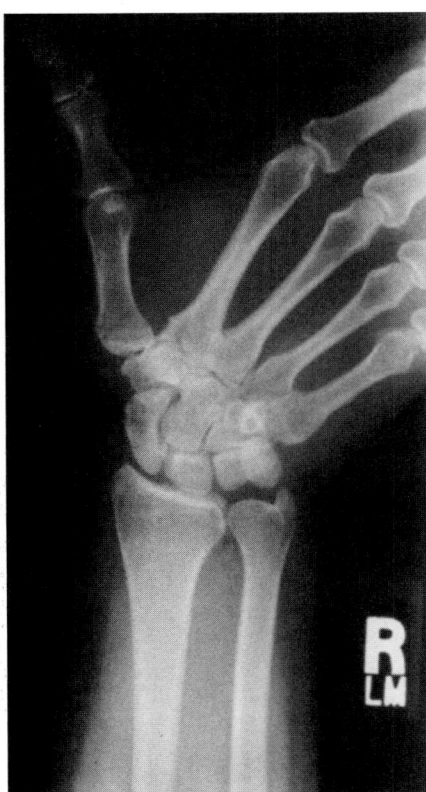

Figure 24A1–11. In ulnar deviation, the scaphoid has assumed a more horizontal position and appears lengthened, whereas the triquetrum has moved to a more distal position on its articulation with the hamate.

phy of the wrist is also an essential element in diagnosis. Our usual views that are taken for problems involving the wrist include five views and then additional special views for other specific problems as found. These include (1) anteroposterior (AP) or posteroanterior (PA); (2) lateral—make sure this is a true lateral to denote carpal instability; (3) carpal tunnel views; (4) AP view with the wrist in ulnar deviation; and (5) closed fist APs or PAs in both pronation and supination. Particularly in flexible individuals who have an increased scapholunate space, a view of the opposite wrist to show this is helpful; in these individuals there is often an increased space physiologically. These views are helpful in identifying fractures of the scaphoid and accentuating a scapholunate gap that may not be apparent in the standard views. The carpal tunnel view allows visualization of the hook of the hamate and demonstrates any calcific deposits in the carpal tunnel. On occasion, additional views, including oblique and AP views in maximum radial and ulnar deviation and lateral views in maximum flexion and extension, are helpful in diagnosing fractures or dislocations of the carpus.

Instability patterns can be identified on the lateral radiograph. In the normal wrist in the neutral position, the axes of the radius, the lunate, and the capitate are co-aligned. Dorsal intercalary segmental instability (DISI) is present when the lunate lies palmar to the capitate but is flexed dorsally (Fig. 24A1–12). Volar intercalary segmental instability (VISI) is present if the lunate lies dorsal to the capitate and is palmar flexed (see Fig. 24A1–12). Either

of these collapsed patterns can be associated with carpal instabilities, and each is discussed later in this section.

There are two main carpal instability patterns, static and dynamic. The static instabilities are those that are present at rest and can be diagnosed on routine AP and lateral radiographs, as mentioned earlier. Dynamic instabilities require certain maneuvers to occur with stress, and motion fluoroscopy is often required for diagnosis.

There are various types of instabilities that are instantly recognizable. The key to recognizing these in static pictures is the lunate and its appearance on the direct lateral film. Certain series describe up to 10 views for evaluation of carpal instability; although a number may be helpful in difficult cases, this can be diagnosed with only two additional views, a lateral in flexion and a lateral in extension. One concept needs to be remembered: With flexion, everything flexes, and with extension, everything should extend.

In general, although many types of carpal instabilities can be found, there are six *classic* types: rotary dissociation of the scaphoid, dorsiflexion instability, volar flexion instability, dorsal carpal subluxation, palmar carpal subluxation, and ulnar translocation. The so-called SLAC (scapholunate advanced collapse) wrist may eventually occur, and its characteristic pattern is remarkably constant in its progressive deformity and degeneration, with the radiolunate articulation almost never affected.

Various oblique views are occasionally helpful but are very inconsistent because the overlap of the multiple bones often distorts rather than clarifies the diagnosis. The ulnar deviation PA view thins and lengthens the scaphoid and is often helpful in diagnosis of fractures of the scaphoid.

The carpal tunnel view is very helpful in a diagnosis of fracture of the hook of the hamate, so often seen in sporting injuries, particularly baseball and golf. Often, stiffness of the wrist with limitation or dorsiflexion prevents this view from being productive. In these cases, a 20-degree to 25-degree view in supination may be helpful, but the computed tomography scan is the most reliable study.

Oblique views to show the pisotriquetral ligament are

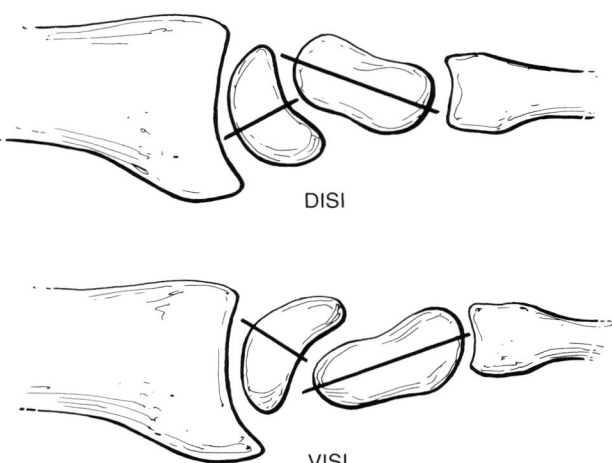

Figure 24A1–12. Patterns of carpal instability. Dorsal intercalated segmental instability (DISI) is present when the lunate lies volar to the capitate but is flexed dorsally. Volar intercalated segmental instability (VISI) is present if the lunate lies dorsal to the capitate and is flexed volarly.

useful in diagnosis of arthritic changes at this particular joint that are often not seen well on the usual positions. Special positions and views are helpful to allow more precise diagnosis of the various articulations as they are found clinically and by history.

Various other radiographic techniques can be used to evaluate additional injuries that are not completely defined by routine radiographs. A bone scan performed 48 to 72 hours after an injury can be helpful in confirming an occult fracture and may be helpful in chronic cases in defining an area of arthrosis. Trispiral tomography is especially helpful for documenting an occult fracture such as a fracture of the hook of the hamate. Motion studies with an imaging intensifier or formal cineradiography will help document abnormal carpal kinematics that is not apparent on static views. We have found it helpful to use cineradiography to create a permanent record in these cases. We routinely study the uninvolved wrist to have it as a normal comparison. Our standard study includes an anteroposterior view with the wrist moving from full radial deviation to full ulnar deviation and a lateral view with the wrist moving from full dorsiflexion to full volar flexion. In difficult cases, we frequently follow this study with an arthrogram, in which contrast material is injected into the radiocarpal joint. We observe to see if there is any abnormal filling from the radiocarpal joint into the midcarpal joint or the distal radial ulnar joint. To complete the study, we then ask the patient to go through the range of motion again and record this later for review.

Additional methods of study include computed tomographic scanning, magnetic resonance imaging (MRI), and, more recently, the three-dimensional scanning techniques. We have occasionally found these methods useful in difficult cases in which a definitive diagnosis could not be made with the preceding studies. This has been the exception rather than the rule, however, and we do not routinely employ these techniques.

Diagnostic Wrist Arthroscopy

Wrist arthroscopy has evolved into an important diagnostic and therapeutic tool. Much of this evolution is attributed to improved arthroscopy instrumentation and better understanding of normal and pathologic wrist anatomy. Wrist arthroscopy is turning into an alternative method of treating triangular fibrocartilage complex tears, ligament injuries, and chondral injuries in athletes.

Imaging techniques of the wrist include standard radiographs, computed tomography scanning, cineradiography, and MRI. MRI has been useful for soft tissue injuries but still has limitations in diagnosing these conditions accurately. Johnstone and associates[73] compared preoperative wrist MRI results with arthroscopy findings in 43 patients. Eight of the 20 preoperative MRI diagnoses were changed. High false-positive MRI readings led the authors to view MRI readings with skepticism. Some authors have found arthrography to be superior to MRI for detecting full-thickness triangular fibrocartilage tears.[34, 124] In general, these techniques fail to visualize structures accurately in three dimensions—something arthroscopy does so well.

Although ancillary studies such as arthrography and MRI may aid in the diagnosis, these confirmatory tests may only increase costs and delay the athlete's return to competition. When to proceed to arthroscopy in an athlete weighs heavily on whether it is the on or the off season, the particular sport the athlete is involved in, and the athlete's competitive level. A case-by-case analysis is generally recommended.

Wrist arthroscopy is performed with the wrist in 8 to 10 pounds of traction using a commercially available traction device. The standard wrist arthroscope is 2.7 mm in diameter and 60 mm long and has a 30-degree viewing angle. A mechanical irrigation pump is generally preferred for better pressure and flow rate. Arthroscopic instrumentation includes graspers, a probe, and a motorized shaver with 2- to 3.5-mm full-radius resectors and burs.

Anatomic landmarks of the wrist should be palpated. The bony landmarks include Lister's tubercle, radial styloid, dorsal lip of the distal radius, ulnar styloid, and the distal radioulnar joint. Soft tissue landmarks include the extensor tendons. Soft tissue landmarks that are at risk during the procedure include the radial artery, the sensory branch of the radial nerve, and the dorsal sensory branch of the ulnar nerve.[120] Because of these at-risk structures, it is important to incise only the skin when making a portal and to spread with a hemostat when dissecting down to capsule. Damage to articular cartilage and small arthroscopic instrumentation is also a risk with a potential economic impact.

Portal placement and the names of the portals are dependent on the surrounding extrinsic extensor tendon compartments (Fig. 24A1–13).[1] The radiocarpal joint uses four primary portals: the 3-4 portal, the 4-5 portal, the 6-R (radial) portal, and the 6-U (ulnar) portal. The 3-4 portal is located 1 cm distal to Lister's tubercle and can be palpated between the extensor pollicis longus tendon (third compartment) and the extensor digitorum communis tendon (fourth compartment). This is the main radiocarpal arthroscopic viewing portal. Instruments must be angled approximately 20 degrees proximally in line with the volar tilt of the distal radius. The scaphoid, the lunate, and their respective radial fossae are best visualized through this portal. Intercarpal and volar radiocarpal ligaments can also be seen.

The 4-5 portal, located between the extensor digitorum communis tendon to the little finger and the extensor digiti minimi tendon, is used to view the midportion of the triangular fibrocartilage complex, the lunate, the lunotriquetral joint, and the volar ulnocarpal ligaments. It is used for instrumentation in ulnar-sided wrist disease.

The 6-R portal is radial to the extensor carpi ulnaris tendon. To avoid injuring the triangular fibrocartilage complex, the proximal border of the triquetrum should be used as a landmark rather than the distal ulna. The dorsal sensory branch of the ulnar nerve is potentially in danger with the use of this portal. This portal can be used for both instrumentation and arthroscopy in ulnar-sided wrist disease.

The 6-U portal, located just ulnar to the extensor carpi radialis tendon, enters the joint through the prestyloid recess next to the ulnar styloid. Like the 6-R portal, the dorsal sensory branch of the ulnar nerve lies in close proximity. This portal provides visualization of the triangu-

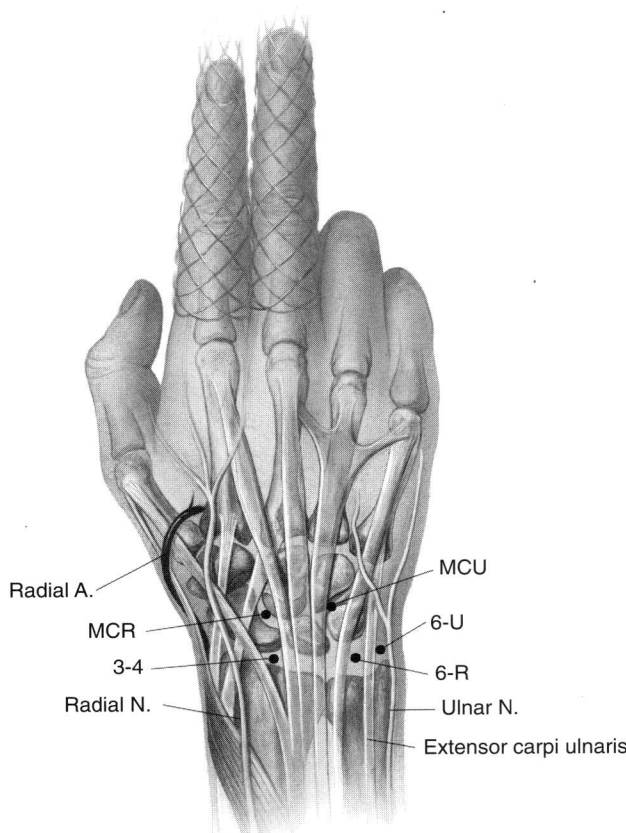

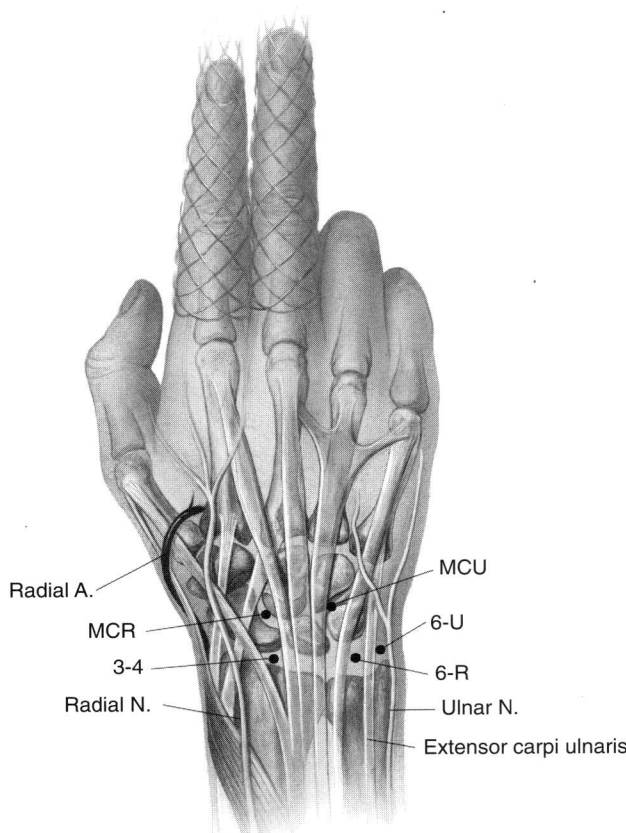

Figure 24A1–13. The 3-4, 6-U, and 6-R portals provide the access and visibility needed for basic diagnostic wrist arthroscopy. The midcarpal (MC) portals provide a view of the midcarpal joint. R, radial; U, ulnar. (From Wrist Arthroscopy: Portals to Progress, as described by Gary Poehling. Andover, Mass, Dyonics Inc., 1989.)

lar fibrocartilage complex and the ulnocarpal ligaments and can also be used for outflow.

Arthroscopy of the midcarpal joints has also been described, using the radial midcarpal portal, the ulnar midcarpal portal, the scaphotrapeziotrapezoid portal, and the triquetrohamate portal. The radial and ulnar midcarpal portals are most commonly used for midcarpal disease and are located 1 cm from the 3-4 and 4-5 portals, respectively. Although rarely used, portals for the distal radial ulnar joint have been described; they are called the distal distal radial ulnar joint portal and the proximal distal radial ulnar joint portal.

Diagnostic wrist arthroscopy should be performed in a systematic fashion so as not to miss any occult disease.[99] It is common to switch arthroscopy portals to view the radial and ulnar aspects of the radiocarpal joint. Creation of the 3-4 portal and the 6-R portal allows visualization of radial scaphoid and lunate fossae and their articulating ends of the scaphoid and lunate. The triquetrum, the ulnar head, and the pisiform can also be seen. The volar radiocarpal ligaments as well as the scapholunate and lunotriquetral ligaments are inspected in a radial to ulnar direction. The triangular fibrocartilage complex should be seen from both sides of the wrist.

Midcarpal disease is viewed through both radial midcar-

pal and ulnar midcarpal portals. The radial midcarpal portal views the distal scaphoid, the lunate, and the proximal pole of the capitate. The distal ends of the lunate and triquetrum and the proximal portions of the capitate and hamate are visualized with the ulnar midcarpal portal. Ligamentous structures viewed through these portals include the palmar scaphotrapezial ligament, the scaphocapitate ligament, the triquetrohamate ligament, and the triquetrocapitate ligament.

Operative Arthroscopy of the Wrist

Disorders of the athlete's wrist include injury to the triangular fibrocartilage complex (TFC); intrinsic ligament injuries, including the scapholunate and the lunotriquetral ligaments; and osseous or cartilaginous injuries.[43, 143]

The most common wrist arthroscopic finding in the athlete is a lesion of the TFC. Palmer divided these findings into type I (traumatic) and type II (degenerative).[106] Type I lesions are usually traumatic as a result of carpus impaction on the distal ulna and involve either a central or a peripheral tear. Peripheral detachment may occur either on the ulnar side (type IB) or on the radial side (type ID). Type II degenerative lesions start with wearing on the TFC, then progressively worsen to include chondromalacial changes of the lunate and triquetrum and eventual ulnocarpal arthritis. Avascularity of the articular disk and the radial margin has led to the proposal to repair ulnar-sided lesions and to débride other lesions. Degenerative lesions with significant evidence of impingement may also require an ulnar shortening procedure.

Débridement of the TFC uses the 4-5 portal for arthroscopy and the 6-R and 3-4 portals for instrumentation.[121] A suction basket and a full-radius shaver are used to remove any loose flaps of cartilage. Ulnar-sided peripheral detachments are repaired using the Tuohy needle technique, which uses the 4-5 portal for arthroscopy and the 6-R portal for instrumentation. A Tuohy needle is introduced through the 1-2 portal, piercing the TFC, and is passed out the dorsal ulnar aspect of the capsule and skin. A 2–0 polydioxanone suture is passed into the needle from radial to ulnar, with hemostats placed on both ends. The Tuohy needle is pulled back into the wrist. The tip is then passed through the articular disk portion and is carried out of the wrist and capsule 3 mm adjacent to the first piercing. This suture end is now brought out through the Tuohy needle. The Tuohy needle is backed out of the wrist. A small skin incision is performed connecting the two suture ends. A hemostat is used to spread down to wrist capsule and avoid damage to the dorsal sensory branches of the ulnar nerve. The suture ends are hooked with a probe and are brought out through this skin incision. With direct visualization of the TFC through the 4-5 arthroscope portal, the suture ends are tied down to the dorsal ulnar capsule. Postoperatively, the wrist is placed in a splint in ulnar deviation, the wounds are checked in 10 to 14 days, and the joint is kept immobilized in ulnar deviation for 1 month. Gentle range of motion exercises are then initiated.

Incomplete intercarpal ligament tears have been seen as a source of mechanical wrist pain. There may be point tenderness over the involved ligament. A lidocaine injection test can be helpful in the diagnosis. MRI and arthrography have shown that asymptomatic wrists can have perforations of the scapholunate and lunotriquetral ligaments, and, therefore, careful delineation between traumatic tears and coincidental findings is best accomplished with a thorough history and physical examination.

Visualization of the scapholunate ligament from the 3-4 portal is performed with débridement carried out through the 4-5 portal. Viewing a suspected lunotriquetral ligament tear is accomplished by inserting the arthroscope in the 4-5 portal and using the 6-R portal for instrumentation. The scapholunate interval is probed and stressed, and if there is any doubt of instability, the interval should be assessed from the ulnar midcarpal portal. Gross instability is evident with obvious gapping of the interval in the radiocarpal joint or the midcarpal joint. Arthroscopically assisted pinning of grossly unstable joints has been reported, but we favor arthrotomy and pinning in these situations, whether acute or chronic.[143]

Wrist arthroscopy of intra-articular distal radius and carpal fractures has gained popularity. Arthroscopy has been helpful in reducing intra-articular distal radius fractures as well as in diagnosing concomitant intercarpal ligament injuries.[45, 119] Arthroscopy has also been used for reduction and internal fixation of scaphoid fractures.[134] Our use of arthroscopy for these fractures is limited, and we still resort to open reduction and internal fixation (ORIF) of these fractures. Osteochondral flaps, chondromalacia, and degenerative arthritis can also be diagnosed and treated effectively arthroscopically.

Wrist Disorders

Carpal Instabilities

Scapholunate Instability

Scapholunate instability or rotary subluxation of the scaphoid is the most common form of carpal instability. It is frequently diagnosed late owing to the patient's own delay in presenting for treatment. Diagnosis can be difficult because of the subtle findings in this condition.

Three ligaments are involved in scapholunate instability: the interosseous scapholunate ligament, the dorsal scapholunate ligament, and the volar radioscapholunate ligament (Fig. 24A1–14), which is the strongest and most important of the three. Anatomic studies have demonstrated that two of the three ligaments must be disrupted for dissociation to occur, and the volar radioscapholunate ligament must be ruptured before complete subluxation can occur.[83, 132]

Clinical Evaluation

The usual history involves a fall or direct blow that causes hyperextension of the wrist. Pain, swelling, and tenderness are noted over the dorsoradial aspect of the wrist, particularly in the anatomic snuffbox. Watson[138] has described a provocative test in which the examiner stabilizes the scaphoid by placing his or her thumb over the volar pole of the scaphoid while the wrist is held in ulnar

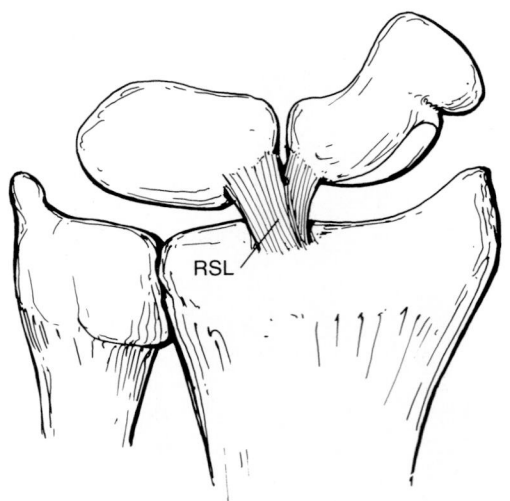

Figure 24A1–14. Volar ligaments. The most important stabilizer of the proximal pole of the scaphoid is the radioscapholunate ligament (RSL). (Illustration by Elizabeth Roselius, © 1985. Reprinted with permission from Taleisnik J: The Wrist. New York, Churchill Livingstone, 1985.)

deviation. As the hand is brought into radial deviation, pain is produced as the force is transmitted to the injured scapholunate ligaments (Fig. 24A1–15).

Radiograph findings may be subtle (Fig. 24A1–16). An

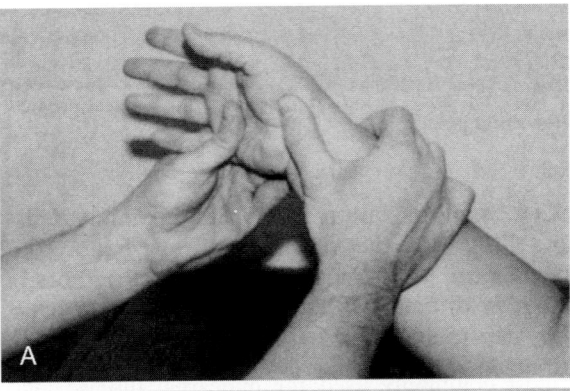

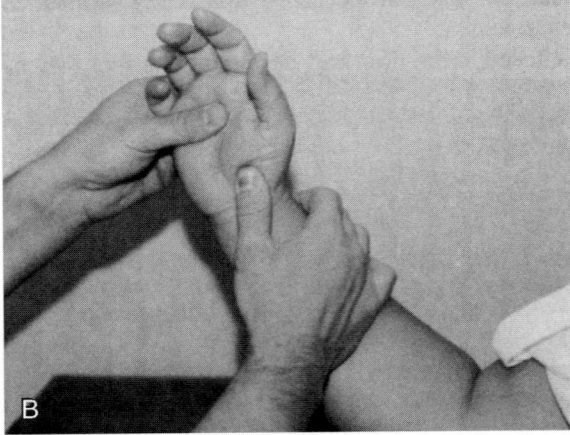

Figure 24A1–15. The Watson test for scapholunate instability. *A,* The scaphoid is stabilized with the thumb over the volar pole. *B,* When the hand is brought from ulnar to radial deviation, pain results.

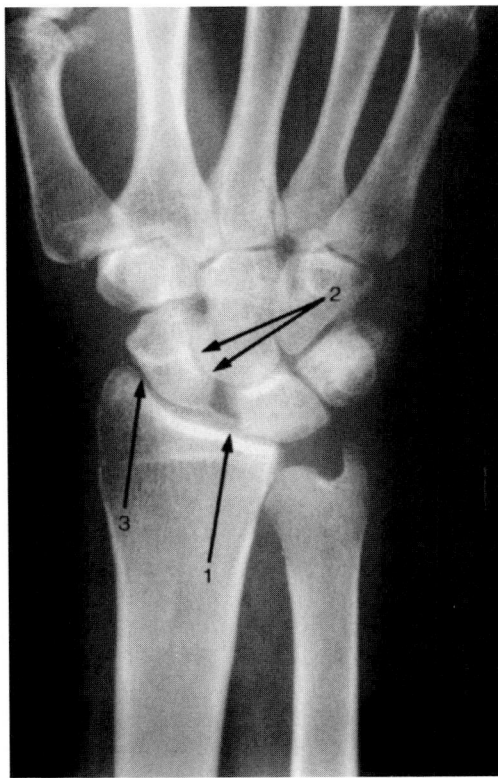

Figure 24A1–16. Radiographic findings of scapholunate dissociation: (1) widening of the scapholunate interval, (2) shortened appearance of the scaphoid, and (3) the "ring sign" of the cortical projection of the distal pole.

AP view in full supination may demonstrate widening of the scapholunate interval. A gap of more than 2 mm is abnormal. The scaphoid will be shortened because it is subluxated into a more vertical position, and a ring sign may be present representing the cortical projection of the distal pole in its more vertical position. The lateral radiograph may reveal a DISI pattern. A scapholunate angle of more than 70 degrees (normal 30 to 60 degrees) is also suggestive of scapholunate dissociation (Fig. 24A1–17).[40] The scaphoid axis is drawn longitudinally through the long axis of the scaphoid transecting the proximal (dorsal) and distal (volar) convexities at each end of the bone. The lunate axis is drawn perpendicular to the proximal and distal articular surfaces of the lunate and should transect the bone into dorsal and volar halves. The angle formed by these two lines is the scapholunate angle, and its normal values range from 30 to 60 degrees.[88]

Special radiographic studies usually are not necessary. If the diagnosis remains in doubt, cineradiography can be helpful in demonstrating the instability.[103] Bone scans and arthrography can aid in localizing the area of injury[68] but are not specifically indicated for scapholunate instability.

Treatment of Acute Injuries

Early treatment of ligament injuries yields the best results. Injuries diagnosed within 3 weeks can be treated as acute,[14] although Linscheid has suggested that acute treatment may be successful for up to 3 months.[88]

Cast immobilization has been recommended by King[77] with the wrist in full supination, mild dorsiflexion, and ulnar deviation. Most authors feel that it is difficult to maintain reduction in a cast. This treatment is probably applicable in cases of suspected scapholunate injury in which actual dissociation has not occurred and radiographic studies are negative.

Closed reduction and percutaneous pinning may be successful, but care must be taken that a complete reduction has been obtained.[104] The wrist should be maintained in dorsiflexion to reduce the proximal pole of the scaphoid while the scapholunate joint is pinned. A Kirschner wire (K-wire) is passed percutaneously through the snuffbox and across the scapholunate joint. A second K-wire may be used to provide additional stability across the scapholunate joint. The wrist should then be gently palmar-flexed to approximate the volar ligaments.[37] A K-wire is then passed across the scaphoid into the capitate for final stabilization. A K-wire across the radiocarpal joint is not necessary. The wires can be removed after 8 to 10 weeks, and a protective splint is then used for an additional 4 weeks.

ORIF offers the obvious advantage that the scapholunate joint is reduced, and direct repair of the ligaments can be accomplished. Most authors recommend a dorsal approach.[104] Repair of the volar ligaments does not appear to be necessary for a good result. Blatt[16] has used a portion of the dorsal capsule as a tenodesis to reinforce acute repairs.

It is particularly important to remember that in patients with acute or chronic scapholunate instability, treatment of any type rarely gives completely satisfactory results. In patients with partial injuries, closed reduction and cast immobilization for 6 to 10 weeks may allow healing. In complete tears with significant displacement, however, we have found it difficult to obtain a satisfactory reduction by closed means. In certain cases, percutaneous pinning with image intensification may allow satisfactory reduction. To allow proper approximation of the torn ends of the ligaments, the scaphoid should be reduced initially with the wrist in dorsiflexion and pinned to the carpals to stabilize

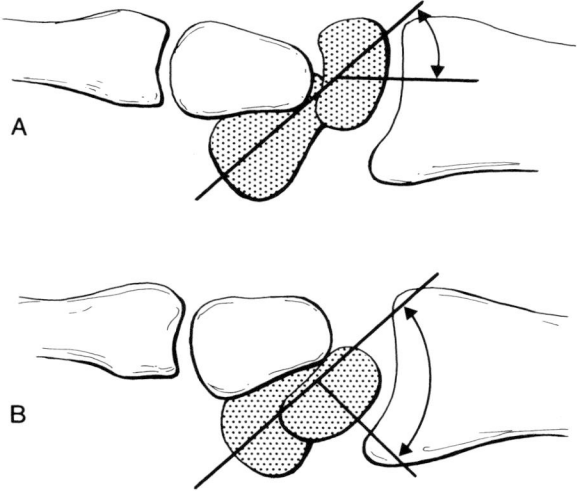

Figure 24A1–17. The normal scapholunate angle (A) is 30 to 60 degrees. A scapholunate angle of more than 70 degrees (B) suggests scapholunate dissociation. (Redrawn from Green DP: Operative Hand Surgery, 2nd ed. New York, Churchill Livingstone, 1988.)

the proximal pole of the scaphoid. Then the wrist is brought into volar flexion to approximate the torn ends of the volar ligaments, and the radioscaphoid joint is pinned in this position. The wrist is then immobilized in a short-arm thumb spica cast. The wires can be removed at 8 weeks and the wrist immobilized for an additional 4 weeks in a short-arm cast. The patient is then fitted with a protective splint, and an active rehabilitation program is started.

Authors' Preferred Method of Treatment. In the majority of cases, we have not felt that a satisfactory reduction could be attained by closed methods. We prefer to treat most patients with open techniques. In our experience, open reduction is best performed through a dorsal approach with repair of the dorsal scapholunate interosseous ligaments. When the ligament cannot be adequately repaired, reinforcement with local soft tissue is carried out. This can be accomplished by using a portion of the dorsal capsule. In addition, a second incision is made on the volar aspect of the wrist to expose and repair the avulsed volar ligaments, which are usually detached en masse. Decompression of the medial nerve can also be accomplished at the same time because associated carpal tunnel syndrome is often present. It is important to remember that the fresh injury may be superimposed on a chronic instability, and soft tissue as well as articular cartilage changes may be encountered. Fixation with K-wires is indicated for temporary stabilization of the scaphoid to the capitate and lunate as well as for stabilization of the radiocarpal joint. The wrist can be immobilized in a neutral or slightly dorsiflexed position in a thumb spica cast for 8 weeks, at which time the pins are removed. A short-arm cast is used for an additional 4 weeks, and then the patient is fitted with a protective splint, and a rehabilitation program is begun. Our rehabilitation program is discussed at the end of this subchapter.

Criteria for Return to Sports Participation. The athlete may be allowed to return to sports activity after he or she demonstrates progress in a supervised rehabilitation program. Normally, 1 to 2 months are necessary to demonstrate significant progress in strength and range of motion. The athlete should be protected by an orthosis such as a silicone or synthetic fiberglass cast during participation in sports. At 6 months, the athlete may be allowed to participate without an orthosis if he or she demonstrates maximum strength and range of motion.

Treatment of Chronic Injuries without Degenerative Changes

Chronic scapholunate instability presents a more complex problem and a greater challenge in management. Chronic instability is defined as an injury that has lasted longer than 3 months. The diagnostic criteria and clinical evaluation for chronic injuries are the same as described previously for acute injuries. Additionally, degenerative changes may be noted on radiographs with loss of the interosseous space at the radiocarpal and intercarpal joints as well as osteophyte formation in the late stages. There is still no consistently reliable and predictable procedure for treatment of chronic injuries.

Blatt[16] uses a dorsal tenodesis technique in which the dorsal capsule acts as a check rein to prevent volar rotation of the distal pole of the scaphoid. Other authors[40, 132] have used tendon grafts to reconstruct the scapholunate ligament or the radioscapholunate ligament. These methods are complex and not consistently reliable.

A variety of intercarpal arthrodeses have been performed to correct late scapholunate instability. These limited wrist arthrodeses attempt to control the subluxation of the scaphoid. Scapholunate joint arthrodesis intuitively seems to be the most appropriate procedure; however, this is a difficult joint in which to attain successful fusion[136] owing to its small size and the significant forces directed across it. The capitate can be included in a scapholunate arthrodesis to increase success in attaining solid fusion by increasing the area of fusion. This, however, results in further loss of wrist motion,[60] primarily palmar flexion. Triscaphe (trapezium-trapezoid-scaphoid) fusion in which the distal pole is stabilized has been popularized by Watson.[138] This prevents subluxation of the proximal pole, but the technique is demanding, and care must be taken that the scaphoid is properly reduced.

The delay in diagnosis may lessen the chance of a successful result, and it is important to remember that a completely successful result almost never occurs. In chronic cases without degenerative changes, various methods of reconstruction of the ligaments may be carried out. We initially used a variation of the procedure described by Dobyns and colleagues[40] to reconstruct the interosseous ligament with a strip of the extensor carpi radialis. We have been relatively pleased with the initial results, although stretching of the structures with widening of the scapholunate interval often occurs. The presence of an interpositional ligament, however, seems to prevent proximal migration of the capitate and the subsequent changes caused by migration. Motion, although decreased in most cases, is usually within a functional range. The primary drawback to this procedure, however, is the technical difficulty in performing the reconstruction of the interosseous ligaments.

In our experience, attempts to perform a scapholunate arthrodesis to stabilize the scapholunate joint are functionally gratifying. Although bony arthrodesis may not occur, it appears that a fibrous union does occur to prevent migration of the capitate. Including the capitate in the fusion increases the chances of obtaining a bony fusion but does result in further restriction of motion. The scapho-trapezial-trapezoid arthrodesis described by Peterson and Lipscomb[112] and popularized by Watson[138] has met with some success in our hands. We are concerned about the increased stress on the other joints, particularly the radioscaphoid joint and the lack of control of the scapholunate interval. We have used a number of these procedures with varied success, but results have improved with more experience.

Authors' Preferred Method of Treatment. At present we are using the procedure described by Blatt, the dorsal capsulodesis, and we have been gratified by the functional results and lack of problems with healing compared with the other procedures described. The goal of the procedure is to reduce the scaphoid from its rotary subluxation and secure it in a reduced position with a strip of the dorsal capsule (Fig. 24A1–18). A dorsal approach to the wrist is made, and a 1-cm strip of dorsal capsule is fashioned based

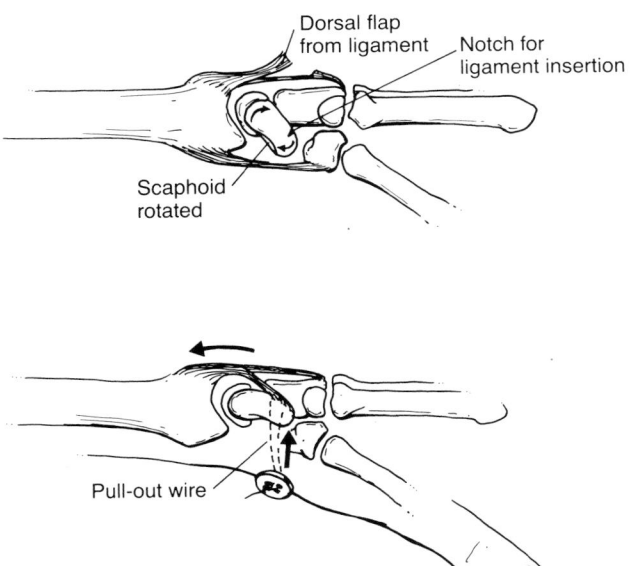

Figure 24A1–18. Blatt's dorsal capsulodesis for chronic scapholunate dissociation. (Illustration by Elizabeth Roselius, © 1988. Reprinted with permission from Green DP: Operative Hand Surgery, 2nd ed. New York, Churchill Livingstone, 1988.)

on the ulnar aspect of the distal radius. This provides a flap of the capsule that will be oriented obliquely across the carpus in line with the long axis of the scaphoid. The scaphoid is reduced by manipulating the scaphoid out of its volar rotated position. The reduction is maintained by passing a K-wire through the distal pole of the scaphoid and into the capitate. An additional K-wire may be passed across the radioscaphoid joint for additional stability. A trough is created in the distal pole of the scaphoid, taking care to make the trough distal to the mid axis. The dorsal flap of tissue is then secured to the trough with a pullout wire over the button on the volar aspect of the wrist. The wrist is immobilized in a thumb spica cast. The K-wires and pullout wire are removed at 8 to 12 weeks. Total cast immobilization lasts for 12 weeks followed by active rehabilitation. We are becoming more pleased with the triscaphe intercarpal fusion through a transverse incision half an inch distal to the radial styloid and a half an inch proximal to the radial styloid to obtain the bone graft. Direct reconstruction with the use of a free graft between the roughened scaphoid and lunate bone surfaces held with bone anchors can be considered. Our rehabilitation program is discussed at the end of the subchapter.

Criteria for Return to Sports Participation. The athlete may be allowed to return to sports activity after he or she demonstrates progress in a supervised rehabilitation program. Normally 1 to 2 months are necessary to demonstrate significant progress in strength and range of motion. The athlete should be protected by an orthosis such as a silicone or synthetic fiberglass cast during participation in sports. At 6 months, the athlete may be allowed to participate without an orthosis if he or she demonstrates maximum strength and range of motion.

Salvage Procedures

In patients with scapholunate instability and established arthrosis, pain will not be relieved by the preceding procedures. Athletes with an advanced stage of arthrosis[2] will probably have already experienced significant limitation of sports activity that is dependent on wrist function. Even with a salvage procedure, they would not be expected to regain their previous level of activity.

A variety of salvage procedures have been suggested. Styloidectomy may be applicable in patients with arthrosis localized to the radioscaphoid joint, but it is often only a temporizing procedure and can compromise later procedures. Occasionally, it can cause increased instability if too much of the styloid is removed. Proximal row carpectomy appears to have relatively good results but does result in decreased grip strength.[61] The procedure must be done before degenerative changes involve the proximal pole of the capitate or the lunate fossa of the radius. Silastic scaphoid replacement carries the risk of silicone synovitis. The implications of this complication are not clear at this time. If this technique is to be used, it should probably be combined with a midcarpal arthrodesis.[137] One should avoid placing K-wires or sutures through the implant if possible because this process may be related to later silicone synovitis. Total wrist arthroplasty is applicable only in persons who are not involved in activities that place heavy stress on the wrist. Wrist arthrodesis is more applicable as a salvage procedure in patients who are athletically active.

Salvage procedures by definition are probably not consistent with maintaining athletic activities. For completeness, however, we briefly cover procedures that can be considered. We have found that the proximal row carpectomy, despite its controversial aspects, has been very useful in allowing preservation of functional wrist motion. It should be performed before degenerative changes are present in the proximal pole of the capitate. This procedure does result in some weakness of grip strength. If the procedure is unsuccessful owing to persistent pain, an arthrodesis can be carried out at a later date. If degenerative changes in the carpus are significant, particularly in individuals desiring to return to heavy activity, wrist arthrodesis is the procedure of choice. Arthroplasty can be carried out to maintain motion but does not hold up with heavy use. Implants with associated intercarpal fusion may be helpful in certain individuals, but again these do not do so well in people requiring heavy or repetitious use of the wrist.

Medial (Ulnar) Carpal Instability

Our appreciation of wrist instabilities on the ulnar aspect of the wrist has increased tremendously over the last decade. In the past, these problems have been more difficult to diagnose and treat because of our lack of knowledge. Recent advances have resulted in an increased awareness and more appropriate management. Patients present with wrist pain and often complain of a painful click, which may be audible or palpable. There may be a history of trauma, but frequently the patient does not recall a specific inciting episode.

Triquetrohamate Instability

The most common ulnar instability is triquetrohamate dissociation. These patients have a characteristic "clunk" that can be audible and palpable. It is reproduced by active motion. Alexander and Lichtman state that the ulnar arm of the arcuate ligament extending from the capitate to the triquetrum is torn, causing the instability.[3] This clunk represents the triquetrum suddenly snapping back and forth over the lunate articulation with ulnar and radial deviation rather than following its normal smooth synchronous course.

Clinical Evaluation. Physical examination may elicit point tenderness over the triquetrum. Plain radiographs usually offer no clues to the pathologic process. A DISI pattern may be present in advanced stages, although a VISI pattern has rarely been noted.[128] Cineradiographs are most useful and demonstrate abnormal motion well.[3] In particular, the lunate can be seen to snap suddenly at the moment the triquetrum reduces on the lunate. An arthrogram should be negative in isolated triquetrohamate instability because the lesion does not involve communication between the radiocarpal joint and the midcarpal joint. When a triquetrolunate lesion coexists, however, with a triquetrohamate instability, the arthrogram will be positive owing to flow of dye through the incompetent triquetrolunate joint. In these cases, the clinical effect of triquetrohamate instability will take precedence over the less severe triquetrolunate lesion.

Triquetrolunate Instability

Clinical Evaluation. Triquetrolunate instability is not as common as triquetrohamate instability. Patients may or may not have a wrist click. Local tenderness can be elicited over the triquetrolunate joint. Reagan and colleagues[115] have described a ballottement test (Fig. 24A1–19) in which the lunate is stabilized by one hand while the other hand shifts the triquetrum in a palmar and dorsal direction. This reproduces the pain the patient has experienced. Plain radiographs are usually not helpful in our experience, although a VISI pattern has occasionally been noted.[84] Measurement of the lunate-triquetral angle has been described,[105] but we have found it difficult consistently to measure this angle accurately. Cineradiography is usually normal, unlike in triquetrohamate instability, in which it is notably abnormal. Arthrograms can be helpful but should be observed closely to determine whether dye flows through the triquetrolunate joint to confirm the site of disease.[23]

Treatment. All patients should have a trial of conservative treatment consisting of immobilization in a splint or cast and an anti-inflammatory medication. Local steroid injection into the involved joint can be helpful. Modification of activities may be necessary after acute symptoms resolve. Athletes who are symptomatic primarily during sports activity can be fitted with a splint to correct triquetrohamate instability.[84] The splint reduces the VISI sag of the proximal row by pushing dorsally on the pisiform (Fig. 24A1–20).

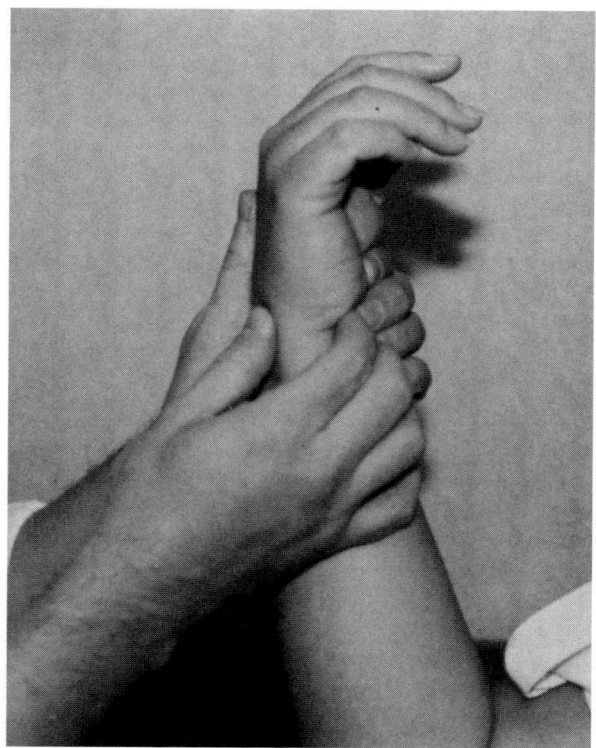

Figure 24A1–19. The ballottement test described by Reagan and colleagues.[115] The lunate is stabilized by one hand while the triquetrum is shifted in a palmar and dorsal direction with the examiner's opposite hand.

Authors' Preferred Method of Treatment. Surgery can be considered in patients who do not respond to conservative treatment. Reconstruction of the ligaments is technically demanding. We prefer to perform an intercarpal arthrodesis of the involved joint. In this procedure we use a dorsal approach between the fourth and fifth dorsal com-

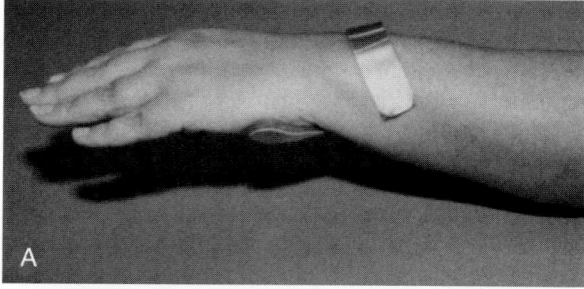

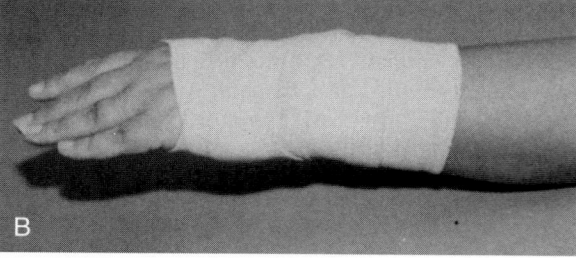

Figure 24A1–20. A splint supporting a wrist with triquetral hamate instability helps to reduce the proximal row by putting pressure dorsally on the pisiform.

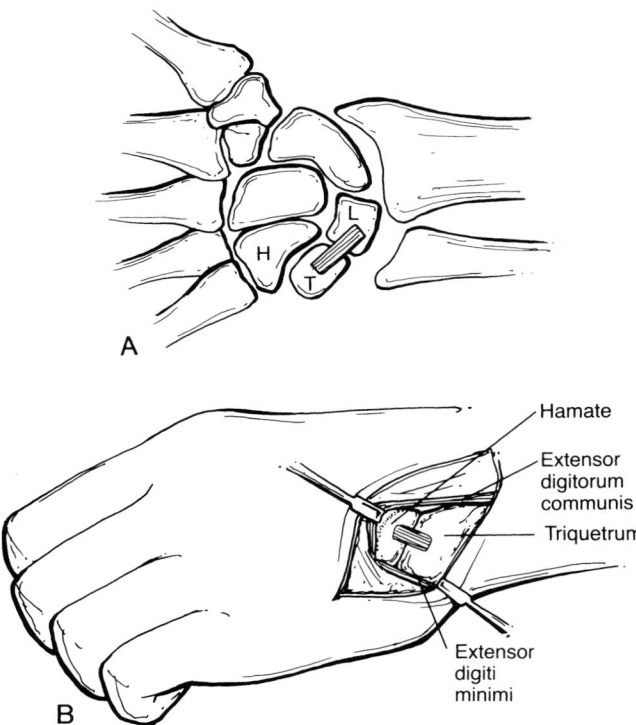

A

Hamate

Extensor
digitorum
communis

Triquetrum

Extensor
digiti
minimi

B

Figure 24A1–21. *A*, Triquetrolunate arthrodesis. *B*, Triquetrohamate arthrodesis. H, hamate; L, lunate; T, triquetrum.

partments. The triquetrohamate and triquetrolunate joints are inspected, and the wrist is stressed by axial compression and deviation to confirm the location of the instability. The triquetrum is then reduced and fixed internally by inserting K-wires across the involved joint. The joint surfaces are denuded, and a trough is created across the joint. The spatial relationship of the joint is maintained by filling the joint space with cancellous bone chips. A corticocancellous graft is taken from the distal radius to fill the trough (Fig. 24A1–21). The wrist is immobilized for 8 weeks in a short-arm cast, after which the pins are removed and a rehabilitation program is initiated. Patients should expect to lose some wrist motion. Usually, range of motion will improve during the first year postoperatively. Proportionally more dorsiflexion than palmar flexion can be expected to be regained.

Criteria for Return to Sports Participation. The athlete may be allowed to return to sports activity after he or she demonstrates progress in a supervised rehabilitation program. Normally 1 to 2 months are necessary to demonstrate significant progress in strength and range of motion. The athlete should be protected by an orthosis such as a silicone or synthetic fiberglass cast during participation in sports. At 6 months, the athlete may be allowed to participate without an orthosis if he or she demonstrates maximum strength and functional range of motion.

Fractures

Scaphoid Fractures

Fractures of the scaphoid are the most common fractures involving the carpal bones.[20] The incidence of this fracture

in college-level football players has been reported to be as high as 1 in 100 players per year.[147] The trauma causing the injury is frequently minor and leads many physicians to discount it as a sprain, resulting in delayed diagnosis. The mechanism of injury is probably forced hyperextension with the wrist in ulnar deviation.[95]

The vascular supply of the scaphoid plays a prominent role in the high incidence of nonunion associated with this fracture. Extraosseous vessels enter the middle and distal portions of the scaphoid.[47] The proximal pole (see Fig. 24A1–3) receives no direct vascular supply but derives its supply from the intraosseous vessels passing retrograde from the waist. This arrangement provides an anatomic basis for the notably high rate of nonunion and avascular necrosis characteristic of proximal pole fractures.

Clinical Evaluation. Patients present with wrist pain localized to the snuffbox. This finding alone should be enough to justify immobilization until a definitive diagnosis is made. Radiographs should include a PA view in neutral and ulnar deviation, a lateral view, and a closed fist view (Fig. 24A1–22). Polytomography is helpful in defining a nondisplaced fracture.[89] A bone scan after 72 hours can also identify a fracture, and a negative bone scan effectively rules out the diagnosis (Fig. 24A1–23).[103]

Factors Affecting Healing. Several factors have been identified as having an adverse effect on healing. Fractures of the proximal pole clearly have a higher incidence of delayed union,[39] nonunion, and avascular necrosis.[34] Russe[122] states that vertical and oblique fractures are potentially unstable and require prolonged immobilization. Uncorrected displacement of more than 1 mm and delay in diagnosis for longer than 4 weeks affect healing adversely.[42] Uncomplicated scaphoid fractures have a union rate of 95% when they are diagnosed early and immobilized.[104]

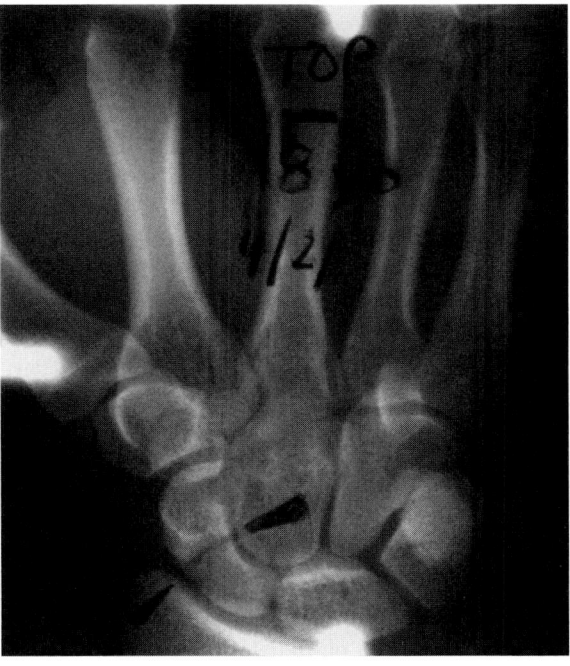

Figure 24A1–22. Scaphoid fracture.

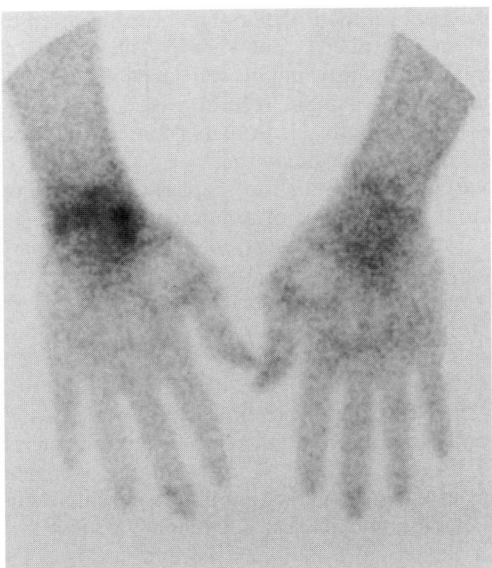

Figure 24A1–23. Bone scan demonstrating increased uptake over the scaphoid.

Treatment

Nondisplaced Fractures. Nondisplaced fractures can be treated by immobilization. There is significant disagreement about the position and type of immobilization. A review of the literature[72, 95, 104] supports placing the wrist in slight (10 degrees) palmar flexion and radial deviation. A recent prospective study gives strong support to using a long-arm thumb spica cast for 6 weeks followed by a short-arm spica cast.[51] This study indicates that healing time is shortened by using a long-arm spica cast initially. In athletes, nondisplaced fractures of the wrist have been effectively immobilized for competition in contact sports in plaster, synthetic, or Silastic casts.[116] If serial radiographs taken monthly demonstrate no progress toward union after 3 to 4 months, consideration can be given to bone grafting or electrical stimulation.[17]

Displaced Fractures. Displaced fractures of more than 1 mm of the scaphoid require accurate reduction by either closed or open methods. Failure to reduce a displaced fracture accurately results in an unacceptably high rate of nonunion.[42] Several studies[78, 115] have reported successful treatment of displaced fractures by closed methods. Attaining and maintaining accurate reduction of a displaced fracture is quite difficult, and open reduction is usually necessary.[104] ORIF can be accomplished by volar approach and fixation with K-wires. Internal fixation by means of the Herbert screw[65] is technically demanding but has the advantage of providing compression and allowing early mobilization. When a displaced fracture of the scaphoid is associated with a dorsiflexion instability, a dorsal approach is necessary to reduce and pin the lunate along with the scaphoid fracture.

Authors' Preferred Method of Treatment. Nondisplaced fractures (less than 1 mm displacement) are treated in a short-arm thumb spica cast using synthetic (fiberglass) casting material. Based on individual factors, athletes may be allowed to participate in their sport if immobilization

does not prevent sport-specific function of the extremity. Immobilization is continued until healing is demonstrated by radiograph, usually within 3 months. The wrist is protected during strenuous use with a rigid splint for an additional 2 months.

If there is no evidence of healing after 6 months, we prefer to proceed with bone grafting and internal fixation as needed. The scaphoid is approached through a volar incision, and accurate reduction is attained. A trough is developed longitudinally across the nonunion with osteotomes and a power bur. A corticocancellous bone graft is harvested from the distal radius through the same incision and placed in the trough. If the fracture is not thought to be sufficiently stable, internal fixation is attained with two smooth K-wires. The extremity is immobilized for 6 weeks in a long-arm thumb spica cast followed by a short-arm thumb spica until healing has occurred. The K-wires are removed before rehabilitation.

Proximal third fractures of the scaphoid are treated similarly but tend to have a higher incidence of avascular necrosis and nonunion. If the proximal fragment is large enough, cases of nonunion are treated by bone grafting as described above. When the proximal fragment is too small for adequate bone grafting and internal fixation, we have excised the proximal fragment and inserted a hand-fashioned spacer of silicone or a soft tissue spacer of capsule or tendon. The wrist is immobilized for 4 weeks in a short-arm cast, and rehabilitation is then begun.

Displaced fractures are treated by open reduction through a volar Russe approach. Any rotary deformity is corrected, and the fracture is stabilized with at least two smooth K-wires. In isolated scaphoid fractures, the K-wires are not placed across the intercarpal joints. The wires are cut off beneath the skin. The extremity is immobilized in a long-arm thumb spica cast for 6 weeks followed by a short-arm thumb spica cast, which is continued until radiographs demonstrate healing. The K-wires are removed, and rehabilitation is initiated.

Criteria for Return to Sports Participation. Following removal of the cast, the athlete is placed on a supervised program of strengthening and range of motion exercises. The wrist is protected with a rigid splint for athletic activities until strength approaches that of the opposite wrist and motion approaches functional range. The wrist is protected for a minimum of 3 months following cast removal on an empirical basis.

Hamate Fractures

Fractures of the hamate usually occur at the hook, and the diagnosis is commonly missed.[113] In athletes, this injury commonly results from the direct force of a bat, club, or racket.[127] Pain can be localized to the hamate hook over the hypothenar eminence. A carpal tunnel view is necessary to demonstrate the fracture radiographically (Fig. 24A1–24). Tomograms and computed tomography scans can aid in diagnosis in questionable cases. Chronic fractures have been associated with rupture of the flexor tendons to the ring and little fingers[4] and with neuropathy of the ulnar nerve.[19]

Treatment. Healing of acute cases is rare even with ORIF.[15] Excision of the hook through the fracture site is

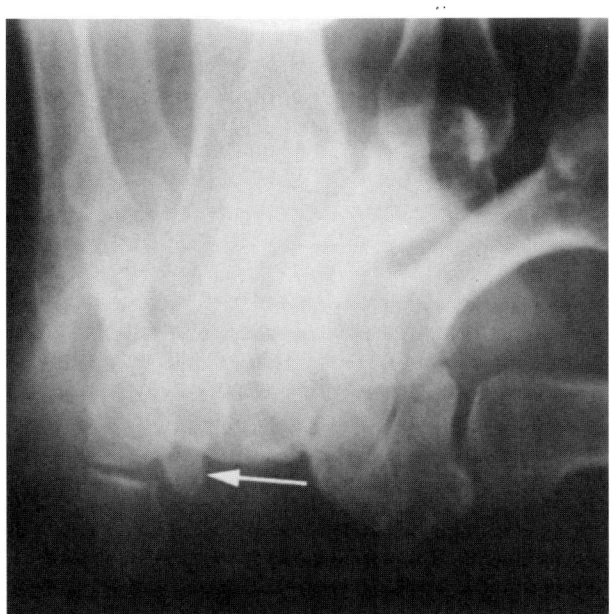

Figure 24A1–24. Carpal tunnel view isolating the hook of the hamate to allow visualization of a fracture.

an effective treatment and allows early return to sports in 6 to 8 weeks.[109] Care must be taken to protect the deep branch of the ulnar nerve during excision.

Fractures of the Body of the Hamate

Fractures of the body of the hamate are less common than hook fractures. They may be associated with dorsal dislocation of the fourth and fifth metacarpals.[92] They are appreciated best on oblique radiographs of the carpus.

Treatment. Nondisplaced fractures heal with cast immobilization for 4 to 6 weeks. Displaced fractures should be reduced and pinned with K-wires.

Authors' Preferred Method of Treatment. Fractures of the hook of the hamate are treated by excision through a palmar incision over the hook. The motor branch of the ulnar nerve is adjacent to the hook and must be identified and protected. The hook is excised through the fracture site, and the base is smoothed. The hand can be splinted until the incisional pain has resolved; vigorous mobilization follows.

See the following discussion on fractures of the body of the hamate for criteria on return to sports participation.

Nondisplaced fractures of the body of the hamate are immobilized in a short-arm cast for 4 to 6 weeks; this is followed by a mobilization program. Displaced fractures of more than 2 cm are treated by ORIF with K-wires. The wrist is immobilized for 4 to 6 weeks in a short-arm cast and then mobilized. The K-wires can be removed at 4 to 6 weeks or left in place until a later date if they are not causing discomfort.

Criteria for Return to Sports Participation. Athletes who have fractures that are treated nonsurgically may return to play immediately. The wrist is protected in a semirigid synthetic cast. Athletes with surgically treated fractures are usually restricted from active participation in

sports until after 4 to 6 weeks of mobilization. Protective splinting is continued for 3 months and thereafter until the wrist has normal strength and range of motion.

Capitate Fractures

Fractures of the capitate resemble fractures of the scaphoid in several ways. The mechanism of injury is variable and can result in different patterns of injury.[2] Fractures can result from a direct blow to the dorsum of the wrist or from forced dorsiflexion or palmar flexion. The wrist is usually found to be swollen with point tenderness over the dorsum at the base of the third and fourth rays. Detection on initial plain radiographs may be difficult, and follow-up radiographs in 7 to 10 days, tomograms, or bone scans may be needed to confirm the diagnosis.[2] Like the scaphoid, the blood supply to the proximal pole of the capitate is retrograde from vessels entering at the waist.[108] This explains the higher incidence of avascular necrosis seen in capitate fractures. Capitate fractures may be associated with fractures of the scaphoid and perilunate dislocations[114]; care should be taken not to overlook the capitate injury in these situations.

Treatment. Nondisplaced fractures can be managed by immobilization. Displaced fractures of more than 2 mm require ORIF with K-wires. Attention should be given to possible avascular necrosis of the proximal pole, although collapse is uncommon. An increased incidence of arthrosis has been noted on late follow-up.[114]

Authors' Preferred Method of Treatment. Nondisplaced fractures are evaluated carefully to ensure the absence of associated fractures of the scaphoid or dislocations of the carpometacarpal joints or perilunate dislocations. Isolated nondisplaced fractures of the capitate are immobilized in a short-arm cast for 6 weeks. The athlete may compete in a semirigid orthosis after the acute pain has resolved. At 6 weeks, the wrist is mobilized and strengthened.

Displaced fractures of more than 2 mm are treated with ORIF with K-wires. The capitate is approached by a dorsal incision, and reduction of the carpometacarpal joints is ensured. These can also be pinned with K-wires if necessary. The wrist is immobilized for 6 weeks in a short-arm cast. The K-wires can be removed at that time or following rehabilitation at the surgeon's discretion. Therapy to regain strength and range of motion is instituted as described later in this chapter.

Criteria for Return to Sports Participation. Athletes with fractures treated nonsurgically may return to play immediately. The wrist is protected in a semirigid synthetic cast. Athletes with surgically treated fractures are usually restricted from active participation in sports until after 4 to 6 weeks of mobilization. Protective splinting is continued for 3 months or until the wrist has normal strength and range of motion.

Pisiform Fractures

Fractures of the pisiform are uncommon and are usually nondisplaced. They usually result from direct trauma to the palm. Tenderness to palpation over the base of the hypothenar eminence suggests a pisiform fracture. These fractures are visualized best on 30-degree oblique AP views or on carpal tunnel views.[48] Pisiform fractures usually heal with immobilization lasting 3 to 6 weeks. Nonunion or malunion that is symptomatic is an indication for excision.[63]

Criteria for Return to Sports Participation. Taping the wrist or using a semirigid synthetic cast usually allows an athlete to resume sports as soon as the acute pain subsides. In rare cases of nonunion, the pisiform can be excised at the end of the athletic season.

Triquetrum Fractures

Triquetrum fractures can result from hyperextension with impingement of the distal ulna on the triquetrum. This typically causes an avulsion fracture from the dorsal cortex, which is demonstrated on a lateral or oblique radiograph of the wrist. The dorsal chip fracture routinely becomes painless after immobilization in a short-arm cast for 3 weeks. The athlete can participate in sports wearing a semirigid cast. Nonunion of a dorsal chip fracture has been noted but rarely causes persistent symptoms.[11]

Criteria for Return to Sports Participation. Athletes can usually participate in sports wearing a semirigid cast. When participation is precluded by a cast, the athlete can resume activity whenever the discomfort lessens to an extent that it does not interfere with sport-specific activity.

Osteochondroses

Lunate Kienböck's Disease

In 1910, Kienböck published an article titled "Traumatic Malacia of the Semilunar Bone"[76] in which he postulated that traumatic lesions of the lunate occurred more frequently than was believed at that time. The cause of this lesion and an accepted treatment have yet to be well established. Kienböck attributed the progressive collapse of the lunate to avascular necrosis, and although this theory is generally accepted, the cause of the lesion remains undetermined. Trauma has been implicated by Peste[111] and Kien-

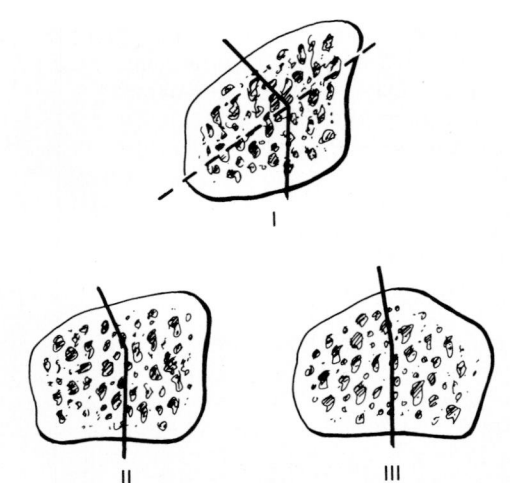

Figure 24A1–26. A lunate with an apical proximal surface (type I) has been implicated as being more susceptible to avascular necrosis and is associated with an ulnar-minus variant. (Illustration by Elizabeth Roselius, © 1988. Reprinted with permission from Green DP: Operative Hand Surgery, 2nd ed. New York, Churchill Livingstone, 1988.)

böck. Many subsequent authors have shared this view.[5, 14, 46, 110] Hulten[69] noted the increased incidence of avascular necrosis of the lunate in wrists that have an ulnar-minus variant in which the articular surface of the ulna is proximal to the articular surface of the radius (Fig. 24A1–25). Axelsson[9] and Gelberman and colleagues[48] have verified this finding. The shape of the lunate was implicated by Zapico,[6] who suggested that a lunate with an apical proximal articular surface is most susceptible to avascular necrosis (Fig. 24A1–26).

Although no single factor can be blamed for Kienböck's disease, avascular necrosis probably results from repetitive compression forces that cause microfractures of the cancellous bone in patients with a vascular or mechanical predisposition.[131] Continued stress prevents healing and leads ultimately to progressive collapse of the lunate and subsequent degenerative changes in the wrist.

Clinical Evaluation. Patients may complain of pain or stiffness. On occasion, symptoms of carpal tunnel syn-

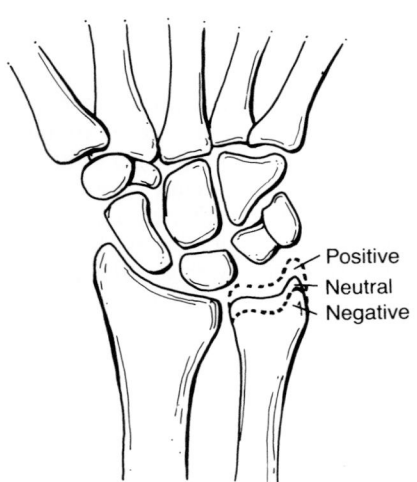

Positive
Neutral
Negative

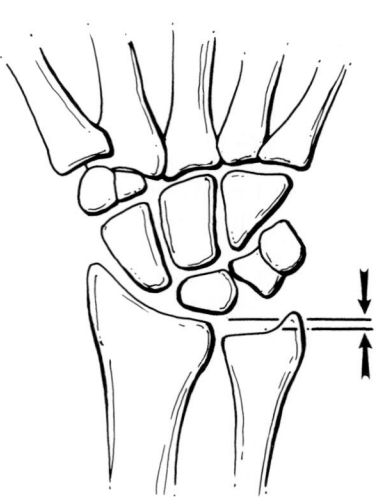

Figure 24A1–25. Ulnar variance. Ulnar-minus variant is associated with an increased incidence of avascular necrosis of the lunate.

drome have been noted.[12] Routine radiographs in the early stages may reveal no changes in the lunate, but the ulnar-minus variant may be noted. Tomography is sometimes helpful to demonstrate early lunate changes. Bone scans may demonstrate increased local uptake of contrast material.[13] Progressive radiograph changes noted include sclerosis, cyst formation, fragmentation and collapse with loss of carpal height, and finally degenerative joint changes throughout.[85] Stahl developed a classification of Kienböck's disease based on the radiographic changes (Fig. 24A1–27).[27]

Treatment. Multiple treatment methods have been suggested for Kienböck's disease. Basically, they can be categorized into two types. The first is an attempt to allow revascularization of the lunate by relieving the compression forces. This is accomplished by lengthening the ulna or shortening the radius in stage I before collapse of the lunate. In stage II, intercarpal arthrodesis may be appropriate. In the more advanced stages III and IV, treatment

methods include excision of the lunate with either soft tissue interposition or silicone replacement arthroplasty, or various types of intercarpal arthrodesis. Salvage procedures used in end-stage disease include proximal row carpectomy and wrist arthrodesis.

Immobilization in stage I was recommended by Stahl,[126] but other authors have noted progression of the disease when this method alone is used.[86, 135] Immobilization with an external fixator has been suggested to unload as well as immobilize the lunate,[85] but no results have yet been reported. Attempts to revascularize the lunate directly with pedicle flaps have been described,[22, 27] but the results so far have been inconclusive.

Ulnar shortening or radial lengthening to correct ulnar-minus variance is based on the theory that correction of this predisposing factor will relieve stress on the lunate and allow healing. Studies have demonstrated good results from these methods.[5, 7] This treatment is logical if it is applied before collapse of the lunate in stage III. Both

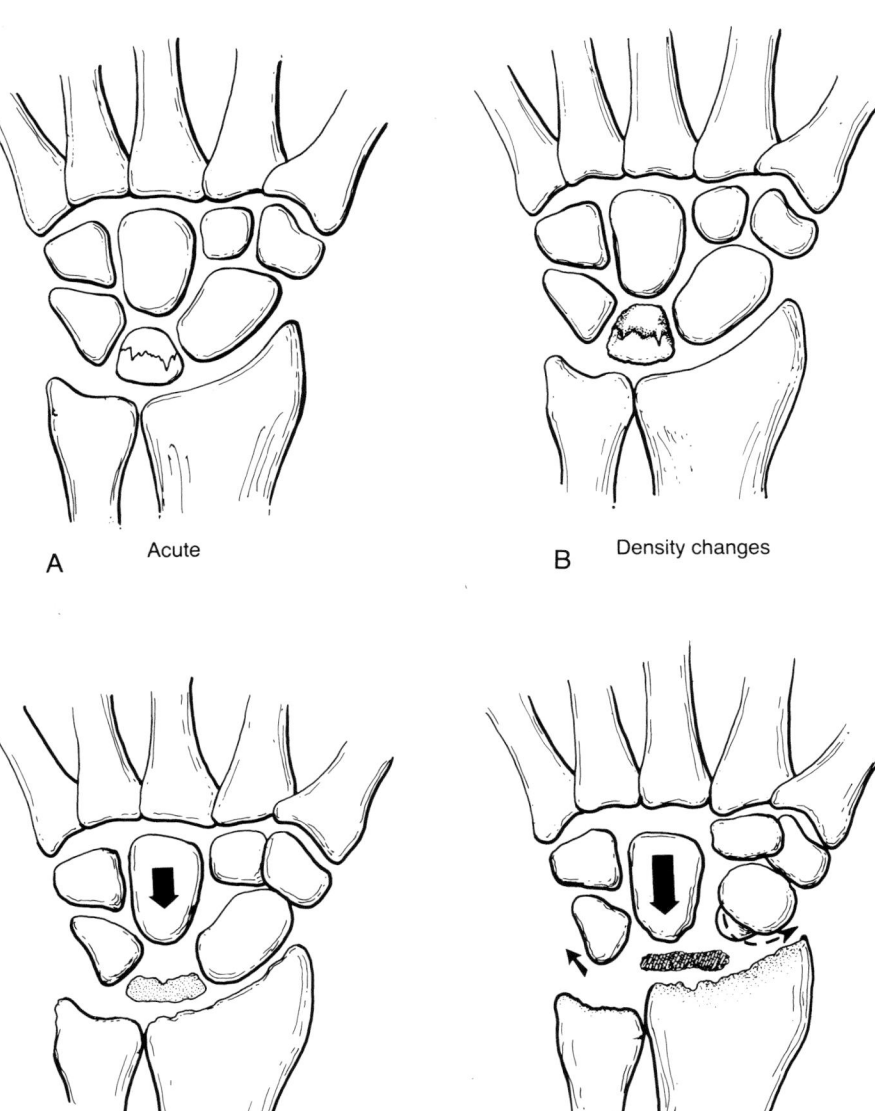

Figure 24A1–27. Modified Stahl's classification of Kienböck's disease. *A,* Stage I: Normal-appearing lunate with a compression fracture demonstrated by a radiolucent line. *B,* Stage II: Sclerosis of the lunate. *C,* Stage III: Collapse of the lunate. *D,* Stage IV: Pancarpal arthrodesis. (Redrawn from Lichtman DM, Alexander AH, Mack GR, Gunther SF: Kienböck's disease—update on silicone replacement arthroplasty. J Hand Surg 7:343–347, 1982.)

A   Acute

B   Density changes

C   Collapse of lunate

D   Pancarpal arthrosis

methods require osteotomy and internal fixation. Ulnar lengthening in addition requires harvesting bone graft from a donor site.

In theory, limited intercarpal fusion will relieve compression on the lunate and prevent further distortion of the normal carpal alignment. This method also has the advantage of preserving some carpal motion, unlike complete carpal arthrodesis. Several different methods have been advocated, including arthrodesis of the lunate to the adjacent carpal bones,[93] capitohamate fusion,[97] and triscaphe fusion.[85] These methods may be combined with lunate arthroplasty to obtain improved results. Lunate excision with or without interposition arthroplasty has been used as a treatment method in patients with stage III lesions in the past. Various tendons and capsules have been used as interposition material with fair results,[8] but this technique has been criticized by others[59] because proximal migration of the capitate is probable.

In end-stage Kienböck's disease with diffuse arthrosis, the previously mentioned procedures will not be adequate to relieve pain. Salvage procedures such as proximal row carpectomy[36] or complete wrist arthrodesis[86] have been used successfully in these instances. These methods, however, obviously sacrifice function to accomplish pain relief.

Authors' Preferred Method of Treatment. Lichtman and colleagues[80] recommended correlating treatment with the radiographic stages of Kienböck's disease as modified from Stahl's original classification (see Fig. 24A1–27). In stage I, the lunate is "decompressed" by procedures to prevent further trauma. This can be accomplished by using a leveling procedure (ulnar lengthening or radial shortening for ulnar-minus variant) or by a scapho-trapezial-trapezoid arthrodesis to decrease the compressive forces on the lunate. In stage II, collapse of the lunate exists, and we have used excision of the lunate and replacement with a silicone prosthesis. Despite the recent concern about silicone synovitis, we have not found this to be a significant problem in lunate replacement arthroplasty. It is important to avoid placing K-wires or suture through the implant. Also, sufficient stability of the implant must be attained at the time of surgery. The arthroplasty may also be combined with methods to reduce shear stress such as radial shortening, ulnar lengthening, or intercarpal arthrodesis.

The procedure is done through a dorsal incision over the lunate. A dorsal flap of capsule based distally is developed, and the lunate is excised with osteotomes and rongeur. The palmar cortex of the lunate is retained to provide volar support. Trials are used to obtain the appropriate size for the implant. There should be a full range of motion of the wrist without subluxation of the implant. The dorsal capsule is closed to provide additional support. If satisfactory stability cannot be attained, silicone arthroplasty should be abandoned, and a tendon interposition should be substituted for the implant.[85] The wrist is immobilized in a short-arm cast for 6 weeks.

With further collapse and associated carpal instability in stage III, we prefer to combine silicone replacement arthroplasty with scapho-trapezial-trapezoid arthrodesis. In stage IV, when advanced perilunate degenerative changes are present, a proximal row carpectomy is useful to maintain wrist motion. A complete wrist arthrodesis is an alternative if extensive arthrosis exists.

Criteria for Return to Sports Participation. Following removal of the cast, the athlete is placed on a supervised program of strengthening and range of motion exercises. The wrist is protected with a rigid splint for athletic activities until its strength approaches that of the opposite wrist and motion approaches the functional range. The wrist is protected for a minimum of 3 months following cast removal on an empirical basis.

Osteochondrosis of the Capitate

Avascular necrosis of the capitate is a rare disease. It was first reported by Destot of France in 1924.[100] In 1942, Jonsson recognized that avascular necrosis of the capitate was similar to Kienböck's disease.[75] The number of reported cases had been fewer than 10 until the 1980s, when this condition began to be recognized more frequently.[2, 18, 21, 66] There are no distinct differences in regard to age, sex, or occupation. Among athletes, this condition is seen more frequently in gymnasts.[100] It is postulated that chronic or repeated trauma is the cause.

Anatomically, the proximal portion of the capitate is supplied by intraosseous vessels flowing in a retrograde direction. Case reports describe the main lesion located anywhere from the isthmus to the proximal portion of the capitate. It is postulated that a microfracture may take place at the isthmus, thereby blocking blood flow to the more proximal portion and causing avascular necrosis.

Clinical Evaluation. Patients complain of gradual onset of pain without a specific episode of trauma. The pain is worse with exercise. Swelling and point tenderness are noted over the dorsum of the wrist, and range of motion is limited primarily in dorsiflexion. Grip strength is typically decreased. Radiographs show avascular changes in the capitate with sclerosis and absorption of bone.

Treatment. Treatment methods are varied and include intercarpal fusion and partial resection of the capitate. Intercarpal fusion is effective in relieving pain but does result in significant loss of motion. Partial resection will preserve motion but may not be as effective in the long term in relieving pain.[93] The limited number of cases reported, however, does not allow any definite conclusions about the appropriate management of these rare lesions.

Authors' Preferred Method of Treatment. We have not treated an athlete for this condition. Murakami and Nakajima[100] reviewed eight patients who were treated by partial resection of the capitate. This was combined with intercarpal arthrodesis in some patients. We agree with their recommendation that, in athletes, intercarpal arthrodesis should be avoided if full range of motion is required for athletic activity.

Criteria for Return to Sports Participation. Reports indicate that recovery in these cases may be prolonged. Return to sports must be judged individually based on reduction in pain and recovery of motion and strength. This appears to be particularly applicable to gymnasts.[100]

Entrapment Neuropathies

Median Nerve Compression (Carpal Tunnel Syndrome)

Carpal tunnel syndrome is the most common entrapment neuropathy associated with sports activities. The carpal

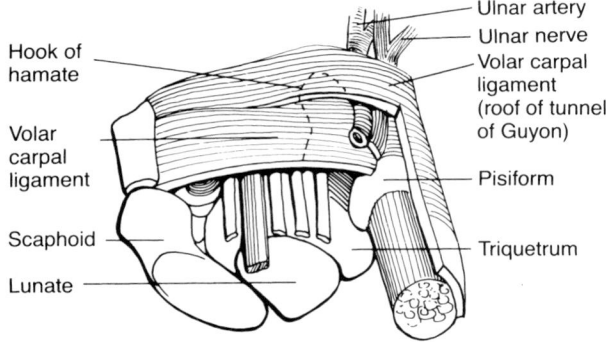

Figure 24A1–28. The carpal tunnel is formed by the transverse carpal ligament volarly and the carpal bones on the floor and the sides. Guyon's canal is formed by the volar carpal ligament (roof), the hamate (lateral wall), and the pisiform (medial wall).

tunnel is a fibro-osseous canal bound volarly by the transverse carpal ligament; the floor and walls are formed by the carpal bones (Fig. 24A1–28). The transverse carpal ligament attaches radially to the scaphoid and trapezium and ulnarly to the pisiform and hamate. The flexor pollicis longus, flexor digitorum profundus, and flexor digitorum superficialis tendons traverse the carpal tunnel along with the median nerve. Before entering the carpal tunnel, the median nerve gives off the palmar cutaneous branch, which passes superficial to the transverse carpal ligament and radial to the course of the median nerve (Fig. 24A1–29). The motor branch to the thenar muscles can vary its anatomic pattern from the median nerve (Fig. 24A1–30).[79] Usually the motor branch comes off distal to the transverse carpal ligament, but occasionally it can branch proximal to it and pass below the ligament or over the ligament. Usually the motor branch comes off on the radial side of the median nerve, but rarely it branches on the ulnar side and passes superficial to the transverse carpal ligament. Appreciation of these anatomic variants by the surgeon is

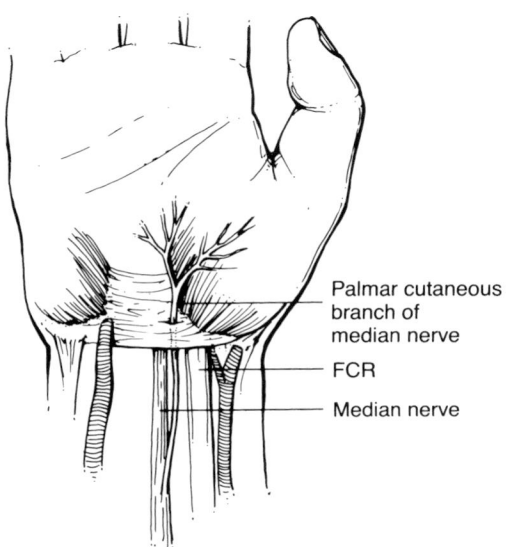

Figure 24A1–29. Palmar cutaneous branch of the median nerve. FCR, flexor carpi radialis.

critical to ensure protection of the motor branch during surgical exposure. The distal branches of the median nerve supply sensation to the thumb, index, and long fingers and to the radial aspect of the ring finger.

Any condition that reduces space in the carpal tunnel can cause compression of the median nerve. Usually, compression is caused by flexor tenosynovitis. Any sports activity that involves repetitive flexion or grasping can provoke symptoms,[80] which include numbness or tingling in the median distribution and aching pain radiating to the forearm, elbow, or shoulder. Pain or paresthesia often awakens the patient at night.[28] Symptoms can be triggered by position (wrist flexion) or repetitive grasping. Frequently, patients complain of clumsiness and loss of dexterity.[56]

Clinical Evaluation. The physical examination should include sensibility, motor, and provocative testing. Two-point discrimination is abnormal (>5 mm) in more advanced cases but can be normal in mild cases. Vibratory sensation may be a more sensitive test for detection of early carpal tunnel syndrome.[52] Motor testing should include observing for thenar atrophy and testing abduction against resistance (abductor pollicis brevis). Provocative tests include those to elicit Phalen's sign and Tinel's sign. Electromyography (EMG) can be used to confirm the diagnosis by demonstrating prolonged motor or sensory latency across the wrist. EMG testing is not necessary for patients who give a typical history and have appropriate physical findings. It is more useful for differentiating carpal tunnel syndrome from cervical radiculopathy.[99]

Treatment. Treatment is discussed in the following section on ulnar nerve entrapment.

Ulnar Nerve Compression (Guyon's Canal Syndrome)

Entrapment neuropathy of the ulnar nerve in Guyon's canal is much less common than carpal tunnel syndrome, but it is particularly apt to occur in cyclists and has been called "handle-bar palsy."[105] The cause in this case is direct pressure, and the syndrome is characterized by paresthesia in the ulnar one and a half digits.

Guyon's canal is triangular and is formed by the volar carpal ligament (roof), the hamate (lateral wall), and the pisiform and pisohamate ligament (medial wall) (see Fig. 24A1–28).[38] The ulnar nerve bifurcates within the canal into superficial and deep branches. The deep branch of the ulnar nerve, along with a branch of the ulnar artery, passes deep to the hypothenar muscles and is the motor branch to the interosseous muscles and adductor pollicis (Fig. 24A1–31). The superficial branch of the ulnar nerve passes superficial to the hypothenar muscles and supplies sensation to the ring and little fingers.[111]

Clinical Evaluation. Symptoms due to compression vary with the location of the lesion. Pressure proximal to the bifurcation of the ulnar nerve will result in both sensory and motor findings. Sensation is decreased in the ring and little fingers. Intrinsic muscle weakness or atrophy may be noted. Tinel's test may cause paresthesias into the little and ring fingers. Conversely, a lesion distal to the bifurcation of the nerve will result in findings limited to either motor

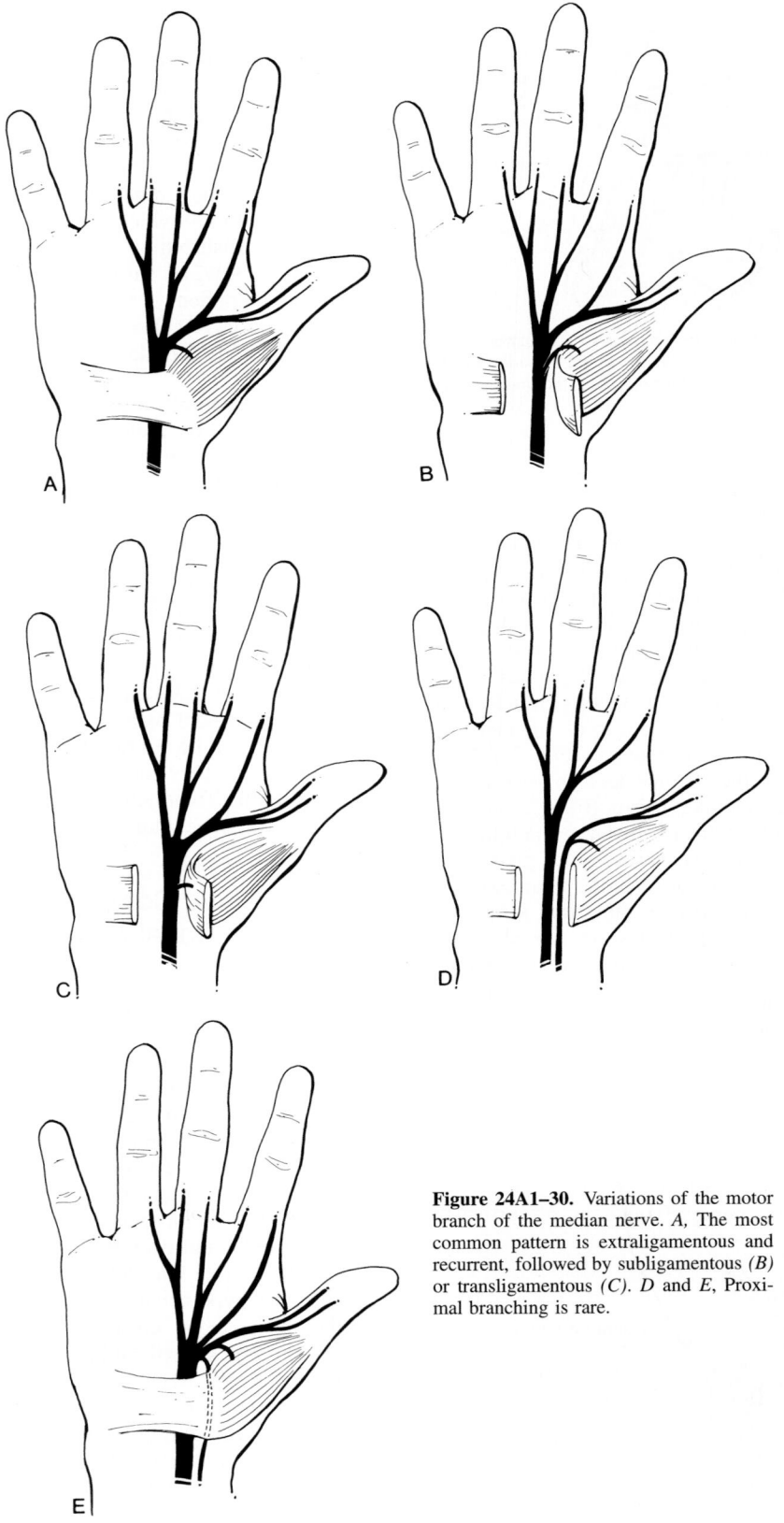

Figure 24A1–30. Variations of the motor branch of the median nerve. *A,* The most common pattern is extraligamentous and recurrent, followed by subligamentous *(B)* or transligamentous *(C). D* and *E,* Proximal branching is rare.

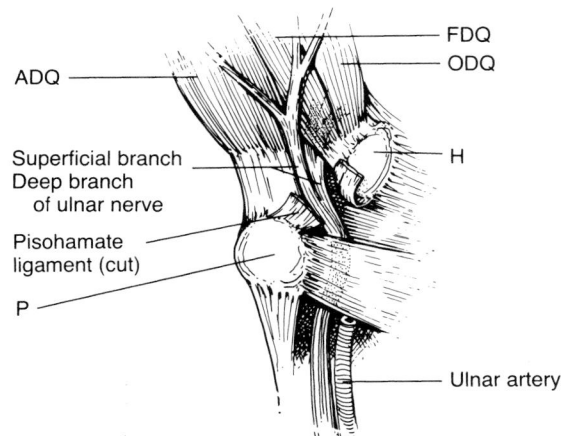

Figure 24A1–31. Branches of the ulnar nerve. ADQ, abductor digiti quinti; FDQ, flexor digiti quinti; H, hamate; ODQ, opponens digiti quinti; P, pisiform.

or sensory changes depending on which branch is affected, the deep motor branch or the superficial sensory branch.

EMG is useful in confirming the diagnosis. EMG will demonstrate denervation potentials in the interosseous muscles. Nerve conduction velocity studies will demonstrate prolongation of the motor latency to the first dorsal interosseous. A difference of over 1 msec is considered significant. These changes aid in localizing the lesion to Guyon's canal as opposed to a more proximal area of compression.

Compression of the ulnar nerve usually has a definite temporal onset related to trauma, which can include acute fractures of the hamate[57] or distal radius[67] as well as the chronic insult seen in bicycle riders. Other causes include anomalous muscles, lipomas, or ganglia in Guyon's canal.[64] Ulnar artery aneurysm or thrombosis can also result in pressure on the ulnar nerve.

Treatment. Conservative treatment consists of splinting, anti-inflammatory medication, and modification of activity. We use an off-the-shelf splint that maintains the wrist in a position of function in slight dorsiflexion. We recommend wearing the splint at night and as tolerated during the day. The splint may be removed as needed for essential activity. Local injection of a corticosteroid into the carpal tunnel or Guyon's canal may be effective. The appropriate technique of injection must be followed to avoid further injury to the nerve.[145] Injection of corticosteroids is frequently transient in effect, and 60% to 90% of patients experience recurrent symptoms.[74] Surgical treatment is indicated in patients who fail to respond appropriately to conservative treatment or when symptoms recur after an initial response.

Authors' Preferred Method of Treatment. Surgical release of the carpal tunnel and Guyon's canal must take into account the anatomic variations in the motor branch and the position of the palmar cutaneous branch and must provide for adequate release. Many approaches have been recommended. We use a slightly curved incision over the axis of the ring finger ray extending from the distal palmar crease to the volar wrist crease. The palmar fascia is exposed and partially excised to provide good exposure of the transverse carpal tunnel, which is then incised with

care to protect the underlying median nerve. The antebrachial fascia proximal to the incision can be released subcutaneously with scissors to ensure that no residual compression remains. The motor branch of the nerve should be identified and avoided. This approach also allows easy access to the volar carpal ligament over Guyon's canal, permitting decompression of the ulnar nerve as well.

We do not routinely release Guyon's canal at the time of carpal tunnel release. In patients with symptoms of ulnar neuropathy or changes in the ulnar nerve documented on EMG, we also release Guyon's canal, but these cases are rare. Epineurectomy is not routinely necessary but may be considered if there is evidence of significant epineural fibrosis. A strip of the transverse carpal ligament is routinely removed to prevent recurrent compression. The skin is closed, and a bulky hand dressing is applied to compress the palm.

Endoscopic carpal tunnel release offers the potential for reduced morbidity and an earlier return to activity; however, this technique requires much more skill from the surgeon, and the risk of neurovascular injury is much greater in the hands of an inexperienced surgeon. Long-term studies are needed to determine the efficacy of this procedure compared with an open carpal tunnel release. We have limited experience with this technique and do not use it on a routine basis.

The wrist is immobilized for 10 to 14 days, during which time the patient is encouraged to use the hand as tolerated and to flex and extend the fingers. The sutures are removed at 10 to 14 days, and the patient is started on a program comprising gentle range of motion of the wrist and massage of the incision to decrease scar formation.

Criteria for Return to Sports Participation. After removal of the sutures, the athlete can return to sport-specific activities as tolerated. Pain in the palm will limit activities that depend on fine manipulation and gripping. A volar splint should be worn or taping of the hand and wrist should be done for athletes who return to sport activity before 8 weeks postoperatively.

Vascular Thrombosis

Thrombosis occurring in the ulnar artery in Guyon's canal[35] and in a persistent median artery in the carpal tunnel[82] will precipitate an acute neuropathy that frequently requires early surgical intervention. Blunt trauma to the palm causing this problem is usually associated with activity in which the hand is used as a hammer. Generally, one or more sensory branches of the ulnar nerve are affected; the median nerve is affected uncommonly.

Clinical Evaluation. Thrombosis of the ulnar artery can present as a tender mass in the hypothenar area. The patient may experience ischemic symptoms of pain and pallor as well as numbness due to compression of the involved nerve. The symptoms may mimic those of carpal tunnel syndrome or ulnar tunnel syndrome, depending on the nerve involved. These thromboses can result from blunt trauma sustained during athletic activity localized to the hypothenar area. Occasionally, such thrombosis occurs with a fracture of the hamate.[26] The diagnosis is suggested by the history. Allen's test will be abnormal with poor filling through the ulnar artery. Doppler ultrasound can help to confirm obliteration of the superficial palmar arch pulse when the radial artery is compressed.[10]

Treatment. The most widely accepted treatment is surgical resection to remove the mass and to perform a sympathectomy.[81] Indirect methods include vasodilators,[147] stellate ganglion block,[32] and chemical clot lysis.[29] Some authors have recommended reanastomosis or vein grafting to re-establish blood flow.[55] Numerous studies have demonstrated that simple resection is curative.[58]

Authors' Preferred Method of Treatment. We prefer surgical resection of the thrombus and ligation of the involved artery. The approach is made through a curved incision parallel to the thenar crease over the fourth metacarpal. This provides access to Guyon's canal or the carpal tunnel as needed. The ulnar nerve is identified and carefully protected. The thrombosed section of the artery is resected, and the proximal and distal stumps of the artery are ligated with nonabsorbable suture. The tourniquet should be deflated to ensure adequate hemostasis and also adequate perfusion of the hand from the radial artery before closure. Ischemia of the hand at this point is the only indication for arterial reanastomosis or vein grafting. Postoperative care involves a standard bulky dressing for 2 weeks before the sutures are removed.

Criteria for Return to Sports Participation. After the sutures are removed, a standard rehabilitation program is begun, emphasizing range of motion and strengthening. We restrict participation in vigorous activity or contact sports for 6 weeks. The athlete may then return to play if he or she demonstrates satisfactory motion and strength. The wrist is protected in a splint or by standard taping of the hand and wrist for 3 months after surgery.

Tendinitis

Tendinitis of the wrist is the most frequent problem in sports that requires medical attention. Symptoms often begin some time after an inciting event, which is usually overuse of some kind.[90] The athlete complains of localized pain that is made worse by activity. Findings include local swelling and pain that is intensified by movement of or tension on the affected tendon. Radiographs are usually negative except in chronic cases, in which calcification rarely may be present in the soft tissues.[144] Calcification is much more common in the supraspinatus tendon of the shoulder.

Flexor Carpi Ulnaris—Flexor Carpi Radialis Tendinitis

Tendinitis of the two wrist flexors is relatively common.[41] It is caused by chronic repetitive trauma. Localized tenderness and swelling are present over the tendon. Pain is increased with passive dorsiflexion or resisted palmar flexion. Crepitus may be noted with movement.

Treatment. Treatment with splinting, anti-inflammatory agents, and temporary restriction of activity is usually successful. Unless the splint prohibits essential activity-

related motion, most athletes can continue with their sport. The wrist is splinted in a neutral position or in slight dorsiflexion. At the end of the athletic season, restriction of the inciting activity usually results in resolution of persistent symptoms. In recalcitrant cases, surgery may be necessary to excise calcific deposits or to lyse adhesions. The flexor carpi ulnaris may require excision of the pisiform in rare cases.[107] The flexor carpi radialis may require decompression of its fibro-osseous tunnel.

Authors' Preferred Method of Treatment. We splint the wrist and, if necessary, restrict the activity causing stress on the tendons. Local heat and anti-inflammatory agents are used as indicated. In difficult cases, we apply a short-arm cast for 2 weeks. Most cases respond to conservative treatment. In rare patients who have recurrent episodes, we perform a tenolysis through a standard volar approach. Following surgery, the wrist is immobilized for 2 weeks. After suture removal a standard rehabilitation program is begun to allow the patient to regain range of motion and strength. The athlete can be expected to progress rapidly.

Criteria for Return to Sports Participation. The athlete can return to sports as soon as full range of motion and strength return, usually within 1 month after surgery. In individual cases, we allow earlier return to sports if the athlete wears a protective splint. Splinting should not be necessary after full motion and normal strength are attained.

Subluxation of the Extensor Carpi Ulnaris

Subluxation of the extensor carpi ulnaris has been noted in athletes.[24] A painful snap over the dorsoulnar aspect of the wrist occurs with pronation and supination. This injury results when the ulnar septum of the sixth dorsal compartment is ruptured, allowing the extensor carpi ulnaris tendon to subluxate in supination and to reduce in pronation.

Treatment. Initial treatment of an acute episode requires immobilization in a long-arm cast with the wrist in pronation and slight dorsiflexion to reduce the tendon.[144] In acute cases, the wrist should be immobilized for 6 weeks. Chronic cases may respond to standard taping of the wrist and hand. If this is unsuccessful, the fibro-osseous tunnel can be reconstructed using a flap of the extensor retinaculum.[125]

Authors' Preferred Method of Treatment. In acute cases (less than 2 weeks since the initial injury), the injury is treated with a long-arm cast, with the wrist in full pronation and slight dorsiflexion. The cast is worn for 6 weeks. Following removal of the cast, a standard rehabilitation program is begun to regain range of motion and strength.

In chronic cases and when treatment of acute cases has failed, we recommend reconstruction of the fibro-osseous tunnel as described by Spinner and Kaplan.[125] The distal ulna is approached by a dorsal longitudinal incision. The dorsal sensory branch of the ulnar nerve should be identified and protected. The extensor retinaculum is exposed, and a flap one-half inch wide is elevated from Lister's tubercle and based adjacent to the extensor digiti minimi (Fig. 24A1–32). The vertical septum forming the dorsal compartment of the extensor carpi ulnaris is released radi-

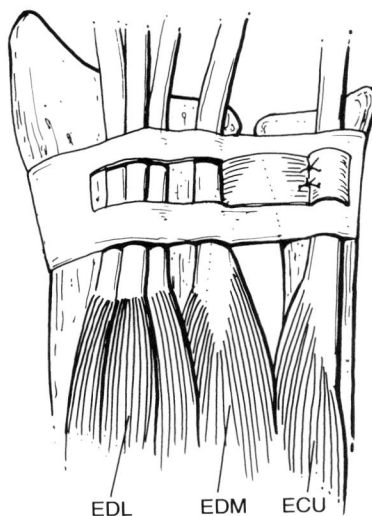

Figure 24A1–32. Extensor carpi ulnaris (ECU) stabilized with a flap of retinaculum. EDL, extensor digitorum longus; EDM, extensor digiti minimi. (Redrawn from Spinner M, Kaplan EB: Extensor carpi ulnaris. Clin Orthop 68:124–129, 1970.)

ally and medially. The flap is then passed beneath the tendon from the radial side and back over the tendon with the synovial side of the flap facing the tendon. The flap is sutured to itself. The tendon is centralized over the ulna. The wrist is immobilized for 3 weeks in a short-arm cast, after which a splint is worn for 3 weeks. The athlete follows the standard rehabilitation program to regain motion and strength.

Criteria for Return to Sports Participation. Whether treatment is surgical or nonsurgical, we allow the athlete to resume active sports when range of motion and strength reach approximately 70% of the levels of the opposite extremity. Protective splinting or a semirigid orthosis is used for 8 weeks or until the athlete attains normal motion and strength.

De Quervain's Disease

De Quervain's disease is a tenosynovitis of the abductor pollicis longus and extensor pollicis brevis at the first dorsal compartment.[25] Sports activities that require repetitive ulnar deviation place an athlete at risk for this syndrome.

Clinical Evaluation. Findings include local swelling and tenderness at the radial styloid. Positive results on the Finkelstein test,[44] in which ulnar deviation of the wrist with the thumb fully adducted causes marked pain, is considered pathognomonic (Fig. 24A1–33). Differential diagnosis includes osteoarthritis of the first carpometacarpal joint and intersection syndrome.

Treatment. Treatment consists of splinting, anti-inflammatory medication, and avoidance of the inciting activity. Local corticosteroid injection at the first dorsal compartment can aid in resolution of the symptoms. In patients in whom inflammation has resulted in thickening and stenosis of the fibro-osseous tunnel, conservative measures may fail.

Resistant cases of de Quervain's disease may require surgical release of the first dorsal compartment. Adequate decompression requires complete longitudinal release on the dorsal aspect. Frequently, there are multiple slips of the abductor pollicis longus, and the extensor pollicis brevis may be in a separate tunnel. Care should be taken that all slips of both tendons are released.[91] Particular attention should be paid to avoid trauma to the sensory branches of the radial nerve either by cutting or by applying undue traction to prevent formation of a painful neuroma. These neuromas can be particularly resistant to treatment and have a poor prognosis.

Authors' Preferred Method of Treatment. Initial treatment consists of splinting or taping to restrict ulnar deviation of the wrist. An oral anti-inflammatory medication is used for 2 weeks. If the symptoms persist, a local corticosteroid injection into the first dorsal compartment is used. The patient should be cautioned that local depigmentation may result from the injection.

Cases that do not respond satisfactorily after 6 weeks of conservative treatment are considered for surgical release of the first dorsal compartment. We perform this procedure through a transverse incision, usually under local anesthesia. Care is taken to release all slips of the abductor pollicis longus and extensor pollicis brevis. The sensory branches of the radial nerve are carefully protected during the procedure. Postoperatively, the hand and wrist are placed in a bulky compressive dressing for 1 week. The thumb is left free, and the patient is encouraged to begin range of motion exercises immediately. Sutures are removed at 10 to 14 days. Range of motion and strengthening exercises are begun.

Criteria for Return to Sports Participation. These patients usually regain strength and range of motion quickly. Taping or splinting can be used as needed for comfort. Athletes can return to their sport as soon as discomfort allows.

Intersection Syndrome

The intersection syndrome is characterized by pain in the area where the abductor pollicis longus and extensor

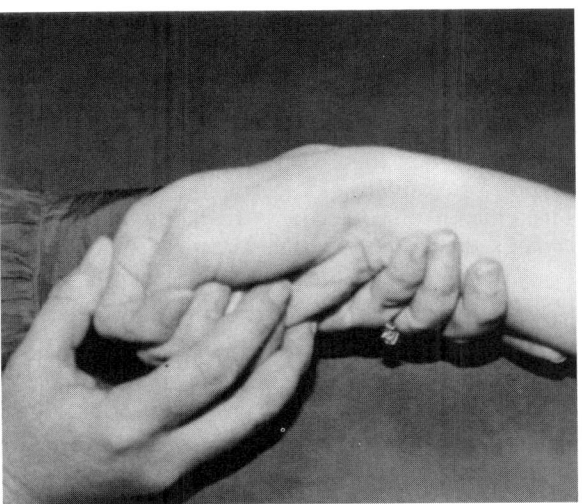

Figure 24A1–33. The Finkelstein test.

pollicis brevis cross over the underlying wrist extensors. This syndrome is common in oarsmen, canoeists, and weightlifters secondary to the repetitive wrist activity required.

Clinical Evaluation. Clinically, there is swelling and tenderness over the dorsoradial aspect of the forearm about 6 cm proximal to Lister's tubercle.[41] Crepitus is the distinguishing finding of this syndrome and may result in an audible squeak.

Treatment. Initial treatment includes splinting in neutral or slight dorsiflexion, anti-inflammatory medication, local heat, and restriction of activity. If symptoms persist, a local injection of a corticosteroid may be helpful. Usually, conservative treatment is successful. In recalcitrant cases, surgical exploration for lysis of adhesions could be considered, but this has not been necessary in our experience.

Protective Splinting

The wrist is exposed in almost all sporting activities and is highly susceptible to injury. Such injuries occur even in sports such as lacrosse and hockey in which padded gloves are worn. The major objective in treating injuries to the wrist is to return the athlete to competition as early as possible while preventing permanent disability. Initially, an athlete's injury must be evaluated by a physician or trainer who is qualified to diagnose and treat the injury. A decision must be made about whether the athlete's injury can be safely protected. Through proper protective splinting, it is possible to allow earlier return to participation in sports while minimizing the risk of recurrent injury. It is the responsibility of the therapist or trainer to fabricate a splint that allows adequate protection from re-injury combined with minimal interference with the functional skills required of each athlete.

Prophylactic taping of a joint has most commonly been done for the ankle. Taping can likewise be used for the wrist in cases of mild injury when only slight restriction of motion is required. Wrist taping does not completely restrict motion but does give support to the wrist for comfort and provides some protection from further injury. A tape adherent is used. An underwrap is optional. The methods of taping vary but usually consist of a figure-of-eight taping technique. The wrist is usually positioned in neutral while it is being taped; however, the wrist can be positioned in hyperflexion, hyperextension, radial deviation, or ulnar deviation, depending on which plane of motion is to be restricted. In general, the wrist is positioned to relax the involved tendons. Radial deviation for de Quervain's disease relaxes the affected extensor pollicis brevis and abductor pollicis longus. In patients with intersection syndrome, the wrist is positioned in hyperextension and radial deviation for taping to relax the wrist extensors and the abductor pollicis longus and extensor pollicis brevis. With subluxation of the extensor carpi ulnaris, the wrist is positioned in ulnar deviation.

Commercial wrist splints that incorporate the distal forearm and wrist can also be used for support (Fig. 24A1–34). Molded orthoplast splints with Velcro fasteners can also be effective as both functional and prophylactic braces in the

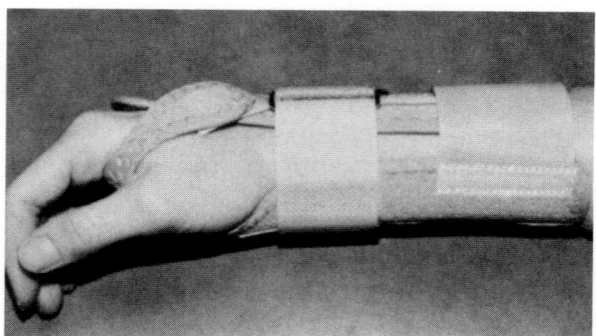

Figure 24A1–34. Commercial wrist splint.

athletic population (Fig. 24A1–35). These splints are easily removed and provide about the same support as taping.

It should be emphasized that regulations for acceptable protective materials vary between high schools and colleges and between school districts. Athletic trainers and attending physicians should familiarize themselves with the local regulations governing these protective materials before using any of the specific products mentioned here.

Rehabilitation

All athletic injuries should be evaluated by a physician, therapist, or athletic trainer before rehabilitation is started. The athlete's status should be documented before the rehabilitation program is started to provide an objective method of determining progress and to assist in the evaluation of the treatment program. Range of motion should be assessed frequently to monitor progress as well as to determine the need for changing the treatment plan (Fig. 24A1–36). Manual muscle testing and sensation testing should be performed.[53] Edema should be assessed by recording circumferential measurements at the wrist. Early mobilization of the injured wrist should be initiated as pain subsides. Active motion is the only modality of hand therapy that has been shown to be of lasting benefit.[94] Active motion should be within pain tolerance.

The use of modalities such as heat, cold, electrical stimulation, and ultrasound may also aid in improving function. Cold is initially used for 12 to 14 hours to reduce the effects of swelling. It may be used in conjunction with

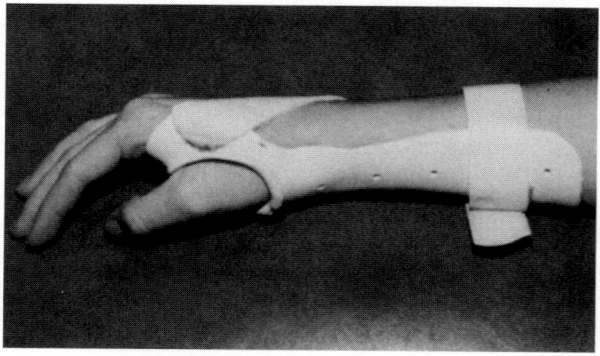

Figure 24A1–35. Orthoplast wrist splint.

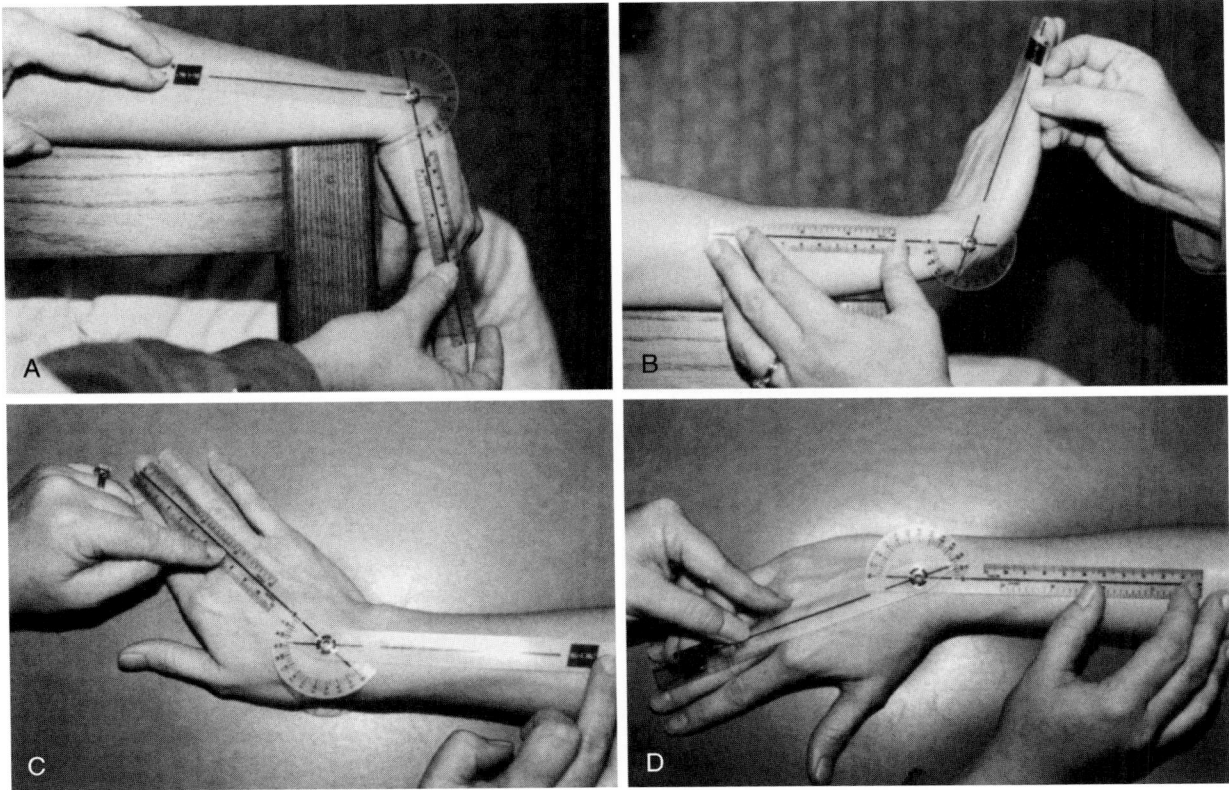

Figure 24A1–36. Range of motion measurements. *A*, Palmar flexion. *B*, Dorsiflexion. *C*, Ulnar deviation. *D*, Radial deviation.

active exercises to improve range of motion. Cold may also be used after exercise for 30 minutes to an hour to reduce the resultant edema. Following the postacute phase, warm whirlpool baths (102°F) can be used. The whirlpool aids in early wrist motion and is used while the athlete performs active exercise. Duration of the treatment is about 15 minutes. Care must be taken to avoid allowing the wrist to assume a dependent position in the whirlpool, which may induce edema to increase. To prevent this, the elbow should be flexed as close to 90 degrees as possible, and the individual should be encouraged to exercise actively. If edema occurs, the temperature of the water may need to be reduced.[53]

Prevention and control of edema are important in the rehabilitation of wrist injuries. Failure to control edema may lead to stiff and painful joints. Methods of controlling edema include:

1. Elevation of the extremity above heart level.
2. Active exercises.
3. Retrograde massage.
4. ICE.
5. Elasticized tape (Coban, 3M Company). This is available in various widths.
6. Compression gloves, which may be off the shelf or custom fitted (Jobst, Toledo, Ohio).
7. Air splints or Jobst intermittent air compression splints.
8. Static splints.[53]

Passive motion is another adjunct used to regain motion.

The benefits of passive exercises in the wrist are probably transient. Overzealous passive exercises may cause increased pain and may be detrimental.[71] Acceptable methods of passive motion include gentle active-assistive exercises, slow deliberate stretching, and joint mobilization techniques after application of heat or cold. Ice should be used until motion is free. Heat should not be used until progress with the use of ice reaches a plateau and there is no increased pain or edema.[53]

Grip strength depends on wrist mobility, stability, and a combination of many muscle groups. Grip is divided into two types: power grip and precision grip.[101] Power grip requires the wrist to be dorsiflexed, thereby providing a mechanical advantage for the long digital flexors. Carpal disease may produce pain that considerably limits functional grip strength. Precision grip is performed with the wrist in any position of volar flexion and dorsiflexion. The thumb is opposed to the fingers, and the intrinsic muscles provide most of the finger movement.

A dynamometer can be used to measure grip strength accurately (Fig. 24A1–37). Grip strength varies according to the size of the object that is grasped and should be evaluated and recorded in five grip spans. Grip strengthening programs should be modified according to the needs of the individual athlete. Strengthening should occur within pain-free limits. Initially, it may be necessary to begin with isometric gripping exercises, gradually increasing these to gentle resistive exercises.

A comprehensive home program is vital to the success of any rehabilitation protocol. Exercises are best done fre-

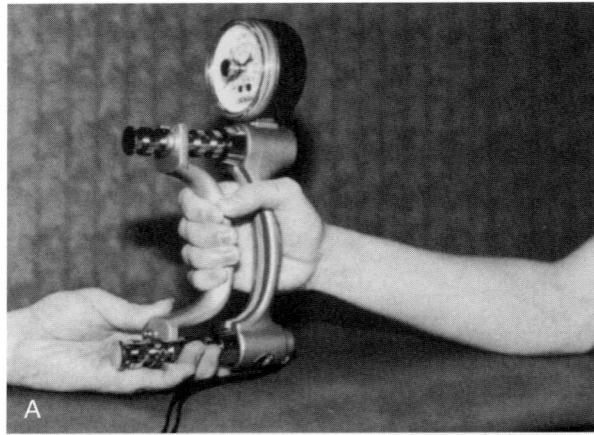

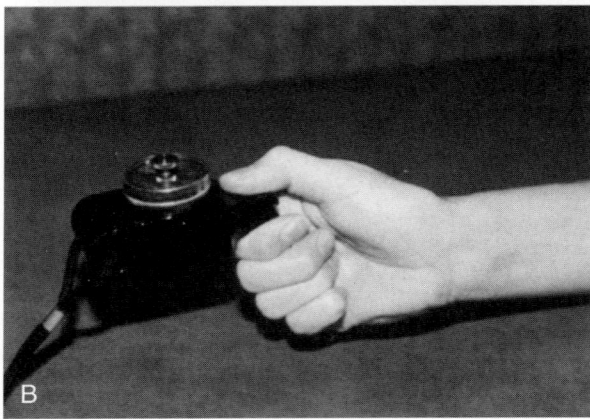

Figure 24A1–37. *A* and *B*, Dynamometer to measure grip strength.

quently throughout the day with a small number of repetitions. Oral, written, and visual instructions can be used. Exercise aids, splints, and modalities can be used as well. Home programs should be reviewed intermittently and altered as needed.

References

1. Abrams RA, Petersen M, Botte MJ: Arthroscopic portals of the wrist: An anatomic study. J Hand Surg [Am] 19:940–944, 1994.
2. Adler JB, Shaftan GW: Fractures of the capitate. J Bone Joint Surg Am 44:1537–1547, 1962.
3. Alexander CE, Lichtman DM: Ulnar carpal instabilities. Orthop Clin North Am 15:307–320, 1984.
4. Alho A, Kanhaanjaa U: Management of fractured scaphoid bones. A prospective study of 100 fractures. Acta Orthop Scand 46:737–743, 1975.
5. Almquist EE, Burns JF: Radial shortening for the treatment of Kienböck's disease—a 5- to 10-year follow-up. J Hand Surg 7:348–352, 1982.
6. Antuna Zapico JM: Malacia del Semilunar [thesis]. Valladolid, Spain, Universidad de Valladolid, Industrias y Editorial Sever Cuesta, 1966.
7. Armstead RB, Linscheid RL, Dobyns JH, et al: Ulnar lengthening in the treatment of Kienböck's disease. J Bone Joint Surg Am 64:170–178, 1982.
8. Atkinson RE, Smith RJ, Jupiter JB: Silicone synovitis of the wrist. Presented at the 40th Annual Meeting of the American Society for Surgery of the Hand, Las Vegas, January 1985.
9. Axelsson R: Behandling av lunatomalaci. Gotenborg (Sweden), Elanders Boktrycker, Aktieboalag, 1971.
10. Barker NW, Fines FH Jr: Arterial occlusion in the hands and fingers associated with repeated occupational trauma. Mayo Clin Proc 19:345–349, 1944.
11. Bartone NF, Grieco RV: Fracture of the triquetrum. J Bone Joint Surg Am 38A:353–356, 1956.
12. Beckenbaugh RD, Shives TC, Dobyns JH, Linscheid RL: Kienböck's disease: The natural history of Kienböck's disease and considerations of lunate fractures. Clin Orthop 149:98, 1980.
13. Bellinghausen HW, Weeks PM, Young LV, et al: Roentgen rounds No. 62. Orthop Rev 11:73, 1982.
14. Blaine ES: Lunate osteomalacia. JAMA 96:492, 1931.
15. Blair WF, Kilpatrick WC, Over GE: Open fracture of the hook of the hamate: A case report. Clin Orthop 163:180–184, 1982.
16. Blatt G: Capsulodesis in reconstructive hand surgery: Dorsal capsulodesis for the unstable scaphoid and volar capsulodesis following excision of the distal ulna. Hand Clin 3:81–102, 1987.
17. Bora FW Jr, Osterman AL, Woodbury DF, et al: Treatment of nonunion of the scaphoid by direct current. Orthop Clin North Am 15:107–112, 1984.
18. Borgeskov S, Christiansen B, Kjaer A, et al: Fractures of the carpal bones. Acta Orthop Scand 37:276, 1966.
19. Bowen TL: Injuries of the hamate bone. Hand 5:235–238, 1973.
20. Boyes JH: Bunnell's Surgery of the Hand, 5th ed. Philadelphia, JB Lippincott, 1970.
21. Brainard CW: J Bone Joint Surg 20:486, 1958.
22. Braun RM: Viable pedicle bone grafts [abstract]. What's New and What's True Orthopaedic Symposium. University of California at Davis, March 1985, pp 28–29.
23. Brown DE, Lichtman DM: The evaluation of chronic wrist pain. Orthop Clin North Am 15:183–192, 1984.
24. Burkhart SS, Wood MB, Linscheid RL: Posttraumatic recurrent subluxation of the extensor carpi ulnaris tendon. J Hand Surg 7:1, 1982.
25. Burman M: Stenosing tendovaginitis of the dorsal and volar compartments of the wrist. Arch Surg 65:752, 1952.
26. Butsch JL, Janes JM: Injuries of the superficial palmar arch. J Trauma 3:505–516, 1963.
27. Chacha PB: Vascularized pedicular bone grafts. Int Orthop 8:117–138, 1984.
28. Cherington M: Proximal pain in the carpal tunnel syndrome. Arch Surg 108:69, 1974.
29. Cho KO: Entrapment occlusion of the ulnar artery in the hand. J Bone Joint Surg Am 60:841–843, 1978.
30. Chuinard RG, Zeman SC: Kienböck's disease: An analysis and rationale for treatment by capitate-hamate fusion. Orthop Trans 4:18, 1980.
31. Chung KC, Zimmerman NB, Travis MT: Wrist arthrography versus arthroscopy: A comparison study of 150 cases. J Hand Surg [Am] 21:591–594, 1994
32. Conn J Jr, Bergan JJ, Bell JL: Hypothenar hammer syndrome: Post traumatic digital ischemia. Surgery 68:1122–1128, 1970.
33. Cooney WP, Dobyns JH, Linscheid RL: Nonunion of the scaphoid. Analysis of the results from bone grafting. J Hand Surg 8:343–354, 1980.
34. Cooney WP: Evaluation of chronic wrist pain by arthrography, arthroscopy, and arthrotomy. J Hand Surg [Am] 18:815–822, 1993.
35. Costigan DG, Riley JM Jr, Coy FE Jr: Thrombofibrosis of the ulnar artery in the palm. J Bone Joint Surg Am 41:702–704, 1959.
36. Crabbe WA: Excision of the proximal row of the carpus. J Bone Joint Surg Br 46:708–711, 1964.
37. Crawford GP, Taleisnik J: Rotary subluxation of the scaphoid after excision of dorsal carpal ganglion and wrist manipulation—a case report. J Hand Surg 8:921–925, 1983.
38. Denman EE: The anatomy of the space of Guyon. Hand 10:69–76, 1978.
39. Dickinson JC, Shannon JG: Fractures of the carpal scaphoid in the Canadian Army. Surg Gynecol Obstet 79:225–239, 1944.
40. Dobyns JH, Linscheid RL, Chao EYS, et al: Traumatic instability of the wrist. Instr Course Lect 24:182–199, 1975.
41. Dobyns JH, Sim FH, Linscheid RL: Sports stress syndromes of the hand and wrist. Am J Sports Med 6:236, 1978.
42. Eddeland A, Eiken O, Hellgren E, et al: Fractures of the scaphoid. Scand J Plast Reconstr Surg 9:234–239, 1975.
43. Ekman EF, Poehling GG: Arthroscopy of the wrist in athletes. Clin Sports Med 15:753–768, 1996.

44. Finkelstein H: Stenosing tendovaginitis at the radial styloid process. J Bone Joint Surg Am 12:509, 1930.

45. Geissler WB, Freeland AE: Arthroscopic management of intraarticular distal radius fractures. Hand Clin 15:455–466, 1999.

46. Gelberman RH, Bauman TD, Menon J: The vascularity of the lunate bone and Kienböck's disease. J Hand Surg 5:272–278, 1980.

47. Gelberman RH, Menon J: The vascularity of the scaphoid bone. J Bone Surg 5:508–513, 1980.

48. Gelberman RH, Salamon PB, Jurist JM, Posch JL: Ulnar variance in Kienböck's disease. J Bone Joint Surg Am 57:674–676, 1975.

49. Gelberman RH, Gross MS: The vascularity of the wrist. Clin Orthop 202:40–49, 1986.

50. Gelberman RH, Panagis JS, Taleisnik J, Baumgartner M: The arterial anatomy of the human carpus. Part I: The extraosseous vascularity. J Hand Surg 8:367, 1983.

51. Gellman H, Caputo RJ, Carter V, et al: A comparison of short and long thumb-spica casts for nondisplaced fractures of the carpal scaphoid. J Bone Joint Surg Am 71:354–357, 1989.

52. Gerstner AL, Omer GE Jr: Peripheral entrapment neuropathies in the upper extremity. J Musculoskel Med 14:29, 1988.

53. Gieck JH, Mayer V: Protective splinting for the hand and wrist. Clin Sports Med 5:795, 1986.

54. Gilford W, Baltar R, Lambrinudi C: The mechanics of the wrist joint. Guy's Hosp Rep 92:52–59, 1943.

55. Given KS, Puckett CL, Kleinert HE: Ulnar artery thrombosis. Plast Reconstr Surg 61:405–411, 1978.

56. Goldner JL: Median nerve compression lesions: Anatomic and clinical analysis. Bull Hosp Joint Dis 44:199–223, 1984.

57. Gore DR: Carpometacarpal dislocation producing compression of the deep branch of the ulnar nerve. J Bone Joint Surg Am 53: 1387–1390, 1971.

58. Goren ML: Palmar intramural thrombosis in the ulnar artery. Calif Med 89:424–425, 1958.

59. Graner O, Lopes EI, Carvalho BC, et al: Arthrodesis of the carpal bones in the treatment of Kienböck's disease, painful ununited fractures of the navicular and lunate bones with avascular necrosis, and old fracture-dislocations of carpal bones. J Bone Joint Surg 48: 767–774, 1966.

60. Green DP: Operative Hand Surgery, 2nd ed. New York, Churchill Livingstone, 1988.

61. Green DP: Proximal row carpectomy. Hand Clin 3:163–168, 1987.

62. Green DP: The sore wrist without a fracture. Instr Course Lect 34: 300–313, 1985.

63. Grundy M: Fractures of the carpal scaphoid in children. Br J Surg 56:523–524, 1969.

64. Hayes CW: Ulnar tunnel syndrome from giant cell tumor of tendon sheath: A case report. J Hand Surg [Am] 3:187–188, 1978.

65. Herbert TJ, Fisher WE: Management of the fractured scaphoid using a new bone screw. J Bone Joint Surg Br 66:114–123, 1984.

66. Hoshi S, Tazawa M, Maeda H: Arterial pattern of the carpus [in Japanese]. Seikei Geka 21:860, 1970.

67. Howard FM: Ulnar nerve palsy in wrist fractures. J Bone Joint Surg Am 43:1197–1201, 1961.

68. Hudson RM, Caragol WJ, Faye JJ: Isolated rotary subluxation of the carpal navicular. AJR Am J Roentgenol 126:601, 1976.

69. Hulten O: Über anatomische Variatonen de Handgelenkknochen. Acta Radiol Scand 9:155–168, 1928.

70. Hunter J, Schneider J, Mackin F, Bell J (eds): Rehabilitation of the Hand. St. Louis, CV Mosby, 1978.

71. Hunter J, Schneider J, Mackin F, Bell J (eds): Rehabilitation of the Hand, 2nd ed. St. Louis, CV Mosby, 1984.

72. Johnson RP: The acutely injured wrist and its residuals. Clin Orthop 149:33–44, 1980.

73. Johnstone DJ, Thoragood S, Smith WH, Scott TD: A comparison of MRI and arthroscopy in the investigation of chronic wrist pain. J Hand Surg [Br] 22:714–718, 1997.

74. Jones KG: Carpal tunnel syndrome. J Arkansas Med Soc 75:58, 1978.

75. Jonsson C: Acta Radiol Scand 23:562, 1942.

76. Kienböck R: Über traumatishe Malazie des Mondbeins, und ihre Folgezustaude: Eufartungsformen und Kompressions Frakturen. Fortschr Roengenstr 16:77, 1910.

77. King RJ: Scapholunate diastasis associated with a Barton fracture treated by manipulation, or Terry-Thomas and the wine waiter. J R Soc Med 76:421–423, 1983.

78. King RJ, Machenna RP, Elnur S: Suggested method for closed treatment of fractures of the carpoid scaphoid: Hypothesis supported by dissection and clinical practice. J R Soc Med 75:860–867, 1982.

79. Lanz U: Anatomical variations of the median nerve in the carpal tunnel. J Hand Surg 2:44–53, 1977.

80. Layfer LF, Jones JV: Hand paresthesias after racquetball. Ill Med J 152:190, 1977.

81. Leriche R, Fontaine R, Dupertuis SM: Arterectomy with follow-up studies on 78 operations. Surg Gynecol Obstet 64:149–155, 1937.

82. Levy M, Pauker M: Carpal tunnel syndrome due to thrombosed persisting median artery. A case report. Hand 10:65–68, 1978.

83. Lewis OJ, Hamshere RJ, Bucknill TM: The anatomy of the wrist joint. J Anat 106:539, 1970.

84. Lichtman DM: The Wrist and Its Disorders. Philadelphia, WB Saunders, 1988.

85. Lichtman DM, Alexander AH, Mack GR, Gunther SF: Kienböck's disease—Update on silicone replacement arthroplasty. J Hand Surg 7:343–347, 1982.

86. Lichtman DM, Mack GR, MacDonald RI, et al: Kienböck's disease: The role of silicone replacement arthroplasty. J Bone Joint Surg Am 59:899–908, 1977.

87. Lichtman DM, Schneider JR, Mack GR, Swafford AR: Ulnar midcarpal instability. J Hand Surg 6:515–523, 1981.

88. Linscheid RL: Scapholunate ligamentous instabilities (dissociations, subdislocations, dislocations). Ann Chir Main 3:323–330, 1984.

89. Linscheid RL, Dobyns JH, Younge DK: Trispiral tomography in the evaluation of wrist injury. Bull Hosp J Dis Orthop Inst 44: 297–308, 1984.

90. Lipscomb PR: Chronic nonspecific tenosynovitis and peritendinitis. Surg Clin North Am 24:780, 1944.

91. Loomis KL: Variations of stenosing tenosynovitis at the radial styloid process. J Bone Joint Surg Am 33:340, 1951.

92. Marck KW, Klasen HJ: Fracture-dislocation of the hamato-metacarpal joint: A case report. J Hand Surg [Am] 11:128–130, 1986.

93. Marek RM: Avascular necrosis of the carpal lunate. Clin Orthop 10: 96–107, 1957.

94. Mayer V, Gieck JH: Rehabilitation of hand injuries in athletes. Clin Sports Med 5:783–793, 1986.

95. Mayfield JK: Mechanism of carpal injuries. Clin Orthop 149:45–54, 1980.

96. Mayfield JK, Johnson RP, Kilcoyne RF: The ligaments of the human wrist and their functional significance. Anat Rec 186:417–428, 1976.

97. McMurty RY, Youm Y, Flatt AE, et al: Kinematics of the wrist. II. Clinical applications. J Bone Joint Surg Am 60:955–961, 1978.

98. Melvin JL, Schuckmann JA, Lanese RR: Diagnostic specificity of motor and sensory nerve conduction variables in the carpal tunnel syndrome. Arch Phys Med Rehabil 54:69, 1973.

99. Miyasaka KC, Rosenwasser MP: Diagnostic wrist arthroscopy. Operative Techniques in Sports Medicine 6:42–51, 1998.

100. Murakami S, Nakajima H: Aseptic necrosis of the capitate bone. Am J Sports Med 12:170–173, 1984.

101. Napier J: The prehensile movements of the human hand. J Bone Joint Surg Br 38:902, 1956.

102. Navarro A: Luxaciones del carpo. An Fac Med Montevideo 6: 113, 1921.

103. Nielsen PT, Hedeboe J: Posttraumatic scapholunate dissociation detected by wrist cineradiography. J Hand Surg [Am] 9:135–138, 1984.

104. O'Brien ET: Acute fractures and dislocations of the carpus. Orthop Clin North Am 15:237–258, 1984.

105. Palmer AK, Levinsohn EM, Kuzma GR: Arthrography of the wrist. J Hand Surg 8:15–23, 1983.

106. Palmer AK: Triangular fibrocartilage complex lesions: A classification. J Hand Surg [Am] 14:594–606, 1989.

107. Palmieri TJ: Pisiform area pain treatment by pisiform excision. J Hand Surg 7:477, 1982.

108. Panagis JS, Gelberman RH, Taleisnik J, Baumgartner M: The arterial anatomy of the human carpus. Part II: The interosseous vascularity. J Hand Surg 8:35, 1983.

109. Parker RD, Berkowitz MS, Brahms MA, Bohl WR: Hook of the hamate fractures in athletes. Am J Sports Med 14:517–523, 1986.

110. Perrson M: Casual treatment of lunatomalacia. Acta Chir Scand 100: 531–544, 1950.

111. Peste: Discussion. Bull Soc Anat 18:169–170, 1843.

112. Peterson HA, Lipscomb PR: Intercarpal arthrodesis. Arch Surg 95: 127, 1967.

113. Polivy KD, Millender LH, Newberg A, et al: Fractures of the hook of the hamate: A failure of clinical diagnosis. J Hand Surg [Am] 10:101–104, 1985.

114. Rand J, Linscheid RL, Dobyns JH: Capitate fractures. A long term follow-up. Clin Orthop 165:209–216, 1982.

115. Reagan DS, Linscheid RL, Dobyns JH: Lunotriquetral sprains. J Hand Surg [Am] 9:502–514, 1984.

116. Reister JN, Baker BE, Mosher JF, Lowe D: A review of scaphoid fracture healing in competitive athletes. Am J Sports Med 13:159–161, 1985.

117. Rockwood CA, Green DP: Fractures, vol. 1. Philadelphia, JB Lippincott, 1975, p 421.

118. Ruby LK: Common hand injuries in the athlete. Orthop Clin North Am 11:819, 1980.

119. Ruch DS, Bowling J: Arthroscopic assessment of carpal instability. Arthroscopy 14:675–681, 1998.

120. Ruch DS, Poehling GG: Diagnostic arthroscopy of the wrist. In Andrews JR, Timmerman LA (eds): Diagnostic and Operative Arthroscopy. Philadelphia, WB Saunders, 1997, pp 193–198.

121. Ruch DS, Poehling GG: Operative arthroscopy of the wrist. In Andrews JR, Timmerman LA (eds): Diagnostic and Operative Arthroscopy. Philadelphia, WB Saunders, 1997, pp 199–205.

122. Russe O: Fracture of the carpal navicular. J Bone Joint Surg Am 42:759–768, 1960.

123. Shea JD, McClain EJ: Ulnar nerve compression syndromes at and below the wrist. J Bone Joint Surg Am 51:1095–1103, 1969.

124. Shionoya K, Nakamura R, et al: Arthroscopy is superior to MRI for diagnosing injuries of the triangular fibrocartilage. J Hand Surg [Br] 23:402–405, 1998.

125. Spinner M, Kaplan EB: Extensor carpi ulnaris. Its relationship to stability of the distal radio-ulnar joint. Clin Orthop 68:124–129, 1970.

126. Stahl F: On lunatomalacia (Kienböck's disease), a clinical and roentgenological study, especially on its pathogenesis and the late results of immobilization treatment. Acta Chir Scand (Suppl) 126:1–133, 1947.

127. Stark HH, Jobe FW, Boyes JH, et al: Fracture of the hook of the hamate in athletes. J Bone Joint Surg Am 59:575–582, 1977.

128. Sutro CJ: Bilateral recurrent intercarpal subluxation. Am J Surg 72:110–113, 1946.

129. Taleisnik J: The ligaments of the wrist. J Hand Surg 1:110–118, 1976.

130. Taleisnik J: Scapholunate dissociation. In Strickland JW, Steichen JB (eds): Difficult Problems in Hand Surgery. St. Louis, CV Mosby, 1982.

131. Taleisnik J: The Wrist. New York, Churchill Livingstone, 1985, p 174.

132. Taleisnik J: Wrist: Anatomy, function, and injury. Instr Course Lect 27:61–87, 1978.

133. Taleisnik J, Kelley PJ: The extraosseous and intraosseous blood supply of the scaphoid bone. J Bone Joint Surg 48:1125–1137, 1966.

134. Taras JS, Sweet S, Shum W, et al: Percutaneous and arthroscopic screw fixation of scaphoid fractures in the athlete. Hand Clin 15:467–474, 1999.

135. Viernstein K, Weigert M: Die Radiusverkurzungsosteotomie bei der Lunatummalazie. Münch Med Wochenschr 109:1992, 1967.

136. Watson HK: Limited wrist arthrodesis. Clin Orthop 149:126–136, 1980.

137. Watson HK, Ballet FL: The SLAC wrist: Scapholunate advanced collapse pattern of degenerative arthritis. J Hand Surg [Am] 9:358–365, 1984.

138. Watson HK, Hempton RF: Limited wrist arthrodesis I: The triscaphoid joint. J Hand Surg 5:320–327, 1980.

139. Watson HK, Ryu J, DiBella A: An approach to Kienböck's disease: Triscaphe arthrodesis. J Hand Surg 10A:179–187, 1985.

140. Weber ER: Biomechanical implications of scaphoid wrist fractures. Clin Orthop 149:83–89, 1980.

141. Weber ER: Concepts governing the rotational shift of the intercalated segment of the carpus. Orthop Clin North Am 15:193–207, 1984.

142. Weber ER, Chao EY: An experimental approach to the mechanism of scaphoid wrist fractures. J Hand Surg 3:142–148, 1978.

143. Whipple TL: The Role of arthroscopy in the treatment of wrist injuries in the athlete. Clin Sports Med 17:623–635, 1998.

144. Wood MB, Dobyns JH: Sports-related extraarticular wrist syndromes. Clin Orthop 202:93–102, 1986.

145. Wood MR: Hydrocortisone injections for carpal tunnel syndrome. Hand 12:62–64, 1980.

146. Yorun Y, McMurtry RY, Flatt AE, Gillespie TE: Kinematics of the wrist. I. An experimental study of radioulnar deviation and flexion-extension. J Bone Joint Surg Am 60:423–431, 1978.

147. Zemel NP, Stark HH: Fractures and dislocations of the carpal bones. Clin Sports Med 5:709–724, 1986.

148. Zweig J, Lie KK, Posch JL, Larsen RD: Thrombosis of the ulnar artery following blunt trauma to the hand. J Bone Joint Surg Am 51:1191–1198, 1969.

2. WRIST INJURIES IN THE CHILD

Richard J. Wyzykowski, MD ■ Jeffrey L. Lovallo, MD ■ Barry P. Simmons, MD

The epidemiology and demographics of childhood and adolescent sports participation have continued to change in recent years, and so has our ability to diagnose and treat the consequent injuries. It is the goal of this chapter to review these changes and provide insight into how to approach wrist injuries among athletes within this age group.

Epidemiology

Children or Little Adults?

In part because of changes in performance levels, training intensity, and a younger age of entry into competitive sports, the distinction between children and adults is becoming less clear. In fact, recent reports and reviews have called attention to the emerging similarities between younger athletes and their adult counterparts.[12, 51, 74, 123, 134]

Dalton has noted that of entrants in a Melbourne marathon in 1991, 190 of 5807 runners were between 7 and 17 years of age. One 7-year-old completed the race in 3 hours, 31 minutes, and a 13-year-old ran it in 2 hours, 55 minutes. Young gymnasts can train for 3 hours or more each day, and runners can run 100 km/week. As of 1992, 50% of males and 25% of females 8 to 16 years of age had participated in organized competitive sports, and over 20 years (1960–1980), childhood sports involvement doubled in the United States.[51] Increasing numbers of children are training at younger ages, and more intensely, as a result of the "catch them young" philosophy.[12, 123] As a result, overuse syndromes are emerging as important elements of sports injury in this population.[74, 134]

Changing Patterns of Injury

Traditionally, child and adolescent athletic injuries have for the most part been comprised of acute injuries including fractures, sprains, contusions, and lacerations. The types and severity of injuries in children and adolescents, however, are changing. Increased and more intensive sports participation at younger ages has led to *more overuse injuries* and *changes in the patterns of acute injury* within this population.

Several excellent reviews have documented the increasing prevalence of overuse injury among younger athletes.[32, 51, 74, 102, 127, 134, 151] Micheli noted that although overuse traditionally has been attributed to breakdown of aged tissue in the "weekend warrior," it now is being seen increasingly in younger populations, and he suggests that the common denominator in overuse injury is too much stress in too short a period of time. He also identified training errors and muscle tendon imbalance associated with the growth spurt as the major factors contributing to this phenomenon.[74, 134, 151] This is echoed by Bylak, who reported that most tennis injuries are caused by overuse of the muscle-tendon unit.[32] These injuries are more common among adolescents, whereas fractures predominate among more skeletally immature athletes.[74]

Others have documented changes in the pattern of acute injury.[54, 198] Deibert and associates detailed the changing patterns of skiing injuries in older versus younger populations over three decades and noted that besides increases in upper extremity fractures overall across all age groups (pediatric +402%, adolescent +202%, adult +35%), pediatric gamekeeper's injuries rose 36%. Stanciu and Dumont documented the changing distribution of scaphoid fractures. They reported 50% of scaphoid fractures as occurring at the waist rather than distal pole, which were more commonly reported in previous studies.[198] The reason for these changes is unclear.

Risk Factors for Injury

Numerous studies have tried to establish risk factors for injury in children and adolescents, but the results have been varied, possibly resulting from referral center biases, nonstandardized definitions of injuries, differences in workup for injury, and inconsistent reporting of injuries by participants.

The type of sport has some influence on risk of injury. Logically one might suspect that activities with more contact might put the athlete at greater risk for injury. Markiewitz and associates noted that more upper extremity injuries occurred among football players as compared with other sports.[126] The association between contact/impact sports and risk for injury has been supported by other studies as well. Bhende and associates reported that hand injuries among pediatric patients reporting to the emergency room were highest among football players, followed by basketball and gymnastics.[19] Chambers' report on orthopaedic injuries among athletes 6 to 17 years of age participating in six organized sports followed the same risk pattern (football > basketball > gymnastics > soccer > baseball > swimming).[39] A review of the literature provided the data in Tables 24A2–1, 24A2–2, and 24A2–3. They serve to summarize the injuries most commonly associated with each sport, the prevalence of reported injuries in various

TABLE 24A2–1
Wrist Tendinitis and Overuse Syndromes in Various Sports

Pathologic Process	Sport
De Quervain's disease	Golf, racquet sports (squash, badminton)
Intersection syndrome	Crew, weightlifting, squash
EPL tendinitis	Squash
ECU tendinitis	Crew, racquet sports requiring snapping at wrist (squash)
FCU tendinitis and pisotriquetral arthritis	Golf, racquet sports, volleyball
Scaphoid stress fracture	Gymnastics
Distal radial stress reaction syndrome	Gymnastics
Distal ulnar stress reaction syndrome	Break dancing
Ulnocarpal impingement	Gymnastics
Scaphoid impingement	Gymnastics, weightlifting
Triquetrohamate impingement	Gymnastics, racquet sports
Repetitive DRUJ injury	Bowling, tennis, gymnastics
Carpal tunnel syndrome	Cycling, badminton, baseball, field hockey, golf, ice hockey, racquet sports, rowing, skiing, rock climbing
Ulnar nerve compression at the wrist	Cycling, racquet sports
Hypothenar hammer syndrome	Judo, karate, lacrosse, volleyball

DRUJ, distal radioulnar joint; ECU, extensor carpi ulnaris; EPL, extensor pollicis longus; FCU, flexor carpi ulnaris.

sports, and the specific prevalence of wrist injuries in each sport respectively.

Gender differences have also been noted when types of injuries and their prevalence are compared. Bylak and Hutchinson examined a population of young tennis players and reported more wrist and hand injuries among females whereas males presented with more shoulder and elbow problems.[32] Weir and Watson reported their data on 266 Irish adolescents 12 to 15 years of age and noted higher injury rates among males, though they also had higher participation rates.

Interestingly, overuse injuries involving the wrist were comparable between sexes.[220] Watson's experience with 6799 children and adolescents during one academic year showed higher injury rates among males, especially fractures, strains, and other miscellaneous injuries, whereas females experienced more sprains.[218] He also noted age-related variation in risk for injury. Males older than 14 years of age had threefold greater risk for injury than younger boys. The opposite, however, was true among females. Those older than 15 years of age were found to be at less risk for injury than younger girls. Age-related differences such as these are detailed by other studies as well.

Among 3500 pediatric and adolescent skiers 3 to 19 years of age, Garrick and Requa found those younger than 10 years of age had the lowest injury rates whereas those 11 to 14 years of age had the highest.[68] In Weir and Watson's study, 12-year-olds had the highest numbers of injures. Blitzer and associates documented a propensity for injuries among adolescent skiers 11 to 16 years of age and implicated poor judgment and suboptimal hand-me-down equipment as contributory in this age range.[26]

TABLE 24A2–2
Prevalence of Musculoskeletal Injuries in Various Sports

Sport	Fractures/ Dislocations	Sprains/ Strains	Inflammation	Contusion	Laceration	Other
Overall	7–31	24–63	1–11	9–43	1–39	7–24
Outdoor soccer	0–61	20–75	5–17	10–36	—	—
Indoor soccer	9	63	—	19	—	—
Skiing	11–65	0–51	—	17–30	—	—
Gymnastics	60	—	—	35	—	—
Roller skating	41–69	9–24	—	10–23	7–12	—
In-line skating	45	19	—	16	14	—
Snowboarding	44	—	—	—	—	—
Volleyball	37	39	—	16	1	—
Weightlifting	7	85	4	0	0	4
Martial arts	1–75	7–28	1	3–36	1–14	3–7
Football	20–45	31–40	—	17–23	—	21
Ice hockey	16–29	21	7	36–42	7	—
Basketball	7–9	47–56	—	15–20	2–9	—
Wrestling	≤1	30	—	—	6	—
Equestrian	43	—	—	39	—	—

Data from references 8, 18, 20, 21, 31, 68, 69, 75, 81, 86, 93, 109, 113, 133, 148, 150, 159, 163, 173, 183, 188, 193, 199, 202, 218, and 227.

Differences in injury risk between competition and practice sessions have also been reported, but there is no consensus. Most authors feel that injury risk is greater during competitive events than during practice sessions.[126, 133, 169, 176, 202] Baxter-Jones and associates have reported similar findings, with the single exception of soccer.[12] In their review of injuries among elite athletes, they noted more soccer-related injuries during games. This contrasts with the findings in the other sports they reviewed, where more injuries occurred during practice sessions. A few authors have suggested that practice sessions present more risk for injury than games. In their review of high school sports, Garrick and Requa reported a higher prevalence of injury related to practice sessions.[70] Similarly, in their review of risk factors associated with injury in high school football, Halpern and associates found that most injuries occurred during practices (especially during the injury-prone preseason), and they recommended controlled, noncontact sessions as a means of prophylaxis.[81]

Increased risk may be a time-dependent phenomenon, and Backx and associates suggest that exposure is the common denominator that helps explain higher practice-related injury rates.[9] Meeusen and Borms implicated exposure time as a risk factor for injury among gymnasts,[132] and Gabel reported increased prevalence of overuse injuries among those gymnasts with more years of experience and heavier practice schedules.[65] This may also help explain the higher injury rates among first-string players in Roser and Clawson's series of football players 9 to 17 years of age.[176] Among soccer players, higher injury rates among more skilled players also appear to be the case.[148] In contrast, Baxter-Jones and associates have found lower rates among elite athletes.[12]

Risk may also be related in part to poor judgment among those participants who possess enough skill to be at risk. As Blitzer points out in adolescent skiers, they are skilled enough to ski fast, but don't yet have the judgment to keep them out of precarious situations.[26] Poor judgment was also addressed by Watson, who reported foul play and recklessness as significant contributors to injury in his study of 6799 school-age children.[218]

As might be expected, therefore, supervision is an important element of prevention. Chambers found twice as many injuries arising from unsupervised activities such as skateboarding,[39] and Kvist and associates reported more injuries during nonorganized sporting activities.[109] In addition, Zaricznyj and associates documented more wrist injuries among participants in nonorganized sports including roller skating, trampolining, and ice skating.[236]

With regard to overuse injury, the two most frequent factors cited are training errors, including lack of cross-training, and the growth spurt. Micheli and others have raised awareness of overuse syndromes in younger athletes, and Table 24A2–4 provides a distillation of the risk factors detailed in their reports.[51, 74, 134, 151] The cause of overuse injury is clearly multifactorial, but Micheli has emphasized training errors as the number one culprit.[74, 134, 151] Training errors not only include doing too much in too short a time but, as Maffulli points out, can be attributed to the transition from varied free play to participation in sports involving repeated focused patterns of activity.[12, 123] Most authors agree that muscle strength-flexibility imbalance associated

TABLE 24A2–3
Wrist Injuries in Various Sports

Sport	Percent
Overall	4–5
Roller skating	39–53
In-line skating	37–56
Skiing	33–38
Football	15–28
Snowboarding	20
Skateboarding	19
Wrestling	6
Gymnastics	6
Weight training	4
Basketball	2–3
Ice hockey	2

Data from references 8, 18, 21, 31, 68, 81, 113, 150, 163, 173, and 202.

TABLE 24A2–4
Risk Factors for Overuse Injury

Intrinsic

Anatomic factors
  Growth (esp. growth spurt)
  Malalignment
  Muscle-tendon imbalance
Physiologic factors
  Associated disease state
  Nutritional factors
  Cultural deconditioning (obesity)
Psychological factors

Extrinsic

Training errors
Equipment (poor quality/poor fit)
Environment (playing surface, gymnastics equipment)

From Gill TJ IV, Micheli LJ: The immature athlete. Common injuries and overuse syndromes of the elbow and wrist. Clin Sports Med 15:401–423, 1996; and Dalton SE: Overuse injuries in adolescent athletes. Sports Med 13:58–70, 1992.

with the growth spurt contributes to adolescent vulnerability.[12, 51, 74, 123, 134, 151]

Biology and Biomechanics of Injury

Wrist Ossification Centers

In order to accurately evaluate radiographs for injury, it is important to have a clear understanding of carpal ossification patterns and their timing of appearance. Fortunately, the appearance and closure of ossification centers in the skeletally immature wrist occur in a predictable pattern with some temporal variation, the details of which are summarized in Table 24A2–5.

One must be cautious using carpal bone age alone to estimate true bone age. Carpenter and Lester showed that carpal bone age may underestimate actual bone age, and is gender dependent. In their study, carpal, distal radius/ulna, and hand bone age determinations lagged behind chronologic age for boys, and in girls carpal and distal radius/ulna age correlated well, but hand bone ages lagged behind

TABLE 24A2–5
Average Ages of Appearance of Ossification Centers and Physeal Closure Around the Wrist*

Bone	Appearance	Closure (yr)
Capitate	2 mo	13–15
Hamate	3–4 mo	13–15
Radius	10–12 mo	16–17
Triquetrum	2–3 yr	13–15
Lunate	3 yr	13–16
Scaphoid	4–5 yr	13–16
Trapezium	4–6 yr	13–16
Trapezoid	4–6 yr	13–16
Ulna	6 yr	15–17

*These values represent averages and do not specifically reflect gender differences.

From Stuart HC, Pyle SI, Cornoni J, Reed RB: Onsets, completions and spans of ossification in the 29 bone-growth centers of the hand and wrist. Pediatrics 29: 237–249, 1962.

actual chronologic age.[37] These variations should be kept in mind while estimating bone age as it applies to determination of growth remaining and remodeling potential.

Effect of Exercise on Growth

Germane to the discussion of injuries among skeletally immature athletes are details regarding the effects of exercise on growth. It is clear from Wolff's law and the effects of zero-gravity environments that weight-bearing has profound effects on remodeling and bone density. In addition, the Hueter-Volkmann principle reminds us that there exists an inverse relationship between compressive forces across the physis and the rate of growth of epiphyseal cartilage.[6] How these principles affect the maturation and growth of bones in athletes is unclear.

Booth and Gould showed in experiments using growing animals that low-intensity training can increase the girth and length of growing bones while low intensity over long periods or high intensity regardless of duration can have the opposite effect.[27] Kiiskinen felt that the shorter long bone lengths seen after moderate and intensive training in young mice were a result of accelerated bone maturation and earlier physeal closure.[106] Simon conducted a series of experiments in rats and proposed a bimodal relationship between the amount of compression across the growth plate and the growth activity of the cartilage in it. Accelerated growth activity was seen with either moderate relief or increase in dynamic loading, but beyond a definable point, excessive relief or increase in compressive force resulted in inhibition of growth activity.

The clinical relevance of these findings for athletes is significant. Delayed bone ages in gymnasts, for example, is well documented. However, the reason for this as well as for higher rates of ulnar positive variance in gymnasts versus controls is not yet clear. In light of the earlier discussion, it is reasonable to suggest that different ulnocarpal and radioulnar loads may cause varying degrees of ulnar overgrowth, radial growth inhibition, or combinations of both.

Adolescent Physeal Risk

In their classic experiments on rats, Bright and associates demonstrated for the first time that cartilage is viscoelastic, and that physeal injury risk correlated closely with pubescence.[29] Failure through the physis was nonuniform in 85% and resulted from shear cracks consequent to subcritical loading, and was often seen after application of only 50% of energy required for failure. Propagation of the crack extended from its origin at the metaphyseal-diaphyseal junction into and through the upper resting and proliferative layers.

During the growth spurt, adolescents are at particular risk for physeal injury. Relative weakness of the physis as compared with the surrounding ligamentous constraints appears to be responsible. Prior to and after the growth spurt, however, the physis resists injury better than ligament, muscle, and tendon, and, therefore, sprains and strains are more common. During the first 4% of tendon strain, collagen becomes tight. In the 4% to 8% range, microtrauma occurs whereby molecular cross-links break, and collagen fibers slide past one another. With continued strain, complete tendon failure ensues.[105] Evaluation of patients with injuries around open physes should therefore be carried out with this age-dependent vulnerability in mind.

Mechanisms and Categories of Injury

In his review of wrist injuries in sports, Howse organized the mechanisms and categories of injury into groups, and this may help the clinician develop an organized approach to evaluation and treatment of these problems.[90] Table 24A2–6 summarizes this information.

Overuse Syndromes

The emergence of overuse injury among younger athletes is a relatively new phenomenon and is apparently multifactorial in origin. Table 24A2–1 details the more common overuse injuries of the wrist. The wrist is the most commonly involved site in cases of overuse syndromes and tendinitis. These injuries occur under tension or shear and are usually the result of repetitive submaximal loading episodes that are well within the physiologic range.[105]

Tendinitis

Tendinitis about the wrist occurs with participation in many different sports. Racquet sports, however, produce proportionately greater inflammatory problems than other

TABLE 24A2–6
Mechanisms and Categories of Wrist Injury in Sports

Mechanisms	
Throwing	
Weight-bearing	
Twist	
Impact	

Categories	Examples
Overuse	De Quervain's, intersection syndrome, ECU tendinitis/subluxation, Lindberg's syndrome, extensor digitorum manus, Kienböck's disease
Neurovascular	Carpal tunnel syndrome, ulnar neuropathy, superficial radial sensory neuritis, hypothenar hammer syndrome
Traumatic	Carpal fractures, carpal instability, TFCC injury, chondral injury
Weight-bearing	Distal radial physeal stress reaction, scaphoid stress fracture, TFCC injury, ulnar impaction syndrome, scaphoid impaction syndrome

ECU, extensor carpi ulnaris; TFCC, triangular fibrocartilage complex.
Adapted from Howse C: Wrist injuries in sport. Sports Med 17:163–175, 1994.

sports. De Quervain's tenosynovitis and inflammation of the second, third, and sixth dorsal compartments are all recognized in adult athletes and are becoming more prevalent among younger athletes. Treatments include rest, activity modification, splints, modalities to decrease inflammation, judicious use of anti-inflammatory agents and occasional steroid injections. A graduated reintroduction to sport is then pursued once the athlete is asymptomatic. During competition, athletes may "play through" their discomfort, but should be encouraged to rest the area in question once the season is over.

Dorsal Wrist Capsulitis or Dorsal Impingement Syndrome

Wrist capsulitis has been recognized among gymnasts for many years and results from repetitive wrist extension impaction during vaulting, handsprings, and balance beam maneuvers. Reports have estimated that the overall loads transmitted during pommel horse routines could be as high as two times body weight,[127] and for back handsprings, maximums reached three times body weight.[107] It is not surprising then that 46% to 87% of gymnasts present with wrist pain during their career. The treatment approach is similar to that of other inflammatory problems. A full recovery can be expected, but the clinician should remain aware of other possible causes for dorsal wrist pain, including osteonecrosis, carpal stress fractures, distal radial and ulnar physeal stress reaction, ligament injuries, chondral injuries, and problems involving the triangular fibrocartilage complex (TFCC; Table 24A2–7). Should pain be persistent, débridement of the dorsum of the scaphoid, lunate, and scapholunate ligament may be indicated.

Impaction Syndromes

Scaphoid impaction syndrome may be seen in athletes who experience repetitive wrist hyperextension and radial deviation stress (e.g., gymnastics, weightlifting), although a single traumatic event may occasionally be contributory. Initial nonoperative management includes splints, rest, ice, anti-inflammatory agents, and occasionally steroid injections. If these are unsuccessful, however, dorsal cheilotomy may be required. Triquetral-hamate impaction results from repetitive hyperextension and ulnar deviation, and should be approached in a similar fashion.[59, 119]

Ulnocarpal impaction may result from repetitive loading of the ulnar side of the wrist, and most often is associated with ulnar positive variance. Plain radiographs are useful in evaluation, although a pronated-grip view may be required to effectively diagnose dynamic ulnar variance.[207] If nonoperative treatment fails (rest, splints, ice, anti-inflammatory agents, and so forth), ulnar shortening osteotomy may be considered. The advantage of an osteotomy is that it preserves ulnocarpal and radioulnar stability, but requires that the TFCC be intact. Wrist arthroscopy is therefore often done prior to osteotomy in order to examine the ulnocarpal joint and débride or repair any associated TFCC injuries.

TABLE 24A2–7
Gymnastic Wrist Injuries

Chronic

Osseous

Distal radius physeal stress reaction—compressive
   Radiographic
   Preradiographic
Distal radius and ulnar physeal stress reaction—traction
Scaphoid impaction syndrome
Lunate impaction syndrome
Scaphoid stress fractures
Avascular necrosis of the capitate
Kienböck's disease
Ulnar abutment syndrome
Triquetrohamate impingement
Acquired Madelung's deformity
Carpal chondromalacia

Soft Tissue

Wrist impingement
Wrist capsulitis
Wrist splints
Triangular fibrocartilage complex tears
Ganglia
Distal radioulnar joint instability
Carpal instability

Acute

Osseous

Scaphoid fracture
Distal radius fracture

Soft Tissue

Contusion
Wrist sprain

Adapted from Gabel GT: Gymnastic wrist injuries. Clin Sports Med 17:611–621, 1998.

Stress Fractures

Few reports exist that describe stress fractures in young athletes. Gabel noted that scaphoid stress fractures have been reported in young gymnasts, but they are rare, and are thought to be related to chronic dorsiflexion stress and forearm fatigue[65] (Fig. 24A2–1). Murakami and Nakajima reported two cases of apparent stress fractures occurring in gymnasts with capitate osteonecrosis, both in gymnasts with 6 years of participation. One patient was 18 years old at presentation and complained of 3 years of wrist pain. Radiographs revealed proximal capitate resorption with a small sequestrum inside. Two years after resection and drilling, the patient returned to gymnastics. The other patient presented at 19 years of age with 1 year of pain, and radiographs showed distal capitate sclerosis with proximal resorption. Four years after resection and drilling, the patient had no pain or tenderness, but experienced some limited range of motion (dorsiflexion 70 degrees, palmar flexion 60 degrees).[143] Israeli reported fatigue fractures of the pisiform in two volleyball players. Presentation was insidious, and physical examination revealed hypothenar soft tissue swelling along with ulnar sensory nerve deficits and intrinsic weakness. The authors recommended a carpal tunnel view or oblique views of the carpus with the wrist hyperextended. Both completely resolved with 6 weeks of immobilization and rest.[95] Bone scans and magnetic resonance imaging (MRI) are useful adjuncts for detecting occult stress fractures.

Acute Injuries

Acute fractures sustained during sporting events are treated no differently than those incurred during nonsport-

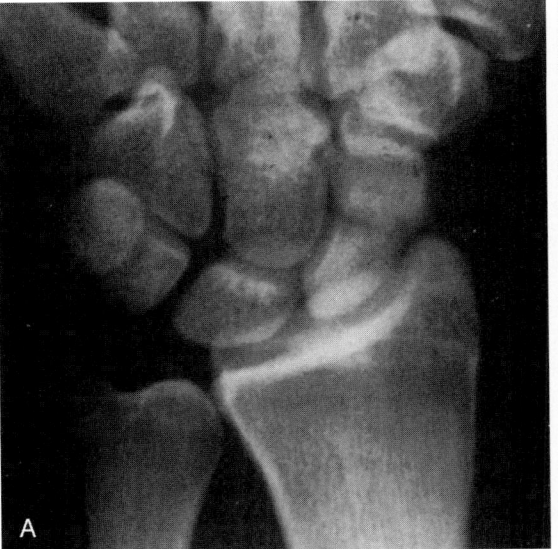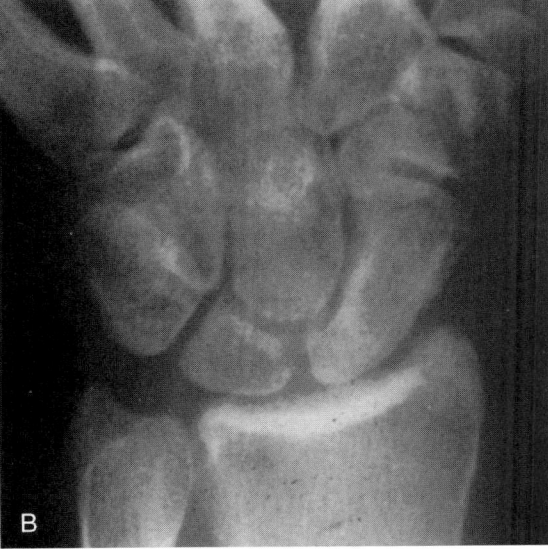

Figure 24A2–1. *A,* This patient was a 17-year-old elite gymnast who had complained of chronic wrist pain for approximately 3 months. Two previous radiographs were normal. This radiograph demonstrates a transverse wrist fracture of the scaphoid consistent with a stress fracture. *B,* Five months later, after volar autogenous bone grafting without internal fixation, there is complete healing of the scaphoid fracture, and the patient has returned to competitive gymnastics.

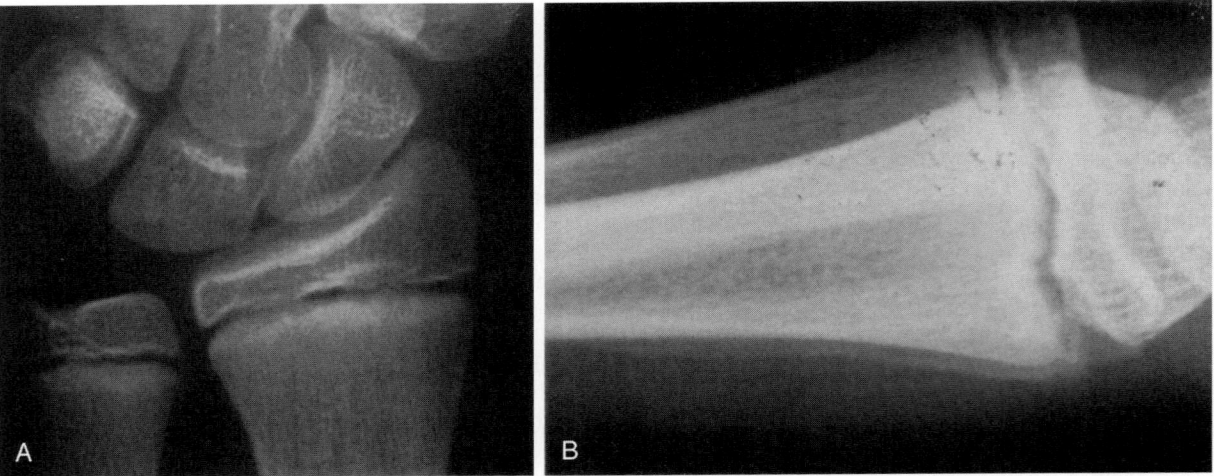

Figure 24A2–2. *A,* This patient was a 14-year-old boy who fell on his outstretched hand while playing soccer. Initial radiographic findings were negative. Physical examination demonstrated tenderness over the distal radius, and he was placed in a short-arm cast. *B,* Four weeks later, volar callus formation is consistent with a nondisplaced Salter I fracture.

ing activities, and will not be emphasized here. However, ligament injuries and a few fractures deserve special mention (Fig. 24A2–2).

Intercarpal Ligament Injury

Scapholunate instability is extremely rare among children and adolescents, and to date, there are only four case reports of scapholunate instability occurring in the skeletally immature carpus.[47, 52, 71, 238] In each case, a dorsal carpal instability pattern was noted, and time to treatment ranged from 4 weeks to 7 years after injury. Techniques included intercarpal stabilization with smooth Kirschner wires, ligament reconstruction with radiocarpal pinning, and two dorsal capsulodeses as described by Blatt.[24] Gerard reported stiffness (dorsiflexion 10 degrees, volar flexion 30 degrees, radial and ulnar deviation 15 and 35 degrees respectively, full pronation-supination), and diminution in power grip strength 8 months after ligament reconstruction and radiocarpal pinning for static deformity thought to have resulted from an injury at 3 months of age.[71] There was no evidence for recurrent carpal collapse, and his 7-year-old female patient was pain free. Zimmerman and Weiland reported their experience with a 13-year-old male seen 6 months after scapholunate injury. He underwent dorsal capsulodesis for static deformity, and 13 months later, the patient had no pain and was able to return to full sporting activities with full grip strength.[238] As might be expected, however, he did lose some motion (dorsiflexion 50 degrees, volar flexion 40 degrees, radial and ulnar deviation 20 and 30 degrees respectively). Cook and associates reported their experience with a 14-year-old male seen 4 weeks after scapholunate injury.[47] He underwent reduction and dorsal capsulodesis for static scapholunate instability, and 12 months later, full range of motion was restored and normal alignment of the carpus maintained. They did not, however comment on complaints of pain. Dautel and Merle performed percutaneous pinning of a 14-

year-old female with dynamic scapholunate instability 9 months after her injury.[52] Six months after pin removal, they noted a persistent scapholunate gap on passive stress views, but the patient was pain free.

Physical examination of patients with suspected scapholunate ligament injury may reveal tenderness and soft tissue swelling over the scapholunate joint dorsally as well as decreased range of motion, and the scaphoid shift test may be positive.

Radiographs may reveal a widened scapholunate interval or an increased scapholunate angle, but when imaging any wrist injury, especially among children and adolescents, it is crucial that comparative radiographs are obtained. Leicht and associates, and Kaawach and colleagues have described and quantitated the normal scapholunate gap seen on anteroposterior radiographs of adolescent and pediatric wrists.[99, 114] Because of incomplete ossification of the scaphoid and lunate, an apparent gap exists that must not be mistaken for scapholunate dissociation (Terry Thomas sign). As the scaphoid and lunate ossify, the apparent gap between the bones decreases. Normative values from these investigations are presented in Tables 24A2–8 and 24A2–9.

Triple injection arthrography and MRI can be helpful adjuncts to plain radiographs, but should be interpreted with caution. In several studies comparing the utility of arthrography, MRI, and arthroscopy in evaluating intra-articular wrist pathology, the preponderance of evidence has shown arthroscopy to be the best diagnostic tool. In one study comparing arthroscopy to triple-injection cinearthrography for detecting tears of the scapholunate ligament, lunatotriquetral ligament, and triangular fibrocartilage as a group, the sensitivity, specificity and accuracy of arthrography were 56%, 83%, and 60%.[221] In Cooney's study[48] comparing arthrography with arthroscopy using arthrotomy as the reference standard, arthrography resulted in four false-positive and three false-negative evaluations for scapholunate ligament tears. Arthrography also resulted in one false-positive and two false-negative evaluations for

TABLE 24A2–8
Scapholunate Distances in Children and Adolescents

Age (yr)	Scapholunate Distances (mm)	
	Range	*Median*
7	7–11	9
8	5–12	8
9	4–9	6
10	2–7	4
11	4–8	5
12	2–6	4.5
13	2–6	4
14	2–7	3
15	2–5	3

From Leicht P, Mikkelsen JB, Larsen CF: Scapholunate distance in children. Acta Radiol 37:625–626, 1996.

lunatotriquetral ligament tears, although there was perfect correlation with arthrotomy in evaluating TFCC pathology. Arthroscopy correlated perfectly with arthrotomy for evaluations of the scapholunate and lunatotriquetral ligaments, although one false-negative examination of the TFCC was noted. He concluded that arthroscopy is a more valuable technique for determining the location, size, and extent of wrist ligament injuries. In the largest study published comparing wrist arthrography with arthroscopy in 150 patients with suspected wrist ligamentous injuries, Chung and colleagues reported the sensitivity, specificity, and positive and negative predictive values of arthrography to be 74%, 56%, 93%, and 21% respectively.[42] In another study, the sensitivity and specificity of MRI compared with arthroscopy for evaluating TFCC pathology were 80% and 70% respectively. For scapholunate ligament pathology, the sensitivity and specificity were 37% and 100%, and for lunatotriquetral ligament pathology, they were 0% and 97%.[98] MRI technology appears to be improving. Scheck and colleagues published their results comparing nonenhanced MRI and magnetic resonance arthrography to arthroscopy,

TABLE 24A2–9
Range of Scapholunate Distances in Children and Adolescents

Age (yr)	Scapholunate Distances (mm)			
	Males		Females	
	Range	Mean	Range	Mean
6	4.2–9.2	6.7	5.8–11.9	8.9
7	3.6–8.6	6.1	5.1–11.1	8.1
8	3.1–9.0	5.6	4.4–10.4	7.4
9	2.5–7.4	5	3.7–9.6	6.6
10	2–6.9	4.4	2.9–8.9	5.9
11	1.4–6.3	3.9	2.2–8.1	5.2
12	0.8–5.8	3.3	1.5–7.4	4.4
13	0.2–5.2	2.7	0.7–6.7	3.7
14–15	0–4.7	2.1	0–6	3

From Kaawach W, Ecklund K, Zurakowski D, Waters P: The 54th Annual Meeting of the American Society for Surgery of the Hand, Poster Session, September 1999, Boston, Mass.

and reported the sensitivity and specificity of MRI as 52% and 34% respectively.[186] Substantial improvement was noted with magnetic resonance arthrography, with reported sensitivity and specificity of 90% and 87%.

Initial treatment of suspected scapholunate ligament injury in the absence of radiographic abnormality involves short- or long-arm cast treatment for 6 weeks, followed by a well-supervised rehabilitation program. Failing these measures, bone scans, arthrography, and MRI may be helpful in ruling out other coincident pathology, but, ultimately, wrist arthroscopy has the greatest advantage of being both a diagnostic tool as well as a therapeutic modality. Several studies have documented the utility of arthroscopic débridement of partial tears in adults,[180, 222, 224] and this has been successfully employed in children and adolescents unresponsive to conservative measures (Peter M. Waters, MD, personal communication). Acute displaced injuries can be treated by either open or arthroscopic reduction with pinning.

If scapholunate alignment is abnormal but reducible, arthroscopy may be performed to rule out any coincident intra-articular pathology. This is followed by open reduction of the scapholunate joint, and capsulodesis as described by Blatt.[24] We prefer to use suture anchors for capsulodesis rather than the pullout sutures originally suggested by Blatt. Treatment of chronic irreducible instability patterns is more controversial, and the choice of procedure should be left up to the individual surgeon. We currently prefer soft tissue reconstruction in the immature carpus and scapho-trapezial-trapezoid arthrodesis in the mature carpus.

Distal Radioulnar Joint and Triangular Fibrocartilage Complex Injuries

Distal Radioulnar Joint Disruption

Distal radioulnar joint (DRUJ) disruption often occurs secondary to a fall, but may also result from hyperpronation, forceful pronation, or repetitive stressful pronation, particularly in athletes who are ligamentously lax. Tennis players, bowlers, and gymnasts are more prone to stress-induced instability while those who play hockey or other contact sports are more likely to have had a specific injury.[119]

Acute distal radioulnar joint disruption most often occurs after a fall onto an outstretched, pronated forearm, resulting in dorsal dislocation or instability. Disruption of the DRUJ while the forearm is supinated results in volar instability. Acute dislocations should be reduced and treated with 6 weeks of long-arm cast immobilization, keeping the forearm fully supinated in the case of dorsal dislocations, and between neutral and fully pronated for volar dislocations. Inability to reduce the joint should prompt a search for interposed material such as the extensor carpi ulnaris tendon. Cases that are recalcitrant to these methods may require a tethering procedure to stabilize the DRUJ.[28, 92, 189, 208]

TABLE 24A2–10
Traumatic Triangular Fibrocartilage Injury Classification (Class 1)

Type	Location
A	Central perforation
B	Ulnar avulsion (± distal ulna fracture)
C	Distal avulsion (carpal attachment)
D	Radial avulsion (± sigmoid notch fracture)

Triangular Fibrocartilage Complex Injuries

Traumatic TFCC tears have been classified by Palmer[155] and are summarized in Table 24A2–10.

Only a single series has been written addressing the management of TFCC injuries in children and adolescents.[204] The ages of the 29 patients at the time of injury ranged from 7.9 to 19.2 years, and the time interval between injury and surgery averaged 2.4 years, suggesting that these injuries are often overlooked in younger patients. The preoperative Mayo wrist scores averaged 79.6, and the authors suggest that the absence of severe wrist symptoms may be partly to blame for delayed diagnosis. The majority of tears in their series were Palmer 1B lesions (79%), and they recommend repair of those as well as 1C and 1D lesions. Palmer 1A lesions should be débrided. Various arthroscopic techniques have been described previously.[14, 225, 235] Excellent results as measured by a Mayo Modified Wrist Score were found in 89% postoperatively, whereas good results were recorded for the rest. The authors stressed that a comprehensive approach should be adopted, and a high index of suspicion should be maintained for other wrist disorders, which should be addressed concomitantly (e.g., DRUJ instability, carpal instability, ulnar styloid nonunion, ulnocarpal impaction syndrome).

Carpal Fractures

Scaphoid Fractures and Nonunion

The prognosis for scaphoid fractures has improved considerably since Gouldesbrough's account appearing in Lancet in 1916.[76]

It is a well known fact that in adults very rarely, if ever, does a fractured carpal bone unite, at any rate to bony union?

The scaphoid is the most commonly fractured carpal bone in children,[144, 229] representing 88% to 89% of all pediatric and adolescent carpal fractures. In most large series, the majority of pediatric scaphoid fractures involve the distal pole (58% to 87%), with fewer waist and even fewer proximal pole fractures reported,[41, 144, 213, 229] although Stanciu suggests that the prevalence of waist fractures may be rising.[198] Of the distal pole fractures reported in the literature, the proportion that is avulsion type ranges from 18% to 44%.[213, 229] Vahvanen documented that 98% of these

avulsions involve the dorsoradial aspect and recommended splint treatment for 3 to 4 weeks.[213] Union can be expected in virtually all pediatric and adolescent scaphoid fractures treated with short- or long-arm thumb spica casting for 6 to 8 weeks, though nonunions have been reported in 1% to 3%, mainly involving waist fractures.[41, 137, 144, 198, 213, 229] Huene reported the results of primary internal fixation of scaphoid fractures in 13 patients, 4 of whom were athletes.[91] He used local anesthesia and a dorsal approach with postoperative splinting only. No casts were required, and the athletes were allowed to return to noncontact sports immediately. Contact sports were allowed after 6 to 8 weeks without joint protection, and all went on to heal with full range of motion. Such an approach is appealing for those athletes needing to return to sport sooner.

Although case reports exist that detail successful nonoperative treatment of established nonunions in children,[228, 158] most authors recommend open reduction with internal fixation and autologous bone grafting.[41, 131, 137, 138, 144, 152, 196] A variety of implants are available and include Kirschner wires, AO screws, Herbert screws, and Acutrak screws (Acumed, Beaverton, Ore). Mintzer and associates reported their experience with the use of Herbert screw fixation and bone grafting for five scaphoid nonunions.[137] In their study, patient age averaged 12.7 years, and the average delay to surgery was 1.4 years. Patients were casted an average of 9 weeks postoperatively followed by protective splinting for 6 weeks. There were no complications and the average time to union was 17 weeks. At an average follow-up of 3.3 years, range of motion and grips strengths were symmetrical, and there were no signs of signs of carpal instability or degenerative change. More recently, Mintzer and Waters published their results of nine pediatric scaphoid nonunions treated by Herbert screw fixation and iliac crest bone grafting and compared them with four others treated using the Matti-Russe procedure.[138] At an average of 6.9 years' follow-up, 11 of the 12 patients had excellent results as measured by the Mayo Modified Wrist Score, and all went to union. They found that postoperative immobilization time may be reduced by using Herbert screw fixation. We recommend a volar approach with distal radius bone graft, avoiding the growth plate for scaphoid nonunions. We routinely use K-wires and try to avoid screw fixation.

Associated Injuries

In Vahvanen's series, 4% (4/108) of scaphoid fractures had an associated distal radius fracture or physeal injury,[213] and other reports exist that document these as well as other associated injuries. Albert and Barre published a report of an 11-year-old child who sustained a Salter-Harris II fracture of the distal radius in association with a scaphoid waist fracture. He was treated in a long-arm thumb spica cast for 3 months with an anatomic reduction and full painless range of motion at final follow-up.[1] Gamble and Simmons reported a case of bilateral scaphoid waist fractures with a Salter-Harris II fracture on one side. He was treated for 10 weeks in bilateral short-arm thumb spicas, and at 3.5-year follow-up, he was radiographically and clinically normal.[66] Anderson reported a case of an 11-year-old boy who sustained a scaphoid fracture and minimally displaced capitate fracture while playing football. He was treated in a short-arm thumb spica cast for 6 weeks and at final follow-up, the fracture was healed and he had full range of motion.[5]

More severe associated injuries exist as well. Peiro and associates reported a case of dorsal transscaphoid perilunate dislocation in a 10-year-old boy who fell from a 5-meter height. After closed reduction and casting for 7 weeks, range of motion therapy was instituted. By 9 weeks, the patient had full and pain-free range of motion. Normal strength was attained by 9 weeks.[157] Compson published his experience with three transcarpal injuries and associated distal radius fractures. One patient was a 13-year-old male who fell 10 feet, and was diagnosed with a distal radius fracture and displaced scaphoid fracture. He was taken to the operating room, underwent closed reduction, and was placed in a cast in wrist flexion and radial deviation. A nondisplaced capitate fracture was identified at that time, and the patient was left in the cast. He developed carpal tunnel symptoms, and underwent release with relief of his symptoms. At 6-month follow-up, the fractures were healed and there was no evidence of avascular necrosis. He also treated a 13-year-old presenting with a buckle fracture of the distal radius along with a scaphoid fracture after a skateboarding accident. He was treated in a thumb spica cast for 6 weeks, but after 3 weeks, a nondisplaced triquetral fracture was noted. At 10 weeks of follow-up, the patient was doing well. The last patient was a 10-year-old who fell off a diving board, sustaining a nondisplaced Salter-Harris II distal radius fracture and a slightly displaced capitate fracture. Four days later, he noted a nondisplaced transverse fracture of the distal pole of scaphoid. He was treated in a short-arm thumb spica for 4 weeks and at 4-month follow-up, the fracture was healed without evidence of avascular necrosis. The patient was asymptomatic. Compson pointed out that the scaphoid and capitate fractures were not visible on the same radiographic view before 3 weeks. He recommended obtaining oblique in addition to anteroposterior and lateral views and maintaining a high index of suspicion for other carpal fractures once one fracture was seen.[46]

Triquetral Fractures

The triquetrum is the second most commonly fractured of the carpal bones in children.[144] In the largest published series of triquetral fractures in children, Letts and Esser reported their experience with 15 patients.[115] They found that these fractures were more common in the 11- to 13-year-old age group and presented with post-traumatic dorsal wrist pain. The mechanism they described involves a combined chisel effect of the ulnar styloid against the hyperextended carpus in patients with ligamentous laxity. The point of maximal tenderness was just distal to the ulnar styloid. Most of these fractures were the dorsal "flake" type fractures, and were amenable to short-arm cast or splint treatment for 3 weeks. Follow-up averaging 4 years was available on 10 patients, and 2 reported pain on wrist hyperextension. These fractures can be difficult to diagnose, and, indeed, in their series, 20% were initially misdiagnosed as sprains or Salter-Harris I fractures of the distal radius or ulna. In cases of incomplete ossification of

the triquetrum, injury to the cartilaginous portion of the bone is not visible on plain radiographs, but when ossification is complete, 45-degree oblique views may be helpful in documenting the fracture.

Capitate Fractures and Nonunion

Isolated capitate fractures are very rare, and no large series are available for review. Wulff and Schmidt reported a capitate fracture in a child whom they treated in a short-arm thumb spica cast for 5 weeks with good results.[229] Two other case reports of isolated capitate fractures in children exist.[73, 234] Young's patient was treated in a short-arm thumb spica for 6 weeks with uneventful healing. Gibbon's report highlighted the difficulty in diagnosing these injuries at presentation but did not give follow-up results.

Nonunion of capitate fractures can occur, but only one report in a child was found. Minami and associates reported a single case of capitate nonunion in a 13-year-old diagnosed 6 months after injury. He presented with wrist stiffness, pain, and dorsal wrist soft tissue swelling and tenderness. Radiographic examination revealed a capitate nonunion, and after iliac crest bone grafting followed by thumb spica casting for 8 weeks, the nonunion was healed. At 2-year follow-up, the patient's range of motion was normal.[136]

Trapezoid Fractures

Two case reports describing isolated trapezoid fractures in children are present in the literature.[144, 229] Both healed with thumb spica casting. Nafie also reported three cases of isolated trapezoid fractures that also healed with casting alone.

Hamate Fractures

Three children with isolated hamate fractures are reported in the literature.[144, 229] At least one of the cases reported by Nafie was a body fracture, but the details of the other were not clear. All of the fractures healed with casting alone.

Fractures of the hamate hook may present with tenderness and soft tissue swelling over the fracture site, and my be accompanied by ulnar sensory deficits and/or intrinsic weakness. These can be difficult to diagnose, but carpal tunnel views, bone scans, and computed tomographic scanning can be helpful imaging techniques. A trial of casting may be successful in promoting healing, but if the patient continues to be symptomatic, excision of the hook may be performed with little morbidity[22] (Fig. 24A2–3).

Pisiform Fractures

No reports of pisiform fractures in children were found in the literature, but presumed fatigue fractures have been reported in two volleyball players in their twenties.[95] With the increased intensity of play among young athletes, however, it is conceivable that this problem may not be exclusive to adult athletes. Both presented with insidious onset

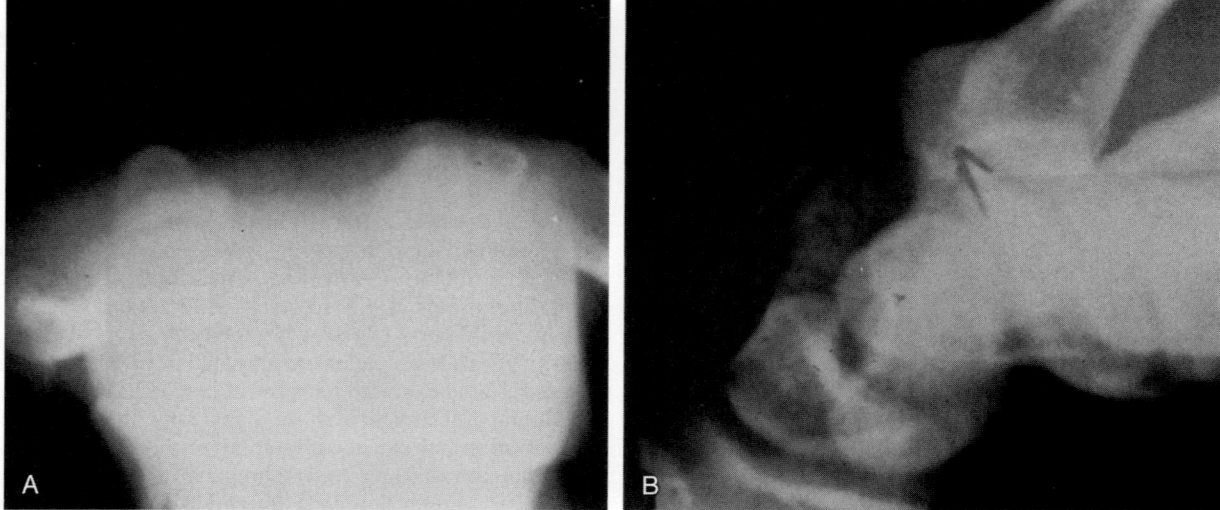

Figure 24A2–3. *A,* The patient was a 19-year-old youth who complained of pain in his ulnar palm (for approximately 3 months) after batting practice. An initial carpal tunnel view was negative for a fracture. *B,* An oblique radiograph demonstrated a hook of hamate fracture. Despite cast immobilization, the fracture remained painful and nonunited. Subsequent excision was required.

of pain, hypothenar tenderness, soft tissue swelling, and ulnar nerve symptoms. Carpal tunnel views and oblique views with the wrist hyperextended were useful in diagnosing these fractures. Both patients had complete symptom resolution with activity modification and immobilization for 6 weeks.

Physeal Injuries/Growth Disturbances

The most common physeal injuries involving the wrist occur at the distal radius and ulna. Of particular relevance to the focus of this chapter are physeal injuries that occur as a result of repetitive sports-related stress.

Distal Radius

Distal radius stress reaction was first described by Carter and colleagues in their report of seven competitive gymnasts and one champion roller skater.[38] The radiographic changes they described included (1) irregular physeal margins (especially the metaphyseal side), (2) flaring of the distal radial metaphysis with spurring on the palmar aspect, and (3) occasional discrete fragmentation within the growth plate. These radiographic features are akin to those seen with rickets. Bone density was normal in their athletes, but bone ages were retarded 1 to 2.5 years. In each case, 3 months of rest led to resolution of the problem. They suggested that the "weakest link" was the hypertrophic layer just above the zone of provisional calcification, and that it is particularly vulnerable during the growth spurt when it is thickest. Further, they theorized that repetitive stress induced temporary metaphyseal ischemia that may prevent cartilage calcification, causing the physis to widen.

Caine and colleagues suggested a spectrum of injury in their report of 60 competitive gymnasts.[33] Initially, the growth plate widens under repeated stress that exceeds tolerance limits. With more prolonged exposure, these loads lead to distal radial physeal fracture, and may affect new bone formation although longitudinal bone growth remains unaffected. With more time, a negative cumulative effect develops that may impair growth. In extreme cases, growth arrest occurs with resultant ulnar positive variance.

Beunen and colleagues[17] offered a different view regarding the etiology of ulnar positive variance associated with "gymnast's wrist." They compared radial maturity with ulnar variance, and found that female gymnasts with ulnar positive variance had earlier union at the epiphyseal-diaphyseal junction. They suggested that ulnar positive variance resulted from accelerated maturation of the ulna rather than premature radial physeal closure. An interesting possibility which arises out of Simons' bimodal theory is concomitant growth retardation of the radius and growth acceleration of the ulna. It may be that different events along with varied wrist positions during those events dynamically load or unload the ulnocarpal and radiocarpal joints differently leading to opposite effects—growth acceleration of the ulna and growth retardation of the radius. Clinical studies have yet to address this idea.

"Gymnast's wrist" is clinically thought to result from repetitive dorsiflexion and axial loading and is typically seen in females between 12 and 14 years of age with heavier training schedules (>35 hours/week).[65] The prevalence ranges between 8% and 42%,[55, 57, 178] and can occur bilaterally in one third of cases.[65] Patients present with dorsal wrist pain that develops after a few hours of working out and becomes more intense as the workout continues. Initially, ice is helpful and allows them to return to practice. As the process progresses, however, this becomes ineffective. Examination reveals painful limitation of wrist range of motion, most often at the extremes of active and passive dorsiflexion. Dorsal impingement and gymnast's wrist are

differentiated by tenderness over the dorsal and volar physis in the latter.

Gabel has suggested a staging system and treatment
strategy, the details of which are as follows.[65] Stage I is
preradiographic, in which the diagnosis is made on clinical
grounds. Avoidance of axial compressive loading events is
prescribed, and after 2 to 4 weeks, if patients have full
pain-free range of motion and are nontender, they may
return to full participation. Stage II consists of four radiographic features including (1) physeal widening, (2) irregular and cystic changes especially involving the metaphyseal
side of physis, (3) beaked distal epiphysis (especially volarly and radially), and (4) an indistinct physeal appearance.
Cast treatment may be necessary to prohibit axial loading
of the limb, and resolution of symptoms is uniformly more
prolonged in this stage versus stage I. Stage III is a relatively late presentation that includes the radiographic
changes noted in stage II, but with ulnar positive variance
in addition. Ulnocarpal impingement may need to be addressed in addition to the physeal source of pain. MRI
confirms the radiographic findings,[40, 56, 96, 191] but does not
provide any additional information regarding treatment. It
may be useful, however, for evaluating wrist pain in the
absence of plain radiographic changes.

Ulnocarpal impingement is fairly common among gymnasts, especially those participating in events that involve
ulnar deviation and pronation such as the pommel horse.[65]
Under normal circumstances, the ulnocarpal joint carries
approximately 15% of the load across the wrist joint, and
with 2.5 mm of ulnar positive variance, this can increase
to 40%.[61, 156]

Gymnasts seem to be particularly at risk for developing
ulnocarpal impingement, especially in the presence of ulnar
positive variance. Examination typically reveals tenderness
in the ulnar snuffbox, passive ulnar deviation tenderness,
and pain with dorsal and volar manipulation while the wrist
is ulnar deviated. Initial management includes nonsteroidal
anti-inflammatory drugs and activity modification. If there
is no improvement, then wrist arthroscopy can be performed in order to débride or repair associated TFCC
lesions. Ulnar shortening osteotomy may be the procedure
of choice if the young athlete exhibits ulnar positive variance.[206] This has the advantage of preserving radioulnar
and ulnocarpal stability but requires an intact TFCC.

An interesting case of presumed secondary ulnocarpal
impingement was reported by Vender and Watson.[214] Their
patient was a 17-year-old with 14 years of gymnastics
experience who presented with a 3- to 5-year history of
ulnar-sided activity-related wrist pain. Her workouts initially lasted 15 hours per week, but during the previous 5
years she had increased her workouts to 25 hours per
week. Examination revealed mild limitations in pronation,
supination, and wrist extension. Synovitis was noted over
the DRUJ, and pain was elicited at the extremes of pronation and supination although there was no tenderness over
the DRUJ. Radiographically, her physes were closed and
she was found to have bilateral Madelung's deformity,
which they felt was acquired in nature. Because her left
DRUJ was incongruent and ulnar positive variance was
evident, matched distal ulnar resection was performed. Unfortunately, no follow-up information was provided.

Distal Ulna

Repetitive injury resulting in distal ulnar physeal injury
is much rarer than that affecting the distal radius. Gerber
and associates reported a single case of distal ulnar physeal
abnormality in a 14-year-old break dancer.[72] Radiograph
examination revealed distal ulnar physeal changes identical
to those seen at the distal radial physis in "gymnast's
wrist" (physeal widening with metaphyseal irregularity).
Six weeks of short-arm cast immobilization resulted in
complete resolution of his symptoms, and repeat radiographs showed evidence of interval healing. Yong-Hing
and colleagues presented another case report of a young
gymnast with distal ulna stress reaction and subsequent
ipsilateral distal radial stress reaction.[233] Pain was noted
with traction but not flexion or extension at the wrist. After
4 weeks in a long-arm cast, the area over the ulna was
nontender, and he was able to resume training 4 months
later. One year later, he had similar symptoms over the
distal radius and radiographs revealed abnormal widening
of the distal radial growth plate, and incipient ulnar growth
plate closure. Four weeks of immobilization led to symptom resolution, but no further follow-up was given.

They felt that the injury was secondary to traction stress,
and attributed it to use of dowel grips.

Osteonecrosis

Kienböck's Disease

Kienböck's disease occurs more often in adolescence,
but reports in the literature detail cases involving children
as well. The goals of treatment are to reduce pain, preserve
wrist motion, promote lunate revascularization, and prevent
carpal collapse and arthritis. Stahl's classification[197] as
modified by Amadio[2] and Lichtman[116] is the most commonly used system today (Table 24A2–11). In general,
treatment is dependent on the stage of disease. Patients
with ulnar negative variance and Lichtman stage I to IIIB
disease may be treated by radial shortening, ulnar lengthening, external fixation combined with curettage and iliac
crest bone grafting, limited carpal fusion (e.g., capitate
shortening combined with capitohamate fusion), or a variety of vascularized bone grafts (Fig. 25A2–4). Patients
with ulnar neutral or positive variance, however, are at
increased risk for ulnocarpal impingement if joint leveling
procedures are used. Triscaphe arthrodesis is favored by
some for stage II to IV disease, whereas proximal row
carpectomy and total wrist arthrodesis are reserved for later
stages (IIIB to IV).

Reports of Kienböck's disease in pediatric and adolescent patients are rare. The largest series available is reported by Nakamura and colleagues and details the treatment of 10 patients (7 patients 9 to 17 years old) with
Lichtman stage II to IV disease.[145] Various treatments including nonoperative methods were used. The authors recommended radial shortening particularly in the presence of
ulnar negative variance. Foster reported 16-month follow-
up results on an 8-year-old female who underwent radial
shortening osteotomy after 8 months of failed nonoperative

TABLE 24A2–11
Classification of Kienböck's Disease*

Stage	Pain	MRI	Fracture Line/ Inc. Density	Lunate Collapse	Carpal Collapse	Arthritis
O	+	+	—	—	—	—
I	+	+	±	—	—	—
II	+	+	+	—	—	—
IIIA	+	+	+	+	—	—
IIIB	+	+	+	+	+	—
IV	+	+	+	+	+	—

*Kienböck's disease can be classified according to radiographic finding. Stages I, II, and III are most likely in the adolescent age group.
MRI, magnetic resonance imaging.

treatment for Lichtman stage III disease.[64] Preoperative ulnar variance was negative, and carpal height ratio was decreased. Three years postoperatively, carpal height and symptoms had improved substantially. Edelson and colleagues reported results that were not so favorable in a 12-year-old female who underwent radial shortening osteotomy.[60] Initial follow-up showed clinical and radiographic resolution of her disease, but 16 months postoperatively, her pain and stiffness returned, and radiographs revealed recurrent lunate sclerosis and collapse. Yasuda and colleagues published an interesting report of temporary scaphotrapezoid pinning after failure of 2 months of splinting in a 12-year-old female with stage IIIB disease.[231] The scaphoid was pinned in a relatively vertical position to unload the lunate, and the wrist was immobilized for 4 months, after which the pins were removed. At 16-month follow-up, her pain had resolved, and range of motion was full with improvement of carpal height. MRI done at that time showed improvement as well.

These reports must all be viewed in light of the fact that the natural history of Kienböck's disease remains unknown, and it is therefore difficult to say whether surgical intervention alters the course of each patient's disease. A case in point is Hosking's reporting of spontaneous clinical resolution of stage III disease in an 8-year-old football player treated with 6 months of immobilization.[88] The patient initially presented with wrist pain, 50% decreased range of motion, tenderness over the lunate, and radiographic evi-

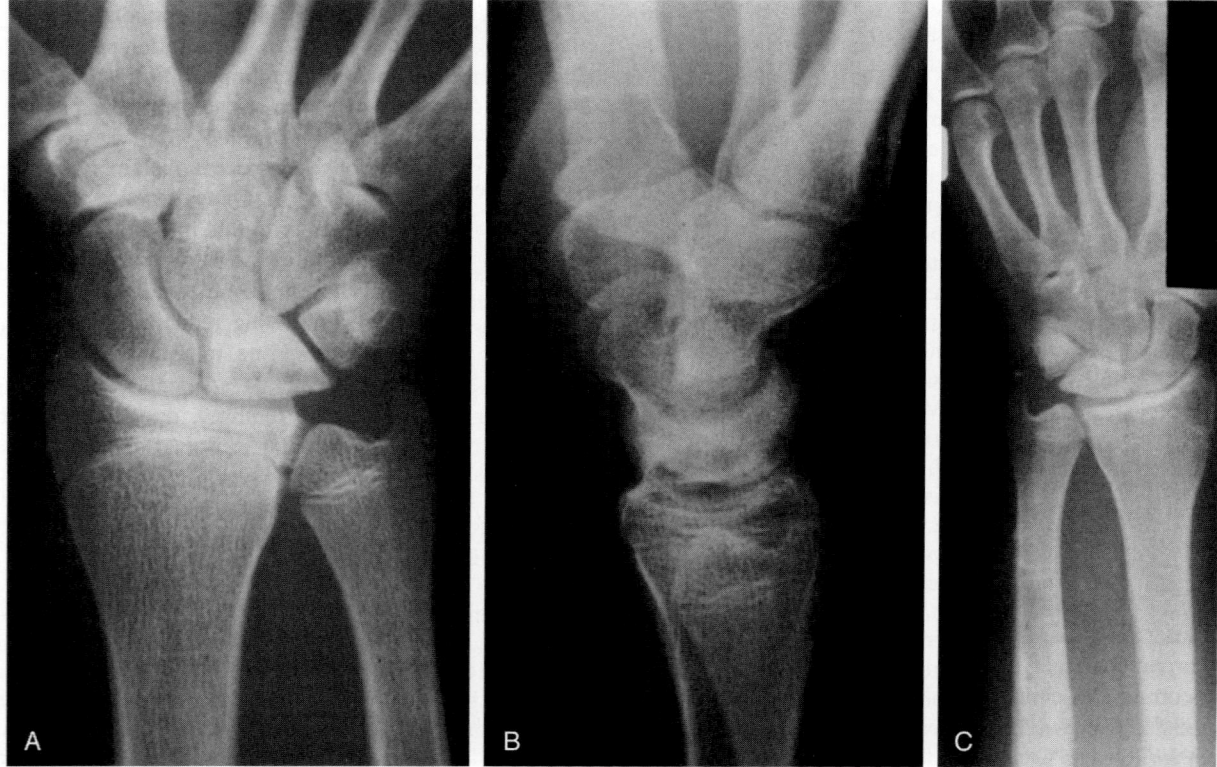

Figure 24A2–4. *A,* Kienböck's disease in a 15-year-old boy who presented with pain after a fall playing basketball. Note that the distal ulna is shorter than the distal radius (negative ulna variance). *B,* Lateral radiograph shows maintenance of carpal height. *C,* Ulnar lengthening in the midshaft resulted in healing of the lunate without collapse.

dence for lunate collapse and ulnar negative variance (-5 mm). At 1-year follow-up, his radiographs were unchanged, but he had complete pain-free range of motion.

Scaphoid Avascular Necrosis

Only a single case of idiopathic avascular necrosis in a child has been reported.[97] The authors treated a 10-year-old who presented with wrist pain and radiographic evidence of scaphoid osteonecrosis. Three weeks of immobilization was not helpful, but at 28 months' follow-up, the patient was asymptomatic and had returned to unrestricted activities. Radiographs, however, revealed unchanged fragmentation of scaphoid and radial subluxation of capitate.

Capitate Avascular Necrosis

As mentioned previously, Murakami and Nakajima reported their experience with two gymnasts who presented with symptomatic capitate osteonecrosis and were presumed to have had stress fractures resulting from repetitive hyperextension injuries.[143] Both patients underwent resection and drilling with resolution of their pain, and one was able to return to gymnastics.

Vascular Problems

A number of vascular disorders have been described in association with sports participation,[7, 172] but most relevant to the wrist is hypothenar hammer syndrome.

Hypothenar Hammer Syndrome

Hypothenar hammer syndrome typically results from repeated injury to the palmar aspect of the wrist and hand,[7, 172, 223] and may involve intimal damage within the ulnar artery, leading to thrombosis or the formation of true aneurysms (involving all the layers of the arterial wall) or false aneurysms (involving only the outer layers). Vasospasm of distal vessels may also occur as a result of increased sympathetic tone after wall injury. Patients present with ischemic symptoms (anisothermia and pain), which may radiate into the forearm. Early on, pain is activity related, and in advanced cases, rest pain and night pain become more prominent. Occasionally, ulnar motor and sensory findings or digital ulceration is present as well.

In the absence of severe changes, activity modification, and use of orthotics and padding may be helpful in relieving or preventing progression of the symptoms. If these methods fail or if changes are severe at presentation, then exploration of the ulnar artery is warranted. The lesion is resected followed by reverse vein grafting to re-establish flow. This is particularly important in the 20% of cases in which the palmar arch is incomplete.[85, 172]

Conclusion

Initial management of wrist pain in pediatric and adolescent patients begins with an effort to classify the problem as related to an acute injury or whether it is attributable to overuse. Evaluation of overuse injuries should include a review of risk factors (see Table 24A2–4), a trial of rest, and if needed, immobilization, followed by rehabilitation and a gradual reintroduction to sport. If the patient fails to gain symptomatic relief with these measures, further diagnostics including plain radiographs, cineradiographs, arthrogram, bone scan, computed tomography, and MRI should be considered. Wrist arthroscopy or an open procedure is warranted if a treatable entity is suspected.

Pediatric and adolescent athletes are indeed becoming little adults, and their injuries are beginning to mirror those of their adult counterparts. Awareness of these newly forming patterns will help the clinician evaluate, treat, and be instrumental, it is hoped, in preventing many of these injuries.

References

1. Albert MC, Barre PS: A scaphoid fracture associated with a displaced distal radial fracture in a child. Clin Orthop 240:232–235, 1989.
2. Amadio PC, Hanssen AD, Berquist TH: The genesis of Kienböck's disease: Evaluation of a case by MR imaging. J Hand Surg [Am] 12:1044, 1987.
3. Amadio PC: Epidemiology of hand and wrist injuries in sports. Hand Clin 6:379–381, 1990.
4. American Academy of Pediatrics Committee on Sports Medicine: Recommendations for participation in competitive sports. Pediatrics 81:737–739, 1988.
5. Anderson WJ: Simultaneous fracture of the scaphoid and capitate in a child. J Hand Surg [Am] 12:271–273, 1987.
6. Arkin AM, Katz JF: The effects of pressure on epiphyseal growth. The mechanism of plasticity of growing bone. J Bone Joint Surg Am 38:1056–1076, 1956.
7. Aulicino PL: Neurovascular injuries in the hands of athletes. Hand Clin 6:455–466, 1990.
8. Backx FJ, Erich WB, Kemper AB, Verbeek AL: Sports injuries in school-aged children. An epidemiologic study. Am J Sports Med 17:234–240, 1989.
9. Backx FJ, Beijer HJ, Bol E, Erich WB: Injuries in high-risk persons and high-risk sports. A longitudinal study of 1818 school children. Am J Sports Med 19:124–130, 1991.
10. Bak K, Boeckstyns M: Epiphysiodesis for bilateral irregular closure of the distal radial physis in a gymnast. Scand J Med Sci Sports 7:363–366, 1997.
11. Barone GW, Rodgers BM: Pediatric equestrian injuries: A 14-year review. J Trauma 29:89–95, 245–247, 1989.
12. Baxter-Jones A, Maffulli N, Helms P: Low injury rates in elite athletes. Arch Dis Child 68:130–132, 1993.
13. Beatty E, Light TR, Belsole RJ, Ogden JA: Wrist and hand skeletal injuries in children. Hand Clin 6:723–738, 1990.
14. Bednar JM, Osterman AL: The role of arthroscopy in the treatment of traumatic triangular fibrocartilage injuries. Hand Clin 10:605–614, 1994.
15. Bernhardt DT, Landry GL: Sports injuries in young athletes. Adv Pediatr 42:465–500, 1995.
16. Berson BL, Passoff TL, Nagelberg S, Thornton J: Injury patterns in squash players. Am J Sports Med 6:323–325, 1978.
17. Beunen G, Malina RM, Claessens AL, and colleagues: Ulnar variance and skeletal maturity of radius and ulna in female gymnasts. Med Sci Sports Exerc 31:653–657, 1999.
18. Bhairo NH, Nijsten MW, van Dalen KC, ten Duis HJ: Hand injuries in volleyball. Int J Sports Med 13:351–354, 1992.

19. Bhende MS, Dandrea LA, Davis HW: Hand injuries in children presenting to a pediatric emergency department. Ann Emerg Med 22:1519–1523, 1993.
20. Bijur PE, Trumble A, Harel Y, and colleagues: Sports and recreation injuries in US children and adolescents. Arch Pediatr Adolesc Med 149:1009–1016, 1995.
21. Birrer RB, Halbrook SP: Martial arts injuries. The results of a five year national survey. Am J Sports Med 16:408–410, 1988.
22. Bishop AT, Beckenbaugh RD: Fracture of the hamate hook. J Hand Surg [Am] 13:135–139, 1988.
23. Bixby-Hammett DM: Pediatric equestrian injuries. Pediatrics 89:1173–1176, 1992.
24. Blatt G: Capsulodesis in reconstructive hand surgery: Dorsal capsulodesis for the unstable scaphoid and volar capsulodesis following excision of the distal ulna. Hand Clin 3:81–102, 1987.
25. Bley L, Seitz WH Jr: Injuries about the distal ulna in children. Hand Clin 14:231–237, 1998.
26. Blitzer CM, Johnson RJ, Ettlinger CF, Aggeborn K: Downhill skiing injuries in children. Am J Sports Med 12:142–147, 1984.
27. Booth FW, Gould EW: Effects of training and disuse on connective tissue. Exerc Sport Sci Rev 3:83–112, 1975.
28. Breen TF, Jupiter JB: Extensor carpi ulnaris and flexor carpi ulnaris tenodesis of the unstable distal ulna. J Hand Surg [Am] 14:612–617, 1989.
29. Bright RW, Burstein AH, Elmore EM: Epiphyseal plate cartilage—a biomechanical and histological analysis of failure modes. J Bone Joint Surg Am 56:668–703, 1974.
30. Bright RW: Physeal injuries. In Rockwood CA, Wilkens KE, King RE (eds): Fractures in Children. Philadelphia, JB Lippincott, 1984, pp 87–115.
31. Brust JD, Leonard BJ, Pheley A, Roberts WO: Children's ice hockey injuries. Am J Dis Child 146:741–747, 1992.
32. Bylak J, Hutchinson MR: Common sports injuries in young tennis players. Sports Med 26:119–132, 1998.
33. Caine D, Roy S, Singer KM, Broekhoff J: Stress changes of the distal radial growth plate. A radiographic survey and review of the literature. Am J Sports Med 20:290–298, 1992.
34. Caine D, Howe W, Ross W, Bergman G: Does repetitive physical loading inhibit radial growth in female gymnasts? Clin J Sport Med 7:302–308, 1997.
35. Calle SC, Evans JT: Snowboarding trauma. J Pediatr Surg 30:791–794, 1995.
36. Campbell RM Jr: Operative treatment of fractures and dislocations of the hand and wrist region in children. Orthop Clin North Am 21:217–243, 1990.
37. Carpenter CT, Lester EL: Skeletal age determination in young children: Analysis of three regions of the hand/wrist film. J Pediatr Orthop 13:76–79, 1993.
38. Carter SR, Aldridge MJ, Fitzgerald R, Davies AM: Stress changes of the wrist in adolescent gymnasts. Br J Radiol 61:109–112, 1988.
39. Chambers RB: Orthopaedic injuries in athletes (ages 6 to 17). Comparison of injuries occurring in six sports. Am J Sports Med 7:195–197, 1979.
40. Chang CY, Shih C, Penn IW, and colleagues: Wrist injuries in adolescent gymnasts of a Chinese opera school: Radiographic survey. Radiology 195:861–864, 1995. Published erratum appears in Radiology 197:319, 1995.
41. Christodoulou AG, Colton CL: Scaphoid fractures in children. J Pediatr Orthop 6:37–39, 1986.
42. Chung KC, Zimmerman NB, Travis MT: Wrist arthrography versus arthroscopy: A comparative study of 150 cases. J Hand Surg [Am] 21:591–594, 1996.
43. Claessens AL, Lefevre J, Beunen G, and colleagues: Physique as a risk factor for ulnar variance in elite female gymnasts. Med Sci Sports Exerc 28:560–569, 1996.
44. Cockshott WP: Distal avulsion fractures of the scaphoid. Br J Radiol 53:1037–1040, 1980.
45. Cohen MS: Ligamentous injuries of the wrist in the athlete. Clin Sports Med 17:533–552, 1998.
46. Compson JP: Trans-carpal injuries associated with distal radial fractures in children: A series of three cases. J Hand Surg [Br] 17:311–314, 1992.
47. Cook PA, Kobus RJ, Wiand W, Yu JS: Scapholunate ligament disruption in a skeletally immature patient: A case report. J Hand Surg [Am] 22:83–85, 1997.

48. Cooney WP: Evaluation of chronic wrist pain by arthrography, arthroscopy, and arthrotomy. J Hand Surg [Am] 18:815–822, 1993.
49. Culver JE, Anderson TE: Fractures of the hand and wrist in the athlete. Clin Sports Med 11:101–128, 1992.
50. Culver JE: Sports-related fractures of the hand and wrist. Clin Sports Med 9:85–109, 1990.
51. Dalton SE: Overuse injuries in adolescent athletes. Sports Med 13:58–70, 1992.
52. Dautel G, Merle M: Scapholunate dissociation in the skeletally immature carpus. J Hand Surg [Br] 22:173–174, 1997.
53. De Boeck H, Van Wellen P, Haentjens P: Nonunion of a carpal scaphoid fracture in a child. J Orthop Trauma 5:370–372, 1991.
54. Deibert MC, Aronsson DD, Johnson RJ, and colleagues: Skiing injuries in children, adolescents, and adults. J Bone Joint Surg Am 80:25–32, 1998.
55. De Smet L, Claessens A, Lefevre J, Beunen G: Gymnast wrist: An epidemiologic survey of ulnar variance and stress changes of the radial physis in elite female gymnasts. Am J Sports Med 22:846–850, 1994.
56. DiFiori JP, Mandelbaum BR: Wrist pain in a young gymnast: Unusual radiographic findings and MRI evidence of growth plate injury. Med Sci Sports Exerc 28:1453–1458, 1996.
57. DiFiori JP, Puffer JC, Mandelbaum BR, Dorey F: Distal radial growth plate injury and positive ulnar variance in nonelite gymnasts. Am J Sports Med 25:763–768, 1997.
58. Dobyns JH, Gabel GT: Gymnast's wrist. Hand Clin 6:493–505, 1990.
59. Dobyns JH, Sim FH, Linscheid RL: Sports stress syndromes of the hand and wrist. Am J Sports Med 6:236–254, 1978.
60. Edelson G, Reis ND, Fuchs D: Recurrence of Kienböck disease in a twelve-year-old after radial shortening. Report of a case. J Bone Joint Surg Am 70:1243–1245, 1988.
61. Ekenstarn FW, Palmer AK, Glisson RR: The load on the radius and ulna in different positions of the wrist and forearm: A cadaver study. Acta Orthop Scand 55:363–365, 1984.
62. Ekman EF, Poehling GG: Arthroscopy of the wrist in athletes. Clin Sports Med 15:753–768, 1996.
63. Fliegel CP: Stress related widening of the radial growth plate in adolescents. Ann Radiol (Paris) 29:374–376, 1986.
64. Foster RJ: Kienböck's disease in an 8-year-old girl: A case report. J Hand Surg [Am] 21:595–598, 1996.
65. Gabel GT: Gymnastic wrist injuries. Clin Sports Med 17:611–621, 1998.
66. Gamble JG, Simmons SC III: Bilateral scaphoid fractures in a child. Clin Orthop 162:125–128, 1982.
67. Garrick JG, Requa RK: Epidemiology of women's gymnastic injuries. Am J Sports Med 8:261–264, 1980.
68. Garrick JG, Requa RK: Injury patterns in children and adolescent skiers. Am J Sports Med 7:245–248, 1979.
69. Garrick JG, Requa RK: Girls' sports injuries in high school athletics. JAMA 239:2245–2248, 1978.
70. Garrick JG, Requa RK: Injuries in high school sports. Pediatrics 61:465–469, 1978.
71. Gerard FM: Post-traumatic carpal instability in a young child. A case report. J Bone Joint Surg Am 62:131–133, 1980.
72. Gerber SD, Griffin PP, Simmons BP: Break dancer's wrist. J Pediatr Orthop 6:98–99, 1986.
73. Gibbon WW, Jackson A: An isolated capitate fracture in a 9-year-old boy. Br J Radiol 62:487–488, 1989.
74. Gill TJ IV, Micheli LJ: The immature athlete. Common injuries and overuse syndromes of the elbow and wrist. Clin Sports Med 15:401–423, 1996.
75. Goldberg B, Rosenthal PP, Robertson LS, Nicholas JA: Injuries in youth football. Pediatrics 81:255–261, 1988.
76. Gouldesbrough: A case of fractured scaphoid and os magnum in a boy 10 years old. Lancet ii:792, 1916.
77. Green DP: Hand injuries in children. Pediatr Clin North Am 24:903–918, 1977.
78. Greene MH, Hadied AM, LaMont RL: Scaphoid fractures in children. J Hand Surg [Am] 9:536–541, 1984.
79. Gumbs VL, Segal D, Halligan JB, Lower G: Bilateral distal radius and ulnar fractures in adolescent weight lifters. Am J Sports Med 10:375–379, 1982.
80. Hagel BE, Meeuwisse WH, Mohtadi NG, Fick GH: Skiing and snowboarding injuries in the children and adolescents of Southern Alberta. Clin J Sport Med 9:9–17, 1999.

81. Halpern B, Thompson N, Curl WW, and colleagues: High school football injuries: Identifying the risk factors. Am J Sports Med 15:316–320, 1987.
82. Hankin FM, Peel SM: Sport-related fractures and dislocations in the hand. Hand Clin 6:429–453, 1990.
83. Hastings H II, Simmons BP: Hand fractures in children. A statistical analysis. Clin Orthop 188:120–130, 1984.
84. Hickey GJ, Fricker PA, McDonald WA: Injuries of young elite female basketball players over a six-year period. Clin J Sport Med 7:252–256, 1997.
85. Ho PK, Dellon AL, Wilgis EF: True aneurysms of the hand resulting from athletic injury. Report of two cases. Am J Sports Med 13:136–138, 1985.
86. Hoff GL, Martin TA: Outdoor and indoor soccer: Injuries among youth players. Am J Sports Med 14:231–233, 1986.
87. Hokan R, Bryce GM, Cobb NJ: Dislocation of scaphoid and fractures capitate in a child. Injury 24:496–497, 1993.
88. Hosking OR: Kienböck's disease in an 8 year old boy. Aust N Z J Surg 59:92–93, 1989.
89. Houshian S, Andersen HM: Comparison between in-line and roller-skating injury. A prospective study. Scand J Med Sci Sports 10:47–50, 2000.
90. Howse C: Wrist injuries in sport. Sports Med 17:163–175, 1994.
91. Huene DR: Primary internal fixation of carpal navicular fractures in the athlete. Am J Sports Med 7:175–177, 1979.
92. Hui FC, Linscheid RL: Ulnotriquetral augmentation tenodesis. A reconstructive procedure for dorsal subluxation of the distal radioulnar joint. J Hand Surg [Am] 7:230–236, 1982.
93. Inkelis SH, Stroberg AJ, Keller EL, Christenson PD: Roller skating injuries in children. Pediatr Emerg Care 4:127–132, 1988.
94. Innis PC: Office evaluation and treatment of finger and hand injuries in children. Curr Opin Pediatr 7:83–87, 1995.
95. Israeli A, Engel J, Ganel A: Possible fatigue fracture of the pisiform bone in volleyball players. Int J Sports Med 3:56–57, 1982.
96. Jaramillo D, Laor T, Zaleske DJ: Indirect trauma to the growth plate: Results of MR imaging after epiphyseal and metaphyseal injury in rabbits. Radiology 187:171–178, 1993.
97. Jensen CH, Leight P: Idiopathic avascular necrosis of the scaphoid in a child. Scan J Plast Reconstr Surg Hand Surg 29:359–360, 1995.
98. Johnstone DJ, Thorogood S, Smith WH, Scott TD: A comparison of magnetic resonance imaging and arthroscopy in the investigation of chronic wrist pain. J Hand Surg [Br] 22:714–718, 1997.
99. Kaawach W, Ecklund K, Zurakowski D, Waters P: The 54th Annual Meeting of the American Society for Surgery of the Hand, Poster Session, September 1999, Boston, Mass.
100. Kahn SJ, Sherry DD: Kienböck's disease—avascular necrosis of the carpal lunate bone—in a 7-year-old girl with dermatomyositis. Clin Pediatr (Phila) 33:752–754, 1994.
101. Kamano M, Fukushima K, Honda Y: Multiple carpal bone fractures in an eleven-year-old. J Orthop Trauma 12:445–448, 1998.
102. Kannus P, Nittymaki S, Jarvinen M: Athletic overuse injuries in children. A 30-month prospective follow-up study at an outpatient sports clinic. Clin Pediatr (Phila) 27:333–337, 1988.
103. Kaplan TA, Digel SL, Scavo VA, Arellana SB: Effect of obesity on injury risk in high school football players. Clin J Sport Med 5:43–47, 1995.
104. Keller CS, Noyes FR, Buncher CR: The medical aspects of soccer injury epidemiology. Am J Sports Med 16:S105–112, 1988.
105. Kiefhaber TR, Stern PJ: Upper extremity tendinitis and overuse syndromes in the athlete. Clin Sports Med 11:39–55, 1992.
106. Kiiskinen A: Physical training and connective tissues in young mice—physical properties of Achilles tendons and long bones. Growth 41:123–137, 1977.
107. Koh TJ, Grabiner MD, Weiker GG: Technique and ground reaction forces in the back handspring. Am J Sports Med 20:61–66, 1992.
108. Koman LA, Mooney JF III, Poehling GC: Fractures and ligamentous injuries of the wrist. Hand Clin 6:477–491, 1990.
109. Kvist M, Kujala UM, Heinonen OJ, and colleagues: Sports-related injuries in children. Int J Sports Med 10:81–86, 1989.
110. Landry GL: Sports injuries in childhood. Pediatr Ann 21:165–168, 1992.
111. Larson RL, McMahon RO: The epiphysis and the childhood athlete. JAMA 196:607, 1966.
112. Larson B, Light TR, Ogden JA: Fracture and ischemic necrosis of the immature scaphoid. J Hand Surg [Am] 12:122–127, 1987.
113. McLatchie GR: Analysis of karate injuries sustained in 295 contests. Injury 8:132–134, 1976.
114. Leicht P, Mikkelsen JB, Larsen CF: Scapholunate distance in children. Acta Radiol 37:625–626, 1996.
115. Letts M, Esser D: Fractures of the triquetrum in children. J Pediatr Orthop 13:228–231, 1993.
116. Lichtman DM, Degnan GG: Staging and its use in the determination of treatment modalities for Kienböck's disease. Hand Clin 9:409, 1993.
117. Liebling MS, Berdon WE, Ruzal-Shapiro C, and colleagues: Gymnast's wrist (pseudorickets growth plate abnormality) in adolescent athletes: Findings on plain films and MR imaging. AJR Am J Roentgenol 164:157–159, 1995.
118. Linder MM, Townsend DJ, Jones JC, and colleagues: Incidence of adolescent injuries in junior high school football and its relationship to sexual maturity. Clin J Sport Med 5:167–170, 1995.
119. Linscheid RL, Dobyns JH: Athletic injuries of the wrist. Clin Orthop 198:141–151, 1985.
120. Lorish TR, Rizzo TD Jr, Ilstrup DM, Scott SG: Injuries in adolescent and preadolescent boys at two large wrestling tournaments. Am J Sports Med 20:199–202, 1992.
121. Lowrey CW, Chadwick RO, Waltman EN: Digital vessel trauma from repetitive impact in baseball catchers. J Hand Surg [Am] 1:236–238, 1976.
122. Maffulli N, Bundoc RC, Chan KM, Cheng JC: Paediatric sports injuries in Hong Kong: A seven year survey. Br J Sports Med 30:218–221, 1996.
123. Maffulli N: Intensive training in young athletes. The orthopaedic surgeon's viewpoint. Sports Med 9:229–243, 1990.
124. Malanga GA, Stuart MJ: In-line skating injuries. Mayo Clin Proc 70:752–754, 1995.
125. Mandelbaum BR, Bartolozzi AR, Davis CA, and colleagues: Wrist pain syndrome in the gymnast. Pathogenetic, diagnostic, and therapeutic considerations. Am J Sports Med 17:305–317, 1989.
126. Markiewitz AD, Andrish JT: Hand and wrist injuries in the preadolescent and adolescent athlete. Clin Sports Med 11:203–225, 1992.
127. Markolf KL, Shapiro MS, Mandelbaum BR, Teurlings L: Wrist loading patterns during pommel horse exercises. J Biomech 23:1001–1011, 1990.
128. Mayfield JK: Mechanism of carpal injuries. Clin Orthop 149:45–54, 1980.
129. Mayfield JK: Patterns of injury to carpal ligaments. A spectrum. Clin Orthop 187:36–42, 1984.
130. Mayfield JK, Johnson RP, Kilcoyne RK: Carpal dislocations: pathomechanics and progressive perilunar instability. J Hand Surg [Am] 5:226–241, 1980.
131. Maxted MJ, Owen R: Two cases of non-union of carpal scaphoid fractures in children. Injury 13:441–443, 1982.
132. Meeusen R, Borms J: Gymnastic injuries. Sports Med 13:337–356, 1992.
133. Messina DF, Farney WC, DeLee JC: The incidence of injury in Texas high school basketball. A prospective study among male and female athletes. Am J Sports Med 27:294–299, 1999.
134. Micheli LJ: Overuse injuries in children's sports: The growth factor. Orthop Clin North Am 14:337–360, 1983.
135. Minami A, Itoga H, Kobayashi M: Kienböck's disease in an eleven-year-old girl. A case report. Ital J Orthop Traumatol 18:547–550, 1992.
136. Minami M, Yamazaki J, Chisaka N, and colleagues: Nonunion of the capitate. J Hand Surg [Am] 12:1089–1091, 1987.
137. Mintzer CM, Waters PW, Simmons BP: Nonunion of the scaphoid in children treated by Herbert screw fixation and bone grafting. A report of 5 cases. J Bone Joint Surg [Br] 77:98–100, 1995.
138. Mintzer CM, Water PW: Surgical treatment of pediatric scaphoid fracture nonunions. J Pediatr Orthop 19:236–239, 1999.
139. Mirabello SC, Loeb PE, Andrews JR: The wrist: Field evaluation and treatment. Clin Sports Med 11:1–25, 1992.
140. Mooney JF III, Siegel DB, Koman LA: Ligamentous injuries of the wrist in athletes. Clin Sports Med 11:129–139, 1992.
141. Moreland MS: Skiing injuries in children. Clin Sports Med 1:241–251, 1982.
142. Morrongiello BA: Children's perspectives on injury and close-call experiences: Sex differences in injury-outcome processes. J Pediatr Psychol 22:499–512, 1997.
143. Murakami S, Nakajima H: Aseptic necrosis of the capitate in two gymnasts. Am J Sports Med 11:170–173, 1983.

144. Nafie SA: Fractures of the carpal bones in children. Injury 18: 117–119, 1987.
145. Nakamura R, Imaeda T, Suzuki K, Miura T: Sports-related Kienböck's disease. Am J Sports Med 19:88–91, 1991.
146. Nelson DE, Bixby-Hammett D: Equestrian injuries in children and young adults. Am J Dis Child 146:611–614, 1992.
147. Nguyen DT, McCue FC III, Urch SE: Evaluation of the injured wrist on the field and in the office. Clin Sports Med 17:421–432, 1998.
148. Nielsen AB, Yde J: Epidemiology and traumatology of injuries in soccer. Am J Sports Med 17:803–807, 1989.
149. Nieman EA, Swann PG: Karate injuries. BMJ 1:233, 1971.
150. Nilsson S, Roaas A: Soccer injuries in adolescents. Am J Sports Med 6:358–361, 1978.
151. O'Neill DB, Micheli LJ: Overuse injuries in the young athlete. Clin Sports Med 7:591–610, 1988.
152. Onuba O, Ireland J: Two cases of non-union of fractures of the scaphoid in children. Injury 15:109–112, 1983.
153. Osberg JS, Schneps SE, Di Scala C, Li G: Skateboarding: More dangerous than roller skating or in-line skating. Arch Pediatr Adolesc Med 152:985–991, 1998.
154. Osterman AL, Moskow L, Low DW: Soft-tissue injuries of the hand and wrist in racquet sports. Clin Sports Med 7:329–348, 1988.
155. Palmer AK: Triangular fibrocartilage complex lesions: A classification. J Hand Surg [Am] 14:594–606, 1989.
156. Palmer AK, Werner FW: Biomechanics of the distal radioulnar joint. Clin Orthop 187:26–35, 1984.
157. Peiro A, Martos F, Mut T, Aracil J: Trans-scaphoid perilunate dislocation in a child. A case report. Acta Orthop Scand 52:31–34, 1981.
158. Pick RY, Segal D: Carpal scaphoid fracture and non-union in an eight-year-old child. Report of a case. J Bone Joint Surg Am 65: 1188–1189, 1983.
159. Pieter W, Zemper ED: Injury rates in children participating in tae-kwon-do competition. J Trauma 43:89–96, 1997.
160. Pino EC, Colville MR: Snowboard injuries. Am J Sports Med 17: 778–781, 1989.
161. Pitner MA: Pathophysiology of overuse injuries in the hand and wrist. Hand Clin 6:355–364, 1990.
162. Posner MA: Injuries to the hand and wrist in athletes. Orthop Clin North Am 8:593–618, 1977.
163. Powell EC, Tanz RR: In-line skate and rollerskate injuries in childhood. Pediatr Emerg Care 12:259–262, 1996.
164. Prager BI, Fitton WL, Cahill BR, Olson GH: High school football injuries: A prospective study and pitfalls of data collection. Am J Sports Med 17:681–685, 1989.
165. Press JM, Wiesner SL: Prevention: Conditioning and orthotics. Hand Clin 6:383–392, 1990.
166. Read JW, Conolly WB, Lanzetta M, and colleagues: Diagnostic ultrasound of the hand and wrist. J Hand Surg [Am] 21:1004–1010, 1996.
167. Recht MP, Burk DL Jr, Dalinka MK: Radiology of wrist and hand injuries in athletes. Clin Sports Med 6:811–828, 1987.
168. Retsky J, Jaffe D, Christoffel K: Skateboarding injuries in children. A second wave. Am J Dis Child 145:188–192, 1991.
169. Rettig AC: Epidemiology of hand and wrist injuries in sports. Clin Sports Med 17:401–406, 1998.
170. Rettig AC, Patel DV: Epidemiology of elbow, forearm, and wrist injuries in the athlete. Clin Sports Med 14:289–297, 1995.
171. Rettig AC: Elbow, forearm and wrist injuries in the athlete. Sports Med 25:115–130, 1998.
172. Rettig AC: Neurovascular injuries to the wrists and hands of athletes. Clin Sports Med 9:389–417, 1990.
173. Risser WL, Risser JM, Preston D: Weight-training injuries in adolescents. Am J Dis Child 144:1015–1017, 1990.
174. Risser WL: Epidemiology of sports injuries in adolescents. Adolesc Med 2:109–124, 1991.
175. Roberts WO, Brust JD, Leonard B: Youth ice hockey tournament injuries: Rates and patterns compared to season play. Med Sci Sports Exerc 31:46–51, 1999.
176. Roser LA, Clawson DK: Football injuries in the very young athlete. Clin Orthop 69:219–223, 1970.
177. Rowe PH: Colles fracture due to weightlifting. Br J Sports Med 13: 130–131, 1979.
178. Roy S, Caine D, Singer KM: Stress changes of the distal radial epiphysis in young gymnasts. Am J Sports Med 13:301–308, 1985.

179. Ruby LK: Common hand injuries in the athlete. Orthop Clin North Am 11:819–839, 1980.
180. Ruch DS, Poehling GG: Arthroscopic management of partial scapholunate and lunatotriquetral injuries of the wrist. J Hand Surg [Am] 21:412–417, 1996.
181. Ruggles DL, Peterson HA, Scott SG: Radial growth plate injury in a female gymnast. Med Sci Sports Exerc 23:393–396, 1991.
182. Ryan JR, Salciccioli GG: Fractures of the distal radial epiphysis in adolescent weight lifters. Sports Med 4:26–27, 1976.
183. Sahlin Y: Sport accidents in childhood. Br J Sports Med 24:40–44, 1990.
184. Sandzen SC: Growth plate injuries of the wrist and hand. Am Fam Physician 29:153–168, 1984.
185. Savoie FH III, Whipple TL: The role of arthroscopy in athletic injuries of the wrist. Clin Sports Med 15:219–233, 1996.
186. Scheck RJ, Kubitzek C, Hierner R, and colleagues: The scapholunate interosseous ligament in MR arthrography of the wrist: Correlation with non-enhanced MRI and wrist arthrography. Skeletal Radiol 26: 263–271, 1997.
187. Schieber RA, Branche-Dorsey CM, Ryan GW: Comparison of in-line skating injuries with rollerskating and skateboarding injuries. JAMA 271:1856–1858, 1994.
188. Schmidt-Olsen S, Bunemann LK, Lade V, Brassoe JO: Soccer injuries of youth. Br J Sports Med 19:161–164, 1985.
189. Scheker LR, Belliappa PP, Acosta R, German DS: Reconstruction of the dorsal ligament of the triangular fibrocartilage complex. J Hand Surg [Br] 19:310–318, 1994.
190. Sherker S, Cassell E: Preventing in-line skating injuries: How effective are the countermeasures? Sports Med 28:325–335, 1999.
191. Shih C, Chang CY, Penn IW, and colleagues: Chronically stressed wrists in adolescent gymnasts: MR imaging appearance. Radiology 195:855–859, 1995. Published erratum appears in Radiology 197: 319, 1995.
192. Shorter NA, Jensen PE, Harmon BJ, Mooney DP: Skiing injuries in children and adolescents. J Trauma 40:997–1001, 1996.
193. Shorter NA, Mooney DP, Harmon BJ: Snowboarding injuries in children and adolescents. Am J Emerg Med 17:261–263, 1999.
194. Simmons BP, Lovallo JL: Hand and wrist injuries in children. Clin Sports Med 7:495–512, 1988.
195. Snook GA: Injuries in women's gymnastics: A five-year study. Am J Sports Med 7:242–244, 1979.
196. Southcott R, Rosman MA: Non-union of carpal scaphoid fractures in children. J Bone Joint Surg [Br] 59:20–23, 1977.
197. Stahl F: On lunatomalacia (Kienböck's disease): Clinical and roentgenographical study, especially on its pathogenesis and late results of immobilization treatment. Acta Chir Scand Suppl 126:1–133, 1947.
198. Stanciu C, Dumont A: Changing patterns of scaphoid fractures in adolescents. Can J Surg 37:214–216, 1994.
199. Strauss RH, Lanese RR: Injuries among wrestlers in school and college tournaments. JAMA 248:2016–2019, 1982.
200. Strickland JW: Considerations for the treatment of the injured athlete. Clin Sports Med 17:397–400, 1998.
201. Stuart HC, Pyle SI, Cornon J, Reed RB: Onsets, completions and spans of ossification in the 29 bone-growth centers of the hand and wrist. Pediatrics 29:237–249, 1962.
202. Stuart MJ, Smith AM, Nieva JJ, Rock MG: Injuries in youth ice hockey: A pilot surveillance strategy. Mayo Clin Proc 70:350–356, 1995.
203. Teitz CC: Sports medicine concerns in dance and gymnastics. Clin Sports Med 2:571–593, 1983.
204. Terry CL, Waters PM: Triangular fibrocartilage injuries in pediatric and adolescent patients. J Hand Surg [Am] 23:626–634, 1998.
205. Thompson GH, Wilber JH, Marcus RE: Internal fixation of fractures in children and adolescents. A comparative analysis. Clin Orthop 188:10–20, 1984.
206. Tolat AR, Sanderson PL, De Smet L, Stanley JK: The gymnast's wrist: Acquired positive ulnar variance following chronic epiphyseal injury. J Hand Surg [Br] 17:678–681, 1992.
207. Tomaino MM, Rubin DA: The value of the pronated-grip view radiograph in assessing dynamic ulnar positive variance: A case report. Am J Orthop 28:180–181, 1999.
208. Tsai TM, Stillwell JH: Repair of chronic subluxation of the distal radioulnar joint using flexor carpi ulnaris tendon. J Hand Surg 9: 289–294, 1984.
209. Tursz A, Crost M: Sports-related injuries in children. A study of

their characteristics, frequency, and severity, with comparison to other types of accidental injuries. Am J Sports Med 14:294–299, 1986.

210. Twellaar M, Verstappen FT, Huson A: Is prevention of sports injuries a realistic goal? A four-year prospective investigation of sports injuries among physical education students. Am J Sports Med 24:528–534, 1996.

211. Ullis K: Wrist injuries in rollerskating. N Engl J Med 301:1350, 1979.

212. Ungerholm S, Engkvist O, Gierup J, and colleagues: Skiing injuries in children and adults: A comparative study from an 8-year period. Int J Sports Med 4:236–240, 1983.

213. Vahvanen V, Westerlund M: Fracture of the carpal scaphoid in children. A clinical and roentgenological study of 108 cases. Acta Orthop Scand 51:909–913, 1980.

214. Vender MI, Watson HK: Acquired Madelung-like deformity in a gymnast. J Hand Surg [Am] 13:19–21, 1988.

215. Verstappen FT, Twellaar M, Hartgens F, van Mechelen W: Physical fitness and sports skills in relation to sports injuries. A four-year prospective investigation of sports injuries among physical education students. Int J Sports Med 19:586–591, 1998.

216. Wagner KT Jr, Lyne ED: Adolescent traumatic dislocations of the shoulder with open epiphyses. J Pediatr Orthop 3:61–62, 1983.

217. Watson AW: Incidence and nature of sports injuries in Ireland. Analysis of four types of sport. Am J Sports Med 21:137–143, 1993.

218. Watson AW: Sports injuries during one academic year in 6799 Irish school children. Am J Sports Med 12:65–71, 1984.

219. Weiker GG: Hand and wrist problems in the gymnast. Clin Sports Med 11:189–202, 1992.

220. Weir MA, Watson AW: A twelve month study of sports injuries in one Irish school. Ir J Med Sci 165:165–169, 1996.

221. Weiss AC, Akelman E, Lambiase R: Comparison of the findings of triple-injection cinearthrography of the wrist with those of arthroscopy. J Bone Joint Surg Am 78:348–356, 1996.

222. Weiss AC, Sachar K, Glowacki KA: Arthroscopic debridement alone for intercarpal ligament tears. J Hand Surg [Am] 22:344–349, 1997.

223. Werner SL, Plancher KD: Biomechanics of wrist injuries in sports. Clin Sports Med 17:407–420, 1998.

224. Westkaemper JG, Mitsionis G, Giannakopoulos PN, Soteranos DG: Wrist arthroscopy for the treatment of ligament and triangular fibrocartilage complex injuries. Arthroscopy 14:479–483, 1998.

225. Whipple TL, Geissler WB: Arthroscopic management of wrist triangular fibrocartilage complex injuries in the athlete. Orthopedics 16:1061–1067, 1993.

226. Whipple TL: The role of arthroscopy in the treatment of wrist injuries in the athlete. Clin Sports Med 11:227–238, 1992.

227. Williams JM, Wright P, Currie CE, Beattie TF: Sports related injuries in Scottish adolescents aged 11–15. Br J Sports Med 32:291–296, 1998.

228. Wilson-MacDonald J: Delayed union of the distal scaphoid in a child. J Hand Surg [Am] 12:520–522, 1987.

229. Wulff RN, Schmidt TL: Carpal fractures in children. J Pediatr Orthop 18:462–465, 1998.

230. Yang ZY, Gilula LA, Jonsson K: Os centrale carpi simulating a scaphoid waist fracture. J Hand Surg [Br] 19:754–756, 1994.

231. Yasuda M, Okuda H, Egi T, Guidera PM: Temporary scapho-trapezoidal joint fixation for Kienböck's disease in a 12-year-old girl: A case report. J Hand Surg [Am] 23:411–414, 1998.

232. Yde J, Nielsen AB: Sports injuries in adolescents' ball games: Soccer, handball and basketball. Br J Sports Med 24:51–54, 1990.

233. Yong-Hing K, Wedge JH, Bowen CVA: Chronic injury to the distal ulnar and radial growth plates in an adolescent gymnast. J Bone Joint Surg Am 70:1087–1089, 1988.

234. Young TB: Isolated fracture of the capitate in a 10-year-old boy. Injury 17:133–134, 1986.

235. Zachee B, De Smet L, Fabry G: Arthroscopic suturing of TFCC lesions. Arthroscopy 9:242–243, 1993.

236. Zaricznyj B, Shattuck LJ, Mast TA, and colleagues: Sports-related injuries in school-aged children. Am J Sports Med 8:318–324, 1980.

237. Zerin JM, Hernandez RJ: Approach to skeletal maturation. Hand Clin 7:53–62, 1991.

238. Zimmerman NB, Weiland AJ: Scapholunate dissociation in the skeletally immature carpus. J Hand Surg [Am] 15:701–705, 1990.

Section B
Hand

1. ATHLETIC INJURIES OF THE ADULT HAND
Thomas J. Graham, MD ■ Daniel J. Mullen, MD

General Concepts

Care of the athlete's hand and wrist injury is not the work of the hand surgeon alone. Every physician who comes in contact with athletes of any level will be expected to care for these injuries. This includes the team physicians for professional or Olympic sports and those volunteering their time on the sidelines of their daughter's or son's scholastic contests.

Often, the first health professional assessing the patient-athlete is uniquely well positioned to assess and possibly to treat the hand or wrist injury. Perhaps he or she saw the play and can better appreciate the mechanism or energy of the situation. The close observer often gets to "lay hands on" the athlete before significant pain and swelling obscure the examination findings. Finally, those associated with team or individual sports may have key insights regarding the patient-athlete and may be able to help determine, for example, whether the athlete is a stoic who will minimize the injury or whether there are secondary issues that may be causing the athlete to emphasize the injury.

Although every sport has individual characteristics that distinguish it from other sports, all sports and all sport positions are hand intensive. The football lineman will relate how important the use of his hands is in dispatching his opponent just as often as the wide receiver will. With the exception of individuals playing certain soccer positions, participants in running events, and athletes involved in single-handed sports, few athletes would dispute that a hand or wrist injury would have a severe impact on their ability to perform optimally. Therefore, those caring for the athlete at any level are charged with understanding the many factors that surround this unique patient population. This includes the pathophysiology as well as the psychology. Being familiar with the epidemiology, the mechanisms of injury, the sport-specific factors, and the equipment issues can enhance the ability of the treating physician to return the athlete to play in the most appropriate manner.

Caring for the athlete's hand and wrist is not just a microcosm of upper extremity surgery. Instead, it demands all the basic tenets of care for this anatomic region and multiplies by the factors of patient expectation, performance demand, and even popular focus on athletics in our culture. Caring for the athlete's hand and wrist is truly a test not only of the physician's skill and intellectual appreciation for the pathologic process but also of the ability to make decisions in the patient's best interest in the face of pressures from many sources. There is also no greater test of outcome than when our interventions are tested at the level demanded by the elite athlete.

Epidemiology

Several epidemiologic studies have revealed that the incidence of hand and wrist injuries ranges from 3% to 25% of all athletic injuries.[9, 25, 130] These injuries are sustained more commonly in younger athletes. When the Cleveland Clinic Sports Medicine group examined their data over a 10-year period, they found that almost 15% of athletes younger than 16 years of age sustained upper extremity injuries.[9]

Concerning the types of injuries encountered in the athletic population, there has been confusion regarding interpretation of the epidemiologic data from many solid studies contributed by experienced centers. Seemingly disparate data reflect the differences in the type of patients seen in different practices. Incidence numbers change dramatically when the focus is placed on hand-intensive, high-velocity collision sports or when the participation level of the athlete is considered.

When Rettig and colleagues selected eight sports for study from their Indianapolis practice, which cares for athletes from all levels of participation, they found that fractures accounted for 55% of the injuries, whereas sprains (21%) and dislocations (7%) were less frequent.[130] These data appear to contradict a study from the Olympic Training Center in Colorado Springs, in which information reported directly to athletic trainers was obtained. In that population, in which hand and wrist injuries accounted for 8.7% of more than 8300 injuries reported, sprains and contusions were more prevalent (59%) than fractures (10%). The explanation for the discrepancies lies in the reporting mechanisms and the referral pattern. Referral practices, especially those with experience in treating the elite athlete, should anticipate a higher percentage of significant injuries such as fractures. Those on the "front lines," such as athletic trainers and team physicians stationed in the training room, field many of the everyday injuries, such as sprains and contusions.

There are excellent studies on the types of injuries encountered in many of the popular sports, just as there are data describing the prevalence of specific injuries in these endeavors. Almost every sport has been analyzed either individually or as a part of a multisport study.[24, 27, 35, 116, 157] As might be expected, American football is usually the sport in which most hand injuries occur. These injuries often reflect the violent contact nature of the sport and include substantial trauma, such as perilunate dislocations.[127]

The nature of the sport, the way in which the athlete uses his or her hand, and the equipment employed in the sport can all affect the injury patterns and frequency. Just as sports such as golf, tennis, and bat handling in baseball put the hamulus at risk for fracture, there are sport-specific risks, such as "dunk lacerations" on the basketball goal, that will be seen by physicians closely associated with a particular sport.[75]

Mechanics of the Hand and Wrist Related to Sports

Study of the intricacies of hand biomechanics is outside the scope of this chapter, but an appreciation of how the hand functions in sports can enhance the physician's ability to treat the athlete. Here again, it is emphasized that care of the athlete's hand is synonymous with the global practice of upper extremity surgery, with specialized additional concerns and demands. A basic understanding of the fine anatomy and mechanics of this area should be supplemented with knowledge of some basic concepts relating to athletic execution.

There have been several attempts to define or classify the mechanisms and mechanical factors influencing sports injuries to the hand. A general scheme was suggested by Mirabello and associates,[103] in which four major mechanisms of injury were proposed: throwing, weight-bearing, twisting, and impact. Amadio predated Mirabello's contribution with a more descriptive classification: hand contact with the ball, hand contact with competitors, stick sports, and a catchment "other" category.[2] Werner and Plancher expanded on Amadio's lead with categories divided by wrist injury potential.[153] They categorized sports by their potential for wrist injury and enumerated some of the more common injuries seen in these pursuits. In addition to "impact" and "racquet, stick, and club" sports, they added a category for "apparatus/external contact sports," which included gymnastics, bowling, rock climbing, and weightlifting.

These papers do not critically analyze the ranges, the directions, and the amounts of force generated or dissipated during specific athletic activities, but they do provide a general basis for understanding. Taking into account that practically any injury can occur in any sport, there are certain motions or equipment interactions that make specific injuries more prevalent in a particular sport. This has treatment and training implications, and it can also lead to changes in technique and technology.

Caring for the Athlete

In caring for the athlete, the physician may be called upon to mediate among several factions with intentions that are often at cross purposes. These include the athlete, the parents, the coaches or the manager, the agents, and the owner or the organization. This reality causes the decision-making process to be more emotionally charged, if not more difficult.

The management questions set forth by Green and Strickland[51] in treating the athlete remain valid today:

1. Is the method of treatment we have selected the most appropriate for this injury, and can it be expected to provide the best long-term result?

2. If this injury had occurred in a nonathlete or during the off-season, would we manage it in basically a similar manner?

3. Are the potential complications of my anticipated treatment method significantly greater than might be expected from a more conservative approach?

4. Will the treatment allow the athlete to return to competition with little risk of re-injury?

5. If re-injury does occur, would it unfavorably influence the prognosis for a satisfactory recovery?

These guidelines are not limited to those caring for the hand; they are sound principles that apply across the spectrum of sports medicine. They are important, however, to recall in connection with injuries to the hand because these injuries are often minimized by everyone involved in the continuum of treatment and return to play, including the patient. Although hand injuries may not have the same media impact as a catastrophic knee injury or neural axis trauma, hand injuries are critically important to the athlete's ability to function effectively. Treating these injuries requires use of the systematic thought process described by Green and Strickland.[51]

A generic approach cannot suffice for the care of the athlete. Athletes at all levels of organized sport, from grade school to the professional or Olympic level, have special concerns. Even those athletes who are not likely to reach the elite levels of performance will be concerned about the effect of injury on their future in a chosen sport. Some physicians will also be called upon to render care to those who are high-performance and high-profile athletes. The concepts of care for these athletes are distinctive, by definition. Elite athletes may have access to almost unlimited resources, and their expectation and functional demands are nearly 100%. There are mitigating circumstances and many interested parties, possibly with opposing points of view. The surgeon must be an expert communicator and documenter. The trainer, the manager/coach, the agent, and the owner will undoubtedly express their views to the physician. Despite the distractions, the guiding principle must be that the athlete is the surgeon's patient.

The lines between conservative and aggressive treatment have been blurred in this population. Is it aggressive or conservative to fix a fracture to ensure anatomic reduction and return a player to service earlier? The care of the elite athlete will introduce the physician to many innovations in technique and technology, as well as to the importance of sport-specific rehabilitation.

Careful communication is essential for those caring for the elite athlete. Confidentiality is of the utmost importance. The physician may be reporting his or her assessment and findings to a skilled trainer or, at times, to a public relations executive for the team. Consideration of these different circumstances is critical in caring for the elite athlete. Finally, remember that the derivation of "fan" is "fanatic." Many of today's sports enthusiasts have not only loyalty but also money invested in the outcome of events. Physicians caring for athletes should try to keep their name out of the media. If a physician's name does appear in the media, the physician should anticipate contact from fans and should refrain from "leaking" any information.

Osseous and Soft Tissue Injuries of the Triphalangeal Digits

Ligamentous Injuries and Dislocations of the Triphalangeal Digits

The dislocation of one of the small joints in the hand is one of the most frequently encountered injuries in athletic medicine. Torsional or rotational stress, angular deviation, and hyperextension of the interphalangeal or metacarpophalangeal joints can occur in any sports activity. All physicians and trainers will see this injury during their careers. Although many hand dislocations are low-level injuries that require only a short duration of treatment and minimally affect the athlete's participation, others can be complicated. Recognition of the pathoanatomy and the severity level along with appreciation of the potential sequelae is the focus for the physician.

Metacarpophalangeal Joint

The architecture of the metacarpophalangeal (MCP) joint of the fingers and thumb is similar. The MCP is a condyloid joint that allows greater freedom of movement than the interphalangeal joints. The special architecture of the articular head promotes motion, including a dumbbell-shaped dome that narrows centrally to accommodate the collateral ligaments. The volar aspect is broader than the dorsal. Additionally, there is a slight ulnar and volar flattening that is accentuated in the more medial rays (Fig. 24B1–1).

With all these osseous factors that promote motion, the surrounding soft tissues are all the more critical in maintaining stability. The collateral ligaments, the volar plate, an accommodating capsule, the deep transverse intermetacarpal ligament, and the tendons all play a role in imparting stability to the MCP joint. These structures form a "box" with interesting static and dynamic characteristics. The volar plate has diagonally oriented fibers, a structure that allows more collapse and expansion, as is understood when one appreciates the nearly universal capability of the MCP joint to hyperextend (Fig. 24B1–2).

The collateral ligaments originate in the well-defined collateral recesses, and they insert along both the epiphysis and the proximal metaphysis of the proximal phalanx. The MCP proper ligament has a more bundled structure and an axial orientation. It is accompanied by the triangular, and thinner, accessory collateral or metacarpoglenoidal ligament, which inserts on the margins of the volar plate (Fig. 24B1–3).

The action of the collateral ligament complex is the basis for several observations and recommendations. The

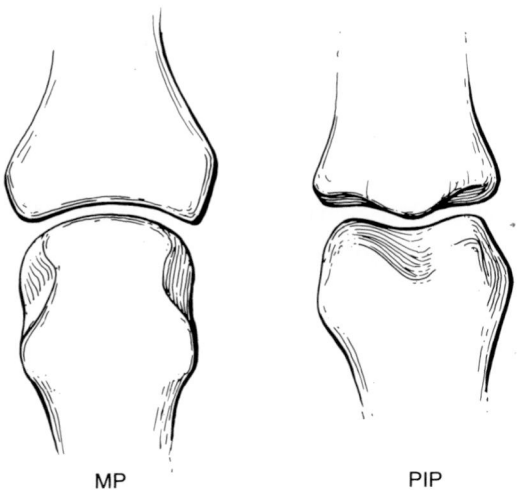

Figure 24B1–1. The metacarpophalangeal (MP) and proximal interphalangeal (PIP) joints are quite different structurally. The PIP joint has a bicondylar configuration, making it inherently more stable than the globular MP joint.

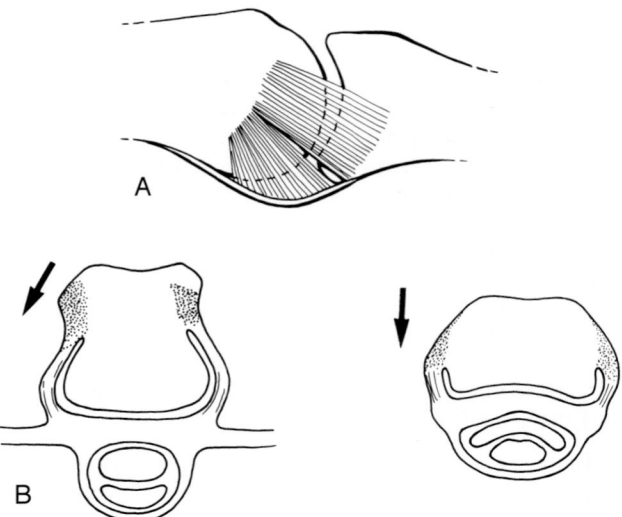

Figure 24B1–3. *A,* In both the metacarpophalangeal and the proximal interphalangeal joints, the collateral ligaments have a cordlike dorsal component and a fan-shaped volar component. *B,* As seen in cross section, the collateral ligaments of the proximal interphalangeal joint *(right)* are more parallel than those of the metacarpophalangeal joint *(left).* (Redrawn from Eaton RG: Joint Injuries of the Hand. Springfield, Charles C Thomas, 1971.)

eccentric configuration of the metacarpal head and the relatively fixed length of the proper collateral cause it to tighten significantly in flexion. This accounts for the restricted abduction-adduction capability of the joint in full flexion, as compared with its lax state in extension. This configuration is the foundation for the "safe position" splinting recommendation. The safe position at the MCP joint is fully flexed because the proper collateral is at its greatest length and thus will not contract (Fig. 24B1–4). The safe position of the interphalangeal joints is in extension, as a result of the regional anatomy at that level.

Finally, the unique relationship of the extensor apparatus to the tissues must be appreciated. Although the extensor can have a rudimentary insertion on the epiphysis of the proximal phalanx in some individuals, it is generally thought to have no bony attachment in the MCP region. Instead, the sagittal bands connect the extensor to the volar plate, which in turn inserts on the volar margin of P1.

Dislocations of the Metacarpophalangeal Joint

Pathologic forces can cause supraphysiologic displacement at the MCP level in one of three directions. First,

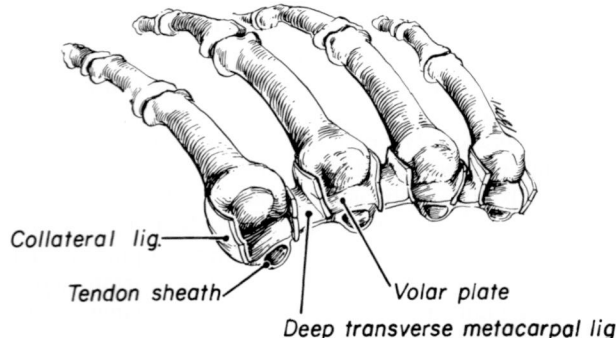

Collateral lig.
Tendon sheath
Volar plate
Deep transverse metacarpal lig.

Figure 24B1–2. Eaton has described the snug, boxlike configuration formed by the collateral ligaments and the volar plates of the metacarpophalangeal joints. Note also the deep transverse metacarpal ligaments, which Eaton has called the *intervolar plate* ligaments. (From Eaton RG: Joint Injuries of the Hand. Springfield, Charles C Thomas, 1971.)

medial or lateral (radial or ulnar) forces can cause collateral ligament attenuation or rupture. Subluxation or dislocation of the MCP joint is relatively uncommon. This is especially true because the central digits are supported or captured by the border digits and thus usually prevented from extreme coronal plane deviation.

Lateral or Coronal Plane Injury. Full-blown lateral or coronal plane injury is rare, but strains of the ligaments and small avulsion or impaction fractures are often seen (Fig. 24B1–5). The fractures can be seen on both sides of the joint, usually in the collateral recess on the metacarpal side and at the dorsolateral margin of the proximal phalanx. Often, the diagnosis of lateral dislocation or subluxation is inferred when an athlete describes the mechanism and manifests the findings of pain and tumescence in the collateral area, accompanied by laxity to specific directional stress.

Spontaneous reduction with reasonable stability is the rule for treatment. Therefore, simple splinting and gradual liberation to play with appropriate buddy taping is the typical course. Rarely, a fracture fragment is large enough or contains enough of the articular surface to warrant either fixation or excision (Fig. 24B1–6). Decisions regarding fracture fixation are based on fragment size, displacement, and residual instability. A symptomatic nonunion can be a late presentation of the problem, although stability of the MCP joint may not be affected. The ectopic calcification or the cortical irregularities often seen in radiographs of a chronic MCP collateral ligament injury can sometimes be confused with those findings seen with an old fracture that has not united (Fig. 24B1–7).

Dorsal Metacarpophalangeal Dislocations. Much has been written and presented about *simple* and *complex* dislocations about the MCP joint, with the most succinct likely being Kaplan's classic contribution.[71] The clinical appear-

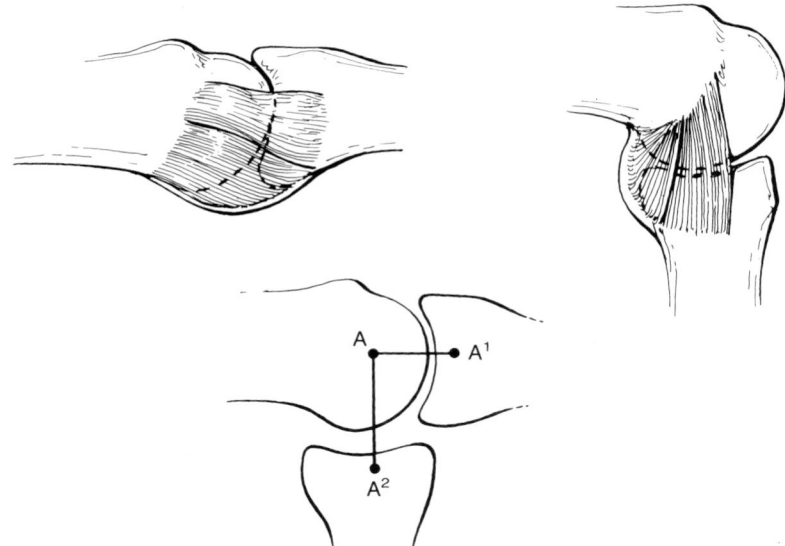

Figure 24B1–4. The shape of the metacarpal head is eccentric, resulting in a cam effect, which makes the collateral ligaments more taut in flexion than in extension. The cam effect is not present in the proximal interphalangeal joint.

ance and the radiographic presentation cannot be considered reliable determinants of pathoanatomy and ultimate treatment course. Many dislocations, however, even complex ones, can be relocated with proper technique. Thus, it is helpful to interpret the term *complex* as "not reducible by appropriate attempt." This distinction can help avoid a

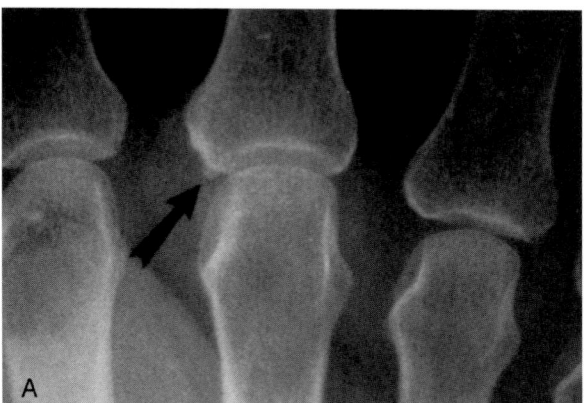

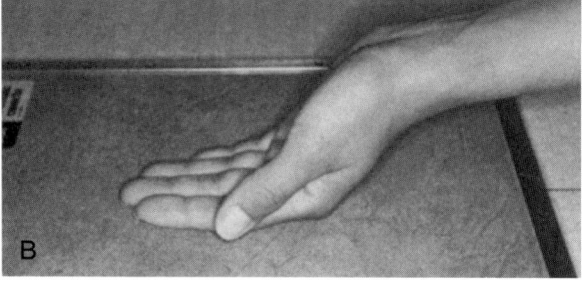

Figure 24B1–5. *A,* Metacarpophalangeal joint collateral ligament injury is occasionally (but not usually) associated with a small avulsion fracture *(arrow). B,* The Brewerton view may be helpful in delineating obscure avulsion fractures of the metacarpophalangeal joint collateral ligaments. The x-ray beam is centered over the metacarpophalangeal joints and is directed 30 degrees from the ulnar side.

trip to the operating room for those dislocations that can be reduced by closed means.

The term *simple* dislocation has historically referred to an MCP joint that is extended about 70 to 90 degrees, although the proximal phalanx is in articular contact with the metacarpal head. It is possible to convert a reducible injury to a potentially unreducible (by closed means) dislocation. Though this result rarely occurs, prolonged or repeated reduction attempts, especially those in which axial traction is the primary component, should be avoided. Typically, longitudinal traction alone will effect a reduction that is both palpable and audible.[98] It is usually immediately satisfying and stable (except in the extremes of hyperextension).

It is sometimes said that the complex dislocation, either in the triphalangeal digits or in the thumb, exhibits "parallelism." This is not always true and can be misleading. What is being described is the relatively axial, yet dorsally translated, arrangement between the metacarpal and the proximal phalanx. In contrast to the simple dislocation, the extreme extension posture at the joint is replaced by a digit that "looks a little funny." The dorsal contour is one clue that can be interpreted along with the historical data. Another clue is a pitting or puckering of the overlying volar skin (Fig. 24B1–8). When sesamoids are present (almost universal in the index finger but exceedingly rare in some rays), their position in the joint can be a sign that reduction may be difficult (Figs. 24B1–9 and 24B1–10).

The blocks to reduction may include several structures, although the dominant issue is the volar plate (Fig. 24B1–11). The volar plate usually remains attached to the base of the proximal phalanx and the flaps dorsal to the metacarpal head. The head is further incarcerated by the flexor digitorum profundus tendon and the lumbrical that takes origin from it. The palmar aponeurosis can add a "collar" around the articular margin. Thus, extensive traction may worsen this situation.

An attempt at closed reduction should be made in all MCP dislocations. This is especially true when the surgeon

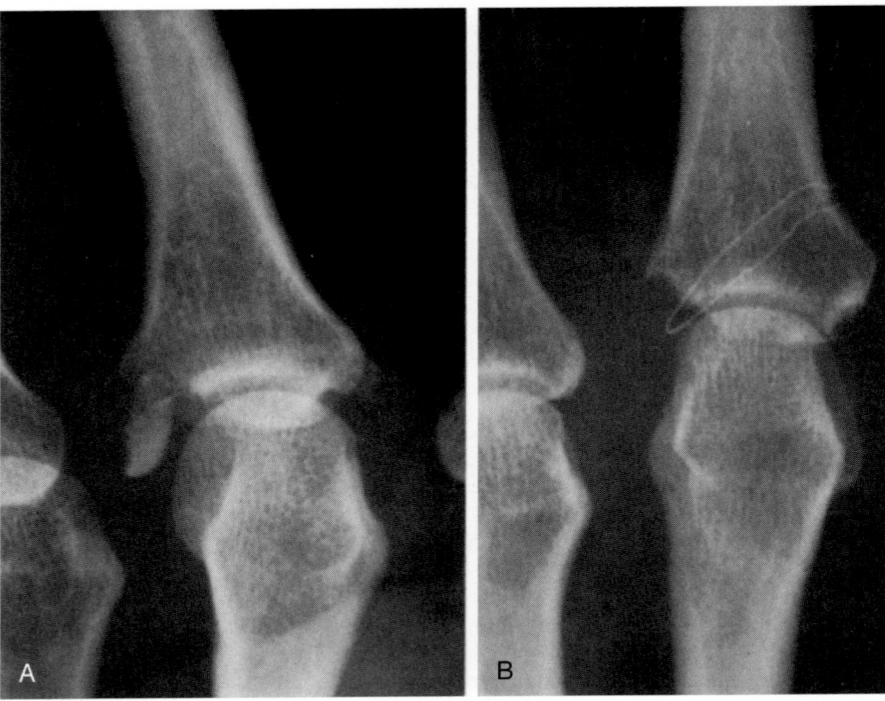

Figure 24B1–6. *A,* An intra-articular corner fracture of the base of the proximal phalanx is a variant of metacarpophalangeal joint collateral ligament injury. *B,* This patient was treated with excision of the fragment and reinsertion of the ligament.

is the initial caregiver and little other manipulation has preceded the patient's presentation to the surgeon. The method of reduction is modified from the recommendations of McLaughlin and Malerich and colleagues[92, 98]:

1. Adequate anesthesia is a must. The choice may depend on venue (emergency room vs. operating room), or it may be dictated by the surgeon's best guess whether the closed reduction will be successful. Regardless, in addition to use of general or regional anesthesia, insufflating the joint area is a must. Capsular tissue was likely torn in the injury, yet the reason for injecting anesthetic agent into the area is twofold. First, it makes the patient more comfort-

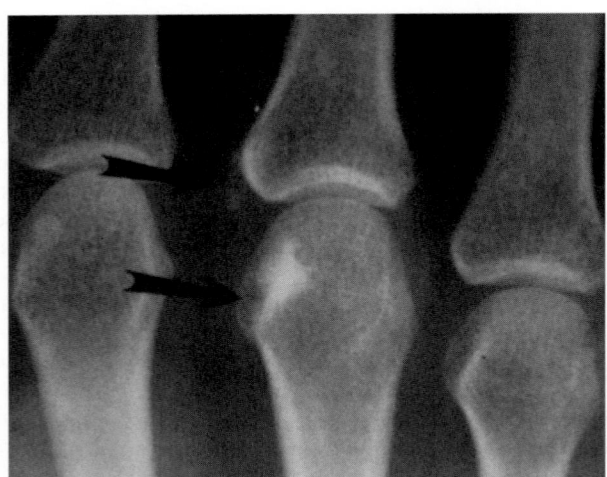

Figure 24B1–7. Patients with chronic metacarpophalangeal collateral ligament injuries may show some cortical irregularity or ectopic calcification on radiography. These injuries cause discomfort for a long period of time and are difficult to treat.

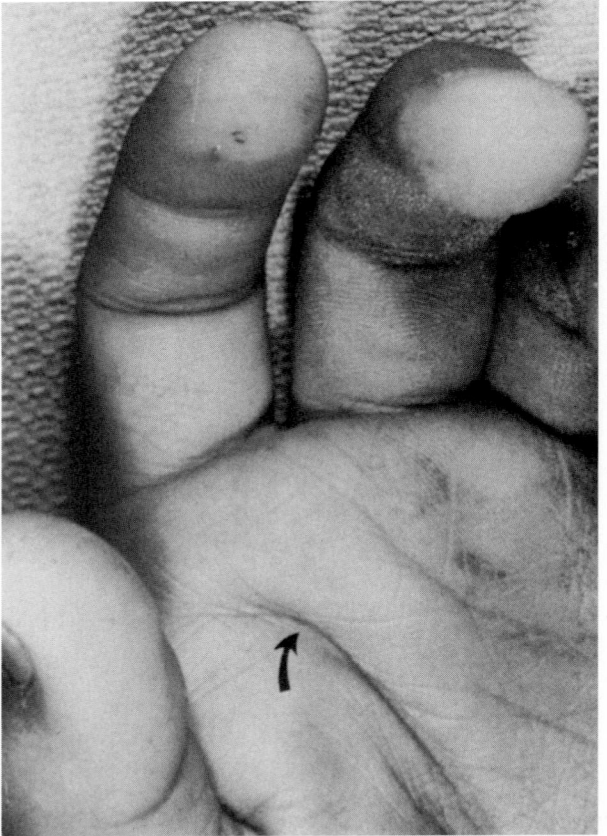

Figure 24B1–8. A consistent finding in patients with complex dislocation of the index metacarpophalangeal joint is puckering of the palmar skin, which may be difficult to see because it lies directly in the distal palmar crease *(arrow).*

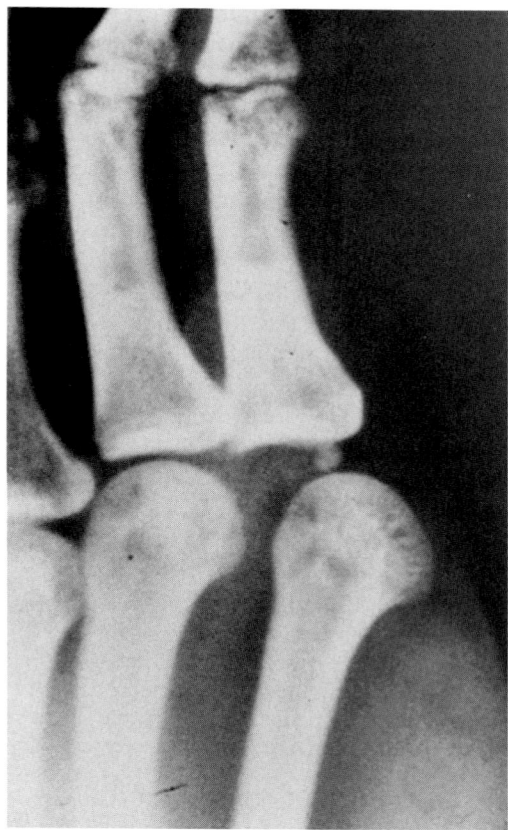

Figure 24B1–9. A pathognomonic radiographic sign of complex metacarpophalangeal dislocation is the presence of a sesamoid in the widened joint space, indicative of interposition of the entrapped volar plate.

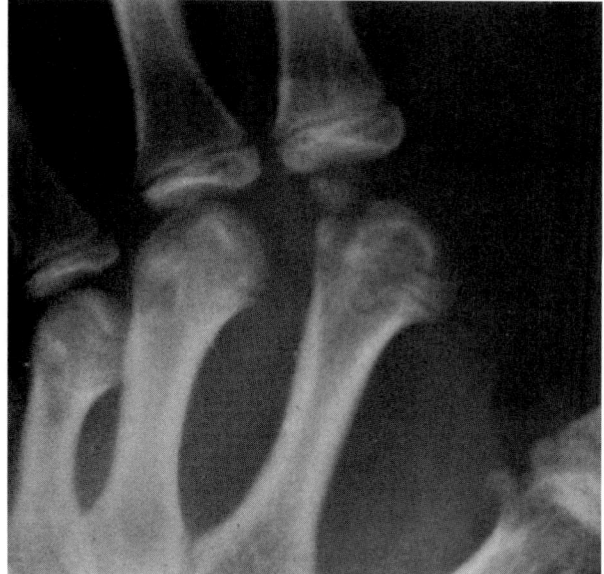

Figure 24B1–10. A concomitant injury sometimes seen with a complex metacarpophalangeal dislocation is a chip fracture of the metacarpal head. This should not be confused with an entrapped sesamoid, as shown in Figure 24B1–9.

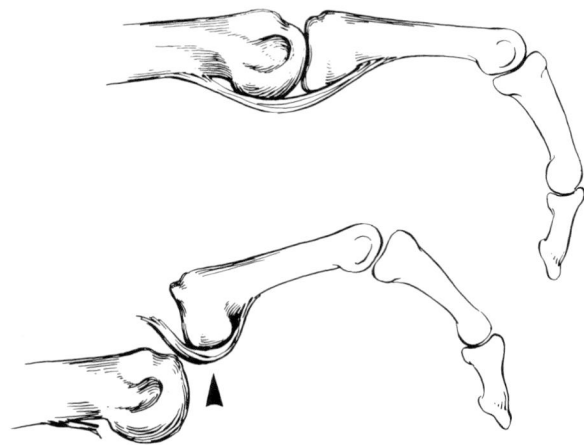

Figure 24B1–11. The single most important element preventing reduction of a complex metacarpophalangeal dislocation is interposition of the volar plate between the base of the middle phalanx and the metacarpal head.

able. Second, it can have the effect of "floating" the volar plate into a more reducible position.

2. Prepositioning for the reduction maneuver is important. Relaxing the flexor system removes or diminishes the cicatrix about the neck of the metacarpal. Therefore, wrist and digital flexion is advocated.

3. The actual reduction maneuver is logical. Hyperextension at the MCP joint is coupled with a move that tries to effect extrication of the volar plate from the joint. This is accomplished primarily by allowing the *dorsal* margin of the proximal phalanx to contact the dorsal margin of the metacarpal head. The phalanx may be slightly translated proximally or distally to "capture" the volar plate. The phalanx is then pushed across the metacarpal articular surface, with care to maintain the dorsal rim contact as long as possible to cause the volar plate to "pop" out of the joint and back into position.

4. Gentle active and passive motion, under the influence of anesthesia, is the sign of success. Radiographs or fluoroscopic images, however, must be obtained to check reduction and to rule out any other impediments to reduction, such as small fracture fragments.

5. Brief splinting (less than 1 week) in the functional or safe position can be followed by a buddy taping regimen to prevent hyperextension, yet promote motion. Depending on the sport, play can be resumed if the likelihood of deformity re-creation is low, or if the hand can be adequately protected from hyperextension forces at the MCP level. Recurrent dislocations are rare at this level, and motion recovery is usually near complete.

If closed reduction is unsuccessful, open reduction can immediately follow if the surgeon has prepared the patient and the venue. There has long been debate concerning the best approach for open reduction. Advocates of volar[70, 98] and dorsal[8, 55, 146] routes both give excellent reasons for their philosophy. Many would argue that the pathologic process is primarily volar, yet the potential complications are also volar. The digital nerve is typically draped over the articular surface of the metacarpal head and is only cell layers below the subdermis upon approach.

Success and safety have dictated that the popular approach to dorsal MCP dislocation is dorsal. The volar plate can usually be pushed out of the joint, permitting reduction. In a minority of cases, the volar plate needs to be split longitudinally to facilitate its extrication. Need for a combined approach should not be thought of as a failure if it is done to increase the margin of safety and to accomplish the surgical goals of reduction. The patient should be prepared for and consent to such an eventuality.

Volar Metacarpophalangeal Dislocations. Volar MCP dislocation is extremely rare, and the mechanics and the anatomy of these injuries are poorly understood.[12, 128, 156, 158] Because these injuries are sometimes seen in conjunction with other forms of major hand trauma, global embarrassment may be necessary for most of these complicated injuries to occur. The tissue that almost always causes difficulty in attaining closed reduction is likely a combination of the collateral ligament, the volar plate, the MCP capsule, and possibly the extensor mechanism.

To reduce a volar MCP dislocation, the steps in reduction of a dorsal dislocation can simply be reversed, with the exception of slight flexion of the wrist and the digits. Open treatment, however, will likely be needed. The need to approach this injury from the volar side is almost a certainty, but the surgeon must be prepared to make a dorsal approach if necessary.

After reduction and brief splinting, motion is encouraged. The rehabilitation phase of treatment may include extensor lag and difficulty in regaining full flexion, but long-term sequelae from the isolated injury are minimal.

Authors' Preferred Method of Treatment. We suggest that almost every player sustaining an MCP dislocation deserves an attempt at closed reduction. After periarticular fracture has been ruled out, reduction can be effected by insufflating the joint with anesthetic and careful manipulation, not only to maneuver the joint into a reduced position but also to attempt to clear any interposed tissue.

If operative intervention is warranted, the dorsal approach provides both adequate access to carry out reduction and the margin of safety required. We have never encountered a case in which reduction could not be accomplished through a dorsal approach with manipulation of an interposed volar plate from the posterior aspect of the joint.

Usually, the reduction is sufficiently stable, and it is feasible to protect the injured joint with splinting or taping. Early return to play, even after open reduction, is reasonable in most sports.

Proximal Interphalangeal Joint Dislocation

The proximal interphalangeal (PIP) joint dislocation, one of the classic injuries in sport, is often called *coach's finger* because it occurs so frequently in almost all athletic pursuits that a coach tends to attempt reduction on the sidelines. The other term for this injury is *jammed finger*, which is a reminder of the spectrum of potential injury, from minor sprain to severe fracture-dislocation, that may present with similar historical and examination findings. This common injury warrants detailed consideration to underscore the logical steps from acute injury and initial "on field" treatment to return to play.

Pathomechanics and Evaluation

The PIP joint is a ginglyotrochlear joint that derives its stability from both the bony architecture and the supporting soft tissues. The articular "fit" is primarily responsible for resistance to rotational forces, direct mediolateral translation, and some element of lateral deviation (see Fig. 24B1–1). The collateral ligaments (accessory and proper), along with the volar plate, provide the most resistance to pathologic forces in lateral deviation (see Fig. 24B1–3). Secondary restraints include the flexor tendon sheath, parts of the extensor apparatus coalescing about the PIP, and the joint capsule.[86, 101] Essentially, this "box" provides multidirectional stability, while permitting well over 120 degrees of motion in most people.

To assess the potential anatomic correlates of injury, careful palpation and provocative testing with directed translational and angulatory stress are recommended. The first clinically relevant observation is whether a periarticular injury at the PIP joint is open or closed. A skin defect in the volar aspect of the PIP flexion crease is likely related to an "inside-out" injury, in which the dermal elements literally tear as the middle phalanx is at its maximum displacement in hyperextension. Many of these open dislocations follow a very similar clinical course to that of closed dislocations, provided that no neurovascular injury or contamination accompanied the injury and that a surgeon has not attempted extensive soft tissue repair about the joint.

The position of the dislocated digital elements may be observed only by the player or the first responder. Because many of these injuries are reduced in the first few seconds after being sustained, the only historical information about the appearance of the digit may come from the patient or a trainer or coach. Swelling is usually global, but tenderness can usually be localized to the volar, lateral, or dorsal areas.

Pathoanatomy and Treatment

PIP dislocations or fracture-dislocations separate into two main types: dorsal and volar. A pure lateral dislocation has been inferred, but injury to the lateral stabilizers is usually an element of one of the major types.[73]

Dorsal Proximal Interphalangeal Dislocations and Fracture-Dislocations

The dorsal PIP dislocation is the most common PIP dislocation and fracture-dislocation. Axial load and hyperextension conspire to force the middle phalanx dorsally and proximally (Figs. 24B1–12 and 24B1–13). Depending

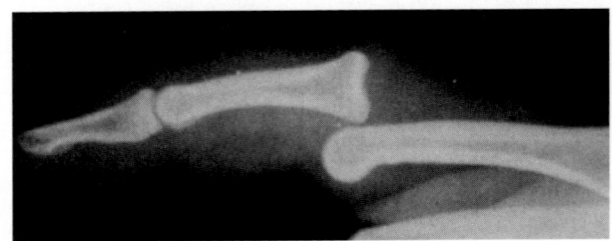

Figure 24B1–12. Dorsal dislocation is by far the most common type of dislocation of the proximal interphalangeal joint.

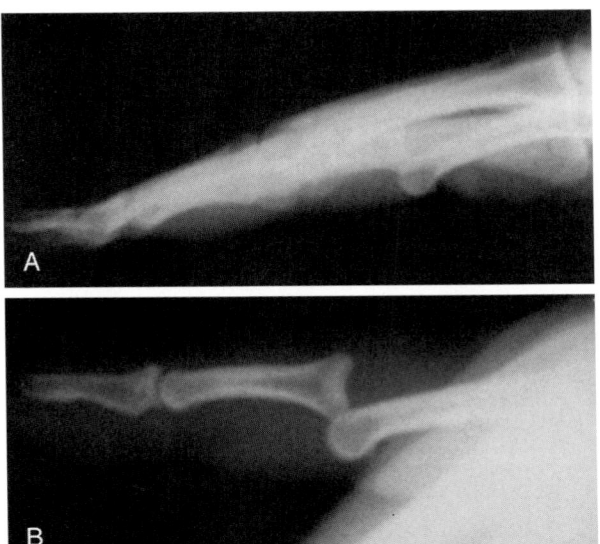

Figure 24B1–13. A lateral radiograph of the entire hand is unacceptable for evaluating injuries of the fingers; a true lateral radiograph of the *individual* digit is mandatory. *A,* In this lateral view of the entire hand, superimposition of the other fingers obscures dislocation of the proximal interphalangeal joint, which is clearly seen in the true lateral view of the involved finger (*B*).

on the magnitude and the direction of forces and on the relationship at the PIP joint throughout its arc, there can be pure soft tissue or combined soft tissue and bone injuries. Often, the herald of this injury after its reduction is a small avulsion fragment "donated" by the volar lip of the middle phalanx and left attached to the volar plate (Fig. 24B1–14). In other patients, the constellation of injury leaves little doubt of the mechanism, because the joint relationship may be unstable and a significant portion of the middle phalanx base may have been fractured.

Classification schemes are often based on the percentage of middle phalanx base fracture. A volar fracture percentage of less than 40% is a stable fracture, whereas unstable fractures are associated with 50% articular involvement. The main concern is whether there is enough bony and soft tissue support to maintain concentric reduction through the normal range of motion. Thus, it is more important to

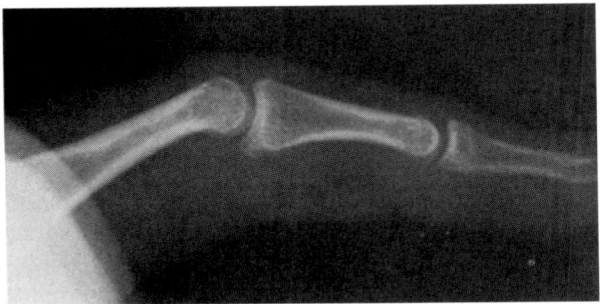

Figure 24B1–14. Small chip fractures avulsed off the base of the middle phalanx by the volar plate are not uncommon after dorsal proximal interphalangeal joint dislocations. These do not affect the routine management of the dislocation and should not be confused with the far more serious fracture-dislocation of the joint, shown in Figure 24B1–15.

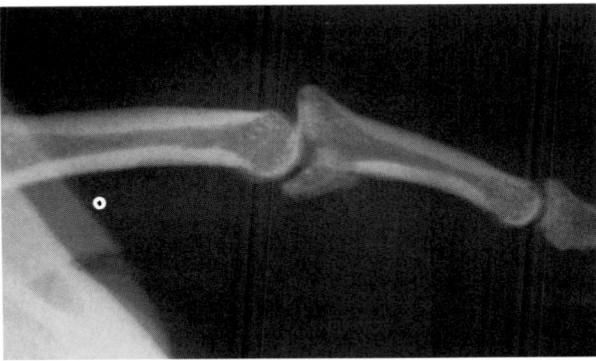

Figure 24B1–15. Fracture-dislocation (more correctly called fracture-subluxation) of the proximal interphalangeal joint. The volar base of the middle phalanx is crushed, usually comminuted, and generally involves 30% or more of the articular surface. The remaining base of the middle phalanx is subluxated dorsally.

be able to recognize the problem fracture-dislocations and to develop treatment plans than it is to measure the amount of the middle phalanx base involved. Furthermore, the morphologic configuration of the fracture and the percentage of articular involvement have an equal role in determining stability (Fig. 24B1–15).

The steps that should be employed to assess whether a PIP dislocation or fracture-dislocation is *stable* or *unstable* should include reduction and arc of motion testing under metacarpal or wrist block anesthesia, provocative stress in lateral and anteroposterior planes, and lateral imaging at various points throughout the arc of motion (Fig. 24B1–16). The examiner's experience will foretell whether a reduced joint will remain that way as it approaches neutral; at times, crepitus of blocked motion implies a fracture even before the injury is imaged. After confident reduction has been attained, while the patient's digit is still anesthetized, it is important to test the range of motion through which

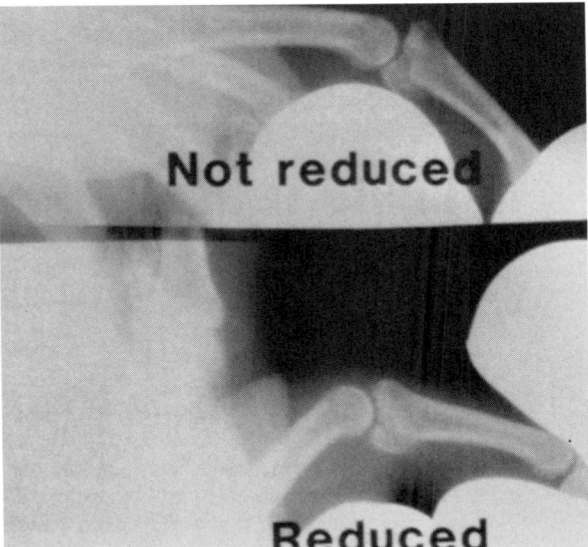

Figure 24B1–16. These two radiographs show the difference between acceptable (*bottom*) and unacceptable (*top*) reductions of a fracture-dislocation of the proximal interphalangeal joint.

the PIP remains stable and to observe the quality of the end points.

It is a great advantage to perform this reduction assessment under fluoroscopic guidance. The behavior of fracture fragments and the joint itself can be appreciated and documented. The injury requires operative intervention if the middle phalanx base splays because of significant impaction injury, if the pilon fracture-dislocation is observed, or if the leading edge of the fracture hinges instead of coapts with the proximal phalanx condyles. Sometimes, the differences are going to be subtle, such as a slight mismatch at the joint expressed as a "V" sign at the dorsal articulation (Fig. 24B1–17).[83]

The majority of these injuries will resume a concentric reduction and will be stable in all but the extremes of

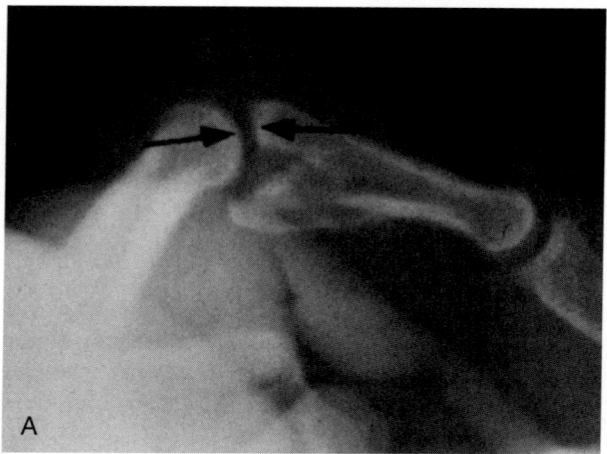

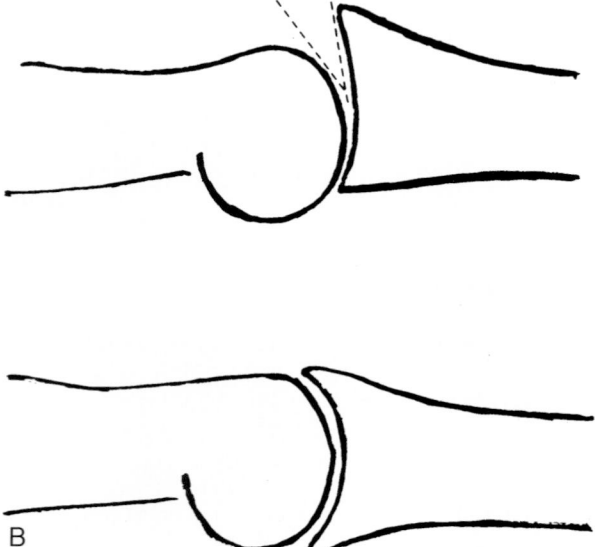

Figure 24B1–17. *A,* The adequacy of reduction of a fracture-dislocation is judged by the congruency between the intact articular portion of the base of the middle phalanx and the head of the proximal phalanx. The volar fragments can be disregarded in a closed reduction if the dorsal aspect of the joint is congruent. Note the impacted articular cartilage centrally *(arrows)*. *B,* Light's V sign *(dotted lines)* is a clear indication that the joint has not been satisfactorily reduced. (*B,* From Light TR: Buttress pinning techniques. Orthop Rev 10:49–55, 1981.)

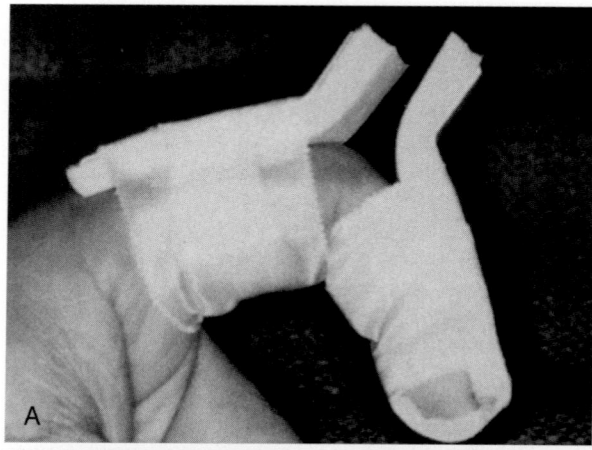

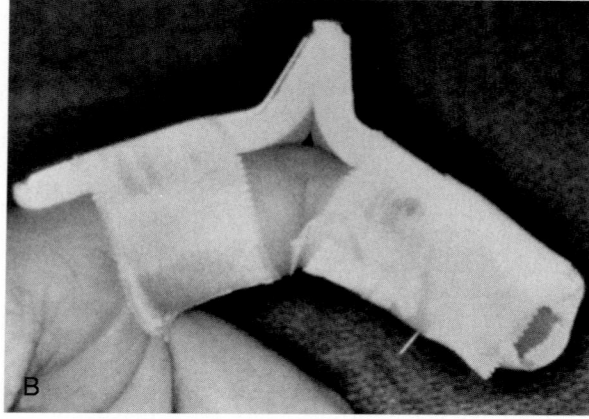

Figure 24B1–18. *A* and *B,* Strong's simpler type of extension block splinting is a bit less secure but is probably a reasonable treatment method in reliable patients. An athlete should certainly not return to competition wearing this type of splint, however.

hyperextension. The fractures will be small avulsion-type injuries from the volar lip of the middle phalanx, and they will be inconsequential in the sense of not involving a significant percentage of the articular surface.

The hallmark of closed treatment of these injuries is dorsal extension block splinting. An essential part of the technique is securing the proximal phalanx to the splint; if it is not secured, the PIP joint extends when the patient flexes the metaphalangeal joint. As the soft tissues or the fracture heals, the PIP joint is gradually allowed to be brought into more extension. Simpler, although less secure, constructs have been designed that achieve the same goal (Fig. 24B1–18). For the select athlete seeking immediate return to play, however, methods such as Strong extension block splinting are not as stable as exchange casting or static dorsal extension splinting (Fig. 24B1–19).

Certain patterns or magnitudes of injury deserve special attention when discussing volar PIP fracture-dislocations: the fracture that represents a large percentage of the articular surface, the pilon-type impaction fracture, and the chronic or unrecognized injury. The discussion of this group of disorders also highlights some of the surgical treatment alternatives available.

Large-Fragment Articular Fractures. There is continuing debate regarding the percentage of volar margin frac-

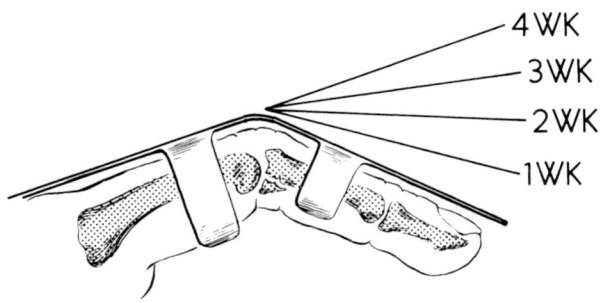

Figure 24B1–19. The dorsal extension splint is gradually straightened at weekly intervals. Its use may be discontinued at 4 weeks.

tures that requires internal fixation. The factors that affect clinical decision-making include the size or percentage of fracture, the reduction that is attainable, and the comminution and additional injuries. Most surgeons would agree that a majority of the 30% margin fractures are stable and that a majority of the 50% fractures are not, yet individual cases vary. If the fragment is large enough that its displacement results in significant incongruity and instability, and if it is large enough to accommodate pins or a minifragment screw, consideration should be given to stabilizing it with such an implant.[46] Our experience is that the fragments can be reduced indirectly through flexion or can be reached through a midaxial incision by reaching around the volar lip with a dental pick. Volar approaches can be contemplated, but the need to dissect within the fibro-osseous theca dissuades many surgeons from this approach. A sound technical algorithm is to reduce the fragment with direct manipulation from a midaxial approach, stabilize it provisionally with a smooth wire, then fix it with a mini–compression screw inserted through the dorsum at the "bare area" of the triangular ligament distal to the central slip insertion. Some authors have suggested dorsal block pinning, in which a smooth wire is driven obliquely into the articular surface of the proximal phalanx to prevent extension of the PIP joint as a means of keeping the joint reduced and keeping larger fragments in an acceptable position while allowing a short arc of motion.[149] Dorsal block pinning has potential problems (e.g., those of intra-articular pin placement) and thus has little or no role in the athlete.

Pilon Fractures. An axial loading injury with intra-articular comminution and displacement, the pilon fracture of the middle phalanx is a complex injury. The fragments are small, and often there is a central, cartilage-bearing fragment that is forced distally into the intermedullary space of the middle phalanx. Interfragmentary fixation, as described earlier, often has little role owing to the small fracture fragment size and the comminution. These fractures may require distraction and ligamentotaxis with or without fragment manipulation. In an effort to avoid extensive surgery at the PIP joint, a small dorsal approach can be employed over the dorsum of the middle phalanx, through which access to the intramedullary canal can be gained through a drill hole distal to the central slip insertion. Proximal "impaction" and fragment manipulation can be done through that portal; a bone graft from the distal radial metaphysis could also be added.

The alternatives for dynamic distraction range from "homemade" fixators to ones that are commercially available. The principles of ligamentotaxis—axial alignment and joint maintenance while permitting motion—are well established.[1, 58, 134] This minimally invasive technique often renders equivalent or better motion gains when compared with lengthy and traumatizing primary PIP surgery. Other options such as volar plate arthroplasty could be entertained if the volar lip of the middle phalanx is too comminuted to support a congruent reduction.

Chronic or Neglected PIP Injuries. A difficult problem becomes worse when the bone becomes friable and the soft tissues contract with the passing of sufficient time before resolution (Fig. 24B1–20). Unfortunately, this is not an uncommon scenario in the athlete, who may conceal a "small injury," such as that of a finger, in favor of more playing time. The chronic fracture-dislocation is an intellectual and technical challenge. The first consideration should be whether sufficient bone and cartilage are available for an attempt at joint salvage.[29, 159] Simple distraction has been used but usually has to be combined with open manipulation.[40, 123] The ultimate salvage technique is volar plate arthroplasty.[33]

Volar Proximal Interphalangeal Fracture-Dislocations

The volar dislocation is rare.[100, 110] The injury is usually sustained when an extended digit is forcibly flexed at the PIP joint.[139] Treatment of this injury is not a simple reversal of the procedures employed for dorsal PIP fracture-dislocations. Although in both disorders the collateral ligament complexes can be injured, the additional soft tissue injuries are often the determinants of outcome. The healing of the volar plate injuries sustained in a dorsal fracture-dislocation is not usually the determinant of ultimate outcome. The extent of disruption and the healing character of the extensor mechanism are key arbiters of the outcome for volar fracture-dislocation (Fig. 24B1–21).[150]

The lateral band can become completely separated from the central tendon as the head of the proximal phalanx herniates through the interval; the lateral band can then become interposed and can block reduction. This can sometimes present as a "closed boutonnière" clinical pattern, discussed in a later section of this chapter. Another pattern of injury that often leads to inferior outcome, a small fracture of the dorsal lip of the middle phalanx, can be associated with disruption of the central slip insertion.

The determining factors of treatment are the ability to achieve and maintain closed reduction, the character of the fracture, and the extent of extensor mechanism disruption. Stable closed reduction should be maintained in a position of PIP extension for approximately 4 weeks. Joint pinning can add predictability to the equation when there is difficulty maintaining the extended posture in a splint or in achieving patient compliance.

As always, large fragment fractures should be treated by open or closed reduction and stabilization.[7] Even when fractures are small but well reduced in extension, transverse pinning of the PIP joint can be entertained. Formal open reduction is a must when the lateral band is blocking

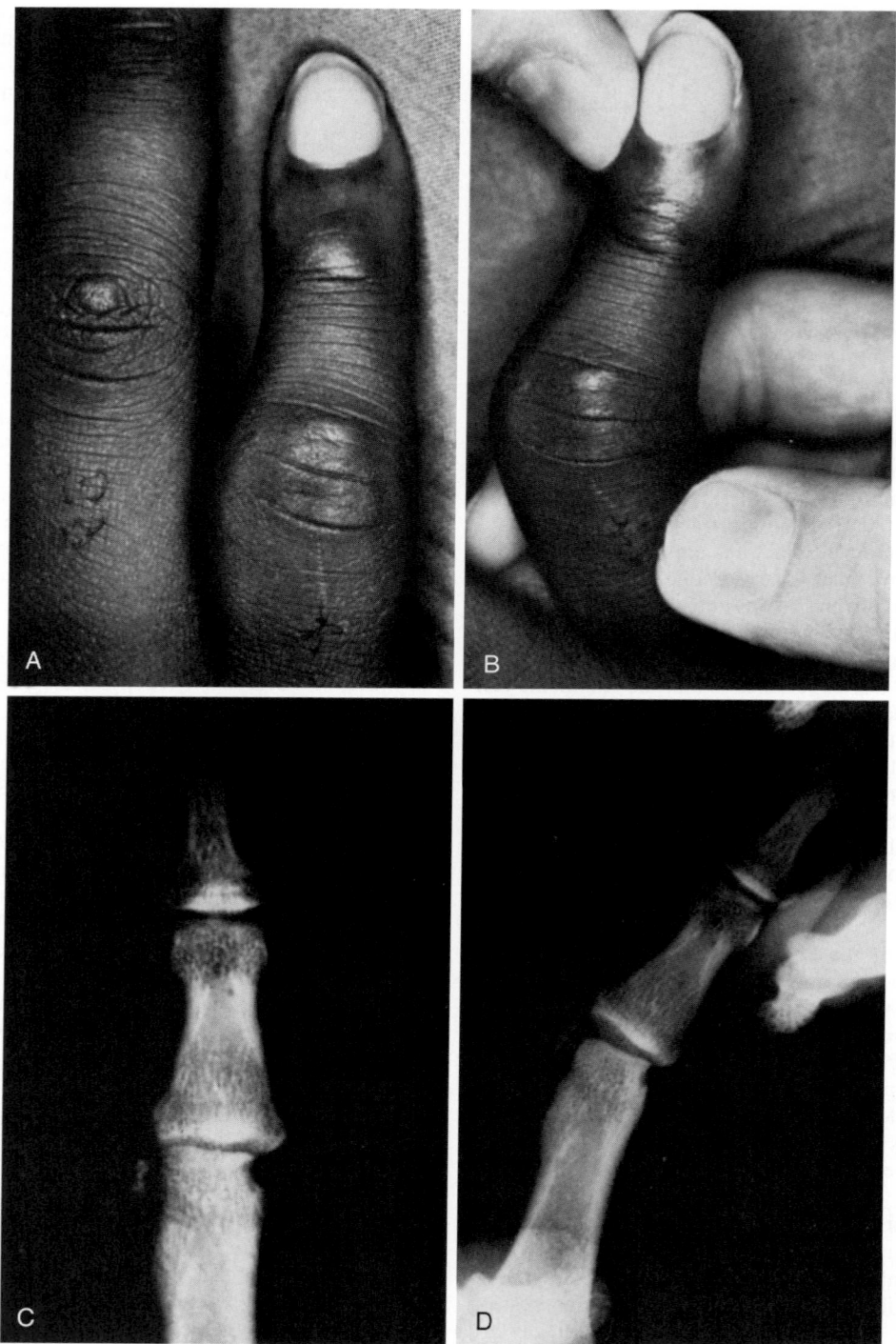

Figure 24B1–20. *A,* The appearance of the little finger of a college basketball player with a 3-year history of chronic problems in the proximal interphalangeal joint. *B,* Instability of the radial collateral ligament was easily demonstrated clinically. *C,* Radiographs showed a small avulsed bony fragment originating from the neck of the proximal phalanx. *D,* Stress radiographs demonstrated distal movement of the avulsed fragment. Late reconstruction of the ligament was done by reinserting the avulsed fragment, and the patient is now a highly paid professional basketball player.

reduction. Primary repair of the rent between the lateral band and the central tendon is advocated. Pinning after open repair is also suggested.

Dynamic distraction can be a helpful adjunct to any primary treatment yet does not substitute for sound primary management. The fixator can neutralize forces across an unstable joint or one in which fixation is tenuous. Some fixators can also assist in alignment and maintenance of joint reduction. Early motion in the volar dislocation may not be as desirable because the injured extensor must be allowed to heal. Fortunately, owing to the greater power of the flexor system, extension contractures are rare.

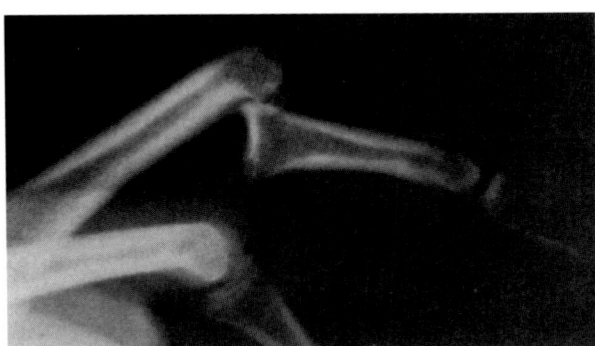

Figure 24B1–21. Volar dislocation of the proximal interphalangeal joint is a relatively uncommon injury. It should be obvious from this radiograph that the central slip must be torn for this injury to occur; therefore, these patients should be treated in the same manner as those with a boutonnière injury.

Authors' Preferred Method of Treatment. For the common dorsal dislocation, the steps of treatment and return to play are relatively simple: rule out fracture, reduce under local block anesthesia, determine the stable range of motion, and splint appropriately. Most PIP dislocations will remain stable in positions from neutral to full flexion, so early motion can be aggressive as long as splinting or taping prevents the extreme of extension. Early return to play is the rule, but adequate protection from re-creation of the injury must be respected.

The rare volar dislocation is a management challenge for those caring for the athlete. Predictably good results can be achieved with full-extension splinting after reduction for a period of 4 to 5 weeks. In the athlete or the sportsman sustaining the injury out of season, this is still the advocated treatment. The elite athlete who is still participating in his or her sport presents a decision-making dilemma. We have tended to advocate open repair, with early motion and a modified splinting/taping regimen for this rare instance. We have encountered this situation in athletes and surgical colleagues whose professions would make them ill suited for lengthy extension splinting. The risk/benefit ratio may point favorably to surgical intervention only in these select individuals.

Distal Interphalangeal Dislocations

A dislocation of the distal interphalangeal (DIP) joint is often seen in ball-handling and contact sports. The deformity in axial alignment is usually obvious externally. Inability to flex actively or to extend the dislocated digit is common. Although the DIP dislocation is almost universally a dorsal dislocation, the status of both the extensor and the flexor systems must be checked thoroughly. Radiographs are imperative to determine the presence or the extent of a fracture, which may be the injury that dictates the ultimate treatment.

The player or sideline personnel reduce most DIP dislocations. Immediate stability with reasonable motion is the rule, not the exception; yet many of these injuries go unrecognized, and late reduction is more difficult. Regardless of the time from initial injury, it is advisable to try to reduce the DIP. Even if a congruous DIP joint lacks some

motion, it is unacceptable to subject a player to accelerated arthrosis by accepting a subluxated or dislocated joint. The open reduction almost always requires the takedown of one or both collateral ligaments. Joint pinning is performed after reduction to stabilize the relationship for 4 weeks, while the PIP joint is left clear for movement. If articular cartilage destruction is noted at the time of attempted reduction and the athlete's career is ending, arthrodesis can be contemplated, but fusion is not well tolerated in the performing athlete. The longer lever arm that arthrodesis puts on the PIP joint may increase the chance of injury at that level. Myriad factors determine the ultimate reconstructive option for the compromised joint in the athletic population, including the athlete's position, longevity of career, and time of season.

Authors' Preferred Method of Treatment. The vast majority of these DIP dislocations will be stable immediately after reduction. Simply watch for open nail bed injuries, fractures, and the occasional flexor or extensor tendon injury. Dislocations in all but the long digit are well protected by buddy taping, so early return to play is reasonable. Low-profile splinting may be used in the more significant injuries or in DIP dislocations of the long finger.

Carpometacarpal Dislocations

The articulation of the rays of the index finger through the small finger at the carpometacarpal (CMC) joints differ; the radial pair are stabilized by stout ligaments, whereas those of the ring finger and the small rays are significantly more mobile. Regardless, a dislocation, or more typically a fracture-dislocation, of the CMC joint is a violent injury. In the athletic realm, stepping on the hand or crushing the hand between two helmets is a typical mechanism.

Isolated CMC dislocation of the fifth or of the fourth and fifth rays may happen as a result of a direct impact or torsional injury. The relatively compliant CMC ligaments can rupture, and the deforming forces, primarily the extensor carpi ulnaris inserting on the dorsoulnar fifth metacarpal base, displace the segment.

When injury is sustained to the lateral digits or the magnitude of injury is sufficiently great, all four metacarpals can dislocate. The translation of the dorsal metacarpal is often accompanied by impaction or avulsion fractures from the metacarpal bases or carpal rims. Larger fragments are usually obvious radiographically and may be amenable to primary fixation. The smaller fragments, however, are often the most troublesome because they block reduction or act as a third body in the partially reduced joint.

When the surgeon sees a "balloon hand" (Fig. 24B1–22), a significant swelling thought to be out of proportion to the time elapsed since injury, a CMC dislocation should be contemplated in the differential diagnosis. Crepitus and gross motion at the CMC joint are not uncommon. Though there may be grades of the injury, such as subtle subluxation, it has been our experience that when it is suspected, a CMC dislocation has usually occurred.

Radiographs can be definitive, yet the snapshot they provide may demonstrate only subtle change or small irregularities in the bony architecture at the CMC level. The lateral or the oblique films are most helpful in these cases. The ultimate diagnosis is made by direct examination,

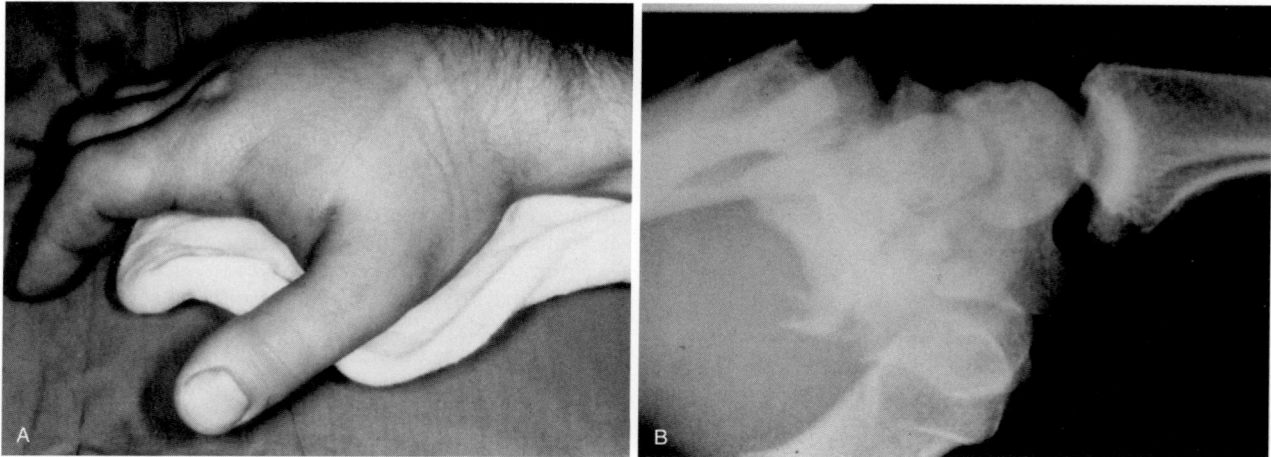

Figure 24B1–22. *A,* The energy needed to cause multiple carpometacarpal joint fracture-dislocations is represented by significant soft tissue swelling resulting in a "balloon hand." *B,* The corresponding lateral radiograph of the wrist is usually the most telling view.

contralateral comparison (especially in cases of isolated fifth ray dislocation), and fluoroscopic examination in selected cases.

Because fairly significant instability is present in many instances, the reduction is often easy to attain. Closed treatment, however, is not adequate because the reduction is not as easily maintained.

Open reduction, inspection of the CMC joint for congruity of reduction, and evacuation of any small fragments are best done through two separate dorsal incisions. Fortunately, these same two dorsal incisions serve as the portals for executing dorsal and volar fasciotomies, which are often needed.

Stabilization of the reduced CMC joints is by pinning, for which there are two general strategies. The first is to engage the metacarpal shafts through percutaneous pinning near the base and then to cross the CMC joint to have the pin rest in the carpus. These pins are directed from the radial and ulnar borders of the hand, securing the lateral and medial rays, respectively. The second pinning technique, collateral recess pinning, relies on intramedullary wires to stabilize the CMC reduction.[76] Pins are started in the collateral recesses or "shoulders" of the distal metacarpals and then travel down the intramedullary canal, cross the reduced CMC joint, and engage the respective carpal bones. This technique provides stable longitudinal fixation and minimizes trauma to the CMC area. These pins are well tolerated and even permit MCP and interphalangeal motion when carefully placed.

Authors' Preferred Method of Treatment. This is a serious hand injury that is often accompanied by concomitant injuries to the skin and the neurovascular structures and also raises the possibility of evolving compartment syndrome. The athlete with a hand injury must be treated by the same principles as any other injured patient. Open reduction through a dorsal approach, with interosseous compartment decompression as needed, is advocated. Inspection of the joint for small fragments of articular cartilage must be carried out. We have had success with intramedullary pinning of the CMC joint with implants (usually 0.045-inch wires) introduced distally through the metacar-

pal collateral recesses. Other pinning methods can be pursued, especially for the border digits.

Tendon Injuries

Injuries to the flexor or extensor systems of the fingers and the thumb can occur in any sport. Aside from open tendon injuries, which are unpredictable and obvious, there are four closed-tendon disorders that present to the sports team physician with sufficient frequency that they deserve special attention. These include the closed boutonnièrre deformity, the traumatic mallet finger, "boxer's knuckle," and flexor digitorum profundus (FDP) avulsion, or "jersey finger."

Closed Boutonnière

The anatomy of the extensor mechanism about the PIP joint is complex (Fig. 24B1–23). The central slip inserts on the epiphysis of the middle phalanx as the lateral bands traverse from volar to dorsal to the axis of rotation about the PIP level. Distal to the PIP joint, the respective lateral bands coalesce to form the terminal tendon and are joined by the spiral oblique retinacular ligaments of Landsmeer, which facilitate conjugate motion at the PIP and DIP joints.

Even in a closed injury, the central slip can be avulsed from the middle phalanx[65] or a rent can develop between the lateral bands and the remainder of the extensor apparatus, or both. When the injured lateral band migrates below the axis of rotation in the process of active PIP joint flexion, it becomes a flexion force at that level and an extensor of the DIP joint. This is the classic boutonnière posture. The sine qua non of the closed boutonnière is the inability to extend the flexed PIP joint actively, yet the ability to maintain the extended posture if the finger is placed there passively.

If detected early (i.e., within 3 to perhaps as long as 6 weeks), a trial of strict extension splinting is recommended (Fig. 24B1–24). The length of extension splinting must be

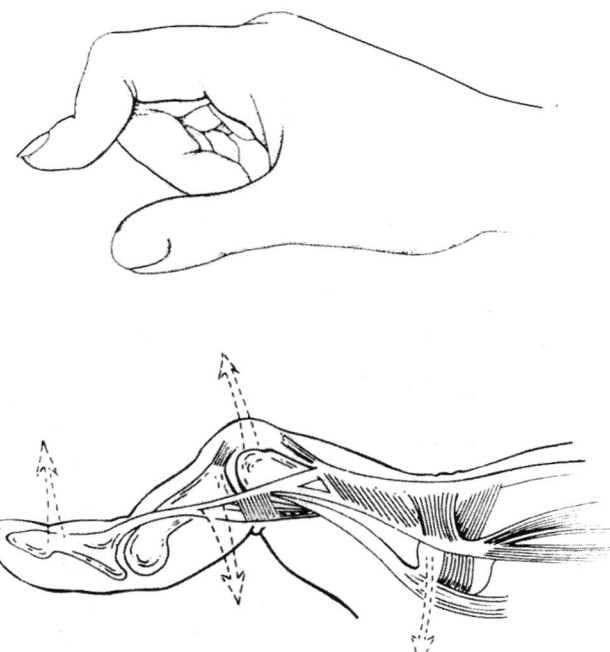

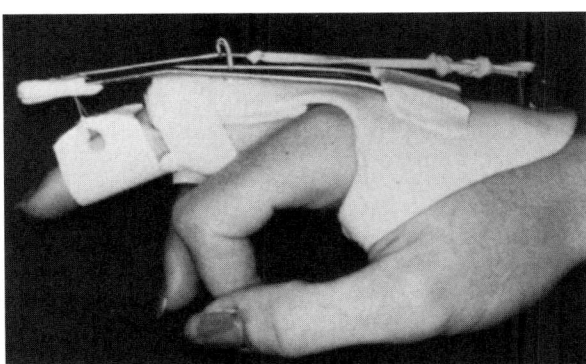

Figure 24B1–25. In longstanding boutonnière deformity, there is frequently a fixed flexion contracture of the proximal interphalangeal joint, which should be corrected with dynamic splinting before surgical repair is undertaken.

Figure 24B1–23. In an established boutonnière deformity, flexion deformity of the proximal interphalangeal joint is caused by loss of active extension through the central slip as well as by the deforming force of the lateral bands, which now pass volar to the axis of the proximal interphalangeal joint. Intrinsic muscle pull through the lateral bands leads to hyperextension of the distal interphalangeal joint.

5 to 6 weeks and must be uninterrupted. For these reasons, some surgeons recommend oblique transarticular pinning to remove the possibility of a single flexion episode negating weeks of healing in extension.

Unfortunately, neglect on the part of the athlete (more often than failure of recognition on the part of the physician) results in a chronic boutonnière deformity. If the deformity is passively correctable, extension splinting with active DIP flexion exercises can be initiated, but results

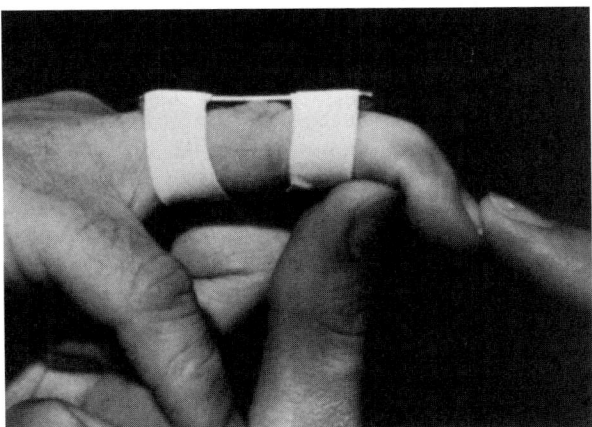

Figure 24B1–24. Appropriate treatment of a boutonnière deformity involves two elements: (1) continuous immobilization of the proximal interphalangeal joint in full extension for 6 weeks and (2) passive stretching of the distal interphalangeal joint into flexion.

vary. The duration of splinting exceeds that for an acute injury; about 6 to 8 weeks will be required. There is no absolute rule regarding the interval tolerated between injury and initiation of splinting; for this reason, it is recommended that all chronic boutonnière deformities undergo a trial of splinting (Fig. 24B1–25).[23]

If the deformity is not supple, aggressive rehabilitation is needed to restore a near-normal arc of motion. Rarely, formal releases will have to be performed at the PIP level to achieve a functional range of motion at that joint. Anatomic reconstruction of the injured extensor mechanism is the first choice if surgical intervention is contemplated for the primary boutonnière deformity. Even in this day of suture anchor use, central slip reinsertion is arduous and unpredictable. Lateral band mobilization and V-Y advancement have also been described.[74]

There are few in-season athletes who can tolerate strict extension splinting for the long periods needed to achieve good results with closed splinting. Thus, it is a challenging dilemma for the physician caring for an elite athlete whether to operate and protect an acute boutonnière deformity or to recommend the nonoperative approach. Many factors must be weighed to tailor the treatment to the individual needs of the patient.

Our bias is always to avoid operation if possible, but the predictability of open repair of an overt closed boutonnière deformity must be considered. Through a dorsal or slightly midaxial approach, the tear in the extensor mechanism can be repaired primarily after the lateral band is reduced back to its position dorsal to the axis of rotation. Pinning of the PIP joint in extension is an option for the potentially noncompliant patient or in special circumstances. The immobilization after operative repair should be approximately 4 weeks, with a graded flexion program to follow.

Authors' Preferred Method of Treatment. As stated, closed treatment is advocated. Only for an elite athlete, when considering the specifics of the situation (the ability to return to participation for playoffs, for example), is open treatment considered.

Pseudoboutonnière

The pseudoboutonnière is another PIP disorder that may be confused with the boutonnièrre deformity. This nomenclature is unfortunate because the pseudoboutonnière really represents a PIP hyperextension injury with likely volar plate disruption.[14] The key finding that differentiates injuries presenting with a flexion contracture at the PIP joint is the absence of compensatory DIP hyperextension in the pseudoboutonnière. Treatment is progressive stretching of the PIP joint; formal volar release is seldom done.

Central Slip Disruption

Like all digital extensors, the central slip inserts on the epiphysis, in this case the epiphysis of the middle phalanx. The central slip can be injured by some closed mechanisms, such as forceful flexion of the extended PIP joint, and potentially by any open injury.

It is challenging to diagnose an isolated central slip disruption if there are no fracture fragments or no PIP dislocation. Often, the ability to extend the finger actively, even without lag, is maintained. A combination of historical evidence and performance of some more advanced examination maneuvers may be the only way to identify the injury acutely. Direct, specific palpation over the dorsal base of the middle phalanx may be the best way to identify the injury. The following clinical tests have been suggested to increase the diagnostic accuracy of identification of a central slip disruption:

- Carducci[18] suggests that an active PIP extension lag of 15 degrees is indicative of central slip disruption when the digit is examined in a position of full flexion of the wrist and metaphalangeal joint. The wrist and metaphalangeal positions place the extensor mechanism at maximal stretch, so the subtle difference in active PIP extension of the injured digit is ascribed to the loss of influence of the central slip.
- In the test proposed by Elson,[36] the injured digit is flexed over a tabletop at the PIP joint, and the middle phalanx is stabilized by dorsal pressure of the examiner's fingers, essentially pinning it against the side of the table. The patient is then asked to extend the DIP joint actively. The ability to extend the DIP joint is thought to be indicative of a central slip disruption. The mechanism is a central slip untethering, which allows the entire extensor mechanism to migrate proximally enough to permit the DIP extension when activated.
- Lovett and McCalla[90] rely on a metacarpal or digital anesthetic block to remove the influence of any pain that may be limiting the full extension at the PIP joint. If simple active extension of the PIP joint after the block demonstrates a lag, or if resisted extension is weak (but not painful), then the central slip injury may be inferred.

If the central slip disruption is diagnosed early (within 3 to 4 weeks, or maybe as late as 6 weeks in some young athletes), immobilization is suggested. A digital splint should keep the PIP in extension but will free the DIP for unrestricted motion. Monitoring of the postimmobilization function and posture will help ensure that a boutonnière deformity is not developing.

The strategy changes when more significant trauma has caused an avulsion or impaction fracture of the articular base of the middle phalanx with separation of the dorsal tubercle (Fig. 24B1–26). While addressing the PIP fracture-

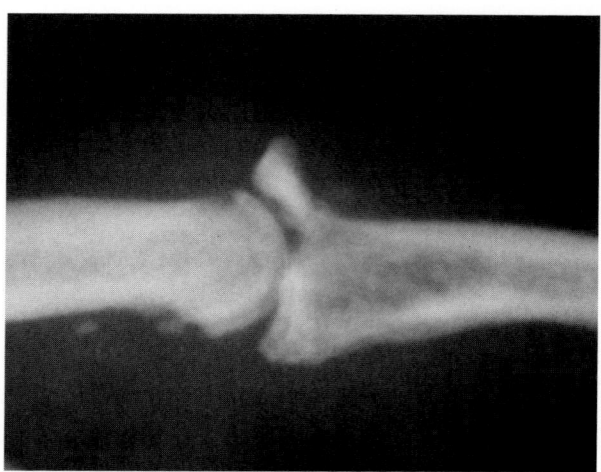

Figure 24B1–26. Occasionally, the central slip may cause a small fragment of bone to avulse off the base of middle phalanx. More commonly, however, the tendon is pulled cleanly off the bone, and the radiograph of a boutonnière lesion usually shows no abnormality.

dislocation, especially the less common volar variant, reconstruction of the central slip should be accomplished.

Authors' Preferred Method of Treatment. The diagnosis is the first key. When the injury is isolated to the soft tissues, splinting is still the preferred method of treatment. If the avulsion is accompanied by a significant bony fragment, or especially a fracture with appreciable intra-articular extension, then operative intervention may yield a more predictable and earlier return to play..

Mallet Finger

Disruption of the terminal extensor at its insertion on the distal phalanx is common in sports. The majority of mallet injuries result from a hyperflexion force on an extended DIP joint, but hyperextension or axial load mechanisms are not uncommon.

The constellation of injuries to the bones and the soft tissues about the DIP usually considered among the mallet family includes simple terminal tendon disruption and more complex fracture-subluxations of the joint (Fig. 24B1–27). Warren and colleagues[151] have described a zone of relative hypovascularity that may be implicated in the development of or susceptibility to a mallet injury.[151]

The basic element in the diagnosis is the inability to extend the DIP joint actively. This is the sine qua non of the mallet injury. The characteristic extensor lag, swelling and tenderness at the site, and certain radiographic findings confirm the diagnosis. Radiographs are suggested in all cases to assess whether there is indeed an accompanying fracture or overt joint subluxation.

Splinting is almost always the treatment for mallet injuries.[44, 143] Practically every study, and the experience of most surgeons, has established that ultimate results with splinting are acceptable and that complications of open treatment are too frequent (Fig. 24B1–28).

If a large dorsal fragment with an attached extensor is present, the basic concepts of fixation are exercised. Even larger fragments, however (approaching 30% to 40% of

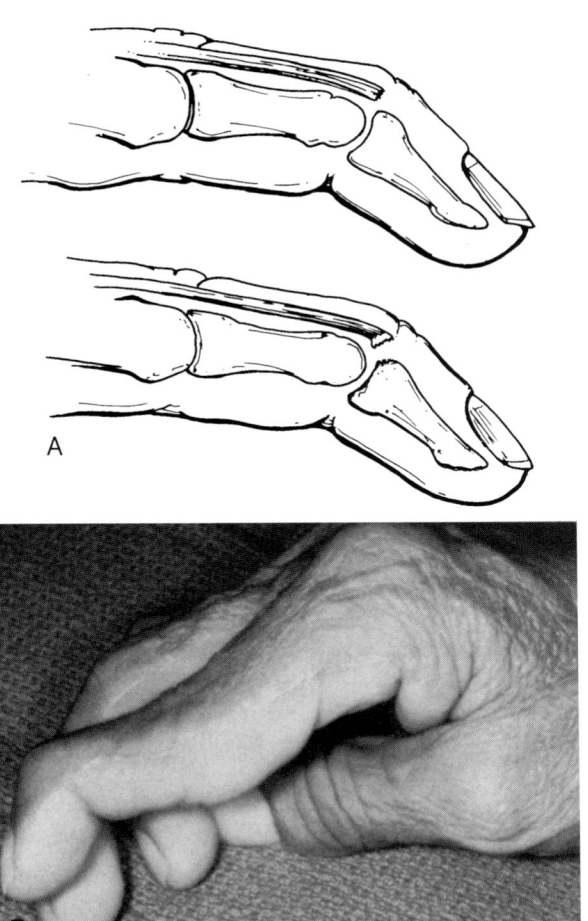

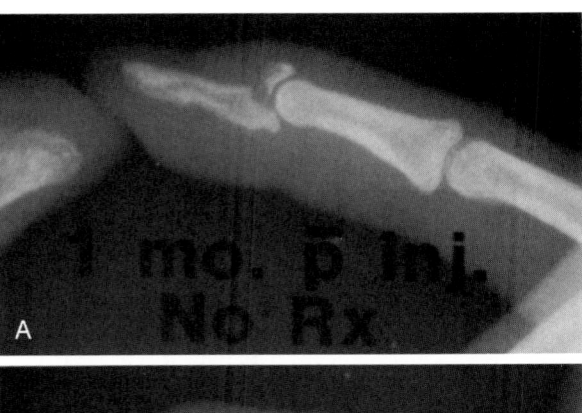

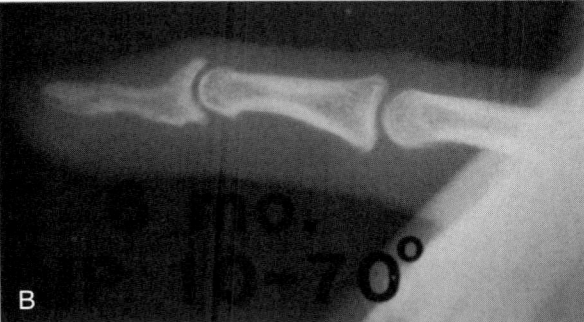

Figure 24B1–28. In our opinion, most mallet fractures should be treated nonoperatively. *A,* This patient, who had received no treatment, was seen 1 month after injury. He was then treated with simple splint immobilization of the distal interphalangeal joint for 6 weeks. *B,* Six months later, there is excellent remodeling of the articular surface. Range of motion in the distal interphalangeal joint is 10 to 70 degrees.

Figure 24B1–27. *A,* The two most common types of mallet finger. The tendon may be avulsed cleanly from the base of the distal phalanx *(top),* or the tendon may pull a small fragment of bone with it *(bottom).* Treatment for these two types is identical. *B,* Severe flexion deformity of the distal interphalangeal joint secondary to a mallet finger may lead to swan-neck deformity. This is particularly likely to occur in patients with lax proximal interphalangeal joints.

splint is selected for day, and the other for night (or shorter intervals can be chosen). The patient must be careful never to allow flexion of the DIP joint when the splints are being changed, but this regimen minimizes the loss of skin sensibility and turgor associated with long-term splinting of a single type. After the initial period of 6 to 8 weeks of 24-hour wear, night splinting is used to maintain the posture as the athlete begins and progresses with flexion exercises.

Authors' Preferred Method of Treatment. Operative intervention, even for late reconstruction of extension lag, has little role in mallet finger management in any patient. The obvious exceptions are mallet fractures, but these fall under the category of intra-articular fracture management. As difficult as it may seem, splinting is the best treatment.

the articular surface), can still be associated with stable or located joints (Fig. 24B1–29). Observation of these injuries under a fluoroscopic imager or plain lateral radiographs of the injury in a reduced position can determine whether the joint can be maintained and whether splinting can be used.

Protection of the in-season athlete for 6 to 8 weeks may present difficulties, particularly in ball-handling sports. This protection is still the first choice for most participants, but the professional or Olympic athlete may present other difficulties. Surgeons should resist the temptation to place a transarticular pin and allow play. The potential complication profile (infection, pin bending or breaking) is devastating. Innovative taping and splinting for game conditions followed by a return to normal extension splinting is a better protocol.

We use a two-splint regimen for almost all patients (Fig. 24B1–30). Both a volar and a dorsal splint are fashioned to provide about 5 to 10 degrees of hyperextension of the DIP joint. The position of the joint and any fracture fragments is verified by a radiograph through the splint. One

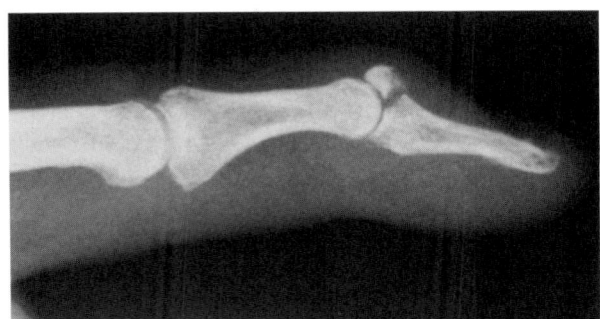

Figure 24B1–29. A mallet finger of bony origin (mallet fracture), typically involving approximately one third of the articular surface, is shown.

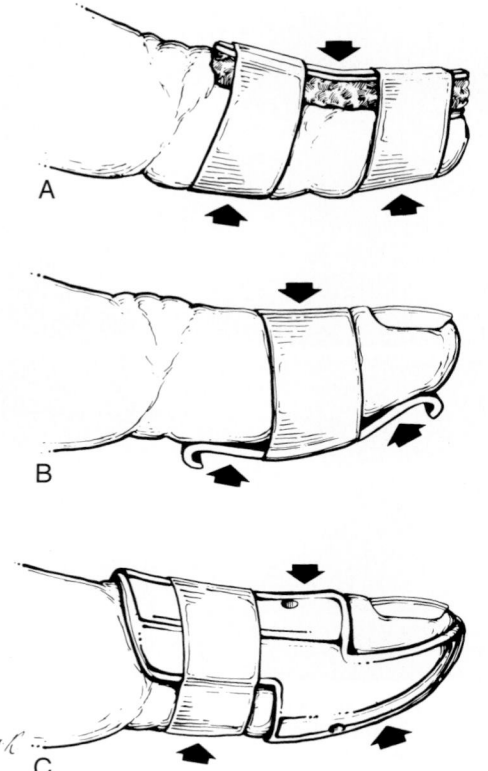

Figure 24B1–30. Several different types of splints have been designed to immobilize the distal interphalangeal joint in full extension. *A*, Dorsal padded aluminum splint. *B*, Volar unpadded aluminum splint. *C*, Stack splint. All three employ a three-point fixation principle.

Resist the temptation to place a buried K-wire across the DIP joint; this would be fraught with potential complications and would have a suboptimal result.

Boxer's Knuckle

Boxing presents many opportunities for injuries to the hand. The consistent impact on many parts of the hand when punching, blocking, and training make the boxer's hand among the most frequently injured in athletics. Disturbing data indicate that the numbers may be escalating and the injuries becoming more severe.[56, 69] Although equipment and training methods may be altered to diminish the likelihood and the severity of injuries, the fact remains that boxing is a uniquely hand-intensive sport in which the fundamental aspects place the hands in harm's way.

All types of hand injuries can be sustained in boxing, including fractures, dislocations, tendon ruptures, and open injuries. One of the most controversial of the sport-specific hand injuries, however, is the boxer's knuckle. It is unclear what the entity truly represents because a spectrum of problems about the MCP joint may be lumped under this definition. A classification or grading system could help address this issue in the future.

The major impact surface for the boxer is the flexed MCP joint. Some elite boxers have told us they have "special punches" in which they preferentially strike with the flexed PIP joint on an extended MCP joint; however,

the vast majority of impacts occur at the MCP joint. Furthermore, the index finger and the long rays are the primary punching tools of the trained boxer. In contrast, an "amateur" who comes into the surgeon's office after a street scuffle usually has a "boxer's fracture" of the fifth metacarpal neck. The trained pugilist usually avoids punching with the ulnar border digits.

Repeated, high-force trauma exposes the MCP joint to an entire spectrum of disorders. The list includes contusion, collateral sprain, and even rupture; extensor tendon or capsular fibrosis; effusion or synovitis; and fracture or dislocation. These disorders are all prevalent in the boxer, but the single entity to which the term *boxer's knuckle* applies is the sagittal band rupture accompanied by subluxation of the extensor tendon.

Pathologic and anatomic factors conspire to cause boxer's knuckle. A major contributor is the lack of protection for the extensor hood when the maximally flexed MCP joint is used for striking. There is little else between the skin and the articular surface to act as a shock absorber during the act of punching. The fine anatomy of the hood at the MCP level is most simply described in terms of the stout extensor tendon centralized over the irregularly shaped metacarpal head (slightly ulnarly inclined, often called the "metacarpal descent") by the investments of the sagittal bands. It has been shown that the sagittal bands invest the extensor, crossing both volar and dorsal to it and interweaving with the fibers from the opposite side.[66] Secondary restraints assisting in the stabilization of the tendon would be considered the juncturae tendinum proximally and the extensor mechanism insertions distally. The sagittal bands originate from the volar plate and the deep transverse intermetacarpal ligaments; thus, the extensor has no true bony insertion at the MCP level.

The terminal or most severe expression of boxer's knuckle is the post-traumatic longitudinal rent in the sagittal band that permits subluxation of the extensor mechanism. This is seen most often in the long ray but can occur in any digit. Rarely, it would be thought of as an acute or a single-event injury, acknowledging that repeated pounding would have introduced microtrauma over a longer period. The subluxation of the extensor is usually ulnarward, reflecting a loss of dorsoradial support; however, the converse can occur.

The clinical presentation is usually an MCP extensor lag, possibly accompanied by a snapping of the extensor tendon over the MCP joint through an arc of flexion and extension. In more advanced cases, the tendon can easily be seen or palpated as it subluxates from a more central position to a more lateral or medial position. When these overt mechanical symptoms are present, the opportunity to control the pathologic cascade with immobilization, restriction of boxing, and medications or injections has expired. Surgery is advocated if the athlete wants to return to sports or simply wants to improve the function of his or her extensor mechanism.

The surgical repair has several germinal elements. First, the approach should not be a direct dorsal longitudinal incision. A crescentic incision with the bias to permit wider exposure of the ruptured sagittal band is advocated. Inspection of the joint should be facile, because it is often clearly visible only after the skin incision. The sagittal band rent usually has a primary longitudinal limb but may also have a deflection either over or away from the tendon in line with its fibers.

The thickened capsule should be débrided, but we would suggest repairing it. Repair could cause undesirable tightness that could lead to loss of flexion. Inability to flex the MCP joint fully is devastating to the elite boxer. Limited extensor tenolysis and preparation of the hood are standard elements of the surgery.

After appropriate centralization, the sagittal band is coapted with absorbable suture, thus minimizing any future irritation that may accompany prominent knots. The final approximation should be done in a position of relative flexion of about 60 degrees. That is the position at which the MCP should be immobilized for 4 to 6 weeks. After the splints are removed, a systematic program for motion recovery is commenced. Boxing activities can be started when a full arc of painless MCP motion is realized and when the tendon position throughout that arc is thought to be stable.

Authors' Preferred Method of Treatment. All factors considered, the chronic symptomatic boxer's knuckle is best treated with surgical exploration and repair. The emphasis is on "symptomatic," because discomfort is as much a part of the constellation of symptoms as the physical aspects. Inspection of the joint and the periarticular tissues can usually be carried out at a time that limits the patient-athlete's missed service days.

Jersey Finger

Jersey finger is the avulsion of the FDP tendon from its insertion on the distal phalanx, an injury that occurs when an athlete gets his or her finger caught in the opposing player's jersey.

The history of the injury is forced extension of a strongly flexed DIP joint. Theories on why this occurs preferentially in the ring finger (more than 75% of cases) have both athletic and anatomic grounding. Many think that the long finger simply slips off the jersey of the competitor, leaving the ring finger to be the next in line to grasp the material in an attempted tackle or takedown.[140] Other anatomic reasons are summarized as follows:

- The common muscle belly of the long, middle, and ring rays makes the ring finger more susceptible.[52]
- The breaking strength of the FDP insertion of the ring finger is significantly less than that of the adjacent digits.[93]
- During grip, the ring finger actually becomes more prominent than the long finger owing to mobility at the CMC base and the relatively long distal phalanx. Additionally, the tendon is tethered by bipennate lumbricals on either side.[16]

The diagnosis is not too challenging to make. Passive examination and radiographs can be used to rule out primary joint disease (e.g., arthrosis) as the reason for limited active flexion of the DIP joint. Loss of active FDP activity results in the characteristic extended posture of the DIP joint, even when the patient attempts to make a fist (Fig. 24B1–31). The inability to activate the DIP joint when the middle phalanx is blocked by the examiner's hand further

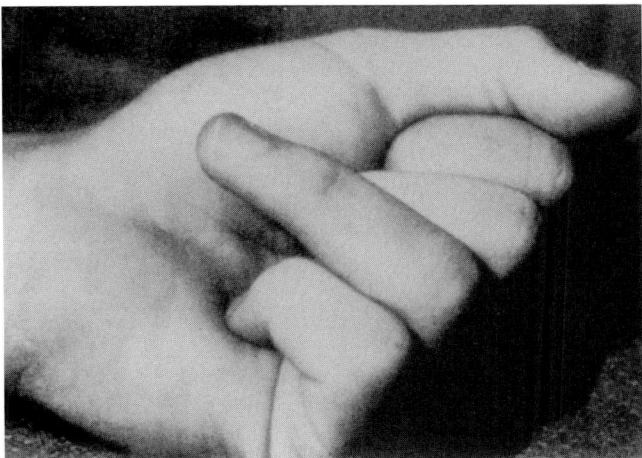

Figure 24B1–31. This patient is attempting to make a fist. Inactivity of the flexor digitorum profundus to the ring finger is evidenced by the inability of the distal interphalangeal joint to participate in the flexion cascade.

confirms the diagnosis (Fig. 24B1–32). When the tendon retracts into the palm, which is frequent, a palpable tender mass adds to the constellation of usual symptoms.

The classification system of Leddy and Packer[81] assists in clinical decision-making for this injury. The system takes into account the germinal anatomic and physiologic factors that have an effect on the ultimate result of treatment. The variables on which the classification system is based include the time between injury and planned intervention, the level of tendon retraction and the implications for the remaining nutritional supply, and the presence or the absence of a bony fragment for the insertion of the FDP. Leddy and Packer[81] provided a four-stage scheme for approaching jersey finger intellectually and clinically, as follows:

- **Type I:** The most frequent and threatening scenario, in which the FDP contracts back to the level of the palm,

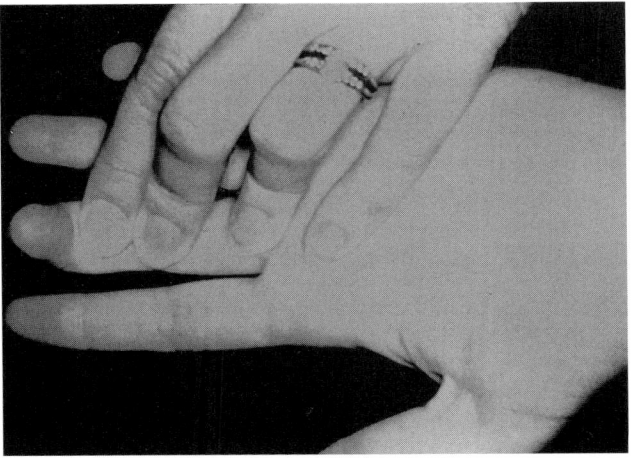

Figure 24B1–32. The flexor digitorum profundus can be tested further by having the patient flex the distal interphalangeal joint while the examiner holds the proximal interphalangeal joint in extension. This patient has a functional flexor digitorum profundus in the long finger.

thus vacating the fibro-osseous theca. All vincular and diffusional blood supply is lost, and significant contraction occurs quickly, making reinsertion arduous. This injury can be one of the most overlooked, yet it is critical to appreciate it early. Reinsertion is usually feasible within the first 1 to 2 weeks. After that period, advancement may be too difficult, and other reconstructive options must be sought. Some younger patients, however, especially those with hyperelastic diathesis, may have tendons that can still be advanced without introducing extreme flexion (Fig. 24B1–33).

• **Type II:** The vincular vessels can sometimes remain intact and tether a retracting FDP tendon within the sheath. This is a bonus because the tendon maintains its nutrition from synovial bathing and from direct vincular blood supply, while also being prevented from contraction. This unusual arrangement may convert to a type I injury at any time. Early reinsertion is again suggested (Fig. 24B1–34).

• **Type III:** Hand surgeons may go through an entire career without encountering a type III FDP avulsion. In these injuries, the tendon avulses a relatively large fragment of bone from the volar metadiaphysis of the distal phalanx. The bone then catches on the A5 or A4 pulley, thus keeping the tendon comfortably within the sheath, with all the benefits that brings. Standard radiographs reveal this finding, but an unusually swollen and ecchymotic pulp is a herald of the type III injury. The usual tenets of fracture fixation can be exercised, but recognizing that

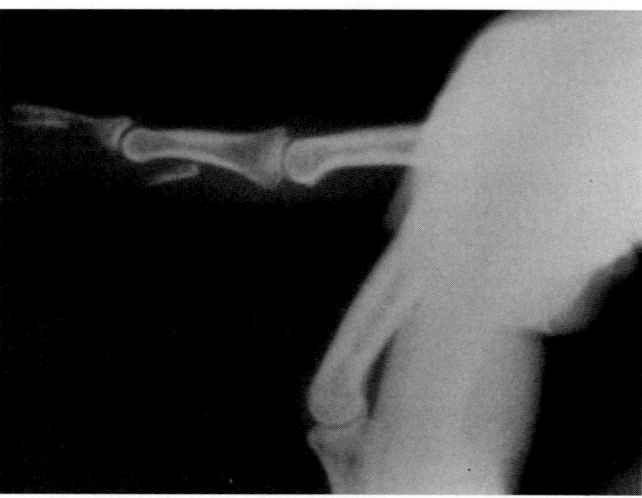

Figure 24B1–34. In a type II flexor digitorum profundus avulsion, the tendon gets hung up at the chiasma of the flexor digitorum superficialis. Occasionally, the tendon may avulse a fragment of bone off the volar cortex of the distal phalanx. (Usually, the fragment is smaller and lies more proximally than is seen in this patient.)

the fragment may be relatively small and friable, simple reinsertion is often a reasonable alternative (Fig. 24B1–35).

• **Type IV:** After Leddy and Packer's original three-part classification in 1977,[81] Leddy and other authors contributed a fourth element to the classification of the jersey finger.[80, 137] The characteristics of the unusual type IV injury are simultaneous fracture at the insertion of the FDP with retraction of the tendon permitted by avulsion from the fractured fragment. There is debate whether this represents a comminuted fracture that simply allows the FDP to retract fully or whether continued contraction of the FDP eventually pulls the tendon from a fragment tethered within the sheath. As for type I injury, reinsertion is usually possible within the first 1 to 2 weeks.

Reinsertion techniques for the avulsed FDP tendon are relatively standard. It is generally favorable to minimize the use of instruments in the interior of the fibro-osseous theca; retrieval of a retracted tendon by passing a pediatric feeding tube through the sheath and into the palm may deliver it. Otherwise, more extensive exposure through a

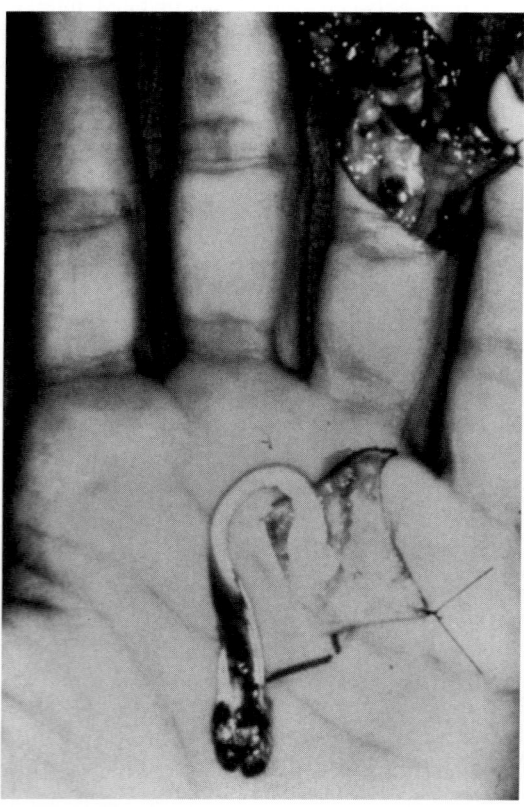

Figure 24B1–33. In a type I flexor digitorum profundus avulsion, the tendon retracts into the palm. Attempted repair after 7 to 10 days may be difficult or impossible.

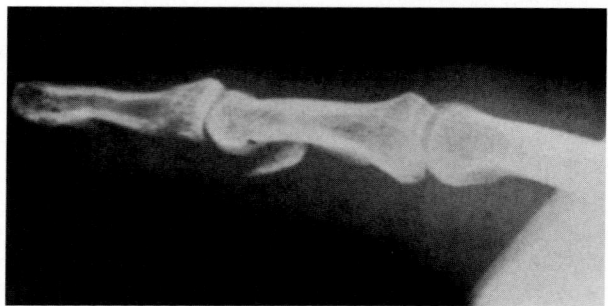

Figure 24B1–35. In a type III flexor digitorum profundus avulsion, a large bony fragment is avulsed by the tendon. This prevents more proximal retraction because the fragment gets hung up at the level of the A4 pulley.

midaxial or Brunner incision will allow the retrieval and passage of the flexor tendon. Distal insertion is usually accomplished with a pullout wire technique. Raising an osteoperiosteal flap at the site of insertion is advocated. The use of suture anchors is now becoming popular, but it may be challenging to achieve proper tensioning of the FDP and to ensure excellent coaptation into the distal phalanx (Fig. 24B1–36).

After reinsertion, a typical flexor tendon program can be initiated, with early passive and active motion at 3 to 4 weeks. Because almost all athletes rely on gripping activity, play may be restricted. Permission to resume competition is usually reserved only for the rare instance when the player can tolerate immobilization in a fist position. Return at the 2- to 3-month mark is the normal projection.

Neglected Flexor Digitorum Profundus Avulsion. There are many reasons why players may not seek care for this and other "minor" hand injuries. The team physician may learn of an FDP avulsion in the end-of-season physicals, only to be informed by the player that it occurred in the season's first contest. Moreover, there are players who, when confronted with the choice of FDP loss versus missing a lengthy period of service, will choose to forego repair. It is imperative to communicate the consequences clearly and to document these conversations.

When confronted with the neglected FDP avulsion, the surgeon should consider the following choices:

• **Late reinsertion:** Extremely unlikely and potentially damaging if extreme flexion is the resulting posture for the postoperative period.

• **Acute single-stage reconstruction:** May be technically feasible if the theca has not collapsed but should be reserved for the rare instance when independent DIP flexion is an absolute necessity.

• **Two-stage flexor reconstruction:** Once a common procedure before primary repair of lacerated tendons was advocated, the techniques of and the experience with this surgery have become less prominent. Very few athletes will submit to even a well-designed plan from an experienced tendon surgeon. This approach probably will be considered too aggressive for the anticipated result.

• **Stabilization:** This is a catchall term for anything from soft tissue imbrication to formal arthrodesis. This is often the best choice for surgical magnitude, minimal rehabilitation, and acceptable result.

• **Forgoing surgery:** This may be the optimal handling of the problem in most cases. The loss of function with the loss of FDP flexion may create little compromise for the player, and the risk-benefit ratio of surgery may be unacceptable. The surgeon should consider excision of the tender palmar mass, the scarred tendon end.

Authors' Preferred Method of Treatment. The gold standard is early recognition and repair. There is little or no role for a plan of delayed addressing of the injury, although a player may lobby for a several-week delay in order to participate in a critical contest.

Unfortunately, most reconstructive options for the chronic injury are arduous for the surgeon and the patient. Results are often disappointing, especially after lengthy rehabilitation. Frankly, we usually dissuade players from

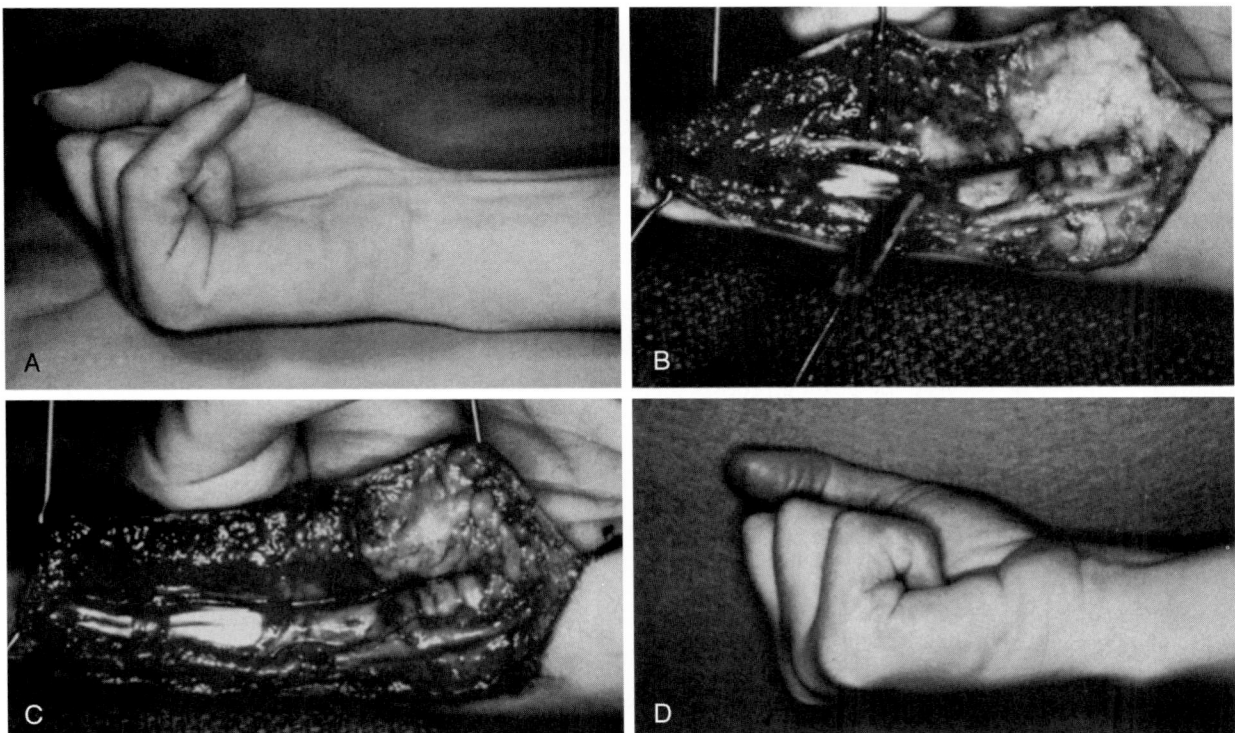

Figure 24B1–36. *A,* Appearance of the small finger after a type II flexor digitorum profundus avulsion. There is absence of flexion in the distal interphalangeal joint and limited flexion in the proximal interphalangeal joint. *B,* Note the hemorrhagic bed at the time of digital exploration and tendon retrieval. *C,* The tendon has been reinserted, preserving the A4 pulley. *D,* The patient had full recovery of active flexion 3 months postoperatively.

embarking on a lengthy and complex reconstructive journey while they are still active. Lack of active DIP flexion is not usually the ultimate limiting factor in an athlete's performance. If it is problematic, then timing of the reconstruction is critical to allow for an extended commitment to rehabilitation before return to play.

Disruption of the Flexor Pulley System

A lesion of the fibro-osseous theca or the flexor sheath is emerging in sports participants. It is almost exclusively isolated to the elite baseball pitcher and the avid rock climber. Attenuation or frank rupture of the elements of the flexor pulley system may result from acute or chronic exposure to forcible contraction of the FDP tendon against extreme supraphysiologic force.

The professional baseball pitcher gets much of his control by the subtle influence on the ball by the distal tip of the long finger. With the angular velocity that the throwing mechanism is known to generate, it is not surprising that the last contact point between the ball and the player is prone to injury. Similarly, flexor system injury may occur when a free climber is supporting his or her body weight with the flexed DIP joint.[47]

Tenderness over the volar and lateral aspects of the middle phalanx is typical of the attenuated pulley system. Additional tenderness along the sheath may accompany the lesion because inflammation or, rarely, bleeding may contribute fullness. The DIP can still be actively flexed, but with some discomfort. A perceived weakness usually accompanies the problem as pain inhibition takes over. The pitcher will see a decrease in velocity of the fastest pitches.

The extreme of the spectrum of injury is overt bowstringing. This usually represents failure of the proximal aspect of the A4 pulley with disruption of the interval "window" between A2 and A4, including the A5 pulley and the first two cruciate pulleys. Rarely, a complete failure of both biomechanically important parts of the sheath, the A2 and A4 pulleys, will occur. To supplement clinical diagnosis, magnetic resonance imaging can be helpful in demonstrating edema and volar translation of the flexor tendons when the scans are taken with applied resistance.[121]

Immobilization, anti-inflammatory medicines and modalities, and rest are the cornerstones of early treatment. Injection can be considered if the inflammatory component of the clinical picture is predominant. The role of injection is somewhat questionable because the healing process that may restore function may be altered. Every player who does not manifest overt bowstringing should receive a trial of conservative therapy. The time course is variable and can be lengthy (up to 3 months) and frustrating. Try to promote patience in the patient.

If the rupture of the flexor pulley system is complete, then reconstruction is indicated. The basic principles of pulley reconstruction include selecting and harvesting the graft (usually the palmaris or the plantaris), wrapping the graft around the flexor tendons and the bone (under the extensor at the A2 level, over the extensor at the A4 level), and securing the graft. Rehabilitation protocols are individualized but include tendon gliding to discourage adhesion and pulley protection to avoid attenuation or rerupture.

Authors' Preferred Method of Treatment. We advocate spending a great deal of time in the evaluation and nonoperative treatment of these injuries. As long as a complete traumatic rupture of the mechanically important pulleys has not occurred, then closed treatment is most likely to yield better results than operative repair.

Digital taping, resting splints, and rehabilitation modalities all may assist in management. We reserve cortisone injection for those patients with definable tenosynovitis in addition to pulley attenuation. If reconstruction is warranted, palmaris grafting and appropriate rehabilitation and protection can be scheduled for the off-season.

Fractures of the Tubular Bones of the Fingers and Thumb

The importance of early fracture fixation cannot be overemphasized in returning an athlete to play. The surgeon caring for the athlete's hand must maintain an understanding of and facility with advanced concepts regarding internal fixation to provide options to his or her patients. This is not to say that conventional closed reduction and immobilization are indicated for a vast majority of sandlot or scholastic athletes. Athletes as a group, and more elite athletes in particular, demand and deserve additional considerations that are now available with recent strides in technique and technology.

It cannot be argued that treatment by closed methods is always successful and introduces only minimal risk for many hand fractures. For this reason, the lines between conservative and aggressive treatment have blurred with respect to the care of the athlete's hand fracture. It may be most conservative to gain anatomic reduction, stabilize a given fracture with compression screws, and then promote early motion and return to play.

Because basic orthopaedic education focuses on the basic elements of skeletal stabilization, fracture care is not discussed extensively here. Instead, several selected injuries are highlighted. These injuries were chosen because of their frequency of presentation and because of their sport-specific characteristics. Patients sustaining these fractures, when managed by innovative techniques, may return to play earlier than was previously possible.

Critical injuries such as intra-articular fractures associated with PIP dislocations, avulsion fractures representing ulnar collateral injuries, and CMC fracture-dislocations were covered earlier in this chapter. The fractures chosen for this special section include the boxer's fracture, fractures at the base of the thumb metacarpal, and spiral oblique fracture of the metacarpal or phalanx.

Boxer's Fractures

When a metacarpal neck fracture is significantly displaced or unstable, or both,[34, 50, 60, 62, 97, 136] an innovative pinning technique can be used to stabilize the fracture in an anatomic position and promote early motion and return to sport. Termed *bouquet pinning* because of the arrangement of the pins in the metacarpal head, this is a technique-dependent but very satisfying procedure that is logical for

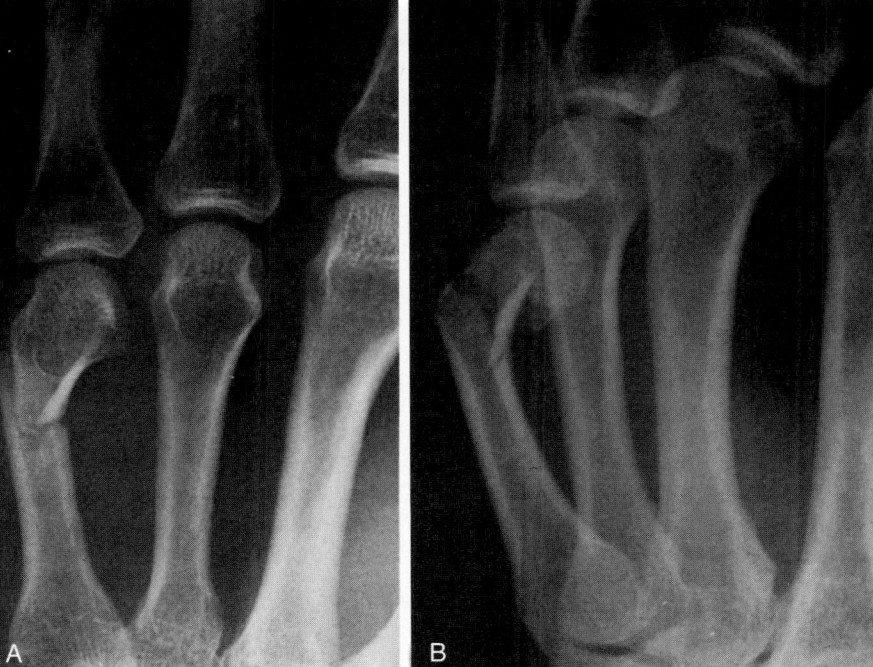

Figure 24B1–37. *A,* Anteroposterior view of a fracture through the neck of the fifth metacarpal with apparent modest angulation. *B,* The same metacarpal fracture seen in a lateral view in 10 degrees of supination. The true amount of angulation is much better appreciated in this view.

use in the athlete or any other individual who wishes rapid return of unrestricted hand function.

To qualify for bouquet pinning, the metacarpal head, or the distal fragment, should be significantly flexed yet reducible (Fig. 24B1–37). This injury would be difficult to control with plaster and would need lengthy immobilization, which may prevent the athlete from play. Bouquet pinning can effect and maintain stable reduction and requires only brief postoperative immobilization.

The technique recapitulates the methods used in stacked intramedullary or Enders pinning[44] for other tubular bone fractures. It can be employed for all triphalangeal digits but is uniquely well suited for the border digits, especially the small ray.[125] The skin is incised over the metacarpal base at the glabrous border. The extensor carpi ulnaris insertion is then elevated to allow access to the small dorsoulnar prominence just distal to the articular surface. A small cortical window is made to allow intramedullary access, and the fracture is provisionally reduced by manipulation.

The sharp points are removed from standard 0.045-inch smooth pins, and the pins are then bent in a gently curved manner. The pins are introduced into the canal and cross the reduced fracture site. They both assist in reduction and stabilize the fracture. Three to four pins are used, depending on canal diameter. They are carefully embedded into the metaphyseal bone of the metacarpal head, and their proximal end is cut short so that it can be placed inside the proximal lip of bone created after cortical perforation (Fig. 24B1–38).

Amazing initial stability is accompanied by rapid healing. The hand may be immobilized in a plaster splint or a simple soft wrap for 2 weeks, after which motion can be started and progressed. Results of this technique, originally described for the noncompliant patient,[54] have been uni-

formly excellent. In our own series of more than 40 bouquet pinnings, we have encountered no complications or nonunions. Many of these patients have been professional athletes, and all have returned to sport at their previous level within 6 weeks.

Bennett's Fracture

More than one fourth of all metacarpal fractures are injuries to the intra-articular base of the thumb.[48] The eponymous classification of Bennett's or Rolondo's fractures may be confusing at times, but the classification essentially describes a comminuted pattern of fracture of more than two parts. The Bennett's fracture is a good model for understanding the deforming forces about the joint.

When the metacarpal shaft is separated from the volar-ulnar lip of the metacarpal's articular surface, the attachment of the volar beak or oblique ligament, the abductor pollicis longus tendon is the primary deforming force. The abductor pollicis longus draws the metacarpal proximally and slightly dorsally. The secondary deforming force is the adductor pollicis. This intrinsic hand muscle's action further accentuates the subluxation at the joint.

Closed manipulation can be attempted or even augmented with percutaneous pins. The reduction maneuver includes longitudinal traction, pronation, and relative extension of the shaft with basilar pressure. If pinning is performed, interfragmentary pins alone will probably be inadequate. Use of a transarticular pin to stabilize the CMC joint and the two components of the articular fracture is advocated (Fig. 24B1–39).

As logical and satisfying as reduction and pinning may be, this treatment will not return an athlete to play in an accelerated fashion. One could argue that in an elite athlete,

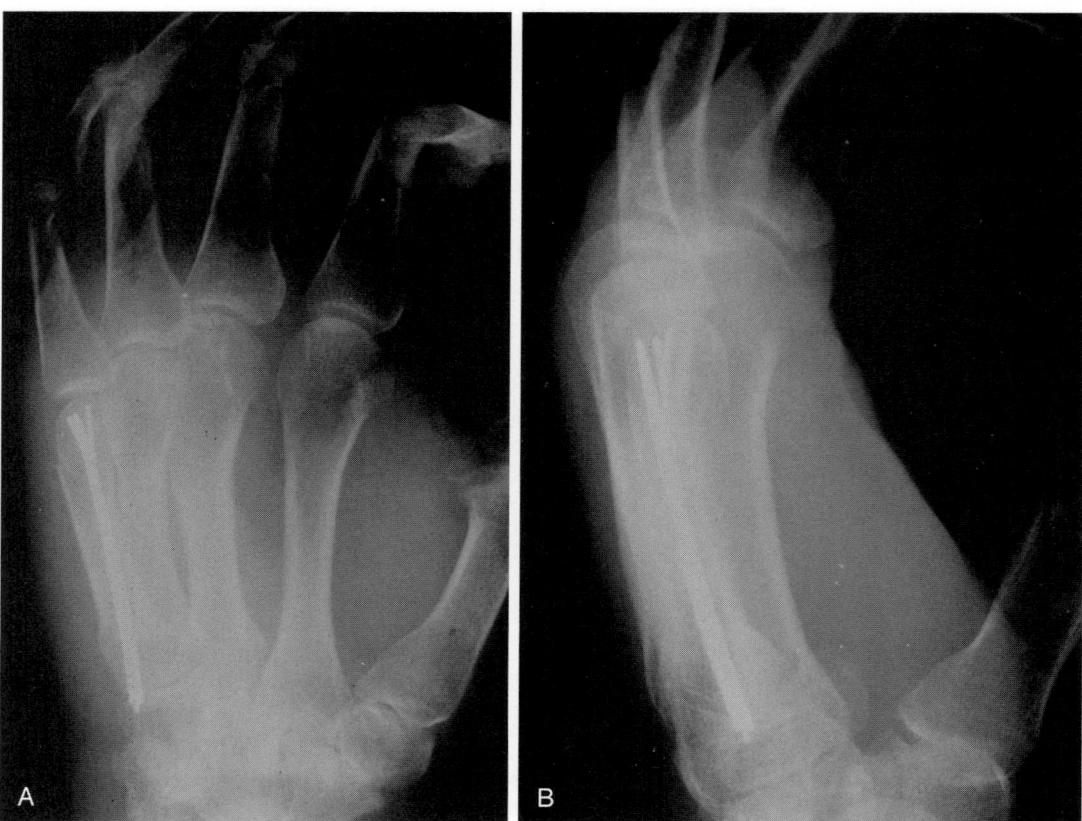

Figure 24B1–38. Termed *bouquet pinning* because of the arrangement of pins in the metacarpal head, this technique can be performed through a small proximal incision and can provide the stability necessary for the athlete's accelerated return to play. *A*, Oblique radiograph; *B*, lateral radiograph.

there would be little benefit to the accepted risk of surgery if rapid return to play were considered the parameter by which success was measured.

For those demanding anatomic reduction and accelerated return to hand-intensive activity, open reduction and internal fixation is predictable and technically feasible. Through a gently curvilinear incision at the thenar base, usually regarded as Wagner's incision, the thenar muscles are elevated, and the capsule is incised. After the hematoma is evacuated, the joint is inspected for additional articular damage and further comminution.

The metacarpal can usually be easily reduced to both the volar fragment and the CMC joint relationships. In some cases, provisional stabilization with small smooth wires, 0.045-inch or 0.035-inch, may be done to check the alignment and to give stability for the ultimate insertion of two minifragment screws. The screws are inserted from dorsal to volar with the usual compression technique (i.e., overdrilling the dorsal cortex). One must be cognizant that the smaller-diameter implants may have lengths only in the range of 20 to 24 mm. This may be too small for some larger athletes. Increase in root diameter of the screw usually accompanies greater length. Delivery of the screw from a slightly different angle may permit fragment engagement.

After 10 to 14 days, the initial plaster thumb spica splint can be exchanged for a removable one as the sutures are discontinued. Gentle interval motion can be started at that time. By 3 to 4 weeks, while checking for clinical and radiographic signs of healing, light strengthening can be started. Ball-handling activities follow motion recovery and effective strength return. Return to play is typically in the third to fourth week for players who can tolerate splint protection (linemen, some hockey players) and 4 to 6 weeks for those who must perform unprotected (quarterbacks, basketball players).

If the metacarpal base fracture is more comminuted (a Rolondo's fracture), the only reasonable surgical option that may have an impact on early return is open reduction and internal fixation. The use of a condylar blade plate to stabilize the multifragmented base and to affix the construct to the shaft may be the only realistic option. The difficulty with some of these fractures should not be underestimated. The goals remain (1) establishment of the articular surface of the metacarpal and its relationship with the trapezium and (2) stabilization of the shaft against the same deforming forces described previously. There will be times when the size and the number of fragments is advantageous for this aggressive treatment and return-to-play plan, but realistic expectation should be exercised on the part of the surgeon, the patient, and the franchise.

Spiral Oblique Fractures of the Tubular Bones

Whether a metacarpal or a phalanx is the bone fractured, subsidence and malrotation can accompany the deformity

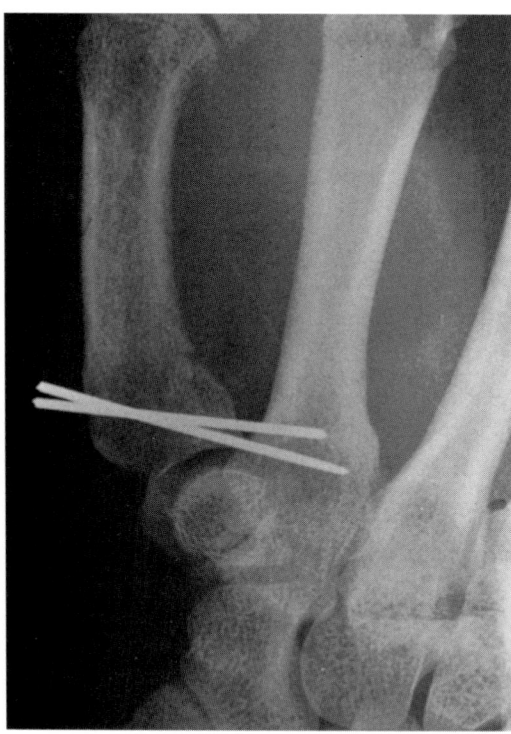

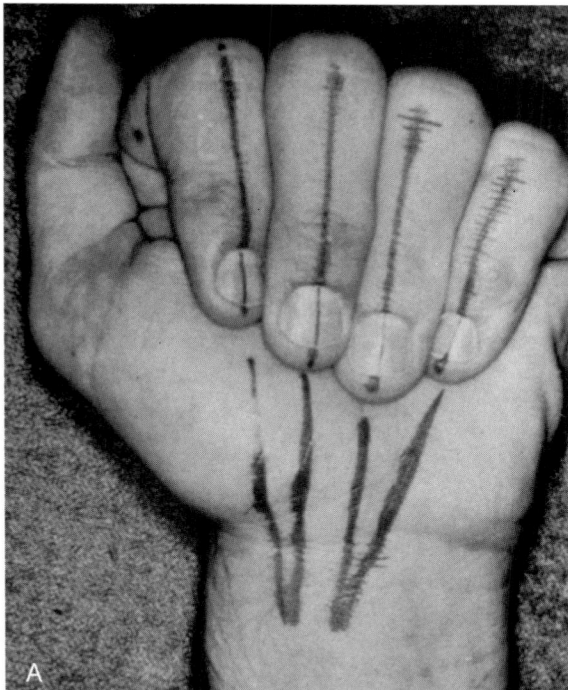

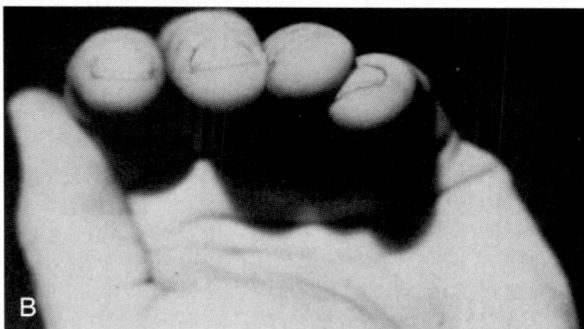

Figure 24B1–39. A reasonable treatment alternative for Bennett's fracture is closed reduction and percutaneous pin fixation. The pins do not necessarily enter the small volar fracture fragment; rather, the intent is to reduce the fracture-subluxation by means of closed manipulation and then to secure the base of the thumb metacarpal to the carpal bones or to the adjacent second metacarpal, as shown here.

(Fig. 24B1–40). The positive element of these fractures is the large surface area for healing if properly coapted, and the negative element is the proclivity to displace when treated by closed means.

In some elite athletes, even an isolated metacarpal fracture of a central ray may cause lost time of service. In almost all athletes, phalangeal shaft fractures will translate into an abbreviated season. The judicious use of internal fixation to stabilize these fractures should be entertained in certain populations. This is especially true when the implant can be interfragmentary screws alone (Fig. 24B1–41) because the bulk of plates is often a deterrent to their use unless a bony defect or an unstable transverse fracture presents.

Although open reduction with internal fixation is the gold standard for osseous stability, the soft tissue component of the fractured hand may preclude this and may instead welcome one of many minimally invasive techniques of stabilization (Fig. 24B1–42). The attitude of the fracture will often declare an obvious "best method" for fixation, but many different techniques for closed reduction and percutaneous pinning are available. The treating physician should be careful not to overuse percutaneous fixation merely to prevent a surgical incision because the price can be nonunion and, thus, a much more difficult problem (Fig. 24B1–43).

Fractures at the neck of a phalanx can sometimes be problematic (Fig. 24B1–44). The pitcher, the rock climber, or any other athlete who relies on full motion and strength

Figure 24B1–40. *A,* When the fingers are flexed, they tend to converge, but not toward a single fixed point, as is sometimes depicted. This is a normal hand. *B,* Maintenance of correct rotational alignment with the fingers semiflexed (as they are in a cast or a splint) is best done by noting the planes of the fingernails as seen end-on. Comparison with the opposite hand is helpful. This hand has no fracture or deformity.

at the interphalangeal joints is best served by anatomic reduction. If adequate reduction cannot be obtained and maintained through closed methods, percutaneous or open fixation may indeed be necessary to maximize the potential for full recovery on return to play (Fig. 24B1–45).

In the area of interfragmentary compression fixation, a few techniques propel the athlete back to earlier play. One of these techniques is meticulous soft tissue handling. For metacarpal-level fractures, double curvilinear or S-shaped skin incisions heal nicely and provide greater exposure than longitudinal incisions of similar length. Avoiding straight dorsal incisions on the digits is also advocated; crescentic incisions should be made that reach the midaxis at their volar extent. We try to avoid extensor-splitting approaches in the athlete, though we have no strong data to support this bias. This is really only an issue at the proximal phalanx level. Careful side-to-side manipulation of the extensor, developed stereognosis, and image intensi-

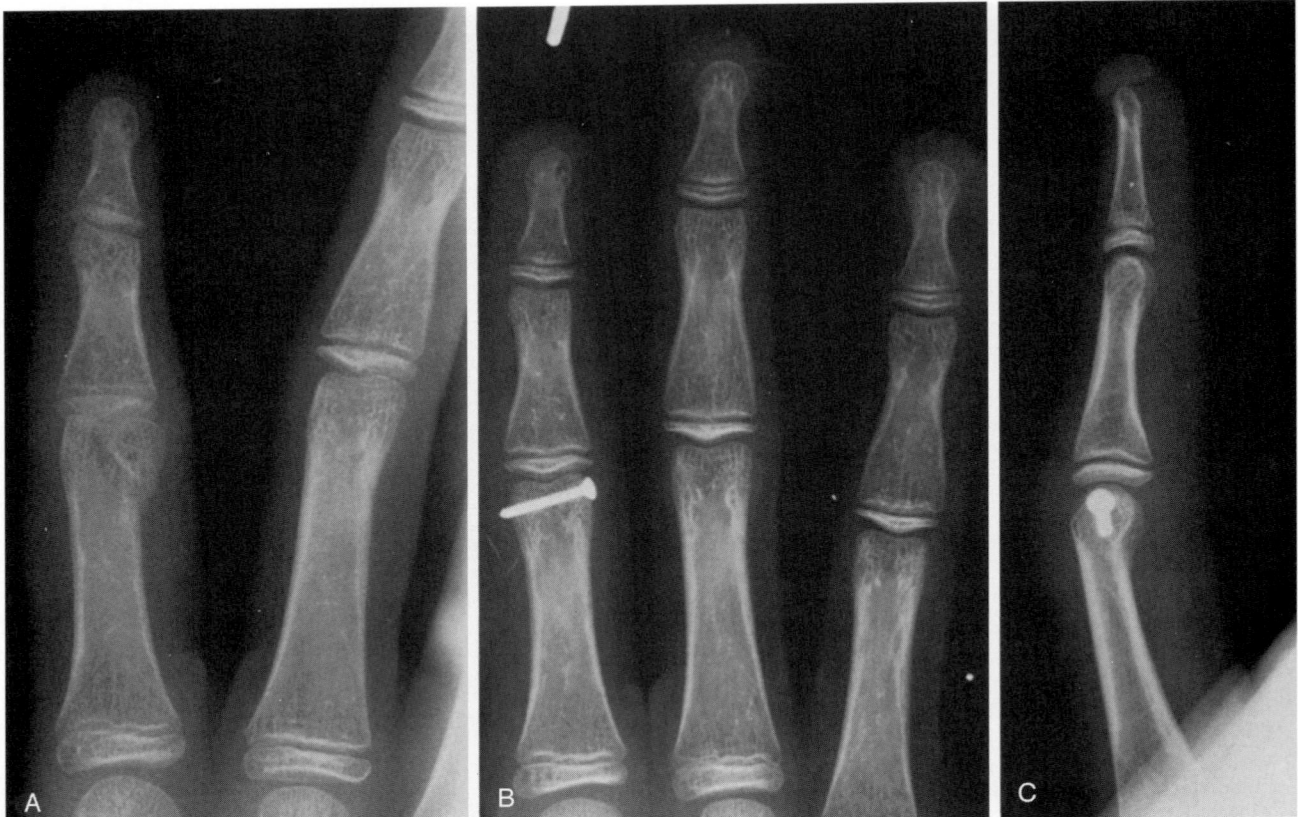

Figure 24B1–41. Displaced condylar fractures virtually always demand internal fixation. *A,* Displaced and rotated fracture of the condyle in a skeletally immature football player. *B* and *C,* Treatment was with open reduction and anatomic restoration of the articular surface with a single 1.5-mm AO screw.

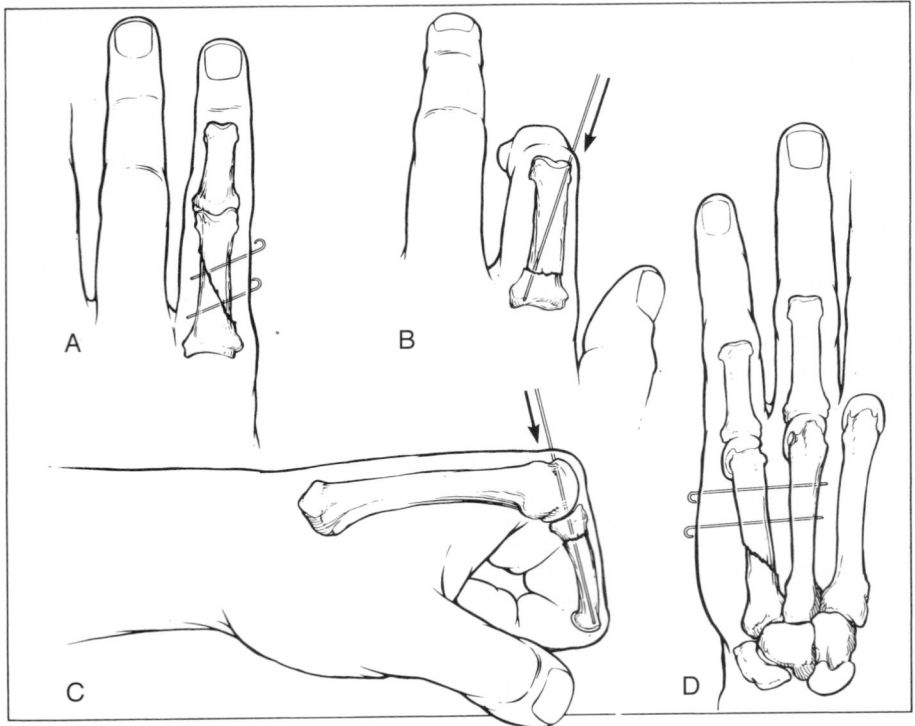

Figure 24B1–42. *A–D,* Four methods of closed reduction and percutaneous pin fixation. (See text for details.)

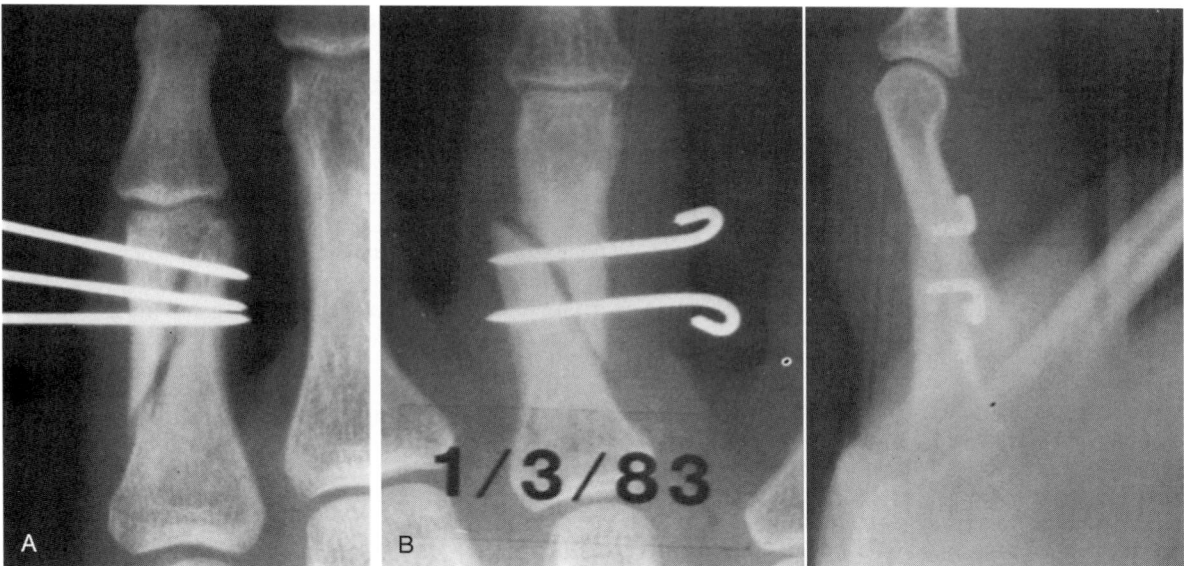

Figure 24B1–43. *A*, Closed reduction and percutaneous pin fixation of a spiral fracture of the proximal phalanx. Reduction is not anatomic, and an unnecessary fracture gap persists. This fracture would have been better managed with open reduction and internal fixation. *B*, Another unsatisfactory closed reduction and percutaneous pin fixation technique. The fracture was not adequately reduced, and pin fixation in this position assured malunion. The closed method should have been abandoned in this patient, and the fracture should have been fixed with open reduction and internal fixation.

fication can allow the experienced surgeon to reduce, provisionally maintain, and ultimately stabilize most of these fractures without extensor disruption.

Extensor mechanism handling must be meticulous. Because many of these athletes are young, the true layer between the extensor tenosynovium and the periosteum can be preserved. Extraperiosteal dissection, with deeper exposure just at the fracture ends for preparation, minimizes undue trauma and promotes healing. The periosteum

can even be closed as a separate layer, but knots should be buried away from the sliding place under the extensor.

The screw size that is most often used is 2.0 to 2.7 mm. Care should be exercised to avoid significant protrusion, especially in the digit, where a screw that is too long may impair tendon and collateral ligament function. The fracture pattern will dictate the ultimate orientation of the screws, but sensitivity to minimize the screw's interference with tendon gliding is a reasonable caveat.

The risks of operation are accepted with the expectation

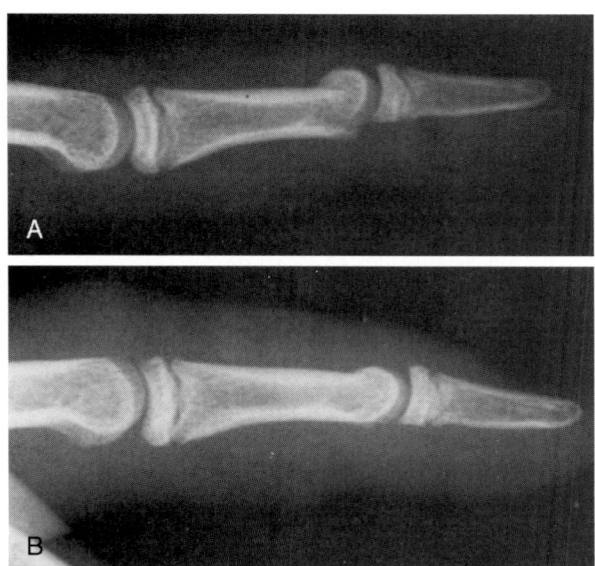

Figure 24B1–44. Fractures through the neck of the proximal or the middle phalanges are classic booby-trap fractures because they are unstable. *A*, Transcondylar fracture of the middle phalanx in a soccer player. *B*, Extension malunion resulted in loss of the subcondylar fossa, which ultimately limited full distal interphalangeal joint flexion.

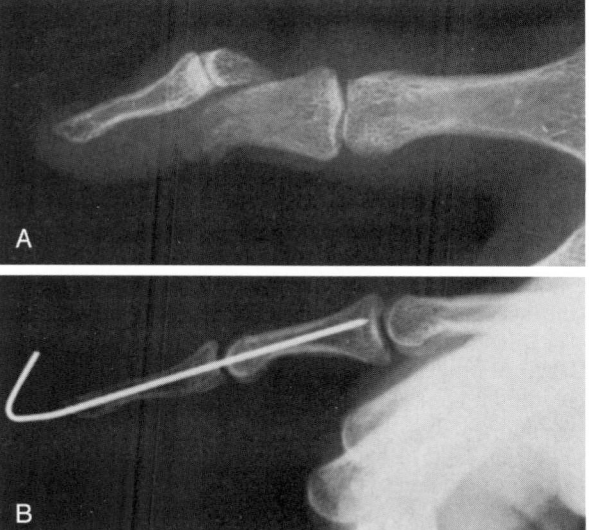

Figure 24B1–45. *A*, This widely displaced fracture through the neck of the middle phalanx was treated with open reduction and internal fixation using a single, longitudinally oriented Kirschner wire. *B*, Because the Kirschner wire crosses the distal interphalangeal joint, return to athletic competition should not be permitted until the pin is removed at 3 weeks.

of benefits to come. Anatomic reduction is a decided benefit, but accelerated return of motion and early return to play are the most important issues for many of these special patients. The level of postoperative dressing may be reduced after internal fixation. If plaster is used, we usually only carry it to the next joint level, if that. Often, a soft bulky dressing allows limited motion.

When the sutures are discontinued at 2 weeks, interval splinting is suggested. Aggressive edema reduction is a key element inasmuch as the hydraulics of a swollen digit are working against motion recovery. We favor night splinting in extension because of the handling of the extensor mechanism and the eventual strength imbalance that always favors the flexors. Active and assisted motion can be pursued at will, but no passive motion is instituted unless there is a motion deficit in later weeks.

At 3 to 4 weeks, motion should exceed 75%, and strengthening can be started. Clinical parameters are often more reliable than following the progress of primary bone healing in this population; when the area of the fracture is nontender and a majority of motion is recovered, sport-specific activities can begin. We target return to sport at 5 to 6 weeks in most athletes, although some have surprised us by returning earlier. It is an advantage if some protection can be afforded against torsional injuries by buddy taping or light splinting.

Authors' Preferred Method of Treatment. There is a balance that must be established when dealing with the athlete with a hand fracture. The central question is whether anatomic restoration, rigid fixation, and early motion yield substantive advantages over nonoperative treatments. There are definite "black-and-white" injuries—severe fractures where operative intervention is absolutely indicated. Likewise, the stable fracture with minimal chance for displacement will continue to be treated by closed methods. It is the "gray area" fracture that brings this central question to the fore.

In our referral practice, in which the treatment of the elite athlete is common, the benefits of operative treatment are carefully considered. The patient must realize the benefit of the surgery and participate in an accelerated rehabilitation program, with return to play earlier than expected with nonoperative treatment.

The Thumb

Patients and physicians alike are familiar with the central role of the human thumb to almost all hand functions. In the specialized world of sports, cylindrical grasp and power pinch needs are often taken to the extreme, whether it is ball or stick handling, grappling with an opponent, or checking the reins. The thumb is exposed to injury because of its unavoidable placement in the most active and demanding of hand tasks.

The thumb manifests a unique osteoarticular column, which differs substantially in its orientation, osteology, mechanics, and function from the triphalangeal digits. It is for this reason that consideration of the injured thumb deserves separate attention. In this section, the common athletic injuries to the thumb and their treatment courses are reviewed.

Ligament Injuries

Because the thumb's primary role is that of a stable and mobile post for pinch and grasp, injury to its soft tissue components can be just as debilitating as fractures. Stiffness is the most frequent and feared complication in soft tissue trauma to the fingers (see the previous section in this chapter on PIP joint dislocation for an example). Conversely, injuries to the ligaments and other supporting structures in the thumb often result in instability. This is the fundamental difference the surgeon must embrace when approaching the constellation of injuries to this member.

Carpometacarpal Dislocation

In the majority of patients, the CMC joint of the first ray is very mobile. Its specialized anatomy allows for the mobility to place the thumb in space, yet becomes stable when the complex set of musculotendinous units, interacting with the static restraints, is activated. Much has been written about this unique anatomy.[64]

Although fractures about the basilar thumb joint are common and will be discussed in subsequent sections, pure soft tissue injuries are infrequent, sometimes difficult to diagnose, and always challenging to treat. Because of the inherent mobility of the joint, there is often a question of where the physiologic boundary of mobility becomes pathologic instability. This is an evaluation that demands contralateral comparison and a diagnosis that is best confirmed with live fluoroscopic stress examination.

The subluxation, rarely a frank dislocation, may present initially as swelling and pain at the basilar joint after a hyperextension or torsional force. It is rare to sustain a CMC dislocation from a direct blow, although a generalized crushing mechanism such as being caught between two helmets or stepping on the flattened hand could create the injury. Radiographs rule out the more frequently encountered Bennett's or Rolondo's fractures.

The athlete is usually too uncomfortable to glean meaningful examination initially. Placement of the hand in a short-arm thumb spica splint is recommended; the interphalangeal joint can be included if desired or if the tenderness is so global that MCP level injury is suspected. Stress examination may be performed under a wrist block, but it is probably advisable to defer that intervention until after the acute phase subsides (5 to 10 days).

The diagnosis is established by demonstrating significant hypermobility to multidirectional stress. It must be compared with the contralateral side. Definitive diagnosis may be elusive in those who maintain a hyperelastic diathesis as a baseline. In those with more limited basilar joint motion, the magnitude of difference will be accentuated.

Even experienced hand surgeons lament the difficulty with interpreting radiographs about the CMC joint of the thumb. The most informative view in our practice is the hyperpronated view of the thumb. This image most clearly demonstrates the relationship between the metacarpal base and trapezium. There is little value to computed tomography scan or magnetic resonance imaging in the evaluation of CMC dislocation without fracture.

Once the surgeon is comfortable with the diagnosis of

CMC dislocation in the athlete, a treatment course must be elected. The optimal treatment is open reduction and pinning, with or without soft tissue augmentation. Though this approach may sound overly aggressive, this injury is undertreated in too many athletes. Closed reduction is unsatisfying, and the ability to control the mobile CMC joint with casting is questionable. Even the addition of percutaneous pinning to closed reduction is likely inadequate in most cases.

The approach is made through a Wagner's incision along the glabrous border of the thenar eminence. Lifting the thenar muscles from the capsule of the CMC joint exposes a patulous soft tissue envelope around the joint; in some cases, a rent is found through which the metacarpal base had herniated. In either event, a T-shaped arthrotomy is made to inspect the joint for articular damage or loose body. While maintaining anatomic reduction of the joint with the thumb positioned in functional anteposition, the surgeon performs pinning with a 0.045-inch or 0.062-inch smooth wire. Care to avoid the thumb extensors and extrinsic abductor is exercised.

Handling the capsule is an important issue. If the injury was recognized early and the capsule was not significantly traumatized, imbrication will be sufficient to augment stability. If there has been significant damage to this structure, augmentation with a tendon, the flexor carpi radialis or the extensor carpi radialis longus, could be elected. Capsular augmentation in the method of Swanson is likely the most familiar to most surgeons. Casting is essential. The pin is left indwelling for 4 to 6 weeks.

Permitting play while the pin is indwelling is inviting disaster. With the exception of perhaps a field goal kicker or track athlete, playing with transarticular pins should be strictly forbidden. After pin removal, playing with a well-molded orthosis, with adequate support at the CMC joint, is feasible. Usually return to play is contemplated after near normal motion recovery and the return of adequate strength. Although sport and position specific, the interval from surgery to play will be between 6 and 10 weeks.

Carpometacarpal dislocation is an elusive entity. It is difficult to diagnose and challenging to treat. It is often a season-ending injury, but could be a career-threatening one if scrutiny and a high index of suspicion are not combined with sound treatment principles. Understanding the entity and accepting the need for operative treatment will maximize ultimate outcome.

Authors' Preferred Method of Treatment. Whether or not the thumb CMC dislocation is accompanied by significant bony injury, we have treated these by operative means. Open inspection of the joint, repair of soft tissues, and stabilization of the joint in a reduced position are the essential steps in the treatment. Later reconstruction will always be more difficult, and the results decrease with time.

Injuries about the Metacarpophalangeal Joint of the Thumb

In theory, MCP joint dislocation and collateral ligament injuries are parts of the same spectrum of injury. Exact mechanisms, magnitudes, and direction of force may differ, but elements of the pathoanatomy are shared. It is useful, however, to separate these two entities and to further subdivide them for clarity. MCP dislocations are distinguished by magnitude or likelihood of closed reduction, expressed as "simple" or "complex" dislocations. Collateral ligament injuries to the radial or ulnar sides are considered separately, though their treatment is similar and is dependent on the degree of attenuation or rupture.

Metacarpophalangeal Dislocation of the Thumb

Like dislocations of the PIP joint, the most common direction of MCP dislocation is dorsal. A hyperextension force, with or without a torsional component, is the likely mechanism. The volar structures, especially the volar plate with its embedded sesamoid bones, become attenuated and may ultimately fail. The fate of the volar plate often determines whether a dislocation will be easily reducible or will require open reduction.

Before expanding on the frequently seen dorsal dislocation, we should mention that volar dislocation of the thumb MCP joint may be encountered. It represents more of a global instability resulting from extensive tearing of the dorsal capsule and even the extensor pollicis brevis tendon.[53, 104, 108, 119] Volar dislocation will most frequently require open treatment, including removal of interposed material, soft tissue reconstruction, and transarticular pin stabilization. In contrast to the long-term effects of a collateral ligament injury, stiffness is the chronic status of a global soft tissue injury resulting in a volar dislocation.

In dorsal MCP dislocations of the thumb, the most important determination is whether the injury is reducible by closed means (simple) or will require open reduction (complex). Many authors maintain that the determination of simple or complex can be made by observational and radiographic assessment alone. The true difference may instead lie in whether the dislocation can be reduced in the hands of an experienced surgeon by closed means. By this modified definition, the "simple" dislocation can be reduced by closed procedures. At times, even those dislocations that manifest some of the characteristics associated with the "complex" variety can be reduced by closed means, thus avoiding a trip to the operating room.

The simple dislocation, or subluxation, is the most striking with regard to physical findings. This is the thumb in which the proximal phalanx assumes a posture essentially 90 degrees to that of the metacarpal axis (Fig. 24B1–46). As vivid as this injury looks, it is relatively easy to reduce, with adequate anesthesia and re-creation of the deforming forces. A wrist block can be supplemented with an "intra-articular" injection (recognizing that the joint in this dislocation is distorted). The hydraulics of the injection may aid in displacing any interposed tissue and facilitate reduction.

One of the characteristics of the "complex" dislocation is the position of the proximal phalanx "parallel" to the metacarpal. It should not be assumed that this condition necessarily rules out closed reduction. The secondary finding of skin dimpling over the volar MCP area and the finding of the sesamoid position atop the metacarpal head

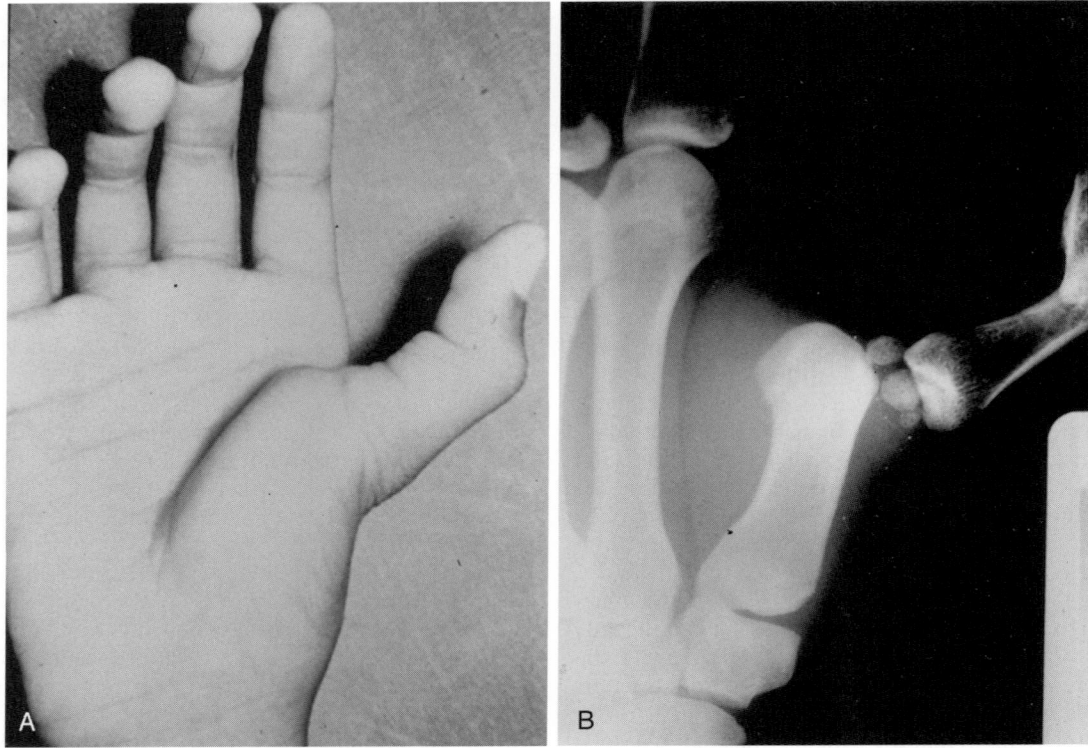

Figure 24B1–46. Clinical *(A)* and radiographic *(B)* images of a dorsal metacarpophalangeal joint dislocation of the thumb. Most often the result of a hyperextension force, dorsal dislocations are far more common than their volar counterparts.

are further heralds of a challenging reduction. These signs should alert the surgeon to the potential difficulty of closed reduction and to the advisability of a transfer from the emergency room to the operating room to attempt the closed procedure. In the complex dislocation, it is sound management to be prepared for open intervention by handling the closed treatment in the operating room.

If the reduction can be attained by closed methods, rehabilitation will be facilitated and return to play accelerated. The surgeon should attempt a closed reduction for almost every patient. This would include insufflating the "joint" with anesthetic to potentially float out the volar plate. The procedure should include hyperextension combined with an attempt to coapt the dorsal rim of the proximal phalanx and the dorsal aspect of the articular surface of the metacarpal head, then "dragging" the base of the proximal phalanx over the articular surface in an attempt to push the volar plate out of the joint. This approach will result in successful closed reduction in a reasonable fraction of these somewhat rare injuries.

It is possible to unintentionally convert a simple dislocation to a complex dislocation that requires open reduction.[41, 98] This potential problem, however, should not deter the initial examiner from attempting closed reduction when the environment has been optimized with relaxation, anesthetic, imaging, and experience. One of the key components to a successful closed reduction is wrist flexion posture to relax the flexor pollicis longus pull. There is no indication to open the successfully reduced dislocation for the purpose of repairing injured volar tissues.

If closed reduction of either the so-called simple or

complex dislocation is achieved, lateral stability should be checked to evaluate the integrity of the collateral ligaments. Anteroposterior translation, flexion, and extension should be checked while the thumb is still anesthetized. This thorough evaluation, with radiographs or fluoroscopic imaging, defines the adequacy of reduction and the stable arc. This will determine the position and length of immobilization.

As in the MCP dislocation of the triphalangeal digits, dorsal and volar exposures are both sound when the surgeon appreciates the pathoanatomy and potential pitfalls. Again, the digital nerves, even more central and subcutaneous in the thumb MCP dislocation, are at significant risk in the volar approach. That is why most surgeons advocate the dorsal exposure. The volar plate can be easily evacuated with a Freer elevator, and any inspection of the joint can be accomplished through this portal.

Often, the closed reduced thumb can be protected for rapid return to play, often within 7 to 10 days. Despite the fact that MCP soreness may linger, recovery of near normal motion and stability is the rule. It is not uncharacteristic to lose 10% of the flexion-extension arc, but this is well tolerated with mobile segments at the CMC and interphalangeal (IP) level.

The need to open the thumb to gain reduction delays the return to play. Thumb spica splinting, including the IP joint, is advisable to allow healing of the dorsal or volar skin incision and other volar tissues. It is reasonable to allow protected return to play at 2 to 3 weeks. The interval could include early mobilization, active and active-assisted motion only, to start at 3 days. Strengthening is deferred until motion recovery has exceeded 75%. Taping or orthosis wear is advisable for the remainder of the season of injury.

Chronic pain can accompany volar plate incompetence.[105, 142] The anteroposterior translation test will reflect the anatomic situation in which the volar plate is avulsed from the metacarpal volar recess and the accessory collaterals may likewise be torn from the margins of the volar plate. Soft tissue reconstruction may be contemplated, but this is a distinctly rare situation.

Authors' Preferred Method of Treatment. We emphasize our philosophy that essentially every patient with a thumb MCP joint dislocation deserves an attempt at closed reduction. This is true despite the presentation of a so-called complex dislocation. Even this category can be successfully treated in at least a subset without a trip to the operating room.

When the thumb MCP joint is irreducible, then we recommend a dorsal approach to open reduction. Again, this provides adequate ability to affect the reduction and inspect the joint and is safer with respect to the digital nerves of the thumb.

Collateral Ligament Injuries of the Thumb Metacarpophalangeal Joint

This topic has been the subject of numerous articles and even chapters in textbooks. This reflects the prevalence of the injury, the likelihood of the injury occurring in almost all sports, and the fact that essentially all surgeons will be asked to evaluate the injured thumb at some time in their career.

Because of the more common athletic posture of cylindrical grasp that leaves the thumb ray exposed for valgus stress, injury to the ulnar collateral ligament is predictably more common than that of the radial counterpart.[17, 32, 63, 106, 138] Some authors suggest, however, that radial collateral ligament injuries to the thumb MCP joint may account for nearly 40% of these injuries.[99] Radial collateral injuries are likely more common than appreciated, yet they represent a relatively small fraction of the total complement of thumb MCP-level disorders. In the senior author's (TJG's) practice, this is statistically true but the injury is usually seen in the ball-handling athlete.

Understanding the anatomy and mechanisms of injury is critical to developing a sound intellectual and technical approach to treatment of MCP soft tissue injuries. Melone and colleagues[99] summarized their clinical and laboratory experience with the anatomy and pathology about this joint as follows:

• The proper collateral ligaments are the main stabilizers of the thumb MCP joint to valgus and varus stress and are the most important structure to repair or reconstruct to return stability to the injured, destabilized thumb MCP joint.
• The accessory collateral ligaments, aponeuroses of the short abductor and adductor and the extensor pollicis brevis tendon, contribute static stability. Repair or reconstruction of these structures is critical in restoring stability when they are significantly compromised.
• Exclusion of the completely ruptured ulnar collateral

ligament from its metacarpal insertion is a uniquely ulnar-sided phenomenon, owing to the difference between the radial and ulnar musculature. There is no radial-sided correlate for the Stener lesion.
• Volar translation or subluxation, seen most vividly on a lateral radiograph of the thumb, is twice as prevalent (86% vs. 44%) in radial collateral injuries as ulnar collateral injuries, respectively. It is thought that the intact radial collateral ligament is a critical stabilizer combating the passive translation of the proximal phalanx volarward on the metacarpal head. This finding is consistent with the concept that global soft tissue injury and intrinsic muscle imbalance accompany radial collateral injuries more often than they accompany ulnar collateral ligament injuries.

Authors' Preferred Method of Treatment. It is surprising to many inquirers that our referral practice operates on fewer than 25% of the ulnar collateral ligament injuries we see resulting from athletic participation. The key for us is testing not only the characteristics of motion and deviation of the injured joint but mostly the quality of the end point.

If there is a strong suspicion of a complete tear of the ulnar collateral ligament, however, we advocate open repair. Interestingly, the rehabilitation programs for those more significantly injured thumbs treated by operative and nonoperative methods are remarkably similar. The predictability of direct inspection and repair outweigh the risks, especially in the elite athlete. Those thumbs with an identifiable Stener lesion should all be treated with open repair.

As far as technique, we have been using intraosseous suture anchors in preference to counterincisions or buttons. Additionally, we are getting away from joint pinning in most reliable patients, which diminishes the articular trauma and removes the risk of pin tract infection or pin breakage. It cannot be emphasized enough that the "complication" of IP joint stiffness can be largely minimized by carefully separating the capsular layer from the extensor mechanism upon closure. This is a technical error that can be easily avoided by understanding the anatomy and careful surgical execution.

In general, radial collateral ligament injuries are less prone to need acute or remote repair/reconstruction. In some ball-handling sports, however, especially basketball, the proclivity to sustain this injury and its effect on play must be considered.

Clinical Concepts: Radial Collateral Ligament Injuries

The first step in the overall approach to the radial collateral ligament injury is to maintain a high index of suspicion. The diagnosis itself is not difficult in this relatively subcutaneous injury, but the examiner may be reluctant to trust his or her intuition because this is not as "publicized" a pathologic process as the ulnar collateral ligament rupture. Tenderness, accentuated deviation to ulnar-directed stress, and inequity of germinal findings in contralateral comparison are the basic components of the diagnosis.

In the experience of the senior author (TJG), the acute radial collateral ligament injury is seldom associated with

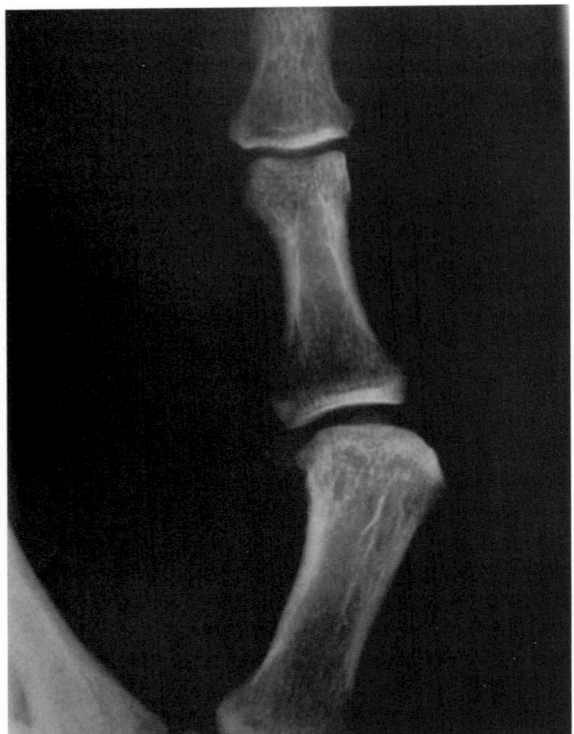

Figure 24B1–47. Patients with chronic instability of the radial collateral ligament of the thumb metacarpophalangeal joint usually present with a tender prominence of the radial aspect of the metacarpal head, which on radiography is seen to be due to volar and ulnar subluxation of the proximal phalanx onto the metacarpal.

bony manifestations, such as avulsion fracture or sesamoid injury. This does not excuse the examiner, however, from obtaining proper radiographs. Irregularity in the form of dystrophic calcification or osteophytosis is sometimes found in the chronic or neglected injury (Fig. 24B1–47).

The entire examination should be geared to two factors common to almost all soft tissue injury evaluation: inventory of injured structures and determination of the extent of ligament incompetence. Assuming the former can be discerned with relative facility by appropriate clinical and radiographic means, the focus is on the difference between a partial and a complete injury.

The proper collateral ligament injury is not usually isolated but is the most easily appreciated manifestation of the pathoanatomy. Palpation should be specific, and stress examination is used to determine which tissues are potentially embarrassed. Rarely, the handling of the thumb will be so painful that paroxysms of withdrawal will devalue the examination before adequate data are gleaned. In this situation, anesthetic block at the wrist level is suggested. Again, the first examiner on the sidelines may have the best shot at determining the extent of the injury before significant tenderness develops.

Some surgeons argue that an incomplete ligament injury, either radial or ulnar sided, can be converted to a complete injury by vigorous examination. It is very likely, however, that if the examination does bring final failure of the last vestige of an attenuated ligament, an operation was indicated anyway.

Like all soft tissue injuries, the treatment of the radial collateral ligament is dictated by the competence of the remaining ligament. There is a distinct difference in comparison with the ulnar collateral ligament (UCL) injury, however. Because the anatomy on the radial side of the joint does not include any soft tissue structures that routinely interfere with direct opposition of the torn ends of the ligament, such as the Stener lesion on the ulnar side, nonoperative treatment has a greater chance of success. In addition, the athlete will experience much less ulnar-directed stress of the thumb MCP joint.

For complete tears, open treatment is still advocated. Reattachment of the avulsed ligament back to (usually) the proximal phalanx through either pullout wire or suture anchor is performed as for ulnar collateral surgery. Joint pinning is the prerogative of the surgeon. Protection in a cast for 4 to 6 weeks is standard. If the athlete has a task through which he or she could play with such protection, then it is not unreasonable to contemplate return during the acute postoperative phase. Players should not return to play with a transarticular pin. After immobilization and pinning has been discontinued, many players can be adequately protected with a playing orthosis or strong taping. Motion recovery exercises should be diligently performed; there is little specific strengthening that is required above normal preparation for return to play.

Clinical Concepts: Ulnar Collateral Ligament Rupture

UCL rupture, also known as UCL sprain, gamekeeper's thumb (Fig. 24B1–48), or skier's thumb, is one of the most common, yet controversial injuries in both sports medicine

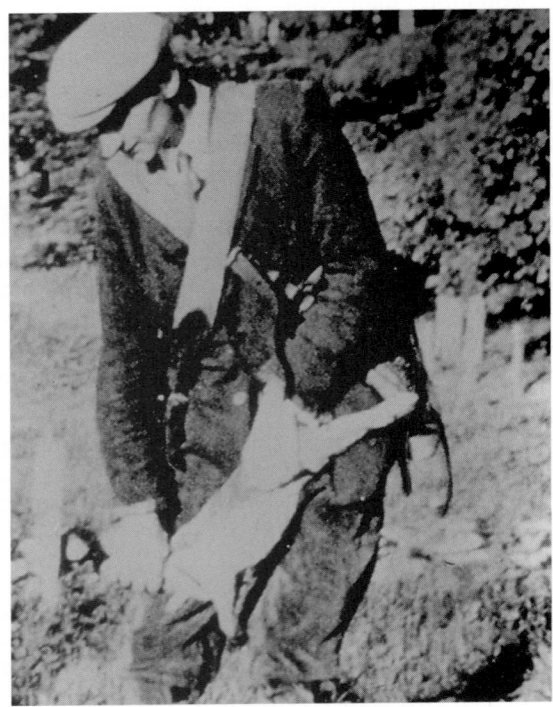

Figure 24B1–48. The "gamekeeper."

and hand surgery. This section summarizes the main concepts and provides a background for treatment of most injuries.

It is helpful to separate the key concepts. These include the subtleties of physical evaluation, the possible components of the diagnostic work-up, and the treatment recommendations matching various grades or extents of ligament injury.

Physical Examination

• Palpation of the ulnar side of the MCP joint immediately after the injury may reveal a tumescence that represents the distal edge of the displaced ulnar collateral ligament, the Stener lesion (Fig. 24B1–49).[141] This subtle finding may only be available in the period before swelling occurs, and thus it is critical to future treatment. Additionally, the player is often more compliant with stress examination directly after the injury, before significant tenderness develops.

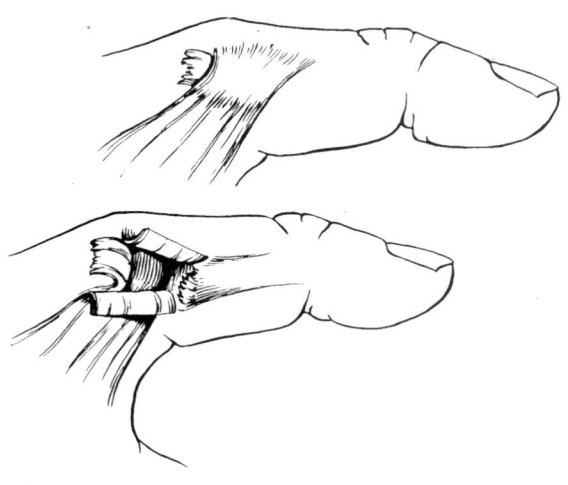

A

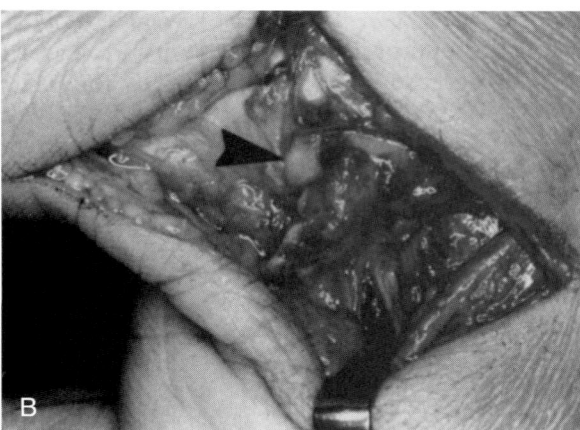

B

Figure 24B1–49. Stener's lesion seen in gamekeeper's (skier's) thumb. *A,* The distal end of the ulnar collateral ligament has been ruptured off the base of the proximal phalanx and is turned 180 degrees, facing proximally. The adductor tendon then becomes interposed between the torn end of the ligament and its site of insertion. *B,* At operation, the torn end of the avulsed ligament is seen end-on, just proximal to the adductor aponeurosis (beneath the *arrow*). Healing cannot occur until the tendon is repositioned into the base of the proximal phalanx.

• Besides palpation for ligament posture and point of maximal tenderness, the stress examination is perhaps the most critical physical examination maneuver. Anesthetic blocking (either local or wrist block) for enhanced examination abilities is a patient- and surgeon-specific decision.[13, 45, 72, 96, 107, 120, 122, 133, 135] Many patients will permit vigorous examination, whereas others will protest significantly, compromising any attempt at information gathering.

• Examination should be conducted by applying abduction or radially directed stress with the MCP joint in both neutral and flexed posture. The latter maneuver essentially isolates the UCL stabilization effect from that of the other ulnar-sided restraints.

• There is continued debate about the magnitude of deviation to radially directed stress that constitutes a UCL rupture versus an incomplete injury. Some investigators note absolute parameters in the range of 30 to 45 degrees[120, 138] or relative deviation compared with the contralateral side,[14] citing a difference of greater than 10 to 15 degrees as an indication of complete tear. It is probably advisable to keep the MCP joint flexed about 40 to 45 degrees and to attempt to reproduce this posture bilaterally.

• As with the absolute magnitude of deviation, the quality of the end point is an important indicator of ligament integrity. This is especially salient when one considers that the athlete may have sustained remote injuries to the thumb MCP joint and maintains an adjusted "baseline" with which he or she functioned well before the index event. For this reason, it is advisable to examine as many thumb UCLs as possible in the course of everyday practice. This will give the surgeon the experience to make the determination between a physiologic and pathologic UCL.

• One helpful adjunct in the diagnosis of UCL rupture is the in-office, low-radiation fluoroscopy unit. Performance of the stress examination under image intensification can yield clues about the behavior of a small bony fragment or depict the MCP relationship in maximal radial deviation (Fig. 24B1–50). Although additional imaging modalities will be discussed in the next section of this chapter, the combination of palpation, stress examination, and fluoroscopic evaluation remain the primary tools for diagnosis in these patients.

Imaging and Evaluation Modalities

• Plain radiographs should be used for all patients to detect the presence and extent of bony injury (Fig. 24B1–51). Injuries to the entire osteoarticular column of the thumb must be ruled out. Likewise, if there is a fracture of the ulnar margin of the proximal phalanx, its character must be assessed (Fig. 24B1–52). As noted by Louis and colleagues,[89] radiographs should predate vigorous examination (with the exception of the on-field assessment). Examination could displace a significant fracture, the only substantive damage an examination could cause. Imaging before embarking on stress evaluation of the swollen, ecchymotic thumb is sound management.

• Arthrography has been employed in several studies to determine the extent of MCP level injury and presence or absence of a Stener lesion.[13, 37, 84, 129, 131, 154] This is

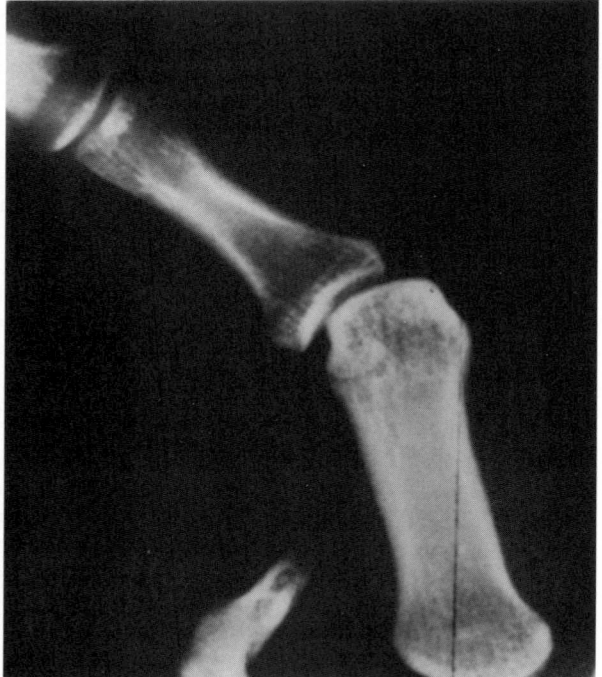

Figure 24B1–50. Stress radiographs of ulnar collateral ligament injuries of the thumb are indicated if complete rupture is not obvious on clinical examination.

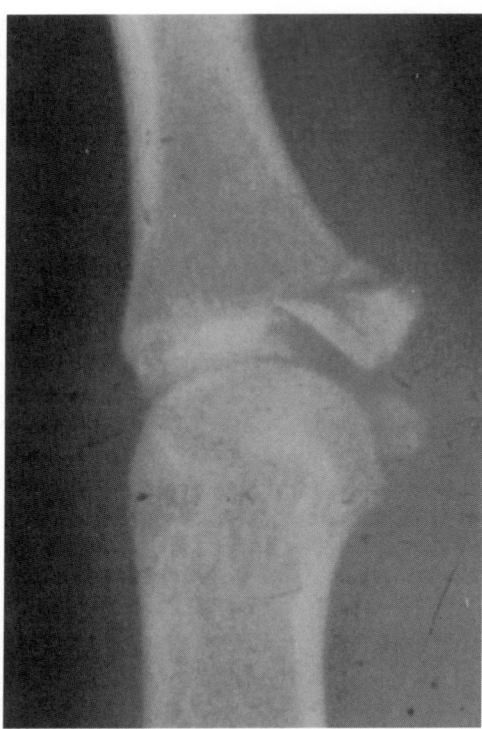

Figure 24B1–52. In a variant of gamekeeper's thumb, a large fracture fragment disrupts a significant portion of the articular surface. Open reduction with anatomic restoration is indicated.

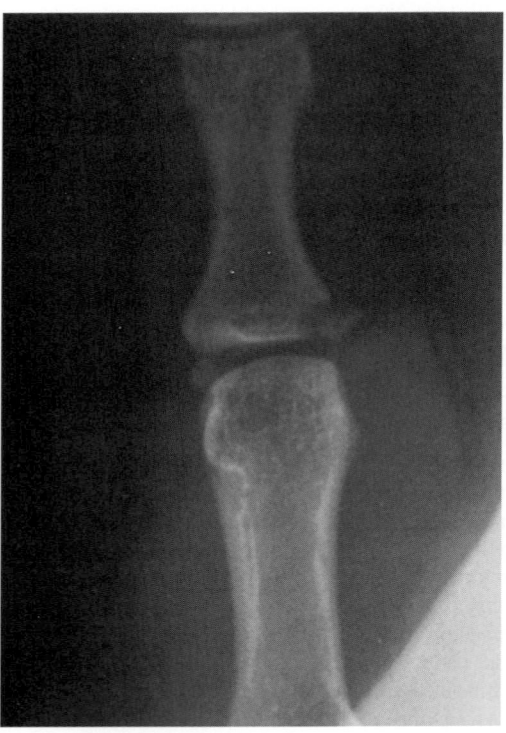

Figure 24B1–51. In a typical fracture seen in gamekeeper's thumb, a small fragment is avulsed by the ulnar collateral ligament.

usually performed by the surgeon, with the benefit of live imaging to see the tracking of the dye. Although there are theoretical advantages of this minimally invasive test, the diagnostic accuracy is unsatisfactory. It is a low risk–low reward maneuver that is best reserved for intellectual, not clinical, satisfaction.

• Magnetic resonance imaging coils, often called "wrist coils," have been designed for interrogation of the small joints and have permitted this modality to be used more effectively for injuries about the hand and wrist. The diagnostic accuracy of magnetic resonance imaging in evaluation of the ulnar collateral ligament injury, however, has not yet reached parity with its successes in the knee, for example.[88] Improvements in this technology could assist the surgeon in key determinations in those cases in which examination was equivocal and a player's season is in jeopardy if an operation is performed.

• Arthroscopy is finding its way into the evaluation and treatment of small joint problems. There are reports of thumb MCP arthroscopy for treatment of osteochondral fracture, and there are implications for diagnosis of a Stener lesion.[148] Perhaps there will be a day in the future when use of the in-office "needle scope" will supplement sound clinical examination in the diagnosis of this and other injuries about the hand.

Treatment

• Partial Tears: Except in the rare instance when circumstances surrounding an elite athlete pressure the medical team to make accelerated treatment decisions, 5 to 10 days of immobilization in a thumb spica splint with re-examination is a sound way to increase diagnostic accuracy. When the examiner is confident that a subtotal rupture or attenuation of the UCL has been sustained, this immobilization can be continued. Special orthoses can be made for the players who can participate effectively with protection. The regimen depends on the severity of the index injury, the premorbid status of the thumb, and the player's individual athletic situation. A reasonable plan, however, may include 2 weeks in a forearm-based thumb spica with the IP joint included, followed by wear of a hand-based orthosis (allowing wrist motion[126]) up to the fourth or fifth week. Taping may be sufficient after that period, but protection for at least the entire season of injury is logical. The athlete may need different splints to wear for practice and game time versus general protection for periods outside of sports.

- Complete Tears: Closed treatment of identifiable complete ruptures of the ulnar collateral ligament of the thumb has been advocated[22]; the more recent philosophy, however, has centered around anatomic repair.[45, 51, 85, 96, 118, 138] Strickland and Green enumerated three compelling reasons to perform this procedure: (1) Because the Stener lesion is present in a significant number of suspected complete tears (50% to 70%), and it is difficult to discern its presence with physical examination and imaging modalities, open treatment is warranted; (2) the operative repair is familiar to most surgeons and can be performed with minimal morbidity and excellent result; and (3) the primary repair is thought to yield superior results to late reconstructive options. A relative indication for open repair may be a fracture of sufficient size or displacement, yet general fracture principles should govern that process of decision making.

- Volar Subluxation: Melone and colleagues[99] found that volar subluxation of the proximal phalanx on the metacarpal may be more characteristic of a global injury about the MCP joint, including embarrassment of the capsule and volar and dorsal supporting structures. These authors concluded that the finding was more prevalent in significant radial complex injuries; yet the finding of volar subluxation related to an ulnar-sided injury may be an indication for open repair because it indicates severe tissue compromise.

Technique for Open Repair of the Thumb Ulnar Collateral Ligament

The basic elements of the reconstruction are shared between the popular techniques. The components include (1) reapproximation of the avulsed ligament to its native insertion; (2) handling of the adductor aponeurosis; and (3) repair of additional soft tissue injury about the MCP joint. These can be accomplished whether a pullout wire or suture anchor[152] (Fig. 24B1–53) is used for the germinal step. The other variable is transarticular pinning in an overreduced position advocated by some authors.[30]

The following tips and potential pitfalls should assist the surgeon undertaking this familiar technique. These suggestions are organized along the steps of the operative procedure.

- Skin Incision: Many approaches have been described, but are essentially variations on the same theme. It is advisable to avoid incisions that cross the dorsum of the MCP

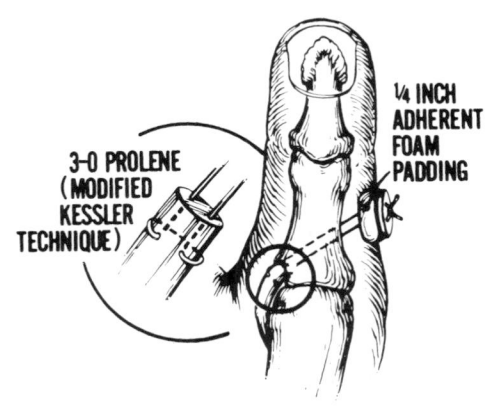

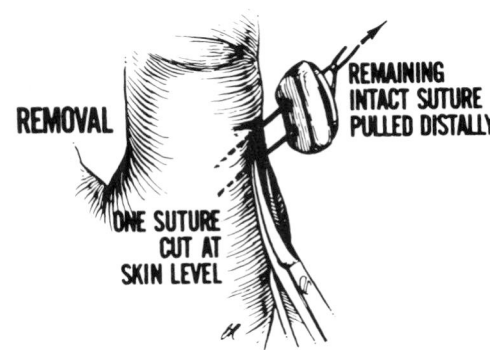

Figure 24B1–53. The preferred pullout technique. Prolene sutures are used because of their ease of use and because removal is less painful than with wire. Removal is accomplished by cutting one end of the suture and pulling through on the other. This type of pullout suture can be used in the hand for any situation in which a ligament or a tendon is sutured into bone. The use of suture anchors is largely replacing this technique.

joint because they can limit access to the important volar interface between the collateral ligament and volar plate; also, additional scarring around the extensors is always a potential problem. Locate the incision in the crease created when the thumb is maximally adducted. The incision is then carried distally at or just volar to the midaxial line. This allows access to all important structures and is actually cosmetic. It is helpful to avoid scarring; many athletes feel that scars provide a target for opponents (this appears particularly true in basketball).

- Aponeurosis Handling: The finding of a ruptured ligament excluded from its bed by the aponeurosis of the adductor confirms the diagnosis and tells the surgeon that the patient would likely have had an inferior outcome if he or she had not chosen surgery. Incising the aponeurosis longitudinally about 2 mm radial to the extensor allows enough tissue to close after repair of the UCL. Advancing the aponeurosis could add a modicum of additional tightness on the ulnar side, as would imbrication of the tissue, and these maneuvers are probably not necessary in the acute situation.

- Bed Preparation: Scarification of the native insertion can be done with a knife, pins, drills, and the like. If a pullout technique will be used, Keith needle drilling obliquely through the juxta-articular proximal phalanx may suffice. Likewise, when a suture anchor is employed, there is some exposure of the metaphyseal trabecular bone. It is probably not useful to "make a trough" in the phalanx, inasmuch as the healing will be at the periosteal level.

- Articular Inspection: Making sure that there was no chondral damage or preexisting arthrosis is the responsibility of the surgeon. This brief step is critical for possible important findings. Chronic findings are just as important to record. Loose body recovery and assessment of osteochondral defects are theoretical advantages of thorough inspection, yet they are found only rarely (Fig. 24B1–54).
- Soft Tissue Repair: Aside from the technique of ligament repair, some significant problems can arise from inadequate closure techniques. The UCL gets much publicity in this regard, but inappropriate handling of the volar plate, capsule, and extensor or adductor mechanisms can cause significant morbidity.

The importance of coapting the volar plate and collateral has been noted previously in this chapter. This is a key step that should be performed; recall the proximity of the radial digital nerve. It is critical to differentiate between the capsule and the extensor mechanism. Sewing all these dorsal tissues together results in IP joint stiffness, though the reasons for this are scarce. Much of the problem is probably the failure to separate the sagittal fibers of the extensor hood from the capsule, thus ensuring that the excursion of the thumb IP joint will be tethered. Passing a Freer elevator under the repair of the extensor and adductor to ensure their freedom from the capsule will nearly eliminate this IP motion loss and may significantly improve the player's ability to perform.

- Pinning: There is no right or wrong answer to the question of whether transarticular pinning should supplement the soft tissue repair. Arguments can be made for both

sides and are supported by the same data (compliance issues, protection through healing phase, and so forth). The additional articular trauma introduced by the pins is a calculated risk, but the specter of sepsis is one of the main arguments against pinning.

A few technical points on pinning can be noted. First, the concept of pinning the MCP joint in an over-reduced position should not be taken to the extreme. Excessive flexion and even articular malalignment can result from supplementary joint stabilization in nonanatomic postures.

Second, ligament reconstruction and tensioning must precede joint stabilization. Perform the soft tissue work first and test it before determining the joint posture and trying to make the fundamental repair conform to it.

Finally, drive the pin from the metacarpal side on the radial border and allow the tip (the leading 1 to 2 mm) to penetrate the ulnar cortex of the proximal phalanx. This is the easiest safeguard against the tragedy of intra-articular pin fracture. If the pin does break, it will invariably fail in the joint. If the distal tip is out of the proximal phalanx, a small counterincision will permit facile removal of one fragment, and the proximal aspect can be removed in the usual fashion. This precludes the need for arthrotomy and potential disruption of the repair.

Tendon Injuries: The Mallet Thumb

The terminal extensor disruption of the thumb extensor pollicis longus (EPL) is not common, especially in the general public. In the sporting world, however, when high forces and eccentric loads are common, this injury presents. There are some real differences between the mallet injury in the triphalangeal digit and that in the thumb. First, the EPL is much more stout at its terminus than the extensor

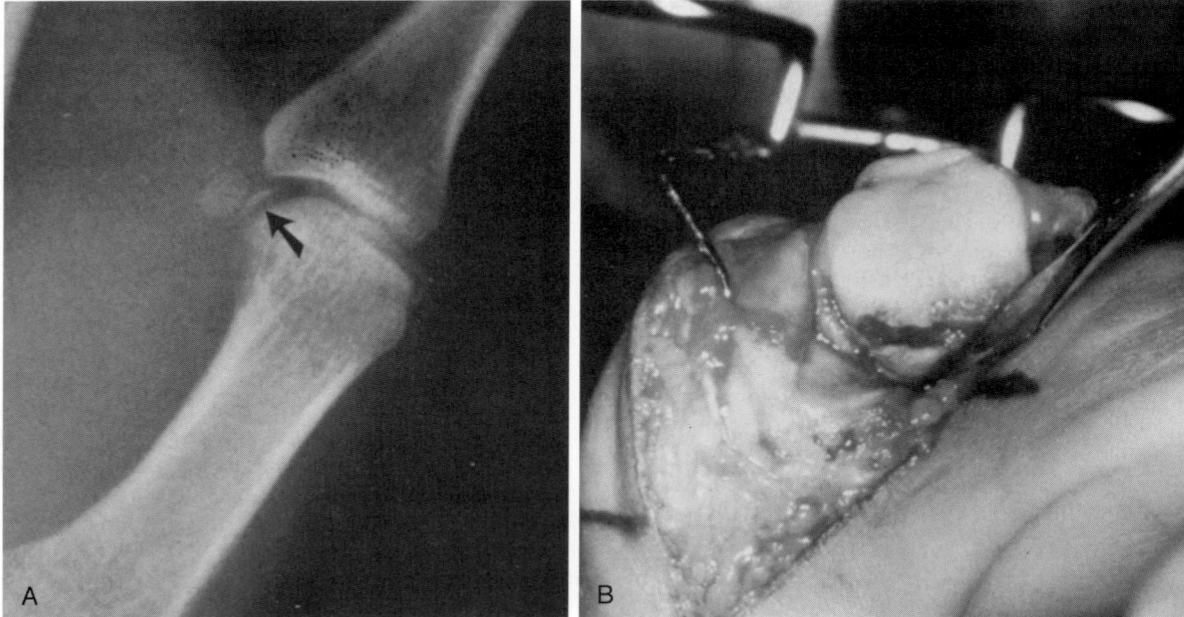

Figure 24B1–54. *A,* A less common fracture seen in gamekeeper's thumb is a shear fracture, visible radiographically on the volar side of the joint. It is important to explore the joint at the time of operation to look for shear fractures or osteochondral defects *(B).*

digitorum communis. The other is the significant range of motion arcs seen at the thumb IP level—some individuals have nearly 90 degrees of extension at the thumb IP and feel that they need to maintain a majority of that motion to remain effective at their sport.

Another distinguishing factor is the mechanism of injury. Typically, mallet thumb results from a very high-energy mechanism and the surgeon has to determine whether it was the collision with another player or between helmets that caused it rather than a simpler axial load against an extended distal phalanx. Fractures often accompany the untethered EPL and may actually be the result of a significant axial load that happened to fracture the area where the EPL inserts.

In any event, more serious consideration should be given to primary repair of the EPL failure. The basic elements of reattachment remain the same, although we have tried to stay away from pullout buttons on the thumb pulp. The EPL is usually of reasonable enough size, and the mobility of the IP joint permissive enough, that a suture anchor can be adequately tensioned. In larger patients who have a massive trauma around the joint, including capsular and collateral tearing concomitant with the EPL avulsion, the joint can be pinned for a period not exceeding 3 weeks. In rare instances when open injury or advanced maceration of the terminal tendon takes place, transposing the EPL to gain greater length for repair can be considered.

There is really not a good position for splinting of an EPL repair that still permits athletic participation. Abduction and relative extension makes the thumb ineffective and vulnerable to further injury, and "taping the thumb in" also presents little protection while rendering the patient-athlete unable to have cylindrical grasp. A period of about 5 to 6 weeks without play may be anticipated in these patients, regardless of treatment plan.

Authors' Preferred Method of Treatment

The extensor pollicis longus is simply more stout than the terminal extensor insertion of the triphalangeal digits. Repair should be considered primarily when the patient typically (contralateral comparison) maintains IP hyperextension. In some patients, a large bony fragment will accompany the tendon, and this is a more facile repair.

Special Categories

Vascular Syndromes

Vascular injuries in the athlete are extremely rare. Sports that require the athlete to endure activities that involve repetitive impacts to the hand and digits pose the greatest risk to the hand in the athlete. Vascular structures typically injured lie relatively superficial in the palm and thus are vulnerable when energy needs to be absorbed in such an area. Typical sports notorious for placing energy absorption demands on the front of the palm include martial arts, catching in baseball, handball, volleyball, lacrosse, and all of the racquet sports.[16, 114, 144, 147] Recognizing these high-risk sports makes it possible to teach modifications in

technique and protective garments and equipment, thus avoiding pathologic sequelae. This section focuses on the anatomy of the vessels of the hand and on the more common vascular syndromes that present in the athletic hand and wrist. These will include the hypothenar hammer syndrome, digital ischemia, ulnar artery thrombosis, and arterial aneurysms. Vascular injuries of more proximal etiology are discussed elsewhere in this volume.

Anatomy of the Vessels of the Hand

The ulnar and radial arteries are responsible for contributing the vast majority of the blood supply to the hand, with varying amounts resulting from a patent median artery. The ulnar artery provides the dominant supply of oxygenated blood to the ulnar three-and-a-half digits, and the radial artery the thumb and radial side of the index finger, with individual variations on this percentage.[21] The two main forearm vessels coalesce in the palm to form two vascular arches (Fig. 24B1–55). The superficial palmar arch is primarily supplied by the ulnar artery, and the deep palmar arch is mainly a tributary of the radial artery; however, each arch receives contributions from both arteries in 80% of individuals. When both arteries contribute to an arch, it is regarded as "complete." Circulation can be compromised with conversion from a complete arch to an incomplete arch by disrupting the flow of either the radial or ulnar artery.

The ulnar artery's supply to the superficial arch eventually branches to the common digital arteries, which further branch out to form the radial and ulnar proper volar digital arteries. Injury to the ulnar artery before it can supply

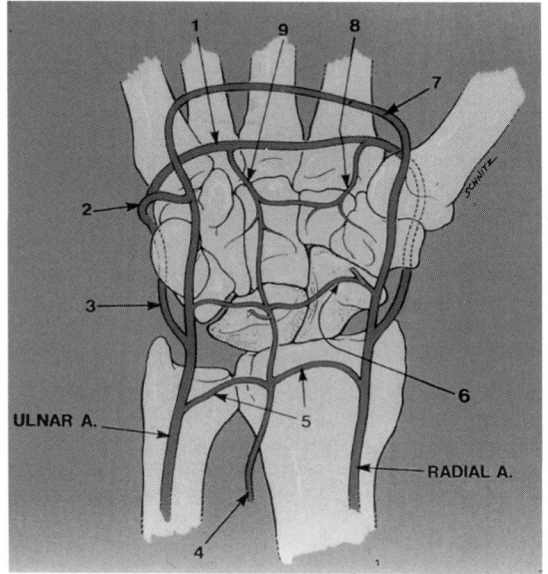

Figure 24B1–55. The two main arteries of the forearm anastomose to form two primary vascular arches in the palm. Most frequently, the ulnar artery will chiefly supply the superficial palmar arch, and the radial artery will chiefly contribute to the deep palmar arch. 1, deep palmar arch; 2, branch of ulnar artery to deep arch; 3, medial branch of ulnar artery; 4, palmar branch of intermediate artery; 5, palmar radiocarpal arch; 6, palmar intercarpal arch; 7, superior palmar arch; 8, radial rec. artery; 9, ulnar rec. artery.

the superficial arch can thus result in significant ischemic consequences. The ulnar artery negotiates the wrist through Guyon's canal, which is bordered by the hook of the hamate on the radial side, the pisiform on the ulnar side, by the pisohamate ligament dorsally, and by a fascial extension of the flexor carpi ulnaris called the volar carpal ligament on the canal's floor. The ulnar artery and its accompanying nerve are in most jeopardy immediately distal to the pisiform because the artery in this area lacks a fascial covering, lies superficial in the palm, and sits in close proximity to the hook of the hamate.[26] Repetitive stress in the form of microtrauma exposes this area of the vessel to potential injury and thus vascular-induced hand pain.[20, 115]

Hypothenar Hammer Syndrome

Long before its description in the athlete, the syndrome resulting from acute and chronic damage to the ulnar artery at the level of the wrist was causing pain and impeding function in a number of people who were using their hands as hammers (Fig. 24B1–56). Von Rosen first described the syndrome of ulnar artery thrombosis in 1934. He wrote that repetitive blunt injury resulted in intimal damage and subsequently causes the arterial thrombosis. Since then, Kornberg postulated that the thrombosis is actually an aneurysm that develops mural thrombi but which maintains a lumen.[79] True aneurysm formation would be attributed to damage in the tunica media with subsequent fusiform dilation of the vessel. False aneurysm formation, however, results from a laceration in a vessel wall that clots off to encapsulate the resulting hematoma. Here, the tunica media is left intact. Since Kornberg's postulate, aneurysms of the ulnar artery at the level of the wrist have been reported in football, basketball, lacrosse, and volleyball.[4, 5, 49, 59, 109] Ulnar artery thrombosis has been reported in baseball, karate, judo, handball, and hockey.[124]

Historically, however, hypothenar hammer syndrome occurs primarily in catching in baseball.[115] The athlete will complain of paresthesias in the ulnar digits, pain in the palm that can radiate into the forearm, and Raynaud's phenomenon.

Examination should focus on negating ulnar neuropathy as the diagnosis by assessing digital sensation, motor function, atrophy, and a Tinel's sign. With arterial etiology, the examiner may auscultate a bruit or palpate a thrill in the case of an aneurysm. The Allen test should demonstrate delayed cutaneous blush upon releasing occlusion of the radial artery. Atrophic and ischemic changes in the fingertips can be seen, and coolness in the fourth and fifth digits is common. Doppler examination, digital plethysmography, digital thermistors, B-mode ultrasonography, and radionuclide flow studies will confirm the diagnosis. Arteriography

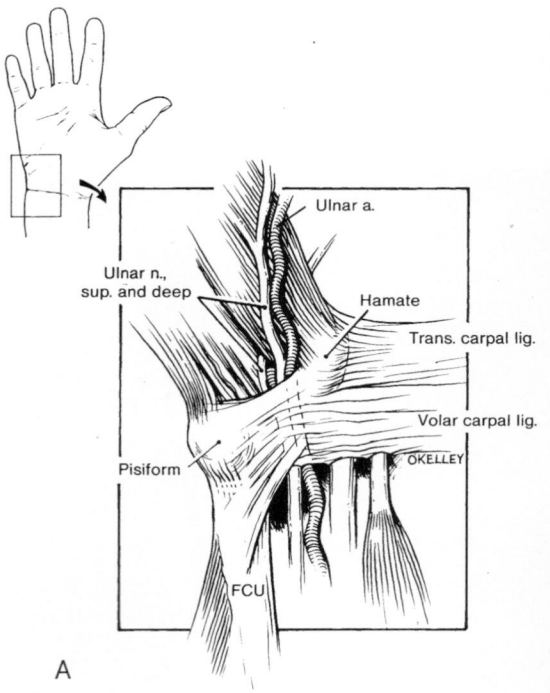
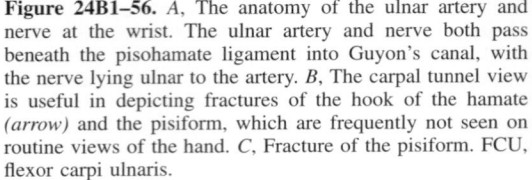
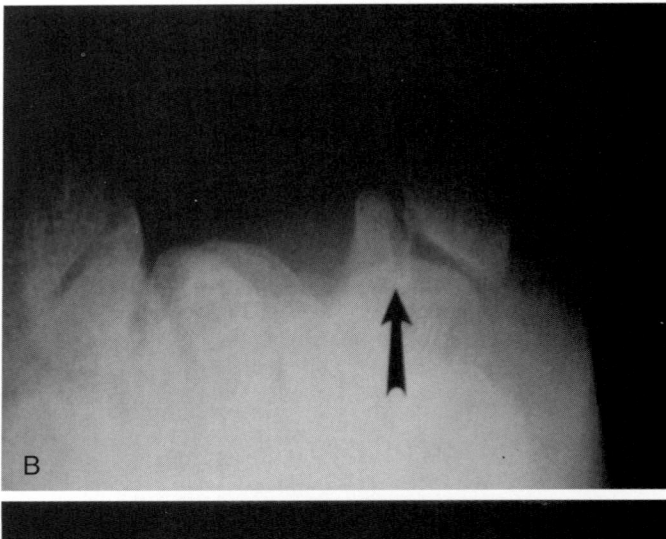
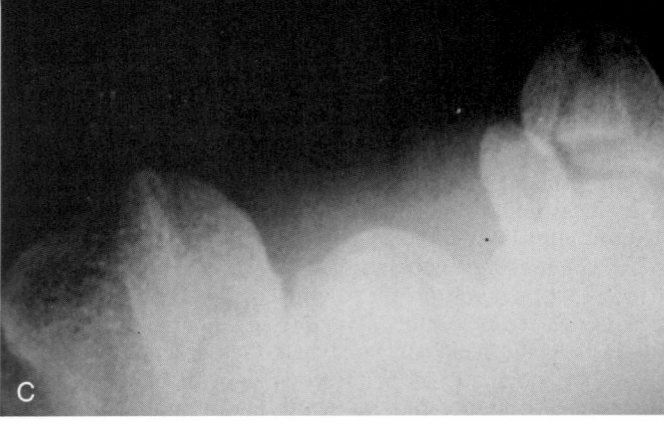

Figure 24B1–56. *A,* The anatomy of the ulnar artery and nerve at the wrist. The ulnar artery and nerve both pass beneath the pisohamate ligament into Guyon's canal, with the nerve lying ulnar to the artery. *B,* The carpal tunnel view is useful in depicting fractures of the hook of the hamate *(arrow)* and the pisiform, which are frequently not seen on routine views of the hand. *C,* Fracture of the pisiform. FCU, flexor carpi ulnaris.

should be reserved for those in whom arterial reconstruction is considered.[77]

Initial treatment should consist of rest followed by increased padding in the vulnerable sections of the hand. Sometimes this can reverse all symptoms; many elite athletes, however, may resist sacrificing any degree of their proprioceptive sensation when incorporating these pads into their gloves, racquets, sticks, and so forth. Cessation of smoking and the use of oral nicotine products can improve circulation. Oral vasodilators, sympatholytic agents, stellate ganglion blocks, and chemical clot lysis have each been tried with success.[68, 78] In severe cases, excision of an aneurysm or thrombosed segment of the ulnar artery with venous grafting performed by a hand surgeon skilled in microsurgical technique may be indicated.[82, 115]

Digital Ischemia

Not unlike hypothenar hammer syndrome, digital ischemia in the athlete is typically a result of repetitive microtrauma to the palm, but at a more distal level. Handball, baseball, karate, softball, Frisbee, football, and volleyball have been reported as sports in which participants have encountered symptomatic digital ischemia.[12, 15, 21, 61, 114, 144, 147] Again, not unlike hypothenar hammer syndrome, catching in baseball still poses what seems to be the highest risk for developing hand pain secondary to this ischemic phenomenon. For at least two reasons, catchers will most often develop ischemic changes at the tip of the index finger of their glove hand. First, the tip of the index finger is the watershed area of digital blood supply between the supply of the ulnar and radial arteries. Second, the main impact of the baseball in a catcher's mitt is in the area of the metacarpal head of the index finger.[91] In a study of 22 minor league catchers, Lowrey reported that 95% had normal Doppler flow measurements in their throwing hand, whereas only 41% had normal flow measurements in their glove hand.[91] Many authors have demonstrated changes in digital perfusion after the addition of padding for the palm in the handball glove and catcher's mitt.[15, 91, 115, 144] In Lowrey's study, all of the 41% of players with normal flow in their glove hand used additional padding, whereas in the abnormal flow group, nearly half of the players did not use any additional padding. The development of symptoms of digital ischemia has also has been shown to correspond with increased accumulated playing time.[144] There have also been reports of baseball pitchers developing ulcerations at the tip of the index finger of their throwing hand.[67]

The athlete will complain of mild pain in the finger, numbness, cold weather intolerance, and paleness of the digit. The physical examination often reveals a finger that is pale, cyanotic, and, in severe cases, has ulcerations forming at the fingertip. The Allen test can be positive. The throwing athlete may also be able to hyperextend the PIP joint of the involved finger, possibly causing Cleland's ligaments to tent the digital artery and impede perfusion. Noninvasive ancillary studies such as thermography, digital ultrasonography, and plethysmography can aid in making the diagnosis. Radionuclide flow studies and arteriography can also show changes in vessel patency.

Initial treatment is again conservative. Smoking and oral nicotine products should be discontinued. Padding is the mainstay of treatment, but many athletes can be reluctant to adhere to a physician's or trainer's recommendations. Catchers will explain that they lose their feel for the ball hitting their mitt and have the tendency to drop more balls. Handball players will respond that they can hit the ball harder with a thinner glove. Nevertheless, it must be stressed that noncompliance with equipment modifications can lead to chronic symptomatology and irreversible ischemic changes that may shorten their athletic career.

Sympatholytic medications can be tried, as well as vasodilating drugs, calcium channel blockers, and topical nitroglycerin ointments and creams. If ulcerations are unresponsive to equipment modifications and pharmacologic therapy, surgical intervention with a digital artery sympathectomy may be indicated.[155] In the case of the throwing athlete with hyperextensibility of the PIP joint, release of Cleland's ligaments in the involved digit on both sides of the finger and/or surgical release of a hypertrophic lumbrical and surrounding vertical septa may facilitate the return to play. Awareness on the part of coaches, trainers, and parents of the at-risk positions in baseball can lead, it is hoped, to the prevention of these vascular syndromes.

Authors' Preferred Method of Treatment. It is of utmost importance to recognize that there are numerous manual manifestations of systemic diseases. It is incumbent on the hand surgeon or sports medicine physician to consider a wide array of underlying disorders when players present with vascular embarrassment. This includes lifestyle decisions such as tobacco use, which is prevalent in some sports.

The cornerstone of care is a systematic work-up of the player's general health and specific hand symptoms. Freely obtaining consultation from experienced parties (radiologists, vascular medicine physicians and surgeons, internists, and so forth) is simply good care.

The Nail

Injury to the fingertip and/or nail bed is by far the most common hand injury for the simple reason that when the hand is withdrawn from potential harm, the ends of the fingers, particularly the longer central fingers, are the last to be removed. Although nail bed injuries rarely cause long-term serious disability for the athlete, they may preclude the quick return to competition if handled improperly.

Anatomy

The nail bed is a collection of the dorsal nail, the intermediate nail, and the ventral nail (Fig. 24B1–57). The dorsal nail is produced by the dorsal roof of the nail fold. The intermediate nail originates from distal to the extensor tendon and extends to the distal lunula. Otherwise known as the germinal matrix, it is the main mass of the nail and is formed from the ventral floor and lateral walls of the nail fold and is intimately related to the dorsal periosteum of the distal phalanx. The germinal matrix is primarily responsible for the growth of a new nail. The terminal edge of the germinal matrix is easily seen just distal to the

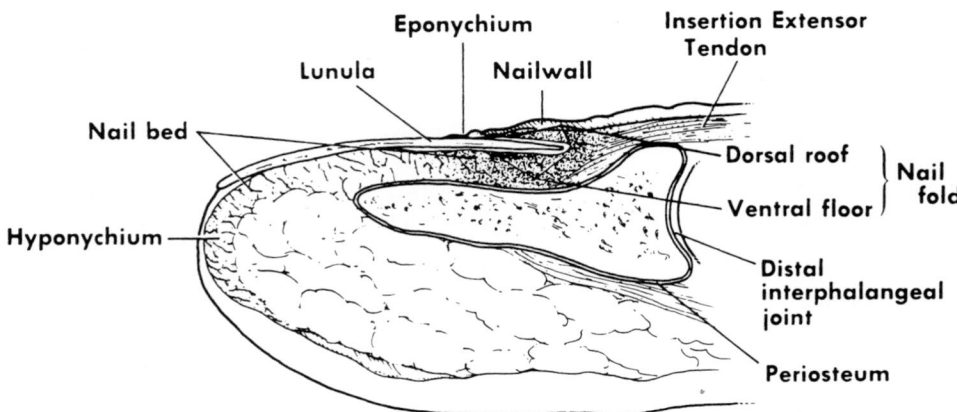

Figure 24B1–57. The anatomy of the nail bed is shown in sagittal section. (From Zook EG, Brown RE: The perionychium. In Green DP, Hotchkiss RN, Peterson WC [eds]: Green's Operative Hand Surgery, 4th ed. New York, Churchill Livingstone, 1999, p 1353.)

cuticle as a blanched, opaque structure that is convex along the distal margin. The third component, the ventral nail, begins at this distal margin of the germinal matrix and extends to the edge of the fingertip. It is otherwise known as the sterile matrix.

Injury Patterns

The athlete can sustain any of five different grades of nail bed injuries. In increasing order of treatment complexity, they are (1) subungual hematoma; (2) simple nail bed laceration; (3) complex nail bed laceration; (4) avulsion of the nail, and (5) complex injury with loss of the nail bed. Regardless of the pattern of injury, immediate repair of the nail to prevent deformity and hasten return to athletic competition is recommended.

Radiographs should be taken to look for phalangeal fractures. The treating physician must remember that stability in the distal phalanx is imperative when providing the optimum environment for nail bed healing (Figs. 24B1–58 and 24B1–59).

Subungual Hematoma

Historically neglected, the subungual hematoma likely represents an injury significant enough to disrupt an underlying vessel. Sometimes an intolerable source of pain for the participating athlete, the accumulating hematoma should be decompressed by trephining the nail plate with either a hand-held battery-powered cautery or even the heated blunt end of a paper clip. Perhaps the most effective and safest technique for relieving the pressure is to "drill" a hole in the nail plate with an 18 gauge needle; usually the surgeon will have to have a syringe attached simply for leverage in twisting the needle.

Either procedure should be done under sterile techniques. The treating physician should be mindful to create a bore in the plate wide enough not to become sealed by the underlying seared blood,[113] but at the same time not injuring the deeper matrix. We have found that these decompressions can be done safely and comfortably without anesthetic. Immediate return to play is allowed.

When the subungual hematoma occupies greater than 25% of the surface of the nail, a likely laceration exists in the matrix. This can only be seen by removing the nail plate and directly examining the matrix. For this we recommend a digital lidocaine block followed by application of a tourniquet. Digital tourniquets can be made by using a Penrose drain or placing a sterile glove on the patient's hand, cutting a hole in the tip of the affected finger, and rolling the latex proximally to the base of the finger. The matrix must be completely inspected and repaired.

Simple Laceration

After digital lidocaine block, tourniquet application, and removal of the nail plate, the simple laceration can be repaired with direct apposition of the lacerated ends under loupe magnification. If the cuticle is also lacerated, we repair this first with 5–0 nonabsorbable monofilament. In the matrix itself, we have found success using 6–0 chromic gut suture, taking care to observe meticulous technique in passing the needle because the matrix is friable and can easily be torn if the curve of the needle is not followed. Replacing the nail plate acts as a biologic splint and protects the repair. When the nail plate is not available, Xeroform (Sherwood Medical, St. Louis, Mo), Adaptic (Johnson & Johnson, Arlington, Tex), artificial nail splints,[117] or metal foil from a suture package should be used to cover the bed and to keep the nail fold open to prevent adhesions.[19]

Complex Lacerations

Higher energy injuries can result in a burst or stellate laceration in the matrix. These higher energy injuries often are associated with underlying distal phalangeal fractures, and thus radiographs should be routine. Nondisplaced fractures can be splinted, but displaced intra-articular patterns should be provisionally fixed with small K-wires for 3 weeks to prevent chronic deformity and early arthritic changes.

The fragments of a burst matrix should be repaired as best as possible. Even fragments not well held with 6–0 chromic gut should be patched in voids as free grafts to maximize the athlete's potential to re-create a complete foundation on which a new nail plate can adhere.

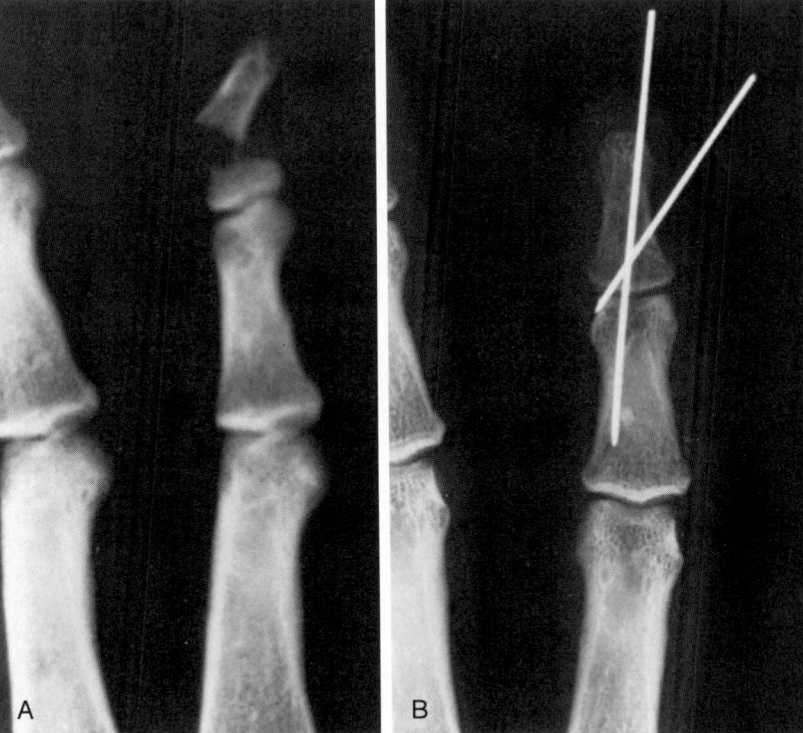

Figure 24B1–58. *A,* A widely displaced fracture through the base of the distal phalanx in a weight-lifter. *B,* This was treated with open reduction and internal fixation with Kirschner wires before the nail bed was repaired.

Avulsions

In this injury pattern, a portion of the sterile matrix often is avulsed with the nail plate. The matrix often can be found still attached to the plate and can thus be incorporated into the repair. No effort should be made to separate the matrix from the undersurface of the nail plate because it is easily friable and can be macerated in the process. Instead, after other lacerations are repaired, the nail plate can be replaced in a manner that allows the avulsed portion of sterile matrix to set in a void as a form of "free" graft. The nail plate itself should be secured to the soft tissue with nonabsorbable sutures either directly or through predrilled holes in the plate.

Complex Injury with Loss of the Nail Bed

In the event that a portion of the nail bed is avulsed and not available for grafting, any small defects can be covered with either a split-thickness skin graft or a reverse dermal graft. If the defect is more substantial, efforts should be made to reconstruct the matrix with a split-thickness matrix graft from another finger[145] or from a toe.[95, 160] The physician should harvest only the most superficial surface of the matrix and avoid any full-thickness defects in the donor nail bed by ensuring that the graft remains thin enough to be diffusely translucent.

Postoperative Care

Each of these wounds should be dressed with Vaseline or bismuth-impregnated gauze cut in the shape of a nail. If the nail plate is available, it can be replaced under the eponychium to prevent adhesions and act as a splint, and may be sewn in with nonabsorbable monofilament in particularly loose stitches. The hand must be elevated for a week, and the dressing can then be removed. Sutures can be removed in 7 days, but the absorbable catgut in the nail bed ought be left alone unless infected. The finger heals quickly, and the nail bed becomes relatively hard and

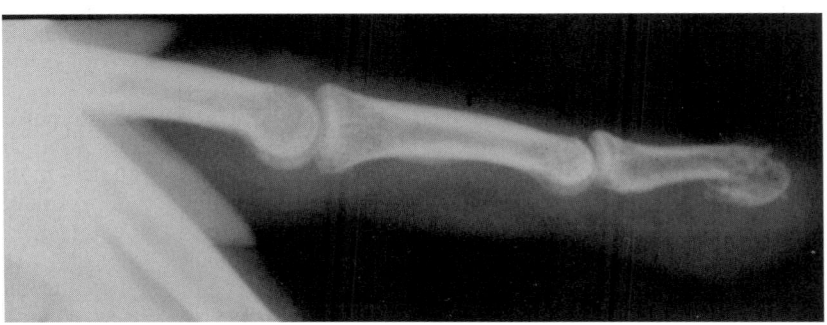

Figure 24B1–59. Inherently stable fractures of the nonarticular portion of the distal phalanx can be treated without internal fixation despite significant nail bed disease. This, however, does not preclude the need for external splinting and a relative delay in returning to athletic participation.

nontender by 2 weeks.[42, 113] It will take another 3 to 6 months before the new nail fully grows back.[3, 42, 113, 132]

Return to Play

The athlete with a nail bed injury will often be pressured by any number of outside sources, in addition to himself of herself, to return to competition immediately. Different athletes will need varying time out of competition, depending on the particular demands placed on their hands and affected digits. We recommend that an athlete can return to play in an AlumaFoam splint immediately if pain free and protected. If the affected digit is critical to optimal performance in the scenario of some elite athletes, we recommend delay in return to play until 2 weeks, or when the nail bed is hardened and not painful. After this time, no nail plate or synthetic splint is typically necessary. A shaft fracture of the distal phalanx may not delay the return to play, but an intra-articular fracture or one requiring pins for 3 weeks will often delay the athlete from returning to elite competition for 4 to 6 weeks, depending on the usefulness of the finger.

Authors' Preferred Method of Treatment

The treatment of nail bed injuries is relatively well documented. The specific problem we have found is the underestimation of injury severity in the athlete. If there is significant subungual hematoma but the nail plate has remained in its folds, decompression with a hypodermic needle used as a "drill" is advocated.

When the nail is avulsed from the folds, especially the proximal fold, we advocate formal nail removal and inspection of the germinal and sterile matrices. At worst, the soft tissue injury, and of course any distal phalanx fracture, can be appropriately addressed. At best, if there is only minimal soft tissue injury, the player can participate without a nail plate without the undue risk of injury.

Nerve Compression Injuries

Compression neuropathies in the athlete result when a limited segment of a peripheral nerve forfeits a portion of its vascular supply in response to a stronger structural element. In the general population, these elements can be intravascular (i.e., hypertension, thrombus, emboli) or extravascular (any adjacent osseous or soft tissue). In the athlete, the offending element is typically inflammatory tissue developing in an area of overuse that compromises a vessel's ability to perfuse peripheral nerve adequately. This inflammatory tissue can result from direct trauma but in the athlete is most likely secondary to repetitive stress producing compression and traction on the nerve and its adjacent tissues.

Focal anatomic locations are notorious for their predisposition for such conditions, and many of these lie in the elbow, forearm, and wrist. Therefore, the care for the athlete's hand demands attention that extends far proximal to the palmar crease. A full neurologic examination on every athlete with complaints about the hand will afford the treating physician the best chance of discovering the true cause of sometimes nondescript symptoms.[38, 39] Knowledge of the anatomy of peripheral nerves, their courses through the upper extremity, and, in particular, the narrow anatomic tunnels through which they pass, is necessary to diagnose and treat the athlete's hand. When discovered early, most of the conditions mentioned in this section can be effectively treated conservatively. On only rare occasions will symptoms be so severe as to preclude a full return to athletic competition.[87]

Compression neuropathies of the upper extremity are well outlined in previous chapters. Compression neuropathies of the hand resulting from disorders that develop distal to the carpus are outlined in this chapter.

Bowler's Thumb

Bowler's thumb is a perineural fibrosis of the ulnar digital nerve of the thumb that may involve the subcutaneous tissues as well as the flexor sheath.[28]

The entity was reported frequently in the early 1970s,[28, 31, 61, 102] but not much more has been written on the topic since then. Nonetheless, it is probably still a very common problem. The bowler will complain of paresthesia in the thumb in the distribution of the ulnar digital nerve, which may either be persistent or, more commonly, associated with pressure. Hyperesthesia and tenderness are also common, and a Tinel's sign may be present over the nerve. The skin itself is often thickened as a result of the frequent pressure and friction over the ulnar margin of the thumb. Although the nerve is often thickened, sometimes the bowler can be mistakenly believed to have a ganglion.

Microtrauma to the ulnar digital nerve is a result of the repetitive gripping and release of the ball. Many experienced bowlers are aware of the symptoms of bowler's thumb and will modify their grip accordingly or have the thumb hole of the ball redrilled to alleviate pressure on the ulnar aspect of the thumb. Decreasing the depth of insertion of the thumb into the thumb hole may also alleviate this problem.[28] When changing grip and delivery do not help, the use of a protective thumb shell, as advocated by Dobyns and associates,[28] is recommended.

Surgical treatment is rarely necessary. Surgical transposition, with or without neurolysis and neurolysis in situ, have all been recommended, with equivocal results.[28, 31, 61, 102] When the nerve is found to be redundant, it is preferable to perform a meticulous dissection of the perineural fibrosis followed by a dorsal ulnar transposition. Regardless of the surgical approach, the bowler cannot resume playing for at least 6 weeks, and the use of a postoperative protective device is recommended for the rest of the bowler's career.

Bowler's finger, a much less common entity, has also been reported.[94] Perineural fibrosis of the dorsal branch of the radial digital nerve of the ring finger can result in a clinical picture analogous to that in the thumb.

Generally, bowler's thumb responds well to conservative treatment. Alternatives in grip and adjustments in delivery, along with a trial of a protective orthosis, are the mainstays of treatment. Surgery is indicated only in refractory cases. Recovery can be long, and recurrence can be frequent.

Handlebar Palsy

In 1975, Smail reported on an entrapment of the motor branch of the ulnar nerve that was associated with long-distance bicycle riding. When riders need to maximize the strength of their pedaling, they lean forward, transferring their weight from their ischia to the palms of their hands. This increase in torque at the pedals has a reactive torque at the palms interfacing with the handlebar. In Smail, who was both the author and the patient, a low ulnar nerve palsy resulted after 2 weeks of riding. His symptoms resolved after a 2-month abstinence from riding. The application of padding to the handlebars or wearing padded gloves can both prevent and help treat this problem (Fig. 24B1–60).[57]

Authors' Preferred Method of Treatment

These player/patients fall into one of two categories: patients with underlying nerve problems and those with sports-specific nerve embarrassment. The first issue is to determine which is the predominant scenario for your patient. When the latter description is most fitting, equipment and technique changes can be effective.

If the neuropathy is advanced and surgical criteria are met, the procedure can usually be done on an elective basis at the conclusion of a season.

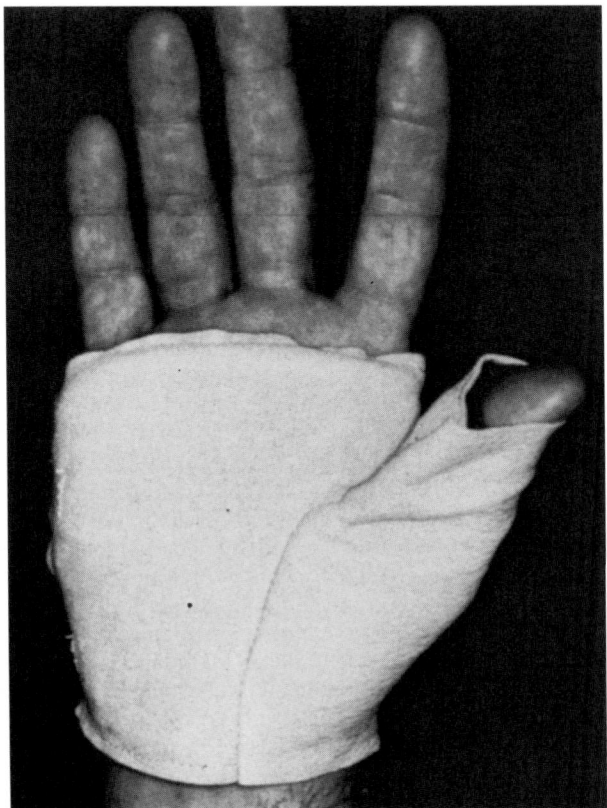

Figure 24B1–60. A prefabricated antivibration glove (Steel Grip, Danville, Ill) may be useful for some athletes, such as cyclists.

Splinting and Rehabilitation

Splinting of the athletic hand injury in competition needs to protect the injured part effectively as well as allow it and the rest of the extremity to function at maximum capacity. The short-term goal of return to play, however, should not supersede the long-term goal of restoration of hand strength and joint mobility.

As emphasized throughout the chapter, the team approach is imperative when managing the injured hand in the athlete. The trainer, physician, and therapist need to work together and communicate to ensure that the athlete's best interests are respected. Furthermore, a clear protocol for activity and management needs to be outlined and coordinated with all members of the treatment team to guarantee that no conflicting agendas interfere with sound medical management. Finally, when developing a management strategy for the injured hand, the treatment team must give attention to the rules drafted by the governing bodies of the particular level of the sport to maintain compliance and eligibility for participation.

This final section of the chapter emphasizes general splinting principles, rules and regulations regarding splints and braces, popular materials for fabrication of splints and braces, and the rehabilitation of the injured hand.

General Principles

Basic tenets must be observed when splinting athletic hand injuries. During the initial phase of injury, static splints keep the injured part at rest in a position that eventually facilitates prompt healing with little additional stress. Only when motion of adjacent uninjured joints does not jeopardize tissue healing can gentle range of motion exercises be commenced. Splints may be designed to allow motion in planes that do not compromise tissue healing while limiting motion in directions that potentially may delay ultimate healing. When joint stiffness is an active or potential problem, dynamic splints can be instituted to facilitate a rapid recovery of active and passive range of motion while continuing to protect the injured tissues.

The quality of the splint is critical to the ultimate success of treatment of the injured athletic hand. It is clear, therefore, that an orthotist properly trained in treatment of athletic hand injuries and sensitive to all their needs can optimize their treatment. Whether these professionals, however, are skilled in the treatment of athletes or not, the higher rule of frequent communication between the orthotist and the physician and trainer always will afford the athlete the most comprehensive care. A good working relationship with the orthotist only makes the treatment team stronger.

Rules and Regulations Concerning Splints and Braces

The physician treating high school or college athletes must be familiar with the rules governing competition in his state or conference. This is not always easy, because considerable confusion exists about what types of splints are allowed to be worn by athletes in competition, especially in football. One of the major reasons for this is that there are at least two major organizations that publish football rules: (1) the National Collegiate Athletic Association (NCAA), which governs most college athletics; and (2) the National Federation of State High School Associations (NFSHSA), which oversees most, but not all, high school competition. For example, Texas does not belong to the NFSHSA, but instead uses the NCAA rules. The confusion stems from two diametrically opposing statements regarding the use of hard splints, as follows.

The NCAA rules[111] state that illegal equipment includes "hard, abrasive or unyielding substances on the hand, wrist, forearm or elbow of any player *unless* covered on all sides with closed cell, slow-recovery foam padding no less than one-half-inch thick or an alternate material of the same minimum thickness and similar physical properties."

The NFSHSA rules,[112] conversely, prohibit any "elbow, hand, wrist, or forearm guard or brace made of sole leather, plaster, metal or other hard substance in its final form, and *even though* covered with soft padding."

Therefore, strict interpretation and enforcement of these rules would make it illegal for a high school player in most states (excluding Texas) to wear any type of hard splint (plaster, fiberglass, or plastic), even if it is covered with foam padding.

Further confusion arises because, in many jurisdictions, the final determination as to what type of splint a high school or college player can wear is left to the discretion of the game officials.

If the athlete is permitted to wear a hard splint, we prefer a standard fiberglass cast for injuries requiring full-time immobilization, and a plastic orthosis for those requiring only protection during practice and games. Both of these must of course be padded during competition. If the athlete is playing under rules that forbid a hard cast, we then prefer the silicone rubber splint originally described by Bassett and coworkers[6] and subsequently popularized by Bergfeld and associates[10] (see description of RTV-11, Table 24B1–1.) These rubber splints are heavy and do not allow the skin to breathe, and therefore they are worn only during practice and games. A plastic orthosis is worn at all other times.

Types of Splints

Adhesive Tape

Athletic trainers are masters with adhesive tape, and it is a delight to watch the speed and efficiency with which a skilled trainer can tape an ankle or wrist. Adhesive tape alone, however, provides very little support, and its functional use in the hand is primarily in the form of buddy taping, in which an injured finger is securely taped to an adjacent normal digit. For the thumb, minimal protection but perhaps some psychological effect can be gained from the use of an adhesive tape thumb spica splint. When taping the thumb or wrist, care must be taken to avoid

wrapping too tightly to avoid swelling of the hand distal to the circumferential tape about the wrist.

Padded Aluminum Splints

These readily available and versatile splints are useful particularly when only a single joint needs to be splinted, for example, the DIP joint for mallet fingers and the PIP joint for boutonniere lesions. The metal part of the splint must be trimmed to eliminate sharp edges, the splint securely taped to the digit, and the entire splint covered with a thin layer of soft padding to prevent injury to other players.

Synthetic Rubber and Plastic Splints

When an athlete is returned to competition with a healing injury that requires protection, this is best provided with a custom-made orthosis designed to protect the injured part. There are many different types of splinting materials available, the various properties and qualities of which are described later. It is neither feasible nor necessary to have all of these materials on hand, for many of the commercially available products have similar characteristics. The therapist, however, must be familiar with the various types of splinting materials and have available materials representing each type.

Materials

An appreciation of the unique characteristics and properties of each material allows the splint maker to determine the optimum type to be used for the support and protection of a particular injured part. Table 24B1–1 lists the material type, trade name, characteristics, and manufacturer of some of the most commonly used splinting materials.

It can be seen that many products with differing characteristics are available and, when used correctly, they can prove valuable and effective in splinting the injured hand of the athlete. Most athletic hand splinting uses low-temperature thermoplastic materials, the majority of which are plastic combined with varying amounts of rubber. A high content of plastic generally gives the material good drapeability and contour, whereas the amount of rubber determines the elasticity and memory. Most low-temperature thermoplastics may be softened at about 160°F by the use of wet or dry heat. Working times vary according to manufacturer, but usually fall between 3 and 6 minutes.

We have found the use of two materials, Polyform and Orthoplast, to be versatile enough for most athletic hand-splinting situations. Polyform, with its high plastic content, has excellent stretching and molding capabilities, producing an exact fit with good contour. When cured, Polyform is quite rigid, with little flexibility. Orthoplast, in contrast, has a higher rubber component, which provides better flexibility and elasticity. These characteristics make Orthoplast the preferred material for larger, more circumferential types of splints, where exacting contour is not so important. Polyflex II and Aquaplast-T are two other splinting materials that may prove useful in specific instances. Polyflex II provides flexibility for circumferential splints

TABLE 24B1–1
Splint Materials

Material	Features	Manufacturer
Splint Materials **Low-Temperature Thermoplastics**		
Polyform (plastic polymer)	Good drapeability with excellent stretch No memory Excellent contourability Excellent rigidity and impact strength	Smith and Nephew Rolyan, Inc. N93 W14475 Whitaker Way Menomonee Falls, Wis 53051
Polyflex (plastic polymer and rubber)	Good draping and contourability Good resilient stretch with slight memory Excellent rigidity—resists fatigue Ideal for larger splints	Smith and Nephew Rolyan, Inc. N93 W14475 Whitaker Way Menomonee Falls, Wis 53051
Orthoplast (transpolyisoprene)	High rubber content Often some stretch with good memory Good rigidity yet lightweight Ideal for circumferential splinting due to flexibility	Johnson & Johnson Products New Brunswisk, NJ 08903
Aquaplast-T nonsticky (polycaprolactone) with surface coating	Clear when heated, enabling control of pressure points over small areas Good conforming qualities Excellent elasticity when heated; good memory with repeated heating Excellent rigidity with small splints	WFR Aquaplast Corporation Post Office Box 327 Ramsey, NJ 07446

Others: Ezeform (plastic polymer), Orthoform (transpolyisoprene), Hexcelite (polymers, filler, and pigment impregnated onto cotton netting), Aquaplast (original sticky) (poly [epsilon] caprolactone), Monorthos (polycaprolactone, other polymers, and pigment), Green Stripe Aquaplast (polycaprolactone, with or without surface coating), Burns Quality Aquaplast (blue stripe), Kay-Splint Series 3 (plastic polymer), K-Splint Isoprene (plastic polymer), Kay Splint I (plastic polymer), JU 1000 Splinting Compound (plastic polymer), MR 2000 Splinting Compound (plastic polymer), RS 3000 Splinting compound (plastic polymer)

High-Temperature Thermoplastics
Vinyl (polyvinyl chloride), Kydex (copolymer of polyvinyl chloride and acrylic), W-Clear (transparent polyester-based orthotic material (copolyester of polyethylene terephthalate)

Material	Features	Manufacturer
Playing Cast Materials		
RTV-11	Liquid-based silicone rubber compound, cured with a catalyst Impregnated with gauze during application Usually padded externally (often with Temperfoam) Requires 3–4 hours to cure completely	General Electric Co. Silicone Rubber Products Div. Waterford, NY 12188
3M Scotchrap	Semirigid support wrap External padding Can be used pending specific regulations for competition	3M Orthopedic Products Div. 6850 S. Harlem Ave. Bedford Park, Ill 60501
Shock-Absorbing Materials		
Neoprene	Closed cell rubber available in variety of thicknesses Retains maximum body heat Provides uniform compression	Local distributor of divers' supplies
Sorbothane	Viscoelastic polymer Elasticity and flowability Can absorb 94% of energy in dynamic load displacement tests High compression resistance	IEM Orthopaedics 251 West Garfield Road Aurora, Ohio 44202
Viscolas	Viscoelastic polymer Has elasticity and flowability Excellent fine-vibration shock absorber High resistance to compression	Chattanooga Corporation Visco-Elastic Products 101 Memorial Drive Post Office Box 4287 Chattanooga, Tenn 37405

Table continued on following page

TABLE 24B1–1
Splint Materials Continued

Material	Features	Manufacturer
Foam Materials		
Polycushion	Soft, closed cell foam with adhesive backing Resists compression well Available in ¼- and ⅛-thickness	North Coast Medical, Inc. 450 Salmar Avenue Campbell, Calif 95008
Temperfoam	Soft, viscoelastic foam product with adhesive back Fluidlike support conforms to hand Resists impact, shock, and vibration	North Coast Medical, Inc. 450 Salmar Avenue Campbell, Calif 95008
Splint Inserts		
Otoform-K (transpolyisoprene)	Paste form of silicone elastomer cured with catalyst Amount of catalyst used will affect firmness of finished rubber mold Good contourability for interfacing splints Good shock-absorbing quality	WFR Aquaplast Corporation Post Office Box 327 Ramsey, NJ 07446
Elastomer (Silastic 382, medical grade)	Liquid-based silicone elastomer cured with a catalyst Produces firm, closed cell rubber mold Excellent contouring for interfacing of splints Good shock-absorbing quality	WFR Aquaplast Corporation Post Office Box 327 Ramsey, NJ 07446
Padded Glove		
Antivibration gloves	Leather or jersey glove with Viscolas insert Available in a variety of sizes and styles	Steel Grip Inc. 700 Garfield Street Danville, Ill 61832

and is more rigid when cured than Orthoplast. It does not, however, have as good a memory. Aquaplast-T has very good elasticity and conformability, in addition to being transparent when heated. This may be beneficial when attempting to splint over small bony areas of the hand that are prone to the development of pressure points. The splint materials should be chosen on the basis of their ability to meet the basic requirements of the injury for which the splint is being fabricated and the experience and preferences of the splint maker.

Some products designed to provide reasonable support to the injured hand and wrist are RTV-11 and 3M Scotchrap. These materials attempt to solve the dilemma of effectively splinting and protecting the injured part while overcoming the restriction on competition resulting from the use of hard devices. RTV-11 is a silicone rubber compound that conforms well and provides better support than some of the previous elastomers (Fig. 24B1–61). Splints made from RTV-11 can be worn without external padding (see Fig. 24B1–61). 3M Scotchrap is applied much like a cast and provides semirigid support. It remains soft enough to be acceptable for competition in most instances, but should be supplemented by an additional layer of padding.

Early protective splinting for return to competition usually requires some type of padding or lining for comfort and shock absorption. Again, a wide variety of materials are available for customizing the splint to the athlete's injury and the needs of the sport. Foam padding has value for lining areas of splints where firm materials may produce excessive pressure and be uncomfortable. Unfortunately, foam substances are not easily contoured around bony

prominences in the hand and usually diminish the protective support provided by the splint. Several types of foam are available in various densities, and most have a peel-off adhesive backing for easy application. We have found the most useful foam linings to be Polycushion, which is supplied in both ¼ inch and ⅛ inch, and Temperfoam, ¼ inch. Polycushion is an excellent, all-purpose, closed-cell foam, used primarily as a splint interface for patient comfort. It can be applied to the splint material before or after fabrication, and the material resists compression well. Temperfoam is a viscoelastic foam that provides fluidlike support and can be contoured to the hand through warmth and body heat, making it quite comfortable. Although it is soft to the touch, Temperfoam is firm on impact, making it a good shock absorber. With the advent of playing cast materials such as RTV-11, Temperfoam has become popular as an external coating that provides the final cushioning that makes the splint acceptable for athletic competition.

Medical-grade silicone elastomers such as Otoform K and Elastomer also provide protective padding and may be useful in the preparation of splints for the injured hands of athletes. Otoform K has a putty-like base and catalyst, whereas Elastomer has a liquid base and catalyst. Both materials may be molded and contoured to a specific area, which can provide an exacting fit. Both materials form flexible rubber molds when they cure, resulting in excellent shock-absorbing capabilities. Elastomer has also been used for playing casts, although it is not as strong and supportive as RTV-11.

Other materials that have gained popularity for their shock-absorbing qualities are Neoprene, Sorbothane, and

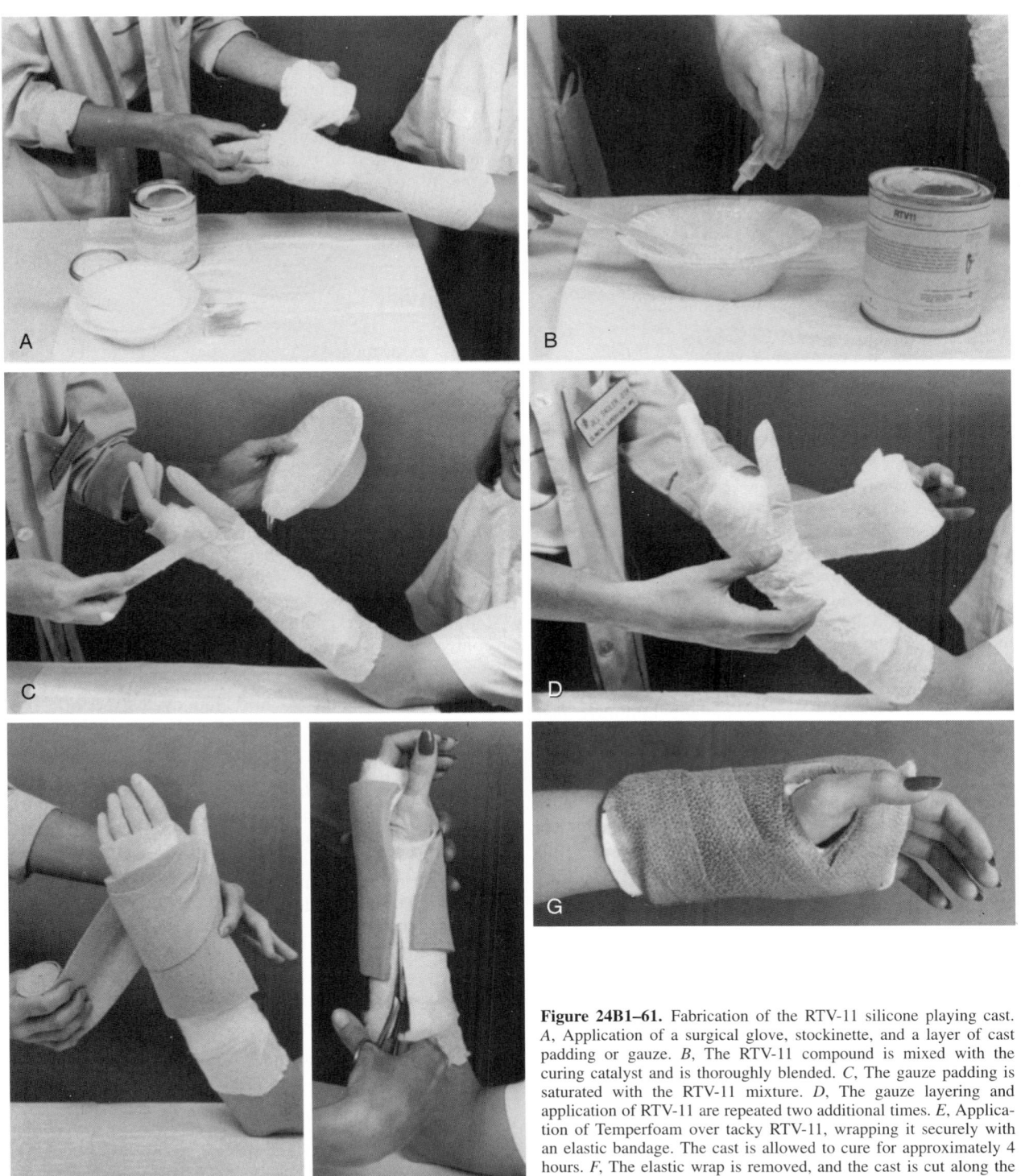

Figure 24B1–61. Fabrication of the RTV-11 silicone playing cast. *A*, Application of a surgical glove, stockinette, and a layer of cast padding or gauze. *B*, The RTV-11 compound is mixed with the curing catalyst and is thoroughly blended. *C*, The gauze padding is saturated with the RTV-11 mixture. *D*, The gauze layering and application of RTV-11 are repeated two additional times. *E*, Application of Temperfoam over tacky RTV-11, wrapping it securely with an elastic bandage. The cast is allowed to cure for approximately 4 hours. *F*, The elastic wrap is removed, and the cast is cut along the noninjured side of the hand and the forearm. *G*, Coban, elastic wrap, or adhesive tape is used to reapply the cast for competition.

Viscolas. Neoprene, which has long been used by wetsuit manufacturers, is a closed-cell rubber material available in various thicknesses. It is usually laminated on both sides to stretch nylon or terry-like materials that provide uniform compressive support while retaining body heat for increased comfort, a quality especially useful in managing compression syndromes and tendinitis. It may be used as an interface for rigid splints, or by itself for custom-made soft splints. Sorbothane and Viscolas are both classified as viscoelastic polymer products. They possess the flowability of a viscous liquid that enables the material to absorb and dissipate impact energies very effectively. Studies have shown Sorbothane to absorb as much as 94% of impact energy during dynamic load-displacement testing. Viscolas is most noted for its ability to absorb vibrations between 90 and 400 cycles/second, the range in which most soft tissue damage occurs. These materials are available in sheets that can be cut to the desired shapes for lining of gloves and splints. A tacky exterior has been created for securing the inserts in position. Both of these products represent important advances in the ability to produce effective splints for the management of athletic injuries as well as for the protection of vulnerable areas of the hand during practice and competition.

Many types of prefabricated antivibration gloves or pads are currently manufactured (Steel Grip), and may be useful for some athletes, such as cyclists (see Fig. 24B1–60).

Choice of Splints

Static splints used as protective devices may be constructed from rigid or flexible materials. Firm splints are employed for protection following ligamentous disruption or bony injury when healing is not complete. Rigid splints that cross the wrist, however, are often impractical for competitive use and may be appropriate only for the athlete whose sport requires minimal use of the hand. Rigid, low-profile splints that are confined to the digits may be suitable for competitive use following ligament injuries of the PIP or DIP joints but do not offer adequate protection for newly healed fractures. Flexible splints are obviously preferred by athletes because they are less restrictive. Although this type of splint may not provide much true protection, they generally provide enough support to help minimize pain and prevent excessive movement.

With contact sports, a wider area of application or more circumferential splints may be indicated in order to provide more support and distribute pressure forces more evenly. Regardless of the splinting program employed for competition, the physician, therapist, and coach must all agree that it will not in any way jeopardize the healing process for a particular injury. Further, it must not risk re-injury that might unfavorably alter the prognosis for the long-term performance of the injured part. Continued protective splinting may be indicated in those situations where the athlete is prone to re-injury.

Rehabilitation

Although minor sprains or strains or even undisplaced stable fractures can be managed by simple protective splinting with the initiation of early motion programs and the expectation of a rapid full recovery, more severe injuries and those that require a protracted recovery often necessitate formal rehabilitation programs. For the most part, these programs should be directed by well-trained sports and hand therapists in an effort to restore maximum joint mobility and extremity strength. Active and passive range of motion programs may be augmented by dynamic splinting or even the use of continuous passive motion machines in a few recalcitrant cases. Specific strengthening programs that employ simple devices such as hand grippers and Silly Putty may be helpful, and exercises designed to maximize

recovery in specific muscle groups may be taught to the patient and supervised by the therapist. Throughout this process, serial recordings of joint motion and measurements of grip and pinch strength help the therapists assess recovery and, when necessary, alter the rehabilitation program. Modalities such as transcutaneous electrical nerve stimulation to modify pain, or functional electrical stimulation in order to augment and retrain injured or unused muscles, may be of value in the rehabilitation of the athlete's hand.

Summary

An assortment of injuries may occur in the hands of athletes during competition or practice. There are no short-cuts to the effective management of these injuries, and sound hand surgical and orthopaedic procedures must be employed. The managing physician should be cognizant of the unique demands and re-injury potential of each injured athlete's sport and playing position before allowing the return to competition. There may be certain calculated alterations of traditional conservative treatment methods to return the athlete to full participation, but these departures should never be made if they run any appreciable risk of compromising the healing or functional result of a given injury. No player's career, no team's record, and no athletic contest is worth permanent deformity or dysfunction of the hand.

Acknowledgments

We thank the two previous authors of this chapter, Drs. David P. Green and James W. Strickland, for their significant contribution to our understanding of the unique manner by which hand and wrist injuries influence the athlete's ability to perform. They have educated countless colleagues with their teachings and writing. We also thank Lyn Camire and Grace Nasrallah for editorial assistance in the preparation of this chapter.

References

1. Agee JM: Unstable fracture dislocations of the proximal interphalangeal joint. Treatment with the force couple splint. Clin Orthop 214: 101–112, 1987.
2. Amadio PC: Epidemiology of hand and wrist injuries in sports. Hand Clin 6:379–381, 1990.
3. Ashbell TS, Kleinert HE, Putcha SM, Kutz JE: The deformed finger nail, a frequent result of failure to repair nail bed injuries. J Trauma 7:177–190, 1967.
4. Aulicino PL, Hutton PM, Du Puy TE: True palmar aneurysms—a case report and literature review. J Hand Surg [Am] 7:613–616, 1982.
5. Axe MJ, McClain EJ: Complete involvement of the ulnar nerve secondary to an ulnar artery aneurysm. A case report. Am J Sports Med 14:178–180, 1986.
6. Bassett FH, Malone T, Gilchrist RA: A protective splint of silicone rubber. Am J Sports Med 7:358–360, 1979.
7. Baugher WH, McCue FC: Anterior fracture-dislocation of the proximal interphalangeal joint. A case report. J Bone Joint Surg Am 61: 779–778, 1979.
8. Becton JL, Carswell AS: The natural history of an unreduced dislo-

cated index finger metacarpophalangeal joint in a child. J Med Assoc Ga 64:413–415, 1975.

9. Bergfeld JA, Weiker GG, Andrish JT, Hall R: Soft playing splint for protection of significant hand and wrist injuries in sports. Am J Sports Med 10:293–296, 1982.

10. Bergfeld JA, Weiker GG, Andrish JT, Hall R: Soft playing splint for protection of significant hand and wrist injuries in sports. Am J Sports Med 10:293–296, 1982.

11. Betz RR, Browne EZ, Perry GB, Resnick EJ: The complex volar metacarpophalangeal-joint dislocation. A case report and review of the literature. J Bone Joint Surg Am 64:1374–1375, 1982.

12. Blacker GJ, Lister GD, Kleinert HE: The abducted little finger in low ulnar nerve palsy. J Hand Surg [Am] 1:190–196, 1976.

13. Bowers WH, Hurst LC: Gamekeeper's thumb. Evaluation by arthrography and stress roentgenography. J Bone Joint Surg Am 59:519–524, 1977.

14. Bowers WH, Wolf J, Nehil JL, Bittinger S: The proximal interphalangeal joint volar plate. I. An anatomical and biomechanical study. J Hand Surg [Am] 5:79–88, 1980.

15. Buckhout BC, Warner MA: Digital perfusion of handball players. Effects of repeated ball impact on structures of the hand. Am J Sports Med 8:206–207, 1980.

16. Bynum DK, Gilbert JA: Avulsion of the flexor digitorum profundus: Anatomic and biomechanical considerations. J Hand Surg [Am] 13:222–227, 1988.

17. Camp RA, Weatherwax RJ, Miller EB: Chronic posttraumatic radial instability of the thumb metacarpophalangeal joint. J Hand Surg [Am] 5:221–225, 1980.

18. Carducci AT: Potential boutonniere deformity: Its recognition and treatment. Orthop Rev 10:121–123, 1981.

19. Cohen MS, Hennrikus WL, Botte MJ: A dressing for repair of acute nail bed injury. Orthop Rev 19:882–884, 1990.

20. Coleman SS, Anson BJ: Arterial patterns in the hand based upon a study of 650 specimens. Surv Med (Sofia) 113:409–424, 1961.

21. Converse TA: Cyclist's palsy. N Engl J Med 301:1397–1398, 1979.

22. Coonrad RW, Goldner JL: A study of the pathological findings and treatment in soft-tissue injury of the thumb metacarpophalangeal joint. With a clinical study of the normal range of motion in one thousand thumbs and a study of post mortem findings of ligamentous structures in relation to function. J Bone Joint Surg Am 50:439–451, 1968.

23. Coons MS, Green SM: Boutonniere deformity. Hand Clin 11:387–402, 1995.

24. Dawson WJ, Pullos N: Baseball injuries to the hand. Ann Emerg Med 10:302–306, 1981.

25. DeHaven KE, Lintner DM: Athletic injuries: Comparison by age, sport, and gender. Am J Sports Med 14:218–224, 1986.

26. Denman EE: The anatomy of the space of Guyon. Hand 10:69–76, 1978.

27. DiFiori JP, Puffer JC, Mandelbaum BR, Mar S: Factors associated with wrist pain in the young gymnast. Am J Sports Med 24:9–14, 1996.

28. Dobyns JH, O'Brien ET, Linscheid RL, Farrow GM: Bowler's thumb: Diagnosis and treatment. A review of seventeen cases. J Bone Joint Surg Am 54:751–755, 1972.

29. Donaldson WR, Millender LH: Chronic fracture-subluxation of the proximal interphalangeal joint. J Hand Surg [Am] 3:149–153, 1978.

30. Dray GJ, Eaton RG: Dislocations and ligament injuries in the digits. In Green DP (ed): Operative Hand Surgery, 2nd ed. New York, Churchill Livingstone, 1988, pp 777–811.

31. Dunham W, Haines G, Spring JM: Bowler's thumb: Ulnovolar neuroma of the thumb. Clin Orthop 83:99–101, 1972.

32. Durham HW, Khuri S, Kim MH: Acute and late radial collateral ligament injuries of the thumb metacarpophalangeal joint. J Hand Surg [Am] 18:232–237, 1993.

33. Eaton RG, Malerich MM: Volar plate arthroplasty of the proximal interphalangeal joint: A review of ten years' experience. J Hand Surg [Am] 5:260–268, 1980.

34. Eichenholtz SN, Rizzo PC III: Fracture of the neck of the fifth metacarpal bone—is over-treatment justified? JAMA 178:425–426, 1961.

35. Ellsasser JC, Stein AH: Management of hand injuries in a professional football team. Review of 15 years of experience with one team. Am J Sports Med 7:178–182, 1979.

36. Elson RA: Rupture of the central slip of the extensor hood of the finger. A test for early diagnosis. J Bone Joint Surg Br 68:229–231, 1986.

37. Engel J, Ganel A, Ditzian R, Militeanu J: Arthrography as a method of diagnosing tear of the ulnar collateral ligament of the metacarpophalangeal joint of the thumb ("gamekeeper's thumb"). J Trauma 19:106–109, 1979.

38. Eversmann WW: Compression and entrapment neuropathies of the upper extremity. J Hand Surg [Am] 8:759–766, 1983.

39. Eversmann WW Jr: Entrapment and compression neuropathies. In Green DP (ed): Operative Hand Surgery. New York, Churchill Livingstone, 1988, pp 1423–1478.

40. Fahmy NR, Kenny N, Kehoe N: Chronic fracture dislocations of the proximal interphalangeal joint. Treatment by the "S" Quattro. J Hand Surg [Br] 19:783–787, 1994.

41. Farabeuf LHF: De la luxation du ponce en arriere. Bull Soc Chir 11:21–62, 1876.

42. Flatt AE: The Care of Minor Hand Injuries, 4th ed. St. Louis, Mosby-Year Book, 1979.

43. Foucher G: "Bouquet" osteosynthesis in metacarpal neck fractures: A series of 66 patients. J Hand Surg [Am] 20:S86–S90, 1995.

44. Foucher G, Binhamer P, Cange S, Lenoble E: Long-term results of splintage for mallet finger. Int Orthop 20:129–131, 1996.

45. Frank WE, Dobyns J: Surgical pathology of collateral ligamentous injuries of the thumb. Clin Orthop 83:102–114, 1972.

46. Freeland AE, Benoist LA: Open reduction and internal fixation method for fractures at the proximal interphalangeal joint. Hand Clin 10:239–250, 1994.

47. Gabl M, Rangger C, Lutz M, et al: Disruption of the finger flexor pulley system in elite rock climbers. Am J Sports Med 26:651–655, 1998.

48. Gedda KO: Studies of Bennett's fractures: Anatomy, roentgenology, and therapy. Acta Chir Scand Suppl 5:193, 1954.

49. Green DP: True and false traumatic aneurysms in the hand. J Bone Joint Surg Am 55:120–128, 1973.

50. Green DP, Rowland SA: Fractures and dislocations in the hand. In Rockwood CA, Green DP, Bucholz RW (eds): Fractures in Adults, 3rd ed. Philadelphia, JB Lippincott, 1991, pp 441–561.

51. Green DP, Strickland JW: The hand. In DeLee JC, Drez D Jr (eds): Orthopaedic Sports Medicine, 1st ed. Philadelphia, WB Saunders, 1994, pp 945–1017.

52. Gunter GS: Traumatic avulsion of the insertion of flexor digitorum profundus. Aust N Z J Surg 30:1–8, 1960.

53. Gunther SF, Zielinski CJ: Irreducible palmar dislocation of the proximal phalanx of the thumb—case report. J Hand Surg [Am] 7:515–517, 1982.

54. Hall RF: Treatment of metacarpal and phalangeal fractures in non-compliant patients. Clin Orthop 73:31–36, 1987.

55. Hall RF, Gleason TF, Kasa RF: Simultaneous closed dislocations of the metacarpophalangeal joints of the index, long, and ring fingers: A case report. J Hand Surg [Am] 10:81–85, 1985.

56. Hame SL, Melone CP: Boxer's knuckle. Traumatic disruption of the extensor hood. Hand Clin 16:375–380, viii, 2000.

57. Handlebar palsy [letter]. N Engl J Med 292:702, 1975.

58. Hastings H, Ernst JM: Dynamic external fixation for fractures of the proximal interphalangeal joint. Hand Clin 9:659–674, 1993.

59. Ho PK, Dellon AL, Wilgis EF: True aneurysms of the hand resulting from athletic injury. Report of two cases. Am J Sports Med 13:136–138, 1985.

60. Holst-Nielsen F: Subcapital fractures of the four ulnar metacarpal bones. Hand 8:290–293, 1976.

61. Howell AE, Leach RE: Bowler's thumb. Perineural fibrosis of the digital nerve. J Bone Joint Surg Am 52:379–381, 1970.

62. Hunter JM, Cowen NJ: Fifth metacarpal fractures in a compensation clinic population. A report on one hundred and thirty-three cases. J Bone Joint Surg Am 52:1159–1165, 1970.

63. Husband JB, McPherson SA: Bony skier's thumb injuries. Clin Orthop 327:79–84, 1996.

64. Imaeda T, An KN, Cooney WP: Functional anatomy and biomechanics of the thumb. Hand Clin 8:9–15, 1992.

65. Imatami J, Hashizume H, Wake H, et al: The central slip attachment fracture. J Hand Surg [Br] 22:107–109, 1997.

66. Ishizuki M: Traumatic and spontaneous dislocation of extensor tendon of the long finger. J Hand Surg [Am] 15:967–972, 1990.

67. Itoh Y, Wakano K, Takeda T, Murakami T: Circulatory disturbances in the throwing hand of baseball pitchers. Am J Sports Med 15:264–269, 1987.

68. Jelalian C, Mehrhof A, Cohen IK, et al: Streptokinase in the treatment of acute arterial occlusion of the hand. J Hand Surg [Am] 10: 534–538, 1985.

69. Jordan BD, Campbell EA: Acute injuries among professional boxers in New York state: A two-year survey. Physician Sportsmed 16: 87–91, 1988.

70. Kaplan EB: Dorsal dislocation of the metacarpophalangeal joint of the index finger. J Bone Joint Surg Am 39:1081–1086, 1957.

71. Kaplan EB: The pathology and treatment of radial subluxation of the thumb with ulnar displacement of the head of the first metacarpal. J Bone Joint Surg Am 43:541–546, 1961.

72. Kessler I: Complex avulsion of the ulnar collateral ligament of the metacarpophalangeal joint of the thumb. Clin Orthop 29:196–200, 1961.

73. Kiefhaber TR, Stern PJ, Grood ES: Lateral stability of the proximal interphalangeal joint. J Hand Surg [Am] 11:661–669, 1986.

74. Kilgore ES, Graham WP: Operative treatment of boutonniere deformity. Surgery 64:999–1000, 1968.

75. Kirk AA: Dunk lacerations—unusual injuries to the hands of basketball players. JAMA 242:415, 1979.

76. Kleinman WB, Grantham SA: Multiple volar carpometacarpal joint dislocation. Case report of traumatic volar dislocation of the medial four carpometacarpal joints in a child and review of the literature. J Hand Surg [Am] 3:377–382, 1978.

77. Koman LA: Diagnostic study of vascular lesions. Hand Clin 1: 217–231, 1985.

78. Koman LA, Urbaniak JR: Ulnar artery insufficiency: A guide to treatment. J Hand Surg [Am] 6:16–24, 1981.

79. Kornberg M, Aulicino PL, Du Puy TE: Ulnar arterial aneurysms and thromboses in the hand and forearm. Orthop Rev 12:25–33, 1983.

80. Leddy JP: Avulsions of the flexor digitorum profundus. Hand Clin 1:77–83, 1985.

81. Leddy JP, Packer JW: Avulsion of the profundus tendon insertion in athletes. J Hand Surg [Am] 2:66–69, 1977.

82. Leriche R, Fontaine R, Dupertuis SM: Arterectomy: With follow-up studies on 78 operations. Surg Gynecol Obstet 64:149–155, 1937.

83. Light TR: Buttress pinning techniques. Orthop Rev 10:49–55, 1981.

84. Linscheid RL: Arthrography of the metacarpophalangeal joint. Clin Orthop 0:91, 1974.

85. Linscheid RL, Grainger RW, Johnson EW: The thumb metacarpophalangeal joint injuries. Minn Med 55:1037–1040, 1972.

86. Liss FE, Green SM: Capsular injuries of the proximal interphalangeal joint. Hand Clin 8:755–768, 1992.

87. Lorei MP, Hershman EB: Peripheral nerve injuries in athletes. Treatment and prevention. Sports Med 16:130–147, 1993.

88. Louis DS, Buckwalter KA: Magnetic resonance imaging of the collateral ligaments of the thumb. J Hand Surg [Am] 14:739–741, 1989.

89. Louis DS, Huebner JJ, Hankin FM: Rupture and displacement of the ulnar collateral ligament of the metacarpophalangeal joint of the thumb. Preoperative diagnosis. J Bone Joint Surg Am 68:1320–1326, 1986.

90. Lovett WL, McCalla MA: Management and rehabilitation of extensor tendon injuries. Orthop Clin North Am 14:811–826, 1983.

91. Lowrey CW, Chadwick RO, Waltman EN: Digital vessel trauma from repetitive impact in baseball catchers. J Hand Surg [Am] 1: 236–238, 1976.

92. Malerich MM, Eaton RG, Upton J: Complete dislocation of a little finger metacarpal phalangeal joint treated by closed technique. J Trauma 20:424–425, 1980.

93. Manske PR, Lesker PA: Avulsion of the ring finger flexor digitorum profundus tendon: An experimental study. Hand 10:52–55, 1978.

94. Manstein CH, Lister GD: Bowler's finger. J Hand Surg [Am] 7: 631, 1982.

95. McCash CR: Free nail grafting. Br J Plast Surg 8:19–33, 1955.

96. McCue FC, Hakala MW, Andrews JR, Gieck JH: Ulnar collateral ligament injuries of the thumb in athletes. J Sports Med 2:70–80, 1975.

97. McKerrell J, Bowen V, Johnston G, Zondervan J: Boxer's fractures—conservative or operative management? J Trauma 27:486–490, 1987.

98. McLaughlin HL: Complex "locked" dislocation of the metacarpophalangeal joints. J Trauma 5:683–688, 1965.

99. Melone CP, Beldner S, Basuk RS: Thumb collateral ligament injuries. An anatomic basis for treatment. Hand Clin 16:345–357, 2000.

100. Meyn MA Jr: Irreducible volar dislocation of the proximointerphalangeal joint. Clin Orthop 158:215–218, 1981.

101. Minamikawa Y, Horii E, Amadio PC, et al: Stability and constraint of the proximal interphalangeal joint. J Hand Surg [Am] 18:198–204, 1993.

102. Minkow FV, Bassett FHI: Bowler's thumb. Clin Orthop 83:115–117, 1972.

103. Mirabello SC, Loeb PE, Andrews JR: The wrist: Field evaluation and treatment. Clin Sports Med 11:1–25, 1992.

104. Miyamoto M, Hirayama T, Uchida M: Volar dislocation of the metacarpophalangeal joint of the thumb—a case report. J Hand Surg [Br] 11:51–54, 1986.

105. Moberg E, Stener B: Injuries to the ligaments of the thumb and fingers. Diagnosis, treatment and prognosis. Acta Chir Scand 106: 166–186, 1953.

106. Mogan JV, Davis PH: Upper extremity injuries in skiing. Clin Sports Med 1:295–308, 1982.

107. Mogensen BA, Mattsson HS: Post-traumatic instability of the metacarpophalangeal joint of the thumb. Hand 12:85–90, 1980.

108. Moneim MS: Volar dislocation of the metacarpophalangeal joint. Pathologic anatomy and report of two cases. Clin Orthop 176: 186–189, 1983.

109. Moussavi SM: Aneurysms and arterial thrombosis of the hand. Vascular Surg 12:294–305, 1978.

110. Murakami Y: Irreducible volar dislocation of the proximal interphalangeal joint of the finger. Hand 6:87–90, 1974.

111. National Collegiate Athletic Association: Illegal Equipment. In Nelson DM (ed): 1988 NCAA Football Rules and Interpretations. Mission, Kan, National Collegiate Athletic Association FR26–FR29, 1988.

112. National Federation Football Rules Committee: Player Equipment. In Schindler D (ed): 1988 Official High School Football Rules. Kansas City, National Federation of State High School Associations 10–12, 1988.

113. Newmeyer WL, Kilgore ES: Common injuries of the fingernail and nail bed. Am Fam Physician 16:93–95, 1977.

114. Nieman EA, Swann PG: Karate injuries. BMJ 1:233, 1971.

115. Nuber GW, McCarthy WJ, Yao JS, et al: Arterial abnormalities of the hand in athletes. Am J Sports Med 18:520–523, 1990.

116. Nutton RW, Guy MJ: Rugby injuries involving the hand. BMJ 1: 414, 1979.

117. Ogunro EO: External fixation of injured nail bed with the INRO surgical nail splint. J Hand Surg [Am] 14:236–241, 1989.

118. Osterman AL, Hayken GD, Bora FW: A quantitative evaluation of thumb function after ulnar collateral repair and reconstruction. J Trauma 21:854–861, 1981.

119. Palmer AK: Injury to the dorsal MCP joint of the thumb. Orthop Rev 11:127–129, 1982.

120. Palmer AK, Louis DS: Assessing ulnar instability of the metacarpophalangeal joint of the thumb. J Hand Surg [Am] 3:542–546, 1978.

121. Parellada JA, Balkissoon AR, Hayes CW, Conway WF: Bowstring injury of the flexor tendon pulley system: MR imaging. AJR Am J Roentgenol 167:347–349, 1996.

122. Parikh M, Nahigian S, Froimson A: Gamekeeper's thumb. Plast Reconstr Surg 58:24–31, 1976.

123. Patel MR, Joshi BB: Distraction method for chronic dorsal fracture dislocation of the proximal interphalangeal joint. Hand Clin 10: 327–337, 1994.

124. Porubsky GL, Brown SI, Urbaniak JR: Ulnar artery thrombosis: A sports-related injury. Am J Sports Med 14:170–175, 1986.

125. Posner MA: Injuries to the hand and wrist in athletes. Orthop Clin North Am 8:593–618, 1977.

126. Primiano GA: Skiers' thumb injuries associated with flared ski pole handles. Am J Sports Med 13:425–427, 1985.

127. Raab DJ, Fischer DA, Quick DC: Lunate and perilunate dislocations in professional football players. A five-year retrospective analysis. Am J Sports Med 22:841–845, 1994.

128. Renshaw TS, Louis DS: Complex volar dislocation of the metacarpophalangeal joint: A case report. J Trauma 13:1086–1088, 1973.

129. Resnick D, Danzig LA: Arthrographic evaluation of injuries of the first metacarpophalangeal joint: Gamekeeper's thumb. AJR Am J Roentgenol 126:1046–1052, 1976.

130. Rettig AC, Ryan RO, Stone JA: Epidemiology of hand injuries in sports. In Strickland JW, Rettig AC (eds): Hand Injuries in Athletes. Philadelphia, WB Saunders, 1992, pp 37–48.

131. Rosenthal D, Murray WT, Smith RJ: Finger arthrography. Radiology 137:647–651, 1980.
132. Rosenthal EA: Treatment of fingertip and nail bed injuries. Orthop Clin North Am 14:675–697, 1983.
133. Sakellarides HT, DeWeese JW: Instability of the metacarpophalangeal joint of the thumb. Reconstruction of the collateral ligaments using the extensor pollicis brevis tendon. J Bone Joint Surg Am 58:106–112, 1976.
134. Schenck RR: Dynamic traction and early passive movement for fractures of the proximal interphalangeal joint. J Hand Surg [Am] 11:850–858, 1986.
135. Schultz RJ, Fox JM: Gamekeeper's thumb. Result of skiing injuries. N Y State J Med 73:2329–2331, 1973.
136. Segmüller G: Fractures of the thumb. In Segmèuller G: Surgical Stabilization of the Skeleton of the Hand. Baltimore, Williams & Wilkins, 1977, pp 126–143.
137. Smith JH: Avulsion of a profundus tendon with simultaneous intraarticular fracture of the distal phalanx—case report. J Hand Surg [Am] 6:600–601, 1981.
138. Smith RJ: Post-traumatic instability of the metacarpophalangeal joint of the thumb. J Bone Joint Surg Am 59:14–21, 1977.
139. Spinner M, Choi BY: Anterior dislocation of the proximal interphalangeal joint. A cause of rupture of the central slip of the extensor mechanism. J Bone Joint Surg Am 52:1329–1336, 1970.
140. Stamos BD, Leddy JP: Closed flexor tendon disruption in athletes. Hand Clin 16:359–365, 2000.
141. Stener B: Displacement of the ruptured ulnar collateral ligament of the metacarpo-phalangeal joint of the thumb. J Bone Joint Surg Br 44:869–879, 1962.
142. Stener B: Hyperextension injuries to the metacarpophalangeal joint of the thumb: Rupture of ligaments, fracture of sesamoid bones, rupture of flexor pollicis brevis. An anatomical and clinical study. Acta Chir Scand 125:275–293, 1963.
143. Stern PJ, Kastrup JJ: Complications and prognosis of treatment of mallet finger. J Hand Surg [Am] 13:329–334, 1988.
144. Sugawara M, Ogino T, Minami A, Ishii S: Digital ischemia in baseball players. Am J Sports Med 14:329–334, 1986.
145. Swanker WA: Reconstructive surgery of the injured nail. Am J Surg 74:341–345, 1947.
146. Tsuge K, Watari S: Dorsal dislocation of the metacarpophalangeal joint of the index finger. Hiroshima J Med Sci 22:65–81, 1973.
147. Vayssairat M, Priollet P, Capron L, et al: Does karate injure blood vessels of the hand? Lancet 2:529, 1984.
148. Vicar AJ: Proximal interphalangeal joint dislocations without fractures. Hand Clin 4:5–13, 1988.
149. Viegas SF: Extension block pinning for proximal interphalangeal joint fracture dislocations: Preliminary report of a new technique. J Hand Surg [Am] 17:896–901, 1992.
150. Wang KC, Hsu KY, Shih CH: Irreducible volar rotatory dislocation of the proximal interphalangeal joint. Orthop Rev 23:886–888, 1994.
151. Warren RA, Kay NR, Norris SH: The microvascular anatomy of the distal digital extensor tendon. J Hand Surg [Br] 13:161–163, 1988.
152. Weiland AJ, Berner SH, Hotchkiss RN, et al: Repair of acute ulnar collateral ligament injuries of the thumb metacarpophalangeal joint with an intraosseous suture anchor. J Hand Surg [Am] 22:585–591, 1997.
153. Werner SL, Plancher KD: Biomechanics of wrist injuries in sports. Clin Sports Med 17:407–420, 1998.
154. Weston WJ: Positive contrast arthrography of the normal mid-tarsal joints. Australas Radiol 13:365–367, 1969.
155. Wilgis EF: Digital sympathectomy for vascular insufficiency. Hand Clin 1:361–367, 1985.
156. Wilhelmy J, Hay RL: Dual dislocation of metacarpophalangeal joints. Hand 4:168–170, 1972.
157. Winge S, Jorgensen U, Lassen Nielsen A: Epidemiology of injuries in Danish championship tennis. Int J Sports Med 10:368–371, 1989.
158. Wood MB, Dobyns JH: Chronic, complex volar dislocation of the metacarpophalangeal joint. J Hand Surg [Am] 6:73–76, 1981.
159. Zemel NP, Stark HH, Ashworth CR, Boyes JH: Chronic fracture dislocation of the proximal interphalangeal joint-treatment by osteotomy and bone graft. J Hand Surg [Am] 6:447–455, 1981.
160. Zook EG: Injuries of the fingernail. In Green DP (ed): Operative Hand Surgery. New York, Churchill Livingstone, 1982, pp 895–914.

2. HAND INJURIES IN CHILDREN

Dina Galvin, MD ■ Jeffrey L. Lovallo, MD ■ Barry P. Simmons, MD

People of all ages in this country have become more sports oriented. There are more televised broadcasts of sporting events than ever before, allowing more people to become interested in sports and also creating multimillion-dollar role models for our nation's children. Kids want to be able to pass like John Elway, jump like Michael Jordan, pitch like Pedro Martinez, and shoot like Wayne Gretzky. Boys and girls are participating in organized sports at an earlier age. With an increase in participation, there is also an increase in sports-related injuries.

According to the National SAFEKIDS campaign, there are more than 3 million children who experience sports and recreation–related injuries each year in the United States. Twenty percent of children participating in sports activities are injured each year, with 25% of these injuries considered serious.[37] In Finland between 1987 and 1991, there were 54,186 sports-related injuries.[25] The sports leading to the highest number of injuries were soccer, ice hockey, volleyball, judo, and basketball.[25] The number of hand and wrist injuries varies from sport to sport but comprises 25% of all sports injuries.[1, 2, 25]

Hands are at risk for injury during sports for several reasons. The hands are exposed in all sports, although their involvement varies from sport to sport. Soccer is played without the use of the hands, so the hand injury rate is lower than in a sport such as basketball in which the hands are continuously exposed. In contact sports such as football, ice hockey, boxing, or judo, the hands can even become weapons, increasing the risk of injury. One football team analyzed over a 15-year period had an average of three significant hand injuries each year.[15] Adolescent football players seem to be affected as commonly as professional players, with 35% of reported injuries in this age group involving the hand and wrist.[42]

Contact can be not only with opposing players but with the equipment used as well. A lot of sports involve the use of sticks or racquets such as field hockey, lacrosse, baseball, and ice hockey. Hands can be struck by these instruments and suffer significant damage. Ice hockey players are reported to have sustained injuries to the upper extremity at a rate of one injury per 2000 hours of play.[44] All sports including speed, contact between players, stick slashing, pucks or balls zooming, or stress loading on the limb can result in high-energy injuries to the hand. These injuries are not always acute injuries but can be chronic injuries as well. Repetitive stress injuries in gymnastics have been reported to range from 17% to 43% of all injuries in gymnasts.[28]

The players, coaches, trainers, and doctors taking care of athletes should all be aware of the potential risks involved in the sport. This chapter emphasizes the type of hand injuries suffered in the pediatric population and their management. Injury to the pediatric hand can result in fractures, dislocations, ligament tears, tendon ruptures, and nerve injuries.

Hand Evaluation

Evaluation of hand injuries begins with a thorough history. It is important to determine the patient's hand dominance, mechanism of injury, time the injury occurred, and any associated injuries. It is also important to determine whether this was an acute or chronic injury, the importance of the hand in their sport, and their level of competition.

On physical examination, the hand should be initially inspected for skin integrity, ecchymosis, visible deformity, and any neurologic or vascular compromise. During the hand examination, each individual tendon and nerve should be tested. The hand should be examined for areas of bony tenderness, crepitus, and instability. Rotational abnormalities should also be identified during the examination. After physical examination has been completed, radiographs should be taken in the anteroposterior, lateral, and oblique planes. By performing a thorough history and examination, the clinician can accurately diagnose the athlete's injury and initiate the appropriate management to minimize the morbidity and shorten the recovery time.

Fractures in the Hand

Digital Fractures

Phalangeal fractures are very common in athletes because exposed digits are subject to crushing, twisting, and bending forces.[6, 19] Phalangeal fractures are most common in ball sports such as baseball, basketball, football, and volleyball where the fingers can get "jammed" by the ball.[2] In the pediatric population, the majority of these fractures involve the physis. The ossific nucleus of the epiphysis appears in both the metacarpals and phalanges by 3 years of age and fuses between 14 and 17 years of age.[41] The presence of open growth plates allows for remodeling. This remodeling occurs only in the plane of motion and will not correct a rotational deformity. Most of the fractures sustained by children can be treated closed, with only 10% to 20% of fractures requiring open reduction.[43]

Evaluation of the fractured digit should include a history of the mechanism of injury, and a thorough physical examination including assessment of the skin integrity, the nail bed, any gross deformity, and rotational alignment. An anteroposterior, lateral, and oblique radiograph of the affected digit should be performed. It is imperative to obtain a true lateral radiograph because condylar fractures are easily misdiagnosed with inadequate radiographs.

Distal Phalanx Fractures

The distal tips of the fingers are most prone to crushing and hyperflexion injuries. A crushing injury to the tip of the finger usually results from contact between two players and often when a shoe or helmet smashes the distal tip of the finger. This results in a tuft fracture of the phalanx and often an injury to the nail. These are often open fractures and should be treated with irrigation and débridement. The nail plate needs to be removed in order to inspect the nail bed. The germinal matrix of the nail bed can get interposed in the fracture site and should be repaired using interrupted 6–0 chromic suture under loop magnification. The finger should be protected with an aluminum splint and buddy taped for 3 to 4 weeks.

Hyperflexion injuries result when the distal aspect of the finger is jammed against another object. This results in either a bony mallet finger in older children or a physeal separation in younger children. In younger children with a physeal separation, the germinal matrix of the nail bed can get interposed and requires open repair using 6–0 chromic suture. This repair should be protected with a splint for 2 to 4 weeks.[20] The bony mallet results from avulsion of the terminal extensor tendon. The distal interphalangeal (DIP) joint will now be held in flexion and be unable to be actively extended. The joint should therefore be splinted in extension and the splint left on for 4 weeks.

Direct trauma to the distal aspect of the finger can also cause a painful subungual hematoma. When the hematoma involves 50% or more of the nail plate, a concomitant fracture and nail bed laceration should be suspected and repaired as mentioned before. Even without a laceration, pressure itself under the nail plate can injure the germinal matrix and as a result may require evacuation. Decompression of the hematoma is achieved by creating a pinpoint hole in the proximal nail plate to allow the blood to escape. This can be done under sterile conditions using a heated paper clip, battery-operated microcautery, or the tip of a No. 11 blade.[29] The fracture should be immobilized for 2 weeks.

Middle and Proximal Phalanx Fractures

Because they are more exposed, the index and small fingers are injured more frequently than the middle and ring fingers. Proximal phalanx fractures occur more frequently than middle phalanx fractures. The middle phalanx is protected by its short length and by the adjacent interphalangeal joints, which absorb most of the force. Fractures of the middle and proximal phalanx are categorized as epiphyseal, diaphyseal, subcondylar, and condylar fractures.

The most common pediatric hand fracture is the Salter-Harris II fracture in the proximal phalanx of the small finger. Physeal fractures of the proximal and middle phalanx should be treated with closed reduction and casting. The injured finger should be immobilized to the adjacent digit in flexion. The border digits should be buddy taped to the adjacent digit to prevent an abduction deformity.

Because these fractures are epiphyseal, they have the greatest potential for remodeling. Twenty degrees of angulation in the plane of motion—dorsal or volar—can be accepted. Care should be taken during the examination of the hand to make sure there is no rotational malalignment.

Malrotation is usually more an issue with diaphyseal than epiphyseal fractures. Torque on the finger or direct compression can produce diaphyseal spiral, oblique, and transverse fractures. Transverse fractures are prone to angulate, oblique fractures to shorten, and spiral fractures to rotate.[29] All types of fractures however, need to be examined for rotational alignment. The finger may look straight when it is extended but may overlap an adjacent finger when a fist is made. Have the patient actively flex the digits and check for nail alignment. All nails when checked should be in the same plane. If the finger demonstrates a rotational deformity, reduction is required. Open reduction is reserved for those cases where rotational control is not restored after closed manipulation. If K-wires are used, they should be left in place 2 to 4 weeks. The finger is immobilized with the adjacent digit for 3 to 4 weeks and then buddy taped another 2 weeks. Most diaphyseal fractures in the pediatric population are nondisplaced because of the thickened periosteum.

Subcondylar phalangeal neck fractures are most common in children between the ages of 5 and 10. These can occur in both the middle and proximal phalanx but are more frequent in the middle phalanx. Dorsal rotation is common with the fragment tethered by the collateral ligaments. At the proximal phalanx, a subcondylar fracture can rotate 90 degrees and entrap the volar plate.[12] A closed or open reduction with K-wires is required. Again, immobilization with the adjacent digit is recommended for 2 to 4 weeks. If the neck fracture is being treated closed, frequent radiographs should be taken to ensure that the fracture does not displace inasmuch as these are unstable injuries. A late open reduction of these injuries is not recommended because of the risk of avascular necrosis. A condylar fossa reconstruction, rather, can be performed for chronic loss of flexion.[43]

Condylar fractures of the head can be either unicondylar or bicondylar. These occur at the articular surface of both the proximal and middle phalanx. In young children, these are osteochondral fractures and have a high risk of avascular necrosis, nonunion, malunion, and loss of motion. Nondisplaced fractures can be treated with cast immobilization but need to be closely monitored. Displaced intra-articular fractures can be treated with closed reduction and percutaneous pinning. Irreducible fractures require open reduction with internal fixation (ORIF). A dorsolateral incision is used when performing an ORIF. Care should be taken to preserve the collateral ligament attachment to the fragment because this is the remaining blood supply to the fracture fragment.[43] The repair should be protected for 3 to 4 weeks. The K-wires are then removed and the finger should be buddy taped to the adjacent digit. The threshold for surgery in both condylar and subcondylar fractures should be low.

Return to athletics after a phalanx fracture is allowed at 2 to 6 weeks, with buddy taping for protection. Return to play can be sooner depending on the sport and the required use of the hand. Some sports will allow participation with a cast but this is not recommended if K-wires are still present.

Thumb Phalanx Fractures

The proximal and distal phalanges in the thumb are subject to the same fracture patterns as the phalanges of the digits: physeal, shaft, subcondylar, and condylar. The same rules of treatment apply. However, there are slight differences in management. Rotation or malrotation is harder to assess in the thumb because there are no other digits in the same plane. However, rotation is also less of a problem in the thumb because of the increased mobility at the carpometacarpal (CMC) joint. In addition, because immobilization cannot be done with any of the adjacent digits, the thumb is immobilized in a thumb spica cast. The most important difference is in treating Salter-Harris III fractures of the thumb proximal phalanx. This is a collateral ligament equivalent in a skeletally immature person. Minimal displacement requires only cast immobilization.

Metacarpal Fractures

Fractures of the metacarpals result from direct impact of the metacarpal heads on an object, classically a closed fist punch. Metacarpal fractures, especially the second, third, and fifth, are commonly associated with boxers and karate enthusiasts.[16, 30] Metacarpal fractures are classified as head, neck, shaft, or base fractures. Because of the transverse palmar arch and the overlap of the metacarpals, injuries in this area are best seen on oblique views of the hand with the forearm placed in 30 degrees of pronation.[29]

Head fractures are intra-articular injuries and most commonly involve the index finger. If more than 25% of the articular surface is disrupted, these need to be surgically reduced in order to restore the normal joint anatomy.[31] Postoperatively these need to be immobilized with the metacarpophalangeal (MP) joints flexed for up to 4 weeks. Excluding the thumb, all of the MP joints should be immobilized in 60 to 90 degrees of flexion with the proximal interphalangeal (PIP) and DIP joints in 10 to 20 degrees of flexion. These positions maintain the length of the collateral ligaments, which helps to minimize the development of joint contractures.[23, 24] Nondisplaced head fractures are treated with cast immobilization with MP flexion.

Neck fractures are some of the most common fractures seen in the hand, especially in the small finger. Although the metacarpal neck fracture is termed a "boxer's fracture," true boxers punch with the radial side of their hands and sustain neck fractures in the second and third metacarpals.[30] Neck fractures tend to have volar angulation at the fracture site as a result of the deforming forces of the intrinsic muscles. The metacarpal head becomes more prominent in the palm of the hand. Too much volar angulation of the fracture not only creates a cosmetic deformity with the loss of the "knuckle" but the presence of the head in the palm can cause pain with gripping or an imbalance to the extrinsic tendons, which can lead to a claw deformity. The amount of angulation tolerated at the fracture site depends on the digit involved. The ring and small fingers have more motion in the CMC joint and that increased mobility will compensate for the angular deformity. Thirty degrees of volar angulation in the ring finger and up to 50 degrees in the small finger therefore can be accepted. The index and middle finger have less motion at the CMC joint so only 10 degrees of angulation is acceptable.[29] These fractures are reduced and kept immobilized in a cast with the MP joints flexed for 2 to 4 weeks (Fig. 24B2–1). After casting, the athlete can return to sports using buddy taping.

No degree of rotational deformity is acceptable. Rotation should be carefully checked on physical examination, and if there is evidence of malrotation, the fracture needs to be surgically treated. Those fractures with a rotational deformity or significant angulation should be treated with closed reduction and percutaneous K-wire fixation. The reduction can be maintained with the use of cross-medullary or intramedullary K-wires.[18] The fixation should be protected for 3 to 4 weeks.

Metacarpal shaft fractures are usually stable injuries and can be treated with cast immobilization for 2 to 4 weeks. Care must again be taken to be sure there is no element of rotational deformity. The same principles apply to the shaft of the metacarpal as to the phalanges in that no rotation is acceptable. A comminuted or severely displaced shaft fracture can be treated with wires, screws, or even a small plate. Reduction and fixation are also required if multiple metacarpal shafts are fractured. Multiple shaft fractures can alter the normal length of the hand and are more likely to rotate. Multiple metacarpal fractures often require ORIF.

Fractures of the proximal metacarpals in the ulnar four digits are usually stable owing to the strong ligamentous attachments at the CMC joints. These can be treated by closed means with cast immobilization for 2 to 4 weeks, again with the MP joints held in flexion.

Thumb Metacarpal Fractures

Thumb metacarpal head, neck, and shaft fractures are similarly treated. Fractures at the base of the thumb in children are classified as physeal, epibasal, Bennett's, and Rolando fractures. Physeal fractures occur through the growth plate at the base of the thumb and are classified by the Salter-Harris classification. Epibasal thumb fractures are extra-articular and are usually transverse or slightly oblique. The fracture is angulated with its apex dorsal. The abductor pollicis longus extends the proximal fragment. Most of these fractures are amenable to closed treatment. Reduction is accomplished by longitudinal traction and pronation of the distal fragment.[5] Thirty degrees of angulation is acceptable in thumb proximal metacarpal fractures (Fig. 24B2–2). A thumb spica cast is recommended for 2 to 4 weeks.

Bennett's fractures are intra-articular, two-part metacarpal base fractures. The mechanism that creates this fracture pattern is usually an axial load on the thumb with the thumb flexed. The Bennett fragment is the smaller of the two fragments, which is the volar ulnar aspect of the metacarpal base. It is held in place by the strong volar oblique ligament, which runs from the fragment to the trapezium. The larger piece is displaced proximally, radially, and supinated by the pull of the abductor pollicis longus. Because of the intra-articular displacement, these fractures require fixation. This can be done either closed or open with wires or screws.

Rolando fractures are three-part intra-articular metacar-

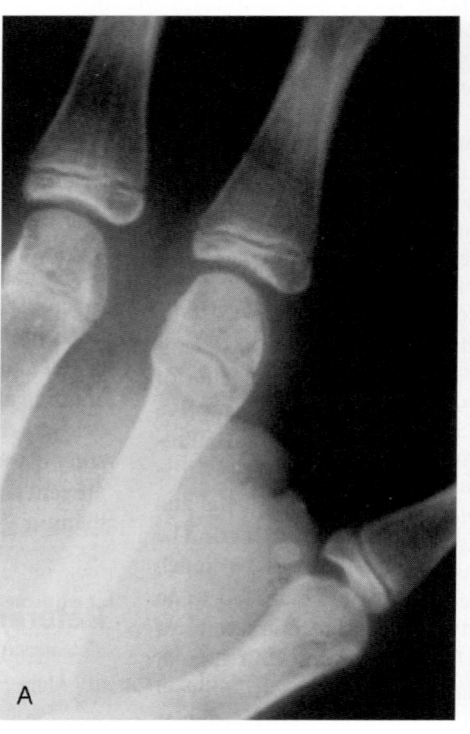
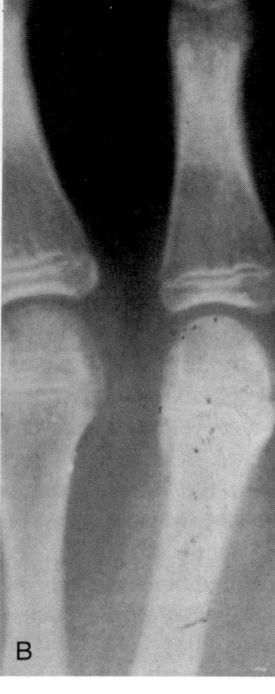

Figure 24B2–1. *A*, This 14-year-old boy injured his right index finger while playing football. Radiographs were equivocal, but on physical examination the patient had a swollen tender distal index metacarpal. *B*, Four weeks following cast immobilization, abundant callus is present, indicating a nonepiphyseal metacarpal neck fracture.

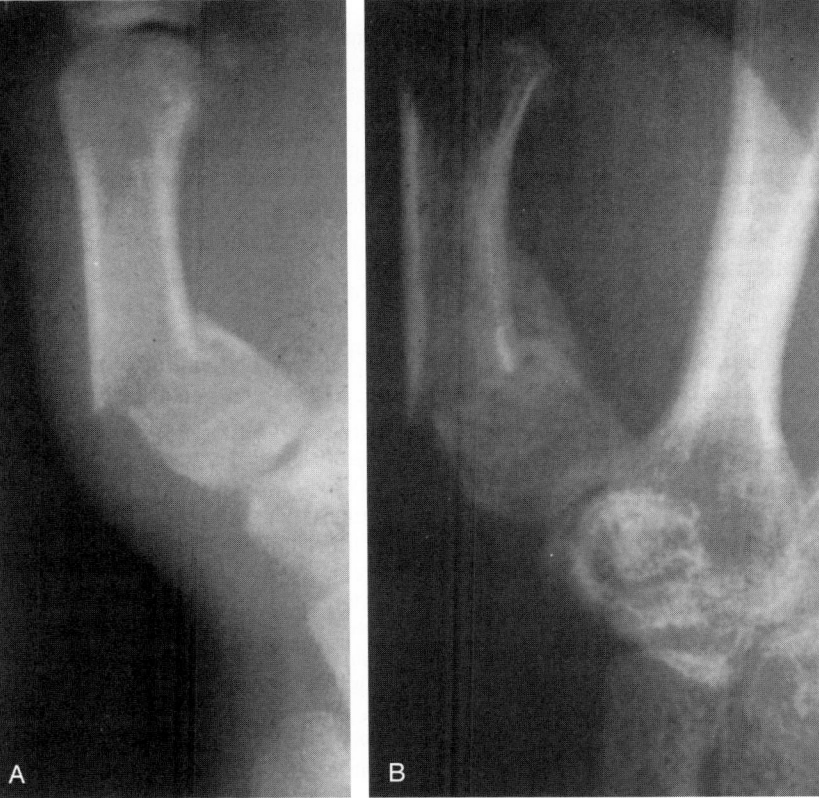

Figure 24B2–2. *A*, This patient was a 17-year-old high school quarterback who struck his right thumb on an opposing player's helmet. The fracture was treated with cast immobilization for 4 weeks. *B*, At 4 weeks, there was abundant callus. Clinically, the patient had a slightly prominent metacarpal but no functional deficit.

pal base fractures usually in a T- or Y-shaped configuration. Open reduction of the articular surface is recommended. Multiple K-wires or a plate to maintain the reduction is necessary. Care must be taken not to devascularize comminuted osteochondral fragments, creating further injury to the articular surface.

Ligament Injuries in the Hand

Ligament injuries in the pediatric population are rare. Fractures, especially the Salter-Harris physeal fractures, are much more common. The tensile strength of ligaments in children is greater than the bone around the growth plate.[38] Therefore, any injury tends to result in a fracture rather than a torn ligament. When a ligament tear does occur in a child, it is usually not in isolation but in combination with a fracture.

Digital Metacarpophalangeal Joint Ligament Injuries

This is a rare injury and when it occurs, it is almost always associated with a fracture. The fracture may involve either side of the MP joint. The injury is a result of a radially or ulnarly deviated force on the digit. If the fracture is nondisplaced, treatment requires cast immobilization with the MP joint flexed for 2 to 4 weeks, followed by buddy taping the finger to the adjacent digit for another 2

to 4 weeks for a total of 4 to 6 weeks of protection. If the fracture is displaced, ORIF with K-wires is required (Fig. 24B2–3). The goal of fixation is to restore the normal articular surface. Postoperatively, the joint is immobilized with flexion of the MP joints for 3 to 4 weeks. The pins are removed at 3 to 4 weeks. The joint should then be protected with buddy taping to the adjacent digit. Return to athletics can be allowed at 4 to 6 weeks with buddy taping.

Gamekeeper's Thumb

Injury to the MP joint of the thumb is much more common than to the other digits. The mechanism is fre-

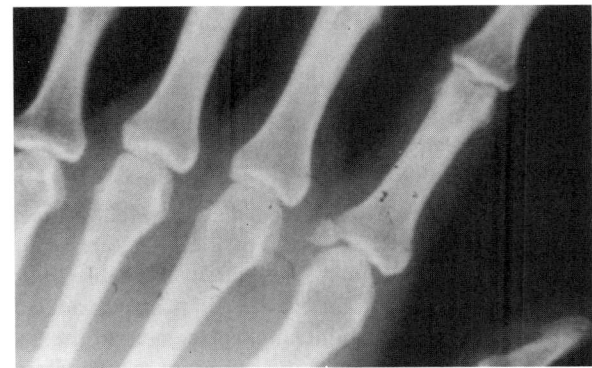

Figure 24B2–3. Displaced intra-articular proximal phalanx avulsion fracture requiring open reduction and internal fixation.

quently a fall onto an outstretched thumb with a radially directed force. Stress is placed on the ulnar side of the thumb, disrupting the ulnar collateral ligament of the MP joint. Campbell in 1955 originally described the clinical signs and symptoms and coined the term *gamekeeper's thumb*. It was frequently an occupational injury of Scottish gamekeepers,[8] although it is a misnomer because the true gamekeeper's thumb was a chronic not acute injury. Today it is more commonly referred to as *skier's thumb*. Falling with a ski pole in the first web space places a valgus force on the abducted thumb that disrupts the ulnar collateral ligament.[11]

The ulnar collateral ligament is made up of two ligaments: the proper collateral ligament, and the accessory collateral ligament. In flexion, the taut proper collateral ligament is the primary joint stabilizer whereas in extension, the accessory collateral ligament is the primary stabilizer to valgus stress on the joint.[21, 34] With a valgus stress on the thumb, one or both of these ligaments may be torn.

Evaluation of a patient with a suspected ulnar collateral ligament tear begins with a thorough history of the mechanism of injury. Radiographs should be obtained prior to any stress testing on the thumb. Radiographs may show a fracture of the metacarpal or proximal phalanx. If either of these bones is fractured, valgus stress testing should not be performed for fear of displacing the fracture. If no fracture is present, stress testing should be done. With the thumb held in 30 degrees of flexion at the MP joint, the examiner places a valgus stress on the thumb to test the integrity of the proper collateral ligament. If there is more than 30 degrees of laxity, or 15 degrees more than the contralateral side, the proper collateral ligament is disrupted. The thumb is then repositioned in extension and a valgus stress is placed by the examiner. If the laxity is now less than 30 degrees or less than 15 degrees different from the other side, the accessory collateral ligament is likely to be intact. If the laxity is still greater than 30 degrees, the accessory collateral is probably ruptured as well. This is important because the rupture of both of these ligaments can lead to displacement of the ligament and the presence of a "Stener lesion."[21]

Stener in 1962 described the displacement of the distal end of the ruptured collateral ligament. The distal stump can then lie proximal and superficial to the adductor aponeurosis.[45] If this occurs, the ligament will not heal back to the bone because of the interposed tissue of the adductor aponeurosis.

Treatment for ulnar collateral ligament tears is based on the ligaments injured. If the accessory collateral ligament remains intact, the proper collateral ligament cannot completely displace and should heal with immobilization. The thumb is placed into a hand-based short-arm thumb spica cast for 4 weeks. The same treatment applies to fractures around the MP joint. The ulnar collateral ligament inserts onto the epiphysis of the proximal phalanx; therefore, in children, a Salter-Harris III fracture is a gamekeeper's equivalent. If it is a nondisplaced fracture, it should be immobilized in a thumb spica cast for 2 to 4 weeks. A displaced fracture on radiographs serves as a marker for the location of the collateral ligament and requires reduction.

If the accessory collateral ligament is torn as well as the proper collateral ligament, the ligament is completely disrupted and may not heal owing to the presence of a Stener lesion. Palpation of a lump on the ulnar side of the MP joint confirms the presence of a Stener lesion.[21, 45] If no lump is palpated (representing the distal stump of the ligament), a Stener lesion may still be present.[21] Therefore, surgery is recommended for thumb injuries when both ligaments are torn (evidenced by instability in flexion and extension) and for displaced Salter fractures. The ligament should be repaired at the site of the tear. This may require an absorbable 4–0 suture if a midsubstance tear occurs in an older adolescent, or more likely a repair back to the bone. This can be performed with the use of a transosseous suture tied over a button on the radial side of the thumb, or with the use of a suture anchor placed directly into the bone.[11] Postoperatively, the thumb is immobilized for 4 weeks in a thumb spica cast. The thumb should be pro-

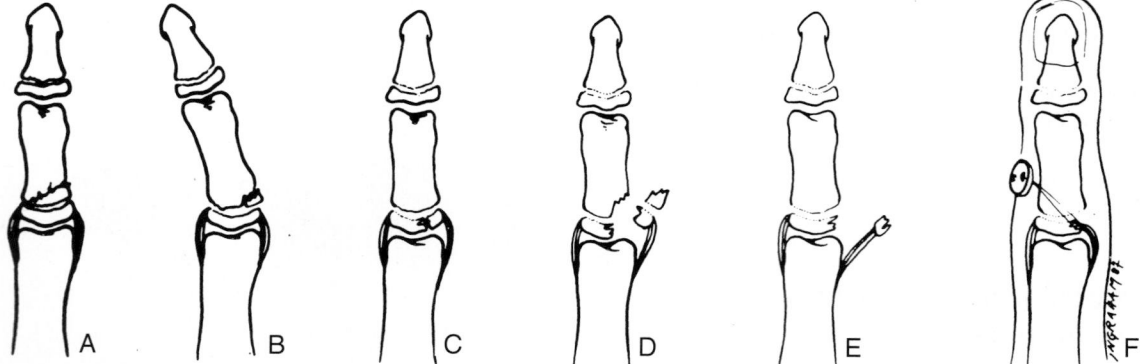

Figure 24B2–4. The spectrum of thumb fractures of the proximal phalanx at the metacarpophalangeal joint level as a result of a radially directed force. The Salter II fractures (*A, B*) are usually seen in the 5- to 11-year-old age group. The remainder occur mainly in adolescents, often in skiing accidents. *A*, Undisplaced Salter II fracture requiring no reduction. *B*, Displaced Salter II fracture requiring reduction. *C*, Minimally displaced Salter III fracture requiring no reduction. *D*, Salter IV fracture in which healing may or may not provide adequate ligamentous stability but would result in a significantly abnormal joint surface. This needs open reduction and K-wire fixation. *E*, Small, significantly displaced Salter III fracture now proximal to the dorsal apparatus (Stener lesion). Left displaced, there would be no significant articular surface abnormality, but severe ligamentous laxity would result. This requires open reduction. If the fragment is sufficiently large, it can be held with a K-wire. *F*, If the fragment is small, it can be removed and the ulnar collateral ligament repaired directly with a pullout suture. The same procedure is used when the ligament tear occurs without a fracture.

tected for 2 to 4 months after surgery during athletic events (Fig. 24B2–4).

Dislocations

Carpometacarpal Joint Dislocations

CMC dislocations are a result of significant trauma and are rare in children except for the thumb CMC joint. These joints have significant intrinsic stability because of the strong ligamentous attachments and the concave-convex bony articulations. Those dislocations seen in the first CMC joint are usually caused by a fall on the outstretched thumb. Fractures may occur in combination with these dislocations, particularly a Salter-Harris III fracture. Treatment is usually closed and reduction is accomplished by longitudinal traction. The reduction should be protected in a short-arm thumb spica cast for up to 4 weeks. Open reduction is reserved for those instances when the reduction is inadequate or unstable. (Fig. 24B2–5).

Metacarpophalangeal Joint Dislocations

The most common dislocation in the hand of a child is the MP joint of the thumb. MP dislocations in the fingers are rare.[41] In the thumb, the MP joint dislocates from a fall or an impaction injury, which causes hyperextension at that joint and a dorsal dislocation. The volar plate ruptures off the metacarpal and may be interposed in the joint. In order to reduce this joint, hyperextension at the MP joint with distally directed pressure applied over the proximal phalanx should be undertaken. The examiner should avoid longitudinal traction with this dislocation because it will further entrap the volar plate and prevent reduction. Distending the joint prior to reduction with 1% lidocaine can help to float the volar plate out of the joint. If the MP joint is irreducible, open reduction with part volar plate extraction is necessary (Fig. 24B2–6).

MP dislocations in the fingers, albeit rare, occur with a hyperextension injury. The index finger is the most commonly affected. The dorsal dislocation of the proximal phalanx can lead to injury to the volar plate and potential entrapment of the volar plate within the joint. Open reduction and extraction of the volar plate is required for these injuries. A volar approach is used with care being taken to avoid injury to the radial digital nerve, which is frequently

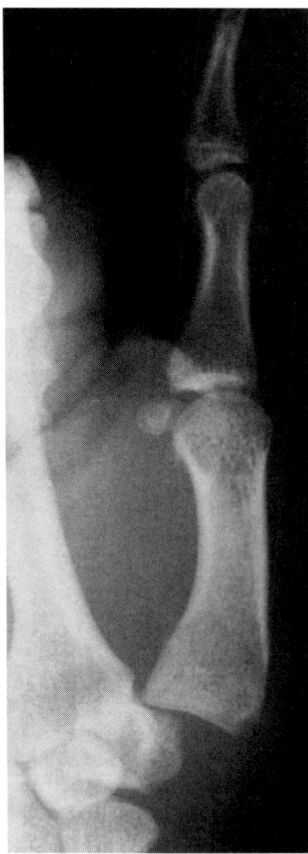

Figure 24B2–5. This thumb trapeziometacarpal joint was initially dislocated at age 15 while the patient was playing football. It was easily reduced on the sidelines and was never immobilized. Two years later, painful chronic subluxation was noted, requiring a flexor carpi radialis tenodesis to stabilize the joint.

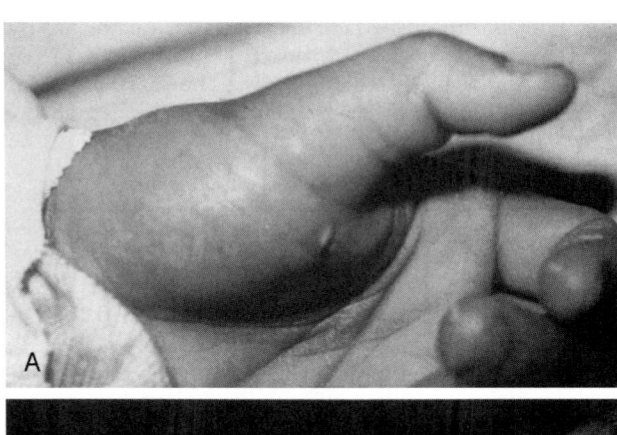
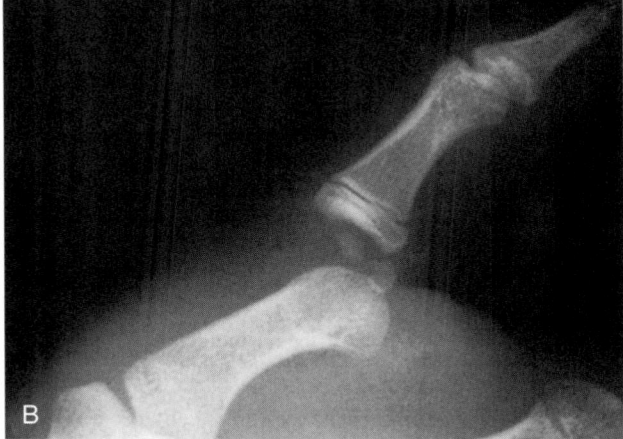

Figure 24B2–6. *A* and *B*, Hyperextension of the thumb metacarpophalangeal joint resulted in this complex dislocation. Interposition of the volar plate often prevents closed reduction.

tented over the metacarpal head. Immediate motion is begun with buddy taping to the adjacent digit.

Proximal Interphalangeal Joint Dislocations

Dislocations of the PIP joint are very common in the child and adolescent athlete. This injury is usually the result of a "jamming" injury with the finger in extension. The PIP joint can dislocate dorsally or volarly. In a dorsal dislocation, which is more common, the volar plate is torn and the middle phalanx dislocates dorsally and proximally. An avulsion fracture may occur on the middle phalanx in association with this injury, usually a Salter-Harris III fracture. The fracture fragment signifies an avulsion of the volar plate (Fig. 24B2–7). Larger fragments may also contain part of the collateral ligaments.[9] Treatment for both types is usually nonoperative. Reduction of a dorsal dislocation is performed by hyperextension with distal pressure applied to the base of the proximal phalanx. If possible, a radiograph should be taken prior to reduction. However, the athlete or trainer often accomplishes reduction on the field. If the PIP joint is stable after reduction, the involved digit is buddy taped to the adjacent digit for approximately 2 to 4 weeks. In those cases where reduction of the dislocated joint is not possible, soft tissue may be trapped in the joint. In dorsal dislocations, the volar plate is usually not entrapped but flexor tendons, collateral ligaments, and joint capsule have all been reported.[19, 46] An open reduction is required to remove the contents of the joint and repair the volar plate.[14] The joint is stabilized with an extension block splint and early motion begun. PIP dislocations are not unstable unless there is a fracture-dislocation. If the joint is stable at 30 or 45 degrees of flexion, a dorsal block extension splint is used with early range of motion. Edema can be controlled by a self adhesive wrap such as Coban. If the fracture dislocation is not stable, which is rare in children, then either ORIF or volar plate arthroplasty is recommended.

In a volar dislocation, the middle phalanx dislocates palmarly and the central slip of the extensor tendon is disrupted. Treatment consists of closed reduction followed by splinting in extension for 3 to 6 weeks, allowing DIP joint flexion. If left untreated, a boutonnière deformity will develop.[19]

Distal Interphalangeal Joint Dislocations

Pure dislocations of the DIP joint are relatively uncommon. When they do occur, they are usually the result of an impaction injury on the extended finger. The dislocation is usually dorsal but volar dislocations can occur. Technique for reduction is similar to PIP dislocations. Dislocations associated with fractures can involve avulsions of the extensor or flexor tendons and require splinting for 4 to 6 weeks.

Tendon Injuries

Mallet Finger

A *mallet finger*, also referred to as *baseball finger*, results from an impaction injury to the tip of the extended finger.[26] It is most common in ball sports. The distal phalanx is forced into flexion upon impact and the distal insertion of the extensor mechanism is disrupted. This may occur with tendon disruption alone or with an avulsion of bone known as a bony mallet. The finger in either instance is then held in flexion at the DIP joint from the unopposed force of the intact flexor profundus tendon. Active extension of the DIP joint is lost. Pure tendon injuries and nondisplaced bony mallets should be treated in an extension splint for 4 to 6 weeks. Open reduction is reserved for those displaced Salter-Harris III fractures in which palmar subluxation persists after attempted closed reduction.[26] In young children, there may be a physeal separation in the distal phalanx that requires open reduction and repair of the germinal matrix.

Boutonnière Deformity

The boutonnière deformity is caused by a rupture of the central slip of the extensor tendon at its insertion into the

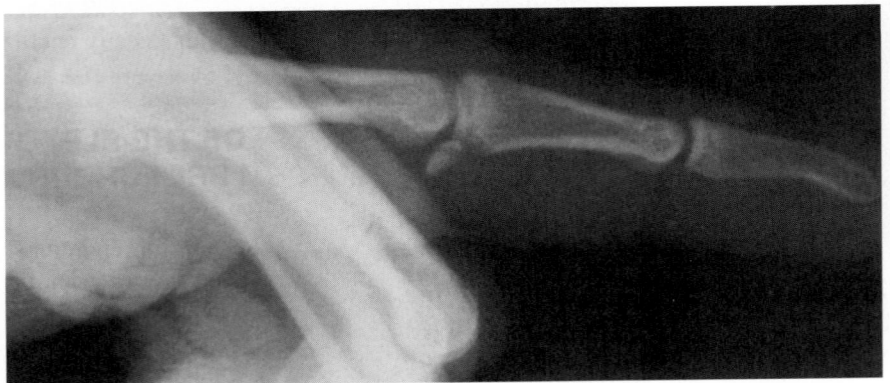

Figure 24B2–7. Axial compression as a result of the fingertip being struck by a ball results in distal interphalangeal joint flexion and proximal interphalangeal joint extension. The "jammed finger" may thus have either a mallet deformity or a proximal interphalangeal injury, usually the latter. This often results in a Salter III fracture from the base of the middle phalanx. Unless the fragment is sufficiently large to result in joint incongruity and subluxation, which is extremely rare in children and adolescents, this should be treated as a soft tissue injury. Although this radiograph shows a large fragment, there is no chronic subluxation, and the patient can be treated nonoperatively; this fragment usually does not block flexion.

middle phalanx. The head of the proximal phalanx is able to then "button hole" through the central slip defect, creating a flexion deformity at the PIP joint. The lateral bands of the extensor mechanism fall below the axis of motion of the PIP joint and retract, causing both a flexion moment at the PIP joint and an extension moment at the DIP joint.[26] Disruption of the central slip of the extensor tendon is caused by a volar dislocation of the PIP joint, or forced flexion of the PIP joint while the finger is attempting to extend. If the PIP joint is concentric on radiograph, the flexion deformity of the PIP joint should be passively correctable despite the athlete's inability to extend the joint. If passive correction is possible, then the PIP joint should be splinted in extension for 4 to 5 weeks. The DIP joint should be left free and flexion and extension of this joint encouraged. If there is a large bony avulsion fragment with joint incongruity, open reduction is indicated. Irreducible volar dislocations require open reduction and removal of the interposed tissue. This can be the lateral band, collateral ligament, or central slip. Chronic boutonnière deformities require surgical reconstruction.[40]

Jersey Finger

Jersey finger is an avulsion of the flexor digitorum profundus tendon insertion. The injury occurs when the digit is forcibly extended while the profundus muscle is under maximal contraction. The finger clenched on an opponent's jersey that gets forcibly extended is a common mechanism in rugby and football, hence the name jersey finger. The ring finger is involved in 75% of cases.[26, 27] The ring finger, although shorter than the middle finger with the hand extended, has the greatest length when the fingers are flexed and therefore is the finger left grasping the jersey. The athlete will be unable actively to flex the DIP joint if the tendon is disrupted. On radiographic examination, a fracture or bony avulsion may be visible. If a bony fragment is avulsed, this serves as a marker for the level of the retracted tendon. Leddy and Packer have described three types of profundus avulsions.[27] In a type I injury, the profundus tendon retracts to the level of the palm. Both the long and the short vincula have been disrupted, interrupting the blood supply to the tendon. This tendon is at risk of contracting and shriveling up because of both the avascularity and the degree of retraction. Therefore, the tendon should be surgically reinserted within 7 to 10 days of injury. This is done through a volar approach. The tendon is repaired by using a transosseous suture secured with a button over the nail plate. Care must be taken not to injure the physis of the distal phalanx.

In a type II injury, the most common type, the tendon retracts to the level of the PIP joint. Only the short vinculum should be disrupted in this injury. With the long vinculum intact, the blood supply to the tendon is preserved. Because some length and blood supply to the tendon have been preserved, surgical repair can usually be done within 6 weeks of injury. If the tendon cannot be repaired, then a free tendon graft is necessary (Fig. 24B2–8). The same volar approach is used as for a type I injury.[27]

In a type III injury, the profundus tendon retracts to the level of the A4 pulley over the middle phalanx. The avulsed bony fragment, if present, is too large in this type of injury to pass through the pulleys. Because minimal retraction has occurred, the long and short vincula are both intact. Treatment consists of open reduction and internal fixation of the large bony fragment or tendon. This can be done with a transosseous suture or suture anchor. Repair may be possible up to 2 to 3 months after injury because of the intact blood supply and tendon length.[27]

Timing of return to sport is dictated by both the type of injury and the age of the patient. Normal return to sport is between 8 and 12 weeks. The button should be left in place for 4 weeks with early passive mobilization.

Sport-Specific Injuries

Several sports are notorious for producing certain types of injuries in the hand that as practitioners we need to be aware of for diagnostic, treatment, and preventive purposes. Hamate fractures are common in racquet sports such as golf, tennis, or baseball, where repetitive contact with the butt end of the racquet can create a fracture.[3] Rupture of the A2 pulley has been reported in rock climbers, where the body weight of the climber is suspended by the flexor tendons.[4] Cyclists can compress the ulnar nerve at Guyon's canal from repetitive pressure on the hypothenar area. Bowlers may injure the ulnar digital nerve of the thumb from the way the thumb is placed in the ball.[13] Skier's thumb refers to injury to the ulnar collateral ligament in downhill skiers. Water skiers can suffer even more serious injuries to their thumbs. The water ski rope can become anchored around the thumb and with the pull from the boat actually avulse the thumb. Avulsion amputations also occur in other sports involved with loops of rope, including rodeo riding.[35] Avulsion of a digit is not exclusive to sports that involve the use of rope. Ring avulsions occur in basketball players who catch their ring on a basket hoop as well as in soccer goalies who catch their ring on the crossbar.[10] Not wearing any jewelry during sports activities is the best way to prevent these types of injuries. Hand protection is imperative to prevent injury in any sport where the hand is at risk for injury, such as wearing hockey gloves to prevent lacerations from a skate blade.

Frostbite

Frostbite injuries can occur during winter sporting activities such as skiing and ice hockey. Frostbite is damage to tissues that occurs as a result of exposure to low environmental temperatures. Mills and associates have classified frostbite into superficial, with injury only to skin, and deep, with damage to the deeper tissues.[33] Most cases of frostbite are superficial and can be treated with rapid rewarming of the hand in a 40°C to 44°C water bath.[32] In children, deeper injury can result in premature closure of the epiphyseal plates. This is caused by direct injury to the chondrocytes in the growth plates.[22] Closure increases in frequency from distal to proximal and can become apparent on radiograph 6 to 12 months following the insult. Brachydactyly can

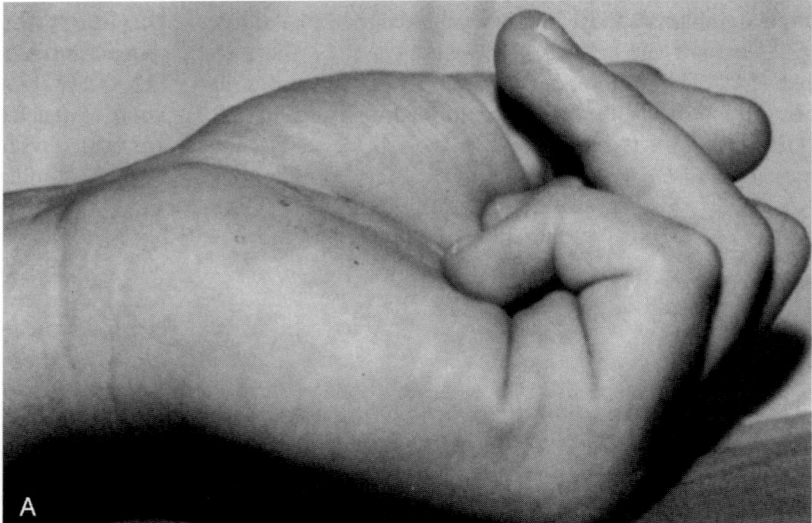

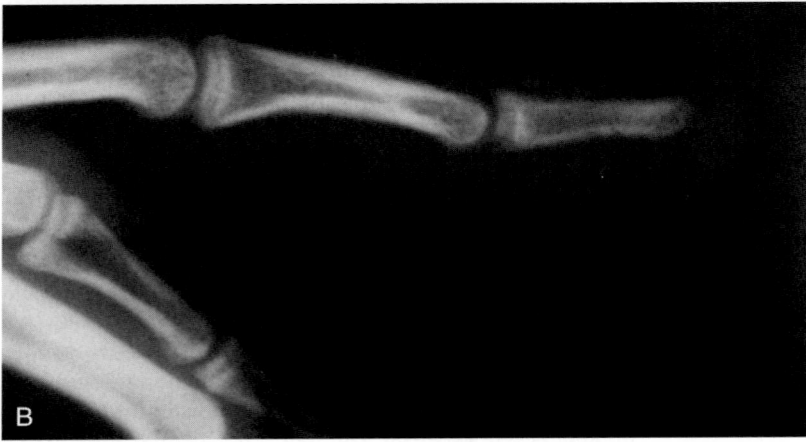

Figure 24B2–8. *A,* A 13-year-old boy presented 6 weeks after a slight sprain to the distal interphalangeal joint of his ring finger while playing football. On examination, the patient was unable to flex the distal interphalangeal joint of his right ring finger. *B.* Lateral radiograph of the involved digit demonstrated a defect in the volar base of the distal phalanx. No fragment was identified in the digit, indicating possible retraction of the tendon into the palm. At surgery, a necrotic tendon was found in the palm, necessitating a free tendon graft.

ensue with mild flexion contractures of the digits.[36] Surgery is rarely necessary for frostbite. When severe deformities result, epiphysiodesis, arthrodesis, or osteotomies may be indicated. The best treatment for frostbite is prevention.

Summary

Hand injuries in sports are very common. The goal of managing all these injuries is to restore normal function to the hand. Early and accurate diagnosis as well as appropriate management are critical in minimizing long-term morbidity. Today there is more pressure to return athletes to competition as quickly as possible. The decision to return players to athletics depends on many variables: their age, hand dominance, type of injury, degree of healing, the required use of the hand in the sport, level of competition, risk involved, and availability of protective devices. Some sports now allow players to participate with casts, thermoplastic splints, and tape. It is important to protect not only the player but also the other athletes. The recommendations made in this chapter are done so in the best interest of the child athlete.

References

1. Allieu Y: The Sportsman's Hand. In Tubiana R (ed): The Hand, vol 2. Philadelphia, WB Saunders, 1988.
2. Amadio PC: Epidemiology of hand and wrist injuries in sports. Hand Clin 6:379–381, 1990.
3. Bishop AT, Beckenbaugh RD: Fractures of the hamate hook. J Hand Surg 13:135, 1988.
4. Bollen SR, Gunson CK: Hand injuries in competition climbers. Br J Sports Med 24:16, 1990.
5. Burton RI, Eaton RG: Common hand injuries in the athlete. Orthop Clin North Am 4:809–838, 1973.
6. Brunet ME, Haddad RJ: Fractures and dislocations of the metacarpals and phalanges. Clin Sports Med 5:773–781, 1986.
7. Capo JT, Hastings H II: Metacarpal and phalangeal fractures in athletes. Clin Sports Med 17:491–511, 1998.
8. Campbell CS: Gamekeeper's thumb. J Bone Joint Surg Br 37:148–149, 1955.
9. Culver JE, Anderson TE: Fractures of the hand and wrist on the athlete. Clin Sports Med 11:101–128, 1992.
10. Curtin J, Kay NRM: Hand injuries due to soccer. Hand 8:93, 1976.
11. Derkash RS, Matyas JR, Weaver JK, et al: Acute surgical repair of the skier's thumb. Clin Orthop 216:29–33, 1987.
12. Dixon GL, Moon NF: Rotational supracondylar fractures of the proximal phalanx in children. Clin Orthop 83:151–156, 1972.
13. Dobyns JH, O'Brien ET, Linscheid RL, et al: Bowler's thumb: Diagnosis and treatment. A review of seventeen cases. J Bone Joint Surg 54:751, 1972.

14. Eaton RG, Malerich M: Volar plate arthroplasty of the proximal interphalangeal joint: A review of ten years' experience. J Hand Surg 5:260–268, 1980.
15. Ellsasser JC, Stein AH: Management of hand injuries in a professional football team. Review of 15 years experience with one team. Am J Sports Med 7:178, 1979.
16. Fahrer M: Anatomy of the karate chop. Bull Hosp Jt Dis 44:189, 1984.
17. Frontera WR: Cyclists palsy: Clinical and electrodiagnostic findings. Br J Sports Med 17:91, 1983.
18. Greene TL, Noellert RC, Belsole RJ: Treatment of unstable metacarpal and phalangeal fractures with tension band wiring techniques. Clin Orthop 214:78–84, 1987.
19. Hankin FM, Peel SM: Sport-related fractures and dislocations of the hand. Hand Clin 6:429–453, 1990.
20. Hastings H, Simmons BP: Hand fractures in children. Clin Orthop 188:120–130, 1984.
21. Heyman P, Gelberman RH, Duncan K, et al: Injuries of the ulnar collateral ligament of the thumb metacarpophalangeal joint: Biomechanical and prospective clinical studies on the usefulness of valgus stress testing. Clin Orthop 292:165–171, 1993.
22. House JH, Fidler MO: Frostbite of the hand. In Green DP, Hotchkiss RN (eds): Green's Operative Hand Surgery, 4th ed, vol 2. Philadelphia, Churchill Livingstone, 1999.
23. James JIP: Fractures of the proximal and middle phalanges of the fingers. Acta Orthop Scand 32:401–412, 1962.
24. James JIP: Common single errors in the management of hand injuries. Proc R Soc Med 63:69–71, 1970.
25. Kujala UM, Taimela S, Antti-Poika I, et al: Acute injuries in soccer, ice-hockey, volleyball, basketball, judo, and karate: Analysis of national registry data. BMJ 311:1465–1468, 1995.
26. Leddy JP: Soft-tissue injuries of the hand in the athlete. AAOS Instruct Course Lect 47:181–186, 1998.
27. Leddy JP, Packer JW: Avulsion of profundus tendon insertion in athletes. J Hand Surg 2:66, 1977.
28. Mandlebaum BR, Bartolozzi AR, Davis CA, et al: Wrist pain syndrome in the gymnast. Am J Sports Med 17:305, 1989.
29. Mastey RD, Weiss APC, Akelman E: Primary care of hand and wrist athletic injuries. Clin Sports Med 16:705–724, 1997.
30. McCowan IA: Boxing injuries. Am J Sports Med 17:305, 1959.
31. McElfresh EC, Dobyns JH: Intra-articular metacarpal head fractures. J Hand Surg 8:383–393, 1983.
32. Mills WJ Jr: Frostbite: A method of management including rapid thawing. Northwest Med 65:119–125, 1966.
33. Mills WJ Jr, Whaley R, Fish W: Frostbite: Experience with rapid rewarming and ultrasonic therapy. Alaska Med 2:114–122, 1960.
34. Minami A, An KN, Cooney WP III, et al: Ligamentous structures of the metacarpophalangeal joint: A quantitative anatomic study. J Orthop Res 1:361–368, 1984.
35. Morgan RF, Nichter LS, Friedman HI, et al: Rodeo roping thumb injuries. J Hand Surg [Am], 9:178, 1984.
36. Nakazato R, Ogino T: Epiphyseal destruction of children's hands after frostbite: A report of 2 cases. J Hand Surg [Am] 11:289–292, 1986.
37. National SAFEKIDS Campaign. Washington, DC, 2000.
38. Ogden JA: Skeletal Injury in the Child. Philadelphia, Lea & Febiger, 1982.
39. Pelligrini VD Jr: Fractures at the base of the thumb. Hand Clin 4: 87–102, 1998.
40. Posner MA, Kapila D: Chronic palmar dislocation of proximal interphalangeal joints. J Hand Surg [Am] 11:253–258, 1986.
41. Rockwood CA, Green DP: Fractures in Children. Philadelphia, JB Lippincott, 1984.
42. Roser LA, Clawson DK: Football injuries in the very young athlete. Clin Orthop 69:219–223, 1970.
43. Simmons BP, Peters T: Subcondylar fossa reconstruction for malunion of fractures of the proximal phalanx in children. J Hand Surg [Am] 12:1079–1082, 1987.
44. Simonet WT, Sim FH: Ice hockey injuries. Am J Sports Med 15: 3, 1987.
45. Stener B: Displacement of the ruptured ulnar collateral ligament of the metacarpo-phalangeal joint of the thumb: A clinical and anatomical study. J Bone Joint Surg Br 44:869–879, 1962.
46. Stern PJ: Stener lesion after lateral dislocation of the proximal interphalangeal joint—indication for open reduction. J Hand Surg 6: 602–604, 1981.

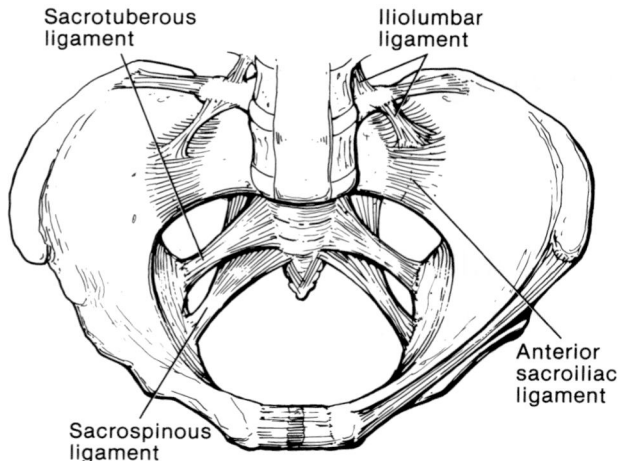

Figure 25A–1. Anatomy of the sacroiliac joints. Note multiple ligamentous reinforcements.

sacrum the forces are transmitted to the fifth lumbar vertebra of the spinal column. In the sitting position, forces are borne through the ischiosacral arch: Weight is transmitted from the ischial tuberosities through the ilia to the sacrum and then to the spinal column.

These two primary arches are augmented by two subsidiary tie arches that connect the arms of the primary arches. The femorosacral arch is joined by a tie arch formed by the bodies of the pubic bones and their horizontal rami. The ischiosacral arch is joined by a tie arch made up of the ischial rami and the inferior pubic rami. The anterior interpubic and arcuate ligaments form an important link in both anterior tie arches. With trauma, the tie arches fail first, followed by the primary arches. The areas most susceptible to injury are the pubic symphysis, the pubic rami, and the areas just lateral to the sacroiliac joints.[58]

The three distinct motions of the pelvis are anteroposterior tilting, lateral tilting, and rotation. Anteroposterior tilting occurs in the sagittal plane around a coronal axis. Anterior tilting is accomplished through the action of the iliopsoas and other hip flexors in conjunction with the extensors of the lumbar spine and is accompanied by an increase in spinal lordosis. Posterior tilting is accomplished through the combined operation of the rectus abdominis, the abdominal obliques, the gluteus maximus, and the hamstring muscles and is accompanied by a decrease in the lumbar lordotic curve.

Lateral tilting takes place in the frontal plane around the anteroposterior axis, and the hip joints act as the centers of rotation. This results in abduction or adduction of the hips, depending on the direction of rotation. Lateral pelvic tilt is controlled by the hip abductors, primarily by eccentric or isometric contraction.

Pelvic rotation occurs in the transverse plane around the vertical axis of the hip joint. Rotation is controlled through the complex interactions of the gluteal muscles, the short external rotators, the upper adductor mass, the pectineus, and the iliopsoas.

The hip is a ball-and-socket, polyaxial joint connecting the lower extremity to the pelvic girdle. The acetabulum forms the bony socket of the hip. A plane taken through

the rim of the acetabulum at its opening intersects the sagittal plane at an angle of 40 degrees and opens anteriorly; with the transverse plane at an angle of 60 degrees, it opens laterally. In other words, the cavity of the acetabulum faces obliquely forward, laterally, and downward.[88, 96] The acetabular surface is lined with hyaline cartilage that is thickened peripherally. The socket is further deepened by a ring of fibrocartilage, the labrum, which attaches around its rim.

The femoral head forms two thirds of a sphere and is slightly flattened superiorly. Its covering of hyaline cartilage is thickest on the mediocentral surface and thinnest at the periphery. Although these differences may influence the transmission of forces through the femoral head, the joint reaction force usually acts on the superior quadrant of the head. The position of the femoral head and neck with respect to the shaft of the femur is characteristically described by two angular relationships—the angle of inclination and the angle of declination. Both are formed during embryonic development and are subsequently modified after birth by the action of the muscles across the joint and the distribution of the forces of gravity.

The angle of inclination is the frontal projection of the angle formed by the long axes of the femoral neck and the femoral shaft. The angle varies with age, sex, and development of the bony skeleton, but in adults it averages between 125 and 135 degrees.[44] The angle of declination is sometimes referred to as the *angle of torsion* or the *angle of anteversion*. It is defined as the projection of the angle between the long axis of the femoral neck and the axis through the femoral condyles in the transverse plane. The angle measures approximately 15 degrees in mature adults.[44] Variations in the angle of torsion will cause compensatory changes in lower extremity rotation to maintain the femoral head within the acetabular cavity. Such changes in rotation may be a predictive factor for the development of conditions such as stress fractures in the lower extremity.[46]

The internal architecture of the femoral neck is made up of cancellous bone arranged in trabecular systems oriented along the principal lines of stress (Fig. 25A–2). Although several of these systems have been described, the

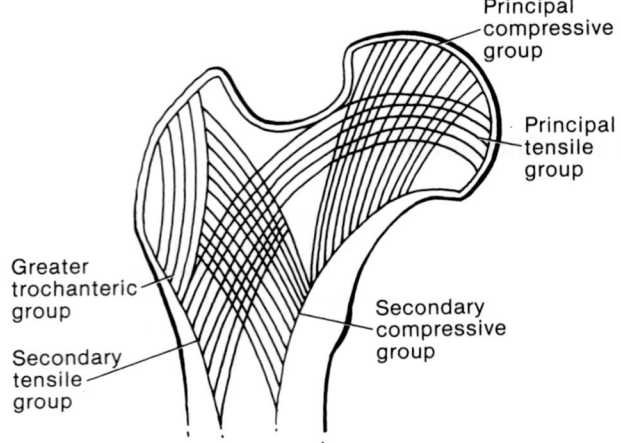

Figure 25A–2. Anatomy of the bony trabeculae of the proximal femur.

two most important are the primary medial (compression) trabeculae and the primary lateral (tension) trabeculae. The medial system arises from the cortical bone of the medial femoral shaft (sometimes known as the calcar) and streams superiorly in layers to the subchondral bone of the superior aspect of the femoral head. This cancellous bone supports the joint reaction force.[88] The lateral system arises from the cortical bone of the lateral femur, crosses the medial system, and ends in the subchondral bone of the inferomedial quadrant of the head. This system develops in response to the forces generated by the abductor muscles and the fascia lata.[81, 88]

Because of its ball-and-socket configuration, the hip has a degree of intrinsic stability unlike that found in other joints. Yet in addition to its inherent stability, the articulation between the acetabulum and the head of the femur retains great mobility. This allows not only the motion necessary for normal ambulation but also performance of a wide range of athletic activities. The hip is capable of motion in three planes: sagittal, frontal, and transverse, the greatest motion occurring in the sagittal plane.[88] During the normal gait cycle, motion of the hip joint takes place in all three planes.[56, 83] It has been suggested that to perform the activities of daily living in a normal manner, hip flexion of at least 120 degrees, abduction of at least 20 degrees, and external rotation of at least 20 degrees are necessary.[57] To participate in sporting activities, significantly greater motion is often necessary.[57]

The forces transmitted across the hip joint during static and dynamic conditions have been measured. During simple one-legged standing, the force transmitted across the hip is 2.6 times body weight.[81] In the normal gait pattern, maximal force occurs during early and late stages of the stance phase.[102] During slow walking, the maximum force is approximately 1.6 times body weight, but this force may be increased up to 3.3 times body weight when speed is increased. Running increases the force to five times body weight during the stance phase and three times body weight during the swing phase. Ascending or descending a ramp further increases the forces across the hip joint.

Soft Tissue Injuries

Contusions

Soft tissue contusions are among the most frequent hip and pelvic injuries sustained by competitive athletes. Contusions result from direct blows to the soft tissue. In general, the mechanism of injury involves collision with another player, the player's equipment (i.e., a football helmet), or the playing surface (i.e., a hockey sideboard). Often, these injuries are minor and can be handled with symptomatic treatment of short duration, with return to competition as symptoms allow.[120]

Because of the varied anatomy of the pelvis, contusions in this region may be superficial, overlying relatively subcutaneous bone, or deep within a large muscle mass.[89] On occasion, significant muscular hemorrhage occurs, resulting in prolonged disability. Slow bleeding may also occur into the tissues surrounding the area of impact. As a result, the

athlete may not experience significant symptoms until the day after the injury.

Injury occurs frequently over the bony prominences of the greater trochanter, the ischial tuberosity, and the pubic rami. When a direct blow to the iliac crest is associated with subperiosteal hematoma and disability, the term *hip pointer* is often used.[4, 64, 89] Unfortunately, this term is confusing and does not properly differentiate between contusions, avulsions, and fractures.

Early treatment for contusions should be directed at controlling deep bleeding with ice, compression, and rest. Radiographs are frequently necessary to rule out fracture. Heat, massage, and vigorous physical therapy should be delayed for 48 hours because they may increase bleeding. Aspirin and other nonsteroidal anti-inflammatory agents may also increase bleeding if they are initiated early. Attempts to aspirate the hematoma have met with only limited success. For adult athletes suffering from a hip pointer due to a contusion—once a fracture has been ruled out clinically—judicious use of a local corticosteroid injection may help alleviate the pain and the disability from this condition and hasten the return to activity.

Treatment of severe muscular contusions is often frustrating. Rehabilitation is aimed at maintaining flexibility and includes strengthening exercises to combat prolonged muscle spasm, disuse atrophy, and decreased range of motion.[120] Muscle use must be restricted until function has returned to normal, however, and return to full competitive activity should be delayed until full strength and coordination have returned. Accelerated treatment or premature return to competition may result in repetitive microtrauma and reinjury, which will prolong disability.

Deep contusions with significant hemorrhage may result in the late complication of myositis ossificans (see later discussion), particularly when a large hematoma forms in the muscles about the pelvis. Severe contusions may also result in bursitis with persistent pain and tenderness in the area of injury. Frequent sites of injury about the hip and the pelvis include the greater trochanter and the ischial tuberosity.[89] Early attempts to control bleeding may limit occurrence of these late sequelae.

Contusion of the sciatic nerve may result after a blow to the buttocks. The athlete experiences pain in the buttocks extending through the back of the thigh and the foot. The pain is nonradicular and frequently corresponds to the entire distribution of the sciatic nerve. Usually, the only treatment required is rest and protection against further injury such as that caused by stretching.[89] Sciatic nerve contusion must be differentiated from gluteal compartment syndrome or crush injury syndrome. Compartment syndrome in this area usually follows a far more severe injury and develops over hours rather than immediately after impact.[106] Compartment syndrome is a surgical emergency, requiring fasciotomy to release the increased intracompartmental pressures to prevent permanent disability.

Myositis Ossificans

Myositis ossificans is a reactive lesion that occurs in soft tissues and periosteum following injury.[55] It is a frequent

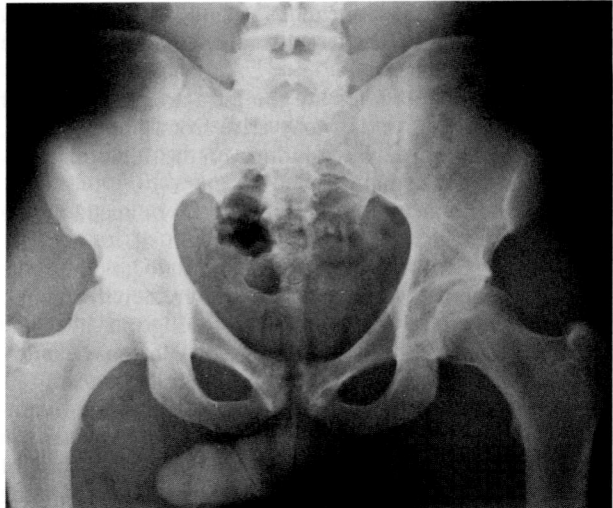

Figure 25A–4. Radiograph demonstrating osteitis pubis.

tendon.[113] Intra-articular cases of snapping hip can be treated with hip arthroscopy, including removal of loose bodies or débridement of the affected labrum and cartilage.[47]

Osteitis Pubis

Osteitis pubis should be considered a possible diagnosis in athletes with pain in the region of the pubis. Although osteitis pubis is a well-recognized entity after surgery of the bladder or the prostate,[6, 7, 125] it has been reported after athletic endeavors as well.[50, 125] It has been reported in long-distance runners, weightlifters, fencers, soccer players, and football players.[62, 125] Athletes with osteitis pubis describe a gradual onset of pain in the pubic region. The pain may radiate into the groin, along the medial aspect of the thighs, or into the abdomen. Tenderness along the subcutaneous border of the pubis is dominant. Passive abduction and resisted active adduction of both lower extremities elicit pain. With continued activity, pain increases, producing spasm in the rectus abdominis and adductor muscles. In severe cases, the athlete develops either an antalgic or a waddling gait.

Early in the course of the disease, bone scans show diffuse increased uptake in the pubis.[120] Radiographic changes may not be visible for 2 to 3 weeks (Fig. 25A–4).[120] Harris and Murray described the typical radiographic features encountered in 37 athletes.[50] These included (1) symmetrical bone resorption at the medial ends of the pubic bones, (2) widening of the pubic symphysis, and (3) rarefaction or sclerosis along the pubic rami. In patients with pronounced cystic changes, the differential diagnosis should include hyperparathyroidism, myelomatosis, sarcoidosis, hemochromatosis, rheumatoid arthritis, and osteomyelitis.[90]

The precise cause of osteitis pubis in athletes remains unclear. Multiple theories have been proposed. Muscle strain with a degenerative reaction at the bony attachment site has been suggested, as have avascular necrosis and

osteochondritis dissecans. Fatigue fracture of the pubis at the symphysis is another possibility, and avulsion of the gracilis attachment at its origin may cause a similar clinical picture.[125] It seems likely that these changes actually represent points along the continuum of a clinical spectrum. The underlying unifying factor is overuse of the adductors and the gracilis.

Clearly, the changes seen in athletes are noninfectious and are probably not secondary to an isolated traumatic incident but rather are caused by repetitive minor trauma and strain. The result is inflammation, periostitis, and bony changes at the pubic origin of the involved muscles. The lesion may be akin to "shin splints" seen at the tibial attachment of the posterior tibialis. Treatment for osteitis pubis centers around rest because the condition is considered self-limited.[90, 109] Anti-inflammatory drugs may hasten recovery, but a 2- to 3-month course of treatment is not unusual. In chronic cases that are unresponsive to conservative therapy, operative treatment may be warranted. Both arthrodesis of the pubic symphysis[2, 90] and local débridement[125] have been described with successful results.

Muscle, Tendon, and Ligament Injuries

Muscular and musculotendinous injuries are perhaps the most frequent athletic-related injuries occurring in the region of the hip and the pelvis. The pelvic ring and the proximal femur are the sites of origin and insertion for several major muscle groups: the insertion of the abdominal muscles on the iliac wing, the origin of the gluteals from the ilium and their insertion on the proximal femur, the origin of the adductors from the pubis, and the insertion of the iliopsoas on the lesser trochanter (Fig. 25A–5). Injury to any of these muscle groups can be quite disabling.

The majority of musculotendinous injuries experienced

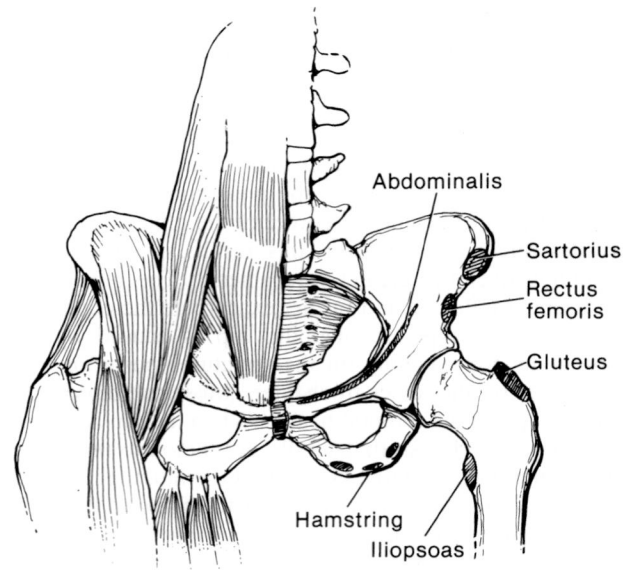

Abdominalis

Sartorius

Rectus femoris

Gluteus

Hamstring

Iliopsoas

Figure 25A–5. Anterior view of the pelvis demonstrating the muscular origins and insertions.

by athletes are acute muscle strains or pulls.[45] Strains are defined as tears, either partial or complete, of the muscle-tendon unit.[17, 45, 103] Muscle strains and tears most frequently result from violent muscular contraction during an excessively forceful muscular stretch.[45] The same mechanism that results in an apophyseal avulsion in adolescent athletes causes a muscular strain or a tear in adults. Both partial and complete tears consistently occur at the musculotendinous junction.[45, 72, 103]

In general, the majority of musculotendinous injuries about the hip can be treated according to well-defined simple guidelines. The program suggested is akin to that devised by Metzmaker and Pappas for apophyseal avulsion injuries[74] and is based on a four-stage plan presented by Sim and Scott.[109] The resulting protocol is divided into five phases (Table 25A–1).

The goal of phase I is to reduce pain and limit bleeding, swelling, and inflammation. The mainstays of treatment during this period are rest, ice, compression, and protection. Ice is applied for 20 minutes every hour and is combined with a compressive wrap. When crutch therapy is combined with compression, the result is greater than when either is employed alone. Spica wraps for groin injuries or abdominal corsets for abdominal injuries provide both compression and protection. During the acute phase, bed rest and positioning are used to rest the affected muscle. Phase I continues until the acute symptoms subside, usually in 48 to 72 hours. Aspirin and other nonsteroidal anti-inflammatory medications are avoided during this time because of their effects on coagulation.

The goals of phase II are to regain range of motion, prevent joint contractures, and limit muscle atrophy. Active and gentle passive assisted range of motion exercises within the limits of pain are initiated. Modalities such as heat, ultrasound, and high-intensity muscle stimulation are added to the regimen. Nonsteroidal anti-inflammatory medication is started at this point to decrease spasm and stiffness, which may arise secondary to inflammation. Protected weight-bearing with crutches or a cane may be used for ambulation until strength and flexibility return.

Phase III is started when a pain-free state of motion is achieved and muscle spasm has subsided. Achievement of normal or near-normal unassisted gait should now be possible. The goals of phase III are to achieve a gradual increase in strength, endurance, and flexibility. Isometric exercises are initiated at various joint angles. Static stretching exercises are used with caution. Well-leg stationary cycling is particularly useful to maintain cardiovascular status as well as flexibility in the affected limb.

Phase IV begins with the initiation of dynamic resistance exercises. These must be done with close supervision. As strength increases before full coordination is attained, there is a tendency toward reinjury. Range of motion is maintained with static and dynamic exercises. Heat and ultrasound are useful before stretching exercises begin. Cryotherapy is used after exercise to prevent reinflammation and muscle spasm. Half-speed straight leg exercises are started as strength returns.

Phase V begins when 70% of strength has returned. Coordination and proprioceptive training are the cornerstones of this final phase. Strength training to regain full normal strength is continued. All strength training should be symmetrical so that strength is maintained in the well limb. Sport- and position-specific agility training is used to regain the skills necessary to participate safely in the athlete's particular sport. Return to participation before full agility and coordination are achieved will lead to reinjury. Specific objective skill tests should be performed before return to full participation is allowed.

External Oblique Strains

The aponeurosis of the external oblique muscle may be injured by forceful contracture of the abdominal muscles while the trunk is forced to the contralateral side. This is a frequent injury in football players making a flying block or tackle or in hockey players who are checked forcefully against the boards. The result is some degree of detachment of the abdominal muscles from their insertion along the anterior and inner portions of the iliac crest. Separation may vary from a few fibers to complete detachment.

Initially, the athlete will experience extreme pain, difficulty in straightening the trunk, and local tenderness along the iliac crest or the superior rim of the inner table. Occasionally, a palpable defect may be felt above the iliac crest. Active flexion to the opposite side will cause pain; this may be a useful means of distinguishing contusion from muscle separation. Pain with active abduction or extension of the thigh when the athlete lies on the contralateral side indicates damage to the gluteal attachments or to the tensor fascia latae and the lateral abdominals.

Initial treatment, as outlined earlier, consists of rest, ice, and compression. Care should be taken to avoid early heat, vigorous massage, or stretching. These should not be instituted sooner than 48 hours after injury. Abdominal binders and taping may be helpful to reduce pain and increase support. Tape is applied over benzoin ointment from below the iliac crest in line with the muscle fibers of the external oblique. Circumferential taping should be avoided because it may restrict breathing. Early rehabilitation exercises should be undertaken within the limits of tolerance. Taping is continued when the athlete returns to activity. In addition, for return to contact sports, the iliac crest should be well padded. Surgical repair to restore anatomic continuity may be required in rare cases.[89, 109]

TABLE 25A–1
Rehabilitation Guidelines for Muscle Injuries

	Goals	Treatment	Time Frame
Phase I	Reduce pain, inflammation, and bleeding	Rest, ice, and compression; crutches prn	48 to 72 hr
Phase II	Regain range of motion	Passive range of motion, heat, ultrasound, EMS	72 hr to 1 wk
Phase III	Increase strength, flexibility, and endurance	Isometrics, well-leg cycling	1 to 3 wk
Phase IV	Increase strength and coordination	Isotonic and isokinetic exercises	3 to 4 wk
Phase V	Return to competition	Sport-specific training	4 to 6 wk

EMS, electrical muscle stimulation.

Sciatic Nerve Entrapment

The sciatic nerve is the major nerve arising from the lumbosacral plexus. It comprises the ventral rami of the fourth and fifth lumbar roots along with the first, second, and third sacral roots. The nerve exits the pelvis through the sciatic notch inferior to the piriformis muscle. The piriformis muscle arises from the anterior surface of the sacrum and the sacrotuberous ligament and inserts into the superior border of the greater trochanter. In 10% of patients, the piriformis muscle splits the sciatic nerve as it exits.[78] The nerve passes along the posterior border of the hip capsule deep to the gluteus maximus and descends near the middle border of the thigh, lying on the adductor magnus. The nerve is purely motor in function, and its two divisions supply all the muscles of the leg as well as the short head of the biceps femoris. The sciatic nerve can become compressed anywhere along its path from the pelvis to the popliteal fossa, but the symptoms produced are usually in the distal extremity.

Piriformis Syndrome. The piriformis syndrome, which causes compression of the sciatic nerve, is a clinical condition that has become more widely recognized as a cause of buttocks and hamstring pain, especially in athletes.[9, 108, 116] Patients usually present with a history of blunt trauma to the gluteal or sacroiliac region with complaints of pain in the lower region of the sacroiliac joint, the greater sciatic notch, and the piriformis muscle occasionally radiating down the posterior aspect of the lower extremity.[99] The pain may also be described as a cramping or a feeling of tightness in the hamstring muscles. Stooping or lifting exacerbates the symptoms.

Diagnosis of piriformis syndrome can be difficult and somewhat controversial. On examination, patients may be noted to have a palpable mass over the piriformis muscle during an exacerbation of symptoms. This mass is markedly tender has been called the pathognomonic sign.[99] Buttocks pain may be exacerbated by hip flexion and passive internal rotation. Results of the straight leg raising test are occasionally positive. It is most important to differentiate this condition from other more common sources of buttocks and lower extremity pain, such as lumbar spine or hip joint disease. Imaging studies of the pelvis and the spine are very important in ruling out other conditions; however, at present, they tend to provide little information that can rule in the diagnosis. Electrodiagnostic studies usually demonstrate normal long latency signals at rest but become abnormal with hip flexion and internal rotation maneuvers.[41]

Treatment of piriformis syndrome initially includes nonoperative modalities. Physical therapy to stretch and massage the piriformis, transrectal ultrasound, local anesthetic or steroid injections, and oral nonsteroidal anti-inflammatory drugs have all been tried, with varying degrees of success. If nonoperative measures fail to provide relief, operative intervention should be considered. Sectioning the piriformis muscle at the tendinous insertion, release of the fibrous bands or compressing vessels, and external neurolysis have been shown to provide relief.[9, 116] Functional loss is minimal because there are several synergistic muscles to the piriformis. One recent report demonstrated 14 patients with piriformis syndrome that was caused by blunt trauma to the gluteal region.[9] All were managed with operative release of the piriformis tendon and sciatic neurolysis after extensive conservative treatment failed. Intraoperative findings revealed adhesions between the piriformis muscle, the sciatic nerve, and the roof of the greater sciatic notch. Results were excellent or good in all patients.

Fractures

Avulsion Fractures

A common injury in the younger athlete is the avulsion fracture (Fig. 25A–6). Although classically considered rare, these injuries have become common among athletic participants,[77] particularly children or young adults[96]; avulsion fractures occur primarily between the ages of 14 and 25 years.[120, 122] They comprised 13.4% of children's pelvic fractures in the Campbell Clinic series.[21]

In the skeletally immature patient, the usual mechanism of injury is either a sudden violent muscular contraction or an excessive amount of sustained muscle action across an open apophysis.[74, 120] As a result, these injuries are most often identified in young sprinters, jumpers, and soccer and football players.[120] Often, there is no history of external trauma. The same mechanism that results in a muscle or tendon strain in an adult can cause avulsion of an apophysis in an adolescent athlete. The apophyseal center is biomechanically susceptible to avulsion injury through the physis by the same mechanism that causes long bone physeal injury.[74] Separation occurs in the cartilaginous area between the apophysis and the bone. Chronic overuse syndromes may present as an apophysitis about the knee similar to that seen in Sinding-Larsen or Osgood-Schlatter disease.

Generally, athletes with pelvic avulsions present with local pain and swelling after an extreme effort. The competitor may recall the specific incident, but, as noted, there is often no history of external trauma. Radiographs are useful in confirming the diagnosis. Comparison views of the contralateral side may be necessary to ascertain the degree of skeletal maturity and the status of the normal apophysis. In patients with old injuries, abundant callus formation should not be confused with malignancy.

The recommended treatment for avulsion fractures of the pelvis has generally been bed rest, a difficult prescription for an athlete of any age; activity modification and limitation may be better tolerated. Metzmaker and Pappas have outlined a five-stage program of progressive rehabilitation for acute avulsion fractures of the pelvis and the hip.[74] Their approach, outlined in greater detail previously, involves (1) rest, using proper positioning to relax the involved muscle groups, combined with the use of ice and analgesics; (2) increased excursion, with the initiation of gentle active and passive range of motion exercises; (3) progressive resistance, beginning when 75% of range of motion is achieved and ending when the involved muscles have regained 50% of their anticipated strength; (4) integration, stretching, and strengthening exercises combined with patterned motions*; and (5) return to competitive activity.

---

*It should be noted that at this point in their recovery, many athletes attempt to return to competitive activity before full integration of muscle function is attained. If this happens, reinjury is likely.

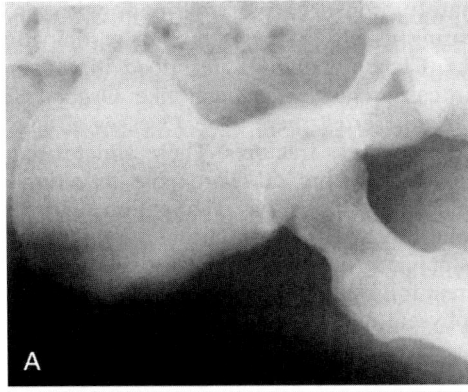

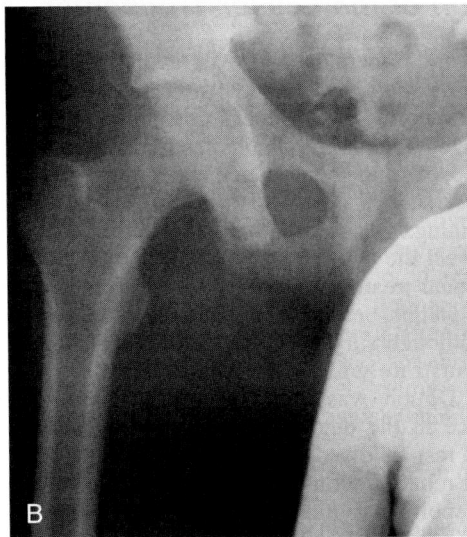

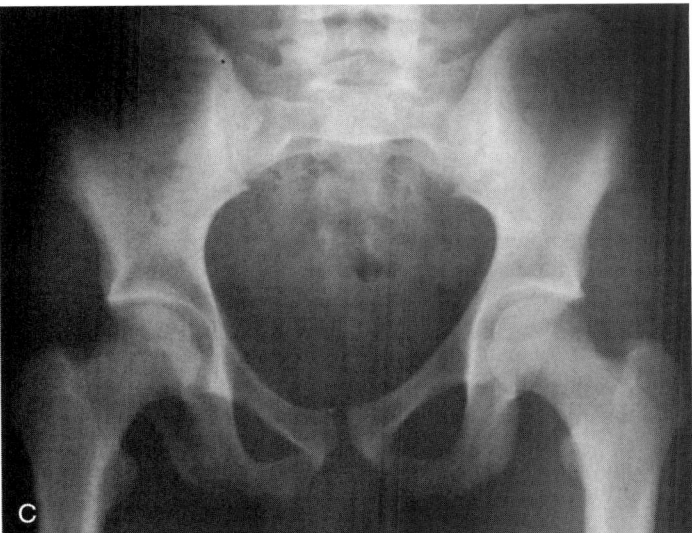

Figure 25A–6. Radiograph showing avulsion fractures of the pelvis. *A*, Anterior superior iliac spine. *B*, Anterior inferior iliac spine. *C*, Ischium.

Surgical intervention with open reduction and internal fixation (ORIF) of avulsion fractures has been described in isolated cases.[21] It has also been advocated by some to avoid functional disability in competitive athletes.[105] The majority of athletes with avulsion fractures of the pelvis and the hip can be treated nonoperatively, however. No advantage has been found for acute surgical intervention in any cases of pelvic avulsion fracture. Therefore, at present, there does not appear to be any indication for ORIF of any of these injuries.

Avulsion of the anterior superior iliac spine (ASIS) occurs when there is a relative overpull of the sartorius muscle during jumping or running. This usually occurs when the hip is extended and the knee is flexed.[21, 58, 98] Clinical findings include local pain, tenderness, and swelling. Attempts to flex or abduct the affected thigh actively elicit pain. Radiographs demonstrate slight displacement of the ASIS; marked displacement is prevented by the fascia lata and the lateral portion of the inguinal ligament.[60, 98, 101] Although Canale and King treated two of their patients with ORIF, they felt that this method had no advantage over nonoperative measures.[21] Patients treated with positioning, protected weight-bearing, and progressive rehabilitation can be expected to return successfully to competition. Acute operative repair does not offer an advantage over conservative care and therefore is not indicated.

Avulsion of the anterior inferior iliac spine (AIIS) is less common than avulsion of the ASIS, both because less stress is generally placed on the AIIS and because it ossifies earlier.[96, 121, 124] This type of fracture occurs with vigorous contraction of the straight head of the rectus femoris muscle, the classic mechanism involved in kicking.[121] After injury, active flexion of the hip causes pain. Radiographs show distal displacement of a fragment of the AIIS. Increased displacement is prevented by the insertion of the rectus through a conjoined tendon and the intact reflected head of the rectus femoris.[21] Contralateral radiographs should be obtained to rule out the possibility of os acetabuli, as noted by Watson-Jones.[121] Although Caudle and Crawford reported an avulsion of the os acetabuli that was successfully treated with ORIF,[23] there are no reports of operative treatment of avulsion fractures of the AIIS. All patients responded to bed rest followed by protected weight-bearing and progressive return to full weight-bearing as tolerated.[21, 23] Treatment as outlined by Metzmaker and Pappas should allow safe return to full participation within 6 weeks.[74] Again, there does not appear to be any indication for acute surgical intervention.

The ischial apophysis appears at the age of 15 years and is one of the last to unite with the bony skeleton (at age 25). It is therefore susceptible to injury for a relatively long period of time.[21, 58] Avulsion is caused by maximum hamstring contraction with the pelvis fixed in flexion and the knee in extension.[1, 10, 70, 76] As a result, injuries to the otherwise. Distinct radiographic findings may not develop until 2 to 4 weeks after the initial injury.[43, 49, 82] Waiting to obtain serial radiographs, although they are important in the characterization of the lesion, should not delay treatment. Bone scintigraphy has proved to be highly sensitive in detecting lesions before they become visible on radiographs.[43, 49, 82] MRI is also very sensitive and should be performed in any patient with the clinical picture of a stress fracture of the femoral neck and with negative radiographic findings (Fig. 25A–8). Imaging studies of the contralateral hip are recommended because of the reported incidence of bilateral stress fractures.[30, 31]

Most approaches to treatment have been based on radiographic characterization of the fracture pattern. In 1965, Devas developed a biomechanical classification of femoral neck stress fractures.[30] He described two types of fracture patterns: transverse and compression. Transverse fractures are more common in older patients and are characterized radiographically by a crack in the superior cortex of the femoral neck. These fractures have a high likelihood of displacement with continued stress. Compression fractures are more common in younger patients, accounting for 50% of fractures in patients younger than 60 years of age in the original series. The early radiographic appearance of these fractures is a "haze" of internal callus along the inferior femoral neck without cortical disruption. Continued stress does not cause displacement.

Ten years after his initial report, Devas redefined transverse and compression injuries as distraction and compression fractures, respectively.[31] He recommended surgical treatment for all distraction injuries and nonoperative treatment for compression fractures only when "good grounds" existed.[31] Pankovich recommended internal fixation for all femoral neck stress fractures as a means of overcoming patient noncompliance.[92]

Blickenstaff and Morris in 1966 presented a descriptive

classification based on degree of displacement.[12, 82] Type I fractures had callus with no fracture line; type II fractures had a definite fracture line but no displacement; and type III fractures were displaced. Blickenstaff and Morris recommended bed rest followed by progressive weight-bearing for type I fractures, plaster immobilization or internal fixation for type II fractures, and reduction and internal fixation for type III fractures. They noted that complications occurred in seven of nine type III fractures.

In 1988, Fullerton and Snowdy presented a classification based on a combination of biomechanical factors and degree of displacement.[43] Their classification also defined the role of bone scintigraphy in the management of femoral neck stress fractures. Bone scan–positive, radiograph-negative lesions were treated with bed rest followed by progressive weight-bearing. In this series, eight fractures with positive bone scan findings healed without subsequent radiographic changes.

Because of the great disability that can arise secondary to displaced femoral neck fractures in young and otherwise healthy athletes, early diagnosis and aggressive treatment are necessary to ensure initiation of treatment before displacement occurs. Therefore, a high index of suspicion is maintained in any athlete who presents with a history and physical findings suggestive of femoral neck stress fracture. If the initial radiographs are negative, mandatory rest and non–weight-bearing ambulation are initiated for 7 days, at which time a bone scan and repeat radiographs are obtained. If both studies are negative, they are repeated after another week. At that time, if they remain negative, a new diagnosis is sought. Athletes with positive bone scan results and negative radiographic findings are treated for a prefracture "stress reaction." This lesion has been described in relation to stress fractures in other long bones. The athlete is kept non–weight-bearing until he or she is pain free. At that time, progressive weight-bearing to the limits of pain tolerance is initiated. Once the patient is bearing full weight with support, cardiovascular training is initiated. Activity levels are increased in small increments as the athlete achieves pain-free function at each level. Radiographs are taken weekly to monitor changes in fracture status. Return to full activity is allowed when there is radiographic evidence of a healed fracture or when bone scan results turn negative.

Nondisplaced fractures on the compression (medial) side are treated with discontinuation of weight-bearing until the patient is pain free. Non–weight-bearing ambulation with crutches is maintained until radiographic evidence of healing is demonstrated. During convalescence, frequent radiographs are obtained to monitor changes in fracture status. If any widening or displacement occurs, the hip is stabilized with internal fixation. If nondisplaced fractures do not respond to bed rest and non–weight-bearing with a reduction in symptoms, consideration is given to stabilization with internal fixation.

For tension-side injuries, an aggressive approach is maintained regardless of the degree of displacement. Owing to the likelihood of displacement with this type of fracture as well as to the extreme nature of complications associated with fracture displacement, internal fixation is performed on an urgent basis. After fixation, a standard

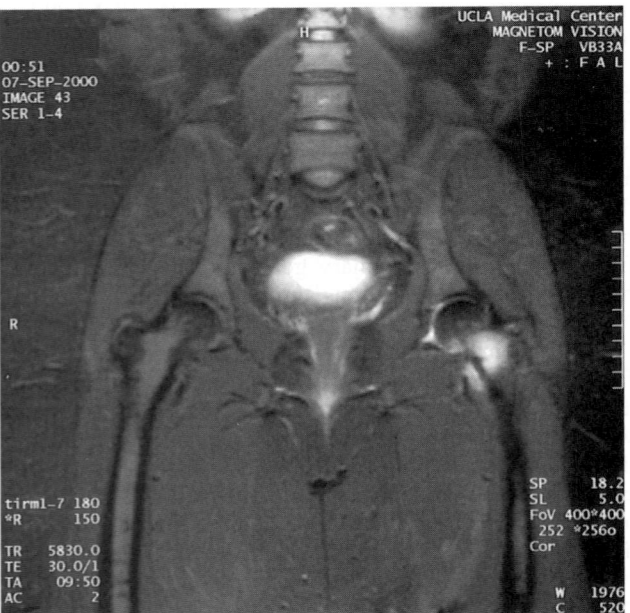

Figure 25A–8. Magnetic resonance imaging of a stress fracture of the femoral neck in a 50-year-old female.

progressive rehabilitation protocol is used. Hardware is generally removed 6 months to 1 year later.

For displaced fractures, immediate anatomic reduction and internal fixation are undertaken. Postoperatively, the athlete is generally kept non–weight-bearing for the first 6 weeks and partially weight-bearing for the subsequent 6 weeks, depending on the nature of the fracture and the fixation. At that time, a program of progressive activity and weight-bearing is started.

Intra-articular Derangements

Hip Dislocation

A simple dislocation of the hip, without associated fractures of the acetabulum or the femoral head, is infrequent but devastating. The hip is an extremely stable joint. A high-energy trauma directed along the axis of the femur when the hip is in the extremes of its normal range of motion is usually necessary to cause dislocation. Prompt reduction using proper technique is the most important factor in decreasing the incidence of late sequelae, particularly avascular necrosis. Reduction after 24 hours has been shown to cause an increase in osteonecrosis and post-traumatic arthritis; reduction within 24 hours, however, has not demonstrated any statically significant improvement in outcome.[3, 15] Because dislocated hips can kink the blood vessels that supply the femoral head, delays of more than 6 hours should be avoided whenever possible.

The majority of traumatic dislocations are posterior; anterior dislocations account for only 8% to 15% of the total.[107, 119] When a hip dislocation occurs, the athlete is immediately disabled, complaining of extreme pain. Any attempt to move the affected hip will increase the discomfort. Hips dislocated posteriorly are characteristically held in flexion, adduction, and internal rotation. In anterior dislocations, the hip is held in flexion, abduction, and external rotation. In addition, the femoral head may be palpable anteriorly.

Attempts at reduction should not be made on the playing field. A careful assessment of associated injuries, including neurovascular status, should be done, and the athlete should then be immobilized and transported to an appropriate center for definitive evaluation and treatment.[86, 119] In the emergency department, a hip trauma series of radiographs is obtained, including anteroposterior and oblique views of the pelvis. Because of the need for rapid treatment, computed tomographic scans are not routinely obtained before reduction.

There are three basic techniques of closed reduction: the Bigelow, the Allis, and the Stimson techniques. In all three methods, hip flexion is used to relax the tightened structures about the hip. The Bigelow and the Allis techniques employ traction to achieve reduction, whereas the Stimson technique is performed with the patient prone and uses gravity. Especially in athletes, in whom the amount of muscle mass and spasm may prevent reduction, general anesthesia is frequently used to ensure adequate muscle relaxation and to reduce the amount of trauma associated with reduction. If closed reduction cannot be achieved, open reduction, usually through a posterior approach, must be performed.

Postreduction radiography and computed tomography may identify previously unrecognized fracture fragments or intra-articular loose bodies. Concomitant acetabular fractures may require ORIF. Because the mechanism of injury frequently involves blunt trauma to the knee, a careful search should be made for associated injury to the ipsilateral knee.

After reduction, the hip should be gently tested to see if it is stable through a full range of motion. If the hip is stable once reduced and there is no evidence of associated fracture, the athlete is placed at rest for 48 hours; an abduction pillow or a knee immobilizer can also be used to help protect the patient. Protected weight-bearing is begun after 48 hours and is continued until the patient is pain free with ambulation, usually after about 2 weeks. The activity level is gradually increased, and by 4 to 6 weeks, the athlete can resume most preinjury activities. It may take up to 3 months to recover muscle strength, provided there were no associated injuries.

As recommended by Epstein, radiographic follow-up is obtained every 3 months for the first year and every 6 months for the next 2 years.[37] MRI may be particularly useful for early diagnosis of postreduction avascular necrosis. Although rare, recurrent instability has been reported and may require open capsulorrhaphy.[85, 107]

Acetabular Labral Tears

The acetabular labrum is a fibrocartilaginous rim that serves to deepen the acetabulum. It is attached to the bony rim of the acetabulum and to the transverse acetabular ligament. The free edge clasps the femoral head beyond its widest diameter, helping to hold the head firmly within the acetabulum. A biomechanical study has shown that the labrum does not significantly participate in load transmission in the hip.[63] The inherent stability of the bony anatomy of the hip joint makes the acetabular labrum less critical to the overall stability of the joint, but there is little doubt that its health is important to the overall function of the joint.

Tears of the acetabular labrum present after a patient has experienced some form of trauma, either modest or severe. Labral tears can also be associated with degenerative disease of the hip. The traumatic event can range from slipping or twisting to hip dislocation.[20, 42] Classic symptoms include painful catching or clicking, although these are not always present. The universal complaint is primarily hip pain, usually discrete episodes of sharp pain precipitated by pivoting or twisting.[42]

Physical examination demonstrates reproduction of the hip pain and possibly a click with manipulation of the hip joint from full flexion, external rotation, and abduction into extension with internal rotation and adduction for anterior labral tears.[42] Bringing the hip from full flexion, adduction, and internal rotation to extension with abduction and external rotation is useful for posterior labral tears.[42] Plain radiographs are essential. Labral tears have been shown to be present in a high percentage of patients with acetabular dysplasia.[33, 86] Radiographs can also show other sources of

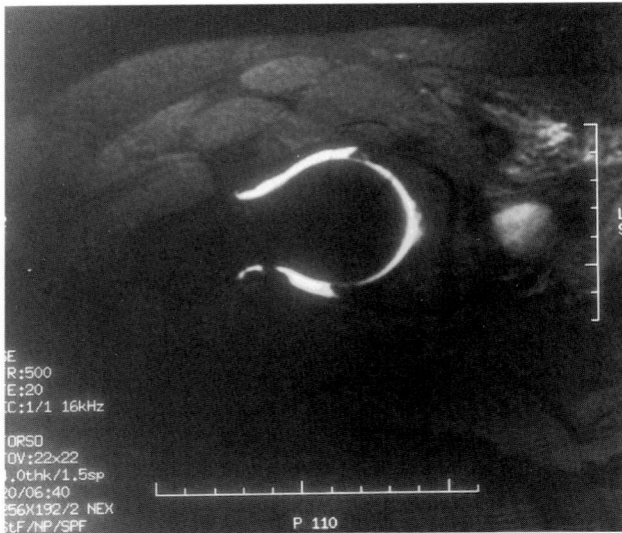

Figure 25A–9. Magnetic resonance arthrogram demonstrating an acetabular labral tear.

intra-articular disease that may account for the symptoms. If no dysplasia or concomitant disease is present, radiographic findings should be normal, because there are no specific findings for labral tears. MRI can be useful in further screening for osteonecrosis, synovial chondromatosis, or other disease. In the detection of acetabular labral tears, magnetic resonance arthrography appears to be the diagnostic test of choice, with reported sensitivities greater than 90% (Fig. 25A–9).[26] Injection of local anesthesia into the hip joint can also be very useful in diagnosing a labral tear.

Treatment of acetabular labral tears begins with a period of protected weight-bearing once the diagnosis has been positively established for 4 weeks. In approximately 13% of patients, symptoms resolve with this regimen.[20] If the pain persists or recurs, surgical intervention should be offered. In most cases of simple labral tears, arthroscopic débridement is the definitive surgical procedure (Fig. 25A–

10). Recent reports of successful arthroscopic débridement of labral tears in professional athletes with relative rapid return to activity have heightened awareness of and interest in this treatment option. The majority of tears are found in the anterior labrum or in the anterior superior labrum and are amenable to arthroscopic débridement.[20]

Avascular Necrosis of the Femoral Head

Avascular necrosis is a poorly understood condition in which the circulation to a segment of the femoral head is interrupted, leading to the death of marrow cells and osteophytes. The resulting necrotic segment usually goes on to collapse and causes progressive arthritis of the hip joint. The causes of avascular necrosis can be traumatic or nontraumatic. Traumatic causes include displaced fractures of the femoral neck and hip dislocation. These events disrupt the blood supply to the femoral head and lead to ischemia, which may progress to necrosis. Nontraumatic causes are not as well defined. Systemic corticosteroid use and heavy alcohol use are the most common underlying factors. Several mechanisms have been proposed to account for nontraumatic avascular necrosis; alteration of circulating lipids and coagulation pathways appears to be the mode of action.[78]

Athletes with avascular necrosis usually present with groin or hip pain that is nonspecific. It is critical to search for predisposing features. Traumatic incidents are common among athletes. It has been reported that traumatic subluxation of the hip has led to avascular necrosis of the femoral head in professional football players.[25] Systemic illnesses that require the use of corticosteroids should also be sought (e.g., asthma). The most important factors in making the diagnosis of avascular necrosis are a high index of suspicion and awareness of the predisposing factors, which are associated with nearly 80% of cases.

On physical examination, hip range of motion and gait should be normal unless the process is advanced. Antero-

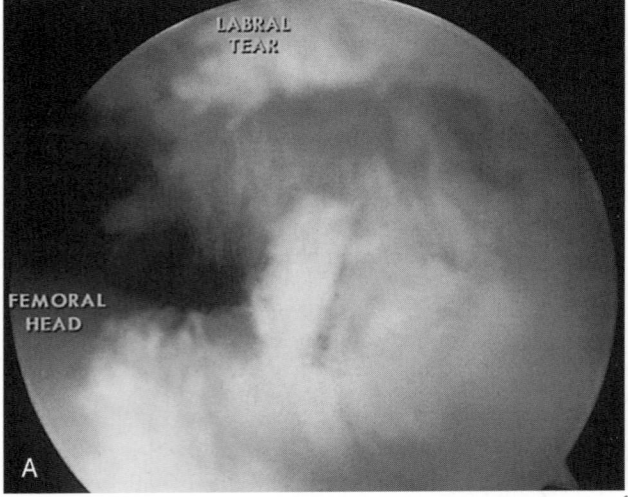
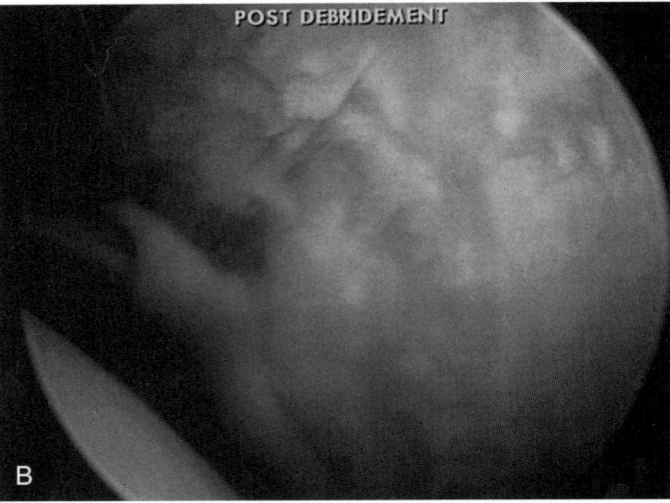

Figure 25A–10. Arthroscopic view of a labral tear before (*A*) and after (*B*) débridement.

posterior and lateral radiographs of both hips are essential. The earliest changes do not occur radiographically until 3 months after the insult. The earliest findings include osteopenia or a mottled appearance of the anterosuperior aspect of the femoral head consisting of patchy areas of sclerosis and lucency. As collapse progresses, the crescent sign appears, representing the collapse of the trabecula beneath the subchondral bone. Secondary degenerative changes can then follow as collapse progresses and arthritis of the joint evolves. If radiographic findings are normal but the disease is still suspected, MRI should be used. This test is very specific and sensitive in detecting avascular necrosis.

Treatment depends on the stage of the disease. Several classification systems have been developed based on either radiographic changes or MRI findings.[40, 114] For early disease, symptomatic treatment and restricted weight-bearing are generally ineffective. Core decompression has been shown to provide good relief of pain in early osteonecrosis, although reports of its success vary considerably.[39, 79, 114] The key element in treating patients with core decompression or core decompression with bone grafting is initiating treatment before collapse of the femoral head. When avascular necrosis has progressed, total hip arthroplasty appears to be the best treatment alternative.

Hip Osteoarthritis

Osteoarthritis of the hip is the end stage of many different disorders. The pathogenesis and the treatment of hip osteoarthritis are beyond the scope of this chapter. It should be considered in the differential diagnosis of hip pain with decreased range of motion. A recent study investigated the link between participation in sports and development of osteoarthrosis of the hip.[117] The investigators performed a case-controlled study of 233 men (up to the age of 49 years) who were recent recipients of a prosthesis for severe idiopathic osteoarthrosis of the hip and 302 men randomly selected from the general population. Men with high exposure (in hours) to sports of all kinds had a relative risk of

developing osteoarthrosis of the hip that was 4.5 times higher than in men with low exposure to sports. Track and field events and racquet sports seemed to be the most hazardous to the hip joint. The authors concluded that long-term exposure to sports among men seems to be a risk factor for developing severe osteoarthrosis of the hip.

Hip Arthroscopy

Arthroscopy of the hip is a developing technique that has found a role in the treatment of certain disorders of the hip. Its usefulness remains limited, however, secondary to the limited accessibility afforded by the hip anatomy and the potential for complications.

Indications. The indications for hip arthroscopy include evaluation of the painful hip for which imaging studies have been unable to produce a diagnosis. It has been shown that hip arthroscopy is able to detect chondral softening, fibrillation, and partial-thickness defects smaller than 1 cm that were not seen on MRI.[36] The authors also showed that osteochondral loose bodies and labral tears were not well demonstrated by MRI but were readily identified and treated at arthroscopy.[36] Once the osteochondral fragments or loose bodies are identified, they can often be treated by arthroscopic removal.[69] Acetabular labral tears can also be treated with arthroscopic débridement.[69] Another indication for hip arthroscopy includes synovitis; biopsy and limited synovectomy can be performed. A role has been suggested for arthroscopy in the management of septic arthritis.[13] Patients with significant degenerative disease do not seem to benefit from arthroscopic débridement.[47]

Technique. Hip arthroscopy can be performed with the patient in the lateral decubitus or the supine position. In the supine position, the patient is placed on a fracture table with a well-padded perineal post, and the hip is abducted 30 degrees (Fig. 25A–11).[46] Traction is applied via the footplate of the fracture table. The key is to apply enough traction to distract the femur far enough to allow the arthroscopic instruments to pass easily into the joint. This is usually 25 to 50 pounds of traction. The image intensifier

Figure 25A–11. The setup for hip arthroscopy. ASIS, anterior superior iliac spine. (From Hunter DM, Ruch DS: Hip arthroscopy. J South Orthop Assoc 5:243–250, 1996.)

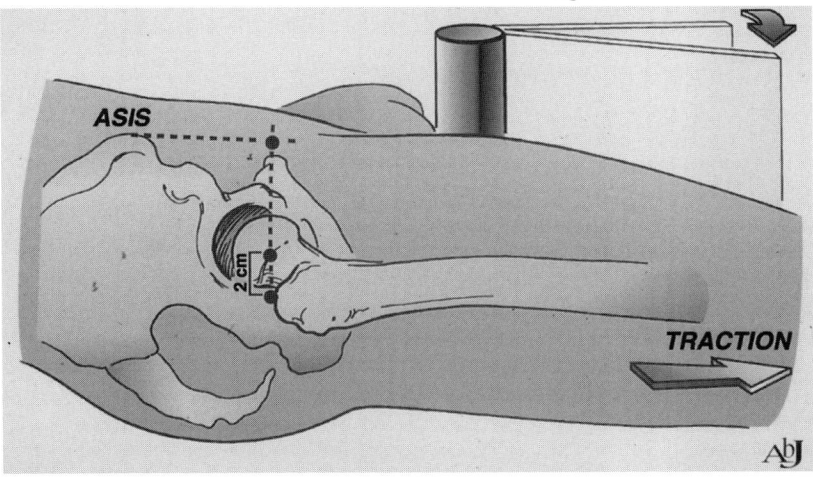

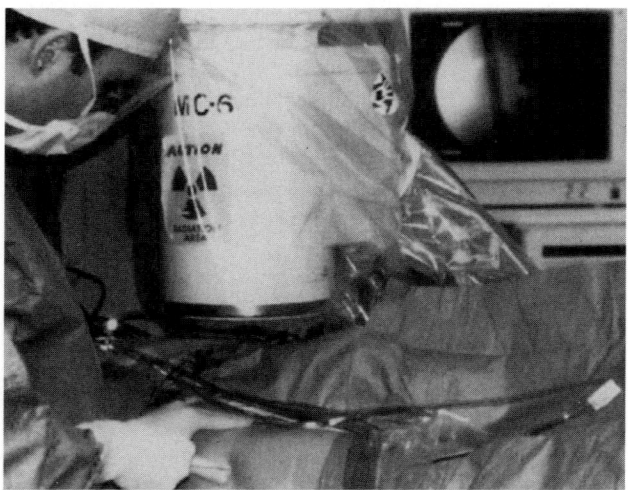

Figure 25A–12. Operating room setup for hip arthroscopy, with a sterilely draped fluoroscope on the side opposite the affected hip. (From Hunter DM, Ruch DS: Hip arthroscopy. J South Orthop Assoc 5:243–250, 1996.)

is used to verify the amount of distraction before prepping and draping. Once adequate distraction has been verified, traction is released, and the patient's extremity is prepped and draped in a sterile fashion. The image intensifier is also draped and is positioned on the side opposite the affected extremity (Fig. 25A–12). Distraction is then reapplied by an assistant and is verified with the image intensifier.

The anterolateral portal is placed first for the introduction of the arthroscope. A 6-inch 18-gauge spinal needle is placed under fluoroscopic guidance at the anterior superior lip of the greater trochanter and is directed perpendicular to a line drawn from the ASIS. Starting as closely as possble to the greater trochanter allows easier passage of the needle under the lateral aspect of the labrum. Once the needle position has been confirmed fluoroscopically, a guidewire is introduced using the Seldinger technique, and the position of the wire is verified. The skin is incised to

accommodate the special hip arthroscopy cannula. The needle is then removed, and a cannulated trocar is introduced over the wire. The blunt end of the trocar is used to create a tract to the capsule, and the sharp end is used to pop through the thick capsule. The cannula for the arthroscope is then passed over this trocar, and again the position of the cannula is verified via fluoroscopy. The camera can then be introduced. The anterolateral portal is best used to visualize areas of avascular necrosis, loose bodies, ligamentum teres avulsion injuries, and acetabular lesions.[68]

The anterior portal is established next. This portal is useful for direct visualization of the superior aspect of the femoral head and is a working portal for instrumentation. This portal is also established using the Seldinger technique. The 18-gauge needle is placed so that it enters the skin at the intersection of a sagittal line drawn distally from the ASIS and a transverse line drawn across the superior margin of the greater trochanter. The needle is directed 45 degrees cephalad and 30 degrees toward the midline, as recommended by Byrd.[19] Once return of outflow through the spinal needle has been established, the wire can be introduced, and the anterior portal can be established. With the shaver in the anterior portal and the arthroscope in the anterolateral portal, visualization and débridement of the majority of lesions can be carried out.

The arthroscope can be switched to the anterior portal. This allows visualization of the medial aspect of the femoral head and also provides better visualization of the acetabulum and the ligamentum teres. The 70-degree arthroscope is routinely used in this portal and allows excellent visualization over the curvature of the femoral head as well as visualization of the labrum and the acetabulum.[51] If a labral tear is detected, the arthroscope may be maintained in the anterior portal, and the labral tear may be débrided through the anterolateral portal.

The posterolateral portal is not routinely used because it has the potential for placing the sciatic nerve at risk.[47] If a third portal is needed, it is useful to place a portal adjacent to the anterolateral portal in line with it but approximately 2 cm more medially (Fig. 25A–13). This allows visualization and débridement of lateral lesions, as

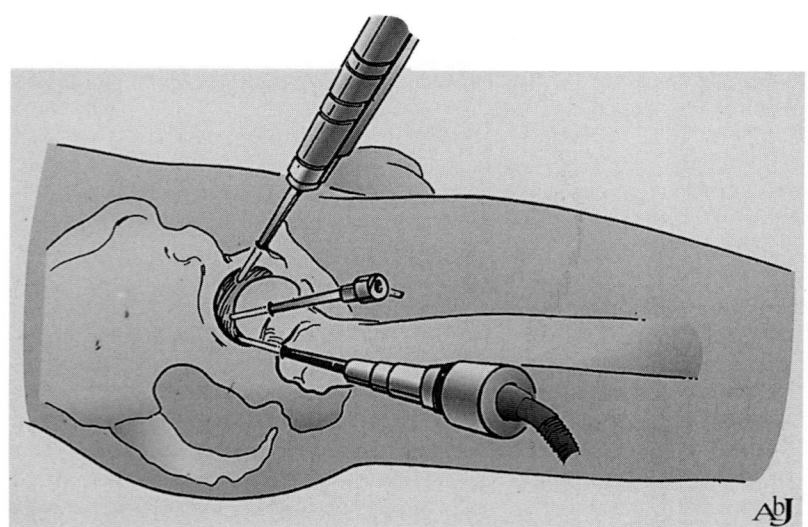

Figure 25A–13. Portal placement for hip arthroscopy. (From Hunter DM, Ruch DS: Hip arthroscopy. J South Orthop Assoc 5:243–250, 1996.)

seen with avascular necrosis and degenerative joint disease, especially in patients with contracted joint capsules that do not allow sufficient distraction.

Complications. Potential complications of hip arthroscopy are not insignificant. Traction-related complications are the most commonly reported.[47, 66] Pudendal nerve neurapraxia and scrotal and labial pressure sores have been related to improper positioning and padding of the perineal post as well as to excessive or prolonged traction of the extremity. These complications can be avoided by ensuring that the perineal post is well padded and properly positioned, by limiting traction on the affected extremity to 50 pounds or less, and by limiting traction time to 2 hours or less.

The most feared complication is damage to the neurovascular structures near the hip. Correct portal placement is essential. Using key anatomic landmarks as described ensures that the sciatic nerve and the lateral femoral cutaneous nerve and artery remain a safe distance from the sharp trocar during portal placement.[66] As mentioned, the posterolateral portal is typically avoided because of the risk it poses to the sciatic nerve.

Damage to the cartilage or the labrum may also occur during portal creation or instrument passage.[66] Obtaining proper distraction of the hip and using meticulous arthroscopic technique can help avoid these complications. Infection is rare, and systemic complications have been reported but are generally infrequent.

Hip arthroscopy can be an effective tool for the management of undiagnosed hip pain or the treatment of loose bodies, labral tears, or synovitis in young patients without advanced degenerative disease. Like arthroscopy of other joints, hip arthroscopy offers diagnostic and therapeutic benefits with minimal invasiveness and shorter recovery periods than for open procedures. As our skills, instrumentation, and understanding of hip disease and injury advance, no doubt the indications for and the usefulness of this technique will also advance.

References

1. Abbate CC: Avulsion fracture of the ischial tuberosity: A case report. J Bone Joint Surg 27:716, 1945.
2. Adams RJ, Chandler, FA: Osteitis pubis of traumatic etiology. J Bone Joint Surg Am 35:685, 1953.
3. Allen WC, Cope R: Coxa saltans: The snapping hip syndrome. J Am Acad Orthop Surg 3:303, 1995.
4. American Medical Association, Subcommittee on Classification of Sports Injuries: Standard Nomenclature of Athletic Injuries. Chicago, American Medical Association, 1966.
5. Antao NA: Myositis ossificans of the hip in a professional soccer player. Am J Sports Med 16:82, 1988.
6. Beach EW: Osteitis pubis. Urol Cutan Rev 53:577, 1949.
7. Beer E: Periostitis and osteitis of the symphysis pubis following suprapubic cystotomies. J Urol 20:233, 1928.
8. Bellabarba C, Sheinkop MB, Kuo KN: Idiopathic hip instability. An unrecognized cause of coxa saltans in the adult. Clin Orthop 355: 261, 1998.
9. Benson ER, Schwitzer SF: Post-traumatic piriformis syndrome: Diagnosis and results of operative treatment. J Bone Joint Surg Am 81:941, 1999.
10. Berry JM: Fracture of the tuberosity of the ischium due to muscular action. JAMA 59:1450, 1912.
11. Blecher A: Über den Einfluss de ParadeMarches auf die Enstehung der Fuss Geschwulst. Med Klin 1:305, 1905.
12. Blickenstaff LP, Morris JM: Fatigue fracture of the femoral neck. J Bone Joint Surg Am 48:1031, 1966.
13. Blitzer CM: Arthroscopic management of septic arthritis of the hip. Arthroscopy 9:414, 1993.
14. Bradshaw C, McCrory P, Bell S, Brukner P: Obturator nerve entrapment. A cause of groin pain in athletes. Am J Sports Med 25: 402, 1997.
15. Brav EA: Traumatic dislocation of the hip: Army experience and results over a twelve-year period. J Bone Joint Surg Am 44:1115, 1962.
16. Brignall CG, Stainsby GD: The snapping hip syndrome: Treatment by Z-plasty. J Bone Joint Surg Br 73:253, 1991.
17. Burkett LN: Causative factors in hamstring strains. Med Sci Sports 2:39, 1970.
18. Butler JE, Eggert AW: Fracture of the iliac crest apophysis: An unusual hip pointer. J Sports Med 3:192, 1975.
19. Byrd JWT: Hip arthroscopy utilizing the supine position. Arthroscopy 10:275, 1994.
20. Byrd JWT: Labral lesions: An elusive source of hip pain. Arthroscopy 12:603, 1996.
21. Canale ST, King RE: Pelvic and hip fractures. In Rockwood CA Jr, Wilkins KE, King RE (eds): Fractures in Children. Philadelphia, JB Lippincott, 1984.
22. Cardinal E, Buckwalter KA, Capello WN, Duval N: Ultrasound of the snapping iliopsoas tendon. Radiology 198:521, 1996.
23. Caudle RJ, Crawford AH: Avulsion fracture of the lateral acetabular margin. J Bone Joint Surg Am 70:1568, 1988.
24. Clancy WG, Foltz AS: Iliac apophysitis and stress fractures in adolescent runners. Am J Sports Med 4:214, 1976.
25. Cooper DE, Warren RF, Barnes R: Traumatic subluxation of the hip resulting in aseptic necrosis and chondrolysis in a professional football player. Am J Sports Med 19:322, 1991.
26. Czerny C, Hoffmann S, Urban M, et al: MR arthrography of the adult acetabular capsular–labral complex: Correlation with surgery and anatomy. AJR Am J Roentgenol 173: 345, 1999.
27. Deal CL, Canosa JJ: Meralgia paresthetica and large abdomens. Ann Intern Med 96:787, 1982.
28. Delagi EF, Perotto A: Anatomic Guide for the Electromyographer, 2nd ed. Springfield, Ill., Charles C Thomas, 1980.
29. DeLee JC: Fractures and dislocations of the hip. In Rockwood CA Jr, Green DP (eds): Fractures in Adults. Philadelphia, JB Lippincott, 1984.
30. Devas MB: Stress fractures of the femoral neck. J Bone Joint Surg Br 47:728, 1965.
31. Devas MB: Stress Fractures. New York, Churchill Livingstone, 1975.
32. Dimon JH III: Isolated fractures of the lesser trochanter of the femur. Clin Orthop 82:144, 1972.
33. Dorrell J, Catterall A: The torn acetabular labrum. J Bone Joint Surg Am 68:400, 1986.
34. Dreinhofer KE, Schwarzkopf SR, Haas NP, et al: Isolated traumatic dislocation of the hip. Long term results in 50 patients. J Bone Joint Surg Br 76:6, 1994.
35. Ecker AD, Woltman HW: Meralgia paresthetica: A report of one hundred and fifty cases. JAMA 110:1650, 1938.
36. Edwards DJ, Lomas D, Villar RN: Diagnosis of the painful hip by magnetic resonance imaging and arthroscopy. J Bone Joint Surg Br 77:374, 1995.
37. Epstein HC: Traumatic dislocations of the hip. Clin Orthop 92: 116, 1973.
38. Ernst J: Stress fracture of the neck of the femur. J Trauma 4: 71, 1964.
39. Fairbank AC, Bhatia D, Jinnah RH, Hungerford DS: Long term results of core decompression for ischemic necrosis of the femoral head. J Bone Joint Surg Br 77:42, 1995.
40. Ficat RP: Idiopathic bone necrosis of the femoral head. Early diagnosis and treatment. J Bone Joint Surg Br 67:3, 1985.
41. Fishman L, Zybert P: Electrophysiologic evidence of piriformis syndrome. Arch Phys Med Rehabil 73: 359, 1992.
42. Fitzgerald RH: Acetabular labral tears. Diagnosis and treatment. Clin Orthop 311:60, 1995.
43. Fullerton LR, Snowdy HA: Femoral neck stress fractures. Am J Sports Med 16:365, 1988.
44. Gardner E, Gray DJ, O'Rahilly R: Anatomy, A Regional Study of Human Structure. Philadelphia, WB Saunders, 1975.

following: specific areas of tenderness, limitation of hip range of motion in all planes, muscle strength, presence or absence of muscle atrophy, and distal neurologic examination findings. Diagnostic considerations include apophyseal injuries, stress fractures, slipped capital femoral epiphysis (SCFE), Legg-Calvé-Perthes disease, and musculotendinous strains, among others. The physical examination often provides necessary information for diagnosis. In addition, both careful history and selective imaging are important for definitive diagnosis. Although standard anteroposterior and lateral radiographs may be diagnostically sufficient, in cases of diagnostic dilemmas, a bone scan, computed tomography, or magnetic resonance imaging (MRI) may be needed to elucidate an unrecognized stress fracture, apophysitis, or other pathologic lesion.

Anatomic Considerations

As Ogden[61] emphasized, understanding the effects of traumatic injury on the skeletally immature hip and pelvis demands a knowledge of the progression of skeletal and vascular growth. The development of the femoral head and neck region into its three separate ossification centers (capital femoral epiphysis, greater trochanter, and lesser trochanter) progressively alters the biomechanics of the proximal femur and thus its injury patterns. The changing vascular pattern of the femoral head and neck greatly influences the risk of occurrence of the many possible complications of trauma to the hip and pelvis, such as avascular necrosis, nonunion, malunion, and possible eventual degenerative disease. On the pelvic side of the hip joint, undisturbed triradiate cartilage growth is crucial for normal acetabular development, and skeletal injuries in this region may have long-term sequelae for the patient in terms of acetabular dysplasia and degenerative hip disease.

There are several apophyses about the hip and pelvis with large muscle attachments, accounting for the frequency of apophyseal avulsion fractures seen in adolescent athletes. These secondary centers of ossification appear between the ages of 11 and 15 years and account for circumferential but not longitudinal growth of the bones.[20, 52] In general, the physis is the weakest structure of the growing skeleton and is most vulnerable to direct trauma and avulsion injuries. Other than SCFE, however, physeal injury in the proximal femur and the acetabulum is a rare occurrence.

Avulsion Fractures

The mechanism of injury is either a sudden violent muscular contraction or an excessive amount of muscle stretch across an open apophysis. There is often no external trauma.[20, 52] The injury occurs most often in adolescent athletes between the ages of 14 and 17 years. A similar overload in an adult would most likely result in a muscle strain. Avulsion fractures are more frequent in males than in females, but this pattern may be changing with the greater frequency of female athletic programs. The most common sites of avulsion fracture are the anterior superior iliac spine (at the origin of the sartorius), the ischium (hamstrings) (Fig. 25B–1), the lesser trochanter (iliopsoas) (Fig. 25B–2), the anterior inferior iliac spine (rectus), and the iliac crest (abdominal muscles). A greater trochanteric avulsion at the insertion of the abductors is extremely rare.[61] These injuries occur in a broad spectrum of individual and team sports, usually in competitive athletes (particularly sprinters, jumpers, and soccer and football players) during the course of an extreme effort. The athlete generally presents with localized swelling, tenderness, and limitation of motion about the site of the avulsion fracture. Pain may be extreme. Radiographs should confirm the diagnosis. On occasion, pelvic inlet, outlet, or oblique views may be necessary to define the lesion and the extent of displacement.

Therapy with bed rest, ice application, and positioning of the limb to lessen the stretch on the affected muscle and apophysis frequently improve the patient's symptoms and decrease the risk of further displacement of the apophysis. Metzmaker and Pappas[52] outlined a five-stage progressive rehabilitation program that was successful in 27 athletes with acute avulsion fractures of the hip and pelvis. The stages are as follows:

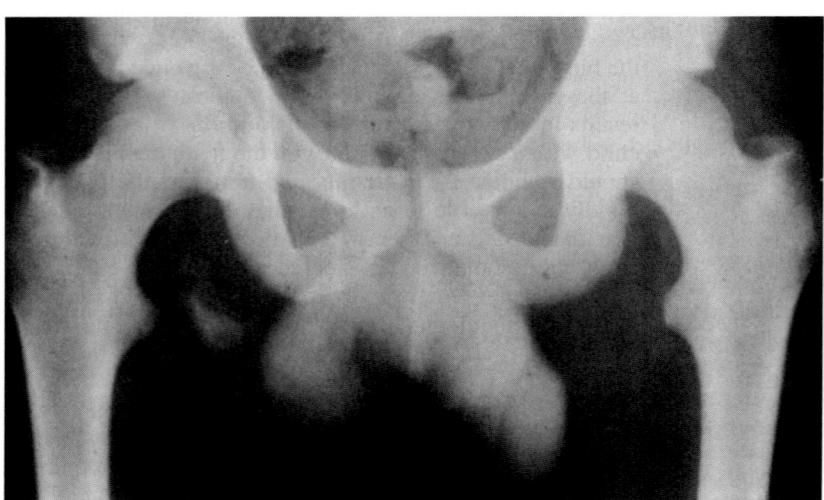

Figure 25B–1. Ischial avulsion fracture caused by forceful hamstring contractures in a track athlete.

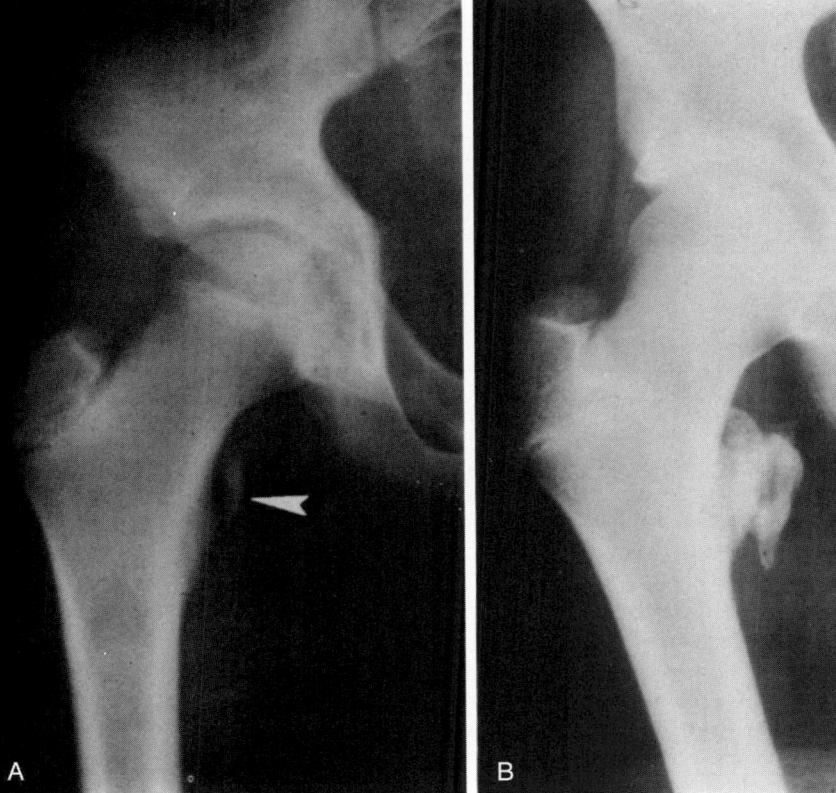

Figure 25B–2. *A,* Avulsion fracture of the lesser trochanter caused by the iliopsoas in an adolescent athlete. *B,* Healing of the bony avulsion, which was treated with observation, rest, anti-inflammatory agents, and physical therapy.

1. *Rest* with positioning to relax the involved muscle group, ice application, and analgesia are initiated at the time of injury.

2. The patient is allowed *gradually to increase the excursion* of the injured musculotendinous unit when pain has subsided.

3. When he or she has obtained full, active range of motion, the athlete institutes a comprehensive *resistive exercise program.*

4. When 50% of anticipated strength has been achieved, the athlete *integrates* the use of the injured musculotendinous unit with the other muscles of the pelvis and lower extremity. This is the stage when the risk of reinjury is high if the patient returns to full participation before normal strength and function are achieved.

5. Only when the athlete has achieved full strength and integration of the injured muscle into the athletic activity is he or she allowed to *return to competitive sports.*

Isokinetic strength testing can be used as a more objective assessment of progress during strength rehabilitation. The great majority of athletes can be successfully treated nonoperatively with a guided rehabilitation program. Rarely, the degree of displacement may be significant enough to lead to either fibrous union or nonunion.[27] This may be associated with chronic pain and functional disability. In these cases, chronic pain may be an indication for excision of the separated apophysis. Early open reduction and internal fixation have been advocated when there is significant displacement of a fragment. Exact surgical indications, however, are unclear. Functional disability in competitive athletes has been described rarely after this injury.[69] We treat our athletes conservatively using a progressive program of isometric strengthening during the early postinjury phase, advancing to resistive isokinetic strengthening before return to competitive sports. Other than circumferential wraps for symptomatic relief, we do not use any special equipment during the athlete's return to sports.

Growth Plate Injuries

Physeal Fractures of Proximal Femur and Acetabulum

Although these injuries are rare in sports,[46] their presence indicates either severe trauma or an associated disease process,[4, 5, 10] and their associated morbidity demands attention. Transphyseal fractures of the femoral neck represent a type I Salter-Harris fracture. In a young child, severe violence is necessary to produce this separation. In the adolescent, this represents one end of the spectrum of SCFE. It may occur with an associated pathologic state such as renal osteodystrophy or hypothyroidism.[10] High-energy fractures may be associated with dislocation of the femoral head from the acetabulum. Emergent, careful open reduction and internal fixation are advocated, using smooth pins across the epiphysis. The risk of premature closure of the epiphysis is high. The results from treatment of this fracture are frequently poor owing to avascular necrosis of the femoral head.[77]

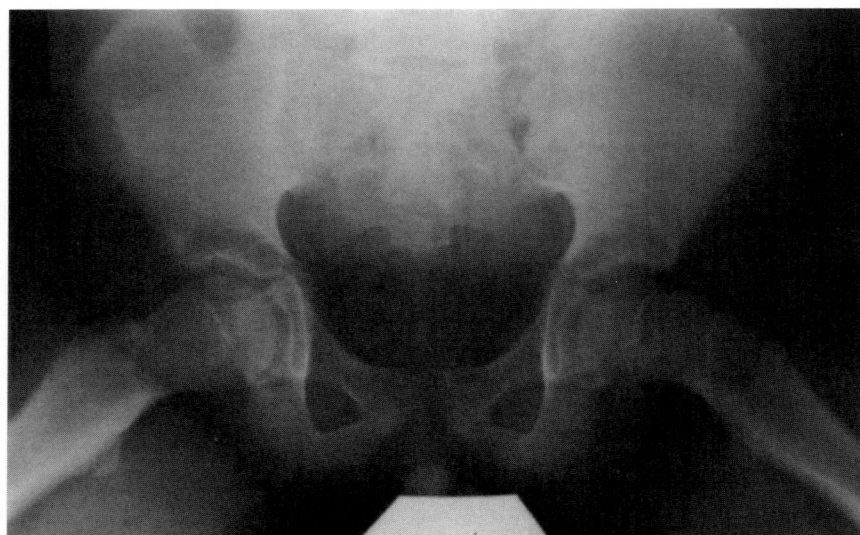

Figure 25B–3. Left slipped capital femoral epiphysis (SCFE) in an athlete who had left groin pain for several weeks. The frog-leg lateral position provides the most sensitive radiographic image for detecting SCFE.

Slipped Capital Femoral Epiphysis

SCFE is the most common hip disorder in the adolescent.[3] This condition represents a mechanical shearing failure of the proximal femoral physis,[11, 15] which results in variable degrees of posterior slippage of the proximal femoral epiphysis and concomitant extension and external rotation of the femoral neck and shaft (Fig. 25B–3). This rarely occurs as an acute fracture associated with a discrete injury. It is usually a chronic microfracturing process of the physis under physiologic loads during the preadolescent and adolescent growth spurts.[30, 81]

Most children who suffer from SCFE are either heavy or rapidly growing.[25, 39, 40] Relative femoral retroversion is an additional strong risk factor.[17] SCFE is more common in males. It rarely occurs before age 9 in girls or age 11 in boys unless there is an underlying endocrinologic disorder. It almost always begins before puberty, but if untreated, the condition can progress until skeletal maturity is attained. The condition is ultimately bilateral in 20% to 50% of cases,[38] although the presentation is rarely simultaneous.

Classification

Historically, SCFE has been classified in terms of both the acuity of the process and the severity of the anatomic abnormality. It is now recognized that it is important, for both prognostic and therapeutic reasons, to characterize a slip qualitatively by its mechanical stability rather than the duration of the symptoms. SCFE is therefore either "stable" or "unstable." By definition, a stable slip allows weight-bearing. An unstable slip is too painful and unstable to allow weight-bearing.[48]

An unstable capital femoral epiphysis represents an acute physeal fracture, with concomitant microscopic instability, risk of osteonecrosis, and malunion.

The patient with a stable SCFE typically has relatively prolonged symptoms that may never have been dramatic and indeed may be minimal.

In addition to the thorough characterization of patients

with SCFE as being in either the stable or the unstable group, it is important to recognize a third category of patients who have had a stable slip for a variable period of time that is suddenly complicated by an acute physeal separation superimposed on a more chronic and more stable physeal deformation.

Characterizing the severity of the anatomic deformity in SCFE is important because the degree of deformity, barring complications,[29] ultimately correlates best with long-term problems, specifically osteoarthrosis of the hip.[3, 11]

Though SCFE has been characterized by the percentage of slipping of the epiphysis (grade 1 to 4), this system is notorious for underestimating the true amount of deformity. It is more accurate to characterize the malposition of the capital femoral epiphysis with regard to the femoral shaft, as seen in the frog-leg lateral view.[73] Even more accurate is employment of the slip angle, which may be determined by computed tomographic scan[17] or biplanar radiography.[68]

Diagnosis

A young athlete with a chronic SCFE will have difficulty with athletic activities. A limp or an external rotation gait may be present. Symptoms are often vague, and pain may not be present at all. When there is a complaint of discomfort, it is usually an aching discomfort that may be located anywhere from the groin proximally to the medial knee region distally. Symptoms are typically worse with physical activity.

SCFE is among the most poorly diagnosed of all pediatric orthopedic conditions, and the diagnosis must be considered in any child between the ages of perhaps 8 and 15 who has any gait abnormality or any symptoms between the pelvis and the tibia. In its early stages, this condition is easily treated by simple in situ pinning and usually has minimal sequelae. If the slipped epiphysis is not diagnosed in a timely fashion[18] and the subsequent deformity becomes severe, the measures needed to treat it are more extreme, and both the surgical risks and the chances of long-term dysfunction are much greater.[3]

Physical examination reveals limited internal rotation. In an acute slip, the hip usually lies in extension, adduction, and external rotation, with any active or passive movements associated with pain. In a chronic slip, which often manifests little or no discomfort during active or passive motion of the affected hip, hip flexion is usually limited. In addition, as the limits of flexion are reached, the hip tends to ride into external rotation as the prominent anterior femoral neck abuts against the anterior acetabulum.

Both anteroposterior and lateral plain radiographs of both hips are crucial to making the diagnosis of SCFE (see Fig. 25B–3). The radiographic diagnosis can be subtle in its earlier stages, but widening and blurring of the proximal femoral physis is an early sign, even before the proximal femoral epiphysis begins its characteristic posterior tilting. At this "preslip" stage, a high-resolution bone scan will show increased uptake at the top of the femoral neck, and MRI will also reveal physeal abnormalities. These supplemental studies are rarely needed for diagnosis if the examining physician includes SCFE in the differential diagnosis.

In a patient with unstable SCFE, there is usually obvious radiographic discontinuity between the anterosuperior portion of the femoral neck and the anterolateral corner of the capital femoral epiphysis. In relatively longstanding, stable cases of slipped epiphysis, the superior neck may remodel rapidly enough to follow the epiphysis as it falls posteriorly. In a very longstanding stable slipped epiphysis, characteristic remodeling of the femoral neck, with bone formation along its posterior aspect, is associated with a variable but characteristic malalignment of the epiphysis with relation to the femoral shaft. The femoral head lies in a position of retroversion in relation to the femoral neck, and the femoral neck itself usually lies in a position of retroversion in relation to the femoral shaft and the knee.

Treatment

If the physis is still open, the first priority in treatment is to stabilize the epiphysis to prevent further slippage. This is most commonly done with a cannulated transphyseal screw. Biplanar image intensification is mandatory for intraoperative control because the direction of slippage of the epiphysis dictates the direction of the internal fixation devices. This is always at some angle to the plane of the femoral neck (*not* in the same plane as the neck) if the device is to cross the physis into the epiphysis at a right angle to the growth plate, as is most desirable biomechanically.[56]

In a stable slip, a single screw usually provides adequate fixation if it is placed ideally through the middle of the physis into the center of the femoral head. If there is any question about the acuity of the slippage, it is probably safer to use two screws (not more than two!).

More severe SCFE, in which the angle of the slippage is 45 degrees or more, is associated not only with dysfunction in the form of limitation of flexion and severe external rotation deformity but also with a significant risk of osteoarthritis owing to anterior impingement. Patients with this much deformity should be considered not only for stabilization but also for a bone realignment procedure in which the epiphysis is realigned into a more physiologic position in the acetabulum.

The problem with realigning procedures is that they are not only technically much more demanding but also more dangerous in terms of the blood supply to the femoral head than are simple stabilization procedures. The choices among realignment procedures include acute manipulative reduction (only to be considered in an acute slip),[12] cuneiform osteotomy,[6, 21] and intertrochanteric osteotomy of the flexion-derotational type.[33, 58] Among the realigning procedures, flexion intertrochanteric osteotomy is probably the most desirable in terms of being not only efficacious but also safe. AO blade plates provide rigid and reliable fixation. Some compensatory deformity is created because the realignment is done in the intertrochanteric region, at a distance of a few centimeters from the true deformity at the top of the femoral neck.

Cuneiform osteotomy is an open reduction of the epiphysis with resection of the posterior reactive bone, allowing gentle anatomic reduction of the epiphysis onto the femoral neck without tension. Some degree of femoral neck shortening may be necessary. Cuneiform osteotomy should be reserved for severe slips, and it may also be safer in cases in which the physis remains clearly open. The literature suggests that cuneiform osteotomy carries a risk of osteonecrosis much greater than that associated with intertrochanteric osteotomy.[6, 21, 68]

Complications

Complications of SCFE may be associated with the condition itself or with the treatment. In a patient with unstable SCFE, avascular necrosis of the femoral head can result from injury to the retinacular vessels at the moment of the acute slip or during reduction maneuvers. With this in mind, the treating physician should be as gentle as possible in dealing with a patient with SCFE. There is no uniform agreement about whether the patient with a severe slippage (greater than 60-degree slip angle) is best treated by means of gentle traction overnight with pinning in whatever position results or by means of a "gentle manipulation" under general anesthesia to bring the knee to a straight-up position. We prefer to keep the patient with a severe acute slipped epiphysis in a comfortable position with the leg on a pillow until he or she can be brought to the operating room (as soon as is practical). We then open the joint through an anterior or anterolateral approach to reduce the deformity under direct vision to the point where the neck and the head start to move as a unit. At this point, if the deformity seems to be reduced to an acceptable position, the epiphysis is pinned in situ. If the deformity is still judged to be so unacceptable that very poor function is likely to result, the epiphysis is pinned as it is, and an acute or a late realignment through the intertrochanteric region is carried out.

Besides osteonecrosis, the other major complication of SCFE is chondrolysis. This destructive process of the articular cartilage is a rare but severe complication that seems to occur as a result of either autoimmune processes or mechanical injury to acetabular cartilage. Chondrolysis rarely occurs in the absence of treatment.

Although chondrolysis can occur in association with

pins or screws that protrude through the femoral head to the acetabulum and that directly abrade the acetabular cartilage,[56, 57, 65] chondrolysis can also occur as a result of impingement of the anterior acetabulum and labrum by the prominent anterior neck or head-neck junction as the hip with SCFE is flexed.[22]

Chondrolysis is diagnosed from the presence of progressive pain and limitation of motion on physical examination, with progressive narrowing of the cartilage space on radiography. It is to be suspected when, after in situ pinning or osteotomy, the patient becomes progressively more uncomfortable instead of more comfortable. If intra-articular protrusion by an implant is the offending mechanism, immediate repositioning of the implant is mandatory. Nonsteroidal anti-inflammatory agents, heavy traction, continuous passive motion, and aggressive physiotherapy may be helpful. Anterior capsulectomy may have a role. Prognosis is guarded, and, in some cases, hip fusion or arthroplasty may ultimately be necessary.

In summary, SCFE is a condition that is usually straightforward and satisfying to treat. The diagnosis, however, must be considered and the appropriate radiographs taken if treatment is to be rendered in a timely fashion. If the diagnosis is made, the young athlete with this condition must cease athletic activities entirely until the slipping epiphysis is surgically stabilized. It must be remembered that the contralateral hip will ultimately slip in 20% to 50% of cases, and follow-up radiographs must at least occasionally show both hips. Any contralateral symptoms must be investigated thoroughly and immediately.

Sports may be possible once the growth plate starts to fuse, although fracture around the screw is possible. The safest course is to limit athletic activity until several months after the internal fixation devices have been removed.

Although implant removal after physeal fusion is not universally recommended, we believe that it is appropriate in the athlete, both to avoid local symptoms and to facilitate future MRI or surgery should either prove necessary. While the open but stabilized physes are closing, noncontact cardiovascular fitness training, lower extremity range of motion exercises, and progressive resistance exercises should be initiated. The implant always remains in place until the growth plate is completely fused, as seen on radiography. After removal of the hardware, activity should be restricted for at least 2 to 3 months to allow bony healing across the pin site. At that point, full athletic activity may resume.

Nonphyseal Fractures

Although these injuries are infrequently caused by skeletal trauma in the athlete,[4, 7, 76, 79] violent trauma or a predisposing pathologic state may result in a pelvic or proximal femoral fracture.

Pelvic Fractures

In Torode and Zieg's[77] series of 141 pelvic fractures in children, five were secondary to sporting events. These injuries are classified as avulsion fractures, iliac wing fractures, simple ring fractures, or unstable ring fractures. Avulsion fractures have already been discussed. Iliac wing and simple ring fractures can be treated nonoperatively; however, type IV injuries with pelvic disruption represent an unstable pelvis that often requires treatment, either by means of open reduction and internal fixation or by means of external fixation. These injuries have a high rate of associated genitourinary, abdominal, neurologic, and other musculoskeletal injuries[7, 76, 79] that need to be addressed when the patient presents to the emergency room.

Return to sports participation by patients with stable pelvic injuries depends on the level of discomfort and the conditioned state of the athlete. Protected weight-bearing as tolerated is allowed for 3 to 6 weeks until the fracture is clinically and radiographically healed. Return to sports is then determined by the time needed to attain full range of motion and lower extremity strength. Isokinetic analysis of strength is helpful in obtaining an objective measurement of strength to lessen the risk of recurrent injury resulting from premature return to competitive sports.

Femoral Neck Fractures

These fractures are classified as transphyseal, transcervical, cervicotrochanteric, or intertrochanteric.[5, 61, 77] They are the result of severe trauma, most frequently from motor vehicle accidents or falls from extreme heights. If any femoral fracture follows minimal trauma, the presence of an underlying pathologic lesion should be suspected.

Displaced femoral neck fractures require immediate reduction to lessen the risk of avascular necrosis. Internal fixation is mandatory for any complete fracture to prevent malunion and nonunion (Fig. 25B–4).

We consider intraoperative anatomic alignment of the femoral neck to be a prerequisite for adequate internal fixation. We routinely use a radiolucent osteotomy table and not a fracture table because we are concerned that strong traction may risk additional vascular injury to the retinacular vessels. Anatomic reduction of the displaced fracture may be achieved by means of gentle traction without direct manipulation of the fragments. Anterior or anterolateral arthrotomy is simple, safe, and very useful. Arthrotomy allows evacuation of a hematoma to decompress the joint. It also enables anatomic reduction of certain difficult fractures without the use of the excessive traction forces that might otherwise be needed.

We prefer internal fixation with two cannulated cancellous screws and washers that are lagged and placed perpendicular to the fracture line. We prefer to avoid crossing the physis with the screws, but if placement within the epiphysis is necessary to stabilize the femoral neck fracture adequately, then we will do so. Although two screws spaced appropriately and placed in parallel with a lag effect are more effective than one screw in stabilizing a displaced femoral neck fracture, the addition of a third screw is virtually never indicated and is usually detrimental. The volume occupied by three screws in the pediatric femoral neck or epiphysis is considerable and may predispose the patient to osteonecrosis. In addition, there is a possibility

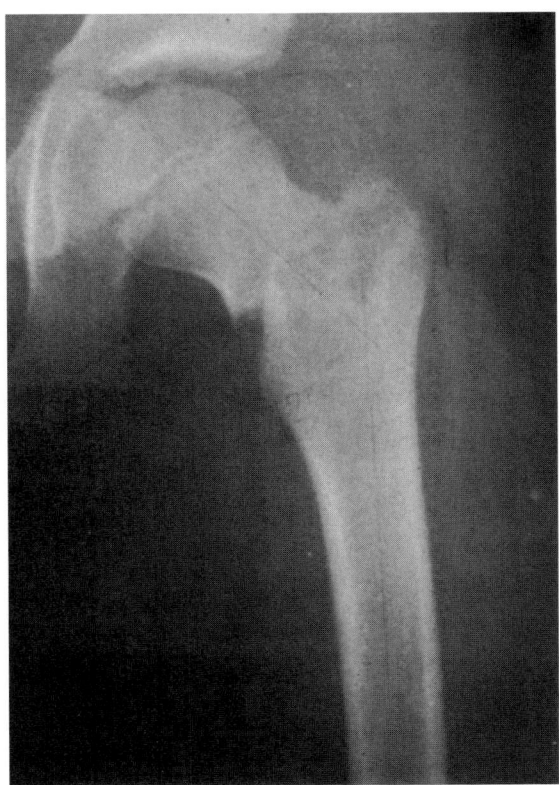

Figure 25B–4. Acute femoral neck fracture requiring emergency reduction anatomically.

that at least one of the three screws may be positioned suboptimally, risking either intra-articular protrusion or actual weakening of osteosynthesis rather than providing the desired further strengthening of the construct. If careful placement of two screws seems not to have provided the desired stability, the use of a supplemental spica cast should be considered.

Bone scans or MRI may be used to monitor the postinjury vascularity of the femoral head. Physiotherapy and protected weight-bearing are instituted as the stability and the healing of the fracture allow. Osteonecrosis of the femoral head must be ruled out via serial radiographs taken for at least 2 years after the surgery, and any signs of osteonecrosis should delay athletic activity until the degree of necrosis and its impact on the function of the hip are determined.

Hardware removal is performed 3 to 6 months after complete union of the fracture, with sports participation allowed 2 to 4 months after screw removal.

Subtrochanteric Femoral Fractures

Subtrochanteric femoral fractures are also a result of a violent injury. Ireland and Fisher[34] noted that 2 of their 20 patients with subtrochanteric fractures were football players. The proximal fragment usually lies in flexion, abduction, and external rotation because of the influence of the iliopsoas, the hip abductors, and the external rotators. In patients younger than 10 years of age, closed reduction,

distal femoral skeletal traction in the 90–90 degree position, and spica casting comprise the standard therapy. In older children and adolescents, open reduction and internal fixation (with a plate or flexible intermedullary rods) is desirable, particularly if acceptable alignment cannot be achieved by closed means. Criteria for return to sports and removal of hardware are similar to those outlined for femoral neck fractures.

Hip Dislocations

Hip dislocations in children are usually posterior (Fig. 25B–5).[78] Classically, the leg is flexed, adducted, and internally rotated on presentation.[60] Hip dislocations in skeletally mature individuals are caused by more severe trauma and are associated with femoral neck and acetabular fractures. A prereduction neurologic examination must be done to evaluate sciatic nerve function. Pretreatment radiography to define the type of dislocation and the associated injuries should be performed. In particular, it is imperative to rule out an associated femoral neck fracture before manipulation. A hip dislocation should be considered an emergency. Closed reduction, under anesthesia if possible, should be performed urgently to lessen the risk of osteonecrosis.

If closed reduction is not possible, unstable, or not anatomic, then an osteochondral fragment or the labrum may be interposed between the femoral head and the acetabular articular cartilage. Emergent MRI or computed tomography may clarify the anatomic lesion (Fig. 25B–6).

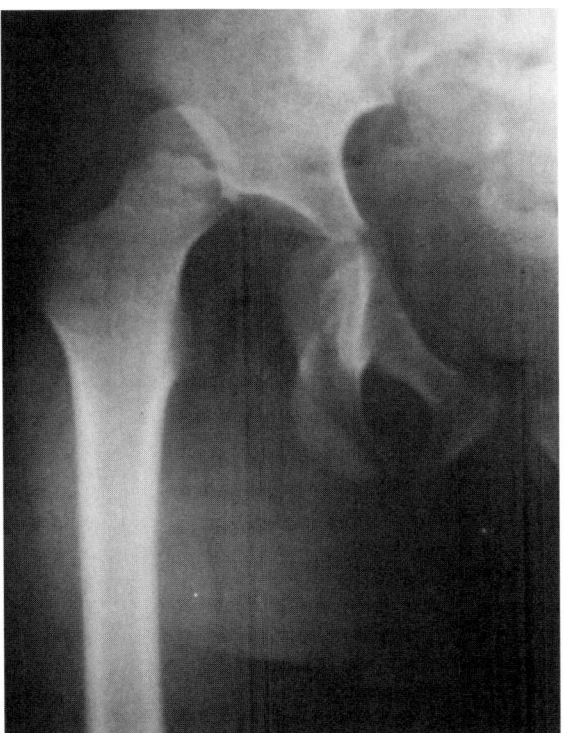

Figure 25B–5. Hip dislocation without a fracture. This is an emergent situation requiring rapid reduction, with the patient under anesthesia if necessary, to lessen the risk of avascular necrosis.

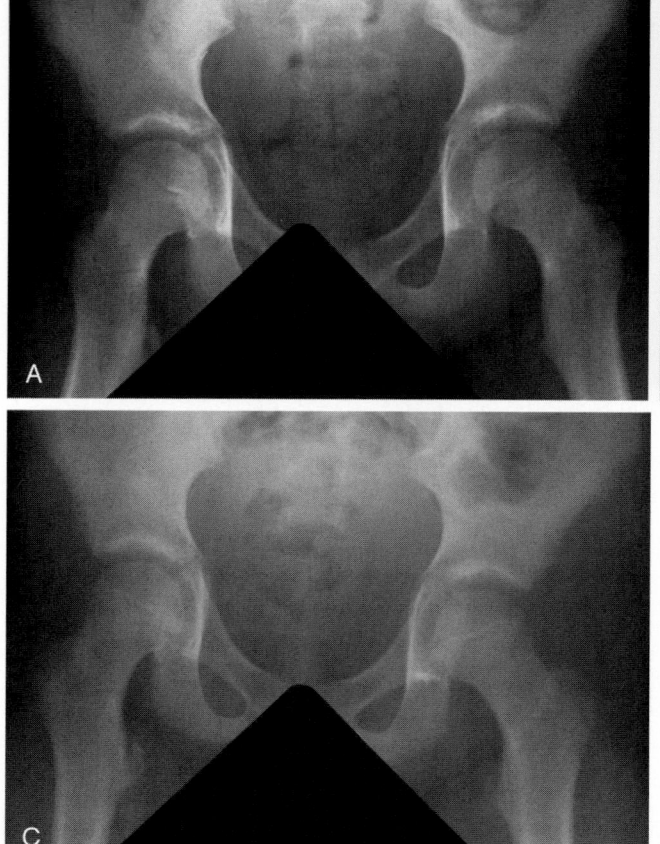

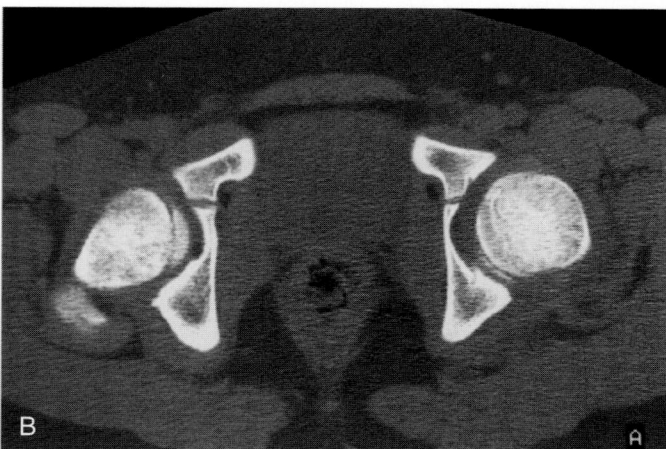

Figure 25B–6. *A,* Image from a 12-year-old boy with nonconcentric reduction of traumatic posterior hip dislocation. *B,* Computed tomography shows interposed osteochondral fragment of posterior acetabular rim and labrum. *C,* Posterior arthrotomy and fixation of the fragment yielded a congruous reduction and a stable hip. Note posteroinferior suture anchor.

In cases in which perfect closed reduction has not been forthcoming, an arthrotomy should be performed through the torn capsule. A posterior approach would therefore be indicated for exploration for treatment of unsatisfactory reduction after a posterior dislocation, and an anterior approach would be indicated for an unsuccessful reduction after an anterior dislocation, with the goal of the arthrotomy being to remove the obstacle to reduction.

Postreduction treatment depends on the stability of the reduction. This may vary from light skin traction for a few days to spica cast immobilization for a period of weeks, with protected weight-bearing on crutches for variable periods of time. In the absence of associated femoral neck or acetabular fractures, the great majority of dislocations are quite stable, and a few weeks of protected weight-bearing is all the treatment that is necessary, though participation in vigorous sports is usually restricted for a minimum of 3 months. Radiography, bone scanning, and MRI are employed to rule out osteonecrosis over the 24 months after the injury. If osteonecrosis of the femoral head has occurred, then individualized treatment, which is beyond the scope of this chapter, is in order.

In the extremely rare but very grave situation in which the traumatic dislocation of an immature hip is associated with a physeal fracture, the best possible treatment would involve stabilizing the physis with screws on top of the femoral neck before the hip is reduced. This initial stabilization of the physis and the head reduces the risk of further damage to the retinacular vessels that would occur if the neck were reduced within the acetabulum and the femoral head left behind. Under any therapeutic circumstances, though, this lesion is nearly universally associated with some degree of osteonecrosis.

Stress Fractures

Stress fractures of the femoral neck are secondary to chronic repetitive microtrauma.[28, 54] This diagnosis should be considered in a competitive runner with persistent discomfort in the groin. The pain is activity related. Female runners may have a history of amenorrhea. Local tenderness in the region of the femoral neck and limited range of hip motion, particularly flexion and internal rotation, may be seen (Fig. 25B–7). Plain radiographic findings may initially be negative. When a stress fracture is suspected clinically, early diagnosis may be made by technetium-99 bone scanning. MRI has been shown to be extremely sensitive in the detection of femoral neck fractures and also allows for evaluation of other soft tissue injuries.[71] Early diagnosis is essential to avoid delays, which could allow for progression to displaced fractures.[36] On diagnosis, immediate cessation of athletic activity is mandatory to pre-

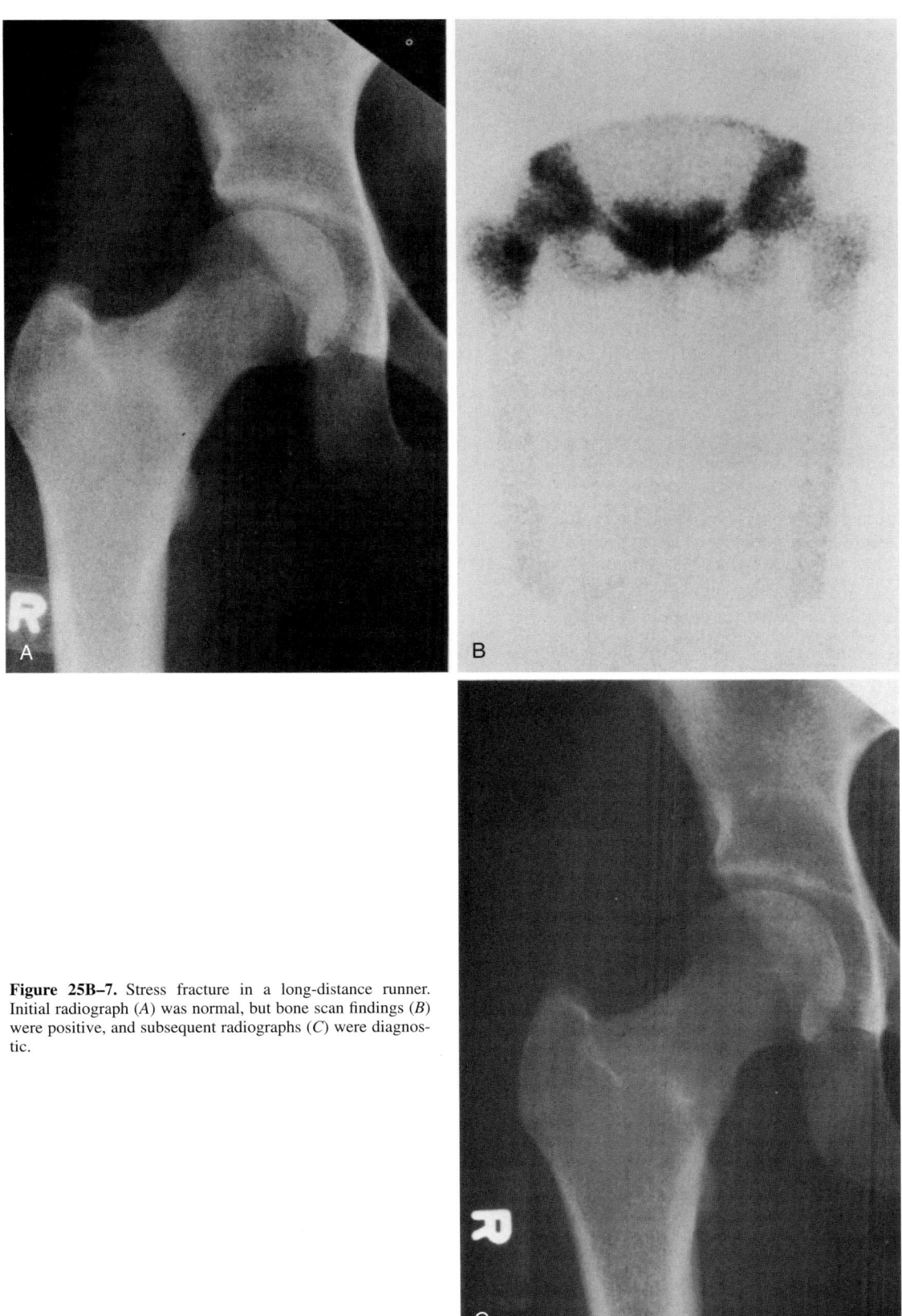

Figure 25B–7. Stress fracture in a long-distance runner. Initial radiograph (*A*) was normal, but bone scan findings (*B*) were positive, and subsequent radiographs (*C*) were diagnostic.

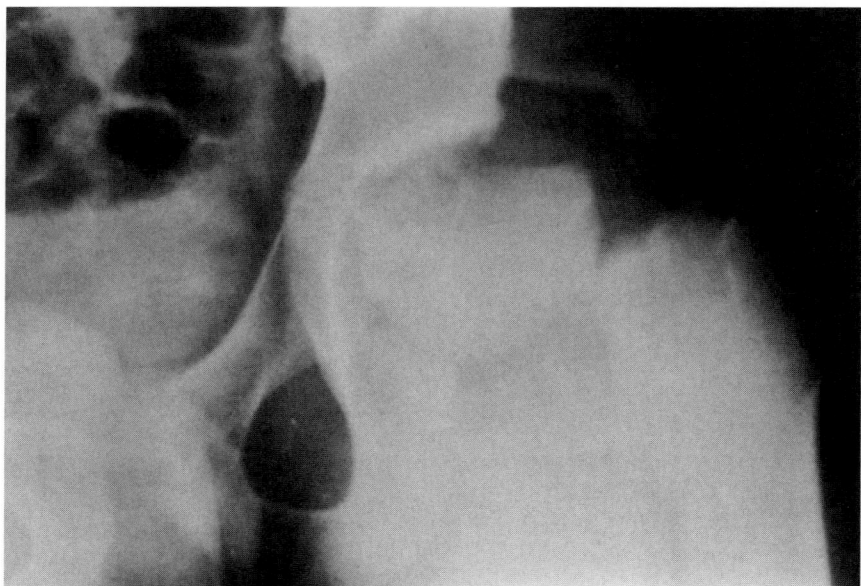

Figure 25B–8. This long-distance runner had a 1-month history of groin pain initially diagnosed as a "pulled muscle." Patient presented emergently with this displaced femoral neck fracture through an area of chronic stress. Open reduction with internal fixation was performed emergently.

vent the disastrous progression of a stress fracture to a displaced femoral neck fracture (Fig. 25B–8).

Devas[19] has identified two types of femoral neck stress fractures. The first is a transverse tension-type stress fracture in the superior portion of the neck that may become displaced. This is more frequently seen in older adolescents and young adults. Internal fixation with threaded pins is recommended before displacement, with its accompanying risks of avascular necrosis and nonunion. The second type is a compression stress fracture in the inferomedial neck that rarely becomes displaced. These fractures frequently can be treated with limited weight-bearing until there is radiographic evidence of callus formation and healing. In younger athletes, these injuries are usually compression stress fractures and are not at risk of displacement. Protected weight-bearing, range of motion exercises, and non-impact-loading cardiovascular conditioning, such as bicycling and swimming, are recommended until healing occurs.

When range of motion is unrestricted, the Trendelenburg test is negative, and activities of daily living are pain free, we consider a return to competitive sports. This must be a graduated, supervised process, with care taken to avoid excessive stress in a relatively deconditioned state, which may cause recurrent injury. We work closely with our physical therapists, sports trainers, coaches, and athletes to outline an individual program of progressive return to sports. Recurrence of symptoms is a clear indication to reduce activity and slow the rehabilitative process.

Stress fractures of the pelvis at the junction of the ischium and the inferior pubic ramus have been described in runners. Bone scan results are positive early, and radiographs taken 2 to 3 weeks after injury reveal periosteal new bone and sclerosis at the junction of the ischium and the inferior pubic ramus. This radiographic appearance may raise concern about a malignant tumor if a stress fracture is not considered in the differential diagnosis. Therapy is similar to that described for femoral neck stress fractures.

Osteitis pubis is an unusual injury that occurs more commonly in long-distance runners but has been described in a variety of athletes.[42] The mechanism of injury appears to be strenuous conditioning of the rectus abdominis and adductor muscles. The individual is tender directly over the symphysis pubis. Bone scans are positive in the symphysis early, and radiographs at 2 to 3 weeks after injury reveal sclerosis on one or both sides of the symphysis pubis. The differential diagnosis includes osteitis secondary to chronic prostatism in males. Rest, heat, and conditioning exercises that do not cause pain are recommended.

Pathologic Fractures and Conditions

A pathologic fracture is a fracture through abnormal bone. When the severity of injury exceeds the trauma that caused the injury, a pathologic lesion or state should be suspected. Similarly, when a rare skeletal injury is present, screening should be done for pathologic conditions. Pathologic conditions present either with an acute fracture through a lesion or with complaints of persistent, activity-related pain similar to symptoms of an overuse injury. Radiographs are necessary for definitive diagnosis. Unfortunately, many busy sports medicine practitioners have seen neoplasms in athletes that have been misdiagnosed and incorrectly treated as sprains or strains. Conditions that may present as pathologic injuries include benign lesions (osteoid osteoma, unicameral bone cysts, fibrous dysplasia), malignant neoplasms (Ewing's sarcoma, osteogenic sarcoma), and endocrinopathies (hypothyroidism, renal osteodystrophy).

Our policy has been to screen our symptomatic athletes radiographically on presentation. We feel that this lessens our risk of inadvertently missing an underlying pathologic condition that is unrecognized clinically (Fig. 25B–9).

Legg-Calvé-Perthes Disease

Legg-Calvé-Perthes disease (or Perthes' disease) is a condition of unknown cause that affects the growth and

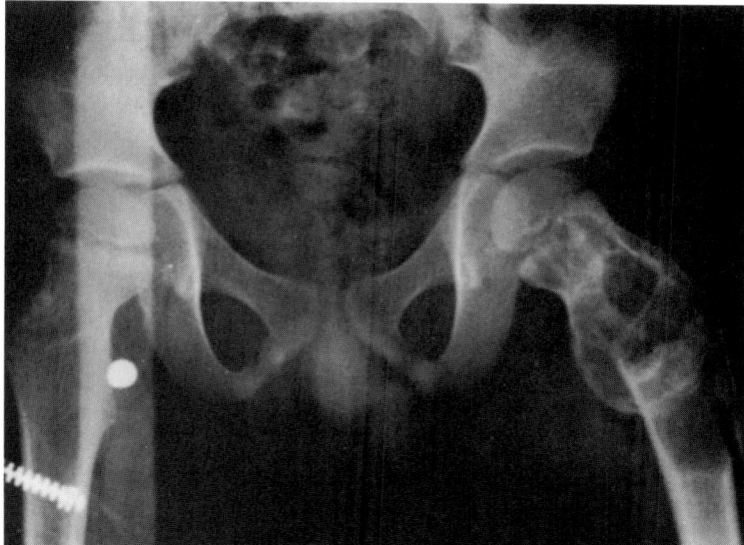

Figure 25B–9. This 8-year-old boy presented with acute pain during a soccer game. In retrospect, it was noted that he had had recurring activity-related pain. Radiographs were diagnostic of a pathologic fracture through a cystic lesion of the femoral neck.

the development of the capital femoral epiphysis; it usually presents between the ages of 4 and 10 years (peak incidence, 5 to 7 years). Its pathophysiology remains incompletely understood and its treatment imperfect. There is an associated circulatory disturbance in the capital femoral epiphysis and a generalized mild retardation of skeletal growth.[14, 44] The search for an underlying etiologic coagulopathy remains controversial.[26] There is a definite male preponderance (4:1), and both hips are involved in at least 20% of cases, though rarely simultaneously. The disease has an extremely variable clinical course but a very characteristic series of radiologic findings.[13, 63]

Diagnosis

The typical patient presents with a history of an intermittent, mildly symptomatic limp of a few weeks' duration. What follows thereafter may range from complete cessation of symptoms to recurring stiffness and pain culminating in early osteoarthritis and permanently disturbed hip function. This frustrating variability in the natural history of the disease seems to depend to a large extent on the age at which the disease begins and the amount of the femoral head that is involved. Younger patients and patients with less than 50% femoral head involvement have the best prognosis.[12, 13, 66] The nature of the primary disorder in Perthes' disease is still uncertain, but it seems not to be primarily inflammatory, neoplastic, or traumatic. The obvious component of hypovascularity during the early stages in the involved part of the epiphysis may be only a secondary finding.[63]

Physical examination at presentation usually reveals a characteristic limitation of internal rotation, extension, and abduction, as noted with any hip condition associated with synovitis. There may be some atrophy of the thigh. Tenderness and swelling are rare. Other joints are characteristically uninvolved (with the occasional exception of the other hip). Some degree of limp is usual.

Radiographs are usually diagnostic (Fig. 25B–10). The sequential characteristic findings are temporary cessation in the growth of the bony epiphysis, a sclerotic appearance of the epiphysis, fragmentation and apparent collapse of the bony epiphysis, and, finally, reossification of the epiphysis with new bone. These radiographic stages are thought to correlate with a circulatory disturbance of the bony epiphysis, with necrosis of the epiphyseal bone followed by reinstitution of the epiphysis by new living bone. The shape of the entire epiphyseal osteocartilaginous model may or may not be disturbed depending on whether the function of the proximal femoral growth plates is disturbed by the disease process. Perthes' disease is primarily a disorder of the bony epiphysis, but it may have secondary effects on the proximal femoral physis and subarticular hemispherical microphysis.

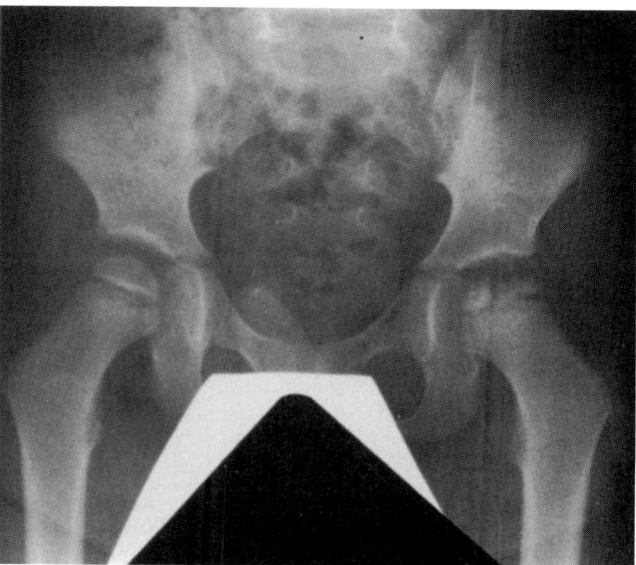

Figure 25B–10. Radiograph of a 5-year-old boy who had chronic groin pain and a limp while playing soccer. Legg-Calvé-Perthes disease frequently presents with activity-related pain.

Arthrography may be necessary to determine the shape of the femoral head during active disease in patients with major femoral head involvement. In the early stages, before plain radiographic findings are present, technetium bone scanning[49] or MRI may be helpful.

Catterall,[13] Salter,[66, 67] and Herring[31, 32] have found that certain radiographic findings are associated with a greater or a lesser risk of femoral head deformation. They have used these parameters as guidelines for instituting treatment: Greater than 50% femoral head involvement is a poor prognostic sign; preservation of the lateral column is a good prognostic sign. Catterall classifies patients into four groups depending on whether the involvement of the epiphysis is 25%, 50%, 75%, or 100%. Salter classifies patients into groups A and B, with A having up to 50% of the femoral head involved and B having more than 50% of the femoral head involved. Salter noted that careful anteroposterior and frog-leg radiographs early in the disease often show the "crescent sign," which he believes is a subchondral fracture with an extent that equals the subsequent extent of maximum resorption of the epiphysis due to Perthes' disease.[67] Herring notes that preservation of the height of the lateral pillar of the femoral head is important prognostically. Twenty-five percent or more collapses of this pillar mandates active treatment.[31, 32] These radiographic prognostic classifications are problematic in that patients in the earliest stages of disease are not classifiable in terms of prognosis; this means that one must make a blind choice in the very early stages between not treating any patients, which means leaving untreated a few who might benefit from it, and treating all of them, which means that containment treatment is used on many who do not need it.

Treatment

The initial aim of treatment[31, 32] in Perthes' disease is to control the symptoms and the disturbed function of the hip joint by instituting restriction of activity, crutches, and perhaps even bed rest with Buck's traction and balanced suspension until the pain and the limitation of motion subside. The second goal of treatment is to prevent deformation of the affected femoral head, because deformation of the femoral head owing to Perthes' disease is a potential risk factor for osteoarthritis in adulthood.[49, 74] If, at the time treatment is instituted, the femoral head is already deformed, the goal of treatment is at least to prevent further deformation and at most to restore the femoral head to a round configuration.

The difficulty in selecting and executing treatment programs for Perthes' disease arises from the fact that there is no agreement on the primary pathophysiology or on the efficacy of different treatment programs. There is general agreement that younger patients and those in whom there is less involvement of the femoral head tend to do better than older patients and those in whom more femoral head is involved. Patients older than 6 years of age in whom more than 50% of the femoral head is involved seem to have the highest risk of osteoarthritis in adulthood; the female gender seems to be an additional risk factor.[49, 74]

There is agreement on treating the stage of synovitis with activity restriction. Further intervention is based on the concept that containment of the anterior and lateral portions of the femoral head in the acetabulum will reduce the tendency toward deformation.[64, 66] The assumption is that uncontrolled growth of the anterior and lateral growth centers in the femoral head is responsible for deformation and that pressure by the interior of the acetabulum on this portion of the femoral head will keep it growing in proportion to the rest of the head. Containment methods, past and present, include (1) ambulatory and nonambulatory abduction casts[64] and braces[65] of various designs, most with a flexion and internal rotation component added; (2) varus intertrochanteric osteotomy[66]; (3) innominate osteotomy[66, 73]; (4) shelf arthroplasty[45]; and (5) Chiari pelvic osteotomy[12] (usually reserved for already deformed and irreducibly subluxated femoral heads). All these containment methods presuppose an aggressive attempt to restore a normal or near-normal range of motion by restricting activity and instituting physical therapy before applying the splints or operative methods. Treatment is continued until the radiographic findings suggest that the involved portion of the femoral head is being covered by at least a rim of new bone.[75] This may require as short a period of time as a few months in a 2- or 3-year-old patient to as long as 2 or 3 years in a patient 10 to 12 years of age.

Most observers agree that noncontainment methods of treatment do not influence the natural course of Perthes' disease. Noncontainment methods have included a variety of unilateral braces, such as the Snider sling, and simple crutches. Even containment devices, such as the Scottish Rite orthosis and the Toronto brace, must be monitored by radiography to be certain that the affected hip is abducted sufficiently to "contain" the lateral portion of the femoral head under the acetabular labrum.

Return to Athletics

Most orthopaedists restrict high-impact athletic activity until Perthes' disease is well into the healing phase on the assumption that loading trauma to the epiphysis negatively affects its growth during this sensitive period. This proscription of sports participation does not apply to patients with apparently mild Perthes' disease involving less than 50% of the femoral head.

The treating physician must be attentive to the patient with healed Perthes' disease because residual deformation of some degree follows in most patients. This deformation may range from mild coxa magna to significant femoral head collapse and joint incongruity. These patients are probably more at risk of an overuse syndrome around the hip than the normal patient, depending on the amount of residual deformation that is present. Younger patients usually tend to do better during the posthealing years because the acetabulum and the femoral head have had more time to remodel. The patient whose Perthes' disease begins in the later years of childhood may be left with a worse situation. The femoral head may heal in an aspherical position, incongruent with an acetabulum that does not have time to remodel before skeletal growth ends. It is this last type of patient that is most prone to develop early osteoarthritis.

In summary, Perthes' disease is often undiagnosed during its active phase. Hip radiographs taken thereafter may show the characteristic femoral head deformities associated with severe Perthes' disease. This radiographic appearance should lead the orthopaedist to advise either restricting activity or instituting active treatment according to the type of deformity present.

Soft Tissue Injuries

Acetabular Labrum Injuries

Hip dysplasia is an extremely important disorder that is frequently undiagnosed in infancy and often first becomes symptomatic in early adolescence.[41, 47, 55] The importance of the timing of symptoms in hip dysplasia (developmental dysplasia of the hip [DDH]) (i.e., appearance in adolescence or early adulthood) lies in the frequency with which it progresses to early osteoarthritis, often in early adulthood to midadulthood.[55] In certain subgroups, particularly females, DDH represents the most common cause of osteoarthritis.[3] Indeed, the flexibility and the good coordination that are often present in a child or an adolescent with DDH lead them into athletic endeavors.

In DDH, the obliquity of the acetabulum causes mechanical overload of the acetabular rim,[41] with secondary acute and chronic damage to fibrocartilaginous acetabular labrum. The acetabular obliquity is sometimes accompanied by valgus deformity of the femoral neck, further loading the acetabular rim. The first symptoms in the child or the adolescent with previously unrecognized DDH may be a result of abductor fatigue as the abductors overwork to attempt to stabilize the mechanically unsound hip. This can manifest as activity-related aching in the area of the greater trochanter. Later, groin pain may predominate, often sharp and transient, sometimes radiating as far down the anterior thigh as the knee. The groin pain occurs as intra-articular mechanics of the joint become more disturbed as the anterior or the anterolateral acetabular labrum stretches or even tears.

The clinical presentation of DDH resulting from overload of the acetabular rim is quite characteristic, although it is infrequently diagnosed as early as it should be. This has been termed the *acetabular rim syndrome* (Fig. 25B–11).[41] Acetabular labral tears are the most common component of this syndrome. It is critical to prevent acetabular labral tears from occurring in DDH because the labral tear disturbs the mechanics of the dysplastic hip, both representing an internal derangement analogous to a torn meniscus in the knee and simultaneously increasing acutely the instability of an already unstable hip. Indeed, acute giving way and locking may occur in the dysplastic hip even without a labral tear, but the symptoms are much more severe—as well as being more damaging to the articular surfaces—in the presence of a torn labrum.

The acetabular rim syndrome and labral tears must be considered if they are to be diagnosed. On physical examination, there is a characteristic impingement test involving acute flexion, adduction, and internal rotation of the hip, which elicits severe anterior hip pain in the patient with an abnormal anterior acetabular rim. The test is extremely sensitive for problems of the anterior acetabular rim,

though it is not absolutely specific to DDH. It may also be positive and symptomatic in patients with anterior impingement from a severe slipped epiphysis.

Another important physical sign often present in adolescent DDH is that of apprehension, experienced when the involved hip is quickly externally rotated from a position of maximum extension and adduction.

Imaging studies are important in diagnosing DDH, and plain radiographs are the gold standard, though they will not directly detect the abnormalities of the soft tissues of the acetabular rim. In an adolescent or a young adult, any hip with a lateral center-edge angle or an anterior center-edge angle of less than 20 degrees is at risk of developing osteoarthrosis.[59] These dysplastic hips should be evaluated and treated by physicians experienced in the treatment of DDH. Gadolinium-enhanced MRI directly images the articular cartilage in the acetabular labrum and is useful for characterizing the location, the size, and the degree of displacement of suspected acetabular labral tears.[47]

If an acetabular labral tear is due to an acute injury and is not associated with DDH, it may be treated well by means of excision of the torn segment through arthroscopy.[8, 50] Arthroscopic débridement of labral tears can be performed with the patient in the supine or lateral positions with good results.[9, 50, 62] Direct repair is usually unproductive, not only because of technical difficulty but also because of the unlikelihood that the sutured labral segment will actually heal. If the torn labrum or the rim fracture is associated with acetabular dysplasia, it is mandatory to correct the acetabular dysplasia surgically by means of pelvic osteotomy if the mechanics of the hip joint are to be normalized and future osteoarthritis prevented.[23, 55, 72]

Chondral Injuries

Chondral injuries of the hip may be seen in association with trauma, such as hip dislocation, or with underlying conditions, such as osteonecrosis or Legg-Calvé-Perthes disease. Patients often present with pain associated with certain motions. The extent of chondral involvement and the status of the articular surface can be assessed with MRI. For acute lesions with an intact articular surface, nonoperative management consisting of protected weight-bearing while maintaining motion can be used to hasten healing. In hinged or loose lesions, chondral resurfacing techniques may be necessary via arthroscopy or surgical dislocation.

Contusions

Contusions, abrasions, and sprains constitute the most common injuries suffered by young athletes.[2, 24, 35] These injuries are frequently minor and can be treated with a brief period of rest, ice, elevation, and return to athletic activity when pain is absent. On occasion, contusions cause significant muscular hemorrhage resulting in prolonged muscle spasm, disuse atrophy, and decreased range of motion. Formal rehabilitation with flexibility and strengthen-

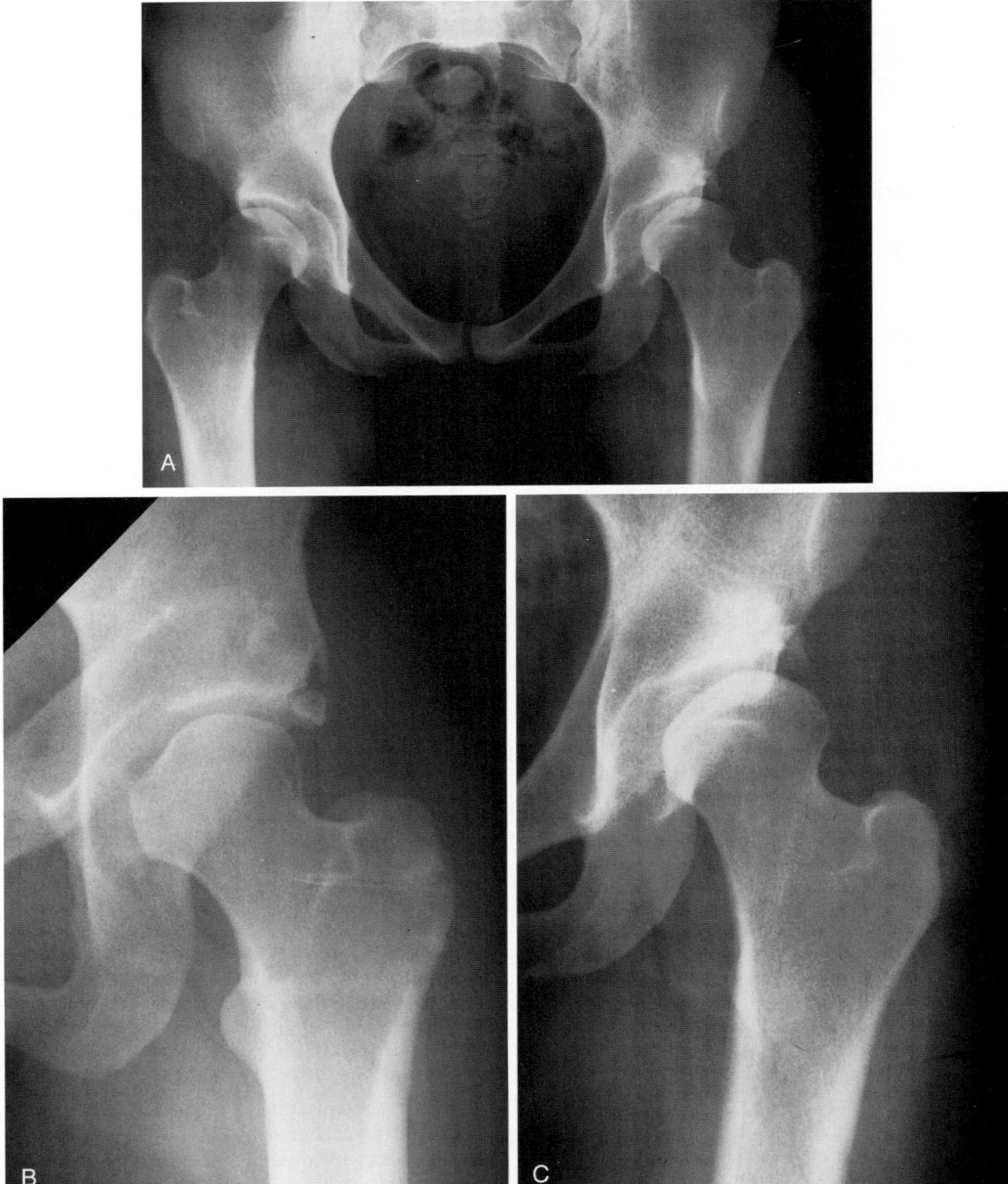

Figure 25B–11. *A,* A 16-year-old field hockey player had a 6-month history of activity-related left groin pain. She experienced sudden onset of severe sharp groin pain while running, followed by inability to bear weight. Radiographs revealed previously undiagnosed acetabular dysplasia, left greater than right, with sclerosis of the left lateral acetabular rim. *B,* The femoral head has acutely subluxated into the acetabular rim fracture site. Arthrotomy at the time of periacetabular osteotomy revealed an associated labral tear. *C,* Postoperative film 2 years after corrective intertrochanteric and periacetabular osteotomies shows a congruous joint and normal bone structure, with spontaneous stable fibrous union of the rim fracture. Strength and motion were normal, and she returned to varsity-level field hockey both in high school and in college.

ing exercises beginning after the acute inflammation has subsided may be necessary. Consideration should be given to the possibility of myositis ossificans[10] if the hemorrhage is severe. The athlete should return to competitive activities only after he or she has regained full strength and coordination. Early unguided return to sports participation may result in repetitive microtrauma that prolongs disability.

Iliac Apophysitis

Clancy and Foltz[16] described a syndrome of iliac crest tenderness on palpation and muscular contraction in the adolescent long-distance runner. These athletes had no history of local trauma but were enrolled in intensive training programs. The radiographic findings were normal. The syndrome seems to be a form of traction apophysitis similar to Osgood-Schlatter disease. Therapy consists of 4 to 6 weeks of rest with adjunctive ice application and anti-inflammatory medication use. Progressive return to sports is initiated with close monitoring of recurrent pain. The condition has also been described in hockey, lacrosse, and football players.[37]

Snapping Hip Syndrome

This entity is most commonly associated with iliotibial band irritation of the greater trochanteric bursa with hip flexion and extension, especially during internal rotation. Athletes frequently describe a sensation of hip dislocation. This entity usually responds to conservative therapy including rest and nonsteroidal anti-inflammatory medication followed by stretching exercises of the fascia lata.[53] Release of the iliotibial band has been performed in the rare athlete who does not respond to conservative therapy.

Athletes may also develop tenosynovitis of the iliopsoas tendon near its insertion at the lesser trochanter. In this condition, the discomfort and the snapping sensation are localized medially along the femoral neck. As with iliotibial band irritation, this entity usually responds to conservative therapy of anti-inflammatory medications, hip abduction and external rotation stretching exercises, and deep heat and ultrasound therapy. If conservative treatment fails, injection of the psoas tendon, under image intensifier control, may be useful. Rarely, release of the iliopsoas tendon sheath may be necessary.[53]

Sprains

As an adolescent approaches skeletal maturity, the ligamentous and musculotendinous structures become more vulnerable to injury. With fusion of the epiphyses and the apophyses, the growth plates no longer form the path of least resistance, and microtrauma and macrotrauma are transmitted through the soft tissue structures. These injuries result either from an acute event of excessive passive stretch or violent muscular contracture against resistance or from a chronic overuse syndrome. If the injury is acute, therapy consisting of rest, ice massage, and progressive flexibility and strengthening exercises when the patient is pain free results in rehabilitation of the musculotendinous injury. If the injury is secondary to chronic overuse, the underlying factor (e.g., improper conditioning, inadequate equipment, or anatomic malalignment) must be identified and addressed to achieve successful therapy.[54]

Differential Diagnosis

In addition to the pathologic conditions that may present as fractures, the clinician treating sports injuries in children should keep in mind medical problems that may present with hip and pelvic pain during athletic activities. These include Perthes' disease, developmental hip dysplasia, toxic synovitis or septic arthritis (with acute pain), and inflammatory synovitis (with chronic pain). Leukemia and neuroblastoma may present with limb pain. Not all "sports injuries" result from trauma, and the sports clinician needs to be ever conscious of the unexpected.

Summary

Hip and pelvic injuries are relatively rare in the young athlete. Contusions and musculotendinous sprains are the most common injuries about the hip and the pelvis. Apophyseal avulsion fractures are also frequently encountered skeletal injuries. Each of these entities can be successfully treated with guided physical therapy after conservative management with rest, anti-inflammatory medications, and ice massage until the patient is pain free. Rehabilitation requires restoration of full joint motion, flexibility, and isokinetic strengthening before return to competitive sports is allowed.

Physeal and proximal femoral fractures are less common entities that are secondary to violent trauma. These injuries are severe and almost always require operative intervention. Femoral neck fractures are associated with a high rate of complications due to avascular necrosis, nonunion, or malunion.

Pelvic fractures usually represent multiple trauma and are frequently associated with genitourinary, abdominal, neurologic, and musculoskeletal injuries. Pathologic pelvic or hip fractures in the skeletally immature athlete are most commonly secondary to benign lesions, such as unicameral bone cysts. All these musculoskeletal injuries require skeletal healing before strenuous rehabilitation can begin. During this phase, we maintain range of motion, isometric strength, and non–weight-bearing cardiovascular fitness. After bony healing, isokinetic strengthening is initiated.

Finally, in children with hip pain during athletic activities, even with antecedent trauma, the sports clinician must screen for SCFE, Perthes' disease, hip dysplasia, toxic synovitis, systemic neoplasia, or an infectious process.

References

1. Allen WC, Cope R: Coxa saltans: The snapping hip revisited. J Am Acad Orthop Surg 3:303–308, 1995.
2. Andrish JG: Overuse syndromes of the lower extremity in youth sports. In Boileau R (ed): Advances in Pediatric Sports Sciences. Champaign, Ill, Human Kinetics, 1984.
3. Aronson J: Osteoarthritis of the young adult hip: Etiology and treatment. Instr Course Lect 35:119–128, 1986.
4. Blatter R: Fractures of the pelvis and acetabulum. In Weber BG, Brunner C, Frueler F (eds): Treatment of Fractures in Children and Adolescents. Berlin, Springer-Verlag, 1980.
5. Boitzy A: Fractures of the proximal femur. In Weber BG, Brunner CH, Frueler F (eds): Treatment of Fractures in Children and Adolescents. Berlin, Springer-Verlag, 1980.
6. Broughton NS, Todd R, Dunn D, et al: Open reduction of the severely slipped upper femoral epiphysis. J Bone Joint Surg Br 70:435–439, 1988.
7. Bryan WJ, Tullos HS: Pediatric pelvis fractures. J Trauma 19:799–805, 1979.
8. Byrd JWT: Labral lesion. An elusive source of hip pain. Arthroscopy 12:603–612, 1996.

athletes; unfortunately, financial considerations have continued to prevent MRI from being considered a routine procedure.

Treatment of femoral stress fractures should be tailored to each patient's clinical presentation. Athletes that have pain during simple ambulation will usually require an initial period of protected weight-bearing ranging from 1 to 4 weeks.[73, 79, 90, 113, 118, 155, 200] Athletes with pain predominantly during running and jumping activities respond well to a period of relative rest, and nonimpact conditioning exercises such as cycling, swimming, and perhaps aqua jogging are allowed if the patient remains asymptomatic.[79] Actual series report resumption of athletic activities, specifically running, on an average of 8 to 16 weeks after onset of pain. This time frame is based on the resolution of symptoms or the appearance of radiographic evidence of the onset of healing. At this time, the literature does not support the concept of surgical prophylaxis for femoral shaft stress fractures.

Authors' Preferred Method of Treatment

Our treatment (Table 26A-1) does not significantly differ from that reported in the literature. Once the diagnosis is made, based on symptoms and a positive bone scan, MRI, or radiograph, treatment is initiated. The historical account of the onset of symptoms makes classification into the initial, intermediate, or late phase a relatively easy matter. Progression from one phase to the next is dependent primarily on time and pain (thigh or groin). We perform serial radiographs on a monthly basis for 3 months to follow the healing response, but we do not depend on these radiographic findings to determine phase progression.

In the initial phase, crutches (toe-touch weight-bearing) are used, with progression to full weight-bearing when the patient can ambulate without pain. During this time, cardiovascular fitness exercises and upper body conditioning are allowed, but lower body exercise is prohibited.

The intermediate phase begins when the patient is off crutches and participation in activities of daily living is pain free. Lower body activities are added to the treatment

regimen, which allows conditioning training in a low-impact mode. Typically, these activities include biking and swimming and are increased in intensity and duration as long as symptoms permit.

Surgery is reserved for displaced fractures of the femoral shaft. Closed intramedullary rodding is the procedure of choice, and a return to activities may proceed as per the protocol outlined for the nonoperative treatment of femoral shaft stress fractures.

There are two criteria for entry into the late phase: (1) A minimum of 6 weeks must have elapsed since the onset of symptoms, and (2) a pain-free, sustained bike ride for 30 to 45 minutes, comparable to a leisurely ride on a flat surface, must be accomplished. Athletes meeting these criteria are gradually allowed to return to running. Light running should initially take place on turf, grass, or a similarly soft running surface. As this becomes increasingly well tolerated, the athlete may return to his or her normal running surface.

Before resuming sports training, a reasonable explanation for this injury is sought. As mentioned previously, female athletes with a history of amenorrhea or oligomenorrhea are placed in a higher-risk category for the development of femoral stress fractures. In addition, any athlete with multiple stress fractures or a history of stress fractures is likewise at high risk of developing more stress fractures in the future. Therefore, we recommend a dual photon absorptiometry scan in all high-risk patients. Patients with a mild-to-moderate risk of fracture are allowed to continue high-impact activities after appropriate medical evaluation. Typically, training error is the most common fault. By and large, stress fractures of the femur occur in runners; therefore, the athlete must understand that rapidly increasing mileage or a marked change in intensity precipitated the injury and must not be repeated. Because stress fractures are secondary to repetitive stress, careful attention is given to those factors responsible for diminishing stress, especially with running. It is beyond the scope of this chapter to evaluate shoewear, orthotics, running surfaces, or running gait, but each plays a role in shock absorption and can be modified to increase its efficiency.

Criteria for Return to Sports Participation

The late phase marks the time when an athlete nears return to full sports participation. Because the majority of these injuries occur during running, the late phase is a running entry protocol (Table 26A-2).

Five miles per week, plus all other activities performed in the intermediate phase, are done initially. At the end of

TABLE 26A-1
Treatment of Femoral Shaft Stress Fractures

| Phase* | Activity Level | | | |
	Crutches	Upper Body Conditioning	Lower Body Conditioning	Running or Training
Initial phase, 2–3 wk	+	+	−	−
Intermediate phase, 3–8 wk	−	+	+	−
Late phase,† 6–12 wk	−	+	±	+

*These phases are based on time from onset of symptoms, and progression from one phase to the next is dependent on resolution of symptoms.
†Obligatory 6 weeks minimum before entry into this phase.
+, Activity used; −, activity not used.

TABLE 26A-2
Running Entry Protocol

Week	Activity	Total Miles per Week
Week 1	Walking	3–5
Week 2	Walking/running	5
Week 3	Running	5

the third week (at the earliest, 9 weeks from the onset of symptoms), if this activity can be done essentially pain free, the runner is permitted to return to half the standard training distance. Gradually, over the next several weeks, instruction is given to increase mileage up to the previous norm.

In other high-impact sports, this same protocol is used, and the athlete then returns to sport-specific training. By gradually increasing the time and the intensity of activity during the next 2 weeks, full participation can be anticipated.

If at any time symptoms recur, the athlete is dropped back to the previous phase for a minimum of 3 weeks and is managed in a similar fashion.

Muscle Strains and Ruptures

Muscle strains and ruptures represent a continuum of injuries that can lead to significant pain and disability, resulting in time being lost to the pursuit of leisure, occupational, and athletic activities.[57] The clinical relevance of muscle strain–related injuries is quite apparent to most sports medicine physicians, with these injuries accounting for up to 30% of a typical sports medicine practice.[28, 103] Strains are best defined as partial or complete tears of the musculotendinous unit.[34] These injuries are generally believed to result from excessive stretching, with failure occurring specifically at the musculotendinous junction.[62] This stretching usually occurs during an eccentric contraction that stretches the already preloaded muscle.[57, 59, 72, 210] Biomechanically, such eccentric contractions have been found to generate forces that are greater than those seen in concentric contractions.[57, 62] When the force and energy absorbed by this action exceed the ultimate tensile strength of the musculotendinous unit, failure occurs.

One of the first studies that addressed the site of injury was done by McMaster in 1933.[125] He stated that failure of a musculotendinous unit did not occur within the tendinous portion. Extensive work done by Garrett and associates[57, 62, 64, 115, 137, 139, 169, 180] showed that this lesion occurred at the musculotendinous junction regardless of the strain rate or the architecture of the muscle. Garrett and associates demonstrated that greater force and energy absorption occurred before failure in contracted muscle compared with nonstimulated muscle.[64] Safran and colleagues reported that isometrically preconditioned muscle required greater forces and an increase in length before failure when contrasted with nonpreconditioned (nonstimulated) muscle.[169] Additional studies have also suggested that athletes engaged in proper strengthening, stretching, and warm-up programs have a decreased incidence of hamstring injuries.[180, 198] Other reports in the literature have implicated poor technique, leg-length inequality, strength imbalances, and adverse neural tension as risk factors for sustaining a hamstring strain.[34, 49, 77, 148, 175, 192, 208] Collectively, these studies give scientific credence to the concept that a routine strengthening and warm-up program can protect a musculotendinous unit from injury. Nonetheless, there continues to be considerable debate regarding this topic, and more scientific work on the effects of athletic training on the musculotendinous junction is needed.

The physiologic properties of the musculotendinous unit are an area in which scientific information can provide insight into the methods of rehabilitation of injured muscle. It has been reported that muscles act according to the predominance of fiber-type content.[71] The fibers of human skeletal muscle can be grouped into two main types. Type I, or slow-twitch, fibers are slow to contract and do not easily fatigue owing to their abundance of aerobic activities. Type II, or fast-twitch, fibers are well suited to activities requiring speed and strength owing to their rapid contractility and capability for glycolysis. Muscles with a large population of type I fibers behave in a more static fashion, whereas type II fibers behave in a rapid or phasic manner[33, 61, 71, 89, 116] and with greater force.[26, 33, 61, 86, 186–188] In the thigh, the quadriceps and the hamstrings both have a higher percentage of type II fibers, as identified by histochemical staining techniques.[42, 59, 89, 153, 178] Therefore, these muscles are best trained by means of high-intensity and rapid activity. When strains of these muscle groups occur, high-intensity and rapid activities are not done in the immediate postinjury state but are gradually restored as pain, inflammation, and collagen repair permit.[138, 140]

After the acute inflammatory phase, early motion is desirable.[25, 107, 211] Early motion should be performed during the healing phase, with the goal of promoting muscle healing and minimizing scar formation while avoiding the risk of re-injury.[172] Therapy usually involves high-speed, low-force isokinetic exercise, as is best suited for type II fiber action. Additionally, isokinetic exercises are performed concentrically (tension when muscles shorten). Eccentric exercises (tension when muscle is elongated) have been shown to generate 20% more force than concentric exercises and are therefore avoided initially.[9, 10, 23, 81, 89, 100]

At the microscopic level, injuries to the musculotendinous unit are characterized by typical histologic changes. In the acute period, a hemorrhagic response occurs and surrounds the injured fibers. During the next 24 to 48 hours, the injured fibers undergo necrotic changes, typified by edema and the presence of macrophages at the site of injury. Inflammatory cells and fibroblastic activity become much more apparent by day 2 and are more notable near the region of the injured fibers, whereas the edematous response is more diffuse.[60, 180] These histologic changes are corroborated by findings seen on CT and MRI of the injured region.[53] MRI has proven to be particularly useful in further evaluating these muscle injuries. Magnetic resonance images of partial tendon tears demonstrate irregular thinning and hematoma at the myotendinous junction. Magnetic resonance, T_2-weighted images of grade I (stretch) injuries show high-signal-intensity edema and hemorrhage surrounding the myotendinous junction, spreading into the adjacent muscle and muscle fascicles, indicative of an acute inflammatory process.[149, 165]

Hamstrings

Hamstring strains and ruptures are the most common strain-related injuries encountered by sports medicine physicians and are the cause of a considerable amount of lost playing time among athletes.[39, 92] The hamstring group

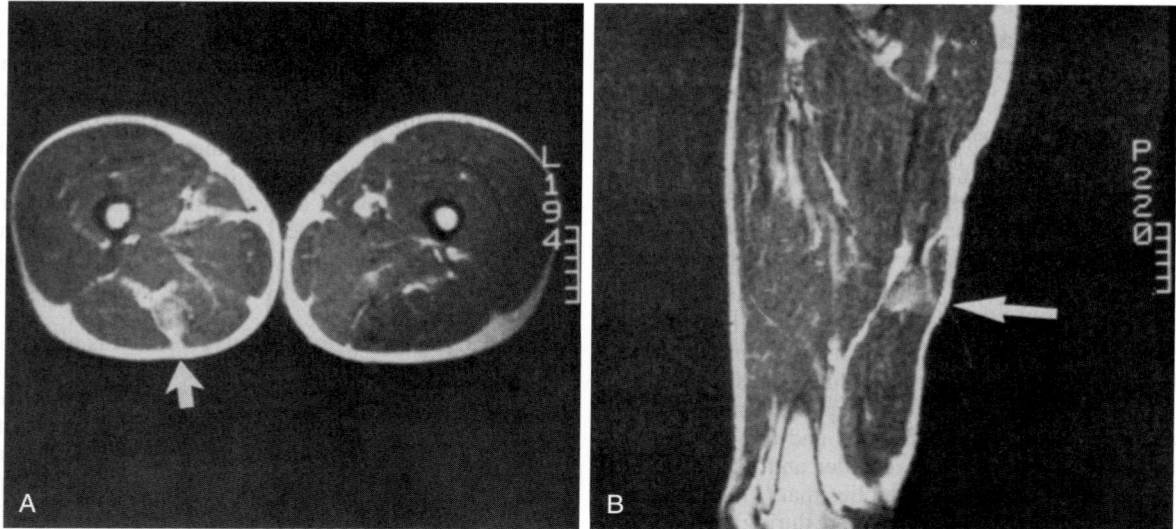

Figure 26A–7. Magnetic resonance image of a partial tear at the middle one third of the semitendinosus. *A*, Transverse view. *B*, Sagittal view.

treatment at present, and the cost of this imaging modality does not justify its routine use in the evaluation of this injury.

The hallmark of treatment for acute muscle strains is the RICE (rest, ice, compression, elevation) regimen. Its primary function is to reduce the inflammatory process and control muscle hemorrhage. After the acute period (lasting 3 to 5 days), most authors recommend a gradually progressive exercise program, including stretching.[39, 67, 77, 105, 140, 151] Patients should be followed for changes in pain, range of motion, and muscle testing and should gradually progress to resistance exercises as pain dictates. One recent study reported considerable success using intramuscular corticosteroid injections for the treatment of severe hamstring strains[108a]; however, we have no personal experience using this particular treatment modality.

The importance of recognizing muscle imbalances between the quadriceps and the hamstrings has been emphasized as a guide to predicting injury and reinjury to the hamstring muscle group.[77, 148] One study showed that rehabilitation of an injured hamstring, achieving a hamstring-quadriceps ratio of 0.55 or greater, resulted in no recurrent injuries. This is in comparison to a recurrence rate of one third in the control group.[77] Therefore, before resumption of normal activity, athletes should have full painless range of motion, restored strength, and correction of all muscle imbalances. This regimen allows most athletes to return to competition in a few days to 2 to 3 weeks.

Authors' Preferred Method of Treatment

The treatment of hamstring strains at our institution varies little from the protocols advocated by most authors. We have used a standard five-phase treatment program with considerable success (Table 26A–4). Essential to the treatment are serial evaluations that include pain scrutiny, range of motion, and muscle testing, either manually or

mechanically. In this manner, treatment can be expeditious, monitored, and changed as necessary.

Initial phase I treatment revolves around institution of the standard RICE protocol and determination of the severity of the strain. If there are no contraindications, we recommend nonsteroidal anti-inflammatory drugs (NSAIDs) acutely for the treatment of all hamstring injuries and then discontinue their use after a brief period. Progression to the next treatment phase is determined by pain relief and function (therapeutic exercises). An attempt is made to classify strains by clinical means, usually during the first 7 to 10 days after injury.

The progression through phase II and ultimately into phases III to V is dictated by the level of pain relief and the functional improvement achieved. The focus of rehabilitation should gradually shift to attaining a balance between promoting muscle regeneration and minimizing scar formation. A supervised rehabilitation program is the best means for achieving this goal. As full range of motion is regained, rehabilitation should progress from isometrics

TABLE 26A–4
Hamstring Treatment Protocol

Phase I

Rest, ice, compression, elevation (RICE)

Phase II

Ice	Stretch ± Isotonics	NSAIDs Condition	Electrical stimulation	Isometrics

Phase III

Ice	Stretch ± Isokinetics*	NSAIDs Condition	± Electrical stimulation	Isotonics

Phase IV

Ice	Stretch	Isokinetics*	Running	Sport-specific training

Phase V

Return to sports

*Concentric high speeds at first, proceeding to eccentric slow speeds.
NSAIDs, nonsteroidal anti-inflammatory drugs.

to isotonics, isokinetics, and finally light running. Continued improvements in strength signify that the athlete is ready for sport-specific training, with a gradual return to full activities shortly thereafter.

A mild or first-degree strain represents injury to a very small area with little hemorrhage and edema and no structural damage. Symptoms can vary from pain and spasms only after workouts to postexercise pain plus pain isolated to high-velocity activities. No objective findings of functional loss can be demonstrated because the integrity of the musculotendinous unit is intact. First-degree strains typically resolve rapidly within days with little loss of sports activity.

A moderate or second-degree strain represents a partial tear of the musculotendinous unit and is associated with a more specific onset of symptoms. An athlete may be able to recall a pop or a tearing sensation within the muscle during activity. Functional loss is usually immediate, although not always; swelling is usually evident and can be followed by circumferential measurements during the first week. A painful palpable mass within the injured muscle belly is present and will not retract on active contraction of the muscle, but contraction increases the pain. All these findings reflect hemorrhage and definite structural damage in the musculotendinous unit. This concept is important because not uncommonly, a "minor" ignored pull ends in a second, much more serious injury.

Severe or third-degree strains represent complete tears and may be difficult to distinguish from second-degree tears during the early stages. Clinically, a mass in the muscle is evident, but it retracts with active muscle contraction, possibly causing skin dimpling; it is particularly noticeable 2 to 3 weeks after injury. It has been our experience that third-degree injuries occur more toward the origin or the insertion of the involved muscle group, and this fact helps differentiate second- from third-degree strains.

Experience has taught us not to try to classify injuries before 24 hours. The more customary first-degree strain is evident within the first 48 hours but may take up to a week to classify. The more severe second- and third-degree injuries usually take longer to classify clinically than their first-degree counterparts. MRI may be useful in this setting because it provides a mechanism by which the injury can be more accurately quantified earlier. This is especially true of tears near the tendinous origin, which in our hands have been more difficult to treat.

Initial phase I treatment of all hamstring injuries revolves around the institution of the RICE protocol. Bagged, crushed ice that conforms to the injured thigh is used, followed by a compression dressing. Rest can be as simple as a temporary cessation of sports. In more severe injuries, in which pain and spasm are more severe problems, crutches and occasionally immobilization in extension for 2 to 3 days may be needed to allow for control of hemorrhage, edema, and pain. Prolonged immobilization is discouraged owing to the potential for detrimental long-term effects.[140] Studies have shown immobilized muscle to have a lower total deformation to failure and lower load to failure when compared with nonimmobilized muscle.[96] In addition, clinical studies conducted by the same authors revealed a 20% decrease in muscle strength after 1 week of immobilization. Crutches are discontinued when the athlete can ambulate without alteration of gait. All strains

are treated in this fashion to minimize the initial injury and the hemorrhage and spasm that inevitably follow.

After phase I treatment, clinical evaluation will uncover the majority of mild first-degree strains; again, the athlete has little or no pain and no objective findings of a hematoma and demonstrates no deficiency on manual muscle testing. These athletes are then advanced to phase IV of treatment. If after the first 24 to 48 hours, a strain cannot be classified or is thought to be a moderate or severe injury, the athlete enters phase II of treatment. This phase lasts 1 to 2 weeks. During this time, most injuries can be classified. Any patient who at the end of this phase shows persistent pain and functional loss must be considered to have a second- or third-degree injury.

In general, phase II treatment consists of early motion by way of protective exercises and passive stretching before and after exercise. A progression of exercises is instituted ranging from isometrics, in different positions at the onset, to isotonics. Application of ice is continued two to three times daily, accompanied by passive stretching in a sitting position. The athlete attempts to bring the chest to the thigh, and this is done in a fashion that elicits only minimal pain (Fig. 26A–8). Each session lasts 15 to 20 minutes.

In addition to ice, light stretching, and compressive wraps or sleeves, adjunctive treatments are instituted. We have found electrical stimulation, transcutaneous electrical nerve stimulation, and anti-inflammatory medicines help-

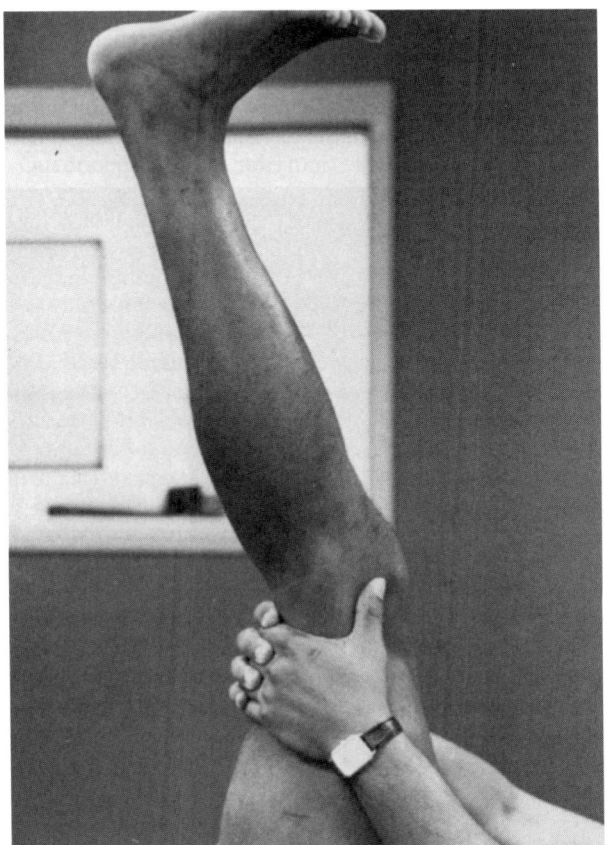

Figure 26A–8. Hamstring stretching is accomplished by active quadriceps contraction. This is also a means to measure hamstring flexibility.

rectus femoris muscle.[184] Athletes with this condition often have a painless soft tissue mass noted on clinical examination and usually no functional deficit or pain elicited with passive knee flexion or quadriceps contraction.

Diagnostic imaging techniques available for quadriceps tendon ruptures and strains include radiography, arthrography, ultrasonography, and MRI.[6, 16, 17, 104, 211] Plain radiographs have normal findings. When evaluating an athlete with a chronic injury, radiographs may be useful in distinguishing a chronic muscle strain from a femoral stress fracture or even myositis ossificans. Chronic rectus femoris strains and proximal strains can be confused with soft tissue sarcomas, underscoring the need for a thorough evaluation and further diagnostic studies when indicated.[45, 52, 83, 184] As with hamstring ruptures, MRI is currently the best imaging modality available for establishing a diagnosis, assessing the severity of the injury, and determining the appropriate treatment and rehabilitation for strains and ruptures (Fig. 26A–10).[121, 211] Routine MRI is not cost-effective for this condition. If a complete tear or an underlying pathologic process is suspected, however, MRI may be warranted.[184]

Treatment of the acute quadriceps muscle strain is similar to that of any other muscle strain and begins initially with standard RICE principles. Most treatment schedules recommend stretching and therapeutic exercise after the first 1 to 3 days, followed by a gradual return to sports.[129,]

[151, 167, 105, 39] Surgical repair is rarely warranted, and the overwhelming majority of these injuries respond well to a structured rehabilitation program. One author suggested a classification of the severity of these injuries that provided guidance regarding the duration and the progression of treatment but made no distinction between strains and contusions of the quadriceps.[167] Most authors recommend the use of NSAIDs initially and then discontinue them once the inflammatory period subsides. As motion improves, the patient is begun on a low-intensity training regimen and is advanced to a high-intensity program as permitted. The goal of therapy is to promote muscle healing and minimize scarring while avoiding the risk of reinjury. When normal strength and flexibility have returned, the athlete may return to all levels of previous activity.

Surgical management has been recommended as an alternative treatment for complete musculotendinous tears of the rectus femoris in the middle or lower third of the thigh.[75, 144] Surgery, if considered, is optimally performed within 7 to 10 days of injury, a time when a complete rupture is difficult to diagnose. In the study by Garrett and associates involving proximal rectus strains, however, conservative therapy failed in 2 of 10 patients, who required delayed surgical excision of fibrous scar tissue in the region of the indirect head of the rectus femoris, with good results.[83] Temple and colleagues also found that some patients benefitted from delayed excision of fibrous scar

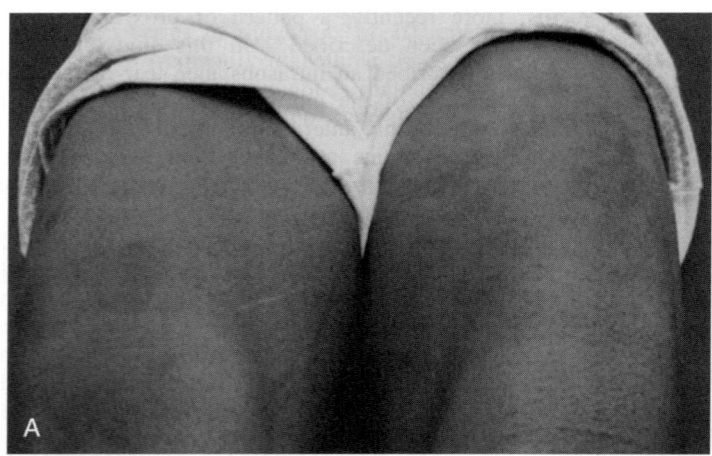
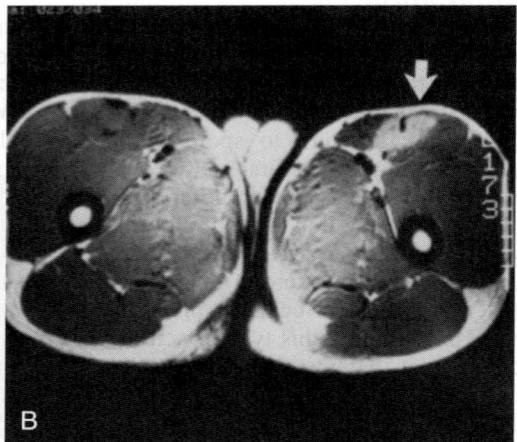
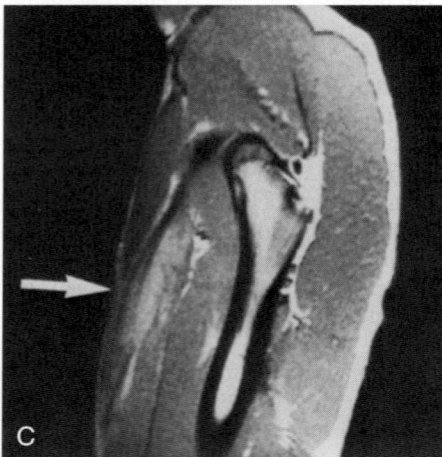

Figure 26A–10. *A*, Photograph of a partial tear of the left rectus femoris in a collegiate defensive back. *B*, Magnetic resonance imaging study, axial view, of both thighs; *arrow* indicates level of injury. *C*, Magnetic resonance imaging study, sagittal view, of the same injury.

tissue.[184] These findings suggest that there may be some role for delayed surgical intervention in certain athletes in whom conservative measures have failed. Potential complications of complete tears of the quadriceps musculature include rerupture, weakness of knee extension with or without an extension lag, and lack of full knee flexion.

Authors' Preferred Method of Treatment

The importance of serial evaluations cannot be stressed enough; they are essential to the treatment process and an injury-free return to athletics. Quadriceps reinjury during this time has been a greater problem in our experience than reinjury of hamstring strains and a lesser problem than reinjury with adductor strains. The physician should routinely reassess the patient's level of pain and examine the injury site for tenderness, knee flexion limitation, and muscle testing. Monitoring these parameters is critical for advancing therapy accordingly while preventing further injury and regression.

Philosophically, our treatment concepts for quadriceps strains are similar to treatment concepts for the hamstrings and employ a five-phase scheme (Table 26A–5). There is justification for this in that both muscle groups have a predominance of type II muscle fibers. Initial treatment for all injuries is phase I (the RICE protocol) for 24 to 48 hours. This minimizes the initial injury and subsequent swelling and allows evaluation time to determine the extent of the strain. The degree of injury can then be classified into one of three groups, based on loss of knee motion as measured with the hip extended or in the prone position. Although not the basis of classification but helpful nevertheless, an assessment is made of the degree of pain, and palpation and manual muscle testing are done on a frequent basis.

Mild or first-degree strains represent a small area of muscle involvement with little hemorrhage, localized by pain but not by palpation and certainly not by a palpable mass or defect. Typical findings are knee flexion to 90

degrees or greater associated with mild symptoms (soreness after exercise) and no functional loss. The hallmark of first-degree strains is a rapid recovery within a few days.

Moderate or second-degree injury represents a partial tear of the musculotendinous unit. Knee flexion is measured in the prone position and is generally 90 degrees or slightly less. Pain is usually more acute, and onset of pain with complaints of rapid loss of function is confirmed by manual muscle testing. One can localize the site of injury, as evidenced by the point of maximum tenderness, and possibly even palpate a mass or a hematoma. At this site, circumferential measurements will disclose a swelling even if it is not evident on inspection; these measurements are followed serially. Active contraction, as well as a passive stretch of this area, causes pain. If a mass is evident, a definite attempt is made to get the athlete to contract the quadriceps actively for observation. In a second-degree injury, mass retraction will not occur.

At times, distinguishing between a second- and a third-degree strain may be difficult because the findings are similar. A third-degree strain—a severe injury—represents a complete tear in the musculotendinous unit. Knee flexion loss is greater, with flexion limited to 45 degrees or less in the prone position. Identification of the site by palpation is generally not a problem. More often than not, it is associated with a mass or a palpable defect. Unlike a second-degree injury, after pain and swelling start to subside, active contraction of the muscle reveals retraction of the mass or the detached muscle segment. This observation may even include dimpling of the skin, but in our experience, this is not readily evident for 10 to 14 days.

During phase I, if a noticeable gait abnormality is observed, crutches are used until the athlete can walk without a limp. Also during this first phase, any athlete complaining of severe pain or in whom a more serious injury is suspected demands close observation, immobilization, and perhaps even bed rest for 48 hours. The potential for compartment syndrome to develop after a muscle strain exists, although it is extremely rare.[18, 93, 99, 157]

All patients with first-degree strains, once identified after phase I, are progressed to phase IV of treatment. Those injuries that are classified as second- or third-degree or are undetermined undergo the phased scheme. Phase II consists of early motion and adjunctive modalities, primarily ice, and progressive resistance exercises. Progression from phase II through phase IV is based on frequent assessments of the degree of pain experienced during exercise and on the following day. If the athlete is slowly taxed with progressive resistance exercises within his or her comfort range, recovery is maximized.

Progression is illustrated by the following example. An athlete who can perform a set of exercises comfortably on a given day is asked to perform the same exercises the next day if he or she is still comfortable and is still able to complete the same exercises; then, on the third day, a more taxing workout is given. This program does not lessen the importance of motion regained in recovery but emphasizes our observation that it follows positive functional gains. Furthermore, any treatment directed at regaining motion will more often than not have a detrimental effect rather than a positive one.

During phase I, bagged, crushed ice that conforms to

TABLE 26A–5
Quadriceps Strain Treatment Protocol

Phase I
Rest, ice, compression, elevation (RICE)

Phase II
Ice   NSAIDs   Electrical stimulation   Isometrics   Isokinetic
  ± Condition   Active stretch

Phase III
Ice   NSAIDs   Electrical stimulation   Isotonics   Isokinetics
  Active stretch   Condition

Phase IV
Ice   Isokinetics   Running   Sport-specific training
  Passive stretching

Phase V
Return to sports

NSAIDs, nonsteroidal anti-inflammatory drugs.

specificity of MRI. MRI is quite useful for determining the integrity of the muscle fibers[14] and grading the severity of muscle strains, making it the imaging modality of choice when evaluating soft tissue injuries.[14, 53, 149] MRI, however, remains prohibitively too expensive for routine use in the treatment of adductor strains, which are self-limiting in the majority of cases. We reserve the use of MRI for evaluating athletes suspected of having a grade III strain, for those with a soft tissue mass but no history of injury, and for athletes with unexplained chronic groin pain in whom appropriate treatment measures have failed. The role of MRI in the evaluation of athletica pubalgia remains unclear at present, and MRI is recommended only as a means of ruling out other potential disorders that mimic this syndrome.[128]

Rest, ice, compression, and elevation followed by a graduated physical therapy program are the mainstays of treatment for patients with acute adductor injuries. NSAIDs can be used in the acute setting to help reduce the inflammatory process. Rest is essential and may include the necessity for crutches for a period of 2 to 3 days in the patient with a mild strain or for as long as 2 to 3 weeks in the patient with a musculotendinous rupture. Before returning to the previous level of activity, the athlete must be placed on a strengthening and stretching program.[78, 127] The need for this program has been substantiated in part by one author's report on a group of high school and college hockey players who showed a power deficit of the injured leg of at least 25% compared with the noninjured extremity.[127] Integral parts of this stretching and strengthening program include both static and dynamic training without load or resistance, isometric exercise with increasing loads, dynamic training with increasing loads, and sport-specific training.[127, 158]

Acute adductor strains that do not respond to appropriate conservative measures can lead to persistent groin pain. Chronic adductor pain can also be the result of adductor tendinitis. Adductor tendinitis differs from an acute strain in that its presentation is insidious groin pain aggravated by sports-related activity. This condition is most frequently seen in soccer and ice hockey players in the third and fourth decades of life. Symptoms can frequently be traced to a previous mild strain that was never appropriately rehabilitated. Another theory suggests that this condition results from microtears occurring over time because of repetitive overload (overuse) of the musculotendinous unit.[1, 117, 201] It has been postulated that these microtears are not large enough to stimulate local bleeding, so the normal physiologic healing response is never initiated.[201] Physical findings do not differ from those found in the acute injury. Most authors suggest a conservative treatment regimen similar to that used for the acute injury.[127, 144, 158] Patients who have not responded to an appropriate period of conservative management may be candidates for selective adductor tenotomy. Several studies in the literature have reported a 81% to 94% rate of good to excellent results in selected cases.[1, 114, 117, 201]

Myositis ossificans is a relatively rare cause of adductor pain in the young adolescent and is seen predominantly in horseback riders and jockeys. It is thought to develop as a result of an acute strain of the adductor longus or after repetitive microtrauma. It responds well to conservative measures and rarely, if ever, requires surgical intervention.

Authors' Preferred Method of Treatment

Although adductor strains are seen as often as other thigh muscle strains, the incidence of severe adductor strains appears to be lower. A rapid return to sport in 1 to 2 weeks has been our norm, thereby negating extensive treatment. Nevertheless, a careful evaluation must be done to identify a more serious injury. Hip flexor function must not be ignored in the examination, because in more serious injuries, it is involved as well as the adductor.

Philosophically, we use a treatment schedule almost identical to that used for hamstring strains, which includes the RICE protocol for 24 to 48 hours, followed by a reassessment of the injury (see earlier description of the authors' preferred method of treatment for hamstrings). Generally speaking, pain resolution is rapid subsequent to phase I, allowing isometric exercises to be started, which are eventually progressed to isotonic exercises (phase II).

The progression from isometric to isotonic exercises illustrates our phased treatment concept. Progression is based on pain control and maintenance of function with therapeutic exercises. If an athlete can perform isometric exercises with little or no pain and the following day has no increase in pain or decrease in function, isotonics are inaugurated. Conversely, if regression is apparent, we advise return to isometrics or possibly a return to phase I. We continue to use ice massage during this interval in conjunction with light stretching as pain permits. Stretching is done initially in the supine position with both hips and knees flexed to 90 degrees and the involved limb lying flat against the table. Passive stretching is dependent on trunk and pelvic rotation away from the injured side, which is primarily controlled by the athlete's tolerance of the pain. As his or her condition improves, the athlete can maintain a comfortable, upright, sitting position. Once in the sitting position with the hip and the knee flexed to 90 degrees and the feet placed sole to sole, further stretching can be accomplished by direct elbow pressure to the knees (Fig. 26A–12). In this way, the same degree of abduction can be obtained bilaterally. Stretching after an acute injury is best done by the athlete because he or she will be able to monitor pain and consequently reduce the risk of additional injury.

Even for patients with more severe strains, isometric exercises can be incorporated into the aforementioned treatment sessions as early as 2 to 3 days after injury. As isometric intensity increases along with the athlete's tolerance, a progressive resistance exercise program is commenced. Isotonic exercises follow isometric exercises and progress to isokinetic training and running (see earlier section on authors' preferred method of treatment for hamstring strains). Again, as pain diminishes and strength and flexibility improve, simulated sporting activities are undertaken before the athlete's actual return to sport.

For complete ruptures of the adductor muscles (excluding avulsion fractures), manifested by a palpable gap with a muscle retraction mass seen during active contraction, surgical repair can be considered. This option may be considered when the injury is primarily tendinous at the pubic attachment, but we still continue to treat these injuries nonoperatively.

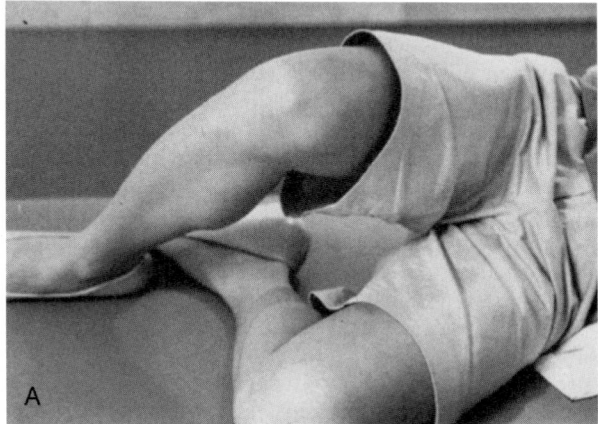
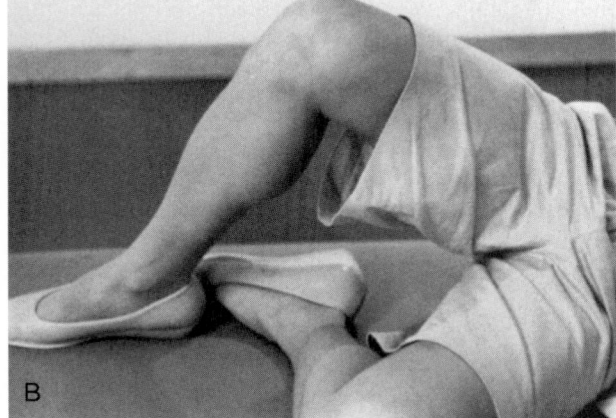
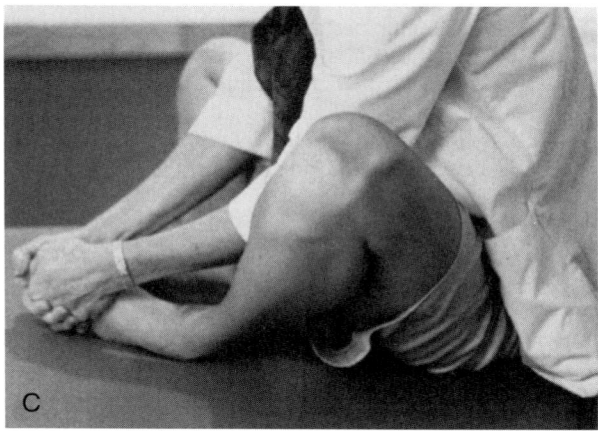

Figure 26A–12. *A* and *B*, Early passive stretch. *C*, Late active stretch.

We have not had any experience with performing an adductor tenotomy for chronic resistant cases of adductor muscle strain, nor have we found it necessary. We admit, however, that this may be a bias based on the type of sporting activities engaged in by our athletic population.

Criteria for Return to Sports Participation

It has been our experience that adductor strains are not as problematic as hamstring and quadriceps strains and are less likely to recur. Criteria for return to sports must include equal flexibility in both lower limbs, isokinetic test results that are within 20% of the results in the uninjured leg, and demonstrable ease and comfort in performing simulated sports activities. Once these goals are achieved, the athlete is fitted with a circumferential thigh girdle and is allowed full sports participation.

Muscle Strains and Nonsteroidal Anti-inflammatories

Reducing the inflammatory changes associated with muscle injuries is the main focus of NSAID therapy in this setting. These drugs have demonstrated their ability to lessen the inflammatory response without adversely affecting the tensile strength or the strength of muscle contraction.[2, 143] Nonetheless, the role of NSAID therapy in the management of muscle strains remains somewhat controversial. Acute musculotendinous injuries are characterized by extravasation of blood into the surrounding tissues and the subsequent recruitment of inflammatory cells, leading to swelling, erythema, pain, and impaired function.[9] This may be the only process, however, whereby the body is able to remove damaged or necrotic tissue. In addition, there is evidence that NSAID use within the first 24 to 48 hours of injury may in fact interfere with the chemotaxis necessary to promote muscle fiber regeneration and may thus result in delayed healing.[37] There is much speculation that the new COX-2 inhibitors will further reduce the risk of frequency of the potential side effects of traditional NSAID use. Obviously, many questions remain regarding the long-term effects of these drugs on the overall healing process and their indications for the treatment of muscle strains. Most authors, however, recommend a brief period of NSAID use immediately after injury and then discontinue their use when the initial pain and the inflammatory response have resolved.[106, 140]

Quadriceps Contusions and Myositis Ossificans

Contusions most commonly result from blunt nonpenetrating trauma.[82] In severe cases, blunt trauma can result in a partial or complete rupture of the quadriceps mechanism, similar to that seen in a muscle strain. In the laboratory model, damage to the muscle secondary to contusions usually results in a characteristic response.[43, 196] After the traumatic event, muscle tissue injury and hemorrhage occur, rapidly followed by an inflammatory response. The absence of hematoma or further edema heralds the gradual resolution of the inflammatory phase. Intense proliferation of myoblasts and fibroblasts ensues. Next in the sequence is the formation of granulation tissue, which eventually matures into dense collagenous scar tissue. In the past, it was believed that the muscle damage occurred deep, adjacent to the bone.[151, 167, 196] Recent animal studies, however, have indicated that the damage may in fact be localized closer to the surface of the muscle, near the site of impact, and then extends deep into the muscle complex.[43]

Athletes with thigh contusions are generally able to recall a particular incident that initiated symptoms, which may or may not have precluded participation in that sporting event. In mild or moderate injuries requiring treatment, it is not unusual for an athlete to have finished their activities that day. As with muscle strains, localized pain, exquisite tenderness, swelling, and the loss of knee flexion are typical findings. With severe injury, an ipsilateral knee effusion may be found. Therefore, examination of the knee must not be ignored. Jackson and Feagin found these injuries to be classifiable at 48 hours based primarily on loss of knee flexion, which had a practical application for treatment.[87] In addition, myositis ossificans should be considered if a firm mass develops at the injury site 3 to 4 weeks after injury.[20]

At the time of injury, roentgenograms are useful only to rule out any bony injury. They may become helpful at 2 to 4 weeks in the evaluation of developing myositis ossificans.[4, 110, 144]

In general, the treatment of quadriceps strains and contusions is similar. One author makes no distinction between quadriceps muscle injuries resulting from overload and those resulting from direct trauma.[167] Ryan and colleagues recommend an initial period of immobilization in flexion followed by early range of motion.[168] One additional exception has been an attempt in quadriceps contusions to speed the resolution of the thigh hematoma. Several methods have been described in the literature to address this concern, including early aspiration of the hematoma, the use of oral proteolytic enzymes or injectable enzymes applied directly to the site of injury, compressive wraps, and immobilization of the hip and the knee in flexion to pain tolerance.[4, 5, 106, 144, 168]

Common to most successful methods of treating quadriceps contusions are an effort to limit the hematoma by the use of the RICE regimen, restoration of knee motion by means of supervised exercises, and restoration of limb function by means of appropriate rehabilitation. This is accomplished in a gradual fashion to accommodate any single athlete's injury regardless of its severity.[87] Most authors recommend an initial period of immobilization for 24 to 48 hours. Motion is then begun and proceeds at the patient's own pace, not assisted by stretching. Isometric exercises are typically used along with gentle, active flexion exercises that are comfortable for the athlete. When flexion of the knee has reached 90 degrees or greater and

a normal gait is evident, a progressive resistance exercise program is initiated. Noncontact sports are encouraged as training before the athlete returns to his or her particular sport.

In three series treated in this fashion, all athletes returned to full participation in sports without surgical intervention, regardless of the severity of the injury.[87, 112, 163] The length of disability varies considerably and appears to depend largely on the severity of the contusion. Several authors have reported an average return-to-play time of 2 to 3 weeks.[112, 168] Other authors have reported considerably longer periods of time, with some athletes requiring as much as 5 to 10 weeks to return to sport.[87, 163]

Two significant complications of quadriceps contusions are compartment syndrome and myositis ossificans. Compartment syndrome of the thigh can result in significant soft tissue damage, permanent disability, and possibly limb loss. By comparison, myositis ossificans has a relatively low morbidity. Physicians treating athletes with quadriceps contusions should be familiar with the signs and symptoms of both these conditions and should begin appropriate treatment when indicated. Both these entities are discussed in further detail.

Authors' Preferred Method of Treatment

The same basic principles of treatment used for quadriceps strains apply equally to quadriceps contusions. The initial treatment, however, differs considerably in regard to our use of early knee immobilization in 100 to 120 degrees of flexion (depending on the patient's level of comfort) within 12 hours of the time of injury, via an adjustable hinged knee brace. We believe that gently stretching the injured muscle causes tamponade of the hematoma at the site of injury, thereby minimizing the size of the hematoma. Ice and a mild compression wrap should also be applied during this time. The affected extremity remains in the brace for 24 hours only and is then removed. Gentle, pain-free active knee flexion is begun at this time along with isometrics and hamstring stretching. The remainder of the treatment program follows our guidelines outlined for quadriceps strain injuries.

Our principle of not using heat modalities is absolute in quadriceps contusions. Many who advocate judicious use of heat admit that a potential problem exists with its use but offer no clear clinical time frame for its safe administration. We have not encountered any problems with the use of ice and have observed at least one case in which ultrasound used 3 weeks after injury in a traditional fashion caused a marked worsening of the condition. Later, this case was associated with the formation of myositis ossificans. The typical situation is an athlete who sustains this injury and at 2 to 3 weeks fails to make progress with knee motion. Therefore, other modalities are tried, most often heat and stretching, to facilitate recovery. The tendency to overtreat must be resisted, because more often than not, it only serves to exacerbate the symptoms and the findings.

We do not recommend, nor have we reviewed, a case in which surgical repair of a complete muscle rupture secondary to a contusion was a viable alternative.

Criteria for Return to Sports Participation

The athlete returns to practice when he or she is pain free, has at least 120 degrees of knee flexion with the hip extended, and performs well with functional testing. The testing criteria are similar to those used for hamstring strains. Circular wraps or thigh sleeves worn with some type of protective padding over the contused site are used when the athlete resumes sporting activity, but the pad must ensure absorption of high-energy impact and must stay in place to be effective.

When this treatment regimen is used from the onset of the injury, we have not found surgery to be necessary, with the majority of athletes able to return to their sport in 2 to 3 weeks.

Compartment Syndrome

Compartment syndrome of the thigh resulting from closed blunt trauma sustained during a sporting event is relatively rare.[40, 161] The majority of cases of acute compartment syndrome result from a direct blow to the anterior thigh, as often occurs during soccer, rugby, and football. There have been case reports, however, of athletes developing an acute anterior compartment syndrome after nontraumatic activities such as weightlifting.[18] Swelling within the fascial compartment results from bleeding of a vessel with subsequent hematoma formation or from increased capillary permeability with resulting third space fluid in the damaged muscle, as may occur after significant trauma. In addition, minor trauma may lead to a compartment syndrome in an athlete with a bleeding dyscrasia; therefore, this underlying cause must always be kept in mind. Elevation of the intracompartmental pressures ensues, leading to muscle ischemia, metabolic and structural deterioration and necrosis of skeletal muscle, and cellular acidosis.

Compartment syndromes can occur in any or all of the three compartments of the thigh. The anterior compartment, however, is involved in the overwhelming majority of cases, corresponding to the location where most contusions occur. The clinical presentation of an impending compartment syndrome of the anterior thigh compartment is frequently indefinite. There have been reports of compartment syndromes of the thigh occurring as late as 7 days after injury, although in general acute compartment syndromes become symptomatic relatively quickly, usually within 24 hours.

Clinically, an athlete with an early anterior compartment syndrome of the thigh will rest the leg with the knee in an extended position to lessen the amount of stretch on the quadriceps muscles. Pain out of proportion to the level of injury is perhaps the most important and consistent sign. The pain is deep, unremitting, progressive, and unrelieved with immobilization.[135] Passive knee flexion exacerbates the pain significantly and is one of the most reliable tests in making the diagnosis. Paresthesias are not uncommon at this time. Sensation over the anterior aspect of the knee and the medial aspect of the lower leg and foot is provided by the saphenous nerve. Diminished sensation in this area

is a more objective finding; however, it occurs infrequently and is suggestive of a more significant level of tissue ischemia.[40, 134, 203] Swelling is frequently difficult to quantitate in the thigh. Motor deficits and loss of pulses are late findings and imply that permanent muscular damage has already taken place.

If a clinician suspects the presence of a compartment syndrome, the diagnosis can be confirmed by measuring compartment pressures. The classic method of determining compartment pressures, and the authors' preferred index, was initially described by Whitesides and colleagues in 1975 and is still the gold standard.[202] Alternative methods of measuring compartment pressures include using a standard electronic arterial-line pressure monitoring system attached to a stopcock, extension tubing, and an 18-gauge needle, or using one of the commercially available compartment pressure measuring devices. Accurate measurements are best taken near the area of injury, often at more than one site, because studies have shown differences in tissue pressure over cephalocaudal distances of as little as 5 cm.[76]

Regardless of the technique used, it is imperative to interpret compartment pressure measurements in light of the degree of soft tissue trauma sustained, the patient's blood pressure, and the clinical signs and symptoms.[135] Human studies have shown a specific relationship between blood pressure and the pressure threshold for physiologic nerve dysfunction.[179] This threshold has been found to range from 10 mm Hg less than the diastolic pressure in healthy muscle to 20 to 30 mm Hg less than diastolic in damaged tissue. This has prompted some authors to recommend these latter measurements as guidelines for decompression.[76, 119, 179] Other authors have recommended fasciotomy when intracompartmental pressures exceed 30 to 35 mm Hg.[120, 133] In general, if clinically there is either a high index of suspicion of an impending compartment syndrome or abnormally increased tissue pressures, fasciotomy of the affected compartment(s) should be conducted in an emergent fashion.

The anterior compartment is most commonly involved. Fasciotomy of this compartment should be performed through a longitudinal incision, and the wounds should be packed open. At 3 to 5 days after decompression, the patient may be returned to the operating room for skin grafting or for delayed closure of the wounds if there is no undue tension. Criteria for return to play are similar to those for quadriceps contusions.

Myositis Ossificans

Myositis ossificans often results from severe compression of muscle tissue against the underlying bone, with injury to the muscle fibers and blood vessels. Clinical experience has shown that this heterotopic bone formation is invariably adjacent to the anterior femur. Its presence reflects a more severe injury but does not necessarily require a specific change in treatment, nor does it appear to alter the ultimate functional result.[87, 112, 163, 168] Simulated laboratory studies have not demonstrated a clear origin of the heterotopic bone that forms in the damaged muscle tissues.[196, 209] Studies have found the incidence of myositis ossificans among military cadets with treated thigh contusions to range from 9% to 20%.[168] In these same series, myositis ossificans was associated with more severe injuries and more commonly with an episode of reinjury.

The differential diagnoses of myositis ossificans should include periosteal osteosarcoma, parosteal osteosarcoma, synovial sarcoma, osteochondroma, juxtacortical chondroma, and infection. The differences between these lesions and myositis ossificans include (1) a history of trauma to the affected site, (2) a course of radiographic stabilization at 3 to 4 months, (3) patient age of younger than 30 years, (4) location of the lesion (anterior thigh), (5) the presence of an intact cortex, (6) a negative alkaline phosphatase level. All these findings are supportive of myositis ossificans. If the clinical appearance warrants a biopsy, a full-thickness biopsy must be obtained. Biopsy specimens confined solely to the cellular, inner layer of the lesion closely resemble the histologic appearance of osteosarcoma. The peripheral zone, however, demonstrates more cellular maturity and a lack of invasion from adjacent tissues—important pathologic criteria for diagnosing myositis ossificans.[197] Usually, it is more appropriate to observe these lesions with serial radiographs.

The radiographic evolution of myositis ossificans parallels its histologic appearance. By the third or fourth week, flocculated densities are seen within the soft tissue mass, and the underlying bone exhibits a periosteal reaction. By 3 to 6 months, the bony mass usually stabilizes or even "shrinks" (Fig. 26A–13). Once mature, these masses may be classified based on their periosteal connection to the femur. There are three basic types of periosteal connections: broad based, connected by a stalk, or no connection at all.[191] Radiographic findings closely parallel those of CT; however, CT may help differentiate immature osteoid in a sarcoma from true ossification in myositis ossificans, and CT may be helpful in determining the size, the density,

and the anatomic location of the lesion. Technetium scans can evaluate early myositis ossificans, but its true value rests in monitoring the maturation of the lesion and determining the appropriate timing of excision.[51, 197] Ultrasonography has also been demonstrated to be useful as a diagnostic tool.[97] It has the ability to detect soft tissue changes that have proved to be precursors of myositis ossificans before the appearance of roentgenographic changes.

The MRI appearance of these lesions varies considerably depending on the level of maturity of the lesion. Early lesions in particular may mimic an aggressive soft tissue sarcoma, whereas more mature lesions have a more benign appearance.[8, 101]

Myositis ossificans rarely alters the athlete's ability to return to play. Occasionally, however, an athlete may remain symptomatic months after the injury, and operative intervention is considered. In this instance, the physician should be aware that surgical management before maturity of myositis ossificans invites disaster. This includes recurrence of bone formation greater than the amount of bone that was excised and a marked increase in the extent of the athlete's disability. It has been suggested that one of the indications for successful surgical excision should be the presence of a mature mass for 6 months if symptoms and disability persist. Surgical technique employs exposure of the entire mass to allow excision in toto, much the same as for an excisional biopsy. Exacting technique, including meticulous hemostasis and atraumatic dissection and excision, are ingredients of a successful surgical procedure.

Authors' Preferred Method of Treatment

We have seen a fair number of athletes who developed myositis ossificans. If treatment is done in an appropriate manner, disability rarely ensues. Occasionally, one may see an athlete with untreated myositis ossificans who has

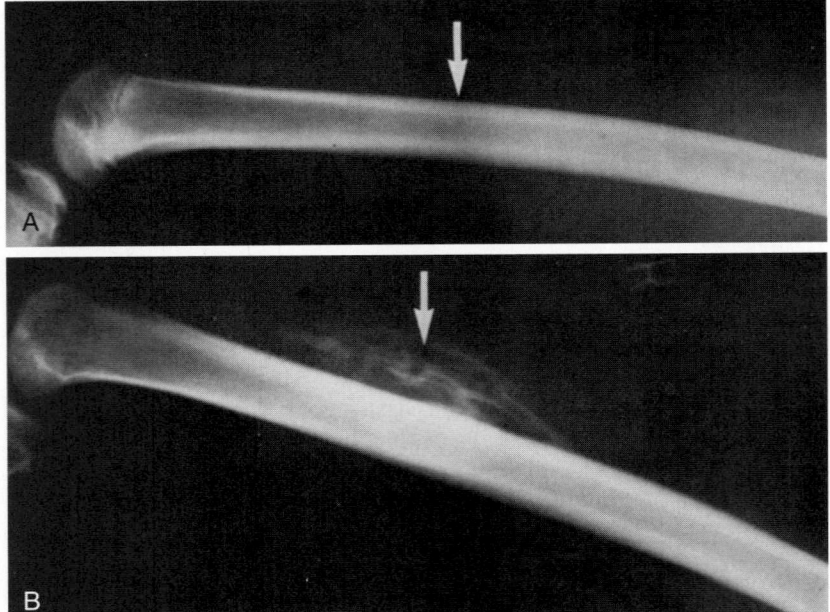

Figure 26A–13. Radiographs of two patients with myositis ossificans, both secondary to an anterior thigh contusion. *A*, Early (3 weeks). *B*, Late (6 weeks).

persistence of loss of motion, a painful bony mass, and significant functional limitation. In this circumstance, we still try conservative means first, and, if these fail, surgical excision of the heterotopic bone is recommended. Surgical excision is not considered before maturation of the bony mass or until a minimum of 6 months (and preferably 12 months) has elapsed since the time of injury.

A routine preoperative work-up is performed, although consideration should be given to obtaining a bleeding profile in athletes who have been on a recent course of NSAIDs. Magnetic resonance or CT-enhanced arteriograms can be helpful in lesions located dangerously close to nearby neurovascular structures. Athletes should be advised to discontinue all NSAIDs 4 to 6 weeks before surgery. Careful surgical technique and gentle handling of the soft tissues are used to avoid unnecessary muscle stripping. Excisional biopsy, followed by splinting, is our routine. Wound drainage is recommended if there is continued bleeding after appropriate hemostatic measures have been performed.

Postoperatively, we have used a knee immobilizer for 3 weeks with partial weight-bearing on crutches, followed by entry into phase II of our treatment protocol (see discussion under quadriceps strains). Anti-inflammatories have demonstrated some promise in the prevention of heterotopic bone formation.[124, 190] The anti-inflammatory drug of choice in this setting is indomethacin. In a very limited number of athletes who underwent surgery, a successful return to athletics was possible. The criteria for return to play are similar to those for quadriceps contusions.

Adductor Canal Syndrome

The adductor canal (Hunter's canal) is an aponeurotic canal in the middle third of the thigh and is bounded anterolaterally by the vastus medialis, medially by the sartorius, and posterolaterally by the adductor longus muscles.[22] The femoral artery, the femoral vein, and the saphenous nerve course through this constrictive space. The pathogenesis of this syndrome is unknown. Direct trauma to the superficial femoral artery at this level may result in an intimal tear and localized thrombosis.[14] Anatomically, compression of the artery by an abnormal musculotendinous band arising from the adductor muscle mass has also been implicated.[194] Saphenous nerve entrapment can occur and seems to be consistent with nerve entrapment syndromes at other sites.[159]

In this extremely rare disorder, the patients are young, athletic, and have no history of arterial disease. These athletes seek medical attention because of gradually worsening lower leg claudication that is exacerbated by activities and relieved by rest. Physical examination findings are essentially normal with the exception of diminished or absent pulses in the involved extremity.

Diagnostic studies that have been useful are an abnormal exercise response (claudication) and a diminished Doppler ankle-brachial index.[194] Although invasive, arteriography is diagnostic for occlusion of the superficial femoral artery at Hunter's canal.[194] An alternative method of diagnosing this lesion that uses arterial pulsatile wave patterns has been described.[108]

Because of its proximity in the adductor canal, saphenous nerve entrapment must be considered in the differential diagnosis of adductor canal syndrome. Clinical features of saphenous nerve entrapment include anterior knee pain and dysesthesias along the saphenous nerve distribution. Evidence supporting nerve entrapment is found by a positive response to an injection of local anesthesia plus corticosteroids, a procedure that may be not only diagnostic but also therapeutic.[159] The clinical distinction between superficial femoral artery occlusion and saphenous nerve entrapment is relatively easy based on their presentations. Additionally, if flow studies are used in the work-up, these two clinical entities should not be confused.

Once the superficial femoral artery has been demonstrated by arteriography to be occluded, treatment consists of exploration of this region. If an aberrant musculotendinous band is found, it is divided. This does not exclude examination of the arterial wall, which may show an intimal tear with localized thrombosis. Arterial continuity is re-established by traditional vascular procedures. If an aberrant musculotendinous band is identified, one author encourages exploration of the contralateral side even if it is asymptomatic.[194]

Authors' Preferred Method of Treatment

In any athlete with symptoms of claudication in the lower extremity, this syndrome should be included in the differential diagnosis and a Doppler ankle-brachial index obtained as the screening procedure. If this test result is positive and reflects diminished flow compared with the normal side, arteriography is recommended.

Assuming that arteriographic findings are positive, surgical intervention would follow, especially if the arterial obstruction is intrinsic in nature. Once normal flow to the vessel is re-established, return to sports depends on the cause of the obstruction and the type of surgical procedure done. No firm guidelines can be given here. In general, if the arterial obstruction was secondary to an aberrant musculotendinous band without arterial injury, rapid return to sports training can be anticipated 7 to 10 days after surgical release. Conversely, if the obstruction involved an intrinsic problem, as in an intimal tear within the vessel, more likely than not a segment of the artery would be excised. Continuity of the vessel would then be re-established by an end-to-end technique or, less likely, by an interposition graft. Obviously, downtime for the athlete will be greater if actual arterial surgery is performed and greater yet if an interposition graft is necessary. Our vascular surgeons advise an athlete not to return the involved extremity to training for 2 to 3 weeks if an end-to-end repair was done and to refrain from training for 6 to 8 weeks if a graft was required. These general time frames assume an uncomplicated postoperative recovery.

Criteria for Return to Sports Participation

An athlete who has had an arterial repair suffers more from deconditioning than from anything selective within a muscle group per se. Therefore, preseason fitness and lower leg strength, power, and endurance evaluations are necessary. With so many variables, no reasonable time frame can be given. What can be offered is a general recommendation that any athlete requiring an arterial repair should wear a protective pad over the adductor canal during training and should not return to contact sports for an empirical 3 months.

References

1. Akermark C, Johansson C: Tenotomy of the adductor longus tendon in the treatment of chronic groin pain in athletes. Am J Sports Med 20:640–643, 1992.
2. Almekinders LC, Gilbert JA: Healing of experimental muscle strains and the effects of nonsteroidal anti-inflammatory medication. Am J Sports Med 14:303–308, 1986.
3. Amendola A, Clatworthy M, Magnes SA: Overuse injuries of the lower extremity. In Herschman E, Mandelbaum EB (eds): Orthopaedic Knowledge Update—Sports Medicine 2. Rosemont, Ill, American Academy of Orthopaedic Surgeons, 1999, pp 365–372.
4. American Academy of Orthopaedic Surgeons (eds): Athletic Training and Sports Medicine. Chicago, American Academy of Orthopaedic Surgeons, 1984, pp 3, 223–234.
5. An HS, Simpson M, Gale S, Jackson WT: Acute anterior compartment syndrome in the thigh: A case report and review of the literature. J Orthop Trauma 1:180–182, 1987.
6. Aprin H, Btoukhim B: Early diagnosis of acute rupture of the quadriceps tendon by arthrography. Clin Orthop 195:185–190, 1985.
7. Arner O, Lindholm A: What is tennis leg? Acta Chir Scand 116:73–77, 1958.
8. Arrington ED, Miller MD: Skeletal muscle injuries. Orthop Clin North Am 26:411–422, 1995.
9. Asmussen E: Positive and negative muscular work. Acta Physiol Scand 28:364–382, 1953.
10. Asmussen E: Observations on experimental muscular soreness. Acta Rheum Scand 2:109–116, 1956.
11. Balaji MR, DeWeese JA: Adductor canal outlet syndrome. JAMA 245:167–170, 1981.
12. Bargren JH, Tilson DH, Bridgeford OE: Prevention of displaced fatigue fractures of the femur. J Bone Joint Surg Am 53:1115–1117, 1971.
13. Basmajian JV: Muscles Alive, 3rd ed. Baltimore, Williams & Wilkins, 1974.
14. Bassett LW, Gold RH: Magnetic resonance imaging of the musculoskeletal system: An overview. Clin Orthop 244:17–18, 1988.
15. Bennell KL, Malcolm SA, Thomas SA, et al: Risk factors for stress fractures in track and field athletes: A twelve-month prospective study. Am J Sports Med 24:810–818, 1996.
16. Berlin RC, Levinsohn EM, Chrisman H: The wrinkled patellar tendon: An indication of abnormality in the extensor mechanism of the knee. Skeletal Radiol 20:181–185, 1991.
17. Bianchi S, Zwass A, Abdelwahab IF, et al: Diagnosis of tears of the quadriceps tendon of the knee: Value of sonography. AJR Am J Roentgenol 162:1137–1140, 1994.
18. Bidwell JP, Gibbons CER, Godsiff S: Acute compartment syndrome of the thigh after weight training. Br J Sports Med 30:264–265, 1996.
19. Black J: Failure of implants for internal hip fixation. Orthop Clin North Am 5:833–844, 1974.
20. Blatz DJ: Bilateral femoral and tibial shaft stress fractures in a runner. Am J Sports Med 9:322–325, 1981.
21. Blecker A: Uber den Einfluss des Parademarsches auf die Entstehung der Fussgeshwulst. Med Kin Berl 1:305, 1905.
22. Blickenstaff L: Fatigue fracture of the femoral neck. J Bone Joint Surg Am 48:1031–1047, 1966.
23. Blix M: Die Lange und die Spannug des Muskels. Skandinavisches Archiv für Physiologie 5:149–206, 1895.
24. Boden BP, Speer KP: Femoral stress fractures. Clin Sports Med 16:307–316, 1997.
25. Booth FW, Gould EW: Effect of training and disuse on connective tissue. In Wilmore JH, Keough JF (eds): Exercise and Sport Sciences Review. New York, Academic Press, 1975, p 105.
26. Bosco C, Komi PV: Mechanical characteristics and fiber composition of human leg extensor muscles. Eur J Appl Physiol 41:275–284, 1979.
27. Bradshaw C, McCrory P, Bell S, Bruker P: Obturator nerve entrapment; a cause of groin pain in athletes. Am J Sports Med 25:402–408, 1997.
28. Branch HE: March fractures of the femur. J Bone Joint Surg 26:387–391, 1944.
29. Breithaupt MD: Zur Pathologie des Menschlichen Fusses. Med Zeitung 24:169, 1855.
30. Brewer BJ: Mechanism of injury to the musculotendinous unit. Instr Course Lect 17:354–358, 1960.
31. Brudvig TJS, Gudger TD, Obermeyer L: Stress fractures in 295 trainees: A one year study of incidence as related to age, sex and race. J Military Med 148:666–667, 1983.
32. Brukner P, Bennell K: Stress fractures in female athletes. Sports Med 24:419–429, 1997.
33. Burke RE, Edgerton VR: Motor unit properties and selective involvement in movement. Exerc Sport Sci Rev 3:31–81, 1975.
34. Burkett LN: Causative factors in hamstring strain. Med Sci Sports Exerc 2:39–42, 1970.
35. Burkett LN: Investigation into hamstring strains: The case of the hybrid muscle. J Sports Med 3:228–231, 1976.
36. Butler JE, Brown SL, McConnell BG: Subtrochanteric stress fractures in runners. Am J Sports Med 10:228–232, 1982.
37. Carter DR, Hayes WC: Bone compressive strength: The influences of density and strain rate. Science 10:1174–1175, 1976.
38. Casperson PC: Groin and hamstring injuries. J Athlet Train 17:43–45, 1982.
39. Clanton TO, Coupe KJ: Hamstring strains in athletes: Diagnosis and treatment. J Am Acad Orthop Surg 6:237–248, 1998.
40. Colosimo AJ, Ireland ML: Thigh compartment syndrome in a football athlete: A case report and review of the literature. Med Sci Sports Exerc 24:958–963, 1992.
41. Cook SD, Harding AF, Thomas KA, et al: Trabecular bone density in menstrual function in women runners. Am J Sports Med 15:503–507, 1987.
42. Coyle EF, Feiring DC, Rotkin TC, et al: Specificity of power improvements through slow and fast isokinetic training. J Appl Physiol 51:1437–1442, 1981.
43. Crisco JJ, Jokl P, Heinen GT, et al: A muscle contusion injury model. Am J Sports Med 22:702–710, 1994.
43a. Cross MJ, Vandersluis R, Wood D, Banff M: Surgical repair of chronic complete hamstring tendon rupture in the adult patient. Am J Sports Med 26:785–788, 1998.
44. Daffner RH, Martinez S, Gehweiler JA: Stress fractures in runners. JAMA 247:1039–1041, 1982.
45. DeSmet AA: Magnetic resonance findings in skeletal muscle tears. Skeletal Radiol 22:479–484, 1993.
46. Devas MD: Stress fractures of the femoral neck. J Bone Joint Surg Br 47:728–738, 1965.
47. Devas MD: Stress Fractures. New York, Churchill Livingstone, 1975, pp 1, 2, 19–27, 113–116.
48. Donald JG, Fitts WT: March fractures: A study with special reference to etiological factors. J Bone Joint Surg 29:297–300, 1947.
49. Dornan P: A report on 140 hamstring injuries. Aust J Sports Med 4:30–36, 1971.
50. Dow S: Reno Orthopaedic Group—Bone densities in elderly runners. Paper presented at the Annual American Medical Jogger's Association Meeting, Dec 9, 1978, Honolulu, Hawaii.
51. Drane WE: Myositis ossificans and the three-phase bone scan. AJR Am J Roentgenol 142:179–180, 1984.
52. Ehman RL, Berquist TH: Magnetic resonance imaging of musculoskeletal trauma. Radiol Clin North Am 24:291–319, 1986.
53. El-Khoury GY, Brandser EA, Kathol MH, et al: Imaging of muscle injuries. Skeletal Radiol 25:3–11, 1996.
54. Elliott BC, Blanksby BA: The synchronization of muscle activity and body segment movements during a running cycle. Med Sci Sports Exerc 11:322–327, 1979.
55. Fitch KD: Stress fractures of the lower limbs in runners. Aust Fam Physician 13:511–515, 1984.
56. Fuller PJ: Musculotendinous leg injuries. Aust Fam Physician 13:495–498, 1984.

57. Garrett WE: Muscle strain injuries. Am J Sports Med 24:S2–S8, 1996.

58. Garrett WE: Strains and sprains in athletes. Postgrad Med 73: 200–214, 1983.

59. Garrett WE, Califf JC, Bassett FH: Histochemical correlates of hamstring injuries. Am J Sports Med 12:98–103, 1984.

60. Garrett WE, Lohnes J: Cellular and matrix response to mechanical injury at the myotendinous function. In Leadbetter WB, Buckwalter JA, Gordon SL: Sports-Induced Inflammation. Park Ridge, Ill, American Orthopaedic Society for Sports Medicine Symposium, 1989, pp 215–224.

61. Garrett WE, Mumma M, Lucaveche CL: Ultrastructural differences in human muscle fiber types. Orthop Clin North Am 14:413–425, 1983.

62. Garrett WE, Nikolaou PK, Ribbeck BM, et al: The effect of muscle architecture on the biomechanical failure properties of skeletal muscle under passive extension. Am J Sports Med 16:7–12, 1988.

63. Garrett WE, Rich FR, Nikolaou PK, Vogler JB: Computed tomography of hamstrings muscle strains. J Med Sci Sports Exerc 21: 508–514, 1989.

64. Garrett WE, Safran MR, Seaber AV, et al: Biomechanical comparison of stimulated and nonstimulated skeletal muscle pulled to failure. Am J Sports Med 15:448–454, 1987.

65. Gibbens MW: March fractures of the neck of the femur. J Bone Joint Surg 27:162–163, 1945.

66. Giladi M, Milgrom C, Stein M, et al: External rotation of the hip: A predictor of risk for stress fractures. Clin Orthop 216:131–134, 1987.

67. Glick JM: Muscle strains: Prevention and treatment. Physician Sportsmed 8:73–77, 1980.

68. Grace JN, Sim FH, Shives TC, Coventry MB: Wedge resection of the symphysis pubis for the treatment of osteitis pubis. J Bone Joint Surg Am 71:358–364, 1989.

69. Grant JCB: Grant's Atlas of Anatomy, 5th ed. Baltimore, Williams & Wilkins, 1962, p 268.

70. Greaney RB, Gerber FH, Laughlin RL, et al: Distribution and natural history of stress fractures in US Marine recruits. Radiology 146: 339–346, 1983.

71. Green HJ, Daub B, Houston ME, et al: Human vastus lateralis and gastrocnemius muscle: A comparative histochemical and biochemical analysis. J Neurol Sci 52:201–210, 1981.

72. Gross RH: Acute musculotendinous injuries. In Delee JC, Drez D Jr (eds): Orthopaedic Sports Medicine: Principles and Practice. Philadelphia, WB Saunders, 1994, pp 131–143.

73. Hallel T, Amit S, Sega D: Fatigue fractures of tibial and femoral shaft in soldiers. Clin Orthop 118:35–43, 1976.

74. Harvey G, Bell S: Obturator neuropathy; an anatomic perspective. Clin Orthop 363:203–211, 1999.

75. Hasselman CT, Best TM, Hughes GC, et al: An explanation for various rectus femoris strain injuries using previously undescribed muscle architecture. Am J Sports Med 23:493–499, 1995.

76. Heckman MM, Whitesides TE Jr, Grewe SR, et al: Histologic determination of the ischemic threshold of muscle in the canine compartment syndrome model. J Orthop Trauma 7:199–210, 1993.

77. Heiser TM, Weber J, Sullivan G, et al: Prophylaxis and management of hamstring muscle injuries in intercollegiate football players. Am J Sports Med 12:368–370, 1984.

78. Henry JH: The hip, part 2. Recognition and treatment of injuries. In Scott WN, Nisonson B, Nicholas JA (eds): Principles of Sports Medicine. Baltimore, Williams & Wilkins, 1984, p 248.

79. Hershman EB, Lombardo J, Bergfeld JA: Femoral shaft stress fracture in athletes. Clin Sports Med 9:11–119, 1990.

80. Hershman EB, Mailly T: Stress fractures. Clin Sports Med 9:183–214, 1990.

81. Hill AV: The series elastic component of muscle. Proc R Soc Lond (Biol) 137:273–280, 1950.

82. Holbrook TL, Grazier K, Kelsey JL, et al: The frequency of occurrence, impact and cost of musculoskeletal conditions in the United States. Park Ridge, Ill, American Academy of Orthopaedic Surgeons, 1984.

83. Hughes C, Hasselman CT, Best RM, et al: Incomplete, intrasubstance strain injuries of the rectus femoris muscle. Am J Sports Med 23:500–506, 1995.

84. Hughston JC: Personal communication, 1978.

85. Hyman AA, Heiser WJ, Kim SE, et al: An excavation of the distal femoral metaphysis: A magnetic resonance imaging study: A case report. J Bone Joint Surg Am 77:1897, 1995.

86. Ivy JL, Withers RT, Brose G, et al: Isokinetic contractile properties of the quadriceps with relation to fiber type. Eur J Appl Physiol 47: 247–255, 1981.

87. Jackson DW, Feagin JA: Quadriceps contusions in young athletes: Relation of severity of injury to treatment and prognosis. J Bone Joint Surg Am 55:95–105, 1973.

88. Jeffrey CC: Spontaneous fractures of the femoral neck. J Bone Joint Surg Br 44:543–549, 1982.

89. Johnson A, Polgar J, Weightman PD, Appleton D: Data on the distribution of fiber types in thirty-six human muscles. J Neurol Sci 18:111–129, 1973.

90. Johnson AW, Weiss CB, Wheeler DL: Stress fractures of the femoral shaft in athletes: More common than expected. Am J Sports Med 22:248–256, 1994.

91. Jones BH, Harris J, Vinhn TN, et al: Exercise-induced stress fractures and reactions of bone: Epidemiology, etiology and classification. Exerc Sport Sci Rev 17:379,472, 1989.

92. Jonhagen S, Nemeth G, Ericsson E: Hamstring injuries in sprinters—The role of concentric and eccentric hamstring muscle strength and flexibility. Am J Sports Med 22:262–266, 1994.

93. Kahan JSG, McClennan SRT, Burton DS: Acute bilateral compartment syndrome of the thigh induced by exercise. J Bone Joint Surg Am 76:1068–1071, 1994.

94. Katz B: The relation between force and speed in muscular contraction. J Physiol 96:45–64, 1939.

95. Kellett J: Acute soft-tissue injuries: A review of the literature. Med Sci Sport Exerc 18:489–500, 1986.

96. Kime RC, Seaber AV, Garrett WE Jr: The effect of position and time of immobilization on the active and passive biomechanical properties of muscle. Paper presented at the 36th Annual Meeting of the Orthopaedic Research Society, February 5–8, 1990, New Orleans.

97. Kirkpatrick JS, Koman LA, Rovere GD: The role of ultrasound in the early diagnosis of myositis ossificans: A case report. Am J Sports Med 15:179–181, 1987.

98. Klafs CE, Arnheim DD: Modern Principles of Athletic Training, 4th ed. St. Louis, CV Mosby, 1977, pp 370–372.

99. Klasson SC, Vander Schilden JL: Acute anterior compartment syndrome of the thigh complicating quadriceps haematoma. Two case reports and review of the literature. Orthop Rev 19:421–427, 1990.

100. Komi PV, Burskirk ER: Effect of eccentric and concentric muscle conditioning on tension and electric activity of human muscle. Ergonomics 15:417–434, 1972.

101. Kransdorf MJ, Meis JM, Jelinek JS: Myositis ossificans: MR appearance with radiologic-pathologic correlation. AJR Am J Roentgenol 157:1243–1248, 1991.

102. Kraus JF: Annual Review of Public Health, 5th ed. Palo Alto, Calif, Annual Review, 1984, p 166.

103. Krejci V, Koch P: Muscle and tendon injuries in athletes. Chicago, Year Book, 1979.

104. Kuivilla TE, Brems JJ: Diagnosis of acute rupture of the quadriceps tendon by magnetic resonance imaging. A case report. Clin Orthop 262:236–241, 1991.

105. Kujala UM, Orava S, Jarvinen M: Hamstring injuries; current trends in treatment and prevention. Sports Med 23:397–404, 1997.

106. Kulund DN: The Injured Athlete. Philadelphia, JB Lippincott, 1982, pp 72, 85, 356–359.

107. Kvist M, Jarvinen M: Clinical, histochemical and biomechanical features in repair of muscle and tendon injuries. Int J Sports Med 3:12–14, 1982.

108. Lee BY, LaPointe DG, Madden JL: The adductor canal syndrome: Description of a case with quantification of arterial pulsatile blood flow. Am J Surg 123:617–620, 1972.

108a. Levine WN, Bergfeld JA, Tessendorf W, Moorman CT: Intramuscular corticosteroid injection for hamstring injuries. Am J Sports Med 28:297–300, 2000.

109. Li R, Zhang S, Chen G, et al: Radiographic and histologic analysis of stress fracture in rabbit tibias. Am J Sports Med 13:285–294, 1985.

110. Liemohn W: Factors related to hamstring strains. J Sports Med 18: 71–76, 1978.

111. Linnell S, Stager J, Blue P, et al: Bone mineral content and menstrual regularity in female runners. Med Sci Sports Exerc 16:343–348, 1984.

112. Lipscomb AB, Thomas ED, Johnston RK: Treatment of myositis ossificans traumatica in athletes. Am J Sports Med 4:111–120, 1976.

113. Lombardo SJ, Benson DW: Stress fractures of the femur in runners. Am J Sports Med 10:219–227, 1982.

114. Lynch SA, Renstrom PA: Groin injuries in sport. Sports Med 28:137–144, 1999.

115. Mair SD, Seaber AV, Glisson RR, Garrett WE Jr: The role of fatigue in susceptibility to acute muscle strain injury. Am J Sports Med 24:137–143, 1996.

116. Markhede G, Nistor L: Strength of plantar flexion and function after resection of various parts of the triceps surae muscle. Acta Orthop Scand 50:693–697, 1979.

117. Martens MA, Hansen L, Mulier JC: Adductor tendinitis and musculus rectus abdominis tendopathy. Am J Sports Med 15:353–356, 1987.

118. Masters S, Fricker P, Purdam C: Stress fractures of the femoral shaft—Four case studies. Br J Sports Med 20:14–16, 1986.

119. Matava MJ, Whitesides TE Jr, Seiler JG III, et al: Determination of the compartment pressure threshold of muscle ischemia in a canine model. J Trauma 37:50–58, 1994.

120. Matsen RA, Wyss CR, Frugmire RB, et al: The effects of limb elevation and dependency on local arteriovenous gradients in normal human limbs with particular reference to limbs with increased tissue pressure. Clin Orthop 150:187–195, 1980.

121. Matsumoto K, Hukuda S, Ishizawa M, Kawasaki T, et al: Partial rupture of the quadriceps tendon (jumper's knee) in a ten-year-old boy. Case report. Am J Sports Med 27:521–525, 1999.

122. Maydl K: Uber subcutane Muskel und Sehnenzerreissungen, sowie Rissfracturen, mit Berucksichtigung der Analogen, durch directe Gewalt enstandenen und offenen Verletzungen. Deutsche Ztschr Chir 17:306–361, 1882; 18:35–139, 1883.

123. McBryde AM: Stress fractures in athletes. J Sports Med 3:2–217, 1975.

124. McMahon JS, Waddell JP, Morton J: Effect of short-course indomethacin on heterotopic bone formation after uncemented total hip arthroplasty. J Arthroplasty 6:259–264, 1991.

125. McMaster PE: Tendon and muscle ruptures. J Bone Joint Surg 15:705–722, 1933.

126. McMaster WC, Walter M: Injuries in soccer. Am J Sports Med 6:354–357, 1978.

127. Merrifield HH, Cowan RFJ: Groin strain injuries in ice hockey. J Sports Med 1:41–42, 1973.

128. Meyers WC, Foley DP, Garrett WE Jr, et al: Management of severe lower abdominal or inguinal pain in high-performance athletes. Am J Sports Med 28:2–8, 2000.

129. Millar AP, Salmon J: Muscle tears. Aust J Sports Med 2:435–438, 1967.

130. Miller WA: Rupture of the musculotendinous juncture of the medial head of the gastrocnemius muscle. Am J Sports Med 5:191–193, 1977.

131. Monteleone GP: Stress fractures in the athlete. Orthop Clin North Am 26:423–433, 1995.

132. Morris J, Blickenstaff L: General considerations and diagnosis and treatment. In Morris J, Blickenstaff L: Fatigue Fractures, A Clinical Study. Springfield, Ill, Charles C Thomas, 1967, p 12.

133. Mubarak SJ, Carroll NC: Volkmann's contracture in children: Etiology and prevention. J Bone Joint Surg Br 61:285–293, 1979.

134. Mubarak SJ, Hargens AR: Compartment Syndromes and Volkmann's Contracture. Philadelphia, WB Saunders, 1981.

135. Naidu SH, Heppenstall RB: Compartment syndrome of the forearm and hand. Hand Clinics 10:13–27, 1994.

136. Nattiv A, Armsey TD Jr: Stress injury to bone in the female athlete. Clin Sports Med 16:197–224, 1997.

137. Nikolaou PK, MacDonald BL, Glisson RR, et al: The effect of architecture on the anatomical failure site of skeletal muscle. Trans Orthop Res Soc 11:228, 1986.

138. Nikolaou PK, MacDonald BL, Glisson RR, et al: Biomechanical and histological evaluation of muscle after controlled strain injury. Am J Sports Med 15:9–14, 1987.

139. Nikolaou PK, Ribbeck BM, Glisson RR, et al: The effect of muscle architecture on the biomechanical failure properties of skeletal muscle under passive extension. Am J Sports Med 16:7–12, 1988.

140. Noonan TJ, Garrett WE Jr: Muscle strain injury: Diagnosis and treatment. J Am Acad Orthop Surg 7:262–269, 1999.

141. Norfray JF, Schlachter L, Kernahan WT, et al: Early confirmation of stress fractures in joggers. JAMA 243:1647–1649, 1980.

142. Norman A, Dorfman HD: Juxtacortical circumscribed myositis os-

143. Obremsky WT, Seaber AV, Ribbeck BM, Garrett WE Jr: Biomechanical and histologic assessment of a controlled muscle strain injury treated with piroxicam. Am J Sports Med 22:558–561, 1994.

144. O'Donoghue DH: Treatment of Injuries to Athletes, 4th ed. Philadelphia, WB Saunders, 1984.

145. Oh I, Harris WH: Proximal strain distribution in the loaded femur. J Bone Joint Surg Am 60:75–85, 1978.

146. O'Neil DB, Micheli LJ: Overuse injuries in the young athlete. Clin Sports Med 7:591–610, 1988.

147. Orava S, Kufala RM: Rupture of the ischial origin of the hamstring muscles. Am J Sports Med 23:702–705, 1995.

148. Orchard J, Marsden J, Lord S, Garlick D: Preseason hamstring muscle weakness associated with hamstring muscle injury in Australian footballers. Am J Sports Med 25:81–85, 1997.

149. Palmer WE, Kuong SJ, Elmadbouh HM: MR imaging of myotendinous strain. AJR Am J Roentgenol 173:703–709, 1999.

150. Parker MG: Characteristics of skeletal muscle during rehabilitation: Quadriceps femoris. J Athlet Train 18:122–124, 1981.

151. Peterson L, Renstrom P: Sports Injuries: Their Prevention and Treatment. Chicago, Year Book, 1986, pp 32–34, 281, 283.

152. Petit HL, quoted by Loos: Uber subkutane Biceps Rupturen. Beitr Klin Chir 29:410–449, 1901.

153. Pipes TV, Wilmore JH: Isokinetic vs isotonic strength training in adult men. Med Sci Sports 7:262–274, 1975.

154. Protzman RR, Griffis CG: Stress fractures in men and women undergoing military training. J Bone Joint Surg Am 59:825, 1977.

155. Provost RA, Morris JM: Fatigue fracture of the femoral shaft. J Bone Joint Surg Am 51:487–498, 1969.

156. Rankin JM, Thompson CB: Isokinetic evaluation of quadriceps and hamstring function: Normative data concerning body weight and sport. J Athlet Train 18:110–113, 1983.

157. Reneman RS: The anterior and lateral compartment syndrome of the leg due to intensive use of muscles. Clin Orthop 113:69–80, 1975.

158. Renstrom PA, Peterson L: Groin injuries in athletes. Br J Sports Med 14:30–36, 1980.

159. Romanoff ME, Cory PC, Kalenak A, et al: Saphenous nerve entrapment at the adductor canal. Am J Sports Med 17:478–481, 1989.

160. Rooser B: Quadriceps contusion with compartment syndrome: Evacuation of hematoma in 2 cases. Acta Orthop Scand 58:170–172, 1987.

161. Rooser B, Bengtson S, Hagglund G: Acute compartment syndrome from anterior thigh muscle contusion: A report of eight cases. J Orthop Trauma 5:57–59, 1991.

162. Rosen PR, Micheli LJ, Treves S: Early scintigraphic diagnosis of bone stress and fractures in athletic adolescents. Pediatrics 70:11–15, 1982.

163. Rothwell AG: Quadriceps hematoma: A prospective clinical study. Clin Orthop 171:97–103, 1982.

164. Roy S, Irvin R: Sports Medicine: Prevention, Evaluation, Management and Rehabilitation. Englewood Cliffs, NJ, Prentice-Hall, 1983, pp 303–304.

165. Rubin SJ, Feldman F, Staron RB, et al: Magnetic resonance imaging of muscle injury. Clin Imaging 19:263–269, 1995.

166. Rupani HD, Holder LE, Espinola DA, Engin SI: Three-phase radionuclide bone imaging in sports medicine. Radiology 156:187–196, 1985.

167. Ryan AJ: Quadriceps strain, rupture and charley horse. Med Sci Sports 1:106–111, 1969.

168. Ryan JB, Wheller JH, Hopkinson WJ, et al: Quadriceps contusions. West Point update. Am J Sports Med 19:299–304, 1991.

169. Safran MR, Garrett WE, Seaber AV, et al: The role of warm-up in muscular injury prevention. Am J Sports Med 16:123–129, 1988.

170. Sallay PI, Friedman RL, Coogan PG, Garrett WE: Hamstring muscle injuries among water skiers: Functional outcome and prevention. Am J Sports Med 2:167–182, 1983.

171. Savoca C: Stress fractures: A classification of the earliest radiographic signs. Radiology 100:519–524, 1971.

172. Sherman WM, Plyley MJ, Vogelgesand D, et al: Isokinetic strength during rehabilitation following arthrotomy: Specificity of speed. J Athlet Train 18:138–141, 1981.

173. Skinner HB, Cook SD: Fatigue failure stress of the femoral neck: A case report. Am J Sports Med 10:245–247, 1982.

174. Slocum DB, James SL: Biomechanics of running. JAMA 205:721–728, 1968.

sificans: Evolution and radiographic features. Radiology 96:301–306, 1970.

175. Stafford MG, Grana WA: Hamstring/quadriceps ratios in college football players: A high velocity evaluation. Am J Sports Med 12:209–211, 1984.
176. Stechow AW: Fussoedem und Rotgenstrahlen. Deutsch Mil Aerzte Zeitg 26:465, 1897.
177. Sterling JC, Edelstein DW, Calvo RD, et al: Stress fractures in the athlete: Diagnosis and management. J Sports Med 14:336–346, 1992.
178. Sutton G: Hamstring by hamstring strains: A review of the literature. J Orthop Sports Phys Ther 5:184–195, 1984.
179. Szabo RM, Gelberman RH: Peripheral nerve compression—etiology, critical pressure threshold and clinical assessment. Orthopaedics 7:1461–1466, 1984.
180. Taylor DC, Dalton JD, Seaber AV, Garrett WE: Experimental muscle strain injury: Early functional and structural deficits and the increased risk for reinjury. Am J Sports Med 21:190–194, 1993.
181. Taylor DC, Meyers WC, Moylan JA, et al: Groin pain in athletes due to abdominal musculature abnormalities. Paper presented to the American Orthopaedic Society for Sports Medicine, June 19–22, 1989, Traverse City, Mich.
182. Taylor DC, Meyers C, Moylan JA, et al: Abdominal musculature abnormalities as a cause of groin pain in athletes. Am J Sports Med 13:239–242, 1991.
183. Tehranzadeh J, Durth LA, Elyaderani MK, Bowers D: Combined pelvic stress fracture and avulsion of the adductor longus in a middle-distance runner: A case report. Am J Sports Med 10:108–111, 1982.
184. Temple HT, Kuklo TR, Sweet DE, et al: Rectus femoris muscle tear appearing as a pseudotumor. Am J Sports Med 26:544–548, 1998.
185. Terrell PN, Davies AM: Magnetic resonance appearances of fatigue fractures of the long bones of the lower limb. Br J Radiol 67:332–338, 1994.
186. Tesch P, Karlsson J: Isometric strength performance and muscle fiber type distribution in man. Acta Physiol Scand 103:47–51, 1978.
187. Thorstensson A, Karlsson J: Fatigability and fiber composition of human skeletal muscle. Acta Physiol Scand 98:312–322, 1976.
188. Tihanyi J, Apor P, Fekete G: Force-velocity-power characteristics and fiber composition in human knee extensor muscles. Eur J Appl Physiol 48:331–343, 1982.
189. Torg JS, Pavlov H, Morris VB: Salter-Harris type III fracture of the medial femoral condyle occurring in the adolescent athlete. J Bone Joint Surg Am 63:586–591, 1981.
190. Tozun R, Pinar H, Yesiller E, Hamzaoglu A: Indomethacin for prevention of heterotopic ossification after total hip arthroplasty. J Arthroplasty 7:57–61, 1992.
191. Tredget T, Godberson CV, Bose B: Myositis ossificans due to hockey injury. Can Med Assoc J 116:65–66, 1977.
192. Turl SE, George KP: Adverse neural tension: A factor in repetitive hamstring strain. Orthop Sports Phys Ther 27:16–21, 1998.
193. Vane JR: Inhibition of prostaglandin synthesis as a mechanism of action for aspirin-like drugs. Nature New Biol 231:232–235, 1971.
194. Verta MJ, Vitello J, Fuller J: Adductor canal compression syndrome. Arch Surg 119:345–346, 1984.
195. Walter NE, Wolf MD: Stress fractures in young athletes. Am J Sports Med 5:165–169, 1977.
196. Walton M, Rothwell AG: Reactions of thigh tissues of sheep to blunt trauma. Clin Orthop 176:273–281, 1983.
197. Wang SY, Lomasney LM, Demos TC, Drane WE: Myositis ossificans and three-phase bone scan. AJR Am J Roentgenol 142:179–180, 1984.
198. Warren GL, Hayes DA, Lowe DA, et al: Materials fatigue initiates eccentric contraction-induced injury in rat soleus muscle. J Physiol 464:477–489, 1993.
199. Waugh RL, Hathcock TA, Elliott JL: Ruptures of muscles and tendons: With particular reference to rupture of biceps brachii with report of 50 cases. Surgery 25:370–392, 1949.
200. Weber PC: Salter-Harris type II stress fracture in a young athlete: A case report. Orthopaedics 11:309–311, 1988.
201. Weinstein RN, Kraushaar BS, Fulkerson JP: Adductor tendinosis in a professional hockey player. Orthopaedics 21:809–810, 1998.
202. Whitesides TE, Haney TC, Morimoto K, Harada H: Tissue pressure measurements as a determinant for the need of fasciotomy. Clin Orthop 113:43–51, 1975.
203. Whitesides TE, Heckman MM: Acute compartment syndrome: Update on diagnosis and treatment. J Am Acad Orthop Surg 4:209–218, 1996.
204. Wiley JJ: Traumatic osteitis pubis: The gracilis syndrome. Am J Sports Med 11:360–363, 1983.
205. Wilcox JR, Moniot AL, Green JP: Bone scanning in the evaluation of exercise-related stress injuries. Nucl Med 123:699–703, 1977.
206. Williams PL, Warwick R: Gray's Anatomy, 36th ed. Edinburgh, Churchill Livingstone, 1980, pp 1053–1054.
207. Wilson E: Stress fractures. Radiology 92:481–486, 1969.
208. Yamamoto T: Relationship between hamstring strains and leg muscle strength: A follow-up study of collegiate track and field athletes. J Sports Med Phys Fitness 33:194–199, 1993.
209. Zaccalini PS, Urist MR: Traumatic periosteal proliferations in rabbits: The enigma of experimental myositis ossificans traumatica. J Trauma 4:344–357, 1964.
210. Zarins B, Ciullo JV: Acute muscle and tendon injuries in athletes. Clin Sports Med 2:167–182, 1983.
211. Zeiss J, Saddemi SR, Ebraheim NA: MR imaging of the quadriceps tendon: Normal layered configuration and its importance in cases of tendon rupture. AJR Am J Roentgenol 159:1031–1034, 1992.

Section B
Pediatric Thigh

Treg D. Brown, MD ■ Michael E. Brunet, MD

Athletes younger than the age of 18 years represent the largest number of sports participants in the United States.[96] Furthermore, athletic participation among these young athletes continues to increase at an astonishing rate. It is estimated at present that more than 30 million children in the United States participate in some form of sports-related activity. In addition, an estimated 16 million of these athletes compete in some type of formal athletic competition.

Unfortunately, as children have become more active in sports, the incidence of injuries in this age group has increased correspondingly. Injuries that were once seen solely in adults are now common among young athletes. Many of the sports that children participate in are the same as those enjoyed by adults (e.g., soccer, baseball, basketball, football). This results in considerable similarity in the various mechanisms of injury seen in these two different athletic populations; however, open growth plates and muscle-tendon units that are unable to keep pace with a rapidly growing skeletal system make these athletes susceptible to a host of injuries not encountered in adults. Strength imbalances and immature bone also play a large role in the often unique presentation of injuries in this young age group.

This chapter discusses diagnosis and management of thigh injuries in the skeletally immature athlete. The recognition that skeletally immature athletes are not simply "small adults" is imperative for the proper treatment of injuries in this active age group. An understanding of the musculoskeletal and physiologic development occurring in the child and the adolescent is also crucial to developing an accurate differential diagnosis and treatment algorithm for these injuries.

Femoral Stress Fractures

Stress fractures of the femur are most commonly seen in athletes participating in activities requiring cyclic loading of the lower extremity. This condition may best be defined as an exaggerated bone remodeling process occurring in response to repeated submaximal loads placed on the bone at that particular site. Ultimately, the resorption rate outpaces the bone's remodeling capacity, and a stress fracture results.

As children and adolescents mature, numerous changes take place anatomically, physiologically, and psychologically. These changes must be considered when evaluating a child suspected of having a stress fracture. The pathophysiology of stress fractures in children and adolescents closely parallels that seen in their adult counterparts, but differences do exist. It appears that the response of the growing skeleton to repetitive stress and training is different from that seen in the fully mature skeleton, with the bone of older individuals being less resistant to fatigue.[100] In addition, children and young adolescents are able to mount a markedly increased osteogenic response to stress and injury relative to their adult counterparts.

Stress fractures are infrequent in children, and femoral shaft stress fractures are rarer still.[31, 93] Hulkko and Orava reviewed 368 stress fractures and found that only 9% occurred in children younger than 15 years of age, 32% occurred in adolescents 16 to 19 years old, and 59% occurred in adults 20 years of age or older.[67] Another study identified 34 stress fractures in 32 skeletally immature patients and found that the femur was involved in only 12%.[153] These findings were further supported in a review of 200 stress fractures occurring in all ages, with 36.5% occurring in the 16- to 19-year-old age group and only 6% in youths 15 years of age or younger.[116] Just as the prevalence of stress fractures in children differs, so do the pattern of injury and the sites most commonly affected.[100] In a review of the literature, Yngve found 23 studies reporting 131 stress fractures in children younger than the age of 14 years and found a difference in the distribution of stress fractures between adults and young athletes.[166] The tibia was found to be involved in 51% of the fractures, the fibula in 20%, and the femur in only 3%. This underscores the relative rarity of femoral stress fractures in the young athlete and should prompt the physician to rule out other possible causes.[93, 153]

The anatomy of the femur lends itself to certain predictable areas of increased force concentration. The shaft of the femur is a long, tubular bone with a predominantly thick cortical rim and an anterolateral bow in the proximal and middle thirds. These two anatomic entities help accommodate stress placed on the femur with standing, walking, and running as well as with all athletic endeavors. The

cortex is in turn covered with a thick periosteal covering. The bowed configuration of the femoral shaft leads to compressive forces across the medial side while the lateral side is under tension during weight-bearing. These forces are most concentrated at the medial aspect of the proximal diaphyseal-metaphyseal junction, making this area particularly susceptible to stress fractures (see Fig. 26A–1).[20] Femoral stress fractures may occur at any site throughout the entire femur, however, including the distal epiphysis (see Fig. 26A–2).[149, 158] If left untreated, they may ultimately progress to complete fracture, resulting in displacement and significant morbidity.[93]

There are several risk factors associated with the development of a stress fracture, including training errors, muscle-tendon imbalance, anatomic malalignment, improper footwear or playing surface, associated disease states, gender and genetic factors, cultural deconditioning, and growth.[6, 44, 115] It has been our experience that a stress fracture can usually be attributed to the presence of two or more of these risk factors. Training errors are the most frequently encountered cause; athletes participating in endurance events, such as runners, are most commonly affected.[100] These errors are most often made in relation to the volume, the intensity, and the progression of the athlete's training. There is little written in the literature pertaining to training progression guidelines for the young athlete. Micheli has empirically found that increasing a young athlete's training level no more than 10% per week poses little risk for development of a stress fracture.[100]

Perhaps the second most commonly encountered risk factor involves the muscle-tendon imbalances that develop in the growing child. Growth is often accompanied by changes in the relative strength and flexibility of agonist or antagonist muscle groups. The subsequent muscle imbalances associated with these changes in strength and flexibility may theoretically lead to asymmetrical stresses on the bones and the joints and may thereby promote the development of stress fractures.[90, 100] This may explain the development of stress fractures in young athletes participating in relatively low-impact activities such as in-line skating.[86, 148]

The incidence of stress fractures in female military recruits has been shown to be consistently greater than in men, suggesting an increased risk of stress fractures among women. There appears to be only a slightly higher risk in civilian women who are athletes compared with men, however.[16, 38] Unfortunately, there are no studies comparing skeletally immature female athletes with their male counterparts. Anatomic malalignment should always be checked for in evaluating a young athlete suspected of having a stress fracture. Leg-length discrepancies, rotational malalignments of the hip, excessive genu varum and genu valgum, and overpronation or cavus foot deformities have all been implicated as potential causative factors in the development of stress fractures and should be considered. Athletes should be asked to bring along their training footwear for inspection. The shoes should be studied for the amount of impact absorption ability remaining, signs of uneven wear, and proper fit. Training on relatively hard playing surfaces causes greater axial loads to be transmitted up the lower extremity and increases the risk of stress fracture. Any preexisting or concomitant illness that could potentially affect the structural integrity of the musculo-skeletal system should also be assessed.

Since 1990, the medical community has become increasingly aware of the prevalence of eating disorders in young athletes and in young females in particular.[109] Among women athletes, there has been found an interrelatedness of disordered eating, amenorrhea, and osteoporosis. This relationship has been referred to as the "female atheIete triad."[11, 24, 109] Athletes deemed at risk of having an eating disorder include those participating in individual sports, sports in which low body weight is perceived as being advantageous (distance running), events in which emphasis is placed on aesthetics (ballet), and sports with weight classes (wrestling). Athletes suspected of having a potential eating disorder, or any at-risk athletes with a stress fracture (particularly those with multiple or recurrent stress fractures), warrant further evaluation.

A rarely mentioned risk factor that has become increasingly common is the "win at all costs" and "play through the pain" mentality among young athletes, coaches, and parents. This promotes the development of numerous overuse injuries, including stress fractures. In addition, the number of children, particularly girls, participating in organized athletics continues to increase, as has the number of year-round sporting leagues. This allows increasing numbers of children to play the same sport virtually year-round with little rest, further promoting the development of stress fractures in this young population.

Children and adolescents with a stress fracture of the femur typically complain of activity-related pain that is initially relieved with rest.[153] The pain usually progresses as the child attempts to continue to play. Ultimately, the pain continues despite the cessation of activities, with rest pain and occasional night pain developing. An antalgic gait and a positive fulcrum test result (Fig. 26B–1) may be noted on examination.[28, 70] The remainder of the examina-

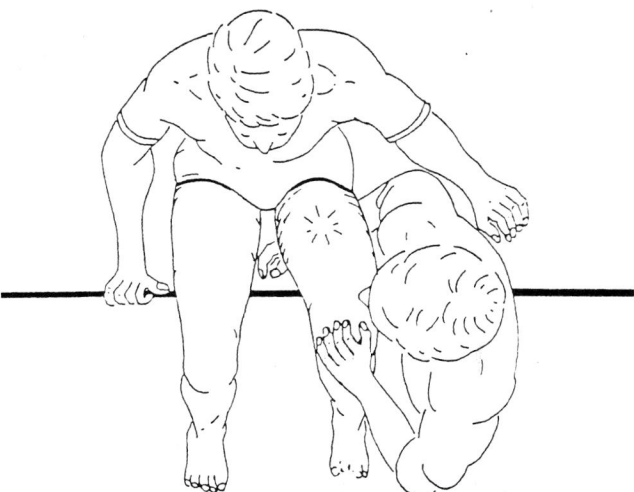

Figure 26B–1. The fulcrum test to evaluate for femoral shaft stress fractures. The examiner's arm (fulcrum) is placed under the distal thigh. Pain produced by applying gentle pressure to the knee is a positive test. (From Johnson AW, Weiss CB, Wheeler DL: Stress fractures of the femoral shaft in athletes—more common than expected. Am J Sports Med 22:248–256, 1994.)

tion may be fairly benign because the femur is surrounded by the muscular quadriceps, adductors, and hamstrings, which often hide any tenderness or swelling that would otherwise be noted. Pain with forced rotation or axial loading are likewise infrequent findings.

Skeletally immature athletes with stress fractures commonly have clinical and radiographic presentations that differ slightly from those seen in adults.[34, 43, 100] This is largely a result of the thick periosteum and the abundant healing response present in this patient population. This abundant healing response should prompt the physician to include infection and tumor in the differential diagnosis of any young athlete suspected of having a femoral stress fracture.[93] There are several tumors commonly mistaken for stress fractures, including eosinophilic granuloma, osteoid osteoma, osteogenic sarcoma, and Ewing's sarcoma.[26, 31, 80, 93] There are several features characteristic of stress fractures that may facilitate their diagnosis; one such feature is an uninterrupted periosteal reaction localized to the cortical surface traversed by the stress fracture. This typically occurs in the absence of frank cortical destruction on plain radiographs. These findings are strongly suggestive of a stress fracture when seen in conjunction with a sharply marginated area of increased uptake on bone scanning and the absence of any soft tissue mass on computed tomography (CT) or magnetic resonance imaging (MRI).[93] Biopsies should be avoided if possible because the surgical defect may delay healing or may precipitate a complete fracture. Furthermore, healing stress fractures and osteosarcomas have similar histologic appearances that can be extremely difficult to distinguish,[26, 93] further supporting the importance of a thorough history and physical examination.[153] A slipped capital femoral epiphysis should also be in the differential diagnosis for any adolescent with nonspecific thigh or knee pain.[121]

Radiography continues to be the initial study recommended for the evaluation of children suspected of having a stress fracture. There is, however, some debate regarding the ability of routine radiography to detect a stress fracture. Estimates of the number of initial radiographs with negative findings for stress fractures have ranged from 10% to 67%.[26, 53, 137] The number of false-negative results, however, appears to be considerably less when athletes 18 years of age or older are excluded.[88, 153] Although the pathophysiology of stress fractures varies little between the adolescent and the adult, the skeletally immature athlete does exhibit a more exuberant healing process, with considerably more periosteal reaction and callus formation than an adult. This abundant healing response results in earlier, more detectable radiographic changes than are seen in their adult counterparts. Nonetheless, these changes may not occur until 1 to 3 weeks after the onset of symptoms, therefore warranting repeat studies if the initial radiographs have negative findings. The physician should look closely for evidence of periosteal reaction, fracture lines, and cortical hypertrophy. Several authors recommend serial radiographs at short intervals if any question exists regarding the diagnosis of a stress fracture; however, this can prolong the anxiety of both the parents and the child who are waiting for a diagnosis and may result in several weeks of unnecessary activity restriction. These concerns have prompted many physicians to proceed to the next level of diagnostic imaging: bone scanning, MRI, and CT. These studies can often provide an immediate confirmation of the diagnosis. Unfortunately, they are more invasive and more costly, which prohibit them from being considered first-line imaging modalities.

The bone scan continues to be considered the gold standard for diagnosing stress fractures.[104] The sensitivity is virtually 100% in athletes, and bone changes can often be detected within 24 to 72 hours of the onset of symptoms. The use of triple-phase technetium diphosphonate scanning has further increased the relative specificity of these scans. In addition, total body bone scans can be helpful in evaluating the entire skeleton for other sites of increased stress, which are commonly present in athletes.[62, 148] Fortunately, the rapid healing response exhibited in the pediatric population often makes bone scan confirmation of stress fractures unnecessary.[153]

Magnetic resonance imaging is an excellent tool for diagnosing stress fractures in young athletes with negative radiographic findings. MRI offers greater overall specificity and sensitivity than bone scintigraphy and radiography. In addition, MRI will often demonstrate abnormalities within 24 hours of the onset of symptoms and is not significantly affected by age or coexisting musculoskeletal abnormalities. MRI is quite useful for visualizing marrow hemorrhage and edema, a characteristically difficult finding to discern on CT. Furthermore, MRI is superior to CT in distinguishing a stress fracture from a suspected bone tumor or an infectious process.[104, 144] Overall, MRI is an excellent imaging modality for the evaluation of suspected stress fractures in young athletes, although financial considerations have prevented MRI from being considered a routine primary imaging modality.

Once the diagnosis of a femoral shaft stress fracture in a child or an adolescent has been established, the treatment varies little from that for adults (Table 26B–1).

The late phase of treatment begins once signs of healing have been demonstrated radiographically and the intermediate phase of treatment is able to be performed without pain. Light running should initially take place on turf, grass, or a similarly soft running surface. As this becomes increasingly well tolerated, the athlete may return to his or her normal running surface.

TABLE 26B–1
Treatment of Femoral Shaft Stress Fractures

Phase*	Activity Level			
	Crutches	Upper Body Conditioning	Lower Body Conditioning	Running or Training
Initial phase, 1–2 wk	+	+	+/–	–
Intermediate phase, 2–6 wk	–	+	+	–
Late phase, 4–10 wk	–	+	+	+

*These phases are based on time from onset of symptoms, and progression from one phase to the next is dependent on resolution of symptoms.
+ = Activity used.
– = Activity not used.

Before sports training is resumed, a reasonable explanation for the causative factor of this injury is sought. The patient with a mild-to-moderate fracture risk is allowed to continue high-impact activities after appropriate medical evaluation. Typically, training error is the most common fault. By and large, stress fractures of the femur occur in runners; therefore, the athlete must understand that a rapid increase in mileage or a marked change in intensity precipitated the injury and must not be repeated. Because stress fractures are secondary to repetitive stress, careful attention is given to those factors responsible for diminishing stress, especially during running. It is beyond the scope of this chapter to evaluate shoewear, orthotics, or running gait, but each plays a role in shock absorption and can be modified to increase its efficiency.

Criteria for Return to Sports Participation

There are no studies in the literature that specifically address when a return to athletics may be expected for children with femoral stress fractures; however, it has been our experience that 6 to 10 weeks is usually sufficient. The late phase of treatment marks the time when an athlete nears return to full sports participation. Because the majority of these injuries occur in running, late-phase treatment should entail a running entry program tailored to the child's or the adolescent's age and level of physiologic development.

The running entry program should begin with 4 miles per week of running plus all other activities performed in the intermediate phase (see Table 26B–1). At the end of the third week (at the earliest, 6 weeks from the onset of symptoms), if these activities can be done essentially pain free, the runner is permitted to return to half of the standard training distance. Gradually, over the next 2 to 3 weeks, instruction is given to increase mileage up to the previous norm. In other high-impact sports, this same protocol is used, and the athlete then returns to sport-specific training. By gradually increasing the duration and the intensity of activity during the next 2 to 3 weeks, full participation can be anticipated. If at any time symptoms recur, the athlete is dropped back to the previous phase for a minimum of 2 weeks and is managed in much the same fashion.

Muscle Strains and Ruptures

Muscle strains and ruptures represent a continuum of injuries that can lead to significant pain and disability, resulting in time being lost from the pursuit of leisure and athletic activities.[45] The clinical relevance of muscle strain–related injuries is quite apparent to most sports medicine physicians, with these injuries accounting for up to 30% of a typical sports medicine practice.[18, 75] The etiology and the pathoanatomy of muscle strains and ruptures of the thigh in children and adolescents vary little from adults, and the reader is referred to Chapter 26A for further review.

At the microscopic level, injuries to the musculotendinous unit are characterized by typical histologic changes.[27,

[47, 111] In the acute period, a hemorrhagic response occurs and surrounds the injured fibers. During the next 24 to 48 hours, the injured fibers undergo necrotic changes, typified by edema and the presence of macrophages at the site of injury. Inflammatory cells and fibroblastic activity become much more apparent by day 2 and are more notable near the region of the injured fibers, whereas the edematous response is more diffuse. These histologic changes are corroborated by findings seen on CT and MRI of the injured region.[49, 120, 129, 135] MRI has proven to be particularly useful in further evaluating these muscle injuries. MRI of partial tendon tears demonstrates irregular thinning and hematoma at the myotendinous junction.[120, 129] T_2-weighted images of grade I (stretch) injuries show high-signal-intensity edema and hemorrhage surrounding the myotendinous junction spreading into the adjacent muscle and the muscle fascicles, indicative of an acute inflammatory process.[120]

In general, in the treatment of a young athlete with a suspected muscle strain, early motion is desirable immediately after the acute inflammatory phase.[27, 45, 77, 111] Early motion should be performed during the healing phase with the goal of promoting muscle healing and minimizing scar formation while avoiding the risk of reinjury.[136] Therapy usually involves high-speed, low-force isokinetic exercise, which is best suited for type II fiber action. Additionally, isokinetic exercises are done concentrically (tension when muscles shorten) rather than eccentrically (tension when muscles elongate) to limit the amount of force generated in the injured muscle.

Hamstring Strains

Hamstring strains are among the most common injuries encountered by sports medicine physicians[28, 36, 72] but are seen less frequently in the skeletally immature athlete. With the arrival of the adolescent growth spurt, however, these injuries appear to occur with increasing frequency. The pathoanatomy, the clinical presentation, and the treatment of these injuries are very similar to adults, but differences do exist. The apophyses in the pelvis and the hip tend to appear later and to fuse later than most epiphyses of the long bones, resulting in skeletally immature athletes being more susceptible to avulsion fractures.[97] These fractures are likely to be due to the tendency for failure to occur at the weaker, open apophysis rather than at the stronger musculotendinous junction. This is particularly relevant when attempting to differentiate a muscle strain from an acute fracture or avulsion in a skeletally immature athlete.

The hamstring muscles in skeletally immature and mature individuals are very similar both anatomically and physiologically. The hamstring muscles consist of the biceps femoris, the semimembranosus, and the semitendinosus muscles, and they span the posterior aspect of the thigh. With the exception of the short head of the biceps, they all have their origins at the ischial tuberosity before spanning two joints: the hip and the knee. The amount of force placed on the hamstrings is therefore dependent on the position of these two joints. In addition, because they pass across two joints, more stresses are placed on these muscles, making them susceptible to injury. The short head

TABLE 26B–2
Muscle Strain Classification

Grade	Features
I	Small disruption of structural integrity at musculotendinous junction
II	Partial tear, some musculotendinous fibers intact
IIIA	Complete rupture of musculotendinous unit
IIIB	Avulsion fracture at tendon's origin or insertion site

of the biceps differs from the other hamstring muscles by taking its origin from the linea aspera of the femur. The remaining hamstring tendons arise from the ischial tuberosity and are in large part responsible for the ischial avulsion fractures seen in young athletes.

There continues to be considerable debate regarding the risk factors associated with hamstring strains, but the exact cause is likely to be multifactorial. Numerous reports in the literature have implicated inadequate warm-up, poor technique, leg-length inequality, strength imbalances, decreased flexibility, adverse neural tension, and fatigue as risk factors for sustaining a hamstring strain.[25, 35, 59, 119, 136, 152, 165] Furthermore, experimental studies have suggested that athletes engaged in proper strengthening, stretching, and warm-up programs have a decreased incidence of hamstring injuries.[140, 156]

Hamstring strains represent a continuum of injuries ranging from minor damage to a few myofibers without loss of structural integrity to a complete tear of the musculotendinous junction.[27] The same classification system may be used for both adult and skeletally immature athletes, with strains being divided into three groups: mild (grade I), moderate (grade II), and severe (grade III) (Table 26B–2).[168] Grade I injuries represent a small disruption of the structural integrity of the musculotendinous unit. Grade II strains are partial tears with at least some of the musculotendinous fibers remaining intact. Grade III tears involve a complete rupture and occur only rarely. Avulsion fractures of the ischial tuberosity or the distal insertion, which are also included in the grade III group, are more prevalent in the skeletally immature.

A combination of hip hyperflexion and simultaneous knee extension has been described as a mechanism of injury for proximal hamstring ruptures in adults[117, 132] but will likely result in an apophyseal avulsion injury in the skeletally immature. These injuries cause severe pain that usually prohibits even simple ambulation. Some authors believe that skeletally immature athletes are relatively inflexible and are therefore more susceptible to avulsion injuries than to actual musculotendinous strains. They attribute this phenomenon to the inability of muscle-tendon growth to keep pace with bone growth in the adolescent.[101] Quite interestingly, others believe that there is increased flexibility during the adolescent growth period, which accounts for the relative paucity of hamstring injuries seen in this age group.[27]

Athletes may present with either an acute or a chronic injury and are often able to recall a specific event that precipitated their complaints. Many athletes with grade I injuries will never seek medical evaluation, whereas most of those with grade II injuries and nearly all with grade III injuries will seek medical treatment immediately after the injury. Similar to their adult counterparts, children and adolescents presenting soon after injury often describe a feeling of sudden onset of pain in the posterior aspect of the thigh during some type of strenuous activity, most commonly while sprinting. When questioned, the young athlete will often relate a history of inadequate warm-up or fatigue associated with the event.[27] Occasionally, the athlete will describe an audible "pop" or a tearing sensation associated with immediate pain, prohibiting further participation and usually causing him or her to fall to the ground or the turf. This type of history is more indicative of a grade II or III injury. Frequently, the pain will subside sufficiently to enable the athlete to ambulate with mild-to-moderate discomfort. Athletes with a more chronic injury often describe a feeling of tightness or an impending "pull," prompting them to limit their training or sports participation. The feeling of tightness may be accompanied by mild pain with activity, ultimately hampering their level of performance.

The physical examination of a young athlete with a hamstring injury does not differ considerably from examination of an adult. Acutely, the athlete may be lying on the ground or the turf grasping the thigh. As the inflammatory phase ensues over the next 24 to 48 hours, the posterior region of the thigh often becomes diffusely swollen and tender in severe strains, with an accompanying area of ecchymosis. At this point, the athlete is frequently unable or unwilling to extend the knee fully secondary to pain, and the injured hamstring is best examined with the patient prone and the knee flexed. It is important to remember that the initial examination will be the most revealing. As the inflammatory process progresses, these clinical findings will become less well delineated.

The posterior thigh is first inspected for any visible deformity or flexion contracture, as may occur from pain and spasm. The entire length of the hamstring muscles should be examined from origin to insertion. Ischial avulsions or complete ruptures of the tendinous origins of the semitendinosus, the semimembranosus, or the long head of the biceps femoris may be accompanied by distal retraction of the hamstring muscles and a visible defect proximally.[68] Similarly, complete tears occurring distally may be accompanied by a visible defect and muscle retraction proximal to the area in question, although this is quite rare. Next, the knee is flexed to 90 degrees, and the entire length of the hamstring is palpated, with particular attention paid to the ischial tuberosity, which is exquisitely tender in the presence of an apophyseal avulsion injury. The hamstring is then palpated while in slight extension. A palpable defect is fairly diagnostic of a complete tear; however, this is extremely rare in this patient population and, if present, is frequently difficult to detect.[131] The patient is then placed in the supine position and, with the hip flexed to 90 degrees, is asked to flex the knee actively against resistance. This will give the examiner some indication of the severity of the injury. Transient sciatica resulting from an acute grade III hamstring strain has been reported in the literature, underscoring the importance of performing a thorough neurovascular examination.[132]

Diagnostic studies are usually unnecessary when evaluating an athlete with a hamstring strain; however, their usefulness has increased with the advent of MRI. The majority of injuries are mild strains or incomplete tears warranting conservative treatment. If a complete tear is suspected clinically, MRI may be useful for further evaluation of the extent of injury and the need for possible surgical repair. For a possible apophyseal injury, routine radiographs are indicated. If the diagnosis of an apophyseal avulsion remains in doubt, CT or MRI may be helpful in confirming the diagnosis and localizing the site of injury.[23, 49] T_2-weighted MRI scans are ideal for the delineation of muscle tears.[33, 41] Acute injuries are represented by areas of high signal intensity on T_2-weighted and short time inversion recovery (STIR) images. Edema and hemorrhage are responsible for these signal changes because they surround the injured myotendinous junction and spread into the adjacent muscle and along the muscle fascicles.[120] T_1-weighted images usually reveal areas of intermediate signal intensity; however, not too infrequently, they appear entirely normal. MRI can also be helpful when evaluating a suspected subacute or chronic avulsion or insertional injury. These injuries may present on plain radiographs as areas of bony rarefaction or even significant bone lysis. These can mimic an infectious or a neoplastic process when there is no clear history of trauma. In addition, one study showed a positive correlation between the amount of cross-sectional involvement of muscle and the time to recovery. At present, the information gained from MRI only infrequently alters the course of treatment, and the cost does not justify its routine use in the evaluation of this injury.

The treatment of grade I, grade II, and most grade III hamstring strains varies little between children and adults. The majority of these injuries will respond to a conservative treatment program predicated on the principles of rest, ice, compression, and elevation (RICE) and a supervised rehabilitation program. There are no studies in the literature specifically addressing the treatment of hamstring strains in the skeletally immature athlete; most reports consist of a mixture of adults and adolescents 12 years of age or older. These studies generally agree that after the acute period (lasting 2 to 4 days), a gradual progressive exercise program should begin, including light stretching. Patients should be followed for changes in pain, range of motion, and muscle testing and should be gradually progressed to resistance exercises as pain dictates. A return to sports activity is generally not allowed until the athlete has achieved full painless range of motion, strength has been restored, and all muscle imbalances have been corrected. This enables most athletes to return to competition in a few days to 2 weeks.

Authors' Preferred Method of Treatment

The treatment of hamstring strains at our institution varies little from the protocols advocated by most authors. We have used a standard five-phase treatment program with considerable success. Initial phase I treatment revolves around the standard RICE protocol and determination of the severity of the strain. If there are no contraindications, we recommend nonsteroidal anti-inflammatory drugs (NSAIDs) acutely for the treatment of all hamstring injuries and then discontinue their use after a brief period. Classification of the strain is performed clinically and can usually be achieved during the first 7 to 10 days after injury. Progression to the next treatment level is determined by pain relief and function (therapeutic exercises).

Phase II treatment consists of early motion by way of protective exercises and passive stretching pre- and postexercise. Isometrics are begun initially and are progressed to isotonics. Passive stretching is performed in the sitting position, with the athlete attempting to bring the chest to the thigh. Flexibility is measured by flexing the hip 90 degrees and maximally extending the knee (see Fig. 26A–8). This is done at each re-evaluation and may serve as an alternative to proprioceptive neuromuscular facilitation if a trainer or a therapist is not available (see Fig. 26A–9). Ice and compressive wraps or sleeves are continued. Phase I and II rehabilitation should focus on reducing pain, swelling, and spasm. We have found transcutaneous electrical nerve stimulation, electrical stimulation, and anti-inflammatory drugs to be helpful adjuncts in achieving this goal.

The progression through phase II and ultimately into phases III to V is dictated by the level of pain relief and the functional improvement achieved. The focus of rehabilitation should gradually shift to attaining a balance between promoting muscle regeneration and minimizing scar formation. A supervised rehabilitation program is the best means for achieving this goal. As full range of motion is regained, rehabilitation should progress from isometrics to isotonics, isokinetics, and finally light running. Continued improvements in strength signify that the athlete is ready for sport-specific training and a gradual return to full activities shortly thereafter.

First-degree strains represent a small focal injury with little hemorrhage and no structural damage. No objective findings of functional loss are present owing to the integrity of the musculotendinous unit. All patients with hamstring strains are initially placed on a phase I treatment protocol (RICE). Immobilization is rarely indicated for this level of injury, although ice can be beneficial when used in the early stages of a muscle strain. There continues to be debate regarding the role of ice in reducing swelling and the inflammatory reaction. Ice has been shown to cause vasoconstriction, which decreases blood flow to the injured area, but this appears to be only temporary and is followed by vasodilation, a phenomenon known as the hunting reaction.[94] Nonetheless, its role as an effective analgesic is well substantiated, supporting its use during the early inflammatory period. We recommend bagged crushed ice, which conforms to the thigh, followed by a compression wrap. After the diagnosis of a first-degree strain is confirmed, the athlete is advanced to phase IV treatment. Mild strains typically resolve rapidly with minimal associated morbidity, and an early return to sporting events can be expected.[14, 138]

Second-degree strains represent a partial tear of the musculotendinous unit and can usually be linked to a particular injury. A painful palpable mass is noted within the muscle belly, which should not retract with active contraction of the muscle. Movement with contraction occurs with grade III injuries (complete tears) and represents a loss of structural integrity. Careful palpation of the muscle's origin and insertion sites is performed to rule out a bony avulsion. Occasionally, in severe grade II and III

injuries, a brief period of immobilization in extension for 3 to 5 days may be needed to allow for control of hemorrhage, edema, and pain. Prolonged immobilization is discouraged because of the potential for detrimental long-term effects.[111] Studies have shown immobilized muscle to have a lower total deformation to failure and lower load to failure than nonimmobilized muscle.[73] In addition, clinical studies conducted by the same authors revealed a 20% decrease in muscle strength after 1 week of immobilization. The use of crutches is dependent on the athlete's level of pain and is usually discontinued once normal gait is resumed. The patient is then sent to physical therapy for phase II treatment, which generally lasts 1 to 2 weeks.

Our indications for surgery in the treatment of hamstring injuries are restricted largely to ruptures of the musculotendinous complex from its origin or its insertion. In the skeletally immature athlete, these injuries most commonly involve bony avulsion of the ischial tuberosity with varying degrees of displacement. Fragments displaced as much as 2 cm or less usually respond to conservative measures as described previously for grade III hamstring strains. Avulsions displaced greater than 2 to 3 cm may lead to weakness and chronic pain, particularly with sitting, and are often better managed by means of early surgical repair. Treatment guidelines for ischial avulsion fractures are discussed in greater detail in Chapter 25.

Complete ruptures of the hamstrings at their distal insertion are usually associated with more serious injuries to the knee joint. Fortunately, these combined injuries are extremely rare in this young age group. When they are present, however, the knee joint should be carefully assessed for additional disease. Posterolateral corner injuries often coincide with avulsion injuries of the biceps femoris from the fibular head and can lead to significant morbidity if misdiagnosed or left untreated. These injuries require repair back to their anatomic insertion site and are discussed in more detail in Chapter 28. These are usually complex injuries, and rehabilitation must be individually tailored to each athlete and his or her injury.

There are very few complications associated with hamstring strains in the adolescent. When properly treated, the young athlete is usually able to return to the previous level of activity. Potential complications include reinjury, fibrosis, residual weakness or pain, and nonunion or malunion of ischial tuberosity fractures. Complications are more frequently associated with grade III injuries and are rarely seen in grade I and II lesions. The most common complication is reinjury, which is frequently the result of an athlete returning to sporting activities too soon. These injuries will often continue to recur if the athlete does not achieve full flexibility and strength before returning to his or her respective sport. Myositis ossificans occurs rarely after a muscle strain and is seen more frequently in association with muscle contusions. Nonunion or malunion has been reported to occur after nonoperative treatment of severely displaced ischial tuberosity avulsions. In some instances, symptomatic bony fragments may require excision.

Criteria for Return to Sports Participation

The primary objective of a sports medicine physician should be to return an athlete to his or her sport in the least amount of time while incurring minimal risk of reinjury. Informing the athlete, the coaches, and the parents of the proposed treatment plan, the rehabilitation program, and the return-to-play criteria during the initial visit is strongly urged. Athletes will often notice considerable improvement in pain and ambulatory function within a few days (usually following phase I and II treatment) and often feel ready to return to play at this point. Waiting until this time to outline the return-to-play timetable will likely lead to frustration and resentment and should be avoided. Furthermore, physicians should not be persuaded by an eager young athlete or parent or an overzealous coach to allow an early return to play. This can result in reinjury and a prolonged rehabilitation and is not in the best interest of the patient. Return-to-play criteria are essentially the same for both nonoperatively and operatively treated hamstring strains and avulsions. We believe that a safe return to sports is possible only after isokinetic testing reveals function to be within 10% to 15% of normal at slow and fast speeds. Muscle imbalances (quadriceps/hamstring strength ratio of less than 50% to 60%) and poor flexibility are often contributing factors to the development of a hamstring strain and should be addressed and corrected before the athlete returns to sports.[27, 136] Functional evaluations are particularly useful in settings where isokinetic testing equipment is not readily available. Sprinting is the most common mechanism of injury and therefore serves as a good functional test. After appropriate stretching and warm-up, the young athlete is asked to sprint 30 to 40 yards three times. In addition, we have the athlete run three figure-of-eights as fast as possible within 10 to 15 yards (depending on the size and the age of the athlete). If these exercises can be done at full speed without discomfort, these tests are considered successful, and the athlete may return to his or her sport.

Quadriceps Injuries

The quadriceps muscle group consists of the vastus lateralis, the vastus medialis, the vastus intermedius, and the rectus femoris. These muscles lie on the anterior aspect of the femur and converge distally, becoming the quadriceps tendon before inserting onto the proximal pole of the patella. It is a relatively homogeneous group of muscles with a common innervation. The rectus femoris differs by originating proximal to the hip joint, functioning as both a knee extensor and a hip flexor. Quite interestingly, the rectus is also the most often injured muscle of this group.[135, 168]

Quadriceps tendons are physiologically similar in skeletally immature and skeletally mature individuals. The muscle fibers are predominantly type II and are best suited for rapid forceful activity.[47] The primary function of the quadriceps is deceleration of knee flexion at heel strike, with simultaneous contraction of the quadriceps and the hamstrings during the support phase of running.[42, 134]

Quadriceps strains and tendon ruptures are the result of eccentric contractions. There is also evidence that a certain subset of these injuries may result from repetitive microtrauma.[143] These injuries usually occur in young to middle-aged men participating in sporting events such as track and field, football, soccer, and basketball.[66, 123] Quadriceps strains tend to occur at the musculotendinous junction.[48, 50, 131] The classic quadriceps strain tends to occur in the distal musculotendinous junction of the rectus. More recently, a pattern of strain involving a previously undescribed muscle-tendon junction within the proximal muscle belly of the rectus has been described.[66] To our knowledge, the incidence of quadriceps strains in young athletes has not been reported; however, 30% of patients (3 of 10) in this study were 16 years of age or younger (two 16-year-olds and one 14-year-old).[66] Although no mention was made of physeal closure or the patient's skeletal age, this study would suggest that these injuries are not uncommon in young adolescents. On the contrary, grade III ruptures of the quadriceps tendon in healthy active adolescents are quite uncommon, being described in the literature predominantly as isolated case reports.[1, 92, 127] Their presence in the skeletally immature is rarer still.[92] The relative infrequency of quadriceps tendon ruptures, partial and complete, in children and adolescents is directly related to the fact that in general healthy tendons do not rupture. Ruptures usually represent a critical degree of degeneration that has taken place within the substance of the tendon. Children and adolescents have healthy tendons with little to no degeneration present. This explains why children more commonly sustain avulsion fractures rather than tendon ruptures.

Young athletes with quadriceps strains usually have a history of acute anterior thigh pain; however, symptoms may be more gradual and may not become evident until after completion of the patient's workout. Some degree of swelling commonly arises, with a mass developing in more severe strains. Measurements of the diameter of the distal thigh are useful for detecting the presence of swelling. Serial measurements may enable the physician to monitor the patient's rate of healing and reassess the level of injury. A mass present at rest usually represents a hematoma and should resolve spontaneously. Masses that occur with muscle contraction may indicate a more severe grade II or III strain. Tenderness on deep palpation in the distal anterior thigh implies that an injury has likely occurred at the rectus muscle–quadriceps tendon junction.[46] Loss of knee flexion is another common finding, and an attempt should be made to determine whether the loss is exacerbated with hip extension. If the loss of knee flexion is greater and more pain occurs with the hip extended than with the hip flexed, there is likely greater involvement of the rectus femoris muscle. If knee flexion and pain are unaffected by hip extension, it is more likely that the vastus medialis, the vastus intermedius, or the vastus lateralis is the injured muscle. Any active contraction of the quadriceps will usually exacerbate the pain.

Chronic rectus strains are another infrequent entity in young athletes. Patients with this condition are frequently unable to recall any specific traumatic event. There is some belief that these injuries represent repeated microtrauma and attrition occurring at the musculotendinous junction of the rectus femoris muscle.[143] There is often a painless soft tissue mass noted on clinical examination. There is usually no functional deficit and no pain elicited with passive knee flexion or quadriceps contraction. These particular injuries can easily be confused with a soft tissue sarcoma, underscoring the need for a thorough history.[32, 37, 143]

Diagnostic imaging techniques available for quadriceps tendon ruptures and strains include radiography, ultrasonography, and MRI.[9, 17, 18, 76, 169] Plain radiographic findings are normal. In a younger athlete with a suspected severe strain or rupture of the musculotendinous junction of the distal rectus femoris, radiographs are helpful in ruling out a proximal pole fracture of the patella. When evaluating an athlete with a chronic nagging injury, radiographs are useful in distinguishing a chronic muscle strain from a femoral stress fracture or even myositis ossificans. On MRI, a chronic rectus strain can easily be confused with a soft tissue sarcoma if the physician is not aware of any previous trauma. In this instance, additional diagnostic studies may be indicated (Fig. 26B–2).[143] As for hamstring ruptures, MRI is currently the best imaging modality for establishing a diagnosis, assessing the severity of the injury, and de-

termining the appropriate treatment and rehabilitation for strains and ruptures.[92, 169] Once again, routine MRI is not cost effective for suspected quadriceps strains. If a complete tear or an underlying pathologic process is suspected, however, MRI is an excellent imaging modality.[143]

Treatment of acute quadriceps strains differs very little from that of any other muscle strain and begins initially with a routine RICE protocol. Most treatment schedules recommend stretching and therapeutic exercise after the first 1 to 3 days followed by a gradual return to sports.[3, 4, 27, 56, 79, 102, 145] Once the initial inflammatory phase has resolved and motion has improved, the patient is begun on a low-intensity training regimen, which is gradually increased as permitted. The treatment protocol is advanced in such a manner as to promote muscle healing and minimize scarring while avoiding the risk of reinjury. When normal

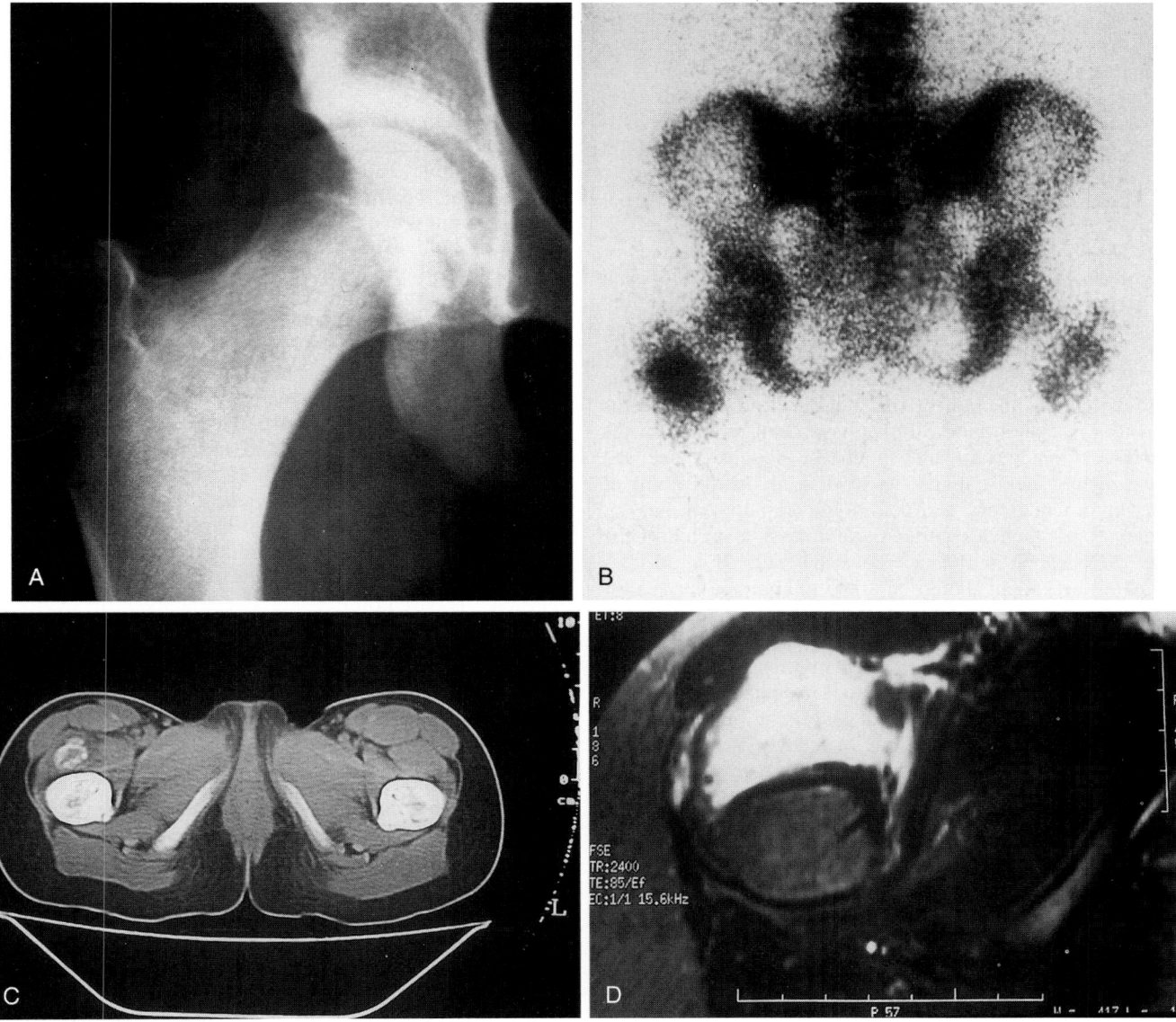

Figure 26B–2. Images from a 15-year-old cheerleader with right hip pain and no history of injury. *A,* Normal anteroposterior radiograph of the hip. *B,* Bone scan demonstrating increased uptake in the metaphyseal region of the proximal femur. *C* and *D,* Computed tomography scan and T_2-weighted magnetic resonance image confirm the diagnosis of a myositis ossificans of the rectus femoris.

strength and flexibility have returned, the athlete may resume all levels of previous activity. The treatment regimen for anterior inferior iliac spine avulsions is similar to that described for severe strains and rarely, if ever, includes surgical intervention.[83] The physician should routinely reassess the patient's level of pain and should examine the injury site for tenderness, knee flexion limitation, and muscle testing. Monitoring these parameters is critical to advancing therapy while preventing further injury and regression.

The degree of injury should be classified as one of three types based on loss of knee motion, as measured with the hip extended or in the prone position. This is perhaps best determined after the initial inflammatory phase has resolved somewhat, usually within the first 5 to 7 days. Although not the basis of classification but helpful nevertheless, assessment of the degree of pain and of tenderness on palpation and manual muscle testing are done on a frequent basis. Mild or first-degree strains represent a small area of muscle involvement with little hemorrhage, localized by pain but not by palpation, and certainly not by a palpable mass or defect. Knee flexion to 90 degrees or greater associated with mild symptoms (soreness after exercise) and no functional loss is a typical finding. The hallmark of first-degree strains is rapid recovery within a few days.

Moderate or second-degree strains represent a partial tear of the musculotendinous unit. Knee flexion is measured in the prone position and is generally 90 degrees or slightly less. Pain is usually more acute, and onset of pain is accompanied by complaints of rapid loss of function, which is confirmed by manual muscle testing. These injuries occur predominantly in the middle to distal third of the thigh; however, more proximal injuries involving the muscle-tendon junction of the indirect head of the rectus and its associated muscle fibers have been reported in the adolescent age group and should be sought.[66] One can localize the site of injury, as evidenced by the point of maximum tenderness, and possibly even palpate a mass or a hematoma. Active contraction and passive stretch of the area in question will exacerbate the pain. If a mass is evident, the patient should be asked to contract the quadriceps actively. By definition, second-degree strains will not demonstrate retraction of the mass. Serial measurements should be made of the thigh's circumference at the site of injury. Measurement is a useful tool for detecting swelling, which is often missed on visual inspection, and quantifies the extent of injury and the rate of recovery.

Unlike in adults, the incidence of severe grade III strains in young athletes is rare, and the need to distinguish them from second-degree strains is infrequent. Grade III injuries exhibit greater loss of knee flexion, with patients typically being unable to flex their knee beyond 45 degrees while in the prone position. A majority of these athletes will have a visible or palpable mass present. Similar to hamstring injuries, avulsion of the origin of the quadriceps (anterior inferior iliac spine) or its insertion should be considered. Unlike second-degree strains, as the inflammatory period and associated swelling subside in grade III injuries, active contraction of the muscle reveals retraction of the mass or the detached muscle segment. Once again, serial examina-

TABLE 26B–3
Quadriceps Strain Treatment Protocol

Phase I

Rest, ice, compression, elevation (RICE)

Phase II

Ice, NSAIDS, electrical stimulation, isometrics, isotonics ± conditioning ± active stretching

Phase III

Ice, NSAIDs, electrical stimulation, isotonics, isokinetics, active stretching, conditioning

Phase IV

Ice, isokinetics, running, sport-specific training, passive stretching

Phase V

Return to sports

NSAIDs, nonsteroidal anti-inflammatory drugs.

tions play an important role in the diagnosis and the management of these injuries.

Authors' Preferred Method of Treatment

Our treatment of quadriceps strains is quite similar to that used for hamstring strains and employs a five-phase protocol (Table 26B–3). This treatment philosophy is predicated on the functional and anatomic similarity of the two muscle groups and the predominance of type II muscle fibers in both. The most commonly injured muscle of the quadriceps group, the rectus femoris, is also the sole biarticular muscle of this group, similar to the biceps femoris hamstring muscle. Treatment for all injuries begins with phase I of the RICE protocol for a minimum of 24 to 48 hours. This minimizes the initial injury and the subsequent swelling and allows time for evaluation to determine the extent of the strain. Frequent re-evaluation cannot be stressed enough; it is essential to the overall treatment process and an injury-free return to athletics. In our experience, quadriceps reinjury during this time has been a greater problem than reinjury of hamstring strains but has been a lesser problem than reinjury of adductor strains. Progression of the treatment program from phase II to phase IV is based on frequent assessments of the degree of pain experienced during exercise and on the following day. If the athlete is slowly challenged with progressive resistance exercises within his or her comfort range, recovery is maximized.

Progression is allowed only after the athlete is able to perform a given set of exercises comfortably on two consecutive days. At that point, the athlete is asked to perform a more taxing workout. Emphasis is placed on our belief that motion regained in the recovery period is a result of positive functional gains. Furthermore, any treatment directed at regaining motion will likely have a detrimental effect rather than a positive one. A detailed outline of our rehabilitation program and criteria for advancement is detailed further in section A of this chapter.

Criteria for Return to Sports Participation

The athlete is allowed to return to practice when he or she is pain free; has a normal range of knee motion within

10 degrees of that of the contralateral side and within 10% of the contralateral leg on isokinetic testing; and performs well on functional testing. Patients are routinely ready to return to competition before the full five-phase program is completed, but more playing time is lost if the late phase is not finished. Return-to-play status is determined using isokinetic appraisal or functional testing, or both, as previously described for hamstring strains. This is an area in which knowledge of the athlete's sport-specific activities is a prerequisite to allowing an earlier return to participation.

It is our practice to use circular wraps or sleeves and, in addition, a protective pad when the athlete resumes training on the practice field or in competition. Using this treatment regimen, we have not found it necessary to operate on any of these injuries. We expect the majority of athletes to return to their sports in an average of 2 to 3 weeks.

Adductor Injuries

Anatomically, the adductors (longus, magnus, brevis), the pectineus, and the gracilis muscles comprise the muscular component of the medial aspect of the thigh. These muscles originate at the symphysis pubis and the inferior pubic rami, travel along the medial aspect of the thigh, and insert on the linea aspera of the femur. The lone exception is the gracilis, which inserts on the medial aspect of the proximal tibia. The tendinous and aponeurotic attachments of the rectus abdominis and internal oblique muscles are also found at or near the adductor's origin. This close proximity often makes it difficult to distinguish the true source of the athlete's pain (see Fig. 26A–11).

Strains and ruptures of the adductor muscles result from repetitive contractions or a single forced contraction of the muscle group while the thigh is in an externally rotated and abducted position. These injuries, commonly seen in young soccer players, occur when two players kick the ball at the same time or during an episode of rapid acceleration.[15, 124] These movements are ubiquitous in sports, and the resultant injuries are quite prevalent in young athletes and become more common with age. These injuries have been thoroughly reported in the literature and occur in ice hockey, soccer, track and field, gymnastics, karate, and horseback riding.[87, 95, 142] As with hamstring injuries, strength imbalances in the adductor group may play a role in predisposing athletes to these injuries.[95]

The patient's recollection of the injury may vary from an insidious onset with progressive pain during intense preseason training, for example, to a sudden, simple, painful event. Less frequently, running straight ahead or cutting may cause a strain of the adductor musculature. The athlete complains of pain in the groin or the medial thigh that is accentuated by passive abduction. There is usually palpable tenderness at the site of the injury, which more often than not represents the musculotendinous unit of the adductor longus muscle.[53, 80] This site can usually be identified by means of palpation along the course of the musculotendinous unit against mild to moderate resistance in adduction. Complete ruptures are rare and are usually associated with bony avulsion of the origin of the adductor muscles. Avul-

sions can be extremely painful and are difficult to examine thoroughly owing to the level of associated tenderness, particularly over the region of the pubis.[116, 128] Although a palpable defect or a large mass may be found distal to the pubis in adults with a complete tendinous rupture, we have not seen a similar finding in the skeletally immature athlete.

Plain radiographs can be helpful in evaluating injuries to the adductor muscle group. Radiographs help differentiate soft tissue injuries from avulsion fractures of the origin of the adductor muscles and late-stage osteitis pubis. In rare cases, myositis ossificans of the adductor longus may also be seen on plain radiographs. Bone scanning can be useful in distinguishing avulsion injuries and early osteitis pubis from the more common musculotendinous injury. Bone scans remain highly sensitive for various pathologic conditions of the pelvis; however, they lack the specificity of MRI. MRI is quite useful for determining the integrity of the muscle fibers and for grading the severity of muscle strains, making it the imaging modality of choice when evaluating soft tissue injuries.[120] MRI remains prohibitively expensive, however, preventing its routine use in the treatment of adductor strains, which are self limiting in the majority of cases. We reserve the use of MRI for athletes suspected of having a grade III strain (see Table 26B–2), those with a soft tissue mass but no history of injury, and those with unexplained chronic groin pain in whom appropriate treatment measures have failed. The role of MRI in the evaluation of "athletica pubalgia" remains unclear at present, and it is recommended only as a means of ruling out other potential disorders that mimic this syndrome.[98]

Rest, ice, compression, and elevation followed by a graduated physical therapy program are the mainstays of treatment most often recommended for acute adductor injuries.[87, 95, 122] Apophyseal avulsion fractures may be treated in a similar manner and rarely require surgery.[83] Rest is essential; crutches may be necessary for 2 to 3 days in the patient with a mild strain or for as long as 2 to 3 weeks in the patient with a musculotendinous rupture. Before returning to the previous level of activity, the athlete must be placed on a strengthening and stretching program.[60, 95] In a study of high school and college athletes with adductor strain injuries who did not undergo a supervised rehabilitation program, a 25% power deficit of the injured leg compared with the noninjured leg was found.[95] Integral parts of the stretching and strengthening program should include both static and dynamic training without load or resistance, isometric exercise with increasing loads, dynamic training with increasing loads, and finally sport-specific training.[123]

Associated Injuries

Chronic adductor tendinitis differs from an acute injury in that its presentation is insidious groin pain aggravated by sports-related activity. This condition may result from a previous mild strain that was never appropriately rehabilitated, however. Another common cause is the development of multiple microtears over time owing to repetitive overload (overuse) of the musculotendinous unit.[2, 87, 159] It has been postulated that these microtears are not large enough to stimulate local bleeding, so the normal physiologic healing response is never initiated.[159] Physical findings are very similar to those found in the acute injury. Most authors recommend a conservative treatment regimen similar to that used for acute injuries.[95] Adult athletes with chronic groin pain localized to the adductor longus that has not responded to conservative measures have shown improvement following selective adductor tenotomy.[2, 87, 159] There are no reports in the literature of surgical intervention being required in the skeletally immature athlete.

Abdominal wall muscle injuries have been increasingly recognized as a source of chronic inguinal or pubic area pain in athletes and should be included in the differential diagnosis.[98] Meyers and colleagues recently coined the term *athletica pubalgia* to describe one particular syndrome that appears to be seen predominantly in the adult population; however, 5% (8) of the patients in their study were of high school age.[98] The majority of these patients have lower abdominal pain with exertion, but a small minority have pure adductor-related pain. Osteitis pubis, "sports hernia," internal snapping hip syndrome, slipped capital femoral epiphysis, stress fractures, inguinal hernias, and obturator nerve entrapment are all commonly mistaken for adductor strains and should be considered in all athletes with chronic groin pain despite appropriate treatment measures.[22, 57, 98, 99, 123, 141] More serious disorders have been encountered in the adult population with chronic groin pain, and their presence in the adolescent athlete should not be discounted. These disorders include inflammatory bowel disease, prostatitis, aseptic necrosis of the hips, infection, endometriosis, and seminoma.[98] The clinician should include all of these in the differential diagnosis when evaluating adductor muscle injuries. Chronic adductor pain is commonly the result of adductor tendinitis and is frequently seen in soccer players and in ice hockey players. The incidence of this injury is relatively low in the skeletally immature athlete, although its presence increases with age, peaking during the third and fourth decades of life.

Myositis ossificans is a relatively rare cause of adductor pain in the young adolescent and is seen predominantly in horseback riders and jockeys. It is thought to develop as a result of an acute strain of the adductor longus or after repetitive microtrauma. It responds well to conservative measures and rarely, if ever, requires surgical intervention.

Authors' Preferred Method of Treatment

Although adductor strains are generally seen as often as other thigh muscle strains, the incidence of severe adductor strains appears to be lower. A rapid return to sport in 1 to 2 weeks has been our experience, thereby negating the need for extensive treatment. Nevertheless, a careful evaluation must be done to identify a potentially more serious injury. Hip flexor function must not be ignored during examination, because in more serious injuries, it is involved as well as the adductor.

Philosophically, we use a treatment schedule almost identical to that used for hamstring strains, which includes the RICE protocol for 24 to 48 hours followed by reassessment of the injury. (See earlier description of the authors' preferred method of treatment for hamstrings injuries.) Generally, pain resolution is rapid following phase I, allowing isometric exercises to be started, which are eventually progressed to isotonic exercises (phase II).

The progression from isometric to isotonic exercises illustrates our concept of treatment phases. Progression is based on pain control and maintenance of function with therapeutic exercises. If an athlete can perform isometric exercises with little or no pain and the following day has no increase in pain or decrease in function, isotonics are inaugurated. If, conversely, regression is apparent, we advise a return to isometrics or possibly phase I treatment. Ice massage should be continued during this interval in conjunction with light stretching, as pain permits. Stretching is done initially in the supine position with both hips and knees flexed to 90 degrees and the involved limb lying flat against the table. Passive stretching is dependent on trunk and pelvic rotation away from the injured side, which is primarily controlled by the athlete's tolerance of the pain.

As his or her condition improves, the athlete can maintain an upright sitting position comfortably. In the sitting position with the hip and knee flexed to 90 degrees and the feet placed sole to sole, further stretching can be accomplished by direct elbow pressure to the knees (see Fig. 26A–12). In this way, the same degree of abduction can be obtained bilaterally. Stretching after an acute injury is best performed by the athlete, because he or she will be best able to monitor for pain and consequently reduce the risk of additional injury. The treatment sessions usually last no longer than 15 to 20 minutes and should include stretching using the sustained hold-relax technique, ice, and possibly electrical stimulation.

Even in patients with more severe strains, isometric exercises can be incorporated into treatment sessions as early as 2 to 3 days after injury. As isometric intensity increases along with the athlete's tolerance, a program of progressive resistance exercises is begun. Isotonic exercises follow isometric exercises and progress to isokinetic training and running. (See earlier section on authors' preferred method of treatment for hamstrings strains.) Again, as pain diminishes and strength and flexibility improve, simulated sporting activities are undertaken before the athlete's actual return to sport.

Adductor avulsion fractures from the pubis are treated nonoperatively and heal without consequence in the overwhelming majority of cases. To our knowledge, a complete rupture of the adductor muscles of an adolescent athlete has not been reported in the literature. This is likely a consequence of the relative weakness of the physis compared with the musculotendinous unit. Injuries therefore appear to result in avulsion fractures rather than complete tears in the skeletally immature athlete. We have not had any experience with performing adductor tenotomy for chronic, resistant cases of adductor muscle strain in the skeletally immature athlete—nor have we found it to be necessary in the literature.

Criteria for Return to Sports Participation

Criteria for return to sports must include equal flexibility in both lower limbs and isokinetic and functional testing similar to that described for hamstring strains. Once these goals are achieved, the athlete is fitted with a circumferential thigh girdle and is allowed full sports participation.

Muscle Strains and Nonsteroidal Anti-inflammatory Drugs

Reducing the inflammatory changes associated with muscle injuries is the main focus of NSAID therapy. It has been demonstrated that these drugs have the ability to lessen the inflammatory response without adversely affecting the tensile strength or the strength of muscle contraction.[5, 112] Nonetheless, the role of NSAID therapy in the management of muscle strains remains somewhat controversial. Acute musculotendinous injuries are characterized by extravasation of blood into the surrounding tissues and the subsequent recruitment of inflammatory cells, leading to swelling, erythema, pain, and impaired function.[4] This may be the only process whereby the body is able to remove damaged or necrotic tissue. In addition, there is evidence that NSAID use within the first 24 to 48 hours of injury may in fact interfere with the chemotaxis necessary to promote muscle fiber regeneration and may thus result in delayed healing.[28] There does not appear to be similar controversy regarding the effectiveness of NSAIDs in the management of mild to moderate pain in the pediatric population.[151] Obviously, many questions remain regarding the long-term effects of these drugs on the overall healing process and the indications for their use in the treatment of muscle strains.

Prevention of Muscle Strains

The role of stretching in the prevention of overuse injuries, muscle strains, and ruptures continues to be a topic of considerable debate. Although intuitively beneficial, stretching has yet to be clinically proven to reduce the rate of strain consistently.[55] Numerous studies have attempted to address this topic, often with conflicting findings.[39, 52, 59, 65, 110, 163] When performed properly, stretching exercises have been shown to improve flexibility.[147] Establishing a direct relationship between increased flexibility and the prevention of muscle strains has remained elusive, however.

It has been our practice to recommend a routine stretching program for all athletes and, in particular, for young adolescents experiencing growth spurts. Theoretically, increased flexibility may decrease the amount of tension developed in the muscle-tendon unit during eccentric contraction. This in turn increases the critical force required to produce a musculotendinous strain or a bony avulsion. Although the benefits are unproven, there is certainly no risk associated with a properly performed stretching program and very likely some benefit. Passive stretching of an injured muscle is not advised and should be avoided to reduce the risk of developing myositis ossificans or extensive scarring.[54]

Quadriceps Contusions and Myositis Ossificans

Contusions most commonly result from blunt nonpenetrating trauma.[64] In severe cases, blunt trauma can result in a partial or complete rupture of the quadriceps mechanism, similar to that seen in a muscle strain. In the laboratory model, damage to the muscle secondary to contusions usually results in a characteristic response.[30, 154] After the traumatic event, muscle tissue injury and hemorrhage occur, followed rapidly by an inflammatory response. The absence of hematoma or further edema heralds the gradual resolution of the inflammatory phase. Intense proliferation of myoblasts and fibroblasts ensues. Next in the sequence is the formation of granulation tissue, which eventually matures into dense collagenous scar tissue. In the past, it was believed that the muscle damage occurred deep, adjacent to the bone[129, 154]; however, recent animal studies have indicated that the damage may be closer to the surface of the muscle, near the site of impact, and may then extend deep into the muscle complex.[30]

Athletes with thigh contusions are generally able to recall a particular incident that initiated symptoms, which may or may not have precluded participation in that sporting event. In mild or moderate injuries requiring treatment, it is not unusual for an athlete to have finished his or her activities for that day. As with muscle strains, localized pain, exquisite tenderness, swelling, and the loss of knee flexion are typical findings. With severe injury, an ipsilateral knee effusion may be found; therefore, examination of the knee must not be ignored. Jackson and Feagin found these injuries to be classifiable at 48 hours based primarily on loss of knee flexion, which had a practical application for treatment.[69] In addition, myositis ossificans should be considered if a firm mass develops at the injury site 3 to 4 weeks after injury.[1, 11]

At the time of injury, radiographs are useful only to rule out bony injury. They may become helpful after 2 to 4 weeks in the evaluation of developing myositis ossificans.[1, 69, 90]

In general, the treatment of quadriceps strains and of quadriceps contusions is similar, although differences do exist. Reports by both Ryan and colleagues and Aronen and associates have recommended an initial period of immobilization in flexion followed by early range of motion.[12, 130] One difference in treatment has been an attempt in quadriceps contusions to speed the resolution of the thigh hematoma. Several methods have been described in the literature to address this, including early aspiration of the hematoma, the use of proteolytic enzymes administered orally or injected directly into the site of injury, compressive wraps, and immobilization of the hip and the knee in flexion to pain tolerance.[1, 2, 66, 90, 130]

Common to most successful methods of treating quadriceps contusions is an effort to limit the hematoma by the use of the RICE regimen, restoration of knee motion by means of supervised exercise, and restoration of limb function by means of appropriate rehabilitation. This is accomplished in a gradual fashion to accommodate the athlete's injury regardless of its severity.[69] Most authors recommend an initial period of immobilization for 24 to 48 hours. Motion is then begun and proceeds at the patient's own pace, not assisted by stretching. Isometric exercises are typically used along with gentle active flexion exercises that are comfortable for the athlete. When flexion of the knee has reached 90 degrees or greater and a normal gait is evident, a progressive resistance exercise program is initiated. Participation in noncontact sports is encouraged as a means of training before the athlete returns to his or her particular sport.

In three series of patients treated in this fashion, all athletes returned to full participation in sports without surgical intervention, regardless of the severity of the injury.[69, 83, 126] The duration of disability varies considerably and appears to depend largely on the severity of the contusion. Several authors have reported an average return-to-play time of 2 to 3 weeks.[82, 130] Other authors have reported considerably longer periods of time, with some athletes requiring as many as 5 to 10 weeks before return to sport.[69, 126]

Two significant complications of quadriceps contusions are compartment syndrome and myositis ossificans. Compartment syndrome of the thigh can result in significant soft tissue damage, permanent disability, and possibly limb loss. In comparison, myositis ossificans is associated with a relatively low morbidity rate. Physicians treating athletes with quadriceps contusions should be familiar with the signs and symptoms of both these conditions and should begin appropriate treatment when indicated. Both entities are discussed in further detail later in this chapter.

Authors' Preferred Method of Treatment

The same basic principles of treatment for quadriceps strains apply to quadriceps contusions. The initial treatment, however, differs considerably in regard to our use of early knee immobilization in 120 degrees of flexion with an adjustable hinged knee brace. It is important to begin bracing the knee within 4 hours of the time of injury. Ice and a mild compression wrap should also be applied during this time. The affected extremity remains in the brace overnight for a period of 24 hours only; then the brace is removed. Gentle, pain-free active knee flexion is begun at this time, along with isometrics and hamstring stretching. The remainder of the treatment program follows our guidelines outlined for quadriceps strains.

Our principle of not using heat modalities is absolute in quadriceps contusions. Many who advocate judicious use of heat admit that a potential problem exists with its use but offer no clear clinical time frame for its safe administration. We have not encountered any problems with the use of ice and have observed at least one case in which ultrasound applied 3 weeks after injury in a traditional fashion caused a marked worsening of the condition. Later, this patient developed myositis ossificans. The typical situation is an athlete who sustains this injury and at 2 to 3 weeks fails to make progress with knee motion. Therefore, other modalities are tried, most often heat and stretching, to facilitate recovery. The tendency to overtreat must be resisted, because more often than not, it only serves to exacerbate the symptoms and the findings.

We do not recommend surgical repair of complete quadriceps muscle ruptures resulting from severe contusions.

Criteria for Return to Sports Participation

The athlete returns to practice when he or she is pain free, has at least 120 degrees of knee flexion with the hip extended, and performs well on functional testing. The testing criteria are similar to those used for hamstring strains. Circular wraps or thigh sleeves worn with some type of protective padding over the contused site are used when the athlete resumes sporting activity, but the pad must be able to absorb a high impact and must stay in place to be effective.

When this treatment regimen is used from the onset of the injury, we have not found surgery to be necessary, with the majority of athletes able to return to their sport in 2 to 3 weeks.

Myositis Ossificans

Myositis ossificans often results from severe compression of muscle tissue against the underlying bone with injury to the muscle fibers and the blood vessels. Clinical experience has shown that this heterotopic bone formation is invariably adjacent to the anterior femur. Its presence reflects a more severe injury but does not necessarily require a specific change in treatment, nor does it appear to alter the ultimate functional result.[69, 82, 126, 130] Simulated laboratory studies have not demonstrated a clear origin of the heterotopic bone that forms in the damaged muscle tissues.[154, 167] Studies have found the incidence of myositis ossificans among military cadets with treated thigh contusions to range from 9% to 20%.[130] In these same series, myositis ossificans was associated with more severe injuries and, more commonly, with an episode of reinjury. The incidence in child and adolescent athletes appears to be markedly lower.[108]

The differential diagnosis of myositis ossificans should include periosteal osteosarcoma, parosteal osteosarcoma, synovial sarcoma, osteochondroma, juxtacortical chondroma, and infection. The differences between myositis ossificans and osteosarcoma often include (1) a history of trauma to the affected site, (2) a course of radiographic stabilization at 3 to 4 months, (3) patient age of less than 30 years, (4) location of the lesion (anterior thigh), (5) presence of an intact cortex, and (6) a negative alkaline phosphatase level. All these findings are supportive of myositis ossificans. If the clinical appearance warrants a biopsy, a full-thickness biopsy must be done. Biopsy specimens obtained solely from the cellular inner layer of the lesion closely resemble the histologic appearance of osteosarcoma. The peripheral zone demonstrates more cellular maturity and a lack of invasion from adjacent tissues, however, which are important pathologic criteria for diagnosing myositis ossificans.[156] Usually, it is more appropriate to observe these lesions with serial radiography.

The radiographic evolution of myositis ossificans parallels its histologic appearance. By the third or fourth week, flocculated densities are seen within the soft tissue mass, and the underlying bone exhibits a periosteal reaction. By 3 to 6 months, the bony mass usually stabilizes or even "shrinks." Once mature, these masses may be classified based on their periosteal connection to the femur. There are three basic types of periosteal connections: broad based, connected by a stalk, or no connection at all.[151] Radiographic findings closely parallel those of CT; however, CT may help differentiate immature osteoid in a sarcoma from true ossification in myositis ossificans. CT may also be helpful in determining the size, the density, and the anatomic location of the lesion. Technetium scanning can evaluate early myositis ossificans, but its true value rests in monitoring the maturation of the lesion and determining the appropriate timing of excision.[155] Ultrasonography has been useful as a diagnostic tool because it can detect soft tissue changes proven to be precursors of myositis ossificans before the appearance of radiographic changes.

The MRI appearance of these lesions varies considerably depending on their level of maturity. Early lesions in particular may mimic an aggressive soft tissue sarcoma, whereas more mature lesions demonstrate a more benign appearance.[13, 74]

Myositis ossificans rarely alters the athlete's ability to return to play. Occasionally, however, an athlete may remain symptomatic months after the injury, and operative intervention is then considered. In this instance, the physician should be aware that surgical management before maturity of myositis ossificans invites disaster. This includes a recurrence of bone formation greater than the amount of bone that was excised and a marked increase in the extent of the athlete's disability. It has been suggested that indications for successful surgical excision should include a mature mass and a minimum waiting period of 6 months if symptoms and disability persist. Surgical technique includes exposure of the entire mass to allow excision in toto, much the same as for an excisional biopsy. Exacting technique, including meticulous hemostasis and atraumatic dissection and excision, is required for a successful surgical procedure.

Authors' Preferred Method of Treatment

We have seen a fair number of athletes who developed myositis ossificans. If treatment is done in an appropriate manner, disability rarely ensues. Occasionally, one may see an athlete with untreated myositis ossificans who has persistence of loss of motion, a painful bony mass, and significant functional limitation. In this circumstance, we still try conservative means first, and, if these fail, surgical excision of the heterotopic bone is recommended. Surgical excision is not considered before maturation of the bony mass or until a minimum of 6 months (and preferably 12 months) has elapsed since the time of injury.

A routine preoperative work-up is performed, although consideration should be given to obtaining a bleeding profile in athletes who have been on a recent course of NSAIDs. MRI- or CT-enhanced arteriograms can be helpful for lesions located dangerously close to nearby neurovascular structures. Athletes should be advised to discontinue all NSAIDs 4 to 6 weeks before surgery. Careful surgical technique and gentle handling of the soft tissues are used to avoid unnecessary muscle stripping. Excisional biopsy followed by splinting is our routine. Wound drainage is recommended if there is continued bleeding after appropriate hemostatic measures have been performed.

Postoperatively, we have used a knee immobilizer for 2 to 3 weeks with partial weight-bearing on crutches, followed by entry into phase II of our treatment protocol (see "Quadriceps Injuries"). Anti-inflammatory drugs have

demonstrated some promise in the prevention of heterotopic bone formation.[84, 150] The anti-inflammatory drug of choice in this setting is indomethacin. In a very limited number of athletes who underwent surgery, a successful return to athletics was possible. The criteria for return to play are similar to those for quadriceps contusions.

Compartment Syndrome

Compartment syndrome of the thigh resulting from closed blunt trauma sustained during a sporting event is relatively rare.[29, 125] The majority of instances of acute compartment syndrome result from a direct blow to the anterior thigh, as often occurs during soccer, rugby, and football. Chronic compartment syndrome has been reported in the literature but is extremely rare and occurs predominantly in the adult population.[118] There has been a case report of an adolescent athlete's developing acute anterior compartment syndrome after a weightlifting session.[19] Swelling within the fascial compartment results from bleeding of a vessel with subsequent hematoma formation or from increased capillary permeability with resulting third space fluid in the damaged muscle, as may occur after significant trauma. Elevation of the intracompartmental pressures ensues, leading to muscle ischemia, metabolic and structural deterioration and necrosis of skeletal muscle, and cellular acidosis. Compartment syndrome can occur in any or all of the three compartments of the thigh; however, the anterior compartment is involved in the overwhelming majority of cases, corresponding to the location where most contusions occur.

The clinical presentation of impending compartment syndrome of the anterior thigh compartment is frequently indefinite. There have been reports of compartment syndrome of the thigh occurring as late as 7 days after injury, although in general acute compartment syndrome becomes symptomatic relatively quickly, usually within 24 hours. Clinically, an athlete with early anterior compartment syndrome of the thigh will rest the leg with the knee in an extended position to lessen the amount of stretch on the quadriceps muscles. Pain out of proportion to the level of injury is perhaps the most important and consistent sign. The pain is deep, unremitting, progressive, and unrelieved with immobilization.[107] Passive knee flexion exacerbates the pain significantly and is one of the most reliable tests for making the diagnosis. Paresthesias are not uncommon at this time. Sensation over the anterior aspect of the knee and the medial aspect of the lower leg and the foot is provided by the saphenous nerve. Diminished sensation in this area is a more objective finding; however, it occurs infrequently and is suggestive of a more significant level of tissue ischemia.[29, 106, 160]

Swelling is frequently difficult to quantitate in the thigh. Motor deficits and loss of pulses are late findings and imply that permanent muscular damage has already taken place. If a clinician suspects the presence of compartment syndrome, the diagnosis can be confirmed by measuring compartment pressures. The classic method of determining compartment pressures, and the authors' preferred index, was initially described by Whitesides and colleagues in

1975 and is still the gold standard.[161] Alternative methods of measuring compartment pressures include (1) using a standard electronic arterial-line pressure monitoring system attached to a stopcock, extension tubing, and an 18-gauge needle or catheter and (2) using one of the commercially available compartment pressure measuring devices. Accurate measurements are best taken near the area of injury, often at more than one site, because studies have shown differences in tissue pressure over cephalocaudal distances of as little as 5 cm.[58]

Regardless of the technique used, it is imperative to interpret compartment pressure measurements in light of the degree of soft tissue trauma sustained, the patient's blood pressure, and the clinical signs and symptoms.[107] Human studies have shown a specific relationship between blood pressure and the pressure threshold for physiologic nerve dysfunction.[139] This threshold has been found to range from 10 mm Hg below the diastolic pressure in healthy muscle to 20 to 30 mm Hg below the diastolic pressure in damaged tissue. This has prompted some authors to recommend these latter measurements as guidelines for decompression.[58, 89, 139] Other authors have recommended fasciotomy when intracompartmental pressures exceed 30 to 35 mm Hg.[91, 105]

In general, if there is either a high index of suspicion clinically of impending compartment syndrome or abnormally increased tissue pressure, fasciotomy of the affected compartment(s) should be conducted in an emergent fashion.[58, 89, 91, 105, 139] The anterior compartment is most commonly involved. Fasciotomy should be performed through a longitudinal incision, and the wounds should be packed open. At 3 to 5 days after decompression, the patient may be returned to the operating room for skin grafting or for delayed closure of the wounds if there is no undue tension. Criteria for return to play are similar to those for quadriceps contusions.

Summary

In summary, injuries are an unavoidable part of athletics. The risk of reinjury can be minimized if the athlete follows the treatment guidelines outlined, including the use of RICE, early mobilization, functional strengthening, and restriction of return to sport until the extremity has been properly rehabilitated.

References

1. Adolphson P: Traumatic rupture of the quadriceps tendon in a 16 year old girl. A case report. Arch Orthop Trauma Surg 112:45–46, 1992.
2. Akermark C, Johansson C: Tenotomy of the adductor longus tendon in the treatment of chronic groin pain in athletes. Am J Sports Med 20:640–643, 1992.
3. Almekinders LC: Anti-inflammatory treatment of muscular injuries in sport. An update of recent studies. Sports Med 28:383–388, 1999.
4. Almekinders LC: Anti-inflammatory treatment of muscular injuries in sports. Sports Med 15:139–145, 1993.
5. Almekinders LC, Gilbert JA: Healing of experimental muscle strains and the effects of nonsteroidal anti-inflammatory medication. Am J Sports Med 14:303–308, 1986.
6. Amendola A, Clatworthy M, Magnes SA: Overuse injuries of the lower extremity. In Herschman EB, Mandelbaum BR (eds): Orthopaedic Knowledge Update: Sports Medicine 2. Park Ridge, Ill, American Academy of Orthopaedic Surgeons, 1999, pp 365–372.
7. American Academy of Orthopaedic Surgeons: Athletic Training and Sports Medicine. Park Ridge, Ill, American Academy of Orthopaedic Surgeons, 1984, pp 3, 223–234.
8. An HS, Simpson M, Gale S, Jackson WT: Acute anterior compartment syndrome in the thigh: A case report and review of the literature. Orthop Trauma 1:180–182, 1987.
9. Aprin H, Btoukhim B: Early diagnosis of acute rupture of the quadriceps tendon by arthrography. Clin Orthop 195:185–190, 1985.
10. Arendt EA (ed): Orthopaedic Knowledge Update: Sports Medicine 2. Park Ridge, Ill, American Academy of Orthopaedic Surgeons, 1999, pp 49–63.
11. Arner O, Lindholm A: What is tennis leg? Acta Chir Scand 116:73–77, 1958.
12. Aronen JG, Chronister R, Ove PN, McDevitt ER: Thigh contusions: Minimizing the length of time before return to full athletic activities with early immobilization in 120 degrees of knee flexion (abstract). Am J Sports Med 18:547, 1990.
13. Arrington ED, Miller MD: Skeletal muscle injuries. Orthop Clin North Am 26:411–422, 1995.
14. Backous DD, Friedl KE, Smith NJ, et al: Soccer injuries and their relation to physical maturity. Am J Dis Child 142:839–842, 1988.
15. Basmajian JV: Muscles Alive, 3rd ed. Baltimore, Williams & Wilkins, 1974.
16. Bennell KL, Malcolm SA, Thomas SA, et al: Risk factors for stress fractures in track and field athletes: A twelve-month prospective study. Am J Sports Med 24:810–818, 1996.
17. Berlin RC, Levinsohn EM, Chrisman H: The wrinkled patellar tendon: An indication of abnormality in the extensor mechanism of the knee. Skeletal Radiol 20:181–185, 1991.
18. Bianchi S, Zwass A, Abdelwahab IF, et al: Diagnosis of tears of the quadriceps tendon of the knee: Value of sonography. AJR Am J Roentgenol 162:1137–1140, 1994.
19. Bidwell JP, Gibbons CER, Godsiff S: Acute compartment syndrome of the thigh after weight training. Br J Sports Med 30:264–265, 1996.
20. Black J: Failure of implants for internal hip fixation. Orthop Clin North Am 5:833–844, 1974.
21. Blatz DJ: Bilateral femoral and tibial shaft stress fractures in a runner. Am J Sports Med 9:322–325, 1981.
22. Bradshaw C, McCrory P, Bell S, Brukner P: Obturator nerve entrapment. A cause of groin pain in athletes. Am J Sports Med 25:402–408, 1997.
23. Brandser EA, El-Khoury GY, Kathol MH, et al: Hamstring injuries: Radiographic, conventional tomographic, CT, and MR imaging characteristics. Radiology 197:257–262, 1995.
24. Brunker P, Bennell K: Stress fractures in female athletes. Sports Med 24:419–429, 1997.
25. Burkett LN: Causative factors in hamstring strain. Med Sci Sports Exerc 2:39–42, 1970.
26. Bush MT: Sports Medicine. In Morrissy RT (ed): Lovell & Winter's Pediatric Orthopaedics, 4th ed. Philadelphia, Lippincott Williams & Wilkins, 1996, pp 1181–1228.
27. Clanton TO, Coupe KJ: Hamstrings strains in athletes: Diagnosis and treatment. J Am Acad Orthop Surg 6:237–248, 1998.
28. Clement DB, Amman W, Tauton JE, et al: Exercise-induced stress injuries to the femur. Int J Sports Med 14:347–352, 1993.
29. Colosimo AJ, Ireland ML: Thigh compartment syndrome in a football athlete: A case report and review of the literature. Med Sci Sports Exerc 24:958–963, 1992.
30. Crisco JJ, Jokl P, Heinen GT, et al: A muscle contusion injury model. Am J Sports Med 22:702–710, 1994.
31. Davies AM, Carter SR, Grimer RJ, Sneath RS: Fatigue fractures of the femoral diaphysis in the skeletally immature simulating malignancy. Br J Radiol 62:893–896, 1989.
32. DeSmet AA: Magnetic resonance findings in skeletal muscle tears. Skeletal Radiol 22:479–484, 1993.
33. DeSmet AA, Best TM: MR imaging of the distribution and location of acute hamstring injuries in athletes. AJR Am J Roentgenol 174:393–399, 2000.
34. Devas MB: Stress fractures in children. J Bone Joint Surg Br 45:528–541, 1963.

35. Dornan PA: A report on 140 hamstring injuries. Aust J Sports Med 4:30–36, 1971.

36. Edstrand J, Gillquist J: Soccer injuries and their mechanism: A prospective study. Med Sci Sports Exerc 15:267–270, 1983.

37. Ehman RL, Berquist TH: Magnetic resonance imaging of musculoskeletal trauma. Radiol Clin North Am 24:291–319, 1986.

38. Ekenman I, Tsai-Fetlander L, Westblad P, et al: A study of intrinsic factors in patients with stress fractures of the tibia. Foot Ankle Int 17:477–482, 1996.

39. Ekstrand J, Gillquist J: The frequency of muscle tightness and injuries in soccer players. Am J Sports Med 10:75–78, 1982.

40. Ekstrand J, Gillquist J: Soccer injuries and their mechanisms: A prospective study. Med Sci Sports Exerc 15:267–270, 1983.

41. El-Khoury GY, Brandser EA, Kathol MH, et al: Imaging of muscle injuries. Skeletal Radiol 25:3–11, 1996.

42. Elliott BC, Blanksby BA: The synchronization of muscle activity and body segment movements during a running cycle. Med Sci Sports Exerc 11:322–327, 1979.

43. Engh CA, Robinson R, Milgram J: Stress fractures in children. J Trauma 10:532–541, 1970.

44. Fitch KD: Stress fractures of the lower limbs in runners. Aust Fam Physician 13:511–515, 1984.

45. Garrett WE Jr: Muscle strain injuries. Am J Sports Med 24:S2–S8, 1996.

46. Garrett WE Jr: Strains and sprains in athletes. Postgrad Med 73:200–214, 1983.

47. Garrett WE Jr, Califf JC, Bassett FH: Histochemical correlates of hamstring injuries. Am J Sports Med 12:98–103, 1984.

48. Garrett WE Jr, Nikolaou PK, Ribbeck BM, et al: The effect of muscle architecture on the biomechanical failure properties of skeletal muscle under passive extension. Am J Sports Med 16:7–12, 1988.

49. Garrett WE Jr, Rich FR, Nikolaou PK, Vogler JB II: Computed tomography of hamstring muscle strains. Med Sci Sports Exerc 21:506–514, 1989.

50. Garrett WE Jr, Safran MR, Seaber AV, et al: Biomechanical comparison of stimulated and nonstimulated skeletal muscle pulled to failure. Am J Sports Med 15:448–454, 1987.

51. Grace JN, Sims JG, Shives TC, Coventry MB: Wedge resection of the symphysis pubis for the treatment of osteitis pubis. J Bone Joint Surg Am 71:358–364, 1989.

52. Grana WA, Moretz JA: Ligamentous laxity in secondary school athletes. JAMA 240:1975–1976, 1978.

53. Greaney RB, Gerber FH, Laughlin RL, et al: Distribution and natural history of stress fractures in US Marine recruits. Radiology 146:339–346, 1983.

54. Gross RH: Acute musculotendinous injuries. In DeLee JC, Drez D (eds): Orthopaedic Sports Medicine: Principles and Practice. Philadelphia, WB Saunders, 1994, pp 131–143.

55. Gross RH: Acute musculotendinous injuries. In Stanitski CL, DeLee JC, Drez D (eds): Pediatric and Adolescent Sports Medicine, vol 3. Philadelphia, WB Saunders, 1994.

56. Gross M, Nasser S, Finerman G: Hip and pelvis. In DeLee JC, Drez D (eds): Orthopaedic Sports Medicine: Principles and Practice. Philadelphia, WB Saunders, 1994, pp 1063–1085.

57. Harvey G, Bell S: Obturator neuropathy: An anatomic perspective. Clin Orthop 363:203–211, 1999.

58. Heckman MM, Whitesides TE Jr, Grewe SR, et al: Histologic determination of the ischemic threshold of muscle in the canine compartment syndrome model. J Orthop Trauma 7:199–210, 1993.

59. Heiser TM, Weber R, Sulliban G, et al: Prophylaxis and management of hamstring muscle injuries in intercollegiate football players. Am J Sports Med 12:368–370, 1984.

60. Henry JH: The hip, part 2. Recognition and treatment of injuries. In Scott WN, Nisonson B, Nicholas JA (eds): Principles of Sports Medicine. Baltimore, Williams & Wilkins, 1984, p 248.

61. Heppenstall RB, Scott R, Sapega A, et al: A comparative study of the tolerance of skeletal muscle to ischemia. J Bone Joint Surg Am 68:820–828, 1986.

62. Hershman E, Lombardo J, Bergfeld JA: Femoral stress fractures in athletes. Clin Sports Med 9:111–119, 1990.

63. Hershman EB, Mailly T: Stress fractures. Clin Sports Med 9:183–214, 1990.

64. Holbrook TL, Grazier K, Kelsey JL, et al: The Frequency of Occurrence, Impact and Cost of Musculoskeletal Conditions in the United States. Park Ridge, Ill, American Academy of Orthopaedic Surgeons, 1984.

65. Hubley-Kozey CL, Stanish WD: Can stretching prevent athletic injuries? J Musculoskel Med 7:21–31, 1990.

66. Hughes C, Hasselman CT, Best RM, et al: Incomplete, intrasubstance strain injuries of the rectus femoris muscle. Am J Sports Med 23:500–506, 1995.

67. Hulkko A, Orava S: Stress fractures in athletes. Int J Sports Med 8:221–226, 1987.

68. Ishikawa K, Koichi K, Mizuta H: Avulsion of the hamstring muscles from the ischial tuberosity. Clin Orthop 232:153–155, 1988.

69. Jackson DW, Feagin JA: Quadriceps contusions in young athletes: Relation of severity of injury to treatment and prognosis. J Bone Joint Surg Am 55:95–105, 1973.

70. Johnson AW, Weiss CB, Wheeler DL: Stress fractures of the femoral shaft in athletes—more common than expected. Am J Sports Med 22:248–256, 1994.

71. Jones E: Skeletal growth and development as related to trauma. In Green NE, Swiontkowski MF (eds): Skeletal Trauma in Children, vol 3, 2nd ed. Philadelphia, WB Saunders, 1998, pp 1–16.

72. Jonhagen S, Nemeth G, Eridsson E: Hamstrings injuries in sprinters—the role of concentric and eccentric hamstring muscle strength and flexibility. Am J Sports Med 22:262–266, 1994.

73. Kime RC III, Seaber AV, Garrett WE Jr: The effect of position and time of immobilization on the active and passive biomechanical properties of muscle. Paper presented at the 36th Annual Meeting of the Orthopaedic Research Society, Feb 5–8, 1990, New Orleans.

74. Kransdorf MJ, Meis JM, Jelinek JS: Myositis ossificans: MR appearance with radiologic-pathologic correlation. AJR Am J Roentgenol 157:1243–1248, 1991.

75. Krejci V, Koch P: Muscle and Tendon Injuries in Athletes. Chicago, Year Book, 1979.

76. Kuivilla TE, Brems JJ: Diagnosis of acute rupture of the quadriceps tendon by magnetic resonance imaging. A case report. Clin Orthop 262:236–241, 1991.

77. Kujala UM, Orava S, Jarvinen M: Hamstring injuries: Current trends in treatment and prevention. Sports Med 23:397–404, 1997.

78. Kulund DN: The Injured Athlete. Philadelphia, JB Lippincott, 1982, pp 72, 356–359.

79. Leadbetter WB: Anti-inflammatory therapy in sports injury. The role of nonsteroidal drugs and corticosteroid injection. Clin Sports Med 14:353–410, 1995.

80. Levin DC, Blazina ME, Levine E: Fatigue fracture of the shaft of the femur: Simulation of malignant tumor. Radiology 89:883–885, 1967.

81. Liemohn W: Factors related to hamstring strains. J Sports Med 18:71–76, 1978.

82. Lipscomb AB, Thomas ED, Johnston RK: Treatment of myositis ossificans traumatica in athletes. Am J Sports Med 4:111–120, 1976.

83. Lynch SA, Renstrim PA: Groin injuries in sport: Treatment strategies. Sports Med 28:137–144, 1999.

84. McMahon JS, Waddell JP, Morton J: Effect of short-course indomethacin on heterotopic bone formation after uncemented total hip arthroplasty. J Arthroplasty 6:259–264, 1991.

85. Mair SD, Seaber AV, Glisson RR, Garrett WE Jr: The role of fatigue in susceptibility to acute muscle strain injury. Am J Sports Med 24:137–143, 1996.

86. Mares SC: Hip, pelvic, and thigh injuries and disorders in the adolescent athlete. Adolesc Med 9:551–569, 1988.

87. Martens MA, Hansen L, Mulier JC: Adductor tendinitis and musculus rectus abdominis tenopathy. Am J Sports Med 15:353–356, 1987.

88. Marymont JV, Lynch MA, Henning CE: Acute ligamentous diastasis of the ankle without fracture: Evaluation by radionuclide imaging. Am J Sports Med 14:407–409, 1986.

89. Matava MJ, Whitesides TE Jr, Seiler JG III, et al: Determination of the compartment pressure threshold of muscle ischemia in a canine model. J Trauma 37:50–58, 1994.

90. Matheson GO, Clement DB, McKenzie DC, et al: Stress fractures in athletes: A study of 320 cases. Am J Sports Med 15:46–58, 1987.

91. Matsen RA III, Wyss CR, Krugmire RB Jr, et al: The effects of limbs with particular reference to limbs with increased tissue pressure. Clin Orthop 150:187–195, 1980.

92. Matsumoto K, Hukuda S, Ishizawa M, et al: Partial rupture of the quadriceps tendon (jumper's knee) in a ten-year-old boy. Case report. Am J Sports Med 27:521–525, 1999.

93. Meaney JEM, Carty H: Femoral stress fractures in children. Skeletal Radiol 21:173–176, 1992.

94. Meeusen R, Lievens P: The use of cryotherapy I sports injuries. Sports Med 3:398–414, 1986.

CHAPTER TWENTY-SEVEN

Thoracolumbar Spine

Section A
Thoracolumbar Spine in the Adult

Frank J. Eismont, MD   ■   Scott H. Kitchel, MD

Thoracolumbar spine injuries in athletes are discussed and written about less commonly than other sports injuries for a number of reasons. First, thoracolumbar spine injuries are relatively uncommon in all athletic participation. Second, most of the injuries to the lumbar spine that do occur are relatively minor and fit into the category of strains or soft tissue injuries. Most of these injuries are self-limited and resolve without specific treatment or coming to the attention of a team physician. Finally, most health care providers with an interest in athletic medicine and sports injuries have little interest in thoracolumbar spine problems.

The frequency of thoracolumbar spine injuries in athletes is difficult to document. As noted by O'Leary and Bosaroo,[45] there are three fundamental reasons for this difficulty: (1) Most athletic injuries occurring in sports occur during practice, when team physicians are not always in attendance. (2) Most athletes are reluctant to document minor injuries. (3) Most thoracolumbar spine injuries are self-limiting and resolve without extensive treatment or time loss from participation.

Available studies that document the epidemiology of thoracolumbar spine injuries in athletes suffer from a lack of prospective data.[33, 71] Accepting these limitations, there are many studies that should be discussed as they relate to the epidemiology of spine injuries in athletes. Keene and associates[33] reviewed the frequency and types of back injuries sustained by intercollegiate athletes in 17 varsity sports during a 10-year period. These investigators found an injury rate of 7 per 100 participants. The injury rates were significantly higher in football and gymnastics. Only 6% of the injuries in this series occurred during competition. The other 94% occurred during preseason conditioning or practice. Injuries were divided into acute back injuries, overuse injuries, and injuries associated with preexisting conditions. Acute back injuries were the most common, with most being muscle strains.

In the British experience, reported by Williams[71] in 1980, it is estimated that spine injuries account for 15% of all injuries sustained in sports in the United Kingdom. In his series, injuries to the thoracic and lumbar spine seemed to be more frequent in automobile racing, horseback riding, parachuting, mountaineering, and weightlifting. There is no other report in the literature correlating a specific sporting activity with an increased incidence of injury to a specific area of the spine.

Many other studies are available that attempt to document the epidemiology of thoracolumbar spine injuries in athletes.[64] All of these are limited by the inclusion of only specific patient subpopulations or participation in only one specific sport. U.S. Air Force Academy injury statistics, collected during a 1-year period, indicate that 9% of all athletic injuries are related to the spine. Ryan[53] reviewed more than 1000 injuries from one professional football team and found that 6% were related to the spine. Snook[59, 60] reviewed musculoskeletal injuries sustained by collegiate wrestlers and female gymnasts and found a 2% and 13% injury rate of the thoracolumbar spine.

In reviewing all of the epidemiologic data available and taking into account the limitations that have been mentioned, it is evident that the incidence of thoracolumbar spine injuries in sports is relatively low. Catastrophic spine injuries with spinal cord injury and long-range neurologic sequelae constitute less than 1% of all sports injuries. Most of these are cervical spine injuries and are not related to the thoracolumbar spine.

Many controversies exist concerning athletic injuries in the thoracolumbar spine. The area of preparticipation screening for congenital anomalies as well as underlying conditions of the spine continues to be intensively investigated. Many centers are looking into the advisability of kinetic muscle testing in an attempt to select individuals who may be at risk for spine injuries. Athletic participation as it relates to the cause of spondylolysis with subsequent spondylolisthesis in the young athlete continues to be controversial at this time.

This chapter discusses athletic injuries of the thoracolumbar spine. Through an understanding of the pertinent anatomy and biomechanics, we address the evaluation, treatment, and return to sports participation of athletes suffering from thoracolumbar spine injuries.

Anatomy

The anatomies of the thoracic and lumbar spines are sufficiently different that they are considered separately. Anatomy is discussed to correlate its practical application with common injury patterns.

Thoracic Spine

The thoracic vertebral column is responsible for the support of the thorax and protection of the thoracic spinal

These muscles provide some stability to the lumbar spine as well as being the primary extensors of this region. The enveloping fascia in the lumbar spine is thicker and stronger than its thoracic counterpart. This fascia has been divided into three distinct layers, which provide stability as well as compartmentalization in the lumbar spine.

The nerve and blood supply of the lumbar spine is functionally identical to that of the thoracic spine. The segmental vessels and the nerves run courses similar to the thoracic spine and provide similar function.

Intervertebral Disk

The intervertebral disk is the fibrocartilaginous structure that forms the articulation between adjacent vertebrae. It provides a strong union, while allowing the degree of intervertebral motion necessary for function. Disks of the various portions of the spinal region differ considerably in size but are basically identical in their organization. They all consist of two components, the outer, laminar fibrous container (or anulus) and the inner, semifluid mass (the nucleus pulposus) (Fig. 27A–4).

The anulus fibrosus is a concentric series of fibrous lamellae. Its major function is to withstand tension from the torsional stresses of the vertebral column as well as the horizontal extensions of the compressed nucleus that it contains. The anulus is attached to the vertebral body through a blending of the fibers with the vertebral periosteum as well as the longitudinal ligaments.

The nucleus pulposus occupies a concentric position within the confines of the anulus. Its major function is that of a shock absorber. The nucleus pulposus exhibits viscoelastic properties under applied pressure, responding with elastic rebound. There is no definite structural interface between the nucleus and the anulus. The two tissues blend imperceptibly.

The disks make up approximately one fourth of the height of the entire spinal column. Moving from cephalad to caudad, the disks become larger in their cross-sectional area as well as thicker when measured from one vertebral end plate to the next. The thoracic disks are heart-shaped compared with the more oval form seen in the lumbar spine.

The blood supply and nutrition of the intervertebral disk is achieved primarily by diffusion from the adjacent vertebral end plates. The anulus is penetrated by capillaries for only a few millimeters. The disk is not inert; the normal disk tissue has a high rate of metabolic turnover. The disk itself has no direct innervation. Sensory fibers are abundant, however, in the adjacent longitudinal ligaments. The pain attributable to disk disease most likely is carried through those fibers.

Spinal Cord and Cauda Equina

In the thoracolumbar spine, it is important to differentiate between spinal cord and cauda equina. The spinal cord typically ends at the thoracolumbar junction, and caudad to that level is the cauda equina. The cauda equina is merely a collection of nerve roots that are traversing the spinal canal until they exit at their appropriate foramen. This differentiation is important because of the differences in structural anatomy and the responses to injury of the spinal cord or cauda equina.

The thoracic spinal cord is generally wider laterally than it is deep in the anteroposterior direction. The cord is smaller in the thoracic region than its cervical counterpart. The average anteroposterior depth found by Elliott[15] was approximately 9 mm. An average anteroposterior vertebral canal diameter is 17 mm. The cord occupies approximately one half of the space available within the vertebral column.

The major function of the thoracic spinal cord is the transmission of nerve impulses, from the periphery to the brain and from the brain to the peripheral muscles. The tapered lower end of the spinal cord is the conus medullaris. From this point caudad, only individual nerve roots exist and are grouped together as the cauda equina. These nerve roots pass caudad until they reach the appropriate level, where they pass out through the vertebral foramen.

The response of the spinal cord to injury is different from the response of the cauda equina. The nerve roots in the cauda equina recover from injury in the same fashion as a peripheral nerve. Injury to the spinal cord is generally irreversible, however, and has permanent consequences. This fact is important when considering injuries of the thoracolumbar spine with associated neurologic deficits.

Biomechanics

The thoracolumbar spine is a complex, three-dimensional structure with coupled motion characteristics.[55] The thoracolumbar spine is capable of flexion, extension, lateral flexion, and rotation. The total range of motion is the result of a summation of the limited movements permitted between the individual vertebra. The musculature and ligaments have key roles in the initiation and control of movements as well as in supporting the bone structures. The individual motions vary considerably in the different vertebral regions. Although all thoracolumbar vertebrae are united in the three-joint system of the intervertebral disk and the two zygapophyseal articulations, the size and shape of the intervertebral disk as well as the shape and orienta-

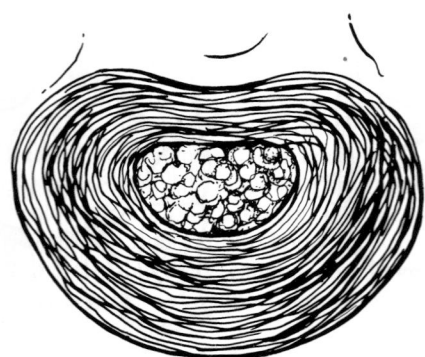

Figure 27A–4. Anatomy of the thoracic disk.

tion of the articular joints determine the types and range of motion available at an individual intervertebral articulation.

The most common movement of the vertebral column is flexion. Flexion requires an anterior compression of the intervertebral disk, along with a gliding separation of the articular facets at the zygapophyseal joint. This movement is limited by the posterior ligamentous complex and the dorsal musculature.

Extension is a more limited motion, producing posterior compression of the disk along with gliding motion of the zygapophyseal joint. Extension is limited by the anterior longitudinal ligament as well as the ventral musculature. The lamina and spinous processes limit extension by direct opposition.

Lateral flexion necessarily is accompanied by some degree of rotation. It involves lateral compression of the intervertebral disk, along with a sliding separation of the zygapophyseal joint on the convex side, whereas an overriding of this joint occurs on the concave side. Lateral flexion is limited by the intertransverse ligament as well as the extension of the ribs.

Rotation is related most directly to the thickness of the intervertebral disk. It involves compression of the anulus fibrosus fibers. Rotation also is limited directly by the geometry of the zygapophyseal joints. The disk limits rotation by resistance to compression in the anulus.

Normal range of motion for the thoracolumbar spine cannot be considered without also considering the synchronous motions of the cervical spine. The entire vertebral column moves as a whole in all planes of motion. The column can rotate approximately 90 degrees to either side of the sagittal plane. Most of this rotation is accomplished in the cervical and thoracic sections. Flexion of 90 degrees is possible, using cervical, thoracic, and lumbar regions. Approximately 90 degrees of extension is also possible, but this occurs primarily in a combination of the cervical and lumbar regions. Lateral flexion, which must be accompanied by some rotation, is allowed to nearly 60 degrees. This is primarily a cervical and lumbar function.

The mobility of the thoracolumbar region is not uniform throughout any of its segments. The upper thoracic spine is impaired greatly in its motion by the rib cage. The articular facets in this region are oriented in the frontal plane. The lower thoracic region allows more flexion and extension because the disk and vertebral bodies progressively increase in size. Also, in the lower thoracic spine, the articular facet joints begin to turn more toward the sagittal plane, permitting greater flexion and extension but limiting rotation. The lumbar region is oriented to allow significant amounts of flexion, extension, and lateral flexion. The zygapophyseal joints are oriented in the sagittal plane, however, locking them against rotation (Fig. 27A–5). This orientation allows a gliding action of the joints that permits the neural arches to separate and approximate during flexion and extension.

The lumbosacral joints change their orientation so that they are midrange between frontal and sagittal planes. This alignment allows some rotation; however, this is limited by the iliolumbar ligaments. The essential function of the lumbosacral joints is to buttress the fifth lumbar vertebra in relation to the sacrum.

Each region of the spine has its own characteristic

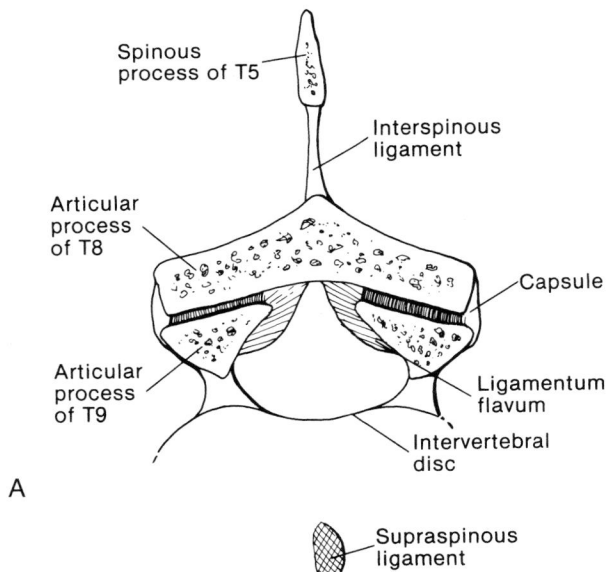

A

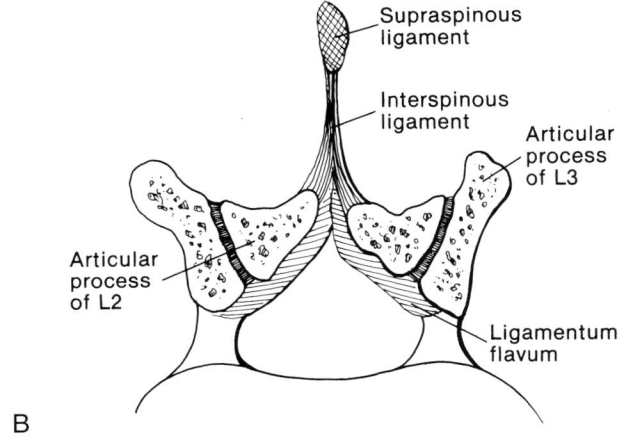

B

Figure 27A–5. Zygapophyseal joints of thoracic *(A)* and lumbar *(B)* spine.

curvature. These curves allow upright posture while maintaining the center of gravity over the major weight-supporting structures of the pelvis and lower limbs. The normal thoracic kyphosis places the thoracic vertebrae posterior to the center of gravity. This kyphosis compensates for the normal cervical lordosis, which allows the head to be held in its erect position. The lumbar lordosis brings the middle of the lumbar spine anterior to the center of gravity, allowing erect posture. The transitional vertebrae between each major spinal segment intersect the center of gravity and appear to be the most unstable regions of the spine. This fact is emphasized by the high incidence of fractures and dislocations in the transitional regions.

The biomechanics of the intervertebral disk emphasize its functional competency. The anulus fibrosis receives most forces transmitted from one vertebral body to the other. It is constructed best to resist tension and shear. This resistance is accomplished by the radial alignment of the progressive lamellae of the anulus. Experimental analysis has shown that different portions of the anulus respond differently to the same degree of tension. It appears that the peripheral anulus has the greatest recovery, whereas the medial sections are more distensible.

The nucleus pulposus is designed best to resist compression forces. It receives primarily vertical forces from the vertebral bodies and redistributes them in a radial fashion to a horizontal plane. The internal pressure of the nucleus distorts the anulus, which, with its resiliency, allows recovery from the pressure.

The tension of the intervertebral ligaments and anulus preloads the disk. This preloading increases stability in the spine. Through this function, the disk must dissipate and transfer the axial thrust necessary to permit erect posture and motion.[46] The spine must act as a flexible boom. The spine is the fulcrum of a first-class lever system.

Clinical Evaluation

Evaluation of the thoracolumbar spine in athletes must follow the same sound principles as any clinical evaluation. The essentials include an accurate, problem-oriented history; spine and lower extremity evaluation; physical examination; and appropriate and specialized diagnostic studies based on the history and physical examination. It is essential that the clinician develop a reproducible standardized method of obtaining the evaluation so that there are no omissions or missing clinical information that would prevent an accurate diagnosis. The injured athlete is highly motivated to return to preinjury activity. The evaluation must lead to a working diagnosis so that treatment may begin and return the athlete to participation as soon as possible.

History

One of the keys to an accurate diagnosis of any thoracolumbar spine problem is a carefully taken history. The athlete generally understates his or her complaints and generally omits any past spine problems or injuries. The history should include the patient's chief complaint, a discussion of the present illness, a past history of any spinal or general orthopaedic problems, and a brief discussion of any family history of back problems.

A commonsense approach is essential in this process. A good clinician allows the athlete to render the story in his or her own words but elicits the important information. History taking varies widely in extent and length of time as the clinical situation dictates. Often, after an acute injury, only a brief history is obtained, but the clinician should return at a later time to obtain a more complete history of any previous problem or injury predisposition. Spending a little extra time obtaining a complete history provides great dividends in understanding the athlete's problem and working toward a correct diagnosis.

The chief complaint must be provided by the athlete. This should key the clinician into a certain line of history taking related to that specific body part. The history of the present illness enlarges on this chief complaint. This history can be obtained from the injured athlete and from other participants who may have witnessed the injury or who were present at the time.

The most common initial complaint in spine problems is pain. It is important to attempt to localize and characterize the pain. The onset of the pain, as related to the time of injury, may provide important information regarding the diagnosis. Diffuse aching pain in the lumbar spine that began the day after an extended workout would lead the clinician into checking for a musculoligamentous type of overuse injury.

The most important part of the history is the present illness. This part of the history should work toward a chronologic development of the spine pain, its character, and any improvement between its onset and the examination of the patient.

The temporal onset of the pain gives the clinician a clue as to the correct diagnosis. Mechanical causes of back pain have a sudden, acute onset. Often the athlete reports that the onset of pain is associated with a specific activity. The pain generally starts immediately or within a few hours. A more insidious onset of pain should alert the clinician to consider medical causes of low back pain.

A history of the duration and frequency of the pain is essential. The clinician should ascertain whether the pain is episodic or more persistent. Most mechanical pain of the thoracolumbar spine is intermittent. The frequency of the episodes varies depending on the exposure of the athlete. The duration of the pain can lead the clinician to an accurate diagnosis. Most muscular strains are relieved within a week. Disk problems generally require longer to resolve.

A history of the quality of the pain itself must be obtained. The quality of the pain and its intensity can be helpful in identifying its source. The patient should be allowed to describe the pain in his or her own words, without being led by the examiner. The intensity of the pain must be ascertained. It is often difficult for the athlete to describe pain intensity; this may be facilitated by asking the athlete to rank the pain on a scale of 0 to 10, with 0 being absence of pain and 10 being the worst pain ever felt.

Localizing the pain to a specific area in the thoracolumbar spine is helpful. The pain may be localized to a specific midline structure or may radiate out from there into the adjacent soft tissues. A key to the evaluation of thoracolumbar spine discomfort is any radiation of the pain. It is especially important to differentiate strictly back pain from pain that may radiate into the leg or foot. Pain that radiates into the lower leg is suggestive of nerve root impingement, such as occurs with disk herniation. The athlete should be questioned carefully about any aggravating or alleviating factors. Generally, mechanical lesions of the thoracolumbar spine improve with supine positioning and worsen with increased activity. Not all thoracolumbar spine movements necessarily exacerbate muscle strain pain. A careful history defines which movements seem to help or aggravate the pain.

Questioning the athlete regarding specific variances in pain related to time of day helps to sort out mechanical disorders from underlying inflammatory problems. In the typical muscle strain injury, the athlete notes that the pain is worse at the end of the day, after he or she has been active. Medical disorders, such as inflammatory arthropathies, cause stiffness in the morning when attempting to get out of bed. During the day, the stiffness lessens. Underlying tumors of the spine or spinal cord generally cause increased pain at night because the pain is increased with recumbency and is more noticeable with the loss of other sensory input while in bed.

A past history of spinal problems is a key to accurate diagnosis. The patient should be asked at several different times in several different ways if he or she has had any previous spine problems. Questions about childhood and adolescence should be included. A preexisting condition of the spine may lead the clinician to an accurate diagnosis because a previous problem may recur or may predispose to a new injury. In this portion of the history, a brief time should be spent discussing any family history of spine problems with the athlete. Familial predisposition to back problems is characteristic of many medical illnesses, including disk degenerative conditions, ankylosing spondylitis, Reiter's syndrome, and other spondyloarthropathies.

As more older athletes become involved with high-demand workout schedules, it is important to remember that these athletes have other social and occupational activities that may contribute to their spine problem. In such an athlete, it is essential to obtain an occupational history to determine what tasks the athlete may be performing at work that may contribute to spine problems. Individuals required to do heavy lifting at their jobs are at risk of developing mechanical low back pain. Review of leisure-time activities is important to look for predisposing causes of the spine problem.

The patient history is the essential foundation on which the remainder of the diagnostic process is constructed. By taking a little extra time and listening carefully to the athlete's description of the chief complaint, the clinician should be able to generate a list of potential diagnoses to direct the remainder of the history taking and physical examination.

Physical Examination

After carefully obtaining the history, a problem-oriented physical examination is the next step in the diagnostic process. Physical examination takes a variety of forms, depending on when the examination is performed. The clinician should never feel limited by time in evaluating acute injuries of the thoracolumbar spine. In the acute setting of an injury to the spine, enough time must be taken to rule out injuries that could produce instability or threaten the neurologic structures before moving the patient.

On the field, management of acute spine injuries must be approached with caution because of the potential neurologic sequelae of inadequate immobilization or transportation of the unstable spine. If there is any question of a spinal column injury with neurologic symptoms, it is important to immobilize the athlete in the position in which he or she was found and not attempt to move the athlete. No attempt should be made to remove equipment, such as a football helmet or part of the uniform. The athlete may be immobilized on a spine board or immobilized without change in body position by a scoop, such as is used by emergency medical personnel. This process takes time and should not be rushed so that there is a minimum risk of increased neurologic injury or manipulation of the spine.

The athlete and the provider are better served by overimmobilizing the injured athlete than by attempting to move him or her in a hurry to allow completion of the athletic event.

A spine board always should be available for transporting the spine-injured athlete. This board often is available because emergency medical personnel are at the scene of the athletic contest. When no medical emergency personnel are on hand, the institution should have a spine board available for transporting these athletes. All athletes with evidence of injury to the spine and neurologic signs or symptoms should be transported immobilized on a spine board. Athletes who have significant pain in the spine secondary to a high-velocity injury should be transported immobilized on a spine board because of the potential for spinal instability, which could lead to neurologic sequelae. Any athlete who is in too much pain to allow mobilization simply on the basis of muscle spasm should be transported on a spine board. It cannot be overemphasized that adequate immobilization and careful transportation prevent possible catastrophic neurologic injury in athletes with spinal column injuries. The clinician should not hesitate to take all the time needed and should have adequate equipment available before any attempt is made to transport the injured athlete.

The essentials of the physical examination of the thoracolumbar spine are no different from those for examination of any other region of the body. The objective of the examination is to show the physical abnormalities that sort out the possible pathologic conditions elicited during the history taking. Essentials include inspection, palpation, range-of-motion testing, and neurologic examination. Inspection of the patient as a whole and of the thoracolumbar spine in particular should be carried out initially with the patient in the standing position and disrobed sufficiently to allow the spine to be seen. The patient should be viewed from behind as well as laterally and anteriorly. From behind, the level of the shoulder should be noted as well as any lateral curvature or cervical scoliosis. The patient should stand with the head centered over the pelvis and feet. Any deviation at one location in the spine must be compensated for by an opposite deviation elsewhere if the patient is standing erect. A list occurs if the thoracic vertebrae are not centered over the sacrum. The list may be measured by dropping a perpendicular line from the first thoracic vertebra and measuring how far this falls to the right or left of the gluteal cleft.

When viewing the patient in the lateral plane, any exaggeration or decrease of the normal spine curvature should be noted. Particularly, any increase in thoracic kyphosis or decrease in lumbar lordosis is significant. The lower extremities should be viewed in the lateral plane. Particular attention should be paid to any flexion or extension deformities of the hips and knees.

Inspection from the front of the patient should include the position of the head and level of the shoulders. It is generally easy to view the iliac wings, and these should be of equal height. There should be no tilt to the pelvis. The skin about the thoracolumbar spine should be inspected, noting the superficial structures. Particular attention should be paid to any skin lesion, such as café-au-lait spots or a tuft of hair over the spine.

After adequate inspection of the thoracolumbar spine, the next step in a complete examination is palpation of the area of tenderness. The primary area of tenderness should be palpated, but because this will cause the patient maximum discomfort, it is wise to palpate certain other anatomic landmarks first. Tenderness should be assessed over the spinous processes at each level. The paraspinal muscles should be palpated looking for tenderness as well as muscle spasm. The sacroiliac joints and the sciatic notches should be palpated for tenderness, and deep palpation of the posterior thighs should be performed.

When an area of maximum tenderness is identified, palpation should be carried out in an attempt to identify the primary structure that is tender at that level. The tenderness may be superficial, such as that seen with the spinous processes or dorsal musculature, or it may be more deep and diffuse, such as that related to a fracture or disk injury. There may be no area of point tenderness in many musculoligamentous-type injuries of the thoracolumbar spine.

Assessing the range of motion of the thoracolumbar spine is important to identify the problem adequately. The absolute range of motion is not of major significance because there is a great deal of individual variance. Range of motion of the lumbar spine should be assessed for flexion-extension and lateral flexion. The reported average range of forward flexion is 40 to 60 degrees. Forward flexion is a complex motion of the lumbar spine, sacroiliac joints, and hip joints. It may be significantly influenced by tightness of the hamstrings if the gauge is the athlete's ability to touch the toes. Extension is considered average at 20 to 35 degrees. There should be approximately 20 degrees of side bending, right and left. Rotation of the lumbar spine is limited and difficult to assess because it occurs in symmetry with the thoracic spine. The major thoracic motion to be evaluated is rotation. With the feet in place, the patient is rotated at the shoulder level. Rotation to nearly 90 degrees can be achieved in the average athlete.

While assessing the range of motion, the patient should be asked to squat in place. This tests not only the general muscle strength of the lower extremities, but also joint function. If the patient is unable to squat, it should be assessed whether this is secondary to pain or some specific decreased function in the lower extremities.

When an athlete with an injury to one of the functional units of the spine attempts to bend or rotate, this motion is inhibited by protective muscle spasm. The lumbar spine may be observed not to have a normal curve in the erect position and not to reverse its lordosis with attempts at flexion. This observation is highly suggestive of protective muscle spasm. If the protective spasm is unilateral and predominantly affects the tissue on one side of the spine, a scoliosis may develop. Scoliosis also may develop from nerve root irritation on one side of the spine, such as occurs with disk herniation.

After the patient has flexed forward fully, it is helpful to observe how he or she regains the erect posture. This gives clues to tissue injury as well as muscle integrity. Normally, the return to the erect position is accomplished by a derotation of the pelvis without changes of spine curvature until the patient has come up to 45 degrees.

During the terminal 45 degrees, the low back resumes its lordosis.

Pain caused by any motion should be noted. Pain precipitated by flexion is a nonspecific finding and may be related to many pathologic conditions. Pain with extension generally is related to an increase of the lordosis forces across the facet joints or stresses in the pars interarticularis; this in turn narrows the foramen where the nerve roots exit the spine and compresses the posterior disk. Pain with hyperextension generally can be related to a pathologic condition involving the facet joints, pars interarticularis, posterior disk structures, or neuroforamen. The pain may be back pain, leg pain, or both. No special significance should be placed on pain with lateral bending. Lateral bending causes ligamentous or muscular stretching and may be restricted in many conditions. In some cases, pain that increases with flexion to the ipsilateral side may be related to articular facet disease or lateral disk protrusion. This should be considered if radicular pain is elicited with lateral bending.

Similarly, limitations of rotation are nonspecific. These limitations may be secondary to muscle spasm within the thoracic spine or simple increases in pain with this motion. A more helpful way of checking rotation is to seat the patient, stabilizing the pelvis and hips. This not only limits the rotation of the spine, but also gives a more specific view of spine rotation, eliminating that from the hips and pelvis.

A neurologic examination of the thoracic and lumbar spine must include sensory and motor evaluation of the thorax and the lower extremities. In the thoracic spine, this evaluation is limited by sensory overlapping and the multiple levels of innervation. Sensation can be assessed most sensitively by light-touch examination of the thorax. Motor examination of the thoracic and paraspinal musculature is difficult in the athlete with thoracolumbar spine problems because of pain and attendant muscle spasm.

Neurologic examination of the lower extremities in the patient with thoracolumbar spine pain is particularly important. Neurologic examination is essential in a patient who complains of any leg pain, numbness, or weakness. This evaluation must include motor strength testing, light-touch sensation, reflex testing, sciatic and femoral nerve tension signs, and assessment of sacral motor and sensory function.

Initial assessment of lower extremity strength can be made in rough terms by asking the patient to squat, then return to an erect position. This rough motor examination can be supplemented by asking the patient to walk first on the heels, then on the toes. Any weakness seen in toe walking is suggestive of weakness in the triceps sura musculature. Difficulty with heel walking is consistent with ankle dorsiflexion weakness.

When this evaluation has been completed, the patient is seated on the table with the legs dangling off the side. Muscle testing in the lower extremities is performed, including the hip flexors, adductors, quadriceps, hamstrings, tibialis anterior, foot everters, extensor hallucis longus, and foot plantar flexors (Table 27A–1). This information is recorded according to the standard nomenclature on a 0-to-5 scale. Any specific deficits are noted.

A sensory examination of the lower extremities is carried out by light-touch testing (Fig. 27A–6). This test is

TABLE 27A–1
Muscle Testing of the Lower Extremities

Nerve Root	Muscle Group	Reflex
L1	Hip flexion	
L2	Hip flexion	
L3	Knee extension	
L4	Foot dorsiflexion	
	Knee extension	Knee jerk
L5	Big toe extension	Posterior tibial
	Foot eversion	
S1	Foot plantar flexors	Ankle jerk
	Knee flexion	

performed most easily by simple light stroking of the thighs and legs in all different dermatomes. Any specific deficit is noted and retested. We do not routinely advocate sharp-dull discrimination or position-sense testing unless other deficits have been found.

Reflex examination of the lower extremities is carried out in the sitting position. This examination should include an evaluation of knee jerks and ankle jerks. The knee jerk reflex is mediated primarily through the L4 nerve root. The ankle jerk is mediated by the S1 nerve root. These reflexes are recorded in the standard 0-to-4 nomenclature.

The patient is asked to lie supine on the examining table for evaluation of nerve root tension signs. The classic test of sciatic nerve irritation is the straight leg raising test.[48] The intent of this test is to stretch the dura and nerve roots, reproducing leg pain. The patient experiences pain along the anatomic course of the sciatic nerve into the lower leg, ankle, and foot. Symptoms should not be produced until the leg is raised to at least 30 to 35 degrees. When the leg

has been elevated beyond 70 degrees, no further stretching of the nerve roots and dura occurs. To be considered positive, the test must reproduce the patient's radicular symptoms. Production of back pain does not indicate a positive result (Fig. 27A–7).

Many other sciatic nerve root tension tests have been described. In the Laseque test,[61] the patient lies supine with the hip flexed to 90 degrees. The knee is extended slowly until the radicular pain is reproduced. This test is likely less specific than the straight leg raising test because hip and knee joints are moved. The bowstring sign[71] is performed with the knee flexed to 90 degrees and the body bent forward to lengthen the course of the sciatic nerve. The examiner's finger is pressed into the popliteal space to increase further the tension on the sciatic nerve. A positive test occurs if the patient's pain increases down the leg. The Milligram test[40] is another sciatic nerve tension sign. The patient lies in the supine position, then raises both extended legs several inches above the examining table. This movement increases intra-abdominal pressure and intrathecal pressure. The patient is asked to hold the position for 30 seconds. The test is positive if the maneuver recreates the radicular leg pain.

Nerve tension signs of the femoral nerve have been described. The most popular names for these tests are *reverse straight leg raising* and *femoral nerve tension sign*. This testing is performed with the patient in the prone position. The knee is flexed to 90 degrees. The hip is extended with the pelvis fixed to the table. Recreation of anterior thigh radicular pain is considered a positive test.

Sacral sensory and motor function is not checked routinely in the athlete unless it is indicated by the history or other portions of the physical examination. To assess this function adequately, evaluation of perianal sensation, sphincter tone, contractility of the anal sphincter, and the superficial anal reflex is required. This reflex is mediated by the S2, S3, and S4 nerve roots. Touching the perianal skin should cause contraction of the anal sphincter and external anal muscles.

The history and physical examination can be modified depending on the circumstances and the individual. The complete history and physical examination cannot be carried out on the field of competition while the competition is delayed. The clinician should never feel rushed when evaluating a patient with a thoracolumbar spine injury, however, and should not consent to move the patient until he or she is convinced there is no evidence of serious injury. Only a small portion of this evaluation may be carried out acutely, and the remainder of it should be done as soon as possible.

The importance of a careful history and physical examination cannot be overemphasized. When this portion of the evaluation is completed, a working diagnosis or differential diagnosis should be established. This diagnosis guides the clinician through the remainder of the evaluation process, including the use of diagnostic testing.

Diagnostic Testing

Evaluation of thoracolumbar spine pain in the athlete frequently includes many radiographic techniques used to

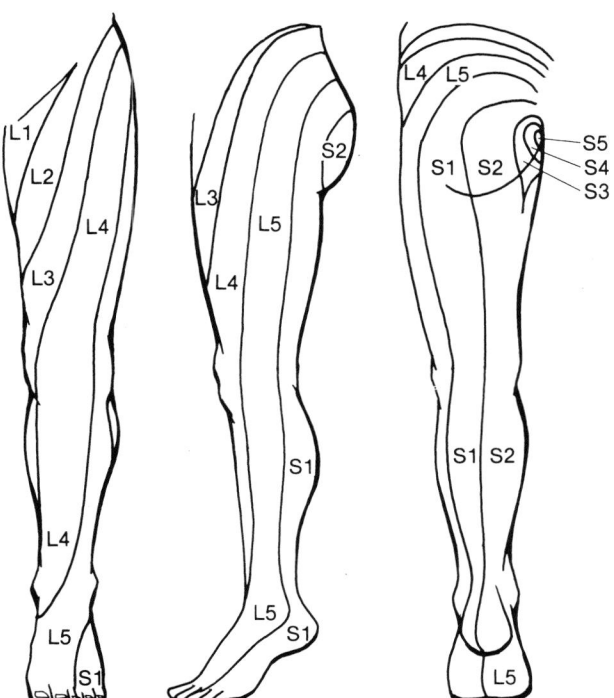

Figure 27A–6. Dermatomal innervation of the lower extremities.

nasts. Bone scans should never be used as a first-line test and should be reserved for specific indications.

Computed tomography (CT) is useful for evaluating abnormalities of the thoracolumbar spine because of its complex three-dimensional, spatial anatomy.[58] CT images not only recreate anteroposterior and lateral radiographs, but also allow cross-sectional imaging in all three planes. CT images best assess bony configuration and structure and show graded shadings of soft tissue, such as ligaments, discs, nerve roots, and fats. CT allows excellent visualization of the paraspinal soft tissues.

CT scanning should be used to confirm clinical findings derived from the history and physical examination. CT is not a tool for primary diagnosis, but rather one for confirmation of this diagnosis when a primary bony abnormality is considered. Many studies[51, 70] have shown that routine CT scanning for thoracolumbar pain is not useful or cost-effective. CT scanning should be directed to the area of pathology and should not be used as a shotgun technique to evaluate the whole spine.

A CT section of the lumbar spine contains different anatomic structures depending on the level of the cross section. Each CT cut is able to assess only one slice of the skeleton. Abnormalities that are not contained in that plane are not viewed by the CT scanner. Figure 27A–16 shows a typical CT scan cross section through the intervertebral disk.

CT scanning of the thoracolumbar spine in the athlete is particularly useful for the diagnosis of bony abnormalities.[52] This examination generally is most useful in the evaluation of significant trauma involving fractures of the thoracolumbar spine in which the question of spinal canal impingement needs to be answered. CT scanning is helpful in the evaluation of tumors of the thoracolumbar spine for localizing the lesion and determining its extent.

The usefulness of CT scanning alone to identify significant disk herniations continues to be questioned. Many clinicians still believe that myelography must be used with CT scans to obtain adequate information about disk pathology. Magnetic resonance imaging (MRI) seems to have

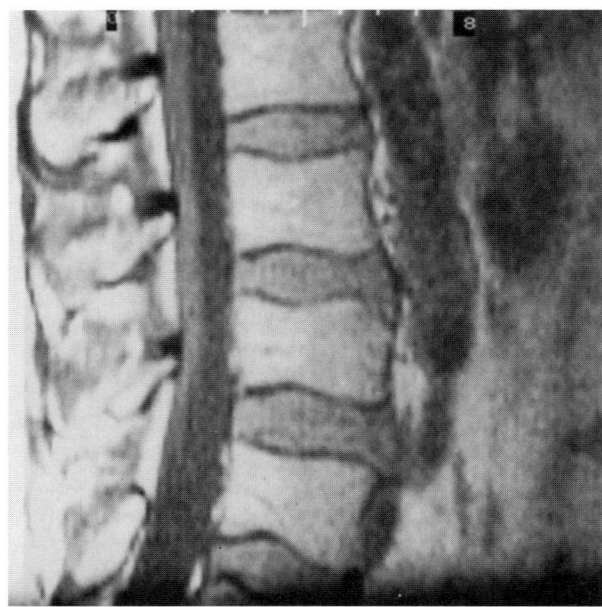

Figure 27A–17. Normal magnetic resonance imaging scan of the lumbar spine.

advantages that supersede those of myelography and CT scanning in the diagnosis of disk pathology.

MRI allows excellent visualization of the soft tissues. As the imaging technology has advanced, MRI has become progressively more useful in the diagnosis of problems of the thoracolumbar spine. MRI is now the imaging modality of choice for all soft tissue injuries of the thoracolumbar spine. MRI also has a role in evaluation of bone injuries when they are causing significant impingement of soft tissue structures, such as the nerve roots.

The principle behind MRI involves the generation of a magnetic field by protons of hydrogen atoms. Hydrogen atoms are the major constituent of water, which is found in varying amounts in all structures of the body. MRI allows visualization of all body structures and is not limited by direct changes in the density of tissues, as are other radiographic techniques. A normal MRI image of the lumbar spine, including the sagittal and transaxial views, is shown in Figure 27A–17. MRI allows visualization of the vertebral column, intervertebral disk, and spinal canal. The axial views show the paravertebral soft tissues, the spinal canal, and the disk or vertebral body.

At this time, MRI is an excellent technique for viewing the spinal canal and soft tissues about the spine, including the nerve roots and intervertebral discs.[20, 44, 47] In injuries commonly seen in the athletic spine, MRI is a superb technique for visualizing disk pathology, nerve root compression, and ligamentous injury associated with hemorrhage. MRI is an excellent technique for characterizing primary changes occurring within the spinal cord or nerve roots, intramedullary tumors, and syringomyelia.

Two other radiographic techniques bear discussion in the evaluation of thoracolumbar spine injuries in the athlete—tomography and discography. In a limited number of patients, tomography presents a useful alternative to CT or MRI, particularly if CT or MRI is not available.

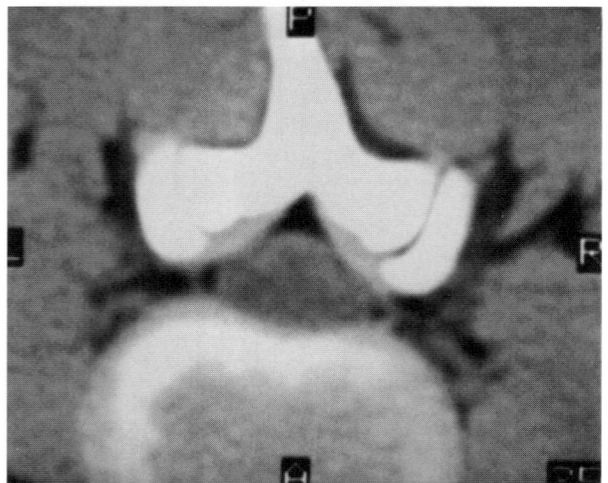

Figure 27A–16. Computed tomographic cross section through intervertebral disk.

Tomographic slices through the vertebral bodies and posterior elements may define bony abnormalities.

Discography is performed by inserting a spinal needle into a disk space, then injecting radiopaque dye.[24, 67] Information is obtained by the radiographic appearance of the dye, the injection pressure used, and the reproduction of the patient's pain during the test. There continues to be controversy at present concerning the validity of discography. Radiographically, it is a sensitive technique to image the internal architecture of the disk when it is combined with CT scanning. The clinical significance of discography must be assessed in conjunction with the patient's pain response when the disk is injected. Discograms rarely are indicated in the management of thoracolumbar spine pain in athletes.

Instrumented kinetic muscle testing of the thoracolumbar spine is used infrequently in athletes. At this time, there are no studies documenting the ability of this technique to evaluate the thoracolumbar spine in athletes. With time and further studies, it is hoped that instrumented kinetic muscle testing may prove to be successful in the rehabilitation of the athletic spine as well as in predicting certain deficiencies that may predispose the athlete to injury.

Specific Injuries of the Thoracic Spine

Injuries to the thoracic spine are rare in athletics. Most cases that do occur are related to high-velocity and high-impact sports. Many injuries deserve consideration and review, however.

Soft Tissue Injuries

The most common injury of the thoracic spine in athletes involves the soft tissues. Soft tissue injuries are either musculoligamentous strains or sprains or contusions related directly to a blow. The key points in the evaluation of soft tissue injuries in the thoracic spine are an accurate, sensitive history and physical examination. The history of the present illness must be stressed to the athlete to ascertain if he or she had a direct blow such as would cause a contusion. In the absence of this information, a history of the pain and its onset is helpful in the evaluation of soft tissue sprains or strains. Often the athlete does not recall any specific inciting event but notes that the pain seems to come on with an increase in activity or a change in the training protocol.

The physical examination should be tailored to the area of tenderness. Inspection of the area for any obvious deformity is the first step. Palpation is helpful in localizing the area of pathology. If this area is large and diffuse, it is more suggestive of muscle strain. If there is a discrete area of tenderness associated with a direct blow, it most likely represents contusion or possible underlying fracture.

Diagnostic testing should be kept to a minimum in the evaluation of soft tissue injuries of the thoracic spine. Plain radiographs are indicated when there is a history of a direct blow or sufficient point tenderness to make the clinician suspicious of an underlying fracture. In the absence of a history or tenderness, plain radiographs of the thoracic spine can be deferred and used only in the evaluation of soft tissue injuries that do not improve with appropriate conservative care.

Ligamentous Strains and Sprains

The treatment of muscle strains of the thoracic spine is similar to that of muscle strains elsewhere in the body. The initial period of inflammation must be controlled to minimize the recovery time; this is accomplished best with cold therapy, such as icing, in the situation of an acute injury. Many injuries may be of insidious onset and are not related to one specific event. When the period of initial inflammation has been controlled, therapy must be directed toward rehabilitation, reconditioning, and return to participation.

Treatment should include stretching to allow return to a normal range of motion as well as muscle strengthening to prevent repeat injury. No specific form of bracing has been reported to be successful in the management of soft tissue sprains or strains of the thoracic spine.

Contusions of the Spine

Contusions of the thoracic spine generally result from a direct blow. The most common mechanism is a football helmet striking directly on the thoracic spine or the paraspinal musculature. Immediate treatment of this sort of injury is icing. The development of significant muscle spasm and subsequent loss of range of motion as well as pain are the aspects that must be considered in treatment. After icing for the initial 48 hours, a program of muscle reconditioning and stretching should be instituted. Depending on the severity of the injury, medications to reduce muscle spasm and inflammation may be helpful.

Rehabilitation and reconditioning of the thoracic spine must emphasize the normal function and motions of this region, which are rotation and lateral flexion and extension. Muscle conditioning and stretching should be targeted at these functions. Initially, isometric muscle contraction is begun while there is still significant pain and loss of range of motion. This isometric muscle contraction is accomplished by having the athlete stand in a door jamb and simulate lateral flexion as well as rotation while standing against the edge of the door, preventing any motion; this should be done only below the threshold of pain. When pain allows, these exercises should be done for 10 seconds with 20 repetitions three times a day. When pain and muscle spasm allow, stretching of the thoracic spine is instituted, again primarily involving lateral flexion and rotation motions. Ballistic stretching is absolutely contraindicated. Lateral stretching is performed in the standing position by flexing the spine laterally while allowing the upper extremity on that side to slide down the lateral aspect of the leg. The position of the hand on the leg is a good gauge of the degree of lateral flexion obtained. Rotational stretching is accomplished in a standing position by rotating the hips and pelvis in one direction while rotating the shoulders and upper trunk in the opposite direction.

Individual flexibility among athletes varies greatly, and no exact guidelines can be given as to how much lateral flexion or rotation can be achieved.

The criteria for return to sports participation after soft tissue injuries of the thoracic spine have not been addressed specifically in the literature. There is no specific method of strength testing that can be done to document adequate rehabilitation. The primary requirements for return to sport are pain control that allows participation and return of sufficient range of motion such that the patient is not risking further injury by splinting of the thoracic spine or inability to protect himself or herself from other sports trauma.

Authors' Preferred Method of Treatment

Our preferred method of treatment for soft tissue injuries of the thoracic spine is initial icing and cold therapy after the acute event. After 48 hours of limiting the inflammatory response, an aggressive rehabilitation program is begun, with muscle strengthening and stretching for range of motion. The athlete is allowed to return to participation as soon as he or she is comfortable enough to engage in workouts and has regained sufficient motion. Protective padding may be used in contact sports in an attempt to make the athlete more comfortable; this varies greatly from one sport to another. In contact sports, the athlete must have regained nearly full motion to be able to protect himself or herself from contact or further injury. In other sports, it may be possible to return to participation with significant deficits of thoracic motion and still compete safely.

Fractures

Three fractures of the thoracic spine occurring in sports bear discussion: fractures of the transverse process or rib bases, compression fractures, and fracture-dislocations.

Fractures of the Transverse Process

Fractures of the transverse processes, or rib bases, in the thoracic spine generally result from a direct blow. This fracture is most likely to occur in contact sports, such as football, or other athletic activities in which collisions may occur. The key portion of the history is the observation or memory of a direct blow to the thoracic spine. The most common mechanism is a football helmet striking posteriorly along the spine. The patient remembers the blow and the immediate onset of pain. This pain may be associated in the acute setting with shortness of breath or painful respirations.

The physical examination reveals tenderness over the area of the fracture. With careful palpation, the clinician may be able to localize the exact site of the fracture. On inspection, the clinician may notice changes in alignment of the spine to allow a more comfortable stance. This alignment change may result in either a scoliosis or a relative kyphosis.

When the area of maximum tenderness has been located, the appropriate diagnostic test is a plain radiograph. Radiographs should be obtained in the anteroposterior and lateral projections. It may be helpful to place a radiopaque marker over the skin at the area of maximum tenderness to allow precise visualization of this area on the radiograph.

If plain radiographs are negative and there is sufficient clinical suspicion based on physical examination, CT scanning may be indicated to determine whether a fracture is present.[50] No other specialized testing is indicated. If a fracture cannot be identified with plain radiographs and CT, further pursuit of this diagnosis with bone scanning or other modalities is rarely indicated.

Treatment and Return to Participation. Treatment options for these fractures consist primarily of local measures. Protection of the area to avoid repeated trauma is universally advocated. This protection may take the form of a flak jacket in a football player or simple padding in other athletes. The fracture pattern is a stable one and does not require any form of bracing or immobilization. The transverse processes and rib bases are enveloped in a series of muscles and fascia that give them good inherent stability. Bracing in most instances only adds to the patient's discomfort.

Rehabilitation of this form of injury is aimed at reducing the discomfort and regaining the normal motion in the thoracic spine. Local measures such as heat and ultrasound may decrease the local soft tissue irritation that accompanies these injuries. As pain allows, a stretching program to regain rotation allows more rapid return to participation. The stretching program must emphasize the normal motions of the thoracic spine. These are primarily rotation, lateral flexion, and, to a lesser degree, flexion and extension. The stretching program is similar to the one outlined for contusions of the thoracic spine. Lateral flexion stretching is done in the standing position by laterally flexing the spine as the hand gradually runs down the ipsilateral leg. This exercise is done on the right and left sides. Rotational lateral stretching is done by rotating the pelvis and hips in one direction while rotating the shoulders and upper trunk in the opposite direction. This must be done in both lateral positions to produce stretching in right and left rotations. True flexion-extension stretching of the thoracic spine is accomplished in the standing position with the thoracic spine and trunk flexed forward over the pelvis, followed by extension of the shoulders. This motion is in concert with motions of the lumbar spine and cannot be isolated to eliminate lumbar spine motion. Protection of the area with padding when the athlete is allowed to return to participation decreases the discomfort should another direct blow be sustained.

Return to participation after these injuries should be guided by the patient's discomfort and range of motion. The radiographic appearance of the fracture often lags behind clinical healing and should not be used as a primary criterion for return to participation. When the athlete has regained normal thoracic motion and is free of pain during activities required by the sport, he or she may be allowed to return to participation. If repeated direct trauma to the area is likely, it should be padded or a protective device should be worn.

Authors' Preferred Method of Treatment. Our preferred method for treating this sort of fracture is initial cold therapy to reduce the local inflammation and soft tissue response. The athlete is initially sore and has significant loss of thoracic motion. When the initial 48 hours has passed, a program of tissue massage, moist heat, and stretching is begun. The intense muscle spasm that accompanies the injuries may be treated with antispasmodic medications. As pain allows, the athlete is allowed to return to participation. In contact sports such as football, the athlete is not allowed to return until the athlete has gained full thoracic motion so that he or she has sufficient ability to protect himself or herself from oncoming players. A specially fitted flak jacket may be worn, or the area can be padded with a combination of soft and rigid materials to provide protection.

Compression Fractures

Compression fractures are the most common fracture in the thoracic region (Fig. 27A–18).[32] This fracture represents a failure of the anterior bone column in compression as a flexion movement is applied to the spine. Most compression fractures occurring in athletics do not produce any posterior comminution of the vertebral body or displacement of bone into the spinal canal, which causes spinal cord injuries. In young athletes, compression fractures require a significant amount of trauma. If no history of significant trauma is present, the practitioner must be suspicious of a preexisting pathologic condition in the vertebral body. This situation may require further evaluation and specialized testing. In older athletes who are just becoming

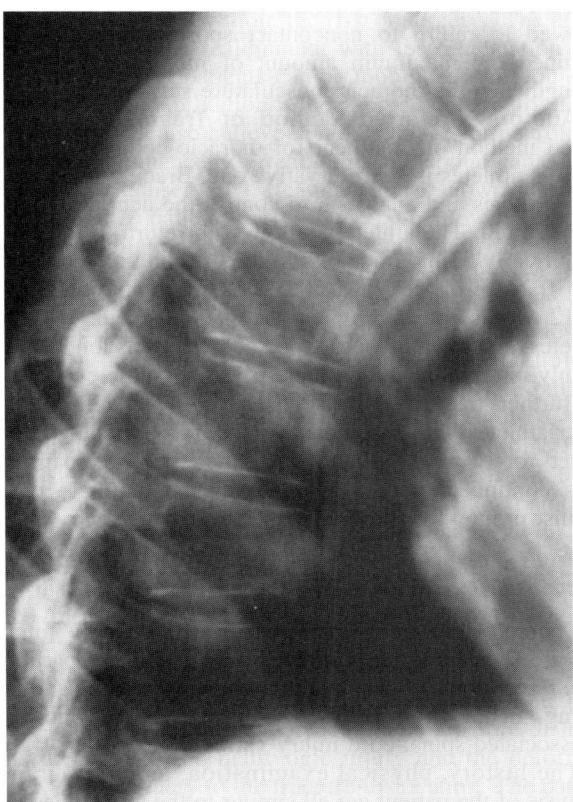

Figure 27A–18. Compression fracture of the thoracic spine.

involved in participation in athletic events, relatively trivial injuries can cause compression fractures in osteoporotic bone.

The key point in the history in an athlete with an acute thoracic compression fracture is the occurrence of the event. Nearly all participants are able to recall an acute event with flexion loading of the thoracic spine or vertical compression of the thoracic spine. In these athletes, a history should be obtained about any transient neurologic deficit that might have occurred. Should there be any history of transient paralysis or paraplegia, it is incumbent on the clinician to evaluate the patient for evidence of an undiagnosed fracture-dislocation or possible soft tissue spinal cord compression or hemorrhage.

On physical examination, the athlete is generally in a protected and mildly kyphotic posture. Percussion over the area of maximum complaint significantly increases the pain. There is a great deal of attendant paraspinal muscle spasm, and the athlete does not allow range-of-motion testing. As in all spinal injuries, it is important to carry out a neurologic examination to eliminate the possibility of spinal cord injury.

Plain radiographs in the anteroposterior and lateral planes make the diagnosis of compression fractures in the thoracic spine. These fractures may be difficult to detect on anteroposterior projection but should be clear on a lateral view (see Fig. 27A–19). The severity of the fracture must be judged according to the amount of compression of the vertebral height. This is done by taking measurements on the lateral radiograph and comparing the measurement of the anterior vertebral body with the height of the body posteriorly as well as the height of the radiograph to rule out two or three contiguous compression fractures; this must be carefully assessed. Many conditions may mislead the clinician into a mistaken diagnosis of acute compression fracture. The most common of these are Scheuermann's kyphosis in young athletes and old compression fractures in older athletes.

Most compression fractures occurring in athletics show less than 25% compression of the anterior vertebral body.[32] As compression of the anterior vertebral body approaches 50%, there are more likely to be associated injuries of the posterior ligamentous structures, or a posterior vertebral body may be forced into the spinal canal.[7] If there is 50% compression of the anterior vertebral body compared with the posterior vertebral height or adjacent anterior vertebral bodies, CT scanning is indicated to evaluate the spinal canal and rule out any spinal canal compromise.

Treatment and Return to Participation. The treatment of thoracic fractures is related directly to the severity. This discussion assumes that the athlete has no evidence of neurologic damage from the compression fracture. All compression fractures of the thoracic spine are painful injuries, and initial management must be aimed at analgesia, prevention of chronic deformity, and fracture healing.

Treatment must be tailored individually to the athlete, the athlete's age, the severity of the fracture, and the sport. In general, compression fractures with less than 25% compression are treated with analgesia, immobilization in a thoracic orthotic device, and exclusion from sports participation until evidence of fracture healing exists. This regimen varies a great deal depending on the patient's age and

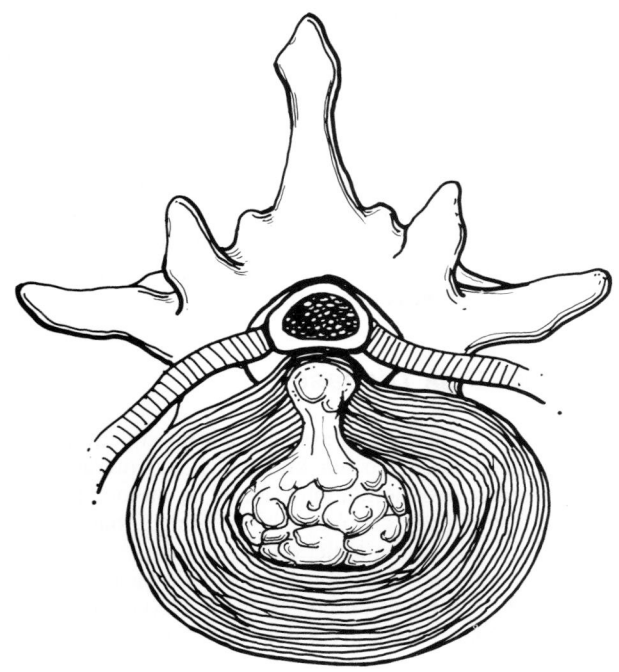

Figure 27A–20. Central thoracic disk herniation.

Treatment and Return to Participation

Treatment of thoracic disk disease requires accurate and correct diagnosis; this has been notoriously difficult to achieve in past years. With the presentation of pain, the disease remains a puzzle, prompting diagnoses of costovertebral joint syndrome, intercostal neuralgia, herpes zoster, or visceral disease. When the patient presents with significant neurologic findings, a diagnosis may be arrived at much more promptly through the use of appropriate diagnostic testing.

The treatment of thoracic disk herniations depends on the clinical syndrome and the disk anatomy. For patients with more lateral disk herniation with a normal neurologic examination and only radicular pain, many authors advocate conservative treatment.[3, 5, 66] Conservative treatment

includes a period of bed rest, the use of analgesics, bracing in a thoracic orthosis, and epidural injections, all prescribed in an attempt to reduce the pain. Surgery is reserved for pain that has not responded to adequate conservative treatment.

The patient with thoracic disk herniation associated with neurologic deficits requires surgical intervention. Many different surgical approaches have been described. Laminectomy with attempted disk excision has been largely discarded because of its poor results.[48] Hulme,[25] in the early 1960s, was the first to report an alternative to laminectomy. He modified the classic costotransversectomy to allow a posterolateral approach to the disk without disturbing the spinal cord. Many authors have further advocated a direct anterior approach to the thoracic disk via thoracotomy with disk removal and fusion. Posterolateral and anterior approaches to the disk appear to offer significantly improved results over laminectomy.

The question of allowing an athlete to return to participation after treatment of thoracic disk disease requires evaluation of the surgical technique used as well as the type of participation required of the athlete. An athlete who has been treated with a posterolateral diskectomy and no fusion should be allowed to return to participation in all athletic endeavors after an adequate rehabilitation program that includes thoracic strengthening and range of motion. After thoracotomy with partial disk excision and fusion, most surgeons do not allow return to contact sports. This judgment is based on the increased risk of adjacent disk injury after fusion and the increased biomechanical requirements of the lever arm in the thoracic region because of the fused segment. When a solid bony fusion has been achieved, however, the athlete could return to all noncontact sports.

Authors' Preferred Method of Treatment and Criteria for Return to Participation

Our preferred method of treatment for a patient with a thoracic disk herniation with no neurologic findings is a period of initial conservative management aimed at reducing the patient's pain. This pain is primarily radicular in nature and should respond to anti-inflammatory medica-

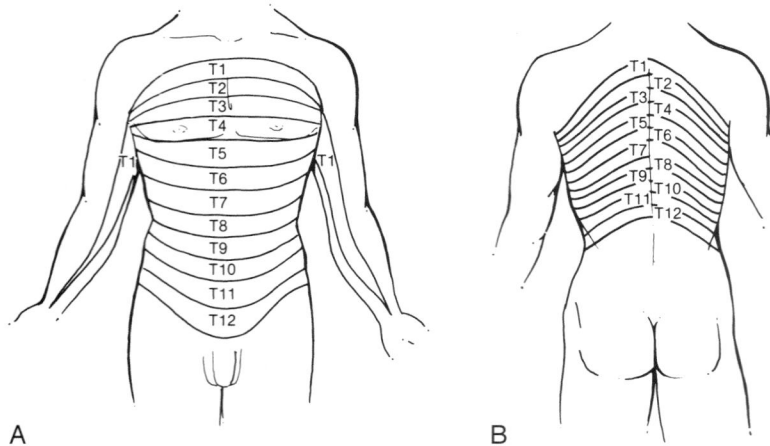

Figure 27A–21. Dermatomal representation of chest wall. *A*, Anteroposterior view. *B*, Posterior view.

tions, physical therapy, bracing, or direct injection therapy. The radicular pain should have decreased in intensity within several days of beginning oral anti-inflammatory medication. If this is not the case, selective nerve blocks should be undertaken to relieve the radicular pain further.

Return to sports participation after treatment for thoracic disk herniation depends on the treatment. After conservative treatment for a lateral herniation, the athlete may return to participation as soon as his or her discomfort has subsided and the athlete has regained sufficient range of motion to protect himself or herself in athletic competition. After surgical treatment for thoracic disk disease with a diskectomy and fusion, the athlete is not allowed to return to contact sports. Return to noncontact participation is allowed as soon as there is evidence of a solid fusion and the athlete has been rehabilitated to regain maximum thoracic motion.

In patients with neurologic findings and a central disk herniation, there is no question that surgical treatment is indicated. We prefer the anterior approach via thoracotomy with disk excision and anterior fusion using a rib, which is removed at the time of thoracotomy. Postoperatively, patients are immobilized in a TLSO until there is evidence of bony fusion. The patient is not allowed to return to contact sports.

Kyphosis and Scoliosis

Deformity in the thoracic spine may be seen in young athletes. This is not the result of athletic participation but may lead to many questions concerning participation in sports by athletes with ongoing spinal deformity and the choice of appropriate treatment for the underlying deformity. Kyphosis and scoliosis are covered together in this section because of their similarities in the athlete.

Scoliosis (Fig. 27A–22) can be classified by its cause, which has been subdivided into congenital, neuromuscular, and idiopathic components. Congenital scoliosis is caused by a defect in the physical structure of the spine that is present from birth. The two major categories are failure of segmentation and failure of formation in the spine. Neuromuscular scoliosis implies scoliosis secondary to any abnormality of neuromuscular function. Examples include poliomyelitis, spinal muscle atrophy, post-traumatic paraplegia, and muscular dystrophies. By far the largest group of scolioses is idiopathic in nature. Although a great deal of research and effort has been put into clarifying the underlying cause of the idiopathic scolioses, no clear positive factors have been identified.

Kyphosis in adolescent athletes similarly may be subdivided into congenital, neuromuscular, and postural types and Scheuermann's disease. Failures of formation or segmentation in the thoracic spine can lead to congenital kyphosis. Similarly, neuromuscular disorders may cause kyphosis, including cerebral palsy, myelomeningocele, syringomyelia, polio, spinal muscle atrophy, and dysautonomia.[76] The leading cause of kyphosis in adolescents is postural kyphosis or juvenile round-back. These are benign conditions of adolescence and should not be confused with Scheuermann's disease, which is a distinct clinical entity with an unknown cause.[1]

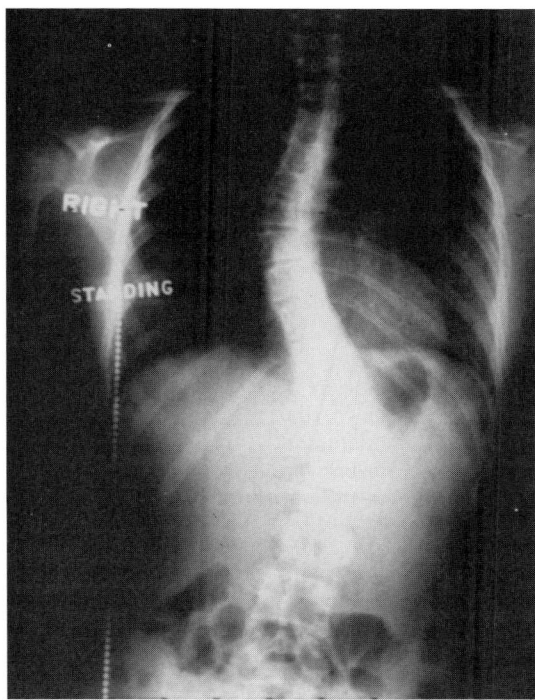
Figure 27A–22. Anteroposterior radiograph of spinal scoliosis.

Adolescent athletes with spinal deformity rarely come to the attention of the clinician as a result of an injury. More likely, questions arise about participation of an athlete with a preexisting deformity, or the deformity may be found serendipitously when an athlete is evaluated for another spinal problem.

Physical examination of the spine in an athlete with a deformity should include all the essentials of a good examination. The first of these is inspection, which may often give a hint of the deformity. In the kyphotic patient, a round back and stooped shoulders may be noted. In a scoliotic athlete, some deformity of shoulder height may be noted, the pelvis may not be level, or there may be a significant thoracic prominence. Palpation of the spine often confirms the presence of a deformity. A neurologic examination should be performed to rule out any associated neurologic changes. Leg length should be evaluated because leg-length inequality may be a cause of spinal deformity.

The diagnosis of spinal deformity is confirmed by plain radiographs of the spine. These films should be obtained with the athlete standing and initially should include the entire spine in anteroposterior and lateral projections. The deformity can be quantified by construction of the Cobb angle (Fig. 27A–23), measuring the maximally tipped vertebrae in scoliosis or the maximally kyphotic vertebrae in kyphosis. No further diagnostic studies are routinely warranted in the initial evaluation of spinal deformity.

Treatment and Sports Participation

Treatment of spinal deformity is beyond the scope of this chapter. It is important, however, for clinicians to have

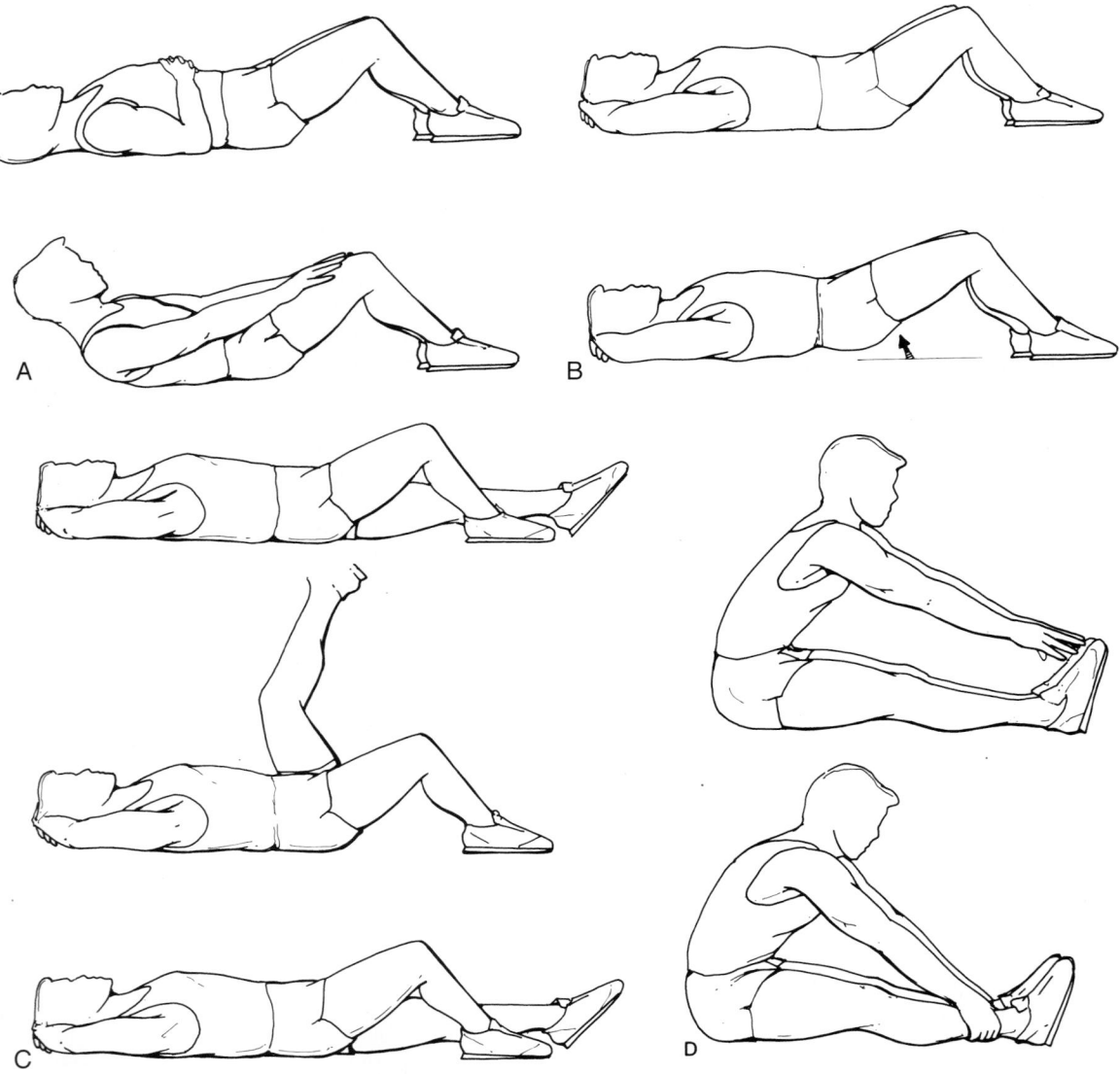

Figure 27A–26. *A*, Half sit-up. *B*, Pelvic tilt. *C*, Straight leg raise. *D*, Hamstring stretch.

for abdominal stretching includes knee-to-chest raises, elbow prop-up, press-ups, and hip hyperextension (Fig. 27A–27). The exact regimen for these exercises must be tailored individually to each athlete. It is essential that the exercises be done at least every day, and they are usually prescribed three times a day for the athlete in the rehabilitation phase. At the initial prescription, the clinician should run through each exercise with the athlete to ensure that none of the exercises increase the athlete's pain. If any exercise seems to exacerbate pain, this exercise is left out of the regimen. Each exercise initially is performed for five repetitions. This number is increased to 15 repetitions as the athlete becomes capable of performing them.

The exercise and stretching regimen for the posterior paraspinal muscles is similar. Strengthening exercises include press-ups, hip hyperextension, and pelvic tilt. Stretching is accomplished through the knee-to-chest raise and single-leg raise.

It is essential that the hamstring musculature not be left

out of any program of lumbar spine rehabilitation and conditioning. Hamstring stretching should be performed with each set of lumbar spine exercises. This should not be ballistic stretching. Hamstring strengthening is important and is accomplished by using a leg-curl machine in the prone position.

Deep tissue massage and manipulation have been advocated by many authors in the treatment of lumbar spine musculoligamentous injuries. This treatment is controversial, but there is no question that in some hands it has beneficial effects. No surgical treatment is indicated for musculoligamentous injuries of the lumbar spine.

Return to sports participation after ligamentous strains and sprains of the lumbar spine requires an individualized program that is set up in light of the requirements of the individual athlete and the particular sport. In general, athletes are allowed to begin light participation and light workouts as soon as their pain allows. As the muscle spasm decreases and the range of motion increases, athletes

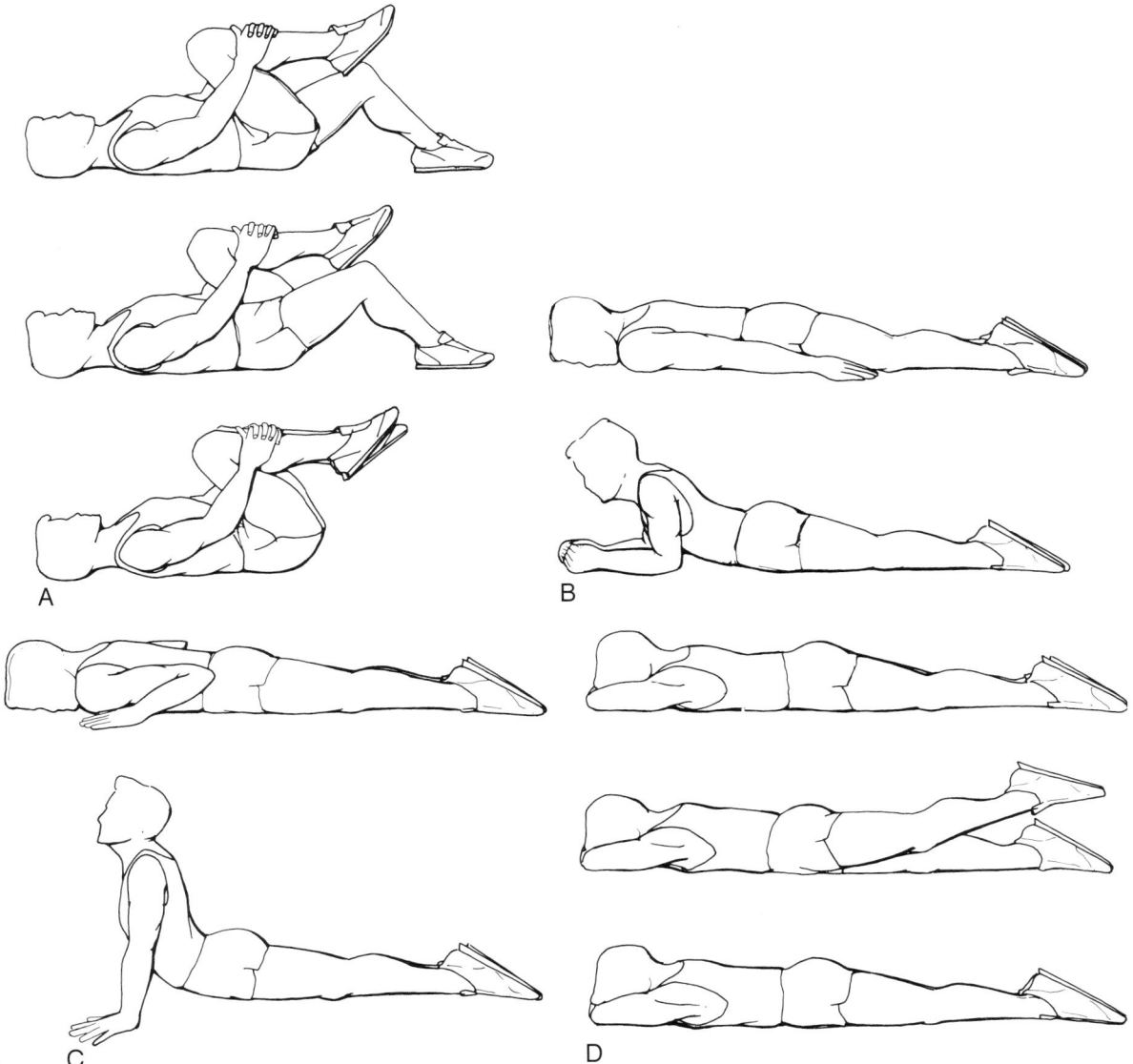

Figure 27A–27. *A*, Knee-to-chest raise. *B*, Elbow prop-up. *C*, Press-up. *D*, Hip hyperextension.

gradually increase their activities and the duration of workouts. Generally, the pain and limitation of motion automatically limit the participants' activities until they are ready to return. In contact sports such as football, the pain need not have resolved completely but should be manageable with modality treatments to allow participation. The range of motion must have returned to a sufficient degree to allow the athlete to protect himself or herself in contact activities. The athlete may be allowed to compete in a lightweight, lumbosacral corset-type brace as an intermediary during return to full participation.

Authors' Preferred Method of Treatment

Our preferred method of treatment for athletes with lumbar spine musculoligamentous injuries is aimed initially at minimizing and decreasing the attendant muscle spasm. In the acute setting, this treatment involves icing, antispas-

modics, and use of a lightweight lumbosacral corset for support. As the muscle spasm is reduced, the patient is begun on modality treatments, including moist heat and an active exercise program emphasizing stretching, abdominal muscle strengthening, and paraspinal muscular strengthening. The athlete is allowed to return to participation as soon as the pain has subsided sufficiently to allow it and adequate motion has been regained to allow protection.

Fractures

Fractures of the lumbar spine are relatively rare in athletes. Fractures occur in only a few athletes with back problems.[34] Fractures of the lumbar spine must be classified in a manner that allows rational treatment based on that classification. Many classification systems are based on mechanism of injury and spine stability.

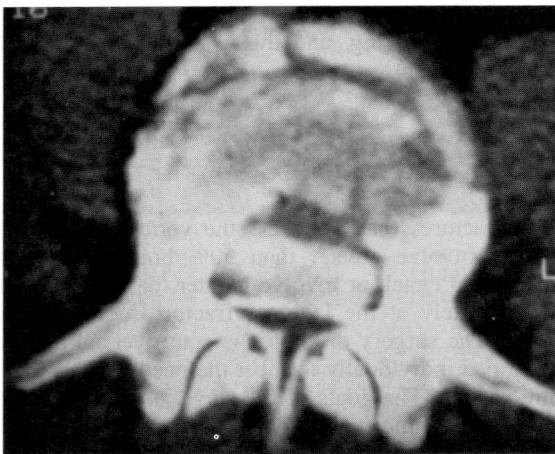

Figure 27A–29. Computed tomographic scan of lumbar burst fracture.

Anterior and Posterior Column Fractures

Flexion distraction injuries of the lumbar spine represent failure of the anterior column under a compressive load in flexion with failure of the posterior column ligamentous structures in distraction. These are fractures that previously have been classified as seat-belt injuries and Chance fractures. These injuries are uncommon in athletic participation. The key to their treatment is the determination of stability or instability caused by the fracture. In general, fractures that involve bony injuries to the posterior, middle, and anterior columns are considered stable and may be treated with bed rest followed by immobilization and bracing. Fractures that involve bony injury to the anterior column with ligamentous or disk injury in the middle and posterior columns are acutely unstable. The criteria for which of these fractures requires surgical intervention are still evolving. This decision is based on the potential instability of the spine created by a ligamentous injury posteriorly. This potential is judged best by the degree of anterior vertebral compression and the divergence of the spinous processes posteriorly. If there is more than 50% compression of the anterior column or greater than a 20-degree acute kyphosis, surgical treatment must be considered.

Fracture-Dislocations

Fracture-dislocations of the lumbar spine (Fig. 27A–30) are the rarest of all sports injuries. These are extremely high-energy injuries that require sufficient force to disrupt all three columns of the spine with subsequent dislocation of one vertebra over another. The injuries often involve damage to the cauda equina, and decision making regarding treatment must take into account the patient's neurologic status. Because of the lack of inherent stability of the lumbar spine compared with the thoracic spine, all fracture-dislocations require surgical stabilization. The treatment of choice is most often a combined anterior and posterior procedure emphasizing open reduction of the spine with instrumentation and fusion to stabilize it. The neurologic status of the patient must be considered, and care must be taken not to disrupt further any damaged nerve roots.

Rehabilitation after fractures requires consideration of the fracture pattern, its stability, and the desired athletic participation of the individual. The overall goal of rehabilitation in all of these injuries is to regain sufficient function to allow the athlete to compete without pain. This involves strengthening the paraspinal and abdominal muscles as well as stretching to maximize the range of motion. After fractures resulting from direct trauma, rehabilitation is centered on protecting the previously fractured area and regaining muscular strength with range of motion. This involves wearing some protective padding over the area if contact is likely. A prefabricated flak jacket or a simple combination of soft and rigid protective padding may be used. When the athlete is sufficiently pain-free to have regained normal range of motion, he or she may be returned to all noncontact activities. Contact activities are not allowed until there is evidence of fracture healing, either by loss of tenderness at the fracture site or by radiographs.

Rehabilitation and criteria for return to sports participation are similar for compression fractures of the lumbar spine, which are treated conservatively with bracing. The athlete must be sufficiently pain-free to allow participation, and there should be radiographic evidence of no further collapse at the fracture level. A vigorous exercise program is begun, including strengthening of the lumbar and abdominal musculature and return of normal lumbar motion. When these goals have been accomplished, the athlete may return to all participation in contact or noncontact sports.

After surgical treatment of lumbar fractures with instrumentation and fusion, rehabilitation is more arduous. It follows a period of 12 weeks of immobilization in a TLSO. Initially, as the athlete is weaned from the orthosis, a program of reconditioning, cardiovascular fitness, and stretching is begun. As long as the patient's pain allows, he or she progresses through the muscle-strengthening and range-of-motion program. When the discomfort has been alleviated, and the athlete has regained maximum motion, the athlete is allowed to return to noncontact sports. After instrumentation and fusion of the spine, contact sports are prohibited.

Authors' Preferred Method of Treatment

Our preferred method of treatment for lumbar spine fractures encompasses the general guidelines given previously. For fractures of the transverse or spinous process resulting from a direct blow, treatment is aimed at reducing the athlete's discomfort and allowing the fracture to heal; this initially involves a period of cold therapy, followed by some analgesics and immobilization in a soft corset or brace. When the discomfort allows, the patient is allowed to begin a cardiovascular fitness program through bicycling in a brace or water exercising. As the pain subsides, a vigorous program of reconditioning and range-of-motion exercises is begun. When normal motion has been resumed, the athlete is returned to participation.

Our treatment of lumbar compression fractures with less than a 50% vertebral height loss is similar to the treatment we use for transverse process and spinous process fractures; this initially involves bracing in a TLSO to prevent further collapse of the fracture or the creation of late deformity.

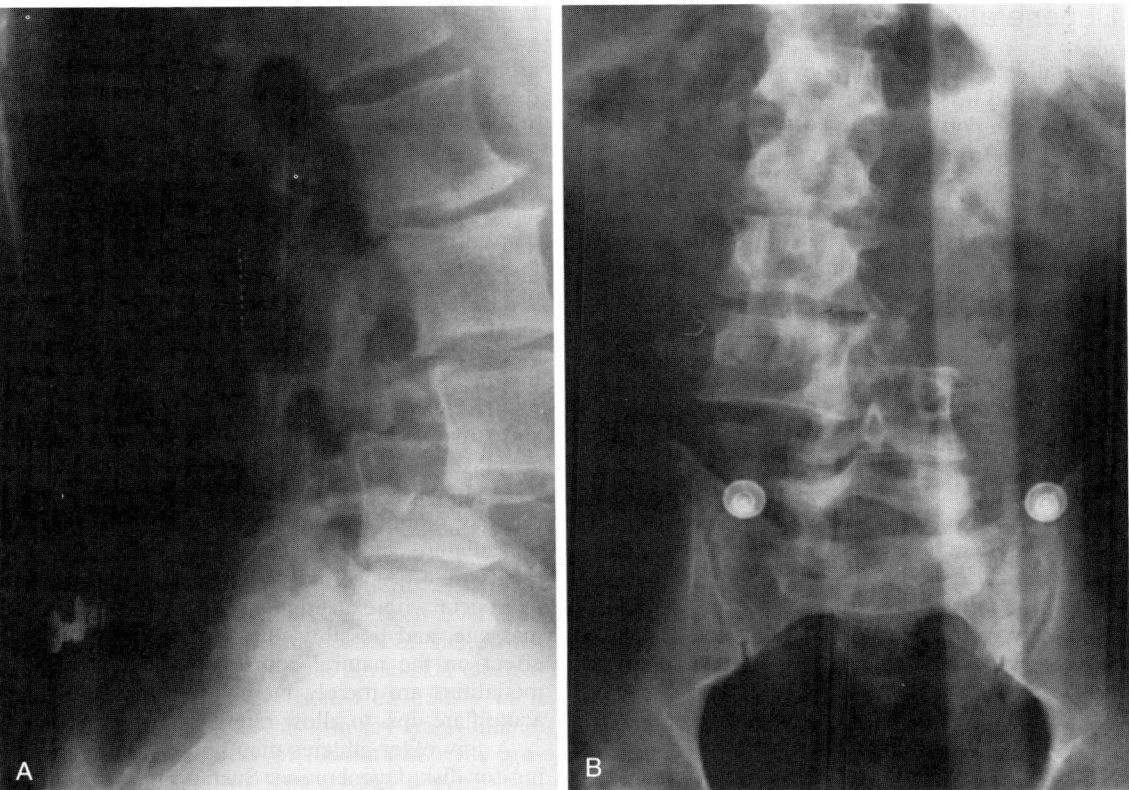

Figure 27A–30. Fracture-dislocation of the lumbar spine. *A*, Side view. *B*, Front view.

Bracing is maintained for a length of time based on the preexisting bone quality and the patient's age. In young athletes with normal bone stock, bracing may be maintained for 4 to 6 weeks. In older athletes with osteoporosis in whom there is a greater chance of deformity, bracing is maintained for 12 weeks. After this period, a rehabilitation and stretching program is begun as outlined earlier. For compression fractures with more than 50% anterior vertebral height loss, we prefer surgical treatment with combined anterior and posterior decompression and stabilization to minimize the number of vertebral bodies fused, followed by mobilization in a TLSO. As previously mentioned, surgical treatment precludes a return to contact sports.

In patients with flexion distraction injuries of the lumbar spine, we individualize the treatment to the exact fracture pattern. The true Chance fracture, or bone injury through all three columns of the spine, can be treated with a TLSO and mobilization of the patient as he or she becomes comfortable. When the posterior column injury is a ligamentous one with the creation of an acute kyphosis greater than 20 degrees, we believe posterior compression instrumentation and fusion is indicated, followed by mobilization in a TLSO.

When a lumbar spine fracture is treated nonoperatively, the patient is allowed to return to full participation. Patients requiring instrumentation and fusion are prohibited from contact sports. Lumbar spine fractures that are treated with instrumentation and fusion require at least three levels of fusion. There is an increased biomechanical lever arm force exerted across the disk space and joints at the levels above and below this instrumented and fused segment. Athletes have an increased risk of injury at those levels, and the prohibition from contact sports is enforced strictly in our patients. In the rare athlete with a lumbar spine fracture-dislocation, we use open reduction and internal fixation with combined anterior and posterior instrumentation and fusion. This treatment precludes the athlete from returning to contact sports. The athlete may return to noncontact sports and recreational activities as function allows.

Lumbar Disk Disease

The continuum of degeneration and herniation of lumbar discs that occurs in all individuals is also present in athletes. The disk represents a living tissue that undergoes loss of water content and degeneration with aging. As the water content is lost, more of the stress in the disk is transferred to the anulus fibrosis, causing radial tears that provide the site for potential herniations as well as localized back pain.

Disk disease is common in athletes and may result from degeneration of the disk with attendant low back pain or disk herniation with radicular symptoms. It is important for the clinician caring for athletes to be able to differentiate the low back pain associated with disk degeneration and radicular leg pain from disk herniation and nerve root compression.

nerve roots is being compressed directly, placing it under tension increases the pain down the leg. For the upper lumbar nerve roots (L2, L3, L4), the femoral nerve root tension sign is a sensitive indicator of nerve root compression. This test is performed with the patient prone on the table by flexing the knee to 90 degrees and extending the hip. This test is considered positive if it reproduces radicular pain down the anterior thigh. Sciatic and femoral nerve tension signs should be tested bilaterally and reported as positive or negative.

Any patient with neurologic findings in the lower extremities or a history of bowel or bladder incontinence should undergo a neurologic evaluation of the sacral nerve roots. This evaluation involves testing sensation around the anus and scrotum in a male; anal sensation is checked in a female. The motor function of the sacral nerve roots is related primarily to the anal sphincter. Sphincter tone should be checked through a rectal examination as well as by asking the patient to contract the sphincter against a finger in the rectum. This portion of the examination often is deferred, but it is an essential part of evaluation of a patient with lower extremity neurologic deficits.

Diagnostic testing for lumbar disk herniations requires a modality that can visualize the lumbar discs, spinal canal, and lumbar nerve roots. Because of this requirement, plain radiographs are of little use in evaluating disk herniation and radicular leg pain with or without neurologic deficits. The mainstays of this evaluation are myelography, CT scanning and MRI (Fig. 27A–32). The standard against which all other tests must be measured continues to be the combination of lumbar myelography with postmyelographic CT scanning. With the evolution of MRI, it appears that this test is a sensitive and specific indicator of lumbar disk problems in young individuals. It is still a matter of preference of the clinician as to whether MRI is undertaken as the initial evaluation or CT scanning is used instead. Myelography generally is reserved for further delineation of a specific lesion and should be used only as a preoperative planning tool.

Treatment. Treatment of lumbar disk herniation in athletes requires appropriate diagnostic studies to arrive at the correct diagnosis as well as a treatment regimen aimed at reducing pain and allowing an early return to athletic participation. The early management of acute disk herniation should involve a program of bed rest in the position of greatest comfort, along with medication to relieve the pain and reduce muscle spasm.

Most athletes find that they are more comfortable in the supine position with a pillow under the knees to flex the hips slightly; this decreases the radicular leg pain. Anti-inflammatory medications help to control pain. In many athletes, it may be necessary to supplement these medications with narcotic analgesics. During this initial period of bed rest and medication, it is important to monitor the patient carefully for evidence of neurologic deterioration. A progressive neurologic deficit may indicate the need for early surgery.

In the athlete who fails to respond to initial conservative treatment of bed rest and analgesics, the next possibility is an epidural injection to ameliorate the sciatica. A combination of steroid medications and narcotics may be injected into the epidural space to relieve the pain and local inflammation. This injection has been controversial in terms of long-term effect, but there appears to be no question that it reduces the acute pain from disk herniation.[69] The epidural injection should not be expected to have any immediate effect on the neurologic deficit.

When the pain has been controlled, either through bed rest and analgesics or by epidural injection, the patient can be mobilized and started on a physical therapy program that emphasizes extension exercises and reconditioning.[19] Failure of conservative treatment is indicated when sufficient pain relief is not achieved or there is evidence of a progressive neurologic deficit. The duration of conservative treatment varies from athlete to athlete.[8] In general, if there has not been sufficient pain relief to allow resumption of day-to-day activities without the use of oral narcotic

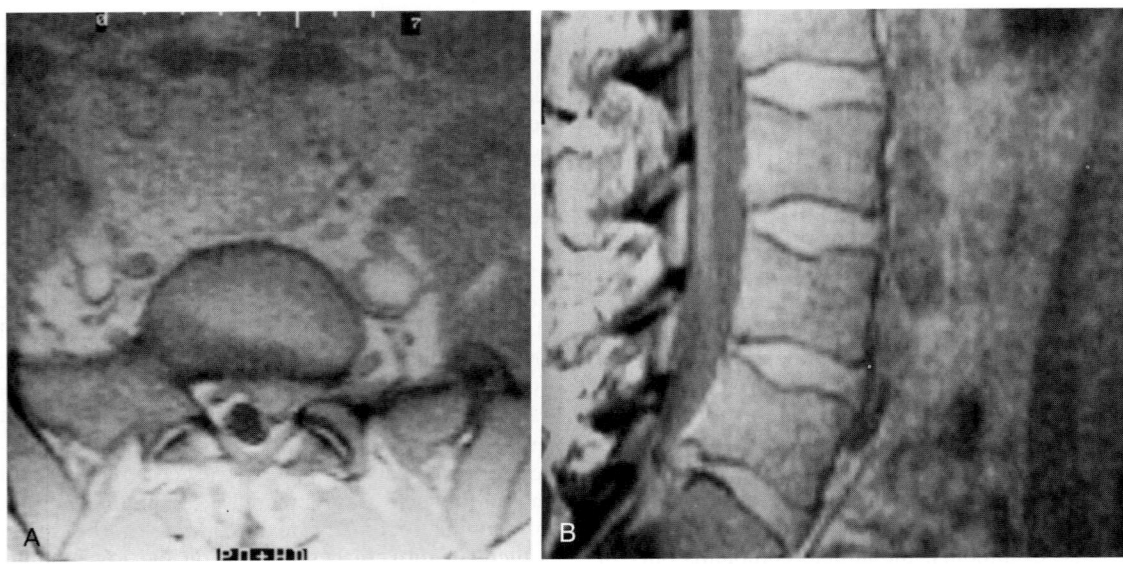

Figure 27A–32. Magnetic resonance imaging scans of lumbar disk herniation. *A,* Axial view. *B,* Sagittal view.

medications within 6 weeks, another source of treatment should be considered.

There are many variations of intervention treatment for lumbar disk herniation, including injection therapy into the disk with an enzyme to attempt to resolve the disk, percutaneous diskectomy with radiographic control, microsurgical diskectomy, and traditional hemilaminotomy with disk excision. Each of these techniques has advocates and detractors in the literature.

Chemonucleolysis with enzyme to dissolve the disk has been largely discontinued in the United States. There are still some advocates of this treatment, but its inferior long-term results and risks of anaphylactic reaction or toxicity have led to a decrease in popularity.

Automated percutaneous diskectomy is a less invasive alternative in the treatment of lumbar disk herniation. Advocates say it is indicated for patients who have a prolapsed, herniated disk without evidence of free fragment herniation.[40] Automated percutaneous diskectomy is contraindicated when sequestered disk fragments are present. It is contraindicated when there is evidence of secondary bony narrowing of the spinal canal associated with disk herniation. This procedure involves placement of a cannula into the disk space through a posterolateral portal. The disk is evacuated with punch forceps and suction or an automated probe. The theoretical advantage of this technique is the lack of an open surgical procedure, an outpatient stay in the hospital, and no direct manipulation of the nerve root or epidural space. The surgical results of this procedure do not compare favorably with open microsurgical diskectomy. Automated percutaneous diskectomy must be approached with caution because it may not result in significant resolution of symptoms and may lead to a second interventional procedure.

Microsurgical diskectomy initially was popularized by Williams in 1978.[72] The guidelines for this technique are avoidance of laminectomy and trauma to the facets; preservation of normal extradural fat; a blunt perforation of the anulus fibrosis; and preservation of healthy, nonherniated intervertebral disk by removing only sufficient disk to relieve compression on the nerve root. Advocates point out that microsurgical diskectomy involves decreased operative time, decreased morbidity, less blood loss, and a shorter stay in the hospital. Microsurgical diskectomy adds the additional risk of a limited exposure and incomplete decompression. The long-term results of microsurgical diskectomy have been excellent and equal to the previous results of traditional laminotomy and diskectomy.

Rehabilitation after lumbar disk herniation must be directed toward return to the type of sports participation desired and to the treatment that has been rendered. If conservative treatment has yielded a satisfactory result in terms of decreased pain and no further neurologic deterioration, the athlete may be started on an exercise regimen that includes extension exercises as well as generalized back conditioning and stretching. When the pain has been relieved sufficiently to allow the athlete to return to participation, the athlete is allowed to return as long as he or she regains normal motion. After surgical diskectomy, the rehabilitation process is longer and more arduous. Initially, the patient is allowed to ambulate on the first postoperative day. Then the athlete is taken through a program involving

progressively longer distances to regain muscle strength and stamina. At 4 weeks after surgery, the athlete is begun on a program of back reconditioning and strengthening, including exercises in flexion and extension as well as a stretching program to restrengthen the back and regain its range of motion. Provided that the athlete has had a good surgical result, at 6 weeks he or she is allowed to return to noncontact sports participation. Return to contact sports participation, specifically football, must be decided on an individual basis. The general criteria are pain relief that allows participation plus a return to normal range of motion. In the case of significant lower extremity neurologic deficits, strength must have been regained in that extremity.

Authors' Preferred Method of Treatment. Our preferred method of treatment for lumbar disk herniation is an initial course of conservative care, combining bed rest in a position of maximum comfort with anti-inflammatory medications and analgesics. If this approach does not lead to significant pain relief by 1 week, an epidural injection combining narcotics and steroid medications is performed. When adequate pain relief has been achieved, the athlete is begun on an exercise program that emphasizes extension exercises, stretching, and muscle restrengthening in the lumbar spine.

Early surgery is reserved for patients with a cauda equina syndrome or the development of a progressive neurologic deficit despite nonoperative treatment. Should either of these conditions be present, surgery is performed as early as possible. In the absence of these problems, the relative indications for surgery include intolerable pain, severe postural list, and persistent pain that compromises the athlete's ability to perform daily tasks and recreational activities. Surgery for these indications must be tempered by the fact that long-term follow-up indicates no better results after surgery than conservative treatment.[68] We do not consider a static neurologic deficit to be an absolute indication for surgery.

In an athlete who meets the criteria for surgery of a herniated lumbar intervertebral disk, open microdiskectomy is our treatment of choice. We believe that this procedure produces the most reliable result, and although some of the other techniques appear promising, no adequate long-term follow-up study has documented their superiority to standard lumbar diskectomy. After microdiskectomy, the athlete should be able to return to any athletic endeavor. The criteria for such a return are based on neurologic recovery as well as rehabilitation of the surgical region in the lumbar spine. The criteria for neurologic recovery require that the athlete have regained sufficient muscle strength and sensation in the affected lower extremity to participate safely. For instance, an athlete with residual peroneal muscle weakness from an L4–L5 disk herniation is predisposed to a possible ankle sprain until those stabilizers of the ankle have been rehabilitated adequately. The criteria for rehabilitation of the lumbar spine are return of adequate motion that allows the athlete to protect himself in his particular sport and pain that has subsided enough to allow him to participate adequately. Typically, our patients return to limited workouts about a month after surgical diskectomy and are allowed to return to full participation at 6 to 8 weeks.

be allowed back into the gym to begin a graduated workout program that included no hyperextension and no impact loading. At the end of another 2 weeks, if the gymnast were still symptom-free, she would be allowed to begin exercises involving impact loading, such as running and landing from a dismount. Assuming that no symptoms returned with this activity, the gymnast would be allowed to return to full participation at the end of another 2 weeks.

The rehabilitation of a patient with long-standing spondylolysis and a relapse of back pain is different because one cannot expect the spondylolytic defect to heal in that individual. The patient is immobilized for a shorter period of time and only to relieve the acute pain and spasm. As soon as the pain has subsided, the patient is begun on a rehabilitation program emphasizing strengthening of the abdominal musculature, spinal range of motion, and hamstring stretching. This is the same treatment program used for a patient with recurrent back pain and evidence of spondylolisthesis.

Rehabilitation after lumbar spine surgery for spondylolisthesis is delayed until there is evidence of solid bone union. At that time, bracing is stopped, and the patient is started on a gradually increasing program of activity. This activity is combined with a program of muscle strengthening and reconditioning for the lumbar spine and abdominal musculature. When that program has begun and there is no recurrence of back pain, a range-of-motion program is initiated to regain the maximum lumbar motion. Return to participation may be limited by the athlete's loss of flexibility and loss of motion secondary to fusion.

The criteria for return to participation with a stress fracture or stress reaction of the pars interarticularis require that the athlete be pain-free and have regained lumbar motion. Despite the desire of these athletes to return to participation, it should be stressed to them that, in these early stages of the disease, there is a chance of bone healing and a chance to prevent possible chronic, long-term spinal problems.

In the athlete with established spondylolysis, return to participation may be much quicker. There is little chance of bone healing in this lesion, and return to sports should be allowed as soon as the pain and spasm have subsided and the athlete has regained motion in the lumbar spine.

Participation in sports should not be limited solely on the basis of spondylolisthesis. There are many documented cases of professional athletes with established spondylolisthesis participating in contact sports. Participation does not appear to represent a risk of progression of the lesion or any neurologic sequelae. Controversy exists about how to manage the athlete with established spondylolisthesis and evidence of progression from one stage to another. At this time, there is no evidence that progression from stage I to stage II spondylolisthesis represents a reason for exclusion from any sporting activity, including contact sports. There is no evidence documenting this progression as an increased risk factor for the development of neurologic sequelae or an acute fracture. These athletes often are limited in sports participation by recurrent episodes of back pain and limitation of function.

Authors' Preferred Method of Treatment

Our preferred method of treatment for stress reaction or stress fractures of the pars interarticularis in the athlete is

cessation of sporting activities and bracing in a lumbosacral orthosis with a small amount of flexion. This approach requires avoidance of all impact loading in the lumbosacral spine as well as all hyperextension activities. Bracing is continued until the athlete is pain-free or for a minimum of 6 weeks. The duration of bracing depends on the amount of pain, the age of the athlete, and the acuteness of the symptoms. In general, a younger athlete with more acute symptoms can be expected to experience pain relief over a shorter interval than an older athlete with more chronic symptoms. During this period of bracing, the athlete is allowed to maintain cardiovascular fitness by bicycling on a stationary bicycle with the brace in place or deep water running. When the pain has subsided, a graduated return to activities is allowed, as outlined earlier in the rehabilitation section.

We treat established spondylolysis and spondylolisthesis in the athlete with acute intervention at the time of back symptoms. Treatment is aimed at reducing the acute pain and spasm and involves short-term immobilization in a lightweight lumbosacral corset, along with the use of antispasmodic and anti-inflammatory medications. Modality treatments and stretching are begun as soon as the athlete is comfortable. Then, as the pain and muscle spasm subside, the athlete is allowed an early return to sporting participation.

Surgical treatment of spondylolisthesis is rare in athletes. Surgery is reserved for patients with spondylolisthesis with associated radicular symptoms or high-grade (grades III or IV) slippage. At this time, we advocate adequate decompressive laminectomy for the patient with radicular complaints associated with in situ fusion from a posterior approach. In surgery for grade III or IV spondylolisthesis, no attempt is made at reduction, but adequate stabilization may require a posterior instrumentation system for rigid internal fixation. Alternatively, a combination of anterior and posterior surgery occasionally is used.

Summary

Serious injuries of the thoracolumbar spine are rare secondary to athletic participation. Most injuries are musculoligamentous strains or sprains. Appropriate conservative management of these injuries with good rehabilitation leads to gratifying results.

As with all athletic injuries, prevention of spinal injuries should be stressed whenever possible. Prevention involves an active preparticipation conditioning program with an emphasis on stretching, strengthening of the abdominal and paraspinal muscles, and counseling about proper technique and body mechanics.

References

1. Aufdermur J: Juvenile kyphosis: Radiography, histology and pathogenesis. Clin Orthop 154:166, 1981.
2. Bedbrook AM: Spinal injuries and tetraplegia and paraplegia. J Bone Joint Surg Br 61:267, 1979.
3. Benson M, Byrnes OP: The clinical syndromes and surgical treatment

of thoracic intervertebral disc prolapse. J Bone Joint Surg Br 57: 471, 1975.

4. Bohlman HH: Traumatic fractures of the upper thoracic spine with paralysis. J Bone Joint Surg Am 56:1299, 1974.
5. Borenstein OG, Wiesel SW: Low Back Pain. Philadelphia, WB Saunders, 1986.
6. Boxau D, Bradford D, Winter R, Moe J: Management of severe spondylolisthesis in children and adolescents. J Bone Joint Surg Am 61:479, 1979.
7. Burke D, Murray D: The management of thoracic and thoracolumbar injuries of the spine with neurologic involvement. J Bone Joint Surg Am 58:72, 1976.
8. Cacayorin ED, Hochhauser L, Petro GR: Lumbar and thoracic spine pain in the athlete: Radiographic evaluation. Clin Sports Med 6: 767–783, 1987.
9. Day A, Friedman W, and Indelicato P: Observations on the treatment of lumbar disc disease in college football players. Am J Sports Med 15:72, 1987.
10. Denis F: Spinal instability so defined by the three-column spine concept in acute spinal trauma. Clin Orthop 189:65, 1984.
11. Dickson J, Harrington P, Erwin W: Results of reduction and stabilization of the severely fractured thoracic and lumbar spine. J Bone Joint Surg Am 60:799, 1978.
12. Dunn HK: Anterior stabilization of thoracolumbar injuries. Clin Orthop 189:716, 1984.
13. Edwards CC, Levine AM: Early rod sleeve stabilization of the injured thoracic and lumbar spine. Orthop Clin North Am 17:121, 1986.
14. Eismont FJ, Currier B: Surgical management of lumbar intervertebral disc disease. J Bone Joint Surg Am 71:1266, 1989.
15. Elliott HC: Cross-sectional diameters and areas of the human spinal cord. Anat Rec 93:287, 1945.
16. Ferguson R, McMaster J, Stanitski C: Low back pain in college football lineman. Am J Sports Med 2:63, 1974.
17. Flesch J, Leider L, Erickson D, et al: Harrington instrumentation and spine fusion for unstable fractures and fracture-dislocations of the thoracic and lumbar spine. J Bone Joint Surg Am 59:143, 1977.
18. Galanta JD: Tensile property of the human lumbar annulus fibrosus. Acta Orthop Scand 100:1–91, 1967.
19. Grutch A: Herniated lumbar disc associated with running. Am J Sports Med 9:155, 1981.
20. Haughton VM: MR imaging of the spine. Radiology 166:297, 1988.
21. Hellstrom M, Jacobsson B, Sward L, Peterson L: Radiologic abnormalities of the thoraco-lumbar spine in athletes. Acta Radiol 31: 127–132, 1990.
22. Herkowitz HN, Samberg LC: Vertebral column injuries associated with tobogganing. J Trauma 18:806–810, 1978.
23. Holdsworth F: Fractures, dislocations and fracture-dislocations of the spine. J Bone Joint Surg Am 52:1534, 1970.
24. Holt EP: The question of lumbar discography. J Bone Joint Surg Am 50:720–726, 1968.
25. Hulme A: The surgical approach to thoracic intervertebral disc protrusions. J Neurol Neurosurg Psychiatry 23:133, 1960.
26. Jackson D: Low back pain in young athletes. Am J Sports Med 7: 364, 1979.
27. Jackson D, Wiltse L, Dingeman R, Hayes M: Stress reactions involving the pars interarticularis in young athletes. Am J Sports Med 9: 305, 1981.
28. Jacobs RR, Asher MA, Snider RK: Thoracolumbar spine injuries. Spine 5:463, 1986.
29. Jacobs RR, Casey MP: Surgical management of thoracolumbar spinal injuries. Clin Orthop 189:22, 1984.
30. Kaneda K, Abunu K, Fijiya M: Burst fractures with neurologic deficits of the thoracolumbar spine: Results of anterior decompression and stabilization with anterior instrumentation. Spine 9:788, 1984.
31. Keene J: Radiographic evaluation of thoracolumbar fractures. Clin Orthop 189:58, 1984.
32. Keene J: Thoracolumbar fractures in winter sports. Am J Sports Med 216:39, 1987.
33. Keene JS, Albert MJ, Springer SL, et al: Back injuries in college athletes. J Spinal Disord 2:190–195, 1989.
34. Koo DW, Fish WW: Spinal cord injury and snowboarding—the British Columbia experience. J Spinal Cord Med 22:246–251, 1999.
35. Kostuck JP: Operative treatment of idiopathic scoliosis. J Bone Joint Surg Am 72:1108, 1990.
36. Krompinger WJ, Fredrickson BE, Mino DE, Yuan HA: Conservative treatment of fractures of the thoracic and lumbar spine. Orthop Clin North Am 17:161, 1986.
37. Letts M, Smallman T, Afanasiev R, Gouw G: Fracture of the pars interarticularis in adolescent athletes: A clinical-biomechanical analysis. J Pediatr Orthop 6:40–46, 1986.
38. Lowe TG: Scheuermann's disease. J Bone Joint Surg Am 72:940, 1990.
39. MacNab L: Backache. Baltimore, Williams & Wilkins, 1977.
40. Maroon JC, Onik G: Percutaneous automated diskectomy: A new method for lumbar disc removal. J Neurol 66:143, 1987.
41. McEvoy RD, Bradford DS: The management of burst fractures of the thoracic and lumbar spine. Spine 10:631, 1985.
42. Micheli L: Low back pain in the adolescent: Differential diagnosis. Am J Sports Med 7:362, 1979.
43. Mixter WJ, Barr TS: Rupture of the intervertebral disc with involvement of the spinal canal. N Engl J Med 211:210, 1934.
44. Modic MT, et al: Magnetic resonance imaging of the spine. Radiol Clin North Am 24:229, 1986.
45. Reference deleted in proof.
46. Panjabi M, Brand R, White A: Mechanical properties of the human thoracic spine. J Bone Joint Surg Am 58:642, 1976.
47. Paushter DM, Modic MT, Masaryk JJ: Magnetic resonance imaging of the spine: Applications and limitations. Radiol Clin North Am 23: 551, 1985.
48. Perot P, Munro DD: Transthoracic removal of midline thoracic disc protrusions causing spinal cord compression. J Neurosurg 31:452, 1969.
49. Rauschning W: Imaging anatomy of the lumbar spine. In Wiesel SW, Weinstein JN, Herkowitz HN (eds): The Lumbar Spine. Philadelphia, WB Saunders, 1990.
50. Reid DC, Henderson R, Saboe L, Miller JD: Etiology and clinical course of missed spine fractures. J Trauma 27:980–986, 1987.
51. Rosenthal DF, Manken HJ, Bauman RA: Musculoskeletal applications for computed tomography. Bull Rheum Dis 33:1, 1983.
52. Rothman SL, Glenn WJ Jr: CT multi-planar reconstruction: 253 cases of lumbar spondylosis. AJNR Am J Neuroradiol 5:81, 1984.
53. Ryan AJ: Medical aspects of sports. JAMA 194:1118–1124, 1965.
54. Saal JS, Saal JA: Management of chronic discogenic low back pain with a thermal intradiscal catheter: A preliminary study. Spine 25: 382–388, 2000.
55. Sances A Jr, Myklebust JB, Maiman DJ, et al: The biomechanics of spinal injuries. Crit Rev Biomed Eng 11:1-76, 1984.
56. Schamm S, Taylor T: Tension signs in lumbar disc prolapse. Clin Orthop 44:163–170, 1966.
57. Silver JR, Silver DD, Godfrey JJ: Injuries of the spine sustained during gymnastic activities. BMJ 293:861–863, 1986.
58. Simen FA, Rothmau RH: Clinical usefulness of CT scanning in the diagnosis and treatment of lumbar spine disease. Radiol Clin North Am 21:197, 1983.
59. Snook GA: Injuries in women's gymnastics: A 5 year study. Am J Sport Med 7:242–244, 1979.
60. Snook GA: Injuries in intercollegiate wrestling: A 5 year study. Am J Sports Med 10:140–144, 1982.
61. Spangfert E: Laseque's sign in patients with lumbar disc herniation. Acta Orthop Scand 42:459, 1971.
62. Stanish W: Low back pain in middle aged athletes. Am J Sports Med 7:367, 1979.
63. Suzuki N, Endo S: A quantitative study of frank muscle strength and fatigability in the low-back-pain syndrome. Spine 8:69, 1983.
64. Sward L: The thoracolumbar spine in young elite athletes: Current concepts on the effects of physical training. Sports Med 13:357–364, 1992.
65. Sward L, Hellstrom M, Jacobsson B, Karlsson L: Vertebral ring apophysis injury in athletes: Is the etiology different in the thoracic and lumbar spine? Am J Sports Med 21:841–845, 1993.
66. Tovi D, Strang RR: Thoracic intervertebral disc protrusions. Acta Orthop Scand 41, 1960.
67. Walsh TR, Weinstein JN, Spratt KF, et al: Lumbar discography in normal subjects: A controlled study. J Bone Joint Surg Am 72: 1081–1088, 1990.
68. Weber H: Lumbar disc herniation: A controlled, prospective study with ten years of observation. Spine 8:131, 1983.
69. White AH, Derby R, Wynne A: Epidural injections for the diagnosis and treatment of low back pain. Spine 5:78, 1980.
70. Williams AL, Haughten VM, Syvertsen A: Computed tomography in the diagnosis of herniated nucleus pulposus. Radiology 135:95, 1980.

71. Williams JDA: Biomechanical factors in spinal injuries. Br J Sports Med 14:14, 1980.
72. Williams RW: Microlumbar diskectomy. Spine 11:851, 1986.
73. Willis TA: Nutrient arteries of the vertebral bodies. J Bone Joint Surg 31:538–541, 1949.
74. Wilson E, Lindseth R: The adolescent swimmer's back. Am J Sports Med 10:174, 1988.
75. Wiltse LL, Jackson DW: Treatment of spondylolisthesis and spondylolysis in children. Clin Orthop 117:92, 1976.
76. Winter RB: Classification and terminology. In: Scoliosis and Other Spinal Deformities. Philadelphia, WB Saunders, 1987.
77. Witt I, Westergaard A, Rosenkliwt A: A comparative analysis of x-ray findings of the lumbar spine in patients with and without lumbar pain. Spine 9:298, 1984.

Section B
Sports Injuries to the Thoracolumbar Spine in Children and Adolescents

William C. Lauerman, MD ■ Benjamin S. Shaffer, MD

Injuries to the thoracolumbar spine and associated back pain represent a relatively small proportion of sports injuries. Approximately 10% of all sports injuries involve the spine, with certain sports (e.g., gymnastics, football, rowing) representing greater risks, particularly to the low back.[25] In our experience, it is not uncommon to see skeletally immature athletes presenting with back pain; indeed, among the children and adolescents in our practice, thoracolumbar spine injuries likely represent 20% to 25% of sports injuries and cases of pain persisting for greater than 1 month.

When considering the pediatric athlete with back pain, it is helpful to be familiar with the prevalence of back pain in a general population of children and adolescents. Although the prevalence of low back pain in children younger than the age of 10 years has been reported to be as low as 1% to 3%, this prevalence increases in teenagers, varying among different researchers but reported to be as high as 20% to 25%.[23] Relatively few of these children or adolescents present for treatment. When involved in organized sports requiring daily training and regular competition, however, the athlete with a complaint of persistent back pain will often visit the trainer or the physician. These complaints may stem from either isolated or repetitive trauma; in many cases, they may not be related to sports participation at all. It is essential, however, to address the athletic component of the pain complaint simultaneously, including timely return to participation, while bearing in mind the prevalence, the differential diagnosis, and the expected response to treatment of pediatric back pain in general.

There are a number of factors predisposing to back injuries and back pain in the growing child and adolescent. Included among these is a skeletally immature spine, including the disk–vertebral body complex, the ligaments, and the musculotendinous unit. The adolescent growth spurt places the soft tissue structures at particular risk, owing to occasional difficulty, or mismatch, between the osseous components of the spine and the soft tissue structures. The disk–vertebral body complex is also unique in the growing child. Before skeletal maturity, the cartilaginous and bony end plates are densely adherent to one another, but the ring apophysis, which extends around the periphery at the margins of the vertebral body and is intimately adherent to the anulus, is at significant risk of injury.[2] In fact, it is injuries to the ring apophysis that frequently present as pediatric disk herniations.

Athletic injuries to the thoracolumbar spine can be broadly grouped into two categories: acute traumatic injuries and chronic or overuse syndromes. Acute traumatic injuries involving fracture or dislocation are exceedingly rare in all age groups, including the skeletally immature, and when seen most commonly involve the cervical spine. These ominous injuries are discussed elsewhere. Neurologic injury in association with injury to the thoracolumbar spine is similarly rare. Acute soft tissue sprain or strain is the most common truly acute injury seen; frequently, on close questioning, it is determined to have been preceded by a prodrome of back pain. Without a doubt, chronic pain, usually representing an overuse syndrome, is the most common complaint bringing the pediatric athlete to medical attention.

Appropriate management of the skeletally immature athlete with a back injury or persistent back pain often requires persistence, diplomacy, and luck. Increasingly, young children are participating in organized sports with schedules for training and competition as well as techniques that may not match the physiology of the growing skeleton. In addition, attention to appropriate training and stretching regimens, including stretching of the neck and the low back, may be lacking; this is particularly true in elementary school children.

Other factors to be considered when evaluating the underage athlete with persistent back pain are the desires or the motivation of the athlete. Although most athletes at all levels enjoy their chosen sport, we occasionally see grade school and, in particular, high school athletes with persistent complaints of back pain who subconsciously or consciously seem to be signaling a desire to move on to a different activity. Factoring this into the management of the pediatric athlete with back pain is important but requires finesse, and suspected lack of enthusiasm should never represent a reason not to evaluate a complaint of pain.[18] Finally, the reaction of the parents to what is all too often a protracted course of low back pain with attendant activity restrictions may add to the clinician's challenge.

Many parents find it unfathomable that a child can have back pain, let alone pain that eludes diagnosis and treatment. Reassuring the family of the relatively common nature of the problem being addressed is frequently quite helpful.

Evaluation

History

History taking is the key to appropriate, rational management of the pediatric athlete with back pain. The goal for the clinician, which should be clearly expressed to the patient and the parents, is primarily symptom-free return to full activity. Although failing to identify a serious underlying cause of the individual's pain is unacceptable, overemphasis on the need for a concrete diagnosis, when one frequently is elusive, can lead to enhanced frustration, needless limitation of activity, and extensive unnecessary imaging studies. History taking begins with inquiry about trauma. It is helpful to attempt to identify a traumatic episode, although, in our experience, these are quite rare. The patient should be asked about the onset of pain, be it acute or insidious, and whether there was any pain before the event or the day in question. Frequently, it becomes clear that there was in fact a relatively long history of gradually worsening pain that culminated on a single day, or in a single game, when the pain was reported. When a traumatic episode has been identified, it is very important to inquire about a history of any transient neurologic signs or symptoms (e.g., inability to move an extremity, whole body numbness or numbness from the waist down, or loss of bowel or bladder control). All these are extremely rare with sports injuries to the thoracolumbar spine but are significant when present.

Most pain complaints are chronic and of insidious onset. A helpful mnemonic to pursue is a CLEAR picture of the patient's pain. C represents the *character* of the pain complaint (e.g., burning, stabbing). L represents the *location* of the pain. Clinical terms such as back, buttocks, hips, or spine frequently mean different things to different people, and it is essential to have the patient accurately define where he or she experiences the pain. This can be difficult, particularly with younger children, but is essential in the evaluation of any persistent complaint. E represents *exacerbation*: What makes the pain worse? This is usually activity, but certain activities and positions may be particularly painful and should be defined. A stands for *amelioration*: What can the patient do to lessen the pain? Night pain is a relatively nonspecific complaint, but, in general, rest should relieve most episodes of musculoskeletal back pain. The child or the adolescent who clearly describes pain that persists or is worse at night needs to be evaluated much more aggressively than the typical teenager with activity-induced back pain. Finally, R stands for *radiation*: Where does the pain go? True radicular pain is seen in only 1% to 2% of children or adolescents with back complaints but, when present, should be identified.[10]

It is important to decide on appropriate evaluation in the context of the severity of the patient's complaints. Pain is truly subjective and therefore impossible to quantify, but certain factors provide insight into the magnitude of the problem. This is particularly true in children and adolescents who, given the choice, will always pursue their preferred activities and rarely recognize secondary gain in the sense that adults sometimes do. It is therefore important to inquire about interference with daily activities. Is the child missing school? Is he or she not participating in sports, either practices or games? Are any medications being used to help with the pain? Anything other than occasional interference with preferred activities represents a more serious problem and is an indication to pursue further evaluation aggressively.

Neurologic symptoms should be defined. The presence of pain or paresthesias down the leg may signify true nerve root compression or irritation. Lhermitte's sign, radiating electric sensations down the back and the legs with forward flexion of the neck, is rare but may represent an underlying intraspinal abnormality masquerading as a sports injury. Similarly, abnormalities of bowel or bladder function are unusual, but relatively thorough history taking to exclude the possibility of cauda equina, including asking about new-onset enuresis, should be pursued.

Although treatment of back pain in this population frequently involves "reinventing the wheel" while waiting for the problem to resolve, it is important to explore what previous treatment has been employed and the patient's response. Activity restriction is a first-line treatment; therefore, a history of activity restriction and whether it was complete or incomplete should be identified. Also important is whether the patient was compliant with the prescribed restrictions. Physical therapy is frequently used, so the clinician should inquire whether therapy has been prescribed, and, if so, what exactly was done. Physical modalities may be helpful, but return to full function typically requires instructing the patient in the use of back exercises. Because a variety of exercise regimens are available, it is important to define which exercises were pursued and the completeness or incompleteness of compliance. A history of medication usage and response is also sought. Finally, the previous use of bracing or casting should be explored. Identifying the type of brace, the regimen prescribed, patient compliance, and whether any sports participation was attempted while in the brace lays the foundation for further attempts at immobilization.

With all but the most short-lived complaints of back pain, a thorough general medical history is essential. This includes a birth history, including the occurrence of any developmental delays, and a family history, both general and of any spinal disorders such as scoliosis or spondylolisthesis. A thorough review of systems should be undertaken and constitutional symptoms such as fever, chills, or weight loss noted. Finally, psychosocial indicators such as depressive symptoms should be identified.

Physical Examination

Examination of the patient with a low back complaint begins with inspection, which cannot be performed adequately unless the patient is in an examining gown that opens in back, is disrobed down to underpants and bra, and has shoes and socks off. Inspection of the skin is performed, and skin lesions such as café au lait spots are identified. Asymmetry of the shoulders, the pelvis, the scapulae, and the skin creases is noted. The Adam's forward bend test—having the child bend forward to touch his or her toes and noting asymmetry of the ribs or the flank—is also carried out. Gait is then observed, including normal gait as well as heel and toe walking. A broad-based gait may signify myelopathy; this may be confirmed by inspecting tandem gait (having the patient heel-toe walk as in a sobriety test).

Palpation of the back is then performed. Palpation helps define exactly where the painful area is, even if it is not tender. Tenderness is noted, including tenderness in the midline, in the paraspinal region, and over the buttocks or the trochanteric bursae. Palpation may also identify a step-off in the lower lumbar spine, possibly signifying spondylolisthesis.

Range of motion of the spine should be tested. Limitation of forward flexion may represent disk disease, although hamstring spasm, which may result in gait abnormality, may also limit forward flexion. Pain on extension of the lumbar spine, particularly with a painful catch, is sometimes evidence of spondylolysis or spondylolisthesis. Hamstring spasm or tightness should be specifically assessed.

Neurologic involvement is exceedingly rare in pediatric patients with back pain but should be considered. Assessment for atrophy or asymmetry of the leg and the foot is undertaken. Light-touch sensory testing, motor strength assessment, and testing of the reflexes are all carried out, with deep tendon reflexes typically being quite brisk in this age group. Upper motor neuron findings such as clonus, Babinski's sign, or asymmetry of the superficial abdominal reflexes should also be sought. Tension signs, particularly the straight leg raising sign, are also assessed, because straight leg raising is a highly sensitive test for disk herniation in this population.[11, 18]

Examination of associated nonspinal areas is also pursued, including the abdominal contents, the hips, and, when indicated, the sacroiliac area (by testing for Faber's or Gaenslen's sign).

Imaging

Radiographic imaging studies are costly, at times time consuming, and sometimes inaccurate in identifying the true source of back pain in all age groups, including children and adolescents. Furthermore, it is relatively uncommon for a radiographic abnormality to alter treatment decision-making significantly, particularly in the early phase of back pain. Decision-making regarding the need for imaging in the pediatric athlete with complaints of back pain is driven, therefore, by a number of factors, including severity and duration of symptoms as well as response to previous treatment. Although rare, a history of acute trauma, particularly in the presence of neurologic signs or symptoms, represents a more urgent scenario for pursuing imaging. There is no cookbook or algorithmic approach to ordering

radiographic testing in the pediatric patient, athlete or not, with back pain. In the acute setting, we frequently find it helpful to employ initial treatment and to assess response. If the patient does not improve, an inexpensive test like plain radiography is employed, and more treatment is undertaken. If no response is seen, then a more sophisticated test may be ordered, and more treatment is employed. It is essential to bear in mind that most diagnoses do not need to be radiographically proven at the time of initial assessment; this includes conditions such as disk herniation and spondylolisthesis. Even more ominous conditions such as tumor or infection, which are discussed later, rarely progress so rapidly that an initial brief period of treatment and observation followed by close re-evaluation would adversely affect the patient's outcome to a significant extent.

Plain radiographs represent the typical first-line test. They are indicated in the pediatric athlete with a true history of acute trauma in whom fracture is suspected. We typically obtain plain radiographs in adolescents with significant symptoms for more than 3 to 4 weeks or, on initial presentation, in the child or the adolescent with severe pain or who is unable to attend school (Fig. 27B–1). The standard plain radiographic series for the lumbar spine includes anteroposterior and lateral views of the lumbar spine as well as a lumbosacral spot view to identify clearly the L5–S1 level. Plain lateral radiography identifies 80%

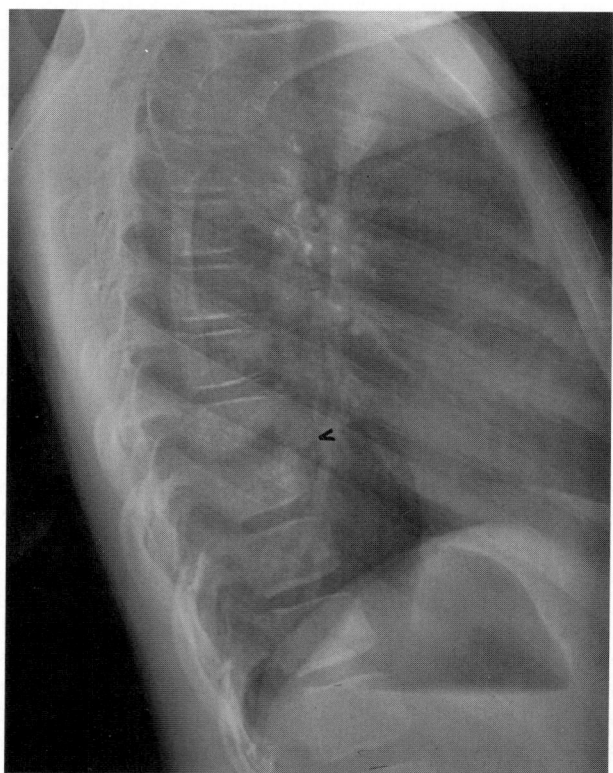

Figure 27B–1. Lateral radiograph from an 11-year-old swimmer with a 2-month history of back pain. Six weeks earlier, he had stopped participating in swimming, and he had been housebound for 1 week before this image was taken. This radiograph demonstrates end plate erosion and vertebral body involvement at T9–T10 *(arrowhead)* consistent with diskitis and vertebral osteomyelitis.

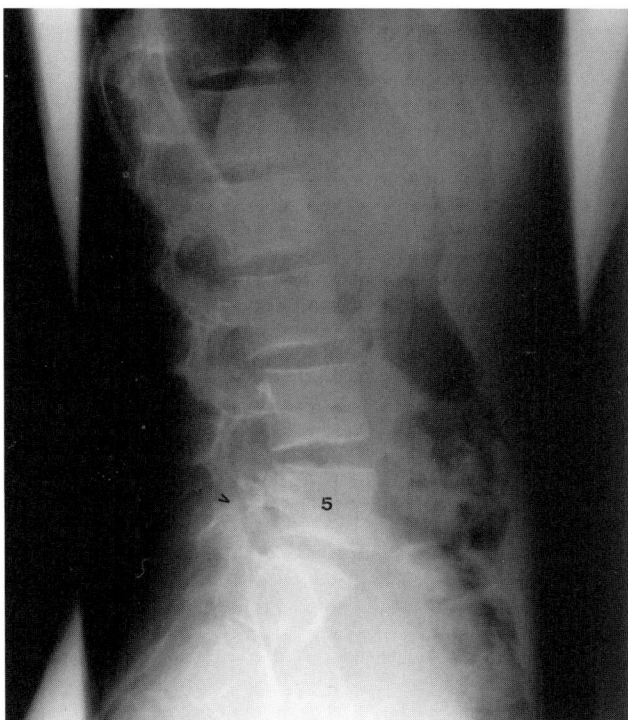

Figure 27B–2. A plain lateral radiograph of the lumbar spine from a 15-year-old soccer player with low back pain for 8 months demonstrates lysis of the pars interarticularis at L5 *(arrowhead)* without spondylolisthesis.

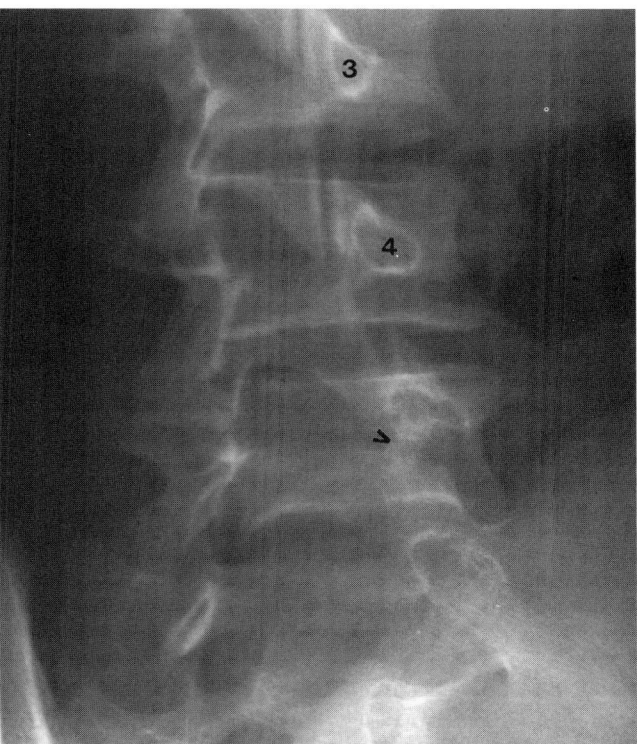

Figure 27B–3. A defect in the pars interarticularis of L5 *(arrowhead)* is seen on this oblique radiograph. The normal bony continuity of the pars (the "neck of the Scotty dog") of L3 and L4 can also be appreciated.

of defects of the pars interarticularis (Fig. 27B–2) and essentially all cases of spondylolisthesis.[7] These views will also identify virtually all significant fractures, such as compression fracture of the vertebral body. If a pars defect is suspected but not identified on the plain views, then oblique views of the lumbar spine are ordered (Fig. 27B–3), but these are not routine in our practice. A standing scoliosis series, including both anteroposterior and lateral views, is ordered if truncal asymmetry or hyperkyphosis is identified on physical examination. It is important to recognize that hyperkyphosis, with or without mild secondary scoliosis, is frequently misinterpreted by primary care practitioners as scoliosis; therefore, all initial scoliosis evaluations should include a lateral radiograph.

Nuclear medicine testing, specifically technetium bone scanning, can be helpful in identifying occult lesions of the spine not seen on plain radiographs. The sensitivity of technetium is enhanced with single photon emission computed tomography (SPECT), which essentially provides tomographic images of the radiotracer in the lumbar spine (Fig. 27B–4). SPECT scanning is currently the test of choice for identifying occult defects of the pars interarticularis.[1] It is also sensitive, although relatively nonspecific, for other bony lesions such as tumors of the posterior elements, apophyseal fractures, and diskitis. Some of these lesions may be missed on magnetic resonance imaging (MRI). Although technetium scanning can be helpful in identifying occult cases of spondylolysis, its efficacy in defining the acuity of the injury is unclear, and in our practice we do not assume that an active area of uptake on a SPECT scan necessarily correlates with an acute defect of the pars.

Computed tomographic (CT) scanning is also helpful in certain circumstances, particularly in the evaluation of spondylolysis.[27] Although not quite as sensitive as SPECT scanning, CT scanning using 3-mm parallel cuts is a sensitive modality for identifying defects of the pars. It is very specific for spondylolysis as well as for differentiating such pars defects from sclerosis of the pars or the pedicle, from tumors such as osteoid osteoma or osteoblastoma, or from apophyseal injuries. In addition, when clinically indicated, CT scanning is the ideal modality for monitoring healing of a defect in the pars interarticularis. In our practice, CT scanning provides the best definition of the bony anatomy of the posterior elements of the lumbar spine.

MRI is commonly employed, although it rarely provides information that is therapeutically significant in these patients. MRI in a pediatric athlete with acute pain is of limited usefulness and should be restricted. Despite the limitations of MRI, we do employ this test initially for patients with clear-cut neurologic signs or symptoms and certainly for those with evidence of deterioration. Similarly, a history of constitutional symptoms would merit early evaluation with MRI. We also routinely use MRI in the pediatric athlete with functionally disabling pain that has interfered with activities for greater than 3 months. Although this point is still early in the disease process, patient and specifically parent expectations tend to be so high that when improvement is not seen, evaluation with a modality as sensitive, as specific, and as noninvasive as MRI is appropriate.

The advantage of MRI is that it is noninvasive, it does

condition has been referred to as lumbar Scheuermann's disease.[3] This condition is commonly seen in association with back pain in young adults and in our practice is occasionally seen in the pediatric athlete.

Chronic overuse syndrome is common in the adolescent athlete with persistent low back pain. This should be, however, a diagnosis of exclusion. Axial low back pain is the typical complaint, with minimal radiation into the buttocks, the thighs, or the legs. Relief with rest and evanescent pain usually responding to activity restrictions are common. Although the authors are opposed to overly aggressive imaging early in the evaluation of a pediatric athlete with back pain, we feel that thorough radiographic evaluation, including plain radiographs, dynamic views, SPECT, and MRI, should be employed before arriving at a final diagnosis of chronic overuse syndrome. This typically occurs over a 6- to 12-month period of evaluation and treatment.

Most pediatric athletes have back injuries or back pain that falls into one of these categories. The remainder, a relatively small subset, are diagnosed with one of the less common causes of back pain in the pediatric population, such as spinal deformities. Adolescent idiopathic scoliosis, although typically described as a painless condition, is often associated with mild-to-moderate complaints of pain (Fig. 27B–7). This condition should only rarely require activity limitation, and the athlete who voluntarily restricts sports participation should be thoroughly evaluated for a cause of pain other than idiopathic scoliosis. Other causes

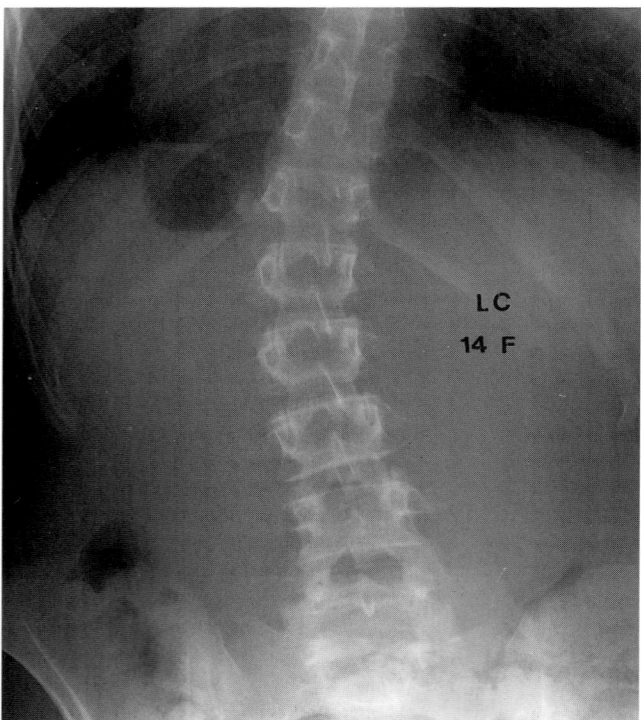

Figure 27B–7. A 14-year-old swimmer had a 6-month history of mild low back pain that did not interfere with her participation in sports. Physical examination suggested scoliosis, which was confirmed on this plain anteroposterior radiograph. Her pain improved with a stretching and strengthening regimen, and the scoliosis, which progressed, was treated with nighttime bracing.

of painful scoliosis include tumors such as osteoid osteoma or osteoblastoma as well as intraspinal lesions. Hyperkyphosis may be painful in the adolescent, and pain is a relatively common presenting complaint of juvenile patients with Scheuermann's kyphosis.

A number of tumors of the spine, although all quite rare, may present with back pain in the child or the adolescent. These include lesions of the posterior elements, such as osteoid osteoma or osteoblastoma; lesions of the anterior column, including eosinophilic granuloma, lymphoma, or primary malignancy such as Ewing's sarcoma; or lesions of the spinal cord or cauda equina, such as ependymoma, astrocytoma, or neuroblastoma (Fig. 27B–8). Pain severity, the presence of pain at rest, and neurologic signs or symptoms serve to differentiate the patient with a tumor and trigger a more aggressive imaging approach.

Infectious conditions of the spine such as disk space infection and vertebral body osteomyelitis are fairly common in the pediatric population, particularly in younger children; the mean age at presentation is 6 to 7 years. A history of constitutional symptoms such as fever, chills, or weight loss may be present, and frequently a history of a recent infection, such as an upper respiratory infection or a skin lesion, is obtained. The presence of pain at rest is also relatively common. Finally, metabolic abnormalities, generalized systemic malignancies such as leukemia or lymphoma, and visceral disorders should be considered.

Management

General

Most pediatric athletes presenting with the new onset of back pain will respond quickly to a series of general measures. In this setting, it is rarely essential to arrive at a specific diagnosis early in the course of the patient's complaints, and in fact it is rarely cost effective to order aggressive imaging of children or adults with recent-onset back pain except in certain circumstances. Most pediatric athletes present with a more chronic course, frequently of insidious onset. These patients should be evaluated for so-called red flags (e.g., a history of significant trauma, as described previously), which are potential indicators of a more serious underlying condition. The presence of incapacitating pain causing the patient to stay home from school or be bedridden might lead to a more aggressive approach to evaluation. Similarly, a history of constitutional symptoms such as unexplained weight loss, fever, or chills or the presence of significant neurologic signs or symptoms also may suggest the need for an expedited approach to imaging.[18]

Unless one of these red flags is present, most patients are begun on a generic management triad of activity restriction, moist heat and stretching, and over-the-counter medication such as acetaminophen or ibuprofen. Effective management of these patients has as its goals both a timely return to full activity with minimal or no pain and identification (in the unusual case) of more serious underlying disease. This requires relatively frequent re-evaluation. We typically bring the pediatric athlete with back pain back

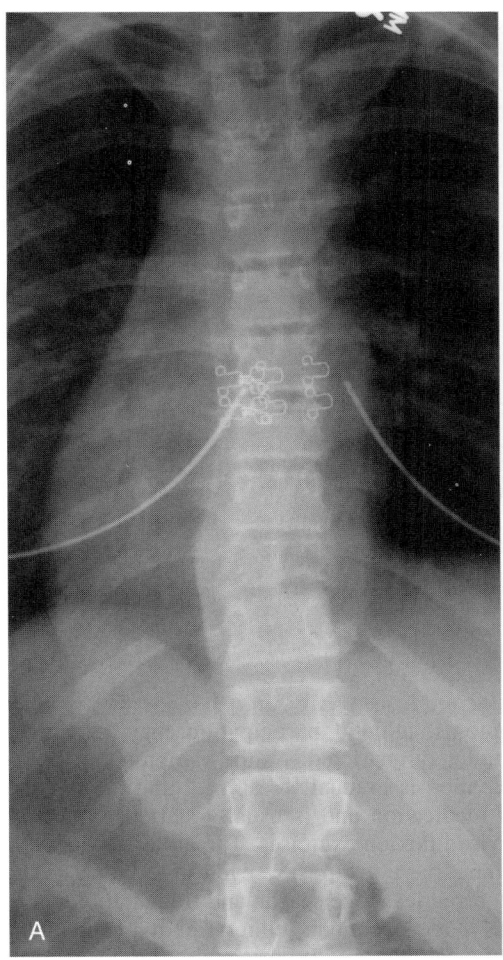

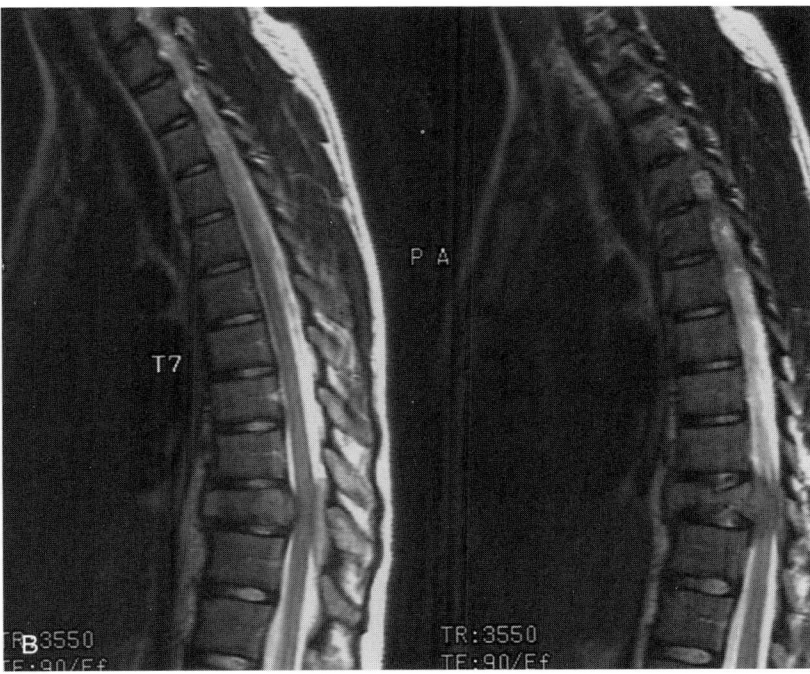

Figure 27B–8. A 14-year-old girl who presented after injuring her back playing soccer complained of diffuse back pain and tingling in her feet. On plain anteroposterior radiography, there is collapse of T10, irregularity of both pedicles, and a prominent soft tissue mass *(A)*. Sagittal magnetic resonance images *(B)* demonstrate a pathologic fracture, proved on biopsy to be caused by lymphoma.

for re-evaluation on a weekly basis for the first 2 or 3 weeks and then every 2 or 3 weeks thereafter until acceptable resolution of the disability has occurred.

In most cases, improvement will be seen either spontaneously or as a result of this treatment. Depending on the duration of the patient's symptoms, their severity, and the rapidity of improvement, the athlete first is allowed to return to his or her daily activities, then is started on a program of back stretching and strengthening exercises under the guidance of a licensed physical therapist to try to avoid recurrences. Once the exercise program has been mastered without recurrence of pain, gradual resumption of athletic activities is allowed. Because pain is a strictly subjective complaint, it is difficult to define objective criteria regarding when the patient can resume specific activities. We find the most useful guideline (which can be applied to individuals who have sustained a "stinger" while playing football or to athletes who have missed 6 months of soccer owing to chronic back pain) to be the presence of a minimal level of pain in an individual who is nontender with a normal range of motion and who is neurologically normal in the affected body part.

Another aspect of the management of the pediatric athlete with ongoing back pain of almost any cause is counseling. The athlete and, in particular, the parents rarely under-

stand that a child can suffer from low back pain. It is imperative that the physician be prepared to reinforce the fact that this is a relatively common problem and frequently involves a prolonged recovery. It also needs to be stressed that although it is exceedingly frustrating for the family, the exact diagnosis in the child or the adolescent with back pain is often unclear.

The appropriate role of imaging studies, in medicine in general and in the evaluation of back pain in particular, is to guide treatment; these expensive tests should therefore be obtained when they can reasonably be expected to have a significant impact on therapeutic decision-making. It has been our experience that with the exceptions noted previously, imaging is rarely helpful in the first 2 to 4 weeks of symptoms. Although no hard-and-fast rules exist, we typically obtain plain radiographs in individuals whose back pain has failed to significantly improve within this time frame. If plain radiographic findings are negative and the pain persists, then we commonly order MRI after 2 to 3 months of symptoms. If this study also has normal findings and symptoms persist for 6 months or longer, we will usually recommend technetium bone scanning. If there is particular concern that occult spondylolysis is the cause of the patient's pain, we will often proceed to SPECT before MRI.

rity, activity restrictions should be based solely on the patient's symptoms, because progressive slippage is very uncommon in the adult population.

Lumbar Disk Injury

In North America, approximately 1% to 2% of clinically significant disk herniations occur in children younger than the age of 18 years. Approximately 50% of patients will describe a history of trauma, and the incidence appears to be equal in boys and girls. Low back pain, stiffness, abnormal posture, and limping are the most common presenting complaints, and leg pain, paresthesias, and subjective weaknesses are present in approximately 25%. Many authors note a prolonged duration of symptoms before diagnosis, lasting from several months to a year.[4, 10]

Three typical findings are seen in the adolescent with a disk herniation. First, there is frequently significant back stiffness, spasm, and postural abnormality. Second is the common absence of any neurologic abnormality. Third is the exceedingly high incidence of a positive straight leg raising test result. The clinician should be aware of the significance of the straight leg raising sign in the pediatric population and its association with disk herniation and should not allow a normal neurologic examination to exclude this diagnosis.[19]

Advanced imaging should be undertaken when 6 weeks of nonsurgical treatment have failed to relieve the disorder, when there is a significant or worsening motor deficit, or when there is any suggestion of bowel or bladder dysfunction typical of cauda equina syndrome (Fig. 27B–11). MRI is the test of choice and will identify and define most disk herniations.[15] The possibility of false-positive findings,

even in this population, should be entertained, and close correlation between the patient's signs and symptoms and the radiographic findings is required before surgical intervention is considered. MRI may not be as accurate as CT scanning in the diagnosis of apophyseal fracture.[12] This variant of disk injury is less common than true disk herniation but is seen occasionally in young patients. The signs and symptoms are similar to those associated with typical disk herniation; when this condition is suspected and the MRI is nondiagnostic, CT scanning is appropriate. Occasionally, a posteriorly displaced fleck of bone at the disk–vertebral body interface will be identified on the plain lateral radiograph; this is an indication to proceed with CT rather than MRI as the next step in diagnosis.[19]

Treatment of the pediatric patient with a lumbar disk herniation virtually always begins with a nonsurgical approach. Our approach, at least initially, is quite similar to that used in adults. An initial period of restricted activity is initiated, including restriction from sports, and we often prescribe nonsteroidal anti-inflammatory medication. Moist heat is also quite helpful in the early postinjury period. Once the patient is able to walk without a limp and has a near-normal range of motion, a more active approach to treatment is initiated. We begin the individual on a program of extension-type low back exercises under the supervision of a physical therapist and allow the patient to resume normal activities, including sports, gradually. Nonsurgical treatment of lumbar disk herniation is a unique challenge in the active athlete when compared with treatment of a more sedentary patient; this is no less true in pediatric athletes. Most, however, will respond to treatment within several weeks, and a return to sports with a good prognosis can usually be predicted.

In those patients who fail to respond, several options are available. A longer period of activity restriction or more stringent restrictions can be initiated. A trial of epidural steroid injections may also be recommended; this is usually highly successful, at least in the short term, in relieving radicular pain. As a final option, surgery may be recommended.

The indication for surgery in the adolescent with a lumbar disk herniation is persistent unacceptable pain despite appropriate nonoperative treatment for a minimum of 6 to 12 weeks.[26] Although adults who qualify as surgical candidates will almost always manifest pain distally into the leg, the adolescent patient often complains primarily of pain in the buttocks and the posterior thigh. Similar to the adult, however, the adolescent should have a positive straight leg raising sign to be considered a good surgical candidate. If these indications are met, then a *confirmatory* neuroradiographic study, usually MRI, should be sought to identify a disk herniation at the appropriate level and on the appropriate side. There is virtually never a role for exploratory surgery in the patient with an MRI scan with negative or unconvincing results. Surgical treatment consists in most cases of hemilaminotomy and diskectomy. Although some authors have advocated fusion in this population, there is no consensus that this offers any short- or long-term advantages. Including fusion in the surgery certainly extends the expense, the duration of hospitalization, and the duration of rehabilitation. The results of surgical treatment have, in some studies, been somewhat disappointing. Although greater than 90% of adults experi-

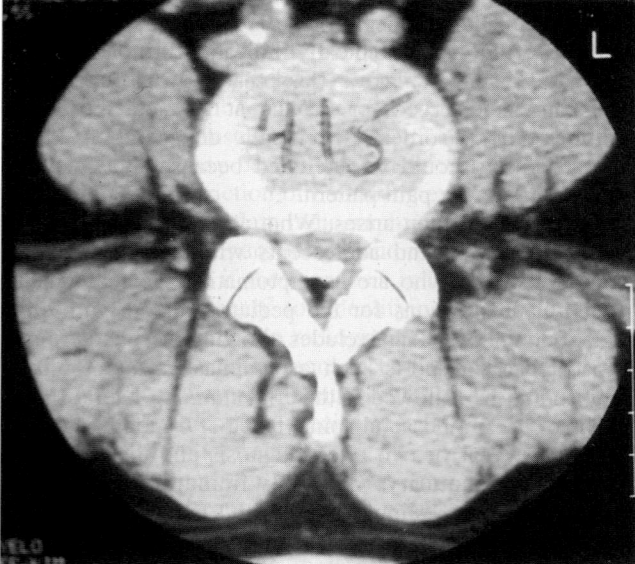

Figure 27B–11. Computed tomographic myelogram through the L4–L5 interspace in an 18-year-old wrestler with a 3-month history of pain in his back and left buttock. A characteristic posterolateral herniation, in the presence of a somewhat narrow spinal canal, leads to marked thecal sac and nerve root compression.

ence complete or near-complete relief of their preoperative sciatica after uncomplicated diskectomy, similarly outstanding results are not seen in adolescents. In the adolescent population, the percentage of patients with long-term complete resolution of symptoms is more on the order of 75% to 80%.[9]

When can the pediatric athlete with a disk herniation return to sports? We allow patients to return to athletics when they have been successfully treated nonsurgically; when they have a near-complete range of motion; when they are nontender; and when they are neurologically normal with a negative straight leg raising sign. Although the time frame may vary, most patients are better in 4 to 6 weeks and are able to return to at least noncontact sports at that time. It is not uncommon for the period before return to a collision sport such as football to be twice as long. One of the goals of surgical treatment is return to full activity, although we typically approach this relatively cautiously. After uncomplicated hemilaminotomy and diskectomy, patients are allowed to return to swimming and riding an exercise bicycle at 2 to 3 weeks, are allowed to begin running at 4 to 6 weeks, and can resume contact sports at approximately 4 to 6 months, if their symptoms allow. Most patients are eventually able to return to full athletic participation.

In addition to frank disk herniation, degenerative disease of one or more lumbar disks is occasionally seen with associated symptoms. This entity has been referred to as juvenile disk disease or lumbar Scheuermann's disease. Radiographic findings are similar to those seen in the thoracic spine in Scheuermann's kyphosis. These include end plate irregularity, Schmorl's node formation, and flattening or wedging of one or more vertebral bodies.[3] Actual kyphosis is rarely seen, but loss of normal lumbar lordosis is quite common. On MRI, disk desiccation at one or more levels is identified in addition to the abovementioned findings. Pathologic changes reflect these radiologic findings.

The prevalence of juvenile disk disease has not been adequately defined. In our practice, it is more common in boys than in girls and is an occasional, although not a common, cause of low back pain in adolescents. These radiographic findings are quite common, however, in young adults with low back pain (Fig. 27B–12).

Patients present with a primary complaint of axial back pain with occasional radiation into the buttocks. Pain radiating distally into the posterior thigh or more distally down the leg is uncommon unless actual herniation of the disk has occurred. Physical findings are relatively nonspecific but include paraspinal spasm and loss of motion. Neurologic testing usually has normal results. The straight leg raising sign will typically be negative, in contrast to disk herniation, in which the straight leg raising sign is almost always positive.

Treatment of a patient with juvenile disk disease depends on the stage at which he or she presents for treatment. In the acute phase, the standard regimen of activity restriction, nonsteroidal anti-inflammatory medications, and moist heat is frequently quite successful. Even when the patient responds readily, we typically pursue an aggressive program of back rehabilitation. The uncertain prognosis for individuals with symptomatic juvenile disk disease, as well as what would appear to be a significant incidence of low back pain in early adulthood, leads us to be fairly cautious in treating adolescents in whom this is identified. We encourage these individuals to continue with a program of very aggressive back stretching and strengthening well beyond their recovery time frame. We also counsel the athlete in clear-cut terms regarding the suitability of various sports and try to guide some individuals toward long-term participation in activities that are somewhat less stressful on the lumbar spine.

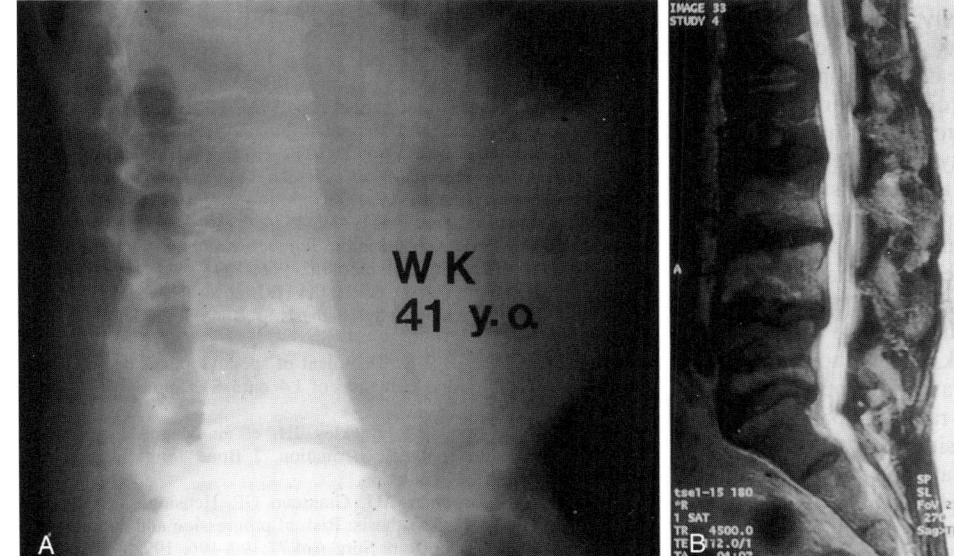
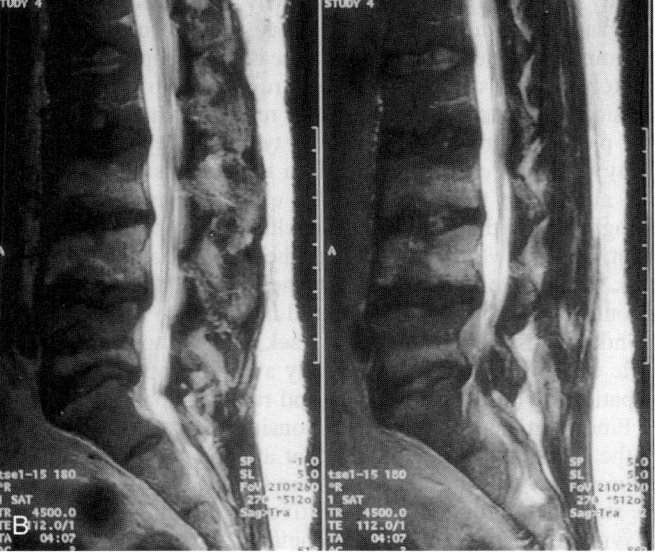

Figure 27B–12. Plain lateral radiograph *(A)* and sagittal T₂-weighted magnetic resonance image *(B)* of a 41-year-old man with chronic low back pain and lumbar Scheuermann's disease.

CHAPTER TWENTY-EIGHT

Knee

Section A
Relevant Biomechanics of the Knee

Bruce D. Beynnon, PhD ■ Robert J. Johnson, MD
Kathryn M. Coughlin, MS

The knee joint is the largest and most complex joint in the human body. The joint capsule and ligaments, which provide structural stability to the knee, are particularly vulnerable to injury by large moments that can be created through the forces acting along the long lever arms of the lower limb. Thus, it is not surprising that the knee is one of the most frequently injured joints. An injury to the knee, such as disruption of the anterior cruciate ligament (ACL), can result in an extensive disability because this injury may alter normal knee kinematics and therefore locomotion. An extensive background in biomechanics or mathematics is not required to understand the fundamental mechanical principles governing the knee joint. Knowledge of knee biomechanics provides an essential framework for understanding the consequences of injury and joint disorders; it aids in the intelligent planning of surgical procedures, serves as the basis for developing objective rehabilitation programs, and describes the effects of different types of orthoses on the knee joint.

The knee joint comprises three independent articulations, one between the patella and femur and the remaining two between the lateral and medial tibial and femoral condyles. The patellofemoral articulation consists of the patella, which has a multifaceted dorsal surface that articulates with the femoral trochlear groove. The tibiofemoral articulations consist of femoral condyles with saddle-shaped tibial condyles and interposing menisci. The posterior aspect of the femoral condyles is spherical, whereas the anterior aspect of the femoral condyles is more flat. Thus, in extension, the flat portion of the femoral condyles is in contact with the tibia, and in flexion, the spherical portion of the femoral condyles is in contact with the tibia.

To the untrained observer, the knee joint may appear to function as a simple pinned hinge (ginglymus) with flexion-extension rotation the only apparent motion between the femur and tibia. The motion characteristics of the knee joint are extremely complex, however, requiring a full six degrees of freedom (three translations and three rotations) to completely describe the coupled, or simultaneous, joint motions (Fig. 28A–1). An example of coupled motion is demonstrated with flexion rotation of the knee from the extended position. With this rotation, there is a coupled posterior movement of the femoral contact regions on the tibial surface in the sagittal plane and an internal rotation of the tibia relative to the femur in the transverse plane. By use of the Eulerian-based coordinate system described by Hefzy and Grood,[69] the translations and rotations can be described in anatomically referenced directions (see

Fig. 28A–1). Although many different types of coordinate systems have been used to describe three-dimensional knee motion, this system is appealing because it allows joint rotation to be expressed in terms familiar to the clinician. Grood and Noyes[63] have applied the three-dimensional coordinate system to the interpretation of various clinical examination techniques and have developed a "bumper model" of the knee joint. This model is useful in describing the soft tissue restraints to anterior-posterior translation and internal-external rotation of the knee joint. In addition, the model can be applied to demonstrate the types of tibiofemoral subluxations that may result when different soft tissue structures are disrupted. Application of this approach may aid in the examination of injuries to the knee ligaments and capsular structures.

This section assumes a working knowledge of the biomechanical terms essential to the description of knee function. For an introduction to basic knee biomechanics, the reader is encouraged to review the work of Frankel,[54] Frankel and Burstein,[55] and Mow and Hayes,[120] along with the definition of biomechanical terms as they apply to the knee presented by Noyes and coworkers[124] and Bonnarens

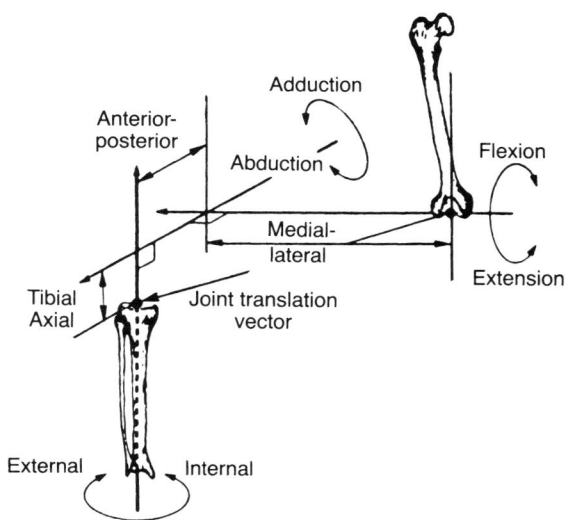

Figure 28A–1. Coordinate system for knee joint rotations and translations. Flexion-extension rotation is about the fixed femoral axis. Internal-external rotation is about a fixed tibial axis. Abduction-adduction is about an axis that is perpendicular to the femoral and tibial axes. The joint translations occur along each of the three coordinate axes. (From Hefzy MS, Grood ES: Review of knee models. Appl Mech Rev 41:1–13, 1988.)

Implantable Force Probe (AIFP), if it is calibrated after implantation. They noted that similar limitations have been reported for other force transducers that operate on the same principle, although the errors associated with other arthroscopic force transducers have not been reported. In addition, Fleming and colleagues[52] determined that the AIFP output is specimen dependent. When the force transducer was removed and reimplanted into the same location, the results were not repeatable. The errors ranged from 4% to 109%. On reimplantation into another location in the same ACL, the percentage errors ranged from 2% to 203%. These findings highlight a need for a more repeatable transducer that will yield relative measurements of ACL stress in vivo. Because stress is directly related to force or strain, several investigators have chosen to measure strain, rather than force, in the ligaments. Fleming and coworkers[15, 46] have shown the accuracy associated with strain measurements in the ACL to be on the order of 0.2% and 0.1% with use of the Hall-effect strain transducer and the differential variable reluctance transducer, respectively.

Strain Measurement of Ligaments

Several investigators have measured ligament displacement, enabling the calculation of strain pattern, to understand the effect of knee joint position and muscle activity on ligament biomechanics.[5, 26, 40, 94, 135, 163] Most of this work has been carried out in vitro, and the results are conflicting.

Edwards,[40] Kennedy,[94] Brown,[26] Berns,[12] Hull,[82] and their associates used mercury-filled strain gauges to measure the length of ligaments at various angles of knee flexion. Henning and colleagues[70] have constructed a device to measure displacement in the ACL in vivo.

Butler and associates[30] and Woo and colleagues[170] have developed optical techniques for mapping surface strains in various tissues. Butler and coworkers[29, 30] used high-speed cameras to record the movements of surface markers and measured both midsubstance and insertion site deformations of soft tissues. These techniques are ideal methods for monitoring surface strains, particularly during high-rate tests, but are not useful for out-of-plane movements or for ligaments such as the cruciates that cannot be directly viewed. They also suffer from the theoretical disadvantage that the tissue of interest has to be exposed and therefore is not in a physiologic state.

Other workers have calculated strain by measurement of the change of ligament attachment length under various applied joint loadings. For example, Wang and colleagues[163] measured the three-dimensional coordinates of pins stuck in a cadaver joint at the palpated origin and insertion points of the major knee ligaments. They recorded the relationship between torque and angular rotation of the femur relative to the tibia. After excision of certain ligaments, the tests were repeated to determine the contribution of these elements to torsional restraint. In the most extensive and elegant studies, Sidles and associates[144] used a three-dimensional digitizer to compute ligament length patterns. In a slightly different approach, Trent and colleagues[157] used pins embedded in the ligament attachments and measured the displacement of one pin relative to the other. In addition, in this study, they located the instant centers of transverse joint rotation. Warren and cowork-

ers[165] also used pins placed at ligament origins but measured displacements with a radiographic technique.

The pins or other markers used as locators of ligament origin generally estimate average ligament strain. This technique may produce confusing results owing both to the difficulty in choosing the center of a ligament insertion and to the changes in strain from place to place within a ligament.

Previous work at the University of Vermont has focused on the measurement of ACL displacement in the in vitro environment by use of the Hall-effect strain transducer and, more recently, a differential variable reluctance transducer, which allow computation of strain.[5, 16, 45, 135] This technique has been applied to the measurement of ACL strain in vivo.[13, 14, 16, 46, 48–50]

Ligament Biomechanics

The primary function of the knee ligaments is to stabilize the knee, to control normal kinematics, and to prevent abnormal displacements and rotations that may damage articular surfaces. Ligaments, the most important static stabilizers, are primarily composed of collagen, the constituent that provides resistance to a tensile load developed along the length of the ligament, with lesser and varying amounts of elastic and reticulin fibers. Cellular elements, ground substance, vascular channels, and nerves are also present. Collagen fibers and their orientation within the tissue are responsible for the primary biomechanical behavior of each of these structures. The fibers of the large distinct ligaments are almost all arranged in parallel bundles, making them ideal for withstanding tensile loads, whereas capsular structures have a less consistent orientation, making them more compliant and not as strong in resisting axial loading.

The ligament insertion sites are designed to reduce the chance of failure by distributing the stresses at the bone-ligament interface in a gradual fashion. This is accomplished by the collagen fibers passing from the ligament into the bone through four distinct zones: (1) ligament substance, (2) fibrocartilaginous matrix, (3) mineralized fibrocartilage, and (4) bone itself.[34] In spite of the transitions, Noyes and colleagues[125] demonstrated that some strain concentration occurs near the ligamentous insertion sites. Later, Sidles and coworkers[143] developed an analytic model of the ACL tibial insertion. They demonstrated that for typical ACL insertion geometry, the transverse pressures are similar to the tensile stress along the ligament.

The knee ligaments can best control motion of the bones relative to each other if the motion takes place along the direction of the ligament fibers. For example, when the knee is loaded in valgus, the medial collateral ligament develops a tensile stress in combination with a compressive force across the lateral compartment of the knee, and a resistance to medial joint opening is provided. Acting alone, ligaments cannot restrain the relative rotation associated with applied torques. The ligament would simply rotate about its bony insertion sites. A second force, usually developed through cartilage-to-cartilage compression, is required. For example, as the knee is loaded with an internal torque, a transverse rotation causes the femoral condyles to ride up the tibial spines (Fig. 28A–4). This combination creates a compressive force across the tibiofemoral contact regions and an oppositely directed tensile force along the cruciate and collateral ligaments. This example may help demonstrate the mechanism by which the ACL interacts with tibiofemoral articular compression to resist an applied internal rotation to the knee joint.

The ability of a ligament to resist applied tensile loading may best be described through examination of the load-elongation curve produced during tensile failure testing of an ACL (Fig. 28A–5). As a tensile load is applied, the ligament elongates; the slope of the measured load-displacement relationship represents the stiffness of the ligament. The steeper the slope of this curve, the stiffer the ligament. In the unloaded state, the ligament fibers are under minimal tension, and the collagen fibers have a wavy pattern. As a tensile load is applied, the wavy pattern begins to straighten out. Initially, little load is required to elongate the ligament. This is characterized by the relatively flat "toe" region of the curve. The change from the toe to the linear portion of the curve represents the change in stiffness that an examiner perceives during a clinical laxity examination when a ligament's "end point" is reached. As the tensile load continues to increase, all the collagen fibers are straightened, and the curve becomes nearly linear. This region of the curve characterizes the elastic deformation of the ligament until the yield point is reached. At this point, there is a sudden loss in the ability

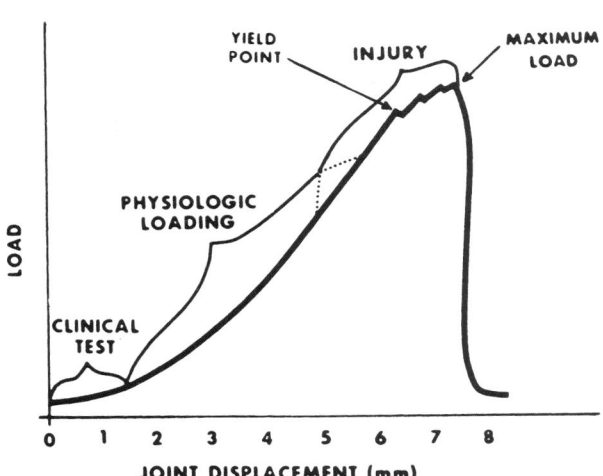

Figure 28A–5. Load-elongation curve for the tensile failure of the anterior cruciate ligament. (From Cabaud HB: Biomechanics of the anterior cruciate ligament. Clin Orthop 172:26, 1988.)

of the ligament to transmit load. If loading continues, a maximum or ultimate failure load is reached, and a sudden drop in load is recorded, representing total failure of the ligament. The area under the load-deformation curve represents the amount of energy absorbed by a ligament during testing. Noyes and associates demonstrated that the characteristics of the ACL's load-displacement curve are dramatically affected by variables such as age,[127] strain rate,[128] and duration of immobilization (disuse).[126] Young adults have a yield point that can be as much as three times greater than that of an older person.[127] Noyes and colleagues[128] also demonstrated the sensitivity of the ACL's load-displacement response to strain rate. ACLs that failed rapidly (0.6 second) demonstrated a 20% increase in load to failure above those that failed at a speed two orders of magnitude slower (60 seconds). The energy stored just before ligament failure was 30% greater in preparations tested at the high strain rate in comparison with those that failed at the slow rate. In addition, any ligament that has been immobilized for even short periods will demonstrate a reduction in ligament strength.[126]

The majority of orthopaedic surgeons who operatively restore the function of the ACL perform an intra-articular reconstruction with autograft material.[4] Noyes and associates[125] characterized the relative strength of the various ligament replacement materials, demonstrating that a 14-mm-wide bone–patella tendon–bone preparation was 168% as strong as the normal ACL, the strength of all other autogenous replacements being less in comparison with the normal ACL. Woo and coworkers[169] have demonstrated that the normal tensile strength of the ACL may be as high as 2500 N, rather than the original 1725 N standard presented by Noyes and associates.[125] This has led some surgeons to use combinations of autogenous graft material in an effort to increase the strength of the ACL replacement. Butler[28] used the primate model to demonstrate that maintaining a vascular supply to an ACL graft produces no material property differences in comparison with a similar free graft 1 year after implantation.

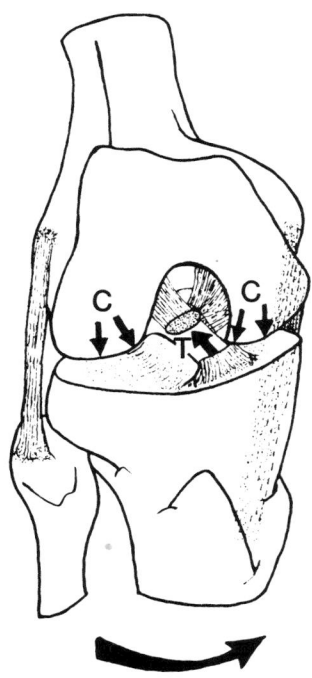

Internal Rotation

Figure 28A–4. Internal rotation of the tibia relative to the femur. The internal rotation causes the femoral condyles to ride up on the tibial spine, producing tension in the cruciate ligaments and a compressive force across the articular surfaces. C, compressive force produced between the tibiofemoral articular surfaces; T, tensile load developed along the anterior cruciate ligament.

is required to determine whether the AROM strain values between extension and 48 degrees are large enough to produce permanent elongation of the reconstructed tissue or failure of the fixation construct. Our findings illustrate that both muscle activity and knee position determine AMB strain at rest and with joint motion.[14] It appears that for AROM, the AMB is strained between the limits of full extension and 48 degrees.[14] These findings are consistent with Henning's in vivo study of two patients with injured ligaments[70] and with the findings of Markolf and colleagues.[107]

A ranked comparison of the different activities evaluated in subjects with normal ACLs, ordered from high to low risk on the basis of peak AMB strain values, is presented in Table 28A–1. These in vivo data may be used in the development of rehabilitation programs after ACL reconstruction.

In vivo strain measurement within the AMB for PROM between 110 degrees and full extension revealed that the ACL reaches positive strain values as the joint is brought into extension and remains at or below the zero strain level between the limits of 11.5 and 110 degrees of flexion when distal leg support loading is used[14] (see Fig. 28A–6). Therefore, continuous passive motion of the knee within these limits should be safe for the reconstructed ACL immediately after surgery when the leg is supported throughout flexion-extension motion without applied varus or valgus loading, internal or external torques, or anterior shear forces. The limits of near extension (0 to 10 degrees), however, can cause small magnitudes of strain (1% or less).[14] We think this should be viewed as a relatively mild constraint to bracing a patient's knee in the fully extended position (0 degrees) or to the use of continuous passive motion during a rehabilitation program.

Our in vivo PROM investigations[13, 14] and previous in vitro studies[5, 45, 137] have shown that the AMB of the ACL is not "isometric." That is, the fiber length does vary as the knee passes through a range of motion[14] (see Fig. 28A–6). The change in length of fibers is least in the AMB[137]; thus, most intra-articular reconstruction procedures now attempt to reattach an ACL graft to the attachment sites of this portion of the ligament. In vivo strain gauge analysis immediately after the fixation of an ACL graft has allowed us to determine whether the graft strain pattern is either similar to the normal ACL or unacceptable.[13] Devices known as isometers have been devised to assist surgeons in identifying optimal attachment sites for an ACL reconstruction. Therefore, the in vivo ACL data[14] for PROM of the joint may serve as important standards by which to accept or to reject isometer measurements of potential reconstruction tunnel placement sites. For PROM, it was observed that the difference between mean peak and mean minimum AMB strain values was 4.2% (range, 3.0% to 7.2%).[14] If this difference is assumed to occur uniformly over the AMB length and the mean length of the AMB is equal to 36 mm,[123] there would be an average change in AMB length of 1.5 mm (range, 1.1 to 2.6 mm). The range of isometer displacement guidelines should be used with two considerations in performing measurements for an ACL reconstruction tunnel placement. First, with repeated PROM of the knee, the surgeon should strive to reproduce the PROM pattern presented in Figure 28A–6.[14] This would require the isometer to measure elongation between 1.1 and 2.6 mm as the knee is brought from 50 degrees (when it should be at a minimum) out to extension. Likewise, as the knee is flexed from 50 degrees to nearly full flexion, the isometer pattern should demonstrate a slight elongation. Second, our data represent useful criteria when they are used with an isometer measurement system that has load-displacement behavior similar to the normal ACL but not with the highly compliant isometer systems available with present ACL reconstruction instrumentation. Our data show

TABLE 28A–1
Rank Comparison of Peak Anterior Cruciate Ligament Strain Values during Commonly Prescribed Rehabilitation Activities*

Rehabilitation Activity	Peak Strain (%)	No. of Subjects
Isometric quadriceps contraction at 15° (30 Nm of extension torque)	4.4 (0.6)	8
Squatting with sport cord	4.0 (1.7)	8
Active flexion-extension of the knee with 45-N weight boot	3.8 (0.5)	9
Lachman's test (150 N of anterior shear load; 30° flexion)	3.7 (0.8)	10
Squatting	3.6 (1.3)	8
Active flexion-extension (no weight boot) of the knee	2.8 (0.8)	18
Simultaneous quadriceps and hamstrings contraction at 15°	2.8 (0.9)	8
Isometric quadriceps contraction at 30° (30 Nm of extension torque)	2.7 (0.5)	18
Stair climbing	2.7 (2.9)	5
Weight-bearing at 20° of knee flexion	2.1 (1.7)	11
Anterior drawer (150 N of anterior shear load; 90° flexion)	1.8 (0.9)	10
Stationary bicycling	1.7 (1.9)	8
Isometric hamstrings contraction at 15° (to −10 Nm of flexion torque)	0.6 (0.9)	8
Simultaneous quadriceps and hamstrings contraction at 30°	0.4 (0.5)	8
Passive flexion-extension of the knee	0.1 (0.9)	10
Isometric quadriceps contraction at 60° (30 Nm of extension torque)	0.0	8
Isometric quadriceps contraction at 90° (30 Nm of extension torque)	0.0	18
Simultaneous quadriceps and hamstrings contraction at 60°	0.0	8
Simultaneous quadriceps and hamstrings contraction at 90°	0.0	8
Isometric hamstrings contraction at 30°, 60°, and 90° (−10 Nm of flexion torque)	0.0	8

*Mean (±1 standard deviation).

that measurements of ACL strain after ACL reconstruction do not correlate with elongation predicted by one type of isometer.[48] It is important to recognize the limitations inherent in isometry systems. Care must be taken in interpreting isometer findings because the measurement is being made in an ACL-deficient knee that may have abnormal kinematics. Because the ACL is not present, a measurement system with normal ACL load-displacement behavior would provide the unique ability to restore normal tibiofemoral joint kinematics. In these circumstances, the isometry measurement will make a potential tunnel placement prediction based on conditions to which the ACL substitute will be exposed once it is implanted.[46] This is not possible with current commercially available isometer systems.

The cruciate ligaments serve several functions as passive stabilizers of the knee. The cruciates guide the knee joint through normal kinematics as demonstrated by the four-bar linkage model. The anterior and posterior cruciates are the primary restraints to corresponding anterior and posterior translation of the tibia relative to the femur. The coupled internal and external tibial rotation that occurs with corresponding anterior and posterior shear loading is controlled in part by the cruciate ligaments and should be considered a significant aspect of the clinical examination. In addition, the cruciates act as secondary restraints to varus-valgus motion of the knee joint. Surgical reconstruction of the anterior cruciate should reproduce the in vivo normal ACL strain biomechanics.

Medial and Lateral Collateral Ligaments and Their Function in Joint Stability

Using the flexibility approach, Warren and associates[165] assessed the restraining action of the medial collateral ligament (MCL) complex in human cadaver specimens. They demonstrated that sectioning of the superficial long fibers of the MCL complex produced a significant increase in valgus rotation of the tibiofemoral joint in experiments performed at 0 and 45 degrees of knee flexion. Sectioning the posterior oblique or deep medial portions of the MCL complex had no significant effect on increasing valgus knee angulation.

These findings were confirmed by the work of Seering and coworkers,[141] who employed the stiffness approach in the study of two human cadaveric specimens. They reported that combined superficial and deep portions of the MCL provided 71% of the resistive valgus restraint in one specimen and 55% in another. Grood and colleagues[66] also applied the stiffness approach to investigate the medial ligament complex and presented results that support the findings of the Warren[165] and Seering[141] groups. In addition, Grood and coworkers[66] demonstrated that the long superficial portion of the MCL complex provided 57% of the valgus restraint at 5 degrees, which increased to 78% at 25 degrees of flexion. The variable restraint behavior with valgus loading was attributed to the restraint provided by the posterior medial capsule, which decreased as the knee was brought from an extended into a flexed position. The same research group[67] studied six intact and MCL-deficient cadaveric knees and found that there is a coupled external rotation associated with abduction in an MCL-deficient knee at extension, 15° of flexion, and 30° of flexion. In contrast, the intact knees studied had a coupled internal rotation associated with abduction. This finding, that is, the presence of a coupled external rotation as opposed to a coupled internal rotation, may be used in physical examination for diagnosis of isolated MCL injuries.

Grood and coworkers[66] applied the stiffness approach to investigate the LCL complex. They demonstrated that in response to varus stress, this complex limits lateral opening of the joint. In response to varus loading, the LCL was found to provide 55% of the total restraint at 5 degrees and 69% at 25 degrees of knee flexion. An increase in the contribution of the LCL to the total varus restraint resulted as the knee was brought from an extended to a flexed position. This change was attributed to a decrease in resistive support provided by the posterior portion of the lateral capsule as the knee was flexed. With the knee joint in full extension, the investigators demonstrated that the secondary restraints (including the cruciate ligaments and the posterior portion of the joint capsule) block opening of the knee joint after the collateral ligaments have been cut.[66] Simulating the forces applied by the dynamic stabilizers (iliotibial tract and biceps muscles) revealed their important contribution to varus stability of the knee in vivo.[66] The contribution of the dynamic stabilizers to overall stability of the knee is difficult to assess because the actual muscle force magnitudes for a specific activity are unknown. In a later investigation, Gollehon and associates[60] applied the flexibility approach to study the contribution of the LCL and deep ligament complex (popliteus tendon and arcuate ligament) to joint stability. They demonstrated that the LCL and deep ligament complex function together as the principal structures resisting varus and external rotation of the tibia.[60] Höher and colleagues[71] conducted a cadaver study and concluded that the LCL and popliteus carry a majority of the force in PCL-deficient knees under a posterior load at high flexion angles. Further, they loaded the popliteus in tension to simulate muscle activation and found that the force in the popliteus complex was significantly greater than the force in the LCL at all flexion angles tested (0 to 90 degrees), in both intact cadaveric knees and PCL-deficient knees. Further research is required to assess the interaction of the popliteus complex when the other surrounding muscles are simulated.

Meniscal Biomechanics

Function of the Meniscus in Load Transmission

Meniscal injury is thought by some investigators to be the most common injury sustained by athletes.[151] The menisci were originally thought to be vestigial structures that served no significant function for the tibiofemoral joint.[98] The meniscus was thought to be an expendable structure, and this concerned Jackson,[88] who reported, "The exact function of the meniscus is still a matter of some conjecture." This perspective prompted many orthopaedists to without compressive joint loading. They determined that isolated lateral meniscectomy did not produce a significant change in the anteroposterior load-displacement behavior of the knee. In addition, the effect of the lateral meniscus on restraining anterior translation of the tibia relative to the femur in the ACL-deficient joint was also evaluated. This portion of the investigation demonstrated that the lateral meniscus does not act as a restraint to anterior translation of the tibia relative to the femur, leading the researchers to suggest that this structure may not behave like the medial meniscus in providing an effective posterior wedge to anterior translation.[100] It is important that the results of these investigations of the meniscus be applied to events that occur without a compressive joint load, such as the swing phase of gait, and not to activities that include compressive joint loading.

The menisci have also been thought to assist with joint lubrication, to provide resistance to extreme joint flexion or extension, and to aid in the damping of impulsive loads transmitted across the tibiofemoral joint. These functions are difficult to characterize biomechanically or to describe with clinical impressions, however.

Patellofemoral Joint Biomechanics

The patellofemoral joint consists of the patella with a multifaceted dorsal surface that articulates with the femoral trochlear groove. It is a key component of the knee extensor mechanism.

In 1977, Ficat and Hungerford[44] characterized the patellofemoral joint as the "forgotten compartment of the knee." A study of patellofemoral joint biomechanics is necessary to understand the pathologic processes, to develop rational treatment regimens, and to understand the effects that various rehabilitation programs have on this joint. For example, an abnormally high compressive patellofemoral joint reaction (PFJR) force produces abnormally high stress across the articular cartilage and is thought to be one of the initiating factors of alterations in articular cartilage metabolism, chondromalacia, and subsequent osteoarthritis[7, 87, 103, 129]; in addition, morphometric abnormalities in the trochlear groove or the dorsal articular surface of the patella in combination with high lateral forces at the patellofemoral articulation have been thought to cause lateral subluxation or dislocation of the patella.[44, 83, 85, 129]

Patellofemoral Contact Area

In the normal knee, the patellofemoral contact area is optimally designed to respond to the increase in PFJR load developed with knee flexion through a corresponding increase in contact area. This helps distribute the contact force while minimizing patellofemoral contact stress.

Goodfellow and colleagues[62] used the dye method to measure patellofemoral contact area in human cadaveric knees subjected to simulated weight-bearing conditions. Area measurements were made at 20, 45, 90, and 135 degrees of knee flexion and are presented in Figure 28A–7. Movement of the knee from full extension to 90 degrees

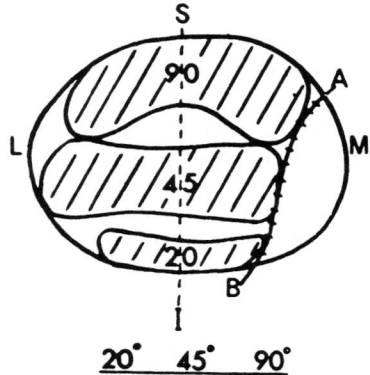

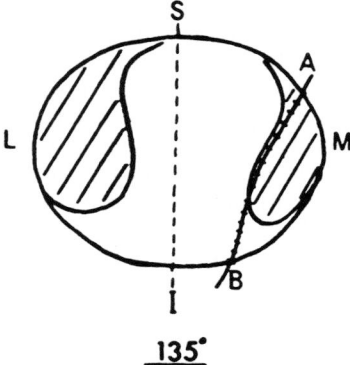

Figure 28A–7. Patellofemoral contact regions at different knee flexion angles. (From Goodfellow J, Hungerford DS Zindel M: Patellofemoral joint mechanics and pathology. J Bone Joint Surg Br 58:287–290, 1976.)

revealed that the contact area on the dorsal aspect of the patella moves in a continuous zone from the inferior to the superior pole of the patella. Continued flexion of the knee to 135 degrees developed two separate contact regions, one on the "odd medial facet" and the other on the lateral aspect of the patella (see Fig. 28A–7). Singerman and colleagues[146, 147] calculated the center of pressure from a 6 degree of freedom patellar transducer in human cadaveric knees and reported that the center of pressure translates superiorly and medially as the knee is flexed to 90 degrees. At flexion angles greater than 85 degrees, the results were somewhat variable, but the center of pressure always moved inferiorly with extension.[146] Huberti and Hayes[78] used pressure-sensitive film to measure the increase of patellofemoral contact area that occurs concurrently with knee flexion (Fig. 28A–8). At a flexion angle of 10 degrees, contact between the dorsal surface of the patella and the trochlea is initiated. The length of the patellar tendon controls when patellar-trochlear contact occurs. In patients in whom the patellar tendon is too long, patella alta may be present, and flexion of the knee greater than 10 degrees may be required to seat the patella adequately in the trochlear groove. With knee movement between extension and 90 degrees, the patella was found to be the only component of the extensor mechanism that contacts the femur, holding the quadriceps tendon away from the femur. With knee motion between 90 and 135 degrees, the quadriceps tendon

Figure 28A–8. Experimental measurement of patellofemoral contact made in human cadaver specimens for the squatting activity with a normal Q angle. Values between 90 degrees and 120 degrees have been extrapolated. *Left,* Contact area; *Middle,* contact pressure; *right,* contact force. (From Huberti HH, Hayes WC: Patellofemoral contact pressures. The influence of Q-angle and tibiofemoral contact. J Bone Joint Surg Am 66:715–724, 1984.)

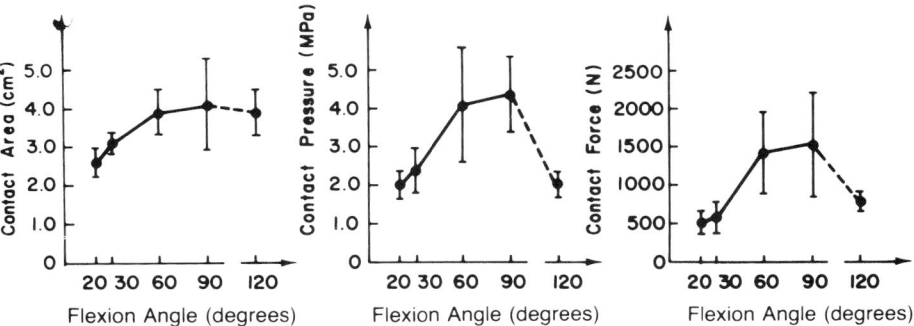

contacts the femur.[159] Once the quadriceps tendon contacts the femur, the compressive PFJR force is divided between contact of the broad band of the quadriceps tendon with the femur and patellofemoral contact.

The interaction between the patellofemoral contact area and PFJR force can be demonstrated with the squatting activity. During this activity, as knee flexion increases, the PFJR force initially increases, while the patellofemoral contact area available for distributing the contact force also increases, effectively distributing the articular contact stress. The opposite situation may occur with knee extension during weight-training programs that apply a weight to the distal aspect of the tibia with the athlete in a seated position. For this activity, the patellofemoral contact area decreases as the PFJR force increases; therefore, the PFJR stress may become high even if light weights are applied to the distal aspect of the tibia. This example may help explain why isotonic or isokinetic exercises through a full range of motion are not advised in the treatment of patellofemoral pain syndromes. Quadriceps exercises extending the knee only through the last 15 to 20 degrees of extension are more likely to be tolerated, as demonstrated by the decrease in PFJR force in Figure 28A–8.

Patellofemoral Force Transmission

The patella transmits force from the quadriceps muscle group to the patellar tendon while developing a large PFJR force. This serves to stabilize the knee against gravity when the joint is in a flexed position and assists in the forward propulsion of the body as the knee is extended during gait. Therefore, the loads developed along the patellar tendon and the PFJR force are a function of both quadriceps force and knee flexion angle. A sagittal plane analysis can be used to demonstrate this. This employs application of statics in a simple engineering approach to describe the forces and moments required to maintain the knee joint in equilibrium. For example, with use of this technique, the quadriceps force (F_{Quads}), the PFJR force, and the patellar tendon force (F_{PT}) may be related at chosen knee flexion angles. Figure 28A–9 is a simplified sagittal plane static representation of the relation between the PFJR and the quadriceps muscle forces. The mass of the upper body (W), assumed to act at the hip joint, is supported by the F_{Quads} developed by the quadriceps muscle groups. The vertical line below the center of mass at the subject's hip joint represents the force vector due to upper body weight, and this falls well

behind the flexion axis of the knee. The distance from the center of mass force vector to the flexion axis of the knee is defined as the moment arm (c). The moment arm is relatively small with the knee near extension. Therefore, the support mechanism provided by the F_{Quads} and the developed PFJR are relatively small. In the right portion of Figure 28A–9, the knee is in a position of greater flexion with an associated increase in the moment arm (c′). To maintain the knee in static equilibrium, the new force (F_{Quads}) generated by the quadriceps must increase significantly. As a result of the increased quadriceps force, the PFJR must also be larger. This model may help explain the mechanism by which both PFJR and F_{Quads} increase during squatting activities.

In the earlier force analysis studies, the patella-trochlea articulation was represented as a frictionless pulley.[7, 44, 84, 116, 118, 119, 131, 134, 149] This assumption was justified on the basis of the low coefficient of friction between the patellofemoral articular surfaces. With use of this approach, the forces developed by the quadriceps muscle group were assumed to be equal to the force developed along the patellar tendon throughout the full range of knee motion, with the direction of the PFJR force defined as the bisector of the angle between the quadriceps and the patellar tendon force vectors. Employing the mechanics principle of static equilibrium, and with the assumption that the patella-trochlea articulation behaves like a frictionless pulley, Reilly and Martens[134] predicted a compressive PFJR force of 0.5 times body weight for level walking. For ascending and descending stairs, the PFJR was estimated to reach 3.3 times body weight.[134] Analysis of the squatting activity revealed that a maximum PFJR of 2.9 times body weight occurred at 90 degrees of flexion.[134] Active extension of the lower leg with a 9-kg boot while the femur was orientated in a horizontal position produced a peak PFJR at 36 degrees of flexion.[134] Maquet[104, 106] questioned the frictionless pulley assumption and demonstrated with a lateral vector diagram of the patellofemoral articulation that the forces in the quadriceps mechanism and patellar tendon can differ and can also vary as a function of knee flexion angle. Several investigators have confirmed Maquet's findings.[1, 17, 27, 41, 77, 158]

In later work performed by Huberti,[77] Van Eijden,[158] Buff,[27] Ahmed,[1] Singerman,[146] and their coworkers, the combined tibia, femur, and patella were evaluated by use of both experimental and theoretical techniques. Because the force values F_{PT} and F_{Quads} are unequal, these researchers have chosen to report results by calculating the ratio between the two force values ($F_{PT}:F_{Quads}$) at selected knee

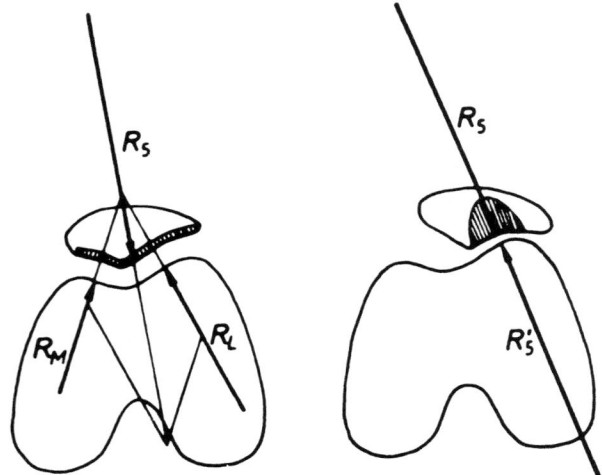

Figure 28A–13. Patellofemoral joint reaction forces for the normal knee *(left)*. The joint reaction force (R_S) is resisted by the lateral (R_L) and medial (R_M) components. In the knee with a lateralized patella *(right)*, the joint reaction force is resisted by the lateral component only (R'_S). (From Maquet P: Mechanics and osteoarthritis of the patellofemoral joint. Clin Orthop 144:70, 1979.)

sor mechanism and prevention of recurrent subluxation of the patella. An evaluation of 116 patients observed for at least 1 year demonstrated this procedure to be a satisfactory method for the prevention of lateral subluxation, with recurrence in only 7% of the cases. Careful attention to the medial transfer of the tibial tuberosity without a posterior displacement was emphasized as the key to successful long-term results.[35] Procedures resulting in some posterior transfer of the tibial tuberosity, such as that described by Hauser, decrease the patellar tendon moment arm and consequently increase the patellofemoral contact stress. Fulkerson and Hungerford[57] have reviewed the clinical and radiologic outcomes of the Hauser procedure and have presented evidence of progressive knee joint degeneration.

Summary

Future research endeavors in biomechanics should continue to perform in vivo strain measurement of the soft tissues surrounding the knee and establish new in vivo measurement techniques, such as pressure or force sensors. In addition, the development of an analytic model that includes both patellofemoral and tibiofemoral articulations will permit the study of injury mechanisms, will allow the investigation of soft tissue reconstruction procedures, and will permit research concerning commonly prescribed rehabilitation activities. Application of the in vivo experimental techniques and analytic models should strive to establish the relationship between the biomechanical behavior of a graft and the resulting biologic properties. Technology, such as an implantable telemetered load sensor, should be designed to allow an optimal match between a rehabilitation regimen and the biologic-mechanical behavior of the graft. Biomechanics research efforts should strive to establish intraoperative techniques and measurements that can accurately provide the surgeon with the ability to reestab-

lish normal joint kinematics during a soft tissue reconstruction procedure. Future clinical biomechanical investigations of surgical procedures should include prospective, randomized, well-controlled, long-term studies that use standardized outcomes to assess the relative effectiveness of the many different soft tissue reconstruction techniques.

References

1. Ahmed AM, Burke DL, Hyder A: Force analysis of the patellar mechanism. J Orthop Res 5:69–85, 1987.
2. Ahmed AM, Burke DL: In vitro measurement of static pressure distribution in synovial joints. Part I. Tibial surface of the knee. J Biomech Eng 105:216–225, 1983.
3. Allen CR, Wong EK, Livesay GA, et al: Importance of the medial meniscus in the anterior cruciate ligament–deficient knee. J Orthop Res 18:109-115, 2000.
4. Ameil D, Kleiner JB, Akeson WH: The natural history of the anterior cruciate ligament autograft of patellar tendon origin. Am J Sports Med 14:449–462, 1986.
5. Arms SA, Pope MH, Johnson RJ, et al: The biomechanics of anterior cruciate ligament rehabilitation and reconstruction. Am J Sports Med 12:8–18, 1984.
6. Bach JM, Hull ML: Strain of the anterior cruciate ligament increases linearly with quadriceps contraction. In Johnson RJ (ed): Skiing Trauma and Safety, vol 12 (ASTM STP 1345). West Conshohocken, Pa, American Society for Testing and Materials, 1999, pp 94–104.
7. Bandi W: Chondromalacia patellae and femora-patellare Arthrose, Atiologie, Klinik, and Therapie. Helv Chir Acta Suppl 11:3–70, 1972.
8. Baratz ME, Fu FH, Mengato R: Meniscal tears: The effect of meniscectomy and repair in intraarticular contact areas and stress in the human knee. Am J Sports Med 14:270–275, 1986.
9. Bargar WL, Moreland JF, Markolf KL, et al: In vivo stability testing of postmeniscectomy knees. Clin Orthop 150:247–252, 1980.
10. Barry D, Ahmed AM: Design and performance of a modified buckle transducer for the measurement of ligament tension. J Biomech Eng 108:149–142, 1986.
11. Bartel DL, Marshall JL, Schieck RA, Wang JB: Surgical repositioning of the medial collateral ligament. J Bone Joint Surg Am 59:101–117, 1977.
12. Berns GS, Hull ML, Patterson HA: Strain in the anteromedial bundle of the anterior cruciate ligament under combination loading. J Orthop Res 10:167–176, 1992.
13. Beynnon BD: The In Vivo Biomechanics of the Anterior Cruciate Ligament: Reconstruction and Application of a Mathematical Model to the Knee Joint [PhD dissertation]. Burlington, University of Vermont, 1991.
14. Beynnon BD, Howe JG, Pope MH, et al: Anterior cruciate ligament strain in vivo. Int Orthop 16:1–12, 1992.
15. Beynnon BD, Fleming BC: Anterior cruciate ligament strain in vivo: A review of previous work. J Biomech 31:519-525, 1998.
16. Beynnon BD, Johnson RJ, Fleming BC, et al: The strain behavior of the anterior cruciate ligament during squatting and active flexion-extension. A comparison of an open and a closed kinetic chain exercise. Am J Sports Med 25:862-863, 1997.
17. Bishop RED, Denham RA: A note on the ratio between tensions in the quadriceps tendon and infra-patella ligament. Eng Med 6:53–54, 1977.
18. Blankevoort L, Kuiper JH, Huiskes R, Grootenboer HJ: Articular contact in a three-dimensional model of the knee. J Biomech 24:1019–1031, 1991.
19. Blankevoort L, Huiskes R: Ligament-bone interaction in a three-dimensional model of the knee. J Biomech Eng 113:263–269, 1991.
20. Blankevoort L, Huiskes R: ACL isometry is not the criterion for ACL reconstruction. Trans Orthop Res Soc 16:203, 1991.
21. Blankevoort L, Huiskes R, de Lange A: Recruitment of the knee-joint ligaments. J Biomech Eng 113:94–103, 1991.
22. Blankevoort L, Huiskes R, de Lange A: Helical axes of passive knee-joint motions. J Biomech 22:1219-1229, 1990.
23. Bylski-Austrow DI, Ciarelli MJ, Kayner DC, et al: Displacements

of the menisci under joint load: An in vitro study in human knees. J Biomech 27:421–431, 1994.

24. Bonnarens FO, Drez D: Biomechanics of artificial ligaments and associated problems. In Jackson DW, Drez D (eds): The Anterior Cruciate Deficient Knee: New Concepts in Ligament Repair. St. Louis, CV Mosby, 1987, pp 239–253.

25. Brattström H: Shape of the intercondylar groove normally and in recurrent dislocation of the patella. A clinical and x-ray–anatomical investigation. Acta Orthop Scand Suppl 68:1–148, 1964.

26. Brown TD, Sigal L, Njus GO, et al: Dynamic performance characteristics of the liquid metal strain gauge. J Biomech 19:165–173, 1986.

27. Buff HU, Jones LC, Hungerford DS: Experimental determination of forces transmitted through the patellofemoral joint. J Biomech 21:17–23, 1988.

28. Butler DL: Anterior cruciate ligament: Its response and replacement. J Orthop Res 7:910–921, 1989.

29. Butler DL, Grood ES, Noyes FR, Sodd AN: On the interpretation of our anterior cruciate ligament data. Clin Orthop 196:26–34, 1985.

30. Butler DL, Grood ES, Zernicke RR, et al: Non-uniform surface strains in young human tendons and fascia. Trans Orthop Res Soc 8:8, 1983.

31. Butler DL, Noyes FR, Grood ES: Ligamentous restraints to anterior-posterior drawer in the human knee. J Bone Joint Surg Am 62:259–270, 1980.

32. Campbell WC: Operative Orthopaedics. St. Louis, CV Mosby, 1939, pp 406, 415.

33. Churchill DL, Incavo SJ, Johnson CC, Beynnon BD: The transepicondylar axis approximates the optimal flexion axis of the knee. Clin Orthop 356:111–118, 1998.

34. Cooper RR, Misol S: Tendon and ligament insertion: A light and electron microscopic study. J Bone Joint Surg Am 52:1-20, 1970.

35. Cox JS: Evaluation of the Roux-Elmslie-Trillat procedure for knee extensor realignment. Am J Sports Med 10:303, 1982.

36. Crowninshield R, Pope MH, Johnson RJ: An analytical model of the knee. J Biomech 9:397–405, 1976.

37. Dandy DJ, Jackson RW: Meniscectomy and chondromalacia of the femoral condyle. J Bone Joint Surg Am 57:1116-1119, 1975.

38. Dandy DJ, Jackson RW: The diagnosis of problems after meniscectomy. J Bone Joint Surg Br 57:349–352, 1975.

39. Daniel D, Malcolm L, Losse G, et al: Instrumented measurement of anterior laxity of the knee. J Bone Joint Surg Am 67:720–725, 1985.

40. Edwards RG, Lafferty JF, Lange KD: Ligament strain in the human knee. J Basic Eng 92:131–136, 1970.

41. Ellis MI, Seedhom BB, Wright V, Dowson D: An evaluation of the ratio between the tension along the quadriceps tendon and the patella ligament. Eng Med 9:189–194, 1980.

42. Fairbank TJ: Knee changes after meniscectomy. J Bone Joint Surg Br 30:664, 1948.

43. Ferguson AB, Brown TD, Fu FH, Rutkowski R: Relief of patellofemoral contact stress by anterior displacement of the tibial tubercle. J Bone Joint Surg Am 61:159–166, 1979.

44. Ficat RP, Hungerford DS: Disorders of the Patellofemoral Joint. Baltimore, Williams & Wilkins, 1977.

45. Fischer RA, Arms SW, Johnson RJ, Pope MH: The functional relationship of the posterior oblique ligament to the medial collateral ligament of the human knee. Am J Sports Med 13:390–397, 1985.

46. Fleming BC, Beynnon BD, Johnson RJ, et al: Isometric versus tension measurements: A comparison for the reconstruction of the anterior cruciate ligament. Am J Sports Med 21:82–88, 1993.

47. Fleming BC, Beynnon BD, Nichols CE, et al: An in vivo comparison of anterior tibial translation and strain in the anteromedial band of the anterior cruciate ligament. J Biomech 26:51–58, 1993.

48. Fleming BC, Beynnon BD, Nichols CE, et al: An in vivo comparison between intraoperative isometric measurement and local elongation of the graft after reconstruction of the anterior cruciate ligament. J Bone Joint Surg Am 76:511–519, 1994.

49. Fleming BC, Beynnon BD, Renstrom PA, et al: The strain behavior of the anterior cruciate ligament during stair climbing: An in vivo study. Arthroscopy 15:185–191, 1999.

50. Fleming BC, Beynnon BD, Renstrom PA, et al: The strain behavior of the anterior cruciate ligament during bicycling. An in vivo study. Am J Sports Med 26:109–118, 1998.

51. Fleming BC, Good L, Peura GD, Beynnon BD: Calibration and application of an intra-articular force transducer for the measurement

of patellar tendon graft forces: An in situ evaluation. J Biomech Eng 121:393–398, 1999.

52. Flemin, BC, Peura GD, Beynnon BD: Factors influencing the output of an implantable force transducer. J Biomech 33:889–893, 2000.

53. Frankel VH, Burstein AH, Brooks DB: Biomechanics of internal derangement of the knee. Pathomechanics as determined by analysis of the instant centers of motion. J Bone Joint Surg Am 53:945–962, 1971.

54. Frankel VH: Biomechanics of the knee. Orthop Clin North Am 2:175–190, 1971.

55. Frankel VH, Burstein AH: Orthopaedic Biomechanics. Philadelphia, Lea & Febiger, 1970.

56. Fukubayashi T, Torzilli PA, Sherman MF, Warren RF: An in vitro biomechanical evaluation of anterior-posterior motion of the knee. J Bone Joint Surg Am 64:258–264, 1982.

57. Fulkerson JP, Hungerford DS: Patellar subluxation. In Disorders of the Patellofemoral Joint. Baltimore, Williams & Wilkins, 1990, p 142.

58. Furman W, Marshall JL, Girgis FC: The anterior cruciate ligament—a functional analysis based on postmortem studies. J Bone Joint Surg Am 58:179-185, 1976.

59. Girgis FG, Marshall JL, Monajem ARSH: The cruciate ligaments of the knee joint. Clin Orthop 106:216–231, 1975.

60. Gollehon DL, Torzilli PA, Warren RF: The role of the posterolateral and cruciate ligaments in the stability of the human knee. A biomechanical study. J Bone Joint Surg Am 69:233–242, 1987.

61. Goodfellow J, O'Conner J: The mechanics of the knee and prosthesis design. J Bone Joint Surg Br 60:358–369, 1978.

62. Goodfellow J, Hungerford DS, Zindel M: Patellofemoral joint mechanics and pathology. J Bone Joint Surg Br 58:287–290, 1976.

63. Grood ES, Noyes FR: Diagnosis of knee ligament injuries: Biomechanical precepts. In Feagin JA Jr (ed): The Crucial Ligaments. New York, Churchill Livingstone, 1988.

64. Grood ES, Stowers SF, Noyes FR: Limits of movement in the human knee. Effect of sectioning the posterior cruciate ligament and posterolateral structures. J Bone Joint Surg Am 70:88–97, 1988.

65. Grood ES, Suntay WJ, Noyes FR, Butler DL: Biomechanics of the knee-extension exercise. J Bone Joint Surg Am 66:725–734, 1984.

66. Grood ES, Noyes FR, Butler DL, Suntay WJ: Ligamentous and capsular restraints preventing straight medial and lateral laxity in intact human cadaver knees. J Bone Joint Surg Am 63:1257–1269, 1981.

67. Haimes JL, Wroble RR, Grood ES, Noyes FR: Role of the medial structures in the intact and anterior cruciate ligament–deficient knee. Limits of motion in the human knee. Am J Sports Med 22:402–409, 1994.

68. Harner CD, Xerogeanes JW, Livesay GA, et al: The human posterior cruciate ligament complex: An interdisciplinary study. Ligament morphology and biomechanical evaluation. Am J Sports Med 23:736–745, 1995.

69. Hefzy MS, Grood ES: Review of knee models. Appl Mech Rev 41:1–13, 1988.

70. Henning CE, Lynch MA, Glick KR: An in vitro strain gauge study of elongation of the anterior cruciate ligament. Am J Sports Med 13:22–26, 1985.

71. Höher J, Vogrin TM, Woo SL, et al: In situ forces in the human posterior cruciate ligament in response to muscle loads: A cadaveric study. J Orthop Res 17:763–768, 1999.

72. Hollis JM, Pearsall AW, Niciforos PG: Change in meniscal strain with anterior cruciate ligament injury and after reconstruction. Am J Sports Med 28:700–704, 2000.

73. Hollis JM: Development and Application of a Method for Determining the In Situ Forces in Anterior Cruciate Ligament Fiber Bundles [PhD dissertation]. San Diego, University of California, 1988.

74. Hollister AM, Jatana A, Singh AK, et al: The axes of rotation of the knee. Clin Orthop 290:259–268, 1993.

75. Howe JG, Wertheimer CM, Johnson RJ, et al: Arthroscopic strain gauge measurement of the normal anterior cruciate ligament. Arthroscopy 6:198-204, 1990.

76. Hsieh HH, Walker PS: Stabilizing mechanisms of the loaded and unloaded knee joint. J Bone Joint Surg Am 58:87–93, 1976.

77. Huberti HH, Hayes WC, Stone JL, Shybut GT: Force ratios in the quadriceps tendon and ligamentous patellae. J Orthop Res 2:49–54, 1984.

78. Huberti HH, Hayes WC: Patellofemoral contact pressures, the influ-

ence of Q-angle, and tendofemoral contact. J Bone Joint Surg Am 66:715–724, 1984.

79. Huckle JR: Is meniscectomy a benign procedure? A long-term follow-up study. Can J Surg 8:254, 1965.

80. Hughston JC, Andrews JR, Cross MJ, Moschi A: Classification of knee ligament instabilities. Part 1. The medial compartment and cruciate ligaments. J Bone Joint Surg Am 58:159–172, 1976.

81. Hughston JC, Eilers AF: The role of the posterior oblique ligament in repairs of the acute medial collateral ligament tears of the knee. J Bone Joint Surg Am 55:923–940, 1973.

82. Hull ML, Berns GS, Varma H, Patterson HA: Strain in the medial collateral ligament of the human knee under single and combined loads. J Biomech 29:199–206, 1996.

83. Hungerford DS, Haynes D: The dynamics of patellar stabilization in knee flexion and rotation. Trans Orthop Res Soc 7:254, 1982.

84. Hungerford DS, Barry M: Biomechanics of the patellofemoral joint. Clin Orthop 144:9–15, 1979.

85. Insall J: "Chondromalacia patellae": Patellar malalignment syndrome. Orthop Clin North Am 10:117–127, 1979.

86. Insall J, Palvoka A, Wise DW: Chondromalacia patellae. A prospective study. J Bone Joint Surg Am 58:1–8, 1976.

87. Insall J, Goldberg V, Salvati E: Recurrent dislocation and the high-riding patella. Clin Orthop 88:67–69, 1972.

88. Jackson JP: Degenerative changes in the knee after meniscectomy. Br Med J 2:525, 1968.

89. Jacob RP: Observations on rotary instability of the lateral compartment of the knee. Acta Orthop Scand Suppl 52:1–31, 1981.

90. Johnson RJ: The anterior cruciate: A dilemma in sports medicine. Int J Sports Med 3:71–79, 1982.

91. Johnson RJ, Pope MH: Functional anatomy of the meniscus. In Symposium on the Athlete's Knee: Surgical Repair and Reconstruction. American Academy of Orthopaedic Surgeons. St. Louis, CV Mosby, 1978, pp 3–13.

92. Johnson RJ, Kettlekamp DB, Clark W, Leaverton P: Factors affecting late meniscectomy results. J Bone Joint Surg Am 56:719–729, 1974.

93. Kapandji IA: The Physiology of the Joints: Annotated Diagrams of the Joints, vol 2. Edinburgh, Churchill Livingstone, 1970.

94. Kennedy JC, Haskins RJ, Willis RB: Strain gauge analysis of knee ligaments. Clin Orthop 129:225–229, 1977.

95. Kennedy JC, Hawkins RJ, Willis RB, Danylchuck KD: Tension studies of human knee ligaments, yield point, ultimate failure, and disruption of the cruciate and tibial collateral ligaments. J Bone Joint Surg Am 58:350–355, 1976.

96. Kennedy JC, Weinberg HW, Wilson AS: The anatomy and function of the anterior cruciate ligament as determined by clinical and morphological studies. J Bone Joint Surg Am 56:223–235, 1974.

97. Kettlekamp DB, Jacobs AW: Tibiofemoral contact areas—determination and implications. J Bone Joint Surg Am 54:349, 1972.

98. King D: The function of semilunar cartilage. J Bone Joint Surg Am 18:1069–1076, 1936.

99. Krause WR, Pope MH, Johnson RJ, Wilder DG: Mechanical changes in the knee after meniscectomy. J Bone Joint Surg Am 58:599, 1976.

100. Levy MI, Torzilli PA, Gould JD, Warren RF: The effect of lateral meniscectomy on motion of the knee. J Bone Joint Surg Am 71:401–406, 1989.

101. Levy MI, Torzilli PA, Warren RF: The effect of medial meniscectomy on anterior-posterior motion of the knee. J Bone Joint Surg Am 64:883–888, 1982.

102. Lewis JL, Jasti M, Schafer M, Wixson R: Functional load directions for the two bands of the anterior cruciate ligament. Trans Orthop Res Soc 5:307, 1980.

103. Maquet PG: Mechanics and osteoarthritis of the patellofemoral joint. Clin Orthop 144:70–73, 1979.

104. Maquet PG: Biomechanics of the Knee. New York, Springer-Verlag, 1976.

105. Maquet PG, Van De Berg AJ, Simonet JC: Femorotibial weight-bearing areas: Experimental determination. J Bone Joint Surg Am 57:766, 1975.

106. Maquet PG: Biomechanics and osteoarthritis of the knee. Société Internationale de Chirurgie Orthopédique et de Traumatologie, 11th Congress, 1969, Mexico.

107. Markolf KL, Gorek JF, Kabo M, Shapiro MS: Direct measurement of resultant forces in the anterior cruciate ligament. An in vitro study performed with a new experimental technique. J Bone Joint Surg Am 72:557–567, 1990.

108. Markolf KL, Bargar WL, Shoemaker SC, Amstutz HC: The role of joint load in knee stability. J Bone Joint Surg Am 63:570–585, 1981.

109. Markolf KL, Burchfield DM, Shapiro MM, et al: Combined knee loading states that generate high anterior cruciate ligament forces. J Orthop Res 13:930–935, 1995.

110. Markolf KL, Graff-Radford A, Amstutz HC: In vivo stability—a quantitative assessment using an instrumented clinical testing apparatus. J Bone Joint Surg Am 60:664–674, 1978.

111. Markolf KL, Meusch JS, Amstutz HC: Stiffness and laxity of the knee—the contributions of the supporting structures. J Bone Joint Surg Am 58:583–594, 1976.

112. Markolf KL, Slauterbeck JL, Armstrong KL, et al: Effects of combined knee loadings on posterior cruciate ligament force generation. J Orthop Res 14:633–638, 1996.

113. Markolf KL, Slauterbeck JR, Armstrong KL, et al: A biomechanical study of replacement of the posterior cruciate ligament with a graft. Part II: Forces in the graft compared with forces in the intact ligament. J Bone Joint Surg Am 79:381–386, 1997.

114. Markolf KL, Wascher DC, Finerman GA: Direct in vitro measurement of forces in the cruciate ligaments. Part II: The effect of section of the posterolateral structures. J Bone Joint Surg Am 75:387–394, 1993.

115. Marshall J, Girgis FG, Zelko R: The biceps femoris tendon and its functional significance. J Bone Joint Surg Am 54:1444–1450, 1972.

116. Matthews LS, Sonstegard DA, Heuke JA: Load-bearing characteristics of the patellofemoral joint. Acta Orthop Scand 48:511–516, 1977.

117. Menschik A: Mechanik des Kniegelenkes. Z Orthop Ihre Grenzgeb 112:481–495, 1974.

118. Morrison JB: The mechanics of the knee joint. J Biomech 3:51–61, 1970.

119. Morrison JB: Function of the knee joint in various activities. Biomed Eng 4:573–580, 1969.

120. Mow VC, Hayes WC: Basic Orthopaedic Biomechanics. New York, Raven Press, 1991.

121. Muller W: The Knee: Form, Function and Ligament Reconstruction. New York, Springer-Verlag, 1983.

122. Nisell R, Nemeth G, Ohlsen H: Joint forces in extension of the knee. Acta Orthop Scand 57:41–46, 1986.

123. Norwood LA, Cross MJ: Anterior cruciate ligament: Functional anatomy and its bundles in rotatory instabilities. Am J Sports Med 7:23–26, 1979.

124. Noyes FR, Grood ES, Torzilli PA: The definitions of terms for motion and position of the knee and injuries of the ligaments. J Bone Joint Surg Am 71:465–472, 1989.

125. Noyes FR, Butler DL, Grood ES, et al: Biomechanical analysis of human ligament grafts used in knee ligament repairs and reconstruction. J Bone Joint Surg Am 66:344–352, 1984.

126. Noyes FR: Functional properties of knee ligaments and alterations induced by immobilization. Clin Orthop 123:210–242, 1977.

127. Noyes FR, Grood ES: The strength of the anterior cruciate ligament in humans and rhesus monkeys: Age-related and species-related changes. J Bone Joint Surg Am 58:1074–1082, 1976.

128. Noyes FR, DeLucas JL, Torrik PJ: Biomechanics of ligament failure: An analysis of strain-rate sensitivity and mechanism of failure in primates. J Bone Joint Surg Am 56:236–253, 1974.

129. Outerbridge RE, Dunlop JAY: The problem of chondromalacia patellae. Clin Orthop 110:177–196, 1975.

130. Paulos L, Noyes FR, Grood ES, Butler DL: Knee rehabilitation after ACL reconstruction and repair. Am J Sports Med 9:140–149, 1981.

131. Perry J, Antonelli P, Ford W: Analysis of knee joint forces during flexed-knee stance. J Bone Joint Surg Am 57:961–967, 1975.

132. Pevsner DN, Johnson JRG, Blazina ME: The patellofemoral joint and its implications in rehabilitation of the knee. Phys Ther 59:869–874, 1979.

133. Quigley TB: Knee injuries incurred in sports. JAMA 171:1666, 1959.

134. Reilly DT, Martens M: Experimental analysis of the quadriceps muscle force and patellofemoral joint reaction force for various activities. Acta Orthop Scand 43:126-137, 1972.

135. Renström P, Arms SW, Stanwyck TS, et al: Strain within the anterior cruciate ligament during hamstring and quadriceps activity. Am J Sports Med 14:83–87, 1986.

136. Salmons S: Meeting report from the 8th International Conference on Medical and Biological Engineering. Bio Eng 4:467–474, 1969.

137. Sapega AA, Moyer RJ, Schneck C, Komalahiranya N: Testing for isometry during reconstruction of the anterior cruciate ligament. J Bone Joint Surg Am 72:259–267, 1990.

138. Seedhom BB: Transmission of the load in the knee joint with special reference to the role of the menisci. Part I. Anatomy, analysis, and apparatus. Eng Med 8:207, 1979.

139. Seedhom BB, Hargreaves DJ: Transmission of load in the knee joint with special reference to the role of the menisci. Part II. Experimental results, discussion, and conclusions. Eng Med 8:220, 1979.

140. Seedhom BB, Dawson D, Wright U: Functions of the menisci—a preliminary study. J Bone Joint Surg Br 56:381, 1974.

141. Seering WP, Pizialli RL, Nagel DA, Schurman DJ: The function of the primary ligaments of the knee in varus-valgus and axial rotation. J Biomech 13:785–794, 1980.

142. Shrine N: The weight-bearing role of the menisci of the knee. J Bone Joint Surg Br 56:381, 1974.

143. Sidles JA, Clark JM, Garbini JL: Fiber anatomy and internal stresses in ligaments and tendons: A general geometric model. Trans Orthop Res Soc 14:250, 1989.

144. Sidles JA, Larson RV, Garbini JL, et al: Ligament length relationships in the moving knee. J Orthop Res 6:593–610, 1988.

145. Simon WH: Scale effects in animal joints. Arthritis Rheum 13:244–256, 1970.

146. Singerman R, Berilla J, Davy DT: Direct in vitro determination of the patellofemoral contact force for normal knees. J Biomech Eng 117:8–14, 1995.

147. Singerman R, Berilla J, Kotzar G, et al: A six-degree-of-freedom transducer for in vitro measurement of patellofemoral contact forces. J Biomech 27:233–238, 1994.

148. Slocum DB, Larson RL, James SL: Late reconstruction procedures used to stabilize the knee. Orthop Clin North Am 4:679–689, 1973.

149. Smidt GL: Biomechanical analysis of knee flexion and extension. J Biomech 6:79–92, 1973.

150. Smillie JS: Injuries to the Knee Joint, 4th ed. Edinburgh, Churchill Livingstone, 1971, p 68.

151. Sonne-Holm S, Fledelius I, Ahn N: Results after meniscectomy in 147 athletes. Acta Orthop Scand 51:303–309, 1980.

152. Strasser H: Lehrbuch der Muskel- und Gelenkmechanik, vol 3. Berlin, Springer-Verlag, 1917.

153. Sullivan D, Levy IM, Shaskier S, et al: Medial restraints to anterior-posterior motion of the knee. J Bone Joint Surg Am 66:930–936, 1984.

154. Tapper EM, Hoover NW: Late results after meniscectomy. J Bone Joint Surg Am 51:517, 1969.

155. Torg J, Conrad W, Kalen V: Clinical diagnosis of ACL instability. Am J Sports Med 4:84–92, 1976.

156. Torzilli P, Greenberg R, Hood R, et al: Measurement of anterior-posterior motion of the knee in injured patients using a biomechanical stress technique. J Bone Joint Surg Am 66:1438–1442, 1984.

157. Trent PS, Walker PS, Wolf B: Ligament length patterns, strength, and rotational axes of the knee joint. Clin Orthop 117:263–279, 1976.

158. Van Eijden TMGJ, Kouwenhoven E, Verburg J, Weijs WA: A mathematical model of the patellofemoral joint. J Biomech 19:219–229, 1986.

159. Van Eijden TMGJ, De Boer W, Weijs WA: The orientation of the distal part of the quadriceps femoris muscle as a function of the knee flexion-extension angle. J Biomech 18:803–809, 1985.

160. Walker PS, Erkman MJ: The role of the menisci in force transmission across the knee. Clin Orthop 109:184–192, 1975.

161. Walker PS, Shoji H, Erkman MJ: The rotational axis of the knee and its significance to prosthesis design. Clin Orthop 89:160–170, 1972.

162. Wang CJ, Walker PS: Rotation laxity of the human knee. J Bone Joint Surg Am 56:161, 1974.

163. Wang CJ, Walker PS, Wolf B: The effects of flexion and rotation on the length patterns of the ligaments of the knee. J Biomech 6:587–596, 1973.

164. Warren LF, Marshall JL: The supporting structures and layers on the medial side of the knee, an anatomical analysis. J Bone Joint Surg Am 61:50–62, 1979.

165. Warren LF, Marshall JL, Girgis F: The prime static stabilizer of the medial side of the knee. J Bone Joint Surg Am 56:665–674, 1974.

166. Watson-Jones OR: Fractures and Joint Injuries, vol 2. Edinburgh, Churchill Livingstone, 1955, pp 769–773.

167. Wascher DC, Markolf KL, Shapiro MS, Finerman GAM: Direct in vitro measurements of forces in the cruciate ligaments. Part I: The effect of multiplane loading in the intact knee. J Bone Joint Surg Am 75:377–386, 1993.

168. Wismans J, Veldpaus F, Janssen J, et al: A three-dimensional mathematical model of the knee joint. J Biomech 13:677–685, 1980.

169. Woo SLY, Hollis JM, Adams DJ, et al: Tensile properties of the human femur–anterior cruciate ligament–tibia complex. The effects of specimen age and orientations. Am J Sports Med 19:217–225, 1991.

170. Woo SLY, Gomez MA, Akerson WH: Mechanical properties along the medial collateral ligament. Trans Orthop Res Soc 8:7, 1983.

Section B
Imaging Sports-Related Injuries of the Knee

Robert O. Cone III, MD

For many years, plain radiography was the mainstay of evaluation of the patient with a sports injury. Plain radiographs remain unparalleled in importance in the diagnosis of fractures and dislocations. The great majority of sports injuries, however, are not visible on plain radiographs and in the past were inferred from the history, the physical examination, and, occasionally, an alignment abnormality on radiography.

X-ray tomography provided an enhancement to plain radiography and was especially useful in evaluating complex fractures and determining the location and the orientation of fracture fragments. Polytomography provided further enhancement of this technique and allowed extremely thin sections and much improved spatial resolution.

Computed tomography (CT) was initially limited to the axial imaging plane, with poor quality of reconstructions in other anatomic planes. The new generation of CT units can now provide high-resolution reconstruction of osseous anatomy in any desired plane and has replaced tomography for detailed evaluation of complex bony injuries.

Diagnostic ultrasound was found to be useful in the diagnosis of cystic lesions about the knee. Radionuclide scintigraphy was useful in the diagnosis of occult bony injuries and stress fractures, which were invisible to plain radiographs.

Contrast arthrography was developed to allow greater specificity in diagnosis of soft tissue injuries within joints. Contrast arthrography became especially important in the knee in identifying meniscal tears. Over the years, knee arthrography became a very sophisticated procedure, requiring a great deal of expertise to perform as well as to interpret.

When magnetic resonance imaging (MRI) was developed, the limitations of knee arthrography were readily exposed, and a staggeringly complex array of previously invisible anatomy and injuries was exposed. Initially, MRI was an obscure study with great promise in unlocking occult abnormalities of the central nervous system. Today, the initials MRI, which cause almost everyone immediately to think of athletic injuries, are a source of great anxiety when spoken to our favorite athlete. MRI has replaced all the complex imaging techniques of the past in the diagnosis of injuries of the knee.[32, 94]

Plain radiography remains a useful initial screening examination and is readily available in almost every office and clinic. Diagnostic ultrasound remains useful in localizing juxta-articular cysts for injection or aspiration. CT remains of value in delineation of complex fracture fragments and occasionally in the localization of loose bodies or osteochondral fragments. Recently, spiral CT arthrography has been shown to be highly sensitive and specific for identification and characterization of meniscal tears.[180] Owing to its invasiveness, CT arthrography is unlikely to have an effect on the use of MRI of the knee in typical cases, although it is likely to replace contrast arthrography completely in the evaluation of those occasional patients who cannot undergo MRI evaluation.

MRI allows unparalleled accuracy in the initial diagnosis of athletic injuries of the knee[37, 60, 71, 90, 125, 138] and provides specific preoperative planning as well as a noninvasive means of postoperative follow-up. Hardware and software improvements are constantly improving the accuracy of the examination as well as decreasing the time and the discomfort associated with an MRI examination. The greatest drawback of MRI has been the high cost of acquiring and maintaining the equipment, resulting in a high cost for the examination. Faster acquisition times have allowed greater patient throughput and have allowed some decrease in cost per examination. Though the financial cost remains high, the advantages of the MRI easily outweigh the costs. Most supplemental imaging examinations are no longer needed. Examinations may be performed on the acutely injured knee during the period when physical examination is difficult and often unreliable, allowing immediate surgical treatment if indicated. Negative arthroscopic findings and surgical explorations have become virtually nonexistent because a clear diagnosis and appropriate surgical plan are available preoperatively.[21, 116, 156] Progressive damage may be minimized by the ability to identify unstable or progressive injuries early in their history. In general, the evaluation of athletic injuries of the knee is synonymous with MRI. Other modalities are described and illustrated when applicable, though for the most part MRI has relegated them to obsolescence.

Magnetic Resonance Imaging

Magnetic resonance imaging is in the midst of rapid evolution and improvement. The physics and complex mathematical permutations being used to produce ever faster and more detailed images are far beyond the scope of this section. In its most simple terms, MRI is a means of constructing images of body tissues based on the concentration and the physical environment of protons within the imaging plane. X-rays and other forms of ionizing radiation are not a part of an MRI examination. Any desired imaging plane may be selected without having to move the patient. A variety of imaging coils are available to determine the size of the area depicted and the resolution of the image. Specific scanning sequences have been developed that allow the examination to be planned to maximize the detail of virtually any desired tissue. Detailed explanation of the nature and the basis of these sequences is extremely long and terrifically complicated. For whatever information about the internal structures of the knee is desired, an MRI sequence is available to demonstrate it or will be soon.

The standard diagnostic MRI examination is a carefully selected group of scan sequences that maximally demonstrate the different tissues of the knee, highlight the differences between normal and abnormal tissues, and provide images in multiple anatomic planes.[37, 38, 125, 154] When one encounters an MRI examination with multiple sheets of film containing numerous images in which the same structures seem to change color from sheet to sheet, this is not an attempt to confuse the nonradiologist but rather a coherent group of images that must be viewed together. Some images will maximally demonstrate fluid signal such as effusions, bone contusions, cysts, and fluid-filled soft tissue defects. Other images may demonstrate hyaline cartilage, fibrocartilage, or fibrous tissue maximally. Identifying fat is important because it is the most prominent component of marrow-containing bone. Some sequences can differentiate joint fluid in an effusion from blood or fat, or both, with considerably different implications based on the nature of the effusion.

In illustrating this section, specific images have been chosen to demonstrate the pathologic processes being discussed with the scan sequence noted. Frequently, the choice of a scan sequence is key to an abnormality being visible that would frequently be invisible with another type of sequence. Occasionally, an MR contrast agent may be injected intra-articularly to demonstrate a specific finding. Previously, this technique was useful for detailed evaluation of cartilage thickness and to confirm chondral defects; however, new scan sequences have for the most part solved this problem.

One situation in which we frequently use intra-articular contrast material and perform an MR arthrographic evaluation is postoperative meniscal repair. In these cases, a T_1-weighted fat saturation image in both sagittal and coronal planes is extremely sensitive in detecting contrast agent passing into the site of meniscal repair. In these cases, we inject a total volume of 20 mL into the joint before MRI. Arthrocentesis is performed identically to the method for knee arthrography but using a 25-gauge, 1.5-inch needle. The injected solution consists of 0.1 mL (0.05 mmole) of contrast agent (i.e., gadopentetate dimeglumine) mixed with 19 mL of sterile normal saline solution and 1 mL of Marcaine (bupivacaine), 0.5%. Before injection of the MR contrast agent, 1 to 2 mL of nonionic contrast agent is injected to verify intra-articular location.

Arthrography

Contrast arthrography[62] of the knee, once the gold standard for diagnosis of internal derangements, has been reduced to a third-line procedure after diagnostic arthroscopy and MRI. There are still specialized situations in which arthrography may be selected to answer a specific question or may be necessary because the availability or the quality of MRI is limited.

Technique

For knee arthrography, the patient is placed in a supine position on a fluoroscopic table with the knee relaxed and a small pad or bolster under the popliteal region. The anteromedial or anterolateral aspect of the knee is prepared with a povidone-iodine solution and is appropriately draped with sterile towels or an eye-hole drape. The superior and inferior poles of the patella are grasped between the thumb and the third digit, and a small skin indentation is made with the nail of the second digit at the level of the midbody of the patella in the indentation between the patellar articular facet and the adjacent femoral condyle. This spot is infiltrated with 1% lidocaine (Xylocaine) with a 25-gauge needle, and the joint is entered with a 22-gauge, 1.5-inch needle. The joint is then aspirated, often aided by gentle pressure on the popliteal and suprapatellar regions. If no joint fluid is aspirated and the needle position is uncertain, a small amount of lidocaine may be injected, which should enter easily with no resistance if the needle position is correct. Contrast agent is then injected under fluoroscopic observation, and if the needle is correctly positioned, it will flow rapidly away from the needle tip with no resistance. For double-contrast arthrography, we use 5 mL of radiographic contrast agent with 0.3 mL of 1:1000 epinephrine and 0.5 to 1.0 mL of 0.5% bupivacaine. Bupivacaine provides a long duration (24 to 36 hours) of intra-articular local anesthesia, which gets the patient past the usual painful stage of contrast-induced synovitis that frequently follows arthrography. The injection is then completed with 30 to 35 mL of room air injected into the joint; the needle is then withdrawn. The knee is passively taken through its range of motion, and the patient is asked to walk across the fluoroscopic suite several times to allow even distribution and coating of the contrast agent.

The patient is then placed in a prone position on the fluoroscopic table, where an immobilization device is fastened around the distal thigh and gently turned so that the medial aspect of the knee lies against the table. The posterior horn of the medial meniscus is profiled by gently raising or lowering the patient's leg. When the meniscus is satisfactorily profiled, the joint is stressed by gently pulling the patient's leg toward the examiner, and a spot radiograph using a 9-on-1 setting is obtained. This sequence is repeated at approximately 10-degree intervals as the patient is rotated through 180 degrees, resulting in a total of 18 spot radiographs of the medial meniscus from the posterior horn to the anterior horn. At this point, the fluoroscopic technique should be increased by 5 kV, and, using the thigh immobilizer for stability, the patient flexes and extends his or her knee while the examiner manually provides resistance against the leg to produce arthroscopic anterior and posterior drawer stress positions, which are spot filmed using a 4-on-1 setting. The radiographic technique is re-

duced to the original setting, and the anchor for the thigh strap, if used, is reversed to the opposite side of the table. Then, starting with the lateral aspect of the knee placed against the fluoroscopic table, the procedure is repeated to produce images of the lateral meniscus. A thin pad under the thigh is often useful to align the lateral meniscus properly.

Proper radiographic technique is critical. Because phototimed spot films are usually too dark to highlight the contrast-coated meniscus, we use a manual technique. Before the examination, 9-on-1 spot films of the midportion of the medial joint space are obtained using 60 kV and 100 mA, varying the time of exposure at incremental steps between 0.05 and 0.1 second. Overhead radiographs are obtained as the final step using the anteroposterior, lateral, hanging lateral, and "sunrise" projections. Meniscal tears are demonstrated by the presence of contrast agent within the substance of the triangular-shaped meniscal images. Normal cruciate ligaments have a smooth, straight-edged border with appropriate stress; lack of this finding suggests a cruciate tear. The articular cartilage of the femoral, the tibial, and the patellar condyles is coated with contrast agent, and chondral defects and cartilage thinning may be visualized.

Air and positive contrast agent may also be identified in a communicating synovial or meniscal cyst. When the presence of a communicating synovial cyst is the only concern, we use an abbreviated single-contrast technique using a mixture of 25 mL of radiographic contrast material, 25 mL of sterile saline solution, and 5 mL of 0.5% bupivacaine in a 60-mL syringe. The joint is entered using the previously described technique, and contrast is injected under fluoroscopic observation until the joint is tense but not uncomfortable for the patient. The knee is then manipulated under fluoroscopic control to demonstrate communication with the cyst. When a popliteal cyst does not fill readily, passive hyperflexion of the knee often induces the contrast agent to enter the cyst. If this maneuver is not successful, we usually have the patient dress and walk around for 10 to 15 minutes and then repeat delayed overhead radiographs in anteroposterior, extended lateral, and flexed lateral positions.

Tomography

Plain tomography is occasionally useful for demonstrating subtle fractures and small intra-articular loose bodies, and postarthrographic tomography (arthrotomography) may be used to demonstrate small osteochondral defects as well as loose bodies.[2] If available, complex motion polytomography is preferable because it provides much thinner sections and fewer artifacts from objects outside the focal plane of the section, but linear tomography can provide acceptable examinations. These techniques have largely been supplanted by CT and MRI, which are less time consuming, require less technical expertise to perform and interpret, and are associated with a much smaller or absent radiation dose to the patient. In general, tomographic examinations achieve optimal quality with use of relatively low-kilovoltage radiographic techniques (60 to 70 kV), and as long a scan arc as possible with the unit. On linear tomographic units, 1-cm spacing of tomographic sections is adequate because the slice thickness customarily used provides overlapping sections. With complex motion polytomography, 5-mm cut spacing is adequate for routine examinations, although in-between cuts at 2- to 3-mm intervals taken over a localized section where a subtle abnormality may be suspected may be useful.

Computed Tomography

Computed tomography is occasionally useful in the evaluation of sports-related injuries of the knee. In the past, the primary problem with CT of the knee was its limitation in regard to the axial anatomic plane owing to the size of the CT gantry. Reconstruction of images acquired in the axial plane into other anatomic planes has long been possible, but the quality and the spatial resolution of these images were often quite poor. Newer CT scanners provide thinner sections with greater resolution and improved software reconstruction. The anatomic detail now available has made linear tomography and polytomography obsolete for the evaluation of complex bony anatomy. High-quality images can now be generated in any plane or as three-dimensional images.

The major flaw of CT remains its inability to differentiate intra-articular soft tissues, limiting its use to evaluation of bony structures. At present, the usefulness of CT is limited to evaluation of complex fractures (e.g., tibial plateau), localization of intra-articular bony loose bodies (e.g., osteochondral fragments) that are not visible on MRI, and evaluation of patellar tracking abnormalities. For high-quality, nonaxial reconstructions, the slice thickness should overlap the slice spacing by approximately 50%. For instance, 3-mm slices spaced at 3 mm will often be quite ragged and of poor quality, whereas 3-mm slices spaced at 2 mm will provide high-quality reconstructions. With the new high-speed spiral CT technology, thickness of sections may be diminished even further to 1 mm or less, and exceedingly high-quality reformations can be created in any desired anatomic plane.

Sonography

Real-time sonography is often useful in evaluating masses about the knee, and especially for confirming the presence of a popliteal cyst.[77] The ability to visualize and evaluate the popliteal artery and vein is frequently useful in the identification of popliteal aneurysms and thrombi within the popliteal vein. A 5- or 7.5-MHz transducer used with a modern real-time sonographic unit provides surprisingly detailed information about anatomy, although to the clinician the pictures frequently seem to resemble ink blots.

The patient is placed in a comfortable position with the area of interest presented to the examiner. The overlying skin is coated with a sonographic gel, which provides good contact between the scan head of the transducer and the patient's skin without causing artifact. With real-time scanning, a palpable mass may be identified. Cystic lesions have a sonolucent (black) appearance with parallel bands of increased signal intensity (back wall enhancement) along their distal border (see Fig. 28B–68). Solid lesions demonstrate a sonodense (white) or complex appearance without back wall enhancement. Large popliteal cysts often contain centrally inspissated contents, resulting in a variably complex appearance. Bones and calcified structures result in complete obstruction of the sound beam with a bright echo at its proximal border and complete absence of signal distally. Pulsations and the tubular configuration identify arteries. Their tubular configuration and accelerated flow identify large veins with manual compression of the calf. Muscles and tendons have a solid appearance with intermediate brightness, and fat appears quite bright (white) on sonographic images. We make extensive use of ultrasound in localizing cystic lesions about the knee for aspiration and therapeutic injection of steroids.

Radionuclide Scintigraphy

Radionuclide scintigraphy[42] using technetium-99m medronate methylene diphosphonate is a useful screening procedure for a variety of abnormalities.[79, 119, 127] In general, the radionuclide provides a reflection of the relative blood flow to an area as well as the degree of bone turnover (osteogenesis and osteolysis). In patients with acute trauma in whom a localized abnormality is suspected, we prefer to use a three-phase technique,[79] centered over the area of abnormality and using a high-resolution collimator. With this technique, the area of interest and the contralateral side, if possible, are centered under the gamma camera while the radionuclide is administered intravenously. When activity is first identified on the camera's persistence monitor, a series of 5-second-long sequential images are gathered for 1 to 2 minutes, resulting in an angiographic series (phase 1), which allows relative differences in blood flow to the area to be evaluated. A summation image (phase 2) is also printed, demonstrating the overall immediate blood flow to the region (blood pool image). The patient is asked to return in approximately 3 hours, at which time static-delayed (phase 3) images of the area of interest or of the whole body, if desired, are acquired. A four-phase technique[42] is occasionally useful, especially for differentiating bone infection from adjacent soft tissue infection; in this case, a 24-hour delayed image (phase 4) is added to the procedure. In the setting of trauma, a delay of at least 24 hours between the time of injury and the radionuclide study is minimal for a diagnostic study.

In interpreting the study, the relative blood flow to the region is compared with that on the contralateral side in the immediate dynamic images. On the immediate static (blood pool) images, relative hyperemia, predominantly of soft tissue origin, can be identified. On the delayed images, increased or decreased activity in the area of interest may be defined. In the setting of trauma, blood flow is usually symmetrical with mild hyperemia demonstrated on the blood pool image, in contrast to increased flow and marked hyperemia in inflammatory and some neoplastic processes. Delayed static images demonstrate markedly increased activity in inflammatory, traumatic, and neoplastic lesions, although occasionally the distribution or shape of the increase (i.e., linear in patients with fractures) may suggest a cause. In an inflammatory process, relatively greater activity in the blood pool images may suggest that the process is localized to the soft tissues, including the synovium, and does not directly involve the bone.

Imaging the Knee

The Menisci

Anatomy

The fibrocartilaginous menisci of the knee appear simple but are functionally complex structures that function pri-

marily to guide motion and direct the transmission of force across the knee joint (Fig. 28B–1).[171, 184] The vascular supply to the menisci[6, 7, 41] is limited to the peripheral 20% and comes from the inferior and middle geniculate arteries. In general, the portion of a meniscus that is 3 mm or less from the meniscocapsular junction may be assumed to be vascularized; the area 3 mm to 5 mm from the meniscocapsular junction may be associated with a blood supply; and the area greater than 5 mm from the periphery is assumed to be nonvascular. This is important in assessment of the suitability of meniscal tears for spontaneous healing or surgical repair, as discussed later in this section. Vascularity is richest in the anterior and posterior horns and least in the midbody of the meniscus. No change in the vascular distribution occurs with chronic tears or degeneration.[171]

Both menisci[36, 98, 171] are C-shaped structures, the medial

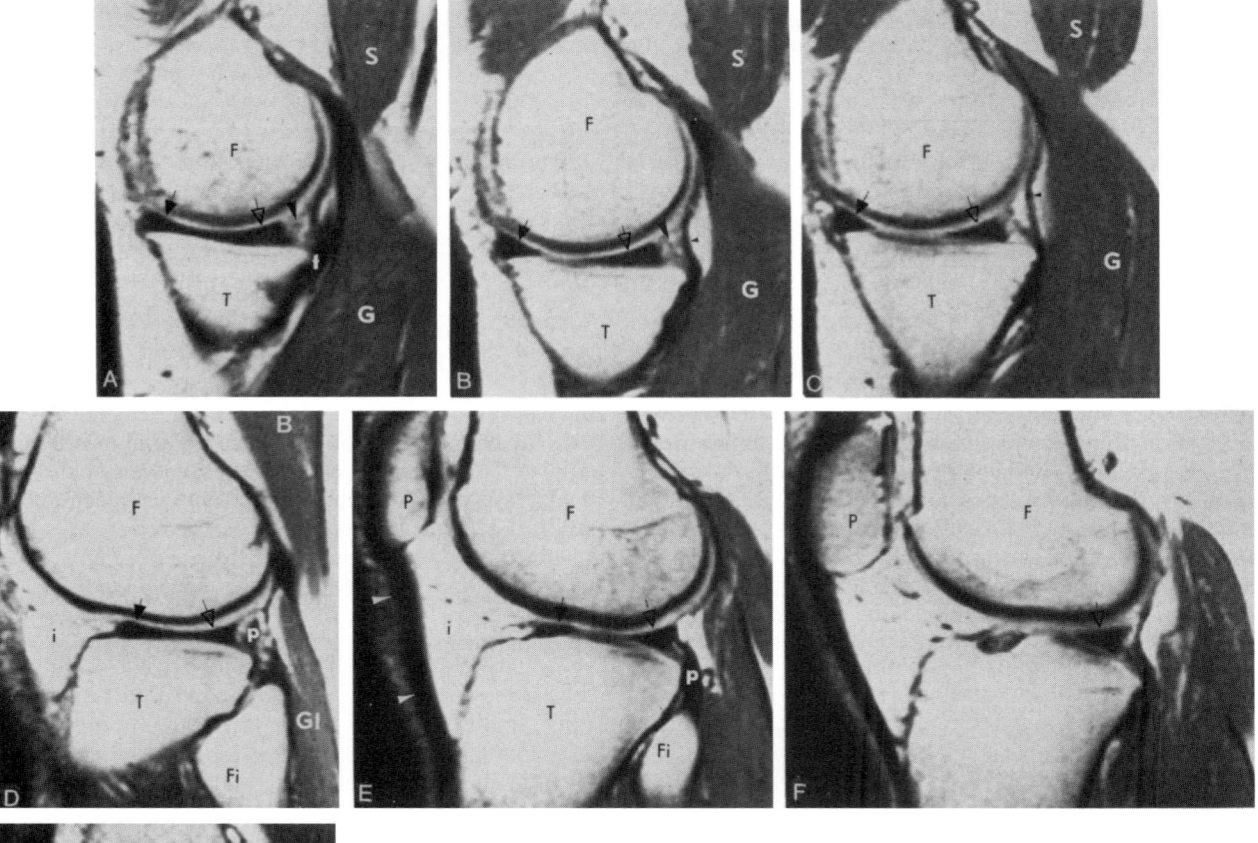

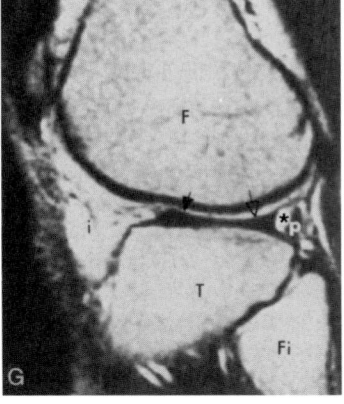

Figure 28B–1. Normal MRI anatomy, sagittal plane. The normal appearance of the medial menisci *(A–C)* and lateral meniscus *(D–G)* are illustrated in sagittal T_1-weighted (2233/30) MR images. In peripheral sections of both the medial *(A)* and lateral *(D)* menisci, the biconcave "bow-tie" configuration is present, whereas the more central images (medial [*B* and *C*], lateral [*E* and *F*]) demonstrate the typical triangular configuration. Both menisci demonstrate a homogeneous dark appearance with "crisp" margins. *G* is a T_2-weighted image (2200/90) at the same level as that in *D* demonstrating the popliteal tendon in its sheath and the superior and inferior struts of the lateral meniscus outlined by joint fluid. B, biceps femoris; F, femur; fi, fibula; G, medial head of gastrocnemius; Gl, lateral head of gastrocnemius; i, infrapatellar fat pad; P, patella, p, popliteal tendon; S, semimembranosus; t, semimembranosus tendon insertion; T, tibia; *black arrows,* posterior (open) and anterior (solid) horns of the menisci; *white arrowheads,* patellar tendon; *large black arrowhead,* fibrovascular meniscocapsular junction; *small black arrowhead,* posterior joint capsule; *, fluid in popliteal tendon sheath.

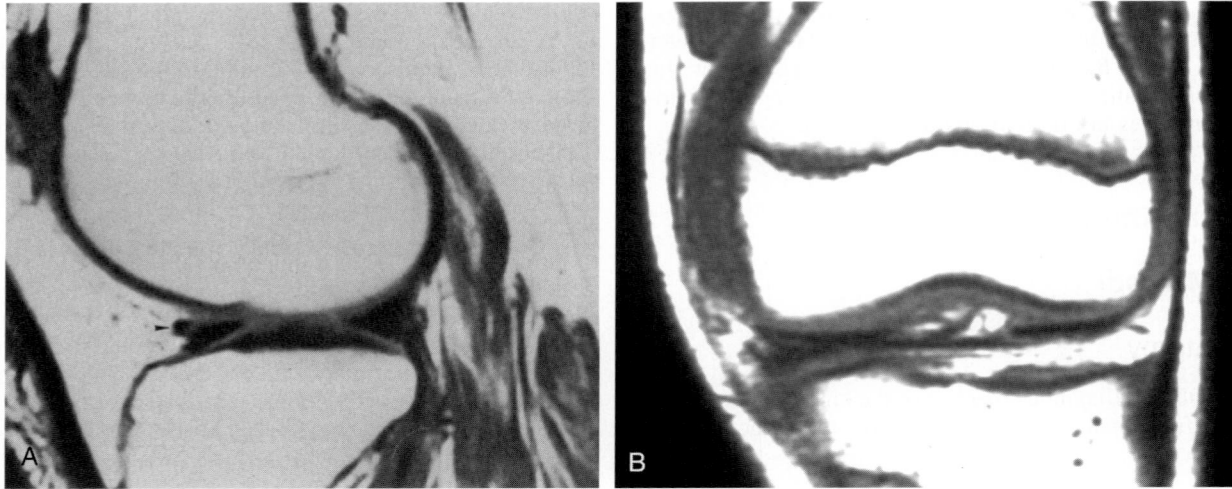

Figure 28B–2. Transverse geniculate ligament (intermeniscal ligament). Sagittal *(A)* and coronal *(B)* T$_1$-weighted (1000/20) images demonstrate the transverse geniculate ligament *(arrowhead)* passing between the anterior horns of the medial and lateral menisci. In the sagittal image, the ligament is closely applied to the anterior aspect of the anterior horn of the lateral meniscus, separated by a thin zone of fat. This appearance may simulate a tear of the lateral meniscus.

meniscus having a slightly greater radius of curvature than the lateral meniscus. The posterior horn of the medial meniscus is larger than the midbody and the anterior horn by about 30% in breadth and height (see Fig. 28B–1*B*), whereas the lateral meniscus demonstrates constant size in all portions. The medial meniscus is tightly bound along its periphery to the medial plateau by the meniscotibial (coronary) and meniscofemoral ligaments. In addition, it is firmly attached to the deep fibers of the medial collateral ligament (MCL) and to the intercondylar portion of the tibia by strong ligaments at the terminations of its anterior and posterior horns. The lateral meniscus possesses similar attachments, although it tends to be somewhat less firmly bound than the medial meniscus. The transverse geniculate ligament (anterior intermeniscal ligament)[124, 131, 186] (Fig. 28B–2) is a structure of variable incidence and thickness that passes between and connects the anterior horns of the menisci. The oblique meniscomeniscal ligament[160] is a

variant intermeniscal ligament that runs obliquely between the anterior horn of one meniscus and the posterior horn of the other. The medial oblique meniscomeniscal ligament passes from the anterior horn of the medial meniscus to the posterior horn of the lateral meniscus, whereas the lateral oblique meniscomeniscal ligament passes from the anterior horn of the lateral meniscus to the posterior horn of the medial meniscus. Both variations pass between the anterior cruciate ligament (ACL) and the posterior cruciate ligament (PCL) as they traverse the intercondylar notch and may be mistaken for a displaced bucket handle meniscal tear. The periphery of the posterior horn of the lateral meniscus is pierced at the meniscocapsular junction by the popliteal tendon and its sheath.[136] At this level, distinct superior and inferior meniscal struts (see Fig. 28B–1*G*) may be identified passing around the popliteal sheath to insert into the lateral capsular ligament. The anterior and posterior meniscofemoral ligaments[5, 124, 186] are accessory

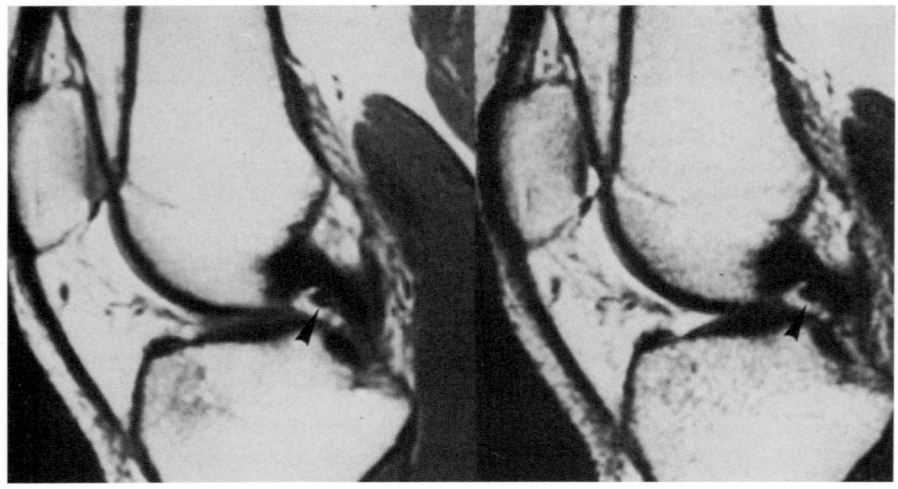

Figure 28B–3. Anterior meniscofemoral ligament (ligament of Humphry). Sagittal intensity windowing (IW) (1200/20) and T$_2$ (1200/65) images through the level of the intercondylar notch demonstrate the anterior meniscofemoral (Humphry's) ligament in cross section anterior to the posterior cruciate ligament.

ligaments that arise from the posterior horn of the lateral meniscus to insert on the lateral border of the medial femoral condyle. The anterior meniscofemoral ligament (ligament of Humphry) (Fig. 28B–3) is typically visualized in sagittal images as a small, dark, circular structure immediately anterior to the anterior border of the PCL at the level of its middle third. The posterior meniscofemoral ligament (ligament of Wrisberg) (Fig. 28B–4) passes from the medial border of the lateral meniscus posterior to the PCL to insert on the medial femoral condyle.

On both arthrograms and MRI, the menisci are homogeneously dark in appearance.[36, 37, 78, 120, 122, 143–145] In younger patients, the periphery of the meniscus, especially the posterior horn of the medial meniscus, may demonstrate a zone of relative hyperintensity related to its vascularized zone (see Fig. 28B–1B). The periphery of the normal meniscus covers the periphery of the tibial articular cartilage and blends smoothly with the adjacent soft tissues at the meniscocapsular junction. The free margins of a normal meniscus are "crisp" with a sharply "penciled" appearance (see Fig. 28B–1). Alterations of the homogeneous dark appearance or sharp smooth margins constitute the most important observations on arthrography or MRI in identifying meniscal tears and degenerative changes.

Meniscal Tears and Degeneration

Meniscal tears and intrasubstance degeneration (mucinous, myxoid, or hyaline) are manifested by a marked increase in signal intensity on T_1- and intermediate-weighted images that is less prominent on T_2-weighted images.[13, 15, 27, 36, 37, 90, 138, 143, 144] The differentiation of these two findings is a major concern in interpreting MRI images of the knee. Tears and meniscal degeneration appear bright

on T_1- and intermediate-weighted images, presumably owing to the adsorption of water onto the surfaces of macromolecules exposed by the tear or degenerative process, resulting in shortening of both T_1 and T_2 relaxation times.[54, 55, 140, 176, 177] This explains the brightness of these changes on T_1 and intensity windowing (IW) images, whereas the variable brightness on T_2-weighted images is apparently related to the presence of free water or joint fluid in the tear or degenerated region.

The grading system for high-intensity signals in the menisci (Fig. 28B–5) proposed by Lotysch and associates[37, 176] provides a useful means for making this distinction. A grade 1 signal (Fig. 28B–5A) is globular and is localized to the center of the meniscus, and there is a distinct zone of dark, low-intensity meniscal substance separating it from all free meniscal edges. This appearance corresponds to histologically identifiable degeneration in the central substance of the meniscus. A grade 2 signal (Fig. 28B–5B) is a linear signal within the substance of the meniscus that does not extend to a free edge. Histologically, this corresponds to a more advanced stage of the abnormality seen in grade 1 with larger bands of mucinous degeneration. A grade 3 signal (Fig. 28B–5C) reaches a free meniscal edge and may have either a linear or an irregular appearance. A grade 3 signal is associated with meniscal tears.

In addition to the grade 3 signal, another critical observation in the identification of meniscal tears is an alteration in the shape of the meniscus (Fig. 28B–6). As previously noted, a normal meniscus has a sharply marginated appearance, the particular shape depending on the level and the orientation of the section (see Fig. 28B–1). Any alteration in this normal appearance, such as a wavy contour, a truncated appearance (Fig. 28B–7), fuzzy edges (Fig. 28B–8), or a loss of normal size relations (see Figs. 28B–7 and 28B–8), should alert one to the likelihood of meniscal disease. One contour variant, an S-shaped fold near the free edge of a meniscus on sagittal images, is termed *meniscal flounce* (Fig. 28B–9).[196] This is a normal variant and not indicative of a meniscal tear; however, because some meniscal tears do demonstrate a flouncelike fold, careful evaluation of the study for other evidence suggesting a meniscal tear is necessary.

Characterization of meniscal tears on MRI follows the same longstanding conventions used in contrast arthrography.[46, 61, 155, 183] Tears may be described as vertical (Fig. 28B–10), horizontal (Fig. 28B–11), oblique (Fig. 28B–12), or complex (Fig. 28B–13). Vertical tears tend to be either concentric (see Fig. 28B–10), in which the defect predominantly parallels the meniscal margin, or radial (see Fig. 28B–8C), in which the tear is oriented tangentially to the free meniscal edge. Horizontal tears (see Fig. 28B–11) course parallel to the plane of the joint and divide the involved portion of the meniscus into superior and inferior portions. Complex tears (see Fig. 28B–13) represent combinations of the previously mentioned patterns. A flap tear (see Fig. 28B–13)[36, 183] occurs when a meniscal tear allows a portion of meniscus to become unstable so that it is displaced from its normal position. The flap fragment may fold over onto the adjacent intact meniscus, displace centrally into the "notch," displace between the weight-bearing portions of the femoral and tibial condyles, or flip peripherally to lie between a collateral ligament and the

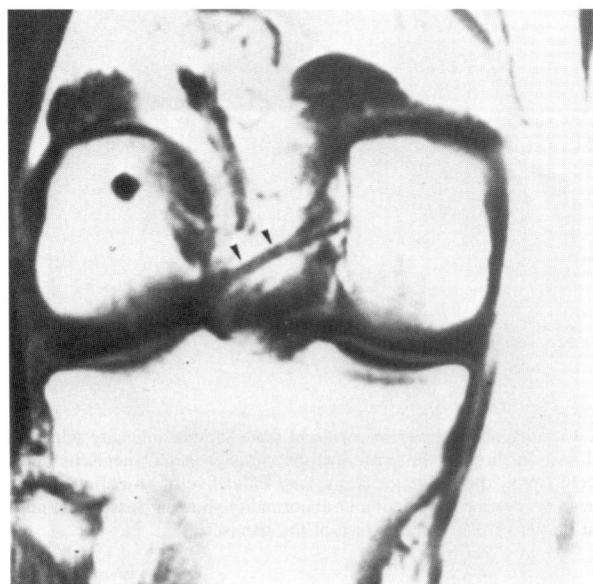

Figure 28B–4. Posterior meniscofemoral ligament (ligament of Wrisberg). Coronal T_1 (600/20)-weighted image through the posterior condylar level demonstrates the posterior meniscofemoral (Wrisberg's) ligament passing obliquely from the posterior horn of the lateral meniscus superomedially to insert on the medial femoral condyle.

Text continued on page 1608

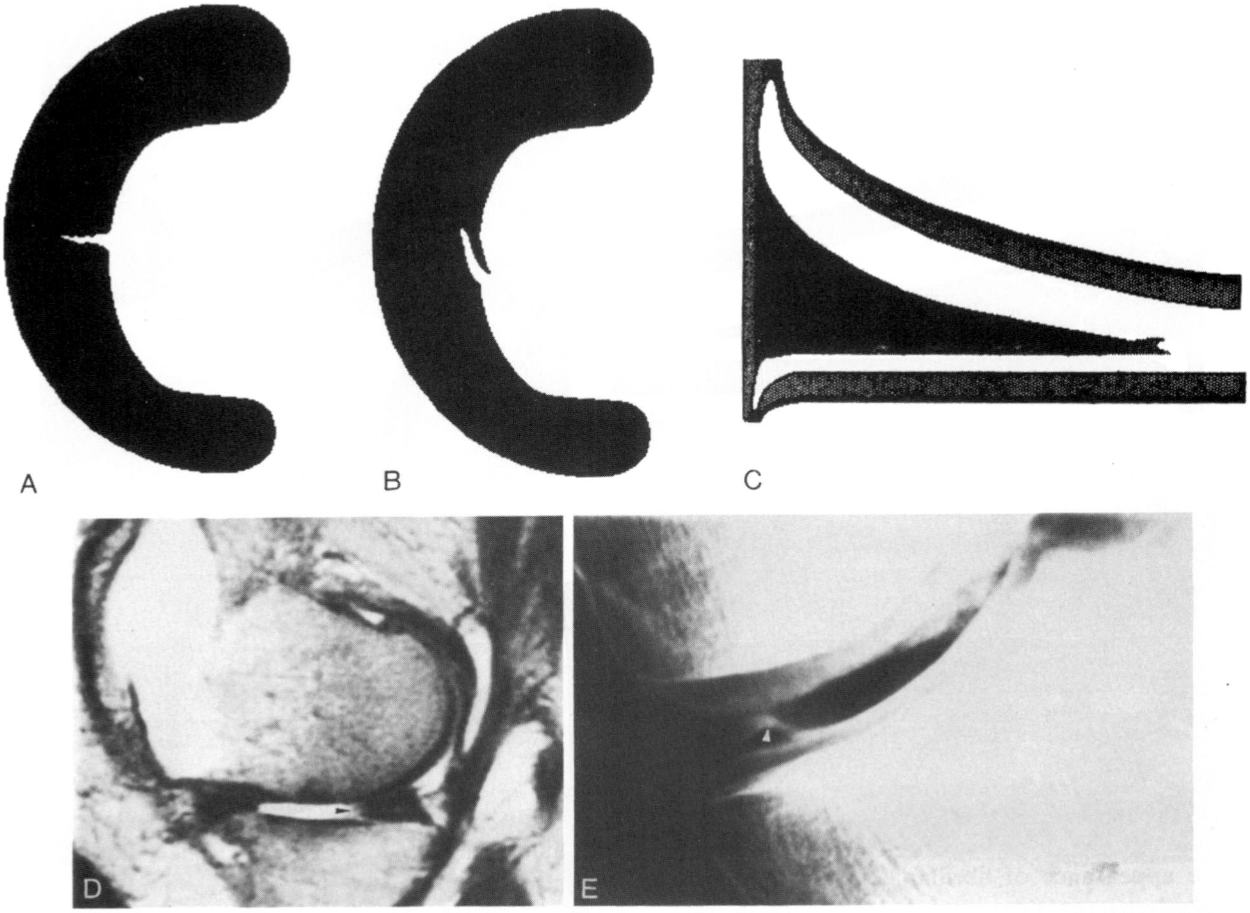

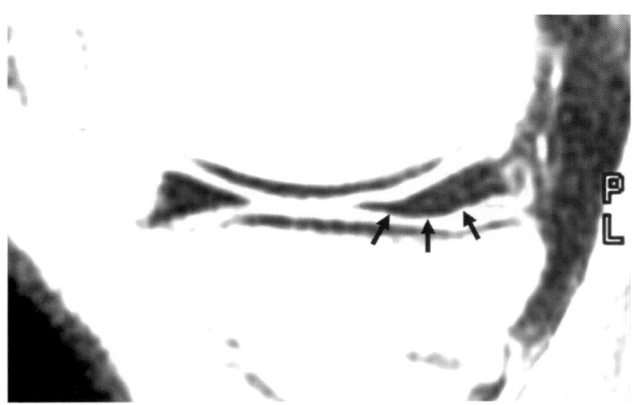

A   B   C

D   E

Figure 28B–8. Abnormalities of the free meniscal edge. Diagrams *(A–C)*, sagittal T$_2$-weighted (2000/90) MR section *(D)*, and arthrographic spot film *(E)* demonstrate abnormalities of the free meniscal edge. Short vertical radial tears *(A)*, "parrot-beak" tears *(B)*, and degenerative fibrillation of the free meniscal edge *(C)* all share similar appearances on MRI and arthrography. MRI changes *(D)* consist of increased signal intensity, often with blunting, of the free meniscal edge *(arrowhead)*. The changes are quite similar with arthrography *(E)*, in which a blunted or "floppy" free meniscal edge is accompanied by localized entrapment (tear) or imbibition (fibrillation) of contrast *(arrowhead)*.

P
L

Figure 28B–9. Meniscal flounce. Sagittal intensity windowing image through the posterior horn of the medial meniscus demonstrates a contour abnormality consisting of a smooth "s" shaped curve *(arrows)* without abnormal meniscal signal. This is a normal variant and does not indicate a meniscal tear.

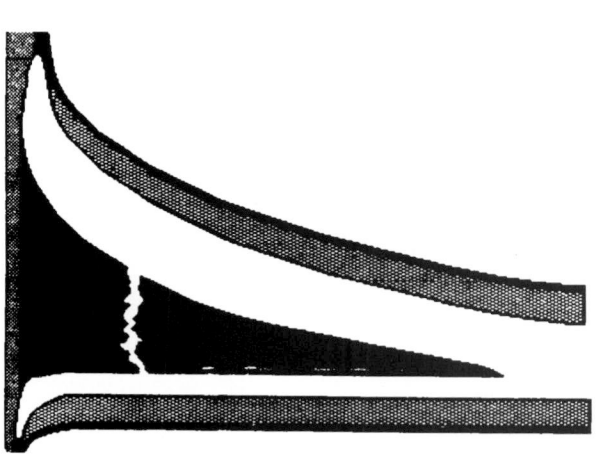

A

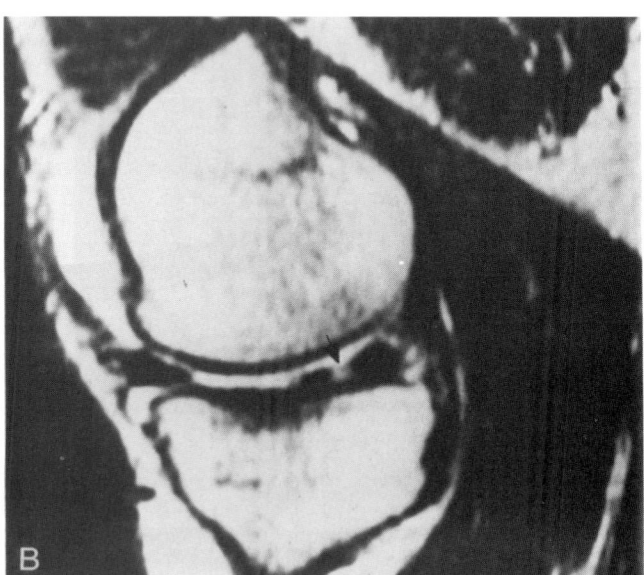

B

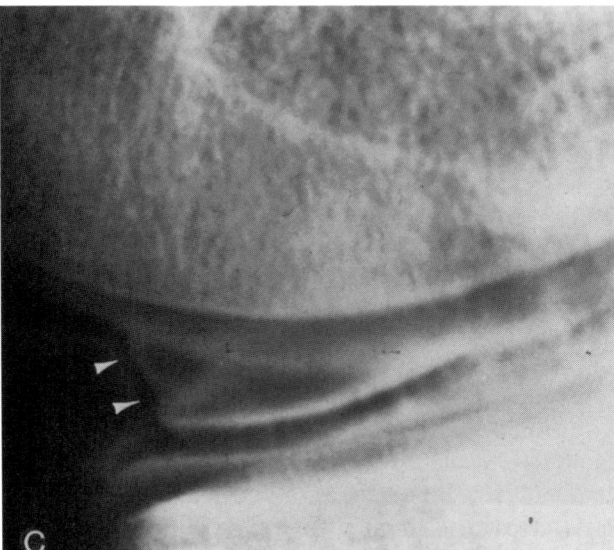

C

Figure 28B–10. Vertical longitudinal concentric meniscal tear. Diagram (A), sagittal T$_2$ (2500/70) MR image (B), and arthrographic spot film (C) demonstrate the appearance of vertical concentric meniscal tears. The tear extends vertically between the superior and inferior meniscal surfaces and is usually of acute traumatic origin.

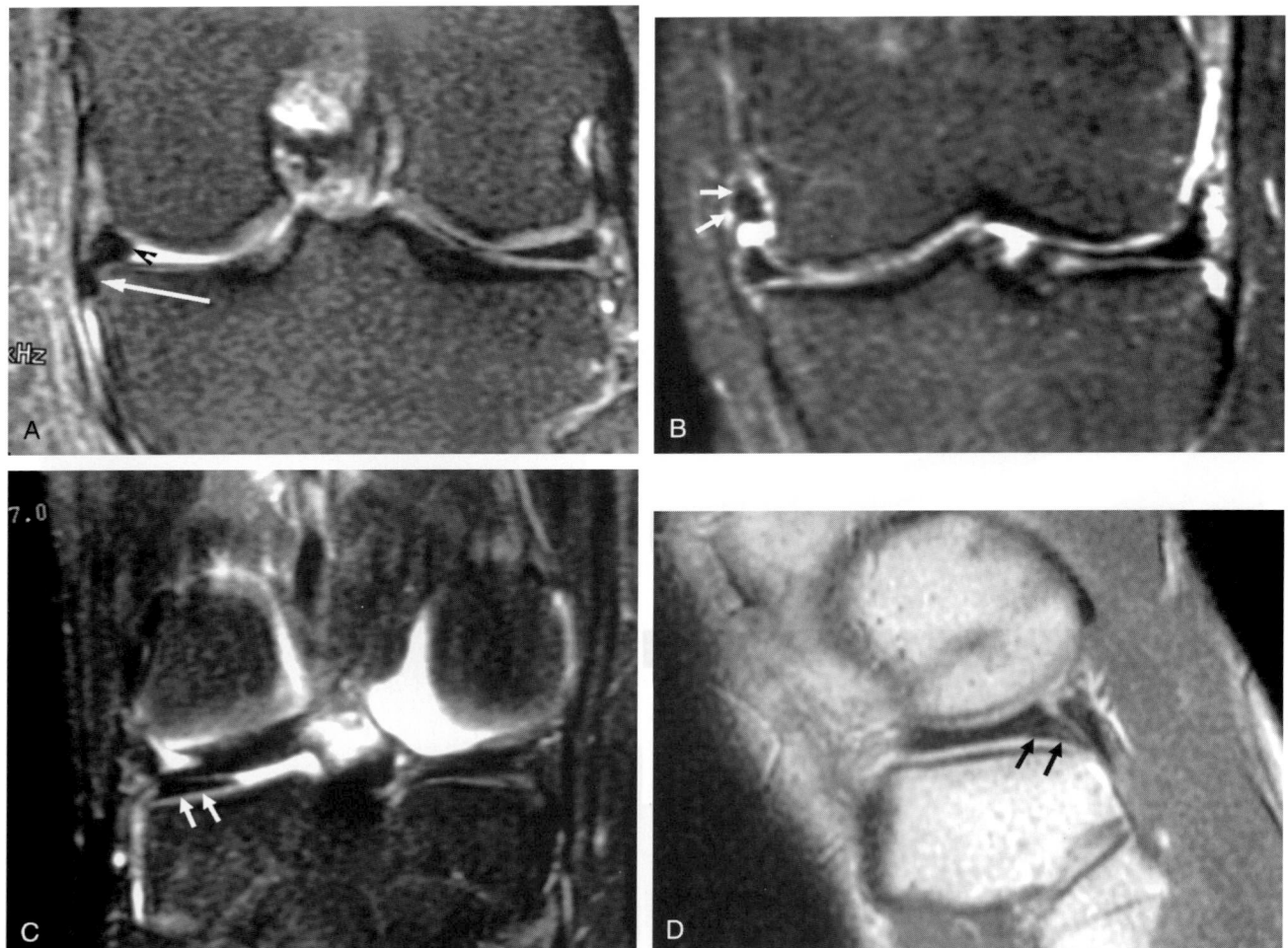

Figure 28B–13. Meniscal flap tears. Coronal T₂ fast spin-echo (FS) *(A–C)* and sagittal intensity windowing *(D)* MRI sections demonstrate common varieties of meniscal flap tears. In *A*, the medial meniscal flap fragment *(arrow)* is displaced inferiorly under the coronary ligament, with the torn free edge of the medial meniscus *(arrowhead)* having a blunted appearance. In *B*, the flap fragment *(arrows)* is displaced superiorly into the medial gutter. In *C* and *D*, lateral meniscal flap fragments *(arrows)* are displaced inferior to the posterior horn of the lateral meniscus.

adjacent femoral or tibial condyle. In the latter instances, the "donor" site of the meniscus is abnormally abbreviated, and some searching may be required to identify the displaced flap fragment.[107]

Bucket handle tears[169, 188] (Fig. 28B–14) are vertical concentric tears in which the inner fragment is displaced toward the midline. "Parrot-beak" tears (see Fig. 28B–8*B*) are small flap tears near the free meniscal edge that are usually small and course obliquely in relation to both the vertical and the horizontal planes. Meniscal tears are seen on MR images as linear or irregular zones of increased signal intensity, frequently with an associated alteration of meniscal contour. In most instances, a tear can be identified by these characteristics and can be described and localized by evaluating multiple contiguous imaging sections. In some circumstances, however, findings may be subtle or indirect, requiring some caution in interpretation.

Description of meniscal tears based on the vascularity of the meniscus at the site of the tear is becoming increasingly more important with the recent advances in arthroscopic meniscal repair.[34, 74] Description of meniscal tears based on the potential for healing of a surgical repair is based on the penetration of vascular structures from the periphery of the meniscus (Fig. 28B–15).[6, 7, 34] In this regard, it is useful to describe meniscal tears in relation to the proximity of the meniscal blood supply. Red-red tears refer to peripheral meniscocapsular separations and tears that lie within 3 mm of the meniscocapsular junction. Red-white tears are 3 to 5 mm from the meniscocapsular junction. White-white tears are greater than 5 mm from the meniscocapsular junction. Red-red tears have a blood supply, may heal spontaneously, and are the best candidates for meniscal repair. Red-white tears may have the potential to heal by means of fibrovascular proliferation.[34] White-white tears are devoid of vascularity and cannot heal spontaneously.

Undoubtedly, rare instances of symptomatic intrasubstance tears, not visible at arthroscopy, do occur.[36] These tears usually demonstrate a grade 3 signal on MRI, though it is certainly possible that grade 2 signal may occur in some instances. At present, there is no reliable way to identify these patients, but a symptomatic patient with a positive MRI signal and negative results on arthroscopy certainly bears close follow-up. A grade 2 signal should be

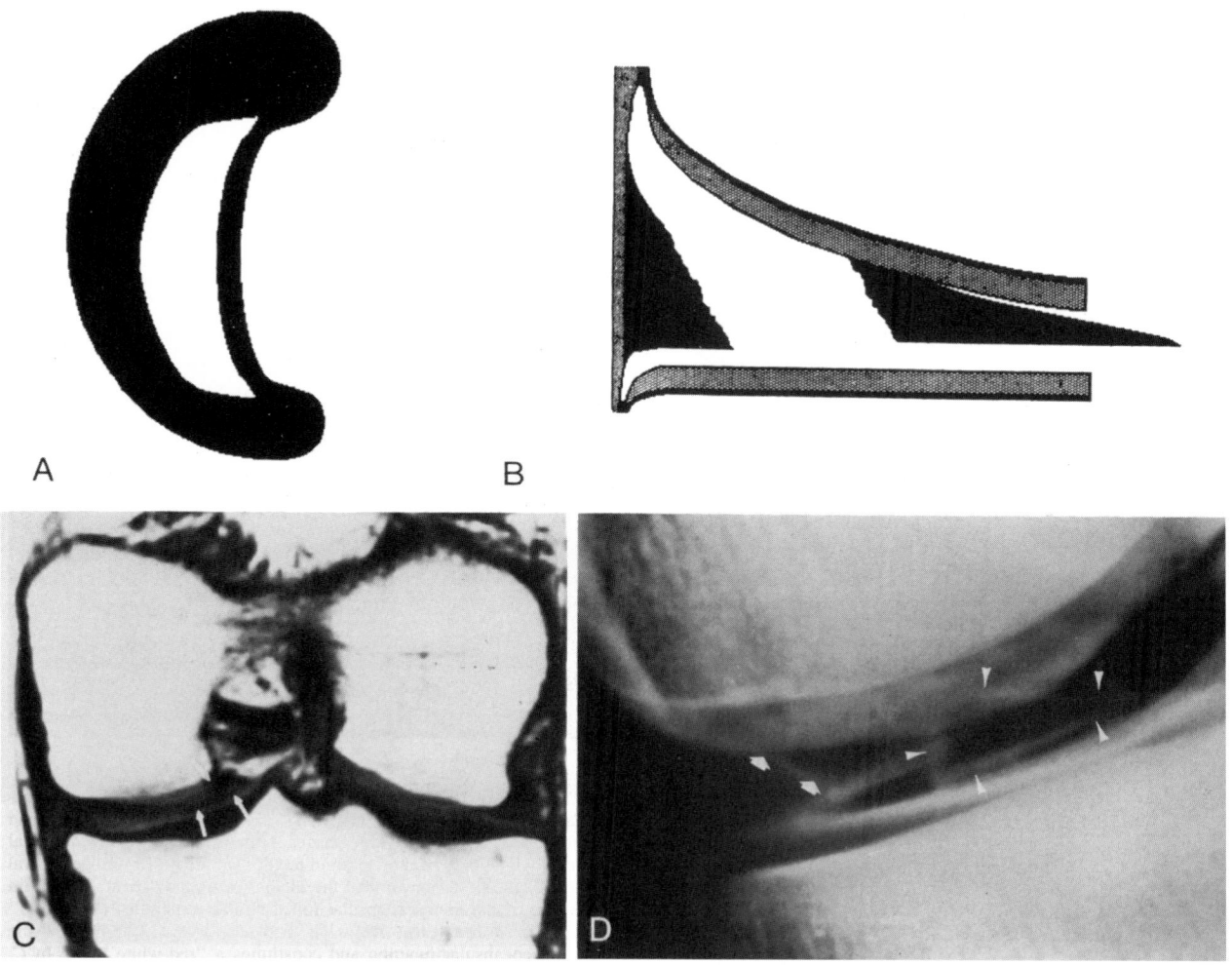

Figure 28B–14. Bucket handle meniscal tear. Diagrams (*A* and *B*), coronal T₁ (900/20) MRI section *(C)*, and arthrographic spot film *(D)* demonstrate typical bucket handle meniscal tears. These tears are a variant of the vertical concentric type of tear in which the central meniscal fragment is displaced inward toward the femoral notch. The centrally displaced fragment is outlined by *arrows* in *C* and by *arrowheads* in *D*. Also in *D*, note that the cleavage plane of the peripheral fragment mimics a normal meniscus, though its small size and abnormally steep superior surface are abnormal.

interpreted with some caution because documented meniscal tears are quite uncommon with this pattern. Peripheral meniscal detachments (Fig. 28B–16) may be quite subtle, and there is usually a zone of higher signal intensity at the periphery of the menisci. A subtle central shift of the dark meniscal tissue, uncovering the peripheral margin of the tibial articular cartilage, may also be present but frequently cannot be appreciated.[126]

In bucket handle tears, the intact peripheral zone of the meniscus may have a shape similar to that of a normal meniscus (see Fig. 28B–14D) but is smaller or has superior and inferior edges of different length.[47, 158, 179] The torn central portion is typically displaced into the intercondylar notch (see Fig. 28B–14). In the sagittal plane, the displaced meniscal fragment[193] is usually identified as a dark structure that tends to lie under and parallel to the PCL (double PCL sign; see Fig. 28B–14).[169, 188] In coronal-oriented images, the fragment usually appears as a dark, triangular structure in the medial or lateral aspect of the notch. Absence of the normal "bow tie" appearance of the meniscus on sagittal MR images has been reported as a reliable sign in bucket

handle tears.[76] The "flipped meniscus" sign (see Fig. 28B–14) occurs when the fragment is flipped anteriorly so that the anterior horn of the meniscus appears enlarged.

Complex or horizontal tears of the posterior horn of the medial meniscus may be manifested by meniscal collapse (see Fig. 28B–13D), in which the posterior horn appears to be of the same size as the anterior horn instead of 20% to 30% larger in height and breadth.[36] Small parrot-beak tears and radial tears (see Fig. 28B–15) of the free meniscal edge may be manifested as a bright "fuzzy" appearance of the edge, identical to the appearance of fibrillar degeneration associated with degenerative joint disease.[27, 61] These tears are difficult to diagnose, as in arthrography, and must be actively searched for to be found.

Several false-positive findings also should be mentioned because they may mimic meniscal tears.[124, 186] The transverse geniculate intermeniscal ligament, which passes between the anterior horns of the medial and lateral menisci, may cause such confusion. In sagittal images of the medial meniscus, a thin zone of fat may lie between the transverse geniculate ligament and the anterior horn of the medial or

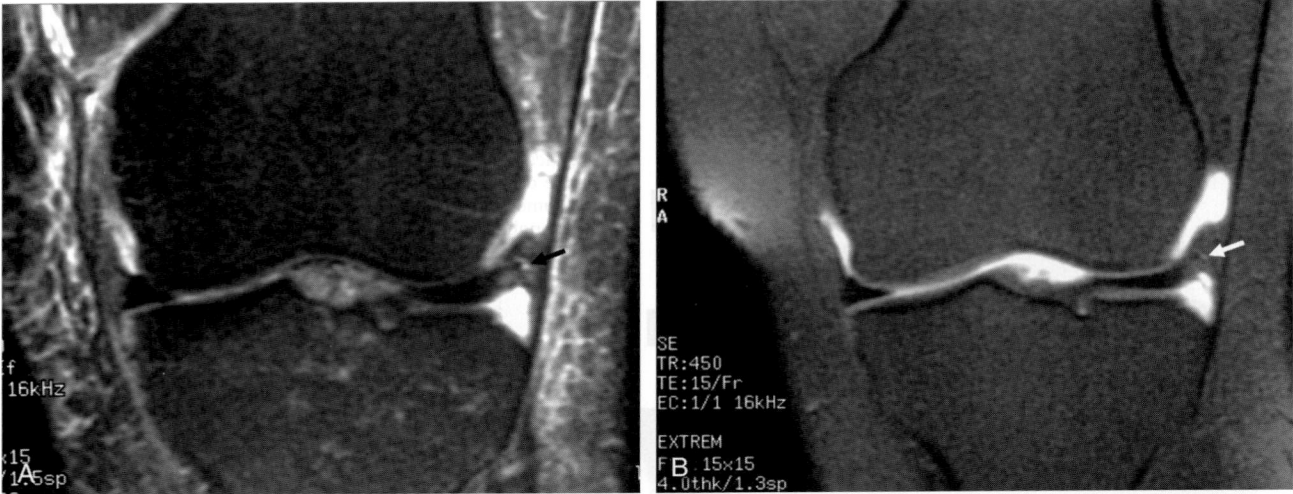

Figure 28B–18. Meniscal repair. Coronal T_2 fat saturation *(A)* and coronal T_1 fat saturation MR arthrogram *(B)* images demonstrate the initial lateral meniscal tear *(A) (arrow)* and complete healing at the site of the tear *(B) (arrow)* 7 months after surgical repair.

after injection and the patient allowed to walk to the MR scanner to allow adequate contrast penetration into meniscal defects. The critical scan sequences are T_1 weighted, in which gadolinium demonstrates high signal. We prefer T_1 fat saturation sequences in the sagittal and coronal planes because the gadolinium contrast will be the only bright signal on these scans.

Discoid Menisci

Discoid menisci[36, 49, 72, 130, 147, 171, 187] are congenital abnormalities in the development of the menisci, resulting in enlargement of all or part of a meniscus.[171] Lateral discoid menisci are much more common than medial discoid menisci. In a review of 985 knee arthrograms, 19 discoid lateral menisci (2%) were identified, and no discoid medial menisci were seen.[72] A variety of classifications of discoid menisci have been proposed based on the arthroscopic, arthrographic, or gross anatomic appearance of the abnormal meniscus. On a functional basis, however, one of the more useful divisions of the discoid lateral meniscus is the differentiation between the complete type and the Wrisberg type.[49] The key difference between these lesions is the presence (or absence) of a normal attachment of the posterior horn of the lateral meniscus to the posterior aspect of the tibial plateau. In the complete type, a normal posterior attachment exists, the meniscus tends to be symmetrically thickened, and there is no associated "click" or "snap" when the knee is flexed or extended. These lesions are frequently asymptomatic, although tears of the posterior horn are more frequent than they are in the normal population, and are the type most typically associated with plain radiographic signs (widened lateral joint space, "squared" lateral femoral condyle, and "cupped" lateral tibial plateau). In contrast, the Wrisberg type of discoid lateral meniscus is characterized by the absence of the posterior attachment of the lateral meniscus to the tibial plateau. This results in hypermobility of the posterior horn, which tends to displace into the intercondylar notch during extension of the knee owing to traction from the ligament of

Wrisberg (lateral meniscofemoral ligament). This results in the snapping knee syndrome as the posterior horn displaces and reduces during flexion-extension motion of the knee. These patients are frequently symptomatic, often presenting with lateral meniscal tears in childhood. Meniscal thickening is most often localized to the posterior horn, and plain radiographic features are typically absent.

In imaging these lesions, plain radiographic features, as noted earlier, have been described but are of limited usefulness because they tend to be quite subjective. Both arthrography and MRI are quite sensitive in identifying discoid menisci. With either of these modalities, the critical observation is the presence of abnormally thickened meniscal tissue interposed into the central intercondylar zone of the medial or lateral compartments.[27, 36, 61] This tissue may be quite thick, in the massive or slab types, or quite thin, in the biconcave type, or it may be localized to a portion of the meniscus (e.g., the posterior megahorn) (Fig. 28B–19).[36] In general, visualization of a meniscus on more than three contiguous 5-mm MRI sections is evidence of abnormal meniscal enlargement. Tears of the discoid menisci are identified and categorized using the same criteria as are used for normal menisci, the presence of a grade 3 signal being the key observation. Depending on the nature of the tear, the presence of a preexisting discoid meniscus may be difficult to identify. MRI identification of a Wrisberg-type discoid lateral meniscus has not been described; however, we have encountered a case in which the posterior horn of the lateral meniscus was contiguous with a thickened ligament of Wrisberg, and a normal posterior insertion could not be seen.

Meniscal Cysts

Meniscal cysts[10, 12, 26, 28, 36, 55, 92, 164] (cystic degeneration) are rather uncommon lesions occurring most frequently within the middle third of the lateral meniscus and least commonly in the medial meniscus, where they tend to occur in the posterior horn.[55, 164] A previous review of 2522 arthrograms reported the incidence of meniscal cysts to be

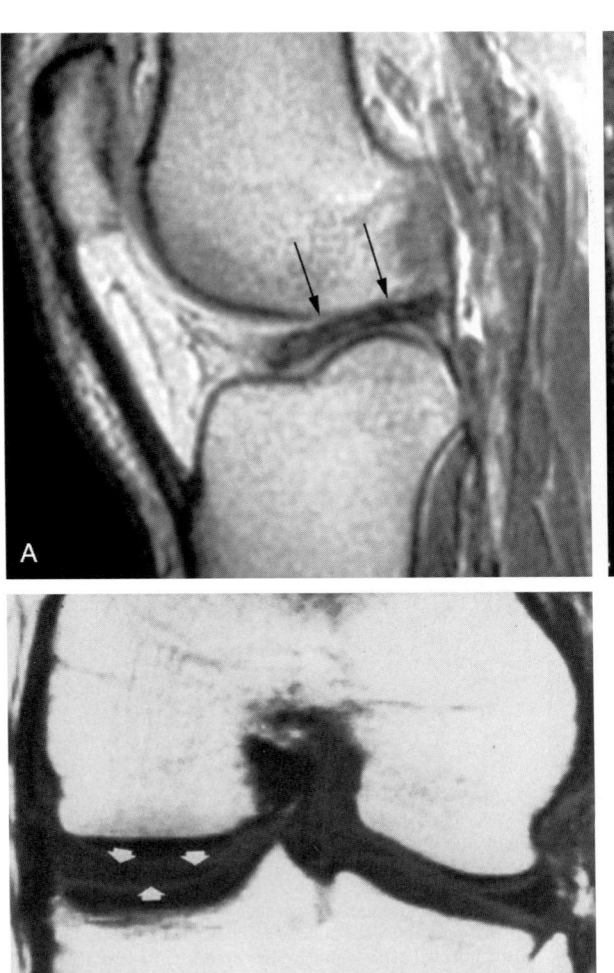

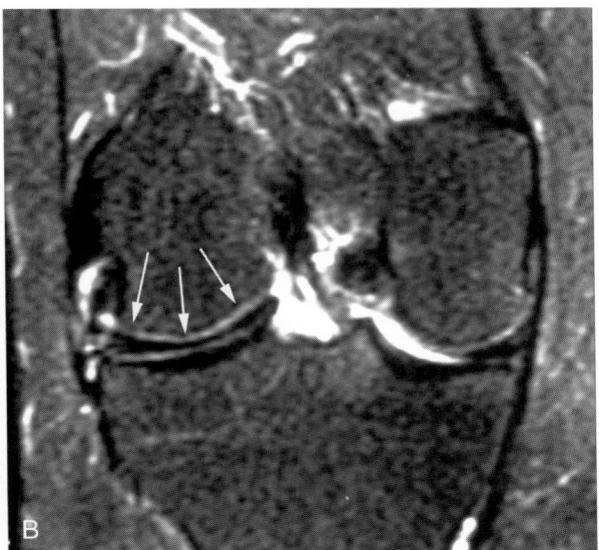

Figure 28B–19. Discoid meniscus. Sagittal intensity windowing *(A)*, Coronal T$_2$ *(B)*, and coronal T$_1$ *(C)* MR images demonstrate congenital discoid menisci. In *A* and *B*, a complete discoid lateral meniscus is demonstrated. Image *B* may mimic a displaced bucket handle meniscal tear if the discoid meniscus is not recognized by analyzing all images. In *C*, a discoid medial meniscus is demonstrated.

1.9% (1.4% lateral, 0.5% medial).[164] This incidence is undoubtedly low because meniscal cysts may not communicate with the joint space, and lesions too small to be noted on physical examination are not infrequently noted on MRI.[28, 36] These lesions appear to be of traumatic origin, compressive force being apparently the most important mechanism.[10, 55] Meniscal cysts are quite frequently associated with horizontal (degenerative) meniscal tears and, on contrast arthrography, are demonstrated as contrast collections in contiguity with a meniscal tear, extending beyond the periphery of the adjacent tibial plateau.[26, 61] CT can also be used to demonstrate a fluid density mass at the level of the joint line, contiguous with the peripheral margin of the meniscus (Fig. 28B–20).

MRI readily demonstrates meniscal cysts as masses contiguous with the periphery of a meniscus displaying the MRI characteristics of joint fluid.[36] That is, these lesions demonstrate intermediate signal intensity on T$_1$- and intermediate-weighted sequences and high signal intensity on T$_2$ sequences (Figs. 28B–21 to 28B–23). The adjacent meniscus is not normal in the presence of a meniscal

cyst (see Fig. 28B–22). This is an important point in differentiating meniscal cysts from less common synovial cysts (ganglion cysts) arising from the joint capsule.[10, 53, 110] A meniscal cyst should be shown to involve the substance of the meniscus in association with either degenerative change or a horizontal cleavage tear of the meniscus. Lateral meniscal cysts tend to be smaller and are localized to the joint line, whereas those arising from the medial meniscus may become quite large (see Fig. 28B–23) and dissect through the capsule, remaining attached to the meniscus by a long thin stalk. Sonography may also be useful in identifying meniscal cysts and may demonstrate the associated tear in some cases.[157]

Imaging the Knee Ligaments

Imaging the ligamentous structure of the knee presented a difficult problem before the advent of MRI. Stress radiographs can imply the presence of collateral and cruciate

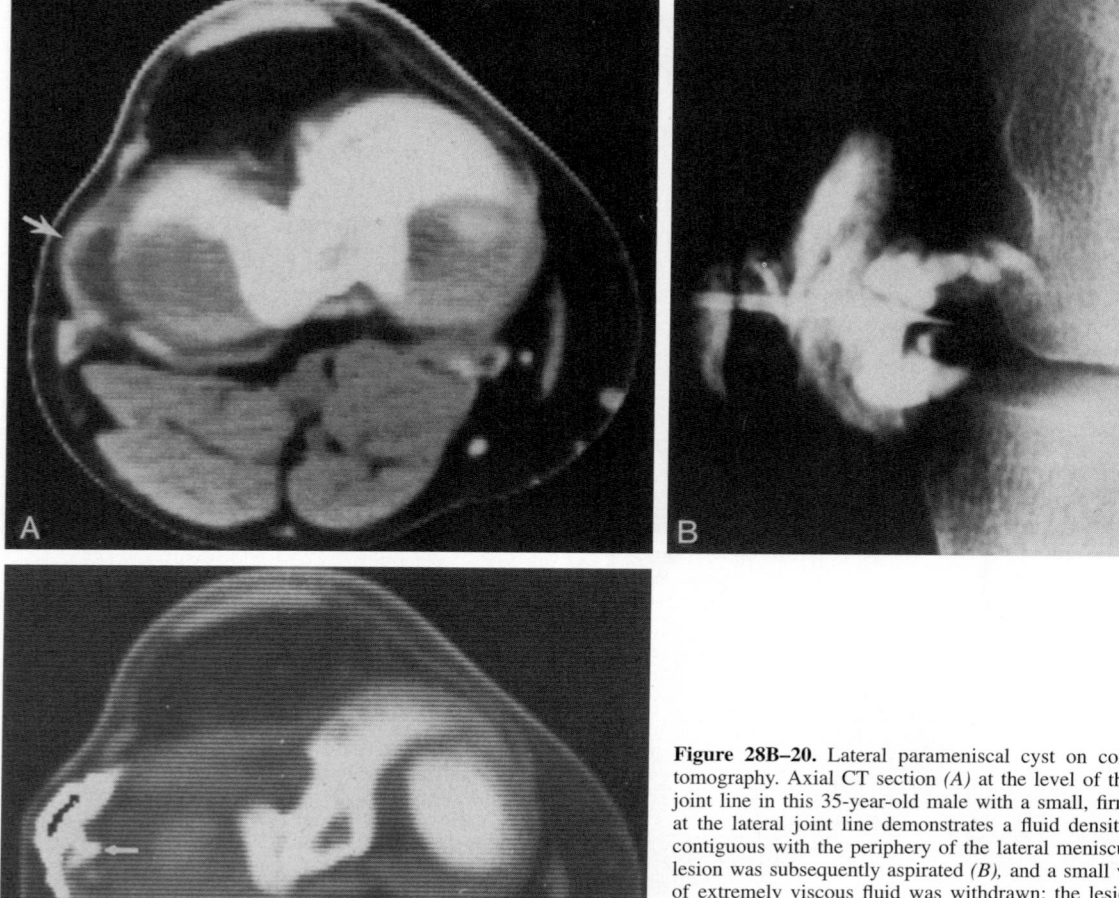

Figure 28B–20. Lateral parameniscal cyst on computed tomography. Axial CT section *(A)* at the level of the knee joint line in this 35-year-old male with a small, firm mass at the lateral joint line demonstrates a fluid density mass contiguous with the periphery of the lateral meniscus. The lesion was subsequently aspirated *(B),* and a small volume of extremely viscous fluid was withdrawn; the lesion was then injected with radiographic contrast. Repeat CT scan *(C)* demonstrates contrast filling the cyst and extending into the substance of the meniscus *(arrow).*

ligament injuries but are frequently misleading. Contrast arthrography, using horizontal beam techniques with appropriate stress and with an experienced arthrographer, can achieve high sensitivity (95%) in identifying complete cruciate ligament tears (Fig. 28B–24*B*).[137] MRI, in contrast, allows direct visualization of these ligamentous structures and has a high degree of sensitivity in identifying pathologic alterations.[90, 109, 124, 138]

The Anterior Cruciate Ligament

The ACL[5, 100, 120, 124, 132] arises from the medial border of the lateral femoral condyle, passes anteriorly, inferiorly, and medially, and inserts into the tibial plateau anterior to the medial portion of the tibial eminence, 8 to 10 mm posterior to the anterior tibial margin. The ligament is approximately 4 cm in length and 1 cm in diameter and is composed of two fiber bundles (anteromedial and posterolateral), which are in turn composed of multiple fascicles.[132] With MRI, the ACL is visualized as a single, moderately dark band or as a collection of two or three discrete bundles separated by higher-intensity zones, which coalesce into a single dark structure near its origin (Fig. 28B–25).[109, 120, 124]

The ACL is best visualized with MRI on T_1- or intermediate-weighted sequences in the sagittal plane. Owing to its oblique course, many prefer to image the ACL in the sagittal plane with the foot rotated 10 to 20 degrees externally. With 5-cm-slice spacing, this foot rotation is essential because occasionally a normal ACL may not be visualized in true sagittal images. With close interslice spacing (e.g., 3 mm), external rotation of the foot is not as important. These images are usually obtained as the first echo (intermediate-weighted; for example, repetition time [TR] 2000 msec, echo time [TE] 20 msec) of a multiecho sequence with the second echo (e.g., TR 2000 msec, TE 80 msec) providing T_2 weighting, which helps to identify hemor-

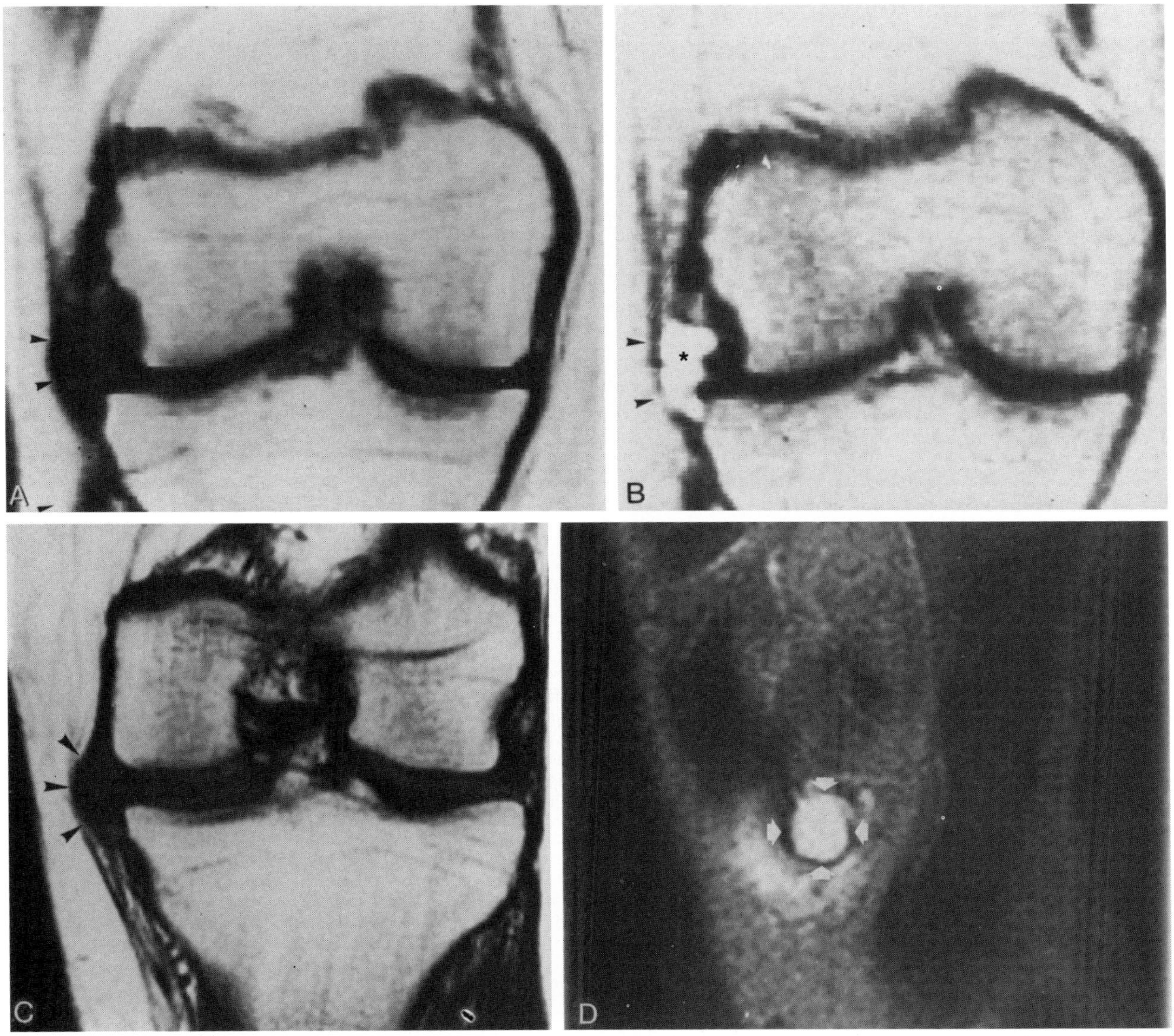

Figure 28B–21. Parameniscal cysts. Coronal *(A)* T$_1$ (400/50) MRI section demonstrates an intermediate density mass along the lateral joint line, which demonstrates the characteristics of fluid *(asterisk)* in T$_2$-weighted sequences *(B,* 2000/120) characteristic of a parameniscal cyst. In another patient, a small medial parameniscal cyst with similar characteristics is shown on coronal *(C)* T$_1$-weighted (600/20) and sagittal *(D)* T$_2$-weighted (2200/80) sequences through the knee.

Figure 28B–22. Lateral parameniscal cyst with tear. Coronal T$_1$ (800/20) MRI section through the anterior horn of the lateral meniscus demonstrates a joint line mass *(arrowheads)* as well as a horizontal cleavage tear *(open arrow)* within the meniscus.

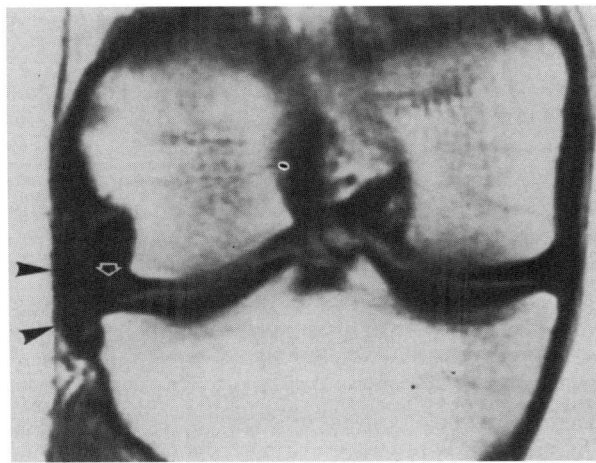

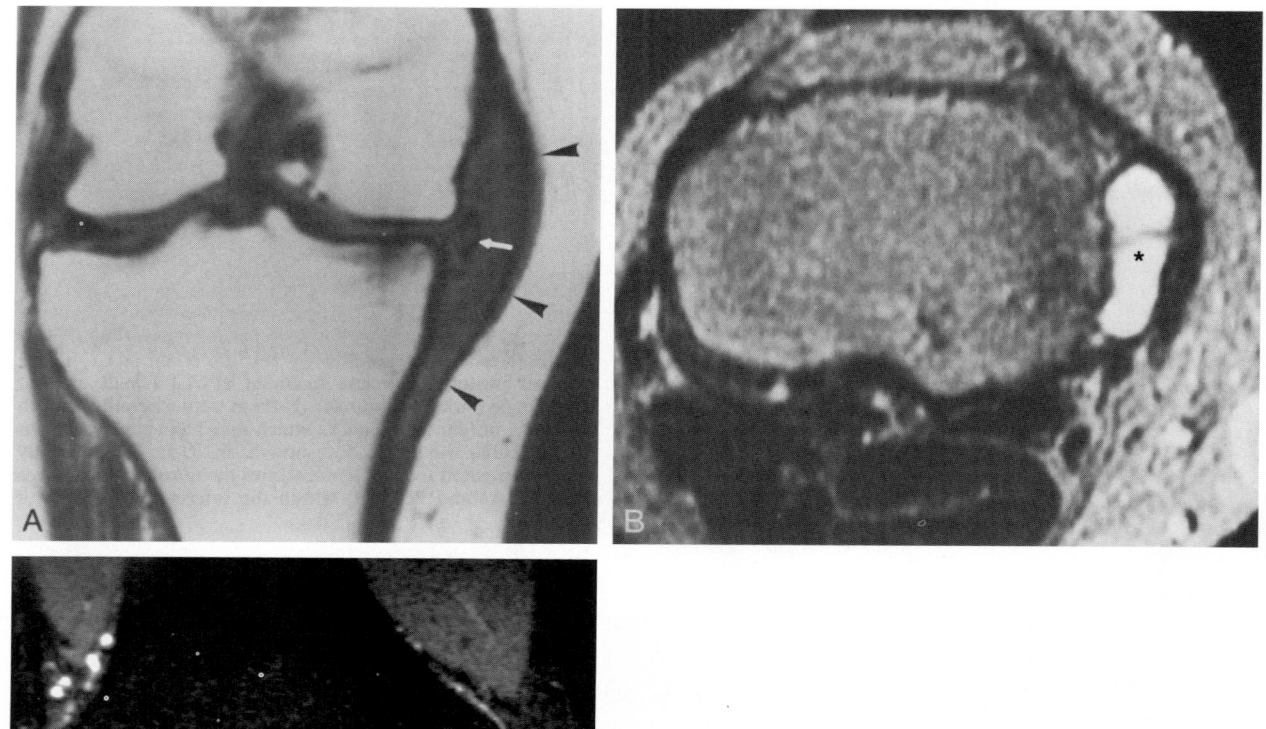

Figure 28B–23. Medial parameniscal cysts. Coronal T_1-weighted (600/20) MRI section *(A)*, axial T_2-weighted (2000/80) MRI section *(B)*, and coronal T_2 fat saturation MRI section *(C)* demonstrate medial meniscal cysts. Note the characteristic large size of the cysts, which displace the superficial band of the tibial collateral ligament *(arrowheads)* as well as the distorted and torn medial meniscus *(arrow)*. Fluid characteristics of the mass *(asterisks)* are demonstrated in the T_2-weighted images.

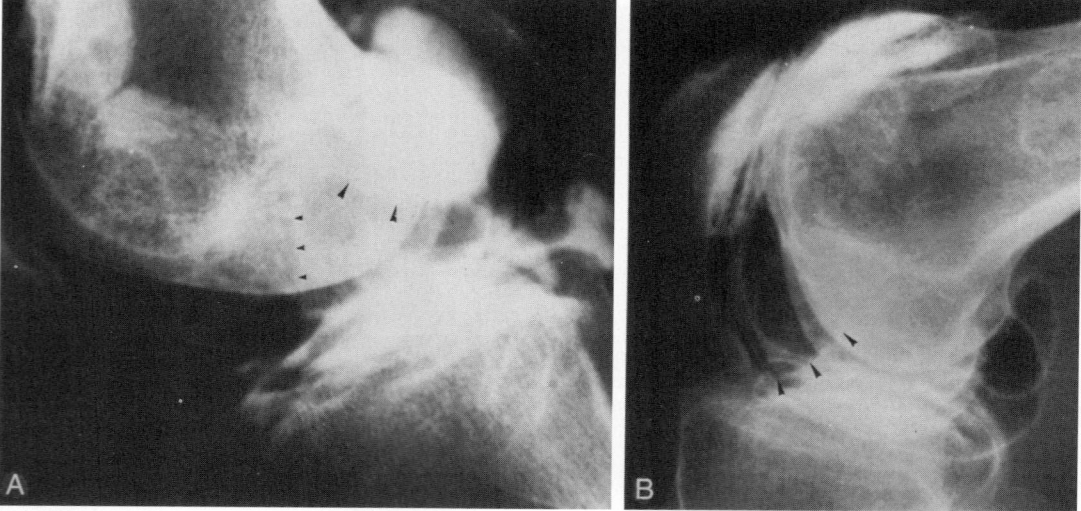

Figure 28B–24. Arthrographic evaluation of the anterior cruciate ligament (ACL). "Hanging" lateral radiographs of the knee obtained during double-contrast arthrography demonstrate the appearance of the normal *(A)* and torn *(B)* anterior cruciate ligament. In *A*, the intact ACL demonstrates a "crisp" straight anterior border *(small arrowheads)*. Slight concave "bowing" of the nonstressed posterior cruciate ligament is normal *(large arrowheads)*. In *B*, the anterior margin of the ACL demonstrates a subtle concave bowing despite the application of appropriate stress.

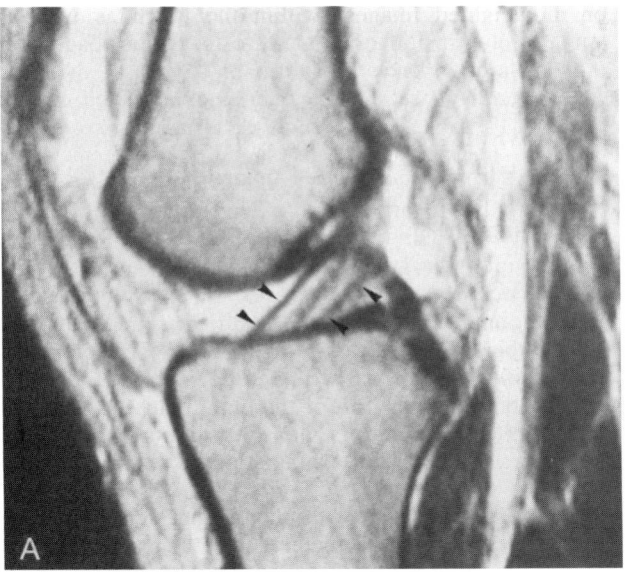
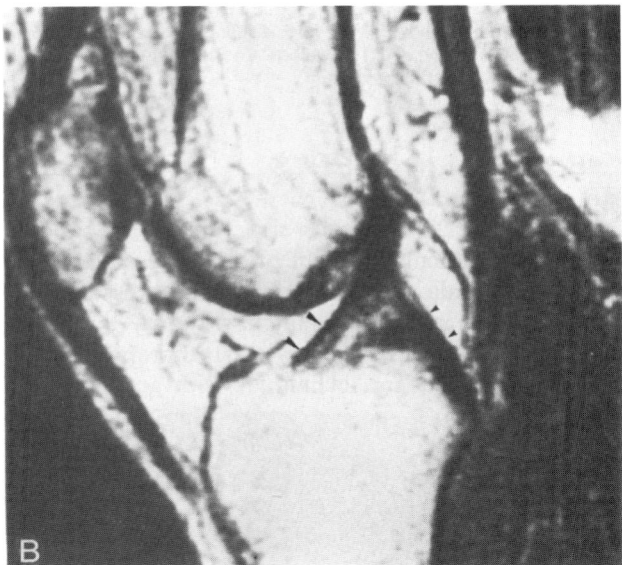
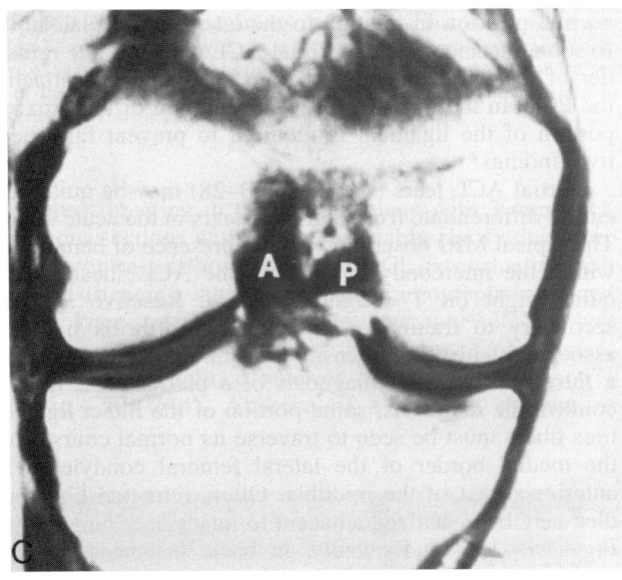

Figure 28B–25. Normal anterior cruciate ligament (ACL). Sagittal T_2-weighted MRI sections in *A* (2200/90) and *B* (2000/80) demonstrate the most common appearances of the normal ACL in the sagittal plane. In *A,* the ACL is sharply outlined by effusion and has the form of three distinct fiber bundles, separated by fat. In *B,* the ACL *(large arrowheads)* and posterior cruciate ligament (PCL) *(small arrowheads)* appear as single dark fiber bundles. Note in both cases the smooth sharp anterior border of the ACL, which may be perfectly straight as in *A* or exhibit a mild, smooth bow as in *B*. In *C,* a coronally oriented T_1-weighted section demonstrates the normal appearances of the ACL (A) and PCL (P) within the intercondylar notch of the femur.

rhage in association with a tear and to distinguish the ligament from surrounding joint effusion. Coronal plane images with T_1 weighting (e.g., TR 800 msec, TE 20 msec) also visualize the ligament in successive sections as it passes through the intercondylar notch.

In evaluating the ACL with MRI, the characteristics of the normal ligament should be considered. The normal ACL (see Fig. 28B–25) should be composed of one or more dark fiber bundles of variable diameter. In some individuals, the ACL may appear as a single thick, dark structure similar to the PCL. In others, more typically females, the ligament may be quite gracile with one or more thin, dark bands being visualized. A smooth, crisp anterior contour to the ligament is an important observation in all intact ligaments. A smooth concave "bow" may be present in mild flexion of the knee, but in all cases the anterior border should be sharply defined. No significant brightening should be present on T_2-weighted images compared with T_1 or IW images. Longitudinally oriented

"bright" zones may be present on T_1 or IW images representing fatty connective tissue between and around ligamentous bands and fascicles[109, 124, 132] (see Fig. 28B–25A); however, this does not brighten with T_2 weighting. Though the sagittal plane is preferred in evaluating the ACL, it is also well seen in sequential sections in the coronal and axial planes (Fig. 28B–26).[59] Often, careful evaluation of all imaging planes clarifies an appearance that is equivocal on sagittal images.

Complete disruption of the substance of the ligament is certainly a highly specific finding in complete ACL tears. In some instances, no vestiges of the ACL can be identified. More frequently, retracted fiber bundles may be identified with a characteristic "coiled spring" or serpiginous appearance (Fig. 28B–27). An irregular or wavy anterior border of the ACL (Figs. 28B–27 and 28B–28) is frequently a useful sign, exaggerated by the presence of adjacent hemorrhage in T_2-weighted images. Frequently, the major portion of the ligament can be identified as a dark band may be identified by its insertion at the anterior margin of the tibia.[3, 135] The infrapatellar plica is usually seen well only in the presence of a torn ACL, and some consider its identification to be presumptive evidence of such a tear.[39, 103] A final pitfall is the normal bowing of the anterior margin of the ACL when it is relaxed. The only protection against this problem is paying careful attention to radiographic positioning and positive findings on both overhead and spot radiographs of the ligament.

Other abnormalities are common in patients with ACL tears, including meniscal tears, medial or lateral collateral ligament tears, avulsions from the lateral margin of the tibia (Segond's fracture, lateral capsular sign), and avulsions at the femoral origin or tibial insertion of the ACL (Fig. 28B–31).[9, 46, 68, 134] Peripheral meniscal tears are exceedingly common in association with ACL tears and are more commonly missed, especially small tears of the posterior horn of the lateral meniscus.[44] Plain radiographs in the lateral projection with anterior stress applied to the tibia have long been used to document ACL instability (see Fig. 28B–31A). The "lateral notch sign" refers to an impaction fracture of the lateral femoral condyle at the site of the normal condylar indentation. This is seen on plain radiographs in association with acute or chronic ACL tears.[9, 65, 112] A homologue or, more accurately, a precursor of the lateral notch sign may be seen with MRI and constitutes an important diagnostic sign in patients with ACL tears.

Frequently, during the examination of acute knee injuries, foci of abnormal signal intensity are noted within the subcortical marrow space of the tibial or femoral condyle. These zones exhibit diminished signal intensity on T_1 or IW images and are associated with "speckled" brightening on T_2-weighted images. These lesions are undoubtedly a manifestation of free hemorrhage between the medullary trabeculae and are probably associated with microfractures of weight-bearing trabeculae.[181] These lesions represent a

new diagnosis uncovered with the advent of MRI, and their nomenclature has not yet become consistent. Thus, these lesions may be referred to as "bone bruises," subcortical trabecular fractures, or subcortical medullary hemorrhage. We have frequently noted subcortical trabecular fractures (bone bruises) in association with acute ACL tears. These, in our experience, are most typically seen on the lateral femoral condyle as a triangular subcortical lesion centered on the normal lateral condylar indentation (incisura) (Fig. 28B–32; see Fig. 28B–54). These bone bruises demonstrate diminished intensity on T_1 or IW images and are associated with T_2 brightening as well as intense enhancement on t_2 fat saturation or short-tau inversion-recovery images. They are usually quite obvious on the coronal T_1-weighted sequence and are easily verified on sagittal images. The importance of these lesions cannot be overemphasized. In our experience, their presence in the location just described is almost pathognomonic for an acute ACL tear. Bone bruises are also seen on the posterior aspect of the lateral tibial condyle in association with acute ACL tears.

On a mechanistic basis, the presence of these lesions is quite predictable. Typically, an ACL tear is the result of valgus angulation at the knee with external rotation of the femur on the fixed tibia. The valgus angulation, in addition to tearing or stretching the MCL, places nearly all the weight-bearing stress on the lateral femoral condyle, which rotates laterally, frequently forcing its midportion on the posterior lip of the lateral tibial condyle. This may result in an impaction fracture (lateral notch sign) if the force is extreme enough, but more frequently it overstresses the subcortical trabeculae of the femoral condyle, yielding a bone bruise centered on the condylar notch. In our experience, follow-up arthroscopy fails to demonstrate any visible abnormality of the overlying articular cartilage. Bone bruises at the posterior margin of the medial femoral condyle (Fig. 28B–33) (contrecoup injury) are also quite com-

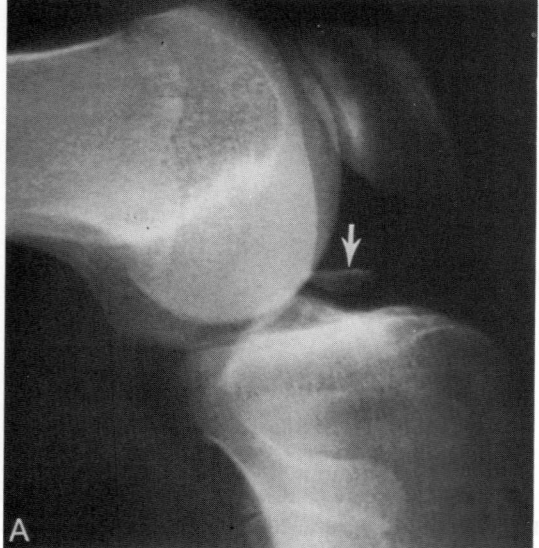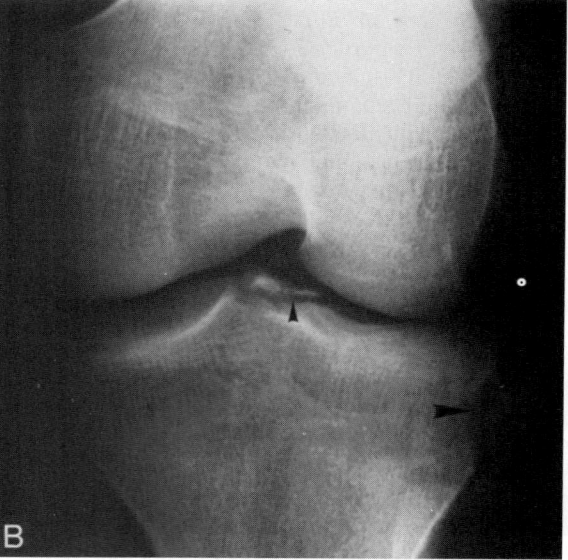

Figure 28B–31. Plain radiographic findings in anterior cruciate ligament (ACL) injuries. In *A,* a lateral radiograph of the knee with anterior stress applied to the tibia demonstrates anterior subluxation of the tibia relative to the femur (radiographic anterior drawer sign) as well as a "flake" fracture from the tibia at the level of insertion of the ACL. In *B,* a Segond fracture is present *(large arrowhead)* as well as a "flake" fracture at the ACL insertion in this patient who also had an associated medial collateral ligament disruption.

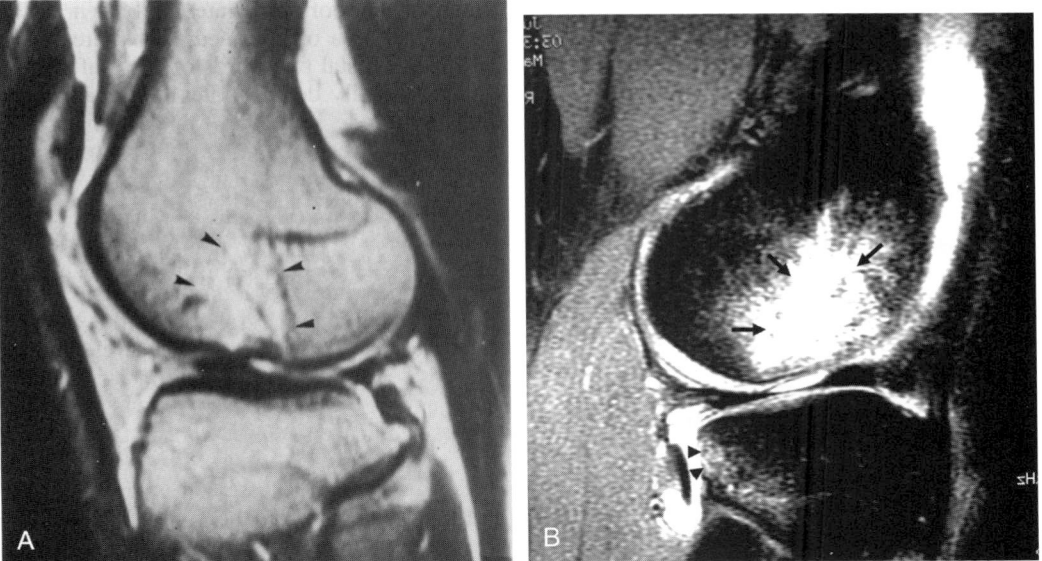

Figure 28B–32. "Bone bruises" in association with anterior cruciate ligament (ACL) tears. Sagittal T₂-weighted (2000/80) MRI section *(A)* through the lateral femoral condyle in this 31-year-old male with an acute ACL disruption demonstrates a triangular-shaped area of T₂ brightening *(arrowheads)* within the medullary bone of the lateral condyle centered at the level of the lateral condylar notch. Despite the presence of apparent indentation of the subchondral bone plate, subsequent arthroscopy demonstrated normal overlying articular cartilage. In another patient with an acute ACL rupture *(B)*, a sagittal IW fast spin MRI image demonstrates intense marrow edema along the posterior lip of the lateral tibial condyle *(arrowheads)* and deep to the lateral femoral incisura *(arrows)*.

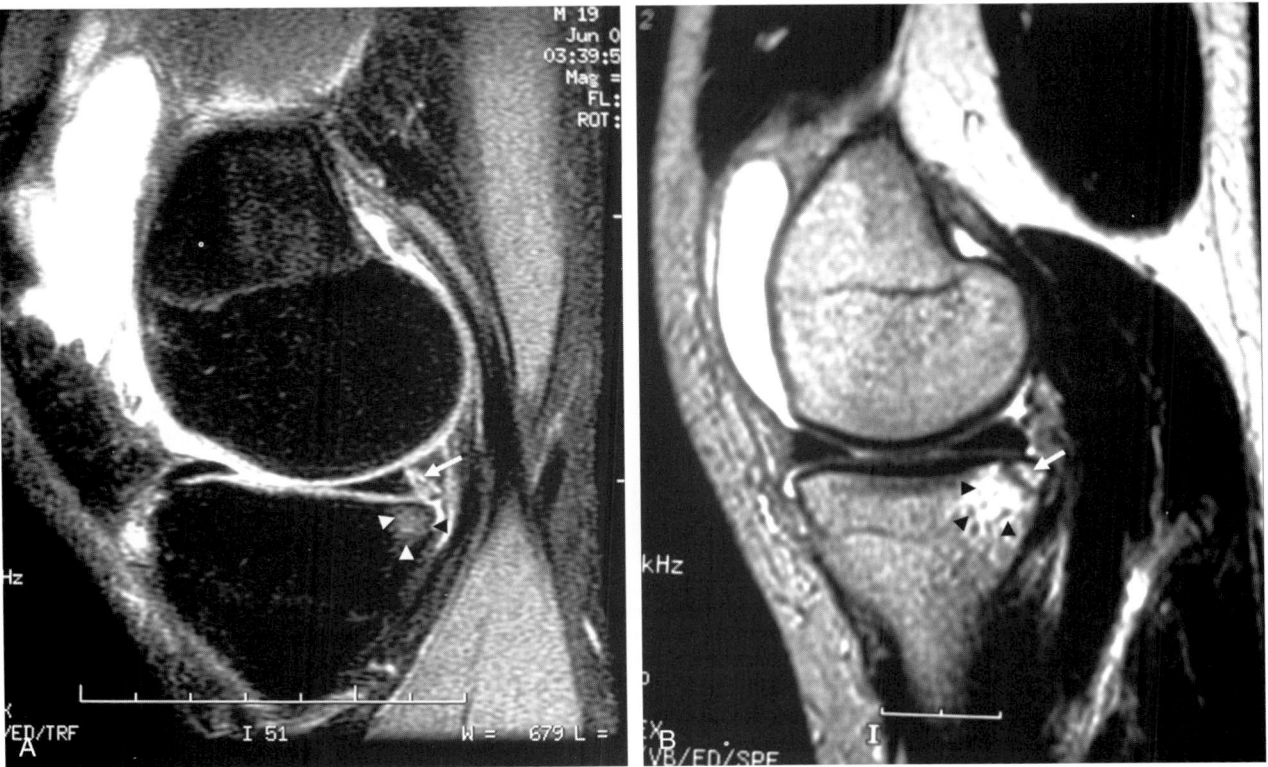

Figure 28B–33. Contrecoup bone bruises. Sagittal intensity windowing (IW) fast spin *(A)* and IW *(B)* images in two patients with acute anterior cruciate ligament ruptures demonstrate contrecoup bone bruises *(arrowheads)* at the posterior lip of the medial femoral condyle. In *A*, a tear of the posterior horn of the medial meniscus *(arrow)* is evident, whereas in B, a nondisplaced fracture of the posterior lip of the medial femoral condyle *(arrow)* can be seen.

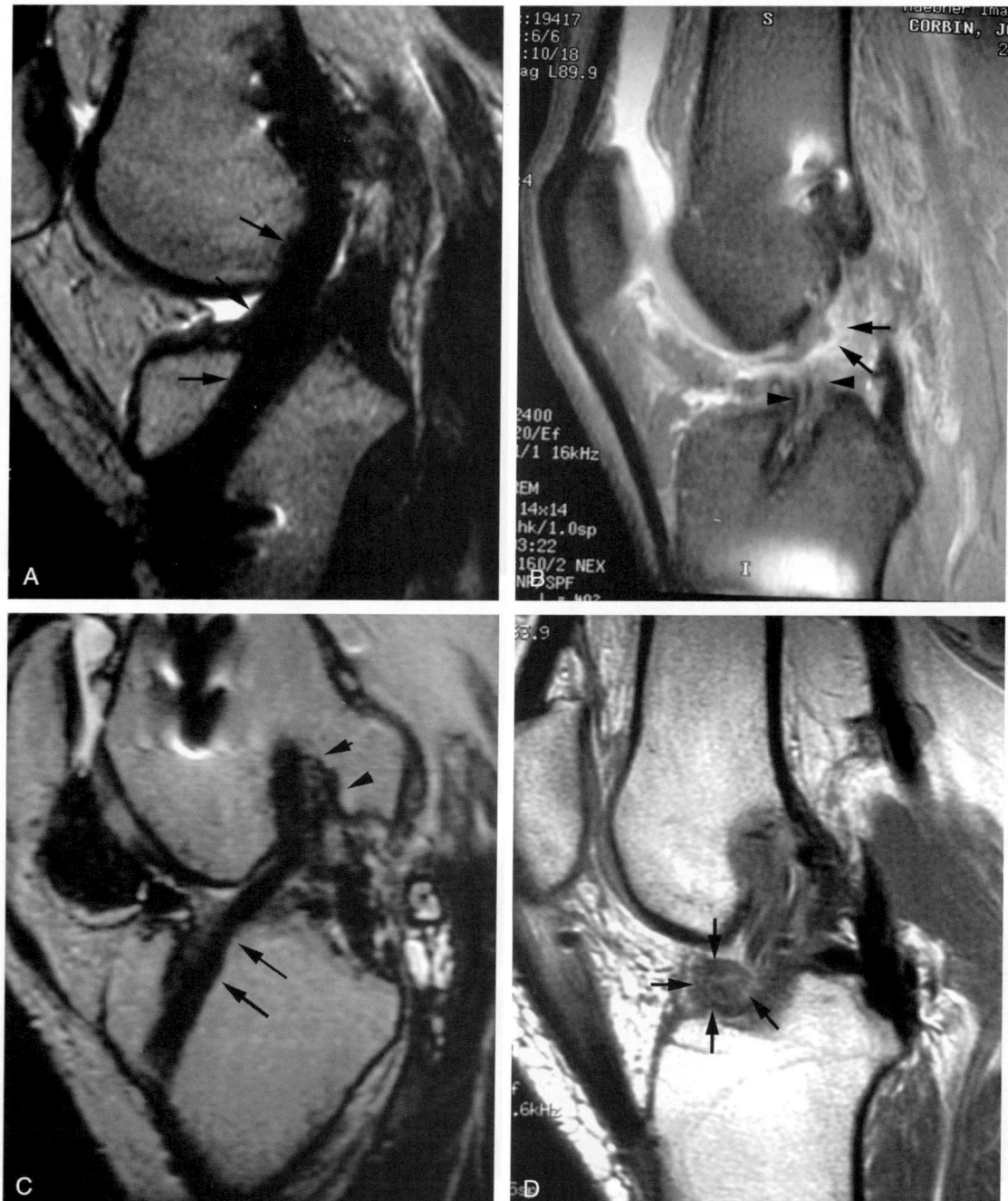

Figure 28B–35. Anterior cruciate ligament (ACL) grafts. *A–D,* Sagittal intensity windowing images obtained along the long axis of the graft demonstrate findings in MRI evaluation of ACL grafts. In *A,* an intact graft *(arrows)* is demonstrated with homogeneous dark signal. In *B,* a rupture of the graft has occurred with the tibial stump *(arrowheads)* visible with hemorrhage and a fluid-filled defect *(arrows)* in the anticipated location of the graft in the notch. In *C,* the femoral *(arrowheads)* and tibial *(arrows)* tunnels are poorly positioned, being too far anterior in both instances. In *D,* the "cyclops" lesion *(arrows)* is demonstrated with a rounded fibrous "mass" anterior to the graft interfering with normal function of the knee.

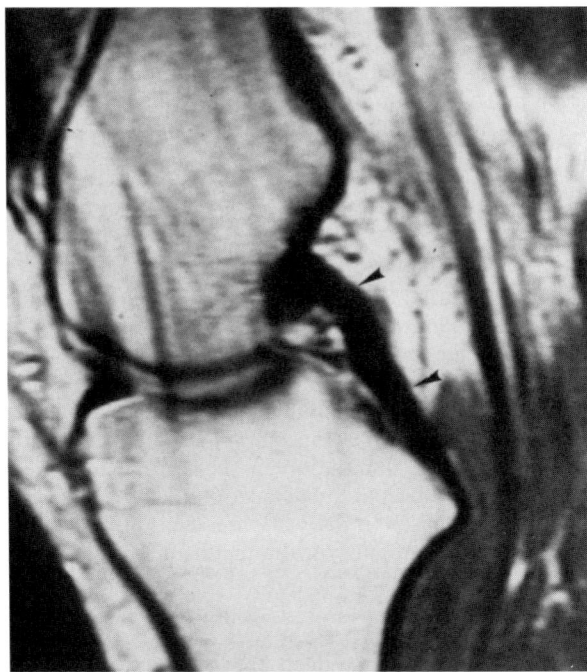

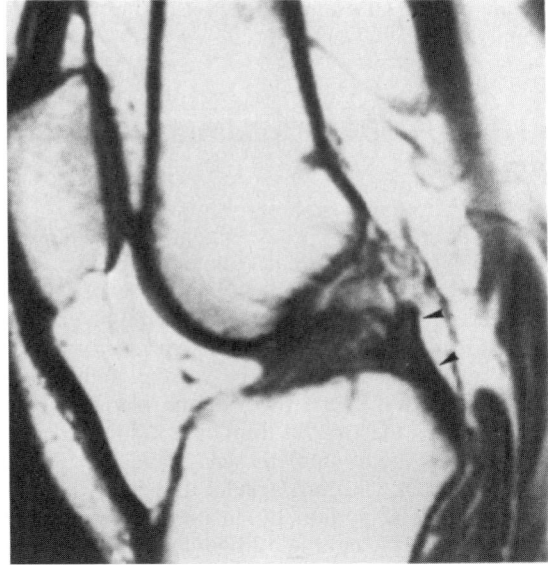

Figure 28B–36. Normal posterior cruciate ligament. Sagittal intensity windowing (2200/30) MRI section through the intercondylar notch demonstrates a normal posterior cruciate ligament. This structure is almost invariably clearly demonstrated and appears as a thick, dark band passing from the lateral border of the medial femoral condyle to the posterior lip of the tibia. Its appearance in the coronal plane is shown in Figure 28B–23C.

Figure 28B–38. Chronic posterior cruciate ligament (PCL) tear. Sagittal T₁-weighted (800/20) MRI section through the intercondylar notch in this 32-year-old female with a long history of PCL disruption demonstrates the residual inferior portion of the ligament *(arrowheads)* overlying the posterior lip of the tibia. Continuity with the medial femoral condyle could not be demonstrated in any images.

mass is less constant than in ACL injuries but, when present, tends to be located near the tibial insertion of the ligament (Fig. 28B–37). T₂ brightening may be apparent in acute injuries but is lacking in chronic injuries. Complete discontinuity of the ligament may be demonstrated (Fig. 28B–38), or an avulsion fracture from the posterior tibial margin may be associated with the PCL insertion.

Categorization of PCL disruptions in regard to interstitial rupture or avulsion is important, as with ACL injuries, because the latter may be amenable to immediate surgical repair, whereas the former are not.

With contrast arthrography, the PCL is almost invariably

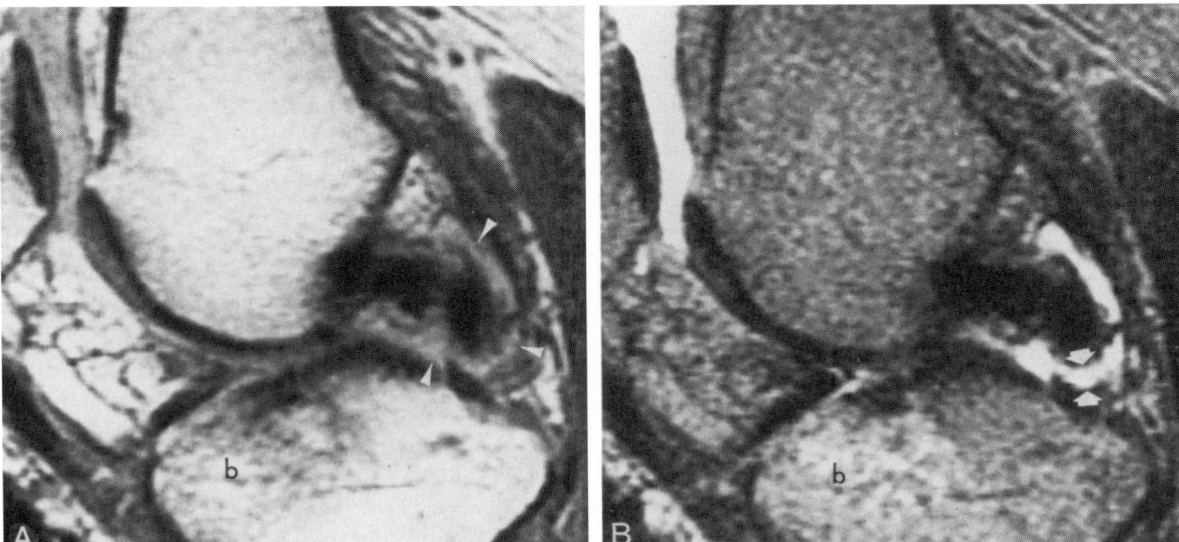

Figure 28B–37. Acute posterior cruciate ligament (PCL) tear. Sagittal intensity windowing (2000/20) *(A)* and T₂-weighted (2000/80) *(B)* MRI sections through the intercondylar notch in this 20-year-old college basketball player demonstrate an acute tear of the posterior cruciate ligament. In *A*, there is a "mass" effect in the posterior aspect of the "notch" *(arrowheads)*, whereas in *B*, discontinuity of the PCL (between *arrows*) is demonstrated; the defect has been filled in with hemorrhage. Also note the presence of a "bone bruise" (b) in the anterior tibial medullary space that brightens considerably on the T₂-weighted image.

readily identified. The same criteria used in evaluating the ACL apply to the PCL.[135]

The Medial (Tibial) Collateral Ligament

The MCL[84, 87, 120, 124, 185] has two primary components. The superficial portion (tibial collateral ligament [TCL]) consists of a strong, flattened, triangular band that arises from the medial epicondyle, immediately below the adductor tubercle, and inserts on the medial surface of the proximal tibia approximately 5 cm below the joint line. The ligament is broadest at the level of the medial meniscus, where it overlies the middle third of the joint space, and gradually tapers both cranially and caudally. The deep portion of the MCL (medial capsular ligament) is separated from the superficial portion by an interligamentous bursa (bursa of Voshell) (see Fig. 28B–41) and is intimately associated with the middle third of the medial meniscus. Superiorly, the deep fibers of the MCL (medial capsular ligament) arise from the medial epicondyle and insert on the tibial articular margin. Anteriorly, the deep fibers of the MCL blend with the medial patellar retinaculum, whereas posteriorly they blend with the capsule to form the posterior oblique ligament.

On MRI,[120, 122, 124] the TCL (Fig. 28B–39) is identified as a thin band of low signal intensity extending from the medial femoral epicondyle inferiorly, in close approximation to the peripheral margin of the medial meniscus, to insert on the medial tibial cortex deep to the cephalic portion of the pes anserinus. A thin zone of fat or fluid

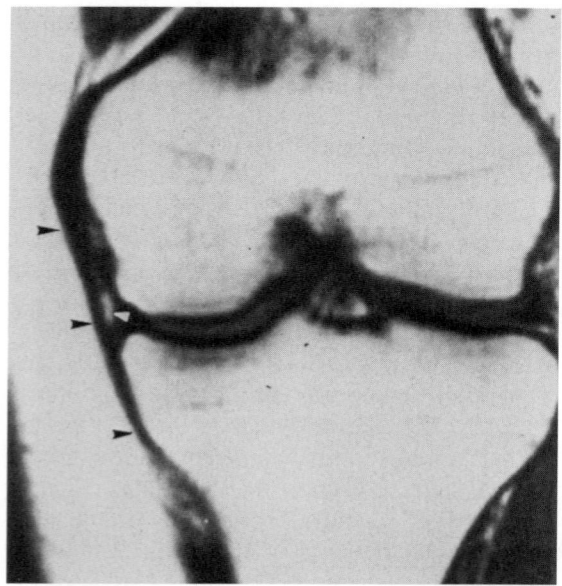

Figure 28B–39. Normal tibial collateral ligament. Coronal T_1-weighted (600/20) MRI section through the midcondylar plane demonstrates the normal appearance *(black arrowheads)* of the superficial layer of the tibial collateral ligament (TCL [medial collateral ligament]). In this patient the fat pad *(white arrowhead),* which parallels the interligamentous bursa (Voshell's bursa) between the deep and superficial layers of the TCL, is quite prominent.

density (Fig. 28B–39) may be identified between the superficial layer and the deep layer as a normal finding in some individuals. With sufficient trauma, usually external rotation and valgus stress, the MCL will be disrupted in a predictable manner.[84, 87, 132] The deep fibers are disrupted first, followed by the superficial fibers, which are followed by the ACL if sufficient force is present. The combination of a complete MCL tear with an ACL tear and a peripheral tear of the medial meniscus is a particularly common and severe football injury that was formerly referred to as O'Donoghue's triad.[134] As opposed to the lateral ligamentous structures and the PCL, the MCL and the ACL tend to tear near their femoral attachments.

On MRI,[124] a complete MCL tear is manifested by hemarthrosis as well as prominent subcutaneous soft tissue swelling and hemorrhage (Fig. 28B–40). This latter finding is manifested by a diminution in the normal high signal intensity in the adjacent subcutaneous fat on T_1-weighted images, but increases in intensity are seen on T_2-weighted images. Loss of contiguity of the ligament is often directly visualized, typically near its femoral insertion. A sprain, or an incomplete tear, of the TCL is present when adjacent subcutaneous edema is present with a visibly intact ligament. Isolated tears of the deep fibers of the MCL (medial capsular ligament) occur and are characterized by localized medial soft tissue swelling associated with an increased amount of fluid in the interligamentous bursa (Fig. 28B–41), often with a medial shift of the meniscus in coronal sections. Meniscotibial (coronary) ligament tears involving the tibial insertion of the MCL may be identified[50] and demonstrate a similar appearance. These deep MCL and coronary ligament tears are often associated with medial meniscal tears. Partial TCL avulsions may also be manifested by a diminution in signal intensity of the marrow underlying the medial femoral epicondyle on T_1 images that brightens on T_2 images, reflecting a subtle partial avulsion injury at the origin of the ligament. A pure avulsion injury with the otherwise intact TCL attached to an avulsed cortical fragment may occur but is rare.

Arthrography[50, 163] is not generally indicated in patients with suspected MCL injuries. If present, however, "gaping" of the medial joint space may be noted when valgus stress is applied to demonstrate the medial meniscus or on plain stress radiographs. Soft tissue swelling may also be noted on spot and overhead radiographs along the medial joint margin. Extravasation of contrast material into either the medial subcutaneous tissues or the interligamentous bursa (see Fig. 28B–41) in isolated deep fiber tears may also be identified, indicating a relatively acute MCL injury.

The Lateral Ligamentous Complex

Acute injuries to the knee resulting in lateral instability are less common and are recognized less frequently than medial instabilities.[50, 120, 124, 137] The major stabilizing structures on the lateral side of the knee are the iliotibial band, the lateral (fibular) collateral ligament, the popliteal tendon (and muscle), the biceps femoris tendon (and muscle), and the lateral capsular ligament (Fig. 28B–42; see Fig. 28B–1D). Isolated injuries in this area may be either

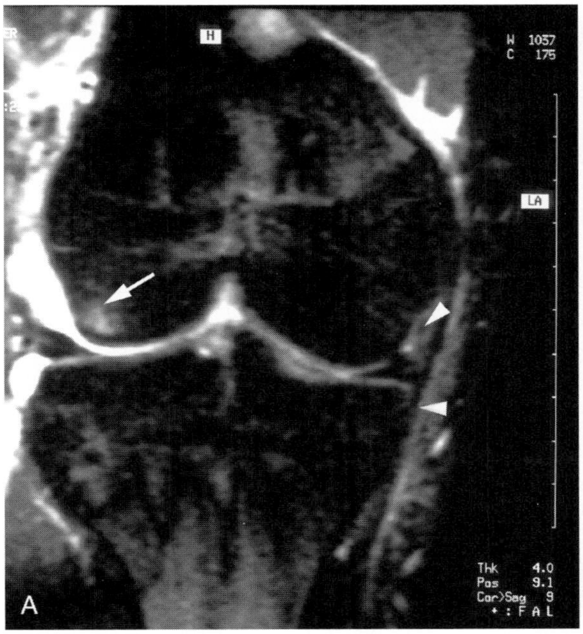

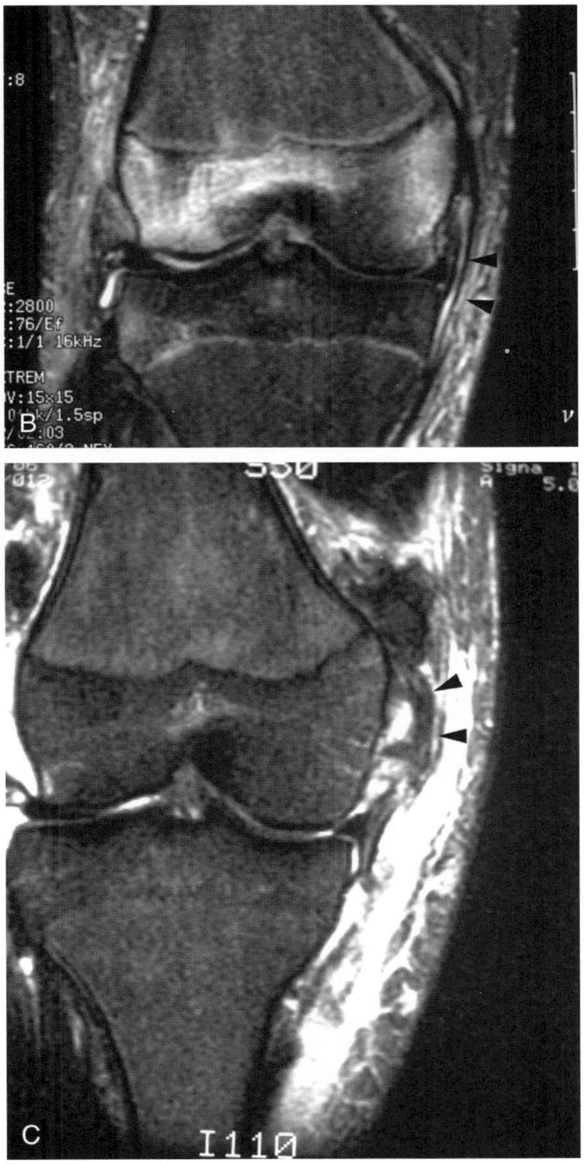

Figure 28B–40. Tibial collateral ligament (TCL) injuries. Coronal T₂ fat saturation MRI images *(A–C)* demonstrate the range of TCL injuries. In *A*, there is soft tissue swelling superficial and deep to an otherwise intact TCL *(arrowheads)*, indicating a grade 1 TCL sprain. The "bone bruise" in the lateral femoral condyle *(arrow)* indicates valgus stress consistent with the mechanism of injury of a TCL sprain. In *B*, there is soft tissue swelling with partial disruption of the TCL *(arrowheads)* typical of a grade 2 TCL sprain. In *C*, a grade 3 lesion *(arrowheads)* is demonstrated with complete disruption of the ligament.

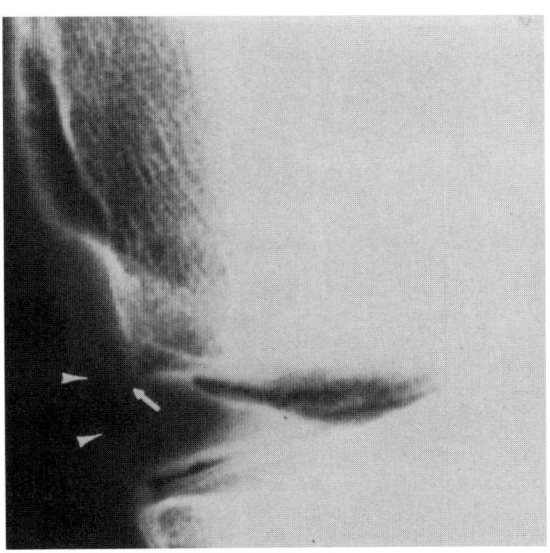

Figure 28B–41. Isolated tear of the medial capsular ligament. This arthrographic spot film of the midportion of the medial meniscus demonstrates a small tear of the superior surface of the meniscus peripherally *(arrow)*. Also note the presence of air in the interligamentous bursa (Voshell's bursa) between the tibial collateral ligament and medial capsular ligament *(white arrowheads)*.

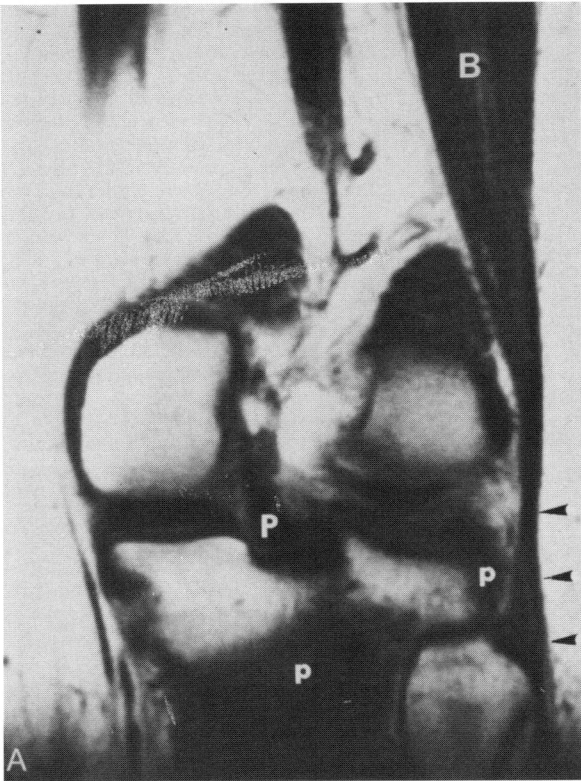

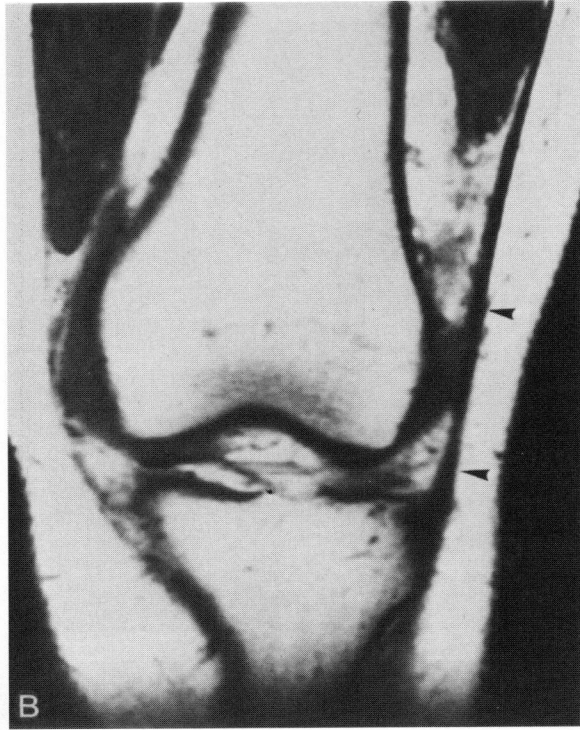

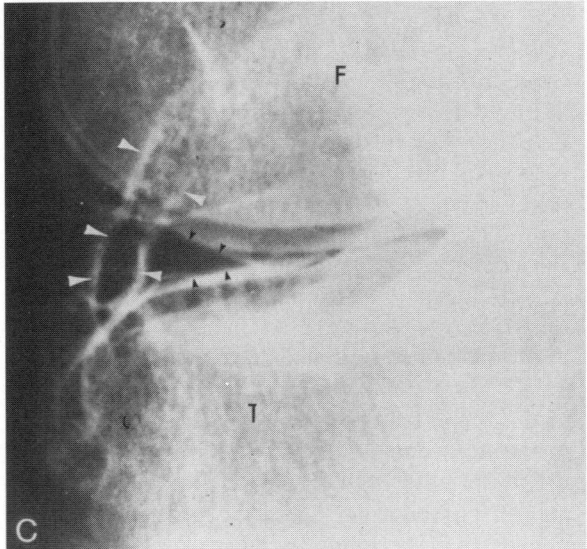

Figure 28B–42. Normal lateral ligaments. Coronal T₁-weighted (800/20) MRI sections through the posterior condylar level *(A)* and anterior condylar level *(B)* demonstrate the major supporting structures of the lateral side of the knee. In *A,* the biceps femoris muscle (B) is shown with its tendon *(arrowheads)* inserting onto the fibular styloid. In *B,* the insertion of the iliotibial band *(arrowheads)* onto Gerdy's tubercle on the anterolateral margin of the tibia is shown. In *C,* an arthrographic spot film of the posterior horn of the lateral meniscus *(black arrowheads)* also demonstrates the course of the popliteal tendon sheath *(white arrowheads).* Also see Figure 28B–1D and E for further detail of the popliteal tendon. B, biceps femoris muscle; F, fibula; p, popliteal tendon and muscle; P, posterior cruciate ligament; T, tibia.

asymptomatic or associated with mild varus instability, though with more extensive disruption, significant instabilities may occur.[85, 93, 151] Anterior and anterolateral tibial subluxation occurs with injuries involving the ACL, middle third capsular ligament, and deep layers of the iliotibial band. Posterolateral tibial subluxation occurs with injuries to the arcuate complex (fibular collateral ligament, arcuate ligament, and popliteal tendon). A particularly severe injury involves an avulsion fracture of the lateral tibial cortex (Segond's fracture) by the middle third of the lateral capsular ligament[124, 137] (lateral capsular sign) in association with tears of the ACL and MCL (see Fig. 28B–31B). These

major structures are all visible on coronal and sagittal MRI images,[120, 124] and although very little has been published about lateral ligament injuries, they are readily visualized.

Primary MRI findings (Fig. 28B–43) are similar to those for injuries of the medial ligaments: subcutaneous hemorrhage and edema, discontinuity of tendinous and ligamentous structures, and cortical avulsion fractures. Deep soft tissue swelling adjacent to the peripheral border of the lateral meniscus may provide evidence of a lateral capsular ligament tear, whereas an avulsion fracture of the fibular styloid may indicate an avulsion of the fibular collateral ligament (Fig. 28B–43). Absence of the popliteal tendon

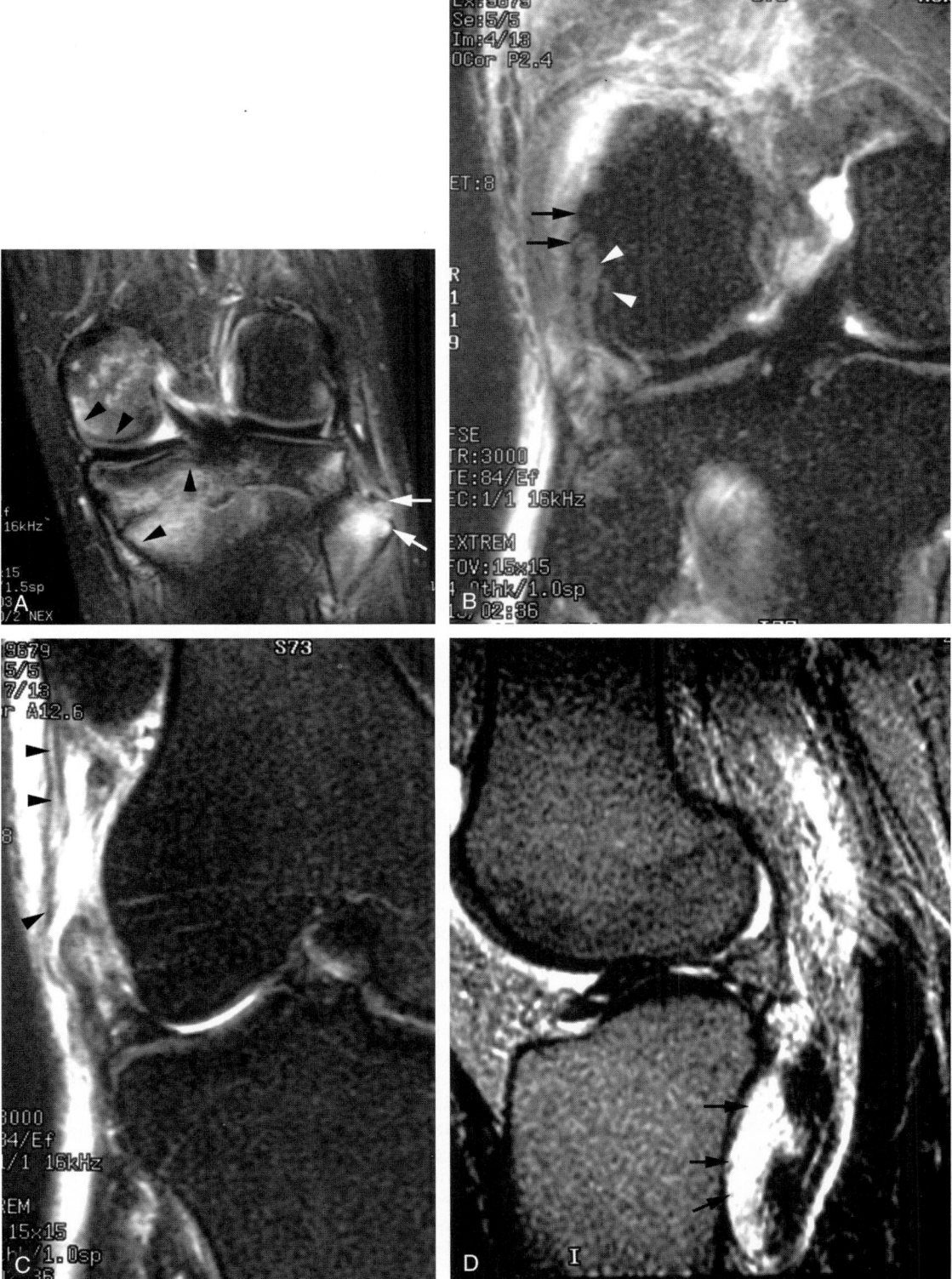

Figure 28B–43. Lateral soft tissue injuries. Coronal *(A–C)* and sagittal *(D)* T$_2$ fat saturation MRI images demonstrate a variety of injuries of the lateral supporting soft tissues. In *A*, there is avulsion of the insertions of the fibular collateral ligament (FCL) and biceps femoris tendon from the fibular styloid *(arrows)*. The contralateral "bone bruises" *(arrowheads)* are indicative of varus stress. In *B*, there have been tears at the femoral origins of the FCL *(arrows)* and popliteus tendon *(arrowheads)*. The image in *C* demonstrates complete rupture of the iliotibial band *(arrowheads)*. In image *D*, there has been avulsion of the tibial insertion of the popliteus muscle *(arrows)*.

within its sheath indicates injury to this tendon, usually in association with hemorrhage and irregularity of the popliteus muscle belly posterior to the proximal tibia. In addition, the popliteus and biceps femoris muscles should be evaluated for evidence of rupture, seen as a wavy muscle contour associated with areas of low or intermediate intensity on T_1- or intermediate-weighted images that increase in intensity on T_2-weighted images. Associated injuries to the ACL and MCL may be present as well as compression fractures or subcortical trabecular fractures of the medial femoral condyle.

Contrast arthrography is not indicated for the evaluation of lateral ligamentous disruptions. If present, however, lateral gaping of the joint space may be noted on application of varus stress to demonstrate the lateral meniscus or with plain radiographic stress views (Fig. 28B–44). In acute injuries (less than 48 hours old), extravasation of contrast agent through lateral capsular ligament disruptions may be noted,[136, 137] but after 48 hours, this sign is unreliable. Iliotibial band friction syndrome is a common cause of lateral knee pain in runners and cyclists. It is characterized by intense pain over the lateral epicondyle area of the femur. The cause is friction between the iliotibial band and the lateral femoral epicondyle, which is most prominent in 30 degrees of flexion. On MR images, bright T_2 signal is noted deep to the iliotibial band. This may be a poorly localized edema pattern or a well-circumscribed fluid collection secondary to adventitial bursa formation and chronic inflammation (Fig. 28B–45).[129]

The Extensor Tendons

The extensor tendons[197] of the knee[57] are the patellar and the quadriceps tendons (Fig. 28B–46). The quadriceps

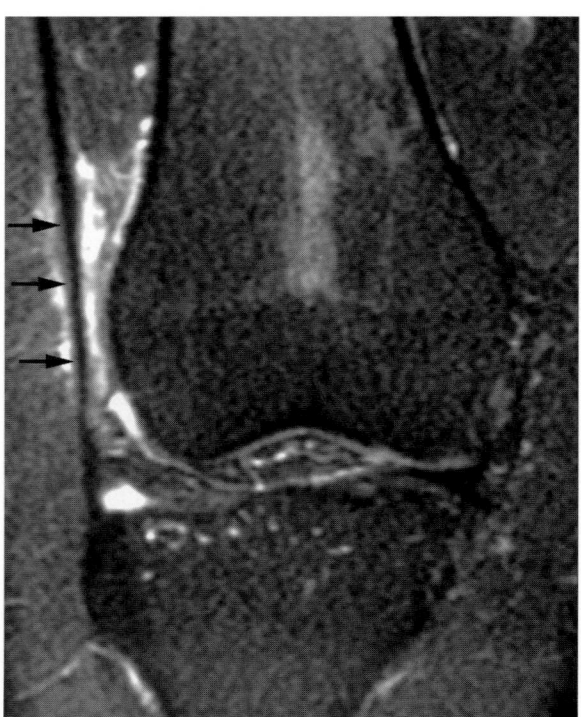

Figure 28B–45. Iliotibial band friction syndrome. Coronal T_2 fat saturation image demonstrates thickening of the iliotibial band *(arrows)* with adjacent soft tissue swelling.

tendon consists of the combined tendinous insertions of the rectus femoris, the vastus medialis, the vastus lateralis, and the vastus intermedius tendons. It inserts into the superior pole of the patella, with some fibers extending over the anterior surface of the patella to join with the patellar tendon. Medial and lateral fascial extensions arising from the vastus medialis and the vastus lateralis form the medial and lateral patellofemoral and meniscopatellar ligaments, which help to provide mediolateral instability for the patella. The patellar tendon arises from the inferior pole of the patella and inserts on the tibial tubercle. It is 5 to 6 cm long and 7 mm thick and varies from 3 cm in width at its origin to 2.5 cm at its insertion. Tears of the patellar or quadriceps tendons[170] (Fig. 28B–47) are uncommon but are readily visualized on MRI.[20, 75, 124, 142] Complete disruptions result in discontinuity of the involved tendon with hemorrhage and edema in the adjacent tissues. In partial injuries,[142] foci of moderately high signal intensity on T_1 images and brightening on T_2- or intermediate-weighted images may be seen within the substance of the involved tendon. Effusions[75] in the infrapatellar or prepatellar bursa may be present. Hemorrhage and swelling may be identified within the quadriceps musculature. We have noted medial retinacular disruptions in association with patellar dislocations in some patients (see Fig. 28B–50B). Sonography has also been shown to be useful in the diagnosis of extensor tendon rupture.[17]

Jumper's knee refers to the clinical syndrome of anterior knee pain with tenderness to palpation over the proximal patellar tendon,[19] which is especially common in athletes who participate in basketball, volleyball, soccer, tennis, and track. The terms *patellar tendinitis* and *patellar tendinosis*

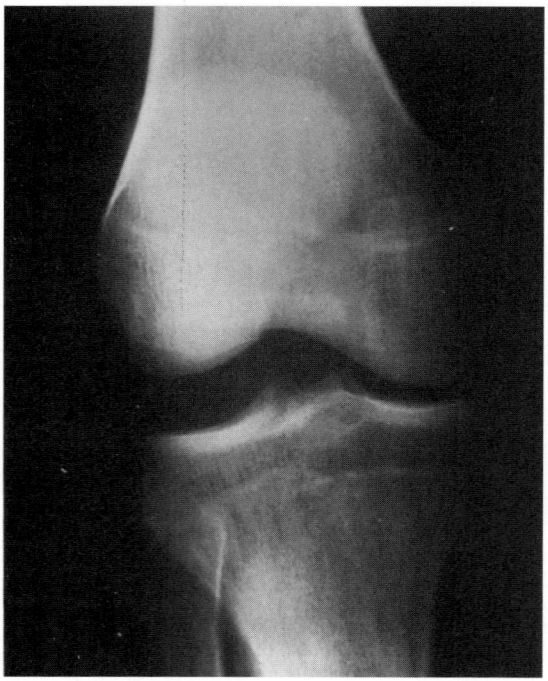

Figure 28B–44. Acute lateral ligamentous disruption. Plain radiograph with varus stress applied to the knee demonstrates lateral joint "gaping" indicating lateral supporting ligament disruption.

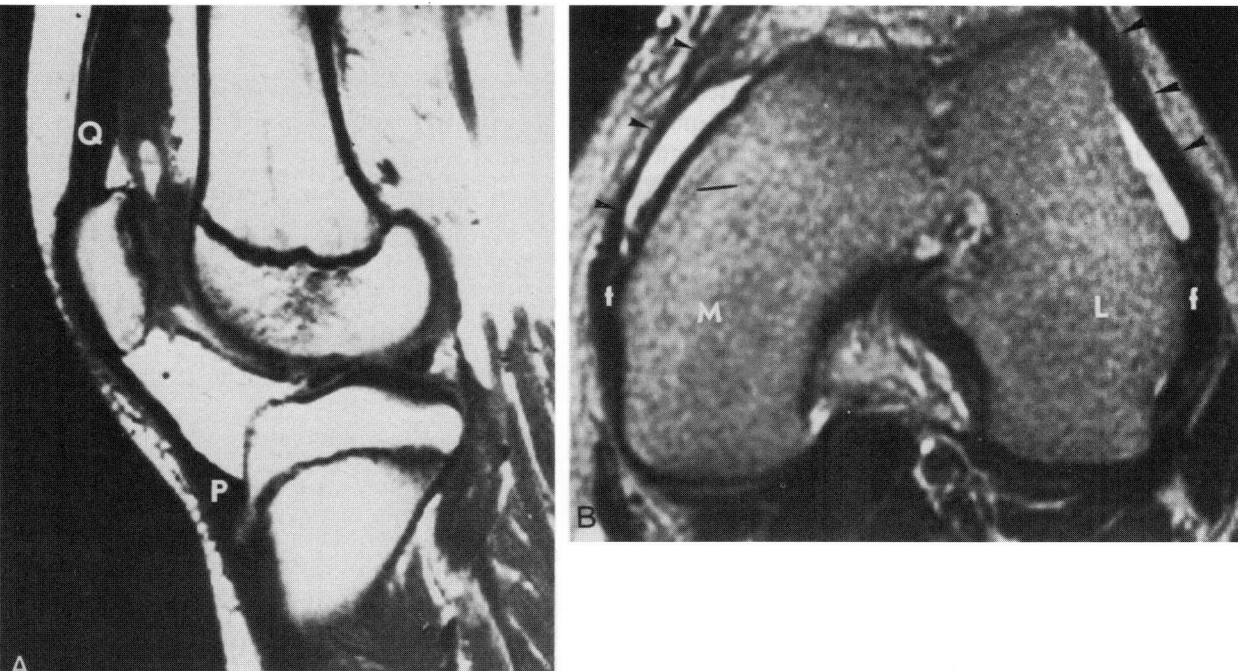

Figure 28B–46. Normal extensor tendons. Sagittal intensity windowing (1300/17) MRI section *(A)* through the midpatellar level demonstrates the normal appearance of the quadriceps (Q) and patellar (P) tendons. Axial T_2 (2000/80) MRI section *(B)* through the femoral epicondylar level demonstrates the medial and lateral patellar retinaculae *(arrowheads)* blending with the origins of the tibial collateral ligament (t) and fibular collateral ligament (f), respectively. The lateral retinaculum (L) is thicker than its medial counterpart (M) and is blended with the fibers of the iliotibial band.

have provided considerable confusion, having been used by different authors to refer to the same constellation of histopathologic and clinical findings.[101] The MRI findings of jumper's knee (Fig. 28B–48)[51, 101, 117] are first seen in the proximal tendon adjacent to its origin from the lower pole of the patella and are limited to the posterior half of the tendon. The proximal tendon is thickened in anteroposterior diameter to 7 mm or greater.[51] Increased T_1 and T_2 signal is present within the tendon as well a loss of definition of the posterior margin of the proximal tendon. Peritendinitis changes may also be present with increased T_2 signal in the adjacent infrapatellar fat pad. With chronicity, changes

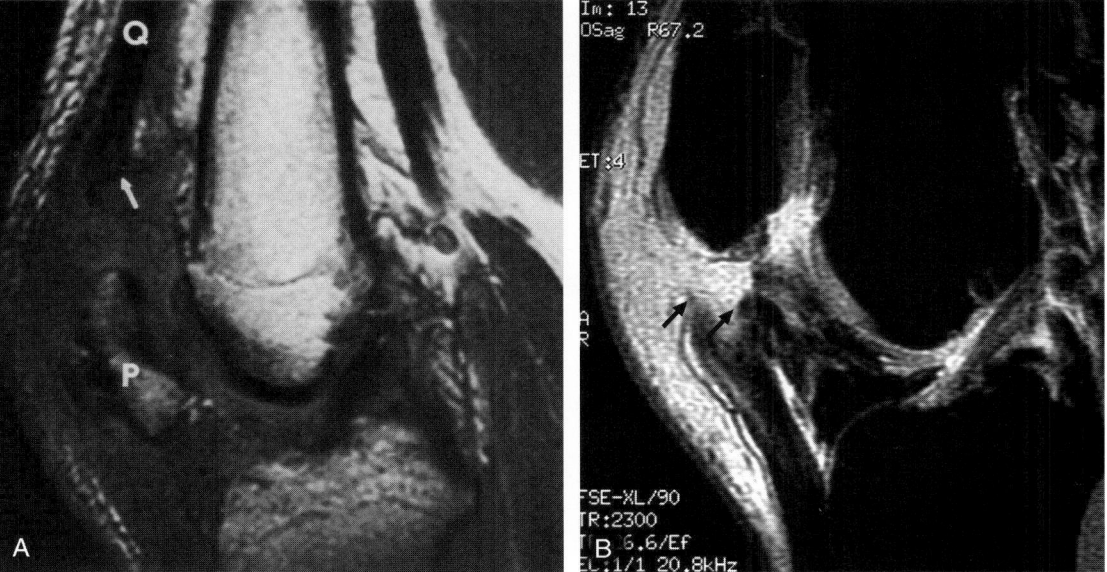

Figure 28B–47. Extensor tendon injuries. Sagittal intensity windowing *(A)* and IW fast spin *(B)* demonstrate complete ruptures of the quadriceps tendon *(A)* adjacent to its patellar insertion *(arrow)* and patellar tendon *(B)* adjacent to its patellar origin *(arrows)*. In both instances, complete disruption of the tendon is demonstrated. P, patella; Q, quadriceps tendon.

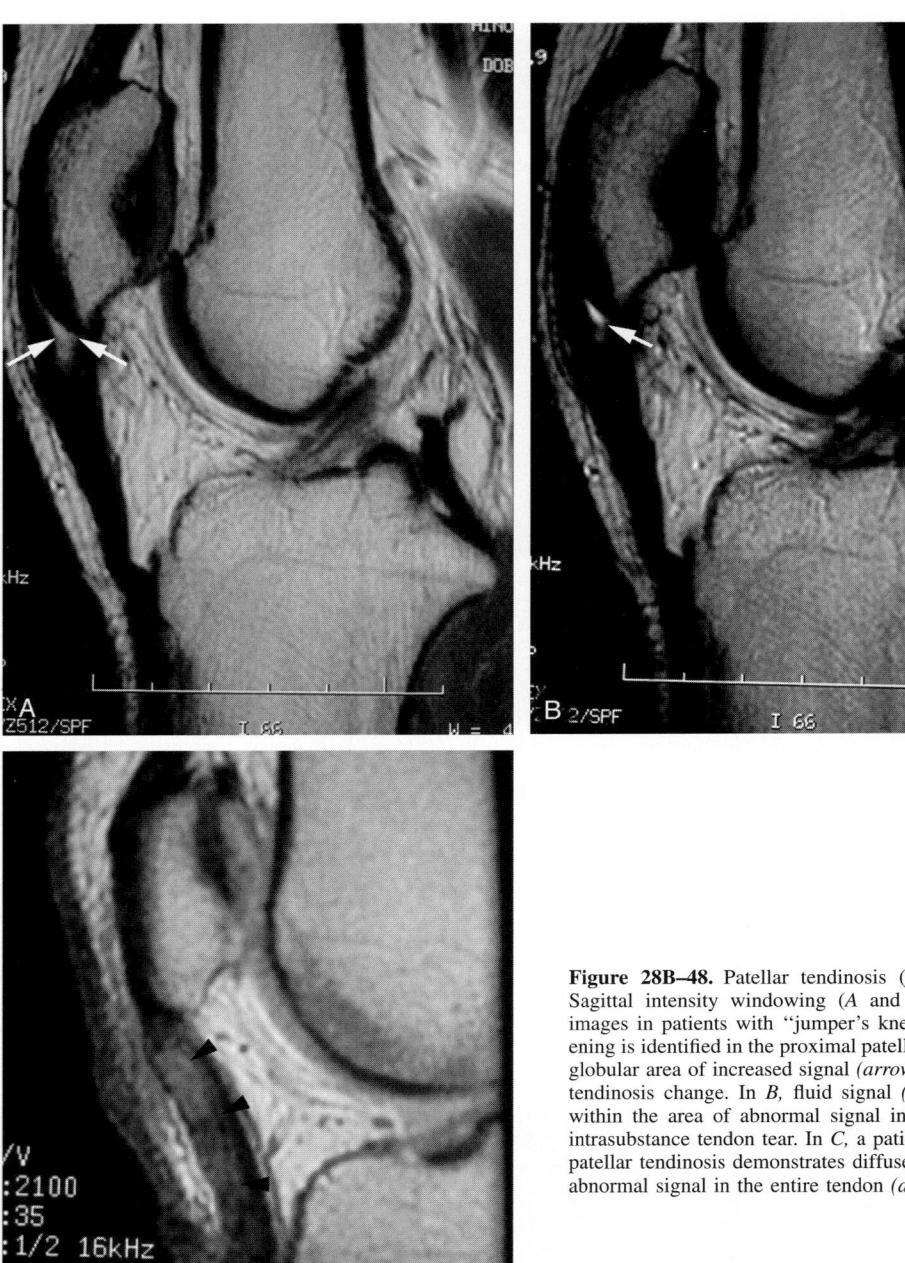

Figure 28B–48. Patellar tendinosis (jumper's knee). Sagittal intensity windowing (*A* and *C*) and T$_2$ *(B)* images in patients with "jumper's knee." In *A*, thickening is identified in the proximal patellar tendon with a globular area of increased signal *(arrows)*, representing tendinosis change. In *B*, fluid signal *(arrow)* is noted within the area of abnormal signal indicating a focal intrasubstance tendon tear. In *C*, a patient with chronic patellar tendinosis demonstrates diffuse thickening and abnormal signal in the entire tendon *(arrowheads)*.

may involve the full thickness of the tendon and may progress distally. Intrasubstance tears and even complete tendon rupture are the end stage of jumper's knee.

Other imaging modalities may provide information in jumper's knee, though none are as sensitive as MRI. Ultrasonography of jumper's knee may demonstrate thickening of the proximal tendon, hypoechoic areas within the tendon, and hyperechogenicity of the peritenon and adjacent fat planes owing to peritendinitis.[43, 101, 128] CT has been reported to demonstrate thickening of the tendon and di-minished attenuation in areas involved in tendinitis or tendinosis.[43] Radionuclide bone scintigraphy may show increased flow as well as increased accumulation of radionuclide at the level of the lower pole of the patella in jumper's knee.[95]

Patellofemoral Dislocation

Acute traumatic dislocation of the patellofemoral joint is a common injury in young athletes. Typically, the dislocation is transient; spontaneous reduction occurs, and the patient is unaware of the nature of the injury.

Likewise, if a swollen and acutely injured knee makes physical examination difficult, the patient may be referred for imaging studies for the evaluation of a possible meniscal tear or a cruciate or collateral ligament injury. The mechanism of injury is a twisting motion of the flexed knee, which is internally rotated on a fixed foot. As a result, the patella is pulled laterally out of the trochlear groove, causing a forceful impact of its medial pole against the anterolateral cortex of the lateral femoral condyle. In virtually all cases, the patella then spontaneously reduces.

The patella is a sesamoid, which increases the efficiency of the extensor mechanism by means of the fulcrum effect. The quadriceps tendon inserts on the proximal pole, with fibers from the rectus femoris continuing distally to form the patellar tendon, which inserts on the anterior cortex of the proximal tibia. The undersurface of the patella forms two facets, which are covered in hyaline articular cartilage and articulate with the medial and lateral facets of the trochlear groove of the distal femur. Though markedly variable, the patellar facets are typically asymmetrical in size, with the lateral facet being larger and flatter and the medial facet being shorter and more vertically oriented. The medial and lateral trochlear facets correspond to the patellar facets. Occasionally, a shallow trochlear groove may be seen, representing a congenital predisposition to patellofemoral instability.

With flexion and extension of the knee, the patella "tracks" along the femoral trochlea, with stability provided by a combination of vertical and horizontal tensile stresses applied to the patella by the quadriceps mechanism (vertical) and the medial and lateral retinacula (horizontal).[18] The lateral retinaculum[64, 174] consists of superficial and deep layers. The superficial retinaculum consists of fibers arising from the iliotibial band and the vastus lateralis fascia. The deep layer consists of three discrete fibrous bands: the transverse ligament, the patellotibial band, and the epicondylopatellar band. The transverse ligament passes transversely from the inner border of the iliotibial band to the lateral pole of the patella. The patellotibial band arises from the patella at the inferolateral margin and inserts on the proximal tibia and the anterior horn of the lateral meniscus. The epicondylopatellar band arises from the superolateral margin of the patella and inserts on the lateral epicondyle of the femur. The medial retinaculum also has superficial and deep layers.[33, 174, 185] The superficial layer arises from the fibers of the sartorius and the vastus medialis muscles, the vastus medialis oblique (VMO) tendon, and the superficial fibers of the MCL.

The deep layer consists of three distinct fascicles: the medial patellofemoral ligament (MPFL), the patellomeniscal ligament, and the patellotibial ligament. The MPFL is the largest and most important medial stabilizer. The MPFL arises from the adductor tubercle of the femur and inserts on the deep surface of the vastus medialis and the vastus intermedius as well as the medial margin of the patella. The patellomeniscal ligament extends from the medial margin of the patella obliquely to insert on the posterior horn of the medial meniscus and the coronary ligament. The patellotibial ligament passes from the medial pole of the patella to the anteromedial aspect of the tibia. Recently,

the importance of the MPFL as the most important static stabilizer of the patella has become evident.[33, 86, 159, 172, 174] By means of its insertion on the undersurface of the VMO, the MPFL serves as a checkrein on the VMO to hold its fibers in an oblique orientation, which allows it to serve as a dynamic stabilizer of the patella.[11, 22, 33] With rupture of the MPFL, the VMO subluxes laterally over the medial femoral condyle, which orients its fibers in a more longitudinal direction and results in a significant loss of its function as a dynamic stabilizer of the patella. For this reason, identification of tears of the MPFL adjacent to its origin at the adductor tubercle (Fig. 28B–49) is the single most important prognosticator of chronic patellofemoral instability after acute dislocation.

MRI is virtually diagnostic in identifying the sequelae of recent transient traumatic patellofemoral dislocation (PFD) as well as in delineating the associated injuries, which may have important prognostic implications. The most useful imaging plane in evaluating this injury is the axial plane. We routinely perform multiplanar gradient-recalled (MPGR) sequences through the patellofemoral joint, but if PFD is suspected, we add a proton-density fat saturation axial sequence. This sequence is more sensitive to fluid and edema and also gives a good look at cartilage. This plane provides information about osteochondral fractures, retinacular disruption, MPFL rupture, and impaction injuries of the lateral femoral condyle and the medial pole of the patella. Coronal T_1 and T_2 fat saturation sequences are useful in demonstrating the characteristic subcortical trabecular fractures (bone bruises) associated with PFD. Sagittal T_2 and proton-density images are useful in identifying elevation of the VMO and provide an additional look at the patellar articular cartilage. Any image may be useful in identifying displaced osteochondral fracture fragments, though there is no sequence, imaging plane, or combination of the two that does not miss a large number of osteochondral fragments.

The possible MRI findings of PFD[35, 102, 104, 172, 182] in the setting of acute trauma are the following:

1. Characteristic subcortical trabecular fracture (bone bruise) on the anterolateral margin of the lateral femoral condyle
2. Irregularity, disruption, inhomogeneity, and increased T_2 signal in the medial patellar retinaculum
3. Impaction injury, which may involve a fracture or a bone bruise at the medial pole of the patella
4. Chondral or osteochondral fracture, usually involving the medial patellar articular facet or the lateral trochlear facet, or both
5. Effusion, hemarthrosis, or lipohemarthrosis
6. Rupture at the origin of the MPFL from the adductor tubercle
7. Elevation of the VMO from the anteromedial femoral cortex, which may be associated with a partial tear of the VMO
8. Displaced osteochondral fracture fragment
9. Lateral subluxation of the patella.

Any or all of these findings may be present.

The femoral bone bruise of PFD is virtually diagnostic (Fig. 28B–50). An area of marrow edema in the anterolateral aspect of the distal femur abutting the inner border of fluid level may be identified, representing a lipohem-arthrosis. These latter findings are strongly suggestive of an associated fracture, and careful evaluation of the patella is recommended.

The significance of rupture of the femoral origin of the MPFL cannot be overemphasized. In anatomic studies, the MPFL has been described as ranging from "wispy" to "thick." In our experience, the MPFL is rarely identifiable on MRI as a distinct structure but rather as an area of soft tissue confluence at the level of the adductor tubercle.

It is the sequelae of MPFL rupture to which we must be sensitive (see Figs. 28B–49 to 28B–51). These include (1) increased T_2 signal overlying the adductor tubercle and (2) elevation or separation of the VMO from the anteromedial femoral cortex. The increased T_2 signal over the adductor tubercle is secondary to hemorrhage and edema associated with the trauma. Certainly, other processes may be associated with edema in this area, but in association with other findings of PFD, the finding is usually quite specific. Loss of the checkrein function of the intact MPFL allows the VMO to separate from its normal position in direct apposition to the anteromedial femoral cortex, usually with increased T_2 signal in this widened space. Occasionally, there may be bright T_2 signal within the VMO muscle belly, indicating a partial muscular tear.

Displaced chondral or osteochondral fragments are common and frequently a frustrating finding on MRI. Owing to their small size and shallow thickness, they frequently blend with other normal tissues in the knee and become virtually invisible even on a good-quality MRI scan. It is extremely frustrating to be presented with a plain radiograph demonstrating a displaced osteochondral fragment that cannot be found on the MRI. Nevertheless, a careful search should be performed in cases in which a donor site is found, and frequently, with careful scrutiny, the fragment may be located. In other instances, the fragment may be discovered on a plain radiograph or CT, and in still others, it is discovered only at arthroscopy. The donor site is typically a localized defect in the patellar or femoral articular cartilage, with marrow edema deep to the donor site.[153] Lateral subluxation of the patella is common after PFD (Fig. 28B–52) and was seen by Lance and associates in 50% of their series. In these cases, the patella will be centered lateral to the midline of the trochlear groove.

Imaging Fractures and Articular Abnormalities

Chondral, Osteochondral, and Subcortical Trabecular Abnormalities

Chondral and osteochondral fractures of the tibial and femoral condyles are not uncommonly associated with acute trauma. Classically, these lesions have been divided into exogenous and endogenous lesions on a mechanistic basis[99, 106]; that is, lesions associated with a direct impact are exogenous, whereas those secondary to rotational, compression, or shearing forces from an adjacent articular surface or avulsion of a tendon or ligament represent endogenous lesions. The lateral notch sign on plain radiographs[9, 112] refers to an endogenous impaction fracture

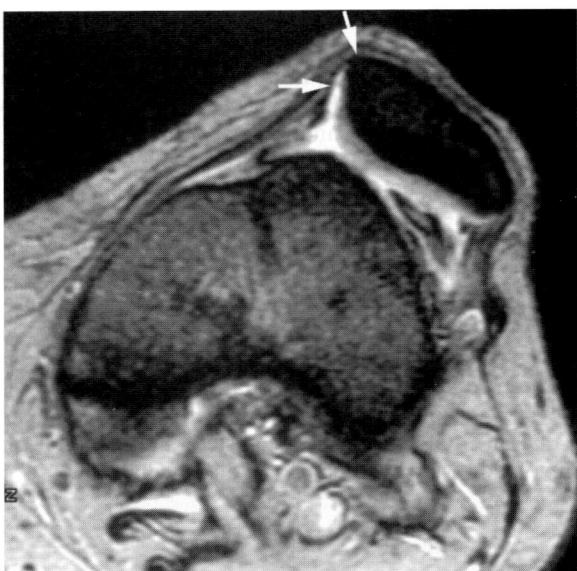

Figure 28B–52. Unstable patellofemoral joint in chronic patellofemoral dislocation. Axial multiplanar gradient-recalled image of the knee in this patient with recurrent patellofemoral dislocation demonstrates spontaneous dislocation of the patella *(arrows)* indicating complete loss of integrity of the normal medial soft tissue supports.

at the normal notch in the lateral femoral condyle associated with an acute or a chronic ACL tear. Endogenous lesions may also be seen on the anterolateral aspect of the lateral femoral condyle or on the inferomedial patellar border in association with patellar dislocations.[123, 152] In children and adolescents, osteochondral fractures are the rule, and pure chondral injuries are quite uncommon, whereas in adults, either type may be encountered.[105, 106] Ipsilateral meniscal tears are commonly associated with

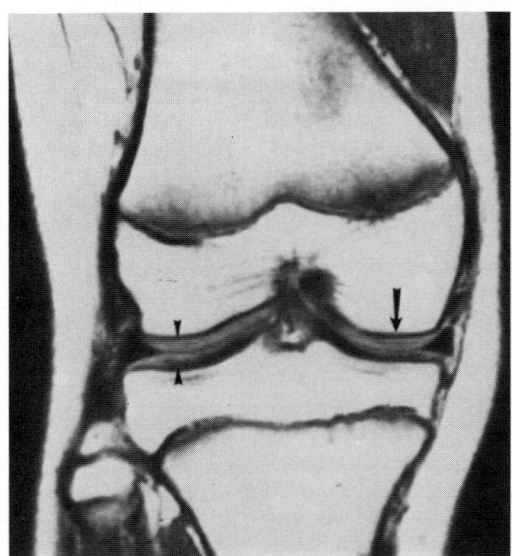

Figure 28B–53. Normal articular anatomy. In this coronal T_1-weighted (600/20) image the midplane of the knee hyaline cartilage (between *arrowheads*) is seen to have intermediate intensity in contrast to the low intensity of fibrocartilage (menisci), the subchondral bone plate *(large arrow)*, and the growth plates.

small chondral and osteochondral fractures of the femoral condyles.[67] With the development of MRI, a new class of lesion, the subcortical trabecular fracture[113, 195] (bone bruise), may be seen in the subchondral trabecular bone in isolation or in association with chondral or osteochondral fractures.

Hyaline cartilage (Fig. 28B–53) is characterized by intermediate signal intensity on T_1- or intermediate-weighted MRI images and by low intensity on T_2-weighted images.[36, 145] The subchondral bone plate (see Fig. 28B–45) is uniformly dark on T_1-, intermediate-, and T_2-weighted images, whereas medullary bone is very bright on T_1- and intermediate-weighted images and moderately bright on T_2

images. Joint fluid, acute hemorrhage, and edema are of intermediate intensity on T_1- and intermediate-weighted images and are very bright on T_2-weighted images. The subcortical trabecular fracture or bone bruise (Fig. 28B–54) has been recognized only with the advent of MRI and is a very common lesion.[67, 113] Presumably, it represents a localized area of acute hemorrhage and edema associated with fracture of the adjacent medullary trabeculae. This lesion is characterized by an area of intermediate or low signal intensity on T_1- or intermediate-weighted images that brightens, often with a speckled pattern, on T_2-weighted images and is typically located adjacent to the subchondral bone plate. Over a period of time, the amount of T_2 bright-

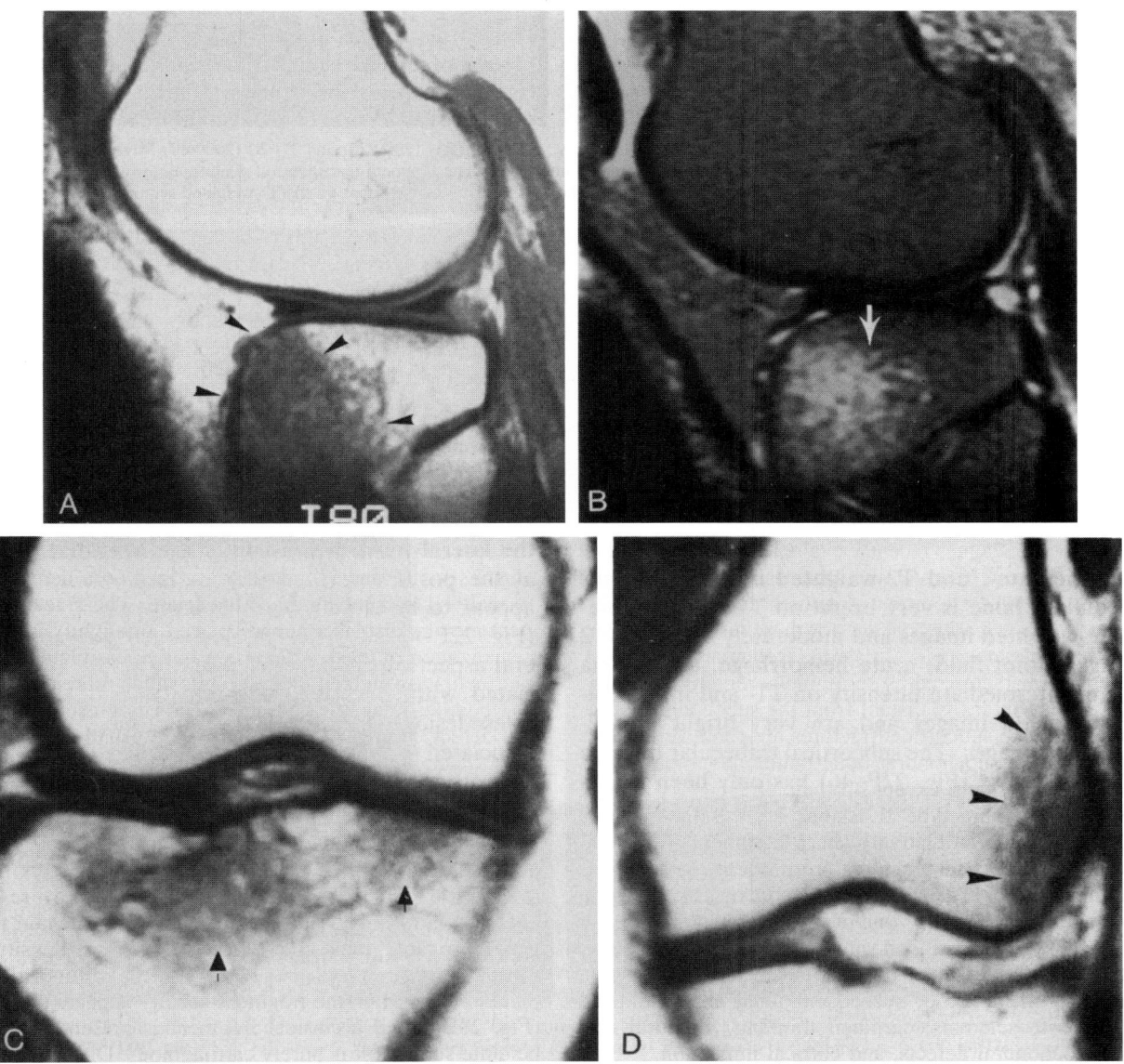

Figure 28B–54. Subcortical trabecular fracture (bone bruise). Sagittal T_1 *(A)* (600/20) and T_2 *(B)* (2500/90) MRI sections through the lateral condylar level demonstrate an area of diminished signal intensity in the anterolateral tibial epiphysis *(arrowheads)*, which brightens on the T_2-weighted sequence *(arrow)* in this 15-year-old girl who received a direct blow to the anterolateral aspect of the knee while playing softball. In *C*, a coronal T_1-weighted (600/20) anterior condylar section demonstrates defects in the medial and lateral tibial epiphysis in this 23-year-old female, who experienced severe pain when landing on her hyperextended knee while playing basketball. In *D*, a coronal T_1-weighted (600/20) section through the anterior condylar level demonstrates a bone bruise on the anterolateral margin of the lateral femoral condyle in this 19-year-old female who suffered a traumatic patellar dislocation. In all of these patients, plain radiographs of good quality were normal.

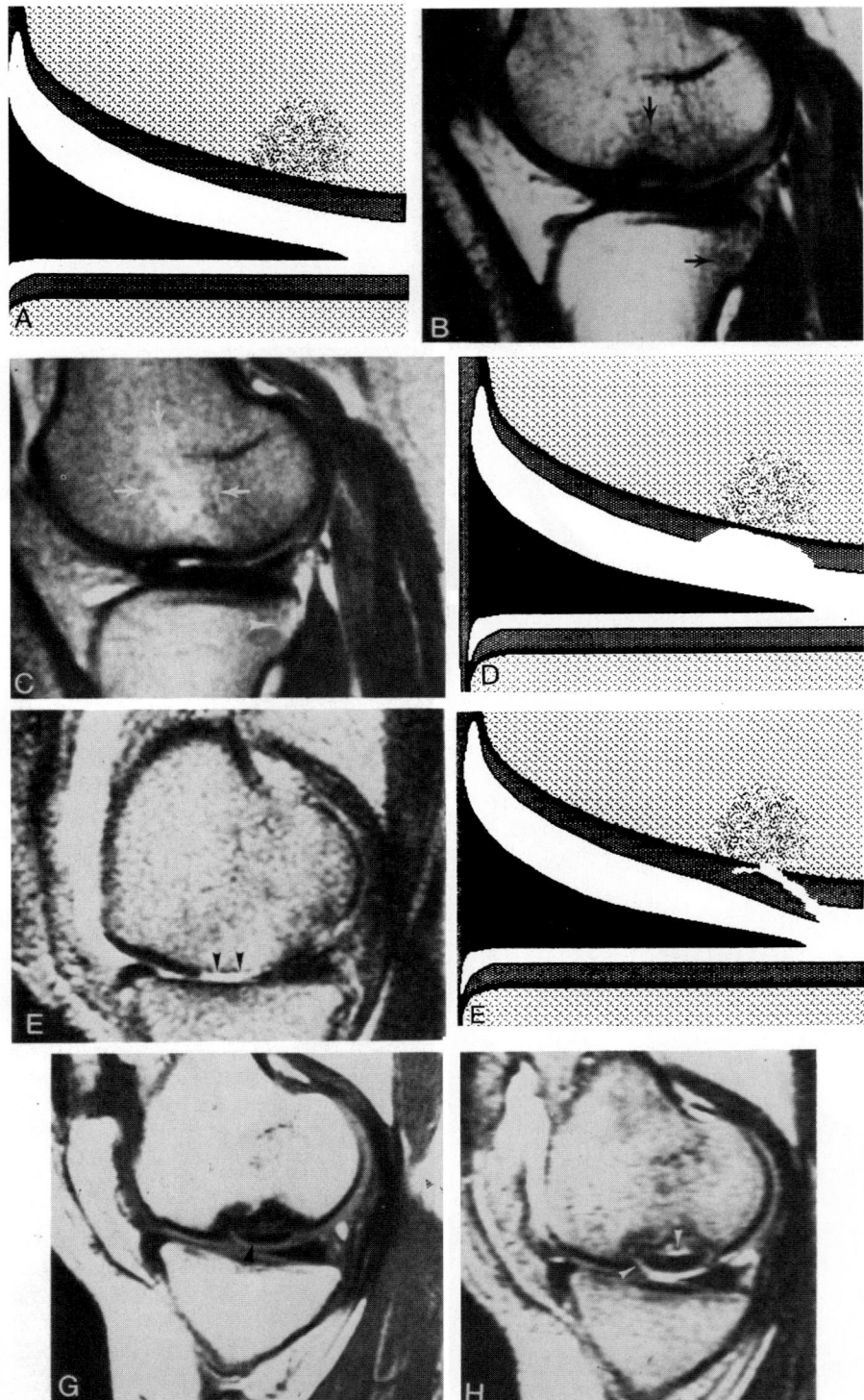

Figure 28B–57. Chondral and osteochondral fractures. Diagram *(A)*, sagittal intensity windowing (IW) (1500/28) *(B)*, and sagittal T$_2$ (1500/80) *(C)* MRI sections demonstrate typical subcortical trabecular fractures (bone bruise) centered on the lateral condylar notch and posterolateral corner of the proximal tibia in this 19-year-old female with an acute anterior cruciate ligament tear. At arthroscopy, the lateral condyle was reported to be normal in appearance without cartilaginous defect. A chondral fracture is shown in *D* and T$_2$-weighted (2000/80) *(E)* sagittal section through the medial femoral condyle. The articular cartilage (dark in this T$_2$ sequence) is stripped from a segment of the intact subchondral bone plate *(arrowheads)*. An osteochondral fracture is demonstrated in the diagram *(F)*, IW (2000/20) *(G)*, and T$_2$-weighted (2000/80) *(H)* sagittal MRI sections through the medial femoral condyle. In *G*, the osteochondral fragment *(arrowhead)* is visualized in the condylar defect, whereas in *H*, joint fluid *(arrowheads)* can be seen between the condyle and the osteocartilaginous fragment.

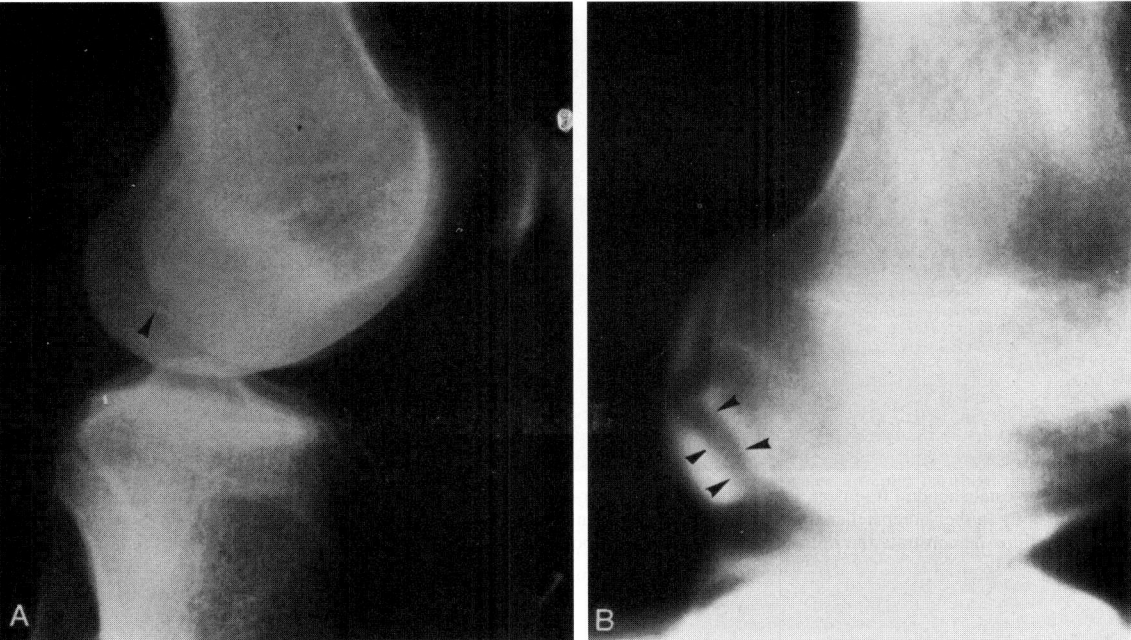

Figure 28B–58. "Tethered" osteochondral fracture. A lateral radiograph of the knee *(A)* in a 27-year-old male who experienced a painful "click" in his knee with extreme flexion demonstrates a thin sliver of bone adjacent to the posterior aspect of the lateral femoral condyle *(arrowhead)*. An arthrotomographic section *(B)* through this area demonstrates an osteochondral fragment *(arrowheads)*, which is "tethered" anteriorly by an intact band of cartilage.

by air; however, it may be invisible if it is lying in a pooled collection of contrast material unless it is associated with a large radiolucent cartilage fragment.[8, 151]

Fluoroscopy (Fig. 28B–60) is often a useful adjunct in

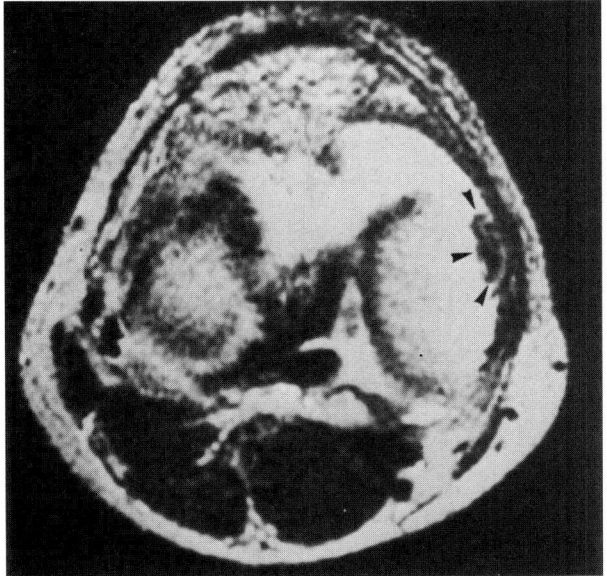

Figure 28B–59. Osteochondral fracture. A T_2-weighted (2000/80) axial section through the inferior condylar level in this 16-year-old male with an acute patellar dislocation demonstrates an osteochondral loose body *(arrowheads)* that has migrated to a position adjacent to the medial femoral condyle. A donor site from the inferomedial aspect of the patella was identified in other sections.

determining whether radiographically visible loose bodies are mobile within the joint or fibrosed in place. CT provides the most sensitive means of all for detecting displaced osteocartilaginous fragments or loose bodies. Pure chondral injuries may be occasionally identified at arthrography but are frequently overlooked or not demonstrated on conventional studies. Chondral defects can be elegantly demonstrated by arthrotomography (see Fig. 28B–58*B*) or computed arthrotomography if they are suspected and appropriately sliced.[161] The inability to scan directly in the coronal or sagittal plane as well as the invasive nature of computed arthrotomography limits its value, especially with the availability of MRI. MR arthrography is quite useful in identifying subtle cartilaginous clefts and in the follow-up of osteochondral fracture repairs (Fig. 28B–61). Bone bruises are, of course, invisible by conventional radiographic means, including CT, but are detectable on high-quality radionuclide scintigrams.[195]

Chondromalacia Patellae

Chondromalacia patellae, characterized by degeneration of the patellar articular cartilage, is a frequent cause of pain and disability in young adults. The etiology of chondromalacia patellae has long been debated, and there are probably several causes, including trauma, anatomic predisposition (excessive lateral pressure syndrome, reflex sympathetic dystrophy syndrome), and primary cartilaginous degeneration.[16, 56, 69, 87, 166] MRI is quite useful in identifying and characterizing the disorder, with axial and sagittal imaging planes providing the most useful information.[146, 198]

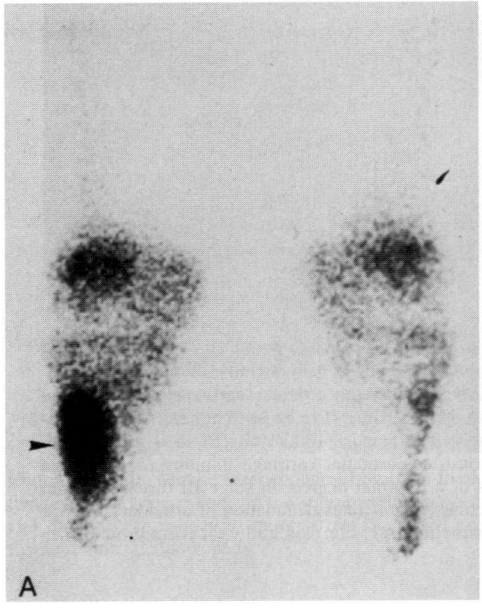
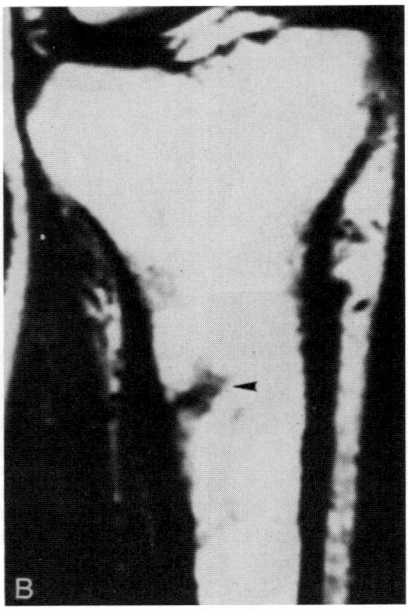

Figure 28B–64. Stress fracture. Radionuclide bone scan *(A)* in this jogger with pain over the proximal tibia demonstrates a focus of markedly increased activity *(arrowhead)* in the proximal right tibial diaphyseal region. After a period of conservative therapy, in which plain radiographs remained normal and the patient's symptoms were not felt to be resolving normally, an MRI study was obtained to exclude the possibility of a subtle neoplasm. A T_1-weighted (600/20) coronal section *(B)* demonstrates the typical appearance of a stress fracture with a horizontally oriented band of diminished intensity *(arrowhead)* within the medullary cavity associated with adjacent cortical thickening.

ening on T_1- and intermediate-weighted images that is associated with inhomogeneous T_2 brightening owing to periosteal and endosteal new bone formation. Avulsion fractures are usually incidental findings on MRI in patients whose symptoms are related to an associated ligament or tendon injury. Typical, uncomplicated stress fractures do not require MRI evaluation, but when the nature of the lesion is equivocal on plain radiographs or when the clinical course is not typical of a stress fracture, MRI is probably the imaging modality of choice to exclude the presence of a neoplasm.

Avulsion fractures are usually readily demonstrated on good-quality plain radiographs and typically are incidental findings with other modalities. With an equivocal lesion, radionuclide scintigraphy[79] is a simple means of verifying the lesion as well as identifying stress fractures that are not visible on plain radiographs.

Osteochondritis Dissecans and the Osteochondroses

Several other lesions, although not sports related, occur in the age groups in which athletic injuries are frequent and may be aggravated by sporting activities. Osteochondritis dissecans[75, 119] (see Fig. 28B–57*F* and *H*) is characterized on T_1- and intermediate-weighted images by an arcuate, frequently serrated zone of low signal intensity enveloping a segment of the subchondral bone plate, often with a subjacent zone of higher signal intensity. The key observation concerns the integrity of the overlying articular cartilage, which may be evaluated on T_2-weighted, MPGR, or MR arthrography images by the presence or absence of joint fluid within the substance of the lesion, as previously described for traumatic osteochondral fractures (see Fig. 28B–61). The value of this observation cannot be overem-

phasized, because fluid within the defect must be associated with cartilage disruption and thus may represent a key surgical indication. This finding can also be identified on contrast arthrography, arthrotomography, and CT arthrography but apparently with less accuracy than in MRI. MR

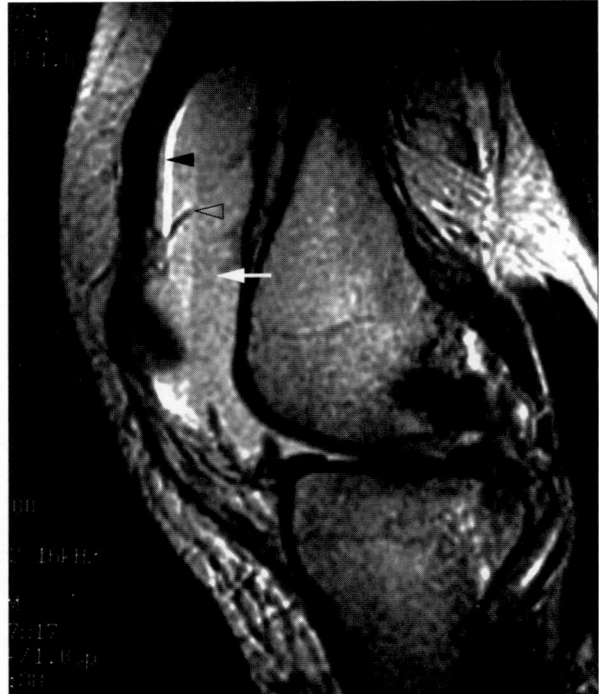

Figure 28B–65. Lipohemarthrosis. Sagittal intensity windowing image demonstrates a large effusion in the suprapatellar pouch with three layers clearly visualized indicating the presence of blood *(arrow),* synovial fluid *(closed arrowhead),* and fat *(open arrowhead)* within the effusion. The presence of fat within the effusion is strongly suggestive of an associated fracture, with release of marrow fat into the joint.

arthrography is relatively new but is probably the most sensitive of all in the identification and the delineation of chondral defects and disruption (see Fig. 28B–61).

Osgood-Schlatter disease[75] is characterized by diminished signal intensity from the marrow of the anterior tibial apophysis adjacent to the insertion of the patellar tendon. Thickening and slight brightening of the signal from the insertion of the patellar tendon may also be seen as well as slight blunting of the inferior margin of the infrapatellar fat pad. Though not yet reported, it is anticipated that Sinding-Larsen-Johansson disease involving the inferior patellar pole at the origin of the patellar tendon would exhibit similar findings. Early in the course of these disorders, conventional radiographic findings are nonspecific; an abnormal bone scan and localized soft tissue swelling on plain radiographs are the only findings. In such a case, if the clinical picture and the physical examination findings leave doubt about the diagnosis, MRI is probably the imaging procedure of choice. Later in the course of these disorders, the plain radiographic findings are usually quite characteristic.

Imaging Effusions, Cysts, and Ganglia

Certainly, a joint effusion is one of the more obvious findings in MRI examinations of the knee.[14] Joint fluid is

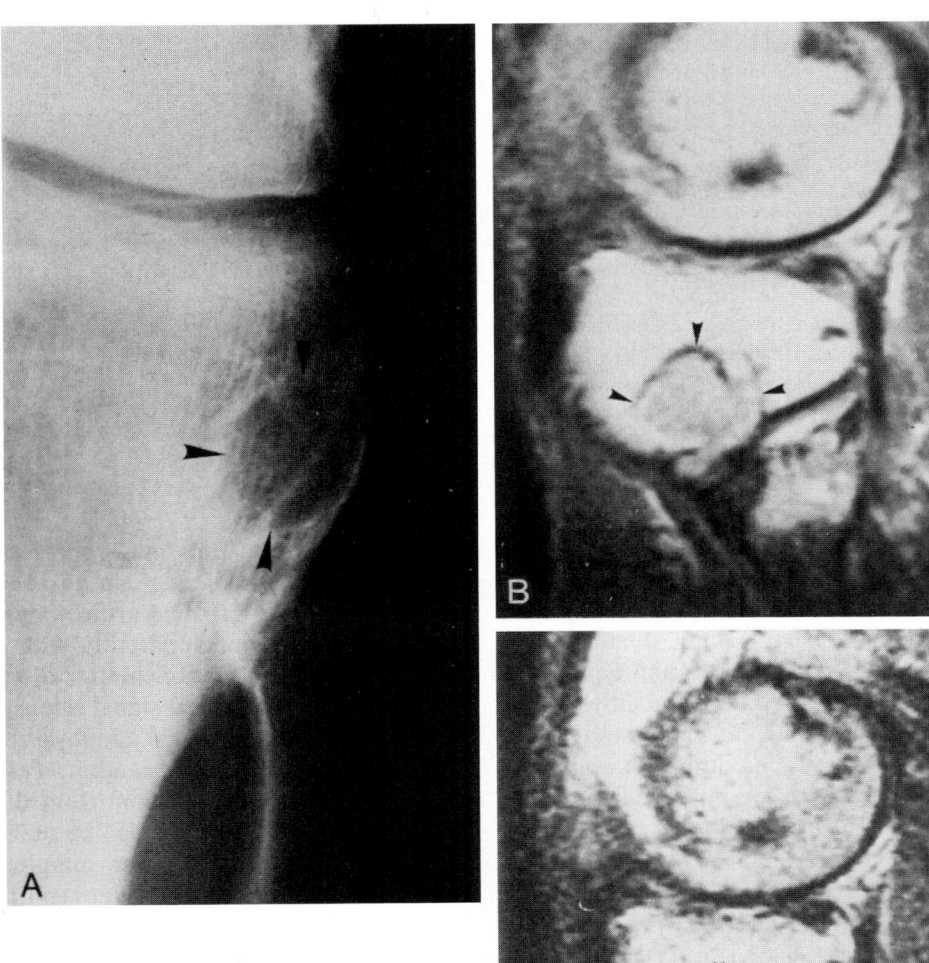

Figure 28B–66. Synovial cyst ("ganglion"). A plain radiograph *(A)* in this patient demonstrates a cystic lesion *(arrowheads)* in the proximal lateral tibia adjacent to the proximal tibiofibular joint. A sagittal intensity windowing (2000/20) *(B)* MRI section through this area demonstrates an intramedullary "mass" of intermediate intensity *(arrowheads).* A sagittal T₂-weighted (2000/80) *(C)* MRI section demonstrates the mass to be of fluid density *(arrowheads)* consistent with an intraosseous ganglion and also highlights another small soft tissue ganglion *(white arrow)* arising from the joint capsule.

characterized by intermediate signal intensity on T_1- and intermediate-weighted images with marked brightening on T_2-weighted images. In addition to indicating the presence of knee joint disease,[29] the presence of an effusion is very often useful in identifying subtle abnormalities such as chondral or osteochondral defects, loose bodies, the contour of the anterior surface of the ACL, and meniscal defects and detachments. In cases of fracture into marrow-containing bone, fat-fluid levels (lipohemarthrosis) may be readily identified (Fig. 28B–65).

Cystic lesions about the knee[92] are common findings that may be related to symptoms owing to their size or location, or they may be incidental findings discovered during evaluation of other abnormalities of the knee. Meniscal cysts (see Figs. 28B–20 to 28B–22), which have already been discussed,[10, 36, 130, 164] consist of various-sized cystic masses originating from the substance of one of the menisci, frequently in association with a tear. Synovial cysts[40, 110, 165] or ganglia (Fig. 28B–66) are fluid-filled masses arising from the joint capsule, a bursa, or a tendon sheath. These lesions are usually associated with disease in the joint or at their point of origin and may dissect along tissue planes or even within the substance of a muscle or adjacent bone. The popliteal cyst[189, 191] (Baker's cyst; Fig. 28B–67) is the most common synovial cyst, usually originating from the posteromedial aspect of the knee at the level of the gastrocnemius-semimembranosus bursa. Direct communication with the posterior capsule of the knee joint is frequently demonstrable, and knee disease, especially tears of the posterior horn of the medial meniscus, is common.[191] These and other synovial cysts become clinically important when they present as palpable masses, are associated with neural or vascular compression, rupture with an associated pseudothrombophlebitis syndrome, or

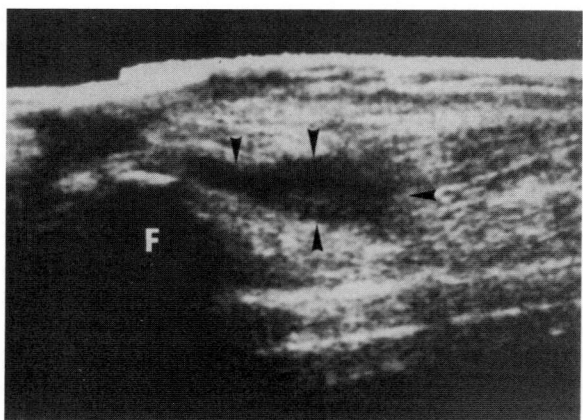

Figure 28B–68. Sonography of a popliteal cyst. Sagittal sonographic section through the popliteal space in this patient demonstrates a sonolucent fluid collection *(arrowheads)* posterior and inferior to the medial femoral condyle (F).

fistulize through the skin. A variety of imaging modalities[14, 77, 164, 165] have been used to evaluate these lesions, including arthrography, CT, sonography, and, recently, MRI. Arthrography (Fig. 28B–67) is certainly the most specific examination when positive, showing filling of a synovial cyst from the joint cavity or extravasation of contrast agent from the cyst in pseudothrombophlebitis syndromes. Arthrography, however, is invasive, frequently requires a great deal of patience to demonstrate cyst communication, and may not show communication in a significant number of synovial cysts. CT is very sensitive in identifying cysts, although some small cysts and intramuscular lesions may be quite difficult to differentiate from soft tissue neoplasms. Sonog-

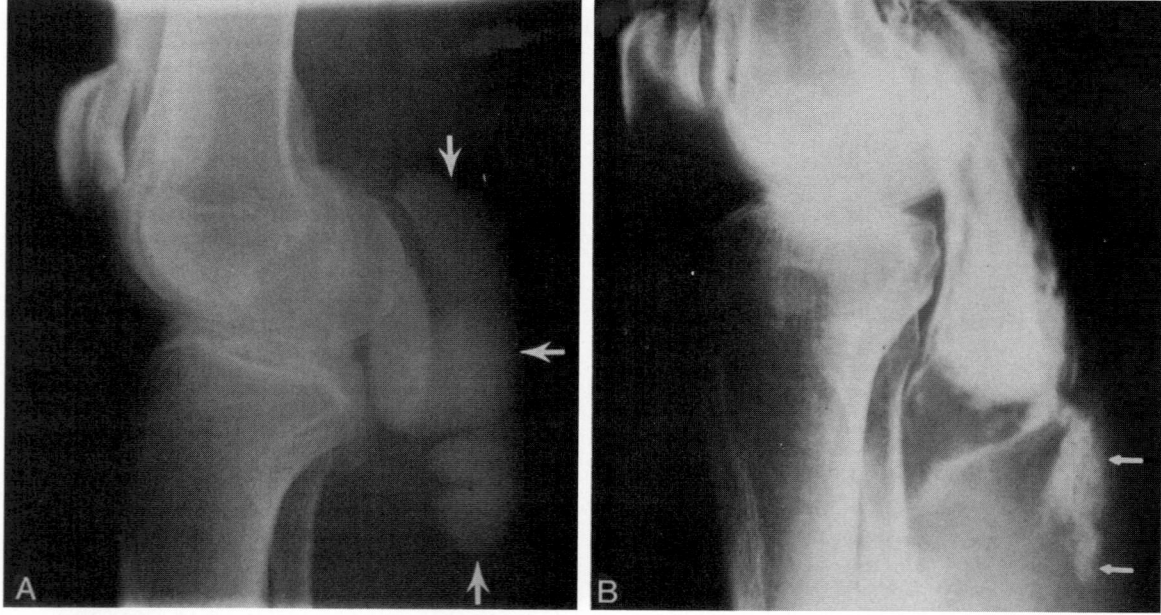

Figure 28B–67. Arthrography of "Baker's cyst." A lateral radiograph of the extended knee *(A)* from a knee arthrogram demonstrates a large popliteal cyst *(arrows)* dissecting inferiorly in the popliteal space. In another patient *(B)* with clinical findings suggestive of thrombophlebitis and a normal venogram of the extremity, arthrography demonstrates extravasation of radiographic contrast *(arrows)* from a large popliteal cyst.

raphy (Fig. 28B–68) is a sensitive, noninvasive, and relatively inexpensive modality that provides a reliable diagnosis in the majority of cases. Occasionally, small or ruptured cysts may be difficult to identify, and cysts with inspissation of their contents may resemble a complex mass. MRI (Fig. 28B–69) can demonstrate synovial cysts of all sizes, usually showing their point of origin, their relationship to adjacent neurovascular structures, intraluminal loose bodies or hemorrhage, and evidence of recent extravasation. These lesions, as with all fluid density lesions about the knee, demonstrate an intermediate density on T_1- and intermediate-weighted images and hyperintensity on T_2-weighted images. Unfortunately, MRI is a very expensive way to demonstrate a synovial cyst, although an abbreviated examination may be tailored to verify these lesions, with a corresponding price reduction.

A final group of liquid density lesions comprises fluid collections within normally located but inflamed or traumatized bursae about the knee (Fig. 28B–70).[73, 110] Bursae lie anterior to the patella (prepatellar bursa) and superficial and deep to the patellar tendon (i.e., superficial and deep infrapatellar bursae), and prepatellar bursitis is a relatively common incidental finding on MRI. Fluid within the bursa between the superficial and deep layers of the MCL secondary to a tear of the deep fibers has already been described (see Fig. 28B–41). Fluid may be seen within the anserine bursa (see Fig. 28B–70C and D), which lies between the pes anserinus (conjoined tendons of semitendinosus, sartorius, and gracilis) and the distal insertion of the TCL and the adjacent medial border of the tibia.[73] Pes bursitis is a common clinical problem that is frequently identified incidentally on MRI or CT. In addition, numerous bursae located about the knee near tendon insertions and ligaments may occasionally be identified.

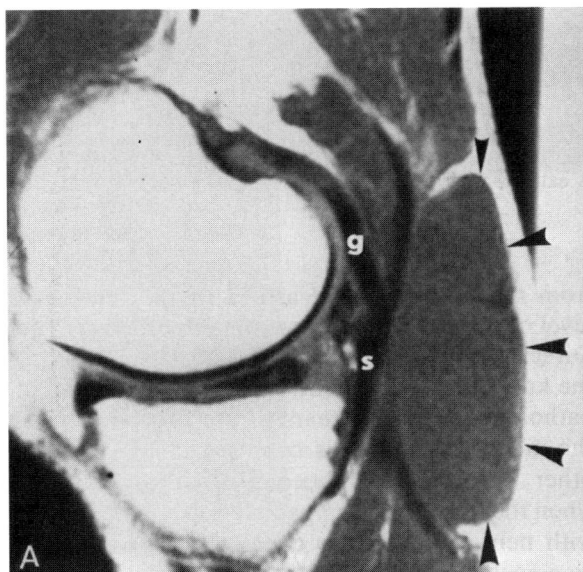

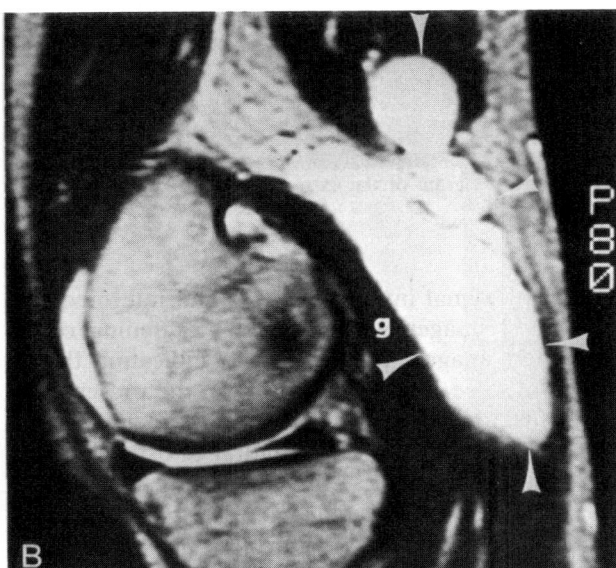

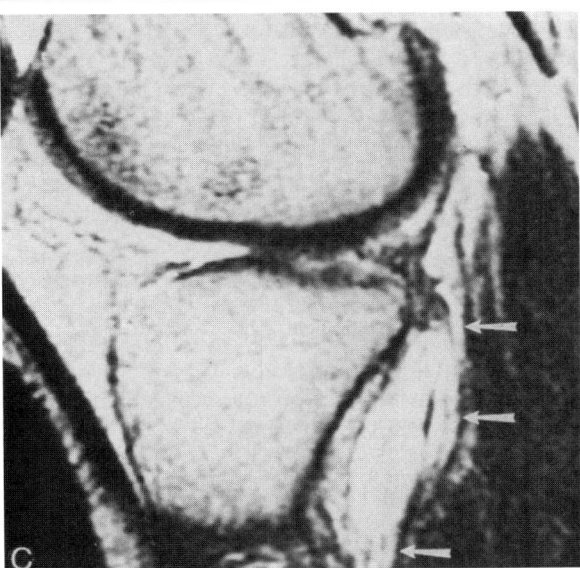

Figure 28B–69. MRI of popliteal cysts. Sagittal intensity windowing (IW) (2000/20) *(A)* and T_2 (2000/80) *(B)* images through the popliteal space demonstrate the typical MRI appearance of synovial cysts. Note on the IW image *(A)* the cyst *(arrowheads)* is of intermediate intensity, similar to that of muscle, whereas on T_2-weighted images *(B)*, the fluid nature of the cyst is readily apparent. In *C*, a T_2-weighted sagittal section (2000/80) through the lateral condylar level demonstrates extravasated cyst fluid *(arrows)* in this 30-year-old male with chronic knee problems who developed posterior peroneal neuropathic problems subsequent to experiencing a sharp "pop" posterior to his knee. g, gastrocnemius tendon; s, semimembranosus tendon.

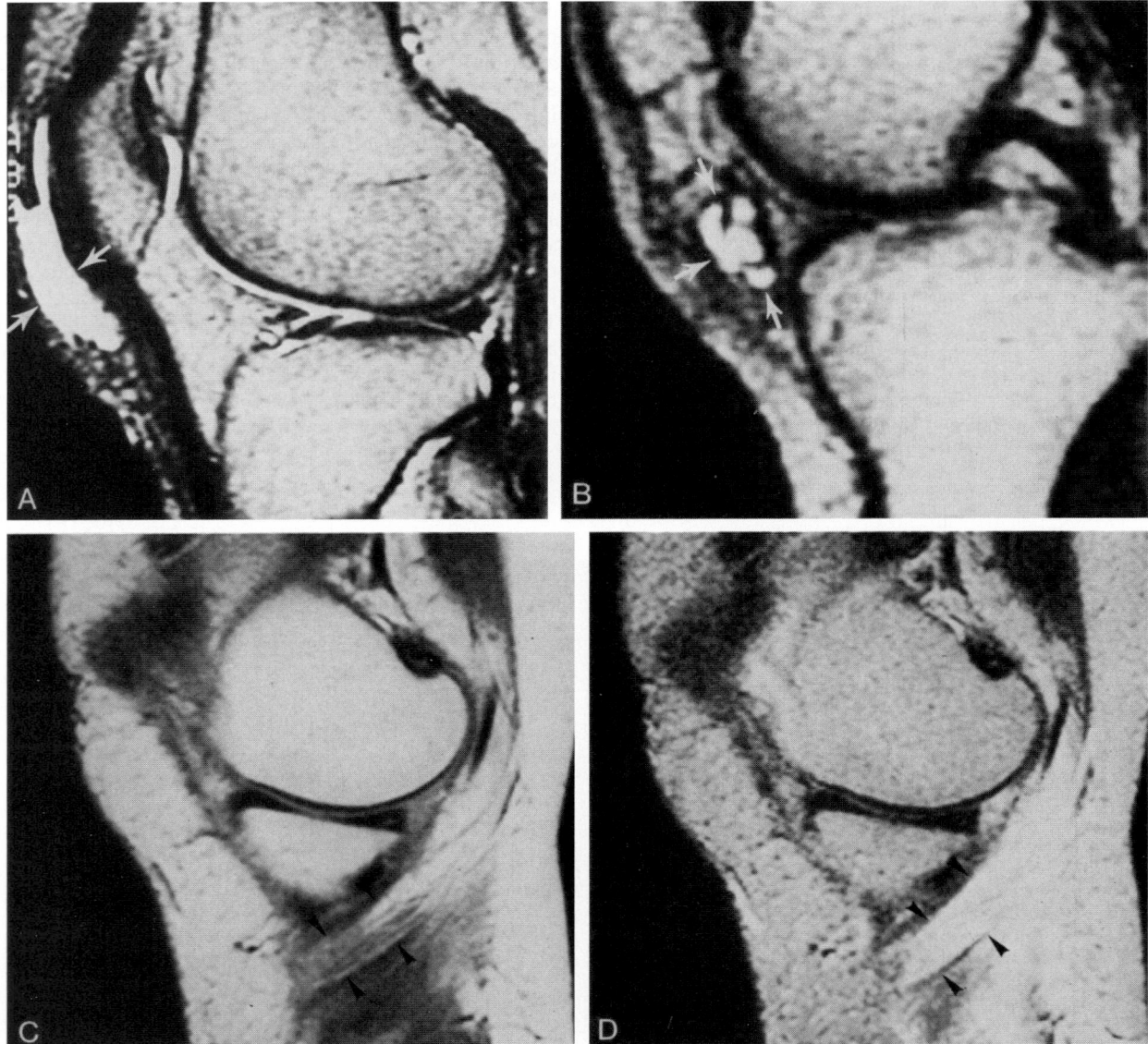

Figure 28B–70. MRI in bursitis. Sagittal T$_2$-weighted (2000/80) midline MRI sections demonstrate prominent fluid collections in the prepatellar bursa *(A)* and in the infrapatellar bursa *(B)* encroaching on the infrapatellar fat pad. Sagittal intensity windowing (2000/20) *(C)* and T$_2$-weighted (2000/80) *(D)* sections at the medial tibial margin demonstrate fluid in the pes anserinus bursa (between *arrowheads*), which markedly brightens on the T$_2$ sequence.

References

1. Ahstrom JP: Osteochondral fracture in the knee joint associated with hypermobility and dislocation of the patella. Osteochondral fracture in the knee joint associated with hypermobility and dislocation of the patella. J Bone Joint Surg Am 47:1491, 1965.
2. Apple JS, Martinez S, Allen NB, et al: Occult fractures of the knee: Tomographic evaluation. Radiology 148:383, 1983.
3. Apple JS, Martinez S, Hardaker WT, et al: Synovial plicae of the knee. Skeletal Radiol 7:251, 1982.
4. Applegate GR, Flannigan BD, Tolin BS, et al: MR diagnosis of recurrent tears in the knee: Value of intraarticular contrast material. AJR Am J Roentgenol 161:821, 1993.
5. Arnoczky SP, Warren RF: Anatomy of the cruciate ligaments. In Feagin JA (ed): The Crucial Ligaments. New York, Churchill Livingstone, 1988.
6. Arnoczky SP, Warren RF: Microvasculature of the human meniscus. Am J Sports Med 10:90, 1982.
7. Arnoczky SP, Warren RF: The microvasculature of the meniscus and its response to injury. Am J Sports Med 11:13, 1983.
8. Ashby ME, Shields CL, Karmy JR: Diagnosis of osteochondral fractures in acute traumatic patellar dislocations using air arthrography. J Trauma 15:1032, 1975.
9. Bach BR, Warren RF: Radiographic indicators of anterior cruciate ligament injury. In Feagin JA (ed): The Crucial Ligaments. New York, Churchill Livingstone, 1988.
10. Barrie HJ: The pathogenesis and significance of meniscal cysts. J Bone Joint Surg Br 61:184, 1979.
11. Bassett FH: Acute dislocation of the patella, osteochondral fractures, and injuries to the extensor mechanism of the knee. In Instructional Course Lectures of The American Academy of Orthopedic Surgeons. St. Louis, CV Mosby, 1976, p 40.
12. Becton JL, Young HH: Cysts of the semilunar cartilage of the knee. Arch Surg 90:708, 1985.
13. Bellon EM, Keith MW, Coleman PE, Shaj ZR: Magnetic resonance imaging of internal derangements of the knee. Radiographics 8:95, 1988.

14. Beltran J, Noto AM, Herman LJ, et al: Joint effusions. Radiology 158:133, 1986.
15. Beltran J, Noto AM, Mosure JC, et al: Knee: Surface-coil imaging at 1.5 T. Radiology 159:747, 1986.
16. Bently G: Articular cartilage changes in chondromalacia patellae. J Bone Joint Surg Br 67:769, 1985.
17. Bianchi S, Zwass A, Abdelwahab IF, Banderali A: Diagnosis of tears of the quadriceps tendon of the knee: Value of sonography. AJR Am J Roentgenol 162:1137, 1993.
18. Blauth M, Tillman B: Stressing on the human femoro-patellar joint. I. Components of a vertical and horizontal tensile bracing system. Anat Embryol 168:117, 1983.
19. Blazina M, Kerlan R, Jobe F, et al: Jumper's knee. Orthop Clin North Am 4:665, 1973.
20. Bodne D, Quinn SF, Murray WT: Magnetic resonance images of chronic patellar tendinitis. Skeletal Radiol 17:24, 1988.
21. Boeree NR, Watkinson AF, Ackroyd CE, Johnson C: Magnetic resonance imaging of meniscal injuries of the knee. J Bone Joint Surg Br 73:452, 1991.
22. Bose K, Kanagasuntheram R, Osman MBH: Vastus medialis oblique: An anatomic and physiologic study. Orthopedics 3:880, 1980.
23. Boven F, Bellemans MA, Guerts J, Potvliege RA: Comparative study of the patello-femoral joint on axial roentgenograms, axial arthrogram, and computed tomography following arthrography. Skeletal Radiol 8:179, 1982.
24. Bradley DM, Bergman AG, Dillingham MF: MR imaging of cyclops lesions. AJR Am J Roentgenol 174:719, 2000.
25. Brandser EA, Riley MA, Berbaum KS, et al: MR imaging of anterior cruciate ligament injury: Independent value of primary and secondary signs. AJR Am J Roentgenol 167:121, 1996.
26. Burgan DW: Arthrographic findings in meniscal cysts. Radiology 101:579, 1971.
27. Burk DLJ, Kanal E, Brunberg JA, et al: 1.5 T surface-coil MRI of the knee. AJR Am J Roentgenol 147:293, 1986.
28. Burk DL, Dalinka MK, Kanal E: Meniscal and ganglion cysts of the knee: MR evaluation. AJR Am J Roentgenol 150:331, 1988.
29. Butler JC, Andrews JR: The role of arthroscopic surgery in the evaluation of acute traumatic hemarthrosis of the knee. Clin Orthop 228:150, 1988.
30. Chan KK, Resnick D, Goodwin D, Saeger LL: Posteromedial tibial plateau injury involving avulsion fracture of the semimembranosus tendon insertion site: Ancillary sign of anterior cruciate ligament tear. Radiology 211:754, 1999.
31. Chan WP, Peterfy C, Fritz RC, Genant HK: MR diagnosis of complete tears of the anterior cruciate ligament of the knee: Importance of anterior subluxation of the tibia. AJR Am J Roentgenol 162:355, 1994.
32. Cheung LP, Li KC, Hollett MD, et al: Meniscal tears of the knee: Accuracy of detection with fast spin-echo MR imaging and arthroscopic correlation in 293 patients. Radiology 203:508, 1997.
33. Conlan T, Garth WP, Lemons JE: Evaluation of the medial soft-tissue restraints of the extensor mechanism of the knee. J Bone Joint Surg Am 75:682, 1993.
34. Cooper DW, Arnoczky SP, Warren RF: Arthroscopic meniscal repair. Clin Sports Med 9:589, 1990.
35. Courneya DL, Spritzer CE, Burk DL Jr, Strong JA: MR imaging of the patellofemoral ligament avulsion: A newly recognized medial retinaculum injury. Radiology 193:289, 1994.
36. Crues JV III, Stoller D: The menisci. In Mink JH, Reicher MA, Crues JV, Deutsch AL (eds): MRI of the Knee. New York, Raven Press, 1993.
37. Crues JV III, Mink JH, Levy TL, et al: Meniscal tears of the knee: Accuracy of MR imaging. Radiology 164:445, 1987.
38. Crues JV III, Ryu R, Morgan FW: Meniscal pathology: The expanding role of magnetic resonance imaging. Clin Orthop 252:80, 1990.
39. Dalinka MK, Garofola J: The infrapatellar synovial fold: A cause for confusion in the evaluation of the anterior cruciate ligament. AJR Am J Roentgenol 127:589, 1976.
40. Dandy DJ: The arthroscopic anatomy of symptomatic meniscal lesions. J Bone Joint Surg Br 72:628, 1990.
41. Danzig L, Resnick D, Gonsalves M, Akeson WH: Blood supply to the normal and abnormal menisci of the human knee. Clin Orthop 172:271, 1983.
42. Datz FL: Bone imaging. In Datz FL (ed): Nuclear Medicine. Chicago, Year Book, 1988, p 72.
43. Davies SG, Baudouin CJ, King JB, Perry JD: Ultrasound, computed tomography and magnetic resonance imaging in patellar tendinitis. Clin Radiol 43:52, 1991.
44. De Smet AA, Graf FK: Meniscal tears missed on MR imaging: Relationship to meniscal tear patterns and anterior cruciate ligament tears. AJR Am J Roentgenol 162:905, 1994.
45. Deizell PB, Schils JP, Recht MP: Subtle fractures about the knee: Innocuous-appearing yet indicative of significant internal derangements. AJR Am J Roentgenol 167:699, 1996.
46. DeLee JC: ACL insufficiency in children. In Feagin JA (ed): The Crucial Ligaments. New York, Churchill Livingstone, 1988.
47. DeSmet AA, Fisher DR, Graf BK, Lange RH: Osteochondritis dissecans of the knee: Value of MR imaging in determining lesions stability and the presence of articular cartilage defects. AJR Am J Roentgenol 155:549, 1990.
48. Deutsch AL, Mink JH: The postoperative knee. In Mink JH, Reicher MA, Crues JV, Deutsch AL (eds): MRI of the Knee. New York, Raven Press, 1993, p 237.
49. Dickhaut SC, DeLee JC: The discoid lateral meniscus syndrome. J Bone Joint Surg Am 64:1068, 1982.
50. El-Khoury GY, Hy U, Berger RA: Meniscotibial (coronary) ligament tears. Skeletal Radiol 11:191, 1984.
51. El-Khoury GY, Wira RL, Berbaum KS, et al: MR imaging of patellar tendinitis. Radiology 184:849, 1992.
52. Feagin JA, Cabaud H, Curl W: The anterior cruciate ligament: Radiographic and clinical signs of successful and unsuccessful repairs. Clin Orthop 164:54, 1982.
53. Feldman F, Singson RD, Staron RB: Magnetic resonance imaging of para-articular and ectopic ganglia. Skeletal Radiol 18:353, 1989.
54. Ferrer-Roca O, Vilalta C: Lesions of the meniscus. Part I. Macroscopic and histologic findings. Clin Orthop 146:289, 1980.
55. Ferrer-Roca O, Vilalta C: Lesions of the meniscus. Part II. Horizontal cleavages and lateral cysts. Clin Orthop 146:301, 1982.
56. Ficat RP: The chondromalacias. In Ficat RP (ed): Disorders of the Patello-Femoral Joint. Baltimore, Williams & Wilkins, 1977, p 170.
57. Ficat RP, Hungerford DS: Normal anatomy: Soft tissue stabilizers. In Ficat RP (ed): Disorders of the Patello-Femoral Joint. Baltimore, Williams & Wilkins, 1977, p 15.
58. Fisher SE, Shelbourne KD: Arthroscopic treatment of symptomatic extension block complicating anterior cruciate ligament reconstruction. Am J Sports Med 21:558, 1993.
59. Fitzgerald SW, Remer EM, Friedman H, et al: MR evaluation of the anterior cruciate ligament: Value of supplementing sagittal images with coronal and axial images. AJR Am J Roentgenol 160:1233, 1993.
60. Fox JM: Magnetic resonance imaging of the knee: A orthopedic surgeon's perspective. In Mink JH (ed): Magnetic Resonance Imaging of the Knee. New York, Raven Press, 1987.
61. Freiberger RH: Meniscal abnormalities. In Freiberger RH, Kaye JJ (eds): Arthrography. New York, Appleton-Century-Crofts, 1979, p 55.
62. Freiberger RH, Kaye JJ: Knee arthrography. In Freiberger RH, Kaye JJ (eds): Arthrography. New York, Appleton-Century-Crofts, 1979, p 55.
63. Friedman RL, Jackson DW: Magnetic resonance imaging of the anterior cruciate ligament: Current concepts. Orthopedics 19:525, 1996.
64. Fulkerson JP, Gossling HR: Anatomy of the knee joint lateral retinaculum. Clin Orthop 153:183, 1960.
65. Garth WPJ, Greco J, House MA: The lateral notch sign associated with acute anterior cruciate ligament disruption. Am J Sports Med 28:68, 2000.
66. Gilbert TJ, Johnson E, Detlie T, Griffiths HJ: Radiologic case study: Patellar dislocation-medial retinacular tears, avulsion fractures, and osteochondral fragments. Orthopedics 16:732, 1993.
67. Gilley JS, Gelman MI, Edison DM, Metcalf RW: Chondral fractures of the knee. Radiology 138:51, 1981.
68. Goldman AB, Pavlov H, Rubenstein D: The Segond fracture of the proximal tibia: A small avulsion that reflects major ligamentous damage. AJR Am J Roentgenol 151:1163, 1988.
69. Goodfellow J, Hungerford DS, Woods C: Patello-femoral joint mechanics and pathology. 2. Chondromalacia patellae. J Bone Joint Surg Br 58:291, 1976.

183. Voto SA: A nomenclature system for meniscal lesions of the knee. Surg Rounds Orthop Oct:34, 1989.
184. Walker PS, Erkman J: The role of the meniscus in force transmission across the knee. Clin Orthop 109:184, 1975.
185. Warren LF, Marshall JL: The supporting structures and layers on the medial side of the knee. J Bone Joint Surg Am 61:56, 1979.
186. Watanabe AT, Carter BC, Teitelbaum GP, et al: Normal variations in MR imaging of the knee: Appearance and frequency. AJR Am J Roentgenol 153:341, 1989.
187. Weiner B, Rosenberg N: Discoid medial meniscus: Associations with bone changes in the tibia. J Bone Joint Surg Am 56:1974, 1974.
188. Weiss KL, Morehouse HT, Levy IM: Sagittal MR images of the knee: A low-signal band parallel to the posterior cruciate ligament caused by a displaced bucket-handle tear. AJR Am J Roentgenol 156:117, 1991.
189. Wilson PD, Eyre-Brook AL, Francis JD: A clinical and anatomic study of the semimembranosus bursa in relation to popliteal cyst. J Bone Joint Surg 20:963, 1938.
190. Wojtys E, Wilson M, Buckwalter K, et al: Magnetic resonance imaging of knee hyaline cartilage and intraarticular pathology. Am J Sports Med 15:455, 1987.
191. Wolfe RD, Colloff B: Popliteal cysts: An arthrographic study and review of the literature. J Bone Joint Surg Am 54:1057, 1972.
192. Woods GW, Stanley RF, Tullos HS: Lateral capsular sign: X-ray clue of a significant knee instability. Am J Sports Med 7:27, 1979.
193. Wright DH, De Smet AA, Norris M: Bucket-handle tears of the medial and lateral menisci of the knee: Value of MR imaging in detecting displaced fragments. AJR Am J Roentgenol 165:621, 1995.
194. Yao L, Lee JK: Avulsion of the posteromedial tibial plateau by the semimembranosus tendon: Diagnosis with MR imaging. Radiology 172:513, 1989.
195. Yao L, Lee JK: Occult intraosseous fracture: Detection with MR imaging. Radiology 167:749, 1988.
196. Yu JS, Cosgarea AJ, Kaeding C, Wilson D: Meniscal flounce MR imaging. Radiology 204:874, 1997.
197. Yu JS, Petersilge C, Sartoris DJ, et al: MR imaging of injuries of the extensor mechanism of the knee. Radiographics 14:541, 1994.
198. Yulish BS, Montganez J, Goodfellow DB, et al: Chondromalacia patellae: Assessment with MR imaging. Radiology 164:763, 1987.

Section C
Factors Predisposing to Knee Injury

Bruce Reider, MD ■ Kenneth J. Mroczek, MD ■ Samuel D. D'Agata, MD

The potential morbidity of knee injuries has led many physicians, trainers, coaches, and athletes themselves to attempt to identify the factors predisposing to these injuries in the hope of minimizing risk. The majority of studies on preventing injury have centered around football in the United States and soccer internationally.

Knee injuries can generally be divided into those caused by an acute traumatic episode and overuse injuries resulting from repetitive forces over time. Overuse knee injuries tend to occur in the extensor mechanism, whereas traumatic injuries include patellar dislocation, meniscal and ligament tears, and osteochondral fractures.

Potential predisposing factors may be divided into external ones, such as shoes, equipment, and playing surfaces, and internal ones, such as loose-jointedness, personality, and lack of conditioning. In this chapter, we review the factors that have been hypothesized or shown to predispose an athlete to knee injury. We hope to eliminate some of the confusion and false speculation that exist in this area. Unfortunately, there are so many potential predisposing factors that it is difficult to eliminate all other variables and prove that a specific factor predisposes to injury. Even when a relationship can be established statistically, it is difficult to prove that a causative relationship exists. Because of these procedural problems, studies on many issues have reached contradictory conclusions.

External Factors

Shoewear

Serious knee injuries in American football players continue to be a major problem. In many instances of ligamentous knee injury, excessive fixation of the foot to the ground has been condemned as a causative factor.[17] Because the foot is fixed, forces that stress the knee in axes other than those of normal motion may result in injury if they exceed the elastic limits of the supporting ligaments.

In the late 1960s and early 1970s, a number of authors blamed long, tenacious cleats for many football injuries and sought to reduce the incidence of knee ligament injuries by instituting their own original cleat modifications.[15, 49, 91, 96, 128] At that time, the conventional football shoe had seven ¾- or ½-inch cleats.[129]

The problem of foot fixation in football was initially addressed by Hanley[51] of Bowdoin College, Maine, in 1965. He attributed rigid fixation to heel cleats and therefore replaced them with a 3-inch-diameter plastic heel disk. These devices were thought to be responsible for the decrease in knee and ankle injuries of Bowdoin varsity football players between 1965 and 1966. Decreases in injuries of Pittsburgh high-school football players were demonstrated by Nedwidek[96] after oblong cleats were substituted for ¾-inch conical heel cleats in 1969.

In 1973, Cameron and Davis[17] reported their use of the swivel shoe to prevent excessive rotational torque in the knee during cutting maneuvers. The shoe they described contained a sealed metallic forefoot turntable to which were mounted four football cleats ⅝ inch in length. The turntable was capable of rotating 360 degrees in either direction but required at least 10 pounds of torque to generate movement. The heel was a cleatless molded platform with a beveled notch to allow skidding. During a common directional change in the swivel shoes, the stance foot rotated with the pelvis, allowing the foot and tibia to follow the femur, thus avoiding torque at the knee or ankle. Cameron and Davis credited the swivel shoe with a decreased incidence of knee and ankle injuries in high-school players in the Durham area. They did not classify these injuries or specify exposure time and did not report whether these differences were statistically significant. This type of shoe was not widely adopted.

The substitution of a "soccer-style" shoe with many short cleats was championed in a series of clinical and laboratory studies by Torg and colleagues.[127–129] Soccer-style shoes with 15 cleats ½-inch in diameter provided an increased effective cleat-tip surface area of 2.8 square inches compared with 0.8 square inch for conventional shoes. The cleat-tip surface area was 3.5 times greater than that provided with conventional shoes, thus decreasing the force through each cleat by a factor of 3.5.[128] In a study of Philadelphia high-school football players, Torg and Quendenfeld[127] determined the effect of shoe type and cleat length on the severity of knee and ankle injuries. On grass surfaces, injuries in players wearing conventional shoes with seven ¾-inch cleats were compared with injuries in those wearing soccer-style shoes with molded soles containing fourteen ⅜-inch cleats (Fig. 28C–1). A marked decrease in severe knee injuries among athletes wearing multicleated shoes was demonstrated. On the basis of these observations, Torg and Quendenfeld recommended that football shoes meet the following specifications: (1) synthetic molded sole, (2) minimum of 14 cleats, (3) cleat diameter of at least ½ inch, and (4) maximal cleat length of ⅜ inch.

To corroborate their findings, Torg and colleagues[129] developed an experimental method to measure the torque necessary to release an engaged shoe-surface interface (Fig. 28C–2). They determined release coefficients for various shoe-surface combinations and came to the following conclusions:

1. The release coefficient varies with the number, length, and diameter of cleats as well as with the type of surface, natural or artificial, wet or dry. These release coefficients varied from a high of 0.55 for conventional ¾-inch football cleats on grass to 0.20 for shoes with the Bowdoin heel on PolyTurf. From their clinical study, Torg

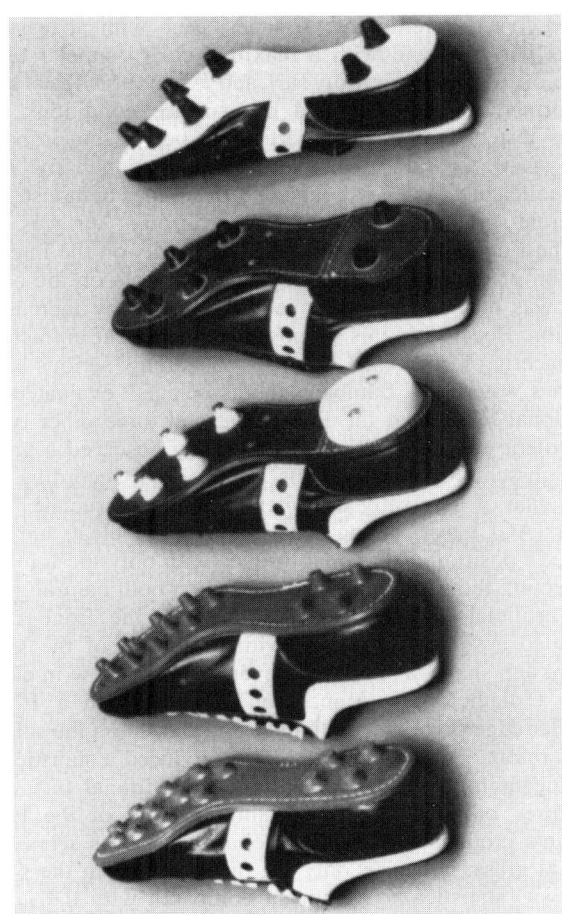

Figure 28C–2. The shoe studies by Torg and colleagues included (from top to bottom): (1) group one prototype, conventional football shoe with seven ¾-inch cleats; (2) group two prototype, conventional seven-posted football shoe with ½-inch cleats; (3) group three prototype, conventional football shoe with Bowdoin heel and five ¾-inch cleats; (4) group 4 prototype, soccer-style shoe with 15 cleats, ½-inch long with ⅜-inch cleat diameter; and (5) group five prototype, soccer-type shoe with 15 cleats ⅜-inch long with ½-inch cleat tip diameter.

and Quendenfeld[127] had concluded that a release coefficient of 0.31 or less was safe.

2. On grass surfaces, conventional seven-posted football shoes with ¾-inch cleats are not safe.

3. The molded sole shoe with 15 cleats ⅜-inch-long with a ½-inch cleat-tip diameter is safe on all surfaces with a nearly constant release coefficient of 0.26 to 0.29.

Their recommendations applied to polyurethane-soled shoes only because they noted in other trials that rubber soles increased the release coefficient, thus limiting their safety. The National High School Athletic Federation has since prohibited the use of the long ¾-inch cleat and has made the ⅜-inch cleat mandatory in high-school competition. The National Collegiate Athletic Association has extensive rules governing football cleats that include prohibition of cleats longer than ½ inch.

Shoe-turf release coefficients for various playing shoes on different surface types were also determined by Culpepper and Niemann[28] at the University of Alabama. They

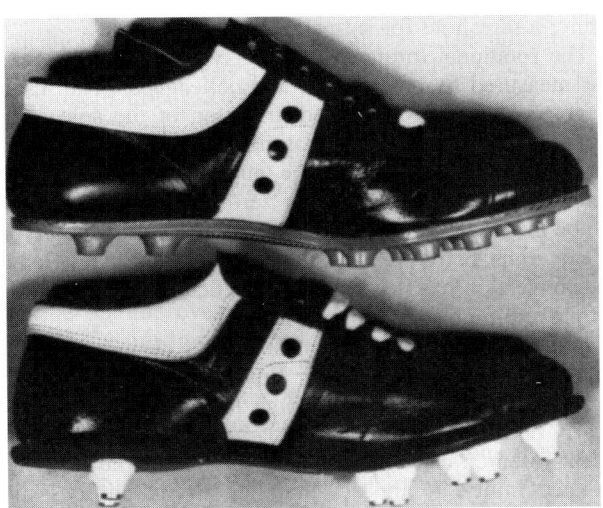

Figure 28C–1. Torg's clinical studies compared injury patterns for soccer-style shoes with fourteen ⅜-inch cleats (above) with those for football shoes with seven ¾-inch cleats (below).

more injuries on all synthetic turf surfaces. Adkinson and associates[1] reported higher injury rates on grass compared with certain synthetic surfaces. In an attempt to compare injury rates on grass with those on one synthetic surface, Keene[73] reviewed the University of Wisconsin football injury data with respect to the use of Tartan Turf. This study found that significantly more serious sprains and torn ligaments occurred on grass than on Tartan Turf. The injuries were not classified according to body part, so it is not known whether knee injuries specifically were significantly more common on grass surfaces. The limitation of their findings is that many of the data were retrospective and historical and thus subject to changes in rules, equipment, style of play, and conditioning programs.

In a comprehensive study,[102] injury rates were determined for National Football League players during games played in stadiums with natural and artificial surfaces during the period 1980 to 1985. Only game-related exposures were considered because most practice sessions were on natural grass, and other parameters of practice sessions were less controlled. Tartan Turf and SuperTurf were excluded from the data analysis because their limited use made comparisons difficult. Thus, the principal comparison was between natural grass and AstroTurf from the database developed by the National Football League's Injury Surveillance Program.

Significant injuries were defined as those that restricted a player's participation for more than 7 days, whereas major injuries kept players out of action for at least 21 days or three games. The authors did not subject their data to traditional analysis for statistical significance, stating "It is not known whether the National Football League injury rates for the various surfaces have equal variances and are normally distributed. Many commonly used statistical models make these two assumptions and may lead to spurious findings for these data." Instead, they developed a "critical interval criterion" to compare the injury rates on the different surfaces. Using this technique, they concluded that a team playing 20 games a season (including four preseason games) on an AstroTurf surface can expect to have one more major knee injury than if it had played all games on grass surfaces. When only knee injuries requiring surgery were looked at, the injury rates per team-game were 0.10 on grass and 0.12 on AstroTurf. As noted, this difference was not analyzed for statistical significance. With use of the critical interval criterion method, however, this would mean one additional surgical knee injury per team for every 50 games, or 2½ seasons, played on AstroTurf instead of grass.

Nicholas and colleagues[99] reported their 26-year experience of game-related events in professional American football. The experience included 18 years of some games being played on artificial turf. No significant difference was found between grass- and turf-related injuries. The number of significant knee injuries (at least two games missed) remained relatively unchanged over time; however, the number of major injuries (at least eight games missed) declined. The authors mention the many limitations of the anecdotal report, including extensive changes in coaches, rules, diagnostic methods, and treatment.

A review of the epidemiologic studies of the impact of artificial turf on American football injuries was published in 1990.[115] The study concluded that play on artificial turf increases the risk for time-loss injuries to the lower extremity by a factor of 1.3 to 1.5 compared with play on natural grass. This did not always result in an additional time loss of one excess injury per team per season.

An update based on the 1980 to 1989 National Football League seasons from the National Football League's Injury Surveillance Program was reported by Powell and Schootman.[103] Once again, only game-related exposures on natural turf and AstroTurf were included for the same reasons; however, this study also analyzed player position, type of play, and severity of injury. The players were divided into linemen, linebackers–tight ends, backs, and special teams players on the basis of similar player tasks and anthropometric characteristics. The types of plays were divided into rushing, passing, and special teams. The severity of injury was classified as category I (missed fewer than three games) or category II (missed at least three games). The concept of incidence density ratio was introduced to allow the determination of the number of injuries attributable to AstroTurf. The incidence density ratio is calculated for both surfaces by dividing the number of injuries on each surface by the number of team-games in each group.

Knee sprains were statistically significantly more prevalent on AstroTurf, accounting for an additional 36 knee sprains during a 10-year period. The most common knee sprain was to the medial collateral ligament (68.2%) followed by the ACL (11%). Certain situations produced an increased risk for injury on AstroTurf. Analysis of knee sprains by position and type of play showed that backs on rushing plays and linemen on passing plays had an increased risk for injury. Linemen on passing plays were at risk for severity category II medial collateral ligament sprains, whereas special teams players demonstrated an increase risk for category II ACL sprains. The authors recognized the limitations of inability to control for many variables, such as player height, weight, injury history, and especially shoe type. The specific situations producing increased risk could in fact be due to these players' wearing certain shoes.

In conclusion, whether artificial surfaces predispose an athlete to knee injury remains open to debate. Many factors, including the shoe-surface interface, need to be considered. It does not appear that artificial turf produces an enormous increase in the incidence of major knee injuries, but it seems likely that artificial surfaces are associated with some increased risk, which is of course significant in human terms.

Internal Factors

Loose-Jointedness

In 1970, Nicholas[98] raised the possibility that loose-jointedness might predispose professional football players to knee ligament injuries. Nicholas performed five tests of ligamentous laxity on 139 football players (Fig. 28C–3). Of the 39 players who had positive test responses in at least three of the five indices of looseness, 28 (72%) sustained a knee ligament injury. Among the remaining

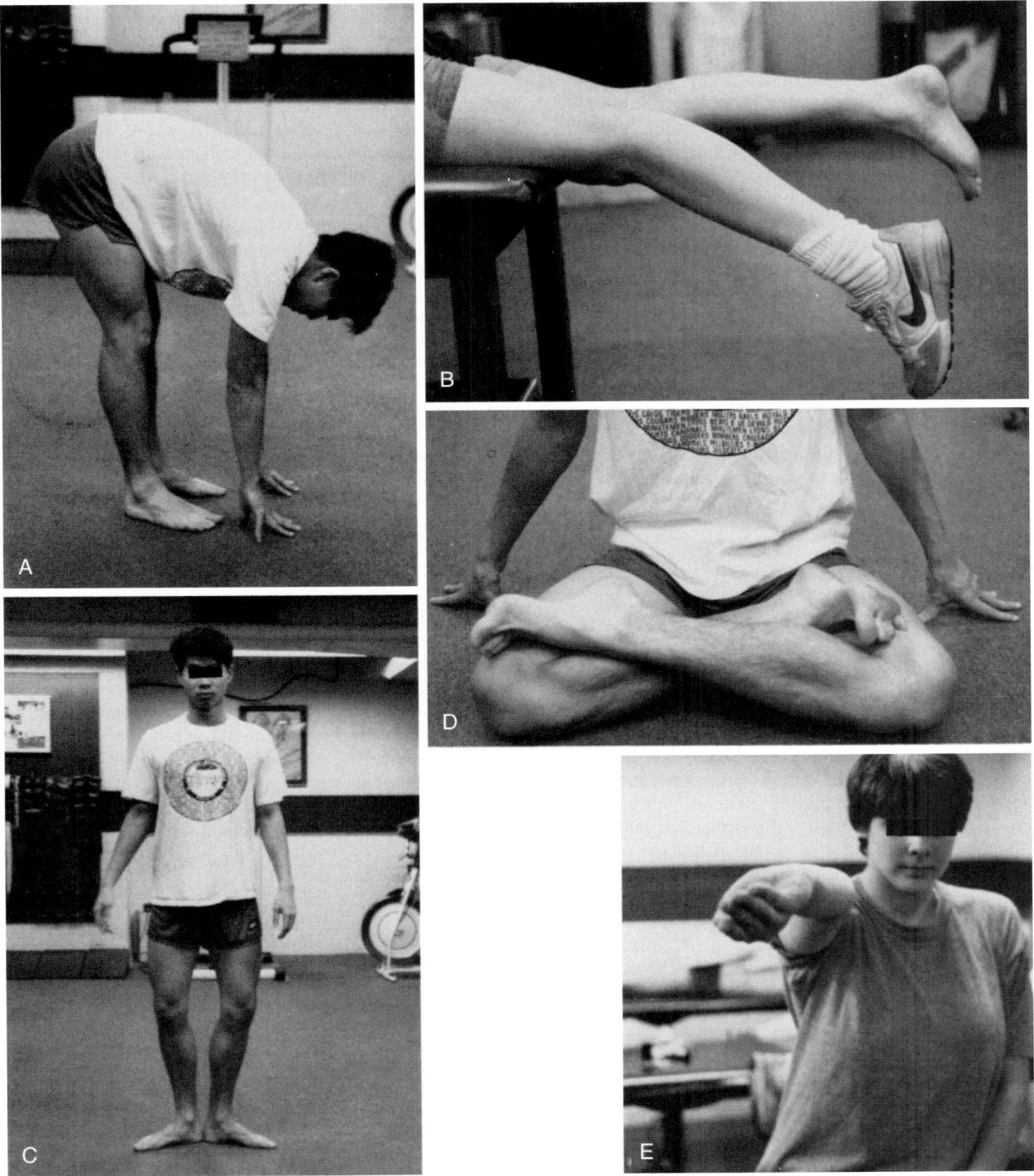

Figure 28C–3. Nicholas used five tests for ligamentous laxity. *A*, The ability to flex the spine so that the palms touch the floor with the knees fully extended is tested. *B*, Recurvatum of the knee of 20 degrees or more is present with the patient prone. *C*, With the knees flexed to 15 to 30 degrees and the hips, the knees, and the ankles turned out to maximum external rotation, the feet form a straight angle of 180 degrees heel-to-heel with the toes out. *D*, Patient has the ability to lie or sit with the knees or the ankles parallel to the floor in external rotation ("lotus position") or in internal rotation of a sufficient degree to permit the legs and the thighs to lie parallel to the floor. *E*, Shoulder flexion, elbow hypertension, and hypersupination of the forearm position the hypothenar eminence to incline cephalad in a vertical plane with the elbows extended and the forearm supinated.

100 players with two or fewer positive indices, only 9% sustained knee ligament injuries; in the group of 50 with no positive indices, only 2 (4%) sustained such injuries. On the basis of these observations, Nicholas concluded that loose-jointedness predisposed a football player to knee ligament injuries. Since the publication of this study, other authors have not been able to confirm Nicholas's conclusions. Kalenak and colleagues[70] in 1975 evaluated 401

college football players by means of traditional joint laxity tests as well as by biomechanical measurement of knee ligament stability. They found no relationship between a player's loose-jointedness and the risk for subsequent knee injury. In addition, they found no correlation between the traditional laxity tests and their biomechanical measurements of knee joint laxity. Other researchers have had similar findings. In 1975, Godshall[42] reported an 8-year study that screened high-school football players with a number of tests, including those espoused by Nicholas. Godshall found no correlation between loose-jointedness and the risk for knee ligament injury. Subsequent studies by Grana and Moretz[46] and Moretz and associates[92] also concluded that there was no correlation between loose-jointedness and a number of different types of injuries. In a large study involving 2300 West Point cadets who participated in a variety of sports as well as additional college and high-school football players, Jackson and associates[65] found no statistical relationship between five joint flexibility indices and subsequent injuries sustained in athletic competition. Thus, despite the initial promise of Nicholas's study, it appears that standard screening tests for joint laxity are not a reliable predictor of susceptibility to knee ligament injury.

Gender

It has often been wondered whether one sex is more vulnerable to injuries, either injuries of certain specific types or injuries in general. This is a difficult question to answer because such a comparison is possible only within the context of a sport in which both men and women participate. Even then, differences in rules, equipment, and training regimens may affect injury risk. The incidence of ACL tears has been reported to be greater in women in many sports including soccer,[6, 10] indoor soccer,[83] basketball,[6, 64, 89] team handball,[93] and volleyball.[37] Possible causes may be divided into intrinsic and extrinsic factors. Intrinsic factors include anatomic, hormonal, and neuromuscular characteristics; extrinsic factors include coaching, training, and conditioning techniques.

Women experience a normal fluctuation in hormones during their menstrual cycles. This has led researchers to investigate whether fluctuations in hormone levels may affect ligament cells and whether the incidence of ACL tears in women varies during the menstrual cycle. Receptors for estrogen and progesterone have been located on both the rabbit and human ACL.[84, 110] Rabbit ACL fibroblast cell cultures have been shown to exhibit significantly decreased collagen synthesis and fibroblast proliferation with increasing estradiol concentrations.[85] Within the physiologic range, an increase in estradiol concentration decreased collagen synthesis by more than 40%. Similar dose-dependent estrogen effects were seen in human ACL fibroblast cell cultures.[143]

The frequency of ACL injuries in relation to different phases of the menstrual cycle was investigated in 28 women who sustained noncontact ACL tears.[137] The authors calculated the number of expected injuries in each of the three phases assuming that there was an equal chance of sustaining an injury on any given day. A higher than expected number of injuries occurred during the ovulatory phase, whereas a lower than expected number of injuries occurred during the follicular phase. This variation may be related to hormone fluctuations, such as estrogen levels, which peak during the ovulatory phase and reach their lowest levels during the follicular phase. Other hormones, such as relaxin, may also play a role. Because this was a retrospective study, the authors had to rely on recall ability and were unable to confirm hormone levels by blood or urine tests. Other limitations were elucidated by Wolman[140] and include the use of oral contraceptives by five participants and the possibility of varying hormone profiles due to the wide age range of the participants.

Huston and Wojtys[60] studied the gender differences in neuromuscular characteristics of athletes and nonathletes. Time to peak hamstring torque was significantly longer in female athletes than in male athletes. In contrast to male athletes, female athletes fired their quadriceps before their hamstrings in response to anterior tibial translation. Analysis of the female athlete group and comparison of the five strongest and weakest on the basis of quadriceps and hamstring peak torque revealed an interesting finding. The strongest athletes exhibited hamstrings-first behavior, whereas the weakest initially fired their quadriceps. The authors hypothesize that proper conditioning programs may reverse muscle recruitment to the more beneficial hamstrings-first pattern.

The effect of a jump training program was reported for 11 female high-school volleyball players.[57] The program included stretching, plyometric exercises, and weightlifting. Performance of the female players before and after the training was compared with that of a male control group. Before training, women exhibited a significantly lower hamstring-to-quadriceps peak torque ratio than that of men; however, after the 6-week program, the hamstring-to-quadriceps ratio was similar to that of the men. The women also increased their vertical jump by 10% while decreasing their peak landing forces.

Rozzi and coworkers[107] measured knee joint laxity and neuromuscular characteristics of healthy collegiate athletes who played soccer, basketball, or both. Although the authors found no difference between the sexes in time to peak torque, female athletes demonstrated greater knee joint laxity, longer time to detect knee joint motion moving into extension, superior single-leg balance ability, and greater electromyographic peak amplitude and area of the lateral hamstring muscle single curve subsequent to landing a jump. The finding of increased laxity is supported by Huston and Wojtys,[60] but it is contradicted by other studies.[3, 136] Rozzi and associates hypothesize that the female athletes may have adopted a compensatory muscle-activation pattern to protect against their increased laxity and proprioceptive defects. Inhibition of this protective mechanism by factors such as fatigue may lead to abnormal forces on the ACL and possible injury. Possibly supporting this theory is a report showing that the isokinetic quadriceps and hamstrings endurance of female athletes was significantly lower than that of male athletes even when it was normalized for weight.[60] Endurance of the athletic population was increased compared with that of nonathletic gender-matched control subjects, however, once again illustrating a possible role for conditioning in reducing the predilection of female athletes for ACL tears.

Differences in anatomic factors within the knee, especially the morphologic features of the intercondylar notch, have been suspected of affecting the female athlete's risk for ACL injury. The studies of intercondylar notch morphology are discussed in a later section.

The increased rate of ACL tears among female athletes in several sports in which both sexes participate is clearly established. The reasons for this difference are probably multifactorial.[52] Some studies suggest that some of the predisposing factors can be modified by training. It remains to be proved whether specific training programs can reduce female athletes' risk for ACL tears.

Muscle Imbalance

There have been attempts to correlate muscle strength and muscle imbalance with knee injury. Klein,[74] in 1974, stated that a strength imbalance between the hamstrings and quadriceps or a total strength imbalance of 10% between the two lower limbs predisposes an athlete to knee injury, an idea also espoused by others.

In a well-controlled prospective blinded study, Grace and colleagues[45] sought to address this issue. Isokinetic testing of the quadriceps and hamstrings was performed in 206 male high-school football players in Albuquerque, New Mexico. Agonist-antagonist imbalance was defined as a deviation of 10% or more from the mean value for a particular side. Strength, power, endurance, and fast and slow times to maximal tension for both quadriceps and hamstrings were measured. Although one in three players had an imbalance of 10% or more, the authors found no consistent relationship between a noted preseason muscle imbalance and the subsequent risk for knee injury. Ipsilateral-contralateral leg imbalance and agonist-antagonist muscle imbalance did not lead to increased knee joint injury either. Increased height and weight were correlated with a higher incidence of knee injury, which was interpreted as being due to the greater mass and resulting momentum leading to greater forces across the knee joint.

Effects of Immobilization and Exercise on Knee Ligament Laxity and Strength

Experimental evidence that exercise may affect knee ligament strength, stiffness, and laxity has raised the possibility that exercise may protect against knee ligament injury in the long term but may predispose to it in the short term. A number of classic studies have found that immobilization decreases ligament strength, whereas activity appears to increase it. Noyes[100] found that 8 weeks of total-body plaster immobilization of primates led to a 39% decrease in maximal failure load and a 32% decrease in energy absorbed to failure of bone-ligament-bone preparations. In addition, he found that the incidence of failure by ligament avulsion increased in the immobilized limbs. Most signifi-

cantly, he found that up to 12 months were required for the complete recovery of ligament strength parameters. Larsen and associates[80] found complete recovery of the strength and elastic stiffness in the rat ACL after only 6 weeks of retraining that followed 4 weeks of immobilization. Furthermore, a transition from avulsion failures to intraligament failures was observed with retraining. Woo and colleagues[141] found an approximately two-thirds reduction in the ultimate load to failure of the immobilized rabbit medial collateral ligament–bone complex. Furthermore, the ligament substance displayed decreased stiffness. Both parameters demonstrated larger reductions after 12 weeks of immobilization compared with only 9 weeks. Histologic evaluation revealed increased osteoclastic activity with bone resorption at the ligament insertion site, which may explain the observed increased failure mode of ligament avulsions. Remobilization for 9 weeks allowed complete recovery of the mechanical properties of the ligament substance but only partial recovery of the ligament-bone junction.

In a review of the literature, Yasuda and Hayashi[142] summarized the effects of immobilization and remobilization on ligaments. Immobilization causes a deterioration in the mechanical properties with a reduction in the cross-sectional area at different rates among various ligaments. Remobilization provides an almost complete restoration of the mechanical properties quickly, but the structural properties of the bone-ligament-bone complex take longer for recovery. Differences in behavior between ligaments, such as the ACL and the medial collateral ligament, may be due to intrinsic differences in their cellular, ultrastructural, biochemical, and biomechanical properties.

Other authors have investigated the effects of exercise on knee ligaments. Tipton and associates[126] noted weakening of the medial collateral ligament after immobilization. When the effects of exercise were examined, Tipton found that chronic endurance exercise increased the strength of the ligament-bone junction of the medial collateral ligament in dogs and rats. He did not find these effects after acute exercise or after chronic spring exercise. Similar increases in strength after chronic exercise were found by Kuei and colleagues[76] in the collateral ligaments of pigs and by Viidik[133] in the ACL of rabbits.

These strengthening effects appear to take time to develop. As mentioned, Tipton found no increase in the strength of rat medial collateral ligament–bone junctions after acute exercise. Weisman and colleagues[135] noticed that in vitro cyclic loading of rat medial collateral ligaments produced stretching out and "softening." Analogous in vivo testing of the medial collateral ligaments of athletes in a number of sports showed an increase in compliance of about 20% in at least one knee of most athletes tested. There was a trend toward a greater change in laxity in athletes who were initially considered "tight-jointed."

Stoller and colleagues[121] noted an increase in the torsional laxity of knees in 13 subjects after a 3.5-mile run. The maximal postexercise increase in laxity was 14%, with a mean recovery time of 52.4 minutes and a standard deviation of 17.8 minutes. The application of a 10-minute ice or ultrasound treatment significantly reduced the postexercise recovery times. Skinner and colleagues[114] tried to relate changes in knee laxity after exercise to muscle fatigue. They tested the laxity of the ACL with use of the KT1000 arthrometer in both knees of a group of 10 highly conditioned U.S. Navy SEALs (Sea, Air, and Land team) after exhaustive exercise. They found a significant increase in ACL laxity in the left knee, which was allowed a half-hour cool-down, but not in the right knee, which was tested immediately after additional isokinetic muscle exercise. They hypothesized that the cool-down period had allowed a decrease in protective muscle tone, which was helping to stabilize the knee. Several of the authors cited have hypothesized that these exercise-related increases in ligament laxity or compliance may predispose to injury, although this has not been proved clinically.

The effect of exercise on anterior-posterior knee laxity was studied by Steiner and colleagues.[120] Knee laxity was measured before and after exercise in weightlifters, basketball players, and distance runners. Measurements of knee laxity were made in 24 weightlifters within 15 minutes of performing squats with an average load 1.6 times body weight for an average of 24 repetitions; 10 female basketball players practiced for 90 minutes, and 12 recreational runners ran a 6.2-mile road race. Nine sedentary office workers served as control subjects. Both posterior and anterior laxity in the basketball players and distance runners increased between 18% and 20%, whereas in the control subjects and weightlifters it remained relatively unchanged. The change in laxity was smaller than the average test-retest variability of the testing device. A subsequent study found a similar 21% increase in anterior laxity after an exercise program on a stationary bicycle.[47]

A female semiprofessional basketball team was observed throughout a typical day to determine whether anterior laxity at 30 degrees of flexion changed according to activity level.[108] Sedentary work did not affect anterior knee laxity; however, after a 150-minute practice session, significant increases were observed. Normal laxity had not been fully restored 90 minutes after practice, but full restoration occurred after 5 hours. In a similar study by Johannsen and associates,[67] anterior laxity after a 30-minute run was still present at 30 degrees of flexion but had resolved at 90 degrees of flexion by 30 minutes after exercise.

The degree of increased laxity from activities of different intensity levels and the time needed to restore normal laxity were further studied by Nawata and coworkers,[95] who measured muscle strength and anterior-posterior knee laxity in two groups of athletes after exercise. The first group consisted of 10 male collegiate volleyball players, and the second group consisted of 10 male triathletes. Knee laxity and muscle strength in the volleyball players were measured before exercise and at 10-minute intervals during running on a treadmill at 7 km/hr. The anterior laxity increased by one third at 20 minutes, remained constant thereafter, and gradually returned to pre-exercise levels by 1 hour after exercise. There was no change in posterior laxity. Because there was no change in muscle strength, the authors concluded that the change in knee laxity was not due to a decrease in muscle strength. The increase in knee laxity after 135-km biking and a 42-km marathon, a mean exercise time of 8 hours and 46 minutes, in the triathletes was similar to that of the volleyball players at 20 minutes. The authors concluded that the magnitude of

change in knee laxity after exercise seems to be fixed, and the threshold to cause this change is low.

The anterior knee laxity in nine healthy female basketball players was measured after a 1-hour exercise session by Sumen and colleagues.[122] A significant increase in anterior knee laxity of approximately 10% was noted. Magnetic resonance imaging examination before and after exercise was also performed. An increase in signal intensity in the ACL after exercise was noted only with three-dimensional gradient-echo T_2 imaging, possibly reflecting an increase in water content from an increase in blood supply to the ACL and surrounding synovium after exercise.

The effect of fatigue on anterior knee laxity was investigated by Wojtys and associates.[139] Ten adults of mixed activity levels were exercised to a fatigue level defined as a 50% decrease in the work output in both the quadriceps and the hamstring muscle groups. After fatigue, the anterior knee laxity by instrument testing increased an average of 32.5%, from 2.08 to 3.33 mm. The authors state that although the effect of temperature is unknown, an increase this large cannot be attributed solely to viscoelasticity but must in part be due to fatigue. Furthermore, fatigue slowed muscle reaction time but did not change the order of recruitment in response to anterior translation.

The effect of weight training and an agility program on anterior tibial translation and neuromuscular characteristics of the knee was studied in 32 healthy volunteers.[138] This controlled study had patients either perform no training or enroll in 6 weeks of weight training or agility training. The weight training was either isotonic or isokinetic and focused on knee flexion, knee extension, and ankle plantar flexion. The agility program consisted of five drills used in ACL rehabilitation, such as cariocas. No difference in anterior laxity was noted in any group after training, except for an increase of 0.83 mm in the isotonic group.

Another goal of Wojtys and colleagues' study was to determine whether the various training programs might affect dynamic knee stability. The authors acknowledged that many factors influence dynamic stability, including muscle reaction time and time to peak torque. The agility training improved both these times, whereas the isokinetic training had mixed results. The authors caution against arriving at comprehensive conclusions from the study because it is based on only two of the many muscle performance indices available.

The fact that immobilization has been shown to produce a long-lasting decrease in ligament strength seems to indicate that a return to sports participation soon after such immobilization might predispose to further ligament injury, although this has not been proved by clinical studies, and there are no clearly established guidelines concerning a safe return to sports after a period of immobilization. Similarly, although laboratory studies show that chronic exercise can strengthen knee ligaments, no specific protocols have been shown to protect clinically against ligament injury. Because in vivo experimental studies must be performed in animal models, it is not known whether the parameters of magnitude and reversibility are the same in humans.

The significance of the short-term effects of exercise on ligaments and their protecting musculature is uncertain because it can be argued that the observed changes may predispose to injury or protect from it. Determining which, if either, effect occurs will require tightly controlled clinical study. It may be easier with large clinical trials to determine whether certain types of training programs can decrease an athlete's risk for knee ligament injury. This possibility is discussed further in the subsequent section on preseason conditioning.

History of Previous Injury

Athletes who have sustained knee injuries are at significant risk for reinjury. In a statistical analysis of high-school football injuries, Pritchett[104] found that knee injuries composed 12.7% of all injuries sustained. The majority of these injuries involved ligaments. A single knee ligament injury increased the likelihood of a subsequent injury to the same knee by a factor of 3. Of patients with patellar injury, 87% reported a subsequent injury to the same knee, and 34% had a patellar injury in the contralateral knee, suggesting a predisposition to patellar injury in these patients.

Pritchett's data did not specify which ligament injuries were associated with increased risk for reinjury. It is likely, however, that many of them were ACL tears, which have been shown to be associated with a high risk for reinjury in young athletes,[92] and not medial collateral ligament injuries, which have not been associated with a high risk for reinjury.[32, 106] The observation that some athletes recover relatively well after an ACL tear has caused many to wonder what additional factors may affect the natural history of ACL tears in the athlete. Factors that have been implicated include activities attempted, protective neuromuscular reflexes, and individual soft tissue differences. It seems clear that individuals with ACL-deficient knees are more likely to experience reinjury if they attempt to participate in sports involving jumping or pivoting, such as basketball, soccer, and football, than if they stick to running, swimming, and cycling.[40, 54, 101] Even in response to the same sports demands, however, some knees seem to hold up better than others.

Knees that recover poorly after ACL rupture have sometimes been called ACL-dependent knees. What factors might make a knee ACL dependent? One possibility is a lack of certain neuromuscular reflexes. Solomonow and associates[116] have shown that stressing of the ACL in the normal knee has a moderate inhibitory effect on the quadriceps while exciting the hamstrings. Similar responses were also seen in patients with ACL damage during loaded knee extension with tibial subluxation, implying that an alternative reflex arc unrelated to ACL receptors was available to maintain joint integrity. Thus, it is possible that patients who do surprisingly well with an ACL-deficient knee may have particularly effective reflex pathways that allow them to prevent anterior tibial subluxation with hamstring contraction. Gait analysis and functional testing of patients with ACL deficiency showed a reduction in the magnitude of the knee flexion moment. This has been called a quadriceps-avoidance gait, inferring a reduction in quadriceps activity.[5, 8] Diminished quadriceps activity along with both an increase in hamstring activity and an alteration in the hamstring firing pattern has been demonstrated in some patients with ACL deficiency by electromyographic analysis.[21, 71, 82, 125]

Functional knee braces, which have been shown to reduce the clinical risk of giving-out episodes even though they have not been proved to stabilize the knee mechanically under high loads, may work by providing additional proprioceptive stimulation to enhance this reflex mechanism. Multiple studies have demonstrated diminished proprioception in the ACL-deficient knee.[7, 9, 11, 25, 87] Beynnon and associates[9] were able to demonstrate a proprioceptive defect, an increased threshold to detection of passive knee motion, in a group of 20 knees with chronic ACL injury compared with the uninjured knee, but they were unable to demonstrate an increase in proprioception with the addition of either a functional brace or a neoprene sleeve. The authors hypothesize that their inability to demonstrate a beneficial effect of braces may be due to a limitation in their testing model or their selection of patients because none of the patients had a history of instability. In another study of ACL-deficient athletes, some of whom had regular instability episodes, Cook and associates[24] found that braces subjectively decreased subluxation episodes and enhanced athletic performance. Biomechanical analysis of these same patients revealed better running and cutting performances braced than unbraced. On the other hand, Branch and associates[14] performed electromyographic analysis of braced ACL-deficient athletes during cutting maneuvers and found no change in the firing pattern of the quadriceps and hamstring muscles.

Other factors may contribute to the ACL dependency of a given knee. One such factor might be individual variations in the relative contributions of the secondary restraints to knee stability. Another factor could be individual variations in the mechanical properties of connective tissue, allowing more severe chronic stretching of secondary restraints. Some knees may also be at greater risk for later reinjury because trauma to the secondary restraints occurred at the time of the ACL tear. It is possible that all these factors contribute to the risk for reinjury in different individuals. We know of no studies that objectively evaluate the relative role of these factors in influencing the risk for reinjury after an ACL tear.

Lack of Preseason Conditioning

It has been proposed that a lack of preseason conditioning may predispose an athlete to football knee injuries. Cahill and Griffith[16] reported the effect of a preseason conditioning program on the incidence and severity of high-school football knee injuries. The program emphasized cardiovascular conditioning, acclimatization to heat, weight training, and flexibility and agility exercises. The authors concluded that this program decreased early season and total knee injuries by 68% and 41%, respectively, and also decreased the severity of these injuries. The beneficial effects were most notable in linemen. Such programs may decrease the risk for knee injury by causing more athletes to train independently and by encouraging coaches to keep players who have not participated in these programs out of contact drills in the early season. Thompson and col-

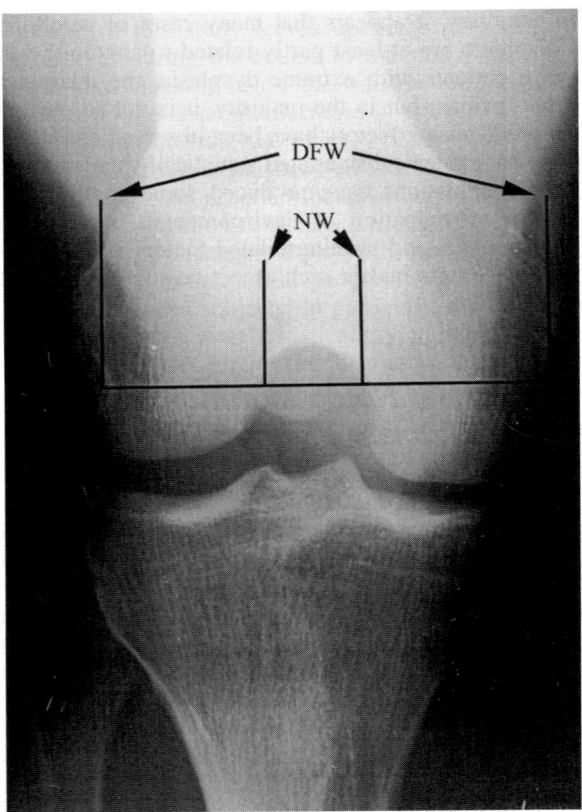

Figure 28C–4. Measured on a tunnel radiograph, the notch width index equals the notch width (NW) divided by the distal femoral width (DFW) at the level of the popliteal groove, parallel to the joint surface.

unilateral, and no ACL tears. Herzog and colleagues[56] also found no difference in NWI or notch width between chronic ACL-deficient knees and a control population. Symmetry of NWI between a subject's knees was shown regardless of sex or ACL status by Teitz and associates.[123] Furthermore, Souryal and Freeman[117] found no difference in NWI between ACL-deficient and ACL-intact knees and only a trend that female athletes had a smaller NWI than that of male athletes.

Lund-Hanssen and coworkers[86] compared radiographic intercondylar notch measurements of 20 female team handball players who had undergone ACL reconstructions with those of 26 uninjured female control subjects of similar age, height, weight, and level of performance. The patients who had undergone reconstruction all had notchplasties and were evaluated on the average of 15 months postoperatively. Because the control population had a high correlation (0.84) between their right and left knees, the authors thought it was appropriate to compare the uninjured knee of the patient who had reconstruction with the control group. The patients who underwent reconstruction had an uninjured knee with a notch width (16.7 mm) and NWI (0.224) significantly smaller than in the control population, who had a notch width and NWI of 18.5 mm and 0.243, respectively. In comparing all patients, a notch width of 17 mm or less produced an odds ratio indicating that a patient was six times more likely to sustain an ACL injury.

Shelbourne and associates[112] measured the intercondylar notch width in a prospective study of 714 consecutive patients who underwent autogenous patellar tendon graft ACL reconstructions. Data collected included height, weight, radiographic width measurements, and intraoperative measurements by arthrotomy. All patients had a reconstruction with a 10-mm graft within a notch that was widened when necessary so that at least a 10-mm-wide space was left for the graft. Female patients had an average notch width of 13.9 mm, which was smaller than the 15.9 mm average for male patients. Both sexes were then stratified into five groups according to height. Women had smaller notch widths compared with those of men of the same height group. The results also indicated that as height increased for both sexes, the femoral bicondylar width increased. The notch width became larger with subsequent height increases only for men, however. The notch width was relatively unchanged with increasing height in women. Therefore, the NWI tended to decrease in taller women, although the absolute notch width might be unchanged compared with short women. As a result, the authors believe that notch width is a more accurate representation than NWI and may help explain the conflicting reports on notch stenosis and its prevalence between the sexes and between ACL-intact and ACL-deficient knees.

In Shelbourne's study, 27 patients subsequently had contralateral ACL tears. When the patients were divided into two groups on the basis of notch width smaller than 15 mm (group 1) or larger than 16 mm (group 2), group 1 had an incidence of contralateral ACL tears almost five times higher than the rate of group 2. There was no difference in tear rates for women and men with the same notch size. In examining the 19 patients who tore their reconstructed grafts, no difference was observed in the retear rates between the two groups. The authors concluded that equal tear rates exist for men and women with equal-sized notches. On the average, they stated that women have narrower notches, which may explain why women have higher primary tear rates. The authors believe that a narrow notch reflects a smaller ACL. They believe that the retear rate was the same for group 1 and group 2 patients because the groups had been equalized by giving all the patients identical 10-mm grafts.

The findings of these studies are all slightly different and do not seem to justify the routine widening of all intercondylar notches at the time of ACL reconstruction surgery; instead, individual evaluation of each case is recommended. Souryal and colleagues[118] noted that young athletes who rupture an ACL through a noncontact mechanism and who have a stenotic intercondylar notch should be "strongly counseled" about their risk of tearing the contralateral ACL. It does not appear that this association is strong enough to warrant routinely counseling these athletes to refrain from further sports participation or performing prophylactic notchplasties in the uninjured knee as the authors suggest.[52] The data of Shelbourne and colleagues[112] suggest that athletes with narrow notches have a 5.9% incidence of a contralateral ACL tear (during an unspecified time); clinicians may wish to share this information with patients who are noted to have a narrow intercondylar notch during primary ACL reconstruction.

Other Anatomic Factors

Anatomic variations of menisci may predispose to knee injury. Ossicles of menisci are rare. They are often mistaken radiographically for loose bodies, but they are actually embodied within the meniscal tissue.[23, 41] They can be considered either primary vestigial sesamoid structures or the result of developmental degenerative metaplasia, perhaps after trauma. These ossicles, which are often in the posterior horn of the medial meniscus, do not necessarily cause symptoms, and therefore the consideration given them as predisposing factors to knee injury is not clearly warranted.

Discoid lateral menisci have been associated with susceptibility to meniscal tear and the "snapping knee syndrome."[33, 75] Not all lateral discoid menisci are symptomatic or cause a snapping knee, however. Dickhaut and DeLee[33] noted that the majority of complete discoid menisci were asymptomatic owing to their normal peripheral attachments. The Wrisberg ligament type, which is attached posteriorly only by the meniscofemoral ligament, is associated with hypermobility of the posterior horn of the lateral meniscus, which typically leads to the syndrome of the snapping knee. These menisci are susceptible to tears.

Conclusion

Factors that may predispose to knee injury may be extrinsic or intrinsic. Extrinsic factors, such as certain football shoes and ski bindings, have clearly been shown to contribute to the risk for injury, whereas the contribution of artificial playing surfaces appears likely. The contributions of intrinsic factors, except for preexisting post-traumatic instability, have been even more difficult to define. This is not surprising when one considers the vast number of factors, such as anatomic variations, tissue types, fitness levels, training techniques, coaching methods, equipment, and playing surfaces, that may influence susceptibility to injury, making a well-controlled study of just one factor difficult to perform. Thus, the results of objective studies should always be supplemented with commonsense guidelines, such as proper conditioning, skilled coaching, and properly fitted equipment, in attempting to minimize knee injuries.

References

1. Adkinson JW, Requa RK, Garrick JG: Injury rates in high school football. Clin Orthop 99:131–136, 1974.
2. Anderson AF, Lipscomb AB, Lindahl KJ, Addlestone RB: Analysis of the intercondylar notch by computed tomography. Am J Sports Med 15:547–552, 1987.
3. Anderson AF, Snyder RB, Federspiel CF, Lipscomb AB: Instrumented evaluation of knee laxity: A comparison of five arthrometers. Am J Sports Med 20:135–140, 1992.
4. Andreasson G, Lindenberger U, Renstrom P, Peterson L: Torque developed at simulated sliding between sport shoes and artificial turf. Am J Sports Med 14:225–230, 1986.
5. Andriacchi TP, Birac D: Functional testing in the anterior cruciate ligament–deficient knee. Clin Orthop 288:40–47, 1993.
6. Arendt E, Dick R: Knee injury patterns among men and women in collegiate basketball and soccer. NCAA data and review of literature. Am J Sports Med 23:694–701, 1995.
7. Barrack RL, Skinner HB, Buckley SL: Proprioception in the anterior cruciate deficient knee. Am J Sports Med 17:1–6, 1989.
8. Berchuck M, Andriacchi TP, Bach BS, Reider B: Gait adaptations by patients who have a deficient anterior cruciate ligament. J Bone Joint Surg Am 72:871–877, 1990.
9. Beynnon BD, Ryder SH, Konradse L, et al: The effect of anterior cruciate ligament trauma and bracing on knee proprioception. Am J Sports Med 27:150–155, 1999.
10. Bjordal JM, Arnoy F, Hannestad B, Strand T: Epidemiology of anterior cruciate ligament injuries in soccer. Am J Sports Med 25: 341–345, 1997.
11. Borsa PA, Lephart SM, Irrgang JJ, et al: The effects of joint position and direction of joint motion on proprioceptive sensibility in anterior cruciate ligament–deficient athletes. Am J Sports Med 25:336–340, 1997.
12. Bowers DK, Martin BR: Impact absorption, new and old Astro Turf at West Virginia University. Med Sci Sports 6:217–221, 1974.
13. Bramwell ST, Requa RK, Garrick JG: High school football injuries: A pilot comparison of playing surfaces. Med Sci Sports 4:166–169, 1972.
14. Branch TP, Hunter R, Donath M: Dynamic EMG analysis of anterior cruciate deficient legs with and without bracing during cutting. Am J Sports Med 17:35–41, 1989.
15. Buchbinder RM, Nappora NJ, Biggs EN: The relationship of abnormal pronation to chondromalacia of the patella in distance runners. Podiatr Sports Med 69:159–162, 1979.
16. Cahill BR, Griffith EH: Effect of pre-season conditioning on incidence and severity of high school football knee injuries. Am J Sports Med 6:180–184, 1978.
17. Cameron BM, Davis O: The swivel football shoe: A controlled study. J Sports Med 1:16–27, 1973.
18. Caraffa A, Cerulli G, Projetti M, et al: Prevention of anterior cruciate ligament injuries in soccer. A prospective controlled study of proprioceptive training. Knee Surg Sports Traumatol Arthrosc 4:19–21, 1996.
19. Cascells SW: The arthroscope in the diagnosis of disorders of the patellofemoral joint. Clin Orthop 144:45–50, 1979.
20. Caylor D, Fites R, Worrell TW: The relationship between quadriceps angle and anterior knee pain syndrome. J Orthop Sports Phys Ther 17:11–16, 1993.
21. Ciccotti MG, Kerlan RG, Perry J, Pink M: An electromyographic analysis of the knee during functional activities. II. The anterior cruciate ligament–deficient and -reconstructed profiles. Am J Sports Med 22:651–658, 1994.
22. Clement DB, Taunton SE, Smart GW, McNicol KL: A survey of overuse running injuries. Physician Sportsmed 9:47–58, 1981.
23. Conforty B, Lotem M: Ossicles in human menisci: Report of two cases. Clin Orthop 144:272–275, 1979.
24. Cook FF, Tibone JE, Redfern FC: A dynamic analysis of a functional brace for anterior cruciate ligament insufficiency. Am J Sports Med 17:519–523, 1989.
25. Corrigan JP, Cashman WF, Brady MP: Proprioception in the cruciate deficient knee. J Bone Joint Surg Br 74:247–250, 1992.
26. Cowan DN, Jones BH, Frykman PN, et al: Lower limb morphology and risk of overuse injury among male infantry trainees. Med Sci Sports Exerc 28:945–952, 1996.
27. Cowan DN, Jones BH, Robinson JR: Foot morphology characteristics and risk of exercise-related injury. Arch Fam Med 2:773–777, 1993.
28. Culpepper MI, Nieman KM: An investigation of the shoe-turf interface using different types of Poly-Turf and Astro-Turf: Torque and release coefficients. Ala J Med Sci 2:387–390, 1983.
29. Dahle LK, Mueller M, Delitto A, Diamond JE: Visual assessment of foot type and relationship of foot type to lower extremity injury. J Orthop Sports Phys Ther 14:70–74, 1991.
30. Dandy DJ, Poirier H: Chondromalacia and the unstable patella. Acta Orthop Scand 46:695–699, 1975.
31. Deibert MC, Aronsson DD, Johnson RJ, et al: Skiing injuries in children, adolescents, and adults. J Bone Joint Surg Am 80:25–32, 1998.
32. Derscheid GA, Garrick JG: Medial collateral ligament injuries in football: Nonoperative management of grade I and grade II sprains. Am J Sports Med 9:365–368, 1981.

cruciate ligament injuries in female athletes [letter; comment]. Am J Sports Med 27:270–271, 1999.
141. Woo SL, Gomez MA, Sites TJ, et al: The biomechanical and morphologic changes in the medial collateral ligament of the rabbit after immobilization and remobilization. J Bone Joint Surg Am 69: 1200–1211, 1987.

142. Yasuda K, Hayashi K: Changes in biomechanical properties of tendons and ligaments from joint disuse. Osteoarthritis Cartilage 7: 122–129, 1999.
143. Yu WD, Liu SH, Hatch JD, et al: Effect of estrogen on cellular metabolism of the human anterior cruciate ligament. Clin Orthop 366:229–238, 1999.

Section D
Meniscal Injuries

1. MENISCAL INJURIES IN THE ADULT
Marc W. Urquhart, MD ■ James A. O'Leary, MD ■ J. Robert Giffin, MD, FRCSC
Freddie H. Fu, MD, DSc

Historical Perspectives

The meniscus was once perceived as a functionless remnant of a leg muscle.[98] Owing to clinical, biomechanical, and basic science investigations over the past 50 years, the meniscus is now understood to play an integral role in the homeostasis of the knee. The meniscus, through its complex interplay with other soft tissue structures in the knee, serves to protect the hyaline articular cartilage.

King[64] was the first to demonstrate the chondroprotective role of the meniscus in his classic experiment on meniscal healing using a canine model. Severe degeneration of the articular cartilage was noted in animals with complete as well as partial meniscectomies involving the posterior meniscal horn. The author concluded that the meniscus functioned in load absorption and contributed to overall joint stability. His study reaffirmed the role of the meniscus in joint lubrication (previously shown by MacConail[70]) and demonstrated the necessity of a peripheral vascular supply for meniscal healing to occur.

Despite this, total open meniscectomy remained the treatment of choice for meniscal injuries for the next 40 years. Furthermore, Fairbank[39] had also reported radiographic evidence to support the weight-bearing function of the meniscus after surveying knee radiographs of 107 patients following meniscectomy. He observed three characteristic radiographic findings now known as "Fairbank's changes": (1) "anteroposterior ridge projecting downward from the margin of the femoral condyle" (i.e., osteophyte formation), (2) "generalized flattening of the marginal half of the femoral articular surface . . . ," and (3) "narrowing of the joint space." The lateral views showed evidence of a "slight sharpening" of the tibial articular surface. These radiographic features were apparent as early as 5 months postoperatively, but they continued to progress over time. Fairbank concluded that these changes were the result of the loss of "circumferential tension" provided by the meniscus that "resists extrusive forces" and shares weight-bearing.

Over the ensuing years, studies regarding the vascularity and ultrastructure of the meniscus have improved our understanding of meniscal injury and healing.[6, 7, 20] Biome-

chanical investigations have furthered the importance of the meniscus in joint stability and load sharing.* Clinical studies have provided long-term follow-up showing the morbidity associated with meniscal injury or partial/complete meniscectomy.†

Epidemiology

The incidence of an acute meniscal tear is as high as 61 per 100,000.[10] It is estimated that 850,000 meniscal procedures are performed in the United States yearly, and nearly double that number are performed worldwide.[10] Given the largely young, active population involved, a delay in the proper identification and treatment of meniscal injuries can have a tremendous socioeconomic impact. Furthermore, it is essential for clinicians to characterize different types of meniscal injuries, so that they can better understand their natural history and appropriately counsel patients regarding various treatment options.

Laprade and associates[68] reported the prevalence of meniscal tears in the knees of 54 asymptomatic patients (25 men and 29 women) using magnetic resonance imaging (MRI). The average age of these patients was 35.3 years, and the prevalence of meniscal tears was 5.6% (medial, 1.9%; lateral, 3.7%). The authors also noted grade II signal changes involving the posterior horn of the medial meniscus in 24.1% of knees; however, their significance was not known. Furthermore, cadaveric studies have shown the prevalence of degenerative meniscal tears to be approximately 60%.[82] Age-related changes do occur, therefore, within the meniscus over time. It is important for clinicians to distinguish these degenerative tears from injuries sustained during sports because the treatment and outcome for patients are different. Sports-related meniscal injuries account for roughly one third of all patients with torn menisci; pivoting sports such as basketball, football, and wrestling are associated with the greatest number of injur-

*See references 5, 8, 9, 11, 17-19, 41, 44, 69, 79, 90, 92, 93, 95, and 106.
†See references 4, 15, 21, 25, 28, 29, 40, 49, 60, 66, 67, 83, 100, 112, and 113.

ies. The medial meniscus is torn more frequently than the lateral meniscus in all sports except for wrestling.[10]

In a multicenter study, Poehling and colleagues reviewed 6039 meniscal tears, identifying patient factors such as gender, age, tear pattern, associated injuries, and treatment.[87] The male-to-female ratio was 2.5:1. The peak incidence of injury for males was noted in the 31- to 40-year-old group. For females, injury incidence peaked in the 11- to 20-year-old group and remained constant into the seventh decade. Two distinct injury profiles were identified. Traumatic tears in the periphery of the meniscus generally occurred in patients younger than 30 years of age. Degenerative tears typically occurred in patients over the age of 30 and had a more complex tear pattern.[33]

The association of meniscal tears with anterior cruciate ligament (ACL) tears is well known. The incidence of meniscal tears with acute ACL tears has been reported to be as high as 90%.[33] Lateral meniscal injuries occur more frequently with acute ACL tears, whereas medial meniscal injuries occur more often with chronic ACL tears.[54]

Current Concepts/Controversies

New Devices

Within the past decade, the primary question regarding meniscal tears has evolved from, "What tears should I repair?" to, "What should I repair the tear with?" The method of how to repair a meniscal tear used to be confined for the most part to one of four techniques: inside-out, outside-in, all-inside, or open. A multitude of orthopaedic devices for meniscal repair have become available over the past decade, providing surgeons with various tools to be used at their discretion (e.g., fibrin glue, arrows, darts, screws).[57, 76] It is beyond the scope of this chapter to discuss all of these individual devices. The orthopaedist using these devices should be aware of their biomechanical strength and rate of absorption as well as with their techniques of insertion. Unfortunately, many of these meniscal repair devices have been released into the market without the benefit of prospective randomized studies comparing their clinical results or outcomes with those of conventional methods of meniscal repair.

Meniscal Reconstruction

Another topic of debate is the role of meniscal reconstruction in treatment of the postmeniscectomized knee. Reconstruction with meniscal allograft, xenograft, and collagen-based prosthetics has been performed.* In addition, controversy still exists surrounding the most accurate method of determining allograft size, as well as the preferred means of graft fixation. MRI studies have demonstrated the potential for graft extrusion that may be related to improper sizing, fixation, or rim preparation.[89] Fixation of the meniscal horns has commonly been accomplished using a bone bridge, bone plugs, or peripheral sutures, or

---

*See references 58, 75, 97, 102, 105, and 111.

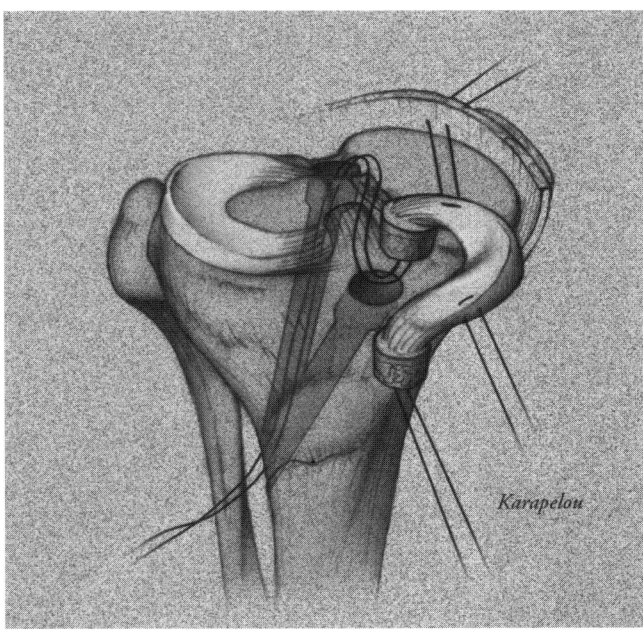

Figure 28D1–1. Meniscal allograft fixation with bone plugs and peripheral sutures. The allograft is inserted through the expanded anteromedial portal. Sutures preinserted through the bone plugs are passed through transosseous tunnels and are tied over a bone bridge on the tibia. Inside-out sutures are then placed peripherally to secure the graft to the capsule. (From Goble M: Meniscal allograft technique. Operative Tech Orthop 10: 220–226, 2000.)

a combination of these methods (Figs. 28D1–1 and 28D1–2).[50] Biomechanical studies have been performed analyzing the graft mobility and load-sharing efficacy associated with various techniques.[84] Radiographic and long-term functional outcome studies are still needed, however, to determine the efficacy of these interventions. Furthermore, follow-up histologic data will add to our understanding of how these grafts interact with the host environment.

Anatomy

Gross Anatomy

The menisci are two semilunar fibrocartilaginous disks interposed between the femoral and tibial condyles (Fig. 28D1–3). The menisci become discernible structures between the eighth and tenth weeks of embryonic gestation. These "C-shaped" structures have a thick peripheral margin that tapers to a thin rim centrally, giving the meniscus a triangular appearance in cross section (Fig. 28D1–4).

Medial Meniscus

The medial meniscus is somewhat semicircular in appearance. It is approximately 3.5 cm in length in the

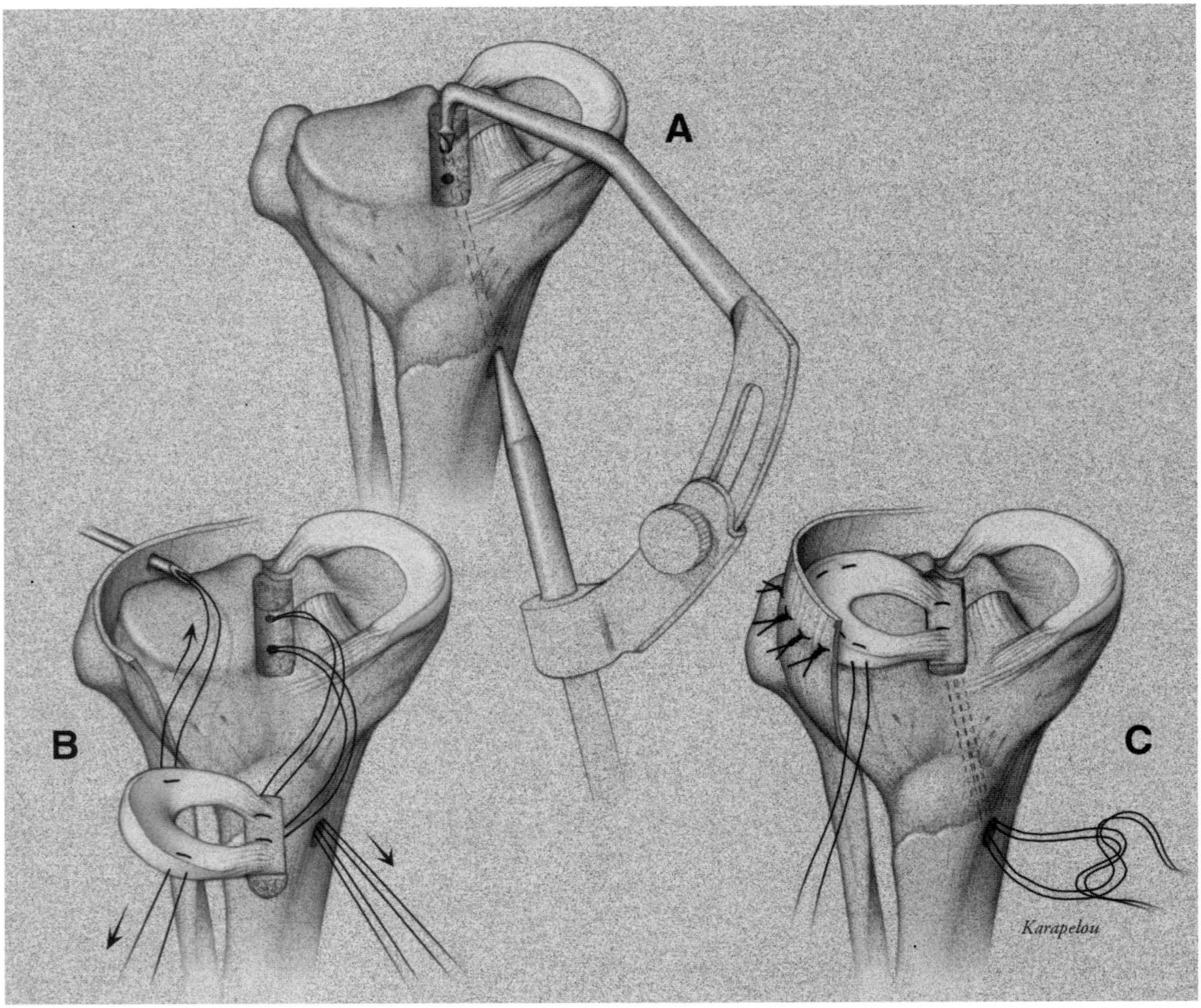

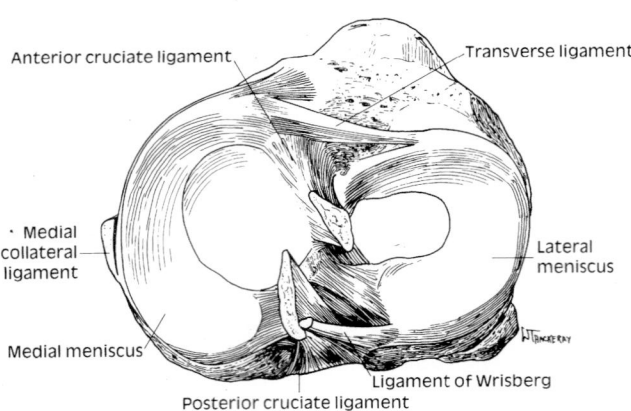

Figure 28D1–2. Meniscal allograft fixation with a bone block and peripheral sutures. *A,* Two transosseous tibial tunnels are placed using an anterior cruciate ligament guide. *B,* The preinserted sutures in the meniscus are passed through the posterolateral capsule. *C,* The preinserted bone block sutures are passed through the tibial tunnels, securing the graft anatomically. (From Goble M: Meniscal allograft technique. Operative Tech Orthop 10: 220–226, 2000.)

Anterior cruciate ligament

Transverse ligament

· Medial collateral ligament

Medial meniscus

Posterior cruciate ligament

Ligament of Wrisberg

Lateral meniscus

Figure 28D1–3. Human knee meniscus as viewed from above. Anterior is on top, medial is to the left, lateral is to the right. (From Warren R, Arnoczky S, Wickiewicz T: Anatomy of the knee. In Nicholas J, Hershman E [eds]: The Lower Extremity and Spine in Sports Medicine. St. Louis, CV Mosby, 1986, pp 657–694.)

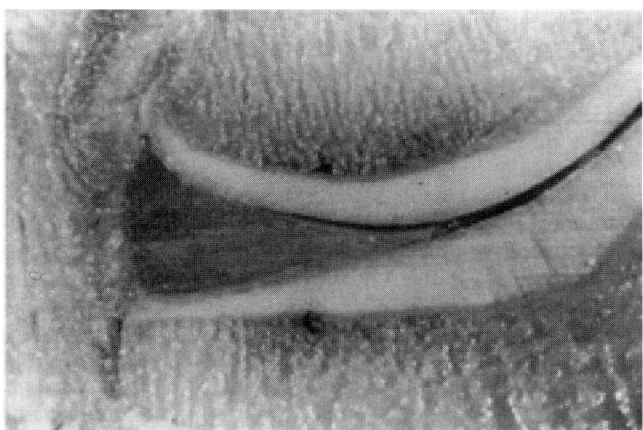

Figure 28D1–4. Coronal section of the medial compartment of the human knee. Femur is above, tibia is below, medial is to the left. (From Warren R, Arnoczky S, Wickiewicz T: Anatomy of the knee. In Nicholas J, Hershman E [eds]: The Lower Extremity and Spine in Sports Medicine. St. Louis, CV Mosby, 1986, pp 657–694.)

anteroposterior dimension and considerably wider posteriorly than it is anteriorly. Its radius of curvature varies, giving it greater length in the sagittal plane than in the coronal plane. The anterior horn is attached to the tibial plateau in the area of the anterior intercondylar fossa, 6 to 7 mm in front of the ACL insertion. An intermeniscal, or "transverse," ligament is present in 64% of individuals; this connects the anterior horn (posterior fibers) of the medial meniscus and the anterior horn (anterior fibers) of the lateral meniscus.[65] The posterior horn attaches to the posterior intercondylar fossa between the attachments of the lateral meniscus and the posterior cruciate ligament (PCL). The medial meniscus is continuously attached to the joint capsule along the entire periphery. The coronary ligament represents the tibial portion of this capsular attachment. At its midpoint, the medial meniscus is firmly attached to the femur and tibia through a robust thickening in the capsule known as the deep medial collateral ligament.

Lateral Meniscus

The lateral meniscus covers a larger portion of the tibial surface than does the medial meniscus. Its radius of curvature remains fairly constant, giving the lateral meniscus an almost circular appearance. The anterior horn is attached anterior to the intercondylar eminence, just posterior and lateral to the ACL attachment with which it partially blends. The posterior horn attaches posterior to the intercondylar eminence, just in front of the posterior end of the medial meniscus. In 50% of individuals, anterior fibers of the posterior enthesis extend to the lateral aspect of the medial femoral condyle, forming the anterior meniscofemoral ligament (ligament of Humphry).[55, 65] In 76% of cases, the posterior fibers of the posterior horn cross posterior to the PCL and attach to the intercondylar fossa of the medial femoral condyle, forming the posterior meniscofemoral ligament (ligament of Wrisberg).[55] The lateral menis-

cus has only a loose peripheral attachment to the capsule, which is interrupted by the popliteus tendon. Lateral meniscal variants, including the most recognized discoid meniscus, have a reported prevalence as high as 16.6% (see "Special Considerations").[43]

Ultrastructure and Biochemistry

Histologically, the meniscus is a fibrocartilaginous structure composed of a network of interlacing collagen fibers and interspersed fibrochondrocytes. Two types of fibrochondrocytes maintain the extracellular matrix (ECM). The superficial layer contains oval or spindle-shaped cells, whereas the deeper layers contain polygonal cells with dendritic projections.[46]

The meniscus is a biphasic structure, having a solid phase of collagen and ECM and a fluid phase of water and electrolytes. The extracellular matrix is composed of 78% water. Its dry weight is 75% collagen, 1% hexosamine, and the remainder noncollagenous proteins and elastin.[38] Type I collagen that is found in bone, tendon, ligament, and fibrocartilage accounts for 90% of the collagen in the meniscus. Lesser amounts of type II, III, IV, V, and VI collagen are also present.[5, 38, 47, 72] In humans, collagen content increases with weight-bearing and joint motion until 30 years of age. The collagen content then remains relatively stable until the eighth decade of life. With aging, the collagen content starts to decrease in the meniscus and there is an associated increase in noncollagenous matrix proteins and hexosamine.[47]

The ultrastructure of the meniscus has been visualized using light and scanning electron microscopy. These studies have shown that the meniscus comprises three structurally distinct layers. A *superficial layer* has a meshlike pattern woven with fine fibrils; a *surface layer* lies just beneath it with randomly oriented collagen fibers; and a *middle layer* with collagen fibers forms a uniform circumferential pattern.[12] In this middle layer, periodic radial fibers ("tie fibers") extend from the periphery into the inner rim and are believed to resist longitudinal splitting of the circumferential fibers.[20, 48, 73] It is this unique framework that allows the meniscus to convert axial loads to circumferential stresses.

Vascularity

During embryonal development, nearly the entire meniscus is vascularized. As an individual approaches 40 years of age, only the peripheral 10% to 30% of the meniscus remains vascularized. The predominant blood supply to the menisci originates from superior and inferior branches of the lateral and medial genicular arteries of the knee.[5, 6, 31, 32] These vessels form a perimeniscal capillary plexus within synovial and capsular tissue. This vascular network is oriented in a circumferential pattern, with radial branches directed centrally.

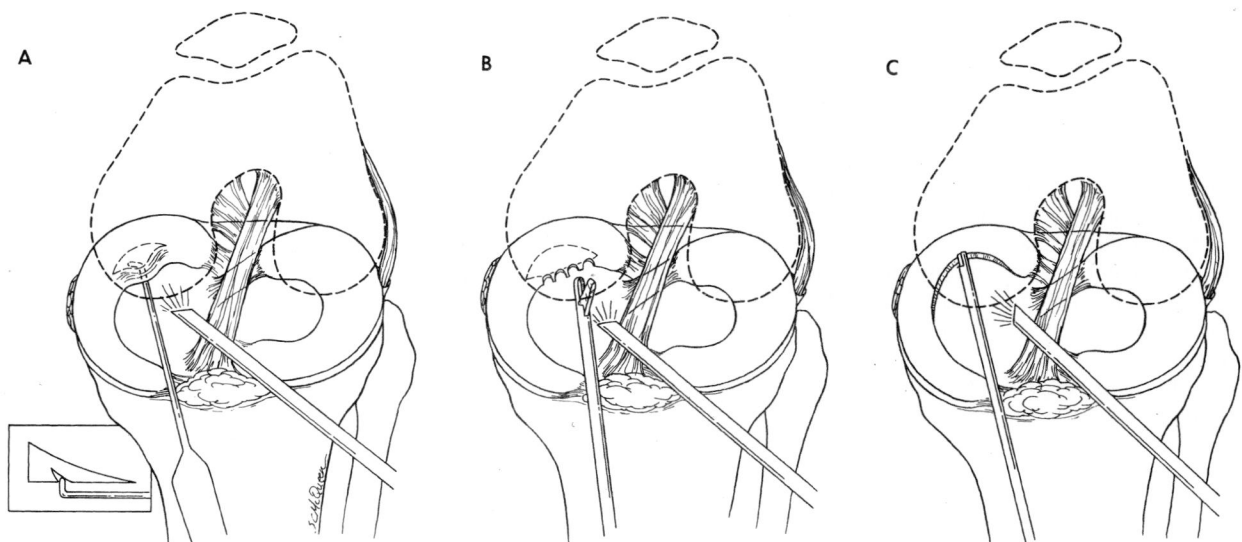

Figure 28D1–6. Resection of a partial vertical longitudinal tear. *A,* Probing the tear to identify the margins and depth. *B,* Resection of the unstable fragment with a basket forceps. *C,* The stable, peripheral rim is contoured with a motorized meniscal resector. (From Phillips BB: Arthroscopy of the lower extremity. In Canale T [ed]: Campbell's Operative Orthopaedics, 9th ed. St. Louis, Mosby, 1998, pp 1470–1561.)

anterolateral portal between the PCL and the medial femoral condyle. Visualization is enhanced further with posteromedial rotation of the tibia relative to the femur. Alternatively, the 70-degree arthroscope can be placed in the posteromedial portal to provide views of tears in this region.

The next step in meniscal repair is preparation of the meniscus. Based on the size and location of the tear, the surgeon must decide whether to implement techniques to enhance meniscal healing. Débridement of the tear with a rasp or motorized resector has been shown to facilitate healing, especially with chronic tears. If the vascularity of the tear bed is in question following débridement, then further healing enhancement techniques should be considered. Arnoczky and coworkers[5] demonstrated the beneficial effects of an exogenous fibrin clot in the repair process of canine meniscal tears in the avascular zone. Abrading the perimeniscal synovium and creating vascular access channels from the vascularized periphery to the edge of the tear are other methods that have been used to improve healing in areas of questionable vascularity.[45a, 53, 97]

The final key step to successful meniscal repair is the anatomical reduction of the meniscus and maintenance of this reduction with the selected suture or device. Vertical mattress sutures have been shown to have greater pullout strength than horizontal mattress sutures because of their ability to encompass more circumferentially oriented collagen bundles of the meniscus.[14a]

The Open Technique

Dehaven reported the earliest series of open meniscal repair using current techniques in the 1980s.[32a] The introduction of arthroscopy had led to improved visualization of meniscal injuries and helped determine which lesions were amenable for repair. Tears ideal for this technique are vertical tears in the posterior horns of the medial or lateral

meniscus at or within 2 mm of the meniscocapsular junction.

For open medial meniscal repair (Fig. 28D1–7A), the incision is made just posterior to the medial collateral ligament (MCL) centered over the medial joint line. The infrapatellar branch of the saphenous nerve is visualized and protected. The sartorius fascia is then incised, allowing the semitendinosus and gracilis to fall posteriorly. The capsule is then incised vertically or obliquely. Transillumination from the arthroscope can be used to guide the approach. The meniscal tear and perimeniscal synovium are abraded, and vertical or horizontal mattress suturing is then performed.

The open approach to lateral meniscal tears (Fig. 28D1–7B) is begun with a vertical incision just posterior to the lateral collateral ligament (LCL). The interval between the iliotibial band and the biceps femoris is then defined. The peroneal nerve is safely protected and remains posterior to the biceps. The lateral head of the gastrocnemius must be dissected free from the posterolateral joint capsule. The capsule is then incised vertically or obliquely. The meniscal tear is rasped and sutured, and then a layered closure is performed.

The clinical success of open meniscal repairs has ranged from 79% to 91% in series with longer than 10 years of follow-up.[33a] Failures were more likely to occur with chronic tears of longer than 6 weeks' duration and with repairs performed in unstable knees. Postoperative MRI has demonstrated persistent high-grade signal changes, which did not correlate well with the clinical outcomes.

The Outside-In Technique

The reported advantages of the outside-in technique are that it avoids a capsulotomy, is performed with readily available materials, and permits easy access to tears involving the anterior and middle horns of the meniscus. The

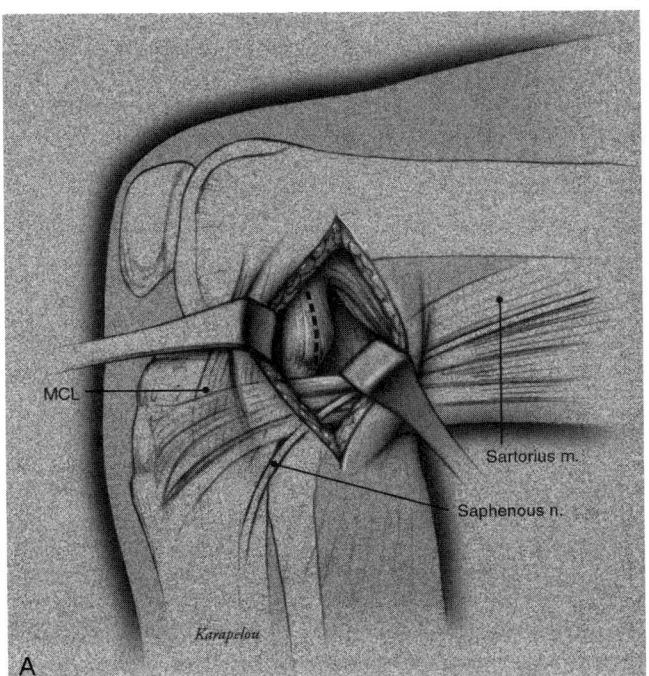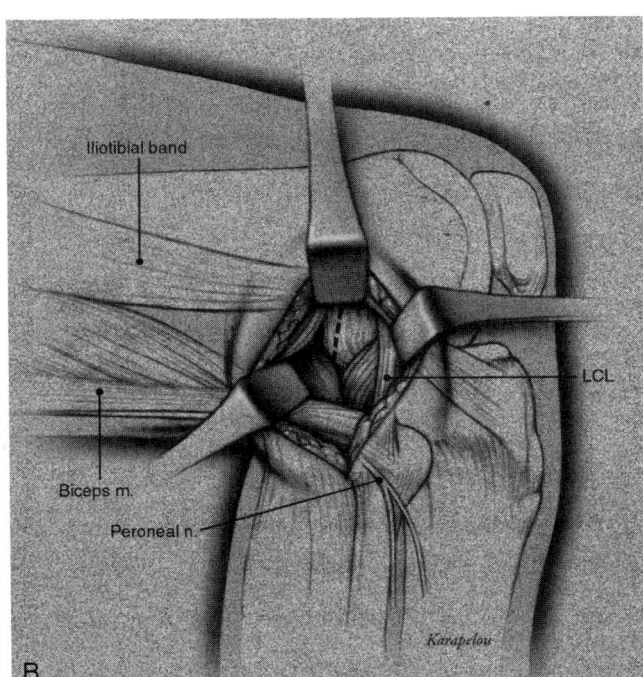

Figure 28D1–7. *A,* Anatomy for medial meniscal repair. *B,* Anatomy for lateral meniscal repair. LCL, lateral collateral ligament; MCL, medial collateral ligament. (From Bottoni CR, Arciero RA: Conventional meniscal repair techniques. Operative Tech Orthop 10:194–208, 2000.)

major disadvantage of this technique is that it does not easily access the posterior horn.[76b, 107a]

The procedure is begun by exposing the capsule in the area of the tear. The edges of the tear are débrided, and the synovium is abraded arthroscopically. A 14- or 16-gauge needle is then introduced from outside the capsule through the meniscal tear, reducing the outer and inner fragments. The 2–0 absorbable suture is then passed through the needle into the joint. The next step can be accomplished using several different methods:

1. A suture retrieval instrument can be inserted in an outside-in fashion parallel to the initial needle insertion site, thereby enabling the free end of the suture to be retrieved and pulled outside the capsule to be tied to the other end of the suture over the capsule.

2. Another suture can be passed via a large-bore needle parallel and adjacent to the first; the intra-articular ends are then pulled out through the anterior portal, and a large "mulberry" knot is tied on each individual end; the knots are pulled into the inner rim of the tear, and the free ends of the suture are tied over the capsule.[107a]

3. Another suture can be passed via a large-bore needle parallel and adjacent to the first; the intra-articular ends are then pulled out through the anterior portal, and these two ends are tied together; the knot is pulled through the meniscus and the free ends of the suture are tied over the capsule.[76b]

4. A wire snare can be passed through a second needle parallel to the first. The suture is passed into the joint through the first needle and is brought out the second via the wire snare, with the free ends tied over the capsule.

The outside-in repair technique has a reported success rate of greater than 90%. The mulberry knots have been shown to be weaker than horizontal and vertical mattress sutures in biomechanical studies, but no reported difference has been shown in clinical outcome.[107a]

The All-Inside Technique

The all-inside technique was introduced in 1991 with the major advantage of decreasing the risk of neurovascular injury.[76a, 80a] It is especially well suited for posterocentral, peripheral meniscal tears. The technique also prevents capsular plication, which could cause knee stiffness and altered meniscal excursion. The major disadvantage is that it is technically demanding, requiring use of a posterior arthroscopic portal, as well as specialized suturing and knot-tying instruments.

A 70-degree arthroscope is used to obtain a "modified Gillquist" view of the posterior compartment. With the knee flexed 90 degrees, the posteromedial or posterolateral portal is established. The meniscus is prepared with a rasp or motorized resector. A curved, cannulated meniscal repair instrument is passed through an arthroscopic cannula and through the edges of the tear. The suture is threaded through the meniscus. Intracapsular arthroscopic knots are then placed on the outer edge of the meniscus.

The Inside-Out Technique

Inside-out meniscal repair was popularized by Henning in the 1980s.[52a] It has the advantages of accessing the anterior two thirds of the lateral and medial menisci. The disadvantages of this technique are that if care is not taken

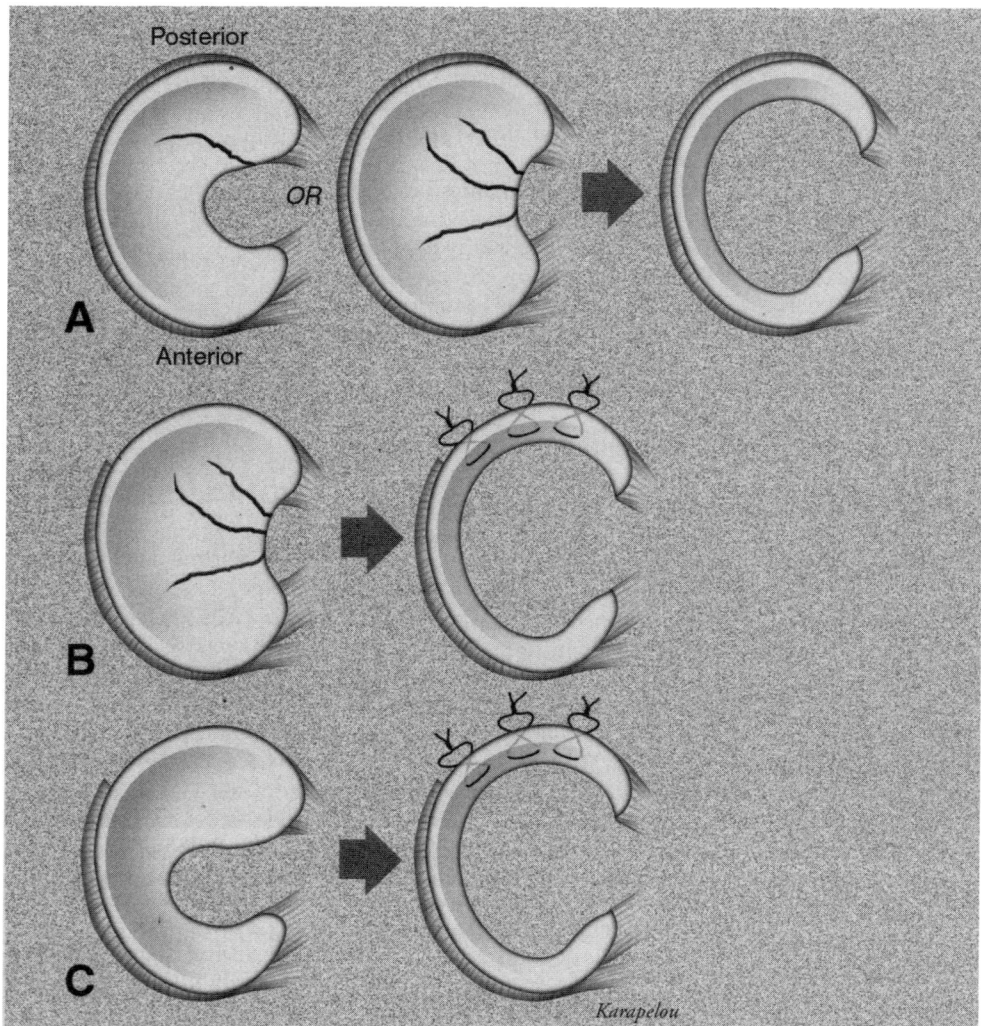

Figure 28D1-9. Technical approaches to lateral meniscal variants. *A,* Partial excision for stable torn discoid meniscus. *B,* Partial excision and peripheral meniscocapsular stabilization for torn unstable discoid meniscus. *C,* Reduction and peripheral meniscocapsular stabilization for unstable discoid meniscus. (From Jordan MR: Lateral meniscal variants. Operative Tech Orthop 10:234–244, 2000.)

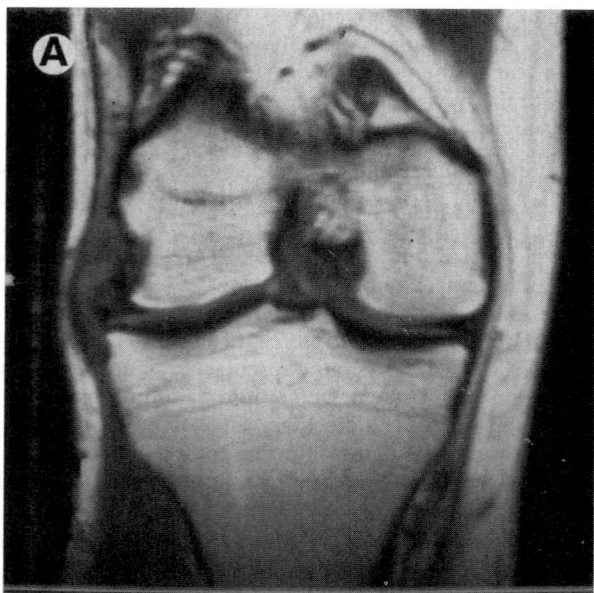
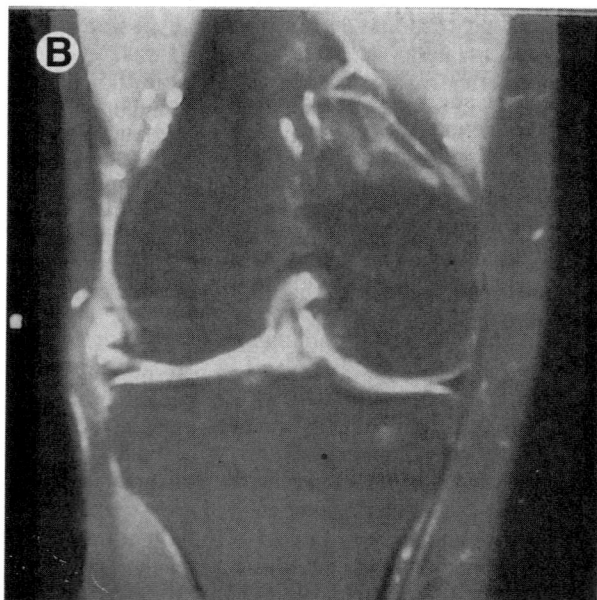

Figure 28D1-10. Magnetic resonance imaging scans of a lateral meniscal cyst. *A,* T$_1$ weighted; *B,* T$_2$ weighted. (From Kim CW, Tontz W Jr, Pedowitz RA: Meniscal cysts. Operative Tech Orthop 10:227–233, 2000.)

Complications of Treatment

Complication rates of knee arthroscopy can range from 0.8% to 8.2%. The most common of these include hemarthrosis, instrument failure, thrombophlebitis, and infection. Complications of meniscal repair occur infrequently, with a reported rate of 1.3%.[96b] The most common complications related to meniscal surgery are failure of repair, neurovascular injury, and arthrofibrosis.

Rates of failure of meniscal repair range from 5% to 29% in the literature.[76b, 97a, 110a] These rates are so variable because "failure" is defined by MRI findings or clinical examination, or is based on repeat arthroscopy. Second-look arthroscopy has revealed that up to 50% of patients with arthroscopically determined failures are asymptomatic.[52b, 100a] Arthrographic or arthroscopic assessment after meniscal repair allows classification of the meniscus into three categories: healed, incompletely healed, or not healed. To minimize failures, one must be prudent in assessing the "reparability" of the tear and in implementing the necessary measures to enhance healing (e.g., fibrin clot). Neurovascular injury is a relatively uncommon complication that can have lasting, deleterious effects. Vascular injury is very rare with the use of a Henning or popliteal retractor. Peripheral nerve injury may result from excessive retraction, laceration, or incorporation of the nerve into the suture loop or fixation. The proximity of the nerve to the capsule, as well as the number of nerve branches, is related to the risk of injury.

The saphenous nerve is the most vulnerable to injury. The incidence of saphenous nerve symptoms following medial meniscal repair has been reported as high as 43%.[96b] Symptoms generally resolve within 3 months unless the nerve has been lacerated or incorporated into the suture. The popliteal artery and vein and the tibial nerve are also at risk with placement of posterior and posterocentral instrumentation. During lateral meniscal repair, the common peroneal nerve, the popliteal artery and vein, and, to a lesser extent, the tibial nerve are at risk. The peroneal nerve should be palpated and, if need be, visualized at this level before meniscal repair is undertaken. The keys to avoiding neurovascular injury are obtaining adequate exposure at the juxtacapsular level with the knee in the appropriate amount of flexion, being cognizant of the neurovascular structures during the surgical approach, and protecting these structures with appropriate retraction.

Arthrofibrosis, or contracture, is another potential complication of meniscal repair. Risk can be minimized by preventing entrapment of the posterior capsule; this can be done by ensuring that the knee is in the appropriate position when the meniscocapsular fixation is implemented. Other complications such as infection and skin breakdown can be decreased with meticulous handling of the soft tissue and avoidance of tying sutures over wide soft tissue bridges.

Anesthesia

Arthroscopic knee surgery traditionally has been performed with general or spinal anesthesia. Local anesthesia with or without intravenous sedation is an effective alternative, particularly with arthroscopic meniscectomies. The use of combinations of 1% lidocaine with epinephrine (1:200,000) and 0.25% bupivacaine hydrochloride (Marcaine) with epinephrine (1:200,000) to infiltrate arthroscopic portal sites, as well as intra-articularly, provides excellent analgesia for up to 2½ hours. Furthermore, it often decreases the need for tourniquet use. With more involved surgeries (e.g., meniscal repair via open incision), regional anesthesia with femoral and sciatic nerve blocks is useful. In our experience, regional blocks reduce the patient's intraoperative discomfort caused by manipulation of the knee with varus or valgus stresses; they also significantly diminish pain during the immediate postoperative period.

The Author's Preferred Technique

Arthroscopic evaluation and treatment is offered to individuals with a history and physical examination consistent with a symptomatic meniscal tear. If the clinical scenario is equivocal, or concomitant articular cartilage injury is suspected, an MRI using the appropriate sequences is obtained. If a reparable lesion is anticipated on the basis of the preoperative work-up, the patient is presented with the idea of meniscal repair and the usual time frame for rehabilitation and recovery. The ideal candidate is compliant and physiologically active and expresses a firm desire and commitment to return to his or her pre-injury activity level. Candidates are not excluded on the basis of age alone. Patients are instructed to avoid any "squatting activities." Most patients receive preoperative physical therapy instruction emphasizing quadriceps function. Patients with concomitant ligamentous injury must undergo preoperative therapy, and their surgery must be postponed until adequate motion and quadriceps function are recovered. Operative consent for meniscal repair versus meniscectomy is obtained, and the patient is counseled about the potential complications of surgery.

The operation is performed under regional anesthesia (femoral and sciatic nerve blocks) or spinal anesthesia. A detailed examination under anesthesia is performed on both knees to detect any motion deficits or ligamentous injury. The procedure is generally performed under tourniquet control with the extremity in a thigh holder. The diagnostic portion of the arthroscopy is performed via the standard anterolateral portal with a 30-degree arthroscope. A thorough, systematic inspection of the synovium, articular cartilage, intra-articular ligaments, and menisci is performed. The suprapatellar space and lateral and medial recesses are viewed to rule out loose bodies. A modified Gillquist view is used to assess the posterior meniscocapsular junction.

The meniscal disease is quantitated and characterized. The tear pattern, length, depth, and distance from the meniscocapsular junction are determined with the use of the meniscal probe. We consider reparable tears to be those that are vertically/longitudinally oriented, with full thickness, and within 3 to 5 mm of the meniscosynovial junction (i.e., the red-red or red-white zone). In young, active patients and in those patients undergoing simultaneous ACL reconstruction, we have extended our indications to include more central tears.

In our experience, meniscal tears longer than 15 mm are unstable and can be displaced with the probe. After the full extent of the tear has been appreciated, the tear is débrided with a 2.5-mm full-radius resector and a double-sided, angled meniscal rasp. The perimeniscal synovium is abraded with the shaver as well. The technique of repair chosen will depend on whether the location of the tear is the anterior third or the posterior two thirds of the meniscus.

Tears in the posterior two thirds of the meniscus are repaired using the inside-out technique. The arthroscope is placed in the ipsilateral anterior portal, and the zone-specific, single-lumen meniscal repair cannula is placed in the contralateral anterior portal. The appropriate cannula will allow for accurate suture placement orthogonal to the meniscal tear and will guide the meniscal needles away from the posterior neurovascular bundle. For medial meniscal repairs, the dissection begins with the knee in 70 to 90 degrees of flexion. The arthroscope is placed through the intercondylar notch to transilluminate the posteromedial capsule. Oftentimes, the shadow of the saphenous vein can be visualized, providing the surgeon with a landmark of where to anticipate the location of the saphenous nerve. A 2-cm vertical incision is made just posterior to the MCL, with one third of the length above the joint line and two thirds below the joint line. The subcutaneous tissue is dissected bluntly to enable identification of the infrapatellar branches of the saphenous nerve. The interval between the pes anserinus and the posteromedial joint capsule is dissected, and a Henning retractor is placed to maintain the interval.

For tears in the posterior two thirds of the lateral meniscus, the knee is placed in 90 degrees of flexion, and a 2-cm incision is placed just posterior to the lateral collateral ligament, with one third of the incision above the joint line and two thirds of the incision below the joint line. The interval between the iliotibial band and the biceps femoris is dissected in a proximal-to-distal direction. Occasionally, for insertion of sutures at the junction of the anterior and middle thirds, the iliotibial band insertion must be partially elevated and repaired. The peroneal nerve is palpated behind the biceps, which will fall posteriorly with the dissection. Next, the interval between the lateral head of the gastrocnemius must be defined. This is best determined by beginning distally, where the gastrocnemius tendon is less adherent to the capsule, and working proximally, where the tendon must be lifted off the capsule with care. The Henning retractor is then placed between the capsule and the lateral gastrocnemius tendon.

The knee is then placed in the proper position—10 to 20 degrees of flexion with valgus stress for the medial repair; or figure-of-four with 45 degrees of flexion for the lateral repair. Double-armed 2–0 polydioxanone sutures (PDS) are passed through the single-lumen catheters into the femoral surface of the inner meniscal fragment. The cannula is used to reduce the meniscus, and the suture is passed through the outer rim and capsule. The needle is advanced 1 cm at a time. As the surgeon is advancing the needle, he or she should call out the orientation of the cannula (e.g., superior for the femoral surface, posterior for the placement of sutures at the posterior portion of the tear). The assistant must be experienced at anticipating the

emergence of the needle. The posterior capsule will bulge before it is penetrated, and the needle tip can be "palpated" with the heavy needle driver that the assistant will use for retrieval. Once the needle tip emerges through the capsule, the assistant orients the Henning retractor to guide the needle away from the neurovascular structures and out of the wound. Once the needle tip has pierced the capsule and the retractor is positioned properly, the assistant tells the primary surgeon to advance. Communication is essential between the primary surgeon ("pitcher") and the fist assistant ("catcher") so that the meniscal repair can be performed efficiently and safely. The other arm of the suture is passed in a horizontal mattress fashion on the femoral surface 3 mm from the first. The two needles are removed from the surgical field and the ends of the mattress suture are clamped. A gentle "tug" on this suture will reduce and elevate the meniscus to facilitate placement of the next horizontal mattress suture on the tibial surface. The sutures are placed approximately 3 to 4 mm from the last with the use of horizontal mattresses that alternate on the femoral and tibial sides; this reduces the meniscus on both the tibial and femoral surfaces. On occasion, if only a few sutures are needed in the case of a short tear, a diverging vertical mattress suture is interspersed between the horizontal mattresses to increase the pullout strength of the repair.

Meniscal tears in the anterior third are managed with an outside-in technique. The meniscus is prepared in a similar fashion with the rasp and motorized shaver. The arthroscope is placed in the contralateral anterior portal, and a 14- or 16-gauge spinal needle is placed percutaneously through the capsule and both ends of the tear. The suture is passed through the needle, and the free intra-articular end is retrieved with a "grabber." A mulberry knot is placed, and the suture is drawn back against the torn fragment to reduce the tear. A second suture is placed in a similar fashion 3 to 4 mm next to the first in a horizontal mattress fashion. Through a small anterior incision, the two ends of the suture are tied down on the anterior capsule. We have alternatively used arthroscopic suture passers and retrievers to perform an outside-in repair, obviating the need for the mulberry knot. In our experience, patients have not demonstrated significant clinical differences.

Once all the sutures are passed and clamped, the knee is taken through an arc of motion from 0 to 90 degrees to ensure that the posterior capsule is not plicated. Arthroscopically, anatomic reduction is confirmed throughout, and if any incongruency is observed, the offending stitch is removed and replaced. The sutures are tied with the knee in 15 to 20 degrees of flexion in a sequential posterior-to-anterior order.

Rehabilitation after Meniscal Repair

Postoperative rehabilitation of the meniscal repair has remained an area of controversy and subjectivity. Historically, postoperative protocols required longer periods of immobilization and non–weight-bearing for up to 6 weeks after meniscal repair. Recent studies have demonstrated no deleterious effects from early, aggressive return to activity.

On the topic of weight-bearing status, some authors

recommend strict non–weight-bearing for 6 to 8 weeks. Others allow partial weight-bearing for varying periods, and some even allow unlimited weight-bearing immediately.

Opinions regarding immobilization are also divergent, some requiring immobilization for up to 8 weeks. Some mandate immobilization in full extension, based on the fact that the posterior horn bucket handle tear reduces to the posterior capsule in extension and separates from the capsule with flexion. Other investigators immobilize the knee in varying positions of flexion. Many have adopted protocols allowing early limited range of motion in a hinged brace.

Currently, our patients follow a five-phase rehabilitation protocol. The initial phase (0 to 4 weeks) allows "toe-touch" weight-bearing, with the knee brace locked in full extension. The hinged knee brace is set to allow 0 to 90 degrees of flexion. Continuous passive motion machines are used to facilitate early motion within this range. Patellar mobilization and straight leg raises are begun immediately. In phase II (4 to 8 weeks), weight-bearing is progressed as tolerated, with the hinged knee brace locked in full extension. Crutches are discontinued when the patient has no extension lag on straight leg raising and exhibits good quadriceps control with the weight acceptance phase of gait. Phase III (8 to 12 weeks) emphasizes strengthening with the use of light weights and high rates of repetition. During this phase, the brace is discontinued; full, unrestricted motion is allowed; and deep squats (more than 90 degrees of flexion) are avoided. Low-impact activities are begun at 12 weeks (phase IV). Swimming, straight-ahead jogging, and use of treadmills/exercise bikes/stair steppers are encouraged. The intensity and duration of these workouts can be increased, with pain and swelling being the limiting factors.

Criteria for Return to Sports

In the final stage of rehabilitation, sport-specific exercises are performed to prepare the athlete for return to competition. Jumping athletes will regain strength and develop endurance by jumping rope and doing workouts on a mini-trampoline. Pivoting and agility drills on varying surfaces will improve proprioception. There is no consensus on when an athlete is ready to return to competition, but the ability to single-leg hop; demonstration of 80% strength of the contralateral quadriceps; and return to full, painless range of motion with no effusion are useful guidelines. In our opinion, bracing is optional. Its main role is to aid in proprioception; therefore, a neoprene knee sleeve provides adequate bracing.

References

1. Ahmed AM, Burke DL: In vitro measurement of static pressure distribution in synovial joints. Part 1: Tibial surface of the knee. J Biomech Eng 105:216–225, 1983.
2. Allen C, Wong E, Livesay G, et al: The importance of the medial meniscus in the ACL-deficient knee. J Orthop Res 18:109–115, 2000.
3. Anderson AF, Lipscomb AB: Clinical diagnosis of meniscal tears. Description of a new manipulative test. Am J Sports Med 14:291–293, 1986.
3a. Annandale T: An operation for displaced semilunar cartilage. Br Med J 1:779, 1885.
4. Appel H: Late results after meniscectomy in the knee joint. A clinical and roentgenographic follow-up investigation. Acta Orthop Scand Suppl 133:1–111, 1970.
5. Arnoczky SP, Adams ME, DeHaven K, et al: Meniscus. In Woo SL-Y, Buckwalter J (eds): Injury and Repair of the Musculoskeletal Soft Tissues. Park Ridge, Illinois, The American Academy of Orthopaedic Surgeons, 1988.
6. Arnoczky SP, Warren RF: Microvasculature of the human meniscus. Am J Sports Med 10:90–95, 1982.
7. Arnoczky SP, Warren RF: Microvasculature of the human meniscus and its response to injury. An experimental study in the dog. Am J Sports Med 11:131–141, 1983.
8. Aspden RM, Yarker YE, Hukins DWL: Collagen orientations in the meniscus of the knee joint. J Anat 140:371–380, 1985.
9. Aspden RM: A model for function and failure of the meniscus. Eng Med 14:119–122, 1985.
10. Baker BE, Peckham AC, Pupparo F, Sanborn JC: Review of meniscal injury and associated sports. Am J Sports Med 13:1–4, 1985.
11. Baratz ME, Fu FH, Mengato R: Meniscal tears: The effect of meniscectomy and of repair on intraarticular contact areas and stress in the human knee. Am J Sports Med 16:1–5, 1986.
12. Beaupre A, Choukroun R, Guidouin R, et al: Knee menisci: Correlation between microstructure and biomechanics. Clin Orthop 208:72–75, 1986.
13. Bird MD, Sweet MB: A system of canals in semilunar menisci. Ann Rheum Dis 46:670-673, 1987.
14. Bird MD, Sweet MB: Canals in the semilunar meniscus. Brief report. J Bone Joint Surg Br 70:839, 1988.
14a. Boenisch UW, Faber KJ, Ciarelli M, et al: Pull-out strength and stiffness of meniscal repair using absorbable arrows or Ti-Cron vertical and horizontal loop sutures. Am J Sports Med 27:626–631, 1999.
15. Bolano LE, Grana WA: Isolated arthroscopic partial meniscectomy. Am J Sports Med 21:432–437, 1993.
16. Bonin M, Carret JP, Dimnet J, et al: The weight-bearing knee after anterior cruciate ligament rupture. An in vitro biomechanical study. Knee Surg Sports Traumatol Arthrosc 3:245–251, 1996.
17. Bourne RB, Finlay B, Papadopoulos D, Andrea P: The effect of medial meniscectomy on strain distribution in the proximal tibia. J Bone Joint Surg Am 66:1431–1437, 1984.
18. Brantigan OC, Voshell AE: The mechanics of the ligaments and menisci of the knee joint. J Bone Joint Surg Am 23:44–66, 1941.
18a. Bronstein R, Kirk P, Hurley J: The usefulness of MRI in evaluating menisci after meniscal repair. Orthopedics 15:149–152, 1992.
19. Brown TD, Shaw DT: In vitro stress distributions on the femoral condyles. J Orthop Res 2:190–199, 1984.
20. Bullough PG, Munuera L, Murphy J, Weinstein AM: The strength of the menisci as it relates to their fine structure. J Bone Joint Surg Br 52:564–570, 1970.
21. Burr DB, Radin EL: Meniscal function and the importance of meniscal regeneration in preventing late medial compartment osteoarthrosis. Clin Orthop 171:121–126, 1982.
21a. Buseck MS, Noyes FR: Arthroscopic evaluation of meniscal repairs after anterior cruciate ligament reconstruction and immediate mobilization. Am J Sports Med 19:489–494, 1991.
22. Cabaud HE, Rodkey WG, Fitzwater JE: Medial meniscus repairs. An experimental and morphologic study. Am J Sports Med 9:129–134, 1981.
23. Cannon WD, Vittori JM: The incidence of healing in arthroscopic meniscal repairs in anterior cruciate ligament reconstructed knees versus stable knees. Am J Sports Med 20:176–181, 1992.
24. Carpenter WA: Meniscofemoral ligament simulating tear of the lateral meniscus: MR features. J Comput Assist Tomogr 14:1033–1034, 1990.
25. Casscells SW: The place of arthroscopy in the diagnosis and treatment of internal derangement of the knee. Clin Orthop 151:135–142, 1980.
26. Cheung LP, Li KCP, Hollett MD, et al: Meniscal tears of the knee: Accuracy of detection with fast spin-echo MR imaging and arthroscopic correlation in 293 patients. Radiology 203:508–512, 1997.

27. Crues JV, Mink J, Levy TL, et al: Meniscal tears of the knee: Accuracy of MR imaging. Radiology 164:445–448, 1987.

28. Dandy DJ, Jackson RW: Meniscectomy and chondromalacia of the femoral condyle. J Bone Joint Surg Am 57:1116–1119, 1975.

29. Dandy DJ, Jackson RW: The diagnosis of problems after meniscectomy. J Bone Joint Surg Br 57:349–352, 1982.

30. Daniel D, Daniels E, Aronson D: The diagnosis of meniscal pathology. Clin Orthop 163:218–224, 1982.

31. Danzig L, Resnick D, Gonsalves M, et al: Blood supply to the normal and abnormal menisci of the human knee. Clin Orthop 172:271–276, 1983.

32. Day B, MacKenzie WG, Shim SS, et al: The vascular supply and the nerve supply of the human meniscus. Arthroscopy 1:58–62, 1985.

32a. DeHaven KE: Peripheral meniscal repair: An alternative to meniscectomy. J Bone Joint Surg Br 63:463, 1981.

32b. DeHaven KE: Meniscal repair. Am J Sports Med 27:242–250, 1999.

33. DeHaven KE: Decision-making factors in the treatment of meniscus lesions. Clin Orthop 252:49–54, 1990.

33a. DeHaven KE, Black KP, Griffiths HJ: Open meniscus repair: Technique and 2- to 9-year results. Am J Sports Med 17:788–795, 1989.

34. DeHaven KE, Collins HR: Diagnosis of internal derangements of the knee. J Bone Joint Surg 57:802–810, 1975.

35. Dervin GF, Paterson RS: Oblique menisco-meniscal ligament of the knee. Arthroscopy 13:363–365, 1997.

36. DeSmet AA, Norris MA, Yandow DR, et al: MR diagnosis of meniscal tears of the knee: Importance of high signal in the meniscus that extends to the surface. AJR Am J Roentgenol 161:101–107, 1993.

37. Escobedo EM, Hunter JC, Zink-Brody GC, et al: Usefulness of turbo spin-echo MR imaging in the evaluation of meniscal tears: Comparison with conventional spin-echo sequence. AJR Am J Roentgenol 167:1223–1227, 1996.

38. Eyre D, Wu J: Collagen of fibrocartilage: A distinctive molecular phenotype in bovine meniscus. FEBS Lett 158:265–270, 1983.

39. Fairbank TJ: Knee joint changes after meniscectomy. J Bone Joint Surg Br 30:664–670, 1948.

40. Fauno P, Nielsen AB: Arthroscopic partial meniscectomy: A long-term follow-up. Arthroscopy 8:345–349. 1992.

41. Frankel VH, Burnstein AH: Biomechanics of internal derangement of the knee. J Bone Joint Surg Am 53:945–962, 1971.

42. Freeman M, Wyke B: The innervation of the knee joint. An anatomical and histological study in the cat. J Anat 101:505–532, 1967.

43. Fujikawa K, Iseki F, Mikura Y: Partial resection of the discoid meniscus in the child's knee. J Bone Joint Surg Br 63:391–395, 1981.

44. Fukubayashi T, Kurosawa H: The contact area and pressure distribution pattern of the knee. Acta Orthop Scand 51:871–879, 1980.

45. Gardner E: The innervation of the knee joint. Anat Rec 101, 1948.

45a. Gershuni DH, Skyhar MJ, Danzig LA, et al: Experimental models to promote healing of tears in the avascular segment of canine knee menisci. J Bone Joint Surg Am 17:1363–1370, 1989.

46. Ghadially FN, Thomas I, Yong N, Launde J-MA: Ultrastructure of rabbit semilunar cartilage. J Anat 125:499–517, 1978.

47. Ghosh P, Ingman AM, Taylor TK: Variations in collagen, noncollagenous proteins, and hexosamine in menisci derived from osteoarthritic and rheumatoid arthritic knee joints. J Rheumatol 2:100–107, 1975.

48. Ghosh P, Taylor TK: The knee joint meniscus: A fibrocartilage of some distinction. Clin Orthop 224:52–63, 1987.

49. Gillies H, Seligson D: Precision in the diagnosis of meniscal lesions: A comparison of clinical evaluation, arthrography, and arthroscopy. J Bone Joint Surg Am 61:343–346, 1979.

49a. Gillquist J, Hegberg G, Oretorp N: Arthroscopic examination of the posteromedial compartment of the knee joint. Int Orthop 3:313, 1979.

49b. Glass RS, Barnes WM, Kells PU, et al: Ossicles of the knee menisci. Clin Orthop 111:163–171, 1979.

50. Goble M: Meniscal allograft technique. Operative Tech Orthop 10:220–226, 2000.

50a. Graf B, Docter T, Clancy W Jr: Arthroscopic meniscal repair. Clin Sports Med 6:525–536, 1987.

51. Gronblad M, Korkala O, Liesi P, et al: Innervation of synovial membrane and meniscus. Acta Orthop Scand 56:484–486, 1985.

51a. Hamada M, Konsei S, Kiyoski K, et al: Usefulness of magnetic resonance imaging for detecting intrasubstance tear and/or degeneration of lateral discoid meniscus. Arthroscopy 10:645–653, 1994.

52. Hamberg P, Gillquist J, Lysholm J: Suture of new and old peripheral meniscus tears. J Bone Joint Surg Am 65:193–197, 1983.

52a. Henning CE: Arthroscopic repair of meniscal tears. Orthopedics 6:1130–1132, 1983.

52b. Henning CE, Clark JR, Lynch MA: Arthroscopic meniscus repair with a posterior incision. Instr Course Lect 37:209–221, 1988.

53. Henning CE, Lynch MA, Clark JR: Vascularity for healing of meniscal repairs. Arthroscopy 3:13–18, 1987.

54. Henning CE, Lynch MA, Yearout KM, et al: Arthroscopic meniscal repair using an exogenous fibrin clot. Clin Orthop 252:64–72, 1990.

55. Humphry G: A Treatise on the Human Skeleton Including the Joints. Cambridge, Macmillan, 1858.

55a. Ikeuchi H: Arthroscopic treatment of the discoid lateral meniscus: Technique and long-term results. Clin Orthop 167:19–28, 1982.

56. Ireland J, Trickey EL, Stoker DJ: Arthroscopy and arthrography of the knee. A critical review. J Bone Joint Surg Br 62:3–6, 1980.

57. Ishimura M, Fujisawa Y: Arthroscopic meniscal repair with fibrin glue. Operative Tech Orthop 10:212–219, 2000.

58. Jackson DW, McDevitt CA, Simon TM, et al: Meniscal transplantation using fresh and cryopreserved allografts. An experimental study in goats. Am J Sports Med 20:644–656, 1992.

59. Jackson DW, Jennings LD, Maywood RM, Berger PE: Magnetic resonance imaging of the knee. Am J Sports Med 16:29–47, 1988.

59a. Johnson LL: Diagnostic and Surgical Arthroscopy: The Knee and Other Joints, 2nd ed. St. Louis, CV Mosby, 1981.

60. Johnson RJ, Kettelkamp DB, Clark W, Leaverton P: Factors affecting late results after meniscectomy. J Bone Joint Surg Am 56:719–729, 1974.

60a. Keene GC, Bickerstaff D, Rae PJ, et al: The natural history of meniscal tears in anterior cruciate ligament insufficiency. Am J Sports Med 21:672–679, 1993.

61. Kennedy J, Alexander I, Hayes K: Nerve supply of the human knee and its functional importance. Am J Sports Med 10:329–335, 1982.

62. Kettelkamp DB, Jacobs AW: Tibiofemoral contact area—determination and implication. J Bone Joint Surg Am 54:349–356, 1972.

63. King D: The healing of semilunar cartilages. J Bone Joint Surg 18:333–342, 1936.

64. King D: The function of the semilunar cartilages. J Bone Joint Surg 18:1069–1076, 1936.

65. Kohn D, Moreno B: Meniscus insertion anatomy as a basis for meniscus replacement: A morphological cadaveric study. Arthroscopy 11:96–103, 1995.

66. Krause WR, Pope MH, Johnson RJ, Wilder DG: Mechanical changes in the knee after meniscectomy. J Bone Joint Surg Am 58:599–604, 1976.

66a. Kurosaka M, Yoshiya S, Ohno O, et al: Lateral discoid meniscectomy: A 20-year follow-up study. Paper presented at the 54th Annual Meeting of the American Academy of Orthopaedic Surgeons, Jan 24, 1987, San Francisco.

67. Lagergren KA: Meniscus operation and secondary arthrosis deformans. Acta Orthop Scand 14:280–287, 1953.

68. Laprade RF, Burnett QM, Veenstra MA, Hodgmen CG: The prevalence of abnormal magnetic resonance findings in asymptomatic knees. Am J Sports Med 22:739–745, 1994.

69. Levy IM, Torzilli PA, Warren RF: The effect of medial meniscectomy on anterior-posterior motion of the knee. J Bone Joint Surg Am 64:883–888, 1982.

70. MacConail M: The function of intra-articular fibrocartilages, with special reference to the knee and inferior radioulnar joints. J Anat 66:210–227, 1932.

70a. Mariani PP, Puddu G: Meniscal ossicle. Am J Sports Med 9:392, 1981.

70b. Martin RC, Brown DE, Zell BK, Lichtman DM: Diagnostic and operative arthroscopy of the knee under local anesthesia with parenteral medication. Am J Sports Med 17:436–439, 1989.

71. Maquet PG, Van de Berg AJ, Simonet JC: Femorotibial weight-bearing areas. J Bone Joint Surg Am 57:766–771, 1975.

72. McDevitt CA, Webber RJ: The ultrastructure and biochemistry of meniscal cartilage. Clin Orthop 252:8–18, 1990.

73. Merkel K: The surface of the human menisci and its aging alterations during age: A combined scanning and transmission electron microscopic examination (SEM, TEM). Arch Orthop Trauma Surg 97:185–191, 1980.

73a. Metcalf RW: Arthroscopic meniscal surgery. In McGinty JB (ed): Operative Arthroscopy. New York, Raven Press, 1991, pp 203–236.

74. Meyers E, Zhu W, Mow VC: Viscoelastic properties of articular cartilage and meniscus. In Nimmi M (ed): Collagen: Chemistry, Biology, and Biotechnology. Boca Raton, CRC, 1988, pp 268–288.

75. Milachowski KA, Weismeier K, Wirth CJ: Meniscus replacement using Hoffa's infrapatellar fat bodies: Initial clinical results. Unfallchirurgie 16:190–195, 1990.

76. Miller MD, Johnson DL: Atlas of meniscal repair. Operative Tech Orthop 10:209–211, 2000.

76a. Morgan CD: The "all-inside" meniscus repair: Technical note. Arthroscopy 7:120–125, 1991.

76b. Morgan CD, Casscells SW: Arthroscopic meniscus repair: A safe approach to the posterior horns. Arthroscopy 2:3–12, 1986.

77. Mow V, Fithian D, Kelly M: Fundamentals of articular cartilage and meniscus biomechanics. In Ewing J (ed): Articular Cartilage and Knee Joint Function. New York, Raven, 1989, pp 1–18.

78. Morrison JB: Bioengineering analysis of force actions transmitted by the knee joint. Biomed Eng 3:164–170, 1968.

79. Mow VC, Arnoczky SP, Jackson DW (eds): Knee Meniscus: Basic and Clinical Foundations. New York, Raven Press, 1992, pp 37–89, 107–115.

80. Mow VC, Holmes MH, Lai WM: Fluid transport and mechanical properties of articular cartilage: A review. J Biomech 17:377–394, 1984.

80a. Mullhollan JS: Inside/inside meniscus repair technique: Sewing and tying through punctures. Paper presented at the 11th Annual Meeting of the Arthroscopy Association of North America, April 1992, Boston.

81. Nicholas JA, Freiberger RH, Killoran PJ: Double-contrast arthrography of the knee. Its value in the management of two hundred and twenty-five knee derangements. J Bone Joint Surg Am 52:203–220, 1970.

81a. Noble J: Lesions of the menisci: Autopsy incidence in adults less than fifty-five years old. J Bone Joint Surg Am 59:480–483, 1977.

82. Noble J, Hamblen DL: The pathology of the degenerative meniscus lesion. J Bone Joint Surg Br 57:180–186, 1975.

83. Northmore-Ball MD, Dandy DJ: Long-term results of arthroscopic partial meniscectomy. Clin Orthop 167:34–42, 1982.

84. Paletta G Jr, Manning T, Snell E, et al: The effect of allograft meniscal replacement on intraarticular contact area and pressures in the human knee: A biomechanical study. Am J Sports Med 25:692–698, 1997.

84a. Peetrons P, Allaer D, Jeanmart L: Cysts of the semilunar cartilages of the knee: A new approach by ultrasound imaging. A study of six cases and review of the literature. J Ultrasound Med 9:333–337, 1990.

85. Peh WCG, Chan JHM, Sek TWH, et al: The effect of using shorter echo times in MR imaging of knee menisci: A study using a porcine model. AJR Am J Roentgenol 172:485–488, 1999.

86. Peterfly CG, Janzen DL, Tirman PFJ, et al: "Magic angle" phenomenon: A cause of increased signal in the normal lateral meniscus on short-TE MR images of the knee. AJR Am J Roentgenol 163:149–154, 1994.

87. Pisani A: Pathognomonic signs for cysts of the knee cartilage. Arch Surg 54:188–190, 1947.

88. Polly DW, Callaghan DD, Sikes RA, et al: The accuracy of selective magnetic resonance imaging compared with the findings of arthroscopy of the knee. J Bone Joint Surg Am 70:192–198, 1988.

89. Potter HG, Rodeo SA, Wickiewicz TL, Warren RF: MR imaging of meniscal allografts: Correlation with clinical and arthroscopic outcomes. Radiology 198:509–514, 1996.

89a. Raber DA, Friederick NF, Hefth F: Discoid lateral meniscus in children. J Bone Joint Surg Am 80:11, 1998.

90. Radin EL, DeLamotte F, Maquet P: Role of the meniscus in the distribution of stress in the knee. Clin Orthop 185:290–294, 1984.

90a. Regan WD, McConkey JP, Loomer RL, Davidson RG: Cysts of the lateral meniscus: Arthroscopy versus arthroscopy plus open cystectomy. Am J Sports Med 5:274–281, 1989.

90b. Rosen IE: Unusual intrameniscal lunulae. Three case reports. J Bone Joint Surg Am 40:925, 1958.

90c. Rosenberg TD, Scott SM, Coward DB: Arthroscopic meniscal repair evaluated with repeat arthroscopy. Arthroscopy 2:14–20, 1986.

90d. Ryu RKN, Ting AJ: Arthroscopic treatment of meniscal cysts. Arthroscopy 9:591–595, 1993.

91. Scott GA, Jolly BL, Henning CE: Combined posterior incision and arthroscopic intra-articular repair of the meniscus: An examination of factors affecting healing. J Bone Joint Surg Am 68:847–861, 1986.

92. Seedhom BB: Transmission of the load in the knee joint with special reference to the role of the menisci. Part I: Anatomy, analysis and apparatus. Eng Med 8:207–219, 1979.

93. Seedhom BB, Hargreaves DJ: Transmission of the load in the knee joint with special reference to the role of the menisci. Part II: Experimental results, discussion, and conclusions. Eng Med 8:220–228, 1979.

93a. Seger BM, Woods GW: Arthroscopic management of lateral meniscal cysts. Am J Sports Med 14:105–108, 1986.

94. Shakespeare DT, Rigby HS: The bucket-handle tear of the meniscus. A clinical and arthrographic study. J Bone Joint Surg Br 65:383–387, 1983.

95. Shoemaker SC, Markolf KL: The role of the meniscus in the A-P stability of the loaded anterior cruciate-deficient knee. J Bone Joint Surg Am 68:71–79, 1986.

96. Shrive NG, O'Connor JJ, Goodfellow JW: Load bearing in the knee joint. Clin Orthop 131:279–287, 1978.

96a. Silverman JM, Mink JH, Deutsch AL: Discoid menisci of the knee: MR imaging appearance. Radiology 173:351–354, 1989.

96b. Small NC: Complications in arthroscopic surgery performed by experienced arthroscopists. Arthroscopy 4:215–221, 1988.

96c. Smillie IS: The congenital discoid meniscus. J Bone Joint Surg Br 30:671–682, 1948.

96d. Smillie IS: Injuries of the knee joint. Edinburgh, Churchill Livingstone, 1973, p 4.

97. Stone KR, Steadman JR, Rodkey WG, Li S-T: Regeneration of meniscal cartilage with the use of a collagen scaffold. J Bone Joint Surg Am 79:1770–1777, 1997.

97a. Stone RG, VanWinkle GN: Arthroscopic review of meniscal repair: Assessment of healing parameters. Arthroscopy 2:77–81, 1986.

98. Sutton JB: Ligaments: Their Nature and Morphology. London, MK Lewis, 1897.

99. Swiontkowski MF, Schlehr F, Sanders R, et al: Direct, real time measurement of meniscal blood flow. An experimental investigation in sheep. Am J Sports Med 16:429–433, 1988.

99a. Symeonides PP, Ioannides G: Ossicles in the knee. Report of three cases. J Bone Joint Surg Am 54:1288, 1972.

100. Tapper EM, Hoover NW: Late results after meniscectomy. J Bone Joint Surg Am 51:517–526, 1969.

100a. Tenuta JJ, Arciero RA: Arthroscopic evaluation of meniscal repairs. Factors that effect healing. Am J Sports Med 22:797–802, 1994.

101. Thompson WO, Thaete FL, Fu FH, et al: Tibial meniscal dynamics using three-dimensional reconstruction of magnetic resonance images. Am J Sports Med 19:210–215, 1991.

102. Toyonaga T, Uezaki N, Chikama H: Substitute meniscus of Teflon-net for the knee joint of dogs. Clin Orthop 179:291–297, 1983.

103. Turner DA, Rappaport MI, Erwin WD, et al: Truncation artifact: A potential pitfall in MR imaging of the menisci of the knee. Radiology 179:629–633, 1991.

104. Vahey TN, Bennett HT, Arrington LE, et al: MR imaging of the knee: Pseudotear of the lateral meniscus caused by the meniscofemoral ligament. AJR Am J Roentgenol 154:1237–1239, 1990.

104a. Vandermeer RD, Cunningham FK: Arthroscopic treatment of the discoid lateral meniscus: Results of long-term follow-up. Arthroscopy 5:101–109, 1989.

105. Veth RPH, Den Heeten GH, Jansen HWB, Nielsen HKL: An experimental study of reconstructive lesions of the meniscus. Use of synovial flaps and carbon fiber implants for artificially made lesions in the meniscus of the rabbit. Clin Orthop 181:250–254, 1983.

106. Walker PS, Erkman MJ: The role of the menisci in force transmission across the knee. Clin Orthop 109:184–192, 1975.

107. Walker PS, Hajek JV: The loadbearing area in the knee joint. J Biomech 5:581–592, 1972.

107a. Warren RF: Arthroscopic meniscal repair. Arthroscopy 1:170, 1985.

107b. Warren RF: Meniscectomy and repair in the anterior cruciate ligament–deficient patient. Clin Orthop 252:55–63, 1990.

108. Watanabe AT, Carter BC, Teitelbaum GP, et al: Normal variations in MR imaging of the knee: Appearance and frequency. AJR Am J Roentgenol 153:341–344, 1989.

108a. Watanabe M, Takeda S, Ikeuchi H (eds): Atlas of Arthroscopy, 3rd ed. Tokyo, Igaku-Shoin, 1979, pp 75–130.

109. Weiss CB, Lundberg M, Dehaven KE, et al: Nonoperative treatment of meniscal tears. J Bone Joint Surg Am 71:811–821, 1989.

110. Wilson A, Legg P, McNeur J: Studies on innervation of the medial meniscus in the human knee joint. Anat Rec 165:485–491, 1969.

110a. Wirth C: Meniscal repair. Clin Orthop 157:153–160, 1981.
111. Wood DJ, Minns RJ, Strover A: Replacement of the rabbit medial meniscus with a polyester-carbon fiber bioprosthesis. Biomaterials 11:13–16, 1990.
111a. Woods GW, Whelan JM: Discoid meniscus. Clin Sports Med 9: 695–706, 1990.
112. Woodyard JE: A long-term survey after meniscectomy. Orthopedics 1:29–39, 1968.

112a. Wroblewski BM: Trauma and the cystic meniscus: Review of 500 cases. Injury 4:319–321, 1973.
113. Yocum LA, Kerlan RK, Jobe FW, et al: Isolated lateral meniscectomy. J Bone Joint Surg Am 61:338–342, 1979.
114. Zimny ML, Albright DJ, Dabezies E: Mechanoreceptors in the human medial meniscus. Acta Anat 133:35–40, 1988.
115. Zivanovic S: Menisco-meniscal ligaments of the human knee joint. Anat Anz 135(suppl):35–42, 1974.

2. MENISCAL INJURIES IN THE SKELETALLY IMMATURE PATIENT

Carl L. Stanitski, MD

Injuries to the menisci are uncommon in school-age patients and are quite rare in children younger than 10 years old whose menisci are morphologically normal. The precise prevalence and incidence of meniscal injuries in skeletally immature patients are unknown. Recent reports of meniscal injuries in school-age patients indicate that meniscal damage does occur as an isolated injury or in conjunction with anterior cruciate ligament (ACL) tears (Fig. 28D2–1).[1, 15, 20, 21, 22]

Anatomy and Development

The menisci are biconcave, C-shaped wedges of fibrocartilage anchored at the intercondylar tibial eminence, tibial coronary ligament, and medial collateral ligament.

The attachment to the lateral collateral ligament is variable. At the end of the 8-week embryonic period, the menisci are adult shaped, and, at birth, they are vascularized throughout. Nine months postnatally, the blood supply recedes centrifugally and continues to do so until 10 years of age, when the adult vascular peripheral pattern is established (Fig. 28D2–2).[9] The lateral meniscus exhibits more developmental variability than the medial meniscus. Despite this variability, Clark and Ogden,[9] in an elegant anatomic study of neonates to preadolescents, demonstrated that at no time in normal development are the menisci discoid in configuration. The menisci have constant meniscal-to-tibial articular surface ratios during development, with intimate maturation of the menisci and their adjoining tibial compartments.

Predominantly type I collagen is arranged circumferen-

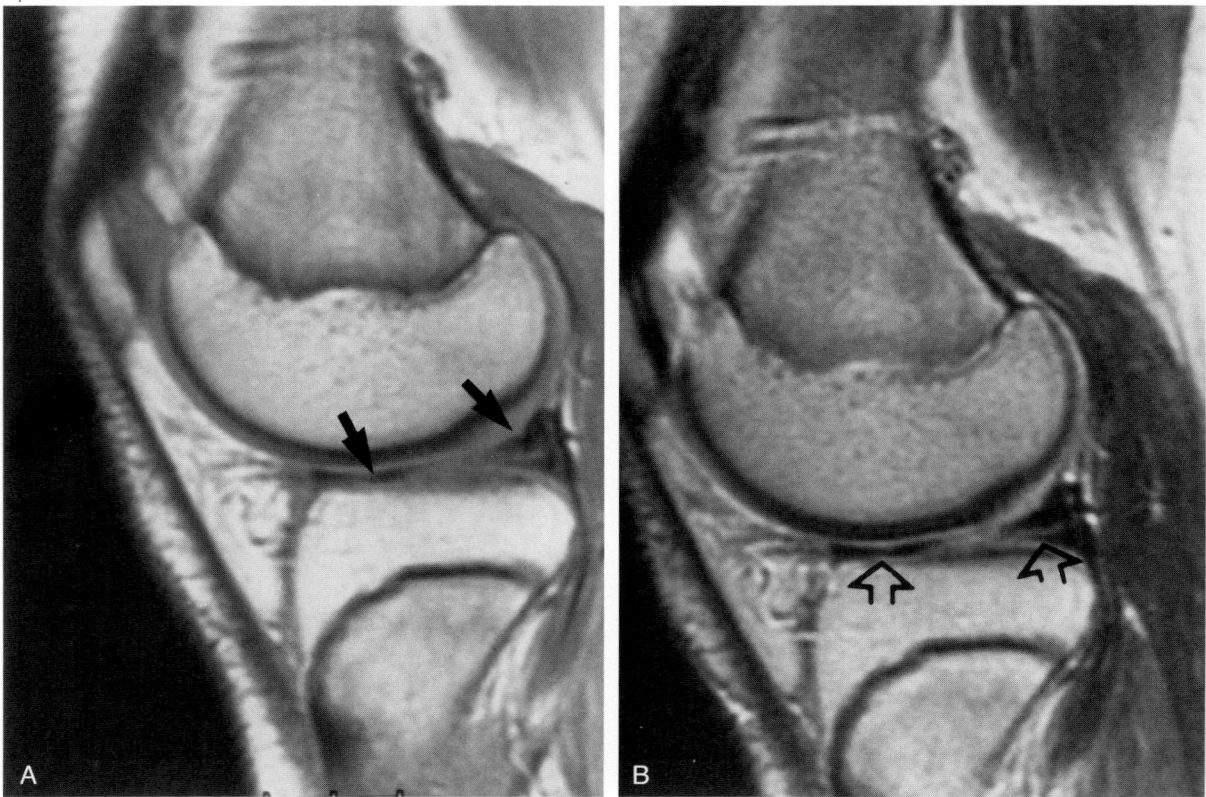

Figure 28D2–1. *A* and *B,* Magnetic resonance image of a torn lateral, nondiscoid meniscus in a 10-year-old soccer player.

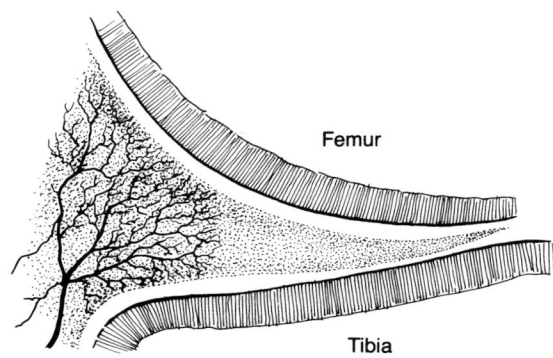

Figure 28D2–2. Meniscal vasculature diminishing from peripheral to central.

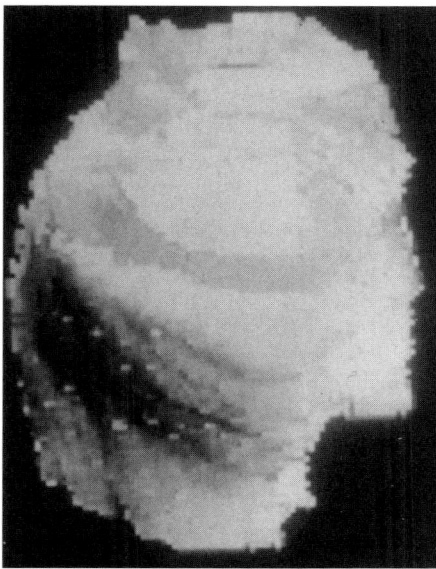

Figure 28D2–3. Three-dimensional dynamic magnetic resonance image. (Courtesy of Dr. Freddie Fu.)

tially in the meniscus with oblique, vertical, and radial fibers present to attenuate hoop stresses and to resist extrusion during weight-bearing. A change in collagen orientation to the adult pattern occurs in response to weight-bearing during early development.[9] Diminished meniscal cellularity is reflected in the conversion of the more chondral-type tissue seen in early childhood to the fibrocartilage adult pattern with further growth.

The menisci function to distribute synovial fluid and as secondary restraints (medial) for knee stability. Their major role is to share weight-bearing loads with the articular and subchondral areas by increasing articular contact area and reducing pressure on the articular cartilage.[6] Seventy percent of the lateral compartment load is borne by the lateral meniscus. Fifty percent of the medial compartment load is carried by the medial meniscus. Vedi and associates[31] recently documented in vivo normal meniscal motion under load conditions using magnetic resonance images (MRIs) of 16 volunteers who were 15- to 18-year-old athletes. The medial meniscus averaged 7.1 mm of anterior horn motion, 3.9 mm of posterior horn sagittal plane motion, and 3.6 mm of transverse plane displacement. The lateral meniscal anterior and posterior horns averaged 9.5 and 5.6 mm of sagittal displacement, respectively, and 3.7 mm of transverse motion. This report of meniscal dynamics reaffirms the preliminary work of Thompson and colleagues,[30] who studied five cadaveric, non–weight-bearing specimens (Fig. 28D2–3). During knee flexion, the lateral horn demonstrates greater movement than the medial, and the anterior horns show greater movement than the posterior, with the least movement seen by the posterior medial meniscal segment. Vedi and coworkers[31] found that the only statistically significant motion difference was in the anterior lateral horn. The minimal radial motion noted within each compartment reflects containment of the meniscus during weight-bearing. They also reported an increase in meniscal vertical height at the periphery in response to the tension generated with weight-bearing. Anteroposterior meniscal motion in response to the cam effect of the femoral condyles during knee flexion maximizes joint congruity, with improved load distribution to the articular surface and subchondral bone.

Clinical Evaluation

Diagnosis of an acute meniscal tear in a youngster may be difficult because of imprecision in relating the injury

mechanism and limited cooperation with the clinical examination due to pain and anxiety. In nonacute cases, classical symptoms of catching, giving way, and locking are often absent. The primary complaint is usually ill-defined pain. Previous symptoms about the knee should be determined. Potential concomitant ACL injury should be sought, particularly when a "pop" is felt at the time of injury. Rapid hemarthrosis onset may be due to an ACL or a peripheral meniscal tear. In a series of children with acute knee hemarthroses, most of the meniscal tears were peripheral and the hemarthrosis source.[28] Delayed onset of a nonhemorrhagic effusion is associated with a meniscal injury not involving the perimeniscal vascular zone.

Tenderness is sought at common sites of injury (e.g., femoral and tibial physes, peripatellar area, tibial tubercle, collateral ligaments, and joint lines). Stability is compared with that in the opposite knee, if uninjured. I find the classic McMurray test of little value in this age group, whose tears are almost always peripheral and not degenerative posterior horn lesions. In my hands, the most accurate physical finding is joint-line tenderness (particularly mid to posterior) with pain exacerbation with varus (medial meniscus), valgus (lateral meniscus), and rotation stress (internal/medial meniscus, external/lateral meniscus) with the knee flexed 30 to 40 degrees. Excellent correlation was seen between these signs and arthroscopically documented meniscal tears, with 92.8% accuracy, 93.3% positive predictive value, 92.3% negative predictive value, 93.3% sensitivity, and 92.3% specificity.[27] In the hands of an experienced surgeon, clinical assessment of meniscal injury in the nonacute setting is highly accurate.

Imaging

Anteroposterior (AP), lateral, skyline, and tunnel-view radiographs are done to rule out unsuspected lesions such

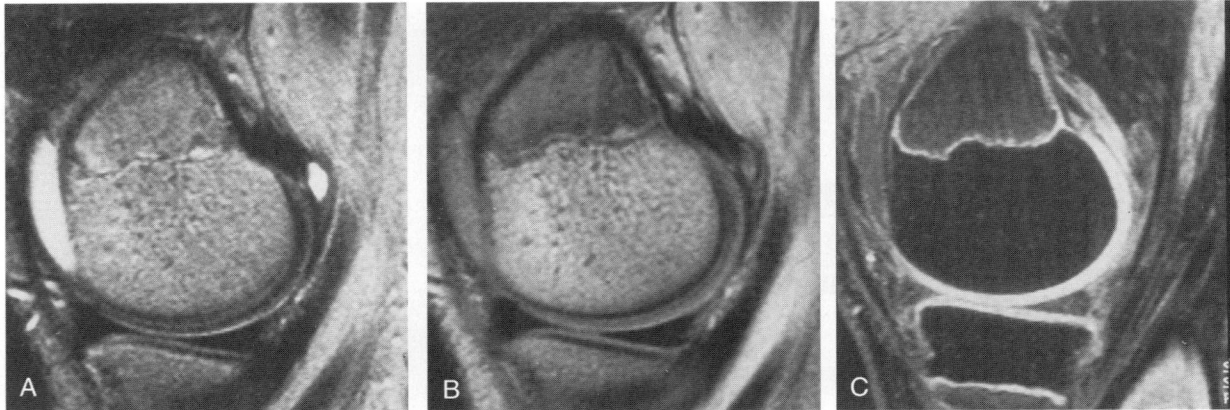

Figure 28D2–4. Three-phase magnetic resonance image of a normal medial meniscus. *A,* T$_2$ image. *B,* Proton density image (meniscus). *C,* Gradient echo image (articular surface—note femoral and tibial physeal definition).

as osteochondral fracture, osteochondritis dissecans, and rare ligament avulsion fracture. These images are almost always normal in cases of otherwise normally shaped menisci. Rapid technical advances have been made in imaging since 1990, but all depend on the sophistication of both the equipment and the interpreter of the images, as well as patient cooperation (Fig. 28D2–4). MRI is an appealing modality because it is noninvasive, uses no ionizing radiation, and has the potential to provide improved resolution of intra-articular soft tissue images. As software and coil size have been modified, imaging time has been dramatically reduced, and the need for sedation or even anesthesia in children has been minimized. The test continues to be expensive. MRI should not be used as a screening procedure because of the significant limitations of the technique in the young patient. Takeda and coworkers[29] reviewed MRI signal intensity and pattern in the menisci of 108 knees in 80 normal, asymptomatic children aged 8 to 15 (average 12.2) years old, using the classification of Zobel and associates,[33] which allows for equivocation for type III signals. Tibial tubercle maturity defined skeletal maturity. In Takeda's study,[29] signal intensity was age sensitive. High signal (grades II and II) was evident in 80% of patients 10 years old or younger, in 65% by age 13, and in 33% at age 15, the latter value approaching the false-positive rate of 29% reported in asymptomatic adults.[8, 18] Two thirds of the patients had positive findings, often grade IIIA (i.e., equivocal extension through the meniscal surface). These authors hypothesized that signal intensity diminution with age was perhaps proportional to reduced peripheral vascularity, particularly in the meniscus posterior horn. Schwartzberg and colleagues[26] reviewed unilateral MRIs of 55 asymptomatic 9- to 15-year-olds who had normal knee examinations. They found that 51% had grade III and 27% had grade II signals in their medial menisci (Fig. 28D2–5). Seven percent had grade III and 7% had grade II signals in their lateral menisci. All children with grade III signals in the lateral menisci also had grade III medial meniscal changes. These authors also cautioned against misinterpretation of MRIs in this age group and emphasized the need for clinical correlation with imaging findings. Several reports relate MRI analysis and arthroscopic findings.[20, 23, 27] In one series, poor correlation was seen between the MRI

reports of radiologists and arthroscopic findings.[27] Significant false-positive and false-negative reports occurred, with only 37.5% accuracy, 50% positive and 50% negative predictive indexes, 50% sensitivity, and 45% specificity noted for interpretations of the radiologist. McDermott and coworkers[20] reviewed 51 patients, 31 adolescent (≥15 years old) and 20 pediatric ones (<15 years old), with suspected meniscal or anterior cruciate disease. Correlation between MRI readings and arthroscopic findings was made. A 100% true-positive correlation was seen for ACL tears in 14 adolescents and a 100% false-positive correlation for two ACL tears in the younger group. A 55% false-positive rate was noted for adolescent meniscal tears. The pediatric group had seven false medial meniscal and five false-positive lateral meniscal tear reports. These authors also cautioned about the accuracy of MRI in meniscal and anterior cruciate ligament disease among the pediatric and adolescent population. Current MRI techniques provide limited information about meniscal tear size and stability or healing potential after repair (Figs. 28D2–6 to 28D2–8).

MRI technology is evolving, and improved images should be forthcoming. MRI should not be used as a screening test. MRI is best ordered by the treating surgeon

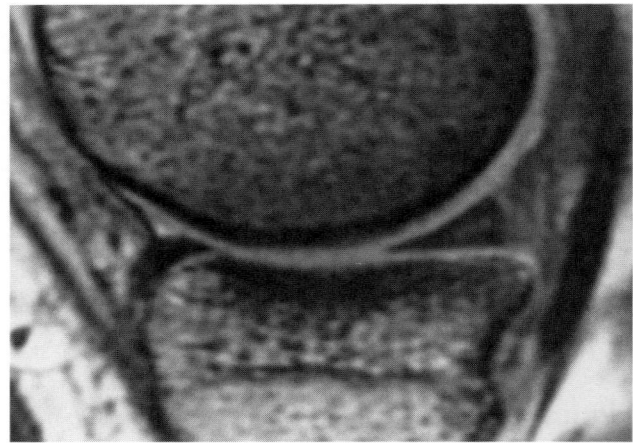

Figure 28D2–5. Grade II medial meniscal change of signal in a normal, asymptomatic 12-year-old girl.

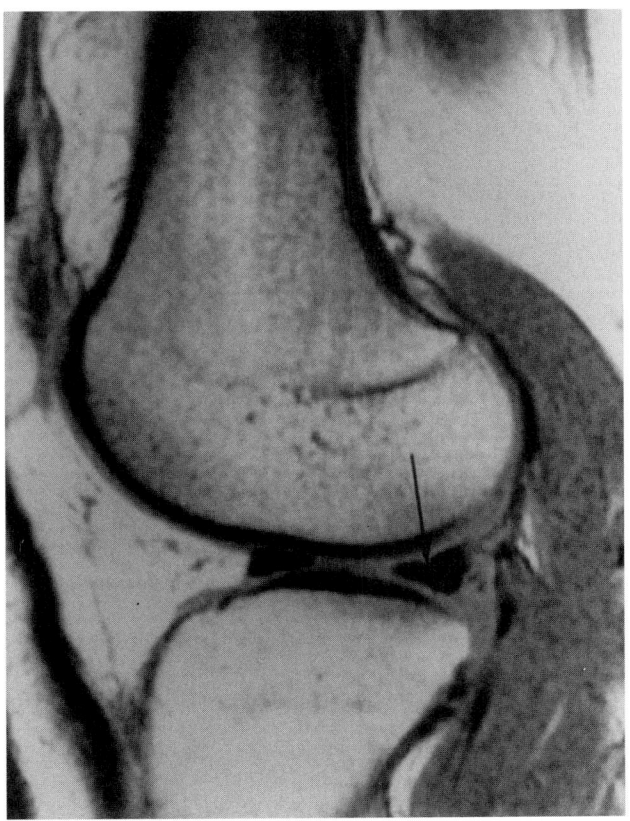

Figure 28D2–6. Undisplaced lateral, nondiscoid meniscal tear *(arrow)* documented at surgery.

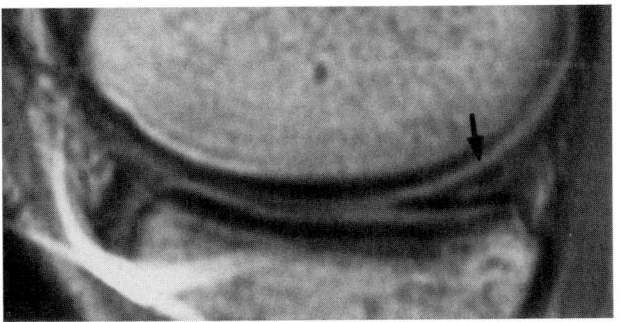

Figure 28D2–7. Grade III meniscal tear *(arrow)* documented at surgery.

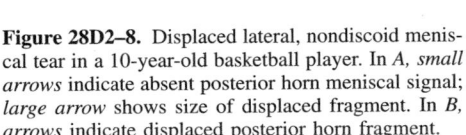

Figure 28D2–8. Displaced lateral, nondiscoid meniscal tear in a 10-year-old basketball player. In *A, small arrows* indicate absent posterior horn meniscal signal; *large arrow* shows size of displaced fragment. In *B, arrows* indicate displaced posterior horn fragment.

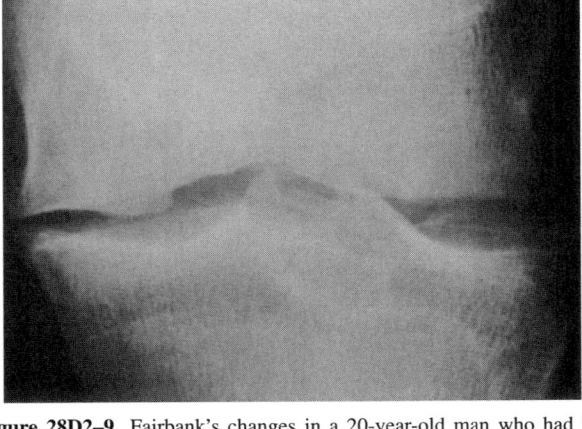

Figure 28D2–9. Fairbank's changes in a 20-year-old man who had had a complete medial meniscectomy at age 10.

following his or her examination. Clinical correlation is mandatory. Clinical evaluation, done by an experienced surgeon in a nonacute setting, is a highly accurate, reliable, and inexpensive method of meniscal injury assessment.

Treatment

The time of ritualistic, unfettered arthrotomy and total meniscal excision for fear of missing a posterior horn tear is past. Dismal outcomes as a consequence of total meniscal extirpation, often without recognition of associated ligamentous instability that led to premature joint overload and development of degenerative arthrosis in the prearthroscopic era, have been well documented (Figs. 28D2–9 to 28D2–11).[6, 12] Meniscal preservation is the current goal to obviate such articular compromise. Annandale[2] reported the first meniscal repair in 1885 by suturing of a torn anterior meniscal tear in a 30-year-old miner who had an excellent functional outcome. More than 6 decades ago, King[17] suggested that based on experimental work in a canine model, longitudinal meniscal tears could heal if communication existed with the meniscal peripheral blood supply. Documentation of the perimeniscal vascular complex by Arnoczky and Warren,[3, 4] using elegant injection

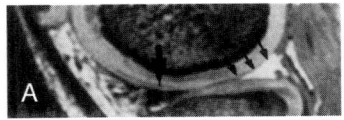

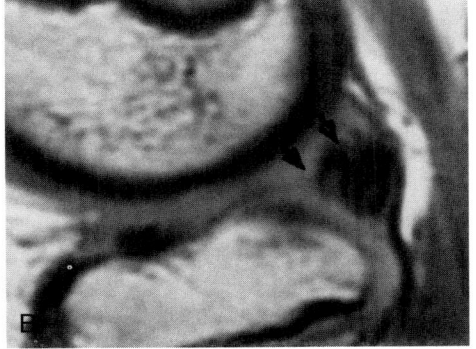

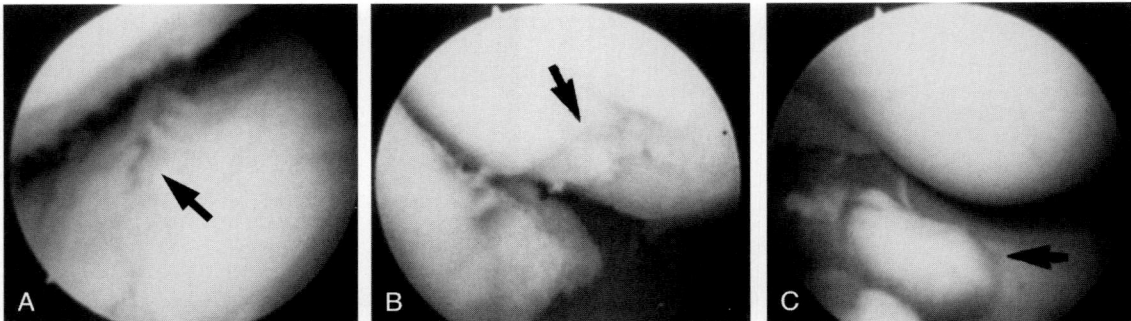

Figure 28D2–10. Arthroscopic views of a 14-year-old boy who had an untreated, unstable lateral meniscal tear for 1 year. *A,* Tibial chondral changes. *B,* Femoral chondral changes. *C,* Tibial osteophyte formation.

studies in elderly cadavers and demonstrating of the ability of the peripheral meniscus to heal in experimental models, provided a physiologic basis for meniscal repair.

These authors[3, 4] believed that peripheral meniscal tears within 3 mm of the meniscosynovial junction had an adequate blood supply for healing. Tears farther than 5 mm from this site were considered avascular unless junctional bleeding was observed at surgery. Tears in the 3- to 5-mm range had inconsistent vascularity. Four vascular zones (0–4) are described. Zone 0 represents the synovial-perimeniscal vascular plexus; 1 equals the vascular "red-red" junction; 2 is the transitional "red-white" zone from vascular to avascular; 3 is the "white-white" avascular zone; and 4 equals the meniscal central free edge. The most common tear is a longitudinal peripheral tear.

I base treatment on a classification scheme I call SAKS, an acronym in which *S* represents the tear's size, site, shape, and stability; *A* is the acuity of the lesion; and *KS* equals knee stability (i.e., ACL and collateral ligament integrity). In a stable knee with an arthroscopically documented acute zone 0 to 1 tear less than 1 cm long that cannot be displaced more than 3 mm, I immobilize the limb in a cylinder cast for 3 weeks. If a similar situation occurs in a chronic setting (i.e., longer than 3 months after injury), I arthroscopically rasp the meniscal tear interface

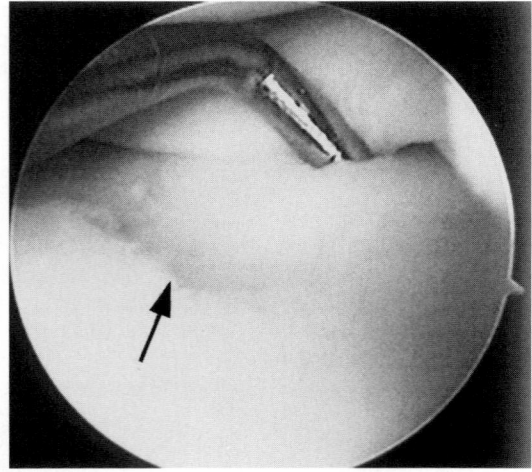

Figure 28D2–11. Tibial articular change *(arrow)* beneath an acute lateral meniscal tear.

and immobilize the limb in a controlled motion brace that limits the arc of motion from 0 to 70 degrees of flexion for 4 weeks. If a displaced tear occurs in zones 0 to 2, is longitudinal, and has a noncomminuted, anatomically reducible inner segment, meniscal repair is done (Fig. 28D2–12). In chronic situations, fragment edge rasping and addition of a fibrin clot are techniques reported to enhance healing.[24] Dowdy and associates[11] studied the effects of post–medial meniscal repair immobilization in a canine model. Animals immobilized in a long-leg cast were compared with nonimmobilized ones after similar meniscal peripheral lesion creation and repair. At 2 and 4 weeks after surgery, collagen at the repair site was histologically equivalent for both groups. At 10 weeks, however, there was twice as much collagen in the nonimmobilized group. These authors suggest that postrepair immobilization is detrimental to collagen production and maturation and recommend a more aggressive rehabilitation program after surgery.

Mintzer and colleagues[21] had a 100% success rate for meniscal repairs in 26 adolescent athletes (29 repairs), 4 with open physes, with an average follow-up of 5 years. More than three fourths (78.5%) of the patients' tears occurred in zones 0 to 1 and had an average length of 2.3 cm. Fifty percent of the patients had a concomitant ACL tear, which was reconstructed at the time of meniscal repair. Twenty-four of the 26 athletes returned to their preinjury level of sport participation.

If the central meniscal fragment is macerated with multiple tears or with tears that cannot be anatomically reduced, repair is not done. Fragment excision is carried out to the stable remaining meniscal rim. No series exists that reports repairs of zone 3 to 4 tears in skeletally immature patients. Rubman and coworkers[25] reported good results for central zone meniscal repairs in adults. Eighty percent of their patients were asymptomatic at an average follow-up of almost 4 years. Seventy-two percent of the cases had concomitant ACL reconstruction at the time of meniscal repair. These authors suggested that such meniscal repairs would be indicated for patients in their second and third decades, with perhaps higher healing potential than for more elderly patients. Questions remain about the ability of repaired menisci to transmit loads because of altered fiber patterns. Unstable tears in zone 4 are excised with preservation of as much stable, intact meniscus as possible. Horizontal and radial tears are uncommon in the school-age population. If

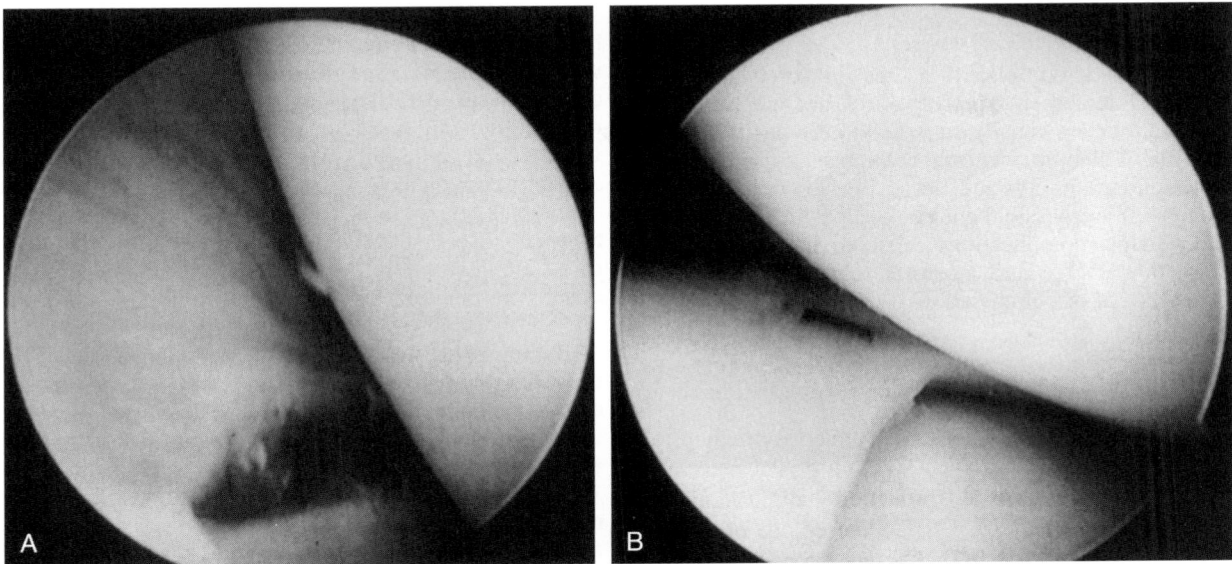

Figure 28D2–12. *A,* Unstable midposterior medial meniscal red-red junction tear. *B,* After repair under arthroscopic control.

such tears occur, the tear is débrided. In horizontal tears, the smaller of the two leaves is resected (Fig. 28D2–13).

Adolescent patients with an unstable knee from a medial collateral injury who also have a peripheral meniscal tear should have meniscal and ligament repair. If the meniscal tear is in a zone not amenable to repair, arthroscopic fragment débridement is done and the collateral ligament injury treated nonoperatively.

MRI evidence of healing after meniscal repair is equivocal because the repair area may be the site of persistent high signal in asymptomatic patients who are without physical signs of incomplete healing.

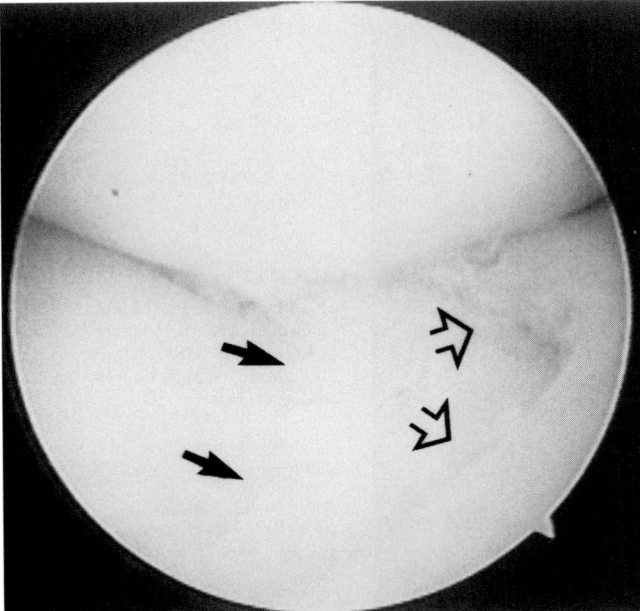

Figure 28D2–13. Horizontal lateral meniscal tear. *Solid arrows,* free edge of inferior leaf; *open arrows,* resected edge of upper leaf.

Patients with what I refer to as an "ACL plus" knee, one with coincident ACL and meniscal tears, should have meniscal preservation by repair, if possible, and concomitant ACL reconstruction appropriate for their skeletal maturity. If knee instability is not addressed and is allowed to persist, repeat meniscal injury and opposite meniscal compartment injury and additional articular compromise follow.

Multiple meniscal repair techniques have been reported.[1, 7, 10, 16, 21] Four broad categories of repair may be used: arthroscopic outside-in, inside-out, or all-inside and formal open methods. Open repair is reserved for combined medial collateral/medial meniscal lesions or for meniscal damage that cannot be approached arthroscopically, an uncommon situation for the experienced arthroscopist. The inside-out technique uses zone-specific cannulas that provide precise suture placement, usually a vertical mattress suture that has double the suture strength of a horizontal stitch. Outside-in repairs use spinal needles placed across the capsule and through the meniscus. A suture is passed through the needle and is brought outside the knee, a knot is fashioned, the suture is reintroduced, and the knot is used for meniscal fragment reduction and fixation. This technique is helpful in situations in which blind suture passage could lead to neural or vascular injury. The all-inside method is an emerging, technically demanding technique. A variety of arthroscopically introduced bioabsorbable meniscal anchors that obviate capsular exposure and external sutures are in use. These devices are sometimes too long or too bulky to use within the confines of a child's knee.[7]

The choice of method of edge preparation of a meniscal tear is based on the tear pattern and acuity. A meniscal rasp stimulates a vascular inflammatory response. In chronic tears, fibrin clot augmentation of the repair site provides a collagen scaffold for vascular invasion and repair.[24]

The reader is referred to standard arthroscopic texts for additional details on meniscal repair.

Complications

Meniscal repair complications are relatively uncommon.[5] A child-adolescent–specific series has not been reported. Infections are usually superficial ones at the capsular suture site. Phlebitis, meniscal re-rupture, arthrofibrosis, arterial (popliteal) injury, and nerve injuries (e.g., saphenous, peroneal) are possible and are dealt with by standard techniques. Most complications relate to neural damage. Portal position choice and attention to suture placement minimize the risk of complications.

Prognosis

Adult meniscal repair outcomes are inversely related to the size and acuity of the meniscal injury and area of reconstruction.[10, 15] In a peripheral tear smaller than 2 cm, clinical failure rates of 10% to 15% are reported. If the tear exceeds 4 cm, 60% failure rates are seen. Repair of a tear within 8 weeks of injury results in a good outcome in 85% of cases, in contrast to only 65% good results in chronic tears that occurred longer than 8 weeks ago. Because the perimeniscal blood supply patterns of 11- to 12-year-old patients are identical to the flow seen in adults, it would seem that these data are transferable to adolescent patients as well. In most reported series, meniscal repair outcomes are better in patients with associated ACL reconstructions. Perhaps this is a function of the postoperative hematoma bathing the meniscal repair site with totipotential cells.[10, 21, 25]

Meniscal Cysts

Meniscal cysts in skeletally immature patients, though uncommon, differ from the degenerative types seen in adults. The cysts are usually lateral and are associated with horizontal or radial meniscal tears. They may be associated with a discoid meniscal tear. Previous data suggested that cyst/meniscal tear frequency was approximately 50% but reflected imaging limitations (arthrography) and diminished visualization (arthrotomy), in contrast to the findings seen at arthroscopy, which define an almost 100% correlation.

Patients complain of pain and may note focal swelling, especially when seated. An effusion is common in chronic cases, along with joint-line tenderness and a palpable cystic mass. This may be hidden by the iliotibial band with the knee in extension and uncovered with knee flexion.[1]

Radiographs are normal except for an associated soft tissue mass. MRI studies define the cyst and meniscal disease (Fig. 28D2–14). Differential diagnoses include discoid meniscus, proximal tibiofibular joint ganglion, lipoma, and extremely rare tumors and vascular malformations.

Cyst decompression and management of associated meniscal disease are done arthroscopically or by mini-arthrotomy.[1, 19] The horizontal meniscal tear's inferior leaf is débrided and the cyst's contents evacuated. This treatment combination usually leads to resolution of the condition. Cyst excision alone, without assessment and management of the associated intra-articular disease, is not indicated. With the current combination procedure, recurrence is uncommon, but patients and their parents need to be cautioned about this possibility.

Summary

Meniscal tears do occur in pediatric and adolescent age groups. These lesions are almost always peripheral in menisci of previously normal morphology. Clinical evaluation by an experienced surgeon provides accuracy in diagnosis. MRI should not be used as a screening technique,

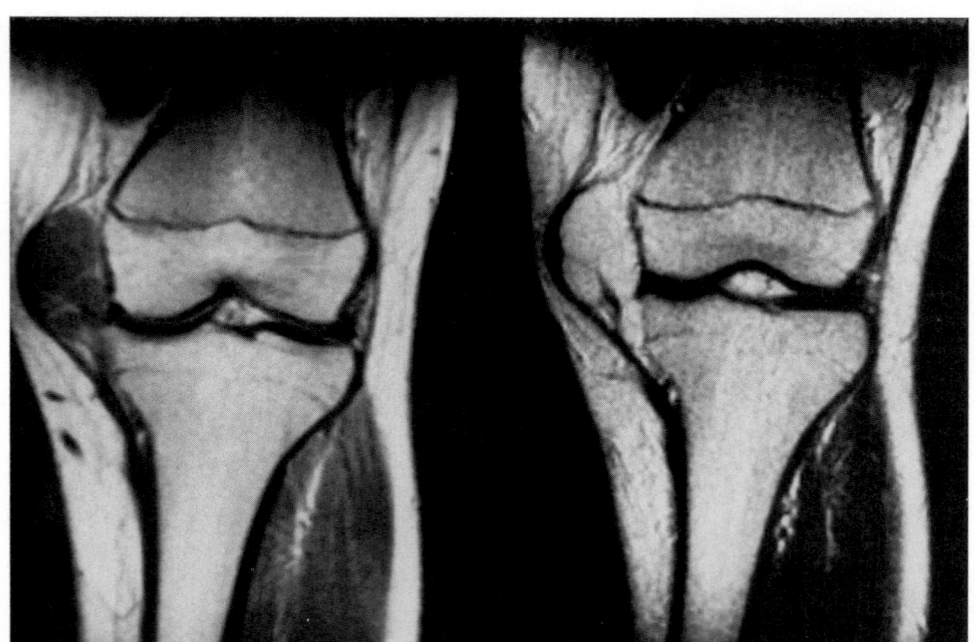

Figure 28D2–14. Magnetic resonance images of a lateral meniscal cyst. A horizontal cleavage tear of the lateral meniscus was seen at arthroscopy.

and clinical correlation is mandatory. High false-positive rates of MRI interpretation in the menisci of normal, skeletally immature patients must be kept in mind.

There is significant evidence that with specific indications and using precise techniques, meniscal salvage and repair procedures allow meniscal tears to heal and function.[1, 4, 10, 11, 21, 24, 25] Meniscal preservation appears to be a major advance in the prevention of premature joint senescence, an all-too-common sequela following total meniscal excision.

Meniscal replacement is receiving attention and is considered experimental and a work in progress at this time.[22] Allograft transplantation is an attractive technique, but the logistics of sterilization (including viral considerations) and preservation, along with the adverse mechanical effects of these methods on the meniscus and storage and size availability, must be solved before meniscal replacement becomes a widespread clinical reality. Laboratory trials have not demonstrated joint mechanics and load-sharing normalization after meniscal transplantation alone. Allografts incorporating subchondral bone fixation in addition to capsular sutures show promise. Molecular biologic processes that allow cell culture of the patient's own tissue for use with tissue engineering techniques to provide a meniscal anlage are a promise on the horizon.[14]

One and one-half decades ago, Ghosh and Taylor[13] reminded us that the meniscus is a "fibrocartilage of some distinction." We should continue to respect it as just that.

Discoid Meniscus

Observation of a discoid lateral meniscus was first recorded by Young in England in 1889; he described "the external semilunar cartilage as a complete disc" in a cadaver dissection.[19] Twenty years later, Kroiss, in Germany, made the first clinical correlation when he associated the snapping knee in childhood with a discoid meniscus.[8] This meniscal anomaly occurs almost exclusively on the lateral side. Discoid medial menisci are extremely rare.

Anatomy

Smillie, in 1948 in Scotland, proposed the first classification of discoid menisci based on his experience with 29 operative cases.[12] He based these types on his theory that the discoid configuration represented an atavistic phenomenon with persistence of a fetally shaped meniscus that had not undergone central absorption.[12] He later retracted his thesis in light of newer data. Kaplan[7] advanced a theory based on his cadaveric and animal dissections and embryologic studies. He felt that at no time during fetal development was the meniscus discoid shaped. He suggested that the lateral tibial plateau meniscal attachments were deficient. Because of the checkrein effects of the ligament of Wrisberg, he felt that abnormal meniscal motion was present, and the lateral femoral condyle caused the meniscus to convert from a normally shaped one to a thickened, ovoid shape. In Japan, Watanabe[18] proposed a tripartite classification that reflected the amount of meniscus covering the tibial plateau and the stability of the meniscus (Fig. 28D2–15). In his scheme, type I covers the plateau completely and type II is an incomplete covering. Normal adult meniscal width is 12 to 13 mm, and its thickness varies from 4 to 5 mm at its periphery, in contrast to the 8- to 10-mm thickness and the 10- to 35-mm width seen with discoid menisci. Type III is most often a normally shaped meniscus, except for a thickened posterior horn that is unstable owing to loss of a posterior tether because of absence of the meniscotibial ligament. He also felt that the ligament of Wrisberg (posterior meniscofemoral) prevented normal meniscal reciprocal motion during flexion and extension and called this variety the "Wrisberg" type (see Fig. 28D2–15). Two meniscofemoral ligaments, specialized segments of the posterior knee capsule, may be present in normal knees—the anterior meniscofemoral ligament of Humphrey and the posterior meniscofemoral ligament of Wrisberg. They occur simultaneously in approximately 70% of normal knees, with 30% of knees lacking one or the other ligament (Fig. 28D2–16). Clark and Ogden,[4] in an elegant study of meniscal formation and development, found that although the lateral meniscus demonstrated greater morphologic variability than the medial one, at no time during development were menisci discoid shaped. Neuschwander and Drez[9] suggested the term *lateral meniscal variant* to identify the type III meniscus and pointed out its nondiscoid shape. In three patients, these authors were unable to document the presence or absence of meniscofemoral ligaments and the role they played in their patients' conditions. None of the classifications addresses

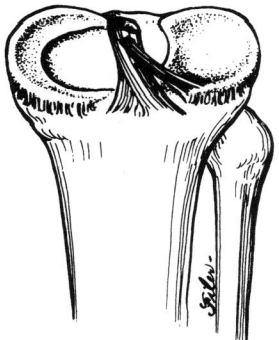 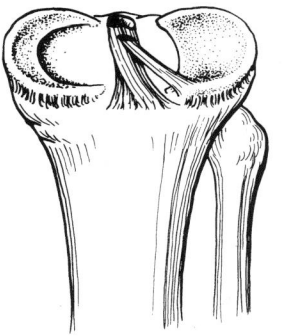 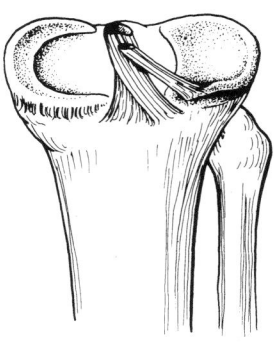

Figure 28D2–15. Watanabe classification of discoid menisci. Type I: stable, complete; type II: stable, incomplete; type III: unstable owing to lack of meniscotibial ligament continuity.

I   II   III

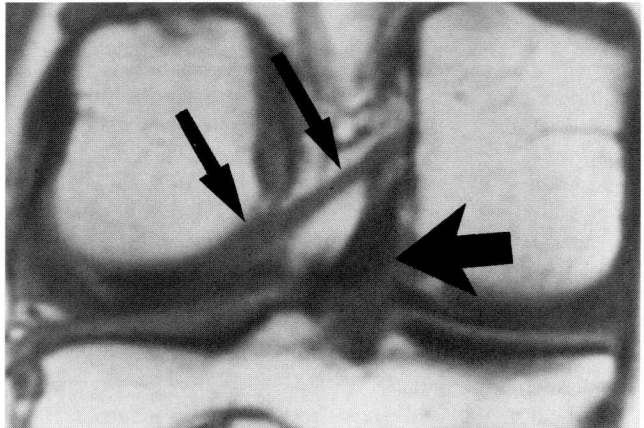

Figure 28D2–16. Magnetic resonance image of ligament of Humphry *(long arrows)* and posterior cruciate ligament *(short arrow).*

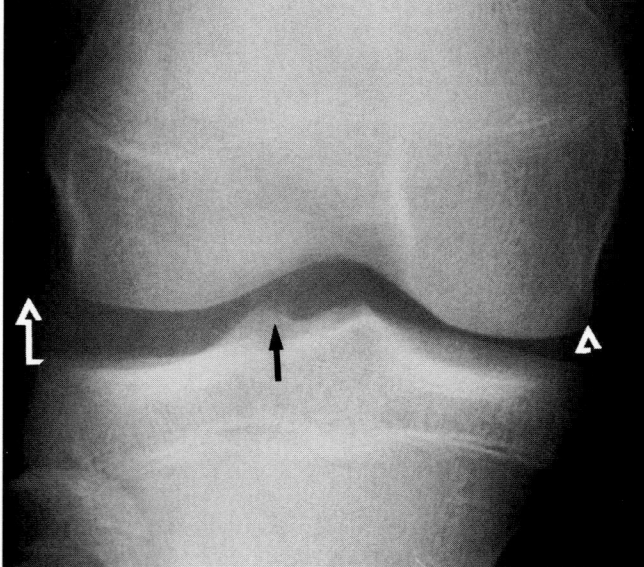

Figure 28D2–17. Radiograph of a 10-year-old girl with a type II discoid lateral meniscus. Note the increased lateral joint space *(open arrows)* and underdevelopment of the lateral tibial eminence *(closed arrow).*

meniscal shape, stability, and continuity. A system suggested by Jordan addresses some of these issues.[6]

The incidence and prevalence of discoid menisci are unknown. Many discoid menisci are asymptomatic. Data reflect methods of detection (e.g., cadaveric dissection versus intraoperative arthroscopic findings). Reported prevalence rates range from 0.4% to 16%, the latter value noted in Asian populations. Type III menisci, uncommon in reported Asian series, are quite rare overall and are most often seen in patients older than 16 years of age. The rate of occurrence of discoid menisci in males and females is equal and bilaterality approximates 10% to 20%.[2, 3]

Clinical Evaluation

The patient may be asymptomatic and may complain only of a bulge noted at the lateral knee. More commonly, the patient has asymptomatic snapping at the lateral knee, usually noted at 3 to 4 years of age. Symptomatic snapping associated with intermittent effusion and mechanical complaints begins at 8 to 9 years of age and is indicative of progressive meniscal instability or tear.

Clinical examination demonstrates snapping with increasing knee flexion, with prominence at the lateral joint line. In symptomatic cases, flexion and extension reproduce the symptoms, and an effusion is noted. Care must be taken not to misinterpret other snapping structures about the knee (e.g., the iliotibial band or pathologic plica) as a discoid meniscus.

Imaging

Routine radiographs are usually normal. In a small percentage of cases, lateral compartment articular space widening and flattening are seen, with or without diminution of the tibial eminences (Fig. 28D2–17). MRI shows a "bow-tie" appearance to the meniscus that is thicker than normal and is seen across the entire lateral compartment with complete and incomplete types (Fig. 28D2–18). MRI may illustrate a tear, but meniscal lesions may also be missed. MRI commonly demonstrates the ligament of Wrisberg, but accurate imaging of the meniscocapsular posterior attachment is purely fortuitous.

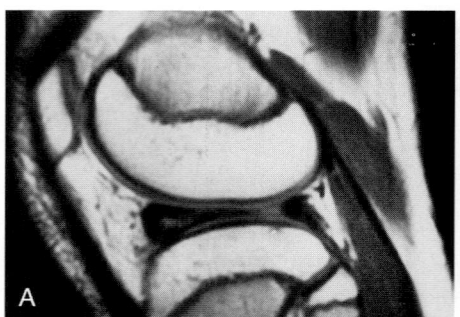
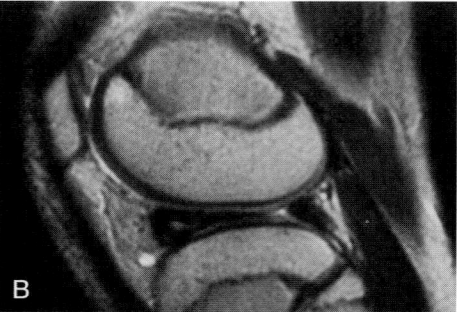
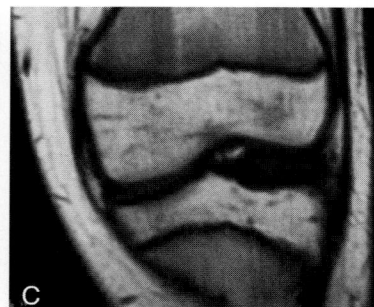

Figure 28D2–18. *A* and *B*, Sagittal magnetic resonance images of a torn posterior horn in a lateral type II discoid meniscus in a 9-year-old girl. *C*, Coronal view of same.

Treatment

Treatment is based on symptoms, meniscal morphology, stability, and pathologic process. Asymptomatic patients whose discoid meniscus is an incidental finding at the time of surgery for another cause require no intervention. For patients whose only complaint (usually parental) is snapping, the parents are informed of the snapping source and the potential need for later treatment. Symptoms other than snapping are usually caused by a radial or horizontal tear in the meniscus, most commonly in the central zone in types I and II. One is faced with management of tissue that is ill formed, poorly vascularized, and potentially unstable. Even after reconstruction, the tissue remaining in types I and II and, rarely, in type III is not normal.

Arthroscopic reconstruction of types I and II is difficult because adequate arthroscopic visualization is prohibited by the large meniscal size, which limits instrument placement and manipulation (Fig. 28D2–19). Arthroscopic surgical experience and facility are necessary for most discoid meniscal reconstructions. Total excision of types I and II was the previous procedure of choice. With the emergence of meniscal preservation and salvage techniques, partial meniscal tear débridement with sculpting of the remainder of the meniscus to a more normal size and shape, while preserving a 6- to 8-mm rim, has come about (Fig. 28D2–20).[3, 5, 15] Some authors suggest partial meniscectomy without contouring.[14] If a peripheral unstable tear is present, meniscal repair is done. Symptomatic type III menisci require stabilization. This can be done arthroscopically or through a miniarthrotomy.[11]

Prognosis and Complications

Outcome analysis of discoid meniscal treatment suffers from retrospective assessment of small numbers of patients of widely varying ages, pathologic processes, and treatments with limited follow-up. Surgical techniques include open and arthroscopic ones by a variety of surgeons. Outcome appears to be related to the remnant of remaining meniscus and its stability. Preliminary overall results are favorable. Series with the longest follow-up place patients in the latter third or early fourth decade of life.[1, 5, 10, 16, 17] Whether satisfactory function will continue or premature joint senescence will ensue is not known. The high rates

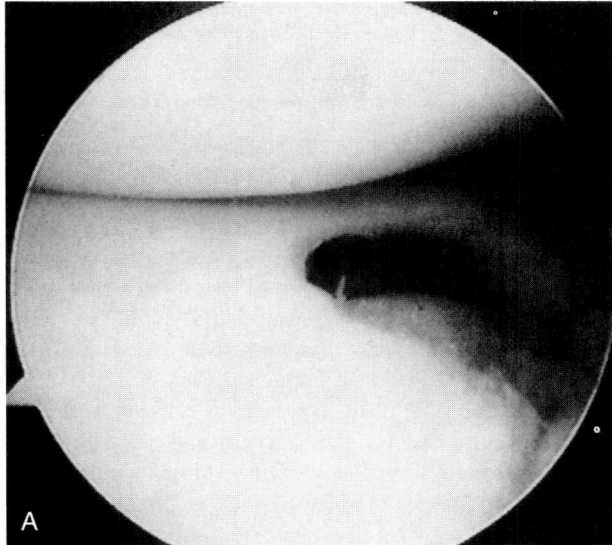

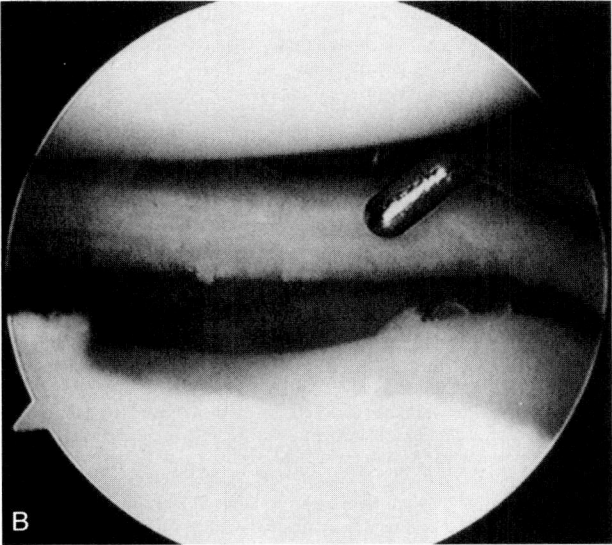

Figure 28D2–20. *A,* Symptomatic type II lateral discoid meniscus. *B,* After sculpting to a more normal shape. (Courtesy of Dr. James Bradley.)

of radiologically evident but clinically minimally symptomatic degenerative joint disease after discoid meniscal excision reported by some authors are cause for concern.[1, 5, 10, 13, 16, 17]

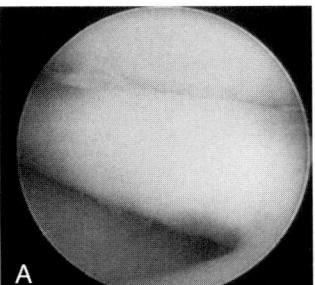
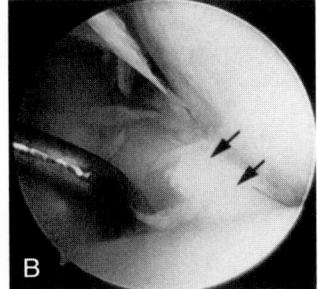

Figure 28D2–19. *A,* Large type II lateral discoid meniscal free edge. *B,* Peripheral tear *(arrows)* with probe retracting central fragment.

References

Meniscal Injuries

1. Andrish JT: Meniscal injuries in children and adolescents: Diagnosis and management. J Am Acad Orthop Surg 4:231–237, 1996.
2. Annandale T: An operation for displaced semilunar cartilage. Clin Orthop 1990:3–5, 1885.
3. Arnoczky SP, Warren RF: Microvasculature of the human meniscus. Am J Sports Med 10:90–95, 1982.
4. Arnoczky SP, Warren RF: The microvasculature of the meniscus and its response to injury. An experimental study in the dog. Am J Sports Med 11:131–141, 1983.
5. Austin KS, Sherman OH: Complications of arthroscopic meniscal repair. Am J Sports Med 21:864–868, 1993.

6. Baratz ME, Fu FH, Mengato R: Meniscal tears: The effect of meniscectomy and of repair on intraarticular contact areas and stress in the human knee. A preliminary report. Am J Sports Med 14:270–275, 1986.
7. Barber FA, Herbert MA: Meniscal repair devices. Arthroscopy 16:613–618, 2000.
8. Boden SD, Davis DO, Dina TS, et al: A prospective and blinded investigation of magnetic resonance imaging of the knee. Abnormal findings in asymptomatic subjects. Clin Orthop 282:177–185, 1992.
9. Clark CR, Ogden JA: Development of the menisci of the human knee joint. Morphological changes and their potential role in childhood meniscal injury. J Bone Joint Surg Am 65:538–547, 1983.
10. DeHaven KE, Arnoczky SP: Meniscus repair: Basic science, indications for repair, and open repair. Instr Course Lect 43:65–76, 1994.
11. Dowdy PA, Miniaci A, Arnoczky SP, et al: The effect of cast immobilization on meniscal healing. An experimental study in the dog. Am J Sports Med 23:721–728, 1995.
12. Fairbank TC: Knee joint changes after meniscectomy. J Bone Joint Surg Br 30B:664, 1948.
13. Ghosh P, Taylor TK: The knee joint meniscus. A fibrocartilage of some distinction. Clin Orthop 224:52–63, 1987.
14. Goto H, Shuler FD, Lamsam C, et al: Transfer of lacZ marker gene to the meniscus. J Bone Joint Surg Am 81:918–925, 1999.
15. Harvell JC Jr, Fu FH, Stanitski CL: Diagnostic arthroscopy of the knee in children and adolescents. Orthopedics 12:1555–1560, 1989.
16. Johnson MJ, Lucas GL, Dusek JK, Henning CE: Isolated arthroscopic meniscal repair: A long-term outcome study (more than 10 years). Am J Sports Med 27:44–49, 1999.
17. King D: The healing of semilunar cartilages. Clin Orthop 1990:4–7, 1936.
18. LaPrade RF, Burnett QM II, Veenstra MA, Hodgman CG: The prevalence of abnormal magnetic resonance imaging findings in asymptomatic knees. With correlation of magnetic resonance imaging to arthroscopic findings in symptomatic knees. Am J Sports Med 22:739–745, 1994.
19. Lonner JH, Parisien JS: Arthroscopic treatment of meniscal cysts. Oper Tech Orthop 5:72–77, 1995.
20. McDermott MJ, Bathgate B, Gillingham BL, Hennrikus WL: Correlation of MRI and arthroscopic diagnosis of knee pathology in children and adolescents. J Pediatr Orthop 18:675–678, 1998.
21. Mintzer CM, Richmond JC, Taylor J: Meniscal repair in the young athlete. Am J Sports Med 26:630–633, 1998.
22. Paletta GA Jr, Manning T, Snell E, et al: The effect of allograft meniscal replacement on intraarticular contact area and pressures in the human knee. A biomechanical study. Am J Sports Med 25:692–698, 1997.
23. Polly DW Jr, Callaghan JJ, Sikes RA, et al: The accuracy of selective magnetic resonance imaging compared with the findings of arthroscopy of the knee. J Bone Joint Surg Am 70:192–198, 1988.
24. Port J, Jackson DW, Lee TQ, Simon TM: Meniscal repair supplemented with exogenous fibrin clot and autogenous cultured marrow cells in the goat model. Am J Sports Med 24:547–555, 1996.
25. Rubman MH, Noyes FR, Barber-Westin SD: Arthroscopic repair of meniscal tears that extend into the avascular zone. A review of 198 single and complex tears. Am J Sports Med 26:87–95, 1998.
26. Schwartzberg R, Lemak LJ, Schwartz ML: MRI of the asymptomatic pediatric knee. Personal communication. Partially presented at the Annual Meeting of the American Academy of Orthopaedic Surgeons, New Orleans, February 1997.
27. Stanitski CL: Correlation of arthroscopic and clinical examinations with magnetic resonance imaging findings of injured knees in children and adolescents. Am J Sports Med 26:2–6, 1998.
28. Stanitski CL, Harvell JC, Fu F: Observations on acute knee hemarthrosis in children and adolescents. J Pediatr Orthop 13:506–510, 1993.
29. Takeda Y, Ikata T, Yoshida S, et al: MRI high-signal intensity in the menisci of asymptomatic children. J Bone Joint Surg Br 80:463–467, 1998.
30. Thompson WO, Thaete FL, Fu FH, Dye SF: Tibial meniscal dynamics using three-dimensional reconstruction of magnetic resonance images. Am J Sports Med 19:210–215, 1991 (discussion 215–216).
31. Vedi V, Williams A, Tennant SJ, et al: Meniscal movement. An in-vivo study using dynamic MRI. J Bone Joint Surg Br 81:37–41, 1999.
32. Veltri DM, Warren RF, Wickiewicz TL, O'Brien SJ: Current status of allograft meniscal transplantation. Clin Orthop 303:44–55, 1994.
33. Zobel MS, Borrello JA, Siegel MJ, Stewart NR: Pediatric knee MR imaging: Pattern of injuries in the immature skeleton. Radiology 190:397–401, 1994.

Discoid Meniscus

1. Aglietti P, Bertini FA, Buzzi R, Beraldi R: Arthroscopic meniscectomy for discoid lateral meniscus in children and adolescents: 10-year follow-up. Am J Knee Surg 12:83–87, 1999.
2. Andrish JT: Meniscal injuries in children and adolescents: Diagnosis and management. J Am Acad Orthop Surg 4:231–237, 1996.
3. Andrish H: The diagnosis and management of meniscus injuries in the skeletally immature athlete. Oper Tech Sports Med 6:186–196, 1998.
4. Clark CR, Ogden JA: Development of the menisci of the human knee joint. Morphological changes and their potential role in childhood meniscal injury. J Bone Joint Surg Am 65:538–547, 1983.
5. Ikeuchi H: Arthroscopic treatment of the discoid lateral meniscus. Technique and long-term results. Clin Orthop 167:19–28, 1982.
6. Jordan MR: Lateral meniscal variants: Evaluation and treatment. J Am Acad Orthop Surg 4:191–200, 1996.
7. Kaplan MJ: "Discoid lateral meniscus of the knee joint: Nature, mechanism, and operative treatment." J Bone Joint Surg Am 39A:77, 1957.
8. Middleton DS: Congenital disc-shaped lateral meniscus with snapping knee. Br J Surg 24:246, 1936.
9. Neuschwander DC, Drez D Jr, Finney TP: Lateral meniscal variant with absence of the posterior coronary ligament. J Bone Joint Surg Am 74:1186–1190, 1992.
10. Raber DA, Friederich NF, Hefti F: Discoid lateral meniscus in children. Long-term follow-up after total meniscectomy. J Bone Joint Surg Am 80:1579–1586, 1998.
11. Rosenberg TD, Paulos LE, Parker RD, et al: Discoid lateral meniscus: Case report of arthroscopic attachment of a symptomatic Wrisberg-ligament type. Arthroscopy 3:277–282, 1987.
12. Smillie IS: The congenital discoid meniscus. J Bone Joint Surg Br 30:671, 1948.
13. Smith CF, Van Dyk GE, Jurgutis J, Vangsness CT Jr: Cautious surgery for discoid menisci. Am J Knee Surg 12:25–28, 1999.
14. Sugawara O, Miyatsu M, Yamashita I, et al: Problems with repeated arthroscopic surgery in the discoid meniscus. Arthroscopy 7:68–71, 1991.
15. Suzuki S: Arthroscopic surgery for discoid meniscus—A report of reoperated cases. Arthroscopy 11:115–118, 1986.
16. Vandermeer RD, Cunningham FK: Arthroscopic treatment of the discoid lateral meniscus: Results of long-term follow-up. Arthroscopy 5:101–109, 1989.
17. Washington ER 3rd, Root L, Liener UC: Discoid lateral meniscus in children. Long-term follow-up after excision. J Bone Joint Surg Am 77:1357–1361, 1995.
18. Watanabe M, Takeda S, Ikeuchi H: Atlas of Arthroscopy. Berlin, Springer-Verlag, 1979.
19. Young RB: The external semilunar cartilage as a complete disc. In Mackay JY, Young RB (eds): Memories and Memoranda in Anatomy. London, Williams and Norgate, 1889, p 179.

Patellofemoral Joint

1. ACUTE DISLOCATION OF THE PATELLA IN THE ADULT

Lee H. Diehl, MD ■ William E. Garrett Jr., MD, PhD

Acute dislocation of the patella in the adult is an entity that both generalist and subspecialist physicians involved in the care of athletes commonly see in the clinic and on the playing field. The appropriate method of treatment for the acute, primary episode of dislocation continues to be debated in the literature. Although the first episode may herald the beginning of a recurring problem in the patient with anatomic predisposition or inadequate treatment, it may also simply be the result of an isolated injury from which the athlete is able to recover and ultimately return to play. The debate regarding treatment of acute patellar dislocation has revolved around the question of anatomic predisposition. Hughston and others published in the early sports medicine literature questioned whether a "normal" patellofemoral joint would ever suffer dislocation and speculated that all affected patients had some degree of predisposition.[17, 28] This position was supported by McManus and Rang, who reported on the natural history of the disorder in children.[45] The successive literature continues to discuss but does not resolve the issue.

Central to the resolution of this controversy is the recognition that two rather distinct patient populations are involved. Both age and anatomy play a role in the initial episode, as well as in the risk of recurrence in some patients. Young age at initial injury has been positively correlated with risk of recurrence, and predisposing anatomic variants have been well categorized.[2, 9, 37] Most physicians, however, now recognize from their own practice that acute patellar dislocation may occur as a traumatic event in a patient with normal patellofemoral alignment, as well as in a patient with preexisting malalignment or other predisposing factors.

Historical references support this division. Gallie in 1924[22] recognized the difference between violent traumatic patellar dislocation in the previously normal knee and that occurring in children or adolescents without "obvious causative traumatism." He contrasted the dislocation by direct violence or abnormal muscular action resulting in "definite rupture" of medial soft tissues, with that felt to be due to abnormal laxity.[22] Cash and Hughston[9] in 1988 recognized these two populations of patients and recorded a 50% lower rate of recurrent instability in the group without a noted predisposition. More recent reports by both Nikku[50] and Atkin[3] also support the dichotomy between occurrence in a predisposed adolescent and that in the normal knee of an adult athlete. What remains unclear about primary acute dislocation in the adult, however, is an estimation of true incidence, an idea of which factors can predict recurrence, and clear guidelines for treatment that will limit resultant functional impairment.

Predisposition to lateral dislocation of the patella falls into the main categories of hypoplasia or dysplasia, malalignment, and congenital or developed contracture or laxity. The examples most commonly cited include hypoplasia of the lateral femoral condyle, patella alta, a shallow trochlea, dysplasia of the patella, hypoplasia of the vastus medialis, an increased Q angle or femoral anteversion, genu valgum, external tibial rotation, and lateralization of the tibial tuberosity. Laxity of the medial retinaculum, tightness of the lateral retinaculum, and contracture of the iliotibial band, as well as pes planus and generalized ligamentous laxity, have also been implicated.[6, 53] Some authors have reported an association with unstable patellar morphology, as described by Wiberg,[69] and other authors have not supported this.[26, 39, 40, 66] Maenpaa and associates[40] followed 75 patients for between 6 and 24 years, after closed treatment for a primary unilateral acute patellar dislocation. They reported a recurrence rate of 49% and felt that radiographically unstable patellar morphology based on Wiberg type, spontaneous reduction, and low-volume hemarthrosis were found to have some prognostic importance for recurrence. Their findings were supported by the theory that less force would be required to displace an already unstable patella, which would result in less intra-articular damage. Stanitski reported in 1995[62] that articular lesions were more than twice as common after acute patellar dislocation among patients who did not have generalized joint laxity. Whether a specific patellar type can be associated with the propensity for patellofemoral instability is inconclusive. In a 1990 study by Vainionpaa,[66] no significance in shape of patella, patellofemoral angle, or presence of patella alta was found. Despite these conflicting results, patella alta is the most consistently associated finding in patellar dislocation. It remains associated, however, in only 30% to 50% of reported cases of acute patellar dislocation in the adult.[3, 30]

The true incidence of acute patellar dislocation in the adult is difficult to discern from the literature. This is primarily due to the lack of population-based prospective studies and a prevalence of retrospective evaluations and case series. The largest North American study to date is that by Atkin and colleagues.[3] They prospectively studied a group of Kaiser Permanente patients from the greater San Diego area of Southern California. The average plan enrollment included more than 360,000 patients, with approximately 1000 of these patients referred each year for evaluation of knee injury. During the 3-year study period, 74 patients from this group were diagnosed with primary patellar dislocation. Broken down by age, at 31 per 100,000, the highest annual risk was noted for patients in the second decade. The average annual risk dropped to 11

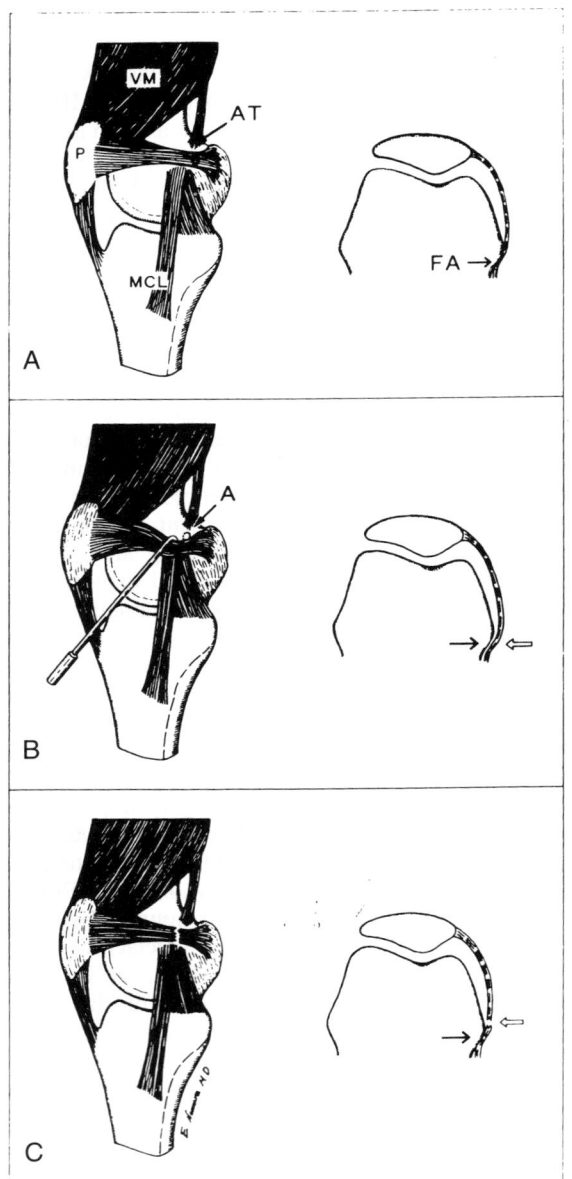

Figure 28E1–4. Schematic diagram of proposed medial patellofemoral ligament injury classification in acute patellar dislocation. *A,* Normal anatomy. *B,* Avulsion-tear type, with disruption/soft tissue discontinuity. (From Normura E: Classification of lesions of the medial patellofemoral ligament in patellar dislocation. Int Orthop 23:260, 1999. © Springer-Verlag.)

to the medial patellar restraining force measured. Desio and associates in 1998[15] sought to improve on the experimental design used by Conlan and conducted their own investigation. Their results were very similar to those of the previous study; they also concluded that the MPFL is the primary restraint to lateral patellar subluxation. They found that it contributed 60% of the restraining power in their study (Table 28E1–1). A third study by Hautamaa and colleagues was a selective release and repair experiment on 17 fresh frozen cadaveric knees, again measuring the individual contributions of the medial and lateral patellar restraints and the individual patellar ligaments. After sequential re-

lease, they added selective repair to their protocol. They found that isolated release of the medial patellofemoral ligament resulted in a 50% increase in lateral patellar displacement. Release of the medial meniscotibial ligament resulted in no added lateral displacement after the medial patellofemoral retinaculum was cut, as long as the MPFL remained intact. Release of the MPFL, however, when preceded by release of the retinaculum and other ligaments, resulted in 75% greater lateral displacement than occurred in the intact state. Additionally, they found that isolated repair of the MPFL restored static lateral stability to the patella. Sandmeier and coworkers in another recent cadaveric study[59] reported results of sectioning medial patellar restraints and demonstrated a substantial restoration of normal patellar tracking after using a gracilis tendon graft to reconstruct the MPFL.[59] Viewed in light of these recent biomechanical studies, it remains unclear why little mention of the medial patellofemoral ligament as a key stabilizing structure can be found in the literature over the preceding 50 years. Furthermore, one must question whether absence of an identifiable MPFL represents a congenital lack,[55] or an attrition of the medial ligamentous structure due to repeated instability of the patellofemoral articulation.[51]

Physical Examination

Acute dislocation of the patella in the adult requires disruption of the medial patellar restraints. Swelling associated with the acute injury is often rapid, and a significant hemarthrosis frequently develops, especially if there is an associated osteochondral fracture. This swelling may mask a persistent lateral subluxation of the patella within the trochlea, which may be noted on physical examination (Fig. 28E1–5). Loose chondral or bony fragments may be palpable in the joint, and attached osteochondral fragments may be palpable in the medial parapatellar retinaculum (Fig. 28E1–6). A thorough palpation of the knee should be performed to detect focal areas of maximum tenderness that suggest soft tissue injury. The examiner may find a palpable defect at the medial patellar margin, tenderness along the course of the MPFL and the other medial retinacular ligaments, or tenderness near the medial femoral epicondyle at the MPFL insertion site. Tenderness at the medial femoral condyle may suggest an injury to the medial collateral ligament of the knee (Fig. 28E1–7). If significant disruption of the VMO insertion has occurred, there may be a palpable defect at its distal insertion, as well as a visible change in its symmetry. A positive apprehension test in 30 degrees of flexion is the classically described examination finding. With or without apprehension, the physician may be able to demonstrate increased medial retinacular laxity, which is not symmetrical with the contralateral knee.

Associated Injuries

Chondral or osteochondral injury is a frequently associated finding in acute patellar dislocation. Incidence of these injuries based on radiographic evidence ranges from 5% to

TABLE 28E1–1
Percent Contribution of the Soft Tissues to the Total Restraining Force at Maximal Patellar Translation at 20 Degrees of Knee Flexion

Specimen	Force in Intact Knee (N)	Restraining Force* (% Contribution)				
		Lateral Retinaculum	*Medial Patellofemoral Ligament*	*Medial Retinaculum*	*Medial Patellotibial Ligament*	*Medial Patellomeniscal Ligament*
1	250	8	41	2	1	35
2	163	7	70	2	1	9
3	125	6	61	3	4	7
4	193	15	47	5	9	16
5	167	9	80	2	1	4
6	177	8	71	1	4	6
7	190	12	51	1	4	16
8	197	16	50	2	1	13
9	178	6	66	12	1	7
Mean	182	10	60	3	3	13
SD	33	4	13	4	3	10
Minimum	125	6	41	1	1	4
Maximum	250	16	80	12	9	35

*The structures were sectioned in the order listed. The contributions of the lateral retinaculum, the medial patellofemoral ligament, the medial retinaculum, the medial patellotibial ligament, and the medial patellomeniscal ligament are given as a percent of the intact load to maximal translation.

From Desio SM, Burks RT, Bachus KN: Soft tissue restraints to lateral patellar translation in the human knee. Am J Sports Med 26:63, 1998. Permission granted by the American Journal of Sports Medicine.

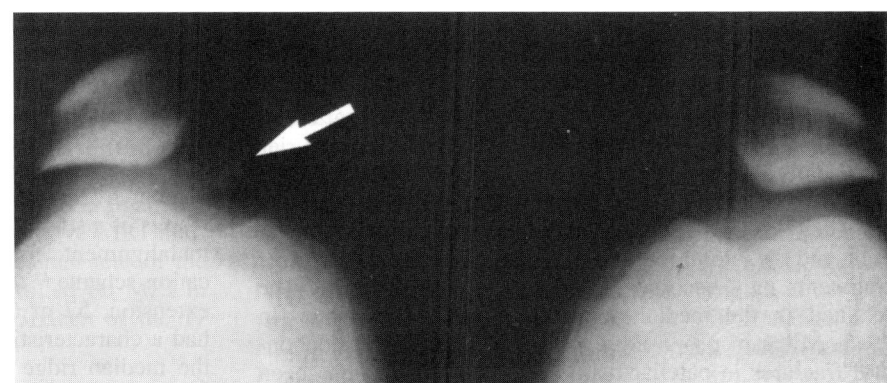

Figure 28E1–5. Patellar dislocation with a large osteochondral fracture *(arrow).*

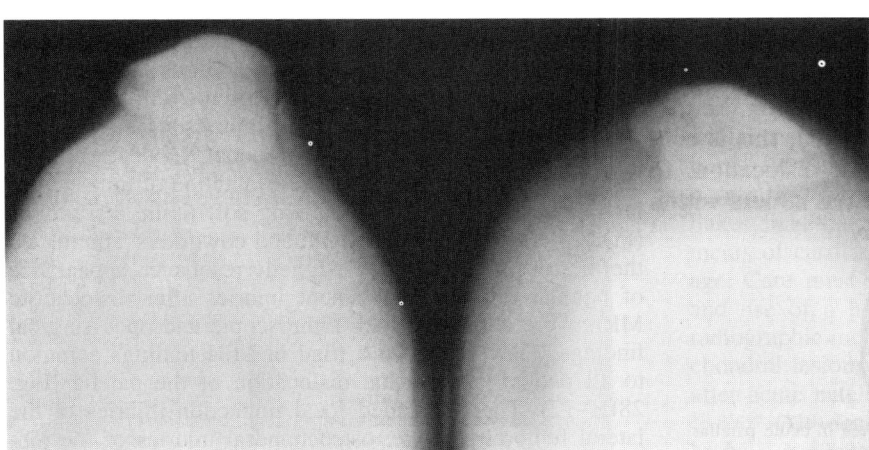

Figure 28E1–6. Axial view shows characteristic avulsion and calcification along the medial edge of the patella.

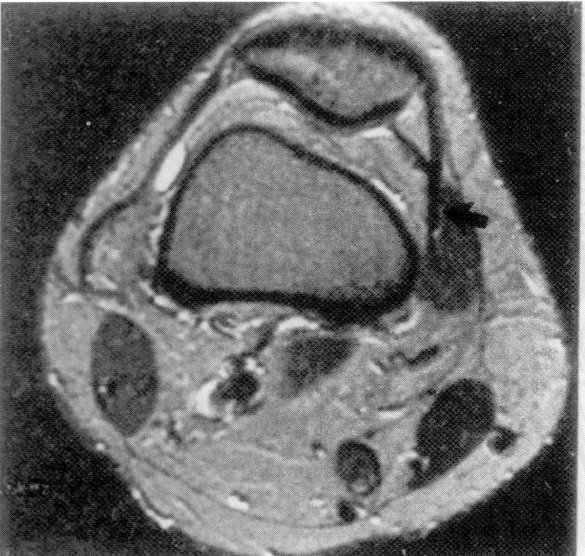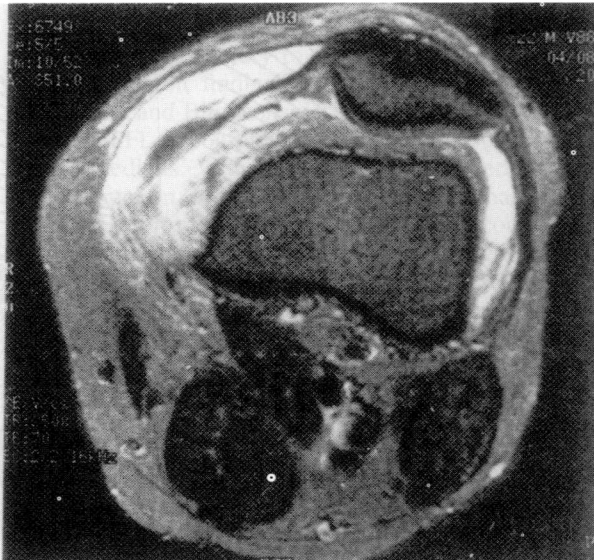

Figure 28E1–11. In the image on the left, the *arrow* points to normal MPFL; image on the right shows avulsion of the MPFL off the medial femoral condyle. (From Boden BP, Pearsall AW, Garrett WE Jr, Feagin JA Jr: Patellofemoral instability: Evaluation and management. J Am Acad Orthop Surg 5:47, 1997. © 1997 American Academy of Orthopaedic Surgeons. Reprinted with permission.)

at arthroscopy in 48 patients sustaining acute initial patellar dislocation. Seventy-one percent had articular damage; only 32% of these lesions had been identified on preoperative radiographs, and only 29% of osteochondral loose bodies were accurately identified. Dainer and Barrack reported similar results, finding articular defects not recognized on preoperative films in 40% of their patients at the time of arthroscopy.[14] These studies would suggest that as many as 6 or 7 of 10 patients sustaining acute dislocation

of the patella will have intra-articular injuries not visualized on plain films. Many authors have cited these statistics as an indication for both MRI and the use of arthroscopy after an episode of acute patellar dislocation.[54, 58, 61, 63]

Treatment

The treatment for an initial patellar dislocation varies between simple immobilization and operative repair or reconstruction. Current evidence from the literature suggests that about half of all adults suffering an acute primary dislocation do reasonably well with nonoperative treatment. The only problem is that this leaves another 50% who do not do as well. Recent studies have shown that many patients with APD are young and active, and there is some evidence that young, active patients suffer a greater degree of prolonged impairment.[3, 12] Some authors have stated that regardless of treatment type, between 30% and 50% of patients will continue to have symptoms of instability or anterior knee pain.[29] Given the multitude of studies of patellar dislocation in the literature, no definitive work yet has recommended for or against conservative or operative treatment.

Nonoperative Management

Nonsurgical treatment usually entails a period of immobilization of between 3 and 6 weeks to allow healing of the disrupted medial supporting structures. No recent studies that guide treatment compare the duration of immobilization and its effect on re-dislocation rate. Similarly, the advancement of range of motion, timing of weight-bearing, use of a patellar restraining brace, and sophistication and

Figure 28E1–12. Classical triad of patellar dislocation injury: Injury of the medial retinacular ligament *(curved arrow)*, osteochondral fracture of the medial patellar facet *(thick solid arrow)*, impaction injury of the lateral femoral condyle *(open arrow)*. (From Quinn SF, Brown TR, Demlow TA: MR imaging of patellar retinacular ligament injuries, JMRI 3:843, 1993. Reprinted by permission of Wiley Liss, Inc., a subsidiary of John Wiley & Sons, Inc.)

aggressiveness of rehabilitation are all variable from physician to physician and from institution to institution. Most of the published studies are nonrandomized and retrospective and involve a mixture of chronic and acute instability. They also involve different methods of immobilization and treatment protocols not applicable to today's standards. The longest-term follow-up studies involve patients enrolled from the 1950s and 1960s; they traditionally included immobilization in a cylinder cast.[23, 40] Re-dislocation or recurrent subluxation rates after nonoperative treatment have been reported to be as high as 48%.[9, 29, 40] Cofield and Bryan[12] reported that in patients considered athletes, at an average of 5 years, 52% remained unable to return to vigorous sports. Even in more recent literature, there is significant variability among both patient population and treatment methods. For example, Maenpaa and Lehto in 1997[40] reported on the long-term follow-up of nonoperative management in 100 patients after acute patellar dislocation. The treatment groups were divided among use of a plaster cast, posterior splint, and bandage or brace. With the duration of follow-up averaging 13 years, only 37% had no complaints after primary conservative treatment, and the re-dislocation rate over the course of the study was 44%. Comparing outcomes of previous studies with those using modern treatment protocols is also difficult. It is generally well accepted now that prolonged immobilization has a deleterious effect on soft tissue strength and joint cartilage. Conversely, mobilization and early range of motion have been shown to result in increased strength of soft tissue repair.[70] Modern rehabilitation techniques currently entail early progressive mobilization and functional training. Even these modern rehabilitation techniques, however, do not appear to make all the difference in ensuring a favorable outcome after an initial patellar dislocation. Garth and Pomphrey[23] reported on an aggressive, modern rehabilitation protocol in 58 athletically active patients. They began a functional rehabilitation program without antecedent immobilization. At the initial visit, patients were instructed in isometric and isotonic quadriceps strengthening, and active and active-assisted range of motion exercises with a stationary bicycle were begun. Patients wore a lateral buttressing knee sleeve initially for ambulation until muscle strength was documented to be at least 80% that of the opposite extremity. They reported a return to full activity generally after 3 to 8 weeks, with resolution of all significant tenderness and return of full isotonic quadriceps strength. Sixty-eight percent of the patients treated after acute patellar dislocation without previous symptoms had good or excellent results, with 30% experiencing impairment in athletics. In a recent study by Atkin and associates[3] examining the early recovery phase, at 6 months, almost 60% of patients continued to have limitations in strenuous activities.[3] These results show that unfortunately, a large percentage of patients are left with recurring problems with patellofemoral pain and instability.

Operative Management

As a group, operative treatment is used to treat osteochondral injury and to re-establish patellofemoral stability.

Stabilization entails procedures that address the specific deficits leading to the persistence of instability. One of four main approaches is used: Repair, reconstruct, release, or realign. Use of a realignment operation assumes that there was an underlying, predisposing malalignment. The use of lateral release entails a belief in the concept of balancing laxity. Repair and reconstruction are appropriate if there is an identifiable soft tissue injury. Arthroscopy is usually adequate for a thorough diagnosis and for treating osteochondral injuries. It may be used alone or in combination with other procedures.

Some authors[33] date the operative treatment of acute patellar dislocation to the late 1800s, when Roux[57] transposed a patellar tendon and fixed it with a screw. Since that time, more than 100 different operations have been described (including a mixture of repair, reconstruction, and realignment procedures), of which none has gained widespread approval and produced uniformly excellent results. In recent reports of operative treatment, rates of recurrence have ranged from 0% to 17%.[7, 14, 27, 34, 41, 66, 71] At first glance, these results appear superior to those attained with nonoperative treatment, but few randomized, truly prospective studies have been done. Follow-up is generally limited, the numbers of patients are small, and the operative methods as well as results are varied. For example, Vainionpaa and colleagues[66] reported the results of open repair in 55 patients followed prospectively after their first patellar dislocation. At 2 years, subjective results were good or excellent in 80%, with a re-dislocation rate of 9%. Sallay and coworkers[58] reported on 16 patients and found 94% to have had the MPFL torn off the femur. Suture repair was performed, and, with an average 3-year follow-up, no recurrences were seen, and 58% of patients returned to their previous sport. Nikku and Nietosvaara in 1997[50] reported results of a prospective, randomized trial of nonoperative versus operative treatment in 176 consecutive patients who had sustained primary patellar dislocation. In the group randomized to operative treatment, patients had individually adjusted procedures, which consisted of a mixture of medial retinacular repair or duplication, adductor magnus tenodesis, and lateral release. In this report of 2-year results, recurrent instability episodes were equivalent, and both function and subjective results were better in the nonoperative group. The authors felt surgery gave no additional benefit, and it remains to be seen whether long-term follow-up will change their findings.

In general, operative indications for treatment of an initial dislocation of the patella in the adult continue to be controversial and less than clear. Several authors[5, 12, 18, 29, 31, 52] have advocated early surgical treatment. The indications, however, varied widely from acute repair to correction of predisposing malalignment. In the current literature, the most commonly cited indications for operative treatment in the adult without predisposing malalignment include the following: patients with evidence of osteochondral loose bodies, patients with large palpable defects in the VMO insertion, those with obvious tears of the medial peripatellar retinaculum, and those with persistent asymmetrical subluxation. Elite athletes and, more recently, patients thought to have an avulsion of the MPFL are also operative candidates.[9, 12, 29, 53, 58]

Operative Methods

Arthroscopy of the knee joint after acute dislocation of the patella is becoming more widely accepted. The main advantage of arthroscopy is the ability to directly inspect the articular surfaces without performance of an arthrotomy. Arthroscopy can be used for the removal of, or facilitate repair of, osteochondral fragments. Current reports in the literature detail the high percentage of chondral and osteochondral injury found at surgery.[14, 67] Many such injuries had not been visualized preoperatively, and others, which were visible during arthroscopy, may not by themselves have mandated operative treatment. Some authors have combined the use of diagnostic arthroscopy with additional procedures such as lateral release and medial retinacular reefing or repair.[20, 50]

The use of lateral release as an adjunct, or as the sole, treatment of acute patellar dislocation is more controversial than in recurrent dislocations. It has been commonly used to bring about a "balanced laxity." When the lateral retinaculum is felt to be too tight, or the medial side (after dislocation) is too loose, cutting the lateral tissues and allowing them to scar in a lengthened position may serve to rebalance the patellofemoral articulation. Lateral release has been shown to be efficacious in reducing abnormal patellar tilt. However, Fulkerson has also noted that retinacular release is inconsistent in relieving lateral patellar subluxation.[20] Several other authors have questioned the efficacy of lateral release in treating patellar dislocation. In clinical studies, Jensen and Roosen[34] found that lateral release provided no advantage over medial capsulorrhaphy alone. Vainionpaa and coworkers[65] found that lateral release led to a medial over-displacement of the patella, and Dainer and Barrack[14] reported an increased rate of re-dislocation after the use of lateral release. In biomechanical studies, Desio and associates[15] showed that the lateral retinaculum provides 10% of the restraining power to lateral displacement of the patella. Cutting the lateral retinaculum, therefore, may actually contribute to lateral dislocation rather than helping to prevent it.

Several authors have used the combination of lateral release and medial plication in relatively large series,[27, 33, 66] and short-term results have been good. Maenpaa and Lehto[40] reported results from a retrospective study that included 177 patients with primary acute patellar dislocation. All patients underwent reefing of the medial capsule, with release of the lateral patellar retinaculum in most. At an average of 4 years' follow-up, subjective results were good or excellent in 77%, with no patients rated poor. Eight percent of re-dislocations occurred after treatment of the primary dislocation. Vainionpaa and colleagues[66] reported on 55 patients treated with medial reefing. Lateral release was added in 37 patients who demonstrated a tight lateral retinaculum, tending to move the patella laterally. Subjective results were 80% good or excellent at 2-year follow-up, with a re-dislocation rate of 9%. Of interest, lateral release was performed in all but one of the cases with re-dislocation. Harilainen and Sandelin[27] reported the 6.5-year follow-up results in a prospective study of 53 patients with primary patellar dislocation, who had been treated with medial retinacular suture repair or reefing and

lateral release. In this longer-term follow-up, they found a 17% re-dislocation rate.

As was previously described, the medial patellofemoral ligament is the major medial restraint to lateral displacement of the patella. Specific mention of repair of this structure after acute dislocation of the patellofemoral joint, however, has been distinctly lacking in the orthopaedic literature over the past 50 years. It may be that this structure was commonly repaired, but not specifically reported, when authors performed medial capsulorrhaphy for acute dislocation. After all, authors such as Vainionpaa[66] did record that 54 of their 55 patients were found to have ruptured the medial retinaculum at surgery. In addition to the recent anatomic and biomechanical studies by Conlan,[13] Desio,[15] Feller,[16] Hautamaa,[28] Nomura,[51] Sandmeier,[59] Spritzer,[61] Quinn,[54] and Sallay and coworkers[58] reported the 2-year results of MPFL repair after acute patellar dislocation. At open surgical exploration, 15 of 16 patients (94%) were found to have tears of the MPFL from its femoral insertion. Direct suture repair, or reattachment with suture anchors, was performed. At minimum 2 years' follow-up, they reported no recurrent dislocations, although 42% of patients still had significant symptoms. It is also important to note that medial reefing may not restore the integrity of the MPFL. Because the ligament commonly tears at its femoral attachment, reefing the patellar attachment alone does nothing to restore continuity.

Gallie in 1924[22] described an extra-articular reconstruction for treatment of patellar dislocation, by fashioning a medial restraint using a strip of fascia lata and anchoring it through tunnels in the superior medial border of the patella and the "most prominent point of the internal condyle." Between 1918 and 1923, he performed the operation seven times with no cases of recurrence. In 1993, Avikainen and Nikku[4] published preliminary results of a new reconstructive technique, described as "adductor magnus tenodesis for patellar dislocation." Of 14 patients, 10 had sustained acute patellar dislocation, and all 10 were noted at surgery to have avulsion of the MPFL from its insertion near the adductor tubercle on the femur. The distal adductor tendon was cut 8 cm proximal to its insertion at the distal femur. After the MPFL and the edge of the vastus medialis retinaculum are attached to the medial femoral epicondyle, the adductor magnus tendon is turned down, redirected anteriorly, and sutured over the vastus medialis retinaculum near the medial border of the patella, thereby augmenting the MPFL (Fig. 28E1–13). At mean follow-up of 6.5 years, they reported one re-dislocation from this group. Nikku and Nietosvaara in 1997[50] used the procedure in six patients, but the results for this subgroup were not separated from those for others.

Taken in summary, the literature suggests that two main groups of patients suffer acute dislocation of the patella—those with, and those without, significant predisposition. It is in the young, athletically active adult without previous history of subluxation who sustains an acute patellar dislocation that surgeons can focus on fixing what's broken. It is clear that some patients do well with nonoperative treatment. There is, however, significant enough incidence of occult intra-articular injury that arthroscopic evaluation should be strongly considered in most patients. More recent anatomic and biomechanical studies, and several

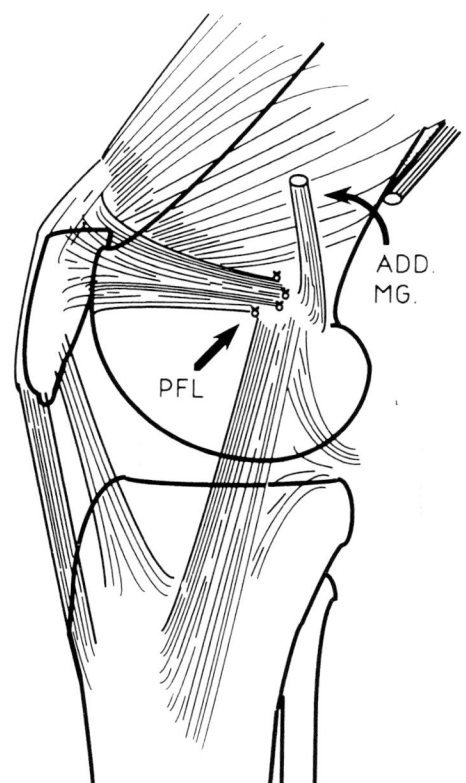

Figure 28E1–13. Schematic diagram showing reattachment of the medial patellofemoral ligament (PFL) to the medial femoral epicondyle, and use of the adductor magnus (ADD. MG.) tendon for reinforcement. (From Avikainen VJ, Nikku RK, Seppanen-Lehmonen TK: Adductor magnus tenodesis for patellar dislocation. Clin Orthop 297:122, 1993.)

small case series, suggest that repairing the main medial stabilizer to lateral translation of the patella, the MPFL, may restore patellar stability. Owing to the lack of long-term, prospective study results, however, it continues to be unclear as to whether operative treatment consistently provides significantly improved outcomes, reliably preventing recurrent subluxation or dislocation.

Rehabilitation and Return to Play

Regardless of initial operative or nonoperative treatment of an acute patellar dislocation, rehabilitation is an important component of long-term recovery and the resumption of normal activities. A structured program should be started, including advancing weight-bearing as tolerated, regaining active and passive range of motion, and beginning closed chain resistance exercises. This type of program is often best established and monitored by a physical therapist or athletic trainer familiar with these injuries. Criteria for return to sports participation should include evidence of adequate healing of the soft tissue injury, and the return of adequate strength to tolerate the demands of play, as well as to protect from recurrent or additional injury. Subjectively, patients should have no complaints of pain, swelling, or sensations of instability. Objectively, they should have no evidence of effusion; should demonstrate a full, pain-free range of motion; should have no tenderness to palpation or apprehension with manipulation of the patella; and should demonstrate adequate quadriceps function. When the quadriceps muscle has regained 80% to 90% of the strength of the contralateral side on functional testing, athletes may begin progressive sport-specific training. When the athlete is able to run and perform cutting maneuvers at full speed without symptoms, he is allowed to resume unrestricted practice and can return to competition. McConnell taping techniques or patellar stabilizing braces have both been commonly used during rehabilitation and when the athlete first returns to athletics.[1, 3, 19] Although these techniques and braces may serve a protective or proprioceptive function, no outcome studies in the literature prove that they reduce the rate of re-dislocation.[11]

Authors' Preferred Method of Treatment

Our recommended treatment for the patient with an initial patellar dislocation depends on his or her age, anatomic factors, activity level or sports participation, and mechanism of injury, and the amount of subluxation and instability remaining in the patella on repeat examination after reduction. Natural history studies suggest that nonoperative treatment is successful in more than 50% of patients. Consideration for operative treatment should, therefore, be tempered by these results. Timing of surgical treatment is important. It is true that surgical treatment does not necessarily have to be done only acutely. However, it may also be true that successful MPFL repair is more predictable when it is done near the time of injury, even though current studies have not addressed this issue. We are more inclined to do acute repair when the patella exhibits significant subluxation or instability, or when the incidence of recurrent dislocation is judged to be high owing to age, athletic participation, or anatomic factors.

Nonoperative Management

In a skeletally immature patient with a valgus alignment, lateral subluxation, and evidence of generalized ligamentous laxity, who has no evidence of significant retinacular tear or intra-articular osteochondral loose body, an initial trial of nonoperative management is our preference. If the patient has a large hemarthrosis, we may aspirate the knee under sterile conditions to evacuate the effusion and to decrease inhibition of the quadriceps. We usually obtain radiographs and an MRI to evaluate for the presence of intra-articular loose bodies. Progressive immediate weight-bearing and discontinuation of crutches as soon as tolerated are encouraged. After the brief initial period of knee immobilization, range of motion exercises and isometric quadriceps activation are begun. The patient may increase knee range of motion based on the level of discomfort rather than according to a set protocol. We usually refer the patient for supervised physical therapy if progress is slow. With regard to bracing during rehabilitation, there continue to be no definitive studies supporting their use. It has, therefore, been our practice to discontinue brace use after the initial period of knee immobilization in the patient with a first-time dislocation. Recurrent dislocators sometimes benefit from the use of a patella-stabilizing brace.

Operative Management

Operative indications vary in the existing literature. The most commonly cited indications include evidence of rupture of the VMO insertion, obvious tears of the medial peripatellar retinaculum, evidence of osteochondral loose bodies, and avulsion of the MPFL from the femoral insertion. Physical examination and radiographic studies help to elucidate these pathoanatomic defects. Palpation for areas of maximal tenderness can help in the detection of peripatellar retinacular defects, distal VMO rupture, or injury near the femoral epicondyle, suggesting avulsion of the MPFL. It can also detect effusion and loose bodies, suggesting osteochondral fragments. Persistent displacement of the patella, effusion, and osteochondral fragments may also be seen on plain radiographs. Studies have shown, however, that plain radiographs are not sufficient for determination of the full extent of injury. For this reason, we usually obtain an MRI study. It remains the most effective diagnostic tool for further evaluating the degree of intra-articular and periarticular soft tissue injury. MRIs can be useful for detecting signal change consistent with injury or frank disruption of peripatellar structures, bone bruises, and loose bodies not visualized on plain radiographs.

Surgical repair of acute patellar dislocation is best performed within 2 to 3 weeks of injury in order to avoid operating through early scar tissue formation. We begin the surgical procedure with a diagnostic arthroscopy to inspect the joint for evidence of soft tissue or capsular injury, and to repair or remove osteochondral or chondral loose bodies. The MPFL is external to the synovial layer and usually is not visible directly by arthroscopy. Repair of MPFL avulsions or VMO insertional tears is performed through a 4- to 6-cm incision just anterior to the medial femoral epicondyle, at the distal edge of the VMO muscle belly. The MPFL is identified confluent with the deep fascia of the VMO, and can usually be demonstrated to have a direct connection to the superior medial border of the patella. In most of these cases, the MPFL can be found to have avulsed off the femur and may be repaired directly by adhering to bone with suture anchors. Complete intrasubstance tears are repaired with permanent suture. Overlying retinacular tears are then repaired with absorbable suture. If the retinaculum and capsule are disrupted near the patella, this is usually clear from the examination and MRI, and repair is performed through a medial parapatellar incision. In patients without a substantial MPFL, we supplement the repair with a hamstring graft from the patella to the femoral attachment site of the MPFL. The retinaculum and VMO are also slightly imbricated in the repair.

We do not routinely perform a lateral release unless there is a history of symptoms and physical evidence of excessive lateral patellar tilt persisting after the medial patellar restraints have been re-established. Similarly, we do not routinely perform any proximal or distal realignment procedures at the same time as the acute repair. These are usually reserved for a separate operation in the patient with an anatomic malalignment and history of patellofemoral subluxation before the dislocation, if the patient continues to have symptoms after repair.

Postoperative treatment consists of progressive weight-bearing as tolerated in a postoperative brace, followed by early range of motion and quadriceps-strengthening exercises. We have found that regaining flexion can be difficult, even if range of motion is started early. Occasionally, manipulation under anesthesia is required. The athlete is allowed to return to sport-specific training when he or she has regained full, nontender, functional range of motion and demonstrates muscular strength equal to 80% to 90% that of the contralateral limb. Return to play follows a demonstration of adequate recovery during functional testing.

Results

Surgical treatment of acute patellar dislocation in the adult can be quite successful in preventing recurrent dislocation, and patients are usually able to return to sports. There are, however, some patients with risk factors for instability or patellofemoral pain, which predate their episode of acute dislocation. Even with successful treatment of the dislocation, many of these patients may continue to have patellofemoral pain and episodes of subluxation. It is certainly best for the surgeon and the patient to understand this preoperatively.

References

1. American Academy of Orthopaedic Surgeons: Athletic Training and Sports Medicine, 2nd ed. Park Ridge, Ill, AAOS, 1991, Chap 21.
2. Arnbjornsson A, Egund N: The natural history of recurrent dislocation of the patella: Long-term results of conservative and operative treatment. J Bone Joint Surg Br 74:140, 1992.
3. Atkin DM, Fithian DC, Maranji KS, et al: Characteristics of patients with primary acute lateral patellar dislocation and their recovery within the first six months of injury. Am J Sports Med 4:472, 2000.
4. Avikainen VJ, Nikku RK: Adductor magus tenodesis for patellar dislocation. Clin Orthop 297:12, 1993.
5. Bassett FH: Acute dislocation of the patella. Instr Course Lect 26:40, 1976.
6. Boden BP, Pearsall AW: Patellofemoral instability: Evaluation and management. J Am Acad Orthop Surg 5:47, 1997.
7. Boring TH, O'Donoghue DH: Acute patellar dislocation: Results of immediate surgical repair. Clin Orthop 136:182, 1977.
8. Bose K, Kanagasuntheram R, Osman MB: Vastus medialis oblique: An anatomic and physiologic study. Orthopaedics 3:880, 1980.
9. Cash JD, Hughston JC: Treatment of acute patellar dislocation. Am J Sports Med 16:244, 1988.
10. Casteleyn PP, Handelberg F: Arthroscopy in the diagnosis of occult dislocation of the patella. Acta Orthop Belg 55:381, 1989.
11. Cherf J, Paulos LE: Bracing for patellar instability. Clin Sports Med 4:813, 1990.
12. Cofield RH, Bryan RS: Acute dislocation of the patella: Results of conservative treatment. J Trauma 17:526, 1977.
13. Conlan T, Garth WP: Evaluation of the medial soft-tissue restraints of the extensor mechanism of the knee. J Bone Joint Surg Am 75:682, 1993.
14. Dainer RD, Barrack RL, Buckley SL, Alexander AH: Arthroscopic treatment of acute patellar dislocations. Arthroscopy 4:267, 1988.

15. Desio SM, Burks RT, Bachus KN: Soft tissue restraints to lateral patellar translation in the human knee. Am J Sports Med 26:59, 1998.
16. Feller JA, Feagin JA Jr, Garrett WE Jr: The medial patellofemoral ligament revisited: An anatomical study. Knee Surg Sports Traumatol Arthrosc 1:184, 1993.
17. Ficat RP, Hungerford DS: Disorders of the Patellofemoral Joint. Baltimore, William and Wilkins, 1977, p 76.
18. Fondren FB, Goldner JL: Recurrent dislocation of the patella treated by the modified Roux-Goldwait procedure. J Bone Joint Surg Am 67:994, 1985.
19. Fu FH, Stone DA. Sports Injuries: Mechanisms, Prevention, Treatment. Baltimore, Williams and Wilkins, Chaps 22, 19.
20. Fulkerson JP: Diseases of the Patellofemoral Joint, 3rd ed. Baltimore, Williams and Wilkins, 1999.
21. Fulkerson JP: Evaluation of the peripatellar soft tissues and retinaculum in patients with patellofemoral pain. Clin Sports Med 8:197, 1989.
22. Gallie WH, Lemesurier AB: Habitual dislocation of the patella. J Bone Joint Surg 575, 1924.
23. Garth WP, Pomphrey M: Functional treatment of patellar dislocation in an athletic population. Am J Sports Med 24:785, 1996.
24. Gilbert TJ, Johnson E, Detlie T, Griffiths HJ: Radiologic case study: Patellar dislocation-medial retinacular tears, avulsion fractures, and osteochondral fragments. Orthopaedics 16:729, 1993.
25. Halbrecht JL, Jackson DW: Acute dislocation of the patella. In Fox JM, Del Pizzo W (eds): The Patellofemoral Joint. New York, McGraw-Hill, 1993, p 123.
26. Harilainen A, Myllynen P: Operative treatment in acute patellar dislocation: Radiological predisposing factors, diagnosis and results. Am J Knee Surg 1:178, 1988.
27. Harilainen A, Sandelin J: Prospective long-term results of operative treatment in primary dislocation of the patella. Knee Surg Sports Traumatol Arthrosc 1:100, 1993.
28. Hautamaa PV, Fithian DC: Medial soft tissue restraints in lateral patellar instability and repair. Clin Orthop 349:174, 1998.
29. Hawkins RJ, Bell RH, Anisette G: Acute patellar dislocations: The natural history. Am J Sports Med 14:117, 1986.
30. Henry JH, Crosland JW: Conservative treatment of patellofemoral subluxation. Am J Sports Med 7:12, 1979.
31. Hughston JC: Reconstruction of the extensor mechanism for subluxating patella. J Sports Med 1:6, 1972.
32. Hunter SC, Marascalco R, Hughston JC: Disruption of the vastus medialis obliquus with medial knee ligament injuries. Am J Sports Med 11:427, 1983.
33. Jarvinen M: Acute patellar dislocation—closed or operative treatment? Acta Orthop Scand 68:415, 1997.
34. Jensen CM, Roosen JU: Acute traumatic dislocations of the patella. J Trauma 25:160, 1985.
35. Kirsch MD, Fitzgerald SW, Friedman H, Rogers LF: Transient lateral patellar dislocation: Diagnosis with MR imaging. AJR 161:109, 1993.
36. Lance E, Deutsch AL, Mink JH: Prior lateral patellar dislocation: MR imaging findings. Radiology 189:905, 1993.
37. MacNab I: Recurrent dislocation of the patella. J Bone Joint Surg Am 34:957, 1952.
38. Madigan R, Wissinger HA, Donaldson WF: Preliminary experience with a method of quadricepsplasty in recurrent subluxation of the patella. J Bone Joint Surg Am 57:600, 1975.
39. Maenpaa H, Huhtala H: Recurrence after patellar dislocation. Acta Orthop Scand 68:424, 1997.
40. Maenpaa H, Lehto MUK: Patellar dislocation: The long-term results of nonoperative management in 100 patients. Am J Sports Med 25:213, 1997.
41. Maenpaa H, Lehto MUK: Surgery in acute patellar dislocation—evaluation of the effect of injury mechanism and family occurrence on the outcome of treatment. Br J Sports Med 29:239, 1995.
42. Makin M: Osteochondral fracture of the lateral femoral condyle. J Bone Joint Surg Am 33:262, 1951.
43. Maldague B, Malghem J: Apport du cliché de profil du genou dans le depistage des instabilites rotuliennes: Rapport Preliminaire. Rev Chir Orthop 71(suppl 2):5, 1985.
44. Maletius W, Gillquist J: Acute patellar dislocation during eccentric muscle testing on the biodex dynamometer. Arthroscopy 10:473, 1994.
45. McManus F, Rang M: Acute dislocation of the patella in children: The natural history. Clin Orthop 139:88, 1979.
46. Milgram JE: Tangential osteochondral fracture of the patella. J Bone Joint Surg 25:271, 1943.
47. Muller W. The Knee. Form, Function, and Ligament Reconstruction. New York, Springer-Verlag, 1982.
48. Murry TF, Dupont J, Fulkerson JP: Axial and lateral radiographs in evaluating patellofemoral malalignment. Am J Sports Med 27:580, 1999.
49. Nietosvaara Y, Aalto K: Acute patellar dislocation in children: Incidence and associated osteochondral fractures. J Pediatr Orthop 14:513, 1994.
50. Nikku R, Nietosvaara Y: Operative versus closed treatment of primary dislocation of the patella. Acta Orthop Scand 68:419, 1997.
51. Nomura E: Classification of lesions of the medial patello-femoral ligament in patellar dislocation. Int Orthop 23:260, 1999.
52. O'Donoghue DH: Treatment of Injuries to Athletes. Philadelphia, WB Saunders, 1962.
53. Orthopaedic Knowledge Update 6: Home Study Syllabus. Park Ridge, Ill, American Academy of Orthopaedic Surgeons, 1999.
54. Quinn SF, Brown TR: MR imaging of patellar retinacular ligament injuries. J Magn Reson Imaging 3:843, 1993.
55. Reider B, Marshall JL: The anterior aspect of the knee: An anatomical study. J Bone Joint Surg Am 63:351, 1981.
56. Rosenberg NJ: Osteochondral fractures of the lateral femoral condyle. J Bone Joint Surg Am 46:1013, 1964.
57. Roux C: Luxation habituelle de la rotule. Rev Chir 8:628, 1888.
58. Sallay PI, Poggi J, Speer KP, et al: Acute dislocation of the patella: A correlative pathoanatomic study. Am J Sports Med 24:52, 1996.
59. Sandmeier RH, Burks RT, Bachus KN, Billings A: The effect of reconstruction of the medial patellofemoral ligament on patellar tracking. Am J Sports Med 28:345, 2000.
60. Seebacher JR, Inglis AE, Marshall Jl, Warren RF: The structures of the posterolateral aspect of the knee. J Bone Joint Surg Am 64:536, 1982.
61. Spritzer CE, Courneya DL: Medial retinacular complex injury in acute patellar dislocation: MR findings and surgical implications. AJR 168:117, 1997.
62. Stanitski CL: Articular hypermobility and chondral injury in patients with acute patellar dislocation. Am J Sports Med 23:146, 1995.
63. Stanitski CL, Paletta GA: Articular catilage injury with acute patellar dislocation in adolescents: Arthroscopic and radiographic correlation. Am J Sports Med 26:52, 1998.
64. Terry GC: The anatomy of the extensor mechanism. Clin Sports Med 8:163, 1989.
65. Vainionpaa S, Laasonen E, Patilala H, et al: Acute dislocation of the patella: Clinical, radiographic and operative findings in 64 consecutive cases. Acta Orthop Scand 57:331, 1986.
66. Vainionpaa S, Laasonen E, Silvennoninen T, et al: Acute dislocation of the patella. A prospective review of operative treatment. J Bone Joint Surg Br 72:366, 1990.
67. Virolainen H, Visuri T, Kuusela T: Acute dislocation of the patella: MR findings. Radiology 189:243, 1993.
68. Warren LF, Marshall JL: The supporting structures and layers on the medial side of the knee: An anatomical analysis. J Bone Joint Surg Am 61:56, 1979.
69. Wiberg G: Roentgenographic and anatomic studies on the femoropatellar joint. Acta Orthop Scand 12:319, 1941.
70. Woo SL-Y, Gomez MA, Sites TJ, et al: The biomechanical and morphological changes in the medial collateral ligament of the rabbit after immobilization and remobilization. J Bone Joint Surg Am 69:1200, 1987.
71. Yamamoto RK: Arthroscopic repair of the medial retinaculum and capsule in acute patellar dislocations. Arthroscopy 2:125, 1986.

2. RECURRENT DISLOCATION OF THE KNEE IN THE ADULT
W. Michael Walsh, MD

Long the stepchild of sports-related knee injuries, injury to the patellofemoral joint has come to be recognized as a common source of knee symptoms and disability in the athlete. As eminent an authority as O'Donoghue[102] stated in the first edition of his classic text, *Treatment of Injuries to Athletes,* that patellofemoral problems "need not be mentioned here." That viewpoint, held by many orthopaedists, had apparently grown out of the teachings of the first half of the 20th century, which stated that patellofemoral disorders were primarily a malady of females. In 1899, Goldthwait published his first (and in 1904 his second) treatise on what he called "slipping patella."[40, 41] In these writings, he portrayed the typical patient suffering from unstable patellas as a somewhat obese, knock-kneed, teen-aged female, certainly not a strapping, muscular male athlete. Though they may seem startling to young orthopaedists of today, these thoughts held sway well into the 1960s.

Primarily through the pioneering work of Hughston[51, 52, 54, 56] and others, our viewpoint has rapidly changed. The consensus among most physicians treating young athletes today is that patellofemoral disorders in both males and females are the most common type of knee disorder encountered in clinical practice. Especially because women both young and old are so much more active in sports than they were only a couple of decades ago, there probably is a preponderance of female patients among those presenting with patellofemoral disorders. The reason for this seems to be related to the inherent differences in the male and female habitus, women having a broader pelvis and more tendency to valgus at the knees. Still, one must remember that the muscular male athlete with normal alignment of the lower extremities may also suffer from an unstable patella.

Classification systems for patellofemoral disorders are almost as numerous as the authors who write about them. Malalignment, subluxation, chondromalacia, excessive lateral pressure syndrome, and other commonly seen terms frequently take on different meanings. Some classification schemes are based purely on radiographic views and measurements.[91, 115] Minkoff and Fein[94] have discussed eloquently the shortcomings of all such efforts. Other classifications hinge on physical findings and clinical test results that may themselves change from time to time in the same patient or may vary widely among examiners. The situation is enough to bewilder the neophyte and dismay the experienced.

Our parlance in this chapter must, therefore, be defined. I believe that if a careful enough search were possible, nearly all patellofemoral disorders would be found to be related to anatomic predisposition. (A patellar fracture from direct trauma would be an obvious exception.) The inherited nature of such a predisposition is confirmed not only by the literature[27, 33, 58, 93] but also by the common clinical experience of finding that the parents or siblings of a patient have had exactly the same type of extensor mechanism disorder. Such a predisposition may involve the bony structures, the soft tissues, or both. Larson[73] categorizes this predisposition further into configurational abnormalities, soft tissue support problems, and malalignment of the extremity. This predisposition determines what I refer to as "malalignment" of the knee's extensor mechanism or, indeed, of the entire lower extremity. Malalignment, even of significant proportions, may lie dormant through an individual's entire life, whereas in others it is associated with symptoms. Those symptoms related to dislocation occur suddenly after a specific traumatic event.

Pertinent Anatomy

It is impossible to discuss patellofemoral disorders without considering the anatomy of the entire lower extremity. Influences on the extensor mechanism may exist from hip to foot. These include both bony and soft tissue structures.

Bony Elements

The anatomy of the entire femur is important in patellofemoral mechanics. The angle of torsion or declination, sometimes called the version angle, indicates the angle of anterior projection (anteversion) or posterior projection (retroversion) of the femoral neck and head. This angle is created by the long axis of the femoral neck and a line drawn through the centers of the two femoral condyles distally when viewed in the transverse plane. Nicholas and Hershman[98] indicate that this angle averages approximately 14 degrees of anteversion in the adult. Using computed tomography (CT), Galland and colleagues[39] defined normal as 11 degrees with a standard deviation of 7 degrees. Further amounts of femoral neck anteversion cause the distal femoral trochlea to face more medially when the femoral neck assumes a neutral position in the hip (Fig. 28E2–1). Additional degrees of femoral neck retroversion cause the opposite effect. In addition, any true excessive torsional deformity from the trochanteric region to the knee

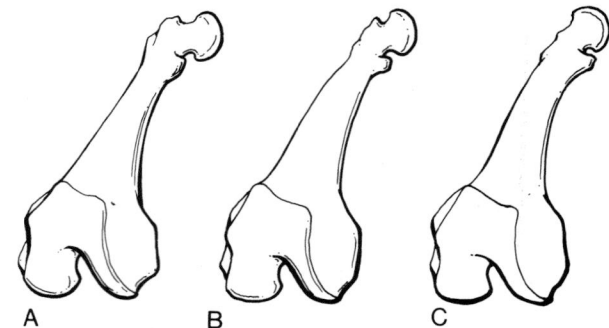

Figure 28E2–1. End-on view of three femurs with different degrees of femoral neck anteversion. Degree of anteversion increases from *A* through *C*. As anteversion increases, the distal femur would tend to face more medially when the hip is in neutral position.

produces a significant alteration in trochlear orientation. When femoral neck anteversion and true internal femoral torsion are present either alone or combined, they are often associated with external tibial torsion. This produces malfunction of the extensor mechanism by tending to displace the patella laterally. Finally, there may be various degrees of true dysplasia of the medial or lateral portions of the femoral trochlea.

Brattström[11] carefully examined the role played by the bony anatomy in patellofemoral dislocation. He found that often "illusory dysplasia" of the lateral femoral condyle resulted from excessive rotational deformity of the femur. Hughston and colleagues[58] reported that normally, at the functional position of 45 degrees of knee flexion, the tangential view of the distal femur shows the lateral femoral condyle approximately 1 cm higher than the medial femoral condyle. This may provide good functional stability for the patella, even when there is severe medial quadriceps dysplasia and an increased quadriceps angle. Computed tomographic techniques exist for quantification of the rotational configuration of the femur.[39, 97]

The bony anatomy of the patella has been described often. Contained within the quadriceps mechanism as a sesamoid bone, the patella is primarily divided into medial and lateral facets by a median ridge. Rarely are the medial and lateral facets of the same size. More commonly, the lateral facet is longer and more sloped, thereby matching the higher and wider lateral femoral condyle. Hughston and coworkers[58] reported that the normal ratio of the lateral facet to the medial facet is 3:2. Wiberg[130] developed the system of classifying patellar shapes into three types based on the relative size of the medial and lateral facets. Reider and colleagues,[105] in a dissection study, showed a high correlation between the Wiberg type and the width of the lateral patellofemoral ligament. They suggested that the lateral patellofemoral ligament had a major influence on creating patellar shape or, alternatively, was itself a reflection of muscle forces occurring during knee development.

In addition to medial and lateral facets, an "odd" facet extending along the most medial portion of the medial facet has been described. This portion of the patella contacts the femur only in deep knee flexion.[34, 42, 59] In addition, there are superior and inferior extensions of the bony patella that are nonarticular and may vary in size. The appearance of the bony patella on radiographs may or may not provide a good impression of the contours produced by the articular cartilage surface. As the knee flexes from full extension, contact between the patella and the femur progresses from a distal to a proximal direction on the patella.[34, 42]

The bony anatomy of the tibia is also important in patellofemoral mechanics. The tibial tuberosity serves as the distalmost attachment of the extensor mechanism. Therefore, variations in its placement influence the quadriceps angle (Q angle) of the knee. The rotational configuration of the tibia and anatomic differences in the frontal plane combine to produce significant mechanical influences. If a tibia has a normal degree of external torsion and a valgus deformity is created in the frontal plane, the Q angle is increased (Fig. 28E2–2). If a tibia has increased external rotation in the proximal segment, the Q angle is also increased, but distal to the tuberosity there may be a varus appearance of the remainder of the leg with varying

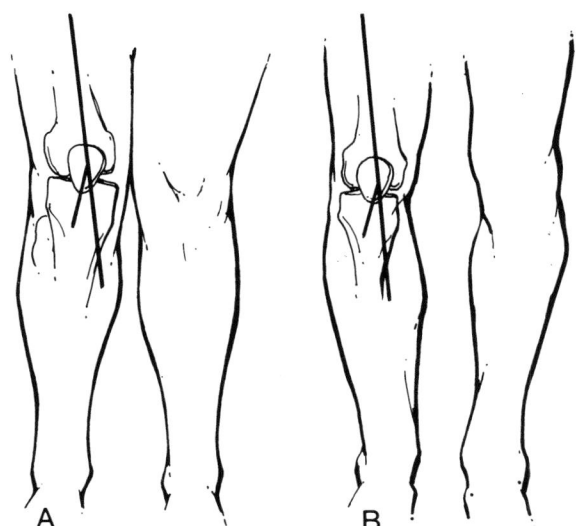

Figure 28E2–2. Legs with increased Q angle. *A* shows valgus configuration. *B* shows a varus leg in which an increased Q angle is secondary to deformity in the proximal tibia. Mechanically, these legs may behave differently.

degrees of true tibial torsion. This leg has far different mechanical problems. These concepts are important in understanding the so-called miserable malalignment syndrome.[65]

The bony anatomy even more distally is important in assessment of the patellofemoral joint. Excessive valgus at the subtalar joint of the foot creates an obligatory internal rotation of the tibia. Conversely, excessive varus at the subtalar joint causes external rotation of the tibia. These anatomic considerations provide the basis of patellofemoral symptoms in some patients with foot deformities and their treatment by correction of such deformities.

Soft Tissue Elements

The quadriceps muscle group comprises several major elements that influence the patellofemoral joint. These are the rectus femoris, the vastus lateralis, the vastus intermedius, and the vastus medialis. Except for the rectus femoris, all these muscles originate from the proximal half of the femur. The rectus femoris originates partly from the pelvis and the anterior hip joint. These four muscles insert in a layered arrangement into the proximal patella[123] at different angles to the long axis of the limb, creating vectors of force on the patella[58, 76, 123] (Fig. 28E2–3). Hughston and associates[58] proposed that the rectus femoris plays a large role in proprioception and therefore in muscular coordination of the limb. They also stated that this muscle may serve as the "command post" for coordinating various actions of the other quadriceps components. The vastus medialis and lateralis contribute to the medial and lateral retinacula by the continuation of their aponeurosis or investing fascia. The retinacula in turn attach to the proximal tibia, thereby providing some direct dynamic input from the medialis and lateralis to the tibia as well as attaching to the proximal patella.

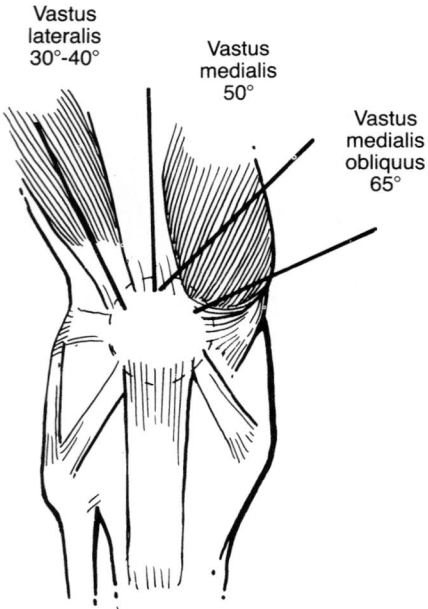

Figure 28E2–3. Various muscular elements of the quadriceps. Different portions attach at different angles to the long axis of the thigh, creating various vectors of force.

Lieb and Perry[76] expanded our concept of the quadriceps mechanism by describing the separate innervation and functional significance of the distal third of the vastus medialis, the vastus medialis obliquus (VMO). These distinct VMO fibers arise from the distal medial intermuscular septum and the adductor tubercle and normally insert into the proximal one third to one half of the medial patellar edge. Functionally, they have nothing to do with extension of the knee but serve a dynamically balancing role against the normally preponderant laterally directed forces on the patella.[84, 108] The VMO fibers normally make an angle of 55 to 65 degrees with the long axis of the thigh. Congenital VMO dysplasia, possibly coupled with secondary atrophy, seems to be one of the prime anatomic factors in producing patellofemoral disorders. Teitge,[122] however, has pointed out the inability to find convincing evidence in the literature to support the belief that the VMO is responsible for patellar stability.

More recently, the concept of a distinct oblique portion of the vastus lateralis, or vastus lateralis obliquus (VLO), has been described. Hallisey and associates[44] state that the VLO originates from the lateral intermuscular septum and inserts in one of three distinct anatomic patterns (Fig. 28E2–4). The VLO can originate beneath the main belly of the vastus lateralis, circling inferiorly and anteriorly to insert obliquely on the vastus lateralis portion of the quadriceps tendon. Second, the fibers of the VLO may not completely join the quadriceps tendon but cross inferiorly to interdigitate with the superficial oblique portion of the lateral retinaculum. Third, the vastus lateralis portion of the quadriceps tendon itself may interdigitate with the superficial oblique fibers of the lateral retinaculum, which then receives the insertion of the VLO without contributing to the patellar tendon. Hallisey and coworkers[44] point out that the surgical significance of this anatomic configuration

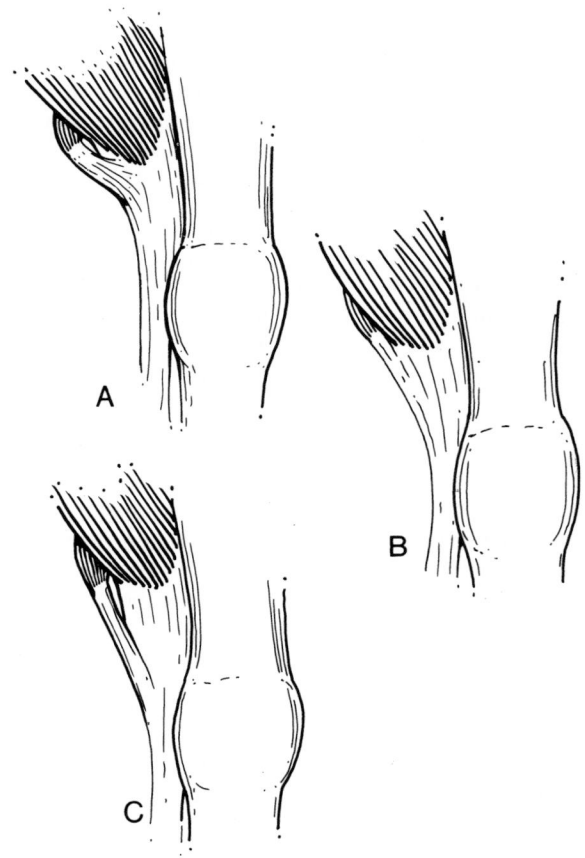

Figure 28E2–4. Variations in insertion of the vastus lateralis obliquus. *A* shows the vastus lateralis obliquus inserting obliquely on the vastus lateralis portion of the quadriceps tendon. *B* shows less distinct insertion blending with the superficial oblique retinaculum. *C* shows vastus lateralis obliquus insertion similar to *A* but with more separate vastus lateralis tendon that does not continue into the patellar tendon.

is that the VLO may be selectively released from the patella without total division of the vastus lateralis itself. They also suggest that a distinct plane of fatty tissue may separate the body of the VLO from the vastus lateralis longus. No separate innervation of this portion of the quadriceps, however, has yet been described.

Terry[123] found that the vastus lateralis longus normally has a 12- to 15-degree angulation to the sagittal plane, whereas Hallisey and associates[44] found that the VLO inserted at an average angle of 48 degrees in males and 38 degrees in women. Clearly, an important laterally directed force is produced by the vastus lateralis on the patella rather than merely a proximal force creating knee extension.

One of the most clinically significant soft tissue elements of the extensor mechanism is the patellar tendon. Taking broad origin from the entire inferior pole of the patella, this tendon tapers to its normal insertion on the tibial tuberosity. In its course, it is normally separated from the anterior proximal tibia by the small but important deep infrapatellar bursa. The deep infrapatellar bursa is an integral part of the extensor mechanism (Fig. 28E2–5). Hughston and associates[58] noted that destruction of this bursa by scarring or other forms of adherence of the patel-

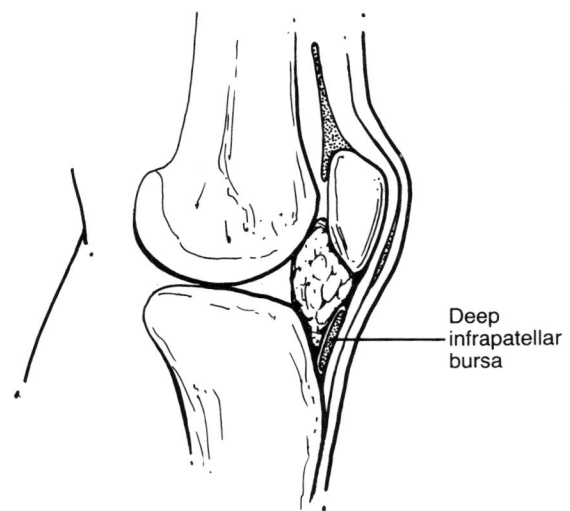

Figure 28E2–5. Deep infrapatellar bursa. The bursa lies between the patellar tendon and the anterior portion of the proximal tibia.

lar tendon to this region causes many problems. Fixation of the patellar tendon insertion more proximally, closer to the tibiofemoral joint, produces less than the normal gliding movement of the tibia about the femoral condyles. Terry[123] also noted that when the knee is in deep flexion, the deep infrapatellar bursa, the fat pad, and the anterior position of the tibial tuberosity prevent impingement between the patellar tendon and the bony structures.

There appear to be different versions of the remaining soft tissue anatomy around the patella. Fulkerson and Gossling,[38] for example, describe a superficial oblique portion of the lateral retinaculum running from the iliotibial band to the patella. This may correspond to the iliopatellar band as described by Terry[123] (Fig. 28E2–6). Fulkerson and

Gossling further describe a deeper and much more substantial transverse lateral retinaculum, the proximal end of which intertwines with the vastus lateralis insertion. The main portion of this deep transverse retinaculum runs directly from the iliotibial band to the lateral patella (Fig. 28E2–7). Since the original description by Kaplan,[67] it has been recognized that there are other soft tissue components that provide some static stability to the patella. Kaplan originally described epicondylopatellar ligaments, which are now more commonly referred to as patellofemoral ligaments. These may be present both laterally and medially (Fig. 28E2–8). Terry[123] suggests that these ligaments are transverse condensations of the medial and lateral retinacula. Fulkerson and Gossling[38] also state that the lateral patellofemoral ligament consists of the proximal fibers of the deep lateral retinaculum. Terry indicates that these ligaments are often thin because of the stress relief provided by their dynamic quadriceps counterparts. Reider and coworkers[105] found a lateral patellofemoral ligament in 13 of their 48 anatomic dissections. Only six of these had a medial patellofemoral ligament (MPFL) as well. One specimen had a medial ligament but no lateral ligament. When present, the lateral ligament ranged in breadth from 3 to 10 mm, whereas the medial varied from 5 to 12 mm. As mentioned earlier, they found a striking correlation between the width of the lateral patellofemoral ligament and the Wiberg shape of the patella. On the other hand, there was a marked negative correlation between the length of the infrapatellar tendon and the width of the MPFL. In other words, in specimens with patella alta, there were much thinner or absent MPFLs.

Numerous studies[13, 21, 31, 47, 100] have documented and

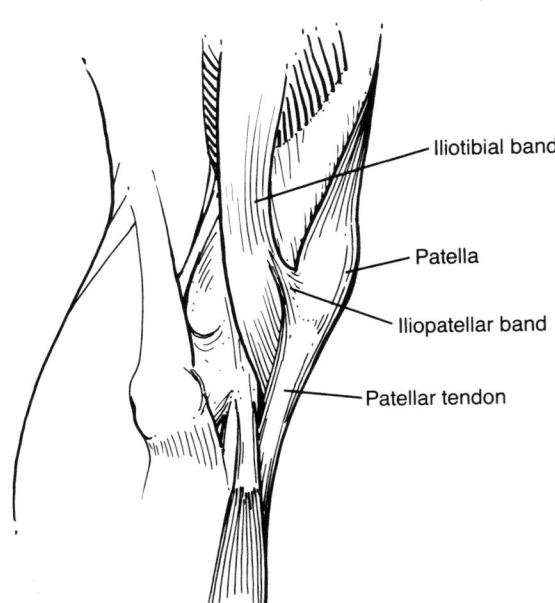

Figure 28E2–6. Lateral structures of the knee: the superficial aspect.

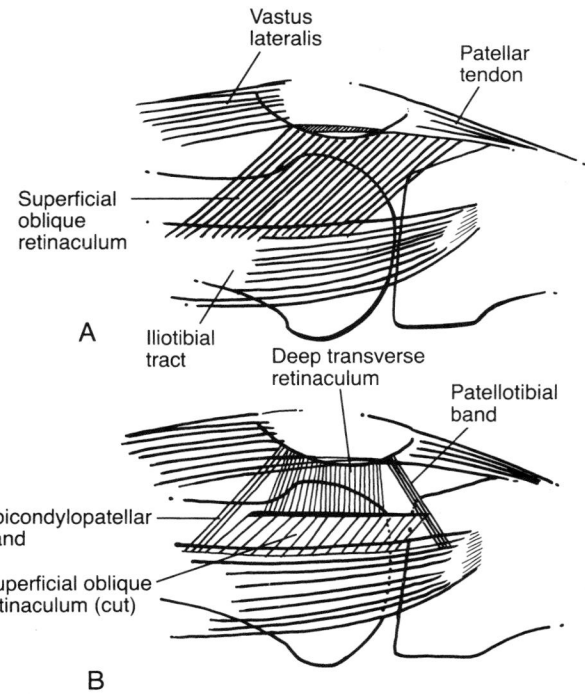

Figure 28E2–7. Lateral anatomy of the knee. *A* shows superficial oblique retinaculum. *B* shows the deep transverse retinaculum with superficial retinaculum removed. (After Fulkerson JP, Gossling HR: Anatomy of the knee joint lateral retinaculum. Clin Orthop 153:183–188, 1980.)

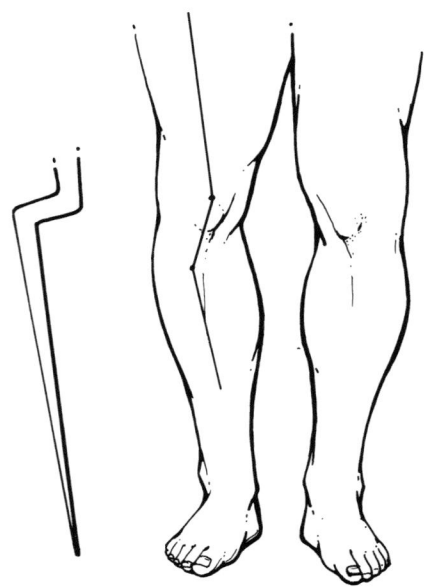

Figure 28E2–11. Miserable malalignment syndrome. The patient shows internal rotational deformity of the femur with inward-looking patellas, external tibial torsion, pronated feet, and a bayonet sign.

fat pad becomes impinged between the patella and the distal femur.

Next, the patient is asked to step slowly up and down a 6-inch step stool. The examiner listens for audible crepitation. The patient is asked whether either the step up or the step down is painful. Normally, this should be a smooth transition from step to floor and back again. In patients with patellofemoral problems, however, both the step up and the step down may lack muscular control. The step up may require a push off from the foot on the floor, leaning forward at the waist to assist the quadriceps, or assistance from the upper extremity by placing the hand on the examination table. The step down may show lack of eccentric control as the foot nears the floor so that the knee actually appears to "give out." The symmetry of the stepping motion is observed. The hip should be in line with the knee and the knee with the foot. The pelvis may tilt owing to gluteus medius weakness, and the patient may look as if he or she is actually side stepping off the stool.

The upright portion of the examination is concluded by observing the patient's angle of gait while walking down the hallway. McConnell points out that a pathologic gait may be viewed as "an attempt to preserve as low a level of energy consumption as possible by exaggerated motions at the unaffected levels."[86] The presence of limping is sought, as are any abnormal movements of the patella as it engages and disengages the trochlea.

The examiner should note whether the patient throws his or her legs in some abnormal fashion, indicating one of the rotational deformities. Hyperextendable knees will assume that posture during the stance phase of walking. McConnell[86] points out that shock absorption through the lower leg then comes from internal rotation of the femur rather than from knee flexion. With this abnormality, hip internal rotation is promoted by the tensor fascia lata, which becomes stronger and tighter from constant recruit-

ment. Consequently, the gluteus medius becomes weak, leading to decreased control of external rotation.[86]

Sitting Examination

Some of the most important observations are made with the patient seated on the examination table with the legs hanging free over the side and the knees flexed to 90 degrees. Even a small effusion may be detected in this position if the knee is not too obese. Obliteration of the normal concavity usually present just medial to the patellar tendon at the joint line indicates the most subtle of joint effusions.

With the patient in this position, one can assess the patellar position by viewing the knee from the lateral aspect (Fig. 28E2–12). The patella should be situated on the distal end of the femur with the proximal patellar pole in approximate alignment with the anterior femur and the anterior surface of the patella facing in essentially the same line as the femoral shaft. Because the patella sits more on the anterior surface than the distal surface of the femur, it faces toward the ceiling, creating a degree of patella alta. Patella baja, or abnormal distal displacement of the patella, is rarely encountered except after overly aggressive surgery on the extensor mechanism or as a complication of other knee surgery if the extensor mechanism is not adequately rehabilitated.

While the patient holds both knees together, the examiner views them from the anterior aspect (Fig. 28E2–13). Although normally positioned patellas face straight ahead, those with both patella alta and lateral tilt appear to be looking up and over the examiner's shoulders toward the ceiling, the so-called grasshopper eyes knee cap.

Attention is directed next to the alignment of the patella and the patellar tendon at its insertion into the tibial tuberosity. Any evidence of an enlarged or a tender tibial tuberosity is noted. Observation for tibial torsion is done by standing above the patient's knees and gazing downward along the tibial tuberosity and the anterior tibial crest. The coronal plane of the lower leg is compared with an imaginary line connecting the medial and the lateral malleoli of the ankle. This will determine the degree of external tibial

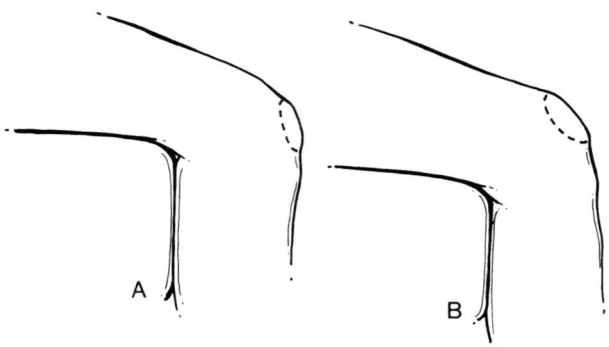

Figure 28E2–12. Examination for patella alta. *A* shows normal patellar position. With the knee flexed over the side of the examination table, the front of the patella appears to face straight ahead. *B* shows patella alta. The patella appears to face the ceiling.

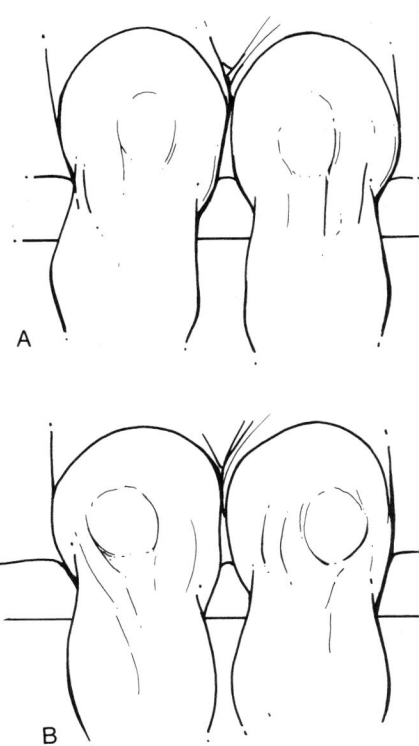

Figure 28E2–13. Examination for patellar position from the front. *A* shows normally positioned patellas. The patellas appear to be centered in the outline made by the soft tissues of the thighs. *B* shows high and lateral posture of the patellas, the so-called grasshopper eyes appearance. When viewed from the front, the patellas appear to be looking up and over the shoulders of the examiner.

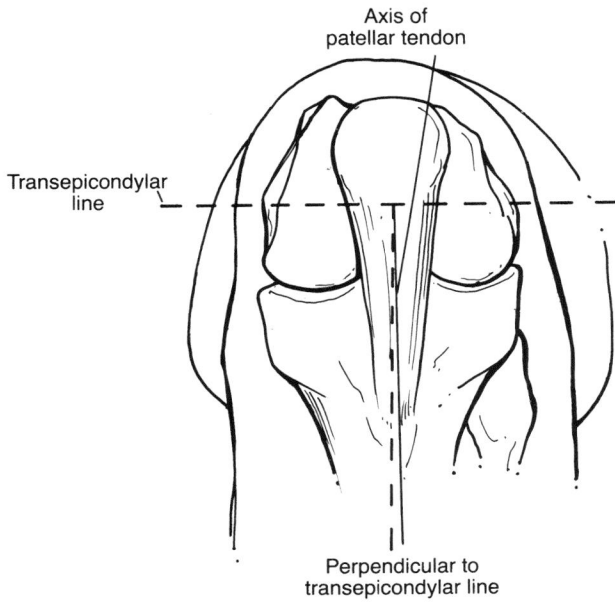

Figure 28E2–14. Tubercle sulcus angle of 90 degrees.[68] With the knee flexed to 90 degrees, the transepicondylar line is assessed. The axis of the patellar tendon is compared with a perpendicular to the transepicondylar line.

torsion. Normal external tibial torsion has been reported to range between 0 and 40 degrees.[39, 98]

Routinely, the quadriceps angle (Q angle) is measured with the patient supine; however, the Q angle can also be assessed with the knee flexed to 90 degrees. Kolowich[68] has described this as the 90-degree tubercle sulcus angle (Fig. 28E2–14). Although measurement of the Q angle in the supine position takes into account the interaction of the distal vector (patella to tuberosity) with the proximal vector (pelvis to patella), the 90-degree tubercle sulcus angle is said to be a more accurate representation of the distal vector alone because most patellas are centered within the trochlea at 90 degrees of knee flexion.[68] The 90-degree tubercle sulcus angle is measured by first palpating the transepicondylar axis of the femur. A line perpendicular to that axis is visualized and compared with a line passing through the center of the patella and the tibial tuberosity. Kolowich and colleagues[68] state that an angle of 0 degrees is normal, whereas an angle of 10 degrees or greater is definitely abnormal. Persistent lateral subluxation of the entire extensor mechanism with the knee acutely flexed may artificially reduce this tubercle sulcus angle, or sitting Q angle, to 0 degrees.

Next, the VMO is assessed, looking not only for its bulk but also for its level of insertion into the patella. The VMO is the main dynamic medial stabilizer of the patella, and it is believed that its sole selective function is patellar alignment[58, 76, 84]; it is no wonder, then, that so much empha-

sis is placed on the function and quality of the VMO. While the patient holds both knees actively at 45 degrees of flexion, the VMO should normally be present as a substantial muscle arising from the adductor tubercle and the medial intermuscular septum, inserting into the upper one third to one half of the patella (Fig. 28E2–15). The more distal its insertion, the greater its biomechanical advantage in stabilizing the patella against lateral forces. In patients with congenital VMO dysplasia, there is a visible or palpable lack of muscular tissue rather than a normal bulk of VMO muscle extending from the adductor tubercle to the proximal medial patella. In the extreme case, this appears to be a substantial "scooped out" or hollow area. Gradations exist between this extreme and normal VMO bulk. Usually, the appearance of the VMO is symmetrical, whether one or both knees are symptomatic, indicating that this is not simply disuse atrophy. In the obese knee, adipose tissue may fill this depression, making dysplasia more

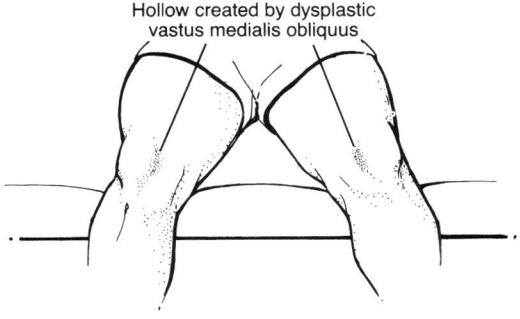

Figure 28E2–15. Vastus medialis obliquus dysplasia with knees held actively at 45 degrees of flexion. Lack of the vastus medialis obliquus is shown by the hollow area adjacent to the proximal medial patella.

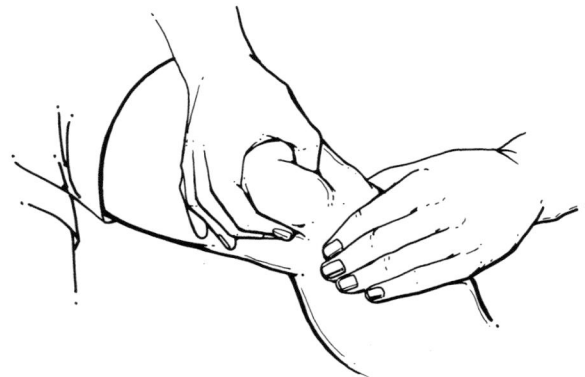

Figure 28E2–20. Palpation for facet tenderness. In this left knee, the patella is displaced medially to allow palpation along the undersurface of the medial facet. Many different structures may be the source of this tenderness.

patellar facet is best palpated by displacement of the patella medially while the knee is flexed to 30 degrees (Fig. 28E2–20). This causes lateral tilting of the patella, thus making the medial edge more accessible to palpation. There are various theories about the source of medial facet tenderness, including degenerative changes of the patellar articular surface and medial capsular pain and synovial inflammation resulting from a chronically malaligned patella. It seems clear that there are many structures between the examining finger and the patella itself that may be the source of pain, making this part of the examination less than specific.

In the patient with an acute patellar dislocation, the entire course of the VMO is palpated. If the VMO has been ruptured from its insertion into the proximal medial patella, a deficit can be palpated that allows invagination of the skin and the soft tissues almost into the interior of the joint.[58, 129] Particular attention should be paid to the region of the adductor tubercle, which is the femoral attachment of the MPFL.

Next, the patella is compressed against the anterior aspect of the femur, both longitudinally and transversely. This may cause crepitation or pain. Traditionally, it has been taught that this painful crepitation represents chondromalacia, but we now know that this is usually not the case.[58, 63] This maneuver is repeated with the knee flexed to 30 degrees over a pillow. Often, both pain and crepitation disappear when the patella is compressed in this position. Symptoms will persist if they are due to true chondromalacia. Their disappearance probably indicates that they originate from a different source than the articular surface.

Close observation of the patella in relation to the femur is continued. McConnell[86] described the patellofemoral joint as principally a soft tissue joint, meaning that its position can be changed by appropriate mechanical means, such as physical therapy. She goes on to describe four components that affect patellar position statically or dynamically: glide, tilt, rotation, and anterior-posterior position.

To measure the glide component, the examiner observes the knee when it is relaxed and in the extended position. In this position, the patella should be sitting in the midline between the two condyles. Statically, the patella may appear normal; once the quadriceps is contracted, however, the patella can be observed to move laterally. Lateral glide is considered significant if the midline of the patella is lateral to the midline of the femur. Kolowich and colleagues[68] have described the "lateral pull sign" to demonstrate this same concept. With the knee in extension, the patient contracts the quadriceps. The examiner observes for movement of the patella in a superior or superolateral direction (Fig. 28E2–21). The patella should be pulled straight superiorly or superiorly and laterally in equal proportions. Excessive lateral displacement represents lateral overpull by the quadriceps and is referred to as an active quadriceps vector.[68] Almost all patients have some degree of lateral glide that requires correction. The amount of glide depends on the tightness of the lateral retinaculum and the relative amount of activity of the VMO compared with the vastus lateralis.

The tilt component is also particularly significant if the deep retinacular structures are tight.[68, 86] The amount of mediolateral tilt is detected by comparing the height of the medial patellar border with the height of the lateral patellar border. The two borders should be level compared with the horizontal. This component has also been described as the "passive patellar tilt test" by Kolowich and colleagues[68] (Fig. 28E2–22). The knee is examined in full extension with the quadriceps relaxed. Standing at the foot of the examination table, the examiner elevates the lateral edge of the patella from the lateral femoral condyle by pressing posteriorly on the medial edge. The patella must remain in the trochlea and not be allowed to subluxate for accurate measurement. Excessively tight lateral restraints will not allow the patella to reach the neutral or horizontal position. Many patients with patellofemoral symptoms show lateral tilting both clinically and radiographically.

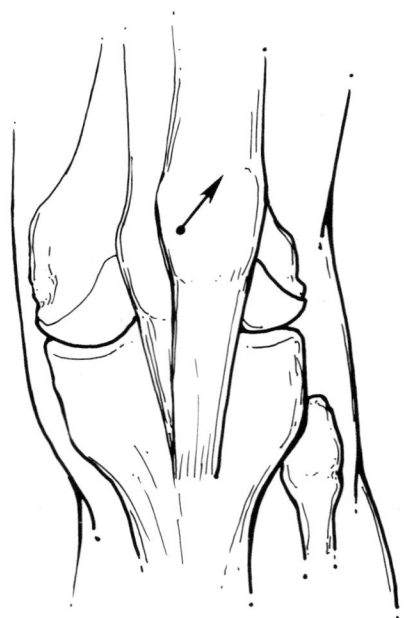

Figure 28E2–21. Lateral pull sign.[68] In this left knee, when the quadriceps is contracted, the patella moves in an exaggerated lateral direction as well as proximally. This also indicates predominance of lateral forces.

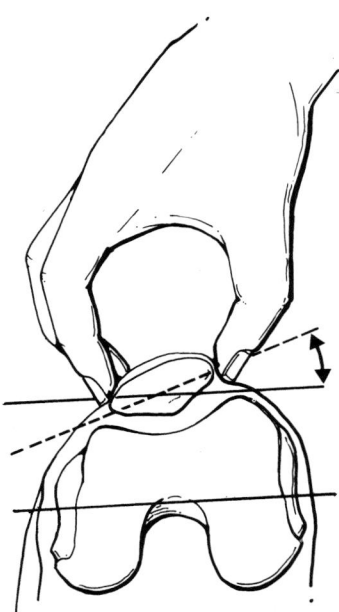

Figure 28E2–22. Passive patellar tilt test. In this left knee, the patella can be tilted so that the lateral edge is well anterior to the medial edge.

The rotational component[86] determines whether there is any deviation of the long axis of the patella from the long axis of the femur. Internal rotation indicates that the inferior pole of the patella is medial to the superior pole; external rotation indicates the opposite situation.

The anterior-posterior component[86] evaluates the position of the inferior pole of the patella relative to the superior pole. The patella is observed while the patient initiates a quadriceps contraction (Fig. 28E2–23). If the inferior pole of the patella tilts posteriorly compared with the superior pole, it can irritate the infrapatellar fat pad. This irritation may cause a sharp stabbing pain medial to the patellar tendon when the knee is in extension or hyperextension as the inferior pole of the patella becomes buried within the fat pad.

Equal in importance to patellar position is assessment of patellar mobility. Mobility may be abnormally *increased* or *decreased.* Assessment is best done by sitting on the side of the examining table with the patient's knee flexed across the examiner's thigh (Fig. 28E2–24). The patient's ankle and foot can conveniently rest on the examiner's other thigh, causing the knee to remain flexed 30 to 45 degrees.[58, 129] The patient's head should remain flat on the examination table, with all muscles, especially the quadriceps, completely relaxed. The examiner's thumbs are positioned along the medial edge of the patella as he or she attempts to push the patella laterally. This maneuver is followed by displacement of the patella medially.

Because there is a wide range of normal retinacular laxity, one must compare mobility not only with the opposite side but also with previously examined knees to determine whether the degree of laxity is pathologic. Carson and associates[14] have described a means of assessing patellar mobility. They state that the patella should displace medially or laterally no more than half the width of the patella. Kolowich and colleagues[68] also describe a test for quantitating the degree of hypermobility with the knee in this position. The patella is divided into four longitudinal quadrants (Fig. 28E2–25). The patella is displaced medially and

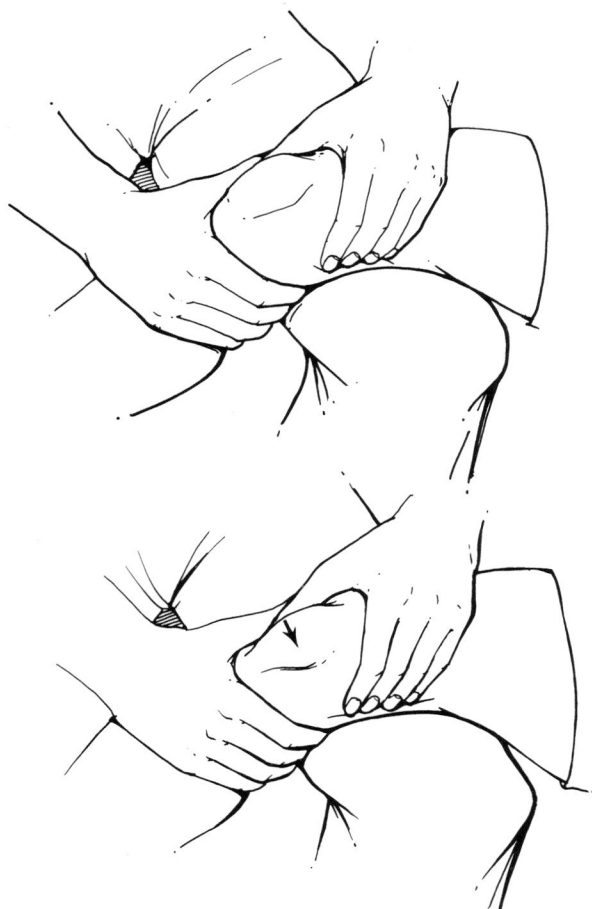

Figure 28E2–24. Hypermobility testing. With the knee flexed approximately 30 degrees over the examiner's leg, firm pressure is exerted along the medial patella to force it over the lateral femoral condyle.

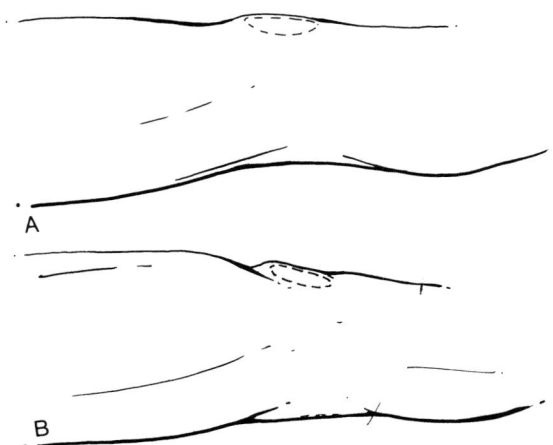

Figure 28E2–23. Abnormal distal tilt of the patella. In *A,* the quadriceps is relaxed. In *B,* the distal patella tilts posteriorly when the quadriceps contracts, potentially creating irritation of the infrapatellar fat pad.

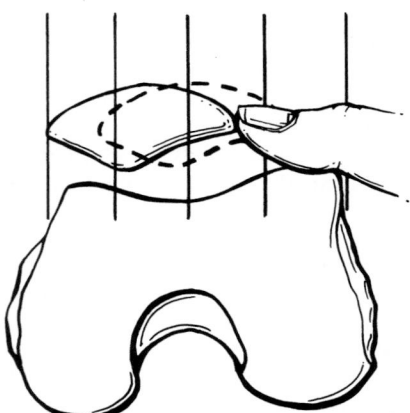

Figure 28E2–25. Assessment of patellar mobility medially and laterally. The patellofemoral joint can be mentally divided into quadrants and patellar mobility assessed in both directions.

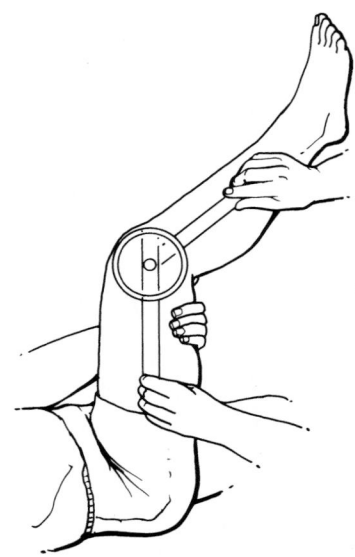

Figure 28E2–26. Measurement of hamstring tightness. With the hip flexed 90 degrees, if the knee will not extend completely, the residual knee flexion angle is measured and recorded as hamstring tightness.

laterally with the examiner's thumb and index finger to determine the amount of parapatellar tightness. A lateral displacement of three quadrants suggests an incompetent medial restraint. A lateral displacement of four quadrants defines a dislocatable patella. A medial displacement of only one quadrant indicates a tight lateral retinaculum and usually correlates with an abnormal passive patellar tilt test. Medial displacement of three or four quadrants suggests a more globally hypermobile patella without tightness of the lateral restraints.[68]

During these maneuvers, one is looking not only for patellar mobility but also for any associated apprehension. If chronic patellar hypermobility is the source of the patient's problems, or if there has been an acute subluxation or dislocation episode, the patient will bolt off the table, telling the examiner not to displace the patella again (see Fig. 28E2–10). The patient may state that this is a familiar feeling when the knee goes out or gives way.

Muscle bulk and tone and flexibility of the quadriceps, hamstrings, and gastrocnemius-soleus group are evaluated. Muscle tone and bulk are compared with tone and bulk on the opposite side. In most instances, it is sufficient to characterize any atrophy as mild, moderate, or severe. Circumference measurements may be done, although these can be misleading because of changes in the relative composition of the limb. Muscle loss accompanied by an increase in adipose tissue may yield a normal circumference measurement despite a marked functional deficit. If measurements are done, they should be carried out at a standard distance above and below a fixed reference point. The patella should not be used for the reference point because the proximal-to-distal location of the patella may vary from side to side. A more appropriate reference point would be the joint lines or Gerdy's tubercle. Tone indicates the turgor of the muscle tissue at rest. Simple palpation with the hand is sufficient to detect changes in resting muscle tone. This may decrease within hours of an injury. In the rehabilitative setting, tone may be more closely correlated with muscular endurance, whereas bulk is more closely linked to strength.

Inflexibility in certain muscle groups is critically important in dealing with the extensor mechanism. Most common is tightness of the hamstrings. With the opposite

leg fully extended on the examination table, the patient flexes the hip to 90 degrees (Fig. 28E2–26). While maintaining the hip at 90 degrees, the patient then tries to fully extend the knee so that the entire leg is pointed straight up toward the ceiling. This indicates reasonable hamstring flexibility in the general population. In certain athletes whose sport places a high premium on flexibility (e.g., dancers and gymnasts), this is a minimum amount of hamstring flexibility. These athletes should be able to bring the entire leg into more flexion at the hip with the leg coming toward the head. Lack of normal hamstring flexibility is shown by an inability to extend the knee fully with the hip flexed to 90 degrees. Another important muscle flexibility measurement is that of the gastrocnemius-soleus group along the posterior calf. With the knee fully extended and the foot in a slightly inverted position, the ankle is passively dorsiflexed as far as possible (Fig. 28E2–27). In normally flexible calves, the foot should come to approximately 15 degrees of dorsiflexion beyond the neutral posi-

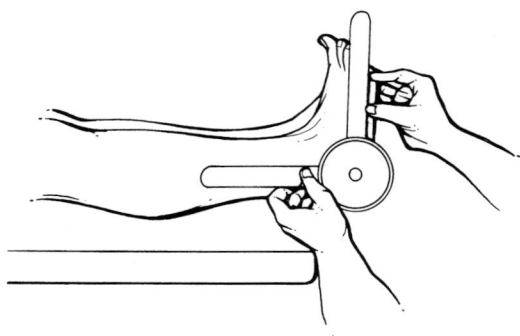

Figure 28E2–27. Measurement for heel cord tightness. With the knee fully extended and the foot slightly inverted, the ankle is dorsiflexed as far as possible. The normally flexible gastrocnemius-soleus complex should allow 15 degrees of dorsiflexion beyond neutral.

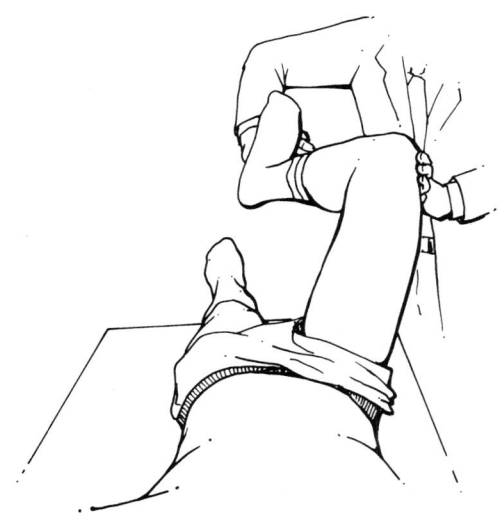

Figure 28E2–28. Examination for hip joint rotation. Excessive internal rotation compared with external rotation indicates increased anteversion of the femur.

tion. Measurements may be repeated with the knee flexed to assess soleus flexibility as opposed to that contributed by the gastrocnemius muscles.

Hip range of motion should also be evaluated with the patient in the supine position (Fig. 28E2–28). With the hip flexed to 90 degrees, internal rotation that exceeds external rotation is an indication of some degree of femoral anteversion. Limited or painful range of motion may indicate a hip disorder masquerading as a knee problem.

Prone Examination

The third and often neglected assessment of flexibility is that of the quadriceps muscle group itself. With the patient in a prone position, the knee is flexed acutely, bringing the heel toward the buttock (Fig. 28E2–29). Lack of knee flexion (that was possible in the supine position) in comparison with the uninjured side, obligatory flexion

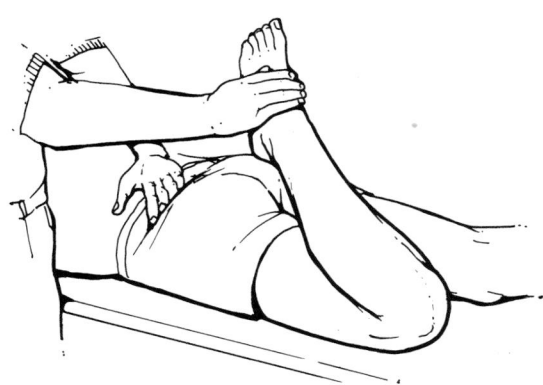

Figure 28E2–29. Measurement of quadriceps flexibility. With the patient prone, the knee is flexed as far as possible. The anterior pelvis rising off the examination table, a sensation of tightness along the anterior thigh, or a lack of knee flexion compared with the opposite side may all indicate quadriceps tightness.

of the hip joint so that the anterior pelvis rises off the examination table, or simply the patient's report of increased tightness along the anterior thigh during this maneuver is an indication of quadriceps muscle tightness. Hip rotation can also be examined in this posture. With the knee flexed to 90 degrees, internal and external rotation can be accurately assessed and compared from side to side.

In summary, patellofemoral disorders require much more skill and time in examination than do other knee problems. The examiner who looks only at the knee of the supine patient has missed many if not most of the important factors that influence the patellofemoral joint. Examination must include both structural and dynamic features extending from the pelvis to the foot.

Diagnostic Studies

Radiography

Radiography of the patellofemoral joint ranks as one of the most-described and -debated yet thoroughly confused issues in all of sports medicine.[15, 24, 32, 94] No fewer than 10 different radiographic views of the patellofemoral joint and their variations have been described, along with a plethora of measurements and calculations that can be extracted from these radiographs. Minkoff and Fein[94] have extensively reviewed all these views and the various indices and measurements obtained from them. They could only conclude the following:

1. A sufficient number of studies exist that show statistically significant correlations between certain radiographic criteria and the existence of patellofemoral disability.

2. Generally, radiographic assessment provides insufficient information to indicate surgery. It merely suggests that an abnormality exists.

3. Radiographic evaluation cannot determine the postoperative elimination of physical signs and patient symptoms. At best, it can demonstrate an improvement in radiographic indices that have been determined to represent the correctness of patellar relations to the trochlea.

4. The most important limitation of radiographic criteria in identifying position disorders is that they do not tell what, if any, operation is indicated nor do they predict what response can be anticipated from the pursuit of nonoperative treatment.

Despite these shortcomings, great emphasis continues to be placed on the axial radiograph of the patellofemoral joint, to such an extent that some classification systems for patellofemoral disorders are based solely on radiographic appearance. For example, Ficat and associates[35] believe that a combination of standard axial radiographs and intraarticular contrast material reveals all patellofemoral disorders, including dysplasias, dislocation or subluxation, excessive lateral pressure syndrome, and degeneration of the cartilage surfaces. Merchant[91] subclassifies patellofemoral dysplasia into lateral patellar compression syndrome and chronic subluxation of the patella based solely on the presence or absence of subluxation on the 30-degree flexed axial view. Galland and colleagues[39] believe that radiography helps define anatomic factors that are either major, minor, or more remote in their influence on the patellofemoral joint.

Regardless of the role each physician assigns to radiography, it is important to obtain radiographs routinely in the athlete who has apparent patellofemoral instability. Standard anteroposterior radiographs of the knee probably offer the least information in these patients. Accessory ossification centers, degenerative joint disease, and other unrelated diagnoses such as bone tumors can be identified in this view. An initial impression regarding the position of the patella (high or low) can also be formed from viewing the anteroposterior radiograph. With a well-centered x-ray beam, the inferior pole of most patellas will rest at about the upper extreme edge of the intercondylar notch shadow (Fig. 28E2–30).

The lateral view is more valuable. The most commonly used information is that relating to an excessively high (patella alta) or excessively low (patella infra or baja) patella. Five techniques for determining this position have been described.[39] The method of Blumensaat is of historical significance only. It related the position of the patella to a line projected along the roof of the intercondylar notch. Later studies showed wide variability in the configuration of the notch, rendering this measurement invalid. For many years, we have used a view credited to Labelle and Laurin in which radiography of the knee is performed with the knee at 90 degrees of flexion (Fig. 28E2–31). These authors pointed out that a line drawn along the anterior femoral cortex passes above the proximal pole of the patella in all but 3% of normal knees. This line also re-creates most closely the position in which we assess patella alta clinically.

There are at least three techniques for assessing patellar

position by measuring various distances on the lateral radiograph.[39] The best known of these is the technique of Insall and Salvati[62] (Fig. 28E2–32). This technique relates the measured length of the patellar tendon to the greatest diagonal measurement of the patella. Insall and Salvati report that the normal ratio is 1.0 ± 20%. Ratios outside the range of 0.8 to 1.2 appear to show definite evidence of patella alta or baja. From the practical standpoint, these measurements are sometimes hard to determine. The upper and lower measuring points for the patellar tendon can be indefinite. The greatest diagonal measurement of the patella can be affected by the often-seen elongated inferior pole of the patella. Marks and Bentley[85] have shown a significant difference in the ratio of the patellar tendon to the patella between "normal" male and female populations.

An alternative technique is that of Blackburn and Peel,[8] which expresses the ratio of the articular length of the patella to the height of the lower pole of the articular cartilage above the tibial plateau (Fig. 28E2–33). Normal values are reported to be between 0.54 and 1.06. In patella alta, the ratio is greater than 1.0.

In addition to patellar position, Malghem and Maldague[82] have described a technique for measuring the depth of the proximal trochlear groove on the lateral knee radiograph (Fig. 28E2–34). They found significant shallowness of the proximal groove in patients with patellar instability. In comparison with the axial approach or CT, the lateral technique has the advantage of providing a full view of the entire trochlear length. These authors felt that it provided recognition of grooves that were normally concave in the middle and distal portions but focally flat in the proximal part. Building on this work, Galland and coworkers[39] defined three types of trochlear dysplasia based on where the

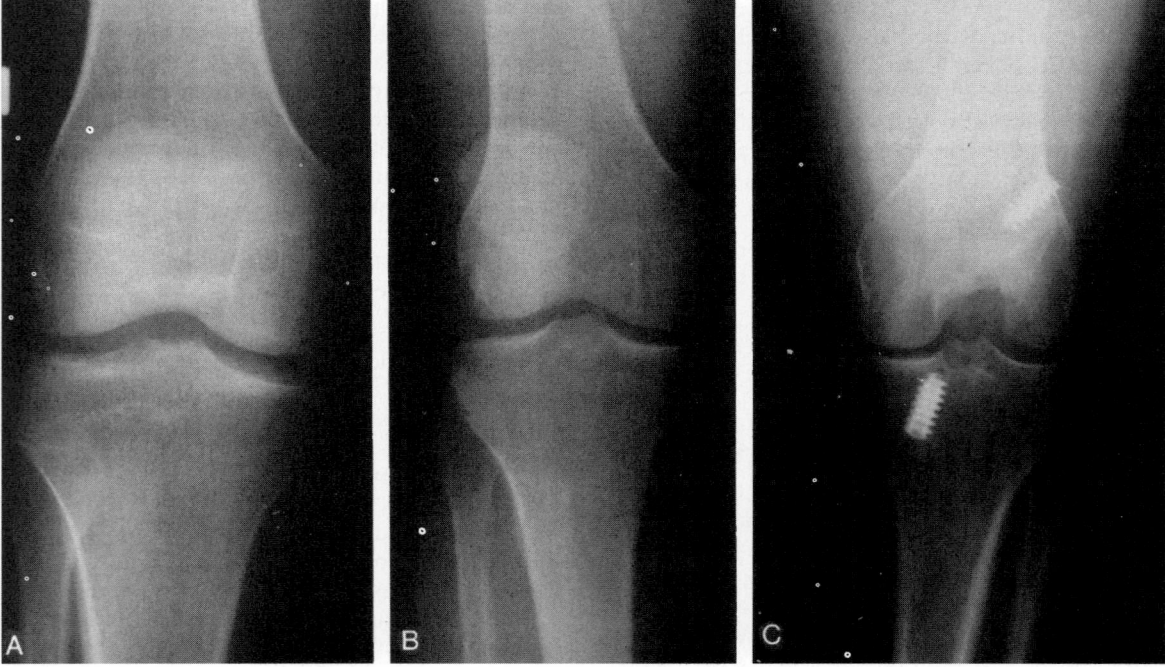

Figure 28E2–30. Anteroposterior radiograph of the knee showing proximal to distal patellar position. *A* shows a normally placed patella with the inferior pole at approximately the top of the intercondylar notch shadow. *B* shows patella alta. *C* shows patella baja, in this case secondary to infrapatellar contracture syndrome.

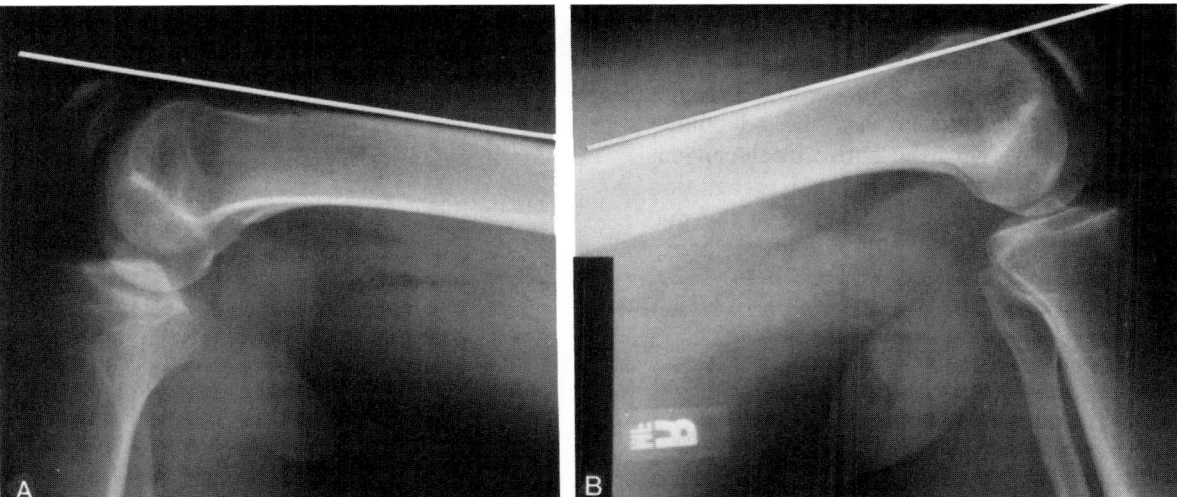

Figure 28E2–31. Lateral radiograph of the knee showing proximal to distal patellar position (technique of Labelle and Laurin). *A* shows the lateral view with the knee flexed approximately 90 degrees. The line projected along the anterior margin of the distal femur is above the proximal pole of the patella. *B* shows patella alta with the proximal pole of the patella above the projected line.

line of the intercondylar groove crossed the shadows of the medial and lateral condyles (Fig. 28E2–35). Remy and colleagues[107] evaluated interobserver and intraobserver reliability in classifying trochlear dysplasia. They found that the "crossing sign" was reliable because the probability of rating a pathologic trochlea as normal was only 3.1%. Classifying types of trochlear morphology, however, was more difficult, with interobserver agreement proving to be only slight and intraobserver agreement only fair.

It has become well established that the traditional sky-

line or sunrise view should be discarded as the preferred axial view of the patellofemoral joint. When the knee is flexed to 90 degrees or beyond, almost every patella will seat normally in the trochlea, providing little specific information about patellofemoral orientation. The most widely used axial views are those described by Merchant and colleagues[90] and Laurin and associates.[74, 75] In Merchant and colleagues' technique, the patellofemoral joint is

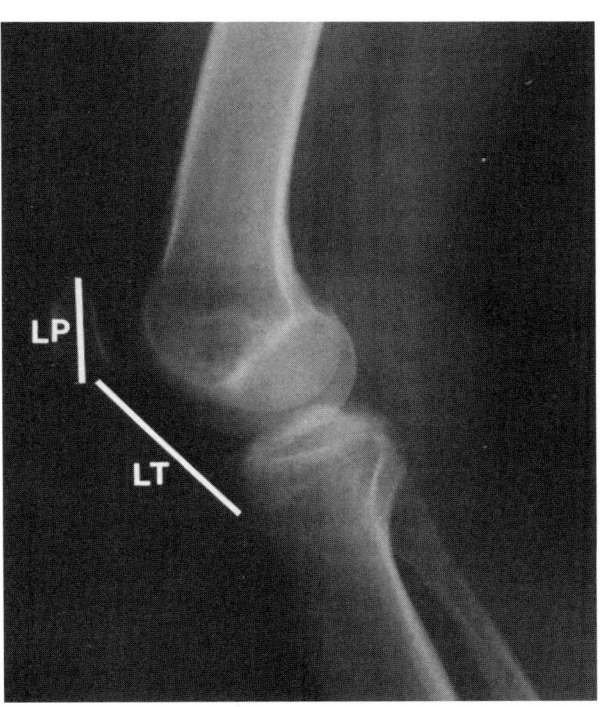

Figure 28E2–32. Assessment of patella alta (technique of Insall and Salvati). The ratio of the longest diagonal of the patella to the length of the patellar tendon should be 1.0 ± 20%.

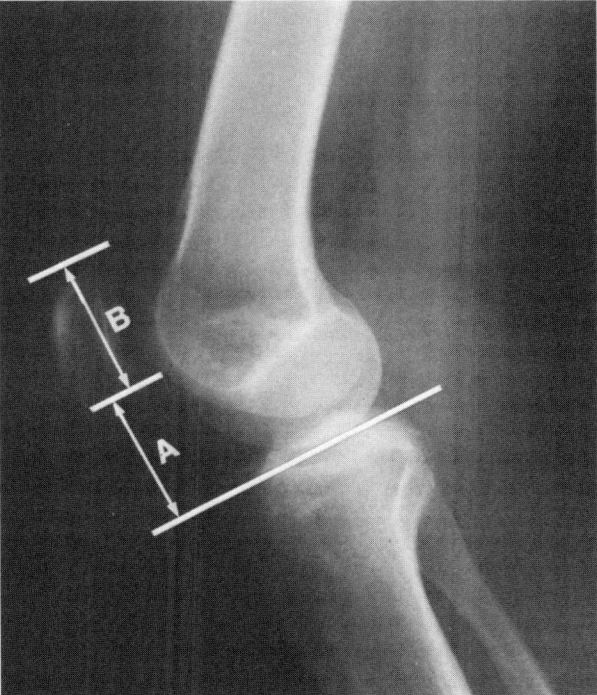

Figure 28E2–33. Assessment of patella alta (technique of Blackburn and Peel). The normal ratio of the articular length of the patella to the height of the lower pole of the articular cartilage above the tibial plateau is between 0.54 and 1.06.

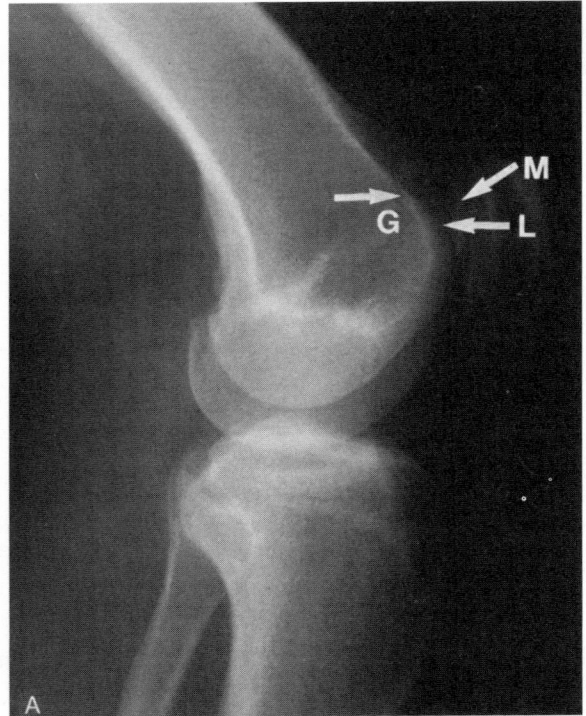

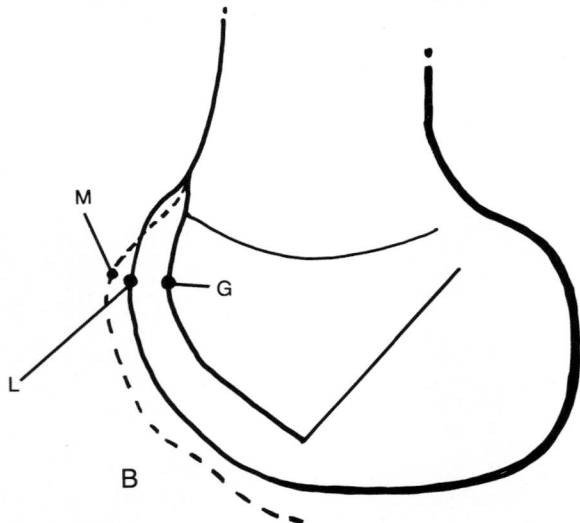

Figure 28E2–34. Measurement of trochlear depth on a lateral radiograph (technique of Malghem and Maldague). *A* shows a lateral radiograph and *B* a diagrammatic representation. Point G is the deepest part of the trochlear groove. Point L is the lateral femoral condyle shadow, and point M is the medial femoral condyle shadow. When measured 1 cm below the upper extent of the groove, the mean depth can be expressed as GM plus GL over 2. The authors found measurements of 2.74 mm ± 1.35 mm in patients with unstable patellas, compared with 5.94 mm ± 1.74 mm in controls.

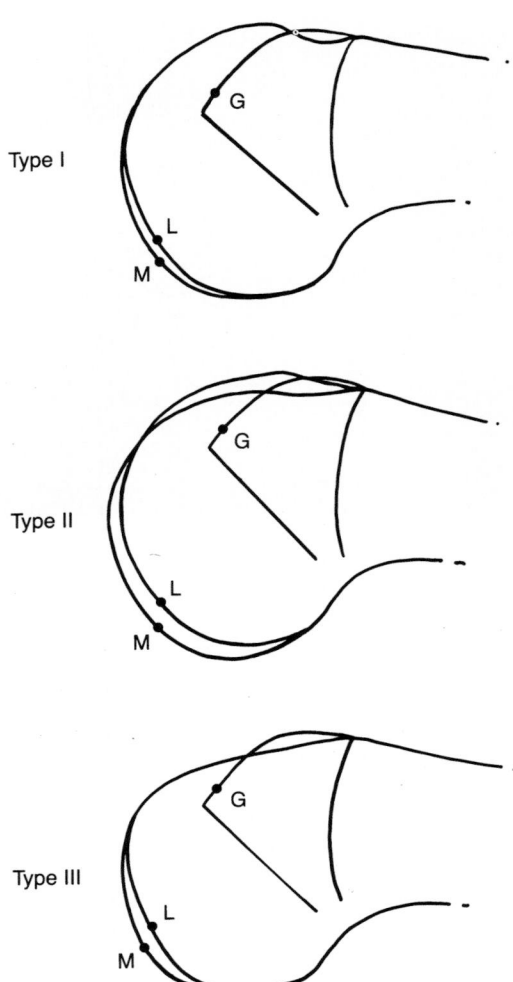

Figure 28E2–35. Femoral trochlear dysplasia.[39] In each, point G indicates the shadow of the trochlear groove, L indicates the outline of the lateral femoral condyle, and M denotes the medial femoral condyle. In type I, the condyles are symmetrical, and a groove line crosses them at the same place in the upper portion of the trochlea. This is the least degree of dysplasia. In type II, the medial condyle is dysplastic. It crosses the line of the trochlear groove at a variable level. In type III, marked dysplasia, the condyles are symmetrical but cross the trochlear groove line at a much lower point. This indicates a flat trochlea.

viewed with knees flexed to 45 degrees (Fig. 28E2–36). The x-ray source is positioned above the knee, with the x-ray plate placed distal to the knees. They originally described the "congruence angle" and the technique of measuring it (Fig. 28E2–37). The average congruence angle in 100 normal subjects was found to be −6 degrees with a standard deviation of 11 degrees. This means that a

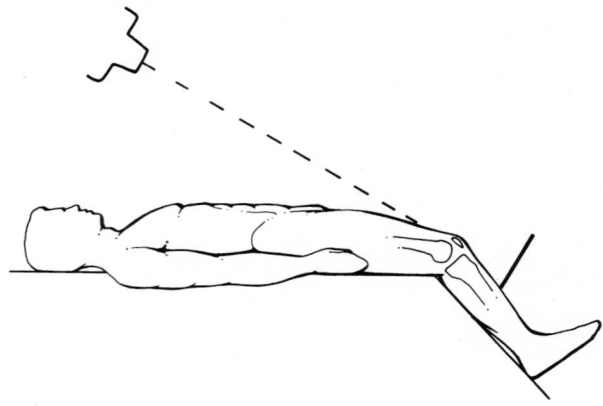

Figure 28E2–36. Axial radiograph (technique of Merchant).

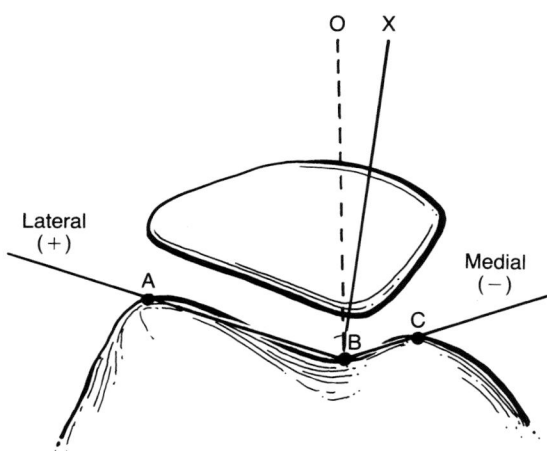

Figure 28E2–37. Congruence angle of Merchant. Line BO is the bisector of angle ABC. Line BX passes through the lowest point on the median ridge of the patella. Angle OBX is the congruence angle. If line BX falls to the medial side of line BO, the angle is expressed as negative degrees. If it falls to the lateral side of line BO, it is expressed as positive degrees.

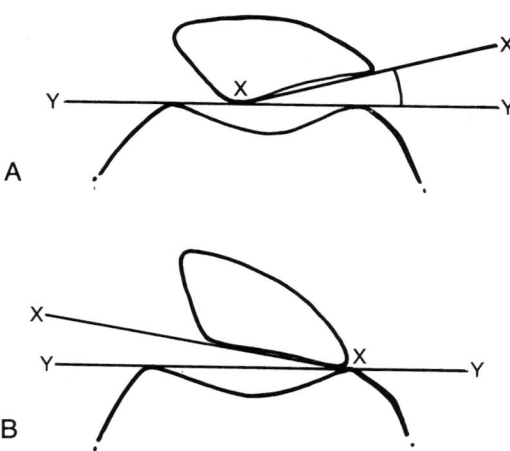

Figure 28E2–39. Measurement of lateral patellofemoral angle.[74] Line YY is drawn across the most anterior portions of the femoral trochea in the axial view of this left knee. Line XX follows the slope of the lateral patellar facet. *A* shows a normal angle in which the angle opens laterally. *B* demonstrates an abnormal angle with the angle open medially. Lines may also be parallel.

congruence angle of greater than + 16 degrees is abnormal at the 95th percentile. Merchant and his coworkers found no correlation between the congruence angle and the degree of patella alta. The average congruence angle for 25 knees with proven recurrent dislocation in their series was + 23 degrees. Merchant[91] and Minkoff and Fein[94] later credited Aglietti with a more accurate definition of the congruence angle. Aglietti found an average congruence angle of − 8 degrees with a standard deviation of 6 degrees.

Laurin and coworkers[74] described a technique in which the knees are flexed to 20 to 30 degrees (Fig. 28E2–38). The x-ray tube is positioned between the ankles with the cassette held proximal to the knees by the patient. On this view, these authors defined a "lateral patellofemoral angle" (Fig. 28E2–39). They indicated that in normal patients, this angle is open laterally, whereas in patients with patellar subluxation, the lines used to define the angle are parallel or open medially. In addition, the patellofemoral index and the measurement of lateral patellar displacement have been

described on the Laurin view[75] (Fig. 28E2–40). Minkoff and Fein[94] have again called into question all such measurements on infrapatellar radiographs, stating that many symptomatic patients have normal indices, and abnormal indices are frequently seen in asymptomatic patients.

We use a version of the Merchant view. A positioning jig is used to obtain some consistency in the angle of knee flexion (Fig. 28E2–41). Despite the use of this jig, the actual degree of knee flexion varies because of differences in body size. Usually, the jig, however, will produce an angle of approximately 30 to 35 degrees of knee flexion on the radiograph. Because of the mentioned shortcomings of all radiographic indices, we do not routinely draw lines and measure angles on every infrapatellar radiograph taken. Lateral patellar tilt and lateral displacement can be noted. Degenerative changes in the patellofemoral joint are easily seen. Osteochondritis dissecans of the patella, accessory ossification centers, and ectopic calcifications in the retinaculum are also seen on the infrapatellar radiograph.

The question arises whether axial radiographs should be taken with the quadriceps contracted or relaxed. Different authors have indicated that quadriceps contraction may either center the patella, thereby reducing a displaced appearance, or increase the appearance of patellar malalignment.[94, 103] Turner and Burns[126] have actually described a technique for obtaining a weight-bearing axial radiograph of the patellofemoral joint (Fig. 28E2–42). In truth, this may make the most sense in creating a dynamic situation within the patellofemoral joint. Its use, however, is not widespread.

Teitge[103] has described an interesting technique for obtaining a stress view of the patellofemoral joint (Fig. 28E2–43). By using a positioning frame with a padded wooden pusher, stress is applied first to the lateral and then to the medial edges of the patella while axial radiographs document the degree of displacement possible. Malghem and Maldague[83] stressed the patellofemoral joint laterally by using forced external rotation of the lower leg (Fig. 28E2–

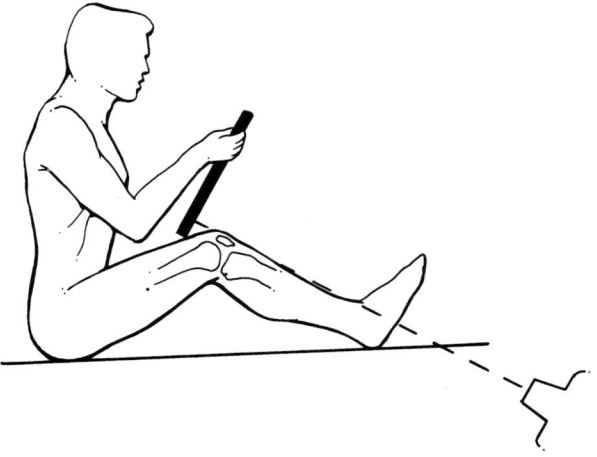

Figure 28E2–38. Axial radiograph (technique of Laurin).

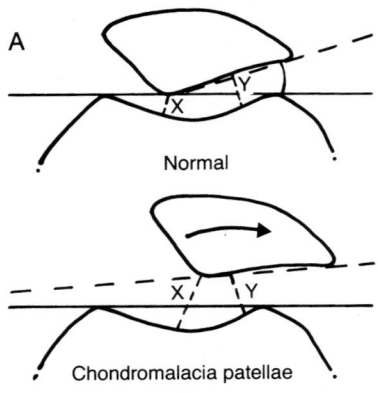

A

Normal

Chondromalacia patellae

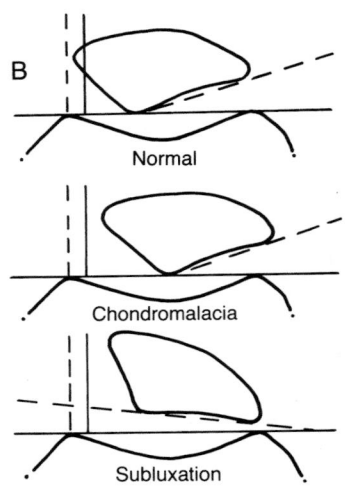

B

Normal

Chondromalacia

Subluxation

Figure 28E2–40. Laurin techniques for measuring patellar position.[75] *A* diagrams the calculation of the patellofemoral index. Distance X is the shortest distance from the medial facet to the medial portion of the trochlea. Y is the shortest distance between the lateral facet and the lateral trochlea. The upper limit of ratio X/Y is 1.6. Higher ratios may indicate chondromalacia. *B* shows the technique for measuring lateral patellar displacement. The position of the patella is compared with the perpendicular with a transtrochlear line. Measurements are valid only at 20 degrees of flexion.

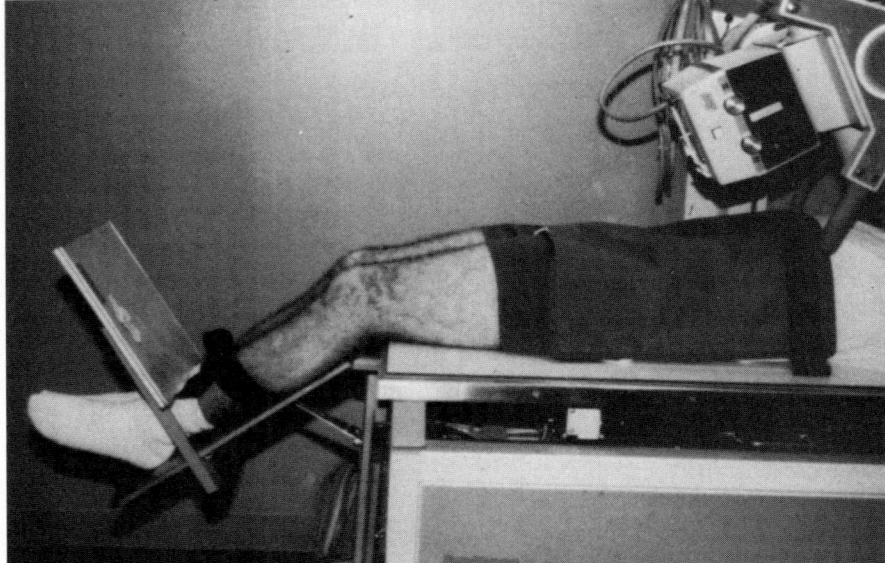

Figure 28E2–41. Cassette-holding jig for modified Merchant view. (Courtesy of Orthopedic Products.)

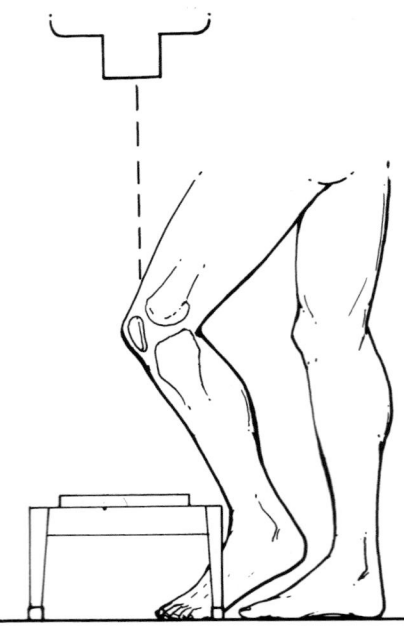

Figure 28E2–42. Technique of weight-bearing axial view described by Turner and Burns.[126]

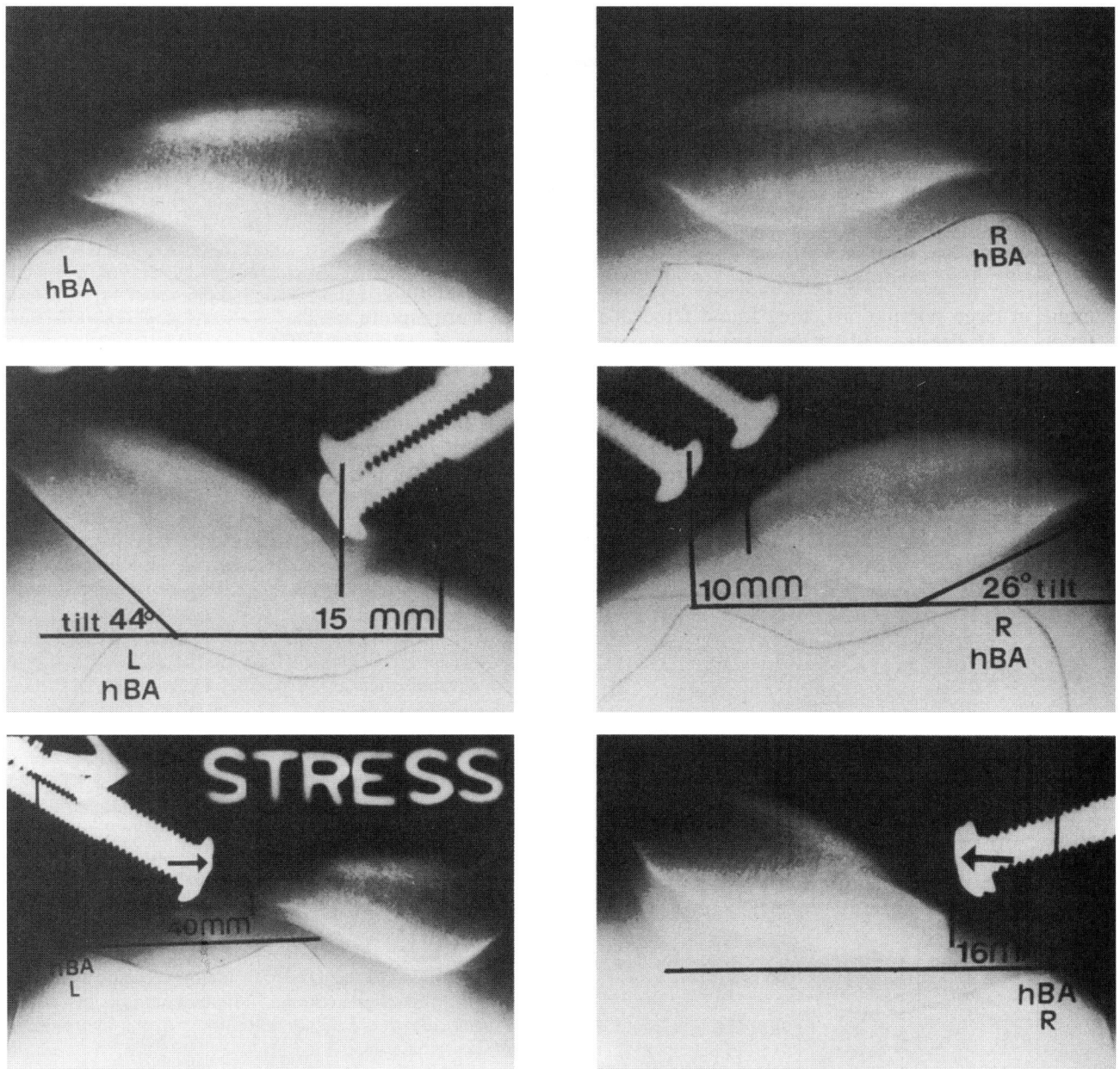

Figure 28E2–43. *Top,* Axial radiographs taken with the Merchant technique show a normal congruence angle and a normal patellofemoral angle. *Center,* Stress radiographs using a quantitative stress device show a 50% (5 mm) increase in lateral excursion of the symptomatic left knee. A difference in lateral tilt is also apparent. *Bottom,* Stress radiographs medially show a complete medial dislocation of the left patella after arthroscopic lateral release. (From *Orthopaedic Knowledge Update.* Park Ridge, Ill, American Academy of Orthopaedic Surgeons, 1990, p 565.)

44). They found this view superior to routine nonstressed views in patients with patellar instability.

With specific regard to patellar dislocation, diagnostic studies should always include plain radiographs. Rarely, one may obtain an infrapatellar view that shows the patella still dislocated laterally (Fig. 28E2–45). Usually, the patella will have relocated in the femoral trochlea, although the radiograph may show excessive lateral displacement. Osteochondral fractures may also be seen (Fig. 28E2–46). In addition to separate osteochondral fragments, there is often a characteristic avulsion fracture or calcification along the medial edge of the patella (Fig. 28E2–47); this is considered pathognomonic for patellar dislocation.

Author's Preferred Method. My standard set of radiographs for a patient with suspected patellofemoral instability includes a standard anteroposterior radiograph, made while the patient is bearing weight if any clinical indication for this exists, and a 90-degree flexed lateral and an axial view of both patellas on the same cassette made as described earlier after the method of Merchant. I use these views for the information they provide on careful visual examination. I do not try to wring a diagnosis from the

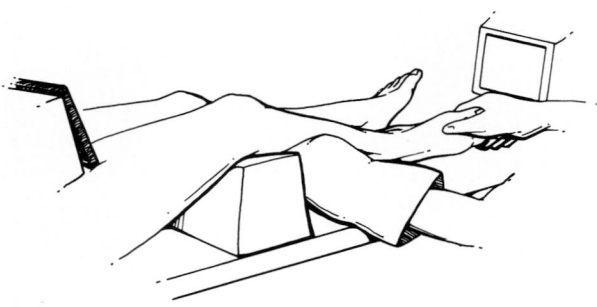

Figure 28E2–44. Technique of 30-degree lateral rotation view of Malghem and Maldague.[83] The patient lies supine on the x-ray table with the right knee flexed 30 degrees over a foam block. The x-ray tube is positioned at the foot and the cassette on the anterior thigh. The examiner applies external rotation to the foot and tibia along with some valgus stress.

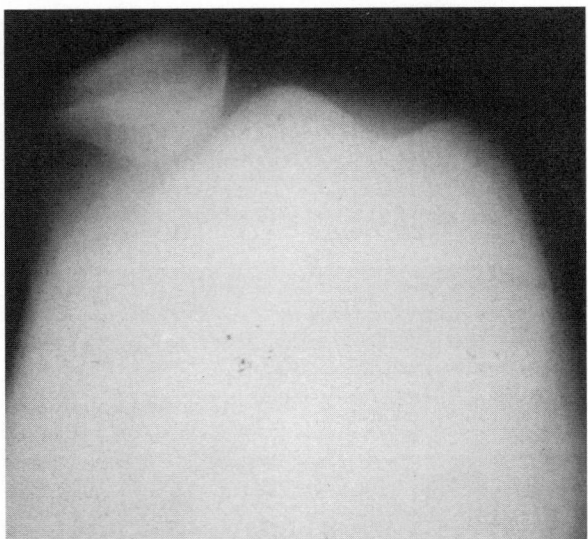

Figure 28E2–45. Patellar dislocation. Infrapatellar radiograph shows the patella still dislocated over the lateral femoral condyle with the knee flexed.

radiographs by constructing and measuring various angles and indices. These radiographs are helpful to me only when they are thoughtfully combined with a detailed history and a careful physical examination.

Computed Tomography

A great deal of interest has been aroused in the use of CT for studying the patellofemoral joint.[30, 39, 61, 115] To a large extent, this interest exists because of the ability of CT to image the knee in greater degrees of extension, including full extension. This eliminates the shortcoming of conventional axial radiographs, which are technically limited by the anterior soft tissues of the lower limb. It has been pointed out that much of the malpositioning and maltracking of the patella takes place in the range of flexion from 0 to 30 degrees. CT has definitely shown that in many cases, the patella in full knee extension rests above the trochlea on the supratrochlear soft tissues.[30, 39] Measurements of congruence angle, lateral tilt, and other indices can be obtained from CT scans just as they can by conventional axial radiographs. Serial CT scans taken at various degrees of knee flexion can also impart some information about the passive tracking of the patella in the trochlear groove.

This technique has been greatly refined by the work of Schutzer and coworkers.[115] They first established two criteria for normal tracking—a patellar tilt angle of less than 8 degrees and a congruence angle of greater than 0 degrees with the knee imaged at 10 degrees of flexion (Fig. 28E2–48). In a study of 54 symptomatic patients and 10 asymptomatic controls, they identified three patterns of "malalignment" (Fig. 28E2–49). Type I was characterized by "subluxation" but no lateral tilting, type II by both subluxation and tilting, and type III by isolated tilting but no subluxation. They felt that type I malalignment was due to an imbalance of longitudinally directed muscle forces without a tight lateral retinaculum. In a patient with type II disorder, the central finding was trochlear dysplasia. Type III corresponded to the excessive lateral pressure syndrome, suggesting that these patients might be candidates for lateral retinacular release. The symptoms in the symptomatic group were not specified, however, and, as Minkoff and Fein[94] have pointed out, no assurance exists that symptoms were correlated to the pattern of malalignment or that

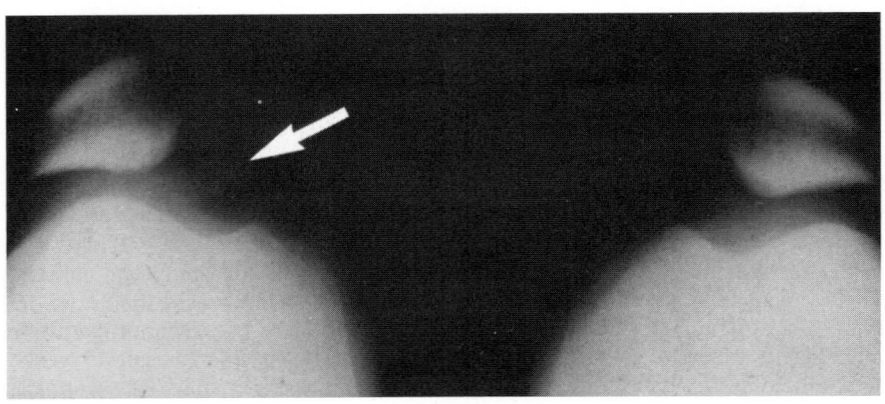

Figure 28E2–46. Patellar dislocation with a large osteochondral fracture *(arrow).*

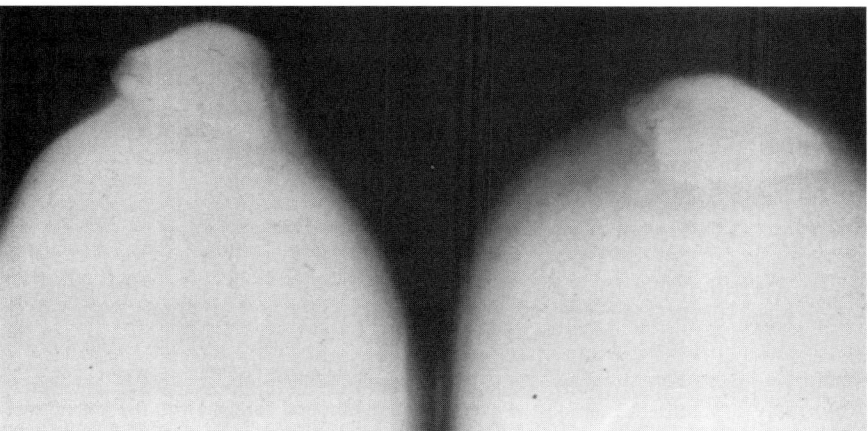

Figure 28E2–47. Axial view shows characteristic avulsion and calcification along the medial edge of the patella.

symptoms could be influenced by specific surgical procedures. In addition, in 22 patients with unilateral symptoms, only 7 of the 22 asymptomatic opposite knees were normal on CT analysis.

Using a combination of CT scans and radiographs, DeJour and colleagues[28] analyzed the factors that they believed were important in patellar instability. Four factors were found to be relevant with symptomatic patellar instability: trochlear dysplasia, quadriceps dysplasia as defined by increased patellar tilt in extension on CT, patella alta, and an increased tibial tuberosity–to–trochlear groove dis-

tance. This last factor can be seen on a CT scan by comparing cuts through the trochlea with those through the tibial tuberosity and measuring the lateral displacement of the tibial tuberosity. The authors state that 20 mm or greater is abnormal. These four abnormal factors appeared in only 3% to 6.5% of control knees.

Despite obvious shortcomings, CT examination may be helpful in understanding the patient with a difficult patellofemoral problem. Not only can it help understand the pattern of maltracking but it also might identify patients in whom all indices are totally normal, prompting a search

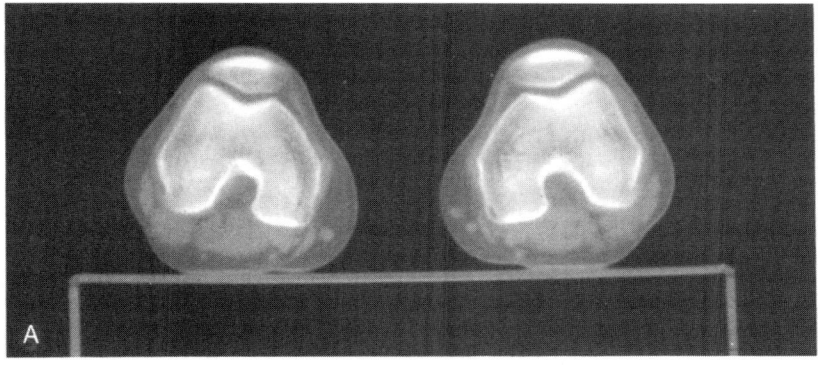

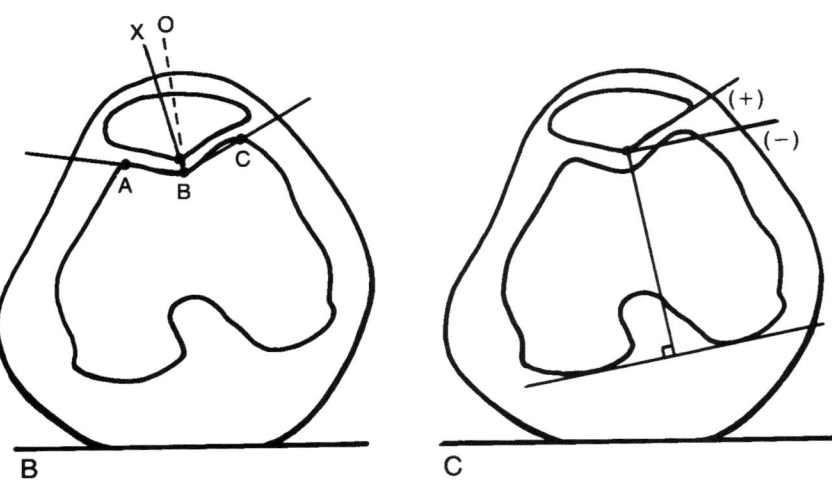

Figure 28E2–48. Normal patellofemoral alignment on computed tomography (CT) scan. *A* shows midpatellar CT cut with knees flexed 10 degrees. *B* shows diagram of congruence angle on the left knee. Normal is greater than 0 at 10 degrees of knee flexion. *C* diagrams the patellar tilt angle measured between a line parallel to the posterior femoral condyles and a line of the lateral facet. Normal is greater than 8 degrees at 10 degrees of knee flexion.

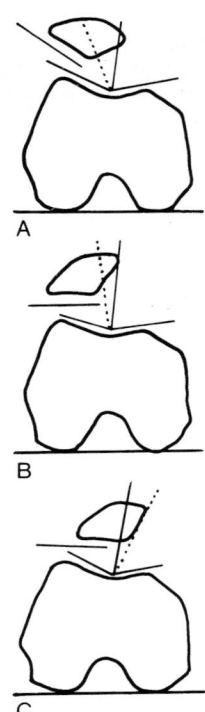

Figure 28E2–49. Three types of abnormal findings on axial computed tomographic scan as described by Fulkerson and Gossling.[38] *A* shows type I, which is lateral subluxation without patellar tilt. *B* demonstrates type II, subluxation with lateral tilt. *C* shows type III, which is lateral tilt without subluxation.

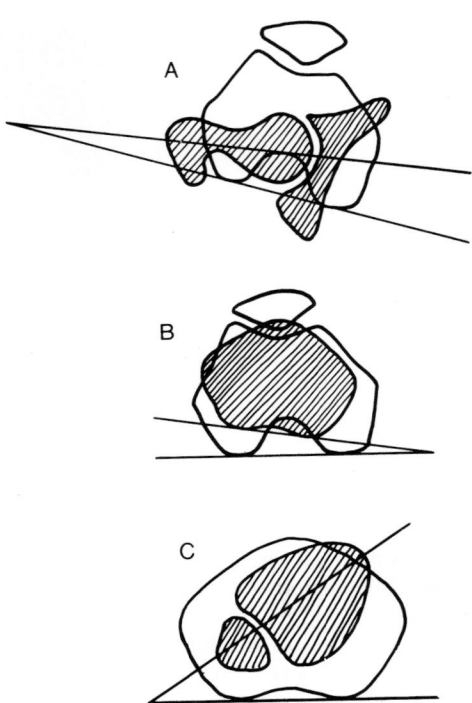

Figure 28E2–50. Technique of measuring rotational alignment with computed tomographic scans. *A* shows the line of the femoral neck (crosshatched) superimposed on the line along the posterior femoral condyles to show rotation in the femur. *B* demonstrates cut-through proximal tibia (cross-hatched) superimposed on the distal femur to show rotational deformity present across the knee joint. *C* demonstrates cut-through transmalleolar area (cross-hatched) superimposed on the proximal tibia, indicating rotation in lower leg.

for other causes of the symptoms. The problems of expense and radiation exposure for these procedures, of course, continue to be significant.

Another use of CT is in the measurement of rotational deformity of the lower extremity (Fig. 28E2–50). It has become apparent that in patients with extreme femoral anteversion and the so-called miserable malalignment syndrome, standard surgical techniques on the extensor mechanism are not likely to be successful. In such individuals, it may even be reasonable to consider derotational osteotomy of the femur. Therefore, determination of femoral rotation becomes even more important. The technique described by Murphy and colleagues[97] seems to have supplanted all previous techniques. They have presented sound geometric reasons for this. Although they have not defined normal values through the use of this technique in large populations, they found femoral rotation of 31 degrees (standard deviation, 4 degrees) in a group of symptomatic patients. Galland and colleagues[39] may have used a different technique but defined normal femoral torsion on CT as 11 degrees (standard deviation, 7 degrees). They also measured rotation in the proximal tibia on CT as well as lateral tibial torsion. In their series, tibial torsion was 33 degrees (standard deviation, 8 degrees). They also demonstrated a method of direct measurement of the lateral displacement of the tibial tuberosity relative to the femoral trochlea, thus imparting an important three-dimensional element to our thinking about extensor mechanism malalignment.

Magnetic Resonance Imaging

The use of magnetic resonance imaging (MRI) has opened other exciting avenues for investigation of the patellofemoral joint. Clearly, pathologic entities such as chondromalacia, other articular cartilage injuries and degeneration, synovial plicae, and patellar tendinitis can be visualized on MRI (Fig. 28E2–51). Studies similar to those made with CT scans can easily be accomplished with MRI without exposure to radiation, although they still obviously involve considerable expense. Shellock and coworkers[118] were among the first to demonstrate the MRI techniques. They imaged the patellofemoral joint in nine different positions from 0 to 32 degrees (Fig. 28E2–52). Special computer software allowed assembly of these images into a "cine-loop" format that produced a pseudodynamic image of the patellofemoral joint. These authors suggested the usefulness of this technique in imaging unstable patellofemoral joints.

Kujala and colleagues[71] later analyzed normal patellar motion in the first 30 degrees of knee flexion using axial MRI in 20 patients without knee symptoms. Their procedure was done with the patient in the supine position, in contrast to Shellock's use of the prone position. Interestingly, when the quadriceps were contracted, the patella moved more medially in half of their subjects and more laterally in the other half. Lateral patellar tilt increased in only one male and one female. They found significant

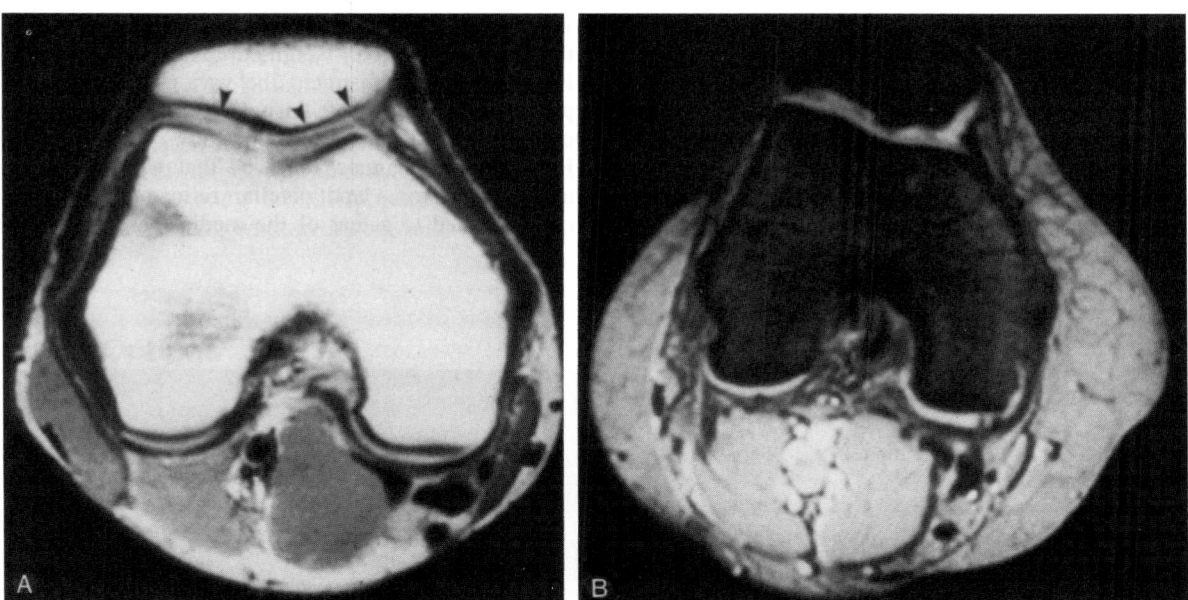

Figure 28E2–51. Magnetic resonance imaging of patellofemoral joint. *A* shows normal, smooth layer of articular cartilage on the patella *(black arrows).* *B* shows presence of irregular chondromalacia of the patella.

differences between males and females, however, suggesting the need for normal values that are sex specific.

More recently, Shellock and associates[117] studied 40 patients with persistent symptoms after arthroscopic lateral release by using their previously described technique of kinematic MRI. Only 2% of these persistently symptomatic patients had normal alignment, whereas 23% had persistent lateral subluxation, 2% had excessive lateral pressure syndrome (by their definition), 63% had medial subluxation,

and 9% showed an unusual pattern of lateral-to-medial subluxation. They addressed in some detail the concept of medial subluxation after lateral release, as proposed by Hughston and Deese.[55] Seventeen of 40 patients with previous unilateral arthroscopic lateral release and persistent medial subluxation actually had medially subluxated patellas on the nonoperated side. This suggests that medial subluxation may have preceded lateral release surgery. They postulated that multiple disordered or uncoordinated

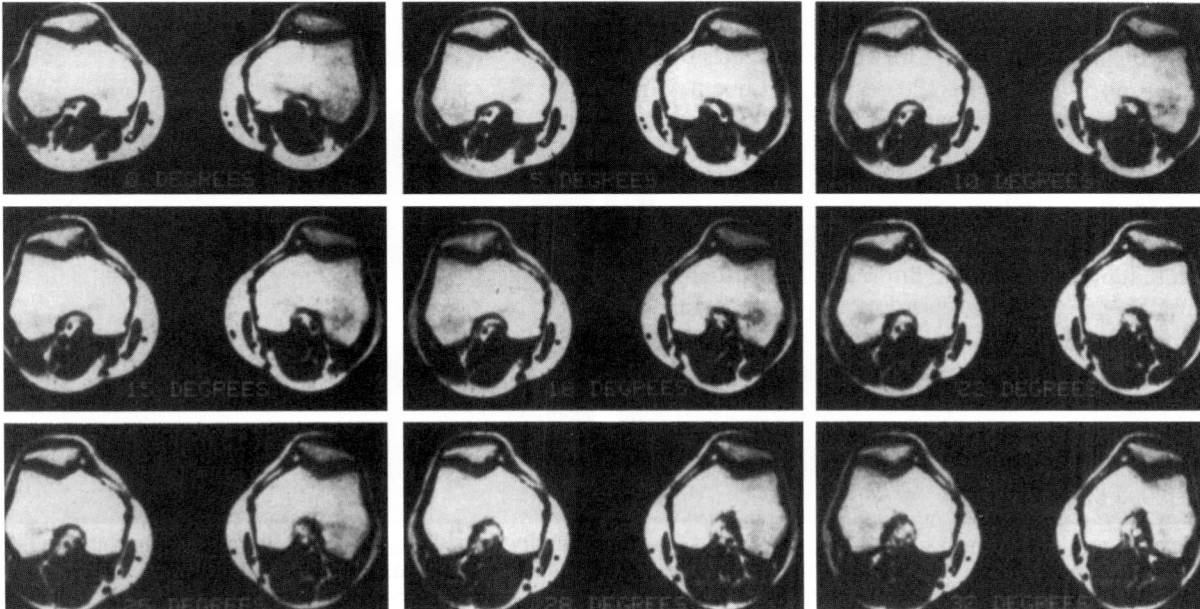

Figure 28E2–52. Five-millimeter axial sections at the same location through the patellofemoral joint of a healthy volunteer with the knees extended and incrementally flexed up to 32 degrees. Note the centralized position of the medial crests of the patellas in relation to the trochlear grooves throughout the range of motion studied. (From Shellock FG, Mink JH, Fox JM: Patellofemoral joint: Kinematic MR image to assess tracking abnormalities. Radiology 168:552, 1988.)

the knee fully extended, the patient is told to flex the knee gently and to roll the hip and leg into slight external rotation over the edge of the table. This helps the last bit of fluid to accumulate in the lateral gutter, allowing it to be removed as the spinal needle is gradually withdrawn. The fluid thus removed from the knee joint should be inspected for the presence of fat globules or, occasionally, small fragments of articular cartilage.

Surgical Treatment

Initial Dislocation

Smillie,[119] Bassett,[5] and O'Donoghue[9] were among the first proponents of surgical repair for initial patellar dislocation. Cofield and Bryan[20] "strongly considered" immediate repair in the presence of an anatomic predisposition to patellar instability or a displaced intra-articular fracture or when the patient was a "serious" athlete. Fondren and colleagues,[37] in reviewing Roux-Goldthwait procedures for recurrent dislocation, used their results to justify immediate surgical repair in patients with initial dislocations. Hawkins and colleagues[48] recommended primary surgical stabilization in patients with predisposing signs such as an increased Q angle or patella alta, even though their numbers were too small for statistical verification. Cash and Hughston[16] hinted that initial surgical treatment might be considered in patients with predisposing physical findings because of the poorer prognosis. Vainionpää and coworkers[127] studied 55 patients prospectively who were suffering their first patellar dislocation. All were treated with open repair. At a minimum 2-year follow-up check, there were good or excellent subjective results in 44 of 55. The redislocation rate was 3% at 1 year and 9% at 2 years. One patient experienced a redislocation 3 years after operation.

Maenpaa and Lehto[80] studied operative versus nonoperative treatment of initial patellar dislocation. Seventeen percent of those undergoing surgical treatment demonstrated osteoarthritic changes. Patients treated nonsurgically who went on to have occasional redislocations of the patella actually showed the lowest incidence of osteoarthritis, at 13%. Strangely, those undergoing nonoperative treatment who did not experience redislocation showed the highest incidence of osteoarthritis, 29%. They believed that their study demonstrated that guided conservative therapy should be the choice for treating patellar dislocation. Nikku and colleagues[99] reported a prospective randomized study of surgical versus nonsurgical treatment for initial patellar dislocation. Other disease was excluded by arthroscopic study. Closed treatment ranged from 3 weeks of immobilization if the patella was dislocatable to a simple brace if it was only subluxable. Operative treatment consisted of repair of the medial retinaculum and additional augmentation of the patellofemoral ligament. The vast majority of patients had an additional lateral release. Follow-up included subjective scales, performance tests, and clinical examination. The subjective result was better in the group undergoing closed repair, whereas the other two methods of evaluation yielded similar results in the two groups. Nine patients in the group undergoing closed repair subsequently under-

went later operation, whereas 12 patients with primary surgery had 15 re-operations.

Thomas[124] performed a critical evaluation of the available emergency medicine literature addressing whether first-time patellar dislocation should be treated surgically or nonsurgically. Seventy-nine papers were identified, of which 74 were irrelevant and three were of insufficient quality. The remaining two papers had significant study weaknesses. The conclusion was that conservative management of primary patellar dislocation was as effective as surgical treatment with a lower complication rate, thus making closed methods the treatment of choice. Sallay and colleagues[113] evaluated acute repair of the MPFL. They found that in their 12 patients, who were observed for a minimum of 2 years after acute repair of the MPFL, there were no redislocations. Four had experienced episodes of "sharp pain" that may have represented subluxation episodes. Although only 58% of the patients had good or excellent results, of the 42% with fair results, all were relegated to that category based primarily on pain and swelling rather than on recurrent instability.

The age of the patient may also affect the decision. Rorabeck and Bobechko,[111] in dealing with 18 children who also had osteochondral fractures with dislocation, found that redislocation occurred in all patients who had the fragment removed but underwent no surgical repair. Cash and Hughston[16] found a decreased recurrence rate when the patient was older than 14 years of age at the time of the initial episode. No patient older than 28 years of age at the time of the initial dislocation had a subsequent redislocation. In their group of 26 patients treated nonsurgically for recurrent dislocation, Crosby and Insall[23] found that dislocations were less frequent with increasing age.

A VMO that has been torn from its patellar insertion provides the most clear-cut situation in which early surgery may help (Fig. 28E2–55). Likewise, the associated disruption of the medial knee ligaments and disruption of the VMO origin and the MPFL from the adductor tubercle[60] are also situations in which early surgical repair can be helpful (Fig. 28E2–56).

If surgical treatment is chosen for the initial patellar dislocation, other decisions must still be made. Should arthroscopic surgery alone be used? Cash and Hughston[16] demonstrated no improvement in results when arthroscopic surgery was used alone compared with nonoperative treatment. Six of 20 patients in the "conservative" group of Hawkins and associates[48] underwent initial arthroscopy, but no definite benefit was demonstrated other than identification and removal of osteochondral fracture fragments. If arthroscopy is done, should isolated lateral retinacular release be considered? Dainer[26] treated 29 acute patellar dislocations with arthroscopy alone. Although lateral retinacular release was done without specific indications on the basis of surgeon's preference alone, those patients having lateral release fared worse. This may speak to the recent evidence that even the lateral retinaculum may have some role in providing medial stability of the patella.[31]

Most authors recommending early surgery suggest direct surgical repair of the damaged tissue. Vainionpää and associates[127] apparently found reparable damage to the medial retinaculum in all cases. The VMO itself may be torn from its origin, from its insertion, or interstitially. The MPFL

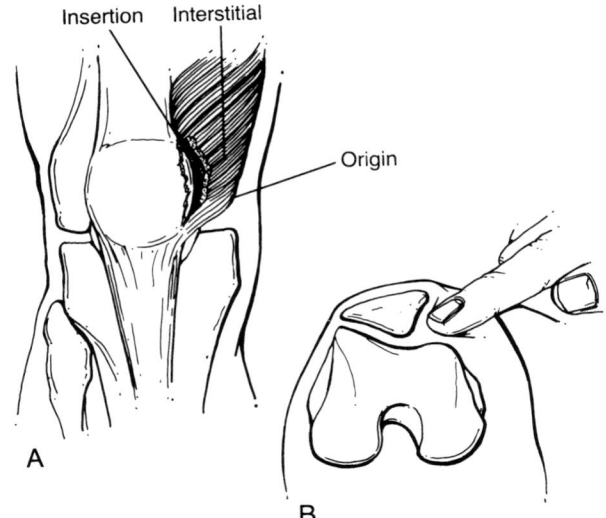

Figure 28E2–55. Rupture of the vastus medialis obliquus muscle with acute patellar dislocation. *A* shows possible sites of vastus medialis obliquus rupture. The majority will be interstitial. Most significant, however, is the insertional rupture, which can be sutured surgically. When insertional rupture occurs, *B* shows how skin and soft tissues can be easily invaginated into the joint through the site of rupture. This should aid in making the diagnosis.

will usually be found torn either at its attachment to the femur or in its midsubstance.

If a repair of the medial structures is undertaken, should the other components of an open extensor mechanism reconstruction be done (i.e., lateral release and transposition of the patellar tendon insertion)? Vainionpää and coworkers[127] carried out lateral release in 37 of their 55 patients. Nikku and colleagues[99] included lateral release in 61 of 70 surgeries done acutely. Obviously, there were strong-enough laterally directed forces to create the dislocation,

and it might seem reasonable that these should be released. With recognition of the contribution of the lateral retinaculum to stability of the patella and with known complications of lateral release (e.g., medial subluxation of the patella), however, careful consideration should be given before adding this to early surgery for acute patellar dislocation.

The distal correction may be just as controversial. Both patella alta and an increased Q angle have been associated with patellar dislocation.[27, 32, 62, 72] Transfer of the tibial tuberosity may seem logical. If this is done, however, one has performed essentially an entire reconstructive procedure when the original intent was to repair only the acutely damaged structures.

Osteochondral fractures should also be discussed in relation to patellar dislocation. In 1943, Milgram[92] first described the mechanism by which osteochondral fractures are created. The shearing of the patellar dislocation and subsequent relocation can fracture either the patella, usually the medial facet, the lateral lip of the trochlea, or both (Fig. 28E2–57). Rorabeck and Bobechko[111] noted this fracture in approximately 5% of all acute dislocations occurring in children. They confirmed the three patterns of fracture location. In their series, fracture fragments were either removed or replaced. Cash and Hughston[16] reported on 29 knees in their series that had osteochondral fragments. Twenty of these were treated in the acute phase with arthroscopic or open removal during surgical repair. None of the fragments appear to have been reattached and internally fixated. Of these 20, only one patient had a poor result. Nine patients in whom osteochondral fragments were visible on radiographs were treated nonoperatively in the series of Cash and Hughston, and five of these had poor results. Osteochondral fractures were also sustained by 14 of 27 patients reviewed by Hawkins and associates.[48] Surgical treatment seems to have consisted only of fragment removal. Ten of these fractures were identified on initial films, one was seen on later films, and three were seen only at the time of arthroscopy. McManus and coworkers,[89] again addressing the problem in children, reported on the removal of three large osteochondral fragments in their 33 patients.

Consequently, even though internal fixation and removal have traditionally been mentioned as treatment options, it appears that removal is the usual choice. Nevertheless, if

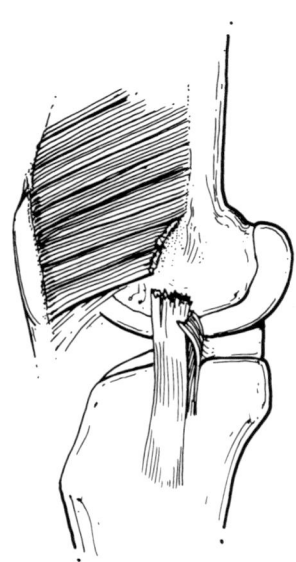

Figure 28E2–56. Rupture of the vastus medialis obliquus combined with medial ligamentous tear. The site of the tear is usually at the confluence of these structures over the medial femoral epicondyle and adductor tubercle.

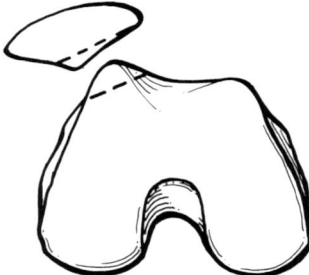

Figure 28E2–57. Mechanism of osteochondral fractures in acute patellar dislocation, axial view of the right knee. Osteochondral fracture of the medial patellar facet or lateral lip of the trochlea can occur with dislocation or relocation of patellar dislocation. Large fracture of the lateral trochlea may affect stability of the patellofemoral joint.

Aglietti and colleagues[1] studied 69 knees with recurrent dislocation treated by a variety of surgical procedures. A lateral release alone gave a 40% recurrence rate. After open realignment, 4% had redislocation but there was pain and swelling in 12% and significant crepitation in 35%. Proximal versus combined proximal and distal realignment yielded similar results. Retensioning of the medial structures and lateral release were effective in reducing the patella. They felt that transposition of the tibial tuberosity, while appealing, did not add evident clinical advantages. On the other hand, Rillmann and colleagues[110] reported on 41 operations in 37 patients consisting only of medialization of the medial third of the patellar tendon with a fragment of tibial tuberosity. They reported no redislocations in 39 knees despite this incredibly simple procedure.

Since recognition of the important role of the MPFL, techniques have begun to emerge addressing this pathologic process. Hautamaa and colleagues[47] believe that proximal realignment should always repair the MPFL and demonstrated the effectiveness of this in restoring balance in cadaver knees. Avikainen and colleagues[4] presented a technique of augmentation of the MPFL with a strip of adductor magnus tendon. There was one redislocation in 14 patients. Muneta and colleagues[96] reconstructed the MPFL with a double-strand gracilis tendon in five and an iliotibial band allograft in one. Sandmeier and colleagues[114] sectioned the MPFL in six cadaver knees and then reconstructed it with gracilis tendon. This "substantially restored" normal patellar tracking.

The theoretical basis of derotational osteotomy of the lower limb is the fact that extensor mechanism malalignment is a three-dimensional deformity. Rotational deformity of the femur and tibia have long been recognized in the situation of the miserable malalignment syndrome.[58, 65] If standard extensor mechanism surgery stands little chance of correcting the problem in a patient with this deformity, then perhaps correction of the rotational deformity might work better. Derotation of the femoral anteversion could be done at either the trochanteric level or the supracondylar level. Correction of excessive external tibial torsion could be done either above the tibial tuberosity, immediately below it, or in the supramalleolar region. Teitge[122] has been the strongest advocate for the role that may be played by derotational osteotomy. Although not specifically dealing with recurrent dislocation of the patella, Delgado and colleagues[29] presented 9 patients with 13 involved extremities that were treated operatively for symptomatic torsional malalignment and associated patellofemoral disease. The patients were 10 to 18 years of age. After an average follow-up of 2 years and 7 months, with a minimum of 18 months, patients had an improvement in gait pattern, extremity appearance, and a marked decrease in knee pain.

As mentioned earlier, attempts to deepen a dysplastic trochlea have been described since the earliest part of the 20th century. Trochleoplasty then fell out of favor until recently, when several reports of current attempts to use this began to appear, especially in the French literature. Thus far, worldwide experience is minimal and its place in the surgical armamentarium is not known. Certainly, violation of the articular cartilage of the trochlea appears to be a major conceptual drawback.

Complications

Significant complications can be encountered with any technique of extensor mechanism reconstruction. These include complications seen early, within approximately 3 weeks after the operation, and those seen late, that is, after approximately 3 weeks. Complications seen early include hemarthrosis, wound hematoma, wound infection, necrosis of skin flaps, nerve palsy or compartment syndrome, and venous complications.

Hemarthrosis has often been mentioned in relation to isolated lateral release. Hemarthrosis may still occur even with open extensor mechanism reconstruction. Hughston and coworkers[58] reported seven patients with hemarthroses in 346 extensor mechanism reconstructions. Careful attention should be given to meticulous hemostasis, particularly in the area of the superolateral geniculate arteries, to prevent this occurrence.

Wound hematoma is an infrequent complication. It is mentioned mainly to differentiate it from hemarthrosis. A collection of blood in the subcutaneous tissues of the wound generally causes far less trouble than a frank hemarthrosis.

As with most orthopaedic procedures, wound infection occurs with some infrequency. Hughston and colleagues[58] reported five superficial infections and one deep infection in 346 operations. DeCesare[27] found three superficial and one deep infection in 67 surgically treated knees. In the 214 patients reviewed, Fielding and associates[36] found 22 superficial infections and two deep ones. Prophylactic antibiotics are considered to minimize this complication.

Although necrosis of a skin flap has been reported mainly in relation to the Maquet procedure, Hughston and coworkers[58] reported three incidents among 346 extensor reconstructions. They emphasized the need to avoid this complication by dissecting through the prepatellar bursa rather than superficial to it.

Compartment syndrome and peroneal nerve palsy have been linked mainly to the Hauser procedure. Wiggins[131] collected six such complications, and Wall[128] reported 11 patients with compartment syndrome following this operation. Wall postulated that bleeding from the anterior tibial recurrent vessels that terminate along the lateral border of the tibial tuberosity was the cause. Two cases ended in above-knee amputations. Others resulted in a range of disability depending on how much delay occurred before appropriate treatment. The most common warning sign was restlessness on awakening in the recovery room or severe unremitting pain in the leg. Milder forms of compartment syndrome can resemble peroneal nerve palsy. Injury to the peroneal nerve itself could conceivably occur. Hughston and colleagues[58] emphasized release of the tourniquet and meticulous hemostasis to avoid this disastrous situation, and Youmans[132] suggested using a postoperative drain and coating the raw bony surfaces with bone wax.

Deep venous thrombosis and potential pulmonary emboli can occur in this as in all lower extremity surgery. Hughston and associates[58] reported thrombophlebitis in three cases and frank pulmonary embolization in two. Fielding and colleagues[36] reported one case of phlebitis and one pulmonary embolus in 377 Hauser procedures.

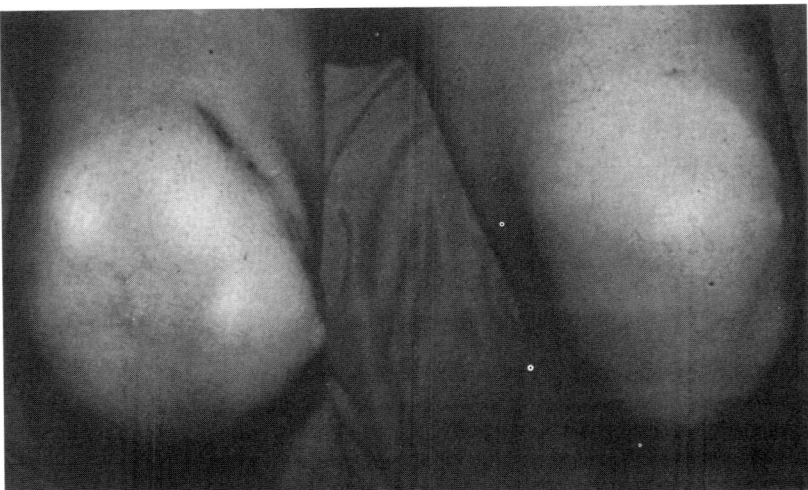

Figure 28E2–59. Medial dislocation of the patella as a complication of extensor mechanism reconstruction. With the right knee flexed, the patella remains completely dislocated over the medial femoral condyle.

Potential late complications include ankylosis, recurrent malalignment/instability, loss of patellar tendon fixation, hardware tenderness, rotational deformities of the limb, nonunion of the tibial tuberosity, and two entities discussed elsewhere, reflex sympathetic dystrophy and infrapatellar contracture syndrome. The true incidence of ankylosis following extensor mechanism surgery is difficult to ascertain. Early loss of motion severe enough to require knee manipulation has been reported in as many as 12% of cases.[58]

It has become much more frequent with current rehabilitative techniques.

Teitge[122] has nicely classified the causes and treatment of complications in patellofemoral joint surgery. His two most common complications leading to further surgery are medial instability of the patella and recurrent lateral instability of the patella. Recurrent extensor mechanism malalignment of all degrees and directions can occur following surgery. Crosby and Insall[23] reported 20% rate of recurrence of lateral dislocation following proximal and distal reconstruction. In their monograph, Hughston and coworkers[58] reported total medial dislocation of the patella a potential postsurgical complication (Fig. 28E2–59). In 1988, Hughston and Deese[55] produced the first report of medial subluxation as a complication in 30 knees. Eighteen of those 30 had no surgery other than a lateral retinacular release. In 1994, Nonweiler and DeLee[101] added five more patients with medial subluxation and described a gravity subluxation test to detect it. Their treatment was reconstruction of the lateral retinaculum. Hughston and colleagues in 1996[53] reported a surgical procedure to correct medial subluxation in 63 patients with 65 affected knees. This included reconstruction of the lateral patellotibial ligament. Teitge[122] likewise reports that his most frequent revision surgery is that of lateral retinacular reconstruction. Excessive patella baja has been reported as a complication primarily of the Hauser procedure,[19, 36, 58] even to the extent of creating patellar abutment against the proximal tibia and an apparent formation of pseudoarthrosis (Fig. 28E2–60). These complications can be minimized only through meticulous surgical technique and attempts to position and balance the patella properly. Teitge[122] contends that such complications result from one of three factors: (1) wrong or incomplete diagnosis; (2) right diagnosis but wrong solution; (3) right diagnosis with right solution but performed poorly or with inadequate materials. The offending tissues may be bony, ligamentous, cartilaginous, or muscular. Correction must address the specific responsible tissue.

When surgery is performed on the patellar tendon and its insertion, fixation of the tendon distally may be lost later. This may result from displacement of internal fixation devices, displacement of bone blocks, or rupture of the patellar tendon, especially when the Roux-Goldthwait technique is used.[43, 58]

Tenderness may occur over the internal fixation hardware in the tibial tuberosity, especially if any degree of anteriorization of the tuberosity has been done. Successful treatment is usually accomplished simply by removing the

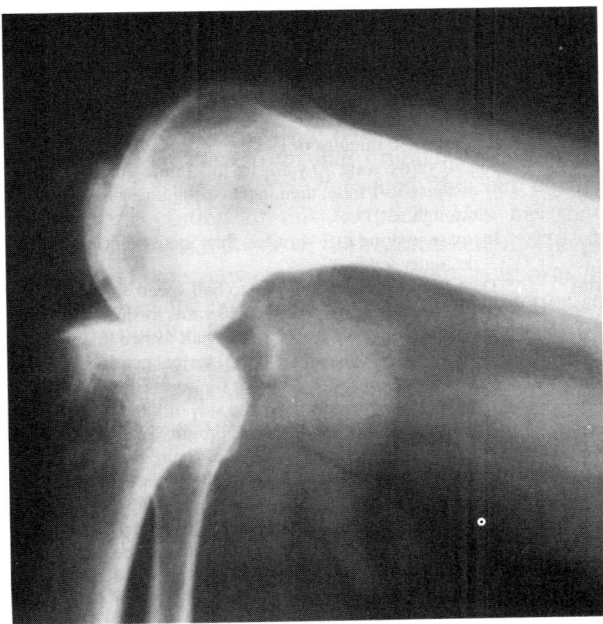

Figure 28E2–60. Patella baja as a complication of the Hauser procedure. The patella has been pulled so far distally as to abut against the proximal tibia.

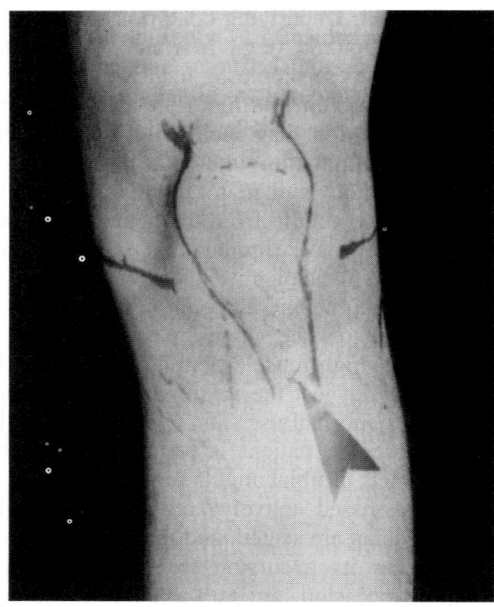

Figure 28E3–8. Increased Q angle due to tibial tubercle lateral development.

is similar to the one causing anterior cruciate ligament (ACL) compromise.

Imaging

Patellar instability is a dynamic process that is difficult to document with routine radiographs. A multitude of spe-

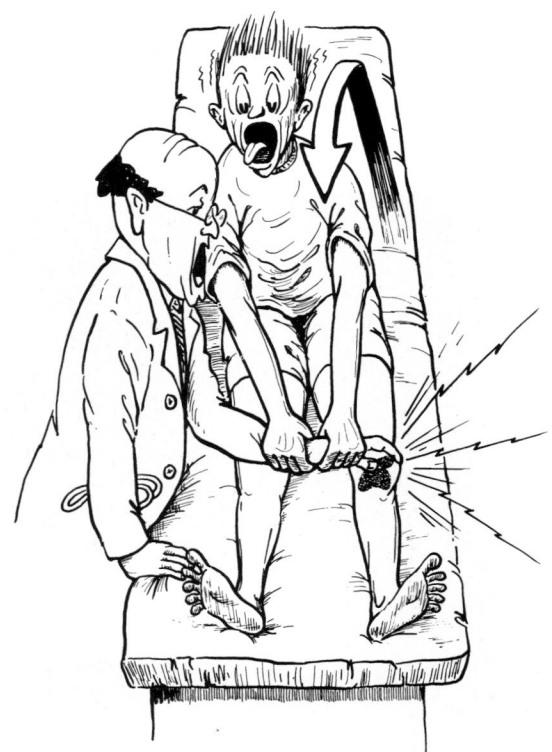

Figure 28E3–9. Apprehension sign. Patient anxiety is due to awareness of unpleasantness associated with patellar dislocation.

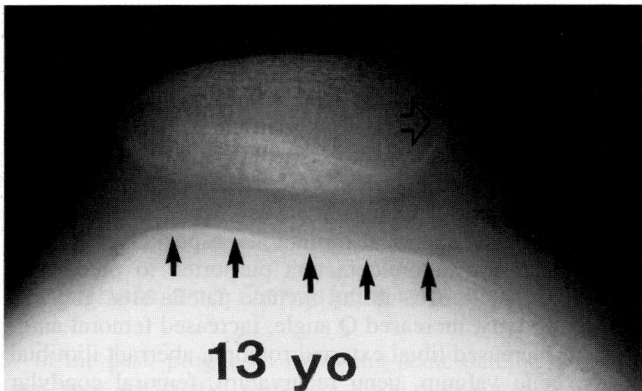

Figure 28E3–10. Undeveloped femoral sulcus and condyles *(solid arrows)* associated with development of a small, vertical medial patellar facet *(open arrow)* in a 13-year-old boy with recurrent patellar instability.

cial radiographic views and measurements are reported, but none is done in the weight-bearing position with the quadriceps contracted.

Routine radiographs should be reviewed for osteochondral injury, loose bodies, and abnormal patellofemoral sulcus relationships (Fig. 28E3–10). One occasionally sees an avulsion fragment at the medial, nonarticulating patellar edge that is the result of previous injury (Fig. 28E3–11). Less commonly, ossification is seen within the previously torn medial patellofemoral ligament (Fig. 28E3–12). The patellar "skyline" view should be done in no more than 20 to 25 degrees of flexion, with the patella pointing straight ahead. In chronic cases, a computed tomographic (CT) scan done in 20 degrees of flexion with the quadriceps relaxed and contracted can give information about patellar tilt, translation, or a combination of tilt and translation. Fulkerson and associates[9, 26] classified CT findings of patients with patellar instability in three categories. Type I had lateral translation; type II had lateral translation plus patellar tilt; and type III had only patellar tilt. Guzzanti and colleagues[12] studied CT evaluations of patellar malalignment done at 15 degrees of knee flexion in 27 adolescents with anterior knee pain but without instability. The quadriceps were contracted and relaxed, and differences of patellar position reviewed between the two states. The

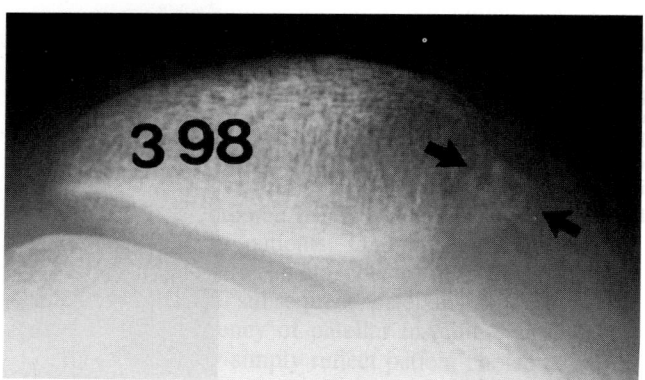

Figure 28E3–11. Healed medial nonarticular avulsion fracture fragment *(arrows)* after an acute patellar dislocation the previous year.

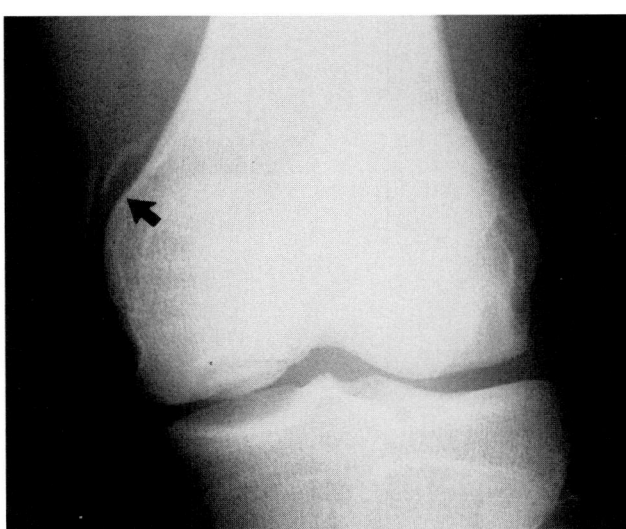

Figure 28E3–12. Ossified medial patellofemoral ligament *(arrow)* in a 17-year-old boy who had dislocated his patella 2 years previously and still complained of patellar instability. Incidental note is made of medial femoral condyle osteochondritis dissecans that was minimally symptomatic.

three Fulkerson categories were seen and, in 11% of cases, the type changed with quadriceps contraction.

The ability to obtain kinematic radiographic images is on the horizon and the technique should have a considerable impact on documenting the spectrum of patellar instability and its genesis.

Nonoperative Treatment

Previous studies have been hampered by their retrospective nature, reporting of varied treatment protocols, lack of return to activity criteria, and lack of data about underlying risk factors for recurrence. Lower extremity rehabilitation should focus on restoration of flexibility, strength, and endurance, with major emphasis on quadriceps function. Because the undersurface of the medialis is the location of an attenuated medial patellofemoral ligament, much commentary is directed toward the necessity for isolated medialis strengthening. No objective data support this thesis. The loss of strength and endurance in the medialis is a reflection of deficiencies present throughout the quadriceps muscle group, and is not a deficit in the medialis alone.

Patellar "stabilizing" braces are commonly used. Although these devices may provide comfort, no objective data document their ability to maintain normal patellar position throughout normal knee motion at functional speeds. Their mechanism of action may be caused by placebo or proprioceptive effects. Taping protocols have been suggested to develop a proprioceptive mechanism that "retrains" the vastus medialis.[19] Recent objective data during functional tasks, comparing outcomes from taping plus rehabilitation with rehabilitation alone, show that taping has no greater efficacy than rehabilitation alone.[17]

Activity modification may be needed and restrictions may need to be placed on participation in athletic events

with high demands for changes of direction. Garth and associates[10] studied a group of patients with recurrent patellar dislocations who were treated with a protective knee sleeve and immediate functional rehabilitation. Forty percent of the patients (30 knees) in their series experienced recurrent patellar instability. Fifty percent of the patients had less than good or excellent results. These authors suggested that their patients younger than 13 years with bilateral instability, multiple joint laxity, and high Q and patellofemoral sulcus angles were at high risk for failure of their nonoperative program. Unfortunately, these characteristics presage a poor outcome with operative management as well.

If the patient fails a well-controlled rehabilitation program, and has persistence of patellar instability, operative management is indicated to prevent progressive articular compromise from recurrent patellar dislocation.

Surgical Treatment

A huge number of types of reconstructive surgical techniques for management of patellar instability have been reported. This plethora of procedures indicates lack of understanding of the factors that need to be addressed to normalize patellar stability. The procedure chosen must be individualized for each patient, taking into account anatomic and physiologic assets and liabilities, and "cookbook" solutions must be avoided. Surgical techniques provide patellar stability by releasing tight lateral structures, improving anatomic alignment, and restoring medial restraint vectors, either alone or in combination with other factors. The goal is to re-establish balance among the patella's four-quadrant cruciform forces. The procedures fall into one of three types: (1) proximal realignment by lateral retinacular release, medial capsular imburcation (including the patellofemoral ligament), vastus medialis transfer, or medial hamstring tenodesis; (2) distal realignment by patellar tendon or tibial tubercle transfer; or (3) combination of proximal and distal procedures.

Lateral retinacular release may be effective to reduce patellar tilt but is not indicated as an isolated procedure for patellar instability, especially for patients with ligamentous laxity. Adequate proximal and distal release of the lateral retinaculum is required. Care must be taken to not provide too vigorous release of the vastus lateralis, which causes imbalance and medial patellar instability. During distal retinacular release, the lateral meniscus should be visualized and protected. Lateral release has a high complication rate.[7, 15, 22] Complications associated with arthroscopic lateral release include total vastus lateralis transection, neuroma and hematoma formation, reflex dystrophy, quadriceps rupture, infection, and phlebitis.

Restoration of an incompetent medial vector requires reapproximation of isometry of the medial patellofemoral and patellomeniscal ligaments as an individual layer augmented by distal transfer of the vastus medialis. Suture of the transferred muscle's tendon into a periosteal cuff of the patella enhances fixation. In skeletally immature patients for whom tibial tubercle transfer is contraindicated because of concern for the occurrence of tibial recurvatum, semitendinosus transfer provides a distal-medial checkrein. Hall and associates[13] report excellent results in 80% of their patients who had a combination medial capsular and vastus medialis advancement with semitendinosus transfer. Similar results were reported by Letts and colleagues[18] at an average follow-up of 3½ years in 29 patients whose average age was 14.4 years at the time of surgery. Use of a cannulated drill over a guide pin drilled under fluoroscopic control (from inferomedial to superolateral) aids in directing the transfer's position with avoidance of the articular surface. Indications for combined lateral retinacular release, medial capsuloplasty, vastus medialis advancement, and semitendinosus tenodesis include skeletal immaturity, major distal patellofemoral and patellotibial malalignment, and patellofemoral sulcus hypoplasia.

The Goldthwaite patellar tendon crossover technique has waned in popularity owing to the procedure's tendency to produce patellar tilt because of the unequal positions of the limbs of transfer.

The distal tibial tubercle transfer proposed by Roux and popularized by Hauser is no longer recommended because it displaces the patella and its tendon distally and posteriorly, increasing patellofemoral contact forces (Figs. 28E3–13 and 28E3–14). The rotational tibial tubercleplasty, interestingly, initially also described by Roux, was later popularized by Elmslie and Trillat and allows reorientation of the patellar tendon axis without distal or posterior positioning (Fig. 28E3–15). Cox[5] reported excellent results from the procedure in 116 U.S. Naval Academy midshipmen involved in vigorous activities. The 88% good or excellent results at 1 year diminished to 68% percent at 7 years postoperatively on further follow-up.[3]

Patients who are skeletally mature with severe patellar articular damage and instability and who require distal realignment may benefit from Fulkerson's modification of the Elmslie-Trillat procedure.[9] The Fulkerson method employs a more sagittal osteotomy that allows medial translation and elevation of the tibial tubercle. The more anterior position improves quadriceps efficiency and diminishes patellofemoral contact forces.

Young children with patellar instability present a multifaceted nature in their condition caused by patellar size, shape, femoral trochlear maldevelopment, lower extremity abnormal biomechanics, ligamentous laxity, and so forth.

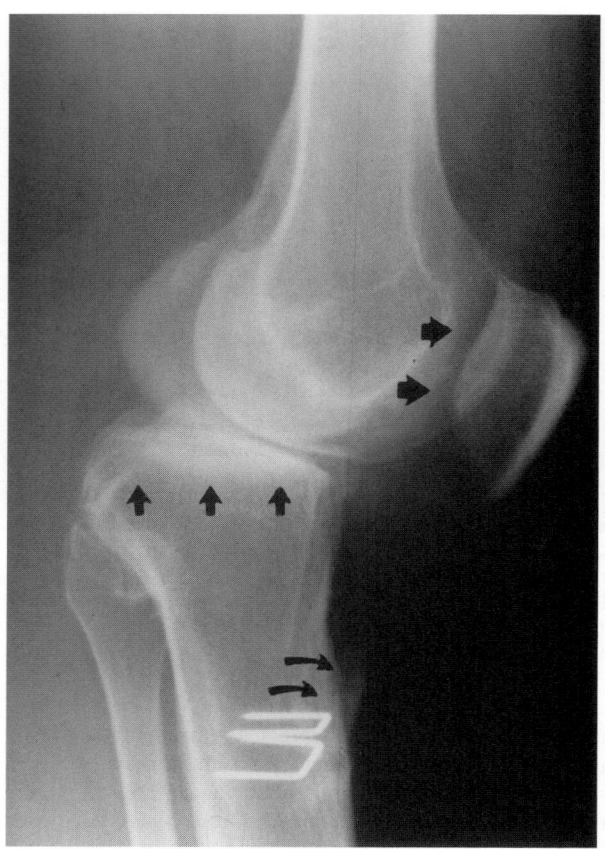

Figure 28E3–14. Patella infra *(large arrowheads)* and tibia recurvatum *(curved arrows)* in a 25-year-old man after a Hauser procedure at age 13. Note early degenerative joint disease *(straight arrows).* (Courtesy of Dr. Jerry Rosenberg.)

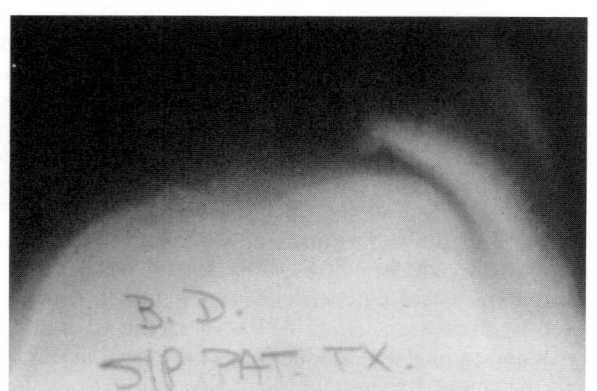

Figure 28E3–13. Patellar malposition after a Hauser patellar tendon transfer.

Soft tissue surgery alone usually does not produce long-lasting results. Adolescents with recurrent patellar dislocations almost always require elements of proximal and distal realignments, depending on the specifics of the individual patient. Patients with patellar instability and marked distal femoral or proximal tibial valgus from congenital or acquired causes may need concomitant femoral or tibial osteotomies, in addition to more routine patellar stabilization methods (Fig. 28E3–16).

Management of patellar instability spawned a multitude of suggested procedures because of the nonspecificity of diagnosis, treatment variations, and dissatisfaction with one particular procedure. Surgical treatment of patellar instability requires a tailor-made operation because of patient uniqueness. Bilateral patellar instability may not be due to identical factors. Preoperative identification of the factors leading to instability allows the surgeon to address each one and to formulate the procedure needed to restore dynamic patellar balance. Generalized ligamentous laxity cannot be overcome by surgery.[28] Patients with abnormal collagen and their parents must be advised accordingly.

Surgical complications include recurrent instability, wound necrosis and infection, saphenous nerve injury, and arthrofibrosis.

Maloccurrences are secondary to misdiagnosis, errors in surgical indications and choice of procedures, and technical errors.

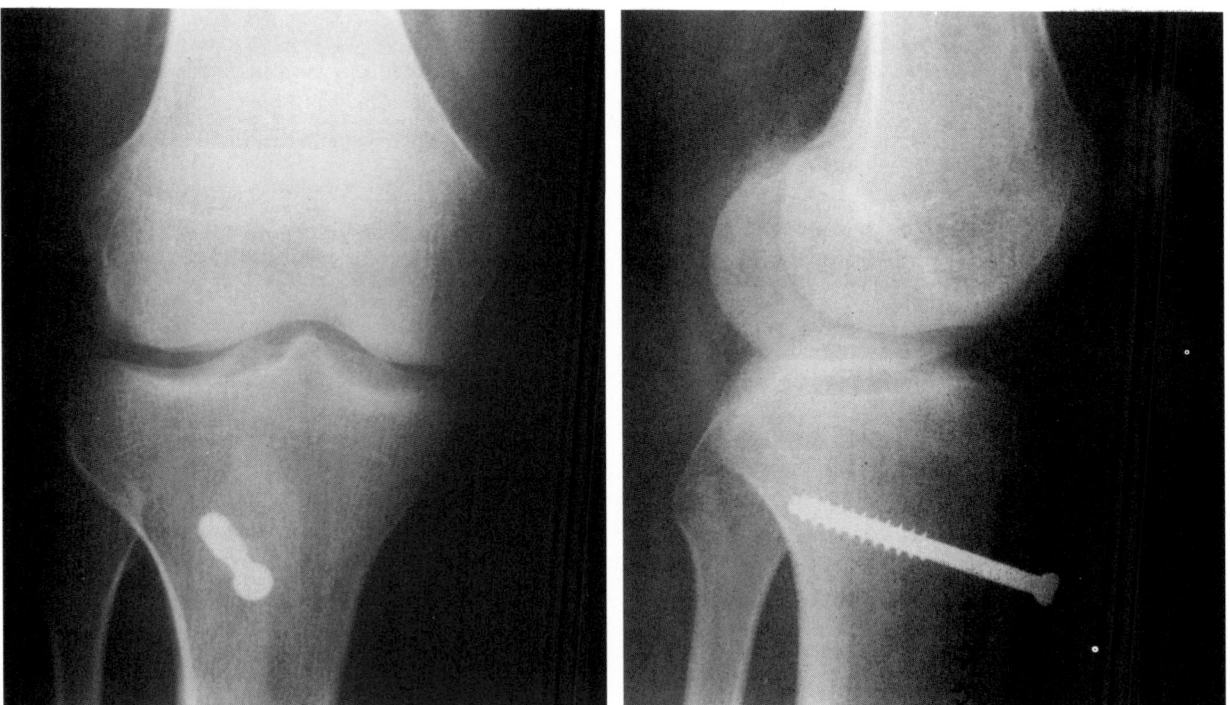

Figure 28E3–15. Elmslie-Trillat transfer.

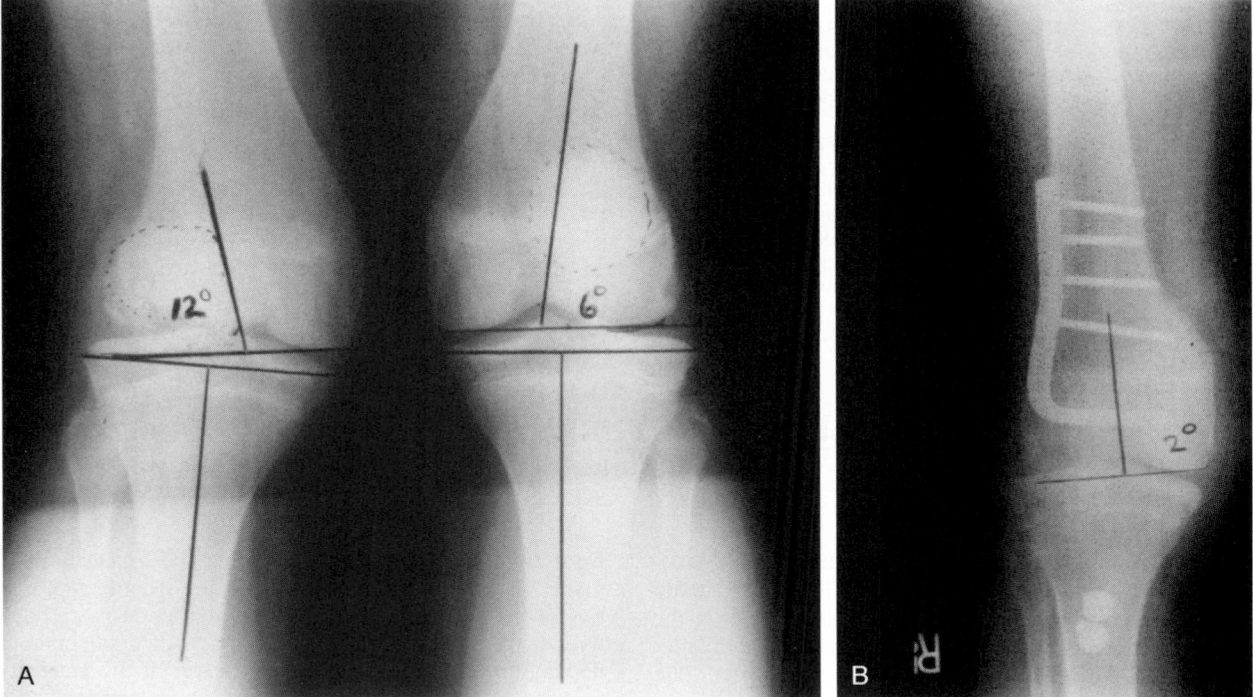

Figure 28E3–16. *A,* Recurrent patellar instability with increased distal femoral valgus in a 16-year-old boy. *B,* Two years after femoral osteotomy, proximal soft tissue realignment, and Elmslie-Trillat tibial tubercle transfer, he is asymptomatic. (Courtesy of Dr. Deborah Stanitski.)

A century and a half ago, Malgaigne noted that "...when I searched along past and present authors for the origins of the doctrines generally accepted today concerning dislocations of the patella, I was surprised to find among them such a dearth of facts with such an abundance of opinions."[8] This observation must be kept in mind during management of patellar instability.

References

1. Atkin DM, Fithian DC, Marangi KS, et al: Characteristics of patients with primary acute lateral patellar dislocation and their recovery within the first 6 months of injury. Am J Sports Med 28:472–479, 2000.
2. Boden BP, Pearsall AW, Garrett WE Jr, Feagin JA Jr: Patellofemoral instability: Evaluation and management. J Am Acad Orthop Surg 5:47–57, 1997.
3. Brown DE, Alexander AH, Lichtman DM: The Elmslie-Trillat procedure: Evaluation in patellar dislocation and subluxation. Am J Sports Med 12:104–109, 1984.
4. Cofield RH, Bryan RS: Acute dislocation of the patella: Results of conservative treatment. J Trauma 17:526–531, 1977.
5. Cox JS: Evaluation of the Roux-Elmslie-Trillat procedure for knee extensor realignment. Am J Sports Med 10:303–310, 1982.
6. Dainer RD, Barrack RL, Buckley SL, Alexander AH: Arthroscopic treatment of acute patellar dislocations. Arthroscopy 4:267–271, 1988.
7. Flandry F, Hughston JC: Complications of extensor mechanism surgery for patellar malalignment. Am J Orthop 24:534–543, 1995.
8. Fulkerson JP, Hungerford DS, Ficat RP: Disorders of the Patellofemoral Joint. Baltimore, Williams & Williams, 1990.
9. Fulkerson JP, Shea KP: Disorders of patellofemoral alignment. J Bone Joint Surg Am 72:1424–1429, 1990.
10. Garth WP Jr, Pomphrey M Jr, Merrill K: Functional treatment of patellar dislocation in an athletic population. Am J Sports Med 24:785–791, 1996.
11. Gross RM: Acute dislocation of the patella: The Mudville mystery. Report of five cases. J Bone Joint Surg Am 68:780–781, 1986.
12. Guzzanti V, Gigante A, DiLazzaro A, Fabbriciani C: Patellofemoral malalignment in adolescents. Computerized tomographic assessment with or without quadriceps contraction. Am J Sports Med 22:55–60, 1994.
13. Hall JE, Micheli LJ, McManama GB Jr: Semitendinosus tenodesis for recurrent subluxation or dislocation of the patella. Clin Orthop 144:31–35, 1979.
14. Hawkins RJ, Bell RH, Anisette G: Acute patellar dislocations. The natural history. Am J Sports Med 14:117–120, 1986.
15. Hughston JC, Flandry F, Brinker MR, et al: Surgical correction of medial subluxation of the patella. Am J Sports Med 24:486–491, 1996.
16. Koskinen SK, Kujala UM: Patellofemoral relationships and distal insertion of the vastus medialis muscle: A magnetic resonance imaging study in nonsymptomatic subjects and in patients with patellar dislocation. Arthroscopy 8:465–468, 1992.
17. Kowall MG, Kolk G, Nuber GW, et al: Patellar taping in the treatment of patellofemoral pain. A prospective randomized study. Am J Sports Med 24:61–66, 1996.
18. Letts RM, Davidson D, Beaule P: Semitendinosus tenodesis for repair of recurrent dislocation of the patella in children. J Pediatr Orthop 19:742–747, 1999.
19. McConnell JS: Training the vastus medialis oblique in the management of patellofemoral pain. Proceedings of the Tenth International World Congress of Physical Therapy, Auckland, New Zealand, 1987.
20. McManus F, Rang M, Heslin DJ: Acute dislocation of the patella in children. The natural history. Clin Orthop 139:88–91, 1979.
21. Nietosvaara Y, Aalto K, Kallio PW: Acute patellar dislocation in children: Incidence and associated osteochondral fractures. J Pediatr Orthop 14:513–515, 1994.
22. Nonweiler DE, DeLee JC: The diagnosis and treatment of medial subluxation of the patella after lateral retinacular release. Am J Sports Med 22:680–686, 1994.
23. Rorabeck CH, Bobechko WP: Acute dislocation of the patella with osteochondral fracture: A review of eighteen cases. J Bone Joint Surg Br 58:237–240, 1976.
24. Sallay PI, Poggi J, Speer KP, Garrett WE: Acute dislocation of the patella. A correlative pathoanatomic study. Am J Sports Med 24:52–60, 1996.
25. Sandmeier RH, Burks RT, Bachus KN, Billings A: The effect of reconstruction of the medial patellofemoral ligament on patellar tracking. Am J Sports Med 28:345–349, 2000.
26. Schutzer SF, Ramsby GR, Fulkerson JP: The evaluation of patellofemoral pain using computerized tomography. A preliminary study. Clin Orthop 204:286–293, 1986.
27. Small NC, Glogau AI, Berezin MA: Arthroscopically assisted proximal extensor mechanism realignment of the knee. Arthroscopy 9:63–67, 1993.
28. Stanitski CL: Articular hypermobility and chondral injury in patients with acute patellar dislocation. Am J Sports Med 23:146–150, 1995.
29. Stanitski CL: Management of patellar instability. J Pediatr Orthop 15:279–280, 1995.
30. Stanitski CL: Patellar instability in the school age athlete. Instr Course Lect 47:345–350, 1998.
31. Stanitski CL, Paletta GA Jr: Articular cartilage injury with acute patellar dislocation in adolescents. Arthroscopic and radiographic correlation. Am J Sports Med 26:52–55, 1998.
32. Vainionpaa S, Laasonen E, Patiala H, et al: Acute dislocation of the patella. Clinical, radiographic and operative findings in 64 consecutive cases. Acta Orthop Scand 57:331–333, 1986.
33. Virolainen H, Visuri T, Kuusela T: Acute dislocation of the patella: MR findings. Radiology 189:243–246, 1993.
34. Woo R, Busch MT: Management of patellar instability in children. Oper Tech Sports Med 6:247–258, 1998.
35. Yamamoto RK: Arthroscopic repair of the medial retinaculum and capsule in acute patellar dislocations. Arthroscopy 2:125–131, 1986.

4. PATELLAR FRACTURES IN THE ADULT

LTC Craig R. Bottoni, MD ■ LTC Dean C. Taylor, MD ■ COL (ret) Robert A. Arciero, MD

Patellar fractures are relatively common injuries constituting about 1% of all skeletal injuries.[4] They are usually the result of significant trauma and are less commonly the result of athletic endeavors. These fractures can be broadly divided into displaced and nondisplaced injuries. The mechanism of injury is either a direct blow or an indirect force applied to the patella through the extensor mechanism. The various fracture patterns are usually representative of the injury mechanism. Both nonoperative and operative management may be employed with good outcomes, depending on the age and activity level of the patient, the fracture pattern, and the amount of displacement. Multiple techniques have been described for the surgical treatment of displaced patellar fractures. The salient points of surgical treatment include anatomic alignment and rigid fixation that will allow early knee motion and rehabilitation.

The views expressed herein are those of the authors and should not be construed as official policy of the Department of the Army or the Department of Defense.

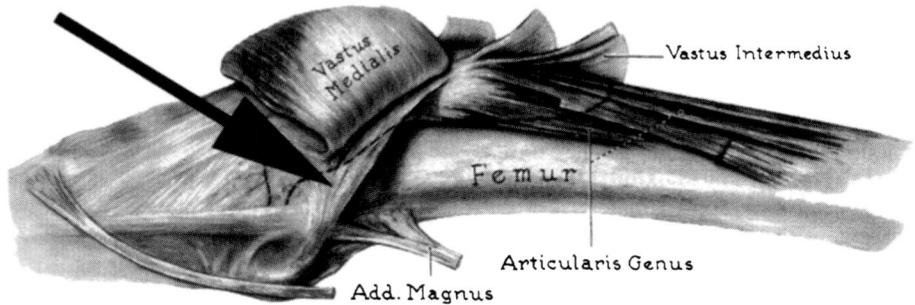

Figure 28E4–1. Anatomy of the distal medial femur. The medial patellofemoral ligament *(arrow)* originates from the proximal medial patella and inserts just distal to the insertion of the adductor (add.) magnus tendon on the medial epicondyle of the femur. (From Anderson JE [ed]: Grant's Atlas of Anatomy, 8th ed. Baltimore, Williams & Wilkins, 1983.)

Anatomy

The patella is the largest sesamoid bone in the body, and its ossification center appears at about 3 years of age. The quadriceps femoris muscle group inserts into the patella through a strong central tendon that actually envelops the patella and then continues to the tibial tubercle. A thin layer of fascia with thick Sharpey's fibers inserts into the patella from the rectus femoris and vastus muscles. The medial and lateral retinacula are extensions of the quadriceps tendon with contribution from deep transverse fibers that originate from the medial and lateral femoral epicondyles. The medial patellofemoral ligament is a thickening of these medial transverse fibers that restrains lateral patellar translation from full extension to 30 degrees when the patella engages the femoral trochlea (Fig. 28E4–1).

The patella articulates with the trochlear groove of the distal femur and undergoes approximately 7 cm of excursion from extension to full flexion. The patellofemoral contact is initiated at about 20 degrees of flexion, and the contact area on the patella moves from distal to proximal with increasing knee flexion. The forces generated across the patellofemoral joint are tremendous, ranging from half of body weight for normal walking to nearly eight times body weight for jumping from a small height.[16] Because of these forces, the articular surface of the patella is the thickest in the body; the average thickness is more than 1 cm.

The posterior articular surface of the patella is divided by a vertical ridge and then again into thirds by two horizontal ridges (Fig. 28E4–2). The lateral facet is larger than the medial. The lower facets articulate first with the trochlear groove in early flexion followed by the middle and then the upper facets. In full flexion, the most medial aspect of the patellar articular surface, designated the crescentic or odd facet, is the main contact point. The apex of the triangular sesamoid is the nonarticulating distal pole. This serves as an insertion site for the patellar tendon.

The vascular supply of the patella is through the anastomosis of the superior, middle, and inferior genicular arteries. The primary arterial supply enters the central and distal patella. Disruption of this supply by injury and subsequent further disruption by surgical dissection can result in avascular necrosis. Rates of 3.5% to 24% have been reported after patellar fracture.[18]

The patella serves two primary functions. It protects the

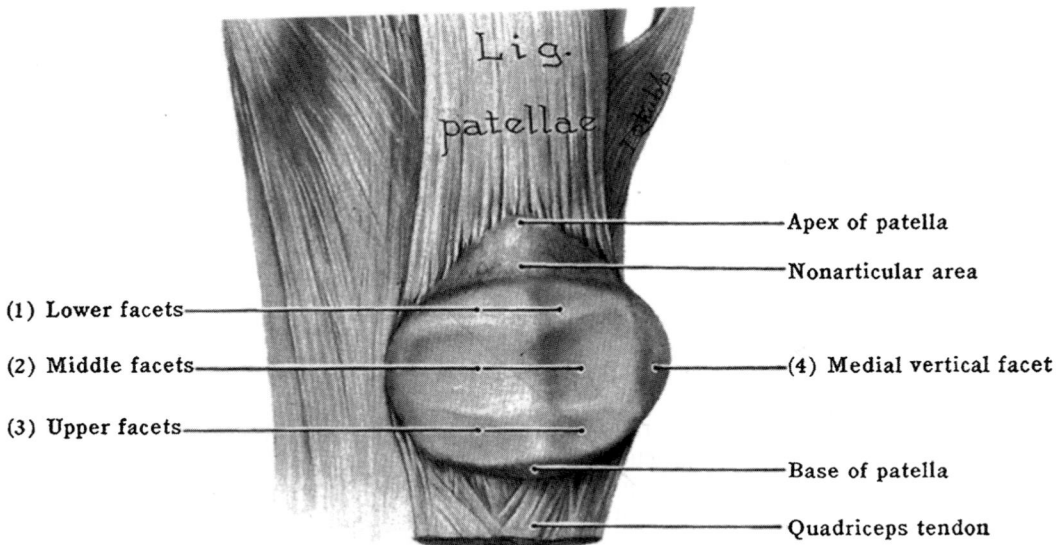

Figure 28E4–2. Anatomy of the patellar articular surface. Note the large longitudinal ridge separating the patella into medial and lateral facets and the smaller medial longitudinal ridge separating the crescentic or odd facet (4). (From Anderson JE [ed]: Grant's Atlas of Anatomy, 8th ed. Baltimore, Williams & Wilkins, 1983.)

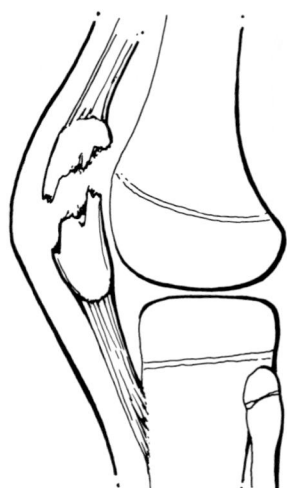

Figure 28E4–7. Diagram of pediatric sleeve fracture demonstrating the large chondral component that may not be evident on radiographs.

to treat these fractures operatively depends on the integrity of the extensor mechanism and the amount of fracture separation, especially the posterior articular surface. Separation of fracture fragments by more than 2 mm and an incompetent extensor mechanism are indications for surgical management.

Nonoperative treatment consists of casting in extension for 4 to 6 weeks. After initial splinting, the fracture is immobilized in a cylinder cast from the ankle to the groin. Weight bearing is allowed as tolerated. Quadriceps exercises are encouraged during casting to limit atrophy. Broström[4] reported 90% good to excellent results in patients treated nonoperatively. A loss of terminal extension or persistent extension lag is not uncommon, but this is rarely a problem. Nonoperative treatment should also be considered in elderly patients who are poor surgical candidates, in the debilitated patient, and in those with poor bone quality. A study on nonoperative treatment of patella fractures displaced by more than 1 cm in elderly patients who were not surgical candidates revealed satisfactory outcome in 9 of 12 patients.[15]

When operative fixation is considered, the goal should be rigid fixation that allows early motion. The technique of patellar fixation is a topic of considerable controversy. Anatomic restoration of the fragments with stabilization by screws or wires gives the strongest construct. With severe localized comminution, however, partial excision with reattachment of the extensor mechanism is a viable alternative. In severely comminuted patellar fractures, primary patellectomy has been advocated to allow earlier motion and quadriceps rehabilitation. Whenever possible, however, preservation of the patella should be attempted.

Skin integrity is an important consideration. Open fractures should be treated with expeditious irrigation and débridement followed by operative fixation if indicated. Timely surgical intervention is recommended if skin abrasions or superficial lacerations are present. Once the lacerations become superficially infected, surgical repair should be delayed 7 to 10 days. Postoperative swelling can also present problems because of the lack of soft tissue coverage over the patella. Skin and subcutaneous necrosis due to swelling can result in a need for skin grafting or flap coverage. Meticulous skin-handling techniques and postoperative elevation should be employed to help prevent these complications. Lacerations should be closely scrutinized for fracture or joint communication.

Both transverse and longitudinal incisions have been advocated to allow exposure and repair of the patella and retinacula. A midline longitudinal incision allows excellent exposure, however, and it does not compromise the skin if future knee operations are required. The retinacular injury usually allows excellent visualization of the articular surface and irrigation of the knee joint. This retinacular exposure can be enlarged to allow better exposure if necessary. Digital palpation of the chondral surface during and subsequent to fixation can ensure anatomic articular surface alignment.

Stabilization of the bony fragments can be accomplished by cerclage wire, tension band techniques, or interfragmentary lag screw fixation (Fig. 28E4–8). Berger first described circumferential (cerclage) wiring to reduce the fragments. Indirect reduction is obtained as compression is applied to the wire. Müller and associates,[13] as part of the AO group, advocated the tension band wiring technique whereby two Kirschner wires are placed longitudinally through the patella. Around these wires, a heavy-gauge (16 or 18) wire is wrapped in a figure-eight fashion and tightened over the anterior surface of the patella (Fig. 28E4–9). The Kirschner wires provide an anchor against which the figure-eight wire is tensioned. Biomechanical evaluation has found that this configuration produces a compression effect on the posterior (articular) surface with knee flexion.[20]

Lag screw fixation of larger fragments can be used alone or in conjunction with tension band techniques. Two large fragments can be rigidly secured with parallel lag screws, or several smaller fragments can be stabilized with lag screws to allow tension banding of the remaining construct. Another technique reported by Berg[2] incorporates the use of cannulated screws through which wire is passed and then secured in a figure-eight fashion. The advantage of this technique is the combination of the compression of the lag screws with the tension band technique while maintaining a low profile. Because of the subcutaneous position of the patella, hardware placed to stabilize fractures often requires subsequent removal after successful stabilization. To avoid hardware complications, heavy-gauge suture has been advocated instead of the wire.[21] Results have been reported to be as good as those with the traditional technique.

Alternative techniques have been described to obtain stable fixation. The use of biodegradable wires and screw compared favorably with conventional fixation in a study by Juutilainen and associates.[7] If comparable fixation can be obtained, the need to remove hardware can be obviated. External patellar fixation was originally described by Malgaigne but abandoned. Liang and Wu[11] reported good or excellent results in 26 of 27 patients treated with an external compression fixator attached by transverse percutaneous pins. No osteomyelitis developed, and 89% of the patients regained knee motion equal to that on the uninjured side.

Long-term results after surgical stabilization have not

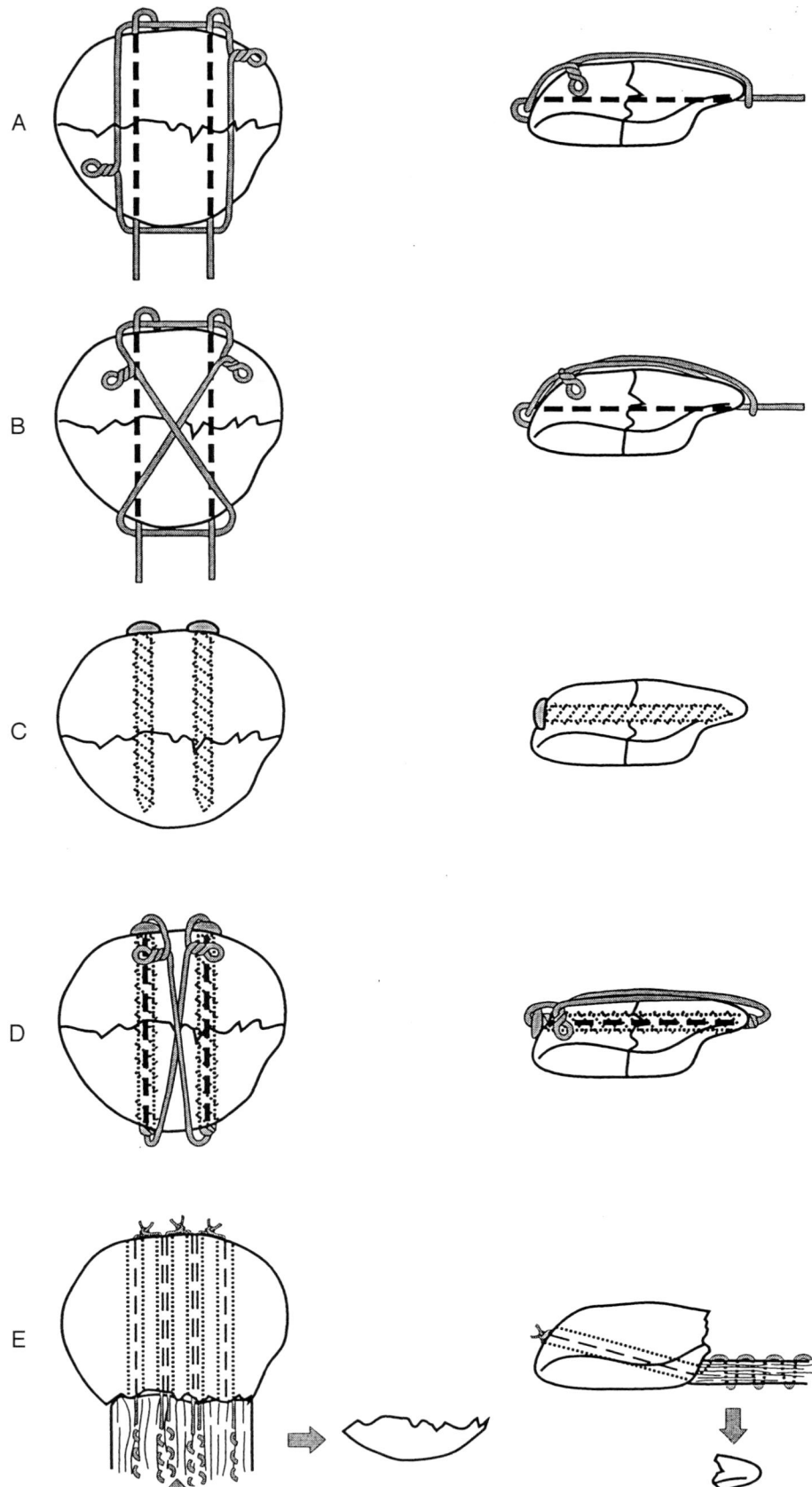

Figure 28E4–8. Techniques of patellar fracture fixation. *A*, Modified tension band wiring in a circular configuration. *B*, Modified tension band wiring technique in a figure-eight configuration. *C*, Lag screw fixation. *D*, Combination cannulated lag screw and tension band wiring. *E*, Partial patellectomy. Note that the tendon is reapproximated at the level of the articular surface of the patella. (From Miller MD, Brinker MR [eds]: Review of Orthopaedics, 3rd ed. Philadelphia, WB Saunders, 2000.)

A

B

C

D

E

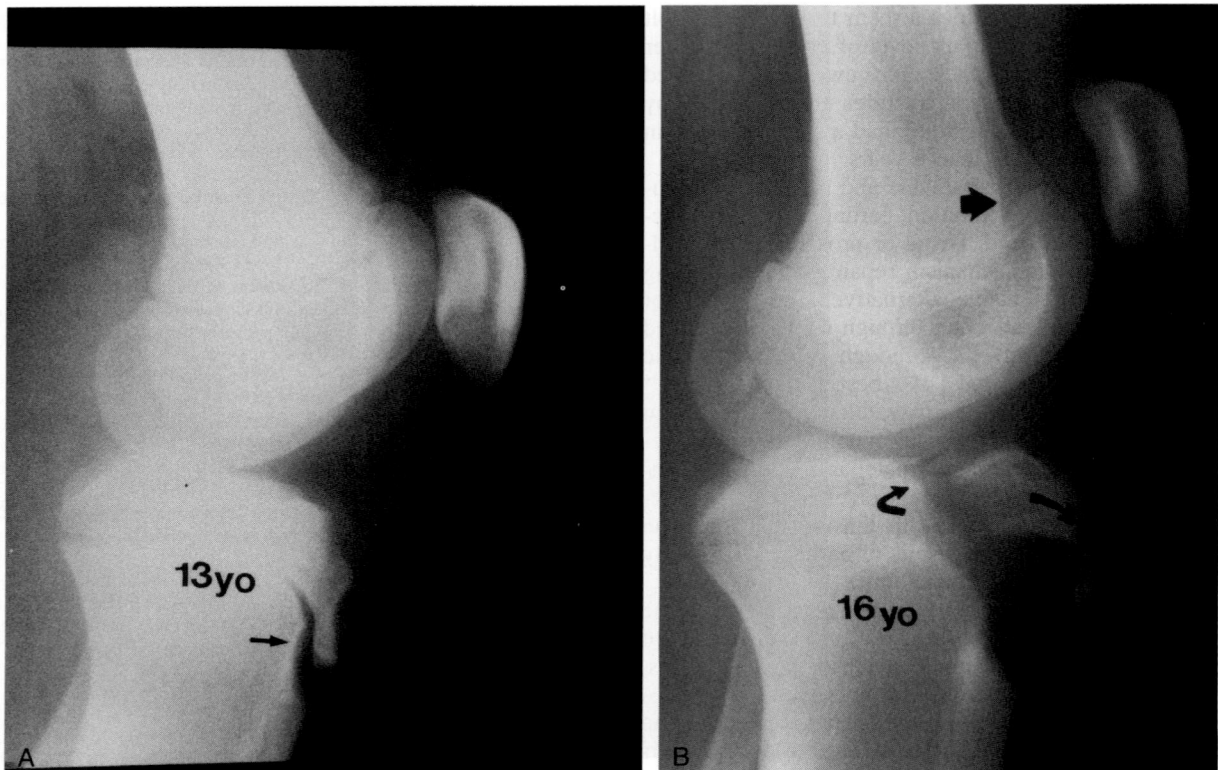

Figure 28E5–1. *A,* Osgood-Schlatter changes (*arrow*). *B,* Type IIIB acute tibial tubercle avulsion fracture 3 years later. Note significant skeletal maturity. *Top arrow* shows patella alta; *curved arrows* show fragment displacement and patellar tendon avulsion fragment.

stage, the ossification center appears within the cartilage tongue. The hallmark of the epiphyseal stage is coalescence of the proximal tibial secondary ossification centers. The bony stage occurs at physiologic epiphyseodesis between the fully ossified tuberosity and the proximal tibial metaphysis that usually occurs in girls at 15 years and boys at 17 years of age. Ogden and colleagues[9] showed three histologic zones within the tubercle growth plate. The proximal tubercle is columnar cartilage; the middle, fibrocartilage; and the distal, fibrous tissue that blends with the perichondrium. Progressive change from fibrocartilage occurs from proximal to distal just before physeal closure. Physiologic epiphyseodesis begins proximally and moves distally to involve the tubercle. The distal residua of columnar carti-

lage predispose the tuberosity to acute avulsion injury just before or during final closure.

The prevalence of preexisting Osgood-Schlatter disorder in patients with an acute tibial avulsion fracture ranges from 12% to 60% in reported series. The mechanism of injury of the two conditions is similar (i.e., traction force across an immature junction), but the rate and magnitude of the force are completely different (Fig. 28E5–1). In the series of Ogden and coworkers,[10] which included 14 patients with 15 acute tibial tubercle avulsion fractures, 9 had Osgood-Schlatter changes radiographically. In 7 patients, the changes were on the contralateral, asymptomatic knee. Three patients with a fracture and concomitant Osgood-Schlatter change had been completely asymptomatic before

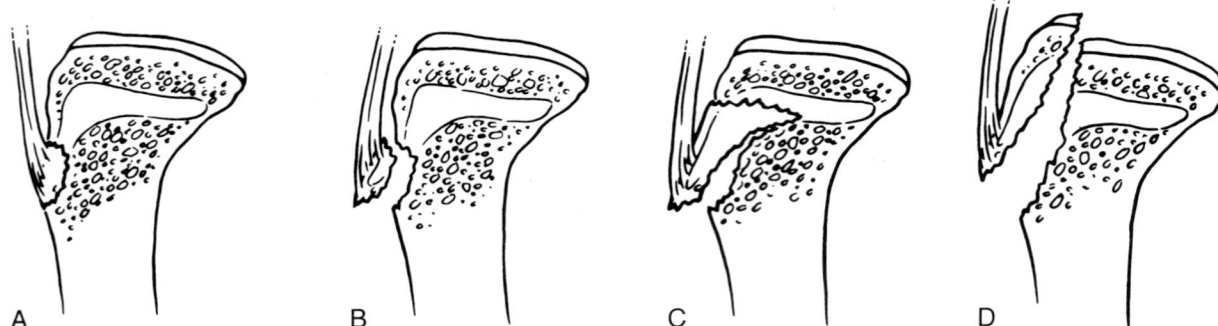

Figure 28E5–2. Watson-Jones classification of acute tibial tubercle avulsion fractures. *A,* Undisplaced. *B,* Displaced without extension. *C,* Displacement with physeal extension. *D,* Displacement with intra-articular extension.

the fracture. Because the equation's denominator is unknown in this extremely common circumstance, that is, the number of athletes with symptomatic and asymptomatic Osgood-Schlatter change, the rare association of an acute tibial tubercle fracture in a patient with Osgood-Schlatter condition seems associative and not causal.

Diagnosis

Physical examination findings reflect swelling, tenderness, and deformity proportional to the injury magnitude. Knee active extension is hindered by pain and the loss of

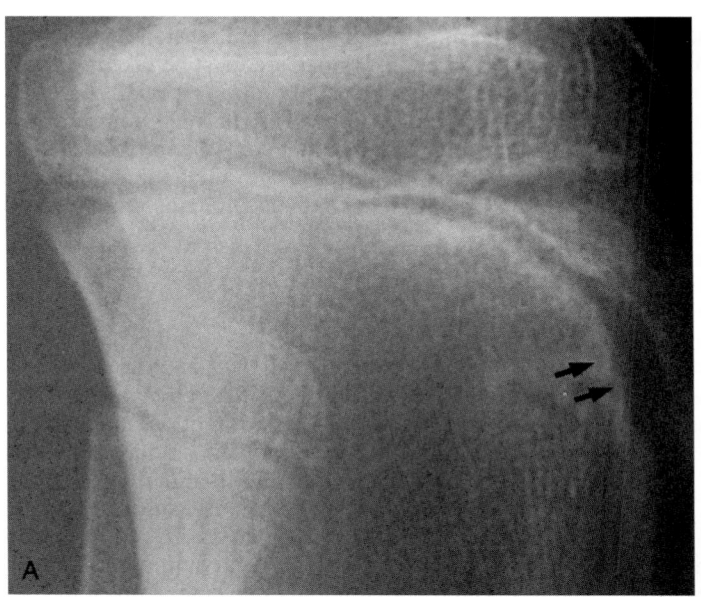

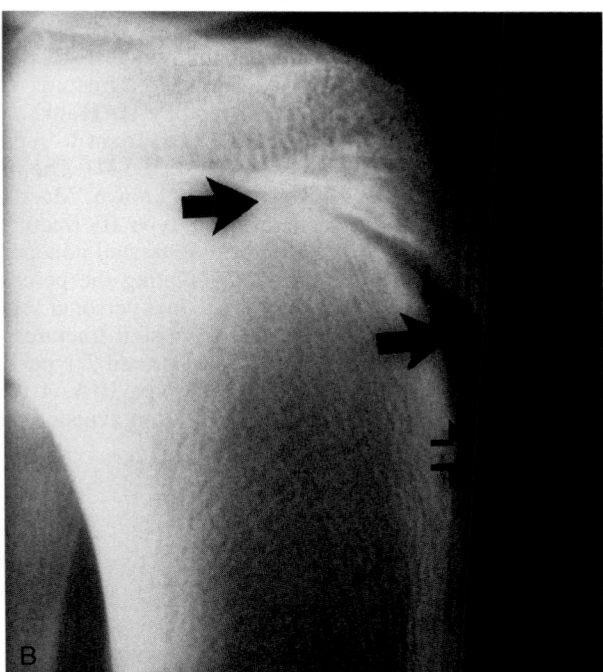

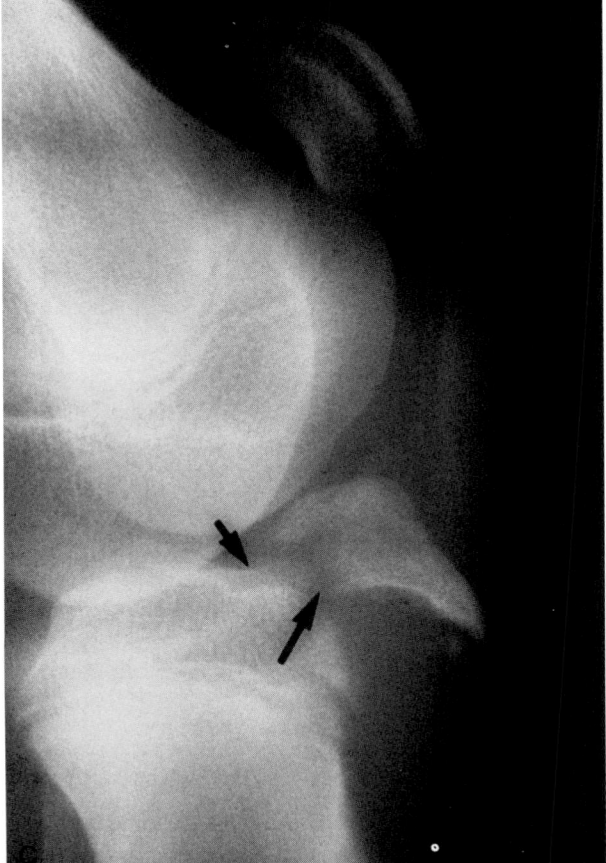

Figure 28E5–3. *A*, Type IA. *B*, Type IIA. Note proximal extension and hinge at closed proximal tibial physis. *C*, Type IIIB. Note patella alta and intra-articular fracture extension.

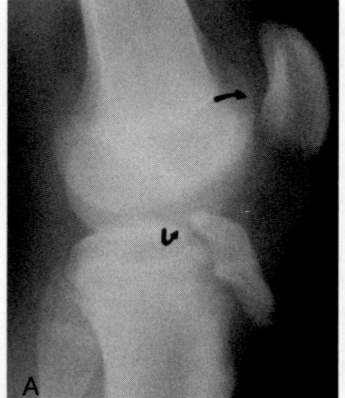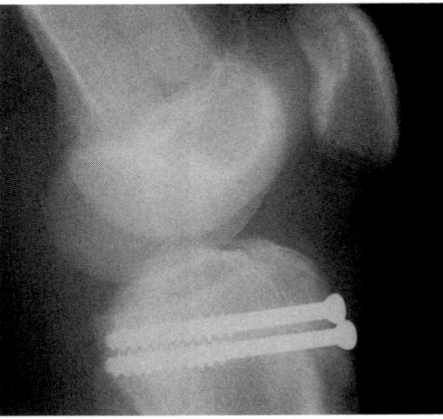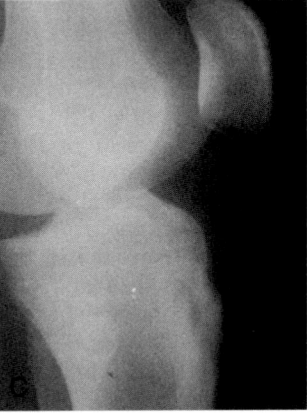

Figure 28E5–7. *A,* Type IIIA fracture in a 15-year-old boy. Note intra-articular extension (*bottom arrow*) and patella alta (*top arrow*). *B,* After open reduction and internal fixation 4 months later. *C,* Follow-up radiograph 2 years after injury with full maturity and no physeal deformity. Hardware site became symptomatic, and hardware was removed 1 year after injury.

gocoele child who developed premature proximal tibial physeal closure, genu recurvatum, and limb length discrepancy.[10]

References

1. Bolesta MJ, Fitch RD: Tibial tubercle avulsions. J Pediatr Orthop 6: 186–192, 1986.
2. Chow SP, Lam JJ, Leong JC: Fracture of the tibial tubercle in the adolescent. J Bone Joint Surg Br 72:231–234, 1990.
3. Ehrenborg G: The Osgood-Schlatter lesion. Acta Chir Scand 288: 1–36, 1962.
4. Falster O, Hasselbalch H: Avulsion fracture of the tibial tuberosity with combined ligament and meniscal tear. Am J Sports Med 20: 82–83, 1992.
5. Frankl U, Wasilewski SA, Healy WL: Avulsion fracture of the tibial tubercle with avulsion of the patellar ligament. Report of two cases. J Bone Joint Surg Am 72:1411–1413, 1990.
6. Lipscomb AB, Gilbert PP, Johnston RK, et al: Fracture of the tibial
7. tuberosity with associated ligamentous and meniscal tears. A case report. J Bone Joint Surg Am 66:790–792, 1984.
7. Mayba II: Avulsion fracture of the tibial tubercle apophysis with avulsion of patellar ligament. J Pediatr Orthop 2:303–305, 1982.
8. Mirbey J, Besancenot J, Chambers RT, et al: Avulsion fractures of the tibial tuberosity in the adolescent athlete. Risk factors, mechanism of injury, and treatment. Am J Sports Med 16:336–340, 1988.
9. Ogden JA, Hempton RJ, Southwick WO: Development of the tibial tuberosity. Anat Rec 182:431–445, 1975.
10. Ogden JA, Tross RB, Murphy MJ: Fractures of the tibial tuberosity in adolescents. J Bone Joint Surg Am 62:205–215, 1980.
11. Pape JM, Goulet JA, Hensinger RN: Compartment syndrome complicating tibial tubercle avulsion. Clin Orthop 295:201–204, 1993.
12. Polakoff DR, Bucholz RW, Ogden JA: Tension band wiring of displaced tibial tuberosity fractures in adolescents. Clin Orthop 209: 161–165, 1986.
13. Ryu RK, Debenham JO: An unusual avulsion fracture of the proximal tibial epiphysis. Case report and proposed addition to the Watson-Jones classification. Clin Orthop 194:181–184, 1985.
14. Watson-Jones R: Fractures and Joint Injuries, vol II, 4th ed. Baltimore, Williams and Wilkins, 1955.
15. Wiss DA, Schilz JL, Zionts L: Type III fractures of the tibial tubercle in adolescents. J Orthop Trauma 5:475–479, 1991.

6. ANTERIOR KNEE PAIN AND PATELLAR SUBLUXATION IN THE ADULT

Peter C. Theut, MD ■ John P. Fulkerson, MD

More than 20 years ago, Ficat and Hungerford characterized the patellofemoral joint as the "forgotten compartment of the knee."[64] With the advent of tremendous interest in sports medicine and with the refinement of both open and arthroscopic surgical techniques, however, this statement is perhaps less accurate today. Although much progress has been made in regard to treatment of the patellofemoral joint, the practitioner is still confronted with difficult clinical presentations. Anterior knee pain is one of the most common problems that an orthopaedist encounters. Despite this fact, few areas in orthopaedics remain as controversial, particularly after the failure of nonoperative measures. Anterior knee pain may be due to injury to underlying carti-

lage, patellofemoral malalignment, trauma, soft tissue disorders, or a combination thereof. This chapter emphasizes a systematic assessment of the patient with anterior knee pain so as to formulate a rational method of treatment.

Anatomy

Osseous Structure

The form of the patella is complex, the details of which are critical to understanding both normal function and disease of the patella. The overall shape is that of a vague triangle with the apex pointing distally. Anthropologic studies have established limits for length varying from 47 to 58 mm, and for width, from 51 to 57 mm. No racial differences have been noted.[49] Grelsamer and associates[94] studied 564 patients and noted three different patellar shape patterns when comparing overall patellar length with length of the articular surface. They described the "Cyrano" patella, in which the nonarticular inferior pole is particularly long[94] (Fig. 28E6–1).

The anterior surface of the patella is slightly convex in all directions. The superior third receives the insertion of the quadriceps tendon. The anterior portion of this tendon continues over the anterior surface to form the deep fascia, which is densely adherent to bone. The middle third reveals numerous vascular orifices, and the inferior third is enveloped by the origin of the patellar tendon.

The posterior surface of the patella can be divided into two parts. The inferior pole is nonarticular and may represent a full 25% of patellar height. The remaining superior portion is covered with hyaline cartilage and is therefore articular. The thickness of the cartilage may reach 4 to 5 mm in the central portion and is the thickest found in the body.[70]

The articulating surface of the patella is divided into

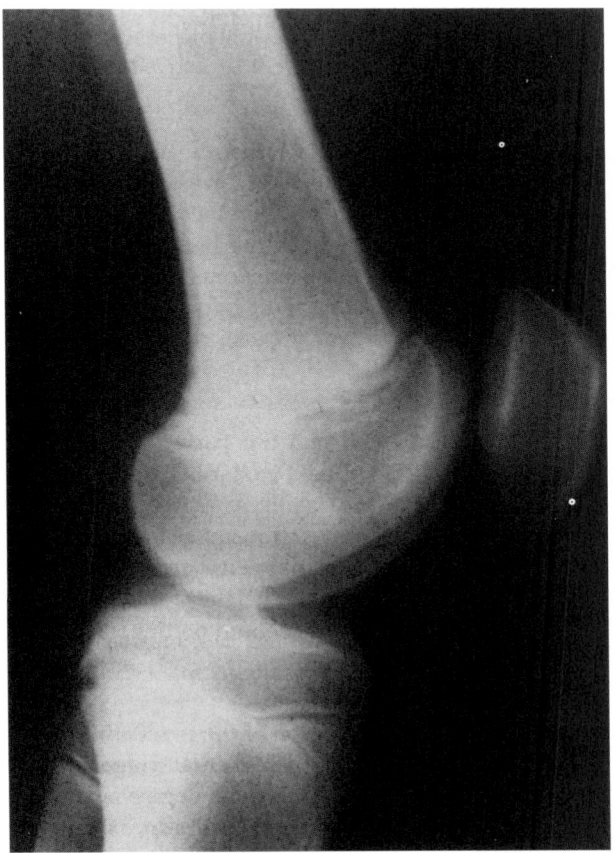

Figure 28E6–1. The "Cyrano" long-nosed patella. (From Fulkerson JP: Disorders of the Patellofemoral Joint, 3rd ed. Baltimore, Williams & Wilkins, 1997.)

medial and lateral facets by a median, or central, ridge that is oriented in the longitudinal axis of the patella. Typically, the lateral facet is larger. However, Wiberg[240] has characterized the different facet configurations ranging from medial/lateral equality to extreme lateral facet predominance. This is also known as the "hunter's cap" patella. A correlation exists between the Wiberg type and the width of the lateral patellofemoral ligament. This may be a manifestation of muscle forces that occur during development.[199]

The medial facet may be divided into the medial facet proper and the smaller "odd" facet located on the medial periphery of the medial facet (Fig. 28E6–2). The odd facet articulates only in deep knee flexion.[112] A purely cartilaginous "secondary ridge" divides these two structures. This ridge conforms to the curve of the lateral border of the medial condyle with the knee in full flexion. There is considerable variation in both the odd facet and the secondary ridge. The shape of the medial facet is variable as well, but it is usually flat or slightly convex.[70]

The lateral facet is both longer and wider, and is concave in both vertical and transverse planes. Different authors have described the presence of three transverse segments delineated by two transverse ridges on both the medial and lateral portion of the facet at the junction of each third. These ridges isolate three segments of different functional significance, as the proximal, middle, and distal third of the patella is brought into contact with progressive flexion.[46, 239] Subchondral bone density is maximal at the proximal lateral facet.[53]

The articular portion of the anterior surface of the distal femur is known as the femoral trochlea, or sulcus. This articulates with the patella and has medial and lateral facets. Proximally, they are in continuity with a shallow groove, conforming to the distal patellar articular surface. Curving distally and posteriorly, this groove deepens to become the intercondylar notch. The junction of the condylar surface with the contiguous trochlear surface is known as the sulcus terminalis. The lateral trochlear facet typically extends more proximally, is larger, and is more prominent anteriorly than the medial trochlear facet (Fig. 28E6–3). There is substantial variability in trochlear depth. The lateral trochlear facet usually functions as a buttress to lateral patellar subluxation, and helps to keep the patella centered in the trochlea from approximately 15 degrees of flexion to full flexion.[70] Hughston and colleagues[111] reported that at 45 degrees of flexion, the lateral condyle is typically 1 cm more anterior than the medial condyle and can contribute to overall lateral stability of the patella despite deficient medial support. Varying degrees of facet dysplasia may exist within the trochlea, either medial or lateral. Apparent lateral facet dysplasia may in fact be "illusory dysplasia" due to rotational deformity of the femur.[20]

The anatomy of the entire femur is critical to patellofemoral mechanics. Femoral version is the angle between the femoral neck and a line between the two femoral condyles as viewed in the transverse plane. Typically, this angle projects anteriorly and is referred to as femoral anteversion. The normal angle is approximately 10 to 15 degrees in the adult. Further increases in this angle can lead to medial rotation of the femoral condyles as the hip assumes a neutral position. True torsion of the femoral diaphysis

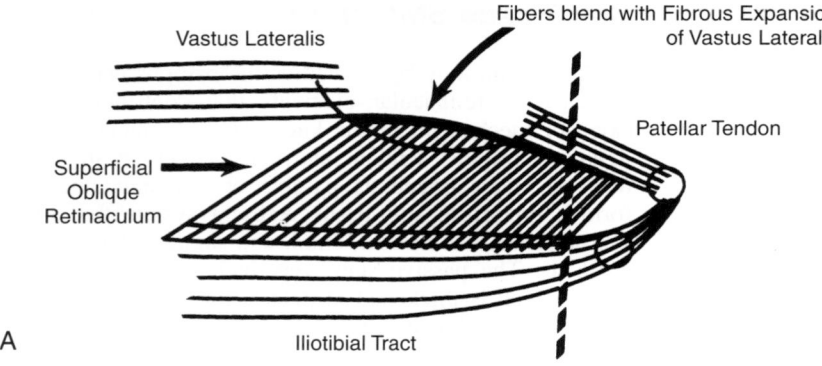

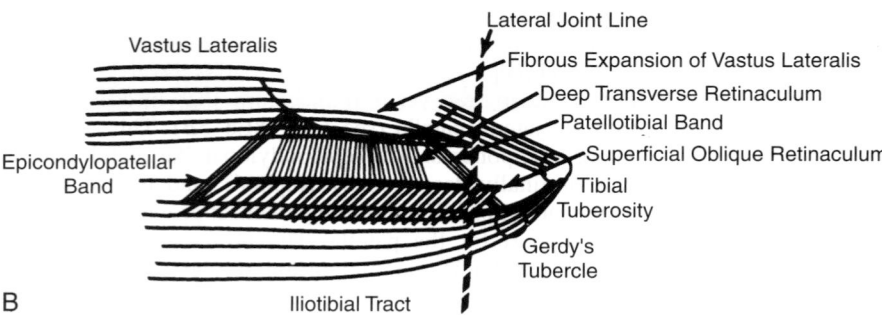

Figure 28E6–5. *A*, Superficial oblique retinaculum. *B*, Deep lateral retinaculum. (From Fulkerson JP: Disorders of the Patellofemoral Joint, 3rd ed. Baltimore, Williams & Wilkins, 1997.)

dense capsular condensation that runs within layer II from near the medial epicondyle at the anterior edge of the superficial medial collateral ligament to the proximal portion of the posterior margin of the medial patella. The vastus medialis obliquus (VMO) inserts into the ligament near its patellar insertion, suggesting a dynamic influence.[59] The functional significance of the MPFL was evaluated by Conlan and coworkers,[37] who used a serial-sectioning technique of the medial soft tissues in cadavers. The MPFL contributed an average of 53% of the total retraining force to lateral displacement of the patella. Desio and associates[48] found the MPFL to be the primary restraint to lateral displacement at 20 degrees of flexion, contributing 60% of the total restraining force. The medial retinaculum is augmented distally by the medial meniscopatellar ligament, which is felt to contribute, on average, 22% of the total restraining force to lateral translation.[37]

There is a delicate balance between the medial and lateral restraints. As the knee flexes, the lateral retinacular structures, along with the iliotibial band, exert a posterolateral force on the patella. If left unchecked by a thinned, deficient medial retinacular support, patellar tilt, lateral subluxation, or dislocation or excessive lateral pressure syndrome[64] may arise.[70]

The rectus femoris and vastus intermedius tendons with peripheral contribution from the vastus lateralis and medialis form the central quadriceps tendon as it inserts into the proximal margin of the patella. The rectus femoris inserts most anteriorly, with the vastus medialis and lateralis in the midportion, and the intermedius more posterior. There is a small potential space between the tendon insertion and the synovial reflection that may be occupied by a fat pad. This thick tendon, greater than 9 mm, provides an alternative graft for cruciate reconstruction (Fig. 28E6–6).[80, 230]

The patellar tendon is 3 cm at the inferior pole of the patella and tapers to 2.5 cm at the tibial tubercle. It is 5 to 6 cm long and 7 mm thick (see Fig. 28E6–6). It serves to extend the knee through the quadriceps musculature, and also to limit the proximal ascent of the patella from the tibia. The retinaculum interdigitates with the patellar tendon both medially and laterally.[70]

The passive stabilizers are somewhat static, but one must remember that the dynamic stabilizers in part affect them. The lateral retinaculum, for example, originates in large part from the iliotibial band, which is also a dynamic stabilizer. The VMO contributes dynamically to the medial retinaculum, and the quadriceps and patellar tendons are obviously under the dynamic influence of the quadriceps musculature.

Dynamic Stabilizers

The quadriceps muscle group is composed of the rectus femoris, the vastus intermedius, the vastus lateralis, and the vastus medialis. Their distal common insertion into the patella comprises the central quadriceps tendon. This layered insertion is described earlier in this chapter. The angle of insertion of the various components of the quadriceps generates different force vectors, and is a very important influence on patellofemoral mechanics.[143, 235]

The VMO has been described by Lieb and Perry.[143] The fibers of the VMO arise from the distal medial intermuscular septum and adductor tubercle and insert into the proxi-

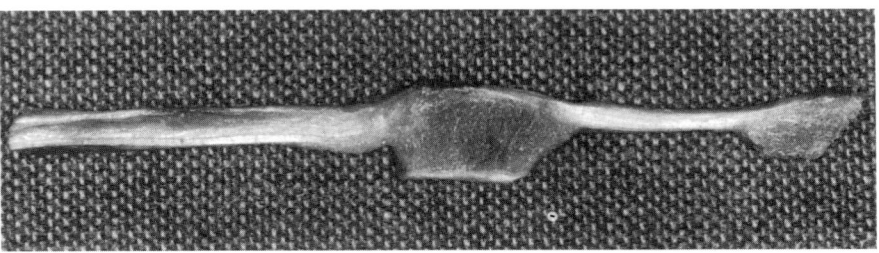

Figure 28E6–6. Central third quadriceps tendon, patella, central third patellar tendon, and tibial tubercle. (From Fulkerson JP: Disorders of the Patellofemoral Joint, 3rd ed. Baltimore, Williams & Wilkins, 1997.)

mal medial patella and the medial patellofemoral ligament. These fibers typically form an angle of 55 to 65 degrees with the long axis of the thigh. The VMO has a separate innervation and functional significance from the main body of the vastus medialis. The VMO functions not as an extensor, but rather as an important dynamic medial restraint to the typically laterally directed forces on the patella.[156] Dysfunction of the VMO, either congenital or acquired, can contribute to lateral patellar instability.

Hallisey and associates[95] have described the vastus lateralis obliquus (VLO) (Fig. 28E6–7). An anatomically distinct group of vastus lateralis fibers is separated from the main belly of the vastus lateralis by a thin layer of fat. These fibers interdigitate with the lateral intermuscular septum in a variable fashion before they insert into the patella. The angle of insertion is variable, averaging 48 degrees in males and 38 degrees in females. The VLO exerts a laterally directed dynamic influence on the patella. The surgical importance of this distinct muscle group is that its fibers may be selectively released during lateral release without violating the main tendon of the vastus lateralis.

The genu articularis is the final muscular component of the quadriceps. This small muscle arises from the distal femur and inserts into the suprapatellar pouch. It functions to retract the suprapatellar pouch in knee extension.

History

When taking a history, it is important to distinguish complaints of pain from those of instability. Patients should be questioned in regard to provocative and palliative factors; the quality, location, and severity of the pain; and any associated radiation of the pain. Deep, aching pain that often worsens with activities such as stair climbing or sitting with the knees bent for an extended period is classical for anterior knee pain. Descending stairs, in particular, can cause anterior knee pain due to the strong eccentric contraction of the quadriceps that is necessary. Sharp pain that reproduces with a given movement or activity may represent an unstable chondral flap. Constant pain with no temporal relation to activity suggests the possibility of complex regional pain syndrome (formerly known as reflex sympathetic dystrophy), referred pain, radicular pain, postoperative neuroma, or malingering. Burning, dysesthetic pain is characteristic of complex regional pain syndrome or may represent a neuroma, especially in the postoperative patient. Pain from disease of the hip joint is often referred to the anterior thigh and may include the knee. Patients should routinely be questioned about, or evaluated for, hip disease. Pain that radiates down the leg, often with burning or paresthesias, is typical of lumbosacral radicular disease.

Patients should be asked to pinpoint carefully the location of their pain. Knee pain diagrams have been shown to predict areas of tenderness on physical examination. Furthermore, 86% of negative patient zones accurately predicted a negative examination. These diagrams can be helpful in the presence of radiculopathy and symptom magnification.[194]

Patients often describe that their knee "gives out," when in fact they have no instability of either the tibiofemoral or the patellofemoral compartment. Often this description is secondary to quadriceps inhibition due to pain, effusion,

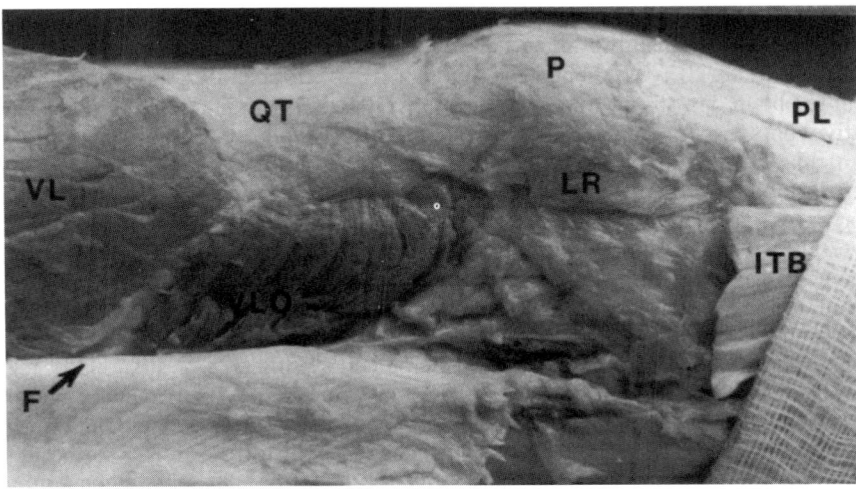

Figure 28E6–7. The lateral musculoretinacular structures that support the patella. F, fat; ITB, iliotibial band; LR, lateral retinaculum; P, patella; PL, patellar ligament; QT, quadriceps tendon; VL, vastus lateralis; VLO, vastus lateralis obliquus. (From Fulkerson JP: Disorders of the Patellofemoral Joint, 3rd ed. Baltimore, Williams & Wilkins, 1997.)

TABLE 28E6–1
Normal Population Q Angle Review

	Supine			Standing	
Author	*Q (Degrees) Angle*	*No. Knees/Age*	*Author*	*Q (Degrees) Angle*	*No. Knees/Age*
Insall et al[115]	14	50/not specified	Woodland	♀ 17.0 ± 0.72	57/20.0
				♂ 13.6 ± .072	69/22.3
Aglietti et al[3]	♀ 17 ± 3	75/23	Fairbank	♀ 23 ± 1.2	150/14.8 ± .1
	♂ 14 ± 3	75/23		♂ 20 ± 1.2	160/14.6 ± .1
Hsu et al[105a]	♀ 18.8 ± 4.7	60/not specified	Horton	♀ 15.8 ± 4.5	50/22.6
	♂ 15.6 ± 3.5	60/not specified		♂ 11.2 ± 3.0	50/22.6
Woodland et al[243]	♀ 15.8 ± .072	57/20.0			
	♂ 12.7 ± .072	69/22.3			

From Fulkerson JP: Disorders of the Patellofemoral Joint, 3rd ed. Baltimore, Williams & Wilkins, 1997.

and colleagues.[137] Their study found a similar decrease in Q angle measurements at 30 degrees of flexion as compared with full extension in both normal subjects and those with anterior knee pain.[137] Nissen and coworkers[171] measured the Q angle at 20 to 30 degrees of flexion with maximum internal, neutral, and external rotation of the tibia. This helps to define the extremes of extensor mechanism malalignment and is important in surgical planning for distal realignment procedures.

It is critical to recognize, however, that most authors feel that an abnormal Q angle does not predict anterior knee pain or patellar subluxation. In studies by Insall[115] and Aglietti,[3] less than half of patients with anterior knee pain had Q angles greater than 20 degrees. Aglietti also showed that those patients with recurrent subluxation did not have statistically significant greater Q angles than control subjects. Fairbank and coworkers[55] were unable to demonstrate a statistically significant difference between Q angles in adolescent males and females with anterior knee pain than in control subjects without anterior knee pain. Several other authors suggest that significant Q angle differences between those with patellofemoral pain and healthy controls cannot be demonstrated.[70, 79, 126, 198] Furthermore, although abnormality of the Q angle may establish that there is malalignment, it is inappropriate to make decisions regarding surgical treatment based on the Q angle alone.[73] Measurement of the Q angle is a traditional component of the patellofemoral examination. The reported range of normal values is wide, however, and it is not predictive of diagnosis or treatment. The benefit of routine measurement of the Q angle remains uncertain.[192]

Sitting Position

Patellar tracking can be evaluated in this position both dynamically and passively, as was previously discussed. With the patient seated at the edge of the examination table, the knee flexed to 90 degrees, and the foot in a neutral position, observe the position of the tibial tubercle relative to the midpatella. The tubercle sulcus angle is the angle created between a line drawn from the center of the tibial tubercle to the inferior pole of the patella and a line

drawn from the femoral sulcus down the tibia perpendicular to the floor (Fig. 28E6–10).[133] With the knee flexed this far, the patella is well centered within the femoral sulcus and therefore provides an accurate location of the position of the sulcus. The position of the foot can affect the location of the tubercle in this test also. The reported normal range of this test is variable. Hughston[111] considered a normal measurement to be 0; Kolowich and associates[133] believe that 10 degrees is the upper limit of lateral displacement. Excessive lateralization of the tubercle with respect to the trochlea has been shown to correlate with an increased incidence of knee pain in women.[167] The 90-degree Q angle is a similar technique to measure distal extensor mechanism malalignment and is simply a measurement of the Q angle at 90 degrees of knee flexion. The reported normal range for this test is −4 to +6 degrees, with values greater than 8 to 10 degrees believed to be abnormal.[79]

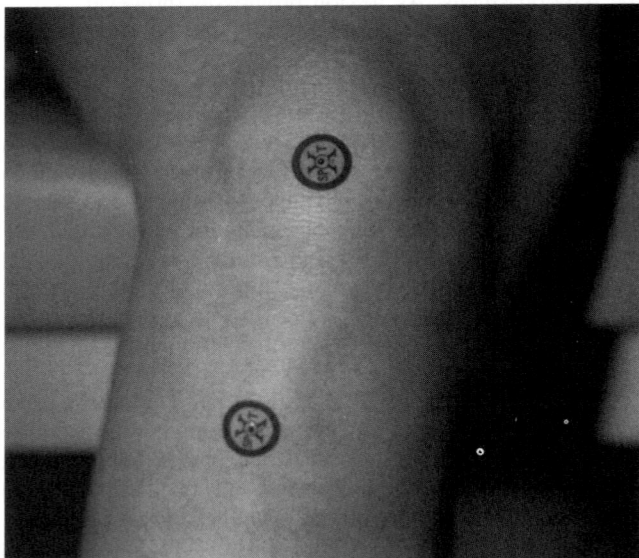

Figure 28E6–10. Seated evaluation of the tubercle sulcus angle. Markers are placed on the center of the patella and the tibial tubercle for purposes of illustration only. (From Fulkerson JP: Disorders of the Patellofemoral Joint, 3rd ed. Baltimore, Williams & Wilkins, 1997.)

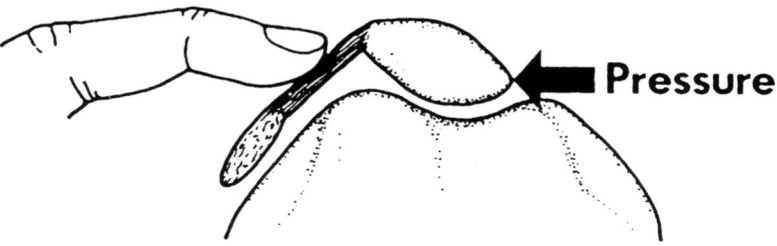

Figure 28E6–11. Place soft tissues under tension before palpation. This helps to limit the pressure transmitted to underlying structures. (From Fulkerson JP: Disorders of the Patellofemoral Joint, 3rd ed. Baltimore, Williams & Wilkins, 1997.)

Supine Position

With the extremity in full extension, one should palpate all structures of the anterior knee. The presence of a ballotable patella should be noted, indicating an effusion. This is an important finding in formulating both a differential diagnosis and a quadriceps rehabilitation plan. It has been shown that as little as 15 mL injected into normal knees can cause reflex inhibition of the quadriceps. The VMO is especially sensitive, with 20 to 30 mL of intra-articular fluid causing reflex inhibition as compared with the 50 to 60 mL that is typically required to inhibit the rectus femoris and the vastus lateralis.[227] This may create a dynamic malalignment that should be addressed during rehabilitation.

The quadriceps muscles and their respective tendon insertions as well as the patellar tendon should be evaluated for tenderness or palpable defects. An extensor lag in this scenario may indicate a quadriceps or patellar tendon rupture. Insertional tenderness of the vastus lateralis is a common finding in excessive lateral pressure syndrome. Tenderness at the inferior pole of the patella, the so-called jumper's knee, represents patellar tendinitis and is common among athletes. The infrapatellar fat pad should be palpated for evidence of inflammation. Note should be made of the size of the VMO. Palpate the medial femoral epicondyle and the medial border of the patella for tenderness of the medial patellofemoral ligament in cases of acute lateral dislocation. The medial and lateral joint lines should be palpated as well to evaluate for potential meniscal disease or tibiofemoral arthrosis.

The medial and lateral retinacular tissues, including the medial parapatellar plica, must be carefully evaluated (Fig. 28E6–11). The peripatellar soft tissues are densely innervated. Neuromatous degeneration has been documented within the lateral retinaculum of patients with patellofemoral malalignment, and may be a primary source of pain.[84] Chronic overload on the retinacular tissues can cause tendinosis, and tendinitis may predominate in the acute setting. In the postoperative setting, reproduction of symptoms by palpation of scars or Tinel's sign may indicate neuroma formation. Saphenous neuritis is characterized by burning pain along the medial side of the knee and can be elicited by palpation of the saphenous nerve just distal to the adductor hiatus[146] (Fig. 28E6–12). Diagnostic injection can be helpful in the diagnosis of localized neuropathic pain. Reflex sympathetic dystrophy, or complex regional pain disorder, may present in the knee as diffuse pain and skin hypersensitivity, particularly to cold. Other classical findings include allodynia, hyperpathia, increased sweating, and skin color and temperature changes.[146]

Patellar tilt is a rotational abnormality in the coronal plane due to shortening of the lateral retinaculum. The vector of the lateral retinaculum is primarily posterior, and excessive tension can cause pain from overload of either the soft tissues or the lateral facet, or both. Tightness of

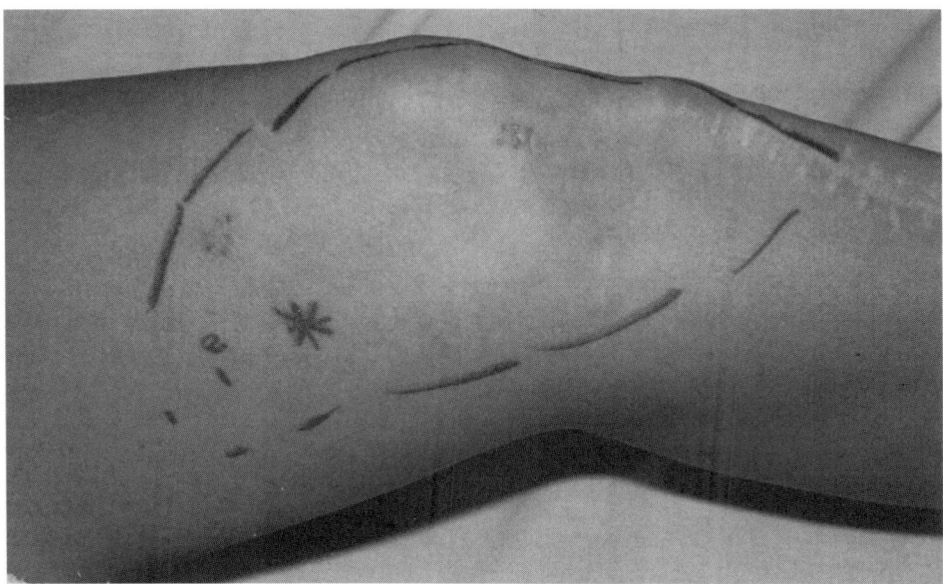

Figure 28E6–12. Patient had saphenous neuritis with hypesthesia as illustrated. (From Fulkerson JP: Disorders of the Patellofemoral Joint, 3rd ed. Baltimore, Williams & Wilkins, 1997.)

the patient to reduce the subluxation actively by quadriceps contraction is considered to be a positive test.[172]

Compression of the patella into the trochlea often causes pain in patients with articular lesions of the patellofemoral joint. It is important to differentiate simple crepitance from pain while doing this because crepitus is frequently found in normal knees.[124] To avoid confusion with retinacular or synovial sources of pain, one should carefully avoid the compression of these structures and also avoid moving the knee through a range of motion during the examination. Instead, the examiner should carefully compress the patella into the trochlea at several points from full extension to full flexion and should assess for any pain at each point (Fig. 28E6–14*A* and *B*). This technique is also important because it provides the examiner with an estimation of the location of the articular disease. Pain that is elicited with compression of the patella into the trochlea early in flexion indicates an articular lesion on the distal pole of the patella or proximal trochlea. As flexion increases, patellofemoral contact becomes progressively more proximal on the patella and distal on the trochlea. This information is crucial if realignment procedures are being contemplated. Avoid confusing patellofemoral disease with a symptomatic plica, which is usually medial to the patella and elicits pain when palpated as a band snapping over the femoral condyle.

Patellofemoral problems are frequently associated with flexibility deficits, and the range of motion of all major lower extremity joints should be evaluated. With the patient supine, a straight leg raise should be performed to assess for potential lumbar radiculopathy. This provides an opportunity to measure the popliteal angle as well, which may reveal tightness in the hamstrings (Fig. 28E6–15). This mandates increased quadriceps force to extend the knee during gait, with subsequently increased patellofemoral joint reaction forces. Active and passive knee range of motion should be noted and compared with the contralateral side. Initial evaluation of the hips should occur with the patient in the supine position. The presence of a hip flexion contracture can result in increased knee flexion during stance (Fig. 28E6–16). This increases the patellofemoral joint reaction force. By evaluating dorsiflexion with the knee extended, tightness of the gastrocnemius can be evaluated. Limited dorsiflexion causes a compensatory increase in subtalar pronation, which prolongs tibial internal rotation and can affect patellofemoral mechanics.

The iliotibial (IT) band and lateral retinaculum interdigitate at the level of the patella.[77, 199] The iliotibial band is displaced posteriorly by knee flexion and can be a causative factor in lateral knee pain. It is best evaluated by Ober's test (Fig. 28E6–17). This test is performed in the lateral position with the contralateral hip down and maximally flexed to stabilize the pelvis. The ipsilateral hip is slowly abducted, is brought into full extension, and then is gently adducted toward the table. Tightness in the IT band may be appreciated; this maneuver may also reproduce anterolateral knee symptomatology, often just proximal to the lateral femoral condyle. Once recognized, a structured stretching program is often therapeutic.

Prone Position

The patient should be evaluated in the prone position as well. The rectus femoris crosses the hip joint. To assess

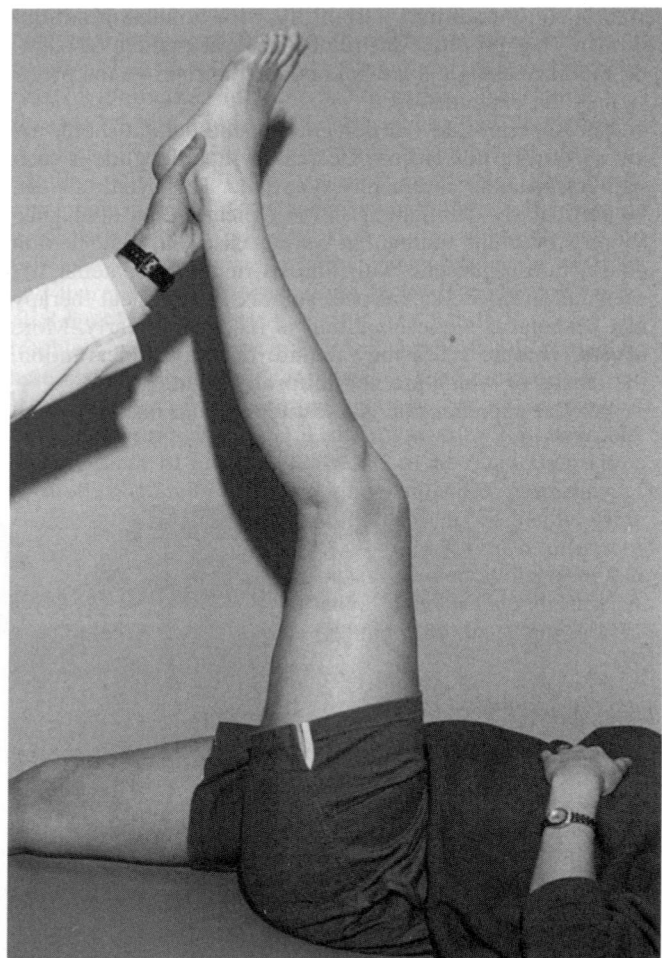

Figure 28E6–15. Straight leg raise evaluates hamstring tightness and potential lumbosacral radiculopathy. (From Fulkerson JP: Disorders of the Patellofemoral Joint, 3rd ed. Baltimore, Williams & Wilkins, 1997.)

appropriately extensor mechanism flexibility, the patient should be prone to stabilize the pelvis and prevent compensatory hip flexion (Fig. 28E6–18). Comparison with the contralateral side should be made and any asymmetries noted. Treating quadriceps inflexibility is critical to restoring proper extensor mechanism function. Patients with patellar tendinitis and persistent postoperative pain often have marked quadriceps tightness that becomes apparent with prone knee flexion.[192] With the patient prone, examination of the hip should continue. Increased internal rotation of the hip may be due to increased femoral anteversion. The relative internal rotation of the femur during gait with increased anteversion moves the trochlea medially and increases the Q angle. Increased anteversion has long been associated with patellofemoral problems despite a lack of studies to support this.[192] Decreased internal rotation of the hip is often seen with hip osteoarthrosis, which can be a referred source of pain to the knee, or may be due to contracture of the hip external rotators.

Miscellaneous

Although patients with patellofemoral problems often have flexibility deficits, some may actually be hypermobile.

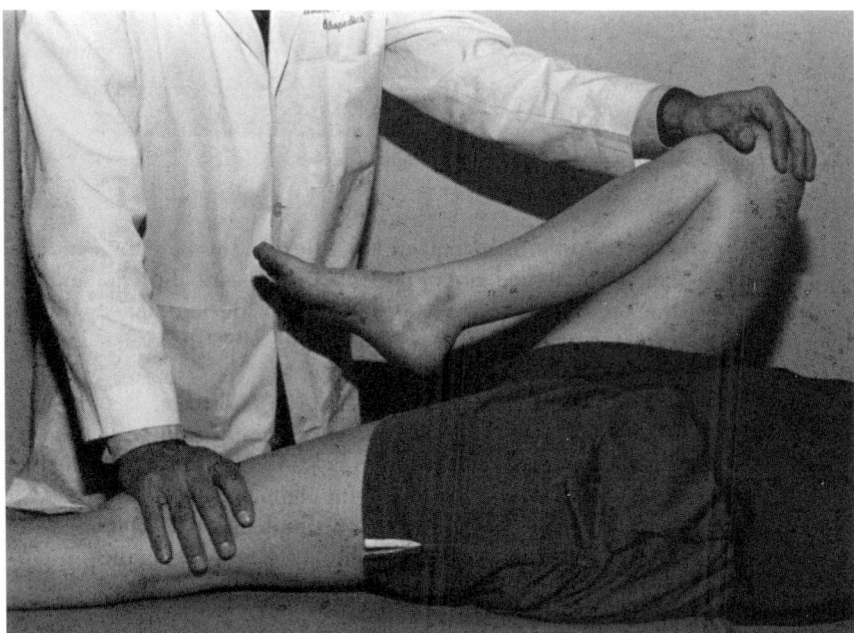

Figure 28E6–16. Evaluate for hip flexion contracture. (From Fulkerson JP: Disorders of the Patellofemoral Joint, 3rd ed. Baltimore, Williams & Wilkins, 1997.)

Patients with systemic hypermobility often have knee, elbow, and fifth metacarpophalangeal joint hyperextension, along with thumb-to-forearm apposition. Patellar dislocation is much more common among hypermobile patients than in age-matched controls, and far fewer sustain articular injury or medial patellar avulsions during dislocation.[205, 229] Ehlers-Danlos or Marfan's syndrome should be considered in cases of marked hypermobility.

A complete examination of the knee includes an evaluation of the status of the cruciate and collateral ligaments. Anterior knee pain is not uncommon with chronic anterior cruciate ligament injuries, and nearly half of patients with chronic posterior cruciate ligament injuries report knee stiffness following prolonged sitting.[184] This is likely due in part to the posterior displacement of the tibial tubercle in the posterior cruciate ligament (PCL)-deficient knee and the subsequent increase in patellofemoral joint reaction forces. Evaluation for meniscal disease and painful osteophytes should be routine as well.

Radiographic Evaluation

We routinely use three views to obtain a complete radiographic evaluation of the knee. These include a standing

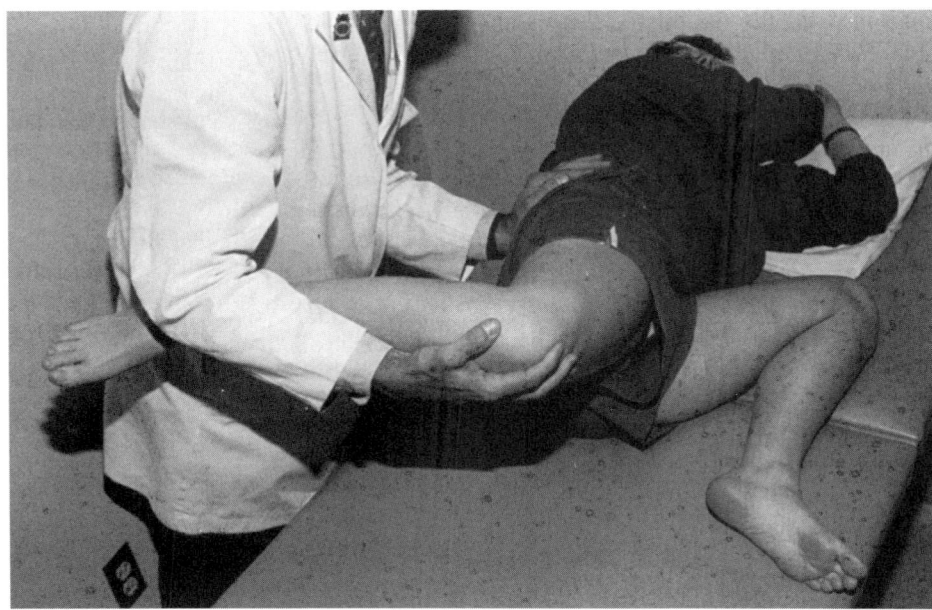

Figure 28E6–17. Ober's test. (From Fulkerson JP: Disorders of the Patellofemoral Joint, 3rd ed. Baltimore, Williams & Wilkins, 1997.)

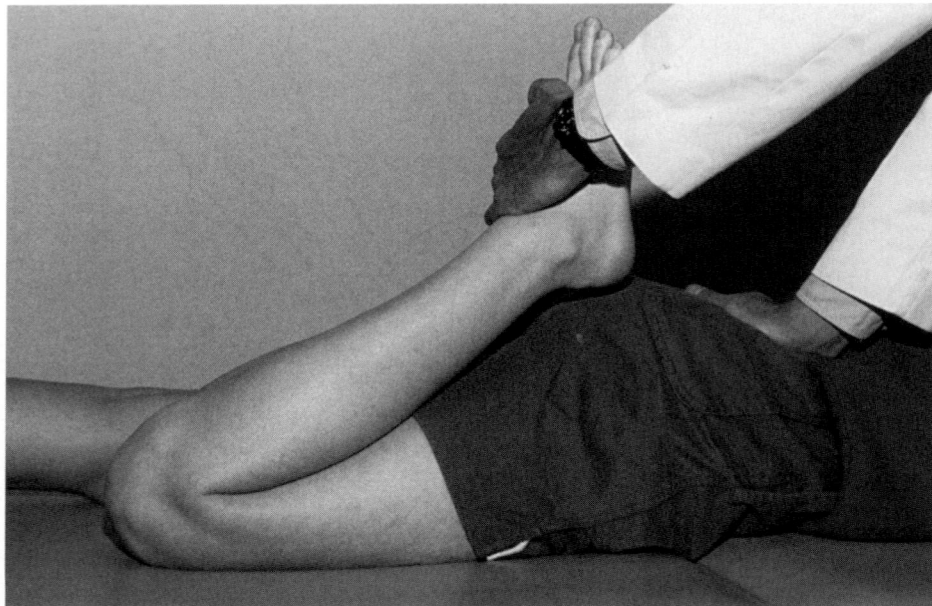

Figure 28E6–18. Test for quadriceps flexibility while the patient is prone. (From Fulkerson JP: Disorders of the Patellofemoral Joint, 3rd ed. Baltimore, Williams & Wilkins, 1997.)

anteroposterior (AP), a 30-degree flexion lateral, and a Merchant axial view. If angular deformity is clinically apparent, weight-bearing AP films on a long cassette that include as much of the lower extremity as possible are indicated. If arthritis is suspected, Rosenberg and associates[202] advocate the use of a 45-degree flexion posteroanterior (PA) view to assess the weight-bearing surface of the tibiofemoral articulation. A 30- or 45-degree knee flexion standing PA view is more sensitive than standard weight-bearing films and correlates better with arthroscopic findings.

Anteroposterior View

One can gain some sense on the AP view of whether the patella appears lateralized or abnormally medial as may be seen in a postoperative patient. The proximal tibiofibular joint should be noted to make sure that the film is a true AP view because rotation can affect the projection of the patella significantly. A bipartite patella is easily seen on this view, as is patella magna or parva and acute fractures.

Lateral View

The lateral radiograph may be taken in the lateral decubitus position or standing with the knee flexed or extended. If flexed views are taken, the amount of flexion should correspond with the axial views. Maldague and Malghem[149, 151] have described the radiographic anatomy of the patellofemoral joint on a precise lateral radiograph with regard to patellar alignment. This interpretation depends on an exact lateral view with precise overlap of the posterior and distal femoral condyles. This often requires fluoroscopy, although an experienced x-ray technician is often able to obtain exact lateral views in the majority of patients.

A major advantage of the lateral view is that it provides information regarding patellar tilt (rotation) with the patient in a weight-bearing position. These views may be obtained at different flexion angles, thus providing a more functional analysis.

Although lateral (or medial) patellar subluxation is best analyzed on axial views, a precise lateral view is an excellent means of obtaining information regarding patellar tilt. The normally aligned patella demonstrates a central ridge that is posterior to the lateral facet. As the patella rotates, the central ridge and lateral facet overlap. The central ridge may actually rotate anterior to the lateral facet in cases of extreme rotation. A classification scheme has been proposed to characterize this, with grade I being normal, and grades II and III representing advancing tilt.[149, 150] Using both extended and 30-degree flexed lateral views, Murray and coworkers[168] found improved sensitivity with regard to patellofemoral pain and previous dislocation, and improved specificity with regard to patellofemoral malalignment, as compared with axial views at 30 degrees of flexion.

The lateral view is also an excellent method for assessing trochlear morphology. This may also be assessed with the axial view; however, this images only one portion of the trochlea while the entire trochlea may be seen on the lateral view. The center of the trochlea will be seen as the most posterior line, and the medial and lateral trochlear facets can be seen separately. Normally, the lateral trochlear line should terminate proximal to the medial trochlear line without crossing the central trochlear line. The distance between the central and lateral trochlear lines at a point 1 cm distal to the upper limit of the central trochlear line should be greater than 5 mm (Fig. 28E6–19). A distance of less than 5 mm represents dysplasia of the lateral trochlear facet.[45] It has been shown that 90% of knees requiring surgery for patellar instability had trochlear depths less than 5 mm, and only 20% of control trochleas were this shallow.[149–152] Murray and associates[168] found that 79% of knees with patellar dislocations had dysplastic trochleae,

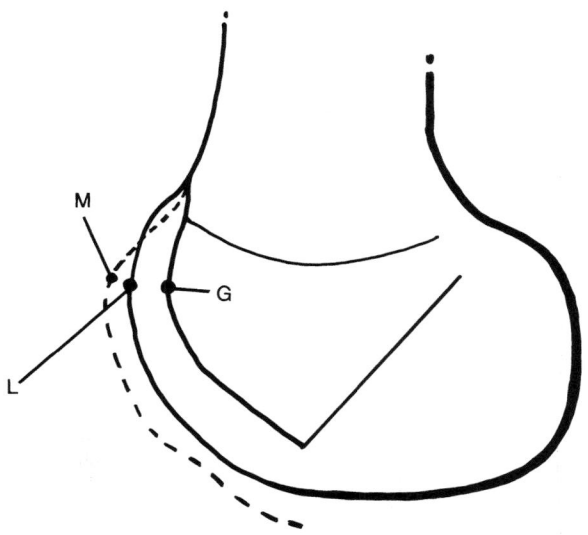

Figure 28E6–19. Measurement of trochlear depth on lateral radiograph (technique of Malghem and Maldague). G, deepest portion of trochlear groove; L, lateral femoral condyle shadow; M, medial femoral condyle shadow.

and only 36% of those with patellofemoral pain demonstrated trochlear dysplasia.

Blumensaat[18] has described the normal relationship of the patella to an anterior prolongation of a dense line that marks the ventral border of the intercondylar fossa (Blumensaat's line) (Fig. 28E6–20). Insall and Salvati[116] dispute Blumensaat's line as an accurate measurement for the position of the patella at 30 degrees of flexion. Their method does not demand a certain degree of knee flexion, and is determined by the ratio of patellar tendon length to greatest diagonal length of the patella. A range of normal is between .8 and 1.[116] Values greater than this indicate patella alta; lesser values are consistent with patella baja. Variations in patellar morphology, however, may diminish

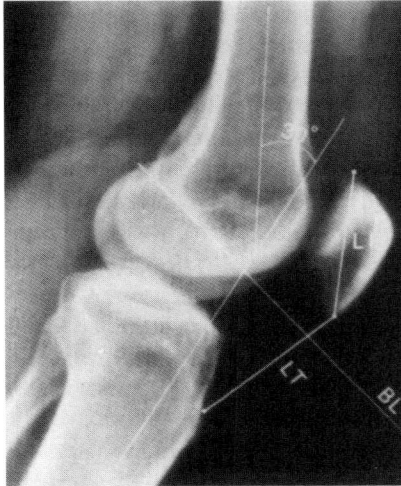

Figure 28E6–20. Lateral radiograph of the knee in 30 degrees of flexion. BL, Blumensaat's line is marked. LP, length of patella; LT, length of patellar tendon. (From Fulkerson JP: Disorders of the Patellofemoral Joint, 3rd ed. Baltimore, Williams & Wilkins, 1997.)

the sensitivity of this measurement because some patellas display a long, nonarticular distal pole. Grelsamer and coworkers[94] have developed a morphology ratio that relates the patellar articular length to the overall patellar length. Blackburne and Peel[15] proposed another modification of this technique using the tibial articular surface as the reference level for patellar height. The ratio of the patellar articular length to the distance between the tibial articular surface and the patellar articular surface is .8 in normal knees flexed at 30 degrees.[15] Bernageau and Goutallier[12] pointed out the importance of describing the patellar articular surface as it relates to the proximal, central trochlea (Fig. 28E6–21A to C).

Axial View

An accurate axial view of the knee gives a great deal of information about the patellofemoral joint. The patella normally enters the trochlea at 10 degrees of flexion, although this is dependent on the length of the patellar tendon. Those with patella alta will obviously engage at later degrees of flexion. The normal patella should be centered within the trochlea, without tilt or subluxation, by 10 to 20 degrees of flexion.[213] Drawbacks to axial radiographs include image distortion and the fact that subtle tracking abnormalities in the first 20 to 30 degrees of flexion are difficult to impossible to detect with axial radiographs. Also, an accurate reference line for determining patellar tilt is not possible with axial radiographs because of the variable anatomy of the femoral trochlea.

Several techniques for obtaining axial radiographs have been proposed (Fig. 28E6–22A to C). The axial view as described by Merchant is preferred.[162] It is taken with the knee flexed 45 degrees and the x-ray beam projected caudad at an angle of 30 degrees from the plane of the femur. The amount of knee flexion can be varied. Techniques that require excessive knee flexion angles may reduce a subluxated patella, creating a false negative. The Ficat technique is accurate but poses an increased risk of radiation exposure to the patient because the beam is directed cephalad. The Laurin technique is performed at 20 degrees of flexion. It also poses an increased radiation exposure risk and is difficult to image clinically.[70, 140, 160] The advantage of this method is that it may detect subtle malalignment that is not apparent at greater degrees of flexion. Laurin showed that the patella is well into the trochlea in 97% of normal individuals by 20 degrees of knee flexion.[140] Some patients, however, have patellofemoral malalignment that can be documented only at this angle of flexion, and not further in flexion as the malaligned patella will eventually centralize. Axial radiographs at 30 degrees of flexion with lateral rotation of the leg may be useful in the assessment of patellar subluxability. This is the tendency for the patella to dislocate with stress or rotation of the knee, as compared with subluxation that occurs when there is displacement of the patella without stress or rotation of the knee.[153]

In the clinical interpretation of axial views, two measurements are helpful—the Laurin lateral patellofemoral angle and the Merchant congruence angle (Fig. 28E6–23A and B). Laurin described criteria for patellar tilt based on

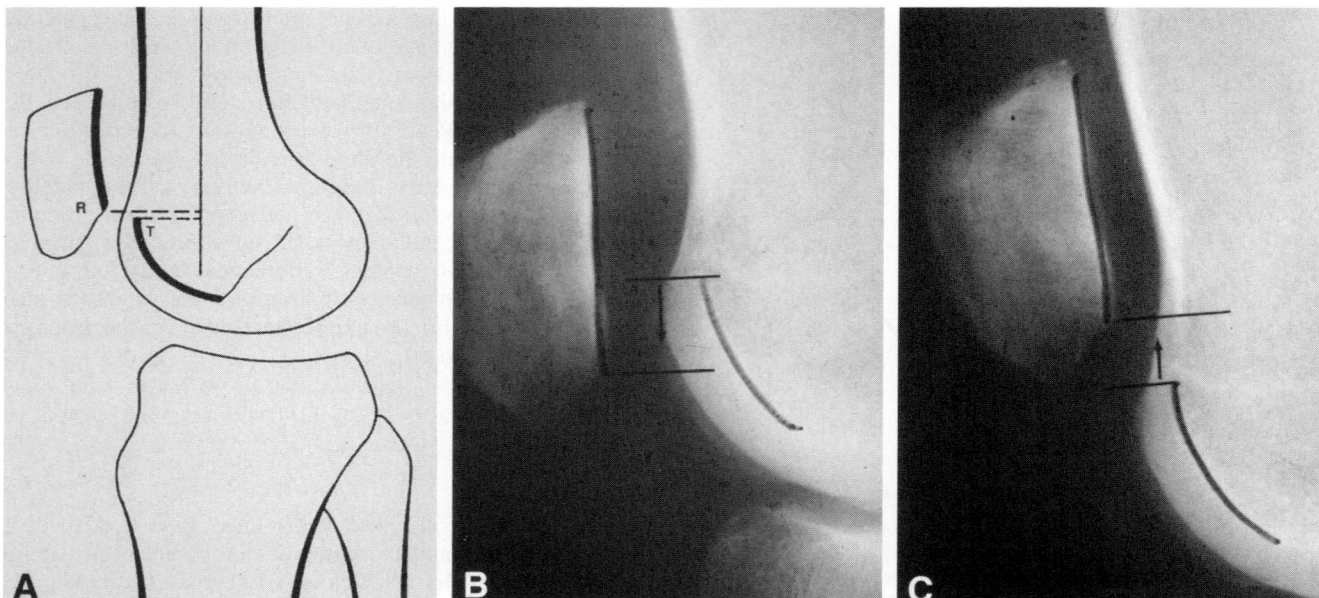

Figure 28E6–21. *A,* Bernageau pointed out the importance of describing the patellar articular surface as it relates to the proximal central trochlea. *B,* Patella infra. *C,* Patella alta. R, Inferior patellar articular surface; T, proximal trochlea. (From Fulkerson JP: Disorders of the Patellofemoral Joint, 3rd ed. Baltimore, Williams & Wilkins, 1997.)

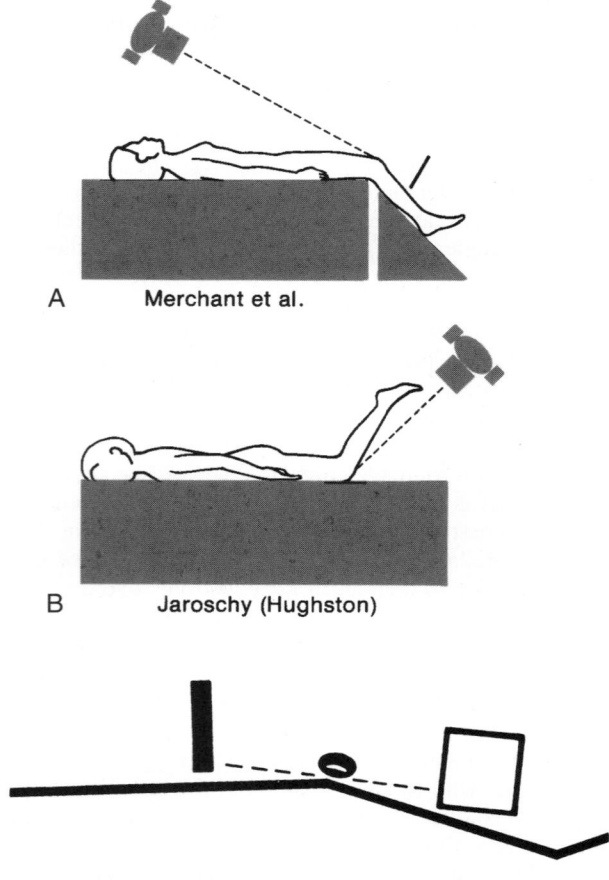

Figure 28E6–22. Techniques for obtaining axial patellofemoral radiographs. *A,* Merchant view. *B,* Jaroschy (Hughston) view. *C,* Laurin view. (From Fulkerson JP: Disorders of the Patellofemoral Joint, 3rd ed. Baltimore, Williams & Wilkins, 1997.)

lines drawn on the lateral patellar facet and the anterior margin of the femoral trochlea.[140] Laurin and colleagues[140] found that 97% of controls had a lateral patellofemoral angle that opened laterally. In those patients with patellar subluxation, 60% had parallel lines and 40% had a medial facing angle. This simple measurement is a good indicator for screening purposes of abnormal patellar tilt.

Merchant's congruence angle is used to assess patellar subluxation. It can be measured from both axial radiographs and computed tomography of the patellofemoral joint. The congruence angle is determined by bisecting the sulcus angle with a neutral reference line. The apex of the median patellar ridge is connected to the lowest point on the sulcus. When this line is medial to the sulcus bisector, the angle is given as a negative value; when lateral, a positive value is assigned. Merchant and coworkers[162] found that normal congruence is −6 ± 11 degrees at 45 degrees of knee flexion. At this amount of flexion, the patellae of most patients will be centralized within the sulcus, including those who demonstrate patellar malalignment at earlier degrees of flexion.

Computed Tomography

To define patellar tracking accurately, computed tomography (CT) offers sequential images at any degree of knee flexion, using the midtransverse patella as a reference. This also provides clear imaging of the posterior femoral condyles (Fig. 28E6–24) and provides a reliable reference plane for determining patellar tilt as compared with a line drawn across the variable anterior femoral trochlear margins.[70] Performing CT of the patellofemoral joint requires careful attention to detail. It is best performed with bolsters in the lateral decubitus position in a manner that

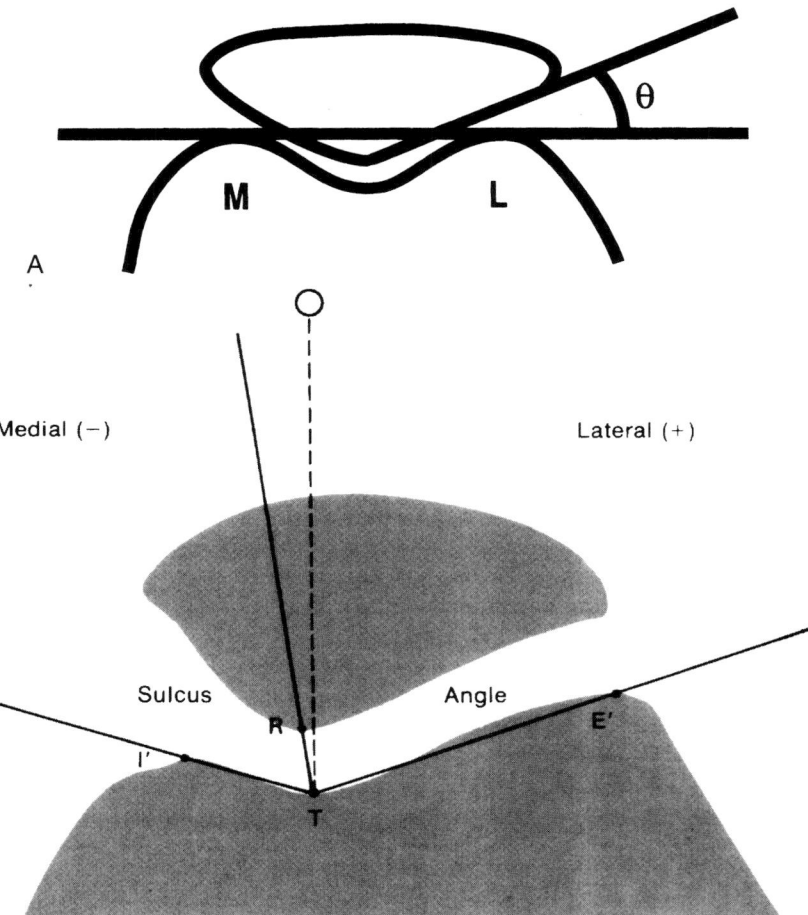

Figure 28E6–23. *A,* The lateral patellofemoral angle of Laurin should open laterally. *B,* Merchant's congruence angle. RT is the line connecting the median ridge to the trochlear depth; TO is the reference line bisecting angle E'TI'. (From Fulkerson JP: Disorders of the Patellofemoral Joint, 3rd ed. Baltimore, Williams & Wilkins, 1997.)

re-creates the patient's normal standing alignment. It is critical to center the beam on the midtransverse patella throughout the study. Tomographic cuts are ideally obtained at 0, 15, 30, 45, and 60 degrees of knee flexion. This allows an evaluation of the patella as it enters the trochlea to a point of maximal contact stress.[70]

Using CT criteria, it is possible to note a variety of different tracking patterns that are not as well defined using standard radiographs. Some patients with patellofemoral

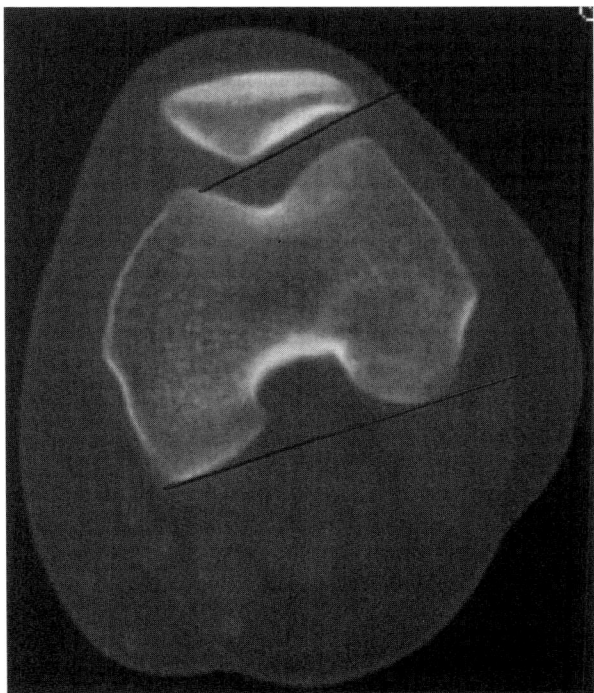

Figure 28E6–24. Computed tomography presents clear imaging of the posterior femoral condyles and provides a reliable reference for determining patellar tilt. (From Fulkerson JP: Disorders of the Patellofemoral Joint, 3rd ed. Baltimore, Williams & Wilkins, 1997.)

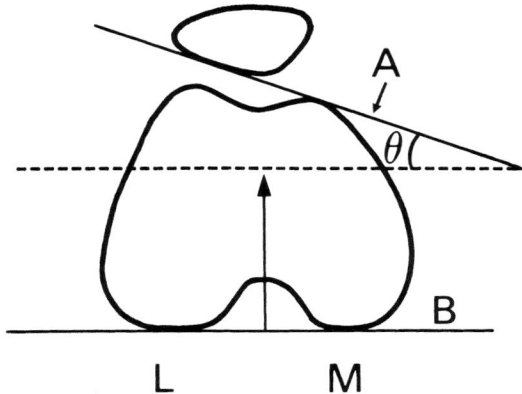

Figure 28E6–25. The patellar tilt angle as referenced off the posterior femoral condyles. (From Fulkerson JP: Disorders of the Patellofemoral Joint, 3rd ed. Baltimore, Williams & Wilkins, 1997.)

promote motion (especially full extension), regain strength, and diminish swelling. Gentle manipulation under anesthesia is sometimes necessary to assist in regaining flexion. Patellar mobilization exercises are critical. If these measures are unsuccessful, then arthroscopic lysis and gentle manipulation are indicated. Débridement of the suprapatellar pouch, medial and lateral gutters, and anterior fat pad should be performed. Once IPCS has progressed to stage II, open débridement is necessary. Through a midline approach, débridement and release of the suprapatellar pouch, along with lateral, and, occasionally, medial retinacular release, are needed. All fibrotic tissue posterior to the patellar tendon should be aggressively released. In late stage II IPCS and in stage III, patella infra will be present, and soft tissue releases will be inadequate to correct the permanent shortening of the patellar tendon.[237] Z-lengthening of the patellar tendon can be performed, or a DeLee tibial tubercle osteotomy may effect an anterior and superior shift of the tubercle.[187]

Criteria for Return to Sports Participation. Before the patient is permitted to return to athletic activities, knee range of motion and strength of the lower extremity should be comparable to those of the opposite limb. The patient should demonstrate well-healed incisions without an effusion. An osteotomy, if performed, should be healed both clinically and radiologically.

Authors' Preferred Method of Treatment. Aggressive physical therapy is instituted for stage I IPCS. Arthroscopy can be helpful early on to débride inflammatory fibrotic tissue throughout the knee. When IPCS follows ACL reconstruction, arthroscopy also provides a means to débride a potential "Cyclops" lesion, and to perform a revision notchplasty if roof impingement is present. If the ACL graft is noted to be grossly malpositioned, it may be need to be excised with plans for a delayed reconstruction. Once stage II IPCS is present, open débridement is performed, with release of parapatellar tendon fibrosis. A meticulous, thorough débridement of any retropatellar tendon fibrotic tissue is critical also. In the presence of patellar arthrosis in stage III IPCS, a modified sagittal plane tibial tubercle osteotomy with a "back-cut" on the lateral tibial cortex provides anteriorization of the tubercle and diminishes contact forces in the patellofemoral joint. (See "Authors' Preferred Method of Treatment" under "Patellofemoral Arthrosis.") Postoperatively, aggressive physical therapy is resumed to maintain restored motion. If an osteotomy is performed, weight-bearing is protected for 6 weeks in a knee immobilizer. Gentle range of motion exercises should still be performed on a daily basis, however.

Patellar Tilt-Compression

Patellar tilt-compression is a form of anterior knee pain without, at least initially, articular breakdown. It is characterized clinically by pain and radiologically by patellar tilt, and leads to two clinical outcomes in many patients: retinacular strain (peripatellar effect) and excessive lateral pressure syndrome, or ELPS[64] (articular effect).[70] Associated patellar subluxation is not present in pure tilt-compression, although it may be present in ELPS. These two disorders are on a continuum; the tilt-compression syndrome will usually proceed through a period of soft tissue

pain related to adaptive retinacular shortening and will eventually lead to patellar arthrosis.[70]

Patients with patellar tilt-compression typically complain of pain instead of patellar instability. This is a critical issue to resolve while taking a history. Patients often experience dull, achy anterior knee pain that is activity related and exacerbated by prolonged knee flexion (sitting or squatting) or resisted knee extension (stair climbing). Pain that is constant in nature is more suspicious for referred pain or neurogenic pain.

On examination, tenderness in the lateral retinaculum is often noted at the insertion of the vastus lateralis near the interdigitation with the lateral retinaculum. Small nerve injury may be present in the lateral retinaculum.[84] Tightness in the lateral retinaculum should be investigated carefully. Medial patellar glide is often diminished to one quadrant or less.[133] The clinician should attempt to raise the lateral edge of the patella past the horizontal plane. Inability to do so is indicative of a tight lateral retinaculum.[79, 133] The medial retinaculum may also be tender as a result of chronic stretching. The presence of a recurrent joint effusion and/or crepitation is somewhat ominous because this may indicate articular surface breakdown at the critical zone (Ficat) and the progression to ELPS (Fig. 28E6–30).

Patellar tilt can be documented with a variety of imaging modalities. Plain films, including both axial and precise lateral views, can be helpful. The lateral patellofemoral angle of Laurin should be noted,[140] and the lateral view should be scrutinized in the manner described by Maldague and Malghem[149] for evidence of patellar tilt. Remember that subtle patellar malalignment may be present only very early in flexion, and cannot be adequately imaged with standard axial views. CT is helpful in this regard because the patellofemoral joint can be imaged at or near full extension.

Indirect signs of excessive lateral pressure due to a tight lateral retinaculum may be seen on plain radiographs (Fig. 28E6–31). The patella may reveal increased subchondral bone density in the lateral facet, with decreased density in the medial facet. Cancellous trabeculae within the patella may become more perpendicular to the lateral facet. These findings can be simply explained by Wolff's law. Relative elongation and flattening of the lateral facet, as seen in the Wiberg type III patella, and hypoplasia of the lateral trochlea are occasionally seen. These findings are likely the result of excessive modulating force during growth. Lateral margin fracture, a distinct entity from a bipartite patella, or

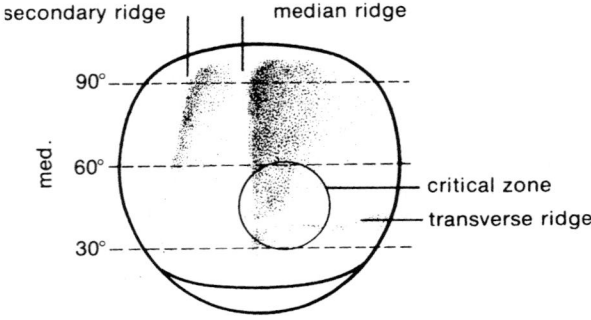

Figure 28E6–30. Ficat's critical zone. (From Fulkerson JP: Disorders of the Patellofemoral Joint, 3rd ed. Baltimore, Williams & Wilkins, 1997.)

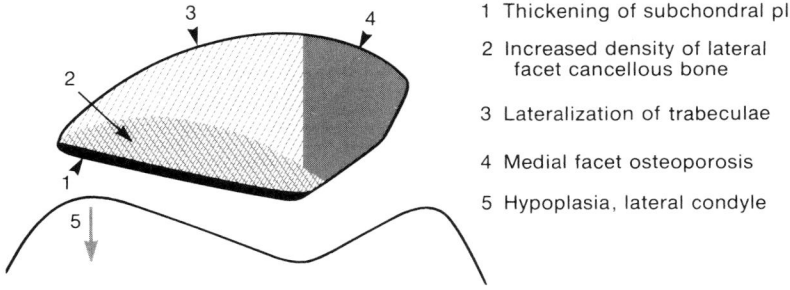

Figure 28E6–31. Indirect radiologic signs of excessive lateral pressure. (From Fulkerson JP: Disorders of the Patellofemoral Joint, 3rd ed. Baltimore, Williams & Wilkins, 1997.)

1 Thickening of subchondral plate

2 Increased density of lateral facet cancellous bone

3 Lateralization of trabeculae

4 Medial facet osteoporosis

5 Hypoplasia, lateral condyle

lateral margin osteophytes are a result of chronic stress from a shortened, tight lateral retinaculum[70] (Fig. 28E6–32).

The mainstay of surgical treatment for patellar tilt is lateral release. Lateral retinacular release has been used for a wide variety of indications, some of which are inappropriate. This has contributed to the poor reputation that this procedure has with many orthopaedists. By adhering to relatively narrow indications, however, such as a painful, tight lateral retinaculum with documented patellar tilt, good results may be obtained. Merchant and Mercer[161] first described lateral retinacular release as an isolated procedure in 1974. Like many earlier reports, the primary indication was patellar subluxation or dislocation. Larson and associates[139] were the first to report on isolated lateral retinacular release for "patellar compression syndrome." They reported that 37 of 45 patients had lessening of pain after the operation, and 10 returned to unrestricted athletic activities. The severity of articular degeneration is a critical factor in the success rate of isolated lateral retinacular release. It is well documented that patients with more severe grades of articular cartilage damage, such as Outerbridge grades III/IV, do not do well over the long term after lateral retinacular release.[34, 177, 180, 216] Shea and Fulkerson[216] reported that 92% of patients with CT-documented patellar tilt and minimal articular degeneration (Outerbridge grade I/II) treated by open lateral release achieved good or excellent results. Only 22% of those with documented tilt and more severe articular change (Outerbridge grade III/IV) achieved good or excellent results. Importantly, they also point out that only 13% of patients without CT evidence of tilt had a good result. They recommend lateral release for patients with anterior knee pain who have failed conservative management with documented patellar tilt with minimal articular degeneration and little to no subluxation.[216] It is important to note that isolated lateral release is not indicated for patellar instability. Several recent reports highlight a late deterioration of good results in patients whose primary diagnosis was instability.[68] This concept will be expanded on in the section on patellar subluxation. Fulkerson and colleagues[82] compared preoperative and postoperative CT scans following lateral release or realignment and found that patellar tilt is consistently improved with lateral release unless advanced articular degeneration of the lateral facet is present, in which case correction is much less. Fulkerson and Schutzer[81] point out several key issues that should be addressed before lateral release: (1) Is there any evidence of referred pain? (2) Is there soft tissue pain around the patella? (3) Is there radiographic or CT evidence of patellar tilt, subluxation, or both at 10 to 20 degrees of knee flexion? (4) Is there evidence of patellofemoral arthrosis? (5) Is it clear that the problem is structural in nature and is not related to any secondary gain or psychiatric issue? (6) Is there any evidence of reflex sympathetic dystrophy?

Kolowich and coworkers[133] also provided clear indications for lateral release. They emphasize the importance of the patellar tilt test in that a negative or neutral degree on this test preoperatively correlated with successful results of lateral release.[133] They place less emphasis on radiographic evaluation, and instead highlight the importance of an accurate, focused physical examination.

A variety of different techniques have been used for lateral release. These include percutaneous, "mini-open," open, and arthroscopic methods. All techniques have the same goal of reducing the posteriorly directed pull of the lateral retinaculum on the lateral patella. Open techniques typically use a 4- to 5-cm incision, and simply divide the lateral retinaculum. Partial excision and Z-lengthening of the retinaculum have been proposed as well.[32, 241] Arthroscopic technique, first described by Metcalf,[163] is common, and most often electrocautery is used to divide the retinacu-

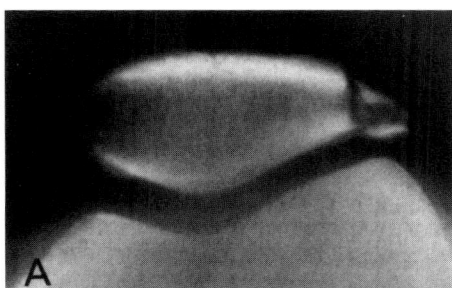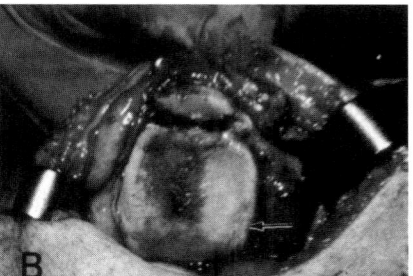

Figure 28E6–32. Radiograph *(A)* and operative view *(B)* of lateral margin fracture, indicating excessive lateral tension. (From Fulkerson JP: Disorders of the Patellofemoral Joint, 3rd ed. Baltimore, Williams & Wilkins, 1997.)

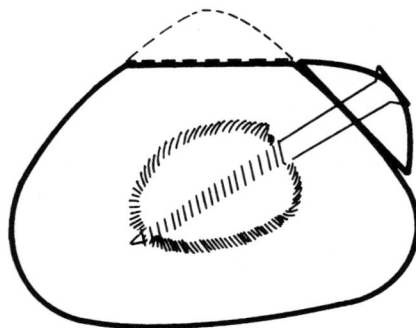

Figure 28E6–36. The Hauser procedure transfers the tibial tubercle in a medial, distal, and posterior direction. (From Fulkerson JP: Disorders of the Patellofemoral Joint, 3rd ed. Baltimore, Williams & Wilkins, 1997.)

cally been used when an isolated lateral release has not been sufficient to restore patellar tracking. Distal soft tissue procedures have been advocated for the skeletally immature patient with patellar instability. The role of proximal realignment and distal soft tissue procedures in the adult with patellofemoral arthrosis is limited. These techniques do have a role in the patient with patellar subluxation, and they will be discussed in the section on patellar subluxation.

Distal realignment procedures typically involve the transfer of the bony insertion of the patellar tendon (the tibial tubercle) and may include a lateral retinacular release. Roux[203] initially described the technique of lateral retinacular release, medial imbrication, and medial displacement osteotomy of the tibial tubercle. The classical medial tibial tubercle transfer was the Hauser procedure first described in 1938.[99] This technique transfers the tibial tubercle in a medial, distal, and posterior directions[72, 194] (Fig. 28E6–36). The posterior displacement, however, decreases the lever arm of the extensor mechanism and leads to increased patellofemoral joint reaction force with a long-term progression to osteoarthrosis.[70, 100]

Elmslie and Trillat modified and popularized a distal realignment procedure based on the technique described by Roux. Cox[41] reported his results of the Roux-Elmslie-Trillat procedure on 116 patients with recurrent patellar subluxation or dislocation followed for at least 1 year. Good or excellent results were noted in 66% of patients, with a 7% recurrence rate.[41] Follow-up was relatively short, but progression of patellofemoral arthrosis was not noted. Importantly, this technique does not posteriorly displace the tibial tubercle. Ideal candidates for pure medialization procedures have anatomic malalignment, minimal articular degeneration, and, primarily, symptoms of instability.[193]

Maquet[154] popularized the anterior transfer of the tibial tubercle initially described by Bandi.[8] This technique provides the important advantage of unloading articular lesions of the patellofemoral joint by increasing the lever arm of the extensor mechanism and thus diminishing patellofemoral joint reaction force. An iliac crest bone graft is used to anteriorize the tibial tubercle, typically about 20 mm. Maquet stated that this reduced compressive forces in the patellofemoral joint by approximately 50% when the knee is flexed to 45 degrees.[155] Complications of the Maquet procedure, however, are potentially severe. They include anterior compartment syndrome and skin necrosis overlying an excessively advanced tibial tubercle. Bessette and Hunter[13] reported their results of a retrospective review of the Maquet procedure with minimum 1-year follow-up. They reported a 40% complication rate, including wound problems, fracture of both the proximal tibia and the osteotomized tubercle, and excessive blood loss and stiffness. They also noted a striking increase in the complication rate when internal fixation was used.[13] The ideal amount of anterior displacement of the tibial tubercle is controversial. Maquet initially described 2 to 2.5 cm of elevation, and this amount of elevation has been supported by others.[182, 196, 197] Different authors, however, report that anteriorization of 1 cm is optimal.[61, 169] Ferguson and coworkers[60] found that little additional decompression of the patellofemoral joint is achieved beyond the first ½ inch of elevation. The length of the tibial shingle is also controversial. Some authors feel that with a shingle length of less than 10 cm, the patella excessively rotates and the superior pole is exposed to high stress concentrations,[169, 182] although others refute this.[11]

Anteromedialization of the tibial tubercle for patellar malalignment was described by the senior author (JPF) in 1983.[72] This procedure combines a lateral release with decompression of the lateral facet by medial and anterior displacement of the extensor mechanism, removal of the lateral tether, and anterior displacement of the patella (Fig. 28E6–37). Anteromedialization of the tibial tubercle most effectively transfers load from the more distal and lateral aspects of the patella onto the proximal, medial articular cartilage.[11, 70] Accordingly, the procedure is most effective when there is osteoarthrosis of the lateral or distal medial facet associated with malalignment. Results of anteromedialization of the tibial tubercle for patellofemoral arthrosis

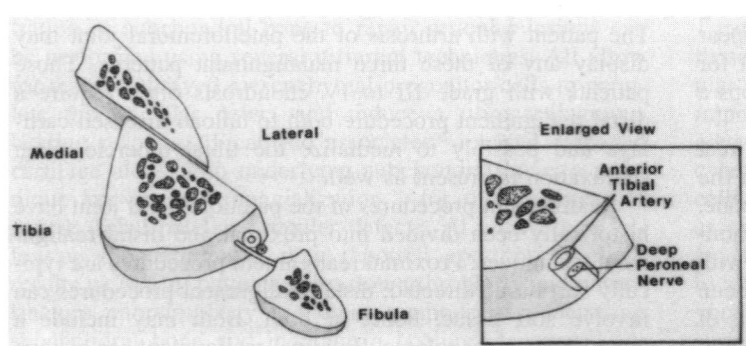

Figure 28E6–37. Anteromedial tibial tubercle transfer along an oblique osteotomy plane, as described by Fulkerson. (From Fulkerson JP: Disorders of the Patellofemoral Joint, 3rd ed. Baltimore, Williams & Wilkins, 1997.)

and/or malalignment have been quite good. Fulkerson and associates[76] reported 93% good and excellent results subjectively and 89% good and excellent results objectively at minimum 2-year follow-up. Seventy-five percent of patients with advanced patellar arthrosis achieved a good result. Serious complications such as skin slough, infection, or compartment syndrome were avoided entirely in 51 consecutive cases.[76] Before anteromedialization of the tibial tubercle is performed, the practitioner should carefully document the nature and location of articular disease within the patellofemoral joint. The location of the articular lesion is critical; Pidoriano and colleagues[190] have demonstrated that those patients with distal and/or lateral articular lesions were significantly more likely to have good or excellent results following anteromedial tibial tubercle transfer. An important finding of this study was that all patients with a central trochlear lesion had poor results.

More recently, anterolateralization of the tibial tubercle has been described.[70, 74] This procedure serves to decompress an overloaded medial patellar facet. The patient typically presents with complaints of pain and/or instability of the patellofemoral joint. Medial patellar subluxation is often present with subsequent medial patellar facet arthrosis. This is usually the result of a distal realignment in which the tubercle is overly medialized, although isolated lateral release can lead to medial subluxation also. Medial patellar facet arthrosis is especially common following a failed Hauser procedure in which the tibial tubercle is medialized and displaced posteriorly.[70, 100] It is critical to note that the instability is medial. This can be documented by a variety of different techniques.[75, 108, 172, 233, 234] Anterolateralization in this scenario provides decompression of the patellofemoral joint and corrects the medial instability if present. Long-term results on this technique are lacking.

Patients with focal chondral lesions of the patellofemoral joint may respond to a wide variety of procedures. Treatment of diffuse and/or severe proximal arthrosis of the patella is very difficult, however. It is in these scenarios that patellectomy or patellofemoral arthroplasty may be indicated. When reviewing the literature in regard to patellectomy, it is important to separate results according to treatment for arthritis, anterior knee pain, or fracture. Arthrosis isolated to the patellofemoral joint definitely predicts a better outcome.[2, 29, 50, 232] Lennox and associates[141] reported long-term follow-up on patellectomy. Only 54% of the patients with osteoarthritis had satisfactory relief of pain, and most had progressive deterioration of function. Ackroyd and Polyzoides[2] reported their results of patellectomy for patients with patellofemoral osteoarthritis. Only 53% of the patients had good results. Feller and Bartlett[58] reported that 15 of 16 patients had arthroscopically documented arthrosis, particularly of the medial compartment and the trochlear groove, following patellectomy. The severity of the arthrosis correlated with the time since patellectomy. Conversely, Baker and Hughston[6] reported very good results with their experience with the Miyakawa patellectomy. This method attempts to maintain a proper length/tension relationship in the extensor mechanism. Loss of extension power following patellectomy is a significant concern. Lennox and colleagues[141] found a 40% quadriceps strength deficit at follow-up in comparison with the contralateral limb. Patellectomy also has significant implications

for total knee arthroplasty, should that become necessary in the future. Kelly and Insall[130] emphasize that alternatives to patellectomy can usually be found. The senior author (JPF) reserves patellectomy as truly a final option when all previous nonoperative and operative measures have failed.

Patellofemoral arthroplasty remains a controversial technique for the treatment of patellofemoral arthritis. Worrell[244] states that resurfacing of the patella should be limited to patients with grade III to IV chondrosis of the patella and poor quadriceps function. In 1955, a metal prosthesis that resurfaced only the patella was introduced.[51] The long-term results of this implant were reported by Harrington,[98] who found that 17 of 24 patients had good to excellent results at 5 years. Of the 3 patients with poor results, 2 had tricompartmental arthrosis at 5-year follow-up. Subsequent designs included a polyethylene patellar button with a metal trochlear component.[16, 31, 147] Several authors conclude that although patellofemoral arthroplasty may be indicated for patients with osteoarthrosis limited to the patellofemoral joint, preexisting patellofemoral malalignment must be corrected during the procedure.[4, 16, 31, 93, 135] The senior author (JPF) has limited experience with isolated arthroplasty of the patellofemoral joint.

Criteria for Return to Sports Participation. Before allowing the patient to return to athletic activities, the surgeon should document normal motion and strength in the operative lower extremity. The patient should not have significant pain or an effusion, and incisions, if present, should be well healed. An osteotomy, if performed, should be healed both clinically and radiologically.

Authors' Preferred Method of Treatment. Surgical treatment of patellofemoral arthrosis is considered after the failure of conservative measures, including quadriceps strengthening, activity modification, and therapy with NSAIDs. Through careful preoperative assessment using physical examination and radiographic findings, the surgeon should be able to formulate a treatment plan. This should take into account the anticipated location and severity of chondral lesions, as well as any existing malalignment. A complete knowledge of previous surgeries is essential.

Arthroscopy of the patient with patellofemoral arthrosis is routinely performed. The arthroscope is used initially through the superomedial portal, as described by Schreiber[212] (Fig. 28E6–38). This provides an excellent view of articular disease in the patellofemoral joint, especially the proximal lesions. These lesions are critical to appreciate because realignment of the tibial tubercle transfers stress to the proximal articular cartilage of the patella. A complete arthroscopic examination of the entire knee is completed through standard anteromedial and anterolateral portals. Loose or fibrillated cartilage can be easily débrided to a stable base arthroscopically. The surgeon should be meticulous in this regard, being careful to maintain all healthy cartilage. Meniscal disease is addressed as indicated. Relatively small, full-thickness articular lesions of the femoral condyles and trochlea are often treated initially with a microfracture technique using specially designed awls to penetrate the subchondral plate.[231] Diffuse articular disease of the knee is perhaps best addressed by total knee arthroplasty, particularly if it is tricompartmental in nature.

If, however, clinical symptoms and documented articular

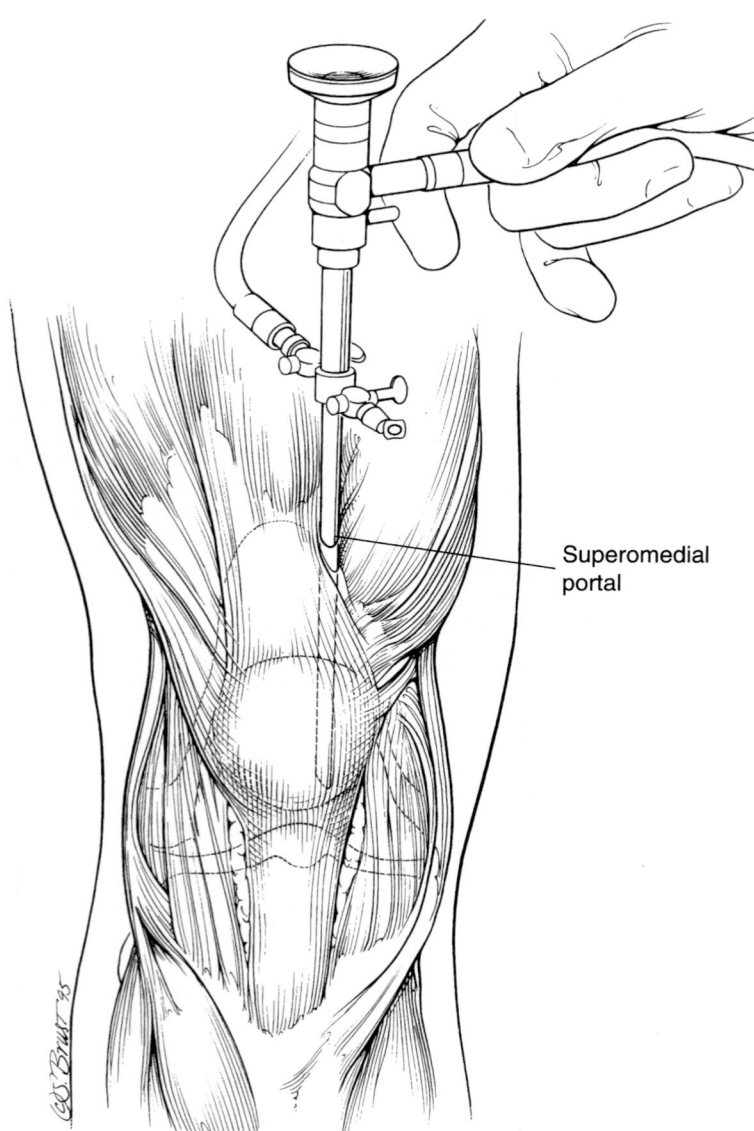

Superomedial
portal

Figure 28E6–38. The superomedial arthroscopy portal, as described by Schreiber. (From Fulkerson JP: Disorders of the Patellofemoral Joint, 3rd ed. Baltimore, Williams & Wilkins, 1997.)

disease are primarily limited to the patellofemoral joint, tibial tubercle realignment is used. Full-thickness lesions of the trochlea are not an absolute contraindication, but the surgeon should realize that results of tibial tubercle realignment are not as good when this lesion is present.[190] At the time of arthroscopy, the surgeon must make a critical assessment as to whether or not tibial tubercle transfer will unload a given articular lesion within the patellofemoral joint and transfer stress to more healthy cartilage. Anteromedialization of the tibial tubercle most effectively transfers load from the more distal and lateral aspects of the patella onto the proximal, medial articular cartilage. Obviously, therefore, the surgeon must document that the proximal, medial patellar cartilage is intact. Most patients with chronic patellar malalignment have distal and lateral facet lesions. Patients with a history of blunt trauma to the flexed knee, however, often have destruction of proximal patellar cartilage and may be less amenable to anteromedial transfer of the tibial tubercle.

An advantage of the anteromedialization procedure described and used by the senior author (JPF)[72] is that the surgeon can alter the obliquity of the osteotomy plane. If malalignment predominates, and articular disease of the distal lateral and/or medial facet is less severe, the osteotomy can be modified to a more coronal plane to effect greater medialization than is attained by anteriorization of the tibial tubercle. Conversely, when malalignment is minimal, yet distal arthrosis is present on the patella, this technique can be modified by making a steeper cut, which allows more anteriorization with less medialization. The osteotomy can approach the sagittal plane in some cases. This is achieved by means of a "back-cut" on the lateral tibial cortex to complete the osteotomy. The maximum anterior transfer that can be accomplished with the traditional anteromedialization is about 17 mm.[83] Use of the "back-cut" technique provides an additional 3 to 5 mm of anteriorization. No bone graft is necessary in either technique.

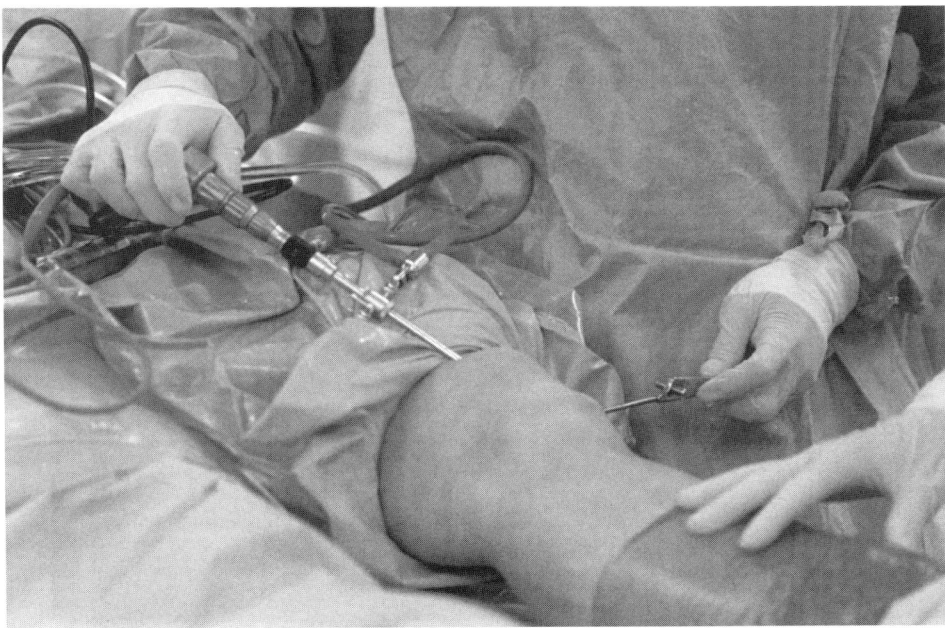

Figure 28E6–39. Routine arthroscopy is performed before anteromedial tibial tubercle transfer. (From Fulkerson JP: Disorders of the Patellofemoral Joint, 3rd ed. Baltimore, Williams & Wilkins, 1997.)

Painful arthrosis of the medial facet may develop when medial subluxation of the patella is present following overzealous lateral release or medialization of the tibial tubercle. This condition may also develop over time following a Hauser procedure. In these scenarios, anterolateralization of the tibial tubercle is used to restore alignment and decompress the medial facet. The surgeon should document that healthy cartilage is present proximally and laterally on the patella because this is the point to which contact stress will be transferred.

Anteromedial Tibial Tubercle Transfer. The patient is positioned supine on the operating room table. A first-generation cephalosporin is administered intravenously be-

fore the procedure is begun. A tourniquet is applied to the proximal thigh, and the lower extremity is prepped from the tourniquet to the toes. A sterile stockinette is secured around the foot and lower leg using a Coban wrap. The lower extremity is then draped in a sterile fashion, and the tourniquet is raised to 250 mm Hg.

Arthroscopy is routinely performed at the outset of anteromedial tibial tubercle transfer, as was previously described (Fig. 28E6–39). Articular disease should be documented on the distal, lateral, and/or medial facet of the patella with preservation of cartilage proximally and medially. The incision for anteromedial tibial tubercle transfer should extend from a point overlying the lateral retinacu-

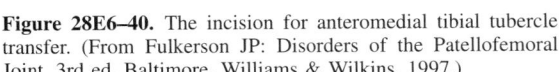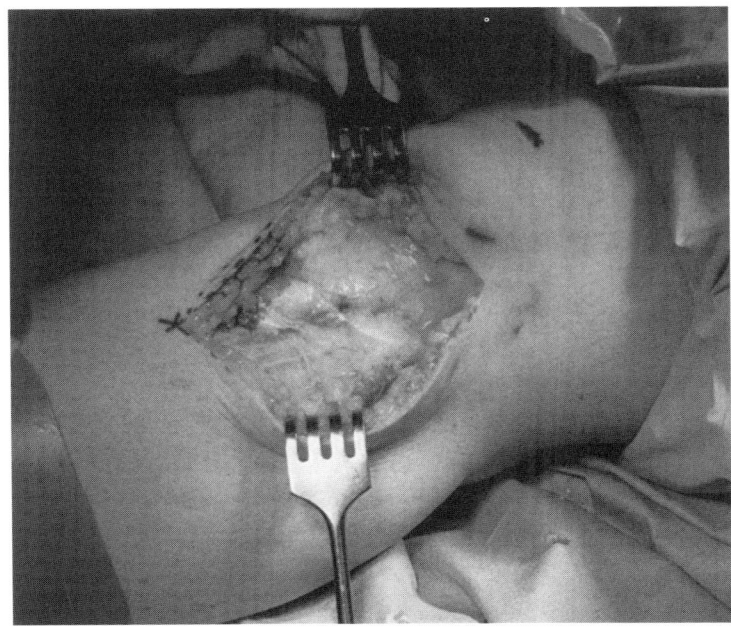

Figure 28E6–40. The incision for anteromedial tibial tubercle transfer. (From Fulkerson JP: Disorders of the Patellofemoral Joint, 3rd ed. Baltimore, Williams & Wilkins, 1997.)

29. Burton VW, Thomas HM: Results of excision of the patella. Surg Gynecol Obstet 135:753–755, 1972.
30. Busch MT, DeHaven KE: Pitfalls of the lateral retinacular release. Clin Sports Med 8:279–290, 1989.
31. Cartier P, Sanouiller JL, Grelsamer R: Patellofemoral arthroplasty. 2–12-year follow-up study. J Arthroplasty 5:49–55, 1990.
32. Ceder LC, Larson RL: Z-plasty lateral retinacular release for the treatment of patellar compression syndrome. Clin Orthop 144:110–113, 1979.
33. Childers JC Jr, Ellwood SC: Partial chondrectomy and subchondral bone drilling for chondromalacia. Clin Orthop 144:114–120, 1979.
34. Christensen F, Soballe K, Snerum L: Treatment of chondromalacia patella by late retinacular release of the patella. Clin Orthop 234:145–147, 1988.
35. Chu CR, Convery FR, Akeson WH, et al: Articular cartilage transplantation. Clinical results in the knee. Clin Orthop 360:159–168, 1999.
36. Coleman BD, Khan KM, Kiss ZS, et al: Open and arthroscopic patellar tenotomy for chronic patellar tendinopathy. A retrospective outcome study. Victorian Institute of Sport Tendon Study Group. Am J Sports Med 28:183–190, 2000.
37. Conlan T, Garth WP Jr, Lemons JE: Evaluation of the medial soft-tissue restraints of the extensor mechanism of the knee. J Bone Joint Surg Am 75:682–693, 1993.
38. Convery FR, Botte MJ, Akeson WH: Chondral defects of the knee. Contemp Orthop 28:100–107, 1994.
39. Cosgarea AJ, DeHaven KE, Lovelock JE: The surgical treatment of arthrofibrosis of the knee. Am J Sports Med 22:184–191, 1994.
40. Cotta H: Zur Therapie der habitullen patellaren Luxation. Arch Orthop Unfallchir 51:256–271, 1959.
41. Cox JS: Evaluation of the Roux-Elmslie-Trillat procedure for knee extensor realignment. Am J Sports Med 10:303–310, 1982.
42. Cox JS: Patellofemoral problems in runners. Clin Sports Med 4:699–715, 1985.
43. Crosby EB, Insall J: Recurrent dislocation of the patella. Relation of treatment to osteoarthritis. J Bone Joint Surg Am 58:9–13, 1976.
44. DeHaven KE, Dolan WA, Mayer PJ: Chondromalacia patellae in athletes. Clinical presentation and conservative management. Am J Sports Med 7:5–11, 1979.
45. Dejour H, Walch G, Neyret P, Adeleine P: La dysplasie de la trochlea femorale. Rev Chir Orthop Reparatrice Appar Mot 76:45–54, 1990.
46. DePalma A: Diseases of the Knee. Philadelphia, JB Lippincott, 1954.
47. Derks WH, deHoose P, vanLinse B: Ultrasonographic detection of the patellar plica in the knee. J Clin Ultrason 14:355–360, 1986.
48. Desio SM, Burks RT, Bachus KN: Soft tissue restraints to lateral patellar translation in the human knee. Am J Sports Med 26:59–65, 1998.
49. DeVriese B: La signification morphologique de la rotule basee sur des recherches antropologiques. Bull Mem Soc Anthrop 4:316, 1913.
50. Dinham JM, French PR: Results of patellectomy for osteoarthritis. Postgrad Med J 48:590–593, 1972.
51. Duncan C, McKeever DC: Patellar prosthesis. J Bone Joint Surg Am 37:1074, 1955.
52. Dye SF, Boll DA: Radionuclide imaging of the patellofemoral joint in young adults with anterior knee pain. Orthop Clin North Am 17:249–262, 1986.
53. Eckstein F, Muller-Gerbl M, Putz R: Distribution of subchondral bone density and cartilage thickness in the human patella. J Anat 180(Pt 3):425–433, 1992.
54. Eckstein F, Putz R, Muller-Gerbl M, et al: Cartilage degeneration in the human patella and its relationship to the mineralisation of the underlying bone: A key to the understanding of chondromalacia patellae and femoropatellar arthrosis? Surg Radiol Anat 15:279–286, 1993.
55. Fairbank JCT, Pynsent PB, Van Poortvliet JA, Phillips H: Mechanical factors in the incidence of knee pain in adolescents and young adults. J Bone Joint Surg Br 66:685–693, 1984.
56. Farr J: Anteromedialization of the tibial tubercle for treatment of patellofemoral malpositioning and concomitant isolated patellofemoral arthrosis. Tech Orthop 12:151–164, 1997.
57. Federico DJ, Reider B: Results of isolated patellar debridement for patellofemoral pain in patients with normal patellar alignment. Am J Sports Med 25:663–669, 1997.
58. Feller JA, Bartlett RJ: Patellectomy and osteoarthritis: Arthroscopic findings following previous patellectomy. Knee Surg Sports Traumatol Arthrosc 1:159–161, 1993.
59. Feller JA, Feagin JA Jr, Garrett WE Jr: The medial patellofemoral ligament revisited: An anatomical study. Knee Surg Sports Traumatol Arthrosc 1:184–186, 1993.
60. Ferguson AB Jr, Brown TD, Fu FH, Rutkowski R: Relief of patellofemoral contact stress by anterior displacement of the tibial tubercle. J Bone Joint Surg Am 61:159–166, 1979.
61. Ferrandez L, Usabiaga J, Yubero J, et al: An experimental study of the redistribution of patellofemoral pressures by the anterior displacement of the anterior tuberosity of the tibia. Clin Orthop 238:183–189, 1989.
62. Ferretti A: Epidemiology of jumper's knee. Sports Med 3:289–295, 1986.
63. Ferretti A, Ippolito E, Mariani P, Puddu G: Jumper's knee. Am J Sports Med 11:58–62, 1983.
64. Ficat P, Hungerford D: Disorders of the Patellofemoral Joint. Baltimore, Williams & Wilkins, 1977.
65. Ficat RP, Ficat C, Gedeon P, Toussaint JB: Spongialization: A new treatment for diseased patellae. Clin Orthop 144:74–83, 1979.
66. Fithian DC, Meier SW: The case for advancement and repair of the medial patellofemoral ligament in patients with recurrent patellar instability. Operative Tech Sports Med 7:81–89, 1999.
67. Fithian DC, Mishra DK, Balen PF, et al: Instrumented measurement of patellar mobility. Am J Sports Med 23:607–615, 1995.
68. Ford DH, Post WR: Open or arthroscopic lateral release: Indications, techniques, and rehabilitation. Clin Sports Med 16:29–49, 1997.
69. Fritschy D, DeGautard R: Jumper's knee and ultrasonography. Am J Sports Med 16:637–640, 1988.
70. Fulkerson J: Disorders of the Patellofemoral Joint. Baltimore, Williams & Wilkins, 1997.
71. Fulkerson JP: Awareness of the retinaculum in evaluating patellofemoral pain. Am J Sports Med 10:147–149, 1982.
72. Fulkerson JP: Anteromedialization of the tibial tuberosity for patellofemoral malalignment. Clin Orthop 177:176–181, 1983.
73. Fulkerson JP: Patellofemoral pain disorders: Evaluation and management. J Am Acad Orthop Surg 2:124–132, 1994.
74. Fulkerson JP: Anterolateralization of the tibial tubercle. Tech Orthop 12:165–169, 1997.
75. Fulkerson JP: A clinical test for medial patella tracking (medial subluxation). Tech Orthop 12:144, 1997.
76. Fulkerson JP, Becker GJ, Meaney JA, et al: Anteromedial tibial tubercle transfer without bone graft. Am J Sports Med 18:490–496; discussion 496–497, 1990.
77. Fulkerson JP, Gossling HR: Anatomy of the knee joint lateral retinaculum. Clin Orthop 153:183–188, 1980.
78. Fulkerson JP, Hungerford DS: Disorders of the Patellofemoral Joint. Baltimore, Williams & Wilkins, 1990.
79. Fulkerson JP, Kalenak A, Rosenberg TD, Cox JS: Patellofemoral pain. Instr Course Lect 41:57–71, 1992.
80. Fulkerson JP, Langeland R: An alternative cruciate reconstruction graft: The central quadriceps tendon. Arthroscopy 11:252–254, 1995.
81. Fulkerson JP, Schutzer SF: After failure of conservative treatment for painful patellofemoral malalignment: Lateral release or realignment? Orthop Clin North Am 17:283–288, 1986.
82. Fulkerson JP, Schutzer SF, Ramsby GR, Bernstein RA: Computerized tomography of the patellofemoral joint before and after lateral release or realignment. Arthroscopy 3:19–24, 1987.
83. Fulkerson JP, Shea KP: Disorders of patellofemoral alignment. J Bone Joint Surg Am 72:1424–1429, 1990.
84. Fulkerson JP, Tennant R, Jaivin JS, Grunnet M: Histologic evidence of retinacular nerve injury associated with patellofemoral malalignment. Clin Orthop 197:196–205, 1985.
85. Fulkerson JP, Wright J, Legeyt M, Cautilli RAJ: Precise criteria of normal and abnormal patellofemoral joint alignment using three dimensional computerized tomography. J Bone Joint Surg 17:1062, 1993.
86. Galloway MT, Noyes FR: Cystic degeneration of the patella after arthroscopic chondroplasty and subchondral bone perforation. Arthroscopy 8:366–369, 1992.
87. Gerbino PG 2nd, Micheli LJ: Bucket-handle tear of the medial plica. Clin J Sport Med 6:265–268; discussion 268–269, 1996.
88. Goldthwait JE: Slipping or recurrent dislocation of the patella: With the report of eleven cases. Boston Med Surg J 150:169–174, 1904.

89. Goodfellow J, Hungerford DS, Woods C: Patello-femoral joint mechanics and pathology. 2. Chondromalacia patellae. J Bone Joint Surg 58:291–299, 1979.

90. Graf BK, Ott JW, Lange RH, Keene JS: Risk factors for restricted motion after anterior cruciate reconstruction [see comments]. Orthopedics 17:909–912, 1994.

91. Grana WA, Hinkley B, Hollingsworth S: Arthroscopic evaluation and treatment of patellar malalignment. Clin Orthop 186:122–128, 1984.

92. Grana WA, Kriegshauser LA: Scientific basis of extensor mechanism disorders. Clin Sports Med 4:247–257, 1985.

93. Grelsamer RP: Patellofemoral arthroplasty. Tech Orthop 12:200–204, 1997.

94. Grelsamer RP, Proctor CS, Bazos AN: Evaluation of patellar shape in the sagittal plane. A clinical analysis. Am J Sports Med 22:61–66, 1994.

95. Hallisey MJ, Doherty N, Bennett WF, Fulkerson JP: Anatomy of the junction of the vastus lateralis tendon and the patella. J Bone Joint Surg Am 69:545–549, 1987.

96. Hangody L, Kish G, Karpati Z, et al: Mosaicplasty for the treatment of articular cartilage defects: Application in clinical practice [see comments]. Orthopedics 21:751–756, 1998.

97. Harner CD, Irrgang JJ, Paul J, et al: Loss of motion after anterior cruciate ligament reconstruction. Am J Sports Med 20:499–506, 1992.

98. Harrington KD: Long-term results for the McKeever patellar resurfacing prosthesis used as a salvage procedure for severe chondromalacia patellae. Clin Orthop 279:201–213, 1992.

99. Hauser EDW: Total tendon transplant for slipping patella. Surg Gynecol Obstet 66:199–214, 1938.

100. Hehne HJ: Biomechanics of the patellofemoral joint and its clinical relevance. Clin Orthop 258:73–85, 1990.

101. Hejgard N, Diemer H: Bone scan in the patellofemoral pain syndrome. Int Orthop 11:29–33, 1987.

102. Henry JE, Pflum FA Jr: Arthroscopic proximal patella realignment and stabilization. Arthroscopy 11:424–425, 1995.

103. Henry JH: Conservative treatment of patellofemoral subluxation. Clin Sports Med 8:261–278, 1989.

104. Hoikka VE, Jaroma HJ, Ritsila VA: Reconstruction of the patellar articulation with periosteal graft. Acta Orthop Scand 61:36–39, 1990.

105. Homminga GN, Bulstra SK, Bouwmeester PS: Perichondral grafting for cartilage lesions of the knee. J Bone Joint Surg Br 72:1003–1007, 1990.

105a. Hsu RWW, Himeno S, Coventry MB, Chao EYS: Normal axial alignment of the lower extremity and load bearing distribution at the knee. Clin Orthop 255:215–227, 1990.

106. Huberti HH, Hayes WC: Patellofemoral contact pressures. The influence of Q-angle and tendofemoral contact. J Bone Joint Surg Am 66:715–724, 1984.

107. Hughston JC: Subluxation of the patella. J Bone Joint Surg Am 50:1003–1026, 1968.

108. Hughston JC, Deese M: Medial subluxation of the patella as a complication of lateral retinacular release. Am J Sports Med 16:383–388, 1988.

109. Hughston JC, Flandry F, Brinker MR, et al: Surgical correction of medial subluxation of the patella. Am J Sports Med 24:486–491, 1996.

110. Hughston JC, Walsh WM: Proximal and distal reconstruction of the extensor mechanism for patellar subluxation. Clin Orthop 144:36–42, 1979.

111. Hughston JC, Walsh WM, Puddu G: Patellar Subluxation and Dislocation. Philadelphia, WB Saunders, 1984.

112. Hungerford DS, Barry M: Biomechanics of the patellofemoral joint. Clin Orthop 144:9–15, 1979.

113. Hungerford DS, Lennox DW: Rehabilitation of the knee in disorders of the patellofemoral joint: Relevant biomechanics. Orthop Clin North Am 14:397–402, 1983.

114. Insall J, Bullough PG, Burstein AH: Proximal "tube" realignment of the patella for chondromalacia patellae. Clin Orthop 144:63–69, 1979.

115. Insall J, Falvo KA, Wise DW: Chondromalacia patellae. A prospective study. J Bone Joint Surg Am 58:1–8, 1976.

116. Insall J, Salvati E: Patella position in the normal knee joint. Radiology 101:101–104, 1971.

117. Insall JN, Aglietti P, Tria AJ Jr: Patellar pain and incongruence. II: Clinical application. Clin Orthop 176:225–232, 1983.

118. Jackson RW, Marshall DJ, Fujisawa Y: The pathologic medial shelf. Orthop Clin North Am 13:307, 1982.

119. Jackson RW, Patel D: Synovial lesions: Plica. In McGinty JB (ed): Operative Arthroscopy. Philadelphia, Lippincott-Raven, 1996.

120. James SL: Chondromalacia of the patella in the adolescent. In Kennedy JC (ed): The Injured Adolescent Knee. Baltimore, Williams & Wilkins, 1979.

121. Jee WH, Choe BY, Kim JM, et al: The plica syndrome: Diagnostic value of MRI with arthroscopic correlation. J Comput Assist Tomogr 22:814–818, 1998.

122. Johnson DP, Wakeley CJ, Watt I: Magnetic resonance imaging of patellar tendonitis. J Bone Joint Surg Br 78:452–457, 1996.

123. Johnson LL: Arthroscopic abrasion arthroplasty historical and pathologic perspective: Present status. Arthroscopy 2:54–69, 1986.

124. Johnson LL, van Dyk GE, Green JR, et al: Clinical assessment of asymptomatic knees: Comparison of men and women. Arthroscopy 14:347–359, 1998.

125. Joyce JJI, Harty M: Surgery of the synovial fold. In Casscels W (ed): Arthroscopy: Diagnosis and Surgical Practice. Philadelphia, Lea & Febiger, 1984, pp 201–209.

126. Kannus P, Nittymaki S: Which factors predict outcome in the nonoperative treatment of patellofemoral pain syndrome? A prospective follow-up study. Med Sci Sports Exerc 26:289–296, 1994.

127. Kaplan E: Some aspects of functional anatomy of the human knee joint. Clin Orthop 23:18, 1962.

128. Keller PM, Shelbourne KD, McCarroll JR, Rettig AC: Nonoperatively treated isolated posterior cruciate ligament injuries. Am J Sports Med 21:132–136, 1993.

129. Kelly MA, Griffin FM: Proximal realignment of the patellofemoral joint. Tech Orthop 12:178–184, 1997.

130. Kelly MA, Insall JN: Patellectomy. Orthop Clin North Am 17:289–295, 1986.

131. Khan KM, Visentini PJ, Kiss ZS, et al: Correlation of ultrasound and magnetic resonance imaging with clinical outcome after patellar tenotomy: Prospective and retrospective studies. Victorian Institute of Sport Tendon Study Group. Clin J Sport Med 9:129–137, 1999.

132. Kim SJ, Choe WS: Pathological infrapatellar plica: A report of two cases and literature review. Arthroscopy 12:236–239, 1996.

133. Kolowich PA, Paulos LE, Rosenberg TD, et al: Lateral release of the patella: Indications and contraindications. Am J Sports Med 18:359–365, 1990.

134. Kosarek FJ, Helms CA: The MR appearance of the infrapatellar plica. AJR Am J Roentgenol 172:481–484, 1999.

135. Krajca-Radcliffe JB, Coker TP: Patellofemoral arthroplasty. A 2- to 18-year followup study. Clin Orthop 330:143–151, 1996.

136. Kramers-de Quervain IA, Biedert R, Stussi E: Quantitative gait analysis in patients with medial patellar instability following lateral retinacular release. Knee Surg Sports Traumatol Arthrosc 5:95–101, 1997.

137. Kujala UM, Dvist M, Osterman K, et al: Factors predisposing army conscripts to knee extension injuries incurred in a physical training program. Clin Orthop 210:203–212, 1986.

138. Kujala UM, Friberg O, Aalto T, et al: Lower limb asymmetry and patellofemoral joint incongruence in the etiology of knee exertion injuries in athletes. Int J Sports Med 8:214–220, 1987.

139. Larson RL, Cabaud HE, Slocum DB, et al: The patellar compression syndrome: Surgical treatment by lateral retinacular release. Clin Orthop 134:158–167, 1978.

140. Laurin C, Dussault R, Levesque H: The tangential x-ray investigation of patellofemoral joint. Clin Orthop Rel Res 144:16–26, 1979.

141. Lennox IA, Cobb AG, Knowles J, Bentley G: Knee function after patellectomy. A 12- to 48-year follow-up. J Bone Joint Surg Br 76:485–487, 1994.

142. Leslie IJ, Bentley G: Arthroscopy in the diagnosis of chondromalacia patellae. Ann Rheum Dis 37:540–547, 1978.

143. Lieb FF, Perry J: Quadriceps function. An anatomical and mechanical study using amputated limbs. J Bone Joint Surg Am 50:1535, 1968.

144. Lindberg U, Lysholm J, Gillquist J: The correlation between arthroscopic findings and the patellofemoral pain syndrome. Arthroscopy 2:103–107, 1986.

145. Lindenfeld TM, Wojtys EM: Operative treatment of arthrofibrosis of the knee. J Bone Joint Surg Am 81:1772–1783, 1999.

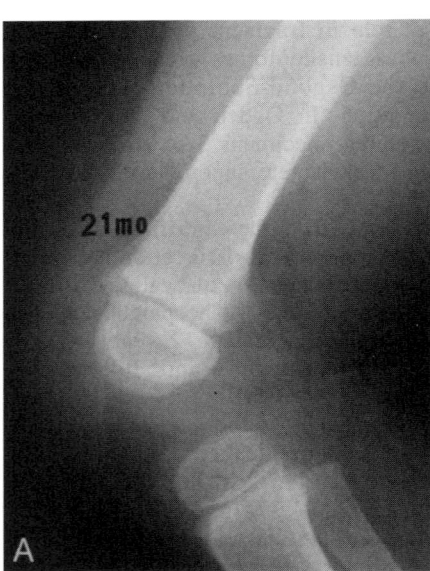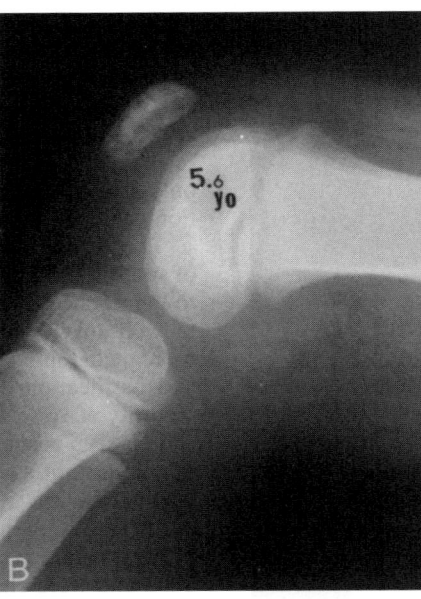

Figure 28E7–11. *A* and *B*, Progressive radiographic appearance of the patella. Note variance of shape and ossification pattern.

graphic tomography, computed tomography (CT) scans, or magnetic resonance imaging (MRI) may be needed to evaluate the fragment–patellar body articular surface relationships in a symptomatic patient. These studies determine if the division is complete (i.e., with intra-articular separation) or if an intact articular mantle is present with fragmentation of the subchondral bone. This subchondral/articular cartilage division is not unlike the situation seen with osteochondritis dissecans.

Treatment depends on symptom acuity and severity. In chronic cases, modification of activity over 3 to 4 weeks may be all that is required. Spontaneous union may occur (Fig. 28E7–14). In acute situations, the pain is secondary to an acute separation between the fragment and the main patellar body. Immobilization with a cylinder cast for 3 weeks usually resolves the pain. In a subacute or chronic case, if symptoms persist, or if acute symptoms occur at the fragment site despite nonoperative measures, surgical excision of the fragment and repair of the quadriceps retinaculum are used for types I and III.[2, 5] Following a brief postoperative period of immobilization for comfort, motion and strengthening exercises are begun. Return to play is predicated on attaining full range of motion, strength, and endurance. A large, type II, completely loose fragment that involves a significant portion of the lateral patella may require internal fixation and grafting or resection, or, if anatomic reduction is not possible, fragment excision is advised (Fig. 28E7–15). Ogata[9] reported results of vastus lateralis release in seven patients with type III and three patients with type II lesions with articular continuity. Clinical results were better in type III than in type II patients. Six of seven type III and none of type II patients went on to radiologic union. Mori and associates[8] reported their results of lateral retinacular excision in 16 knees of 15 patients, seven with type II and nine with type III bipartite patellae. All had arthroscopically documented intact articular surfaces. These authors felt that excessive tension of the lateral retinaculum predisposed the lesion to not heal. All of their patients demonstrated limited patellar mobility preoperatively. A strip of lateral retinaculum 0.5 to 1.0 cm wide and 6 to 8 cm long was removed. All patients had resolution of tenderness at the fragment. Seventy percent of patients had radiographic union within 4 months, and 94% were united by 8 months. Functional scores were excellent or good in all patients. The common theme of these papers is reduction of lateral retinacular tension. The poorer results seen in Ogata's type II patients may be due to the large fragment size and the limited direct vector applied by the vastus lateralis in contrast to type III lesions.

An acute, inferior patellar pole ("sleeve") fracture may be confused with a type I bipartite patella. This fracture occurs in 8- to 12-year-old children involved in jumping, or after acute knee flexion following a fall. Its name is derived from the cuff of unossified patella and articular cartilage that is avulsed, a kind of sleeve of tissue. The

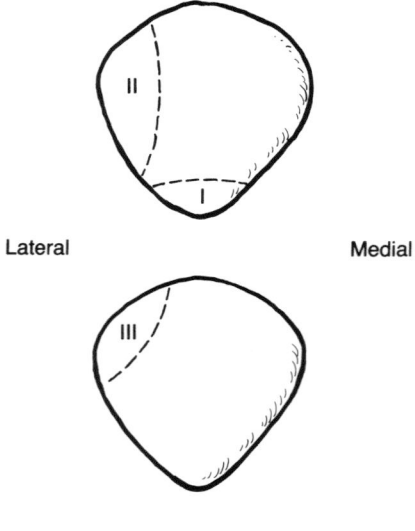

Figure 28E7–12. Saupe's classification of bipartite patellae.

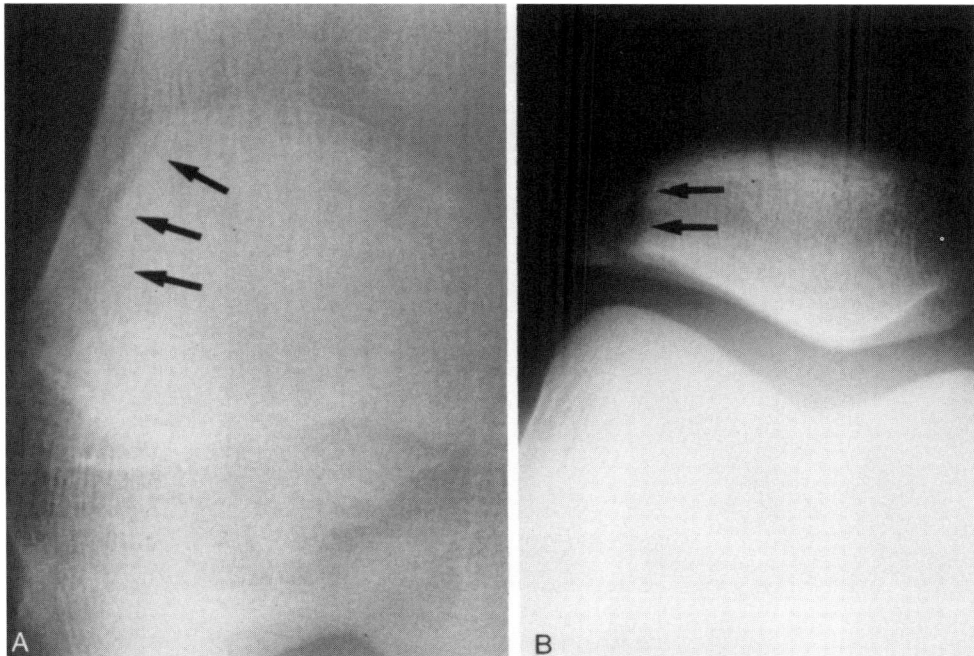

Figure 28E7–13. Acute fracture. Note irregularity and displacement.

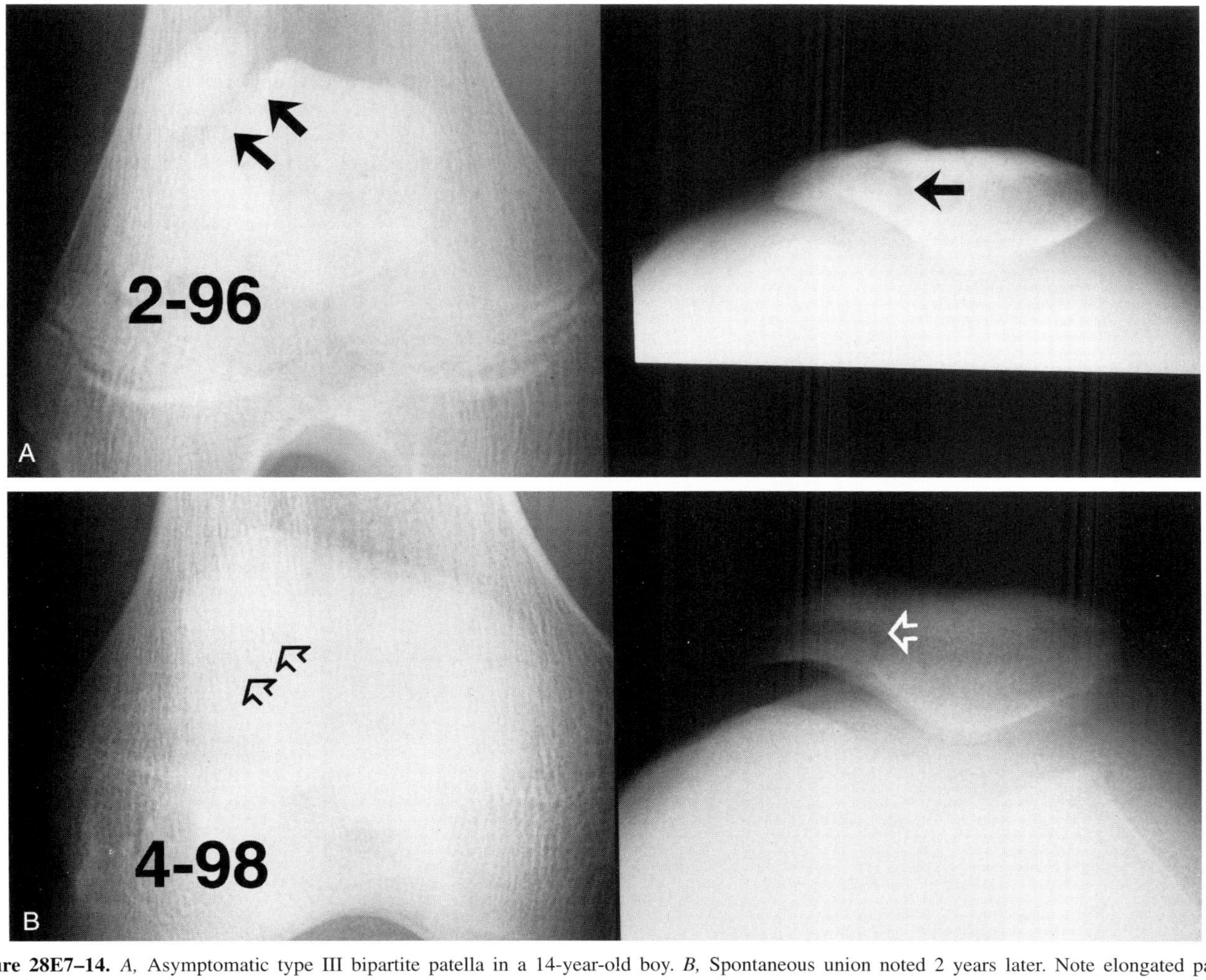

Figure 28E7–14. *A,* Asymptomatic type III bipartite patella in a 14-year-old boy. *B,* Spontaneous union noted 2 years later. Note elongated patellar lateral facet.

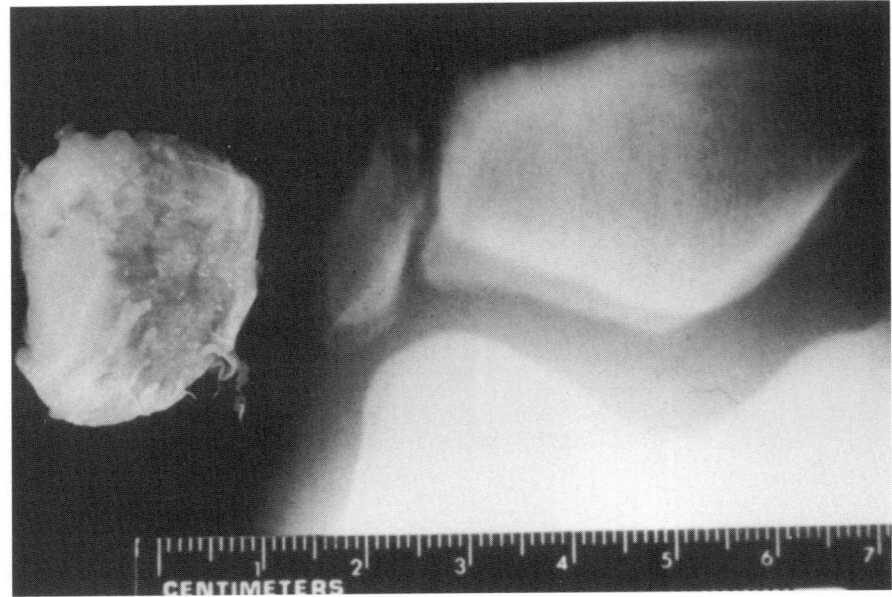

Figure 28E7–15. Chronically symptomatic separated Saupe type II bipartite patella and surgical specimen. There was no history of significant knee trauma.

fracture is much more common at the inferior patellar pole but can occur at the proximal pole as well. Because most of the distal patella and fragment is chondral and is not well visualized radiographically, the diagnosis is often missed, or it is dismissed as a small chip fracture (Fig. 28E7–16). Patients complain of severe pain and giving way of the knee. Marked tenderness is present at the fracture, and a gap may be palpated. Patella alta is often seen with displaced fractures, along with an extensor lag and hemarthrosis. Radiographs show soft tissue swelling and a fracture fragment with varying degrees of ossification and displacement. Treatment depends on the amount of displacement, which may be difficult to determine on routine radiographs because of the nonossified nature of the fragment. In cases with uncertainty about the fragment, MRI is helpful.[1] Minimally displaced fractures are treated by immobilization for 3 to 4 weeks. Displaced fractures are treated by open reduction and fixation to restore articular

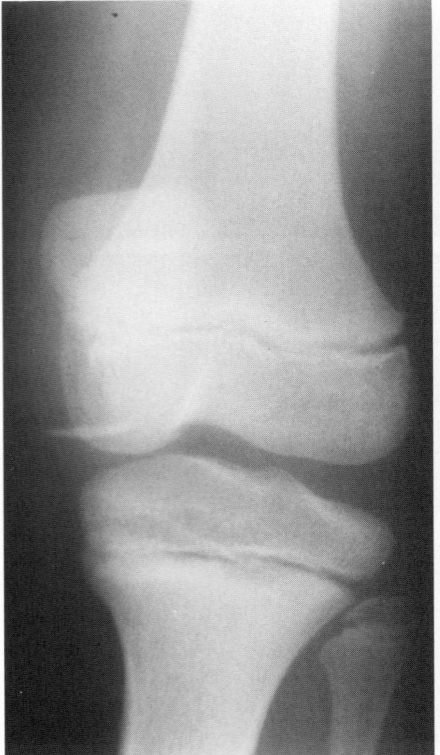
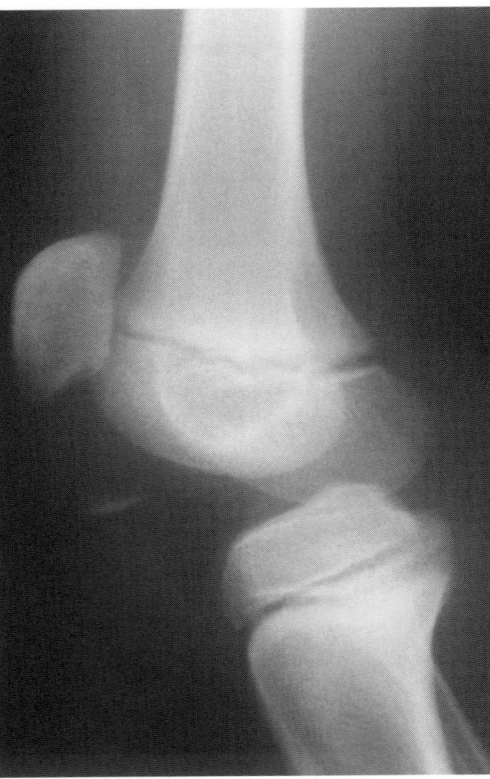

Figure 28E7–16. *A* and *B,* "Sleeve" fracture of the patella. Note patella alta and appearance of a small "chip" fragment in the patellar tendon that represents the inferior border of the ossified patellar fragment.

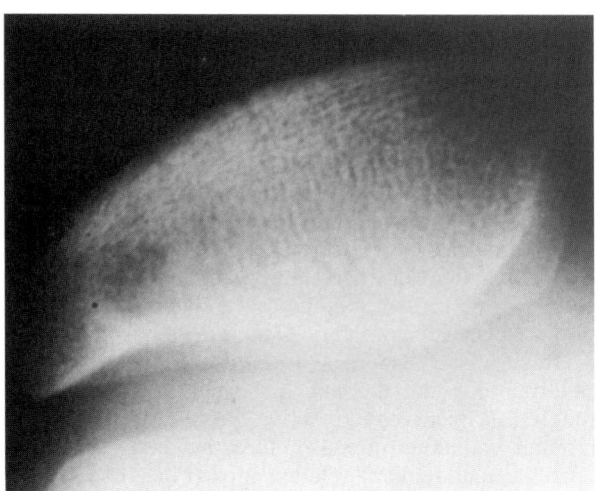

Figure 28E7–17. Dorsal defect of the patella. The patient was asymptomatic, and the knee was nontender at this site.

congruity and extensor mechanism isometry. Fracture fixation can be done by direct suture or internal fixation.

The rare dorsal patellar defect is another incidentally noted patellar roentgenographic curiosity (Fig. 28E7–17). In a review of 1349 consecutive knee radiographs, Johnson and Brogdon[7] found 13 lesions in 12 patients (1%). Although 10 of their 12 patients were female, most studies cite a higher male preponderance. The defect is most often located in the dorsal superolateral patella. The defect has been noted to resolve spontaneously with growth and may be a normal variant of ossification.[13] Van Holsbeeck and colleagues[14] analyzed 2286 knee radiographs and noted six patients with dorsal defects, four of whom had an associated bipartite patella. These authors suggested that the defect is a stress-induced anomaly of ossification caused by traction forces of the insertion of the vastus lateralis with patellar subluxation. Goergen and colleagues[4] reviewed dorsal patellar defects in seven patients, two of whom were symptomatic. Arthrograms in four patients were normal. Haswell and coworkers[6] reviewed cases of patellar defects from 3 centers and described 16 cases, of which 3 patients were symptomatic. Twelve of the sixteen patients were between the ages of 10 and 19 years. Defects averaged 9 mm in diameter (range, 4 to 26 mm). Biopsies in two patients showed the cartilage to be intact and demonstrated normal bone repair without inflammation. At follow-up, spontaneous resolution of the defect occurred in three of five untreated patients.

Benign lesions such as stress fractures, osteoid osteoma, or subacute osteomyelitis must be considered in the differential diagnosis. Osteochondritis dissecans lesions are located in a significantly different position than dorsal patellar defects, that is, convex, inferior (below the transverse central axis), and medial. Dorsal defects of the patella are radiologic curiosities that resolve spontaneously, not unlike nonossifying fibromas; although they occasionally cause a diagnostic puzzle, these defects require little intervention.

Anterior Knee Pain

Over a millennium ago, Galen[7] noted, "The patella covers the condyles of the underlying bone in well-suited depressions—some call this bone the knee cap, some the millstone." Anterior knee pain, especially in adolescent patients, is often perceived as a millstone about the treating orthopedist's neck. Complaints about the anterior knee have been called the "low back pain of knee surgeons." Most past data concerning anterior knee complaints represent a series of mixed diagnoses and a broad spectrum of ages (usually adults) among patients whose problems occurred following direct knee trauma. This section focuses on the commonly encountered condition of anterior knee complaints in adolescents.

The term *chondromalacia patellae* first appeared in published form in 1922 as used by Koenig. Karlson credits Aleman[2] with the first use of the term in his (Aleman's) laboratory as early as 1917. "Chondromalacia patellae" was first quoted in the English literature by Kulowski in 1933.[15] All of these authors used the term to refer to gross articular patellar changes seen intraoperatively or at postmortem examination.[2, 4, 15]

During the past several decades, the meaning of *chondromalacia patellae* has been changed to refer to an ill-defined clinical entity of anterior knee pain attributed to a deranged patellar articular surface. This knee ache commonly occurs during the teenage years in two types of patients: active athletes involved in jumping or kneeling sports; and nonathletic, inactive, often overweight adolescents, commonly girls.[31, 32, 33, 36]

The true cause of this adolescent nontraumatic anterior knee pain is unknown. Theories of minor knee and patellar malalignment, altered patellar blood flow, quadriceps retinacular stress and neuroma formation,[8] imbalanced muscle firing sequence between medial and lateral quadriceps muscles,[34] and overuse from sports have been offered as explanations for this condition. The cause of this discomfort appears to be multifactorial. The condition should be referred to as *idiopathic* anterior knee pain and efforts directed to identify causative factors.

History and Physical Examination

The patient usually complains of vague, poorly localized, anterior knee discomfort. When asked to indicate the focus of this discomfort, he or she encompasses the entire front of the knee with his or her hand, a maneuver I refer to as the grab sign (Fig. 28E7–18). I find this sign helpful to differentiate this type of anterior knee pain from other disorders in which the focus of discomfort is very specifically indicated. Patients commonly complain of discomfort following prolonged sitting (theater sign), with stair ascent and descent, and with increased levels of activity, although the latter is an inconsistent symptom. They may complain of a feeling of locking of the knee, but on further questioning, this is more a feeling of catching or pseudo-locking with no true mechanical block. This feeling may be associated with a sensation of knee instability and giving way, perhaps secondary to reflex quadriceps inhibition. Complaints of occasional joint swelling are common, although they are not often well documented by other observers. Some patients also complain of pain about the distal hamstrings. Anterior knee complaints are usually bilateral

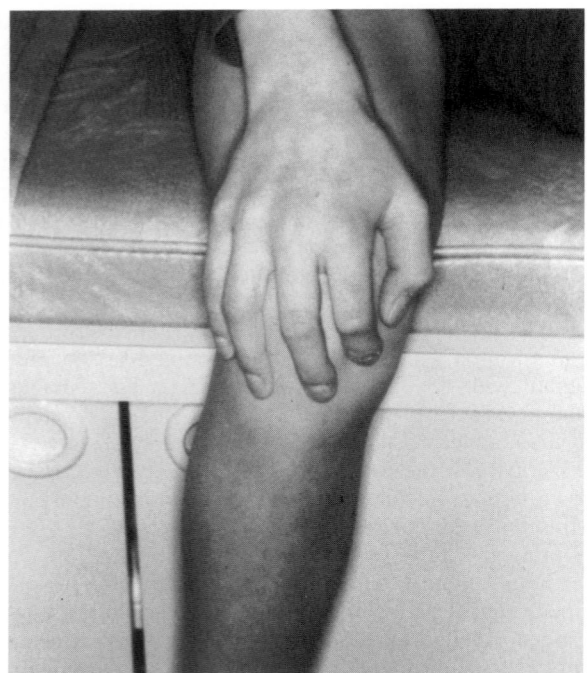

Figure 28E7–18. "Grab sign"—nonspecific localization of anterior knee pain.

with varying side-to-side intensity. Growth rate should be determined and is especially important during the time of peak height velocity.

An accurate assessment of the patient's training program is essential to rule out overuse factors as having a significant etiologic role. Running stadium steps, using stair-climbing exercise equipment, running up and down hills, and performing deep squats with or without weights are all important stress factors at the patellofemoral joint. Previous knee injury or surgery and rehabilitation should be explored in an effort to better understand the starting point of a patient's complaints. Program compliance may also be assessed. The knee may act as a target for somatization of complaints to avoid school, work, or athletics, so functional versus true organic disease must be kept in mind, especially in adolescents. Vague, nonanatomic complaints combined with incapacitating pain, especially of a burning type, out of proportion to any injury or physical findings, should alert the physician to the possibility of reflex sympathetic dystrophy. An important cautionary finding in patients with adolescent knee pain is a parent (usually a mother) who talks more than the patient. The surgeon must be wary of this scenario.

Physical examination is done with the patient appropriately dressed, not merely with slacks rolled above the knee or skirt hiked above the patella. The physical examination must take into account the entire lower extremity in stance and gait. Hip examination is a part of any knee evaluation to rule out a hip disorder such as slipped capital femoral epiphysis, with referred pain to the knee. Knee pain is hip pain until proven otherwise. One must differentiate joint-line tenderness from retinacular tenderness. Anterior joint-line tenderness commonly occurs in patients with patellar disorders in contrast to mid-to-posterior joint-line tender-

ness characteristic of true meniscal disease. Quadriceps, hamstring, and calf muscle tone, definition, and flexibility should be assessed (Fig. 28E7–19). The physical examination provides a measure of the patient's cooperation, interest, and capability of following directions of treatment protocols. A patient who is a true "motor moron" with limited kinesthetic sense, or a truculent, misanthropic adolescent not interested in an effort at improvement, is often unmasked during this process. Range of motion, knee joint stability, patellar tracking stability, focal tenderness, and presence of an effusion are assessed on physical examination. Patients with "ordinary" anterior knee pain are without effusion, and tenderness is diffuse. Patellar tracking is best observed with the patient seated and the knee put through full passive and active ranges of motion. The physician maintains direct en face, hands-on observation of patellar and femoral relationships (Fig. 28E7–20). Patella alta and patella infra are easily recognized by this method. Much has recently been made of the concepts of patellar tilt and patellar glide. Although important components of patellar motion, normal values for these entities have not been agreed upon, and no data have been published specific to children. The patella follows a toroidal course within the femoral groove. Its motion is not simply flexion and extension but more like a bobsled running in a chute.

Patellofemoral crepitus is not necessarily an indicator of intra-articular disease. Abernethy and colleagues[1] examined 123 medical students younger than age 25 and found asymptomatic patellofemoral crepitus in more than 60%.

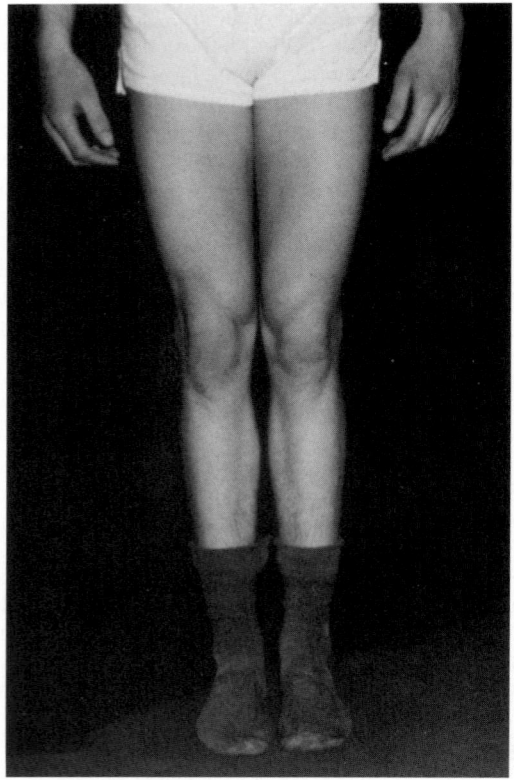

Figure 28E7–19. Excellent quadriceps and calf definition in a high-level athlete.

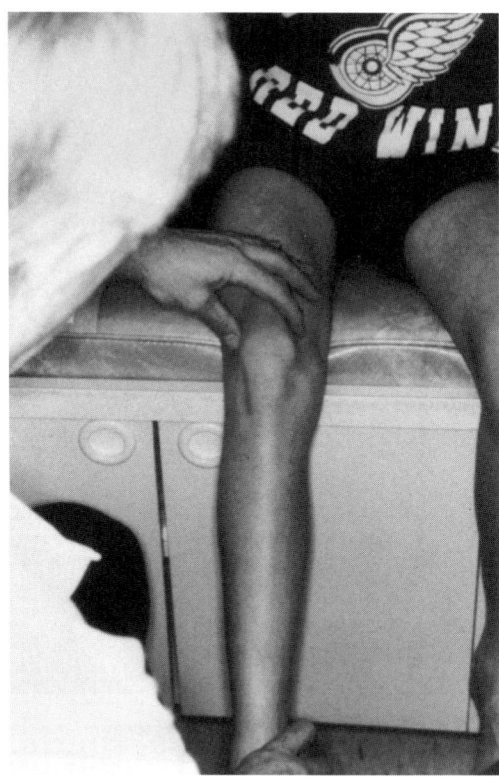

Figure 28E7–20. Direct clinical examination of patellar tracking.

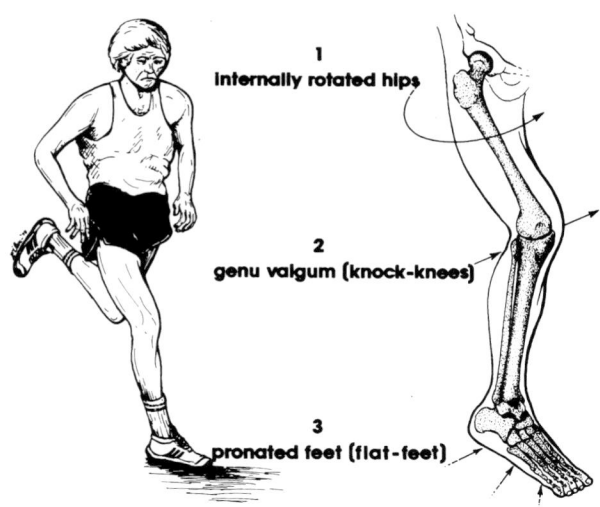

Figure 28E7–21. "Miserable malalignment syndrome," which can manifest itself as anterior knee pain.

Only 29% of the patients had previous transient patellofemoral discomfort. Only 3% had chronic anterior knee pain that limited activity. Articular surfaces are usually pristine in young patients with crepitus. The cause of such sounds in this age group remains enigmatic.

Attempts to elicit patellar tenderness when the patella is displaced laterally or medially while the knee is fully extended (Perkins' sign) may be misleading in patients if synovitis is present and the synovium is trapped on the undersurface of the patella. A variety of patellar compression tests with or without quadriceps contraction can produce significant discomfort in previously asymptomatic normal patients. Excessive patellar mobility as evidenced by patient apprehension is a sign of patellar instability. Remote factors that can affect patellofemoral articulation range from excessive femoral or tibial rotation and abnormal foot and ankle mechanics, primarily excessive pronation, to the miserable malalignment syndrome (Fig. 28E7–21).

Imaging

Anteroposterior, lateral, tunnel, and skyline (patellar tangential) radiographs provide information about patellar size, shape, and position.

A variety of skyline views are described to ascertain the relationship between the patella and its femoral trochlear groove. Brattstrom determined the sulcus angle to measure femoral trochlear depth. Merchant and colleagues[21] suggested a technique with the knee in less flexion to assess the congruence angle. If the patellar articular ridge is lateral to a line central and perpendicular to the sulcus, the congruence angle is positive; if medial, the angle is negative. In 100 consecutive patients, Merchant and associates[21] found an average congruence angle of minus 6 degrees with a standard deviation of 11 degrees. They believed a congruence angle of greater than 16 degrees was abnormal at the 95% confidence limit. No significant difference was seen related to gender, age, laterality, or patella alta in 75 of those patients without patellar instability. Twenty-five patients with proven recurrent patellar dislocation had an average congruence angle of plus 22 degrees. Laurin and coworkers[16] described a roentgen tangential view made with the knee flexed at 20 to 30 degrees with the patient supine. A line between the superior femoral condyles and the lateral patellar facet margin forms the lateral patellofemoral angle (Fig. 28E7–22). The normal angle is open laterally and, in cases of abnormal patellar tilt, the lines are parallel or open medially. They felt that the measurement was helpful in assessing patients with patellar tilt or subluxation, but it was not useful in patients with knee pain alone without evidence of instability. These axial patellar views are highly position-dependent, and care must be taken to ensure reliability and reproducibility. Unfortunately, they are also static assessments, whereas most symptomatic patellar abnormalities occur dynamically.

Maldague and Malghem[19] suggest doing a tangential view of the patella with the quadriceps relaxed, and then a repeat view with the quadriceps contracted, to assess the more dynamic relationships of the patella. Difficulty with positioning may limit the effectiveness of such views. Schutzer and colleagues[28] found no significant differences between radiographs taken with or without quadriceps contractions. Fulkerson and colleagues[6, 7] and others[10] documented the benefit of the use of CT scans of the patellofemoral joint following lateral release or realignment procedures. These authors advocated CT scans as part of the analysis of complex cases, especially those that have failed to improve following previous surgery, and specifically found it helpful to evaluate patellar tilt with or with-

At times of mild recurrence of symptoms, the patient is encouraged to continue a maintenance program emphasizing hamstring and quadriceps flexibility and strength. Return to this program usually allows resolution of symptoms. If the patient is unresponsive to a well-monitored program, one must question the accuracy of the diagnosis and search for other causes of symptoms, including emotional and nonorthopedic sources of pain.

Quadriceps open-chain exercises incorporating long arc extension should be avoided because they produce excessive patellofemoral loads. Full squat exercises with free weights or use of a weight machine requiring knee hyperflexion and rapid extension should also be avoided because of the high patellofemoral joint reaction forces that are generated.

Anterior knee pain appears to be a disorder awaiting the invention of the arthroscope. Arthroscopy is a useful technique for diagnosis and treatment of patellar instability. It should have little role in treatment and diagnosis of nonspecific knee pain. Goodfellow[9] suggested that arthroscopic intervention for idiopathic anterior knee pain was no more rational than using skull burr holes to treat a headache. Lateral retinacular release should be reserved for patients with documented patellar tilt and lateral patellar facet overload. Lateral retinacular release, even when done arthroscopically, carries a significant complication rate.[29, 37] Tibial tubercle elevation to diminish patellofemoral contact forces is contraindicated in skeletally immature patients. Patellectomy for anterior knee pain alone should be condemned, especially in skeletally immature patients. Dimi-

nution in quadriceps force and abnormal knee cosmesis are sinister sequelae of patellectomy.[11]

"Chondromalacia patellae" is an inaccurate, nonspecific term and should not be equated with anterior knee pain. If the patient has pain at the anterior knee, that is what it should be called—idiopathic anterior knee pain—until a satisfactory cause is established. Diagnostic efforts should focus on identifying specific causes of the pain, be they patellar instability, intra-articular disorders, overuse, referred pain, or other causes. Diligence in history taking, physical examination, and various imaging studies is required. Not all knee pain that is unexplained should be written off as chondromalacia patellae[12, 26] (Fig. 28E7–24).

Idiopathic anterior knee pain is usually self-limited and most common and most intense during periods of rapid growth, with the majority of normal lower extremity growth focused about the knee. Nonoperative management by a variety of methods, including nonspecific ones, allows resolution of symptoms in the great majority of patients. An important factor in the treatment of anterior knee pain patients is reassurance of the patient and family of the nonfatal nature of these complaints and the eventual excellent outcome without degenerative knee joint sequelae. Athletes participating in sports requiring high-demand repetitive tasks are best managed by a modified training schedule, participation in a rehabilitation program, and an enhanced understanding of the nature of the condition. These techniques will go a long way toward allowing the athlete to continue sports. There is no evidence that idiopathic adolescent anterior knee pain leads to the develop-

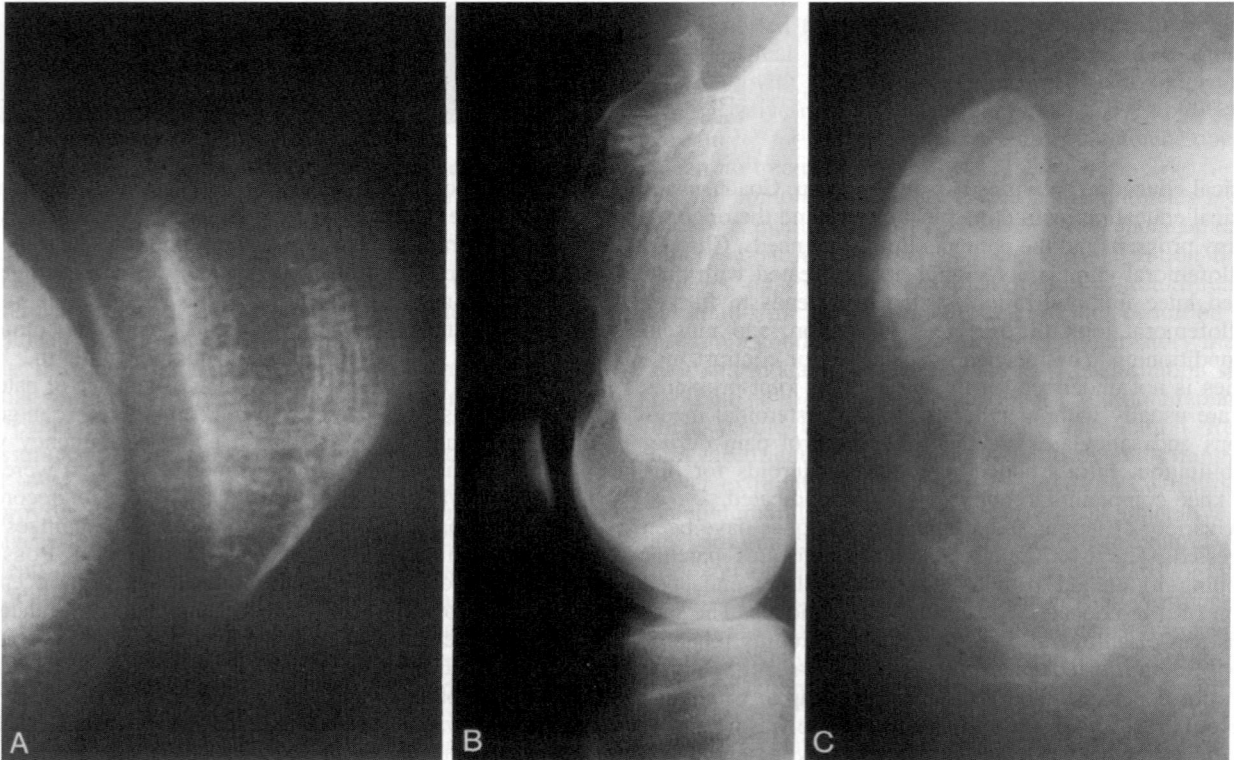

Figure 28E7–24. Anterior knee pain caused by *(A)* patellar stress fracture, *(B)* osteochondroma with quadriceps impingement, and *(C)* patellar aneurysmal bone cyst.

ment of progressive articular malacic changes, early joint senescence, or patellofemoral arthritis.

Plica

The synovial anatomy of the knee was first studied in detail with cadaveric dissections by Fullerton in 1916 and Mayeda in 1918 and arthroscopically by Iino in 1939.[1] The knee is thought to be formed in three compartments, and synovial folds or plicae represent remnants of these compartments' divisions.[2, 3, 5] Normal plicae are well-vascularized, thin, pliable synovial folds. The infrapatellar or anterior plica is located in the femoral notch traversing from the end of the articular femoral surface to the tibial plateau in the sagittal plane. It is commonly called the *ligamentum mucosum* and may be mistaken by an unsophisticated arthroscopist for the anterior cruciate ligament (Fig. 28E7–25). The anterior plica is occasionally thickened and forms a septum between the lateral and medial compartments that makes arthroscopic viewing difficult. The suprapatellar plica is present in the superior portion of the suprapatellar pouch, extending laterally from the medial capsule (Fig. 28E7–26). It may create a septum, sometimes fenestrated, across the entire pouch. The medial patellar plica is a very common finding, and it varies in width, length, and thickness. This medial patellar shelf varies in morphology and may be a complete band or one that is fenestrated or duplicated (Fig. 28E7–27). This shelflike structure courses from the superior patellar or midpatellar medial capsule to the medial fat pad. The medial plica is occasionally contiguous with a suprapatellar one. A rare lateral plica that travels from the superior or midlateral capsule to the lateral tibial plateau completes the array (Fig. 28E7–28).

The plicae may become edematous, thickened, and hyalinized and may cause impingement symptoms. The proposed pathophysiology occurs from one of two inciting

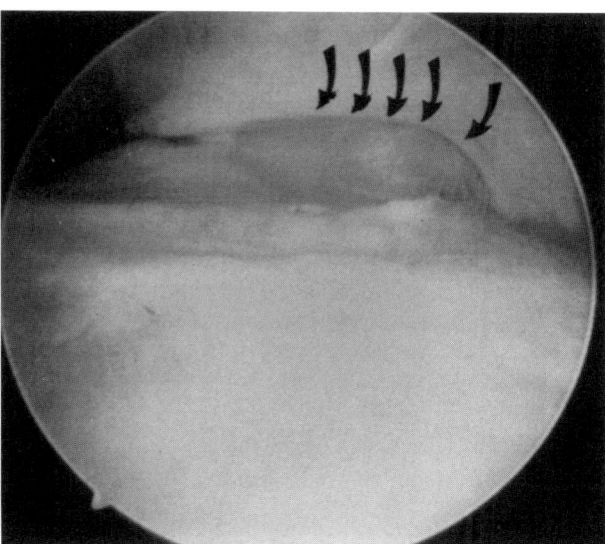

Figure 28E7–26. Normal suprapatellar plica.

mechanisms: direct trauma to the synovium or overuse from task-specific demands accompanied by minor aberrancies of patellofemoral mechanics. The resultant hemorrhage, edema, and progressive fibrosis cause a thickened pathologic plica that becomes a space-occupying lesion and acts like a bow-string that may abrade surrounding tissues (Fig. 28E7–29). Pathologic plicae are reported in 5% to 10% of cases requiring arthroscopic surgery. Disease has not been associated with the anterior plica.

The clinical history is one of nonspecific anterior knee pain. Most patients complain of a popping or snapping sensation during a specific arc of knee flexion. Pain may become progressive with increased levels of activity, especially ones requiring knee flexion and extension. A previous history of a direct blow to the knee with a transient asymptomatic period may be a factor in as many as 50% of cases. A significant increase in sports training may cause overuse and symptoms, especially after activities necessitating squatting or kneeling.

Physical examination findings are limited. There is local tenderness when the cordlike plica along the medial or lateral parapatellar area is palpated. A palpable snap or pop is elicited during knee flexion from 40 to 60 degrees. Medial or lateral patellar translation with the knee in 20 to 30 degrees of flexion may reproduce the pain as the knee is brought from flexion to extension, with associated internal tibial rotation. Knee effusion is rare and, if present, should cause consideration of other diagnoses. Patellar instability should be ruled out. Anterior joint-line tenderness may be seen and should not be misinterpreted as meniscal in origin.

Imaging studies are not particularly helpful. Routine radiographs are normal. There are no specific, reproducible criteria for pathologic plica diagnosis by MRI.

Differential diagnoses include conditions that cause snapping or popping about the knee such as meniscal tears, discoid menisci, loose bodies, and patellar instability. The diagnosis of pathologic plica is usually one of exclusion after the more common considerations are assessed.

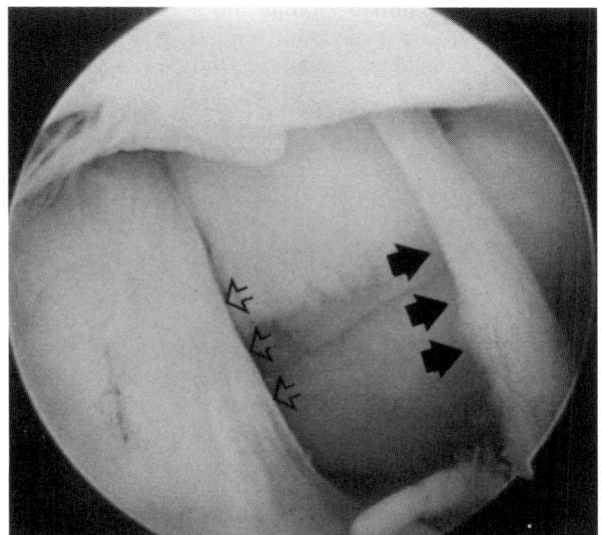

Figure 28E7–25. Ligamentum mucosum *(dark arrows)* and anterior cruciate ligament *(open arrows).*

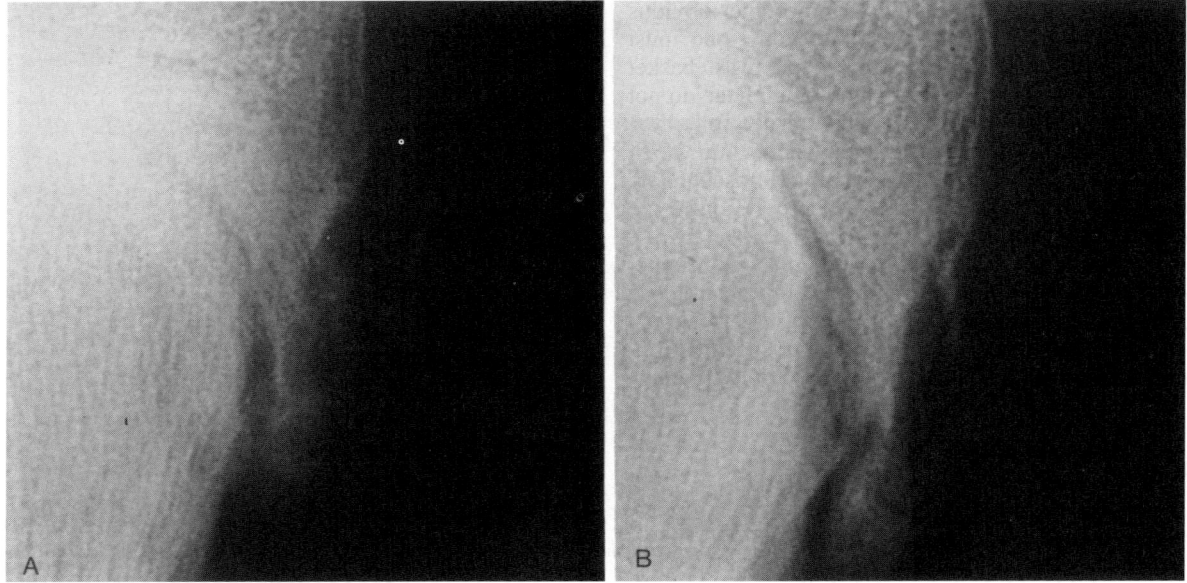

Figure 28E7–32. *A* and *B*, Healing chronic tubercle avulsions.

On clinical examination, there is exquisite tenderness with swelling at the tubercle. In older children (early teens), tenderness is often seen at the patellar tendon and peripatellar areas as well. Bilateral prominence of the tubercle may be present but, commonly, only one side is symptomatic (Fig. 28E7–33). Diminished hamstring, quadriceps, and lower extremity flexibility is usually seen. In very rapidly growing children, patella alta is also seen.

Varied patterns of tubercle ossification are seen radiographically, depending on the patient's age and skeletal development. Tubercle fragmentation is common, as is partial fragment coalescence (Fig. 28E7–34). In as many as 50% of the cases reviewed by Krause and coworkers,[7] a discrete ossicle had formed, separate from the tubercle.

Associated soft tissue swelling was a constant finding, regardless of the tubercle's configuration in their series.

Radiographs are done for diagnostic completeness. One must not be lulled into complacency by the seemingly obvious and mundane diagnosis, especially in unilateral cases. D'Ambrosia and MacDonald[3] warned about pitfalls of OSD diagnosis and reported two cases of clinically obvious OSD, which, in retrospect, turned out to be osteomyelitis of the tubercle in one case and an arteriovenous malformation (AVM) in the other. Concurrent disease may be present in patients with OSD and benign and malignant conditions masked by the more common and apparent appearance of OSD symptoms and signs. OSD and slipped capital femoral epiphysis may coexist in that the conditions

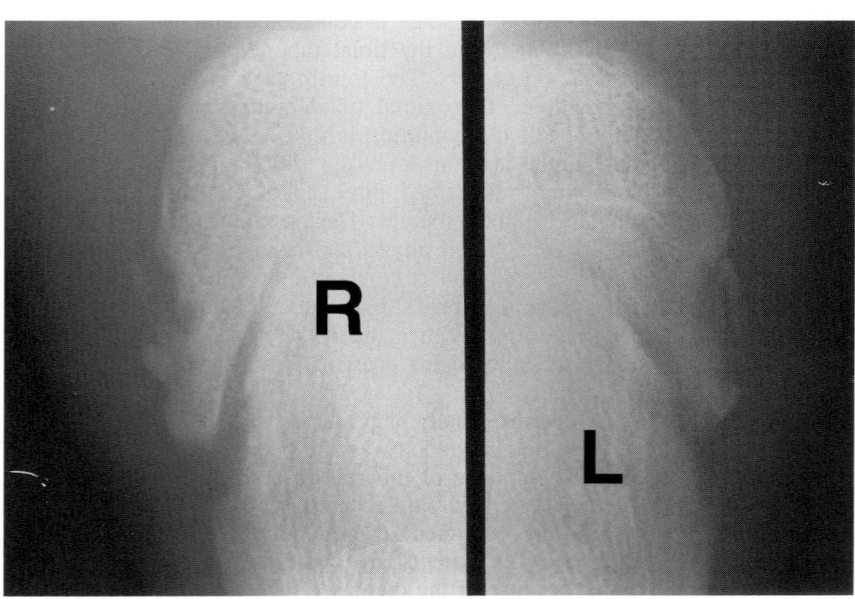

Figure 28E7–33. Bilateral Osgood-Schlatter disease changes. Only the left side was symptomatic.

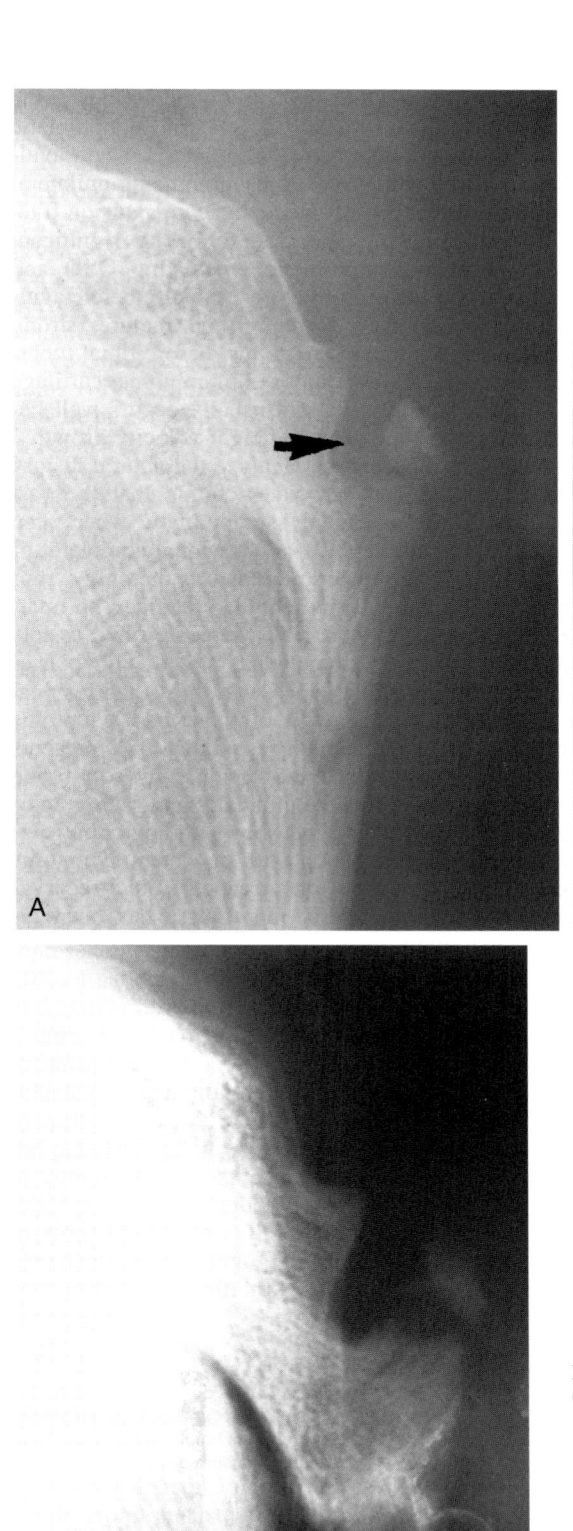

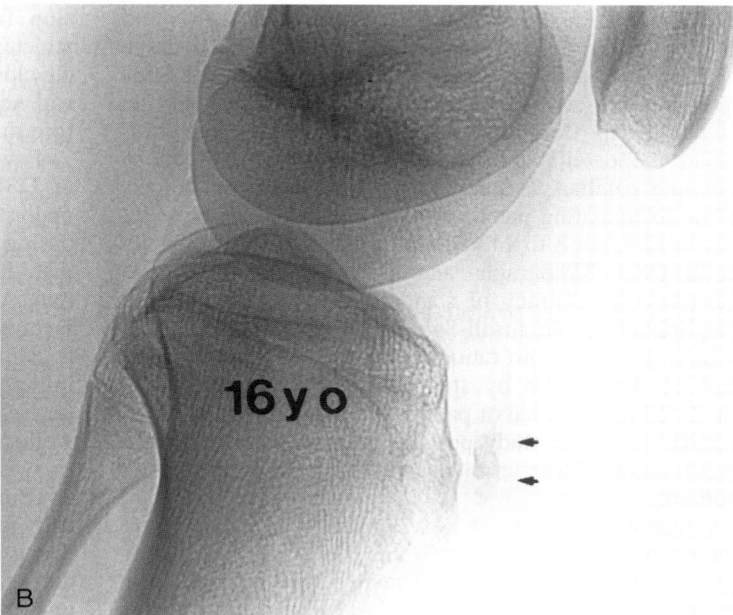

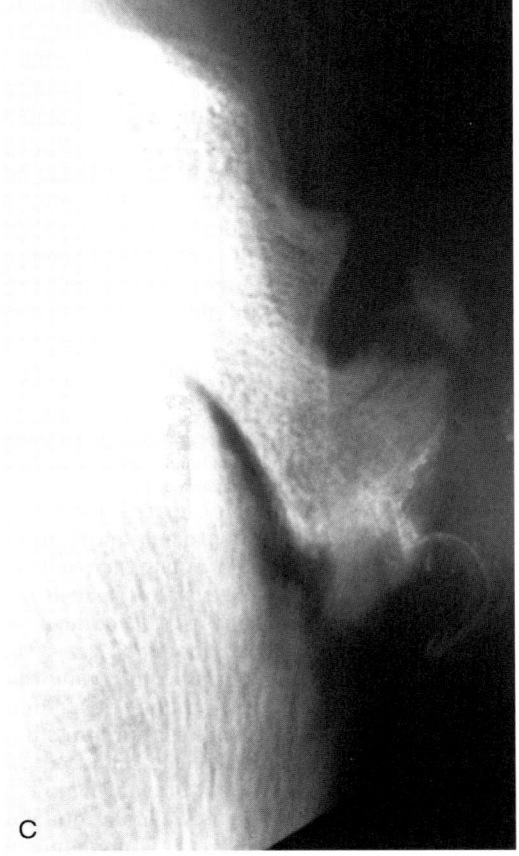

Figure 28E7–34. *A* and *B,* Varied amount of fragmentation and ossicle formation (*arrowheads*). *C,* Fracture through Osgood-Schlatter disease ossicle after acute trauma.

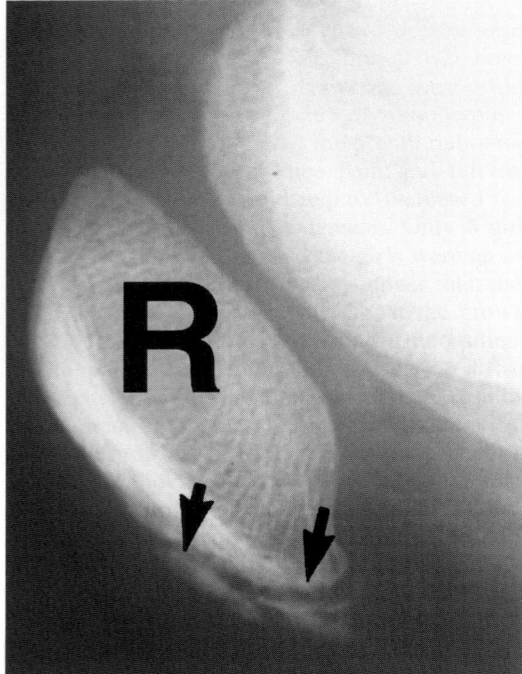

Figure 28E7–38. Sinding-Larsen-Johansson changes (*arrows*) in a symptomatic 11-year-old basketball player.

find tibial tubercle prominence and tenderness in the slightly older child (Fig. 28E7–40). One needs to rule out patellar sagittal alignment abnormalities (e.g., patella alta, patella infra) and limited hip or knee motion that causes increased anterior knee stress. Radiographs are usually normal except for varying amounts of calcification or ossi-

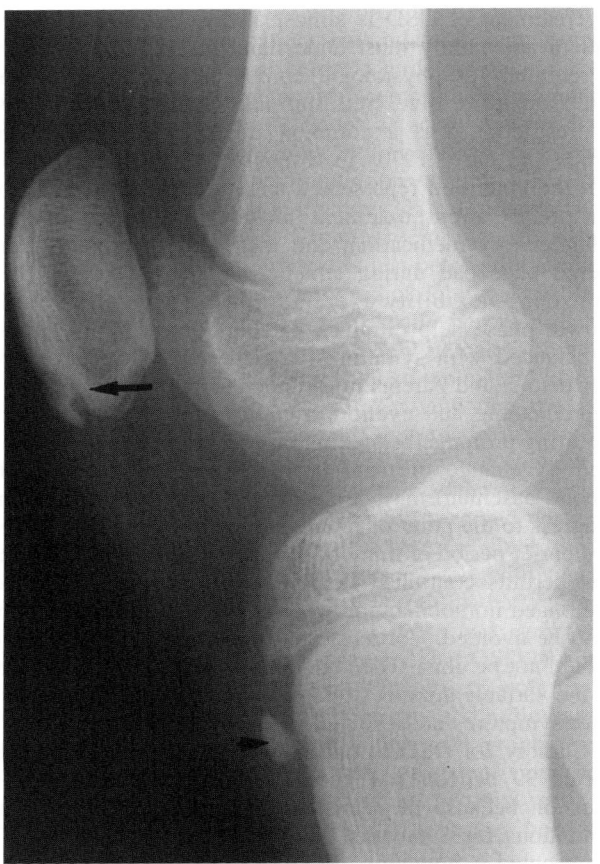

Figure 28E7– 40. Concomitant Sinding-Larsen-Johansson (*long arrow*) and Osgood-Schlatter (*short arrow*) changes. The 12-year-old patient had symptoms at the patellar inferior pole. He was asymptomatic at the tibial tubercle.

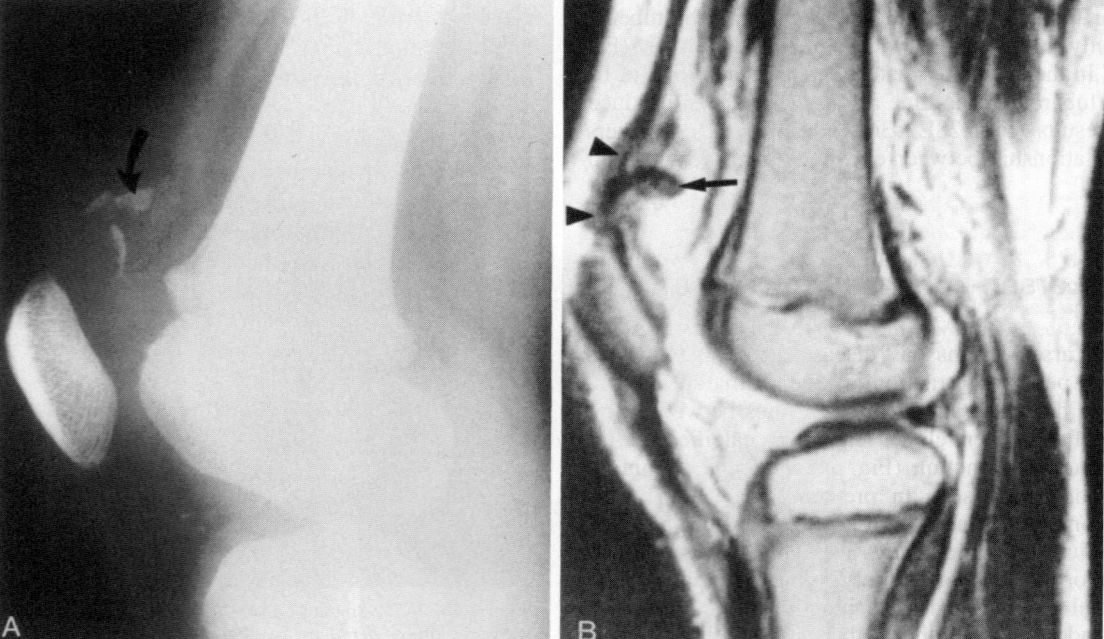

Figure 28E7–39. *A,* Proximal pole "sleeve" fracture. *B,* Magnetic resonance image of lesion showing that a significant part of the fragment is cartilaginous. (Courtesy George W. Gross, M.D.)

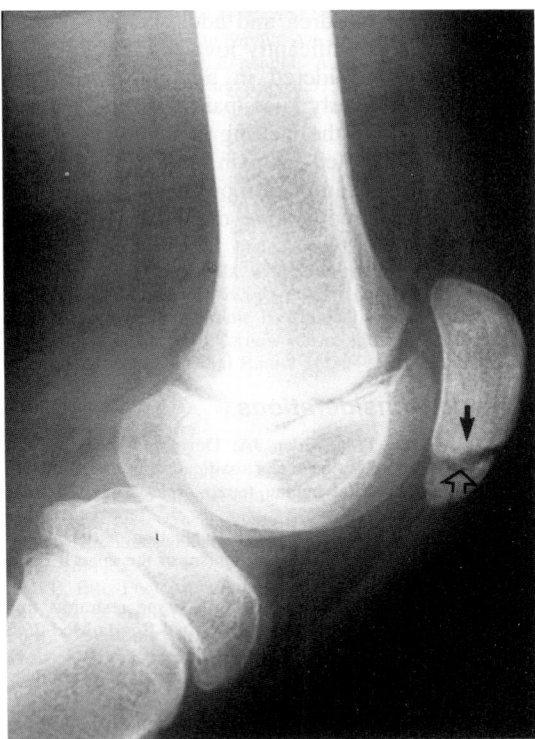

Figure 28E7–41. Type I bipartite patella.

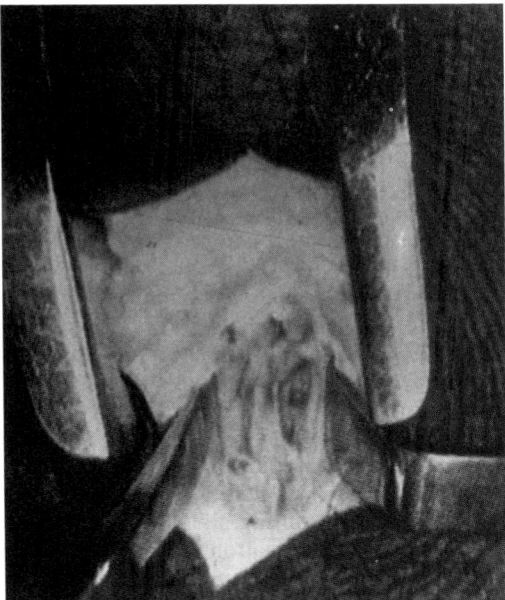

Figure 28E7–42. "Jumper's knee" with necrotic intratendinous debris in a 16-year-old basketball player.

fication at the patella–patellar tendon junction. Similar findings may also be seen in asymptomatic patients.

Differential diagnosis includes type I bipartite patella and patellar stress or sleeve fractures (Fig. 28E7–41).[2] In more mature adolescents, jumper's knee, a chronic, proximal patellar tendinitis, may occur, especially in athletes involved in sports requiring repetitive eccentric quadriceps loading.[4]

As in Osgood-Schlatter condition, treatment consists of explaining the time course of 12 to 18 months required for resolution and the variable symptoms seen during that time. Patients, parents, and coaches, as well as athletic education teachers, need to be aware of these issues. The condition resolves without sequelae and intervention is minimal. Ice massage, use of anti-inflammatory medication, and a knee sleeve or pad will usually allow continued sports participation.

In an older child with a jumper's knee, similar initial treatment is provided. Karlsson and colleagues[4] quantified, by ultrasound, patellar tendon involvement in jumper's knee. Lesions larger than 20 mm usually required surgical débridement of the necrotic, inflamed area (Fig. 28E7–42). Steroid injection into the tendon is condemned because of the high potential for tendon rupture after injection.

Reflex Sympathetic Dystrophy

Katz and Hungerford[5] described 36 adult patients with knee symptoms associated with reflex sympathetic dystrophy (RSD) and suggested that the disorder was an exaggerated sympathetic autonomic response. Surgery or injury at the patellofemoral joint triggered the symptoms in two thirds of their patients. National surveys of complications of arthroscopic surgery showed an inordinately high prevalence of RSD associated with patellofemoral joint procedures.[1, 2] Despite these publications emphasizing the emerging recognition of lower extremity RSD, the diagnosis is still not commonly considered in the differential diagnosis of knee pain.

Numerous recent publications have also pointed out the increased frequency with which RSD is seen in children.[3, 4, 6] Despite these writings, when Wilder and associates[6] reviewed 70 patients younger than 18 years old (average 12.5 years) with RSD, they found an average delay of 1 year from symptom onset to diagnosis. The diagnosis is usually not made until manifestations of the disorder become florid, a stage in which treatment is more difficult.

RSD is marked by a disproportionate pain response, with autonomic sequelae affecting skin, muscles, vessels, and bone. Three classic temporal stages are described: acute, onset less than 3 months; dystrophic, onset 3 to 6 months; and atrophic, onset greater than 6 months. The acute stage manifestation is primarily pain out of proportion to the initiating event. Stiffness, pain, swelling, and osteoporosis are manifestations of the dystrophic phase. The atrophic stage is characterized by continued pain, skin and nail changes, cyanosis, and bone demineralization. Gradations exist in any one patient during a particular phase, depending on the disorder's magnitude and duration.

Clinically, patients complain of pain out of proportion to the magnitude of the initiating event. An absence of expected improvement with specific treatment for the previous condition should raise the question of RSD. With careful questioning, the history is often suggestive of RSD before the surgery that accelerated the complaints. Many authors comment on the conversion-like response seen in RSD as a response to academic, athletic, social, and famil-

adolescent athletes. Retrospective study of incidence and duration. Am J Sports Med 13:236–241, 1985.
9. Mital MA, Matza RA, Cohen J: The so-called unresolved Osgood-Schlatter lesion: A concept based on fifteen surgically treated lesions. J Bone Joint Surg Am 62:732–739, 1980.
10. Ogden JA, Southwick WO: Osgood-Schlatter's disease and tibial tuberosity development. Clin Orthop 116:180–189, 1976.
11. Ogden JA, Tross RB, Murphy MJ: Fractures of the tibial tuberosity in adolescents. J Bone Joint Surg Am 62:205–215, 1980.
12. Osgood RB: Lesions of the tibial tubercle occurring during adolescence. Clin Orthop 286:4–9, 1993.
13. Rosenberg ZS, Kawelblum M, Cheung YY, et al: Osgood-Schlatter lesion: Fracture or tendinitis? Scintigraphic, CT, and MR imaging features. Radiology 185:853–858, 1992.
14. Schlatter C: Verletzungen des Schnabelformingen Fortsatzes der oberen Tibiaepiphyse. Beitr Klin Chir Tubing 38:874–878, 1903.

Sinding-Larsen-Johansson Disease

1. Batten J, Menelaus MB: Fragmentation of the proximal pole of the patella. Another manifestation of juvenile traction osteochondritis? J Bone Joint Surg Br 67:249–251, 1985.

2. Grogan DP, Carey TP, Leffers D, Ogden JA: Avulsion fractures of the patella. J Pediatr Orthop 10:721–730, 1990.
3. Johannson S: En forut icke beskriven sjukdom i patella. Hygiea 84:161–162, 1922.
4. Karlsson J, Kalebo P, Goksor LA, et al: Partial rupture of the patellar ligament. Am J Sports Med 20:390–395, 1992.
5. Sinding-Larsen A: A hitherto unknown affection of the patella. Acta Radiol 1:171–174, 1921.

Reflex Sympathetic Dystrophy

1. Cooper SL: Reflex sympathetic dystrophy following knee surgery. Am J Sports Med 15:525, 1987.
2. DeLee J: Reflex sympathetic dystrophy following arthroscopic surgery. Arthroscopy 1:214, 1985.
3. Dietz FR, Mathews KD, Montgomery WJ: Reflex sympathetic dystrophy in children. Clin Orthop 258:225–231, 1990.
4. Forster RS, Fu FH: Reflex sympathetic dystrophy in children. A case report and review of literature. Orthopedics 8:475–477, 1985.
5. Katz MM, Hungerford DS: Reflex sympathetic dystrophy affecting the knee. J Bone Joint Surg Br 69:797–803, 1987.
6. Wilder RT, Berde CB, Wolohan M, et al: Reflex sympathetic dystrophy in children. Clinical characteristics and follow-up of seventy patients. J Bone Joint Surg Am 74:910–919, 1992.

8. PATELLOFEMORAL TENDINOPATHY
Jon Hyman, MD ■ Scott A. Rodeo, MD ■ Thomas Wickiewicz, MD

Anatomy and Structure of the Extensor Mechanism

The extensor mechanism of the knee begins proximally with the quadriceps muscles and continues distally as the quadriceps femoris tendon, the patella, and the patellar tendon, which then inserts into the tibial tubercle (Fig. 28E8–1). The patella is a sesamoid bone within the knee

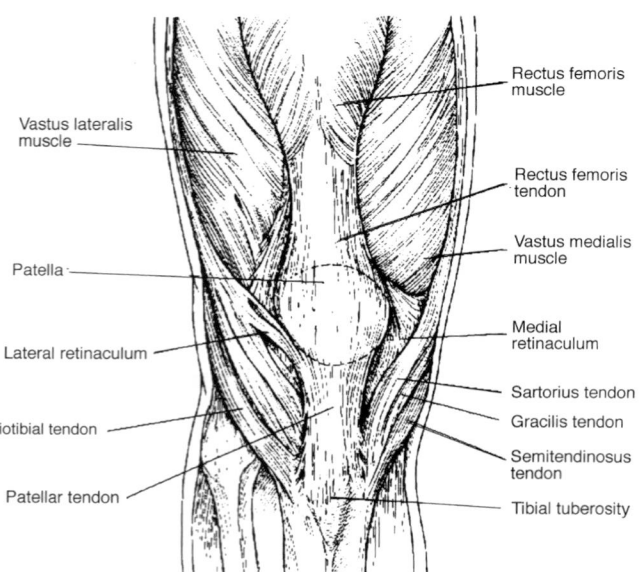

Figure 28E8–1. Normal anatomy of the extensor mechanism of the knee. (© 1996 American Academy of Orthopaedic Surgeons. Reprinted from the *Journal of the American Academy of Orthopaedic Surgeons*, Volume 4(6), 287–296 with permission.)

extensor tendon complex. The medial and lateral retinacula blend into the tendon on their respective sides. In the sagittal plane, the width of the tendon as it attaches to the patella proximally usually averages 4 mm and is generally less than 7 mm.[22] The mean thickness of the tendon increases distally and approaches 5 to 6 mm at its insertion into the tibial tubercle.

The patellar tendon receives its blood supply primarily from the vessels in the infrapatellar fat pad and retinacular structures.[6] The infrapatellar fat pad contributes vessels to the posterior aspect of the tendon via anastomoses from the inferior medial and inferior lateral geniculate arteries.[66] The anterior part of the tendon receives blood vessels from retinacular branches of the inferior medial geniculate and recurrent tibial arteries. These vessels originate at the proximal and middle portions of the tendon and travel distally. The connective tissues at the origin and the insertion of the patellar tendon are relatively avascular.[79] These avascular regions, composed histologically of fibrocartilage, are common sites of rupture.

The quadriceps tendon receives multiple vascular anastomoses. Descending branches of the lateral circumflex femoral artery, branches of the descending geniculate artery, and branches of the medial and lateral superior geniculate arteries all provide blood supply to the quadriceps tendon. The distribution of the vascular network within the quadriceps tendon is somewhat heterogeneous, particularly at the musculotendinous regions. There is an avascular area in the deep part of the quadriceps tendon measuring about 1.5 × 3 cm.[74]

Similar to most tendons, water constitutes approximately 70% of the wet weight of the tendons about the knee, and collagen composes about 70% of the dry weight.[66] Although a subpopulation of small-diameter collagen fibrils is present, tendons contain predominantly large-diameter

Figure labels: Rectus femoris muscle, Rectus femoris tendon, Vastus medialis muscle, Medial retinaculum, Sartorius tendon, Gracilis tendon, Semitendinosus tendon, Tibial tuberosity, Vastus lateralis muscle, Patella, Lateral retinaculum, Iliotibial tendon, Patellar tendon (greater than 100 nm) collagen fibers, of which 90% are type I collagen and fewer than 10% are types III, IV, V, and VI, collectively. Elastin, proteoglycans (principally decorin), and other noncollagenous glycoproteins make up the remaining tendon matrix.[23]

Biology and Biomechanics of the Extensor Mechanism

Recent studies have furthered understanding of the relationship between the biologic structure and the underlying biomechanical properties of tendon. The material properties of tendon are determined principally by collagen. Tissue strength correlates positively with total collagen content, density of stable (pyridinoline) cross-links, collagen organization, and fibril diameter. Tensile strength correlates inversely with type III collagen content and the proteoglycan-collagen ratio. The ability of tendon to resist plastic deformation (creep) is related to the content of small-diameter collagen fibrils, and the ability to resist high tensile loads is related to the content of large-diameter fibrils. Other factors that can affect the material properties of tendon include the collagen crimp (Fig. 28E8–2) and the elastic fibers.[31]

Ascending stairs is estimated to generate a force within the patellar tendon of approximately 3.2 times the body weight.[72] Forces generated in the quadriceps muscles during active knee extension are transferred in a convergent fashion via the extensor mechanism (patellar tendon and retinaculum) to the proximal tibia. The greatest forces in the tendon occur with the knee at approximately 60 degrees of flexion.[30] The extensor mechanism force ratio is the patellar tendon force (distal) divided by the quadriceps tendon force (proximal). This ratio is greater than 1.0 at knee flexion angles of less than 45 degrees.[30] At these smaller flexion angles, the distal pole of the patella articulates in the trochlea. Because the patellofemoral contact area is more distal, the quadriceps tendon has a mechanical advantage during active knee extension through small flexion angles.[30] At flexion angles of greater than 45 degrees, the force ratio is less than 1.0. As knee flexion increases, the patellofemoral contact stress increases proximally, giving the patellar tendon a mechanical advantage during active extension.[30] It is then that the patellar tendon sustains relatively greater stress compared with the quadriceps tendon.[66] The position of the knee when load is applied directly relates to the risk of tensile failure in the quadriceps tendon (flexion < 45 degrees) or the patellar tendon (flexion > 45 degrees).[102] The degree of flexion of the knee at the time of injury therefore plays a role in determining the site of failure of the extensor tendon unit.

It has been shown that the deformation (strain) due to tensile load is much less in the midsubstance of the patellar tendon than in the insertion sites of the tendon.[98] At peak load before failure, the end-region strain at the insertion site is approximately three to four times that in the midsubstance.[98] In addition, there is a corresponding decrease in collagen fiber stiffness at the insertion site compared with the midsubstance region.[66] These observed patterns of force transfer may in part explain why the quadriceps and patellar tendons more commonly rupture near their respective insertion sites rather than in the midsubstance of the tendons. Other factors that affect the pattern of injury are type and rate of the applied load and the patient's age.[31, 34]

Metabolic Disorders Affecting Tendons

Both systemic and local metabolic derangements have been shown to affect tendinous tissue around the patella. These alterations in the biochemical composition and the biomechanical properties can induce pathologic changes in the insertion site and the midsubstance of the tendon. Normal, healthy tendon rarely fails within its substance; ruptures usually occur at the muscle-tendon junction or at the tendon-bone junction.[69] The occurrence of midsubstance rupture of the patellar or quadriceps tendon should prompt consideration of the presence of an underlying tendon disorder (Table 28E8–1).

A common cause of intrinsic tendon weakening in sports medicine is the use of local or systemic corticosteroids.

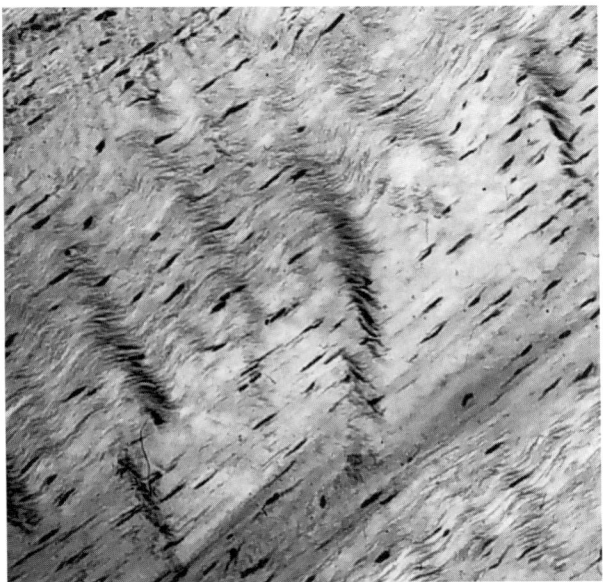

Figure 28E8–2. Histologic features of a normal patellar tendon with typical collagen crimp pattern.

TABLE 28E8–1
Conditions Associated with Occult Tendinopathy

Hyperparathyroidism
Calcium pyrophosphate deposition
Diabetes mellitus
Steroid-induced tendinopathy
Fluoroquinolone-induced tendinopathy
Osteomalacia
Chronic renal insufficiency
Gout
Uremia
Systemic lupus erythematosus
Rheumatoid arthritis

Experimental studies have demonstrated that local corticosteroid injections can impair healing of ligament, probably by inhibition of the inflammatory phase of healing.[95] Bilateral patellar tendon rupture has been reported following local steroid injections.[16] Steroid injections are generally only considered when symptoms have not responded to conservative treatment (generally, for longer than 3 months) and imaging studies do not demonstrate a pathologic abnormality in the tendon. Steroids should not be directly injected into tendons.

Fluoroquinolone antibiotics (e.g., ciprofloxacin) have also been associated with tendon ruptures, possibly owing to pathologic alterations in tendon extracellular matrix.[67, 96] Tendons may also be weakened by abnormal deposition of metabolic products. Deposition of calcium pyrophosphate can occur in the gastrocnemius and quadriceps tendons in chondrocalcinosis of the knee and may contribute to knee pain.[99] Patellar tendon rupture has been reported in hyperparathyroidism and systemic lupus erythematosus.[8] Dystrophic calcification occurs in hyperparathyroidism with deposition of calcium hydroxyapatite and urate crystals in tendon, which may weaken the tendon. Pathologic alterations in tendon matrix with resultant tendon weakening also may occur in gout, renal failure, rheumatoid arthritis, and systemic lupus erythematosus.[8, 10, 17, 58] In these conditions, tendon weakening probably occurs as a result of the basic disease process as well as the frequent associated use of corticosteroids.

Bilateral quadriceps tendon ruptures have been reported in association with gout and renal failure[10, 58] but can also occur with trauma. Bilateral patellar tendon ruptures can likewise occur in the setting of acute trauma or in association with an underlying metabolic disorder. Abnormal deposition of proteoglycan and hyaluronic acid in tendon has been reported in hypothyroidism.[36, 60]

Pathologic changes also occur at tendon entheses or in the underlying bone in several metabolic conditions. Monosodium urate deposits (tophi) often occur at the patellar tendon insertion in gout, resulting in pain and swelling.[26] A similar enthesopathy has been described in calcium pyrophosphate deposition disease (chondrocalcinosis).[99] Pathologic changes at the patellar tendon insertion have been reported in association with isotretinoin (a retinoid used to treat severe cystic acne) treatment.[82] Retinoids have been found to result in skeletal hyperostoses and proliferation of new bone at tendon insertions, such as the patellar tendon.[77]

Conditions that affect bone strength may affect tendon insertions, causing activity-related pain. Avulsion of the patellar tendon from its tibial insertion has been reported in Paget's disease, in which there is rapid bone turnover and remodeling.[52] Renal disease and primary or secondary hyperparathyroidism weaken bone owing to resorption. Ruptures of the patellar tendon insertion have been reported in these conditions. Similarly, synovial proliferation in rheumatoid arthritis can cause bone erosions and weaken tendon insertions. All these conditions may increase the susceptibility of knee tendons to injury, and recognition of such underlying abnormalities is important to provide proper treatment and to advise the patient properly to prevent recurrent injury.[77]

Pathophysiology of Tendon Injury

Overuse tendon injuries around the knee, occurring as a result of repetitive microtrauma, most commonly involve the patellar tendon. The adaptive and reparative ability of tendon can be exceeded when the tendon is strained repeatedly to 4% to 8% of its original length. Such repetitive strain can result in microscopic or macroscopic injury to collagen fibrils, noncollagenous matrix, and the microvasculature, resulting in inflammation, edema, and pain. It is currently felt that the earliest pathophysiologic alteration occurs in the paratenon, which surrounds the tendon, resulting in peritendinitis (also called paratenonitis) (Table 28E8–2). There is inflammatory cell infiltration, tissue edema, and fibrin exudation in the paratenon. If the basal reparative ability of the tendon is overwhelmed by continued overload, the inflammation can become chronic with resulting proliferation of synovial cells, fibroblasts, and capillaries, which eventually leads to fibrosis and thickening of the paratenon.[77]

The term *tendinitis* implies the presence of inflammatory cells and is technically a histopathologic, not a clinical, diagnosis. Intrinsic tendon degeneration (tendinosis) is histologically devoid of inflammatory cells and is a pathophysiologic process, clearly distinct from tendinitis. The clinical picture of pain, swelling, and physical limitation related to tendons is more correctly referred to as *tendinopathy*.

Tendinosis is thought to result from tendon overload and chronic peritendinitis. It appears that tendons go through acute, recurrent, subchronic, and chronic phases of peritendinitis before actual degeneration develops. The cellular mechanisms by which acute or chronic inflammation leads to tendon degeneration are poorly understood. An experimental model in rabbits demonstrated that chronic inflammation of paratenon results in tendinosis.[9] It must be noted, however, that a causal link between chronic peritendinitis and tendinosis has not been conclusively established. A popular model is that tendon degeneration occurs owing to failure of the cell matrix to adapt to excessive load.[56] This suboptimal tendon healing response may be directly related to impaired metabolic activity owing to the release of inflammatory mediators and cytokines in the setting of altered cellular function from repetitive tendon overload.

Tendinosis involves histopathologic alterations to cells, collagen fibers, and noncollagenous matrix components. This process affects the entire tendon architecture. Angiofibroblastic hyperplasia occurs, consisting of proliferation of fibroblasts and new capillaries. Various histologic abnormalities are found, with the most common being collagen fragmentation and mucoid degeneration with glycosaminoglycan deposition (principally chondroitin sulfate).[64] Inflammation is notably absent in tendinosis.[37] The result of such pathologic alterations is decreased tensile strength of the tendon. Furthermore, degenerative tendon with diminished vascularity cannot heal subclinical injury with microfailure of tendon fibers. The result is progressive loss of functional tendon fibers, which increases the load on the remaining tendon, thus increasing its susceptibility to progressive failure.[77]

TABLE 28E8–2
Classification of Tendon Disorders

New	Old	Definition	Histologic Findings	Clinical Signs and Symptoms
Paratenonitis	Tenosynovitis Tenovaginitis Peritendinitis	Inflammation of only the paratenon whether or not lined by synovium	Inflammatory cells in paratenon or peritendinous areolar tissue	Cardinal inflammatory signs: swelling, pain, crepitation, local tenderness, warmth, dysfunction
Paratenonitis with tendinosis	Tendinitis	Paratenon inflammation associated with intratendinous degeneration	Same as above, with loss of tendon, collagen fiber disorientation, scattered vascular ingrowth but no prominent intratendinous inflammation	Same as above, with often palpable tendon nodule, swelling, and inflammatory signs
Tendinosis	Tendinitis	Intratendinous degeneration due to atrophy (aging, microtrauma, vascular compromise)	Noninflammatory intratendinous collagen degeneration with fiber disorientation, hypocellularity, scattered vascular ingrowth, occasional local necrosis, or calcification	Often palpable tendon nodule that can be asymptomatic, but may also be point tender; swelling of tendon sheath is absent
Tendinosis	Tendon strain or tear	Symptomatic overload of the tendon with vascular disruption and inflammatory repair response	Three recognized subgroups: each displays variable histologic characteristics from purely inflammation with acute hemorrhage and tear to inflammation superimposed upon preexisting degeneration, to calcification and tendinosis changes in chronic conditions. In the chronic stage, it may be 1. Interstitial microinjury 2. Central tendon necrosis 3. Frank partial rupture 4. Acute complete rupture	Symptoms are inflammatory and proportional to vascular disruption, hematoma, or atrophy-related cell necrosis. Symptom duration defines each subgroup: A. Acute (<2 weeks) B. Subacute (4–6 weeks) C. Chronic (>6 weeks)

Recent studies have identified several factors that are probably important in the development of tendon degeneration. Tissue hypoxia due to poor vascularity (which may be intrinsic or a result of overuse injury to the microvasculature) results in impaired metabolic activity. Other factors that may affect the ability of tendon to adapt to repetitive loading include age, immobilization, hormones (such as estrogen), and drugs. (Corticosteroid injections and fluoroquinolone antibiotics can lead to pathologic matrix alterations.) Extrinsic factors that may contribute to tendon overuse injury include joint instability, malalignments (such as excessive hindfoot pronation, genu valgum, increased femoral anteversion), decreased flexibility, muscle weakness and imbalance, and excessive body weight. The type of loading (tension, compression, or shear), the pattern of load (concentric or eccentric), and the magnitude of force also affect the response of the tendon to repetitive loading.[31]

Pathologic changes can also occur at the site of tendon attachment to bone. In the skeletally immature child, tensile overload often results in pathologic alterations at the apophysis, resulting in apophysitis. The most common site of apophysitis around the knee occurs at the tibial tuberosity (Osgood-Schlatter disease). Histologically, avulsion of small areas of the ossification center is found. Insertion tendinopathy can also occur in adults, in which the pathologic alterations include collagen fragmentation with disorganization and thickening of the fibrocartilage zone of the insertion.

Clinical Aspects of Patellofemoral Tendinopathy

Tendon injuries about the knee are common and can occur as a result of both acute macrotrauma and repetitive microtrauma. These injuries often cause disabling symptoms and require treatment. Approximately one third of sports injuries seen at outpatient clinics involve the knee.[33] The highest incidences of knee injury are in sports that involve repetitive jumping or significant running and pivoting, such as soccer, basketball, volleyball, and long-distance running. The most common patellofemoral tendon injuries are quadriceps tendon ruptures, patellar tendinitis, patellar tendon rupture, and Osgood-Schlatter disease.

Quadriceps Tendon Rupture

Epidemiology

Ruptures of the quadriceps tendon generally occur in patients older than 40 years of age and occur three times more often than patellar tendon ruptures. These injuries are seldom seen in younger patients. Unilateral quadriceps tendon ruptures occur approximately 15 to 20 times more frequently than do bilateral ruptures.[14] Most ruptures occur transversely within 2 cm of the superior pole of the patella and often progress diagonally (distally and horizontally) into the medial and lateral retinacula. Males more commonly sustain ruptures of the extensor mechanism tendons.[87]

Mechanism of Injury

Failure of the tendon most frequently occurs during an eccentric contraction. The usual mechanism is a violent reflex contraction of the muscle that is initiated against body weight with the knee in a partially flexed position.

With high external loads applied to the the knee, a flexion moment predominates, despite forceful quadriceps contraction. It has been shown, however, that the normal tendon is able to tolerate very high tensile loads.[69] In addition, quadriceps tendon fibers interdigitate among separate bone lamellar systems (osteons or bone marrow spaces) of the patella, which suggests that the tendon insertion is very strong.[15] The site of rupture often appears to be through a degenerative area within the tendon and therefore occurs in an older population, usually older than 40 years of age. In healthy younger individuals, although rare, the rupture is usually due to direct trauma. Iatrogenic tendinopathy has also been observed. DeLee and associates have reported rupture of the quadriceps tendon after harvest of a central-third patellar tendon graft for anterior cruciate ligament reconstruction.[20] Direct steroid injection can also weaken tendon.[92] Tendon degeneration due to a systemic disease tends to occur bilaterally and may precipitate bilateral tendon rupture[55] (see Table 28E8–1).

Clinical Assessment

Acute quadriceps tendon rupture causes immediate onset of pain and moderate swelling. A "pop" is sometimes felt or heard. Pain is sometimes present before the rupture. When the tendon is completely torn, the patient is usually unable to extend the knee against resistance, unless the retinacula are partially intact. In a chronic partial rupture, the patient may complain of difficulty climbing stairs and of giving way during walking. In some cases, the patient is able to walk with the knee in full extension. A palpable defect may be found just above the proximal pole of the patella with subcutaneous hematoma in a complete tear.

It is imperative to rule out concomitant ligamentous injury when assessing tendinopathy about the knee. A careful examination with the patient under anesthesia is one diagnostic tool that should not be overlooked. An incomplete tear without a distinct episode of direct trauma may initially be misdiagnosed. Careful examination is required to diagnose an incomplete tear because there may not be a palpable tendon defect, and full knee extension may still be possible. An accurate medical history is essential, with particular attention paid to past and present medical problems and medications (including injections or surgery) because quadriceps tendon rupture may be associated with systemic disease.[77] Occasionally, tears in patients with systemic diseases are first seen by nonorthopaedic surgeons and physicians, and the injury may be mistaken for neurologic paralysis.[62]

Radiography

Plain radiographs may show patella baja, avulsion of small bone fragments from the superior pole of the patella, calcification within the quadriceps tendon, or a suprapatellar bony spur. The "tooth sign," which is a degenerative bony spur at the superior pole of the patella seen on a tangential view, has been reported in association with quadriceps tendon degeneration[71] and quadriceps and patellar tendon ruptures.[41] This radiographic sign is not necessarily associated with tendon rupture, however. Lateral radiographs of the uninjured knee may be obtained to evaluate patellar height.

Extravasation of dye from the suprapatellar pouch during arthrography is useful in diagnosing a complete tear.[5] Ultrasonography has been shown to demonstrate focal tendon degeneration or partial tears of the tendon. Bianchi and coworkers studied 29 cases of quadriceps rupture diagnosed with ultrasonography and demonstrated a high degree of sensitivity and specificity.[11] Because it is simple and cost-effective, ultrasonography may also be useful for serial examinations to follow tendon healing. With the currently available technology, the principal drawback of ultrasonography is that it is highly operator dependent.

Of the various imaging modalities available, magnetic resonance imaging (MRI) is the most sensitive, specific, and accurate in the evaluation of tendon injuries owing to its superior soft tissue resolution. In the setting of a quadriceps tendon rupture, MRI demonstrates focal tendon discontinuity, increased signal intensity within the tendon, altered tendon structure, and evidence of patella baja[48] (Fig. 28E8–3). The patellar tendon may appear lax because of loss of tension in the extensor mechanism. Because it is tomographic, MRI can accurately depict the exact width and thickness of the tear as well as preexisting pathologic changes within the tendon, such as underlying chondromucoid degeneration or cyst formation.[86] MRI also allows

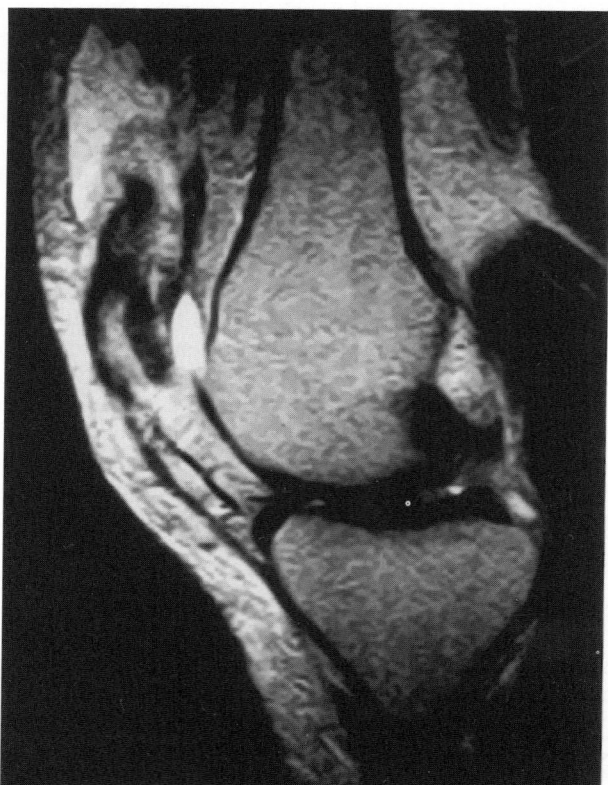

Figure 28E8–3. Magnetic resonance imaging, sagittal view, of a knee with late quadriceps tendon rupture, demonstrating some loss of patellar height, loss of normal tendon architecture, and abundant proximal scar tissue.

visualization of all other intra-articular and extra-articular structures around the knee. Zeiss and colleagues used MRI to evaluate normal and ruptured quadriceps tendons and reported that the normal quadriceps tendon has a laminated appearance with either two (30%), three (56%), or four (6%) layers.[101] Incomplete ruptures were seen as focal discontinuities of individual layers, with other layers remaining intact.[77]

Nonoperative Treatment

Conservative treatment may be indicated for an incomplete tear; however, there is little information in the literature to guide patient selection or to provide information on expected outcomes. If MRI demonstrates a small partial-thickness tear, and knee extension strength is well preserved compared with the uninjured side, nonoperative treatment may be recommended. Following acute injury, ice, compression, elevation, and anti-inflammatory medication are prescribed. The leg should be placed in a long-leg splint with the knee fully extended. Aseptic aspiration of the hematoma may be helpful for both diagnostic and therapeutic purposes. Relatively rigid immobilization is preferred once the initial swelling has resolved. The leg is placed in a cylinder cast or a removable double-upright hinged brace in full extension for 4 to 6 weeks. Straight leg raising isometric exercises may be started immediately. During the first 4 weeks, the patient is restricted to partial weight-bearing and then progresses to full weight-bearing in extension. Between 4 and 6 weeks (based on the size of the tear), the hinges on the brace are opened to allow restoration of normal gait. The brace is discontinued after 2 weeks of ambulation with the hinges open, as long as active leg control, strength, and gait are adequate and documented.

After 4 to 6 weeks in full extension in the cast or the brace, protected active flexion exercises are begun with a gradual restoration of full flexion over the next 2 to 4 weeks. Aggressive attempts to increase knee flexion rapidly should be avoided, because the healing tendon is still remodeling and may stretch excessively. A recommended goal is to achieve 90 degrees of flexion within 2 weeks of cast removal. Progressive resistance exercises for the quadriceps are then begun, starting with closed chain isotonics and progressing to isokinetic exercises. Full participation in sports activities should be avoided for at least 4 months after the injury. If conservative treatment of an incomplete tear is elected, healing should be carefully monitored to detect development of a complete rupture. If there is evidence of delayed healing or progressive rupture, early surgical intervention is recommended because delayed repair may be associated with inferior results.[77]

Surgical Treatment

In complete ruptures, the most optimal overall outcomes generally result from immediate repair. Several surgical techniques for repairing the ruptured tendon have been described. The particular repair technique chosen may be guided by surgeon preference, the extent of retraction of the torn tendon, and the length of the residual tendon attached to the patella. Direct repair to the patella is possible for most acute tears. A midline longitudinal incision is used to expose the torn tendon. The tendon stumps are débrided of any necrotic, degenerative, and inflammatory tissue. If there is sufficient tendon proximally and distally, which occurs infrequently, an end-to-end repair can be performed with multiple No. 2 and No. 5 nonabsorbable mattress sutures. A tendon-grasping suture, such as a Kessler or Bunnell configuration, is used to ensure a secure repair. The retinaculum is also repaired carefully with multiple interrupted nonabsorbable sutures. After the repair is complete, knee range of motion, tension on the repaired tendon, patellar position, and tracking are carefully evaluated. The position of flexion at which there begins to be significant tension on the repair is carefully noted; this degree of flexion will be used to determine the limits of active flexion in the early postoperative period and should be made clear to the treating physical therapist.

Typically, the quadriceps tendon ruptures 1 to 2 cm proximal to the tendon insertion onto the proximal pole of the patella, with or without avulsion fragments of the patella. Often, a small amount of vastus intermedius tendon will remain attached to the superior pole of the patella. In such a case, the tendon stump is débrided of any necrotic, degenerative, and inflammatory tissue. A small horizontal trough is made at the proximal pole of the patella with a rongeur or a high-speed bur. If a small stump of tendon remains on the patella, the trough should be made deep to the stump, and the stump can then be used for augmentation of the repair. Anterior placement of the trough should be avoided because it may induce superior patellar tilt. Several sets of heavy (No. 5) nonabsorbable sutures are passed through the tendon in a Kessler or Bunnell configuration. Two parallel longitudinal drill holes are made in the patella. These drill holes enter into the trough and exit over the inferior pole of the patella. The sutures from the tendon are then passed through these holes. The tendon is reduced to the superior pole of the patella, and the sutures are tied with the knee in full extension. Care should be taken to tie the knots behind the patellar tendon at the inferior pole, so that the risk of skin and tendon necrosis can be lessened. The retinaculum is meticulously repaired using nonabsorbable suture. Adequate hemostasis is confirmed.

Chronic ruptures may be difficult to treat because of contraction of the tendon, degeneration of the residual tendon, and muscle atrophy from prolonged disuse. The tendon is mobilized by releasing adhesions to the surrounding soft tissues, the skin, and the underlying femur.[39] Rarely, to mobilize the central tendon it may be necessary to detach the vastus medialis or vastus lateralis muscles from the tendon. The muscles are then repaired back to the tendon after the tendon has been repaired to the patella. Quadriceps tendon lengthening using a Z-plasty or a V-Y technique may be required to aid in tendon mobilization.[77]

Several techniques are available to aid in repair of a retracted tendon. Techniques described by Scuderi[81] and Codivilla[83] can be used to close the intertendinous gap. Augmentation materials such as strips of fascia lata autograft or allograft, semitendinosus and gracilis tendon, or synthetic materials can be used as well. Levy and associates reported favorable results in four cases of quadriceps tendon repair with a Dacron vascular graft.[57] Circumferential suturing or wiring may also be used for protection of the repair. A heavy No. 5 nonabsorbable suture or 5-mm Mersilene tape is passed through the proximal aspect of the patellar tendon along the inferior pole of patella and then through the quadriceps tendon above the repair site. In this way, a circumferential loop is created and will serve to stress-relieve the repair site. An 18-gauge wire may also be used, with placement through a drill hole in the tibial tubercle. The wire should be removed after 8 weeks. The authors do not favor the use of wire and prefer instead to bury knots of heavy, nonabsorbable suture.

Postoperative Rehabilitation

Protection of the repair during the early healing phase is the first essential component of postoperative rehabilitation. The limb is placed into a hinged double-upright brace. Limited weight-bearing in full extension is allowed immediately in most cases. Typically, toe-touch weight-bearing is done in the first week, followed by 2 to 8 weeks of full weight-bearing in a brace locked in extension. If the repair is tenuous, non–weight-bearing may be prescribed initially, with the knee immobilized for the first 6 to 8 weeks. If the patient is felt to be potentially noncompliant, immobilization in a long-leg cast for the first 3 weeks with the knee in full extension can be considered. Generally, however, a hinged brace is used so that protected early motion may begin. Full weight-bearing is allowed once the patient has regained adequate motor control of the limb. Ambulation out of the brace is allowed when sufficient muscle strength and greater than 90 degrees of flexion have been achieved. The brace is usually worn for a total of 6 to 8 weeks.

Early active flexion is allowed within a range that does not place high stress on the repair (this is determined intraoperatively by flexing the knee until the gap begins to form at the repair site). Up to 90 degrees of flexion may be possible following immediate repair of acute quadriceps tendon ruptures. Early limited motion will provide some mechanical load to the tendon. There is extensive basic and clinical evidence that load can enhance tendon healing.[4, 7, 28, 90] Motion will also prevent immobilization-induced articular cartilage degeneration. Continuous passive motion may be used in the first 3 to 4 weeks to aid in early motion. Only passive extension is allowed during the initial 6 weeks. Isometric quadriceps contractions and straight leg raising exercises may begin immediately for acute repairs. After 6 weeks, active extension exercises are begun. Initially, only the weight of the leg is used for quadriceps exercises. A progressive strengthening program is then followed, with progression to isotonic and isokinetic exercises. Electrical stimulation for the quadriceps may be useful. Active, active-assisted, and passive range of motion exercises are also progressed after the 6-week point. Strenuous sports or occupational activities are not allowed until 6 months after surgery.[77]

If a delayed repair has been performed or if the repair is felt to be tenuous, the postoperative rehabilitation must be modified appropriately. Straight leg raising exercises

and limited weight-bearing may be approached more cautiously. Restoration of range of motion will also be slower in this setting.

Clinical Outcomes

Overall, the results following quadriceps tendon rupture are superior to those following patellar tendon rupture.[53, 87] Following acute repairs and appropriate rehabilitation, most patients achieve normal gait, full quadriceps strength, and satisfactory flexion (120 to 130 degrees). Some terminal flexion, perhaps 10 to 20 degrees, may be lost owing to shortening of the tendon by 1 to 2 cm.

Secondary ruptures are rare after the repair. The principal factor in determining outcome is the length of time between injury and surgery. Chronic quadriceps tendon rupture is associated with disuse atrophy of the muscles of the injured leg, retraction of the quadriceps, and knee joint contracture. Age is also a factor, with better overall results reported in younger patients.[53] Older patients often have preexisting patellofemoral degenerative joint disease, which can be more symptomatic during the rehabilitation process. Delayed quadriceps tendon repair is often associated with persistent quadriceps weakness and extensor lag.

Authors' Preferred Method of Treatment

Direct repair of the acutely torn quadriceps tendon is rarely possible; the authors, therefore, essentially always attempt to repair the tendon directly to bone. A vertical midline incision is used. The tendon ends are identified and freed from any early adhesions, and the torn end of the tendon is débrided back to healthy tendon. Retinacular tears should also be exposed and débrided, if necessary, in preparation for suture repair. Heavy, nonabsorbable sutures (No. 5) are then woven through the proximal tendon with a tendon-gripping configuration (such as Kessler, Bunnell, or Mason-Allen stitch). A trough is made at the superior pole of the patella at the tendon attachment site using a bur or a rongeur. Two parallel longitudinal drill holes are made in the patella, and the sutures are passed through these holes so that they exit over the inferior pole of the patella. The tendon is reduced to the trough, and the sutures are tied over the inferior pole. Care must be taken not to shorten the tendon excessively. Patellar position and tracking should be evaluated before securing the repair sutures. The knot may be brought to one side so that it is not prominent over the front of the knee. The retinaculum is repaired using No. 0 absorbable sutures, though care must be taken not to overtighten the tissue, because this can lead to restricted range of motion postoperatively. After the repair is secured, the knee is brought through a range of motion, and the position of flexion at which there begins to be significant tension on the repair is carefully noted; this degree of flexion will be used to determine the limits of active flexion in the early postoperative period and should be pointed out to the treating physical therapist.

Late repair of the quadriceps tendon may require the

use of augmentation techniques as well as extensive mobilization, or even lengthening, of the retracted tendon. Adhesions between the tendon and the surrounding soft tissues are released. The Scuderi technique, as described earlier, is recommended for delayed repairs. A V-Y technique or Z-plasty lengthening may be necessary in cases with marked tendon retraction. A significant defect at the repair site may also be augmented with semitendinosus and gracilis tendons. The repair may be protected with a circumferential suture passed proximal and distal to the repair site. This suture loop construct transfers stress from the repair site to the periphery.[77]

Complications

The most common complications after surgery include an inability to achieve full knee flexion and residual weakness of the extensor mechanism. A residual extensor lag may occur following delayed repair. Infection and wound problems can occur, particularly when there is poor soft tissue coverage over the tibial tubercle or if the wound closure is under tension, both of which may occur if augmentation materials are prominent at the repair site. Kirschner wire fixation, which has been used in the past, is not recommended because of the risk of infection. Patellar tilt may be induced if the retinacular repair is not balanced, and excessive patellofemoral contact stress may result from excessive shortening of the extensor mechanism. Excessive tightness of the repair may even induce patella infra, which can have detrimental consequences.[53] Superior patellar tilt may be induced if the trough at the superior pole of the patella is placed anteriorly. These complications can be avoided by careful assessment of patellar position during the repair. Recurrent rupture through the repair site is uncommon.

Patellar Tendinitis (Jumper's Knee)

Epidemiology

Blazina first described the clinical entity of "jumper's knee."[12] Patellar tendinitis (tendinopathy) is a common condition affecting the proximal attachment of the patellar tendon to the distal pole of the patella and is found particularly in those engaged in sporting activities such as basketball, volleyball, and soccer. Activities with repetitive jumping predispose to patellar tendinitis, which is why this condition is often called jumper's knee.[93] Patellar tendinitis does not occur only in jumping athletes, however. It can occur as a result of any activities in which repeated extension of the knee is required.[77]

The greatest incidence of this type of patellar tendinopathy is seen from the late teen years into the 30s, although this condition may occur in older individuals. Martens and coworkers reported that volleyball and soccer were the most common sports involved.[65] Blazina and associates reported that patellar tendinitis usually occurred in tall individuals,[12] and Lian and colleagues found a significant difference in body weight between patient and control

groups in their study of volleyball players with jumper's knee.[59] This condition has also been reported in association with several pathologic conditions (e.g., rheumatoid arthritis and gout). Sinding-Larsen-Johansson disease is sometimes described in association with patellar tendinitis; however, the former condition is extra-articular osteochondrosis, more accurately termed traction apophysitis, which is described in another section of this chapter.

Mechanism of Injury

The precise pathomechanics of this type of patellar tendinopathy has not been well described. The injury is thought to result from chronic overuse injury of the patellar tendon. Repetitive microtrauma or a single macrotraumatic event may initiate the underlying pathologic process. Johnson and coworkers suggested that patellar tendinitis may represent an impingement of the distal patellar pole on the middle third of the patellar tendon in flexion because the fibers of the tendon do not all insert directly at the patellar apex but continue over the anterior surface of the patellar apex.[34] These authors supported their hypothesis with MRI evaluations of patellar tendinitis and felt that such a mechanism would explain the characteristic site of the lesion and explain why surgical release of the tendon at the patellar apex is often beneficial.[77] Laduron and colleagues described another type of impingement that occurred between the deep fibers of the patellar tendon and the lateral part of the femoral trochlea when the knee is fully extended.[51]

The anatomic factors that have been related to patellar tendinitis are numerous and include patella alta, abnormal patellofemoral tracking, patellar instability, chondromalacia, Osgood-Schlatter disease, and mechanical malalignment or leg length inequality.[50] The relationship of such factors to patellar tendinitis remains to be clarified. Other studies have characterized factors during the jumping motion that are associated with patellar tendinitis. Lian and associates found that volleyball players with jumper's knee demonstrated better performance in jump tests than uninjured athletes, particularly in jumps involving eccentric force generation, presumably resulting in greater stress on the patellar tendon.[59] Richards and coworkers studied lower extremity movement biomechanics in 10 elite volleyball players and concluded that the likelihood of patellar tendon pain was related to high forces and rates of loading in the knee extensor mechanism, combined with large external tibial torsional moments and deep knee flexion angles.[76]

The pathologic abnormality in this condition appears to be an area of tendon degeneration (tendinosis) within the proximal patellar tendon (Fig. 28E8–4). Histologically, the tissue is characterized as angiofibroblastic hyperplasia (Fig. 28E8–5) with fibroblast proliferation, new blood vessel formation, chondromucoid deposition, and collagen fragmentation. The gross and microscopic appearances are similar to that seen in chronic lateral epicondylitis. Of note, inflammatory cells are typically absent in surgical biopsy specimens; however, inflammation in the paratenon (peritendinitis) may be evident in the early phases of the condition. Very little histologic confirmation is available for early cases because surgery is rarely indicated at this stage.

When the semitendinosus and gracilis tendons are used for augmentation of the repair, they are placed through a transverse drill hole in the patella and through a drill hole in the tibial tuberosity.[40, 54] These tendons are then sutured to the patellar tendon. Other options for augmentation include distal reflection of a strip of the central third of the quadriceps tendon or use of fascia lata.[77]

Chronic ruptures are more difficult to treat owing to proximal retraction of the extensor mechanism and muscle atrophy. The quadriceps tendon is mobilized by releasing any adhesions to the surrounding soft tissues. The vastus intermedius tendon may need to be mobilized from adhesions to the underlying femur. Preoperative traction may be useful in cases with severe proximal retraction. A Steinmann pin is placed transversely through the patella, and traction is applied with progressively increasing weight over 2 to 4 weeks. Traction should be continued until normal patellar height is restored and there is at least 90 degrees of flexion. Once the patella has been restored to its anatomic position, the patellar tendon repair or reconstruction is carried out as the second stage. Patellar traction has also been described using an Ilizarov fixator, with which olive wires are placed vertically in the patella and then connected to a tibial frame. The wires are tensioned 1 mm per day to pull the patella distally.[32] Advantages of this technique are that it allows knee motion and weight-bearing on the injured leg during the period of traction. The tendon repair site can also be protected by the Ilizarov frame postoperatively, with gradual transfer of stress to the healing tendon being accomplished by removing the traction. In cases of severe patellar retraction, a Z-lengthening or V-Y lengthening of the quadriceps tendon may be required to correct patellar height.

Because the tissue quality of the remaining tendon in chronic cases is often inferior, augmentation of the repair or patellar tendon reconstruction is often indicated. There are several options for augmentation and reconstruction. As described earlier, semitendinosus and gracilis tendons can be used. These tendons are useful for augmentation if there is some remaining patellar tendon; however, they are insufficient for use as a sole replacement for an irreparable tendon. An Achilles tendon allograft with a calcaneal bone block[13] and a patellar allograft[97] have been used for patellar tendon reconstruction. A trough is made at the tibial tubercle to receive the calcaneal bone block, which is then secured with two cancellous screws. Care is taken to recreate a normal Q angle when choosing the site for attachment of the bone block to the tibial tuberosity. The tendinous portion of the allograft is divided into three strips, the central third of which is passed through a 9-mm wide longitudinal tunnel in the patella. This central slip of tendon then emerges proximally through a small slit in the quadriceps tendon and is sutured to it with No. 2 nonabsorbable sutures. The medial and lateral thirds of the allograft tendon are passed proximally and are sutured to the medial and lateral retinacula with No. 2 nonabsorbable sutures. Care is taken to avoid producing an imbalance in the tension in the medial versus the lateral retinaculum when suturing the allograft to the retinaculum. The allograft is also sutured to any remaining native patellar tendon. Appropriate graft length is determined by assuring that the knee will flex to 90 degrees and by evaluating the Insall-Salvati ratio.

Intraoperative radiography may be helpful to confirm appropriate patellar height.[77]

Reconstruction can also be performed using a patella–quadriceps tendon autograft.[97] The graft is taken from the central third of the quadriceps tendon, with an attached bone block from the proximal patella. The length of tendon harvested is determined by the length of the normal patellar tendon. The bone block is fixed to a bony trough at the tibial tubercle with a 4-mm cancellous screw. A small horizontal trough is made at the distal pole of the patella with a rongeur or bur. Heavy nonabsorbable (No. 5) sutures are placed into the tendon using a locking suture configuration, such as a Kessler, a Mason-Allen, or a Bunnell stitch. Two longitudinal drill holes are made in the patella, taking care to avoid entering the graft donor site in the proximal patella. The sutures are passed from the tendon into the drill holes, exiting over the superior pole of the patella. The tendon is reduced to the trough in the inferior pole of the patella and is then tied with the knee in full extension. The tendon graft is then sutured to the patellar tendon remnant. The bone that was removed to create the trough in the tibial tuberosity is used to graft the defect in the superior pole of the patella, and the quadriceps tendon donor site is sutured.[77]

Reconstruction of the patellar tendon can also be performed using a bone–patellar tendon–bone autograft from the contralateral knee, as is occasionally used for anterior cruciate ligament reconstruction. A cancellous screw is used at the tibial tuberosity to secure the graft in a trough at that site. On the patellar side, fixation is achieved similarly, but the bone plug is wedge shaped. This plug is then compressed into a matching trough on the patella, which is made with an obliquely oriented surface. A screw is inserted at an orientation of 45 degrees to the axis of the patella, thus avoiding violation of the articular surface of the patella. Alternatively, the graft can be harvested with a bone plug from only the tibial side, creating a bone–patellar tendon graft. This graft is then used as described earlier for a patella–quadriceps tendon autograft. Reconstruction using a bone–patellar tendon–bone allograft has also been reported and represents another option for chronic ruptures.[13]

There are several other special circumstances in which repair or reconstruction of the patellar tendon may be required. Use of the central third of the patellar tendon for anterior cruciate ligament reconstruction has been associated with postoperative rupture of the remaining patellar tendon. This injury can usually be treated by means of direct repair. Direct repair may be difficult if rupture occurs at the tibial attachment, however, and in this setting reconstruction may be required. Sleeve fracture of the patella, an injury that occurs in skeletally immature children, involves avulsion of a small portion of the bony inferior pole of the patella with a large attached piece of articular surface. If not recognized and reduced early, these injuries can result in formation of ectopic bone between the inferior patella and the patellar tendon with a resultant extensor lag. Treatment at that point requires excision of the ectopic bone and repair of the patellar tendon to the patella.[77]

Infrapatellar contracture syndrome can also occasionally require patellar tendon reconstruction. Paulos and associates described this complication following anterior cruciate ligament reconstruction.[73] There is fibrosis in the infrapatellar fat pad and anterior knee capsule resulting in patellar tendon contracture and patellar entrapment. Often, in this setting, substantial loss of motion occurs, and anterior knee discomfort ensues. Early treatment includes arthroscopic lysis of adhesions, removal of the fibrotic infrapatellar tissue, manipulation, and aggressive range of motion exercises. Open capsular and retinacular releases are sometimes required to restore full range of motion. In advanced cases, complete reconstruction of the patellar tendon may be required. The procedures and the principles described earlier for treatment of chronic patellar tendon rupture apply in this setting. Shortening of the quadriceps tendon and Z-lengthening of the contracted patellar tendon may also be required in this setting. Additionally, the surgeon may consider substitution of the pathologic tissue with use of a patellar tendon allograft.

If the patient has a history of previous infection and all attempts at repair and reconstruction have failed, the final salvage for chronic extensor mechanism disruption is knee arthrodesis. Several techniques are available for knee arthrodesis, including plate fixation, external fixation, and intramedullary implantation. The recommended position is 0 to 5 degrees of valgus and 10 to 15 degrees of flexion. The patella may be left intact, or the patellar articular surface may be resected.

Postoperative Rehabilitation

Postoperative rehabilitation is influenced by the perceived strength of the repair site. For acute repairs, weight-bearing as tolerated is allowed in a double-upright hinged brace with the knee in full extension. The brace is worn for 6 to 8 weeks following surgery. When a secure repair is achieved, the affected leg can be mobilized immediately after surgery using a continuous passive motion machine. Mobilization is continued for approximately 2 weeks until an arc of motion of at least 90 degrees is achieved. Active flexion and passive extension exercises are begun by the second week. Flexion is accomplished to the point at which there is tension on the repair, as determined intraoperatively. Straight leg raising exercises are allowed immediately following surgery. At 6 weeks postoperatively, active assisted extension exercises are initiated. Range of motion exercises and progressive resistance exercises for the quadriceps are performed with a physical therapist.[77]

Postoperative rehabilitation will be more gradual following repair or reconstruction of a chronic rupture. Weight-bearing and flexion exercises are delayed for 2 weeks. Partial weight-bearing is prescribed for the first 4 weeks, after which the patient may progress to weight-bearing as tolerated. Straight leg raising may be delayed for 2 weeks. Active extension exercises are allowed at 6 weeks, but resistance exercises are delayed until 12 weeks postoperatively.[77]

Clinical Outcomes

Generally, good results have been reported following surgical treatment. There are a few reports on the long-term outcome of patellar tendon repair in athletes.[21, 41] Kuechle and Stuart reported on six patients, all of whom were able to achieve their preinjury level of sports participation at an average of 18 months after injury.[47] One important factor that appears to influence functional recovery is restoration of normal patellofemoral tracking. Care should be taken to balance the patella appropriately and to avoid shortening the patellar tendon to avoid late patellofemoral pain. Inferior results have been reported following delayed surgery owing to muscle atrophy, proximal retraction of the extensor mechanism, and knee joint contracture.[77]

Authors' Preferred Method of Treatment

Ideally, repair within the first 2 weeks of injury is best for acute patellar tendon ruptures. The repair is performed with heavy sutures placed through drill holes in the patella, as described. Midsubstance ruptures are repaired directly with heavy sutures and are augmented with semitendinosus tendon passed through either the distal quadriceps tendon or a transverse drill hole in the patella and then through a drill hole in the tibial tuberosity. Ruptures at the tendon attachment site on the tibial tuberosity, which are uncommon, are repaired with sutures through drill holes and are augmented with semitendinosus tendon.

Our first choice for patellar tendon reconstruction of a chronic rupture is to use a patella–quadriceps tendon autograft,[97] as described earlier. If this tissue is unsuitable for use as a graft, we would recommend a patellar tendon allograft. Use of tissue from the contralateral knee is recommended if allograft is not available or if the patient refuses use of allograft tissue. Augmentation with both semitendinosus and gracilis tendons together is recommended for reconstructions performed for chronic rupture.

Complications

The complication rate and the need for reoperation following patellar tendon repairs appear to be greater than following quadriceps tendon repair. Secondary ruptures, although uncommon, are seen more frequently following patellar tendon repair as compared with quadriceps tendon repair. Patellar malalignment with abnormal patellar kinematics appears to be the most frequent complication following patellar tendon repair. Lateral patellar tilt may be induced if the retinacular repair is not balanced, and excessive patellofemoral contact stress may result from excessive shortening of the extensor mechanism. Patella infra may occur owing to entrapment of the patellar tendon by fibrosis in the infrapatellar fat pad and can cause significant pain and loss of flexion.[73]

Residual weakness of the extensor mechanism and inability to achieve full knee flexion are also common complications after surgery. A residual extensor lag may occur following delayed repair. Infection and wound problems can occur, especially if there is poor soft tissue coverage over the tibial tubercle or if the wound closure is under

22. el-Khoury GY, Wira RL, Berbaum KS, et al: MR imaging of patellar tendinitis. Radiology 184:849–854, 1992.

23. Frank C, Woo SY, Andriacchi T, et al: Normal ligament: Structure, function and composition. In Woo S, Buckwalter JA (eds): Injury and Repair of the Musculoskeletal Soft Tissues. Park Ridge, Ill, American Academy of Orthopaedic Surgeons, 1988, pp 45–101.

24. Fritschy D: Jumper's knee. Operative Tech Sports Med 5:150–152, 1997.

25. Fukui N, Cho N, Tashiro T, et al: Anatomical reconstruction of the patellar tendon: A new technique with hamstring tendons and iliotibial tract. J Orthop Trauma 13:375–379, 1999.

26. Gerster JC, Landry M, Rappoport G, et al: Enthesopathy and tendinopathy in gout: Computed tomographic assessment. Ann Rheum Dis 55:921–923, 1996.

27. Green JS, Morgan B, Lauder I, et al: The correlation of bone scintigraphy and histological findings in patellar tendinitis. Nucl Med Commun 17:231–234, 1996.

28. Hannafin JA, Arnoczky SP, Hoonjan A, et al: Effect of stress deprivation and cyclic tensile loading on the material and morphologic properties of canine flexor digitorum profundus tendon: An in vitro study. J Orthop Res 13: 907–914, 1995.

29. Hogh J, Lund B: The sequelae of Osgood-Schlatter's disease in adults. Int Orthop 12:213–215, 1988.

30. Huberti HH, Hayes WC, Stone JL, et al: Force ratios in the quadriceps tendon and ligamentum patellae. J Orthop Res 2:49–54, 1984.

31. Hyman J, Rodeo SA: Injury and repair of tendons and ligaments. Phys Med Rehabil Clin N Am 11:267, 2000.

32. Isiklar ZU, Varner KE, Lindsey RW, et al: Late reconstruction of patellar ligament ruptures using Ilizarov external fixation. Clin Orthop 322:174–178, 1996.

33. Jarvinen M: Epidemiology of tendon injuries in sports. Clin Sports Med 11:493–504, 1992.

34. Johnson DP, Wakeley CJ, Watt I: Magnetic resonance imaging of patellar tendinitis. J Bone Joint Surg Br 78:452–457, 1996.

35. Johnson GA, Tramaglini DM, Levine RE, et al: Tensile and viscoelastic properties of human patellar tendon. J Orthop Res 12:796–803, 1994.

36. Josza L, Szederkenyi J: Mucopolysaccharide content of the human aorta in hypothyroidism. Endokrinologie 50:116–122, 1966.

37. Kannus P, Jozsa L: Histopathological changes preceding spontaneous rupture of a tendon. A controlled study of 891 patients. J Bone Joint Surg Am 73:1507–1525, 1991.

38. Karlsson J, Kalebo P, Goksor LA, et al: Partial rupture of the patellar ligament. Am J Sports Med 20:390–395, 1992.

39. Katzman BM, Silberberg S, Caligiuri DA, et al: Delayed repair of a quadriceps tendon. Orthopedics 20:553–554, 1997.

40. Kelikian H, Riashi E, Gleason J: Restoration of quadriceps tendon function in neglected tear of the patella tendon. Surg Gynecol Obstet 104:200, 1957.

41. Kelly DW, Carter VS, Jobe FW, et al: Patellar and quadriceps tendon ruptures—Jumper's knee. Am J Sports Med 12:375–380, 1984

42. Kennedy JC, Willis RB: The effects of local steroid injections on tendons: A biomechanical and microscopic correlative study. Am J Sports Med 4:11–21, 1976.

43. Khan KM, Bonar F, Desmond PM, et al: Patellar tendinosis (jumper's knee): Findings at histopathologic examination, US, and MR imaging. Victorian Institute of Sport Tendon Study Group. Radiology 200:821–827, 1996.

44. King JB, Perry DJ, Mourad K, et al: Lesions of the patellar ligament. J Bone Joint Surg Br 72:46–48, 1990.

45. Krause BL, Williams JP, Catterall A: Natural history of Osgood-Schlatter disease. J Pediatr Orthop 10:65–68, 1990.

46. Kretzler JE, Curtin SL, Wegner DA, et al: Patella tendon rupture: A late complication of a tibial nail. Orthopedics 18:1109–1111, 1995.

47. Kuechle DK, Stuart MJ: Isolated rupture of the patellar tendon in athletes. Am J Sports Med 22:692–695, 1994.

48. Kuivila TE, Brems JJ: Diagnosis of acute rupture of the quadriceps tendon by magnetic resonance imaging. A case report. Clin Orthop 262:236–241, 1991.

49. Kujala UM, Kvist M, Heinonen O: Osgood-Schlatter's disease in adolescent athletes. Retrospective study of incidence and duration. Am J Sports Med 13:236–241, 1985.

50. Kujala UM, Osterman K, Kvist M, et al: Factors predisposing to patellar chondropathy and patellar apicitis in athletes. Int Orthop 10:195–200, 1986.

51. Laduron J, Shahabpour M, Anneert J, et al: Use of dynamic US and MR imaging in the assessment of trochleotendinous knee impingement syndrome. RSNA 79th Scientific Assembly and Annual Meeting, 1993, London.

52. Lapinsky AS, Padgett DE, Hall FW: Disruption of the extensor mechanism in Paget's disease. Am J Orthop 24:165–167, 1995.

53. Larsen E, Lund PM: Ruptures of the extensor mechanism of the knee joint. Clinical results and patellofemoral articulation. Clin Orthop 213:150–153, 1986.

54. Larson RV, Simonian PT: Semitendinosus augmentation of acute patellar tendon repair with immediate mobilization. Am J Sports Med 23:82–86, 1995.

55. Lauerman WC, Smith BG, Kenmore PI: Spontaneous bilateral rupture of the extensor mechanism of the knee in two patients on chronic ambulatory peritoneal dialysis. Orthopedics 10:589–591, 1987.

56. Leadbetter WB, Mooar PA, Lane GJ, et al: The surgical treatment of tendinitis. Clinical rationale and biologic basis. Clin Sports Med 11:679–712, 1992.

57. Levy M, Goldstein J, Rosner M: A method of repair for quadriceps tendon or patellar ligament (tendon) ruptures without cast immobilization. Preliminary report. Clin Orthop 218:297–301, 1987.

58. Levy M, Seelenfreund M, Maor P, et al: Bilateral spontaneous and simultaneous rupture of the quadriceps tendons in gout. J Bone Joint Surg Br 53:510–513, 1971.

59. Lian O, Engebretsen L, Ovrebo RV, et al: Characteristics of the leg extensors in male volleyball players with jumper's knee. Am J Sports Med 24:380–385, 1996.

60. Likar I, Robinson R, Likar L: Glycosaminoglycans and hormones: Mesenchymal response in endocrinopathies. In Varma RS (ed): Glycosaminoglycans and Proteoglycans in Physiological and Pathological Processes of Body Systems. Basel, Karger, 1982, pp 412–439.

61. Lindy PB, Boynton MD, Fadale PD: Repair of patellar tendon disruptions without hardware. J Orthop Trauma 9:238–243, 1995.

62. MacEachern AG, Plewes JL: Bilateral simultaneous spontaneous rupture of the quadriceps tendons. Five case reports and a review of the literature. J Bone Joint Surg Br 66:81–83, 1984.

63. Maffulli N, Binfield PM, Leach WJ, et al: Surgical management of tendinopathy of the main body of the patellar tendon in athletes. Clin J Sport Med 9:58–62, 1999.

64. Maffulli N, Khan KM, Puddu G: Overuse tendon conditions: Time to change a confusing terminology. Arthroscopy 14:840–843, 1998.

65. Martens M, Wouters P, Burssens A, et al: Patellar tendinitis: Pathology and results of treatment. Acta Orthop Scand 53:445–450, 1982.

66. Matava MJ: Patellar tendon ruptures. J Am Acad Orthop Surg 4: 287–296, 1996.

67. McGarvey WC, Singh D, Trevino SG: Partial Achilles tendon ruptures associated with fluoroquinolone antibiotics: A case report and literature review. Foot Ankle Int 17:496–498, 1996.

68. McLaughlin H, Francis K: Operative repair of injuries to the quadriceps extensor mechanism. Am J Surg 91:651, 1956.

69. McMaster PE: Tendon and muscle ruptures: Clinical and experimental studies on the causes and location of subcutaneous ruptures. J Bone Joint Surg 15:705–722, 1933.

70. Micheli LJ, Slater JA, Woods E, et al: Patella alta and the adolescent growth spurt. Clin Orthop 213:159–162, 1986.

71. Nance EP Jr, Kaye JJ: Injuries of the quadriceps mechanism. Radiology 142:301–307, 1982.

72. Nordin M, Frankel VH: Biomechanics of the knee. In Nordin M, Frankel VH: Basic Biomechanics of the Musculoskeletal System. Philadelphia, Lea & Febiger, 1989, pp 115–134.

73. Paulos LE, Wnorowski DC, Greenwald AE: Infrapatellar contracture syndrome. Diagnosis, treatment, and long-term followup. Am J Sports Med 22:440–449, 1994.

74. Petersen W, Stein V, Tillmann B: Blood supply of the quadriceps tendon [in German]. Unfallchirurg 102:543–547, 1999.

75. Podesta L, Sherman MF, Bonamo JR: Bilateral simultaneous rupture of the infrapatellar tendon in a recreational athlete. A case report. Am J Sports Med 19:325–327, 1991.

76. Richards DP, Ajemian SV, Wiley JP, et al: Knee joint dynamics predict patellar tendinitis in elite volleyball players. Am J Sports Med 24:676–683, 1996.

77. Rodeo S, Izawa K: Diagnosis and treatment of knee tendon injury. In Garrett W (ed): Textbook of Sports Medicine (in press).

78. Rosenberg ZS, Kawelblum M, Cheung YY, et al: Osgood-Schlatter

lesion: Fracture or tendinitis? Scintigraphic, CT, and MR imaging features. Radiology 185:853–858, 1992.

79. Scapinelli R: Studies on the vasculature of the human knee joint. Acta Anat 70:305–331, 1968.

80. Scott SH, Winter DA: Internal forces of chronic running injury sites. Med Sci Sports Exerc 22:357–369, 1990.

81. Scuderi C: Ruptures of the quadriceps tendon: Study of twenty tendon ruptures. Am J Surg 95:626, 1958.

82. Scuderi AJ, Datz FL, Valdivia S, et al: Enthesopathy of the patellar tendon insertion associated with isotretinoin therapy. J Nucl Med 34:455–457, 1993.

83. Scuderi C, Schrey EL: Quadriceps tendon ruptures. Arch Surg 61: 42, 1950.

84. Selvanetti A, Massimo C, Puddu G: Overuse tendon injuries: Basic science and classification. Operative Tech Sports Med 5:110–117, 1997.

85. Sen RK, Sharma LR, Thakur SR, et al: Patellar angle in Osgood-Schlatter disease. Acta Orthop Scand 60:26–27, 1989.

86. Siebert CH, Kaufmann A, Niedhart C, et al: The quadriceps tendon cyst: An uncommon cause of chronic anterior knee pain. Knee Surg Sports Traumatol Arthrosc 7:349–351, 1999.

87. Siwek CW, Rao JP: Ruptures of the extensor mechanism of the knee joint. J Bone Joint Surg Am 63:932–937, 1981.

88. Stanish WD, Rubinovich RM, Curwin S: Eccentric exercise in chronic tendinitis. Clin Orthop 208:65–68, 1986.

89. Stanitski CL: Knee overuse disorders in the pediatric and adolescent athlete. Instr Course Lect 42:483–495, 1993.

90. Tanaka H, Manske PR, Pruitt DL, et al: Effect of cyclic tension on lacerated flexor tendons in vitro. J Hand Surg [Am] 20:467–473, 1995.

91. Testa V, Capasso G, Maffulli N, et al: Ultrasound-guided percutaneous longitudinal tenotomy for the management of patellar tendinopathy. Med Sci Sports Exerc 31:1509–1515, 1999.

92. Unverferth LJ, Olix ML: The effect of local steroid injections on tendon. J Sports Med 1:31–37, 1973.

93. Walsh WM: Patellofemoral joint. In DeLee JC, Drez DD (eds): Orthopaedic Sports Medicine: Principles and Practice. Philadelphia, WB Saunders, 1994, pp 1163–1248.

94. Webb LX, Toby EB: Bilateral rupture of the patella tendon in an otherwise healthy male patient following minor trauma. J Trauma 26:1045–1048, 1986.

95. Wiggins ME, Fadale PD, Barrach H, et al: Healing characteristics of a type I collagenous structure treated with corticosteroids. Am J Sports Med 22:279–288, 1994.

96. Williams RJ III, Attia E, Wickiewicz TL, et al: The effect of ciprofloxacin on tendon, paratenon, and capsular fibroblast metabolism. Am J Sports Med 28:364–369, 2000.

97. Williams RJ III, Brooks DD, Wickiewicz TL: Reconstruction of the patellar tendon using a patella–quadriceps tendon autograft. Orthopedics 20:554–558, 1997.

98. Woo S, Maynard J, Butler D, et al: Ligament, tendon and joint capsule insertions to bone. In Woo S, Buckwalter JA (eds): Injury and Repair of the Musculoskeletal Soft Tissues. Park Ridge, Ill, American Academy of Orthopaedic Surgeons, 1988, pp 133–166.

99. Yang BY, Sartoris DJ, Resnick D, et al: Calcium pyrophosphate dihydrate crystal deposition disease: Frequency of tendon calcification about the knee. J Rheumatol 23:883–888, 1996.

100. Yu JS, Popp JE, Kaeding CC, et al: Correlation of MR imaging and pathologic findings in athletes undergoing surgery for chronic patellar tendinitis. AJR Am J Roentgenol 165:115–118, 1995.

101. Zeiss J, Saddemi SR, Ebraheim NA: MR imaging of the quadriceps tendon: Normal layered configuration and its importance in cases of tendon rupture. AJR Am J Roentgenol 159:1031–1034, 1992.

102. Zernicke RF, Garhammer J, Jobe FW: Human patellar-tendon rupture. J Bone Joint Surg Am 59:179–183, 1977.

9. KNEE EXTENSOR MECHANISM INJURIES IN ATHLETES

LTC Craig R. Bottoni, MD ■ LTC Dean C. Taylor, MD ■ COL (ret) Robert A. Arciero, MD*

Extensor mechanism injuries are common injuries in athletes. The quadriceps muscle group, through its insertion into the tibial tubercle, produces knee extension during running to propel the leg forward. During the landing from a jump, the eccentric activation of the quadriceps decelerates the body and dissipates the force. At the bottom of this motion, the quadriceps muscle group in conjunction with the gastrocsoleus muscles contracts to initiate another jump. The complex interaction of these muscles with the patella, the largest sesamoid bone in the body, results in tremendous forces across this joint. During knee flexion, the patella articulates in the femoral trochlea to maintain proper alignment of these forces as well as to increase the mechanical leverage of the quadriceps on the tibia. The excessive forces and complexity of this system can result in a variety of injuries.

Anatomy

The quadriceps femoris, the largest muscle group in the body, consists of four muscles with a common insertion into the tibial tubercle. Three of the muscles, the vastus lateralis, vastus medialis, and vastus intermedius, take their origin from the femur and cross the knee joint. The rectus femoris has two "heads" that originate from the ilium of the pelvis (Fig. 28E9–1). The direct head takes its origin from the anterior inferior iliac spine, and the reflected head originates from the anterosuperior acetabulum and anterior capsule of the hip joint. This muscle inserts into the patella through a strong central tendon and spans both the hip and knee joints. Because of this configuration, the rectus femoris is both a strong knee extensor and a weak hip flexor.

The common quadriceps tendon inserts into and then envelops the patella. The insertion of the tendon into the superior pole of the patella is a trilaminar structure. It then continues as the patellar tendon into the tibial tubercle. The patella acts to increase the moment arm of the quadriceps, thus giving added leverage to the muscle group in extending the knee. The quadriceps muscles, their common tendon, and the patellofemoral articulation are subjected to tremendous loads with athletic activities, especially repetitive jumping. Normal ambulation results in compressive forces up to one-half body weight across the patellofemoral joint.[40] Forces greater than eight times body weight have been recorded in the extensor mechanism with jumping.[40] Disorders of the patellofemoral joint are covered in detail in subsequent chapters.

Although not part of the quadriceps group, a small muscle, the articularis genu, originates on the anterior thigh just proximal to the knee joint and deep to the vastus intermedius. It retracts the superior joint capsule with knee

*The views expressed herein are those of the authors and should not be construed as official policy of the Department of the Army or the Department of Defense.

lesions leading to presenile spontaneous gangrene. Am J Med Sci 136:567, 1908.

15. Burnstein DB, Fischer DA: Isolated rupture of the popliteus tendon in a professional athlete. Arthroscopy 6:238–241, 1990.

16. Clancy WG: Tendon trauma and overuse injuries. In Leadbetter WB, Buckwalter JA, Gordon FL (eds): Sports-Induced Inflammation. Park Ridge, Ill, American Academy of Orthopaedic Surgeons, 1990, pp 609–617.

17. Cohn AK, Mains DB: Popliteal hiatus of the lateral meniscus. Am J Sports Med 7:221–226, 1979.

18. Colson JH, Armour WI: Sports Injuries and Their Treatment. Philadelphia, JB Lippincott, 1975, p 56.

19. Dandy DJ: Anatomy of the medial suprapatellar plica and medial synovial shelf. Arthroscopy 6:79–85, 1990.

20. Darling RC, Buckley CJ, Abbott WM, Raines JK: Intermittent claudication in young athletes: Popliteal artery entrapment syndrome. J Trauma 14:543–552, 1974.

21. Dashefsky JH: Fracture of the fabella. A case report. J Bone Joint Surg Am 59:698, 1977.

22. Dawn B: Prepatellar bursitis: A unique presentation of tophaceous gout in a normouricemic patient. J Rheumatol 24:976–978, 1997.

23. Dupont J: Synovial plicae of the knee. Controversies and review. Clin Sports Med 16:87–121, 1997.

24. Edwards JC, Green T, Riefel E: Neurilemoma of the saphenous nerve presenting as pain in the knee. A case report. J Bone Joint Surg Am 71:1410–1411, 1989.

25. Ehrenborg G: The Osgood-Schlatter lesion. Acta Chir Scand [Suppl] 288:1, 1962.

26. Ehrenborg G, Engfeldt B: The insertion of the ligamentum patella on the tibial tuberosity. Some changes in connection with the Osgood-Schlatter lesion. Acta Chir Scand 121:491, 1961.

27. Estwanik JJ, Bergfeld JA, Collins HR, et al: Injuries in interscholastic wrestling. Physician Sportsmed 8:111–121, 1980.

28. Falk GD: Radiographic observation of incidence of the fabella. Bull Hosp J Dis 24:127, 1963.

29. Fisk GD Jr, Hockhausen M: Lacerations in the popliteal artery due to blunt trauma. Am J Surg 97:651, 1957.

30. Flanigan DP, Burnham SJ, Goodreau JJ, Bergan JJ: Summary of cases of adventitial cystic disease of the popliteal artery. Ann Surg 189:165–175, 1979.

31. Flowers MJ: Tibial tuberosity excision for symptomatic Osgood-Schlatter disease. J Pediatr Orthop 15:292–297, 1995.

32. Franco V, Cerullo G, Gianni E, et al: Iliotibial band friction syndrome. Operative Tech Sports Med 5:153–156, 1997.

33. Gardiner JS, McInerney VK, Avella DG, Valdez NA: Injuries to the inferior pole of the patella in children. Orthop Rev 19:643–649, 1990.

34. Green NE, Allen BL: Vascular injuries associated with dislocation of the knee. J Bone Joint Surg Am 59:236–239, 1977.

35. Gruel JB: Isolated avulsion of the popliteus tendon. Arthroscopy 6:94–95, 1990.

36. Hamming JJ, Vink M: Obstruction of the popliteal artery at an early age. J Cardiovasc Surg 6:516, 1965.

37. Hardaker WT, Whipple TL, Bassett FH III: Diagnosis and treatment of the plica syndrome of the knee. J Bone Joint Surg Am 62:221–225, 1980.

38. Henler DE: Saphenous nerve entrapment caused by pes anserine bursitis mimicking stress fracture of the tibia. Arch Phys Med Rehabil 72:336–337, 1991.

39. Ho G, Su EY: Antibiotic therapy of septic bursitis. Arthritis Rheum 24:905–911, 1981.

40. Ho G, Tice AD: Comparison of nonseptic and septic bursitis. Arch Intern Med 139:1269–1272, 1979.

41. Ho G, Tice AD, Kaplan SR: Septic bursitis in the prepatellar and olecranon bursa. Ann Intern Med 88:21–27, 1978.

42. Hohlbaum J: Die Bursa suprapatellaris und ihre beziehungenzun Kniegelenke. Ein Beitrag zum Entwicklung der Angeboren Schleimbeutal. Bruns Bietr Kin Chir 128:481–498, 1923.

43. Houghton GR, Ackroyd CE: Sleeve fractures of the patella in children. A report of three cases. J Bone Joint Surg Br 61:165–168, 1979.

44. Hunter LY, Louis DS, Ricciardi JR, O'Connor GA: The saphenous nerve; its course and importance in medical arthrotomy. Am J Sports Med 7:227–230, 1979.

45. Iino S: Normal arthroscopic findings in the knee joint in adult cadavers. J Jap Orthop Assoc 14:467–523, 1939.

46. Ishikawa K, Mishima Y, et al: Cystic adventitial disease of the popliteal artery. Angiology 12:357, 1961.

47. Jackson RW, Marshall DJ, Fujisawa Y: The pathologic medial shelf. Orthop Clin North Am 13:307–312, 1982.

48. Jakob RO, Hassler H, Staeubli HU: Observations on rotary instability of the lateral compartment of the knee. Experimental studies on the functional anatomy and the pathomechanism of the true and the reverse pivot shift sign. Acta Orthop Scand [Suppl] 52:1–32, 1982.

49. Jakob RP, Gumppenberg SV, Engelhardt P: Does Osgood-Schlatter disease influence the position of the patella? J Bone Joint Surg Br 63:579–582, 1981.

50. Jeffreys PE: Genu recurvatum after Osgood-Schlatter disease. J Bone Joint Surg Br 47:298–299, 1965.

51. Johansson S: En forut icke beskriven sjukdom i patella. Hygiea 84:161–166, 1922.

52. Jones RE, Smith EC, Bone GE: Vascular and orthopaedic complications of knee dislocations. Surg Gynecol Obstet 149:554–558, 1979.

53. Joyce JJ, Harty M: Surgery of the synovial fold. In Casscells W (ed): Arthroscopy: Diagnosis in Surgical Practice. Philadelphia, Lea & Febiger, 1984, pp 201–209.

54. Justis EJ: Nontraumatic disorders. In Crenshaw AH (ed): Campbell's Operative Orthopaedics, 7th ed. St. Louis, CV Mosby, 1987, pp 2252–2254.

55. Kaalund S: Endoscopic resection of the septic prepatella bursa. Arthroscopy 14:757–758, 1998.

56. Kaplan EB: The iliotibial tract. J Bone Joint Surg Am 40:817–832, 1958.

57. Kalenak A: Saphenous nerve entrapment. Operative Tech Sports Med 4:40–45, 1996.

58. Kerlan RK, Glousman RE: Tibial collateral ligament bursitis. Am J Sports Med 16:344–346, 1987.

59. Kerr DR: Prepatellar and olecranon arthroscopic bursectomy. Clin Sports Med 12:137–142, 1993.

60. Kinnard P, Levesque RY: The plica syndrome. Clin Orthop 183:141–143, 1984.

61. Knight JM, Thomas JC, Maurer RC: Treatment of septic olecranon and prepatellar bursitis with percutaneous placement of a suction/irrigation system. Clin Orthop 206:90–93, 1986.

62. Koch RA, Jackson DW: Juxta-articular hemangioma of the knee associated with a medial synovial plica. Am J Sports Med 9:265–267, 1981.

63. Kover JH, Schwalbe N, Levowitz BS: Popliteal aneurysm due to osteochondroma in athletic injury. N Y State J Med 70:3001–3003, 1970.

64. Krause BL, Williams JPR, Catteral A: Natural history of Osgood-Schlatter disease. J Pediatr Orthop 10:65–68, 1990.

65. Kristenson RU: Pseudoarthrosis between a patellar tendon ossicle and the tibial tuberosity in Osgood-Schlatter's disease. Scand J Med Sci 6:57–59, 1996.

66. Kujala UM, Kzist M, Heinonen O: Osgood-Schlatter's disease in adolescent athletes. Retrospective study of incidence and duration. Am J Sports Med 13:236–214, 1985.

67. Kurosaka M: Lateral synovial plica syndrome. A case report. Am J Sports Med 20:92–94, 1992.

68. Larson RL, Jones DC: Dislocations and ligament injuries of the knee. In Rockwood CA Jr, Green DP (eds): Fractures in Adults, vol. 1, 2nd ed. Philadelphia, JB Lippincott, 1984, p 1480.

69. Larson RL, Osternig LR: Traumatic bursitis and artificial turf. J Sports Med 2:183–188, 1974.

70. Larsson LG, Baum J: The syndrome of anserina bursitis: An overlooked diagnosis. Arthritis Rheum 28:1062–1065, 1985.

71. Last RJ: The popliteus muscle in the lateral meniscus. J Bone Joint Surg Br 32:93–99, 1950.

72. Lazert GD, Rapp I.H: Pathogenesis of Osgood-Schlatter disease. Am J Pathol 34:803, 1958.

73. Leavitt RY, Bressler P, Fauci A: Buerger's disease in a young woman. Am J Med 80:1003–1005, 1986.

74. Levine J, Kashyap F: A new conservative treatment of Osgood-Schlatter disease. Clin Orthop 158:126–128, 1981.

75. Levowitz DS, Kletschka HD: Fracture of the fabella. Report of a case. J Bone Joint Surg Am 37:876–877, 1955.

76. Lie JT: Thromboangiitis obliterans (Buerger's disease) and smokeless tobacco. Arthritis Rheum 31:812–813, 1988.

77. Lippitt AB: Neuropathy of the saphenous nerve as a cause of knee pain. Bull Hosp J Dis 52:31–33, 1993.

78. Love JW, Whelan TJ: Popliteal artery entrapment syndrome. Am J Surg 109:620, 1985.
79. Lundell C, Kadin S: The jogger's aneurysm: Unusual presentation of popliteal artery trauma. Cardiovasc Intervent Radiol 4:239–241, 1981.
80. Lynch MC: Tibia recurvatum as a complication of Osgood-Schlatter's disease: A report of two cases. J Pediatr Orthop 11:543–544, 1991.
81. Magora F, Aladjemoff L, Tannenbaum J, Magora A: Treatment of pain by transcutaneous electrical stimulation. Acta Anaesthesiol Scand 22:589–592, 1978.
82. Mann RA, Hagy JL: The popliteus muscle. J Bone Joint Surg Am 59:924–927, 1977.
83. Martens M, Libbrect P, Burssens A: Surgical treatment of the iliotibial band friction syndrome. Am J Sport Med 17:651–654, 1989.
84. Matsumoto K, Sinsuke H, Ogata M: Juxta-articular bone cysts at the insertion of the pes anserinus. J Bone Joint Surg Am 72:286–290, 1990.
85. Mayeda T: Veberdastrangartige Gebril in der Kneigelenk Hoehle (chorda cava articularis genu). Mitt met sak Kaiserl University of Tokyo 21:507–553, 1918.
86. Mayfield GW: Popliteus tendon tenosynovitis. Am J Sports Med 5:31–36, 1977.
87. McCoy GF, Hannon DG, Barr RJ, et al: Vascular injury associated with low-velocity dislocations of the knee. J Bone Joint Surg Br 69:2, 1987.
88. McDonald PT, Easterbrook JA, Rich NM, et al: Popliteal artery entrapment syndrome: Clinical noninvasive and angiographic diagnosis. Am J Surg 139:318–325, 1980.
89. McGinty J: Arthroscopic surgery in sports injuries. Orthop Clin North Am 11:787–799, 1980.
90. Medlar RC, Lyne ED: Sinding-Larsen-Johansson disease. Its etiology and natural history. J Bone Joint Surg Am 60: 1113–1116, 1978.
91. Mital MA, Matza RA, Cohen J: The so-called unresolved Osgood-Schlatter lesion. J Bone Joint Surg Am 62:732–739, 1980.
92. Mital MA, Hayden J: Pain in the knee in children: The medial plica shelf syndrome. Orthop Clin North Am 10:713–722, 1979.
93. Mozes MA, Ovaknine G, Nathan H: Saphenous nerve entrapment simulating vascular disorder. Surgery 77:299–303, 1975.
94. Murayama K: Entrapment of the saphenous nerve by branches of the femoral vessels. J Bone Joint Surg Am 73:770–772, 1991.
95. Muse GL, Grana WA, Hollingsworth S: Arthroscopic treatment of medial shelf syndrome. Arthroscopy 1:63–67, 1985.
96. Mysnyk MC, Wroble RR, Foster BT, Albright JP: Prepatellar bursitis in wrestlers. Am J Sports Med 14:46–54, 1986.
97. Nauer L, Aalberg JR: Avulsion of the popliteus tendon. Am J Sports Med 13:423–424, 1985.
98. Nielubowicz J, Rosnowski A, Pruszynski B, et al: Natural history of Buerger's disease. J Cardiovasc Surg 21:529, 1980.
99. Noble CA: The treatment of iliotibial band friction syndrome. Br J Sports Med 12:69–73, 1978.
100. Noble CA: Iliotibial band friction syndrome in runners. Am J Sports Med 8:232–234, 1980.
101. Noble HB, Hajek MR, Porter M: Diagnosis and treatment of iliotibial band tightness in runners. Physician Sports Med 10:67–74, 1982.
102. Noon GP, Zamora JL, Pratt CM, et al: Popliteal vein pseudoaneurysm: A case report. Surgery 96:5, 1984.
103. Nottage WM, Spaque NF, Auerbach BJ, Shahriaree H: The medial patellar plica syndrome. Am J Sports Med 11:211–214, 1983.
104. O'Dell JR, Linder J, Martin RS, Moore GF: Thromboangiitis obliterans (Buerger's disease) and smokeless tobacco. Arthritis Rheum 30:1054–1056, 1987.
105. O'Donoghue DH (ed): Treatment of Injuries to Athletes, 4th ed. Philadelphia, WB Saunders, 1984.
106. O'Donoghue DH: Injuries to the knee. In Treatment of Injuries to Athletes, 4th ed. Philadelphia, WB Saunders, 1987, pp 470–471.
107. Ogden JA, Southwick WO: Osgood-Schlatter's disease and tibial tuberosity development. Clin Orthop 116:180–189, 1976.
108. Orava S: Iliotibial band friction syndrome in athletes. Br J Sports Med 12:69, 1978.
109. Osgood RB: Lesions of tibial tubercle occurring during adolescence. Sci J 148:114, 1903.
110. Pancoast HK: Radiographic statistics of the sesamoid independent of the gastrocnemius. Univ Penn Med Bull 22:213, 1909.
111. Patel D: Arthroscopy of the plica-synovial folds and their significance. Am J Sports Med 6:217–225, 1978.
112. Patel D: Plica as a cause of an anterior knee pain. Orthop Clin North Am 17:273–277, 1986.
113. Patel D: Synovial lesions: Plicae. In McGinty JB (ed): Operative Arthroscopy. New York, Raven Press, 1991, pp 361–372.
114. Pipkin G: Lesions of the suprapatellar plica. J Bone Joint Surg Am 32:363–369, 1950.
115. Pipkin G: Knee injuries: The role of the suprapatellar plica and suprapatellar bursa in simulating internal derangement. Clin Orthop 74:161–176, 1971.
116. Renee JW: The iliotibial band friction syndrome. J Bone Joint Surg Am 57:1110–1115, 1975.
117. Rich NM, Collins GJ, McDonald PT, et al: Popliteal vascular entrapment: Its increasing interest. Arch Surg 114:1377–1384, 1979.
118. Rich NM, Spencer FC: Vascular Trauma. Philadelphia, WB Saunders, 1978, p 125.
119. Richmond JC, McGinty JB: Segmental arthroscopic resection of the hypertrophic mediopatellar plica. Clin Orthop 178:185–189, 1983.
120. Rignault DP, Pailler JL, Lunel F: The functional popliteal entrapment syndrome. Int Angiol 4:431, 1985.
121. Robert JM: Fractures and dislocations of the knee. In Rockwood CA Jr, Green DP, Wilkins K (eds): Fractures, vol 3. Philadelphia, JB Lippincott, 1984.
122. Romanoff ME, Cory PC, Kalenak A, et al: Saphenous nerve entrapment at the adductor canal. Am J Sports Med 17:478–481, 1989.
123. Ropes M, Bauer W: Synovial Fluid Change in Joint Disease. Cambridge, Mass, Harvard University Press, 1953, p 121.
124. Rose DJ, Parisien JS: Popliteus tendon rupture. Clin Orthop 26:113–117, 1988.
125. Rosenthal RK, Levine DB: Fragmentation of the distal pole of the patella in spastic cerebral palsy. J Bone Joint Surg Am 59:934–939, 1977.
126. Rovere GD, Ada DM: Medial synovial shelf plica syndrome. Treatment by intraplical steroid injection. Am J Sports Med 13:382–386, 1985.
127. Rudo HD, Noble HB, et al: Popliteal artery entrapment syndrome in athletes. Physician Sportsmed 10:105, 1982.
128. Sagel J: Fractures of the sesamoid bones. A report of two cases. Am J Surg 18:507–509, 1932.
129. Sakakibara J, Watanbe M: Arthroscopy study of Iino's band (plica synovialis mediopatellaris). J Jap Orthop Assoc 50:513–522, 1976.
130. Schlatter C: Verletbungen des Schnabelformigen forsatzes der oberen Tibiaepiphyses. Beitr Klin Chir 38:874, 1903.
131. Scotti DM, Sadhu VK, Heimberg F, O'Hara AE: Osgood-Schlatter's disease, and emphasis on soft tissue changes in roentgen diagnosis. Skeletal Radiol 4:21–25, 1979.
132. Sharrard WJ: Aetiology and pathology of beat knee. Br J Indust Med 20:24–31, 1963.
133. Shields L, Mital M, Cave EF: Complete dislocation of the knee: Experience at the Massachussetts General Hospital. J Trauma 9:192–215, 1969.
134. Sinding-Larsen MF: A hitherto unknown affliction of the patella in children. Acta Radiol 1:171–173, 1921.
135. Sisto BJ, Warren RF: Complete knee dislocation. Clin Orthop 198:94–101, 1985.
136. Stanish, WD, Rubinovich RM, Curwin S: Eccentric exercise in chronic tendinitis. Clin Orthop 208:65–68, 1986.
137. Staubli HU, Birrer S: The popliteus tendon and its fascicles at the popliteus hiatus: Gross anatomy and functional arthroscopy evaluation with and without anterior cruciate ligament deficiency. Arthroscopy 6:209–220, 1990.
138. Stell IM: Management of acute bursitis: Outcome study of a structural approach. J R Soc Med 92:516–521, 1999.
139. Strover AE: An arthroscopic technique of demonstrating the pathomechanics of the suprapatellar plica. Arthroscopy 7:308–310, 1991.
140. Stuart TP: A note on a variation in the course of the popliteal artery. J Anat Physiol 13:162, 1879.
141. Sutker AN, Jackson DW, Pagliana JW: Iliotibial band syndrome in distance runners. Physician Sportsmed 9:69–73, 1981.
142. Sutro CJ, Pomerantz MM, Simon SM: Fabella (sesamoid in the lateral head of the gastrocnemius). Arch Surg 30:777, 1935.
143. Terry GC, Hughston JC, Norwood LA: The anatomy of the iliopatellar band and iliotibial tract. Am J Sports Med 14:39–45, 1986.
144. Thijn CJ, Hillen B: Arthroscopy and the medial compartment of the patellofemoral joint. Skeletal Radiol 76:292–293, 1986.
145. Tindel NL: The plica syndrome. Orthop Clin North Am 23:613–618, 1992.

plus arthroscopic debridement and arthroscopic debridement alone. Arthroscopy 5:25–32, 1989.

12. Bobic V: Arthroscopic osteochondral autograft transplantation in anterior cruciate ligament reconstruction: A preliminary clinical study. Knee Surg Sports Traumatol Arthrosc 3:262–264, 1996.

13. Bocanegra TS, Weaver AL, Tindall EA, et al: Diclofenac/misoprostol compared with diclofenac in the treatment of osteoarthritis of the knee or hip: A randomized, placebo controlled trial. J Rheum 25:1602–1611, 1998.

14. Bradley JD, Brandt KD, Katz BP, et al: Comparison of an anti-inflammatory dose of ibuprofen, an analgesic dose of ibuprofen, and acetaminophen in the treatment of patients with osteoarthritis of the knee. N Engl J Med 325:87–91, 1991.

15. Brady LP: Hip pain. Don't throw away the cane. Postgrad Med 83: 95–97, 1988.

16. Brand RA, Crowninshield RD: The effect of cane use on hip force. Clin Orthop Rel Res 147:181–184, 1980.

17. Breinan HA, Minas T, Hsu HP, et al: Effect of cultured autologous chondrocytes on repair of chondral defects in a canine model. J Bone Joint Surg Am 79:1439–1451, 1997.

18. Brittberg M, Lindahl A, Nilsson A, et al: Treatment of deep cartilage defects in the knee with autologous chondrocyte transplantation. N Engl J Med 331:889–895, 1994.

19. Brittberg M, Nilsson A, Lindahl A, et al: Rabbit articular cartilage defects treated with autologous cultured chondrocytes. Clin Orthop 326:270–283, 1996.

20. Buckwalter JA, Lohmander S: Operative treatment of osteoarthrosis: Current practice and future development. J Bone Joint Surg Am 76: 1405–1418, 1994.

21. Buckwalter JA, Mow VC: Cartilage repair in osteoarthritis. In Moskowitz RW, Howell DS, Goldberg VM, et al (eds): Osteoarthritis, Diagnosis and Medical/Surgical Management, 2nd ed. Philadelphia, WB Saunders, 1992, pp 71–107.

22. Buckwalter JA, Rosenberg LC, Hunziker EB: Articular cartilage: Composition, structure, response to injury, and methods of facilitation repair. In Ewing JW (ed): Articular Cartilage and Knee Joint Function: Basic Science and Arthroscopy. New York, Raven Press, 1990, pp 19–56.

23. Campbell CJ: The healing of cartilage defects. Clin Orthop 64: 45–63, 1969.

24. Cartilage Repair Registry: Genzyme Tissue Repair. Cambridge, Mass, ABT Associates, 1997.

25. Chandler EJ: Abrasion arthroplasty of the knee. Contemp Orthop 11:21–29, 1985.

26. Chang RW, Falconer J, Stulberg SD, et al: A randomized controlled trial of arthroscopic surgery versus closed-needle joint lavage for patients with osteoarthritis of the knee. Arthritis Rheum 36:389–396, 1993.

27. Childers JC Jr, Ellwood SC: Partial chondrectomy and subchondral bone drilling for chondromalacia. Clin Orthop 144:114–120, 1979.

28. Coltier MA, Haugland LM, Bellamy J, et al: Effects of Holmium: YAG laser on equine articular cartilage assessment. Arthroscopy 9: 536–546, 1993.

29. Coutts RD, Woo SL-Y, Amiel D, et al: Rib perichondral autografts in full-thickness articular cartilage defects in rabbits. Clin Orthop 275:263–273, 1992.

30. Coventry MB, Ilstrup DM, Wallrichs SL: Proximal tibial osteotomy: A critical long-term study of eighty-seven cases. J Bone Joint Surg Am 75:196–201, 1993.

31. Creamer P: Intra-articular corticosteroid treatment in osteoarthritis. Curr Opin Rheum 11:417–421, 1999.

32. Crolle G, D'Este E: Glucosamine sulfate for the management of arthrosis: A controlled clinical investigation. Curr Med Res Opin 7: 104–109, 1980.

33. Davis MA, Ettinger WH, Neuhaus JM, et al: Sex differences in osteoarthritis of the knee: The role of obesity. Am J Epidemiol 127: 1019–1030, 1988.

34. Deal CL, Moskowitz RW: Nutraceuticals as therapeutic agents in osteoarthritis. The role of glucosamine, chondroitin sulfate and collagen hydrolysate. Rheum Dis Clin North Am 25:379–395, 1999.

35. Delafuente JC: Glucosamine in the treatment of osteoarthritis. Rheum Dis Clin North Am 26:1–11, 2000.

36. DePalma AF, McKeever CDE, Subin DK: Process of repair of articular cartilage demonstrated by histology and autoradiography with tritiated thymidine. Clin Orthop 48:229–242, 1966.

37. Dickinson JA, Cook SD, Leinhardt TM: The measurement of shock waves following heel strike while running. J Biomech 18:415–422, 1985.

38. Dixon AS, Jacoby RK, Berry H, et al: Clinical trial of intra-articular injection of sodium hyaluronate in patients with osteoarthritis of the knee. Curr Med Res Opin 11:205–213, 1988.

39. Dougados M, Nguyen M, Listrat V, et al: High molecular weight sodium hyaluronate (Hyalectin) in osteoarthritis of the knee: One year placebo-controlled trial. Osteoarthritis Cartilage 1:97–103, 1993.

40. Dovante A, Bignamini AA, Rovati AL: Therapeutic activity of oral glucosamine sulfate in osteoarthrosis: A placebo-controlled double-blind investigation. Clin Ther 3:266–272, 1980.

41. Ettinger WH, Burns R, Messier SP, et al: A randomized trial comparing aerobic exercise and resistance exercise with a health education program in older adults with aerobic knee osteoarthritis: The Fitness Arthritis and Seniors Trial. JAMA 277:25–31, 1997.

42. Felson DT: Epidemiology of hip and knee osteoarthritis. Epidemiol Rev 10:1–28, 1988.

43. Felson DT: Epidemiology of osteoarthritis. In Brandt KD, Doherty M, Lohmander LS (eds): Osteoarthritis. Oxford, Oxford University Press, 1998, pp 12–22.

44. Felson DT: The epidemiology of osteoarthritis: Prevalence and risk factors. In Kuettner KE, Goldberg VM (eds): Osteoarthritic Disorders. Rosemont, Ill, American Academy of Orthopaedic Surgeons, 1995, pp 13–24.

45. Felson DT, Anderson JJ, Naimark A, et al: Obesity and knee osteoarthritis. The Framingham study. Ann Intern Med 109:18–24, 1988.

46. Felson DT, Naimark A, Anderson JJ, et al: The prevalence of knee osteoarthritis in the elderly: The Framingham osteoarthritis study. Arthritis Rheum 30:914–918, 1987.

47. Felson DT, Zhang Y, Anthony JM, et al: Weight loss reduces the risk for symptomatic knee osteoarthritis in women. The Framingham study. Ann Intern Med 116:535–539, 1992.

48. Ficat RP, Hungerford DS (eds): Disorders of the Patello-femoral Joint. Baltimore, Williams & Wilkins, 1977, pp 194–243.

49. Fisher NM, Gresham GE, Abrams M, et al: Quantitative effects of physical therapy on muscular and functional performance in subjects with osteoarthritis of the knees. Arch Phys Med Rehabil 74:840–847, 1993.

50. Friedman MJ, Berasi CC, Fox JM, et al: Preliminary results with abrasion arthroplasty in the osteoarthritic knee. Clin Orthop 182: 200–205, 1984.

51. Fuller JA, Ghadially FN: Ultrastructural observations on surgically produced partial-thickness defects in articular cartilage. Clin Orthop 86:193–205, 1972.

52. Garrett JC: Osteochondral allografts for reconstruction of articular defects of the knee. AAOS Instr Course Lect 47:516–522, 1998.

53. Ghadially FN, Thomas I, Oryschak AF, et al: Long-term results of superficial defects in articular cartilage: A scanning electron-microscope study. J Pathol 121:213–217, 1977.

54. Ghazavi MT, Visram F, Davis AM, et al: Long-term results of fresh osteochondral allografts for posttraumatic osteochondral defects of the knee. Orthop Trans 19:454, 1995.

55. Grande DA, Pitman MI, Peterson L, et al: The repair of experimentally produced defects in rabbit articular cartilage by autologous chondrocyte transplantation. J Orthop Res 7:208–218, 1989.

56. Gross AE: Fresh osteochondral allografts for post-traumatic knee defects: Surgical technique. Oper Technique Orthop 7:334–339, 1997.

57. Gross AE: Use of fresh osteochondral allografts to replace traumatic joint defects. In Czitrom A, Gross AE (eds): Allografts in Orthopaedic Practice. Baltimore, Williams & Wilkins, 1992, pp 67–82.

58. Hangody L, Kish G, Karpati Z, et al: Mosaicplasty for the treatment of articular cartilage defects: Application in clinical practice. Orthopedics 21:751–756, 1998.

59. Haupt JB, McMillan R, Wein C, et al: Effect of glucosamine hydrochloride in the treatment of pain of osteoarthritis of the knee. J Rheum 26:2423–2430, 1999.

60. Hawkey CJ: COX-2 inhibitors. Lancet 353:307–314, 1999.

61. Henderson EB, Smith EC, Pegley F, et al: Intra-articular injections of 750 kD hyaluronan in the treatment of osteoarthritis: A randomized single center double-blind placebo-controlled trial of 91 patients demonstrating lack of efficacy. Ann Rheum Dis 53:529–534, 1994.

62. Hoikka VE, Jaroma JH, Ritsila VA: Reconstruction of the patellar

articulation with periosteal graft. Acta Orthop Scand 61:36–39, 1990.

63. Homminga GN, Bulstra SK, Bouwmeester PS, et al: Perichondral grafting for cartilage lesions of the knee. J Bone Joint Surg Br 72:1003–1007, 1990.
64. Hurley MV, Scott DL: Improvements in quadriceps sensomotor function and disability of patients with knee osteoarthritis following a clinically practicable exercise regime. Br J Rheumatol 37:1181–1187, 1996.
65. Ike RW, Arnold WJ, Rothschild EW, et al: Tidal irrigation versus conservative medical management in patients with osteoarthritis of the knee: A prospective randomized study. Tidal Irrigation Cooperating Group. J Rheumatol 19:772–779, 1992.
66. Insall J, Falvo KA, Wise DW: Chondromalacia patellae: A prospective study. J Bone Joint Surg Am 58:1–8, 1976.
67. Insall JN, Joseph DM, Msika C: High tibial osteotomy for varus gonarthrosis: A long-term follow-up study. J Bone Joint Surg Am 66:1040–1048, 1984.
68. Johnson-Nurse C, Dandy DJ: Fracture-separation of articular cartilage in the adult knee. J Bone Joint Surg Br 67:42–43, 1985.
69. Johnson LL: Arthroscopic abrasion arthroplasty In McGinty JB, Caspari RB, Jackson RW, Poehling GG (eds): Operative Arthroscopy, 2nd ed. Philadelphia, Lippincott-Raven, 1996, pp 427–446.
70. Johnson LL: Arthroscopic abrasion arthroplasty historical and pathologic perspective: Present status. Arthroscopy 2:54–69, 1986.
71. Johnson LL, Uitvlugt G, Austin MD, et al: Osteochondritis dissecans of the knee: Arthroscopic compression screw fixation. Arthroscopy 6:179–189, 1990.
72. Kaplan L, Uribe JW, Sasken H, et al: The acute effects of radiofrequency energy in articular cartilage: An in vitro study. Arthroscopy. 16:2–5, 2000.
73. Keating EM, Faris PM, Ritter MA, et al: Use of lateral heel and sole wedges in the treatment of medial osteoarthritis of the knee. Orthop Rev 22:921–924, 1993.
74. Kerrigan DC, Todd MK, Riley PO: Knee osteoarthritis and high-heeled shoes. Lancet 351:1399–1401, 1998.
75. Kirkley A, Webster-Bogaert S, Litchfield R, et al: The effect of bracing on varus gonarthrosis: J Bone Joint Surg Am 81:539–548, 1999.
76. Komistek RD, Dennis DA, Northcut EJ, et al: An in vivo analysis of the effectiveness of osteoarthritis knee brace during heel-strike gait. J Arthroplasty 14:738–742, 1999.
77. Korkala O, Kuokkanen H: Autogenous osteoperiosteal grafts in the reconstruction of full-thickness joint surface defects. Int Orthop 15:233–237, 1991.
78. Laine L, Hawkey C, Harper S, et al: Effect of the specific inhibitor (C-2SI) rofecoxib on ulcer formation: A double-blind comparison with ibuprofen and placebo. Gastroenterology 116(4 pt 2):G60986, 1999.
79. Lane JG, Amiel ME, Monosov AZ, et al: Matrix assessment of the articular cartilage surface after chondroplasty with the Holmium:YAG laser. Am J Sports Med 25:560–569, 1997.
80. Lane NE, Buckwalter JA: Exercise and osteoarthritis. Curr Opin Rheumatol 11:413–416, 1999.
81. Leach R, Baumgard S, Broom J: Obesity: Its relationship to osteoarthritis of the knee. Clin Orthop 93:271–273, 1973.
82. Levy AS, Lohnes J, Sculley S, et al: Chondral delamination of the knee in soccer players. Am J Sports Med 24:634–639, 1996.
83. Lohmander LS, Dalen N, Englund G, et al: Intra-articular hyaluronan injections in the treatment of osteoarthritis of the knee: A randomized double-blind, placebo-controlled multicenter trial. Ann Rheum Dis 55:424–431, 1996.
84. Lorentzon R, Alfredson H, Hildingson C: Treatment of deep cartilage defects of the patella with periosteal transplantation. Knee Surg Sports Traumatol Arthrosc 6:202–208, 1998.
85. Lussier A, Cividino AA, McFarlane CA, et al: Viscosupplementation with hylan for the treatment of osteoarthritis: Findings from clinical practice in Canada. J Rheumatol 23:1579–1585, 1996.
86. Matsuno H, Kadowaki KM, Tsuji H: Generation II knee bracing for severe medial compartment osteoarthritis of the knee. Arch Phys Med Rehabil 78:745–749, 1997.
87. Matthews LS, Goldstein SA, Malvitz TA, et al: Proximal tibial osteotomy: Factors that influence the durations of satisfactory function. Clin Orthop 229:193–200, 1988.
88. McAlindon TE, Valley MPL, Gulin JP, et al: Glucosamine and chondroitin for treatment of osteoarthritis: A systematic quality assessment and meta-analysis. JAMA 283:1469–1475, 2000.
89. McDermott AG, Langer F, Pritzker KP, et al: Fresh small-fragment osteochondral allografts: Long-term follow-up study on first 100 cases. Clin Orthop 197:96–102, 1985.
90. McGinley BJ, Cushner FD, Scott WN: Débridement arthroscopy: 10-year follow-up. Clin Orthop Rel Res 367:190–194, 1999.
91. Mendelson S, Milgrom C, Finestone A, et al: Effect of cane use on tibial strain and strain rates. Am J Phys Med Rehabil 77:333–338, 1998.
92. Minor MA, Hewett JE, Webel RR, et al: Exercise tolerance and disease related measures in patients with rheumatoid arthritis and osteoarthritis. J Rheumatol 15:905–911, 1988.
93. Moseley JB Jr, Wray NP, Kuykendall D, et al: Arthroscopic treatment of osteoarthritis of the knee: A prospective, randomized, placebo-controlled trial. Results of a pilot study. Am J Sports Med 24:28–34, 1996.
94. Noyes FR, Stabler CT: A system for grading articular cartilage lesions at arthroscopy. Am J Sports Med 17:505–513, 1989.
95. Odenbring S, Egund N, Lindstrand A, et al: Cartilage regeneration after proximal tibial osteotomy for medial gonarthrosis: An arthroscopic, roentgenographic, and histologic study. Clin Orthop 277:210–216, 1992.
96. O'Driscoll S: Current concepts review: The healing and regeneration of articular cartilage. J Bone Joint Surg Am 80:1795–1812, 1998.
97. O'Driscoll SW, Keeley FW, Salter RB: The chondrogenic potential of free autogenous periosteal grafts for biological resurfacing of major full-thickness defects in joint surfaces under the influence of continuous passive motion: An experimental investigation in the rabbit. J Bone Joint Surg Am 68:1017–1035, 1986.
98. Ogata K, Yasunaga M, Nomiyama H: The effect of wedged insoles on the thrust of osteoarthritic knees. Int Orthop 21:308–312, 1997.
99. Ogilvie-Harris DJ, Jackson RW: The arthroscopic treatment of chondromalacia patellae. J Bone Joint Surg Br 66:660–665, 1984.
100. Outerbridge HK, Outerbridge AR, Outerbridge RE: The use of a lateral patellar autologous graft for the repair of a large osteochondral defect in the knee. J Bone Joint Surg Am 77:65–72, 1995.
101. Peterson L, Minas T, Brittberg M, et al: Two to nine year outcome after autologous chondrocyte transplantation of the knee. Clin Orthop Rel Res 374:212–234, 2000.
102. Praemer AP, Furner S, Rice DP: Musculoskeletal Conditions in the United States. Rosemont, Ill, American Academy of Orthopaedic Surgeons, 1999, p 182.
103. Praemer AP, Furner S, Rice DP: Musculoskeletal Conditions in the United States. Park Ridge, Ill, American Academy of Orthopaedic Surgeons, 1992.
104. Pridie KH: A method of resurfacing osteoarthritic knee joints [abstract]. J Bone Joint Surg Br 41:618–619, 1959.
105. Raffa RB, Friderichs E, Reimann W, et al: Opioid and nonopioid components independently contribute to the mechanism of action of tramadol, an "atypical" opioid analgesic. J Pharmacol Exp Ther 260:275–285, 1992.
106. Rainsford KD: Profile and mechanisms of gastrointestinal and other side effects of nonsteroidal anti-inflammatory drugs. Am J Med 107:27S–35S, 1999.
107. Rand JA: Role of arthroscopy in osteoarthritis of the knee. Arthroscopy 7:358–363, 1991.
108. Rand JA, Gaffey TA: Effect of electrocautery on fresh human articular cartilage. Arthroscopy 1:242–246, 1985.
109. Rao JK, Mihaliak K, Kroehke K, et al: Use of complementary therapies for arthritis among patients of rheumatologists. Ann Intern Med 131:409–416, 1999.
110. Raskin JB: Gastrointestinal effects of nonsteroidal anti-inflammatory therapy. Am J Med 106:3S–12S, 1999.
111. Ravaud P, Moulinier L, Giraudeau B, et al: Effects of joint lavage and steroid injection in patients with osteoarthritis of the knee: Results of a multicenter, randomized, controlled trial. Arthritis Rheum 42:475–482, 1999.
112. Rindone JP, Hiller D, Collacott E, et al: Randomized controlled trial of glucosamine for treating osteoarthritis of the knee. West J Med 172:91–94, 2000.
113. Rosenstein ED: Topical agents in the treatment of rheumatic disorders. Rheum Dis Clin North Am 25:899–918, 1999.
114. Salter RB: The biologic concept of continuous passive motion of synovial joints: The first 18 years of basic research and its clinical application. Clin Orthop 242:12–25, 1989.

115. Saski T, Yasuda K: Clinical evaluation of the treatment of osteoarthritic knees using a newly designed wedged insole. Clin Orthop Rel Res 221:181–187, 1987.

116. Siemenda C, Brandt KD, Heilman DK, et al: Quadriceps weakness and osteoarthritis of the knee. Ann Intern Med 127:97–104, 1997.

117. Simon LS, Lanza FL, Lipsky PE, et al: Preliminary study of the safety and efficacy of SC-58635, a novel cyclooxygenase 2 inhibitor. Arthritis Rheum 41:1591–1602, 1998.

118. Steadman JR, Ridkey WG, Singleton SB, Briggs KK: Microfracture technique for full-thickness chondral defects: Technique and clinical results. Oper Technique Orthop 7:300–304, 1997.

119. Stone KR, Walgenbach A: Surgical technique for articular cartilage transplantation to full-thickness cartilage defects in the knee joint. In Miller M (ed): Operative Techniques in Orthopaedics. Philadelphia, WB Saunders, 1999.

120. Superio-Cabuslay E, Ward MM, Lorig KR: Patient education interventions in osteoarthritis and rheumatoid arthritis: A meta-analytic comparison with nonsteroidal anti-inflammatory drug treatment. Arthritis Care Res 9:292–301, 1998.

121. Thal R, Danziger MB, Kelly A: Delayed articular cartilage slough: Two cases resulting from holmium:Yag laser damage to normal articular cartilage and a review of the literature. Arthroscopy 12:92–94, 1996.

122. Tohyama H, Yasuda K, Kaneda K: Treatment of osteoarthritis of the knee with heel wedges. Int Orthop 15:31–33, 1991.

123. Trauner KB, Nishioka NS, Flotte T, et al: Acute and chronic response of articular cartilage to holmium:Yag laser irradiation. Clin Orthop Rel Res 310:52–57, 1995.

124. Troum OM, Lemoine C: Conservative management of the osteoarthritic knee. Curr Opin Orthop 11:3–8, 2000.

125. Turner AS, Tippet JW, Powers BE, et al: Radiofrequency (electrosurgical) ablation of articular cartilage: A study in sheep. Arthroscopy 14:585–591, 1998.

126. Vangsness CT, Smith C, Marshall GJ, et al: The biological effects of carbon dioxide laser surgery on rabbit articular cartilage. Clin Orthop Rel Res 310:48–51, 1995.

127. Vangsness CT: Overview of treatment options for arthritis in the active patient. Clin Sports Med 18:1–11, 1999.

128. Vangsness CT, Ghaderi B: A literature review of lasers and articular cartilage. Orthopedics 16:593–598, 1993.

129. Yasuda K, Sasaki T: The mechanics of treatment of osteoarthritic knee with a wedged insole. Clin Orthop Rel Res 215:162–172, 1987.

130. Zukor DJ, Oakeshott RD, Gross AE: Osteochondral allograft reconstruction of the knee: II. Experience with successful and failed fresh osteochondral allografts. Am J Knee Surg 2:182–191, 1989.

131. Zukor DJ, Paitich B, Oakeshott RD, et al: Reconstruction of posttraumatic articular surface defects using fresh small-fragment osteochondral allografts. In Acbi M, Regazzoni P (eds): Bone Transplantation. Berlin, Springer-Verlag, 1989, pp 293–305.

2. ARTICULAR CARTILAGE LESIONS AND OSTEOCHONDRITIS DISSECANS OF THE KNEE IN THE SKELETALLY IMMATURE PATIENT

Carl L. Stanitski, MD

Osteochondritis dissecans (OCD) is a lesion of subchondral bone that results in subchondral delamination and sequestration with or without articular mantle involvement. Sir James Paget[17] first described the lesion in two patients more than a century and a quarter ago. One patient was a girl who broke thick pieces of wood over her knee. The other patient was an athletic schoolboy "with many blows and strains to his knee from sports." Paget differentiated OCD from an acute osteochondral fracture and noted that the process involved an avascular sequestrum without evidence of inflammatory change. Twenty years later, Koenig[13] coined the term *osteochondritis dissecans* to reflect his concept that the process involved inflammatory dissection of the fragment despite his lacking evidence for such a sequence. He later realized that his concept was in error and recanted his view, but the term has persisted.[6, 14] Initially described in adults, OCD has come to be recognized in skeletally immature patients as well.

Epidemiology

OCD is classified by age or maturity status into the following groups: juvenile, with wide-open distal femoral physes; adolescent, with closing distal femoral physes; and adult, with fully closed distal femoral physes. Juvenile OCD's peak prevalence is during the preteen years, and it is rare among children younger than 10 years old. The condition is seen more commonly in males than females, with a 5:3 ratio. Bilaterality is reported in 20% to 25% of cases.[22] In bilateral cases, the lesions are usually not equal in terms of either size or symptoms (Fig. 28F2–1).[7]

The lesion characteristically involves the lateral poste-rior portion of the medial femoral condyle in 70% to 80% of cases. The classification described by Aichroth[2] is commonly used to identify the involved site. The so-called extended classic lesion involves the medial femoral trochlea as well (Fig. 28F2–2).[9] Lateral condylar involvement is seen in 15% to 20% of cases, most often in the inferocentral segment, with significant weight-bearing surface involvement (Fig. 28F2–3). Patellar lesions occur in 5% to 10% of cases and are almost always located in the inferomedial area (Fig. 28F2–4).[11] Femoral trochlear OCD is quite rare.

Etiology

Multiple theories have been proposed about the etiology of OCD, most of them centered on trauma—either an initial, acute macrotrauma followed by repetitive microtrauma or persistent microtrauma alone at a vulnerable area.[2, 5, 12, 13, 17, 20] Injection studies of the distal femoral subchondral zone show it to possess a rich microvasculature. Exogenous trauma, usually due to sports accidents, has been implicated in OCD by many authors. A significant number of cases (>50%), however, have also been seen with no history of antecedent trauma, athletic or otherwise. The acute trauma, when it occurs, appears to be incidental and not causative. Fairbanks[12] suggested that chronic impingement of the medial tibial eminence during tibial internal rotation caused the lesion. This thesis fails to account for lesions at other sites and the fact that tibial eminence impingement is not seen during normal walking or running gait. Review of OCD cases showed no relationship between abnormal tibial eminence morphology and OCD. Aichroth[2]

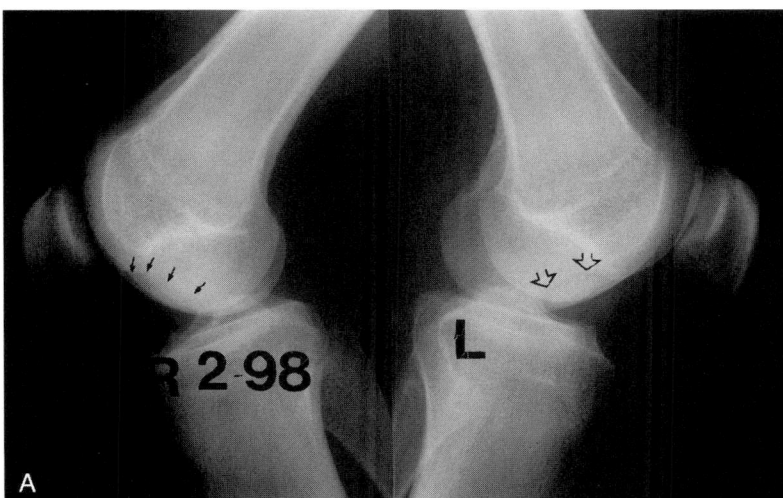

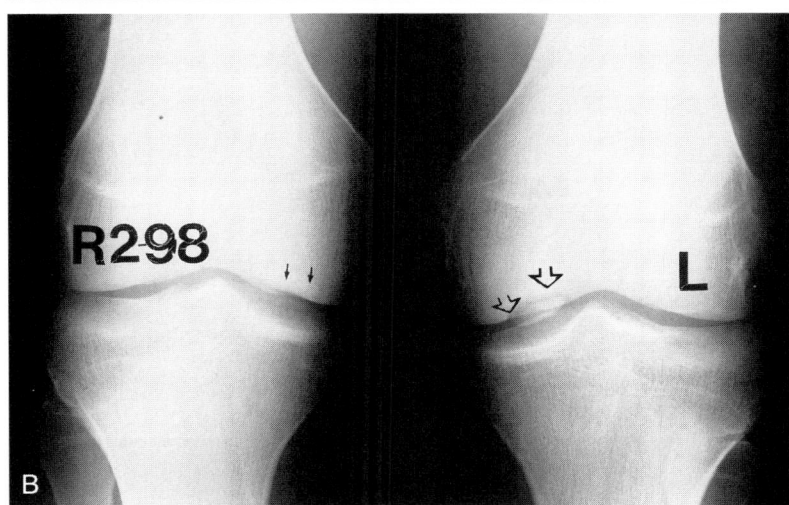

Figure 28F2–1. *A* and *B,* Bilateral, asymmetrical osteochondritis dissecans with a healed right lesion (*small arrows*) and an unhealed, unstable left lesion (*open arrows*) in a 17-year-old tennis player.

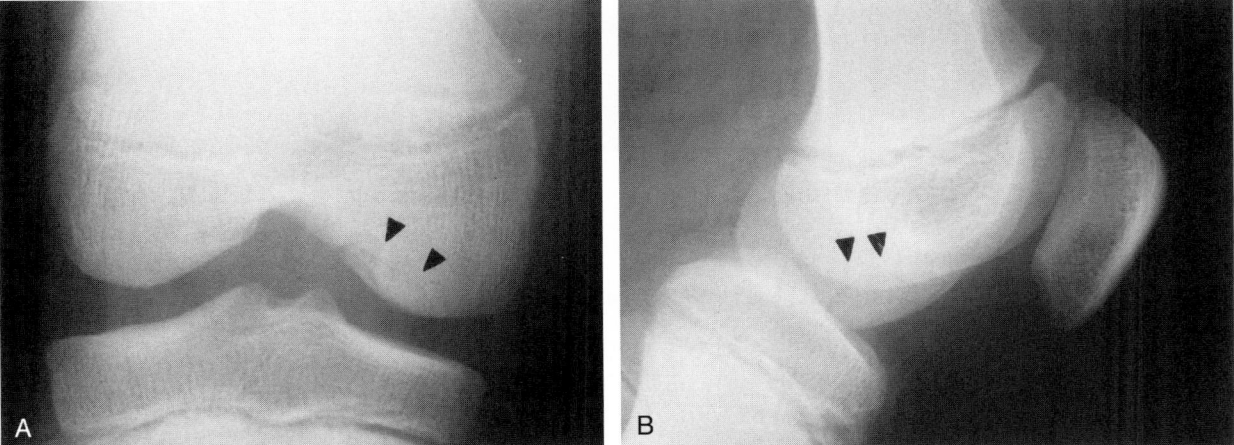

Figure 28F2–2. Extended classic lesion of the medial femoral condyle with trochlear involvement. *A,* Anteroposterior view; *B,* lateral view.

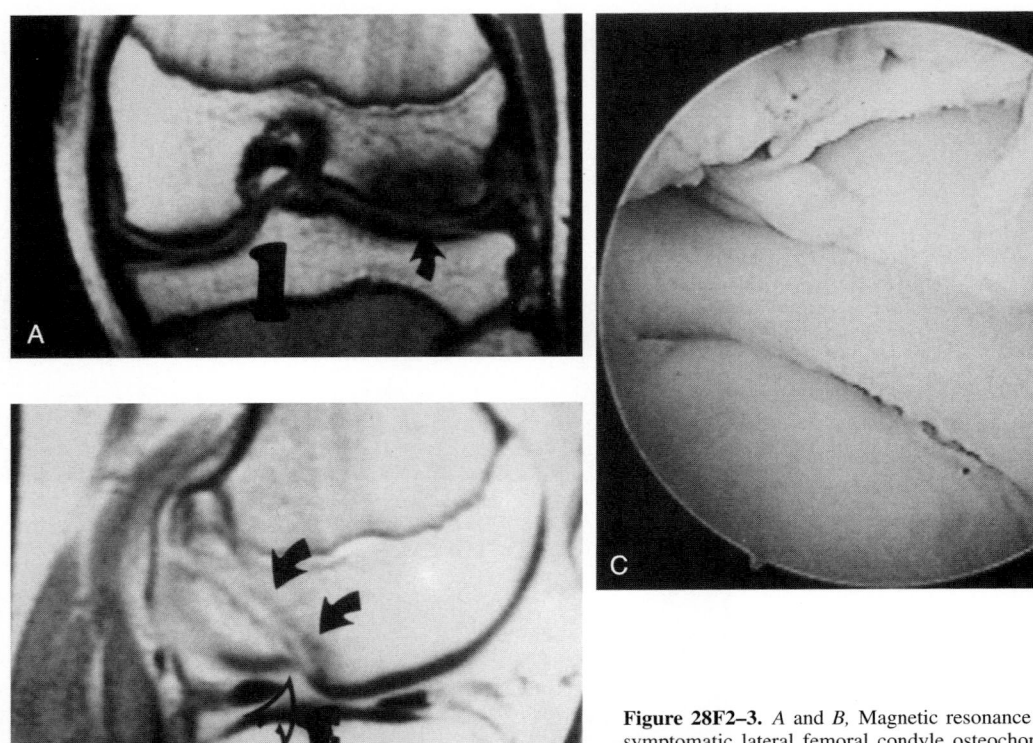

Figure 28F2–3. *A* and *B*, Magnetic resonance imaging (MRI) of symptomatic lateral femoral condyle osteochondritis dissecans in a 15-year-old hockey player. *C*, Arthroscopic view showing fragment displacement not appreciated on the MRI.

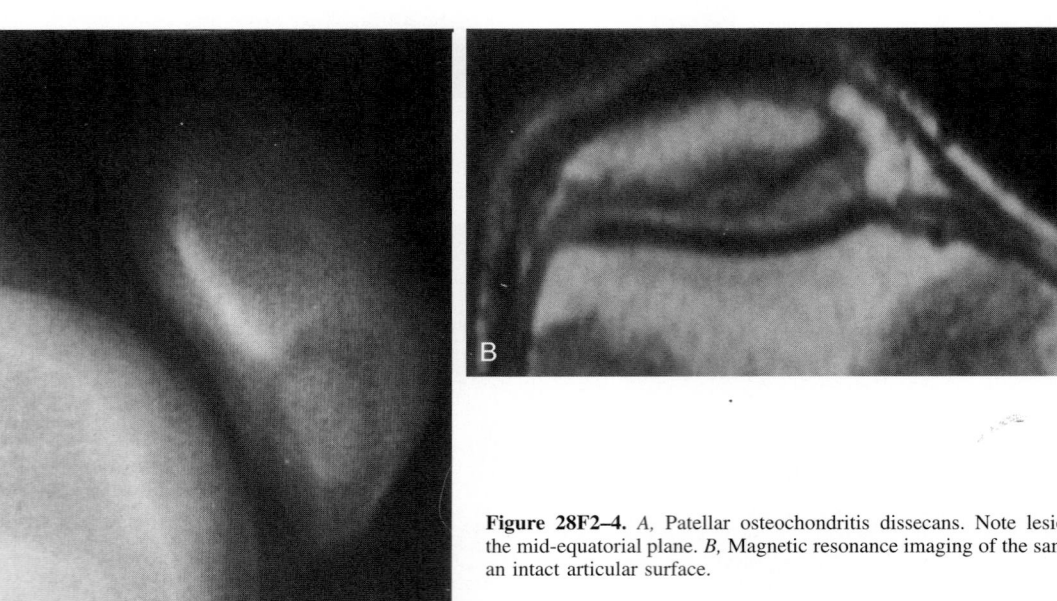

Figure 28F2–4. *A*, Patellar osteochondritis dissecans. Note lesion location below the mid-equatorial plane. *B*, Magnetic resonance imaging of the same patient showing an intact articular surface.

produced OCD-like lesions experimentally in rabbits after subchondral and articular fragment formation. Lesions that were stabilized healed, but those with tenuous or no stabilization developed, not surprisingly, avascular, unstable lesions. Rehbein,[20] using a canine model subjected to repetitive microtrauma, produced lesions that were histologically similar to OCD lesions seen in humans. Analysis of surgically removed loose bodies resulting from human OCD shows avascular, necrotic bone, with articular cartilage overgrowth and no inflammatory response.

Pathophysiology

It appears that after a precipitating insult at a vulnerable site, subchondral avascularity occurs with alteration of the attendant articular cartilage basilar growth. Attempts at revascularization occur, and, in some circumstances, this creeping substitution is successful in restoring the subchondral architecture, especially in juvenile cases. In most situations, however, the repair is inadequate, and an avascular centrum is established, with associated continued disruption of the articular cartilage union. A modulus mismatch between the architecturally inadequate lesion and the surrounding articular surface and subchondral zones occurs, leading to a subchondral fracture with further disorganization of the centrum. Persistent avascularity, along with hostile mechanical forces at the subchondral nonunion, leads to articular surface compromise with a full-thickness fracture. Synovial fluid intrusion at the junction of the subchondral centrum limits healing. With progressive nonunion and loss of fragment stability, a loose body is the result in the most complex cases.

Natural History

Outcomes depend on a multitude of circumstances. Patient maturity is a major predictive factor. Juvenile cases have a high (65% to 75%) healing potential. The prognosis in adolescent cases is not so clear-cut, and the outcome is unpredictable.[9, 10, 22, 24, 25] About 50% go on to heal, and the other half continue along the more adult path of nonresolution. In the skeletally mature, the rate of healing is markedly reduced, with most patients developing clinical and radiographic evidence of premature degenerative joint disease.[24]

Additional prognostic factors include duration of the disorder, size and site of the lesion (especially relative to weight-bearing surface), fragment stability, and articular surface status.

Clinical Evaluation

The patient with OCD is usually otherwise healthy and presents complaining of nonspecific, poorly localized knee pain that is sometimes related to activity. Complaints of knee swelling and stiffness are also noted. Mechanical complaints of locking or catching, indicative of fragment instability, are uncommon. A history of incidental knee trauma is often noted but usually is not specifically related to the current complaints. Family history is most often negative. Patients with underlying medical conditions such as chronic renal disease or malignancies who are undergoing chemotherapy present with OCD-like lesions, but these appear to act like true avascular necrosis without natural resolution. They do not show the spontaneous reparative sequence seen with true juvenile and adolescent OCD (Figs. 28F2–5 and 28F2–6).

The findings on clinical examination reflect the status of the lesion. An antalgic gait is often seen. Wilson[26] described a sign related to his thesis that impingement of the medial tibial eminence on the lesion caused the patient to walk with the leg externally rotated to avoid the impingement. Pain was produced on tibial internal rotation with the knee extended and was relieved with tibial external rotation. In a personal series of 28 patients, 14 with juvenile and 14 with adolescent OCD, only 3 of 14 juvenile patients (21%) and 4 of 14 adolescent patients (28%) with medial femoral OCD had a positive Wilson's sign. All patients had resolution of their pain with fragment resolution (Fig. 28F2–7).

Effusion and synovitis are seen in cases of unstable lesions. Loss of range of motion from loose fragment impingement is uncommon. Diminished thigh girth and muscle definition reflect the chronicity of the condition. Focal tenderness to direct palpation of the lesion (Axhausen's sign[5]) is seen in patients with subchondral insta-

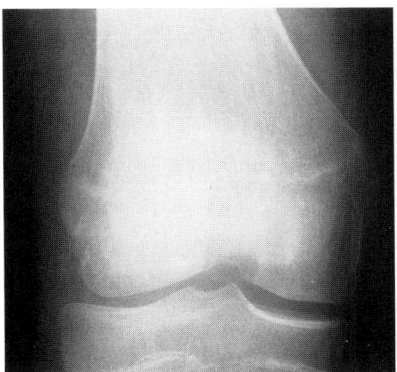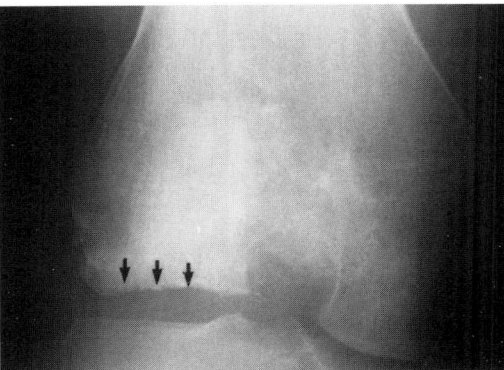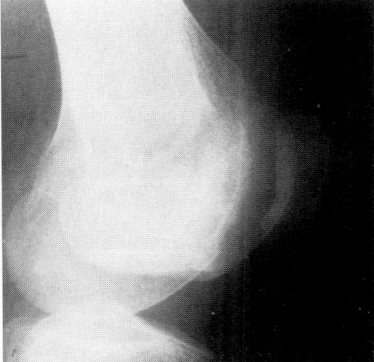

Figure 28F2–5. Medial femoral condylar osteochondritis dissecans–like changes in a 14-year-old girl, 3 years after renal transplantation. *Arrows* point to persistent subchondral irregularity.

bility of the lesion and is a helpful clinical index of progressive healing as the sign abates.

Imaging

Routine radiographs are diagnostic, especially the tunnel view, which places the femoral condyles in greater profile than the anteroposterior view (Fig. 28F2–8). The femoral lesion is classically located posterior to the midline on the sagittal view. An arc of subchondral lucency of varying size is seen. Subchondral sclerosis at the lesion's margin usually indicates a longstanding situation, which, I feel, reflects progressive development of a nonunion of the fragment. Differential diagnoses include an acute osteochondral fracture, normal accessory ossification centers (especially in children younger than 9 years old) (Fig. 28F2–9), true avascular necrosis, and epiphyseal dysplasia. Clinical correlation eliminates most of these potential diagnoses.

Magnetic resonance imaging (MRI) allows further eval-

uation of the centrum and its subchondral junction (Fig. 28F2–10). Increased signal from fluid at the interface is indicative of delayed union. Current MRI techniques have limitations in detecting articular cartilage changes within the lesion.[23]

Some authors recommend static bone scanning to monitor lesion healing. Despite multiple repeated scans, this type of scintigraphy has a poor predictive index. Persistence of nucleotide activity has been observed long after lesion resolution. Other authors[18] reported the use of quantitative technetium bone scanning to identify regional perfusion at the lesion. The predictive index for healing was high in juvenile patients (≤12 years old) but had less accuracy in adolescents, the group who most needed such predictability.

Arthroscopic Diagnosis and Classification

Arthroscopy has revolutionized the diagnosis and management of a myriad of knee disorders, including OCD.

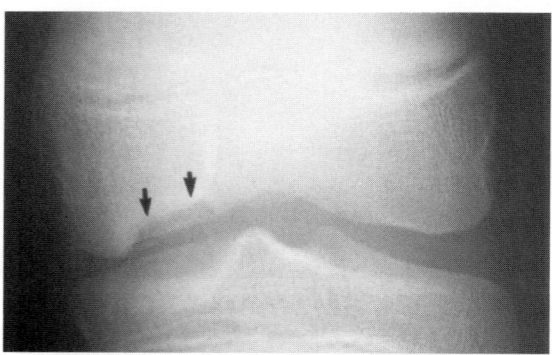
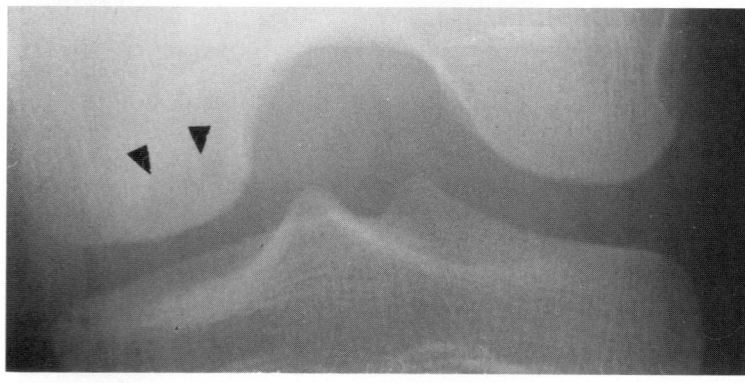
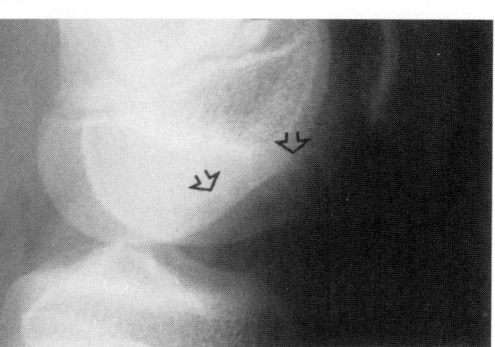
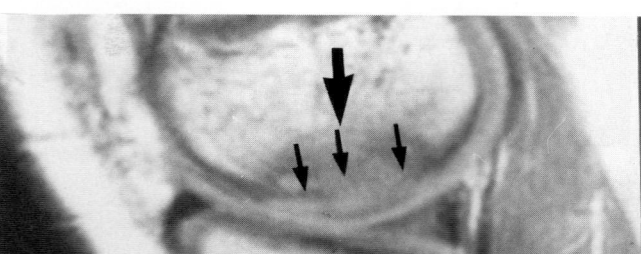
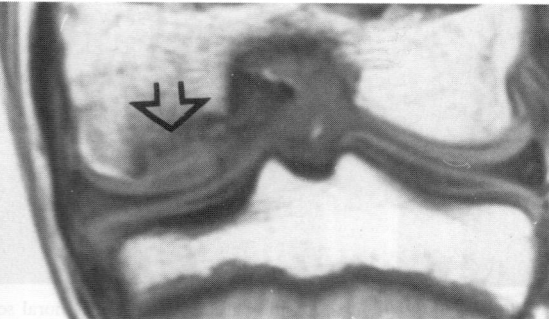

Figure 28F2–10. *A,* Radiographs of a 12-year-old soccer player with symptomatic medial femoral osteochondritis dissecans. *B,* Magnetic resonance imaging shows loss of articular surface continuity *(small arrows).* Arrows indicate the osteochondritis dissecans fragment subchondral junction.

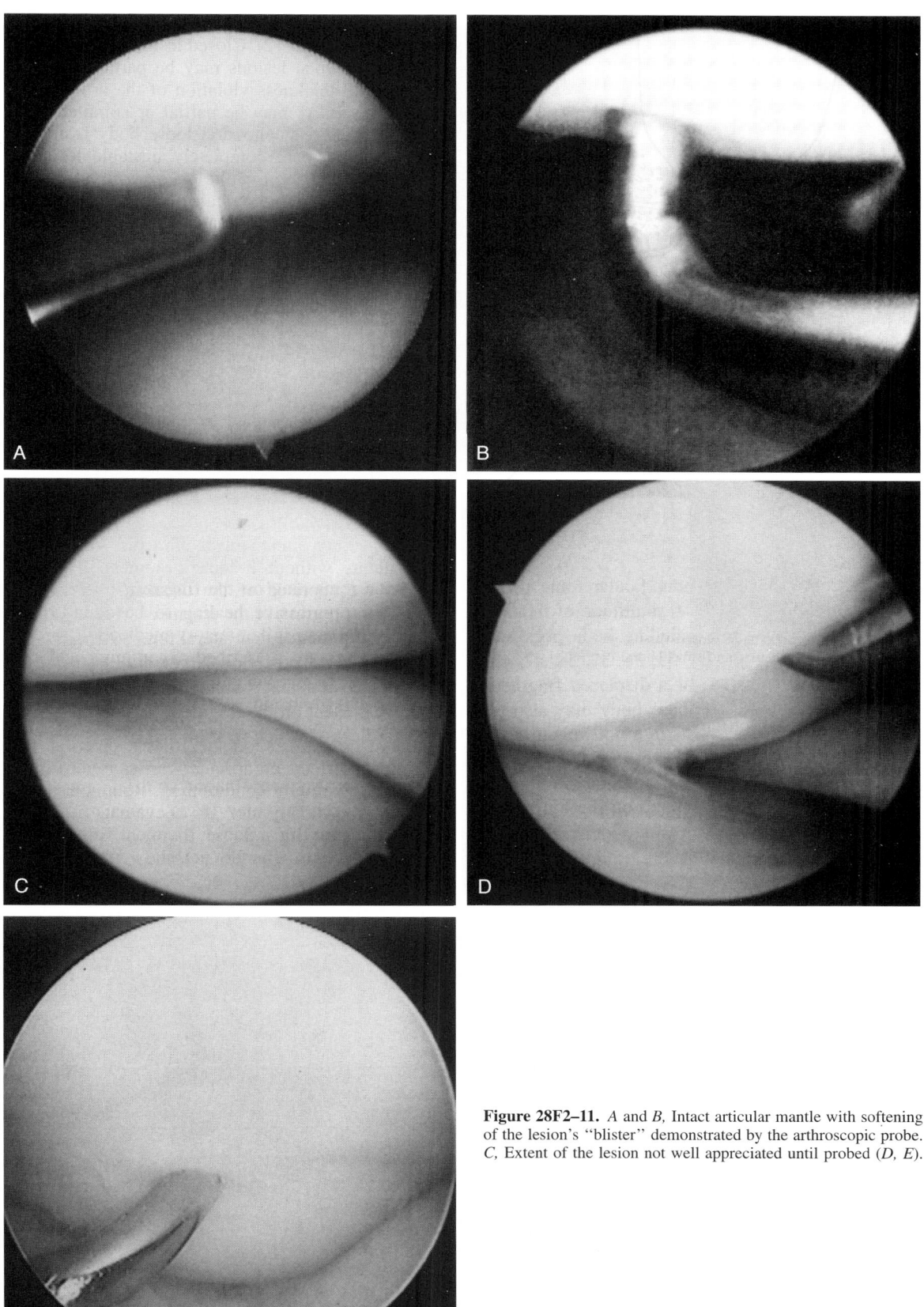

Figure 28F2–11. *A* and *B*, Intact articular mantle with softening of the lesion's "blister" demonstrated by the arthroscopic probe. *C*, Extent of the lesion not well appreciated until probed (*D, E*).

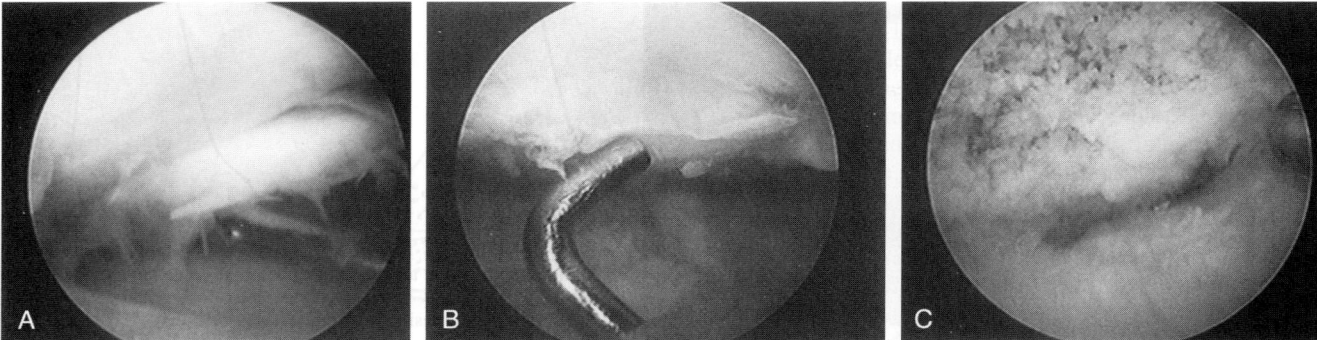

Figure 28F2–15. *A,* Completely open, unstable lesion from lateral femoral osteochondritis dissecans. *B,* Attempted reduction after crater preparation. Note nonanatomic condition due to fragment articular surface growth. *C,* Fragment bed after débridement and drilling. Note punctate vascular channels.

for vascular ingress to promote fragment revascularization and union. Either an antegrade or a retrograde approach may be used. Because antegrade drilling violates an intact articular surface, I prefer the retrograde technique.[16, 19] The retrograde approach is also easier for posterior lesions. A cannulated anterior cruciate ligament guide is helpful for orientation and K-wire or drill insertion. The procedure is done using combined arthroscopic and fluoroscopic controls (Fig. 28F2–16). The subchondral centrum is drilled to just below the subchondral articular margin. Depending on the size of the lesion, three to five channels are made. This technique can be used in a skeletally immature patient because the entry point of the drill or K-wire is in the epiphysis, and the physis is avoided.

Postoperatively, patients are allowed full, active range of motion with closed chain, progressive-resistance exercises. Partial weight-bearing with crutches is done for 3 to 4 weeks, depending on the size of the lesion. Touch-down partial weight-bearing is allowed, to unload the limb and diminish articular compressive forces produced by the knee flexion required for non–weight-bearing gait. Achieving patient compliance is often difficult with this crutch program because of the minimally invasive nature of the procedure and the rapidity of patient recovery. Outcomes have been uniformly good.

In Situ Fixation

Closed, unstable lesions are stabilized with antegrade or retrograde in situ fixation. At arthroscopy, these lesions have an intact articular surface that is ballotable. When the lesion is probed, a sensation is reproduced that is not unlike

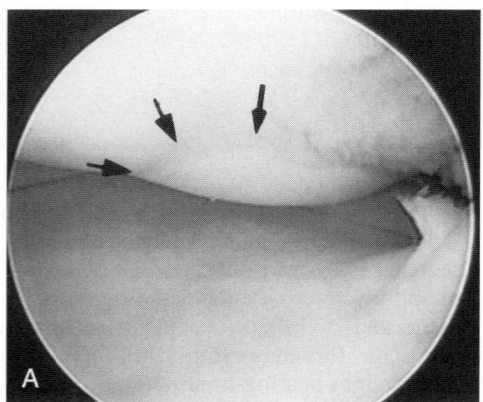

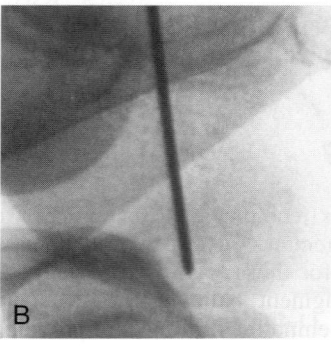
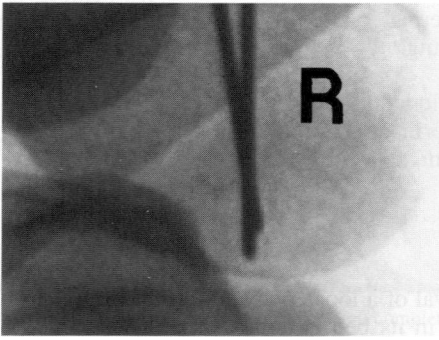
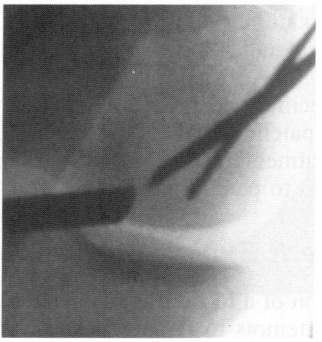

Figure 28F2–16. *A,* Closed, stable, symptomatic right medial femoral condylar lesion in a 17-year-old basketball player with bilateral osteochondritis dissecans. Note extent of articular "blister" (*arrows*). *B,* Retrograde drilling of the lesion centrum using arthroscopic and fluoroscopic control.

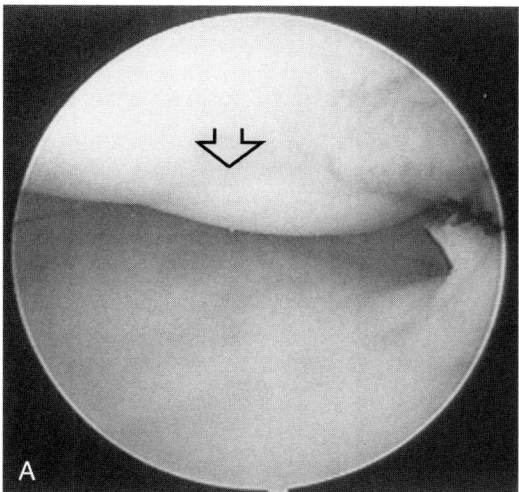

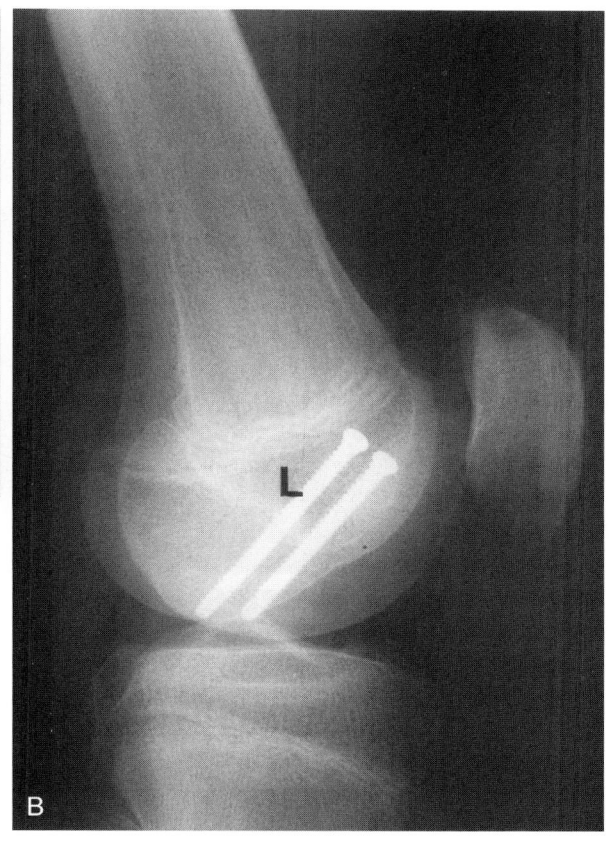

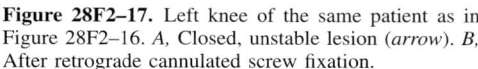

Figure 28F2–17. Left knee of the same patient as in Figure 28F2–16. *A,* Closed, unstable lesion (*arrow*). *B,* After retrograde cannulated screw fixation.

the indentation caused by squeezing a Ping-Pong ball. Stabilization of the lesion results from the mechanical fixation and from the channels provided for neovascularization. A variety of fixation devices may be used, including threaded pins, cannulated screws, bone pegs, and bioabsorbable devices. As with in situ drilling, I prefer the retrograde approach with compression fixation, if possible (Figs. 28F2–17 and 28F2–18). The postoperative rehabilitation program is the same as that described earlier. Removal of the metallic fixation devices is recommended after fragment union is complete because some settling of the fragment may occur with penetration of the implant into or through the articular surface. Outcomes are directly related to the size and site of the lesion. In general, lesions of the lateral femur are larger and involve a greater portion of the weight-bearing area.

In Situ Bone Grafting and Fixation

In patients with closed, unstable lesions, retrograde bone grafting may be performed with the use of matchstick grafts placed through prepared tunnels to just above the articular-subchondral junction, with or without adjunctive metallic internal fixation. In the uncommon case of a partially open, partially unstable lesion, arthroscopic débridement of the subchondral epiphyseal lesion is done, autogenous bone graft is packed into the crater, the articular surface is reduced, and the fragment is internally fixed. After débridement, guide pins for cannulated screw fixation

can be placed antegrade through the epiphysis and skin in preparation for retrograde screw insertion after grafting and fragment reduction. If antegrade fixation is used, an adequate subchondral countersunk position for the fixation is needed to prevent articular erosion. Bioabsorbable fixation devices have been associated with a significant percentage of complications from persistent sterile synovitis and effusion thought to be related to response to byproducts of the implant's degradation. Postoperative rehabilitation is similar to that noted earlier, but the period of crutch-protected partial weight-bearing is extended to 6 to 8 weeks, depending on the size and location of the lesion.

Open Reduction with Internal Fixation

Patients with large, unstable, tenuously attached or totally displaced osteochondral fragments are candidates for open reduction with internal fixation (ORIF). The fragment must be considered salvageable. The precise criteria for determining lesion salvageability have not been determined. In general, the fragment must have a smooth articular surface and an adequate (>3 mm) subchondral base and must be anatomically reducible in its original bed (Fig. 28F2–19). The crater is prepared by débridement of any fibrous tissue to bleeding bone, and bone graft is inserted to make up any voids. The fragment is then reduced and fixed. Fixation can be done antegradely or by the combined antegrade and retrograde approaches described in the previ-

12. Fairbanks H: Osteochondritis dissecans. Br J Surg 21:67, 1933.
13. Koenig F: Über freie Körper in den Gelenken. Dtsch Chir 27:90, 1888.
14. Koenig F: Tagung deutsche Gesellschaft für Chirurgie. Langenbecks Arch Klin Chir 142:1926.
15. Marandola MS, Prietto CA: Arthroscopic Herbert screw fixation of patellar osteochondritis dissecans. Arthroscopy 9:214–216, 1993.
16. Matelic TM, Stanitski CL: Operative treatment of osteochondritis dissecans in situ by retrograde pinning. J Orthop Tech 3:17–24, 1995.
17. Paget J: On the production of some of the loose bodies in joints. St Barth Hosp Rep 6:1, 1870.
18. Paletta GA Jr, Bednarz PA, Stanitski C, et al: The prognostic value of quantitative bone scan in knee osteochondritis dissecans. A preliminary experience. Am J Sports Med 26:7–14, 1998.
19. Paletta GA Jr, Stanitski CL: Juvenile osteochondritis dissecans of the knee. Tech Sports Med 6:268, 1998.
20. Rehbein F: Die Entstehung der Osteochondritis dissecans. Arch Klin 265:69, 1950.
21. Rey Zuniga JJ, Sagastibelza J, Lopez Blasco JJ, et al: Arthroscopic use of the Herbert screw in osteochondritis dissecans of the knee. Arthroscopy 9:668–670, 1993.
22. Schenck RC Jr, Goodnight JM: Osteochondritis dissecans. J Bone Joint Surg Am 78:439–456, 1996.
23. Schneider T, Fink B, Jerosch J, et al: The value of magnetic resonance imaging as postoperative control after arthroscopic treatment of osteochondritis dissecans. Arch Orthop Trauma Surg 117:235–239, 1998.
24. Twyman RS, Desai K, Aichroth PM: Osteochondritis dissecans of the knee. A long-term study. J Bone Joint Surg Br 73:461–464, 1991.
25. Williams JS Jr, Bush-Joseph CA, Bach BR Jr: Osteochondritis dissecans of the knee. Am J Knee Surg 11:221–232, 1998.
26. Wilson JN: A diagnostic sign in osteochondritis dissecans of the knee. J Bone Joint Surg Am 49:477–480, 1967.

Section G

High Tibial Osteotomy in the Anterior Cruciate Ligament–Deficient Knee with Varus Angulation

Frank R. Noyes, MD ■ Sue D. Barber-Westin, BS ■ Richard Simon, MD

Proximal tibial osteotomy has gained wide acceptance since the publication of early investigations as a treatment option for patients with unicompartmental osteoarthritis of the knee and varus deformity of the lower extremity.[9, 21, 30, 39, 46, 56, 61, 63, 66, 138] The rationale for the procedure stems from the hypothesis that a varus deformity results in abnormal loads on the medial tibiofemoral joint, leading to arthritic progression of that compartment.[13, 20] In patients with unicompartmental arthrosis, the procedure corrects the mechanical abnormality and redistributes the loads onto the lateral tibiofemoral joint.[14, 20]

Varus angulation and unicompartmental arthrosis secondary to meniscectomy, articular fracture, joint instability, or injury in younger patients often present the most difficult challenge to successful restoration of lower limb function. These patients are not candidates for total knee replacement and usually wish to remain physically active. Generally, authors have reported that high tibial osteotomy (HTO) provides beneficial results when it is performed early in the course of the arthrosis process in younger individuals.[49, 91, 125] There are questions, however, about the level of physical activity that should be pursued after an HTO because progression of the underlying knee arthrosis can be expected.

An added complexity in the varus-angulated knee with medial compartment arthrosis is the presence of anterior cruciate ligament (ACL) deficiency. Patients who have these combined abnormalities often experience pain, swelling, "giving way," and functional limitations that sometimes result in a truly disabling condition.[117] There may also be an associated deficiency of the lateral and posterolateral ligamentous structures that adds to the varus angulation and clinical symptoms. In these symptomatic knees, many questions arise concerning treatment recommendations and the role of osteotomy. Can the HTO be expected to diminish symptoms reliably and allow increased physical activity for a long enough time (before the eventual return of symptoms) to warrant performing the procedure? Is an ACL reconstruction necessary, and if so, when should it be performed relative to the HTO? When should surgical reconstruction of associated ligamentous deficiencies of the lateral collateral ligament (LCL) and posterolateral structures be undertaken? Undoubtedly, the complexity of arriving at a correct diagnosis of all existing abnormalities and determining the correct treatment plan make these patients some of the most difficult patients with knee problems facing the clinician.

Many authors have described various surgical procedures for a valgus-producing tibial osteotomy, and it is not our intent to repeat their commendable works.* Rather, the objectives of this chapter are to present an evaluation and treatment plan for younger patients with ACL-deficient varus-angulated knees. We present our clinical results and those of other authors on the role of a proximal HTO in these knees. The following areas are discussed:

1. The clinical evaluation, the diagnosis, and the classification of the abnormalities present in the ACL-deficient varus-angulated knee
2. The role of gait analysis in understanding the pathophysiology and the preoperative planning
3. The decision-making criteria needed for treatment of varus-angulated, ACL-deficient knees, particularly those with associated lateral and posterolateral ligamentous injury
4. Our preferred HTO operative technique and postoperative rehabilitation program
5. Recommendations on what is realistic in terms of patient outcomes, sports participation, and occupational activities after HTO

We caution that final conclusions on the results of surgi-

_____
*See references 20, 25–27, 50, 57, 58, 65, 71–74, 81, 86, 87, 94, 95, 126, 132, 136, 137, 143, and 147.

cal treatment for these complex problems should be withheld until long-term results are known. Our treatment rationale is given with the qualification that changes in philosophy and surgical indications will occur as more data become available for critical scientific analysis. The primary objective of this chapter is to address the indications for ligament reconstruction and tibial osteotomy and what can be expected in terms of a realistic outcome after these procedures.

Evaluation and Classification

Causes of Varus Angulation

To devise a rational treatment program, the clinician must first diagnose correctly all abnormalities of the knee joint that are present. Areas of assessment include the underlying tibiofemoral osseous alignment, abnormal knee motion limits, abnormal knee joint positions (subluxation), and specific ligamentous defects. Table 28G–1 shows the various factors that may affect the overall varus alignment of the knee joint. To simplify the clinician's task in logically diagnosing abnormal alignment and ligamentous deficiencies, we have coined the terms *primary, double-varus,* and *triple-varus* knee.

The clinician must first define the primary tibiofemoral geometry of the lower limb, regardless of any ligamentous deficiencies that may be present. This definition is based on the underlying physiologic tibiofemoral osseous alignment and the tibiofemoral geometry at the knee joint.[32] In the varus-angulated ACL-deficient knee, an underlying physiologic tibiofemoral genu varum is often present. A loss of the medial meniscus or damage to the articular cartilage of the tibial and femoral surfaces adds to the overall varus alignment. For example, a patient who has a physiologic varus mechanical axis (MA) of 3 degrees and a loss of 3 mm of the medial tibiofemoral articular cartilage actually has an overall varus tibiofemoral alignment of 6 degrees.[32]

As the tibiofemoral weight-bearing line (WBL) at the knee joint shifts onto the medial tibiofemoral compartment, a tendency is created for greater loads to be placed on the

TABLE 28G–1
Causes of Varus Angulation in the Anterior Cruciate Ligament–Deficient Knee

Tibiofemoral Alignment or Geometry	Knee Motion Limits	Knee Joint Position	Ligament Deficiency	Comments
Primary varus Physiologic tibiofemoral varus alignment	—	—	—	Medial displacement of weight-bearing tibiofemoral line
Narrowing or loss of medial joint cartilage, meniscus	↑ varus or adduction rotation	↓ separation of medial tibiofemoral compartment	Pseudolaxity or slackness of medial ligament structures	Effect on varus alignment more pronounced when preexisting physiologic varus alignment is present
Added lateral ligament or soft tissue deficiency Double varus	1. ↑↑ varus or adduction rotation 2. Often coupled with lateral tibial translation for secondary support, intercondylar eminence against lateral femoral condyle	1. Separation of lateral tibiofemoral joint on standing 2. Varus thrust on stance phase due to lateral condylar lift-off 3. Lateral tibiofemoral joint space compressive forces are insufficient; tension develops in lateral soft tissues	1. Lateral collateral ligament, lateral capsule, iliotibial tract (femorotibial portion) 2. Amount of joint opening depends on slackness of lateral soft tissue restraints 3. Absence of ACL secondary restraint to varus angulation	1. Weight-bearing tibiofemoral line shifts far enough medially to produce separation of the lateral tibiofemoral joint during walking, sports activities 2. Under states of maximal muscle contraction (quadriceps, biceps femoris), sufficient compressive forces may exist to prevent lateral condylar lift-off

Added posterolateral ligament complex deficiency
Triple varus
	1. ↑↑↑ varus or adduction rotation
	2. Varus recurvatum in extension
	  a. ↑ external tibial rotation
	  b. ↑ extension (hyperextension)
	3. ↑ external tibial rotation in flexion
		1. ↑ separation of posterolateral aspect tibiofemoral joint produces varus recurvatum on standing, walking
		2. Varus recurvatum thrust if hamstrings and gastrocnemius do not prevent knee hyperextension
		3. Posterior subluxation of lateral plateau with external tibial rotation
			Above, plus posterolateral capsule, arcuate-popliteal complex
			Knee hyperextension increases with associated damage to ACL and PCL (partial to complete)
				Gait training required to teach patient not to walk with varus recurvatum thrust, maintaining 5 degrees of knee flexion on stance phase
				Knee hyperextension with physiologic slackness to ACL, PCL may be present without actual injury to cruciates allowing varus recurvatum

ACL, anterior cruciate ligament; PCL, posterior cruciate ligament.

If anterior knee pain or patellofemoral arthrosis is present, the patient may not wish to contract the quadriceps muscle to maintain the few degrees of knee flexion during the stance phase. This results in a hyperextended knee position and a markedly abnormal gait. In this state, the quadriceps muscle undergoes marked atrophy because the patient is literally not using this muscle during most gait activities. It is exceedingly important to correct this type of gait abnormality before any consideration is given to surgical reconstruction of the lateral and posterolateral ligamentous structures (Fig. 28G–3), as described previously.[112] If this gait abnormality persists postoperatively (reduced or absent quadriceps activity with knee hyperextension), the likelihood exists that large ligament tensile forces will eventually cause stretching and failure of the reconstructed ligamentous structures, because the knee tends to assume the abnormal varus recurvatum position.

It is well known that the patient's complaint of medial joint-line pain may not show a correlation with the amount of medial compartment arthrosis that is present.[48, 60, 116] In the early stages of medial compartment arthrosis, the patient usually complains of medial pain with sports activities but rarely experiences pain with activities of daily living. When medial joint-line pain occurs with daily walking, there is a strong probability that extensive articular cartilage damage exists, often with exposed subchondral bone. Loss of the medial meniscus is the major risk factor for arthritic progression of the medial compartment.[34, 62, 116] We particularly caution our athletically active patients with physiologic varus-angulated ACL-deficient knees to avoid totally any activities that may result in a giving-way injury that may damage the medial meniscus and to undergo ACL reconstruction to protect a functional medial meniscus. Further, we have advocated repair of complex meniscus tears extending into the avascular zone to avoid removal and, in effect, near-total meniscectomy.[131]

If pain from medial compartment arthrosis is of moderate intensity preoperatively, there is a strong likelihood that this symptom will continue after HTO and ACL reconstruction, particularly in patients who engage in athletic activities. Therefore, the patient should not expect that an HTO will completely eliminate pain, although pain may temporarily diminish after the procedure. The symptom of swelling with activity carries, in our experience, a poor prognosis. We previously reported that swelling with any athletic activity in the chronic ACL-deficient knee correlated with time elapsed since the original injury and the presence of radiographic osteoarthritic changes.[116] Again, this symptom may be present after any operative procedure and may limit the safe return to athletic activities.

Physical Examination

A comprehensive physical examination of the knee joint is required (Fig. 28G–4). We pay particular attention to the following: (1) patellofemoral abnormalities, including extensor mechanism malalignment that is accentuated by increased external tibial rotation and posterolateral tibial subluxation; (2) detection of medial tibiofemoral crepitus on varus loading as an indicator of early articular cartilage damage before the presence of radiographic changes (statistically significant, $P < .01$ correlation with overall knee score[114]); (3) palpation to detect tenderness indicating inflammation of the lateral supporting soft tissues; (4) detection of gait abnormalities during walking and jogging; and (5) careful examination of the motion limits and subluxations of the affected knee compared with the opposite knee. We have reported elsewhere the methods for recording the results of knee examination motion limits and subluxations.[111, 116]

The specific diagnosis of the abnormalities that produce a varus angulation in the frontal plane is shown in Table 28G–2. The clinical test for LCL insufficiency is based on the varus stress test performed at 0 and 30 degrees of knee flexion. The patient's thigh rests against the examining table, and the examiner places the finger and thumb on the medial and lateral tibiofemoral compartments. The examiner must estimate the amount (in millimeters) of joint opening, from the initial closed contact position of each tibiofemoral compartment to the maximal opened position.

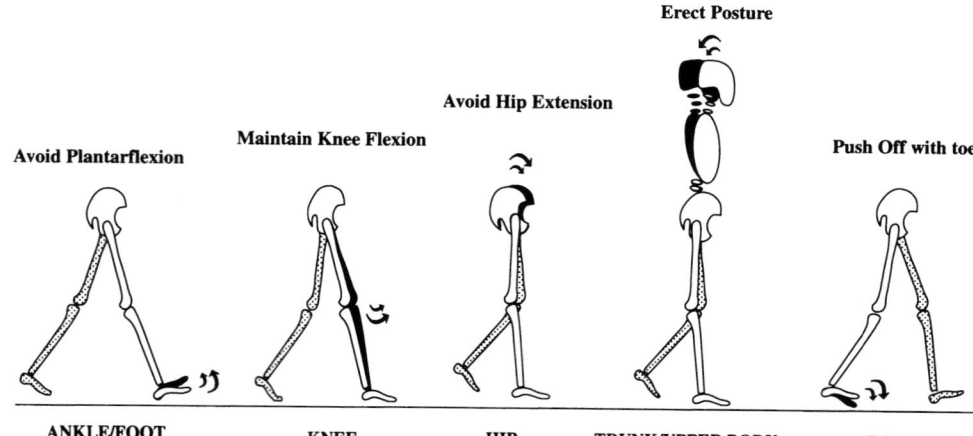

Erect Posture

Avoid Hip Extension

Maintain Knee Flexion

Avoid Plantarflexion

Push Off with toe

ANKLE/FOOT   KNEE   HIP   TRUNK/UPPER BODY   TOE

Look for Patellofemoral pain/rotational instabilities with knee flexion

Avoid medial-lateral body sway

Figure 28G–3. Graphic representation of gait abnormalities observed in patients before retraining. Shaded anatomic structures represent the correct, retrained positions at trunk, upper body, hip, knee, foot and ankle, and toes. (From Noyes FR, Dunworth LA, Andriacchi TP, et al: Knee hyperextension gait abnormalities in unstable knees. Recognition and preoperative gait retraining. Am J Sports Med 24:35–45, 1996.)

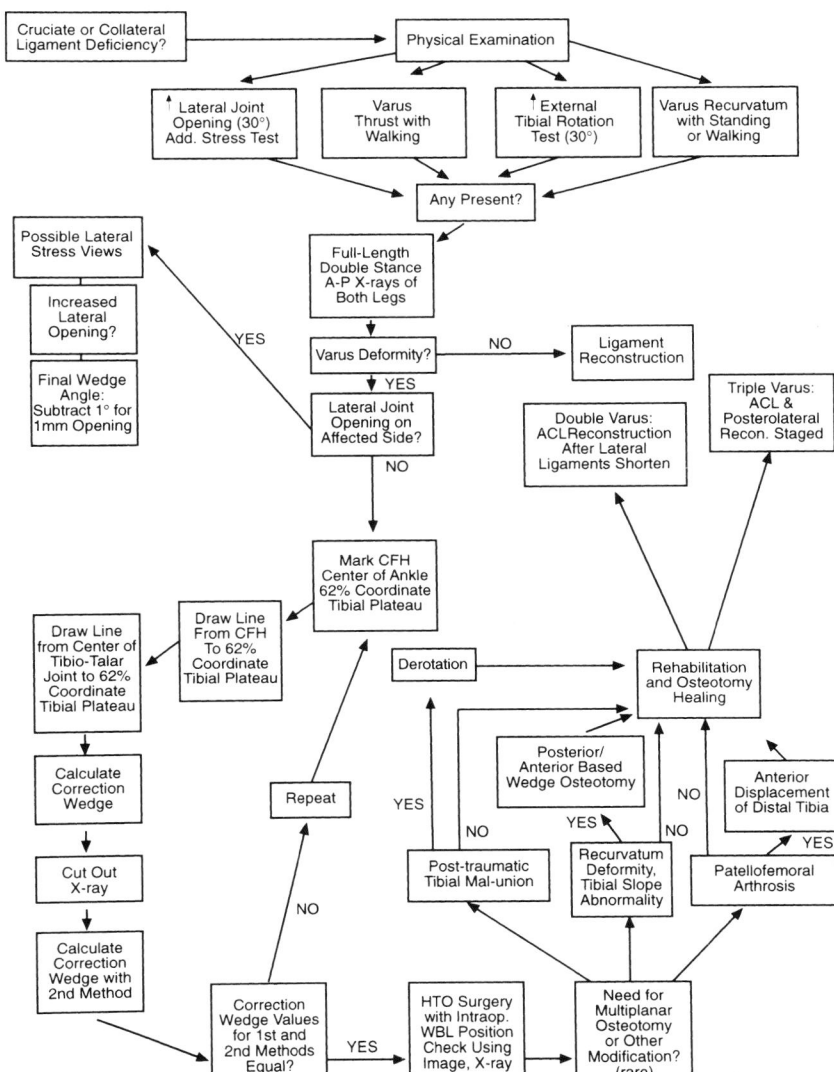

Figure 28G–4. Algorithm for diagnosis and treatment of young athletic patients with varus angular alignment and injury to the lateral ligaments and soft tissues. ACL, anterior cruciate ligament; CFH, center femoral head; HTO, high tibial osteotomy; WBL, weight-bearing line. In the second method, measure angle of tibial radiograph cut at level of osteotomy to achieve 62% coordinate on the tibial plateau. (Modified from Dugdale TW, Noyes FR, Styer D: Preoperative planning for high tibial osteotomy: The effect of lateral tibiofemoral separation and tibiofemoral length. Clin Orthop 274:246–264, 1992.)

The motion involves a constrained varus-valgus rotation, avoiding internal or external tibial rotation, to open the respective tibiofemoral compartment from the initial closed position.[120] Note that it is incorrect to measure only the degrees of varus or valgus rotation; for example, the degrees of varus alignment may be due both to narrowing of the medial tibiofemoral compartment and to opening of the lateral tibiofemoral compartment. Rather, the examination is based on the increase (in millimeters) in the specific tibiofemoral compartment compared with that of the opposite normal knee. Frequently, there is an increase in medial joint opening compared with the opposite knee that represents pseudolaxity. The increased medial joint opening is due to medial tibiofemoral joint narrowing and collapse. With a varus stress, the medial joint opening returns the limb to a more normal alignment, and there is no true medial ligamentous damage. The primary and secondary restraints that resist lateral joint opening have been published.[41, 42] The amount of varus rotation that occurs depends on the flexion angle at which the test is conducted

and the involvement of the secondary restraints (Table 28G–3).

The tests for abnormal increases in external tibial rotation are based on the biomechanical data presented in Table 28G–3. Sectioning of the posterolateral structures, including the LCL, resulted in a mean value of 13 degrees of increased external tibial rotation at 30 degrees of knee flexion.[42] The limits of tibial rotation are dependent on the flexion angle and the ligaments involved.

We use the tibiofemoral rotation test to diagnose posterior tibial subluxations in a qualitative manner after ligament injury.[111] The tibia is first positioned at 30 degrees of knee flexion and neutral tibial rotation (Fig. 28G–5A). The position of the anterior aspect of the medial and lateral tibial plateaus is determined by palpation in reference to the femoral condyles. The tibia is next rotated externally to a maximum position, and again the positions of the medial and lateral tibial plateaus are palpated. The examiner determines whether there is any increase in external tibial rotation, paying particular attention to the tibial tuber-

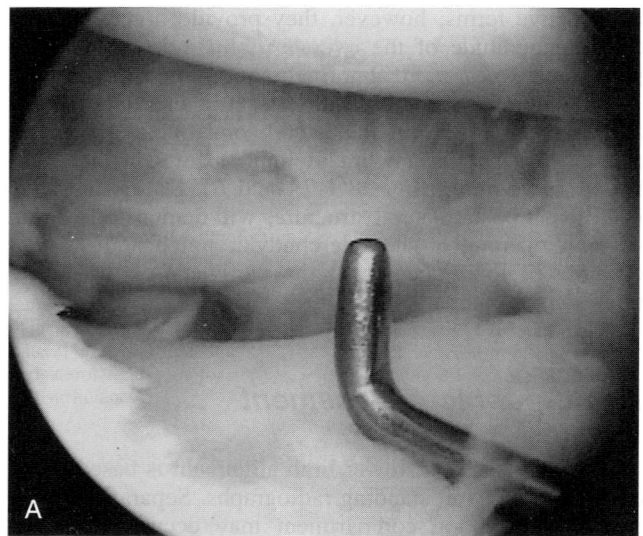

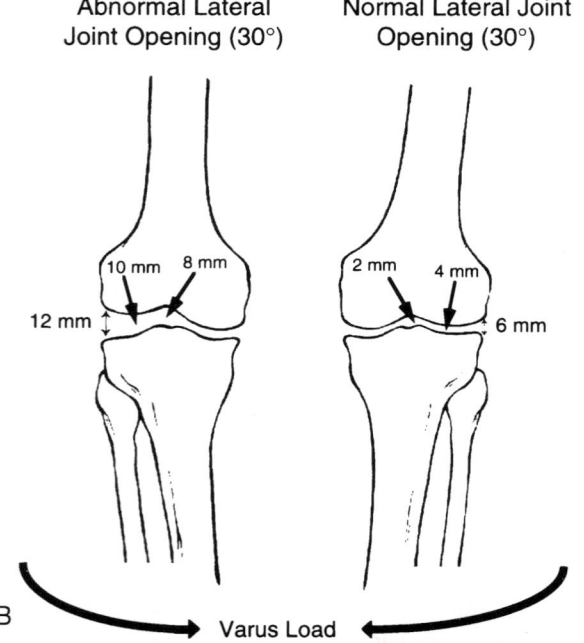

Figure 28G–7. *A,* In the arthroscopic gap test for determining the amount of lateral joint opening, a calibrated nerve hook is used to measure the millimeters of joint space. *B,* In knees that have insufficient posterolateral structures, 8 mm of lateral joint opening will be measured at the intercondylar notch and 12 mm or more will be measured at the periphery of the lateral tibiofemoral compartment. (From Noyes FR, Barber-Westin SD, Hewett TE: High tibial osteotomy and ligament reconstruction for varus angulated anterior cruciate ligament-deficient knees. Am J Sports Med 28:282–296, 2000.)

flexed to 5 degrees to avoid the abnormal varus recurvatum position. The use of a single-stance radiograph is not recommended because of the increased lateral joint opening that occurs with deficient lateral ligament restraints. We and other authors have addressed the steps that must be taken to arrive at a valid assessment of lower limb alignment by radiographic means.[32, 48, 85] Standard double-stance full-length radiographs with the patient contracting the hamstrings and quadriceps muscles may also help ensure

that both tibiofemoral compartments are in contact. It is imperative that simultaneous medial and lateral tibiofemoral contact occur (or that appropriate calculations are made to subtract the lateral compartment opening), so that the true osseous tibiofemoral alignment can be determined.[32] It is the osseous alignment that is corrected by the osteotomy; an overcalculation of the degrees of varus alignment to be corrected can occur if abnormal lateral joint opening is present on the radiographs but is not taken into consideration. The varus alignment may also be due entirely to separation of the lateral tibiofemoral compartment, contradicting an HTO. It is also important to look for the "teeter" effect described by Kettlekamp and co-workers, in which simultaneous contact of the medial and lateral tibiofemoral joints is impossible owing to obliquity of the medial tibial plateau resulting from arthrosis.[75] This indicates that the overall limb alignment will probably remain in a varus position after HTO and that the goals of osteotomy in reducing pain may not be achieved. The measurements that we make on the radiograph include the mechanical axis and the tibiofemoral WBL. We believe that the intersection of the WBL and the tibial line is the most accurate method of determining the angular alignment and the angular correction required.[32]

Gait Analysis

The presence of varus angulation alone is not sufficient to justify a corrective tibial osteotomy. Rather, the symptoms, medial tibiofemoral arthrosis, and functional limitations are the primary indicators of a valgus-producing osteotomy. Gait analysis allows the detection of (1) patients with abnormally high knee adduction moments who are at increased risk of progression of medial tibiofemoral arthrosis due to excessive loading in that compartment; (2) patients with predicted (calculated) abnormally high tensile forces in the lateral soft tissue restraints who are at increased risk of stretching out these tissues owing to lateral condylar liftoff with activity, having lost the stabilizing effect of the lateral tibiofemoral compartment; and (3) patients with abnormally high knee adduction moments who will have a less than desirable outcome from an HTO. Many studies have documented that the external moments about the knee joint and the corresponding tibiofemoral compartment loads are markedly influenced by individual gait characteristics and gait adaptations that occur after injury.* Patients with ACL deficiency may show a decrease in the magnitude of the external flexion moment (quadriceps reduction gait) or an increase in the external extension moment (hamstrings protective muscle force).[7, 10] A high adduction moment may be anticipated because of the varus angulation; however, it is also known that the moments and the loads on the knee joint cannot be reliably predicted from the static alignment of the lower limb measured on radiographs. The alignment of the foot markedly influences the knee adduction moment. Patients with toe-in, or less-than-normal external axial rotation of the foot during stance phase, tend to have a higher knee adduction moment (Fig. 28G–8).[146]

---

*See references 3–7, 10, 19, 31, 45, 59, 69, 92, 93, 129, and 146.

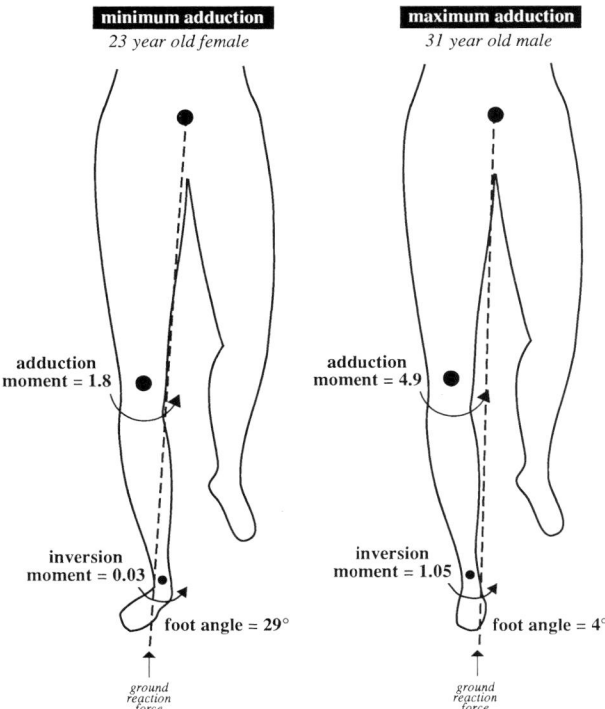

Figure 28G–8. An example of the results of gait analysis is shown for two patients, one with a toe-in position during walking and one with a toe-out position during walking. The rotational position (toe-in or toe-out) of the foot is related to the inversion moment at the ankle during stance phase.[146] There is a significant positive correlation between inversion moment at the ankle and adduction moment at the knee.[120] Patients who have a low inversion moment at the ankle usually have a low or normal adduction moment at the knee. Walking in an increased toe-out position may tend to reduce the adduction moment at the knee.

We recently reported on the results of gait analyses in 32 patients with ACL deficiency and varus angulation.[118] A force plate and an optoelectronic system were used to measure forces and moments of the lower limb and the knee joint. Knee joint loads and ligament tensile forces were calculated using a previously described mathematical model.[133] The majority of patients (20 of 32) had an abnormally high magnitude of the moment, tending to adduct the affected knee (Fig. 28G–9). The calculated medial tibiofemoral loads were excessively high in 21 of 32 patients ($P < .01$). Fifteen of 32 patients had predicted abnormally high lateral ligament tensile forces ($P < .05$). The adduction moment showed a statistically significant ($p < .05$) correlation with predicted high medial tibiofemoral compartment loads and high lateral ligament tensile forces ($P < .01$). We interpreted these findings as indicating a shift in the center of maximal joint pressure to the medial tibiofemoral compartment with a corresponding increase in the lateral ligament tensile forces to achieve frontal plane stability. These phenomena are illustrated in Figures 28G–10 and 28G–11. If the muscle forces are not sufficient to maintain lateral tibiofemoral compressive loads, tensile forces develop in the lateral soft tissues. The data indicate the likelihood, in knees with high lateral ligament tensile forces, that separation of the lateral tibiofemoral joint occurs with condylar liftoff during periods of the stance phase.

The magnitude of the flexion moment (which is related to quadriceps muscle force) was significantly lower in 15 of 32 patients ($P < .05$), and the extension moment (related to hamstring muscle force) was significantly higher in 16 of 32 knees ($P < .05$). These findings indicate a gait adaptation to diminish quadriceps muscle activity and enhance hamstring muscle activity to provide dynamic anteroposterior stability of the knee joint.[10] Following ACL reconstruction, these gait adaptations are lost with resumption of a normal knee flexion moment.

Equally important in the abnormal results was the finding that approximately one third of the patients had normal or low adduction moments and corresponding normal-to-low medial tibiofemoral compartment loads. These patients had gait characteristics or adaptations that tended to lower medial tibiofemoral loads despite the varus angulation of the knee joint. Gait analysis, therefore, allowed identification of patients with a potentially better overall prognosis; the adduction moment and the medial tibiofemoral loads were not excessively high, and an HTO would result in a substantial lowering of the loads placed on the medial tibiofemoral joint.

Markholf and coworkers reported that the absence of lateral tibiofemoral compartment loads with lateral condylar liftoff had a marked effect on reducing joint stability.[89] Further, we have encountered varus-angulated knees with insufficient lateral ligamentous structures in which multiple ligamentous reconstructive procedures failed, and an HTO was required before further soft tissue reconstructive procedures could be done. We believe that the explanation for this clinical finding is that the knees have decompensated from a gait adaptation standpoint, and that excessively high lateral tensile forces are placed across deficient lateral ligament tissues (Fig. 28G–12). Gait analysis predicts which knees would be at higher risk for failure of lateral ligament reconstructive procedures, potentially affecting the treatment options.

Biomechanical Effect of Combined Medial Meniscal Loss and Varus Alignment on Medial Compartment Loads

The overall tibiofemoral alignment and the integrity of the medial meniscus play a paramount role in the forces, the contact area, and the peak pressures experienced in the medial compartment of the knee joint. Hsu and associates reported the results of a two-dimensional static analysis of anatomic and biomechanical factors that act on the knee joint by using a special computer program based on the theory of a rigid-body spring model.[51] In a series of 120 normal subjects, the normal mechanical axis was found to be 1.2 degrees varus; the distal femoral anatomic valgus was 4.2 degrees; the normal force at the knee joint was 94.3% ± 5.4% body weight; shear force was − 0.9% ± 2.9% body weight pointing medially; and joint peak pressure was 3.8% ± 1.2% body weight/mm. Most interesting, when one-legged stance was simulated, 75% ± 12% of the knee joint load passed through the medial compartment. The medial plateau contact area, during one-legged stance,

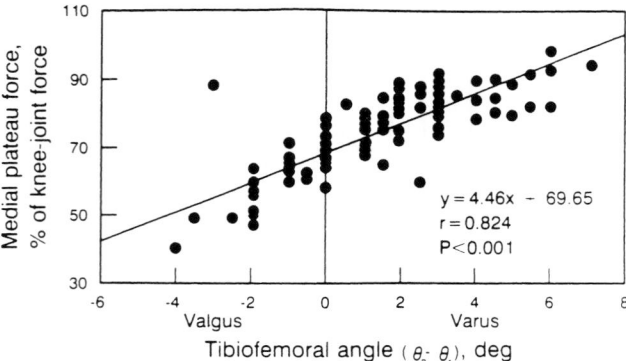

Figure 28G–13. Correlation by Hsu and colleagues between tibiofemoral angle ($\theta_2-\theta_1$) and medial plateau force (percentage of knee joint force) among 120 subjects studied. (From Hsu RW, Himeno S, Coventry MB, et al: Normal axial alignment of the lower extremity and load-bearing distribution at the knee. Clin Orthop 255:215–227, 1990.)

would result in 90% of the knee joint force passing through the medial compartment. These data also support the theoretical basis of the proximal tibial valgus osteotomy. Correction of a tibiofemoral angle of 6 degrees of varus with an osteotomy to 4 degrees of valgus will lower the percentage of knee joint force on the medial plateau from 90% to 50%. This analysis, however, is based on static alignment; the actual loading of the medial tibiofemoral joint also depends on dynamic conditions (i.e., gait characteristics), as defined earlier in this chapter. The actual amount of overcorrection to a valgus alignment is usually stated to be between 3 and 5 degrees,[32] resulting in a WBL intersection between 62% and 66% of the tibial plateau.

It is obvious that valgus alignment and a functioning medial meniscus are quite important in load transmission and load sharing between the medial and lateral knee joint compartments. Loss of the medial meniscus results in an initial doubling of the contact stress, and a varus angulation of 8 degrees would approximately double the medial plateau force (static analysis[51]). Loss of the meniscus with varus alignment in addition to ACL deficiency would result in drastic alterations in the load transmission characteristics of the joint. This would then in turn affect the tissue remodeling and the wear and lubrication properties of the articulating surfaces. Intuitively, the correction of any or all of these maladies would be beneficial to the overall integrity of the knee joint. It is hoped that in the future, meniscus transplantation will become a successful and safe procedure, eliminating the need for HTO in all but the more severely malaligned states. Additionally, we believe that successful meniscus repair techniques preserve meniscal function and may prevent the double- and triple-varus knee syndrome.

Preoperative Planning of Tibial Osteotomy

To provide a satisfactory clinical result, HTO must restore a valgus alignment to the lower extremity and redis-

tribute the tibial plateau forces toward the lateral compartment of the knee. It is assumed that narrowing and obliquity of the medial tibiofemoral joint have not progressed so far that they prevent closure of the lateral tibiofemoral joint—otherwise the HTO would not be indicated.[191] The most common method of preoperative planning involves selecting a correction wedge angle that is equal to the amount of angular deformity and adding it to the amount of overcorrection desired. Although authors disagree on the optimal postoperative alignment, they appear to agree that at least some overcorrection is necessary.[1, 9, 21–23, 37, 44, 48, 56, 57, 64] Several variables, including muscle and ligament forces,[86, 102] joint compartment loads,[45] adduction moment magnitude,[6, 44, 54] upper body positioning,[29, 69] and walking speed,[7, 150] obviously cannot be quantified from the static analysis of plain radiographs. Consequently, static radiographs cannot be used to predict the magnitude of medial compartment loads. Harrington, using gait analysis to study tibial plateau force distribution, found no direct correlation between the angular deformity measured on plain radiographs and the distribution of the forces across the knee joint.[45] However, he concluded that joint forces tend to be highest and centered most medially during the midstance phase of gait. It is probable that the preoperative measurement of the external moments on the knee during gait, along with the tibiofemoral angulation, will allow a more scientific approach to both the identification of patients who will benefit from tibial osteotomy and the amount of correction to be obtained at surgery. Until such advanced techniques are readily available, preoperative planning using static analysis remains a general clinical approximation that may have considerable inherent error.

The results of our studies indicate that determination of the WBL at the knee joint represents the most precise method of preoperative planning.[32] Fujisawa and colleagues also expressed postoperative alignment in terms of the position of the WBL by dividing the tibial plateau in halves from 0% to 100% medially and from 0% to 100% laterally, with 0% corresponding to the center of the tibial plateau.[37]

A WBL crossing the knee lateral to the 75% coordinate has the potential for a liftoff of the medial femoral condyle (Fig. 28G–14).[77] Unicondylar weight-bearing resulting from distraction of the medial compartment is undesirable and could result in rapid lateral compartment deterioration, gradual medial collateral ligament failure, and a possible progressive valgus deformity.[69] In many reports, a relatively broad range of postoperative alignment, as defined by the tibiofemoral angle or the mechanical axis angle, has been considered acceptable. The WBL–tibial intersection depends on two separate variables: the final mechanical axis angle and the femoral and tibial lengths of the patient. An example is given in Figure 28G–11 of the postoperative mechanical axis, in which any excess of 186 degrees would result in a WBL position lateral to the 75% coordinate.

We use two methods to determine the correction wedge on preoperative radiographs. First, the centers of the femoral head and the tibiotalar joint are marked on the full-length radiograph. The selected WBL coordinate of the tibial plateau is identified and marked. This is usually placed at between 62% and 66% of the tibial width, which allows the WBL to pass through the lateral tibiofemoral compartment, providing a 3- to 4-degree angular overcor-

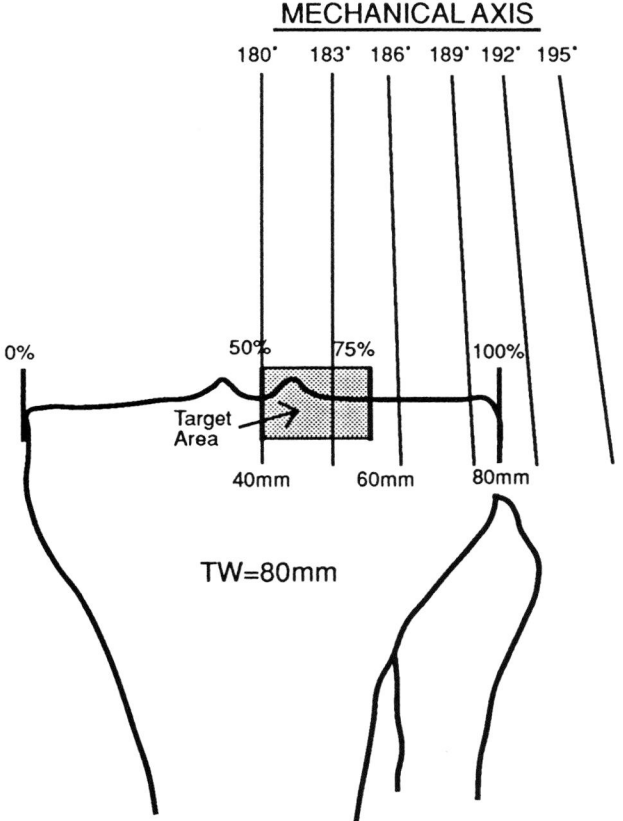

Figure 28G–14. The weight-bearing line positions are shown for different degrees of the mechanical axis. In this example, a correction beyond 186 degrees results in a weight-bearing line lateral to the desired target area. The authors prefer to use the weight-bearing line intersection on the tibia to more accurately determine the osteotomy correction at surgery. TW, tibial width. (From Dudgale TW, Noyes FR, Styer D: Pre-operative planning for high tibial osteotomy: Effect of lateral tibiofemoral separation and tibiofemoral length. Clin Orthop 271:105–121, 1991.)

rection. One line is drawn from the center of the femoral head to the tibial coordinate, and a second line is drawn from the center of the tibiotalar joint to the tibial coordinate (Fig. 28G–15). The angle formed by the two lines intersecting at the tibial coordinate represents the angular correction required to realign the WBL through this coordinate.

The second method of determining the correction wedge involves cutting the full-standing radiograph horizontally through the line of the superior osteotomy cut (Fig. 28G–16). A vertical cut of the lower tibial segment is then made to converge with the first cut at the level of the medial cortex. The distal portion of the radiograph is aligned until the center of the femoral head, the selected WBL coordinate point on the tibial plateau, and the center of the tibiotalar joint are all colinear. With the radiograph taped in this position, the angle of the wedge formed by the overlap of the two radiographic segments is measured and compared with the value obtained using the first method. The mechanical axis is measured to determine the angular correction. If there is a discrepancy between the two correction wedge angles, the procedures should be repeated.

Surgical Techniques for High Tibial Osteotomy

Osteotomy, or correction of limb deformities, is one of the oldest of orthopaedic procedures. Volkman is credited with writing the first report in 1875 on osteotomy performed on the tibia.[145] The operation gained acceptance only slowly because it was deemed dangerous; it was known that fractures of the tibia were sometimes associated with arterial injuries. Jackson in 1958 is given credit for first describing tibial osteotomy as a safe and effective procedure designed to treat degenerative arthritis of the knee.[61] Today, the two most frequently used techniques for correcting varus deformity are the opening and the closing tibial wedge osteotomies.

Dome osteotomy was advocated by Maquet in 1976 for patients who required greater than 15 degrees of correction in whom there was a limited amount of bone in the tibia proximal to the tibial tubercle to allow adequate correction.[84] Today, however, the majority of patients with exces-

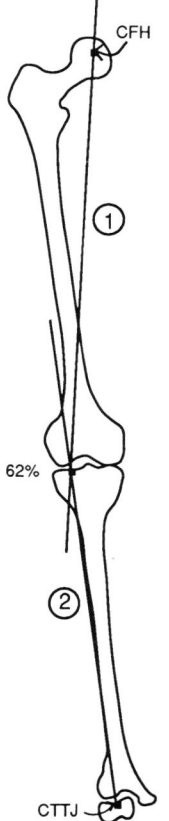

STEPS:

① Draw line from CFH to 62% coordinate

② Draw line from CTTJ to 62% coordinate

Angle formed by the two lines equals the angle of correction required to result in weightbearing line through the 62% coordinate

Figure 28G–15. Graphic depiction of the first method used to calculate the correction angle of a high tibial osteotomy using a full-length anteroposterior roentgenograph of the lower extremity. The lines from the centers of the femoral head (CFH) and tibiotalar joint (CTTJ) converge in this example at the 62% coordinate. This provides the angle of correction, which will result in a weight-bearing line passing through the 62% coordinate. The surgeon selects the percent coordinate in the target area desired (see text for details). (From Dudgale TW, Noyes FR, Styer D: Pre-operative planning for high tibial osteotomy: Effect of lateral tibiofemoral separation and tibiofemoral length. Clin Orthop 271:105–121, 1991.)

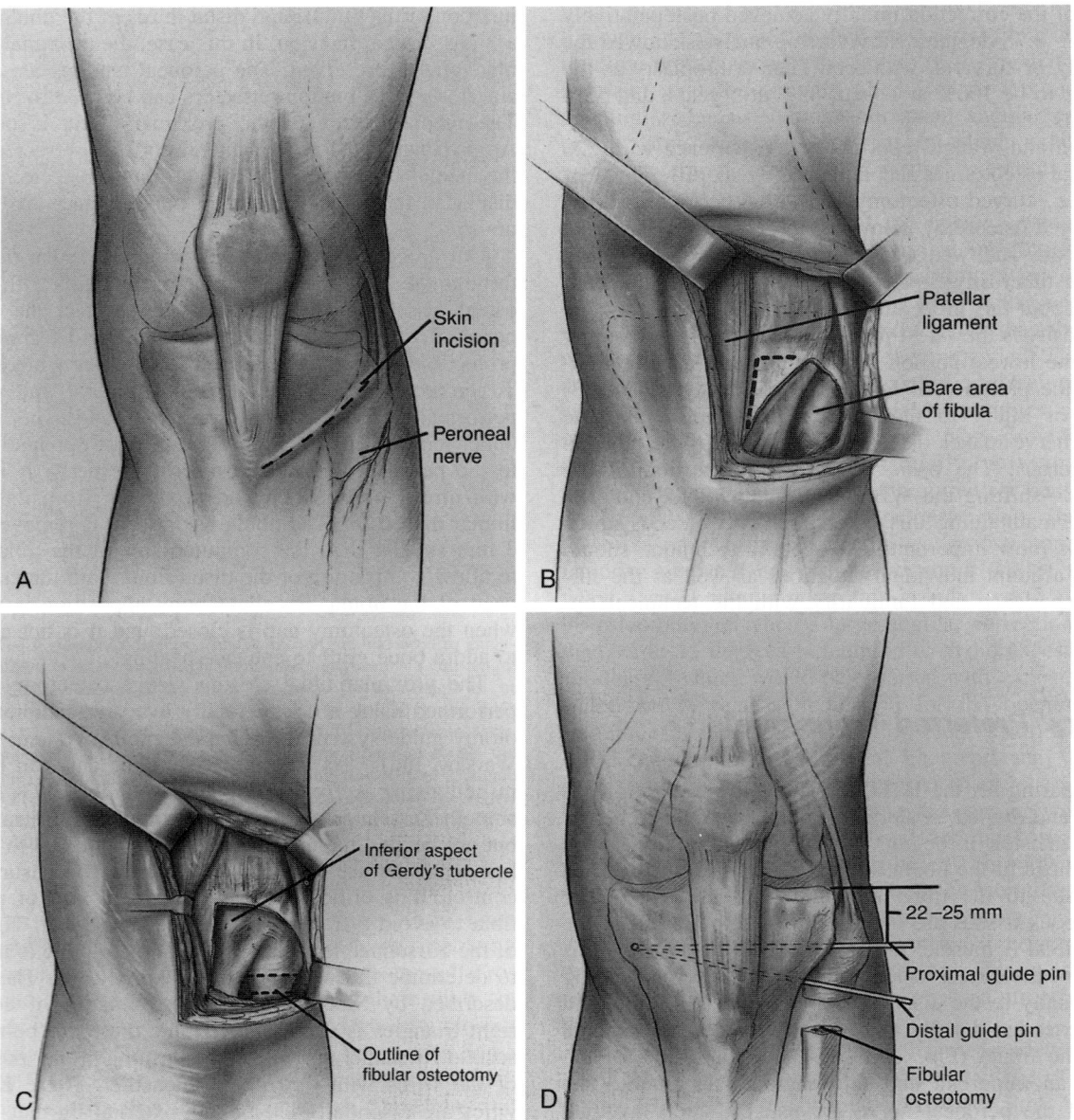

Figure 28G–17. *A,* An oblique skin incision is used in high tibial osteotomy, extending from the bare area of the fibula head to the tibial tubercle. *B,* A dome-shaped fascial incision is made from the lateral border of the patellar tendon to the edge of Gerdy's tubercle and extends to the bare area of the fibula. The anterior tibialis musculature is carefully dissected from the tibia subperiosteally and then reflected distally. *C,* The proximal fibula is subperiosteally dissected, and the peroneal nerve is identified and protected in preparation for the proximal fibular osteotomy. A wedge of bone is osteotomized with the micro-oscillating saw and osteotome and then removed. The posterior periosteum of the fibula is preserved. *D,* The proximal guide pin is placed parallel to the joint and 2.5 cm from it. The width of the proximal tibia is determined by measuring the length of this pin. The preoperative planning notes are consulted to determine the starting point for the distal guide pin with reference to the proximal pin, which has been computed for the desired angle of correction. The distance between the two guide pins is essentially the width of the base of the osteotomy wedge. The pins are inserted under image control either freehandedly or using a calibrated osteotomy guide, which is the authors' preferred technique.[11] (From Noyes FR, Roberts CS: High tibial osteotomy in knees with associated chronic ligament deficiencies. In Jackson DW [ed]: Master Techniques in Orthopaedic Surgery, Reconstructive Knee Surgery. New York, Raven Press, 1995, pp 185–210.)

slope would result in a loss of normal knee extension and would place higher forces on an ACL reconstruction. A decrease in the tibial slope (resulting in an anterior portion of the tibia sloping distally) would produce hyperextension of the knee and would place high forces on a PCL reconstruction.

An alignment guide rod (rigid 3- to 4-mm rod, 1 m in length) is positioned over the center of the femoral head (determined by the image intensifier) and the center of the tibiotalar joint to determine the newly corrected WBL intersection at the tibial plateau. A large single staple may be placed across the lateral tibial osteotomy site for provisional fixation. During this procedure, the lower limb is axially loaded to maintain contact and to maintain closure of both tibiofemoral compartments. The knee is kept at 5 to 10 degrees of flexion, avoiding any hyperextension.

The alignment guide rod represents a new WBL, which should agree with preoperative calculations. If necessary, additional bone may be removed from the osteotomy cuts to adjust the WBL as required. Rigid fixation of the osteotomy is achieved using an L-shaped five-hole buttress plate. Two 6.5-mm cancellous screws are placed in the proximal tibia, and two or three cortical screws are placed distal to the osteotomy (Fig. 28G–18). If needed, a short-threaded 6.5-mm cancellous screw can be placed in a lag fashion from proximal to distal across the osteotomy site into the medial aspect of the proximal tibial bone for additional compression of the medial aspect of the osteotomy. The final WBL determination is made using the rigid rod as a plumb line, as noted previously. The tourniquet is released, and hemostasis is obtained. The fascia of the anterior compartment musculature is loosely reattached to the anterolateral aspect of the tibial border. A Hemovac drain is used for 24 hours. We currently perform our HTO as an outpatient procedure, with the patient leaving the hospital 12 to 23 hours after surgery. Deep venous thrombosis prophylaxis is maintained by the use of antithrombotic stockings, sequential compression boots (begun intraoperatively and continued postoperatively until discharge from the hospital), and aspirin.

Rehabilitation after High Tibial Osteotomy

The protocol for rehabilitation following HTO is shown in Table 28G–4. The program includes immediate range of motion (0 to 90 degrees), quadriceps isometrics, straight leg raises, patellar mobilization, and electrical muscle stim-

ulation.[105] For the first week after surgery, ice, mild compression, and elevation are used to prevent edema and swelling. Patients are ambulatory for short periods of time but are instructed to elevate their limb, remain home, and not resume usual activities. The prophylaxis for deep venous thrombosis includes intermittent compression stocking boots the first night after surgery, antiembolism stockings, ankle pumps, and aspirin (600 mg once a day for 3 weeks).

A Bledsoe (Grand Prairie, Tex) long-leg brace is worn for the first 8 postoperative weeks. Patients are allowed toe-touch weight-bearing for the first 3 weeks to prevent excessive forces at the osteotomy site. Weight-bearing is gradually increased to full by the eighth to tenth postoperative week if radiographs demonstrate adequate healing and maintenance of the HTO position. The protocol emphasizes quadriceps, hamstring, hip, and gastrocnemius-soleus musculature strengthening. Closed chain exercises and stationary bicycling are begun at the fifth postoperative week, and weight machine exercises are begun at the seventh to eighth postoperative week. Excessive use of bicycling and weight machines is not allowed in patients with articular cartilage damage. By the ninth to twelfth postoperative week, other aerobic conditioning exercises are begun as appropriate, including swimming, ski machine workout, and walking.

Patients who also require posterolateral reconstruction are allowed to begin immediate knee motion but are maximally protected against undue joint loads to prevent failure. Patients are warned to avoid knee hyperextension and varus loads, which could place excessive forces on the posterolateral reconstruction. A Bledsoe postoperative brace is worn locked at 0 degrees of extension at all times except for range of motion exercises done four times daily for the first 4 weeks to protect the posterolateral reconstruction.

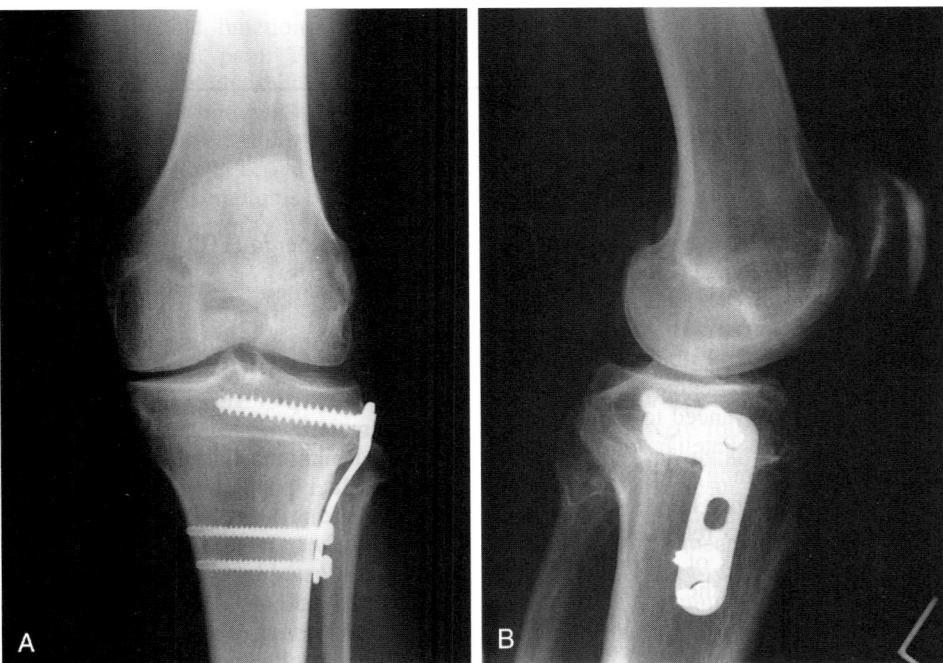

Figure 28G–18. Anteroposterior *(A)* and lateral *(B)* radiographs show the postoperative appearance after proximal tibial osteotomy, fibular osteotomy, and internal fixation. (From Noyes FR, Barber-Westin SD, Hewett TE: High tibial osteotomy and ligament reconstruction for varus angulated anterior cruciate ligament–deficient knees. Am J Sports Med 28:282–296, 2000.)

82. Levy IM, Torzilli PA, Warren RF: The effect of medial meniscectomy on anterior-posterior motion of the knee. J Bone Joint Surg Am 64:883–888, 1982.

83. MacIntosh DL, Welsh RP: Joint debridement—A complement to high tibial osteotomy in the treatment of degenerative arthritis of the knee. J Bone Joint Surg Am 59:1094–1097, 1977.

84. Maquet P: Valgus osteotomy for osteoarthritis of the knee. Clin Orthop 120:143–148, 1976.

85. Maquet P: The biomechanics of the knee and surgical possibilities of healing osteoarthritic knee joints. Clin Orthop 146:102–110, 1980.

86. Maquet P: The treatment choice in osteoarthritis of the knee. Clin Orthop 192:108–112, 1985.

87. Maquet PGJ: Osteotomy. In Freeman MAR (ed): Arthritis of the Knee. Clinical Features and Surgical Management. Berlin, Springer-Verlag, 1980, pp 148–183.

88. Markolf KL, Bargar WL, Shoemaker SC, et al: The role of joint load in knee stability. J Bone Joint Surg Am 63:570–585, 1981.

89. Markolf KL, Kochan A, Amstutz HC: Measurement of knee stiffness and laxity in patients with documented absence of the anterior cruciate ligament. J Bone Joint Surg Am 66:242–253, 1984.

90. Matthews LS, Goldstein SA, Malvita TA, et al: Proximal tibial osteotomy. Factors that influence the duration of satisfactory function. Clin Orthop 229:193–200, 1988.

91. Morrey BF: Upper tibial osteotomy for secondary osteoarthritis of the knee. J Bone Joint Surg Br 71:554–559, 1989.

92. Morrison JB: Bioengineering analysis of force actions transmitted by the knee joint. Biomed Eng 164–170, 1968.

93. Morrison JB: The mechanics of the knee joint in relation to normal walking. J Biomech 3:51–61, 1970.

94. Morscher E: Pathophysiology of posttraumatic deformities of the lower extremity. In Hierholzer G, Muller KH (eds): Corrective Osteotomies of the Lower Extremity. Berlin, Springer-Verlag, 1985, pp 3–37.

95. Muller KH, Muller-Farber J: Indications, localization and planning of posttraumatic osteotomies about the knee. In Hierholz G, Muller KH (eds): Corrective Osteotomies of the Lower Extremity. Berlin, Springer-Verlag, 1985, pp 195–223.

96. Muller W: Kinematics of the cruciate ligaments: In Feagin JA Jr (ed): The Crucial Ligaments: Diagnosis and Treatment of Ligamentous Injuries About the Knee. New York, Churchill Livingstone, 1988, pp 217–233.

97. Myrnerts R: Failure of the correction of varus deformity obtained by high tibial osteotomy. Acta Orthop Scand 51:569–573, 1980.

98. Myrnerts R: High tibial osteotomy with overcorrection of varus malalignment in medial gonarthrosis. Acta Orthop Scand 51:557–560, 1980.

99. Myrnerts R: Knee instability before and after high tibial osteotomy. Acta Orthop Scand 41:561–564, 1980.

100. Naudie D, Bourne RB, Rorabeck CH, et al: Survivorship of the high tibial valgus osteotomy. A 10- to 22-year followup study. Clin Orthop 367:18–27, 1999.

101. Nguyen C, Rudan J, Simurda MA, et al: High tibial osteotomy compared with high tibial and Maquet procedures in medial and patellofemoral compartment osteoarthritis. Clin Orthop 245:179–187, 1989.

102. Nissan M: Review of some basic assumptions in knee biomechanics. J Biomech 13:375–381, 1980.

103. Noyes FR, Barber SD: The effect of a ligament augmentation device on allograft reconstructions for chronic ruptures of the anterior cruciate ligament. J Bone Joint Surg Am 74:960–973, 1992.

104. Noyes FR, Barber SD, Mooar LA: A rationale for assessing sports activity levels and limitations in knee disorders. Clin Orthop 246:238–249, 1989.

105. Noyes FR, Barber SD, Simon R: High tibial osteotomy and ligament reconstruction in varus angulated, anterior cruciate ligament–deficient knees. A two- to seven-year follow-up study. Am J Sports Med 21:2–12, 1993.

106. Noyes FR, Barber-Westin SD: Surgical reconstruction of severe chronic posterolateral complex injuries of the knee using allograft tissues. Am J Sports Med 23:2–12, 1995.

107. Noyes FR, Barber-Westin SD: Surgical restoration to treat chronic deficiency of the posterolateral complex and cruciate ligaments of the knee joint. Am J Sports Med 24:415–426. 1996.

108. Noyes FR, Barber-Westin SD: Treatment of complex injuries involving the posterior cruciate and posterolateral ligaments of the knee. Am J Knee Surg 9:200–214, 1996.

109. Noyes FR, Barber-Westin SD, Hewett TE: High tibial osteotomy and ligament reconstruction for varus angulated anterior cruciate ligament–deficient knees. Am J Sports Med 28:282–296, 2000.

110. Noyes FR, Barber-Westin SD, Roberts CS: Use of allografts after failed treatment of rupture of the anterior cruciate ligament. J Bone Joint Surg Am 76:1019–1031, 1994.

111. Noyes FR, Cummings JF, Grood ES, et al: The diagnosis of knee motion limits, subluxations, and ligament injury. Am J Sports Med 19:163–171, 1991.

112. Noyes FR, Dunworth LA, Andriacchi TP, et al: Knee hyperextension gait abnormalities in unstable knees. Recognition and preoperative gait retraining. Am J Sports Med 24:35–45, 1996.

113. Noyes FR, Mangine RE, Barber SD: The early treatment of motion complications after reconstruction of the anterior cruciate ligament. Clin Orthop 277:217–228, 1992.

114. Noyes FR, Matthews DS, Mooar PA, et al: The symptomatic anterior cruciate–deficient knee. Part II: The results of rehabilitation, activity modification, and counseling on functional disability. J Bone Joint Surg Am 65:163–174, 1983.

115. Noyes FR, McGinniss GH, Grood ES: The variable functional disability of the anterior cruciate ligament deficient knee. Orthop Clin North Am 16:47–67, 1985.

116. Noyes FR, Mooar PA, Matthews DS, et al: The symptomatic anterior cruciate–deficient knee. Part I: The long-term functional disability in athletically active individuals. J Bone Joint Surg Am 65:154–162, 1983.

117. Noyes FR, Munns SW, Andriacchi TP, et al: The double-varus and triple-varus anterior cruciate insufficient knee: Gait analysis and surgical correction [abstract]. Trans Am Orthop Soc Sports Med 11:41, 1985.

118. Noyes FR, Schipplein OD, Andriacchi TP, et al: The anterior cruciate ligament–deficient knee with varus alignment. An analysis of gait adaptations and dynamic joint loadings. Am J Sports Med 20:707–716, 1992.

119. Noyes FR, Stabler CL: A system for grading articular cartilage lesions at arthroscopy. Am J Sports Med 17:505–513, 1989.

120. Noyes FR, Stowers SF, Grood ES, et al: Posterior subluxations of the medial and lateral tibiofemoral compartments. An in vitro ligament sectioning study in cadaveric knees. Am J Sports Med 21:407–414, 1993.

121. Noyes FR, Torvik PJ, Hyde WB, et al: Biomechanics of ligament failure II. An analysis of immobilization, exercise and reconditioning effects in primates. J Bone Joint Surg Am 56:1406–1418, 1974.

122. Noyes FR, Wojtys EM: The early recognition, diagnosis and treatment of the patella infera syndrome. In Tullos HS (ed): Instructional Course Lectures. Park Ridge, Ill, American Academy of Orthopaedic Surgeons, 1991, pp 233–247.

123. Noyes FR, Wojtys EM, Marshall MT: The early diagnosis and treatment of developmental patella infera syndrome. Clin Orthop 265:241–252, 1991.

124. Odenbring S, Egund N, Knutson K, et al: Revision after osteotomy for gonarthrosis. A 10–19 year follow-up of 314 cases. Acta Orthop Scand 61:128–130, 1990.

125. Odenbring S, Tjornstrand B, Egund N, et al: Function after tibial osteotomy for medial gonarthrosis below aged 50 years. Acta Orthop Scand 60:527–531, 1989.

126. Ogata K: Interlocking wedge osteotomy of the proximal tibia for gonarthrosis. Clin Orthop 186:129–134, 1984.

127. Olmstead TG, Wevers HW, Bryant JT, et al: Effect of muscular activity on valgus/varus laxity and stiffness of the knee. J Biomech 19:565–577, 1986.

128. Pope MH, Johnson RJ, Brown DW: The role of musculature in injuries to the medial collateral ligament. J Bone Joint Surg Am 61:398–402, 1979.

129. Prodromos CC, Andriacchi TP, Galante JO: A relationship between gait and clinical changes following high tibial osteotomy. J Bone Joint Surg Am 67:1188–1194, 1985.

130. Rinonapoli E, Mancini GB, Corvaglia A, et al: Tibial osteotomy for varus gonarthrosis. A 10- to 21-year follow-up study. Clin Orthop 353:185–193, 1998.

131. Rubman MH, Noyes FR, Barber-Westin SD: Arthroscopic repair of meniscal tears that extend into the avascular zone. A review of 198 single and complex tears. Am J Sports Med 26:87–95, 1998.

132. Rudan JF, Simurda MA: High tibial osteotomy. A prospective clinical and roentgenographic review. Clin Orthop 255:251–256, 1990.
133. Schipplein OD, Andriacchi TP: Interaction between active and passive knee stabilizers during level walking. J Orthop Res 9:113–119, 1991.
134. Scuderi GR, Windsor RE, Insall JN: Observation on patellar height after proximal tibial osteotomy. J Bone Joint Surg Am 71:245–248, 1989.
135. Seal PV, Chan RNW: Tibial osteotomy for osteoarthrosis of the knee. A five to ten year follow-up study. Acta Orthop Scand 46:141–151, 1975.
136. Sim FH, Frassica FJ, Merkel KD, et al: Knee ligaments in osteoarthritis of the knee. In Feagin JA Jr (ed): The Crucial Ligaments: Diagnosis and Treatment of Ligamentous Injuries About the Knee. New York, Churchill Livingstone, 1987.
137. Slocum DB, Larson RL, James SL, et al: High tibial osteotomy. Clin Orthop 104:239–243, 1974.
138. Smillie IS: Upper tibial osteotomy. J Bone Joint Surg Br 43:187, 1961.
139. Stuart MJ, Grace JN, Ilstrup DM, et al: Late recurrence of varus deformity after proximal tibial osteotomy. Clin Orthop 260:61–65, 1990.
140. Sundaram NA, Hallett JP, Sullivan MF: Dome osteotomy of the tibia for osteoarthritis of the knee. J Bone Joint Surg Br 68:782–786, 1986.
141. Surin V, Markhede G, Sundholm K: Factors influencing results of high tibial osteotomy in gonarthrosis. Acta Orthop Scand 46:996–1007, 1975.
142. Tjornstrand BE, Egund N, Hagstedt BV: High tibial osteotomy: A seven year clinical and radiographic follow-up. Clin Orthop 160:124–135, 1981.
143. Torgerson WR, Kettelkamp DB, Igou RA, et al: Tibial osteotomy for the treatment of degenerative arthritis of the knee. Clin Orthop 101:46–52, 1974.
144. Vainiopaa S, Laike E, Kirves P, et al: Tibial osteotomy for osteoarthritis of the knee. A five to ten-year follow-up study. J Bone Joint Surg Am 63:938–946, 1981.
145. Volkman R: Osteotomy for knee joint deformity. Edinburgh Med J 794, 1875.
146. Wang JW, Kuo KN, Andriacchi TP, et al: The influence of walking mechanics and time on the results of proximal tibial osteotomy. J Bone Joint Surg Am 72:905–909, 1990.
147. Waugh W: Tibial osteotomy in the management of osteoarthritis of the knee. Clin Orthop 210:55–61, 1986.
148. Westrich GH, Peters LE, Haas SB, et al: Patella height after high tibial osteotomy with internal fixation and early motion. Clin Orthop 354:169–174, 1998.
149. Windsor RE, Insall JN, Vince KG: Technical considerations of total knee arthroplasty after proximal tibial osteotomy. J Bone Joint Surg Am 70:547–555, 1988.
150. Zarrugh MY: Kinematic prediction of intersegment loads and power at the joints of the leg in walking. J Biomech 14:713–725, 1981.

Section H
Medial Ligament Injuries

1. MEDIAL LIGAMENT INJURIES IN THE ADULT

Peter A. Indelicato, MD ■ Russell C. Linton, MD

Since Brantigan and Voshell's pioneering work on the anatomy and function of the medial ligaments about the knee, there has been much controversy concerning these structures.[5, 6] The anatomy and function were early sources of controversy. Even after the three-layer concept described by Warren and Marshall[64] and advocated by Müller[38] became widely accepted, the importance of each ligament and layer in resisting valgus loads was disputed.[16, 21, 28, 29, 33, 43] Slocum and colleagues[54, 55] described rotatory instabilities and identified the functional deficits that allowed not only uniplanar but also abnormal rotational motion in the knee with torn ligaments.

O'Donoghue[44, 45] advocated operative repair of medial ligamentous disruptions because he thought that any clinically recognizable medial instability would not recover well without surgery. The type of surgical repair or reconstruction to be used was also argued. Some authors repaired only the superficial medial collateral ligament, whereas others made sure all torn structures were repaired, reefed, or advanced.[2, 8, 27–30, 39, 45] Chronic anteromedial rotatory instability (anteromedial tibial subluxation) was addressed with procedures that included the Nicholas five-one reconstruction,[39] posteromedial fascial sutures,[54, 55] and pes anserine transfers.[11, 18, 42]

In the 1970s, however, excellent results were reported for nonoperative treatment of grade II isolated medial collateral lesions.[12, 13, 19] Controversy about instabilities of lesser grade then focused more on the areas of immobilization and rehabilitation as more investigators found that equal stability and earlier return to athletic competition resulted with nonoperatively treated grade II tears.[3, 22, 24–26, 57, 66] At this time, grade III tears were uniformly repaired with open surgery.

More recently, isolated grade III medial instabilities (abduction rotational instabilities) have been found to have the same long-term results when they are treated nonoperatively as when they are surgically repaired.[15, 31] Indelicato[31, 32] found that following a rigid protocol to rule out cruciate and meniscal disease, good and excellent results could be expected in more than 90% of the athletes. Not only were long-term results equal, but this form of treatment allowed an earlier return to sports. Several authors still argue this work and advocate surgical repair,[29, 30, 35, 38] but prospective studies by Sandberg and colleagues[51] and Jones and associates[34] support Indelicato's work.

Combined injuries involving multiple ligaments have been less controversial in that most studies have shown poor results without surgical repair or reconstruction.[8, 15, 37, 44, 45, 54, 60] A new controversy may be starting, however, about whether the medial collateral ligament needs to be primarily repaired when it is damaged along with complete disruption of the anterior cruciate.[53]

Controversy aside, the medial collateral ligament is the most commonly injured ligament about the knee.[15] The incidence of this injury is probably higher than reported because many grade I sprains are never seen by physicians.

Each structure does not act independently but instead works synergistically with other components of the knee in resisting abnormal loads. It is impossible to create an experimental model that can take into account all the dynamic and static forces that occur with medial compartment injury. The next section of this chapter briefly discusses the biomechanics and the functional role of these anatomic structures.

Biomechanics

Biomechanical studies of the medial capsuloligamentous complex have centered on the various components' resistance to strain and the healing properties of the medial collateral ligament. The medial ligament's main function is to resist valgus and external rotation forces of the tibia in relation to the femur. Slocum and colleagues[55] described this as anteromedial rotatory instability (anteromedial tibial subluxation) or a shift of the central pivot of the knee in the posterolateral direction.

The three functional units of the medial complex consist of the anterior parallel fibers of the superficial medial collateral ligament, the deep medial collateral ligament, and the posterior oblique ligament. The cruciates also resist abduction loads. Kennedy and Fowler[36] found that the first ligament to be disrupted with an abduction load is the deep medial collateral ligament (midthird capsular ligament). Müller[38] thought of the ligaments as triangles, those with the shorter sides having less "elastic reserve" and therefore rupturing sooner (i.e., the posterior oblique before the superficial medial collateral).

Warren and colleagues[63] found that the long parallel anteriormost fibers (4 to 5 mm) of the superficial medial collateral are the primary restraint on abduction and external rotatory loads on the medial side of the knee in their cadaveric models. This study was conducted with varying degrees of knee flexion and selective cutting in different sequences of the posterior oblique, deep middle-third capsular ligament, and superficial medial collateral ligament. They found 5 to 7 mm of increased medial joint opening and a 200% to 300% increase in rotation after sectioning the superficial medial collateral when the posterior oblique and deep medial collateral had previously been cut. No significant valgus or rotation occurred when the superficial anterior parallel fibers were intact.

Grood and associates[21] agree that the superficial medial collateral is the primary restraint and the posterior oblique and cruciates are secondary restraints to pure abduction loads. Their studies also showed only a 5-mm increase in medial joint opening after complete transection of the superficial medial collateral ligament. This increase was small because of the low forces applied during clinical testing and because the secondary restraints blocked further opening even when the primary restraint was sectioned. The superficial medial collateral was found to be responsible for 57% of medial stability at 5 degrees of knee flexion and for 78% at 25 degrees of flexion. The deep medial collateral accounted for 8% at 5 degrees and 4% at 25 degrees, and the posterior oblique accounted for 18% and 4%, respectively. These investigators also showed that axial rotation may cause an examiner to overestimate medial

instability on clinical evaluation. The cruciates are more important in resisting abduction stresses in hyperextension but constitute a lesser percentage of restraint than the superficial medial collateral because of their closeness to the center of rotation and their resulting mechanical disadvantage.

A study by Inoue and colleagues[33] on dogs found that the increase in functional abduction instability resulting from an isolated medial collateral injury is probably less than the 78% reported by Grood and associates.[21] These investigators found that an experimental model restricting axial rotation and anterior-posterior translation placed too much emphasis on the medial ligaments. With 5 degrees of freedom, the anterior cruciate played a larger role in resisting abnormal abduction stress. This finding, in their minds, explained why there are so many good results in patients with isolated medial ligament disruptions, whatever the treatment, when the anterior cruciate is intact.

One must keep in mind that ligament disruption in the knee is a continuum of progressive damage frequently involving more than one ligament at a time. It is possible that subclinical damage can occur to either cruciate ligament once there is complete disruption of the superficial medial collateral ligament.

Biomechanical studies on healthy medial ligaments have dealt mainly with the subject of immobilization. Frank and associates[17] found that unsutured medial collateral ligaments healed with scar formation rather than true ligamentous regeneration. This scar contracted between 3 and 14 weeks but later stretched out to leave some pathologic medial laxity. This scar tissue was biomechanically inferior to normal ligament and showed increased cellularity, less total collagen, and more type III (immature) collagen. The bone-ligament-bone posthealing stress to failure results in these patients were consistently inferior to results in control subjects. These investigators did find that controlled motion did not harm the quality of the scar.

Woo and colleagues[66] found a time-dependent inverse relationship between immobilization and mechanical properties. Immobilization led to decreased stiffness of the ligament with increased osteoclasts and fibrous tissue at the tibial insertion of the anterior parallel fibers. Postimmobilization stress showed consistent rupture of the ligament-tibia interface. Normal integrity of the distal medial collateral ligament–bone insertion was not restored until 1 year after remobilization.

Hart and Dahners[24] found that all healed medial collateral ligaments, whether sutured or allowed to scar in, were more lax than those in uninjured control subjects. Tension to failure results showed more strength for ligaments treated after injury with controlled motion. Häggmark and Eriksson[22] showed that immobilization also had a detrimental effect on the knee musculature. They found atrophy of type I collagen fibers and a decrease in succinate dehydrogenase activity (oxidative capacity or endurance work) in mobilized knees after ligament surgery. The subject of immobilization is also discussed in the section on rehabilitation.

Clinical Evaluation

Ideally, a physician present on the sidelines of an athletic event can observe an injury as it occurs and examine the knee immediately, before the onset of muscle spasm. In most situations, however, this is not possible. The physician must then rely on a careful history, a thorough physical examination, and special diagnostic tests as indicated.

History

How and when the patient was hurt should be ascertained in the history. The mechanism of injury and the position of the knee when it was injured should be elicited as descriptively as possible. As stated previously, lesser grade medial collateral injuries can occur with noncontact valgus, external rotation injuries such as occur in skiing. A grade III medial collateral disruption, however, almost necessitates a lateral blow to the lower thigh or upper leg, as occurs in football. Other important points are the presence or absence of pain, the ability to ambulate immediately and later, the time at onset of swelling, the sensation of a pop or tear, the presence of a deformity (e.g., patellar dislocation), and the immediate site of tenderness.

Hughston and colleagues[27] found that 50% of athletes with grade III injuries could walk into the office unaided by external support. In actuality, some grade I or grade II sprains are usually more painful than grade III injuries. Therefore, absence of severe pain and ability to ambulate do not rule out a severe injury. The immediate onset of swelling also indicates a hemarthrosis secondary to a torn cruciate, a patellar dislocation, an osteochondral fracture, a peripheral meniscus tear, or an incomplete ligamentous sprain. The absence of swelling does not mean that the injury is mild because a large capsular rent can cause escape of fluid into the soft tissues.

The past history, including any previous injury or instability, should also be obtained. Reference to the preseason physical findings is ideal.

Physical Examination

Sprains of the medial collateral can be classified as mild, moderate, or severe. O'Donoghue[45] classifies them as follows:

Mild sprains have a few torn fibers but no loss of ligamentous integrity. The patient has minimal symptoms, possibly with a small, localized hematoma, and can be treated symptomatically.

Moderate sprains are incomplete tears with no pathologic laxity, and the fibers are still apposed. Fiber apposition is the main criterion for ligamentous healing.

In severe sprains, there is loss of integrity of the ligament, with much swelling and ecchymosis. Abnormal motion or pathologic laxity exists with severe sprains.

Pathologic laxity is then graded according to the amount of joint opening that occurs with displacing forces as 0 (normal), I (1 to 4 mm), II (5 to 9 mm), or III (10 to 15 mm).[27] On physical examination, grade I and grade II are found to have definite end points, but grade III tears have a soft, mushy end point (or no end point) to abduction stress.

Physical examination should begin with a careful exami-nation of the uninjured knee and then of the injured knee. Inspection for ecchymosis, localized edema, and effusion should be done first. Point tenderness can accurately identify the surgical location of the lesion in 78% of cases, and localized edema can identify the tear in 64%.[27] Patellar tenderness, apprehension, and medial retinacular tenderness are sought because patellar dislocation is associated with valgus injuries. Hunter and colleagues[30] found a 9% to 21% incidence of damage to the extensor mechanism (vastus medialis tearing) with medial ligament injury. Of 40 patients, 18 had laterally displaceable patellae on stress radiographs preoperatively, but in only 7 of 40 patients could vastus medialis obliquus tenderness be separated from medial collateral ligament tenderness preoperatively.

Abduction stress testing is then done with varying degrees of knee flexion. Even with a complete medial disruption, there will be no abduction instability when the knee is in full extension if the posterior capsule and posterior cruciate are intact. The "gold standard" for medial instability is a stress test performed at 30 degrees of knee flexion. This test should be done with the foot in external rotation because an extra grade of instability can be perceived if the examination allows the tibia to move from internal to external rotation as a load is applied. In larger patients, this degree of flexion (30 degrees) can easily be achieved by resting the thigh on the table and dropping the foot over the edge of the table a few inches. Anteromedial tibial subluxation (described elsewhere) is then evaluated by an anterior drawer test with the foot in external rotation and the knee flexed to 90 degrees and an anterior pull on the proximal calf to palpate laxity. This test should produce no more than a grade I laxity (less than 5 mm of anterior displacement) if the anterior cruciate ligament is intact.

Perhaps the most important part of the examination is the evaluation of the cruciates because a combined injury requires such drastically different treatment. An immediate examination on the sidelines can be up to 95% accurate in identifying cruciate lesions if it is performed before the onset of muscle spasms. A Lachman test is most critical because a pivot shift cannot always be elicited when gross medial instability is present. Severe abduction instability removes the medial support or pivot axis necessary for the pivot shift. A thorough knee examination for lateral and posterior instability (described elsewhere in this chapter) should also be done. A hip examination should be performed in all patients, but especially in adolescents, and a neurovascular examination is needed in all athletes with knee pain.[62]

Diagnostic Studies

Anteroposterior, lateral, and patellofemoral radiographic views should be obtained for all patients with knee injuries. These films should be inspected for fractures, lateral capsular signs (Segond's fracture), ligamentous avulsions, loose bodies, old Pellegrini-Stieda lesions (Fig. 28H1–4), and evidence of patellar dislocation. Stress radiographs are invaluable in adolescents to differentiate epiphyseal injuries from medial collateral injuries (Fig. 28H1–5). In a skeletally mature patient, however, stress radiographs usually do not add to the accuracy of the diagnosis.[31]

TABLE 28H1–1
Knee Rehabilitation Program

Begin	Stages of Program	End
Time of injury	1. Ice for >20 minutes, every 2 waking hours	48 to 72 hours after injury
	2. Compression with elastic wrap	Unsupported ambulation
	3. Elevation when not ambulating	Swelling gone
	4. Crutches, non–weight-bearing on involved side	Painless weight-bearing
	5. Isometric quadriceps contractions (painless—minimum of 5 minutes 3 times a day)	Return to participation / More than 90 degrees of painless active range of motion
	6. Knee immobilizer at 5 to 15 degrees of flexion	
Swelling stabilized	Active range of motion in whirlpool	0 to 120 degrees of painless active range of motion
0 to 30 degrees of painless active range of motion	Short arc (0 to 30 degrees) DeLorme quadriceps isotonic exercises	More than 90 degrees of painless active range of motion
0 to 90 degrees of painless active range of motion	0 to 90 degrees of DeLorme quadriceps isotonic exercises	10 repetitions of weightlifting equaling 33% body weight + 20 pounds
Isotonic lift, 35 pounds	Isokinetic exercises (Cybex II or Orthotron at 180 degrees/second)	Torque output equal to opposite site
After 2 days of isokinetics	Straight-line jogging on level surface	Return to full participation
After attaining 75% normal jogging speed	45-degree cutting; 20-yard figure eights	Able to do at least 75% normal jogging speed
After 75% speed with 45-degree cuts and 20-yard figure eights	90-degree cutting; 10-yard figure eights	Return to full participation
After 75% speed with 90-degree cuts and 20-yard figure eights	Noncontact football drills	Return to full participation
Full noncontact activity; attained isokinetic goals; all drills at 100% speed	Full football activity; no taping; no bracing	Return to full participation

From Derscheid GL, Garrick JC: Medial collateral ligament injuries in football. Nonoperative management of grade I and grade II sprains. Am J Sports Med 9: 365–368, 1981.

were unable to operate on several grade III lesions. To their surprise, they found no better results in the group receiving operative treatment of isolated medial ligament injuries than in the nonsurgical group. With combined ligament injury, however, the nonoperative results were overwhelmingly poor; 78% of their patients with grade III medial lesions were found to have combined instability. The authors concluded that patients with grade III isolated abduction instability must undergo a thorough examination to rule out concomitant cruciate ligament tears.

Fetto and Marshall's findings led to several prospective studies to investigate the nonoperative treatment of grade III isolated medial collateral ligament tears. Indelicato[31] found objectively stable knees in 15 of 16 patients treated

operatively and in 17 of 20 patients treated nonoperatively for isolated third-degree ruptures. His treatment included 2 weeks in a cast at 30 degrees of flexion and then 4 weeks longer in a cast brace with hinges that allowed motion from 30 to 90 degrees. Most patients in both groups had a trace of valgus abduction at 2 to 3 years of follow-up. Subjective scoring of results and earlier return to activity were higher in the patients in the nonsurgical group, leading to good and excellent results in 90% of these patients and in 88% of the surgically repaired group. Again, a rigid protocol was used to exclude anterior cruciate and meniscal disease, and those patients treated with early motion returned to football 3 weeks earlier than immobilized patients did.

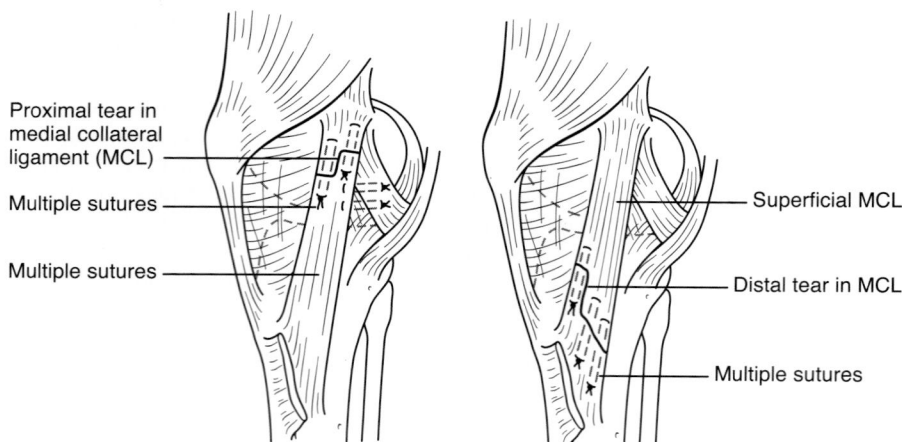

Proximal tear in medial collateral ligament (MCL)

Multiple sutures

Multiple sutures

Superficial MCL

Distal tear in MCL

Multiple sutures

Figure 28H1–7. Intrasubstance superficial medial ligament tears repaired with a combination of approximating and tension-relieving sutures.

Sandberg and colleagues[51] and Jones and colleagues[34] also reported on cast and cast brace treatment of grade III medial disruptions. They agreed with Indelicato that nonoperative treatment of these lesions is justified after ensuring that the injury is isolated. Jones and his group studied 24 high-school football players who returned to competition an average of 34 days after injury. Instability was reduced to grade 0 or I in all patients by 29 days. They also found no increased incidence of reinjury to the knee during the following spring.

The study by Sandberg and associates also included patients with anterior cruciate injuries. At 33 months of follow-up, all of the patients with isolated medial lesions were satisfied with their results. Only 35 of 89 patients with combined anterior cruciate–medial collateral ligament lesions were satisfied with nonoperative treatment, however. The authors noted that these 35 patients had a less positive pivot shift on average than the dissatisfied patients and that the results of treatment of combined injuries tended to deteriorate with time.

A study by Reider[48] reported the results in 35 athletes who were treated with early functional rehabilitation of isolated tears of the medial collateral ligament. The athletes were monitored for more than 5 years. Nineteen patients were able to return to full, unlimited sports in fewer than 8 weeks after their injury. Of the 19 football players, 16 were able to return to the sport within 4 weeks after the injury.

Kannus,[35] on the other hand, has not found 90% + good to excellent results with nonoperative treatment of grade III medial collateral injuries. His paper studied 54 patients with grade II and 27 patients with grade III lesions with a 9-year follow-up. Patients with grade II injuries averaged 92 on the Lysholm scale, whereas 66 was the average score of patients with grade III lesions. He found degenerative changes on radiographic examination with chronic stretching of the other ligaments about the knee. He thought that because these injuries deteriorated with time, they must need early operative repair. Critical examination of his patients, however, reveals that 16 of 27 had greater than 2 + on the Lachman test, and 10 of 27 had anterolateral rotatory instability at follow-up. These observations probably indicate an associated anterior cruciate lesion that was originally not detected, accounting for the poor long-term functional ratings of his patients.

The treatment of significant anteromedial tibial subluxation has filled the pages of orthopaedic literature in the past. As stated earlier, we do not believe significant anteromedial tibial subluxation can exist without a significant tear of the anterior cruciate ligament. Slocum and colleagues[55] found that the late functional deficits of anteromedial tibial subluxation included abduction instability, rotatory instability, vastus medialis weakness, lateral patellar subluxation, decreased joint motion, and degenerative joint disease.

Several procedures were used in the past to decrease anteromedial tibial subluxation, including the Nicholas five-one reconstruction,[39] popliteal advancement,[56] and fascial suture of the posteromedial corner.[8, 54, 55] The pes anserinus transfer was the procedure probably most used for this condition.[11] This transfer was found biomechanically to act as a medial sling and to increase internal rotation

forces dynamically about the knee.[42] In long-term follow-up, however, these surgeries failed when the injuries were associated with anterior cruciate lesions, especially if a meniscectomy had been done previously.[18]

Surgery has always been the treatment of choice for significant anteromedial tibial subluxation. Most authors now agree that for an acute anterior cruciate–medial collateral ligament disruption, some sort of intra-articular cruciate reconstruction must be done along with repair of the medial structures.[14, 38] Chronic anteromedial tibial subluxation is also best treated with anterior cruciate ligament reconstruction. The remaining chronic medial laxity in this combination can then be addressed by proximal and distal advancement of the superficial medial collateral, advancement of the whole medial capsular complex,[44] or posteromedial advancement and augmentation.[29, 38] Again, isometry of the advancement-augmentation as well as full range of motion of the knee must be achieved without pulling out or loosening of the surgically achieved fixation.

Rarely, a special situation may exist in some patients in whom there are insufficient medial collagenous structures to obtain satisfactory repair. Müller[38] reconstructs the superficial medial collateral with a portion of the pes tendons under these circumstances. The reader is referred to the works of Grana and Gimple[20] and Aragona and colleagues[1] for other possible options.

Complications of medial collateral ligament ruptures are rare in the literature, but several are discussed here. Residual pain can occur even after grade I sprains.[7] This pain is usually nearer the femoral origin, possibly because of a small neurovascular bundle there.[38] A radiograph may disclose residual calcification (Pellegrini-Stieda lesions). Treatment consists of anti-inflammatory agents or an injection. Atrophy, arthrofibrosis, and patellofemoral complaints are becoming less frequent with newer nonoperative protocols including early motion and strengthening. Infection is always a possibility with surgery, as is damage to the saphenous vein or nerve posteromedially.[50] Long-term instability or degenerative problems have most often been associated with missed or unrecognized cruciate lesions and previous meniscal excision. Proper early diagnosis and meniscal preservation should avoid these complications. Surgical treatment of combined anterior cruciate–medial collateral lesions in general shows less frequent return of full range of motion and poorer functional results than similar surgery for isolated cruciate reconstruction or medial collateral repair.[53, 67] Robins demonstrated that when damage occurs to the proximal half of the medial collateral ligament in combined anterior cruciate–medial collateral ligament tears, recovery of motion may be a problem, and therefore an aggressive program should be designed that focuses on regaining full extension.

Postoperative Care, Rehabilitation, and Return to Competition

The importance of postoperative rehabilitation and exercise has been stressed by Stewart[58] for many years. Separating the "treatment" from the "rehabilitation" in the nonoperative care of medial collateral ligament sprains is at times difficult. The advent of rehabilitative bracing has allowed control of valgus and rotational stresses while allowing range of motion. Whereas rehabilitation began when the cast was removed in the past, athletes can now exercise to regain motion and strength while soft tissue damage itself is healing.

There is no one perfect rehabilitation protocol that will work with every athlete. Several general guidelines should be followed, allowing individual adaptations along the way.[37] Steadman,[57] Bergfeld,[4] O'Connor,[43] and Cox[10] have had excellent success with their individual protocols for nonoperative treatment of grade I and grade II medial collateral injuries and either operative or nonoperative treatment of grade III disruptions. Wilk[65] published a complete rehabilitation program for collateral ligaments of the knee. The reader is referred to his work for details.

In general, lesser grade sprains are treated in a knee immobilizer with crutches for initial pain relief. Isometric exercises are begun immediately, and range of motion exercises out of the brace are started as soon as the athlete is pain free. Pain usually disappears in several days with grade I sprains but may last 10 to 14 days in patients with grade II to grade III pathologic laxities. Weight-bearing is begun as tolerated. Progressive isotonic resistance exercises to the thigh musculature are started when range of motion is 75% of normal. With the more severe grade II sprains, a controlled motion brace is used initially, limiting flexion

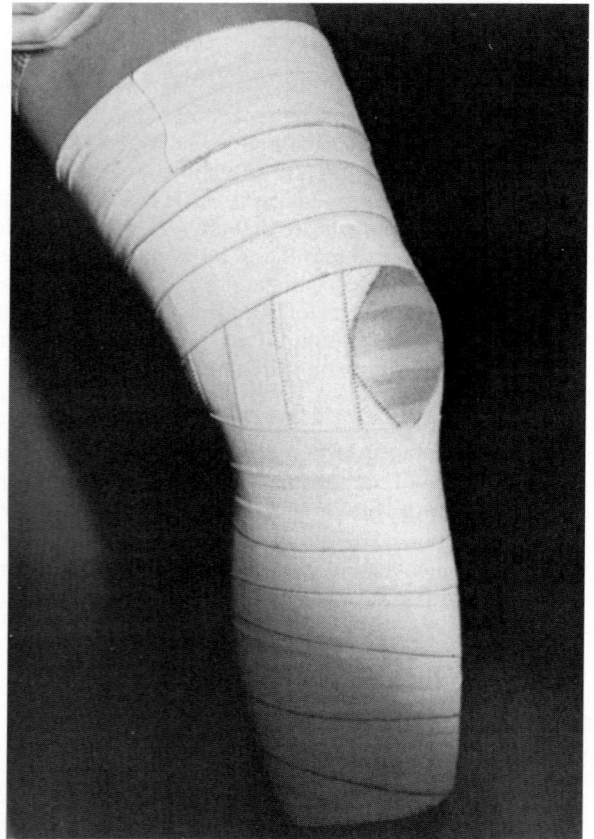

Figure 28H1–8. Anteromedial view of knee with protective taping applied. This athlete had a grade II ligament sprain and was returned to college football action in 3 weeks with his knee taped.

to 30 to 90 degrees. Patients with complete grade III sprains are treated with a cast brace for 2 weeks and then switched to a controlled motion device. Bicycling is used to help regain motion once the patient is out of the brace. Crutches are discarded when the athlete regains 40% of strength as tested isokinetically.

It appears that the location of the damage (proximal versus distal) plays a role in the morbidity of the recovery. Simply stated, the more proximal the lesion, the more likely the patient will encounter some difficulty regaining or maintaining full extension. If reconstruction of the anterior cruciate ligament is undertaken, special attention is necessary to prevent postoperative loss of full extension when a coexisting tear of the proximal superficial medial collateral ligament is present.

Isokinetic exercises are then added, and when the injured leg regains 60% of its normal strength, straight-ahead jogging is begun. When 80% strength is reached, agility drills in a functional brace and sprinting are started. Cutting and pivoting are added slowly. The patient can return to contact drills in a functional brace or appropriately taped (Fig. 28H1–8) when 90% of normal strength in the hamstrings and quadriceps is obtained as tested isokinetically. There should also be no effusion and no more than a trace of painless opening to valgus stress at 30 degrees of knee flexion. Even after return to competition, leg exercises should continue until a total return of strength is achieved.

If an effusion develops along the way, the protocol is held at that stage until the swelling dissipates. On isolated occasions, a few days in a knee immobilizer and an anti-inflammatory medicine are needed. Exercises should not be done isokinetically through a range of motion that is painful to the patient because this will elicit reflex quadriceps inhibition, and no progress will be made in gaining strength. If the effusion continues or strength gains do not occur, the patient should be carefully re-evaluated to rule out loose bodies or meniscal or cruciate disease. Pain at the posteromedial corner, representing semimembranosus tendinitis, is another source of postoperative pain found in up to 10% of patients using isokinetic machines in rehabilitation.

Rehabilitation of a combined anterior cruciate–medial collateral lesion should be geared more toward treatment of the cruciate lesion and therefore is outside the scope of this chapter.

Authors' Preferred Method of Treatment

Before a logical approach to treatment can be made, it is essential to know the proper diagnosis. The same mechanism of injury (valgus or external rotation) can cause medial collateral, anterior cruciate, or meniscal tears and patellar dislocations. It is necessary to rule out concomitant injuries before treating an "isolated" valgus pathologic laxity.

If the patient has no effusion, grade I or grade II pathologic valgus laxity only, and good results on clinical examination indicating intact cruciates, we do not routinely order MRI or insist on arthroscopy of the knee. Knees with any grade of pathologic valgus laxity with an effusion or with a clinically indeterminable cruciate status on examination need an MRI study or an examination under anesthesia with arthroscopy. Patients with grade III laxities need an MRI evaluation because capsular tearing could have occurred and leaked the effusion. Some patients request arthroscopy of the knee in lieu of MRI or vice versa. Once the diagnosis has been decided, we can begin treatment.

We treat grade I and grade II medial collateral ligament sprains with a knee immobilizer and crutches until the pain has subsided. During the first 48 hours, we also use ice, compression, and elevation as much as possible. Quadriceps setting exercises and straight leg raises are begun immediately with the immobilizer on.

As the pain dissipates, we begin passive range of motion exercises out of the brace 7 to 10 times daily for 5 to 10 minutes at a time. The patient supports the injured leg with the well leg, letting gravity bend the knee while sitting on the side of the table, and slowly raises and lowers the good leg. The crutches and knee immobilizer are discontinued when the patient has enough motion and strength in the knee to walk without a limp. The motion is gradually increased and the athlete is allowed to start bike riding and progressive resistance exercises. Straight leg raises with weights are advanced to hamstring and quadriceps exercises with light weights and then to isokinetic exercises. When 60% of normal strength has been achieved, the patient is allowed to jog straight-ahead with the knee taped. Jogging can be initiated on a trampoline to reduce knee stress. When 80% strength has been obtained, agility drills are started. The athlete can return to contact sports whenever agility drills equivalent to those needed in the sport can be performed.

In some grade I sprains, return to sports takes only a few days because no motion and minimal strength are lost with short-term immobilization. Grade II sprains are more variable, depending on the time needed for the initial pain to dissipate. The average is 2 to 3 weeks, and we allow players to return when they no longer have pain with valgus stress, even if slight pathologic laxity is present clinically.

The method of treating complete ruptures (grade III) of the medial collateral ligament has evolved during the past 15 years. The older method involved holding the knee in 30 degrees of flexion for 2 weeks followed by allowing a range of motion from 30 to 90 degrees of flexion in a brace. The brace would be a prefabricated, commercially available one with locking hinges for compliant patients or a fiberglass cast brace for the unreliable ones. Rehabilitation would progress as described before with early emphasis placed on gaining extension once the patient was out of the brace. With the longer period of immobilization, return of muscle tone can take up to 9 weeks even for college athletes. Today, we prefer to place the leg in a commercially available splint in full extension for 2 weeks. After this, we encourage a full pain-free range of motion with no limitations in either extension or flexion. The splint is usually no longer necessary after 3 or 4 weeks. Independent walking without crutches is not allowed until the patient can demonstrate a limp-free gait. Our criteria for return to sports are the same as those listed earlier—at least 80% strength by isokinetic testing, ability to perform noncontact agility drills, and no pain with valgus stress.

The knee is taped or placed in a functional brace when the player returns to sports that same season. The brace becomes optional the following season.

This protocol is delayed in patients with any grade of sprain if increasing pain or an effusion develops in the knee. Patellofemoral pain must be watched for, and if it is present, the exercise protocol should be adjusted to remove any exercise that aggravates this type of pain. Isokinetic exercise can usually be continued, but the speed or range of motion of the machine must be adjusted.

Acute combined anterior cruciate–medial collateral lesions are treated with a bone–patellar tendon–bone reconstruction of the anterior cruciate. Intraoperatively, after the anterior cruciate ligament has been reconstructed, the knee is flexed 30 degrees and stressed with a valgus load. If there is residual medial instability (2+ or greater), the middle-third capsular, the posterior oblique, and the superficial medial collateral ligaments are repaired as anatomically as possible. In a midsubstance tear, each suture is placed carefully, and the knee is motioned after each stitch to make sure the repair does not restrict motion or tear out. If a proximal or distal disruption occurs, the superficial medial collateral is reattached with a suture anchor or a screw with a soft tissue washer to its isometric origin of insertion. Again, care is taken to ensure that a full range of motion exists after securing the metal fixation because postoperative stiffness is three to four times more common after combined repair than after reconstruction of the cruciate ligament alone.[53] With assurance of adequate fixation and a full range of motion at surgery, the patient is placed in a continuous passive motion machine and an unlocked brace postoperatively. MRI can locate the tear in the medial collateral ligament, diminishing the need for large surgical exposures. Ideally, MRI can be used to predict which pattern of torn medial collaterals will heal without repair and which need to be addressed operatively.

Because we believe that chronic anteromedial tibial subluxation of significant degree cannot occur without considerable anterior cruciate disease, we believe that the treatment of such a lesion should be based primarily on intraarticular cruciate reconstruction. If residual medial instability exists after cruciate reconstruction, a proximal and distal advancement of the superficial medial collateral should be done, keeping in mind that the medial ligaments should be repaired isometrically at surgery. Reefing of the posterior oblique ligament can also be added. Special care is taken with this procedure because extension can be limited if the posterior medial structures are reefed too tightly. We have usually found that cruciate reconstruction alone benefits these patients. Although a small amount of objective abduction instability is observed at follow-up, functional stability is good, and arthrofibrosis occurs less frequently.

References

1. Aragona J, Parsons JR, Alexander H, Weiss AB: Medial collateral ligament replacement with a partially absorbable tissue scaffold. Am J Sports Med 11:228–233,1983.
2. Bartel DL, Marshall JL, Schieck RA, Wang JB: Surgical repositioning of the medial collateral ligament: An anatomical and mechanical analysis. J Bone Joint Surg Am 59:107–116, 1977.
3. Bassett, FH, Beck JL, Walker GA: A modified cast brace: Its use in

nonoperative and postoperative management of serious knee ligament injuries. Am J Sports Med 8:63–67, 1980.

4. Bergfeld J: Functional rehabilitation of isolated medial collateral ligament sprains: First-, second-, and third-degree sprains. Am J Sports Med 7:207–209 1979.

5. Brantigan OC, Voshell AF: The mechanics of the ligaments and menisci of the knee joint. J Bone Joint Surg 23:44–66, 1941.

6. Brantigan OC, and Voshell A: The tibial collateral ligament: Its function, its bursae and its relation to the medial meniscus. J Bone Joint Surg Am 25:121–131, 1943.

7. Casscells SW: Tibial collateral ligament strain. Clin Orthop 76:123–124, 1971.

8. Collins HR: Reconstruction of the athlete's injured knee: Anatomy, diagnosis, treatment. Orthop Clin North Am 2:207–230, 1971.

9. Cooper RR, Misol S: Tendon and ligament insertion. A light and electron microscopic study. J Bone Joint Surg 52:1–20, 1970.

10. Cox JS: Symposium: Functional rehabilitation of isolated medial collateral ligament sprains. Injury nomenclature. Am J Sports Med 7: 211–213, 1979.

11. D'Arcy J: Pes anserinus transposition for chronic anteromedial rotational instability of the knee. J Bone Joint Surg Br 60:66–70, 1978.

12. Derscheid GL, Garrick JG: Medial collateral ligament injuries in football. Nonoperative management of grade I and grade II sprains. Am J Sports Med 9:365–368, 1981.

13. Ellsasser JC, Reynolds FC, Omohundro JR: The non-operative treatment of collateral ligament injuries of the knee in professional football players. An analysis of seventy-four injuries treated non-operatively and twenty-four injuries treated surgically. J Bone Joint Surg Am 56: 1185–1190, 1974.

14. Feagin JA: The Crucial Ligaments: Diagnosis and Treatment of Ligamentous Injuries about the Knee. New York, Churchill Livingstone, 1988.

15. Fetto JF, Marshall JL: Medial collateral ligament injuries of the knee: A rationale for treatment. Clin Orthop 132:206–218, 1978.

16. Fischer RA, Arms SW, Johnson RJ, Pope MH: The functional relationship of the posterior oblique ligament to the medial collateral ligament of the human knee. Am J Sports Med 13:390–397, 1985.

17. Frank C, Woo SL, Amiel D, et al: Medial collateral ligament healing. A multidisciplinary assessment in rabbits. Am J Sports Med 11: 379–389, 1983.

18. Freeman BL, Beaty JH, Haynes DB: The pes anserinus transfer. A long-term follow-up. J Bone Joint Surg Am 64:202–207, 1982.

19. Ginsburg JH, Ellsasser JC: Problem areas in the diagnosis and treatment of ligament injuries of the knee. Clin Orthop 132:201–205, 1978.

20. Grana WA, Gimple K: Reconstruction of traumatic complete loss of the medial collateral ligament: A case report. Clin Orthop 160: 153–157, 1981.

21. Grood ES, Noyes FR, Butler DL, Suntay WJ: Ligamentous and capsular restraints preventing straight medial and lateral laxity in intact human cadaver knees. J Bone Joint Surg Am 63:1257–1269, 1981.

22. Häggmark T, Eriksson E: Cylinder or mobile cast brace after knee ligament surgery. A clinical analysis and morphologic and enzymatic studies of changes in the quadriceps muscle. Am J Sports Med 7: 48–56, 1979.

23. Hamada M, Shino K, Mitsuoka T, et al: Chondral injury associated with acute isolated posterior cruciate ligament injury. Arthroscopy 16:59–63, 2000.

24. Hart DP, Dahners LE: Healing of the medial collateral ligament in rats. The effects of repair, motion, and secondary stabilizing ligaments. J Bone Joint Surg Am 69:1194–1199, 1987.

25. Hastings DE: The non-operative management of collateral ligament injuries of the knee joint. Clin Orthop 147:22–28, 1980.

26. Holden DL, Eggert AW, Butler JE: The nonoperative treatment of grade I and II medial collateral ligament injuries to the knee. Am J Sports Med 11:340–344, 1983.

27. Hughston JC, Andrews JR, Cross MJ, Moschi A: Classification of knee ligament instabilities. Part I. The medial compartment and cruciate ligaments. J Bone Joint Surg Am 58:159–172, 1976.

28. Hughston JC, Barrett GR: Acute anteromedial rotatory instability. Long-term results of surgical repair. J Bone Joint Surg Am 65: 145–153, 1983.

29. Hughston JC, Eilers AF: The role of the posterior oblique ligament in repairs of acute medial (collateral) ligament tears of the knee. J Bone Joint Surg Am 55:923–940, 1973.

30. Hunter SC, Marascalco R, Hughston JC: Disruption of the vastus medialis obliquus with medial knee ligament injuries. Am J Sports Med 11:427–431, 1983.

31. Indelicato PA: Non-operative treatment of complete tears of the medial collateral ligament of the knee. J Bone Joint Surg Am 65: 323–329, 1983.

32. Indelicato PA, Hermansdorfer J, Huegel M: Nonoperative management of complete tears of the medial collateral ligament of the knee in intercollegiate football players. Clin Orthop 256:174–177, 1990.

33. Inoue M, McGurk BE, Hollis JM, Woo SL: Treatment of the medial collateral ligament injury. I: The importance of anterior cruciate ligament on the varus-valgus knee laxity. Am J Sports Med 15: 15–21, 1987.

34. Jones RE, Henley MB, Francis P: Nonoperative management of isolated grade III collateral ligament injury in high school football players. Clin Orthop 213:137–140, 1986.

35. Kannus P: Long-term results of conservatively treated medial collateral ligament injuries of the knee joint. Clin Orthop 226:103–112, 1988.

36. Kennedy JC, Fowler PJ: Medial and anterior instability of the knee. An anatomical and clinical study using stress machines. J Bone Joint Surg Am 53:1257–1270, 1971.

37. Miller WE: Kinesiology. Part VI. Psychologic and neurologic aspects of kinesiology. Am J Sports Med 10:250–252, 1982.

38. Müller W: The Knee: Form, Function and Ligament Reconstruction. New York, Springer-Verlag, 1983.

39. Nicholas JA: The five-one reconstruction for anteromedial instability of the knee. Indications, technique, and the results in fifty-two patients. J Bone Joint Surg Am 55:899–922, 1973.

40. Norwood LA Jr, Andrews JR, Meisterling RC, Glancy GL: Acute anterolateral rotatory instability of the knee. J Bone Joint Surg Am 61:704–709, 1979.

41. Noyes FR, Grood ES, Tarzill PA: The definitions of terms for motion and position of the knee and injuries of the ligaments. J Bone Joint Surg Am 71:465–472, 1989.

42. Noyes FR, Sonstegard DA: Biomechanical function of the pes anserinus at the knee and the effect of its transplantation. J Bone Joint Surg Am 55:1225–1241, 1973.

43. O'Connor GA: Functional rehabilitation of isolated medial collateral ligament sprains. Am J Sports Med 7:209–210, 1979.

44. O'Donoghue DH: Reconstruction for medial instability of the knee. J Bone Joint Surg Am 55:941–954, 1973.

45. O'Donoghue DH: Treatment of acute ligamentous injuries of the knee. Orthop Clin North Am 4:617–645, 1973.

46. Pope MH, Johnson RJ, Brown DW, Tighe C: The role of the musculature in injuries to the medial collateral ligament. J Bone Joint Surg Am 61:398–402, 1979.

47. Price CT, Allen WC: Ligament repair in the knee with preservation of the meniscus. J Bone Joint Surg Am 60:61–65, 1978.

48. Reider B, Sathy MR, Talkington J, et al: Treatment of isolated medial collateral ligament injuries in athletes with early functional rehabilitation. A five-year follow-up study. Am J Sports Med 22: 470–477, 1994.

49. Ritter MA, McCarrol J, Wilson FD, Carlson SR: Ambulatory care of medial collateral ligament tears. Physician Sportsmed 11:47, 1983.

50. Rorabeck CH, Kennedy JC: Tourniquet-induced nerve ischemia complicating knee ligament surgery. Am J Sports Med 8:98–102, 1980.

51. Sandberg R, Balkfors B, Nilsson B, Westlin N: Operative versus nonoperative treatment of recent injuries to the ligaments of the knee. A prospective randomized study. J Bone Joint Surg Am 69:1120–1126, 1987.

52. Schwellnus MP: Skeletal muscle cramps during exercise. Physician Sportsmed 27:109–115, 1999.

53. Shelbourne KD, Baele JR: Treatment of combined anterior cruciate ligament and medial collateral ligament injuries. Am J Knee Surg 1: 56–58, 1988.

54. Slocum DB, Larson RL, James SL: Late reconstruction procedures used to stabilize the knee. Orthop Clin North Am 4:679–689, 1973.

55. Slocum DB, Larson RL, James SL: Late reconstruction of ligamentous injuries of the medial compartment of the knee. Clin Orthop 100:23–55, 1974.

56. Southmayd W, Quigley TB: The forgotten popliteus muscle. Its usefulness in correction of anteromedial rotatory instability of the knee. A preliminary report. Clin Orthop 130:218–222, 1978.

57. Steadman JR: Rehabilitation of first- and second-degree sprains of the medial collateral ligament. Am J Sports Med 7:300–302, 1979.

58. Stewart MJ: Rehabilitation in athletes. Instr Course Lect 16:45–48, 1959.
59. Tegner Y, Lysholm J: Rating systems in the evaluation of knee ligament injuries. Clin Orthop 198:43–49, 1985.
60. Thompson WO, Thaete FL, Fu FH, Dye SF: Tibial meniscal dynamics using three-dimensional reconstruction of magnetic resonance images. Am J Sports Med 19:210–215, 1991.
61. Torg JS, Conrad W, Kalen V: Clinical diagnosis of anterior cruciate ligament instability in the athlete. Am J Sports Med 4:84–93, 1976.
62. Towne LC, Blazina ME, Marmor L, Lawrence JF: Lateral compartment syndrome of the knee. Clin Orthop 76:160–168, 1971.
63. Warren LA, Marshall JL, Girgis F: The prime static stabilizer of the medical side of the knee. J Bone Joint Surg Am 56:665–674, 1974.
64. Warren LF, Marshall JL: The supporting structures and layers on the medial side of the knee: An anatomical analysis. J Bone Joint Surg Am 61:56–62, 1979.
65. Wilk KE, Andrews JR, Clancy WG: Nonoperative and postoperative rehabilitation of the collateral ligaments of the knee. Operative Tech Sports Med 4:192–201, 1996.
66. Woo SL, Gomez MA, Sites TJ, et al: The biomechanical and morphological changes in the medial collateral ligament of the rabbit after immobilization and remobilization. J Bone Joint Surg Am 69:1200–1211, 1987.
67. Zarins B, Rowe CR: Combined anterior cruciate–ligament reconstruction using semitendinosus tendon and iliotibial tract. J Bone Joint Surg Am 68:160–177, 1986.

2. MEDIAL LIGAMENT INJURIES IN CHILDREN

Mark A. Erickson, MD ■ Gregory A. Schmale, MD

As children begin to play organized sports at younger ages, the spectrum of sports injuries broadens and more injuries previously thought to be adult in nature are now being seen in children. This chapter is designed to review the pertinent anatomy as well as describe the particular physical examination findings and the basic diagnostic and treatment alternatives for injuries to the medial knee in the active child and adolescent. The literature is replete with descriptions of adult sports injuries involving the medial knee; however, few studies focus on injuries to children and skeletally immature adolescents. We will attempt to make special note of studies that include the truly pediatric population, including studies of adults only when appropriate. A rudimentary differential diagnosis for medial knee symptoms presenting as a sports-related problem in the skeletally immature patient is presented.

Anatomy

The distal femoral epiphysis is the first secondary ossification center to appear in the body, being present at birth. The distal femoral physis is a large and undulating growth plate, making it most susceptible to injury (Fig. 28H2–1). The proximal tibial epiphysis first forms at approximately 2 months of age. An additional ossification center in the proximal tibia appears at the tibial tubercle between 9 and 14 years of age. By about age 15, these two tibial ossification centers have fused. The distal femoral and proximal tibial physes close at a mean age of 14 years in girls and 16 years in boys.

Warren and Marshall described the medial structures about the knee as lying in three discrete layers. Layer I includes the deep or crural fascia, layer II the superficial medial collateral ligament (MCL) and ligaments of the posterior medial corner, and layer III the deep MCL and knee capsule.[76] The posterior oblique ligament has been described as merging with the fibers of the superficial MCL, being just superficial to the semimembranosus complex.[21, 26] The superficial MCL has its origin over a broad region of the medial femoral epiphysis, extending to the physis, inserting on the metaphyseal proximal tibia just distal to the physis. The deep MCL extends from epiphy- seal distal femur to epiphyseal proximal tibia (Fig. 28H2–2). The distal femoral physis remains extracapsular and extrasynovial throughout. The capsule of the knee joint extends superior to the physis anteriorly as a result of the suprapatellar pouch; however, it doubles back on itself to attach to the epiphyseal anterior femur (Fig. 28H2–3). Posteriorly, the knee capsule also originates from the epiphyseal femur. The physis of the proximal tibia is also extracapsular and extrasynovial throughout.[5]

All of the ligaments and cartilage structures of the knee develop from a mesenchymal cell mass that begins to differentiate around week 8 of embryonic development. The menisci develop from this same tissue, which organizes into semilunar rings. A discus shape is not thought to be an embryonic precursor to all menisci but may appear later as a result of changes resulting from hypermobility of what was previously a normally developing meniscus.[20, 40]

History and Physical Examination

Obtaining a thorough history of the patient's knee complaint(s), including identification of any precipitating event, a mechanism of injury and whether it was relatively low or high energy, is essential. The presence of any subsequent swelling and/or recurrent locking, popping, or giving way may point toward intra-articular disease. Determining the duration and intensity of symptoms, whether there are activities that typically cause a flare, and if there are any other accompanying symptoms such as swelling, limp, or generalized malaise will help narrow the differential diagnosis.

The physical examination of the child's knee with symptoms suggestive of a medial injury should begin with careful observation of gait. Asymmetry in foot progression angles, the presence of an antalgic versus Trendelenburg gait, and the presence of any lateral thrust can all help narrow the diagnosis, and may in fact point toward the hip as the culprit (Fig. 28H2–4). Examination of the normal knee to establish a standard for comparison should precede that of the injured knee. This helps reassure the child that the examiner is careful and competent before what may

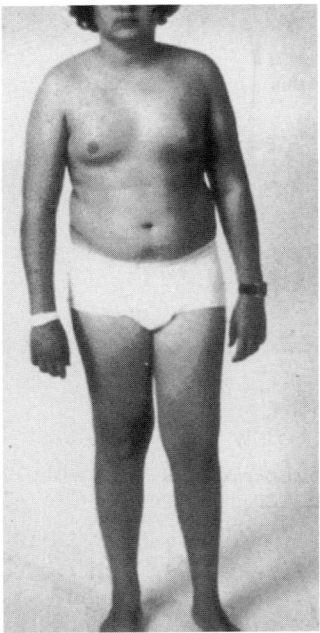

Figure 28H2–4. Subtle findings during the observation of gait may help localize the pathologic process. Note the slight asymmetry in foot progression in this adolescent presenting with knee and thigh pain. Slipped capital femoral epiphysis can mimic knee pain and commonly presents with an antalgic gait and an outward foot progression angle.

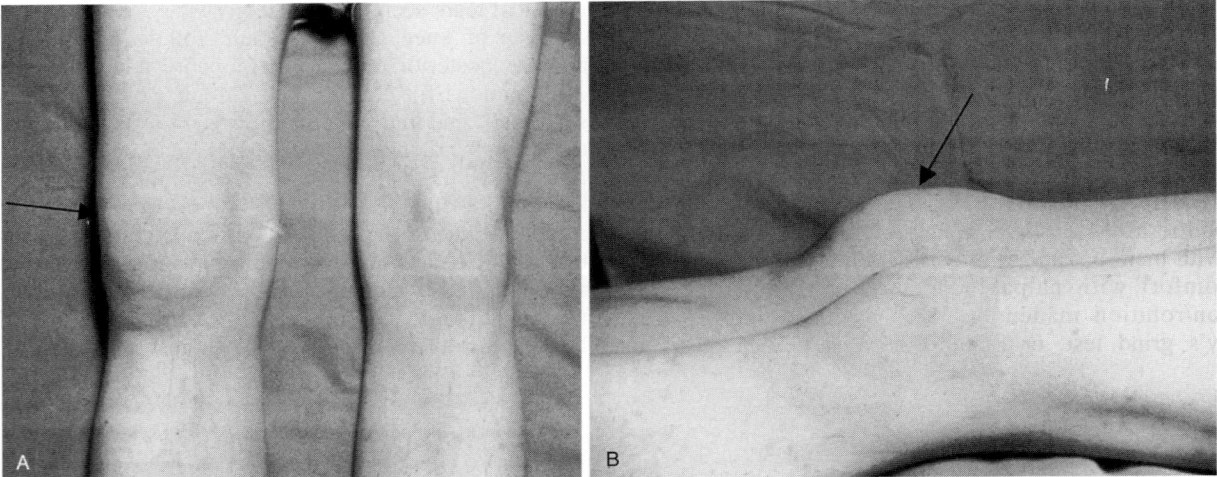

Figure 28H2–5. *A* and *B,* A knee effusion (*arrows*) is highly suggestive of a significant intra-articular injury.

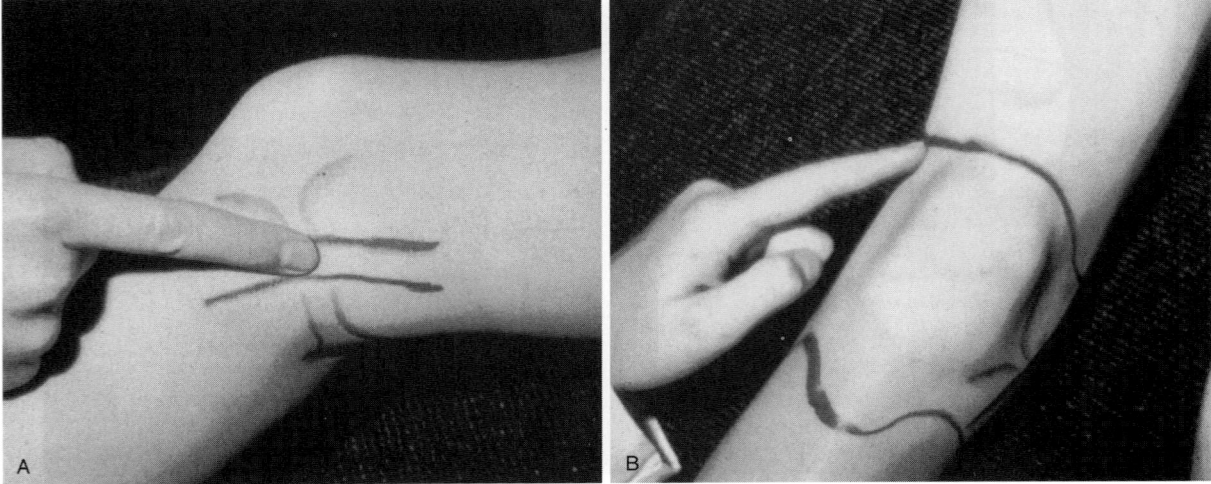

Figure 28H2–6. *A,* Particular attention should be paid to anatomic landmarks during the physical examination. This allows for specific examination, such as of joint-line tenderness. *B,* Note that the distal femoral physis is at the same level as the proximal pole of the patella.

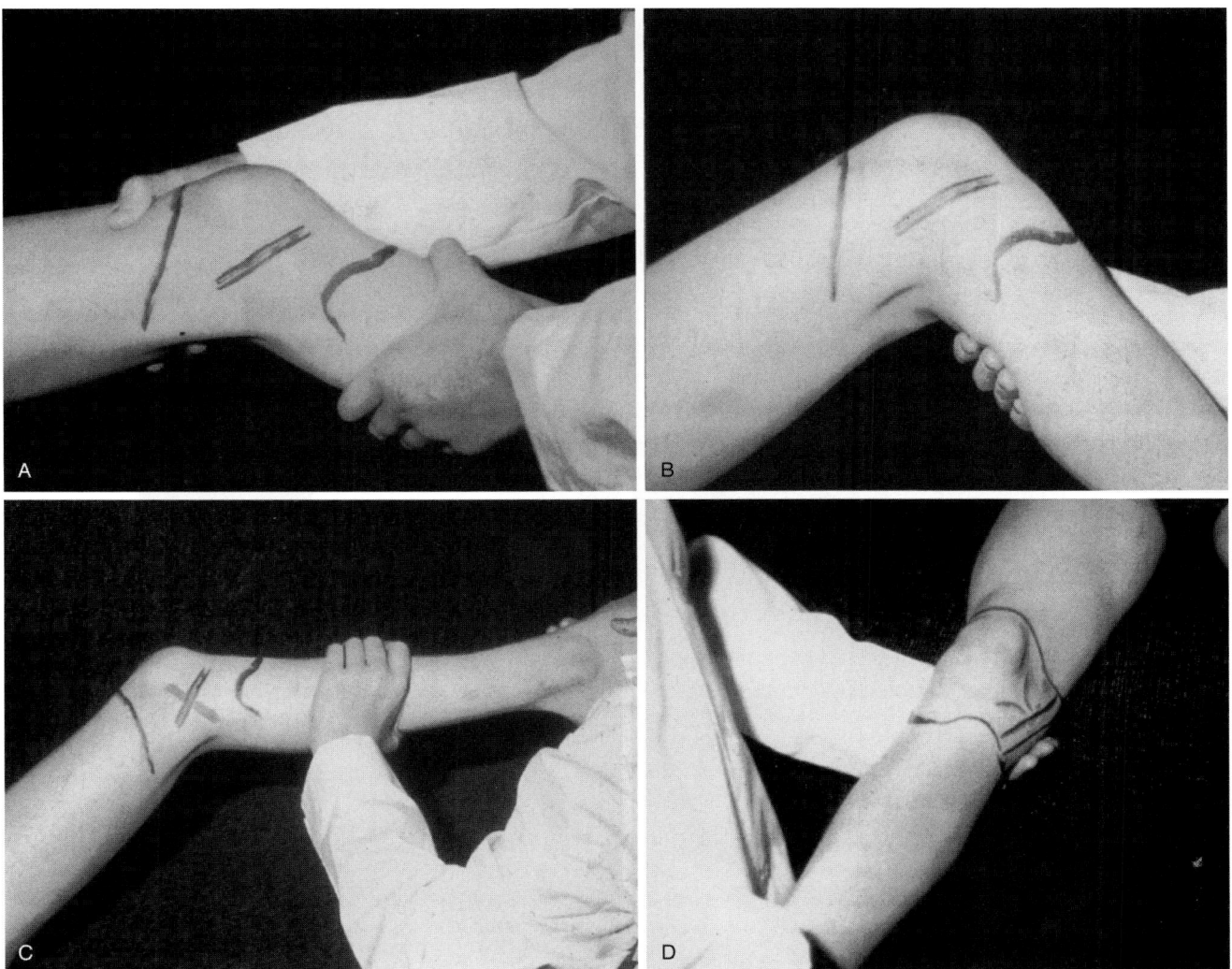

Figure 28H2–7. Examinations to assess ligamentous stability. *A,* Lachman's test. *B,* Anterior drawer test. *C,* Posterior sag test. *D,* Valgus stress test.

injury but a potential injury to the ACL and posteromedial corner (posterior capsule, posterior oblique ligament or posterior fibers of the superficial MCL, and semimembranosus complex) as well.[27] In a knee with a tense effusion, aspiration of the joint using sterile technique with infusion of local anesthetic may help make the examination more tolerable. The presence of fat in the aspirate would be consistent with an intra-articular fracture. Stress radiography would then be helpful to determine whether medial opening with a valgus stress is due to ligamentous deficiency or fracture, or both (Fig. 28H2–8). Such an examination might best be carried out under a general anesthetic with the benefit of intraoperative fluoroscopy.[31]

Examination of the hip for any asymmetry or abnormalities in the range of motion should be included. Loss of abduction with discomfort at the end point might suggest Legg-Calvé-Perthes disease, whereas excessive external rotation with a loss of internal rotation would be consistent with a slipped capital femoral epiphysis. Both these conditions might present as medial knee pain with limp (Fig. 28H2–9).

Further work-up of the child with medial knee pain should include at least anteroposterior and lateral radiographs of the knee in question, to help rule out fracture (Fig. 28H2–10). Hip radiographs should also be obtained if hip disease is suspected after the physical examination. Comparison views with the unaffected knee may help identify pathologic joint space narrowing or widening when a discoid meniscus is suspected. The use of additional studies such as magnetic resonance imaging (MRI) to help make or confirm a diagnosis has received mixed review in the literature. Stanitski has demonstrated that the clinical acumen of the treating orthopaedist is the most sensitive and specific method of coming to a diagnosis.[68] MRI has better than 90% sensitivity and specificity for the detection of cruciate deficiencies, and better than 80% for meniscal tears when these injuries are suspected by an orthopaedist.[19, 53] These numbers drop markedly when the population studied includes the asymptomatic patient or the patient referred for MRI by the nonorthopaedist.[9, 45, 72] The ability of MRI to detect chondral lesions of the patella, distal femur, or proximal tibia is only around 50%.[67]

nearly 1000 patients seen with knee injuries at a trauma center during an 8-year period, Clanton reported pure ligamentous injuries in only 9. Six of the nine had avulsion fractures, four of which involved the intercondylar eminence, and two, the collateral ligaments. The remaining three patients had midsubstance ligamentous disruptions.[14]

Hughston describes a population of patients who, while playing high school or college sports, received a blow to the outside of the knee and sustained significant injury to the soft tissues of the medial knee. In many of these patients, not only were the superficial and deep MCL disrupted but also the ACL and posteromedial structures (insertion of the semimembranosus and posteromedial capsule) as well.[26] The extent of injury is dictated by the energy of the impact, which can often be deduced from a careful history. Examination directed toward determining the extent of valgus instability should include tests of medial opening with a valgus stress in 30 degrees of knee flexion (abduction stress test), and in full extension. An awake examination should be attempted, focusing on the normal knee to establish a baseline for comparison. Care in testing of the affected side to limit the effects of spasm may be unsuccessful, though any single event of wide opening on repeat examinations suggests a severe injury.[26]

Patients with marked medial opening (greater than 1 cm at the joint surface) with valgus stress and discomfort while in 30 degrees of knee flexion have a grade III injury or complete disruption of the superficial and deep MCL. Inasmuch as the ACL and structures present in the posteromedial corner also contribute to stability of the knee in 30 degrees of flexion, grade III instability would call the competency of these structures into question.[26, 65] The presence of a concomitant ACL disruption may be confirmed by increased excursion on Lachman's test, or a positive pivot shift test.[26] Discomfort and maximal opening of only 5 to 10 mm along the joint surface during this examination suggests an incomplete, or grade II, injury to the MCL. An abnormal abduction stress test in full extension suggests a PCL injury.[26] Again, in the skeletally immature patient, physeal fracture should be suspected and is not uncommonly associated with severe ligamentous injuries to the medial knee.

Diagnostic Testing and Treatment Alternatives

MRI may be employed to better delineate the extent of any medial injury, though physical examination may be the most sensitive in determining the extent of knee injury.[68] Again, biplanar radiography should be employed to ensure that no fractures exist, inasmuch as concomitant physeal distal femur fracture and medial ligamentous injury are not uncommon.[7, 14, 71] Numerous studies support the nonoperative treatment of the isolated MCL injury,[18, 30, 34, 38, 71] though in the case of severe medial injury with instability to valgus stress in full extension, repair of the medial and posteromedial structures as well as any ACL deficiency has been advocated.[26] Some have argued that an isolated grade III MCL disruption in the skeletally immature deserves a reconstruction, because persistent laxity is often

the result of conservative treatment, though this view is certainly in the minority.[36–39]

Meniscal Injuries or Abnormalities on the Medial Side of the Knee

Meniscal Tear

Mechanisms of Injury and Physical Examination

Though relatively uncommon in comparison to the frequency of this injury in adults, numerous studies and case reports describe meniscal tears in the skeletally immature. Unlike adults, however, the frequency of medial meniscal tears is similar to that of lateral tears.[1, 51, 60, 64, 74, 78, 79] The mechanisms of injury for medial meniscal tears may include longitudinal loading of a flexed knee that is undergoing simultaneous torsional stress. It is not uncommon, however, for there to be no recollection of an inciting traumatic event for children, especially if they are younger than 13 years of age.[52] Meniscal injury is often followed by development of an acute effusion. Mechanical symptoms, such as locking, popping, catching, or giving way are often noted in the history of a meniscal injury. A loss of motion is the hallmark of a knee with a meniscal tear; it may be noted in the history as well as the physical examination. The most common complaint in this group is of pain.[64, 74, 79]

On examination, an effusion may be palpable. Examination of both knees while the heels are held at the same level up off of the examination table may reveal a loss of extension. Marked anterior discomfort with this test may suggest an incarcerated meniscus. Likewise, a loss of full flexion would be suspicious for meniscal injury, especially if the extreme of flexion is accompanied by discomfort. Joint-line tenderness is typically seen with meniscal injury.[56, 74, 79] Pain with varus stress may signify a medial meniscal tear, whereas marked opening with valgus stress may not only be suspicious of an MCL injury, but a medial meniscal tear as well. Rotational maneuvers while flexing or extending the knee, with the examiner's fingers along the joint line, may reproduce popping or painful catching in the knee with a medial meniscal injury. These tests may be performed sitting (Steinman's test), supine (McMurray's test) or prone (Apley's grind test). Younger patients with meniscal tears, however, may not respond to these provocative tests.[56]

Imaging Studies and Treatment Options

There are a variety of imaging techniques that may be useful in working up the patient suspected of having a medial meniscal tear. An unusual widening along the medial joint line in a weight-bearing anteroposterior radiograph of the knee may suggest a medial meniscal tear. Arthrograms have been employed to detect meniscal tears, though this test may not be as sensitive as MRI. MRI has been shown to have sensitivities of between 79% and 100%, specificities of 46% to 92%, and accuracy of between 38% and 91% for the detection of medial meniscal tears.[4, 19, 29, 33, 41, 48, 57, 68] Again, MRI performed without good clinical suspicion of a medial meniscal injury is less specific than that performed in the setting of medial knee injury consistent with a medial meniscal tear.[9, 68] This is especially important when treating the skeletally immature, inasmuch as a higher incidence of grade 3 signal changes have been noted in asymptomatic children (60% of patients younger than 13 years of age, 30% older than 14 years of age) than has been reported in asymptomatic adults (25%).[45, 46, 72] Diagnostic arthroscopy is an excellent technique for the detection of meniscal tears and is currently the gold standard against which all other techniques are compared (Fig. 28H2–11).

Treatment options for the skeletally immature with meniscal injury are evolving slowly. Many early papers on discoid meniscus and meniscal tears in children advocated total meniscectomy as a simple, effective treatment with few sequelae.[2, 24, 28, 60, 77] Aichroth noted a pseudomeniscus or small peripheral rim on three of four second-look arthroscopies after total lateral meniscectomy for a discoid meniscus, suggesting some degree of regenerative potential for children undergoing a meniscectomy.[2] However, many long-term follow-up studies have cautioned against total meniscectomy in children.[1, 8, 49, 74, 79, 80] Adults who underwent meniscectomy as children often experience an increased incidence of mechanical symptoms in the knee as well as knee instability.[1, 74, 79] Radiographs of such patients often show the Fairbanks changes associated with osteoarthritis: flattening and widening of the femoral condyle as well as narrowing of the joint line.[17] As a result, current recommendations for the treatment of meniscal tears in children are to preserve whatever meniscus is salvageable through repair, performing limited partial meniscectomies when absolutely necessary. Mintzer has shown excellent outcomes 5 years after repair of meniscal tears in patients younger than 17 years of age, suggesting that higher rates of healing can be obtained in children than in adults.[51] In the setting of an ACL deficiency undergoing reconstruction, meniscal tears in children deserve an attempt at repair, when feasible.[6, 75] Certainly all red-on-red and red-on-white tears in isolation deserve an attempt at repair in children. Repair techniques are similar to those employed in adults, including inside-out and outside-in arthroscopic methods, as well as the use of limited open techniques[6, 12] (Fig. 28H2–12). The results of meniscal repairs in children have been good, with the best results seen in the setting of an ACL reconstruction.[51, 62] Arthroscopic partial meniscectomy, when repair is not an option, has the advantages of quicker rehabilitation, shorter hospital stay, fewer complications, and better subjective functional results when compared with total meniscectomy[25, 50] (Fig. 28H2–13).

A laboratory study in dogs showed that leaving a torn meniscus untreated has fewer sequelae for the affected knee than does a total meniscectomy. Weiss and Dehaven outline a number of criteria for leaving meniscal tears without partial excision or repair: Vertical longitudinal tears and partial-thickness split tears may all be observed if stable with probing. It is unclear whether radial tears 5 mm in length or less would do better with observation or débridement.

Discoid Meniscus

Physical Examination

Discoid menisci are much more common laterally than medially,[16, 32, 54, 66] though there are numerous case reports of discoid medial menisci.[3, 13, 15, 54, 58, 70] The incidence of discoid medial menisci is estimated to be less than 0.3%.[15] A "snapping knee" syndrome is often seen in children with discoid menisci,[5] though many patients have pain or loss of motion as their presenting complaint.[3, 24, 54, 55, 70] The origins of discoid menisci are discussed in greater detail in Chapter 28I2. In short, it is thought that the thickened

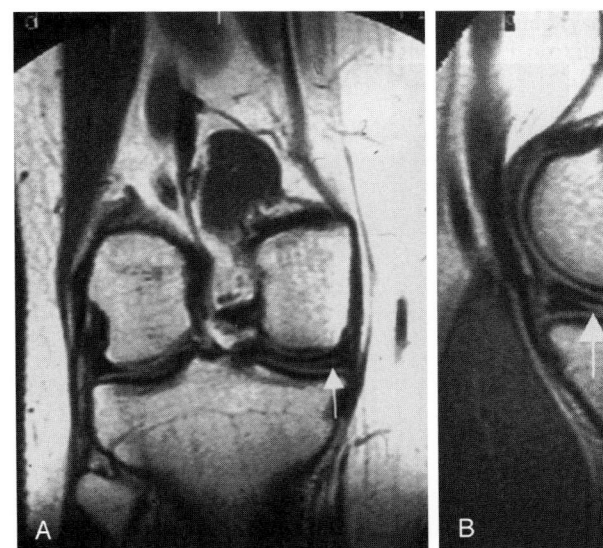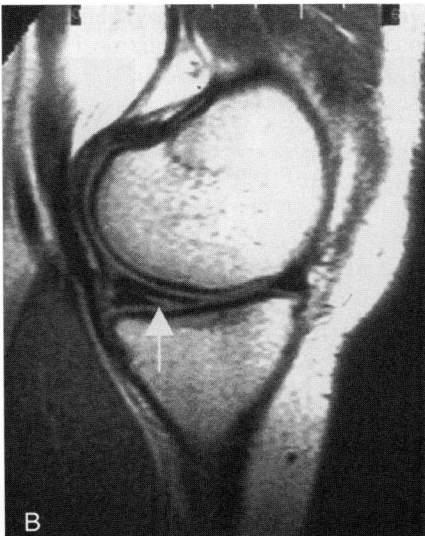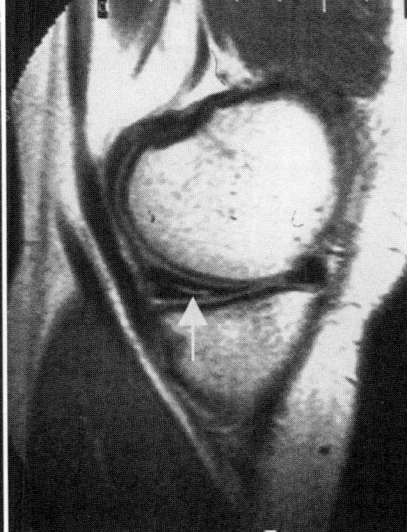

Figure 28H2–11. *A* and *B,* Magnetic resonance imaging can be quite helpful when used appropriately. This 14-year-old was found to have a medial meniscal tear (*arrow*) at the time of surgery, consistent with the findings on magnetic resonance imaging.

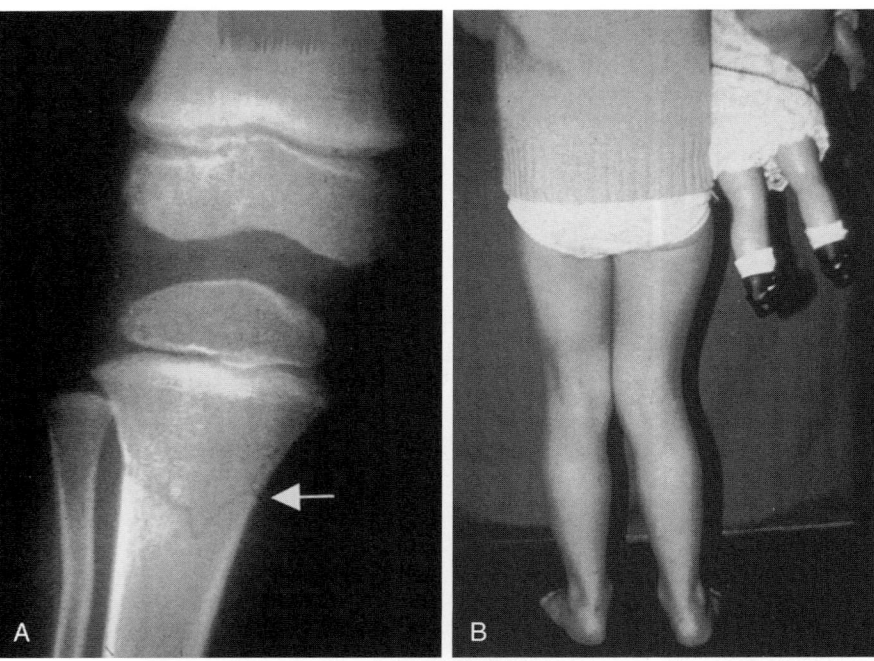

Figure 28H2–20. *A,* Proximal tibial metaphyseal fractures (*arrow*) are commonly associated with valgus deformity subsequent to fracture healing. *B,* Clinically, these deformities are quite apparent. The best treatment is observation with expectant gradual correction over several years.

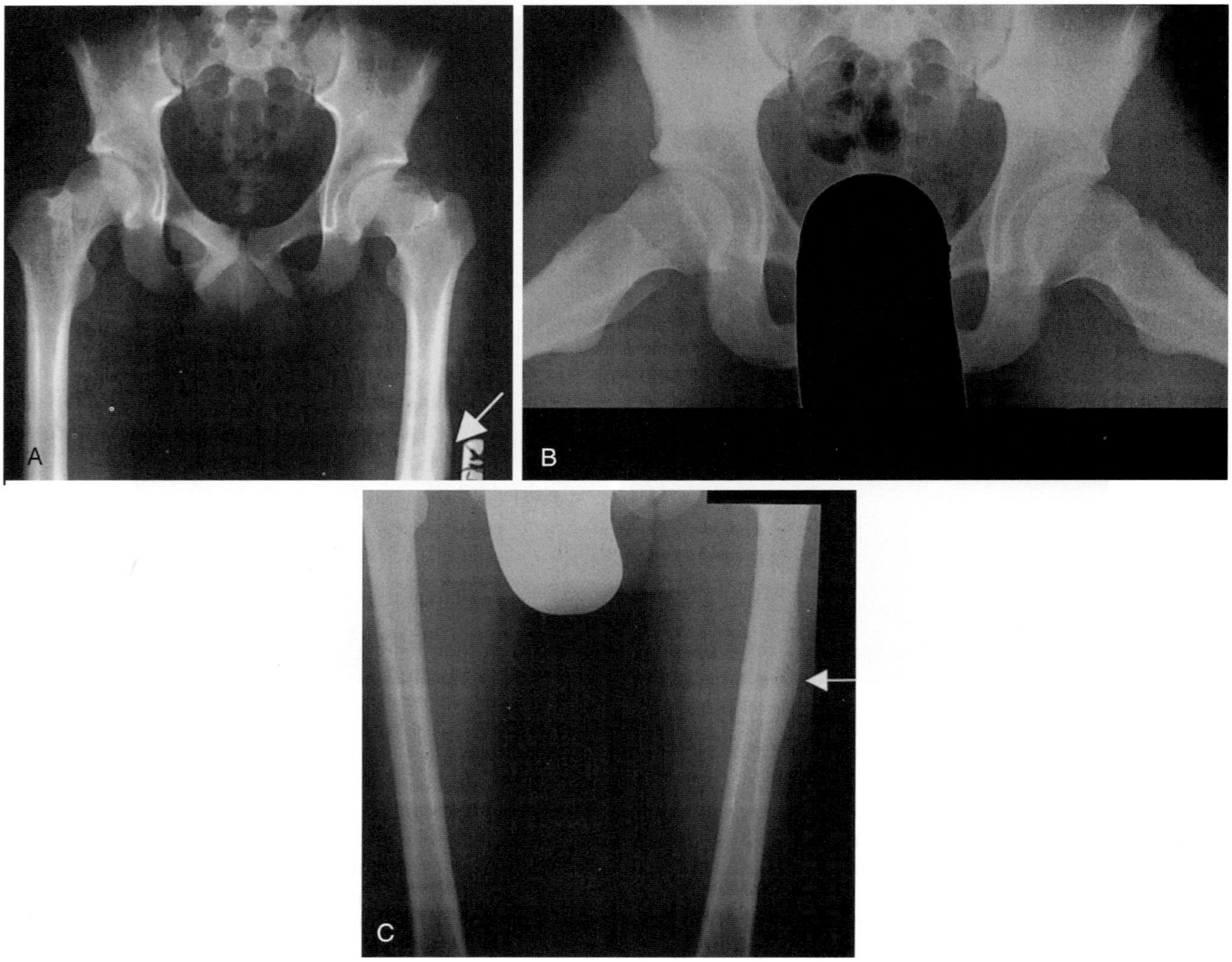

Figure 28H2–21. *A* to *C,* Hip and thigh pain may be referred to the knee. Note the reactive bone (*arrows*) in the diaphyseal region of the femur in this child, who presented with thigh and knee pain.

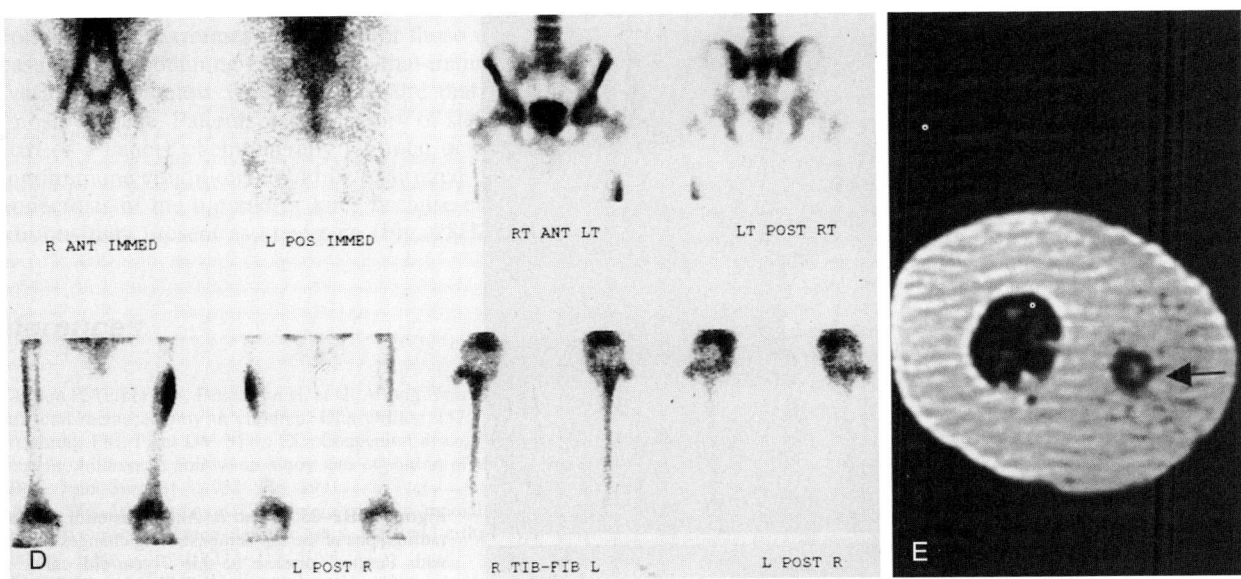

R ANT IMMED   L POS IMMED   RT ANT LT   LT POST RT

D   L POST R   R TIB-FIB L   L POST R   E

Figure 28H2–21 *Continued. D,* Bone scan demonstrates markedly increased uptake in the same region but no other areas of increased uptake. *E,* Computed tomographic scan demonstrates a focal nidus, consistent with the eventual diagnosis of osteoid osteoma.

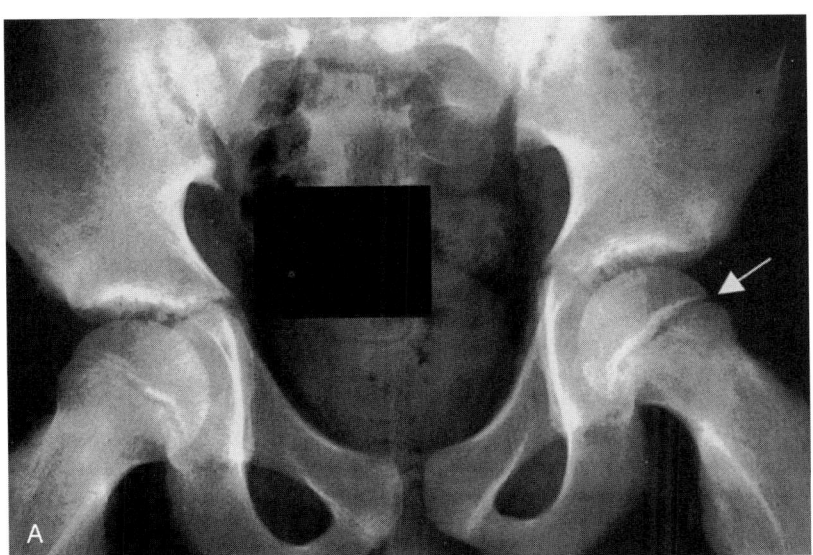

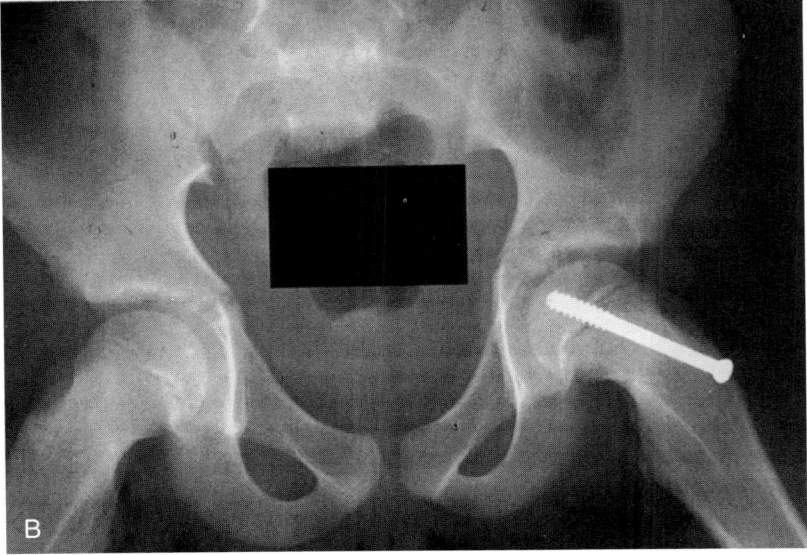

Figure 28H2–22. The hip joint should be scrutinized carefully in any skeletally immature child presenting with knee pain or injury. *A,* Anteroposterior radiograph of a 12-year-old athlete with thigh and knee pain. Note the changes seen in the proximal femoral physis. This is a mild slipped capital femoral epiphysis. *B,* This should be treated surgically with in situ pinning.

tears in athletes: A comparison of clinical and magnetic resonance imaging investigations. Am J Sports Med 25:7–12, 1997.

54. Nathan PA, Cole SC: Discoid meniscus. A clinical and pathologic study. Clin Orthop 64:107–113, 1969.
55. Pellacci F, Montanari G, Prosperi P, et al: Lateral discoid meniscus: Treatment and results. Arthroscopy 8:526–530, 1992.
56. Rang M: Children's Fractures. Philadelphia, JB Lippincott, 1974.
57. Raunest J, Oberle K, Loehnert J, et al: The clinical value of magnetic resonance imaging in the evaluation of meniscal disorders. J Bone Joint Surg Am 73:11–16, 1991.
58. Richmond DA: Two cases of discoid medial cartilage. J Bone Joint Surg Br 40:268, 1958.
59. Riseborough EJ, Barrett IR, Shapiro F: Growth disturbances following distal femoral physeal fracture-separations. J Bone Joint Surg Am 65:885–893, 1983.
60. Ritchie DM: Meniscectomy in children. Aust N Z J Surg 35:239–241, 1966.
61. Robert M, Khouri N, Carlioz H, et al: Fractures of the proximal tibial metaphysis in children: Review of a series of 25 cases. J Pediatr Orthop 7:444–449, 1987.
62. Rubman MH, Noyes FR, and Barber-Westin SD: Arthroscopic repair of meniscal tears that extend into the avascular zone. Am J Sports Med 26:87–95, 1998.
63. Salter RB, Harris WR: Injuries involving the epiphyseal plate. J Bone Joint Surg Am 45:587–622, 1963.
64. Schlonsky J, Eyring EJ: Lateral meniscus tears in young children. Clin Orthop 97:117–118, 1973.
65. Shelbourne KD, Davis TJ, Patel DV: The natural history of acute, isolated, nonoperatively treated posterior cruciate ligament injuries. A prospective study. Am J Sports Med 27:276–283, 1999.
66. Smillie IS: The congenital discoid meniscus. J Bone Joint Surg Br 30:671, 1948.
67. Speer KP, Spritzer CE, Goldner JL, et al: Magnetic resonance imaging of traumatic knee articular cartilage injuries. Am J Sports Med 19:396–402, 1991.
68. Stanitski CL: Correlation of arthroscopic and clinical examinations with magnetic resonance imaging findings of injured knees in children and adolescents. Am J Sports Med 26:743–744, 1998.
69. Stanitski C, Harvell JC, Fu F: Observations on acute knee hemarthrosis in children and adolescents. J Pediatr Orthop 13:506–510, 1993.
70. Stern A, Hallel T: Medial discoid meniscus with cyst formation in a child. J Pediatr Orthop 8:471–473, 1988.
71. Sullivan JA: Ligamentous injuries of the knee in children. Clin Orthop 255:44–50, 1990.
72. Takeda Y, Ikata T, Yoshida S, et al: MRI high-signal intensity in the menisci of asymptomatic children. J Bone Joint Surg Br 80:463–466, 1998.
73. Torg JS, Conrad W, Kalen V: Clinical diagnosis of anterior cruciate ligament instability in the athlete. Am J Sports Med 4:84–93, 1976.
74. Vahvanen V, Aalto K: Meniscectomy in children. Acta Orthop Scand 50:791–795, 1979.
75. Warren RF: Meniscectomy and repair in the anterior cruciate ligament-deficient patient. Clin Orthop 252:55–63, 1990.
76. Warren LF, Marshall JL: The supporting structures and layers on the medial side of the knee. J Bone Joint Surg Am 61:56–62, 1979.
77. Washington ER, Root L, Liener UC: Discoid lateral meniscus in children. J Bone Joint Surg Am 77:1357–1360, 1995.
78. Williams JS, Abate JA, Fadale PD, et al: Meniscal and nonosseous ACL injuries in children and adolescents. Am J Knee Surg 9:22–26, 1996.
79. Wroble RR, Henderson RC, Campion ER, et al: Meniscectomy in children and adolescents. Clin Orthop 279:180–189, 1992.
80. Zaman M, Leonard MA: Meniscectomy in children: A study of fifty-nine knees. In Proceedings of the British Orthopaedic Association. J Bone Joint Surg Br 60:436–437, 1978.
81. Zionts LE, MacEwen GD: Spontaneous improvement of post-traumatic tibia valga. J Bone Joint Surg Am 68:680–687, 1986.

Section I
Lateral and Posterior Instabilities of the Knee

1. LATERAL AND POSTEROLATERAL INSTABILITY OF THE KNEE IN ADULTS

Roger V. Larson, MD ■ Edwin Tingstad, MD

The incidence of injuries to the lateral and posterolateral structures of the knee is not known with any degree of accuracy because injuries to these structures, particularly posterolateral structures, often go undetected.[2, 6, 7, 15, 27, 28] Injuries involving the lateral structures are considered rare and have received relatively little attention in the literature concerning knee ligament injuries.[3, 13, 15, 24, 88] Instability of the posterolateral corner (PLC) is becoming a commonly recognized cause of residual symptoms, however, after anterior cruciate ligament (ACL) or posterior cruciate ligament (PCL) reconstruction.[69, 79] It is accepted that isolated ruptures of the PCL generally do not cause functional instability and are managed best by nonoperative treatment.[1] When functional instability is present in a patient with an injured PCL, the situation is usually not an isolated PCL injury but a combined ligamentous injury frequently involving the PLC.[42] Posterolateral instability of the knee in combination with PCL insufficiency is frequently the cause of functional instability, and the management of this instability requires addressing not only the PCL injury, but also the associated PLC injury.[1, 13, 42, 58] Injury to the lateral and posterolateral structures is seen commonly with injur-ies to the ACL. A poor functional result after ACL reconstruction is frequently the result of unrecognized or untreated lateral or posterolateral instability.[79]

Generally, it is accepted that the results of PCL reconstruction are not as good as the results of ACL reconstruction. Several reasons have been postulated as to why PCL reconstruction techniques do not restore normal laxity or motion patterns to the postoperative knee, including recognized anisometry of a normal PCL and the inability to reconstruct the PCL with a single graft; fairly high constant daily forces on a normal PCL; the use of inadequate grafts; and, perhaps most importantly, the failure to recognize and address associated injuries that may coexist, including injury to the posterolateral structures of the knee.[58] Because isolated PCL ruptures generally do not cause functional instability and can be managed nonoperatively, the presence of functional instability usually is due to associated laxity often of the PLC.

When PCL laxity coexists with posterolateral instability, normal laxity and motion patterns cannot be restored by PCL reconstruction alone.[22] Because this is often the situation in a PCL-injured knee that requires surgery, it frequently is necessary to address laxity of the lateral and posterolateral structures simultaneously. When posterolateral laxity is present associated with PCL insufficiency, normal motion patterns cannot be restored by PCL reconstruction alone, but these patterns can be restored by combined PCL and PLC reconstruction. The strain on an intra-articular PCL graft can be reduced and the environment for survival enhanced if an appropriate extra-articular backup procedure to address the lateral and posterolateral deficiencies is added to the intra-articular PCL reconstruction.[19, 22, 81]

Anatomy of Lateral Collateral Ligament and Posterolateral Corner

The anatomy of the lateral collateral ligament (LCL) and particularly the PLC of the knee is complex and variable.[35, 38, 72, 74, 82] The overall functional and clinical significance of the various structures in this region are not understood completely. Baker and colleagues[6] defined the arcuate ligament complex as the ligamentous complex consisting of the LCL, arcuate ligament, popliteus muscle and tendon, and lateral head of the gastrocnemius. These constituents form a sling that functions statically and dynamically to control external tibial rotation relative to the femur. The popliteofibular ligament (PFL) is important as a static restraint to external tibial rotation.[56, 74] The biceps

femoris tendon and iliotibial band (ITB) contribute to the stability of the lateral and posterolateral aspects of the knee.

Seebacher and colleagues[72] divided the PLC into three layers (Fig. 28I1–1). The first layer consists of the ITB and biceps femoris tendon. The second layer consists of the quadriceps retinaculum and lateral patellofemoral ligament. The third layer is believed to be the most important and contains the LCL, fabellofibular ligament, PFL, popliteus muscle and tendon, and arcuate ligament complex (Fig. 28I1–2). Significant anatomic variability exists in the structures of the third layer. The arcuate and fabellofibular ligaments are present in approximately 67% of patients. The fabellofibular ligament is present alone in 20% of cases and usually is identified by radiographic evidence of a large fabella. The arcuate ligament is present alone in the remaining 13% of the population as suggested by the absence of the fabella or its cartilaginous remnant. Each of these important anatomic structures is discussed separately.[9, 18, 19, 72]

Iliotibial Band

The ITB runs between the supracondylar tubercle of the femur and Gerdy's tubercle on the proximal tibia.[7, 18, 19, 72] The ITB is an important stabilizer of the lateral compartment. The most important portion of this structure acts as an accessory anterolateral ligament.[39] With flexion of the knee, the ITB becomes tight and moves posteriorly, ex-

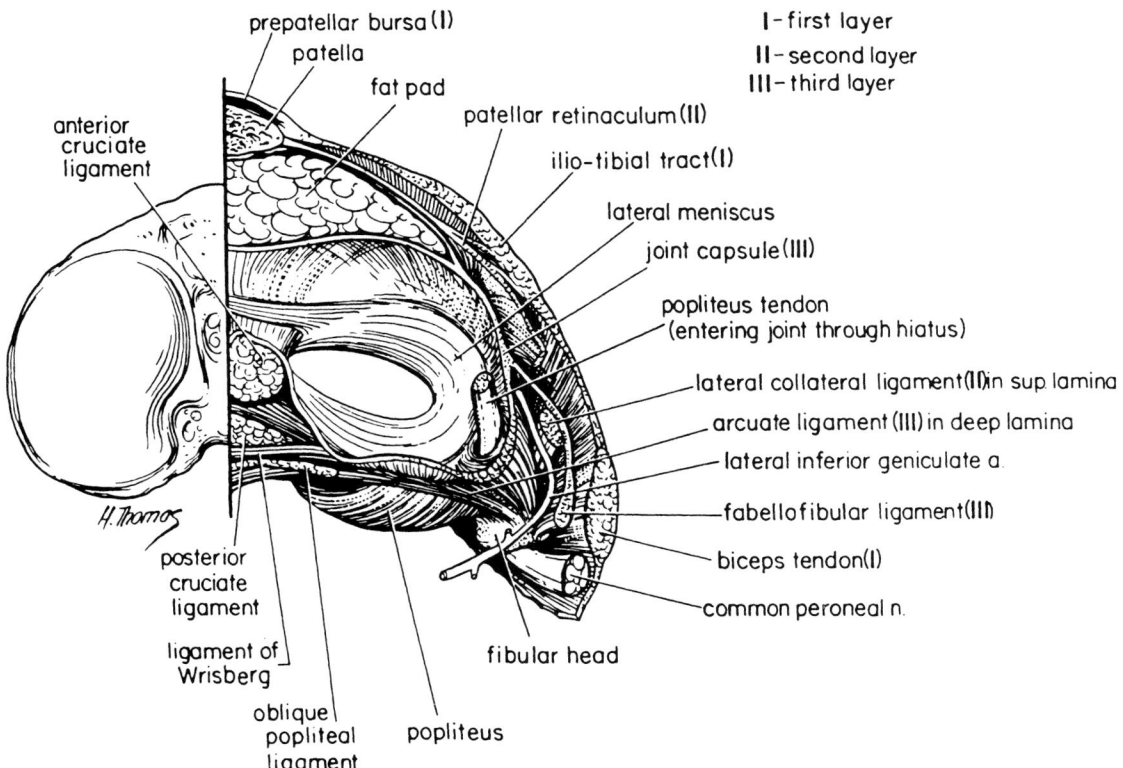

Figure 28I1–1. Coronal section of the knee illustrates the three-layer concept of the anatomy of the posterolateral structures as described by Seebacher and colleagues. (Adapted from Seebacher JR, Inglis AE, Marshall JL, Warren RF: The structure of the posterolateral aspect of the knee. J Bone Joint Surg Am 64:536–541, 1982.)

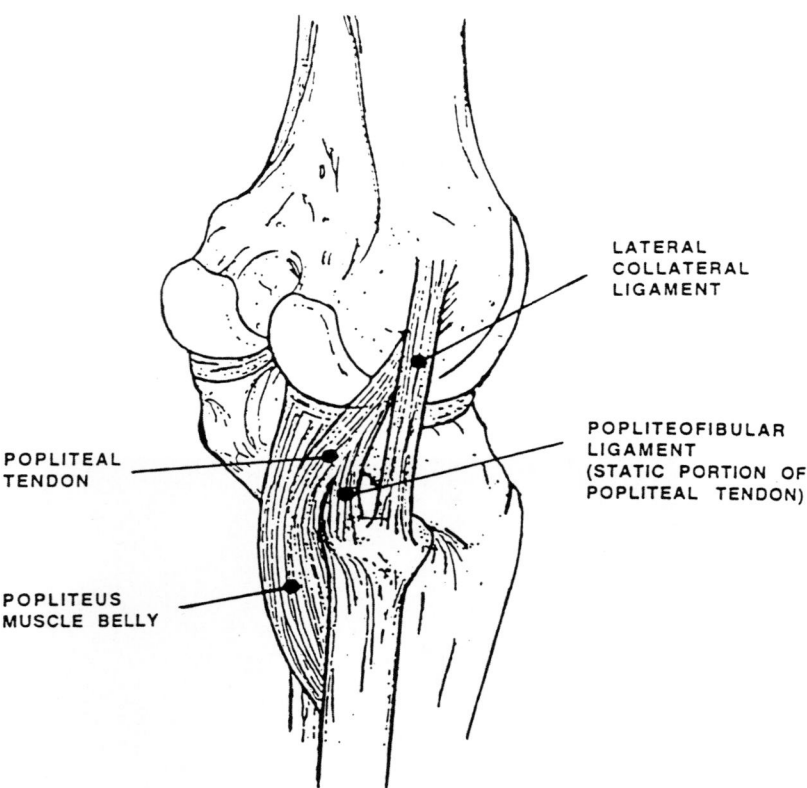

Figure 28I1–5. The relationship between the lateral collateral ligament, the popliteal tendon, and the popliteofibular ligament.

to be present in more than 90% of knees.[56, 74] Because of its dynamic and static restraints, the PFL is a vital component of any reconstruction procedure of the PLC.[9, 86, 87, 89, 90, 92]

Arcuate Ligament

The arcuate ligament is quite variable. This ligament spans the junction from the fibular styloid process to the lateral femoral condyle. The arcuate ligament reinforces the posterolateral capsule and covers the popliteus. The arcuate ligament possesses a medial and a lateral limb, and this Y-shaped ligament is composed of the lateral portion of the popliteus tendon and the fascial condensation over the posterior surface of the popliteus muscle. The fabellofibular or short collateral ligament may be present in conjunction with the arcuate ligament, adding to the variability of this structure and its contribution to posterolateral stability (Fig. 28I1–6).[32, 38, 72, 84]

Biceps Femoris

The biceps femoris muscle tendon complex is described by Terry and LaPrade[84, 85] and consists of a long and a short head with numerous arms. The tendon of the biceps femoris courses primarily posterior to the ITB, inserting primarily into the fibular head. This complex also sends strong attachments to the ITB, Gerdy's tubercle, the LCL, and the posterolateral capsule. In conjunction with the ITB,

the biceps femoris acts as a powerful dynamic external rotator of the tibia and contributes as a lateral stabilizer of the knee (Fig. 28I1–7). Injuries to the biceps femoris complex occur frequently in combination with injuries to the PLC.[15, 34] Substance stretch injuries or avulsion from attachment sites is encountered.[34]

Additional Structures

The middle third of the capsular ligament blends with the capsule over the LCL and inserts slightly posterior to Gerdy's tubercle. This structure is mostly a secondary restraint to varus stress. The lateral head of the gastrocnemius provides varying degrees of dynamic posterolateral stability and blends with the arcuate ligament. The lateral meniscus, which is stabilized by a portion of the popliteus tendon, contributes to lateral stability by creating a concave surface on the otherwise convex lateral tibial plateau; this contributes significantly to the stability of the lateral compartment (Fig. 28I1–8). The posterior capsule is attached proximally to the lateral femoral condyle and is covered by the lateral gastrocnemius and plantaris. The distal capsular attachment is complex. The popliteus muscle and aponeurosis blend into the tibial attachment lateral to the PCL, whereas the distal corner is stabilized to the fibula by the arcuate, popliteofibular, and fabellofibular ligaments.

Biomechanics of the Lateral and Posterolateral Structures

The structures of the lateral and posterolateral knee function primarily to resist varus rotations, posterior tibial

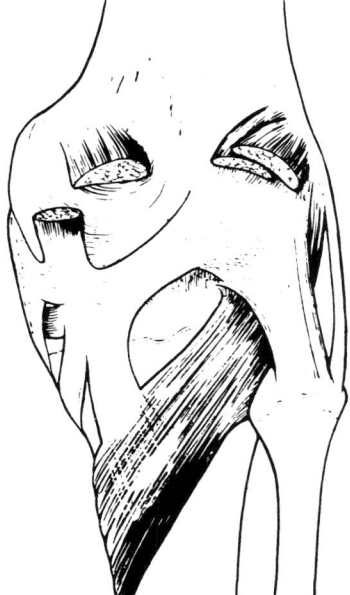
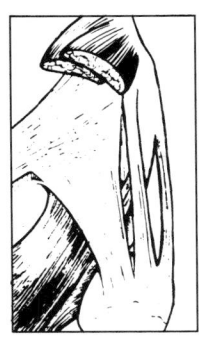
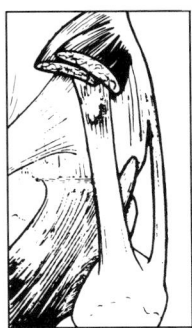

Figure 28I1–6. Variations of the arcuate complex. (From Jakob RP, Staubli HU [eds]: The Knee and the Cruciate Ligaments. Berlin, Springer-Verlag, 1992.)

translation, and posterolateral tibial rotation.* The lateral ligamentous structures of the knee differ from the medial structures in that the lateral structures are stronger and more substantial and are subjected to greater forces during the normal gait cycle. During the stance phase, the medial compartment is under compression in most knees, whereas

*See references 20, 25, 33, 36, 55, 64, 65, 67, 81, and 91.

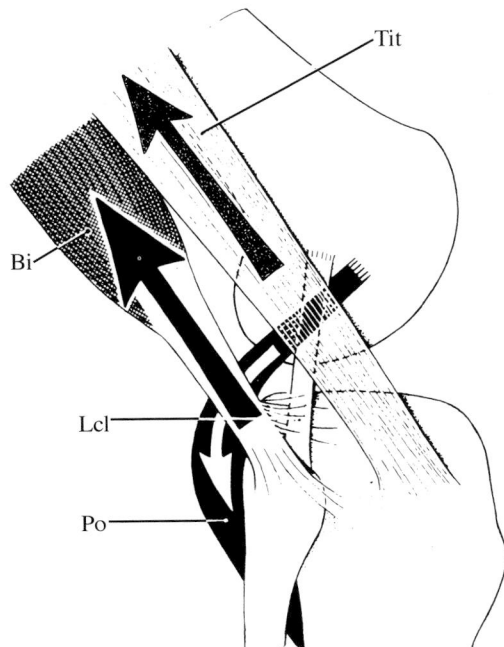

Figure 28I1–7. The dynamic stabilizing function of the iliotibial tract, the biceps femoris, and the popliteus muscles. (From Muller W: The Knee: Form, Function and Ligamentous Reconstruction. New York, Springer-Verlag, 1983.)

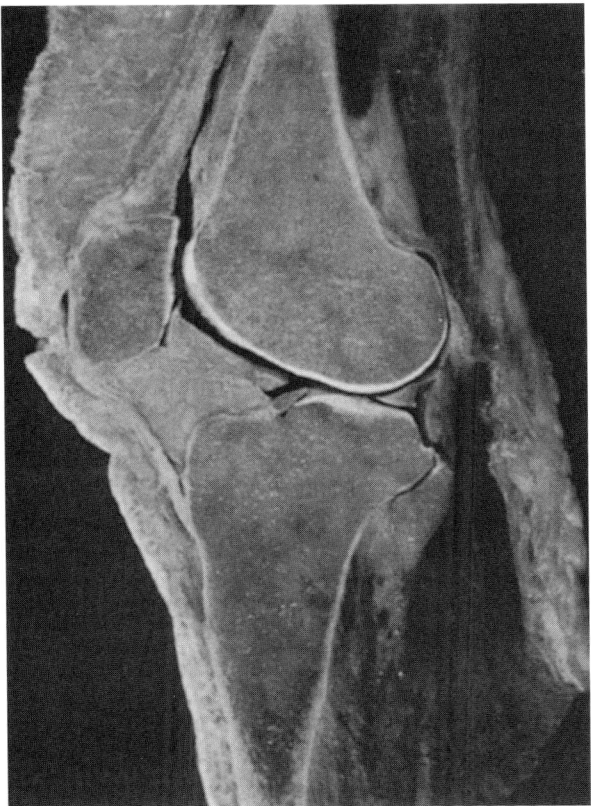

Figure 28I1–8. Sagittal section through the lateral compartment shows how the lateral meniscus adds to the stability of the compartment by its concave shape. (From Jakob RP, Hassler HI, Staubli HU: Observations of rotatory instability of the lateral compartment of the knee. Acta Orthop Scand 191:6–27, 1981.)

Clinical Evaluation of Lateral and Posterolateral Instability

Physical Examination

Patients who have injured the lateral and posterolateral structures of the knee joint often have injuries to other stabilizing structures of the joint, most often the ACL or PCL. A complete knee examination is essential to include all aspects of tibial femoral alignment and stability as well as patellofemoral stability. Evaluation of neurovascular structures is important because 12% to 29% of patients with acute PLC injuries have peroneal nerve injuries.[6, 88]

Posterolateral instability often has a component of varus laxity, particularly if the injury to the PLC was by a varus mechanism. Varus laxity is not essential to the diagnosis of posterolateral instability, however.[46] The most important physical finding with posterolateral instability is increased external tibial rotation present at 30 degrees and 90 degrees of knee flexion. This instability can be shown by the Dial test, in which the femur is stabilized, and the tibia, ankle, and foot are externally rotated and compared with the normal side at 30 degrees and 90 degrees of flexion (Fig. 28I1–11).[54] If more than 5 to 10 degrees of increased external tibial rotation can be shown, an injury to the PLC can be presumed.[58] This PLC injury can be present with or without significant injury to the PCL or ACL.[2] Usually the increase in external rotation is significantly greater than 5 degrees with PLC injuries and often is increased considerably when coupled with an injury to the PCL.

Other Specific Tests for Posterolateral Instability

Posterior Tibial Translation. Posterior tibial translation (Fig. 28I1–12) is assessed at 30 degrees and 90 degrees of knee flexion. The position of the anterior tibia relative to the femoral condyles is noted and compared with the opposite extremity. With PCL injuries, a loss of the normal anterior step-off is seen most notably with the knee flexed to 90 degrees.[20] Isolated posterolateral injury results in a detectable increase of posterior tibial translation at 30 degrees but not at 90 degrees. PCL injuries combined with PLC injuries result in increased posterior tibial translation at 30 degrees and 90 degrees with the translation being

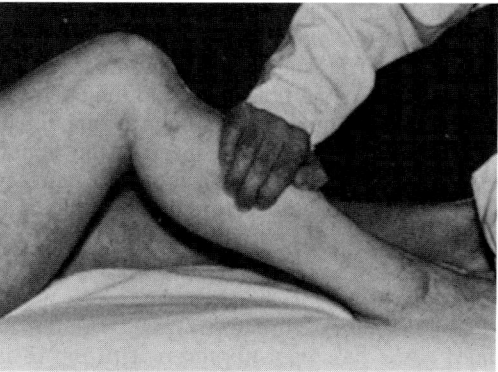
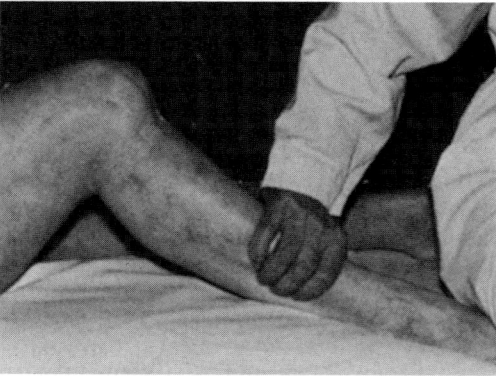
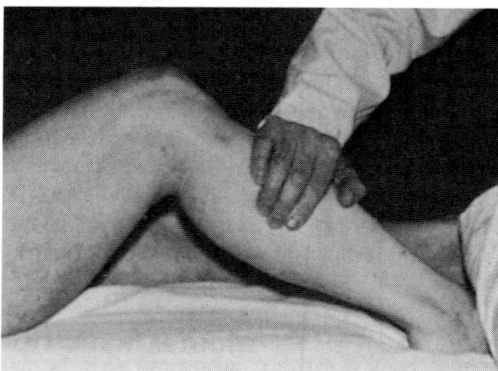

Figure 28I1–12. Posterior drawer sign in severe posterolateral rotatory instability in neutral rotation (*top*) is 2 +; in external rotation (*center*), 3 +; and internal rotation (*bottom*), 0. (From Jakob RP, Hassler H, Staubli HU: Observations on rotatory instability of the lateral compartment of the knee. Acta Orthop Scand 191[suppl]:1–32, 1981.)

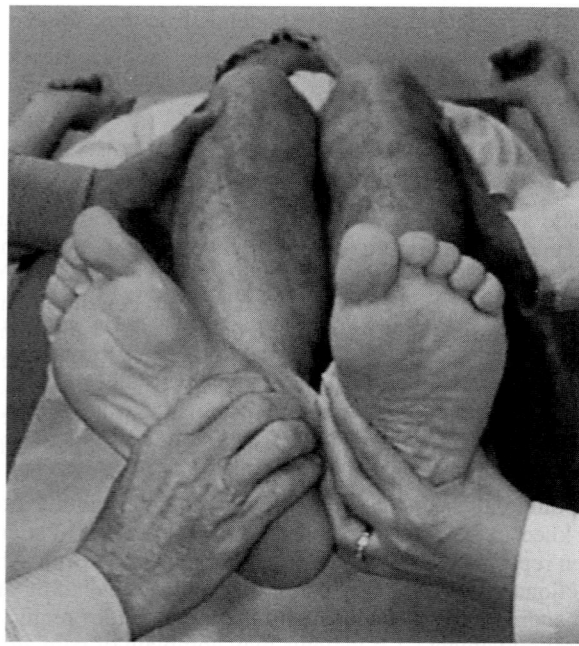

Figure 28I1–11. The Dial test is used to identify and quantitate posterolateral laxity. The foot and the ankle are externally rotating bilaterally, and the thigh-foot angle is compared. A side-to-side difference of greater than 5 degrees indicates injury to the posterolateral corner.

generally greater than 10 mm. Stress radiography can be helpful in delineating and documenting the extent of posterior tibial laxity (Fig. 28I1–13).[24, 31, 52, 58, 80]

The varus-valgus stress test, also termed the *adduction-abduction stress test*, evaluates the integrity of the collateral ligament complex. This test generally is performed with the knee at 0 degrees of flexion and 30 degrees of flexion. The normal amount of laxity with varus stress testing is 7 degrees and quite variable; it is essential to compare the injured knee varus with the normal knee.[2] The LCL is the primary restraint to varus rotation, and, if it is intact, there should not be an increase from the normal knee. An increase in varus laxity indicates an injury to the LCL, and progressively greater varus laxity is created with additional injury to the popliteus tendon and other structures of PLC.[47] Increased varus laxity at full extension indicates injury not only to the lateral and posterolateral structures but also to the cruciate ligaments.

Posterolateral Drawer Test. The posterolateral drawer test was popularized by Hughston and Norwood[30] as a means to assess the amount of external tibial rotation and posterior tibial translation in relation to the lateral femoral condyle (Fig. 28I1–14).[30] The knee is flexed 80 degrees, while the hip is flexed 45 degrees. The foot is held in place by the thigh of the examiner. A posterior drawer test is performed in external, neutral, and internal rotation. Differences in rotation are assessed by noting the prominence of the condyles. A positive drawer test in internal

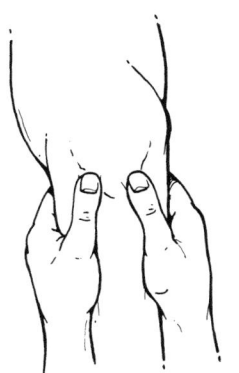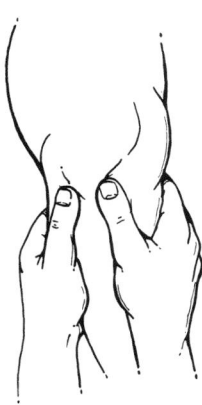

Figure 28I1–14. The posterolateral drawer test is performed with the patient lying supine on the examining table with the hip flexed 45 degrees and the knee flexed to 80 degrees. The foot is held in place by the thigh of the examiner. The posterior drawer test is performed in neutral, external, and internal rotation. Differences in motion, rotation, or prominence of the medial and lateral condyles of the tibial plateau are noted. In patients with posterolateral rotatory instability, the examiner detects rotation of the lateral tibial plateau externally. Posterior translation is greatest with external rotation of the tibia relative to the femur. (From Hughston JC, Norwood LA: The posterolateral drawer test and external rotation recurvatum test for posterolateral rotatory instability of the knee. Clin Orthop 147:82–87, 1980.)

and neutral rotation is consistent with an injury to the PCL. PCL injuries typically are graded 1 to 3 in 5-mm increments based on the degree of translation from the normal anterior position of the tibia in relation to the femur.[60] Patients with PLC injuries have increased external rotation of the lateral tibial plateau and posterior translation of the tibia near full extension. This posterior translation is greatest in external rotation. The posterolateral drawer test has been shown to have variable sensitivity for PLC injuries ranging from 70% to 75%.[5, 6, 15]

External Rotation Recurvatum Test. For the external rotation recurvatum test, the patient is placed in a supine position with knees and hips fully extended. The great toe and foot are lifted together, while encouraging the patient to relax the quadriceps. In patients with posterolateral rotatory instability (PLRI), the involved knee goes into relative hyperextension and varus, and the increased external rotation can be seen by the apparent lateral rotation of the tibial tubercle (Fig. 28I1–15). Alternatively, the test may be performed by extending the knee gradually by lifting the heel and palpating the PLC for evidence of hyperextension. This test has variable sensitivity ranging from 33% to 94%.[15, 34]

Reverse Pivot Shift Test. The reverse pivot shift test has been described in several ways. Most commonly, the test starts with the knee flexed at 90 degrees. The knee is brought slowly into extension while applying an axial load and valgus stress with the foot in external rotation. In the flexed starting position, the tibia is subluxed posteriorly in patients with PLRI. The tibia reduces with a shift or jump as the knee is brought into extension (Fig. 28I1–16). This reduction is thought to occur by the action of the ITB.[42, 57] Typically, this shift occurs at 20 to 30 degrees of flexion. This shift must be distinguished from a true pivot shift test, in which the test is initiated in extension, and the

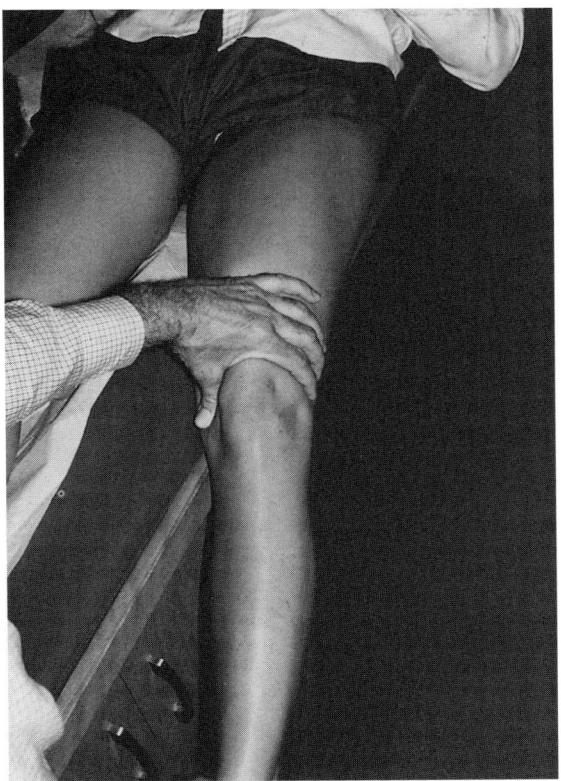

Figure 28I1–13. A varus/valgus stress test should be done to identify and quantitate laxity of the collateral ligaments. It is helpful to place the thigh on a table to control tibial rotation better while performing this test, particularly in patients with combined cruciate instability.

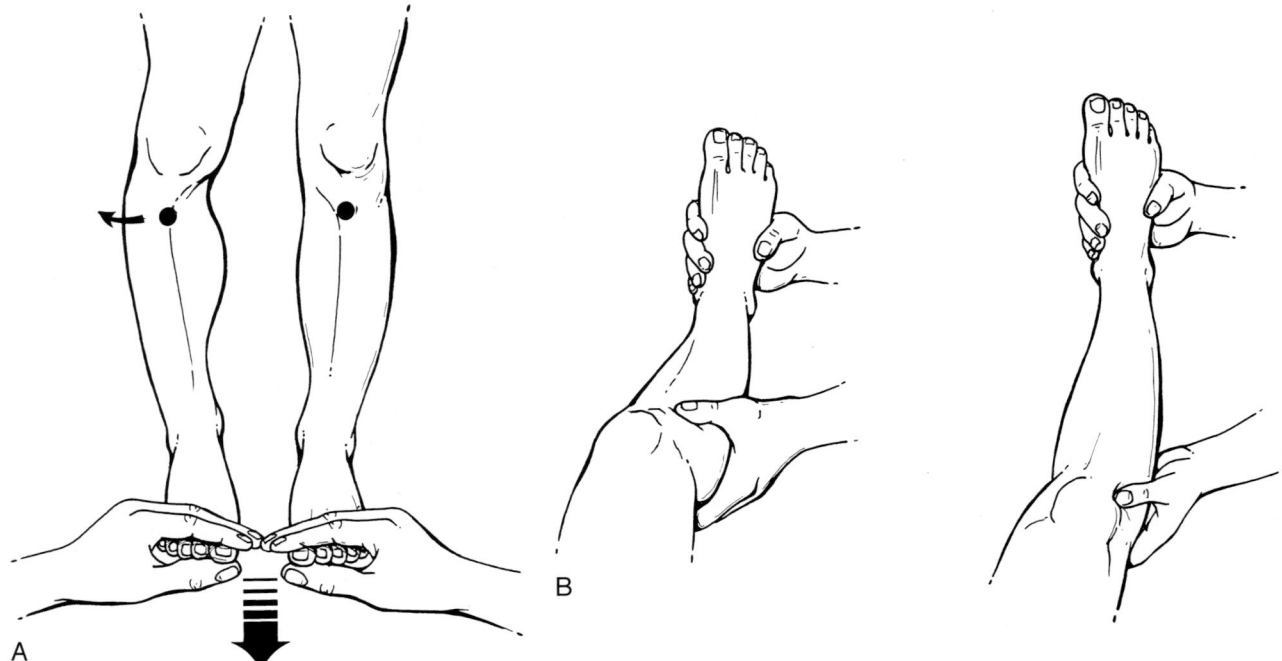

Figure 28I1–15. *A,* External rotation recurvatum test. Both legs rest on the examining table as the patient lies supine. The examiner grasps the great toe on each side and lifts both feet as the patient is encouraged to relax the quadriceps muscles. With posterolateral rotatory instability, the knee goes into a relative appearance of hyperextension-varus, while the tibia rotates simultaneously externally and the tibial tubercle moves laterally. *B,* The test may be performed with the examiner holding the heel of the foot in his or her hand and gradually extending the knee from 30 degrees of flexion while the opposite hand palpates the posterolateral aspect of the knee to detect hyperextension. (*A,* from Jakob RP, Hassler H, Staubli HU: Observations on rotatory instability of the lateral compartment of the knee. Acta Orthop Scand 191[suppl]:1–32, 1981; *B,* from Hughston, JC, Norwood LA Jr: The posterolateral drawer test and external rotational recurvatum test for posterolateral rotatory instability of the knee. Clin Orthop 147:82–87, 1980.)

anterior subluxation of the tibia is reduced as the knee is taken into flexion (Fig. 28I1–17).

The reverse pivot shift test has been described as being initiated in extension, then determining if the subluxation that occurs at 20 to 30 degrees of flexion is anterior or posterior.[2] Specificity of this test is low, particularly under anesthesia, in that 35% of noninjured patients exhibit a positive reverse pivot shift. Findings must be compared with a normal contralateral knee.[14, 33]

Shelbourne and colleagues[76] described a dynamic shift test in which the hip is maintained at 90 degrees of flexion; while the knee is extended slowly, the hamstrings and gravity keep the tibia subluxed posteriorly until knee flexion reaches approximately 20 degrees, when the tibia reduces with a clunk, the dynamic shift. This test is similar to the reverse pivot shift test.

Ninety Degrees Flexion Posterolateral Subluxation Test. Albright and Brown[3] described the 90 degrees posterolateral subluxation test as a feeling of the patient that the tibia is subluxed posteriorly on the lateral femoral condyle. The sense of subluxation is increased as the externally rotated leg is flexed at 90 degrees with a valgus stress. The patient notes that this causes discomfort in the PLC, which is relieved by release of external rotation.

Other Tests for Posterolateral Rotatory Instability. Combinations of the previously mentioned tests commonly are used. The posterolateral external rotation test is performed at 30 degrees and 90 degrees of knee flexion in the supine position. A combination of rotation and posterior

translation forces is applied to the tibia. Subluxation at both flexion angles indicates a combined PCL and PLC injury.[43] The standing apprehension test uses weight-bearing through the slightly flexed knee to recreate a "giving way" sensation. The thumb of the examiner is used to push on the lateral femoral condyle, while the patient slightly flexes the knee. Increased internal rotation of the condyle in relation to the fixed tibia along with a giving way sensation was thought to be 100% sensitive in a group of 15 patients with PLRI. Instrumented testing has been developed but not widely used for PLRI and at this time remains a research tool.[7, 17, 73]

Summary

Physical examination of a patient with suspected lateral and posterolateral injury needs to include a full assessment of the knee starting with mechanical alignment and gait observation to detect any hyperextension or varus thrust. The cruciate and collateral ligaments need to be assessed as well as the PLC. The Dial test is simple to perform and is the most well-accepted means for assessing and quantitating posterolateral laxity. To quantify and follow objectively patients treated for posterior, varus, and posterolateral laxity, it is likely to become essential to record posterior laxity at 30 degrees and 90 degrees of flexion by stress radiography, to quantify varus laxity with stress radiographs, and to document increased external tibial rotation with the Dial test. If these measures are recorded

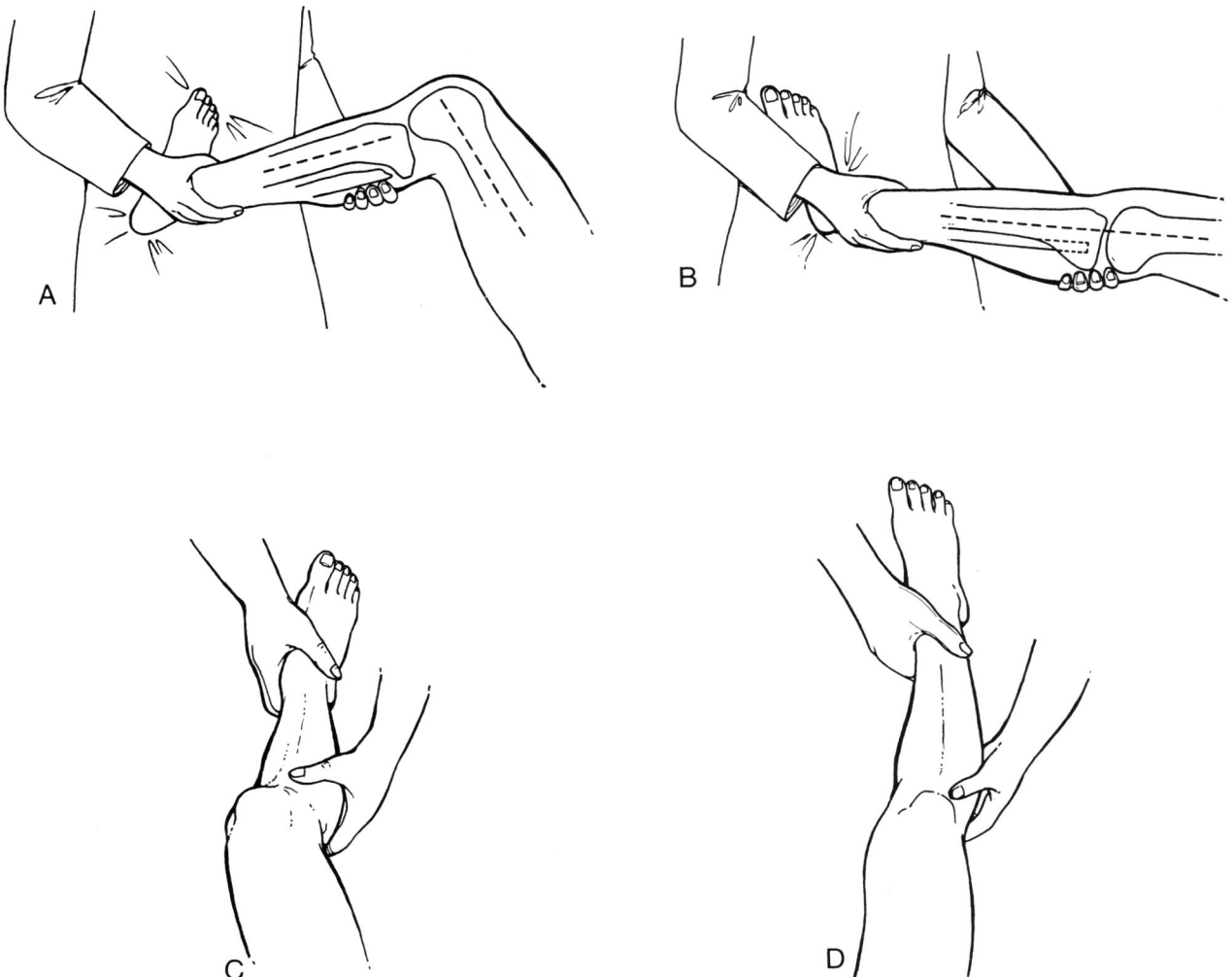

Figure 28I1–16. *A* to *D,* Reversed pivot shift test. The patient lies supine on the examining table. To test the right knee, the examiner, facing the patient, lifts the foot and ankle with his or her right hand, resting it on the right side of his or her pelvis. The left hand supports the lateral side of the calf with the palm on the proximal fibula. The examiner bends the knee to 70 to 80 degrees of flexion. In patients with posterolateral rotatory instability, at this position external rotation of the foot causes the lateral tibial plateau to subluxate posteriorly in relation to the lateral femoral condyle. This is perceived as a posterior sag of the proximal tibia. As the examiner now allows the knee to extend, he or she leans slightly against the foot, transmitting an axial and valgus load to the knee. As the knee approaches 20 degrees of flexion, the lateral tibial plateau reduces from its posterior subluxated position, and a jerklike shift is appreciated. If the test is begun with the tibia in the reduced position in full extension and neutral rotation, rapid flexion to 10 degrees produces the jerklike phenomenon as the tibia subluxates with external rotation relative to the lateral femoral condyle. (From Jakob RP, Hassler H, Staubli HU: Observations on rotatory instability of the lateral compartment of the knee. Acta Orthop Scand 191[suppl]: 1–32, 1981.)

preoperatively, objective parameters are available for comparison with postoperative results.

Radiographic Evaluation

Routine radiographs in all cases of suggested lateral or posterolateral instability should include flexion and extension weight-bearing views, a lateral view of the involved knee, and patellofemoral views of both knees.[70] Radiographs often are normal in cases of posterolateral instability, but they may show several abnormalities, including a proximal fibular tip avulsion fracture or fibular head fracture. Avulsion of Gerdy's tubercle has been observed with ITB injuries.[34] Evidence of associated injuries occasionally

can be found such as tibial plateau fractures, tibiofemoral dislocation, PCL avulsion fractures, Segond's fracture,[73] or tibial spine fractures. Avulsion fractures at other ligament or tendon insertions can be seen.

In cases of chronic PLRI, evidence of patellofemoral or tibiofemoral degenerative changes may be observed. Most commonly, the tibiofemoral involvement is most advanced in the lateral compartment.[34] Lateral tibial osteophytes may be seen along with evidence of joint space narrowing and subchondral sclerosis of the tibial plateau. Stress radiography can be helpful in delineating the degree and direction of laxity.[52, 80] Varus and valgus stress radiographs can be obtained as well as radiographs with defined anterior and posterior forces applied to the tibia to identify and quantitate cruciate laxity (Fig. 28I1–18).

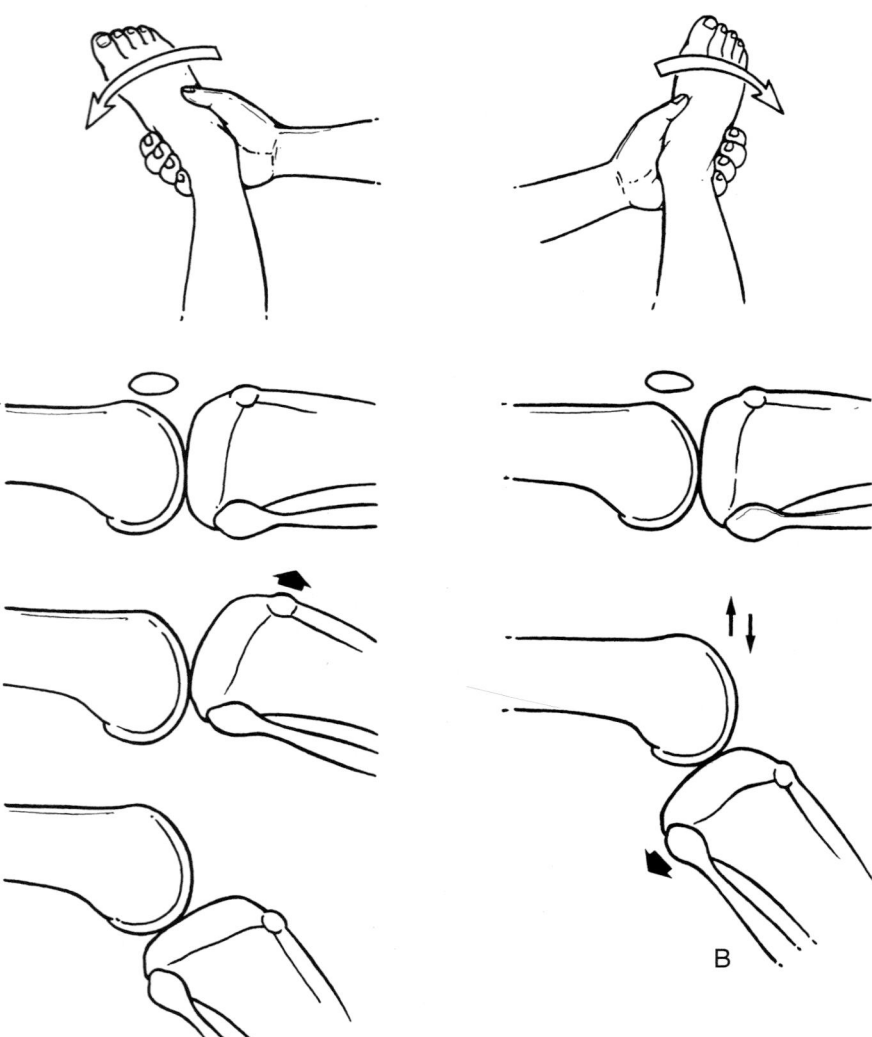

Figure 28I1–17. *A*, In the true pivot shift test, the lateral tibial plateau shifts from a reduced position in extension into anterior subluxation in slight flexion and reduces again at 30 degrees of flexion. *B*, In the reversed pivot shift test, the lateral tibial plateau falls from a position reduced in extension into posterior subluxation and flexion. (From Jakob RP, Hassler H, Staubli HU: Observations on rotatory instability of the lateral compartment of the knee. Acta Orthop Scand 191[suppl]:1–32, 1981.)

Magnetic Resonance Imaging of Lateral and Posterolateral Structures

Magnetic resonance imaging (MRI) has been shown repeatedly to be helpful for defining the complex anatomy of the PLC.[44, 53, 71, 83, 94] Particularly in the acutely injured and painful extremity, MRI may be the most comprehensive means to assess the entire knee joint. Surgically verified lesions of the PLC can be identified predictably.[44] Specific structures, such as the LCL, short head of the biceps tendon, and lateral capsular attachments, can be defined accurately greater than 90% of the time. Injuries to the PFL are not as reliably predicted, however.[34, 40, 44] Associated meniscal and cruciate injuries can be visualized to assist in surgical planning. Comparisons between acute and chronic PLRI imaging have not been done, but several authors believe MRI is a useful adjunct in both settings.[23, 44, 71, 94] The use of standard imaging sequences as well as a coronal oblique series that includes the entire fibular head and styloid is recommended. In conjunction with a comprehensive history and physical examination, MRI can add consistently useful information to help in the surgical planning for knees with injuries to the lateral and posterolateral structures.

Arthroscopic Evaluation

The intra-articular assessment of the PLC structures is often extremely helpful. Visualization of the middle one third of the capsule, the coronary ligaments, and the popliteomeniscal fascicles is possible. Excessive varus laxity can be appreciated by noting a "drive-through" sign when viewing the lateral compartment with a varus stress on the knee (Fig. 28I1–19). The lateral meniscus has been described as translating medially with adduction stress and laterally with abduction stress with injuries of the popliteomeniscal components of the popliteus complex.[88] Careful fluid management and awareness of possible fluid extravasation are needed in an acutely injured or capsular-deficient knee. Arthroscopy allows evaluation of the cruciate ligaments, menisci, and articular surfaces that may require treatment simultaneously.

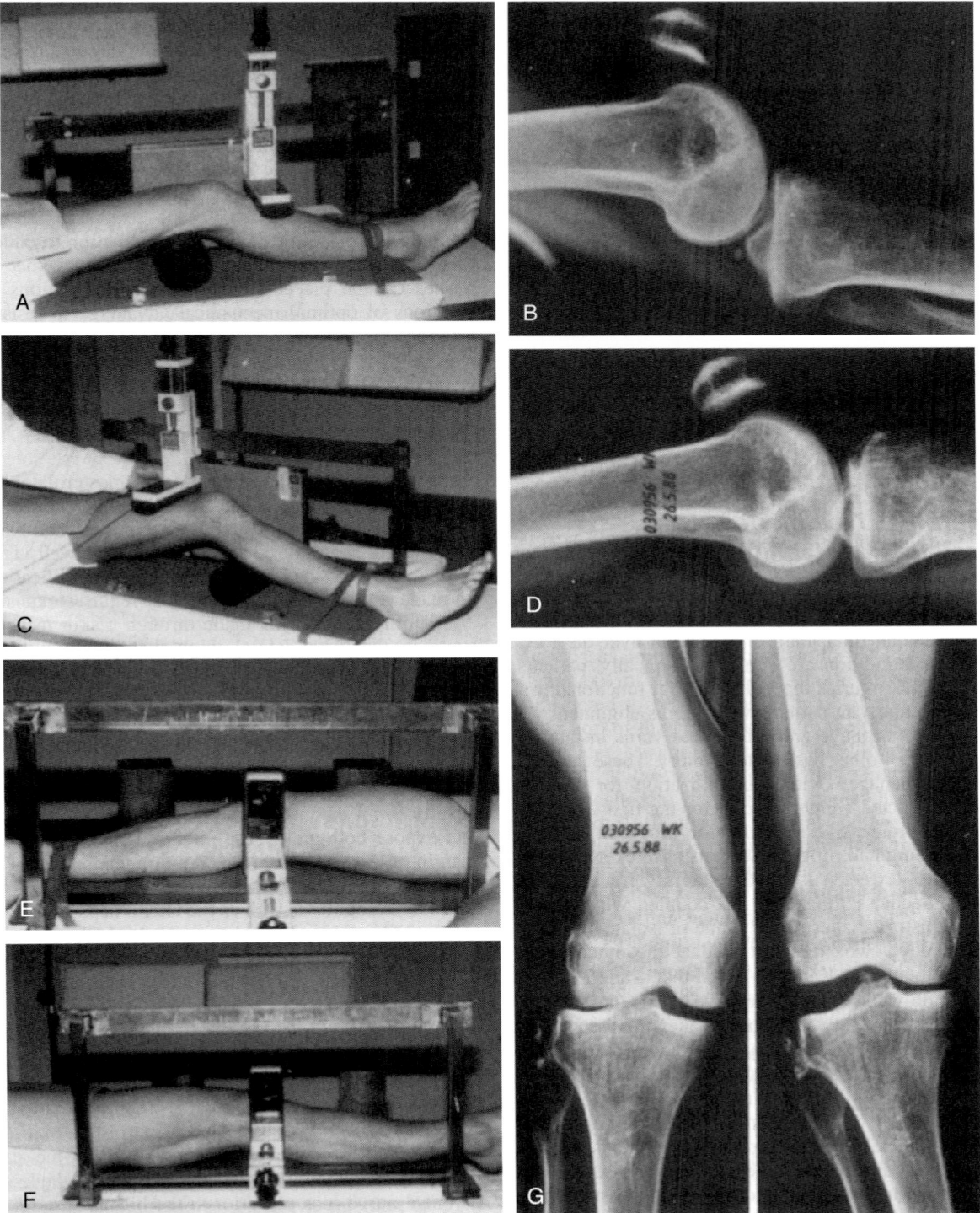

Figure 28I1–18. Stress test radiography performed with the patient under anesthesia. *A* and *B*, Stress weight 15 kilopascals. Posterior drawer near extension. *C* and *D*, Anterior translation (Lachman's test). *E* to *G*, Varus-valgus stress. *H*, In the 0-degree flexion position, the extent of the posterior translation is more marked than in extension. There is marked posterior-posterolateral instability compared with the opposite knee. (From Jakob RP, Staubli HU [eds]: The Knee and the Cruciate Ligaments. Berlin, Springer-Verlag, 1992.)

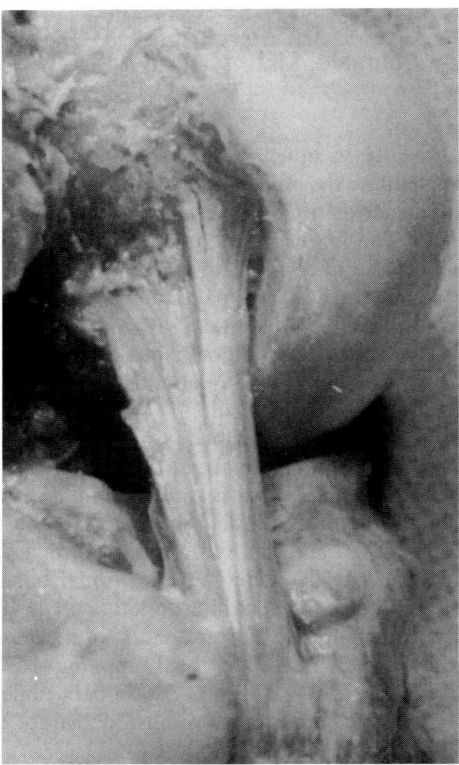

Figure 28I2–2. Anatomic specimen demonstrating the course of the posterior cruciate ligament. Note the broad origin from the medial femoral condyle and the epiphyseal tibial insertion. (From Covey DC, Sapega AA: Anatomy and function of the posterior cruciate ligament. Clin Sports Med 13:509–518, 1994.)

functional components: the iliopatellar and iliotibial tract.[63] The biceps femoris muscle complex consists of a long head and a short head, having five and seven insertions about the knee, respectively.[106] The second layer consists of the patellar retinaculum and patellofemoral ligaments laterally, and the lateral head of the gastrocnemius more posteriorly. The first two layers are adherent along the lateral border of the patella. The third and deepest layer consists of two leaves, divided by the lateral inferior geniculate vessels. The more superficial leaf includes the lateral collateral ligament, extending from the lateral distal femoral epiphysis to the lateral aspect of the proximal fibular epiphysis. More posteriorly, the fabellofibular ligament courses from the posterolateral distal femoral epiphysis to lateral proximal fibula as well. The deeper leaf consists of the meniscotibial/coronary and arcuate ligaments. The arcuate ligament extends from the posterolateral corner of the distal femoral epiphysis down to the fibular head, between the more lateral fabellofibular ligament and the more posterior popliteus muscle, crossing over and interdigitating with the more oblique popliteus muscle-tendon junction.[15] The popliteus muscle originates from the posteromedial corner of the proximal tibia, extending up as a fanlike structure into the popliteus space, dividing into aponeurotic and tendinous insertions (Fig. 28I2–5). The more medial aponeurotic broad insertion is onto the posterior distal femoral epiphysis as well as on the posterior coronary ligament, which anchors the posterior horn of the lateral meniscus to the

tibia. The tendinous insertion passes through a hiatus in the coronary ligament, coursing through the knee joint to its insertion onto the posterolateral distal femoral epiphysis.

More medially and superiorly, the oblique popliteal ligament runs from the distal femoral epiphysis and capsule overlying the lateral femoral condyle to the posteromedial corner of the knee and the insertion of the semimembranosus complex.

Functionally, these three layers are not easily isolated, nor are injuries confined to specific layers. Hughston defined an arcuate ligament complex as a more functional unit supporting the posterolateral corner of the knee.[42] The fibular collateral ligament, tendinous and aponeurotic portions of the popliteus, and the lateral head of the gastrocnemius make up much of the arcuate complex. With the inclusion of the more medial oblique popliteal ligament, the arcuate complex is truly an arch extending over the posterior and posterolateral knee.

Terry has described the mid–third capsular ligament as the deepest layer of joint capsule extending from the lateral distal femoral epiphysis to the lateral proximal tibial epiphysis.[106] Also described are three fascicles, which may serve to stabilize further the lateral meniscus. These are the posterior-superior, posterior-inferior, and anterior-inferior popliteomeniscal fascicles, which form the border of the popliteal hiatus and stabilize the posterior horn of the lateral meniscus to the popliteus tendon.

History and Physical Examination of the Injured Knee

As described in Chapter 28H2, obtaining a thorough history of the patient's knee complaint(s), including identification of any precipitating event and the mechanism of injury, as well as determining whether it was a relatively low- or high-energy mechanism of injury, is essential. The presence of any subsequent swelling and/or recurrent locking, popping, or giving way may point toward intra-articular pathology. Determining the duration and intensity of symptoms, whether there are activities that typically cause a flare, and if there are any other accompanying symptoms such as swelling, limp, or generalized malaise will help narrow the differential diagnosis.

The physical examination of the child's knee with symptoms suggesting a lateral injury should begin with careful observation of gait. Asymmetry in foot progression angles, the presence of an antalgic versus Trendelenburg gait, and the presence of any medial or lateral thrust can all help narrow the diagnosis, and may in fact point towards the hip as the culprit. Examination of the normal knee to establish a standard for comparison should precede that of the injured knee. This helps reassure the child that the examiner is careful and competent before what may be perceived as a potentially painful examination. After establishing a baseline range of motion and stability to anterior, posterior, varus, and valgus stresses, the examiner may turn attention toward the knee in question. Localized swelling and ecchymosis may help point to the site of injury. The presence of an intra-articular effusion suggests a significant ligamentous or meniscal injury, or fracture.[22, 86, 101] Quadri-

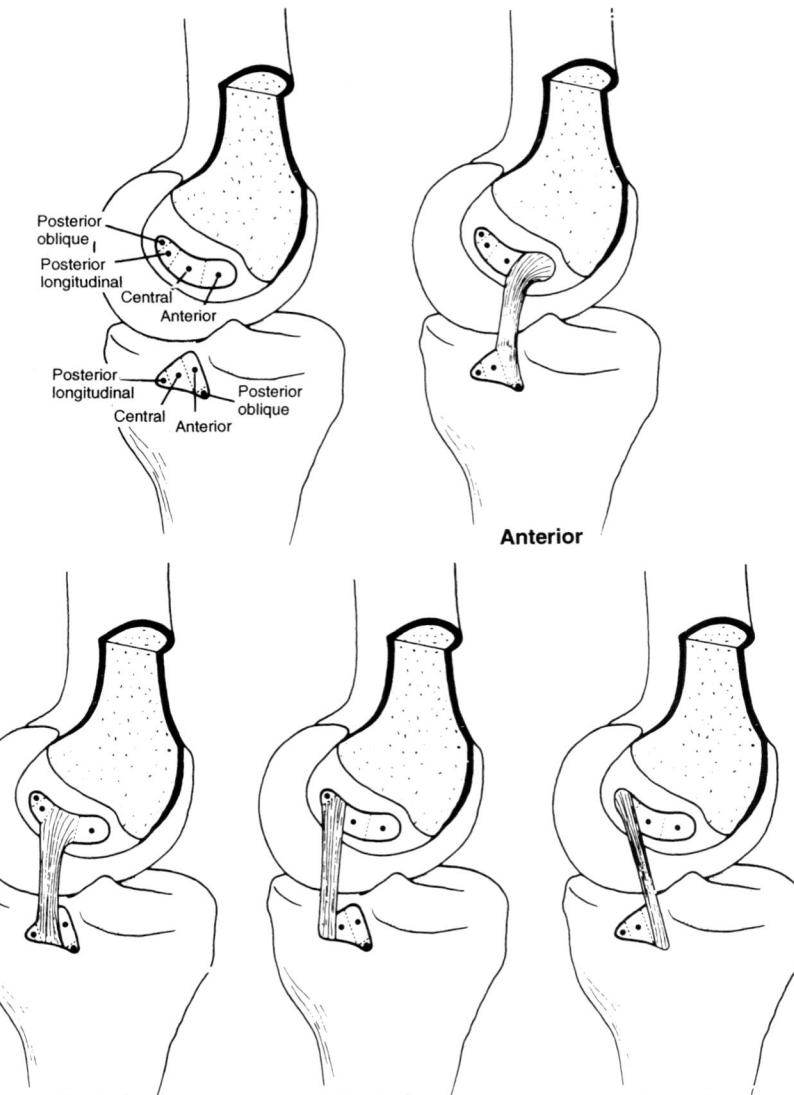

Anterior

Central

**Posterior
Longitudinal**

**Posterior
Oblique**

Figure 28I2–3. The posterior cruciate ligament has been described as having four functional regions or bands (anterior, central, posterior longitudinal, and posterior oblique). (From Covey DC, Sapega AA: Anatomy and function of the posterior cruciate ligament. Clin Sports Med 13:509–518, 1994.)

ceps atrophy has been noted in knees with longstanding meniscal deficiencies.[21, 41]

Joint line tenderness and a loss of flexion or extension with discomfort at the extremes of motion in children is consistent with meniscal injury, as it is in adults.[77] Discomfort with palpable or audible popping during flexion/rotation maneuvers such as McMurray's test, Apley's grind test, or Steinmann's test also suggest a meniscal pathology,[58, 61, 77] although Rang has noted that children commonly pass these provocative tests despite having meniscal tears seen at arthroscopy.[83]

Tests of knee stability should follow. Lachman's test and the posterior drawer test are probably the most sensitive examinations for anterior and chronic posterior laxity, respectively, and thus are straightforward tests for function of the anterior cruciate ligament (ACL) and PCL (Fig. 28I2–6).[109] In the acutely injured knee, the abduction stress test (hip extended, valgus force across the knee) in full extension may be the most sensitive test for PCL deficiency in the presence of concomitant medial injury. Numerous authors emphasize the PCL as the central stabilizer of the knee.[17, 44, 47] Its greatest impact on knee stability occurs when the knee is in 90 degrees of flexion.[21, 66, 80, 115] Thus tests of knee stability that reveal posterior laxity in 90 degrees of knee flexion would be the most sensitive for PCL disruption (posterior drawer, sag test, quadriceps active test). Isolated posterolateral corner injuries would result in increased external rotation and lateral opening with varus stress in 30 degrees of flexion, as the tibia rotates externally on the intact PCL and ACL (Fig. 28I2–7). Less external rotational instability would be seen in such a knee at 90 degrees of flexion, as a result of the influence of an intact PCL. Rotational instabilities in 90 degrees of flexion would suggest a disrupted PCL *and* disrupted structures in the posterolateral corner. Knees with such combined injuries would also have similar increased rotational instability isolated injuries to the posterior cruciate ligament in athletes. J Bone Joint Surg Br 77:895–900, 1995.

98. Silverman JM, Mink JH, Deutsch AL: Discoid menisci of the knee: MR imaging appearance. Radiology 173:351–354, 1989.
99. Smith CF, Van Dyk GE, Jurgutis J, Vangsness CT Jr: Cautious surgery for discoid menisci. Am J Knee Surg 12:25–28, 1999.
100. Speer KP, Spritzer CE, Goldner JL, et al: Magnetic resonance imaging of traumatic knee articular cartilage injuries. Am J Sports Med 19:396–402, 1991.
101. Stanitski CL: Correlation of arthroscopic and clinical examinations with magnetic resonance imaging findings of injured knees in children and adolescents. Am J Sports Med 26:743–744, 1998.
102. Stanitski C, Harvell JC, Fu F: Observations on acute knee hemarthrosis in children and adolescents. J Pediatr Orthop 13:506–510, 1993.
103. Sullivan JA: Ligamentous injuries of the knee in children. Clin Orthop 255:44–50, 1990.
104. Sutker A, Jackson D, Pagliano J: Iliotibial band syndrome in distance runners. Physician Sportsmed 9:69, 1981.
105. Takeda Y, Ikata T, Yoshida S, et al: MRI high-signal intensity in the menisci of asymptomatic children. J Bone Joint Surg Br 80: 463–466, 1998.
106. Terry GC, LaPrade RF: The posterolateral aspect of the knee anatomy and surgical approach. Am J Sports Med 24:732–739, 1996.
107. Tria A: Ligaments of the Knee. New York, Churchill Livingstone, 1995.
108. Torg JS, et al: Natural history of the posterior cruciate ligament-deficient knee. Clin Orthop 246:209–216, 1989.
109. Torg JS, Conrad W, Kalen V: Clinical diagnosis of anterior cruciate ligament instability in the athlete. Am J Sports Med 4:84–93, 1976.
110. Torisu T: Avulsion fracture of the tibial attachment of the posterior cruciate ligament. Indications and results of delayed repair. Clin Orthop 143:107–114, 1979.

111. Torisu T: Isolated avulsion fracture of the tibial attachment of the posterior cruciate ligament. J Bone Joint Surg Am 59:68–72, 1977.
112. Trickey EL: Injuries to the posterior cruciate ligament: Diagnosis and treatment of early injuries and reconstruction of late instability. Clin Orthop 147:76–81, 1980.
113. Vahvanen V, Aalto K: Meniscectomy in children. Acta Orthop Scand 50:791–795, 1979.
114. Vandermeer RD, Cunningham FK: Arthroscopic treatment of the discoid lateral meniscus: Results of long-term follow-up. Arthroscopy 5:101–109, 1989.
115. Veltri DM, Deng XH, Torzilli PA, et al: The role of the cruciate and posterolateral ligaments in stability of the knee. A biomechanical study. Am J Sports Med 23:436–443, 1995.
116. Veltri DM, Warren RF: Isolated and combined posterior cruciate ligament injuries. J Am Acad Orthop Surg 1:67–75, 1993.
117. Warren RF: Meniscectomy and repair in the anterior cruciate ligament-deficient patient. Clin Orthop 252:55–63, 1990.
118. Washington ER, Root L, Liener UC: Discoid lateral meniscus in children. J Bone Joint Surg Am 77:1357–1360, 1995.
119. Watanabe M: Arthroscopy of the knee joint. In Helfet AJ (ed): Disorders of the Knee. Philadelphia, JB Lippincott, 1974, p 145.
120. Williams JS, Abate JA, Fadale PD, et al: Meniscal and nonosseus ACL injuries in children and adolescents. Am J Knee Surg 9: 22–26, 1996.
121. Woods GW, Whelan JM: Discoid meniscus. Clin Sports Med 9: 695–706, 1990.
122. Wroble RR, Henderson RC, Campion ER, et al: Meniscectomy in children and adolescents. Clin Orthop 279:180–189, 1992.
123. Zaman M, Leonard MA: Meniscectomy in children: A study of fifty-nine knees. J Bone Joint Surg Br 60:436–437, 1978.
124. Zionts LE, MacEwen GD: Spontaneous improvement of post-traumatic tibia valga. J Bone Joint Surg Am 68:680–687, 1986.
125. Zobel MS, Borrello JA, Siegel MJ, Stewart NR: Pediatric knee MR imaging: Pattern of injuries in the immature skeleton. Radiology 190:397–401, 1994.

Section J
Anterior Cruciate Ligament Injuries

1. ANTERIOR CRUCIATE LIGAMENT RECONSTRUCTION IN THE ADULT
Michael J. D'Amato, MD ▪ Bernard R. Bach, Jr., MD

Basic Science

Anatomy

On the ultrastructural level, the anterior cruciate ligament (ACL) is composed of longitudinally oriented fibrils of collagen tissue ranging from 20 to 170 μm in diameter.[24] The mean diameter of these fibrils and the cross-sectional area increase from proximal to distal. Throughout the ligament, the percentage of total cross-sectional area occupied by collagen remains nearly constant.[24] Bundles of collagen fibrils make up subfascicular units, which are surrounded by a thin band of loose connective tissue called the endotenon. Several subfasciculi are grouped together to make up a collagen fasciculus. The fasciculus is surrounded by an epitenon, which is much denser than the endotenon. Surrounding the entire ligament is paratenon, which blends with the epitenon (Fig. 28J1–1).[11, 86] On histologic evaluation, the ligament is composed of fibroblasts surrounded by a matrix consisting primarily of type I collagen with a small amount of type III and type VI collagen near the insertion sites.[6, 24]

The cruciate ligaments are covered by a synovial fold that originates at the posterior inlet of the intercondylar notch and extends to the anterior tibial attachment of the ACL. Thus, the cruciate ligaments, although intra-articular, are extrasynovial.[11] The predominant blood supply of the cruciate ligaments is the middle genicular artery, which leaves the popliteal artery and directly pierces the posterior capsule.[12] Branches of the artery form a periligamentous plexus within the synovial sheath surrounding the ligament. This plexus, in addition to providing the nutritional requirements of the ACL, is the source of the hemarthrosis typically seen after an ACL injury. The osseous attachments of the ACL contribute little to its vascularity.[13] There is also a contributing blood supply from the fat pad through the inferior medial and lateral genicular arteries that may play a more important role when the ligament is injured.[13]

Innervation of the ACL is provided by a branch of the tibial nerve, the posterior articular nerve.[167] It arises from the tibial nerve in the popliteal fossa, wraps around the popliteal artery and vein, penetrates the posterior capsule, and forms the popliteal plexus. Branches of this plexus course through the synovial lining of the cruciate liga-

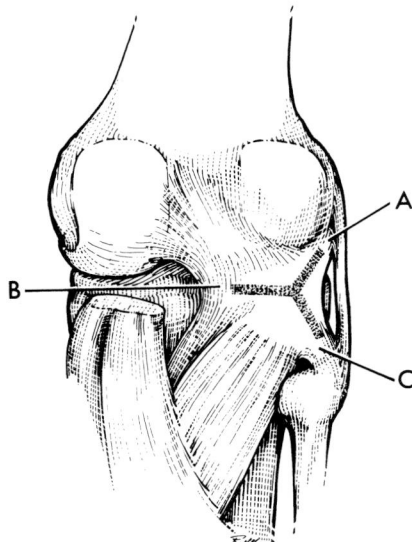

Figure 28I2–5. The multiple insertions of the popliteus muscle. A, Lateral femoral condyle; B, posterior horn of the lateral meniscus; C, head of the proximal fibula. (From Basmajian JV, Lovejoy JF Jr: Functions of the popliteus muscle in man. A multifactorial electromyographic study. J Bone Joint Surg Am 53:557–562, 1971.)

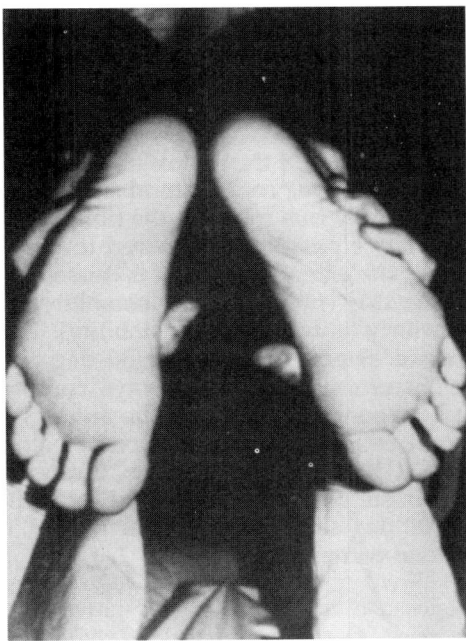

Figure 28I2–7. The tibial external rotation test. This test should be performed with the knee in 30 degrees and 90 degrees of flexion. Patients with a significant posterolateral injury will have excessive external rotation of the tibia on the femur when compared with the uninjured limb. (From Bowen MK, Warren RF, Cooper DE: Posterior cruciate ligament and related injuries. In Insall J [ed]: Surgery of the Knee, 2nd ed. New York, Churchill Livingstone, 1993.)

in 30 degrees of knee flexion, as well as a positive sag test, quadriceps active test, and posterior drawer test in 90 degrees of knee flexion.[116]

In a knee with a tense effusion, aspiration of the joint using sterile technique with infusion of local anesthetic may help make the examination more tolerable. The presence of fat in the aspirate would be consistent with an intra-articular fracture. Stress radiography would then be important to determine whether medial opening with a varus stress is due to ligamentous deficiency or fracture, or both. Such an examination might best be carried out under a general anesthetic with the benefit of intraoperative fluoroscopy.[51]

Examination of the hip for any asymmetry or abnormalities in the range of motion should be included. Loss of abduction with discomfort at the end point might suggest Legg-Calvé-Perthes disease, whereas excessive external rotation with a loss of internal rotation would be consistent with a slipped capital femoral epiphysis. Both of these conditions might present as knee pain with limp.

Further work-up of the child with knee pain should include anterior-posterior and lateral radiographs of the knee in question, to help rule out fracture, as well as an anterior-posterior pelvic radiograph, to rule out occult hip pathology. Comparison views with the unaffected knee may help identify pathologic joint space narrowing or widening when a discoid meniscus is suspected. The use of additional studies such as magnetic resonance imaging (MRI) to help make or confirm a diagnosis has received

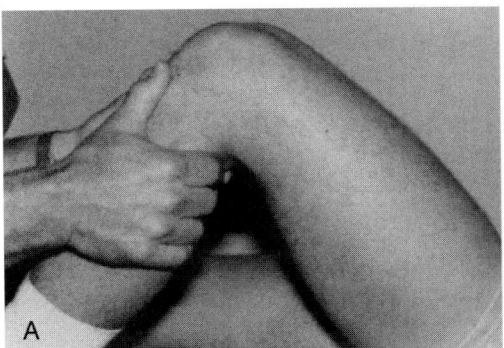
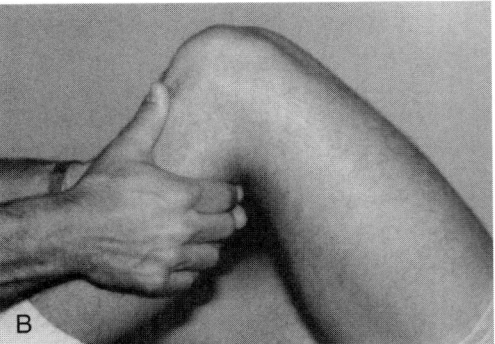

Figure 28I2–6. A and B, Posterior drawer test. In a test with a positive result, the tibial step-off is lost when a posteriorly directed force is applied to the knee flexed to 90 degrees. This is suggestive of a posterior cruciate ligament injury. (A and B from Shelbourne KD: Posterior cruciate ligament injuries. In Reider B [ed]: Sports Medicine: The School-Age Athlete. Philadelphia, WB Saunders, 1991.)

mixed reviews in the literature. Stanitski has demonstrated that the clinical acumen of the treating orthopaedist is the most sensitive and specific method of coming to a diagnosis.[101] MRI has better than 90% sensitivity and specificity for the detection of cruciate deficiencies, and better than 80% for meniscal tears when these injuries are suspected by an orthopaedist.[26, 77] These numbers drop markedly when the population studied includes the asymptomatic patient or the patient referred for MRI by the nonorthopaedist.[12, 64, 105] The ability of MRI to detect chondral lesions of the patella, distal femur, or proximal tibia has been demonstrated to be around 50%.[100]

Injuries to the Posterior Cruciate Ligament and Posterolateral Corner

Injuries to the PCL and posterolateral knee may be combined or isolated. Three major mechanisms of injury are thought to contribute to PCL injuries. Hyperextension injuries, which may be accompanied by a partial or complete ACL tear, possibly as a result of a transient knee dislocation, can result in PCL disruption. Dashboard-type flexed knee injuries, seen in motor vehicle accidents or in athletic events where an athlete falls onto or is struck with high energy on his or her flexed knee, can also produce PCL disruptions. Posteriorly directed torsional forces on the knee may also cause PCL disruption.[112]

The PCL provides its greatest contribution to knee stability in 90 degrees of flexion.[29, 30, 77, 112] As the PCL resists posterior subluxation of the tibia on the femur, tests that attempt to posteriorly subluxate the tibia on the femur or observe resting posterior subluxation on the femur with the knee in flexion can be effective. A posterior drawer test in 90 degrees of knee flexion may show no firm end point in the case of PCL rupture. Although some have suggested that uninjured meniscofemoral ligaments of Wrisberg or Humphries, or both, seen in greater than 70% of the population, may provide somewhat of a firm end point and mask a PCL disruption. An intact arcuate ligament complex may also prevent isolated posterior subluxation in the PCL-deficient knee.[43] Observation of the injured knee including comparison in profile of the knees in 90 degrees of flexion may reveal a sag in the PCL deficient knee, which is an indicator of resting posterior subluxation (Fig. 28I2–8).[50] With the patient's heels resting on the examination table and knees flexed to 90 degrees, at least one of the examiner's fingers should be able to be placed on the anterior tibial plateau. Inability to palpate such a ledge on the anterior joint line suggests posterior subluxation, especially if a difference exists when compared with the contralateral side (Fig. 28I2–9). Because the quadriceps is often uninjured in this setting, having the patient attempt to extend the knee from this 90 degrees flexed position with the heel fixed to the examining table may correct posterior subluxation. This "quadriceps active test" was described by Daniel, and was found to be 98% sensitive for PCL disruption in both acute and chronically injured knees (Fig. 28I2–10).[21] Mild laxity to abduction or external rotation at 30 degrees of knee flexion would be increased at 90 degrees of knee flexion in the presence of a PCL in-

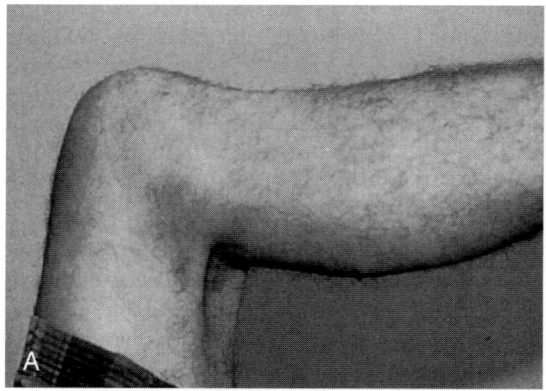
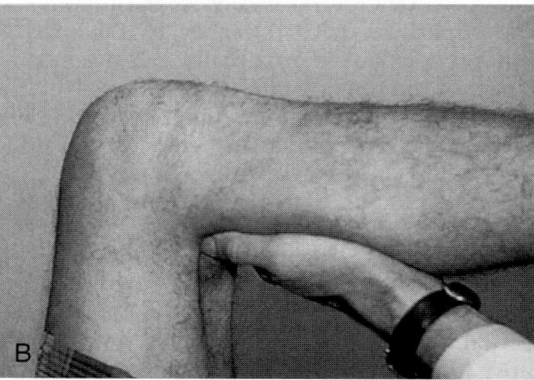

Figure 28I2–8. Posterior sag sign. *A,* Posterior subluxation of the tibia on the femur is noted with the hip and the knee flexed to 90 degrees. *B,* Anteriorly applied force reduces the subluxation, suggesting a significant injury to the posterior cruciate ligament. (*A* and *B* from Swenson TM, Harner CD: Knee ligament and meniscal injuries. Current concepts. Orthop Clin North Am 26:529–546, 1995.)

jury.[31, 34, 115] PCL injuries do occur in isolation, though combined injuries are probably more common.[108] It is the combined injuries that tend to result in more problematic instability and infrequent return to sports and prior activity levels if not surgically treated.[85]

Isolated Injuries to the Posterior Cruciate Ligament

The isolated PCL injury does not routinely necessitate operative intervention. Any suspicion of transient knee dislocation requires a careful assessment of the vascular status of the limb. This may include an arthrogram, ankle-brachial indices, or serial examinations in an inpatient setting. Many authors describe conservative treatment of isolated PCL injuries with early aggressive physiotherapy to rehabilitate the quadriceps as a dynamic stabilizer of the knee.[96, 97, 108] However, Bianchi showed that despite achievement of 99% of normal contralateral quadriceps strength at an average of 6 years from PCL disruption, 65% of patients continued to have symptoms limiting activity.[11] Those patients farther out from their injury also had greater evidence of osteoarthritic change in the patellofemoral and medial compartments of the knee on radiography.

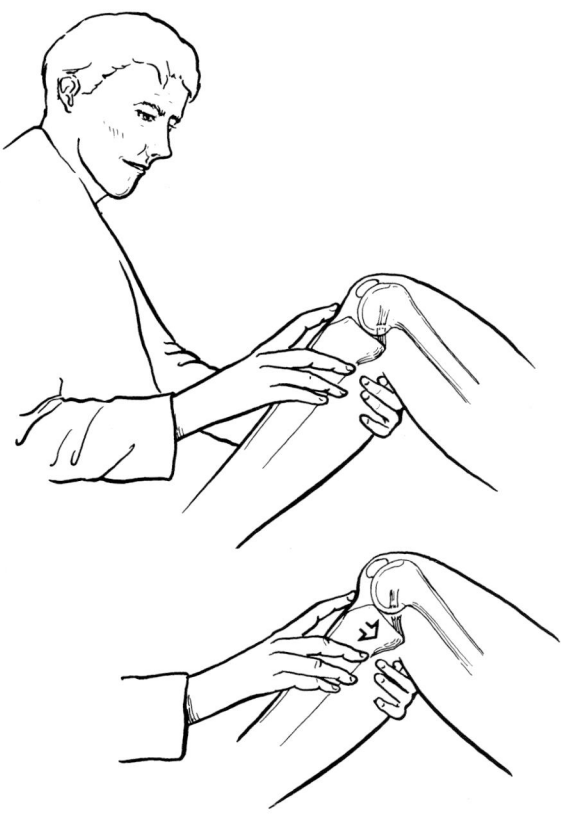

Figure 28I2–9. A ledge or step-off should be palpable along the anterior joint line in a normal knee. In the posterior cruciate ligament–deficient knee, posterior subluxation of the tibia leads to a loss of this ledge. (From St. Pierre P, Miller MD: Posterior cruciate ligament injuries. Clin Sports Med 18:199–221, 1999.)

Operative fixation of PCL avulsion fractures with or without truly osseous fragments is indicated. Frank describes a displaced purely cartilaginous fragment avulsed by the PCL, resulting in instability in a child.[28] Minimally displaced avulsion fractures may progress to nonunion and posterior instability, suggesting the importance of internal fixation. Multiple case reports of avulsion fractures off of both the tibia and femur in the region of the PCL attachments have been described in children. Despite fixation of such fragments, McMaster has noted persistent posterior laxity hypothesized to be a result of PCL stretch or posterior capsular injury, or both.[73] Methods of fixation of avulsed fragments have included the use of screws, wires, and suture, and may be performed open or via arthroscopic assistance.[73, 74, 110, 111]

Midsubstance tears of the PCL are rarely seen in the skeletally immature. As a child approaches skeletal maturity, and the physes of the distal femur and proximal tibia and fibula begin to close, the incidence of purely ligamentous midsubstance PCL injuries rises (Fig. 28I2–11). Also, as the energy of injury increases, the likelihood of a purely ligamentous injury would also rise. This is a result of a greater increase in bending strength seen in bone than in ligament as the rate of deformation increases.[13] For those with symptomatic posterior or multidirectional instability caused or contributed to by PCL insufficiency, numerous techniques for reconstruction using autologous or allogenic tendon and one or two incision arthroscopically assisted techniques have been described, each with good early results.[17, 57, 59] Hughston describes repair of the PCL, augmented in those knees that remained unstable despite PCL repair.[45] Results of this form of treatment were mixed, with 13 of 20 knees at 5 to 16 years' follow-up having good objective results, and 7 of 20 with fair or poor results. As a result, reconstruction of a deficient PCL is the treatment of choice.

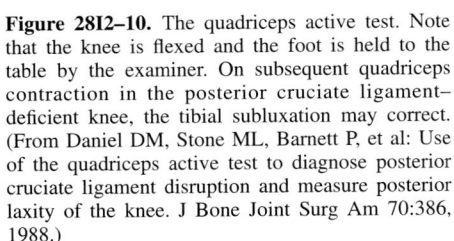

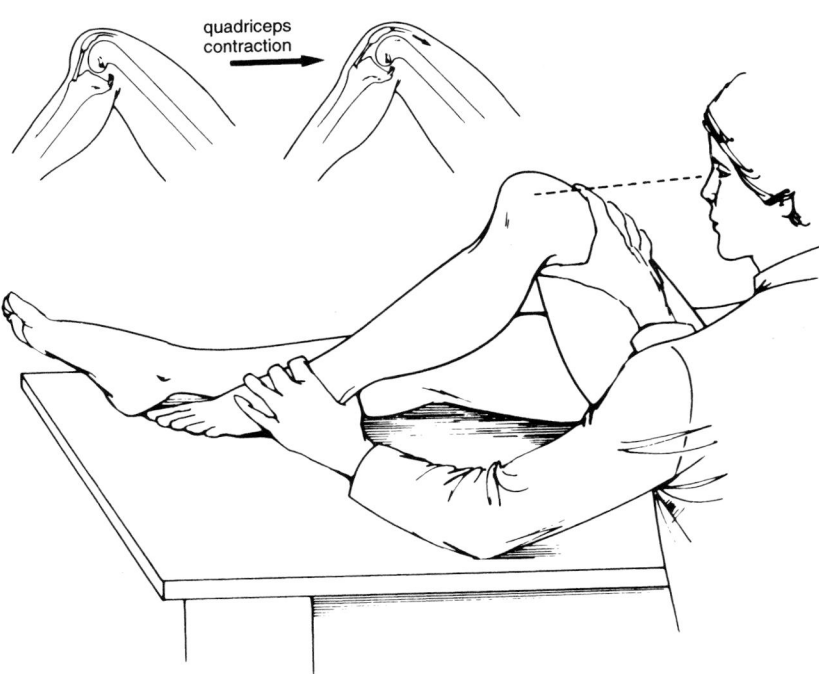

quadriceps contraction

Figure 28I2–10. The quadriceps active test. Note that the knee is flexed and the foot is held to the table by the examiner. On subsequent quadriceps contraction in the posterior cruciate ligament–deficient knee, the tibial subluxation may correct. (From Daniel DM, Stone ML, Barnett P, et al: Use of the quadriceps active test to diagnose posterior cruciate ligament disruption and measure posterior laxity of the knee. J Bone Joint Surg Am 70:386, 1988.)

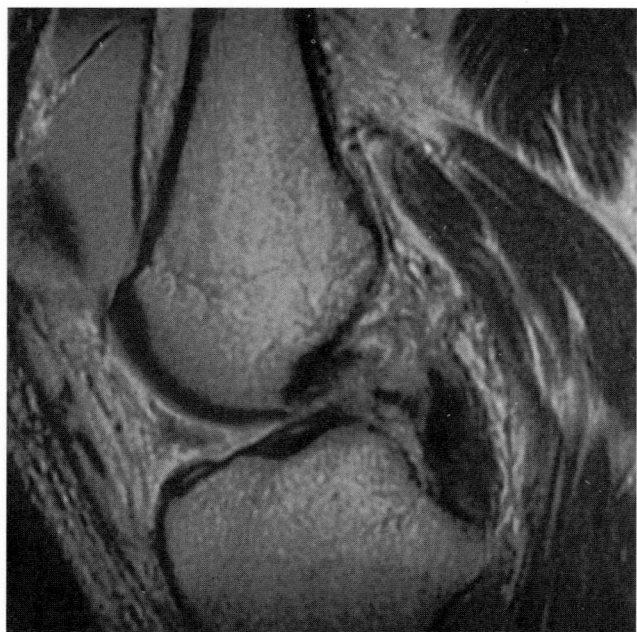

Figure 28I2–11. Magnetic resonance image of the knee demonstrating a midsubstance posterior cruciate ligament tear. (From St. Pierre P, Miller MD: Posterior cruciate ligament injuries. Clin Sports Med 18:199–221, 1999.)

Injuries to the Posterolateral Corner

Though no specific reports on posterolateral corner injuries in the skeletally immature were identified in review of the literature, adolescents as young as 14 years are often included in adult studies and so this literature will be briefly discussed. The mechanism(s) of injury for posterolateral corner injuries are hypothesized to include posteriorly directed forces onto the anteromedial tibia of a hyper-

extended knee, as well as significant varus stress beyond rupture of the lateral collateral ligament.[20, 44, 116] These mechanisms of injury are suggestive of a cruciate injury as well, more commonly PCL than ACL.[53] Car bumper injuries and football tackling are common scenarios for these injuries.[116] Symptoms may include pain with stair walking as well as simple posterior and posterolateral giving way with push-off in an extended knee position such as standing or walking.[47] Football linemen may have difficulty setting up to block, whereas sprinters may have difficulty pushing off from the starting blocks. Pain is more commonly perceived at the medial joint line as opposed to the lateral.[46, 66] A varus thrust with ambulation is also often seen.[66]

LaPrade correlated physical examination findings with injuries of the posterolateral corner (Fig. 28I2–12).[66] An abnormal reverse pivot shift was associated with injury to the fibular or lateral collateral ligament, popliteal complex, and mid–third lateral capsular ligament. Abnormal posterolateral external rotation at 30 degrees of knee flexion was associated with injuries to the fibular collateral ligament and lateral gastrocnemius tendon, whereas an abnormal adduction stress test in 30 degrees of knee flexion was associated with injury to the arcuate ligament.

Conservative treatment of grade III posterolateral corner injuries is not recommended, especially where combined with cruciate insufficiencies, because disabling instability or "functional disability" will result.[85, 108] Grade II posterolateral corner injuries may do well when treated conservatively. Kannus reported 11 patients with grade II sprains after an average of 8 years following injury. Nine of the 11 had returned to activities at pre-injury levels, none had progressed in their degree of postinjury instability, and none had gone on to osteoarthritis by radiographic examination.[85] In the 12 patients with grade III sprains to the posterolateral corner treated conservatively, the results were much poorer. Two lateral meniscectomies between injury and follow-up had been perfomed, 9 of 12 had to decrease their activity level, and 2 had to change occupations. Fol-

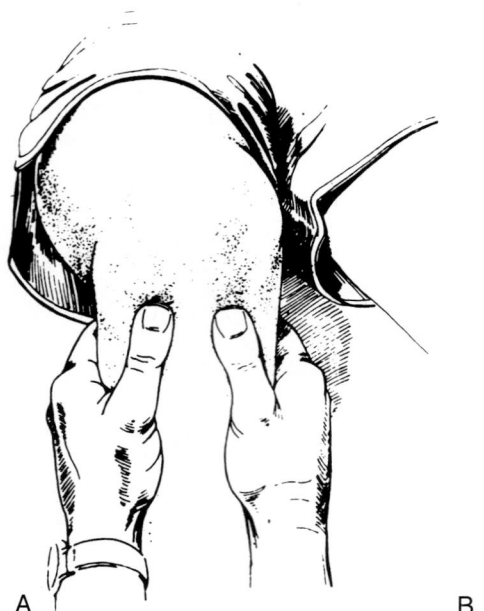
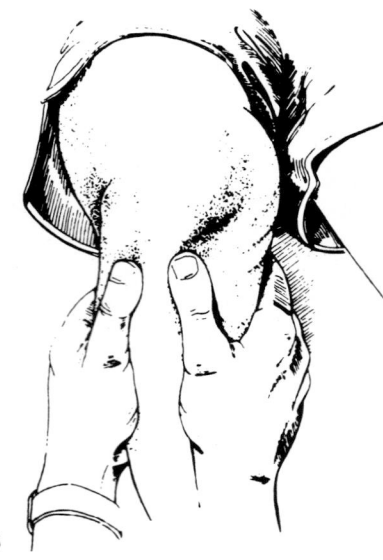

Figure 28I2–12. Posterolateral drawer test. *A,* A posteriorly directed force is applied to the proximal tibia with the knee in 90 degrees of flexion. *B,* In a positive test, the lateral tibial plateau subluxates posteriorly on the femoral condyle. (From Hughston JC, Norwood LA: The posterolateral drawer test and external rotation recurvatum test for posterolateral rotatory instability of the knee. Clin Orthop 147:82, 1980.)

A   B

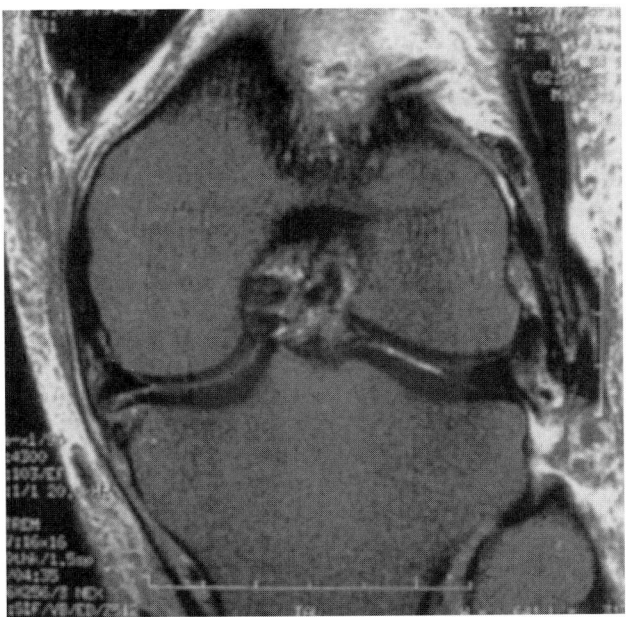

Figure 28I2–13. Magnetic resonance image of the knee demonstrating a complex posterolateral corner injury. Note the lateral collateral ligament and biceps tendon tears. (From Shelbourne KD, Klootwyk TE: Low-velocity knee dislocation with sports injuries. Treatment principles. Clin Sports Med 19:443–456, 2000.)

low-up knee instabilities were mild to severe. Half showed development of post-traumatic osteoarthritis by radiographic examination. In Torg's report of 29 patients with combined multidirectional instability including PCL disruption, at a mean 5 years' follow-up, 14 patients had good or excellent functional results. They returned to their prior level of sporting activity with only occasional mild instability. Fifteen patients had fair or poor functional results, experiencing an inability to return to pre-injury sports because of frequent pain or instability or significant discomfort with activities of daily living. In this latter group of unreconstructed knees in patients with fair or poor function, over half had moderate radiographic evidence of osteoarthritis.[108]

For grade III posterolateral corner injuries, reconstruction of the posterolateral corner or PCL, or both, is recom-

mended (Fig. 28I2–13). Because most posterolateral corner injuries include injuries to elements of the arcuate complex, advancement of this complex as a single unit has been advocated by many. After determination that the insertions of the fibular collateral and fabellofibular ligaments on the fibula as well as the attachment of the mid–third capsular ligament on the tibia are all intact, repair of individual structures that are torn should be performed. Following repairs, advancement of the arcuate complex proximally on the posterolateral femur with a bone block has been described by many.[5, 46, 80] For those injuries accompanied by distal tears, autograft or allograft reconstructions of the posterolateral corner may be the best form of treatment.[80]

Discoid Lateral Meniscus

Approximately 3% of people of western European descent and up to 17% of persons of Korean and Japanese descent may have discoid lateral menisci.[48, 60] These often present with a "snapping" knee, though pain and loss of motion are the more common symptoms.[2, 7, 23, 37, 81, 118] The discoid meniscus may be complete, incomplete, or a Wrisberg-type, as described by Watanabe (Fig. 28I2–14).[119] The complete discoid meniscus may cover the whole lateral tibial plateau, with posterior extensions down the proximal tibia. The incomplete discoid lateral meniscus may have some central and medial tibial plateau left uncovered, though the margins of the meniscus are typically described as much larger than those of a normal meniscus. The Wrisberg-type is a more normally shaped meniscus that lacks the usual posterior attachments to the tibial plateau inasmuch as the posterior half of the coronary ligament normally found medial and lateral to the popliteal hiatus is missing. This produces a more mobile lateral meniscus, allowing anterior subluxation of the posterior horn of the lateral meniscus. The meniscofemoral ligament(s) would be the only stabilizing structures for this type of meniscus, loosely fixing the posterior horn to the posterior femur.

The origin of discoid menisci is not certain. It was incorrectly labeled "a persistent fetal state" by Smillie in 1948. Gray and Kaplan have shown that at no time during normal fetal development are the medial or lateral meniscus discoid in shape.[33, 55] Kaplan has hypothesized that the

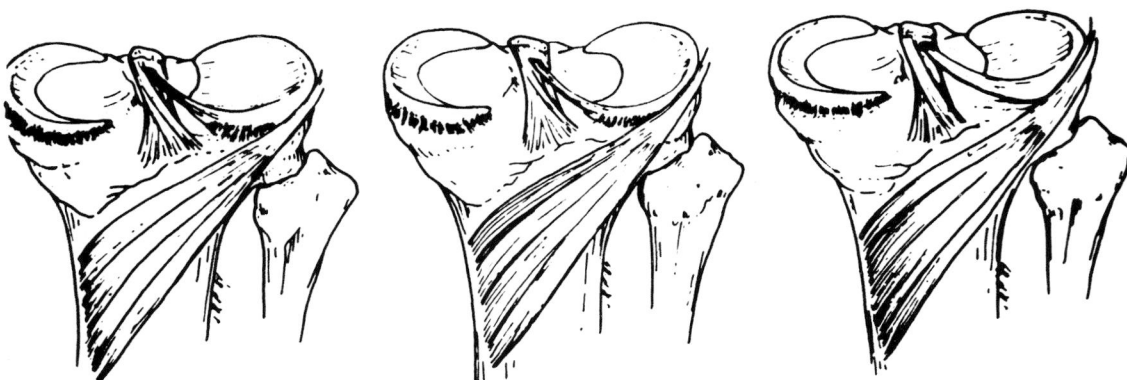

Figure 28I2–14. Three types of discoid lateral meniscus have been described: complete (*left*), incomplete (*center*), and Wrisberg's (*right*).

discoid shape is a result of response to stimulation seen with hypermobility. However, this explanation reveals only part of the story because many discoid menisci are not hypermobile, having adequate posterior attachments. The shape may merely represent a congenital malformation of the meniscus.[121] A history of minor trauma with a painful stiff knee and positive provocative tests for meniscal injury should suggest the diagnosis of discoid meniscus. The diagnostic test of choice is MRI.[98] It has sensitivity and specificity for discoid menisci of better than 80%. Though arthrography has been used with good success in the past, it is an unnecessarily invasive test with the availability of such excellent imaging alternatives as MRI (Fig. 28I2–15).[35]

Treatment of the symptomatic discoid meniscus should begin with a trial of conservative management. Quadriceps and hamstring strengthening with avoidance of hyperflexion or flexion and rotation may allow for symptoms to subside. A return to prior activity may then be attempted. Persistent mechanical symptoms, loss of motion causing a limp or limiting activity would be indications to proceed cautiously with arthroscopy. "Caution" is the best word to guide any thought of operative treatment of the symptomatic discoid meniscus.[99] Débridement of torn and incarcerated fragments of meniscus may help reduce symptoms. Saucerization has been described by multiple authors as a method of converting the discoid meniscus to a more normal—and, it is hoped, less problematic—shape.[24, 29, 113, 121] Often, discoid menisci are noted to have horizontal cleavage tears resulting in a degree of instability that may be reduced by resection of either the inferior or superior leaves, together with saucerization.[4] Hayashi has reported that maintaining a rim of only 6 to 8 mm at the periphery

of the meniscus minimizes the risk of reoperation.[37] Suture fixation of a subluxating posterior horn has been reported, with good short-term success.[81, 121] Total lateral meniscectomy has been described as having the best results for discoid lateral menisci, though follow-up into adulthood is rarely seen in these studies. Total meniscectomy in children is likely a short-term fix at best, with pain, early osteoarthritis, instability, and cutback in activities often seen in adults who underwent meniscectomy as children.[1, 70, 114, 122] Aichroth described a regenerated meniscal rim after total meniscectomy on check-back arthroscopies in two of five patients, though it is not clear that such remnants would perform any of the normal meniscal functions.[2]

Meniscal Injuries or Abnormalities on the Lateral Side of the Knee

Meniscal Tear

Mechanisms of Injury and Physical Examination

Though relatively uncommon in comparison with the frequency of this injury in adults, numerous studies and case reports describe meniscal tears in the skeletally immature. Unlike adults, however, the frequency of lateral meniscal tears may be more on the order of the frequency of medial tears.[1, 75, 87, 94, 114, 120, 122] The mechanisms of injury for lateral meniscal tears may include longitudinal loading of a flexed knee that is undergoing simultaneous torsional stress. Acute tear of a lateral meniscus with anterior cruci-

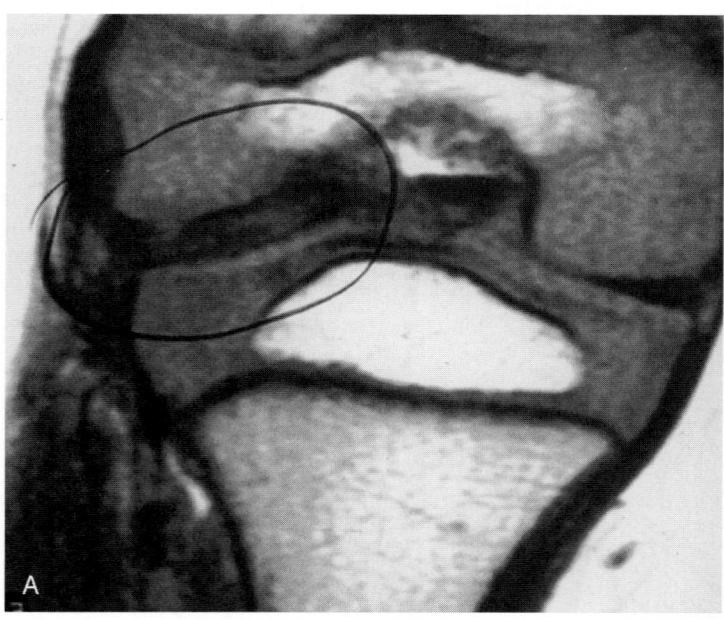

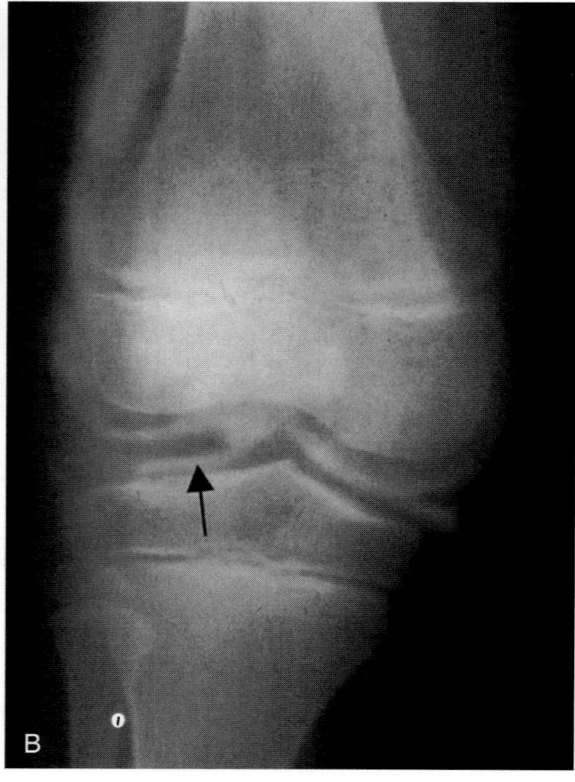

Figure 28I2–15. *A,* Magnetic resonance image of the knee demonstrating a discoid lateral meniscus. *B,* Arthrogram of the knee demonstrating a discoid lateral meniscus *(arrow).*

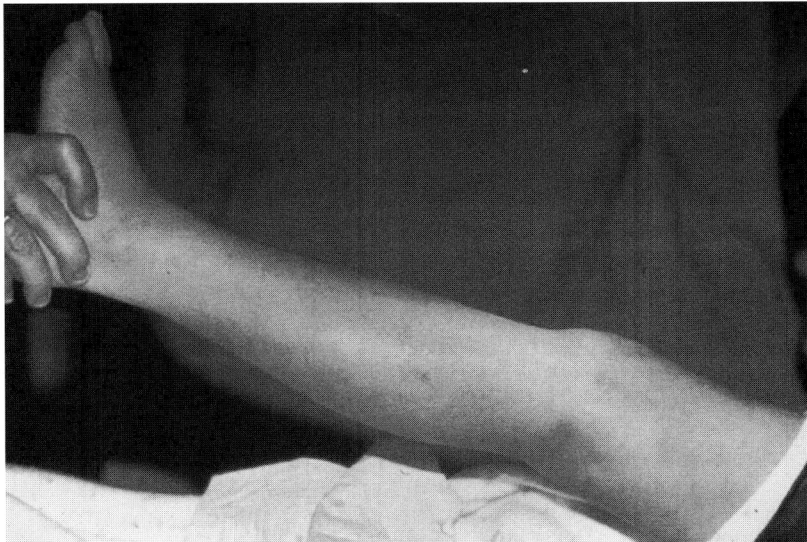

Figure 28I2–16. The lack of full extension is a typical finding in patients with a discoid meniscus.

ate and medial collateral ligament disruptions has been described as resulting from a severe valgus stress on an athlete's knee. It is not uncommon, however, for there to be no recollection of an inciting traumatic event for children, especially if they are under age 13 years.[76] Meniscal injury is often followed by the development of an acute effusion. Mechanical symptoms, such as locking, popping, catching, or giving way are often noted in the history of a meniscal injury. A loss of motion is the hallmark of a knee with a meniscal tear; it may be noted in the history as well as the physical examination. The most common complaint in this group is of pain.[94, 114, 122]

On examination, an effusion may be palpable. Examination of both knees while the heels are held at the same level up off of the examination table may reveal a loss of extension (Fig. 28I2–16). Marked anterior discomfort with this test may suggest an incarcerated meniscus. Likewise, a loss of full flexion would be suspicious for meniscal injury, especially if the extreme of flexion is accompanied by discomfort. Joint line tenderness is typically seen with meniscal injury.[83, 114, 122] Pain with valgus stress may signify a lateral meniscal tear, whereas marked opening with valgus stress may not only be suspicious of an MCL injury, but a medial meniscal tear as well. Rotational maneuvers while flexing or extending the knee, with the examiner's fingers along the joint line, may reproduce popping or painful catching in the knee with a meniscal injury. These tests may be performed sitting (Steinman's test), supine (McMurray's test) or prone (Apley's grind test). Younger patients with meniscal tears may not respond to these provocative tests, however.[83]

Imaging Studies and Treatment Options

A variety of imaging techniques may be useful in working up the patient suspected of having a lateral meniscal tear. An unusual widening along the lateral joint line in a

weight-bearing anteroposterior radiograph of the knee may suggest a lateral meniscal tear. Arthrograms have been employed to detect meniscal tears, though this test may not be as sensitive as MRI (Fig. 28I2–17). In athletes of unspecified ages, MRI has been shown to have sensitivity of between 50% and 96%, specificity of 80% to 98%, and accuracy of between 78% and 94% for the detection of lateral meniscal tears.[6, 26, 49, 52, 56, 69, 77, 84] In children, three studies (each with populations under 30 patients in number) revealed MRI to have sensitivities of 50% to 100% and specificities of 45% to 95% for unspecified meniscal injuries.[62, 125] Again, MRI performed without good clinical

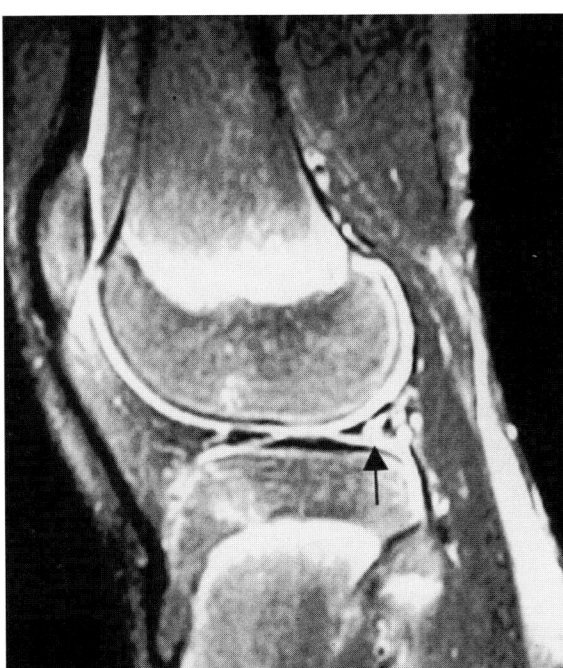

Figure 28I2–17. Magnetic resonance image of the knee demonstrating a lateral meniscus tear (*arrow*).

suspicion of a meniscal injury is less specific than that performed in the setting of a lateral knee injury consistent with a lateral meniscal tear.[12] This is especially important when treating the skeletally immature because a higher incidence of grade 3 signal changes has been noted in asymptomatic children (60% of patients younger than 13 years of age, 30% older than 14 years of age) than has been reported in asymptomatic adults (25%).[64, 65, 105] Diagnostic arthroscopy is an excellent technique for the detection of meniscal tears, and is currently the gold standard against which all other techniques are compared.

Treatment options for the skeletally immature with meniscal injury are evolving slowly. Many early papers on discoid meniscus and meniscal tears in children advocated total meniscectomy as a simple, effective treatment with few sequelae.[2, 37, 48, 87, 118] Aichroth noted a pseudomeniscus or small peripheral rim on three of four second-look arthroscopies after total lateral meniscectomy for a discoid meniscus, suggesting some degree of regenerative potential for children undergoing a meniscectomy.[2] However, many long-term follow-up studies have cautioned against total meniscectomy in children.[1, 10, 70, 114, 122, 123] Adults who underwent meniscectomy as children often experience an increased incidence of mechanical symptoms in the knee as well as knee instability.[1, 114, 122] Radiographs of such patients often show the Fairbanks changes associated with osteoarthritis: flattening and widening of the femoral condyle as well as narrowing of the joint line.[25] As a result, current recommendations for the treatment of meniscal tears in children are to preserve whatever meniscus is salvageable through repair, performing limited partial meniscectomies when absolutely necessary. Mintzer has shown excellent outcomes 5 years after repair of meniscal tears in patients younger than 17 years of age, suggesting that higher rates of healing can be obtained in children than adults.[75] In the setting of an ACL deficiency undergoing reconstruction, meniscal tears in children deserve an attempt at repair, when feasible.[8, 117] Certainly all red-on-red and red-on-white tears in isolation deserve an attempt at repair in children. Repair techniques are similar to those employed in adults, including inside-out and outside-in arthroscopic methods, as well as the use of limited-open techniques (Fig. 28I2–18).[8, 16] The results of meniscal repairs in chil-

dren have been good, with the best results seen in the setting of an ACL reconstruction.[90] Arthroscopic partial meniscectomy, when repair is not an option, has the advantages of quicker rehabilitation, shorter hospital stay, fewer complications, and better subjective functional results when compared with total meniscectomy.[38, 72]

A laboratory study in dogs showed that leaving a torn meniscus untreated has fewer sequelae for the affected knee than does a total meniscectomy. Weiss and Dehaven outline a number of criteria for leaving meniscal tears without partial excision or repair: Vertical longitudinal tears and partial-thickness split tears may all be observed if stable with probing. It is unclear whether radial tears 5 mm in length or less would do better with observation or débridement.

Physeal Fractures about the Lateral Knee

Mechanisms of Injury and Physical Examination

Physeal fractures about the knee are not uncommon, constituting about 1% of all pediatric fractures.[9] High-energy trauma (as seen in motor vehicle collisions, pedestrian or bicycle versus car accidents) is typically the cause, with the distal femoral or proximal tibial physis failing before failure of surrounding ligaments. Concomitant ligament injury in the presence of physeal fracture can occur, however, and may be overlooked.[9, 14, 103] On the femoral side, the fabellofibular ligament, lateral collateral ligament, MCL, ACL, and PCL all attach to the distal femoral epiphysis. Thus strong forces across the distal femur would be more likely to cause failure across the weak physis than through the stronger ligaments, commonly producing Salter-Harris type II and III fractures of the distal femur. On the tibial side, these ligaments attach to the epiphyseal proximal tibia, except for the superficial MCL, which attaches to the metaphyseal proximal tibia. Again, failure through the weaker proximal tibial physis may produce tibial spine avulsion fractures, or Salter-Harris I, II, III, or IV fractures of the proximal tibia.

Diagnosis and Treatment

Obtaining a history of the traumatic event is critical in establishing a mechanism of injury, which often suggests the diagnosis. After examination of the uninjured extremity is performed to establish baseline physiologic laxity, a careful examination of the injured extremity is conducted and should include observation, palpation, and mild stress testing. Initial examination need not include ranging of the injured limb. Any deformity noted is suggestive of fracture. A marked effusion within the first 24 hours suggests fracture or a major intra-articular injury.[36, 102] Palpation should include the course of the MCL, the joint lines, the physes, and the metaphyseal regions above and below the knees. Sites of tenderness suggest injury. Determination of the distal neurovascular status is essential because popliteal artery injuries can occur with fractures about the knee.[83, 92]

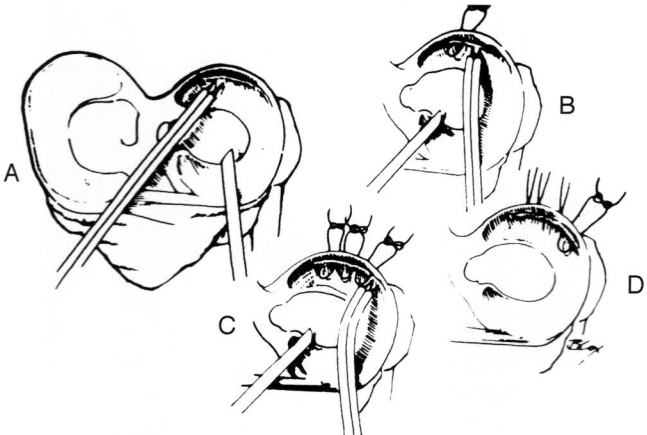

Figure 28I2–18. *A* to *D*, Repair techniques in children parallel those used in adults. This drawing demonstrates the arthroscopic inside-out technique.

In the absence of gross deformity and with a low suspicion for fracture, careful stress testing can be performed after biplanar radiographs are obtained. The abduction and adduction stress tests performed with the hip in mild extension and the knee in both full extension and 30 degrees of flexion should be attempted. If not tolerated by the patient, aspiration of hemarthrosis followed by sterile injection of a local anesthetic may make the examination more tolerable. The presence of fat in the bloody aspirate is suggestive of fracture. Stress radiographs may then be performed more comfortably, under the direction of and with the participation of the examining physician. A general anesthetic may be optimal for performing stress radiography. If the diagnosis remains unclear, diagnostic arthroscopy or MRI of the knee may be employed.

Treatment of fractures must include stabilization. Extraphyseal fractures may be treated nonoperatively as long as minimal displacement and angulation exist. Splinting followed by long-leg casting or single leg hip-spica casting may provide adequate immobilization for healing. The most common distal femoral physeal fractures are Salter-Harris II and III fractures, though all five types of Salter-Harris fractures may occur about the knee (Fig. 28I2–19).[86, 92] Growth arrests in these physeal fractures about the knee are common; thus an anatomic reduction should be sought and careful follow-up pursued.[86] For Salter-Harris II fractures with adequate metaphyseal spikes, extraphyseal fixation of the metaphyseal fragment with screws or Kirschner wires may be adequate. If the fragment is small, smooth Kirschner wires crossing the physis may be necessary, to be removed at approximately 4 weeks after injury. For Salter-Harris type III fractures, anatomic reduction and

fixation of the epiphyseal fragment with purely epiphyseal screws is optimal.

Fractures of the proximal tibia may be purely metaphyseal or may extend into the physis. Salter-Harris I and II fractures of the proximal tibia are not uncommon. Displacement with these fractures can lead to popliteal artery injury and require careful evaluation. Any hint of abnormal arterial function after reduction of these fractures, by such tests as ankle-brachial indices compared with the noninjured side, suggests the need for angiography to better study the vascular inflow to the leg. Treatment of these proximal tibial physeal fractures should include anatomic reduction and stabilization with smooth pins that cross the physis, to be removed in 4–6 weeks. The risk of growth disturbance is high, approaching 40% in two studies.[88] Valgus alignment from overgrowth of the proximal medial tibia also commonly occurs after complete and greenstick fractures of the proximal tibial metaphysis.[88] Once apparent, the safest treatment for the malalignment is probably observation because the deformity may slowly correct over a number of years.[124] For the child approaching skeletal maturity with persistent valgus deformity, medial proximal tibial epiphysiodesis may be an appropriate treatment alternative. Osteotomy of the proximal tibia in the face of valgus overgrowth commonly results in recurrence of the deformity, and is not recommended.[88]

Iliotibial Band Friction Syndrome

Though more commonly seen in adult runners, skiers, bicyclists, and military personnel, iliotibial band friction syndrome has been seen in adolescent patients performing similar activities.[18, 63, 85, 104] Pain in the region of the lateral femoral epicondyle is a common complaint, often occurring after a sudden change in a training program. As the iliotibial band inserts on Gerdy's tubercle of the anterolateral proximal tibial, a knee in 30 degrees of flexion maximizes contact between the iliotibial band and the lateral condyle of the distal femur.[79] A positive Ober's test combined with marked tenderness about the lateral epicondyle of the distal femur would support the diagnosis (Fig. 28I2–20). Ober's test is performed with the patient in the decubitus postion having the affected leg up. The affected hip and knee are flexed to 90 degrees; the hip is then abducted and extended. From this position, adduction of the hip is difficult in a patient with a tight iliotibial band.[91]

Treatment of iliotibial band friction syndrome is conservative in most cases. Rest, a change in training regimen, use of nonsteroidal anti-inflammatory drugs and local modalities such as ice, and stretching of a tight iliotibial band are all useful elements of a treatment program. Injections of steroids may also provide relief in recalcitrant cases. In a report of treatment of over 2000 cases of iliotibial friction band syndrome, Aronen reported better than 99% resolution from a two-phase approach to treatment. The first phase focused on modalities and rest, lasting approximately 3 days, and the second phase focused on gradual return to activity.[3]

When conservative treatment fails, a surgical approach may be adopted. Martens described resection of a triangular

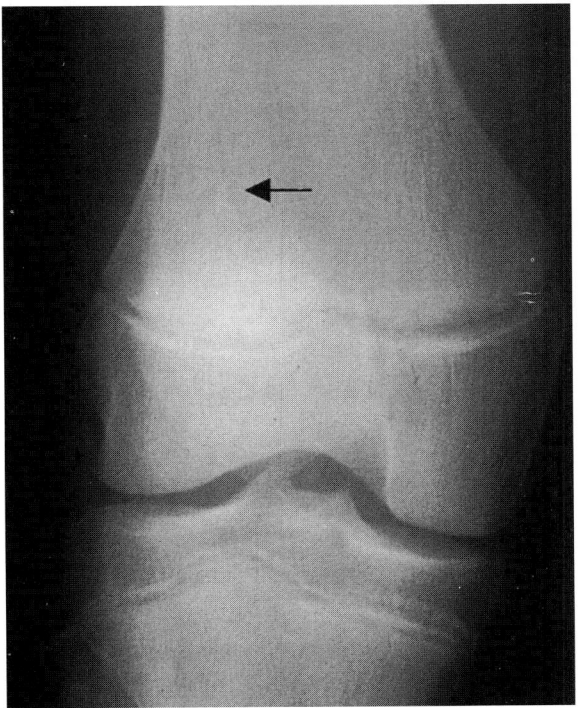

Figure 28I2–19. Salter II fractures that are minimally displaced, such as this one (*arrow*), can be treated with immobilization in a cast.

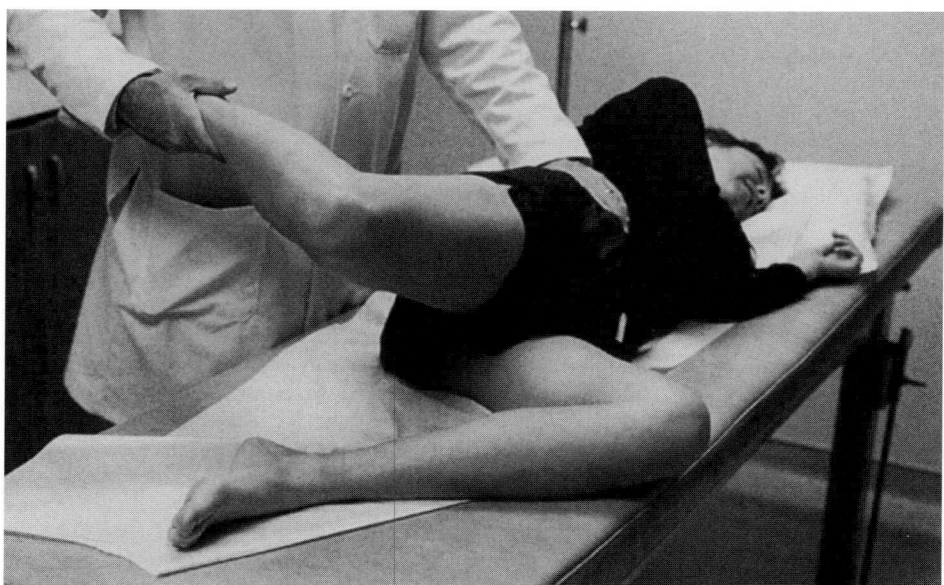

Figure 28I2–20. Ober's test. The patient is placed in the decubitus position with the affected side up. The affected hip and knee are then flexed. From this position, the hip is then abducted and extended and is allowed to adduct. If the iliotibial band is tight, it will be difficult to adduct the hip below a neutral position. (From Safran MR, Fu FH: Uncommon causes of knee pain in the athlete. Orthop Clin North Am 26:547–559, 1995.)

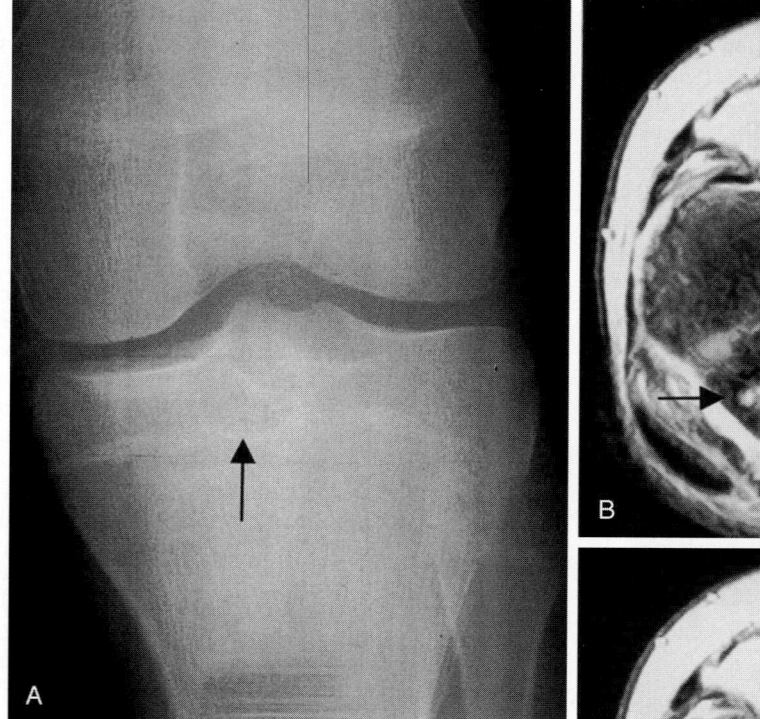

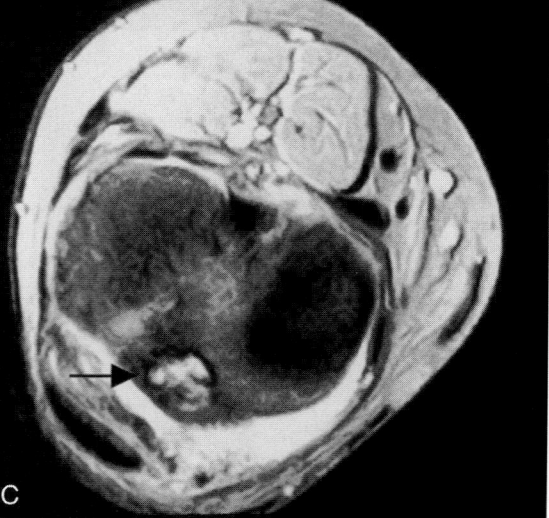

Figure 28I2–21. A, Anteroposterior radiograph of the knee in a 15-year-old athlete who presented with knee pain. Note the lytic lesion in the proximal tibial epiphysis (*arrow*). B and C, Magnetic resonance imaging shows a discrete lesion contained within the epiphysis (*arrows*). Final pathologic examination demonstrated a chondroblastoma.

segment of the posterior portion of the iliotibial band in the region of the lateral femoral epicondyle in 23 patients with resistant iliotibial band friction syndrome. Return to activities averaged 7 weeks, and all returned to their previous level of sports activity.[71] Nobel, Aronen, and Holmes each described similar procedures with uniformly good results.[3, 40, 79]

Conditions about the Knee Mimicking Trauma

The prevalence of truly sports-related injuries to the knee vastly outnumbers that of the following conditions,

which may mimic trauma. However, delaying the diagnosis in the case of a tumorous condition or a slipped capital femoral epiphysis may be disastrous. Both Joyce and Lewis have written about tumors of the lower extremity that were initially diagnosed as sports-related injuries.[53, 67] A common theme among the patient histories in both studies was of an initial traumatic event followed by persistent or intermittent symptoms about the knee, which did not include mechanical symptoms. Joyce and Mankin describe how careful physical examination and plain films including the joint above and below the knee would have suggested a nontraumatic condition in 75% of their patients, all of whom proceeded to unnecessary arthroscopy (Fig. 28I2–21). They

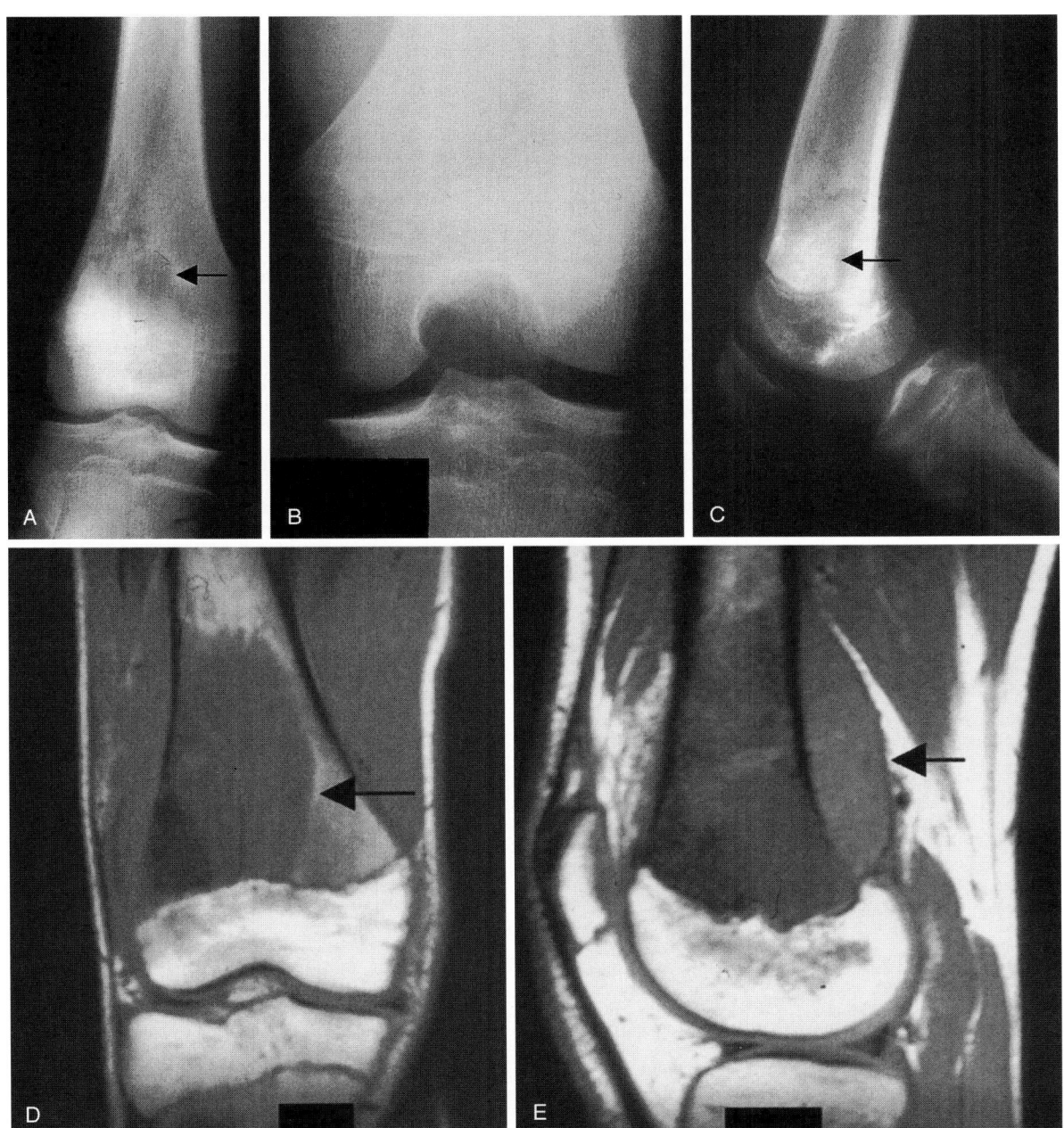

Figure 28I2–22. *A* to *C,* Anteroposterior and lateral images of a metaphyseal lesion in the distal femur (*arrows*) of a 15-year-old with knee pain. *D* and *E,* Magnetic resonance imaging demonstrates the extensive metaphyseal involvement (*arrows*) as well as soft tissue extension posteriorly. Final pathologic diagnosis was osteosarcoma.

also caution against using an arthroscope for biopsy of extrasynovial lesions, as such biopsies may contaminate the knee joint as they cross into a new compartment. Lewis and Reilly described 36 patients who presented to their primary physicians with orthopaedic problems from what appeared to be sports-related injuries (Fig. 28I2–22). Fifty percent of these patients were found to have malignant lesions about the knee. Seventy percent of this group had undergone either arthroscopy, arthrography, or both before their diagnosis of the malignant tumor.

Pain referred to the knee may arise from pathology in the mid-shaft of the femur or the hip joint. Two of Joyce and Mankin's patients had tumors found far from the knee, in the diaphyseal femur. After radiographs of the affected limbs were repeated to include the diaphyseal femur, the diagnoses were made.

Afflictions of the hip joint commonly present as knee pain, though typically medial pain as opposed to lateral. Preadolescents must always undergo a careful hip examination to rule out hip disease, of which slipped capital femoral epiphysis or Legg-Calvé-Perthes disease would be two of the more common hip pathologies masquerading as a knee injury. The findings on examination would include loss of medial rotation for those with a slipped capital femoral epiphysis, and loss of abduction as well as medial rotation with discomfort at the extremes of motion for those with Perthes disease. Again, obtaining radiographs that include the joint above and joint below would help ensure that the correct diagnosis is made. Patients with a history of steroid therapy as part of a cancer chemotherapy regimen or treatment of an autoimmune condition should be examined carefully for osteonecrosis of the hip and or knee because each of these conditions may present as knee pain.

References

1. Abdon P, Turner MS, Pettersson H, et al: A long-term follow-up study of total meniscectomy in children. Clin Orthop 257:166–170, 1990.
2. Aichroth PM, Patel DV, Marx CL: Congenital discoid lateral meniscus in children. A follow-up study and evolution of management. J Bone Joint Surg Br 73:932–936, 1991.
3. Aronen J, et al: Practical conservative management of iliotibial band syndrome. Physician Sportsmed 21:59–69, 1993.
4. Auge WK II, Kaeding CC: Bilateral discoid medial menisci with extensive intrasubstance cleavage tears: MRI and arthroscopic correlation. Arthroscopy 10:313–318, 1994.
5. Baker C, Norwood L, Hughston J: Acute posterolateral instability of the knee. J Bone Joint Surg Am 65:614–618, 1983.
6. Barronian AD, Zoltan JD, Bucon KA: Magnetic resonance imaging of the knee: Correlation with arthroscopy. Arthroscopy 5:187–191, 1989.
7. Bellier G, Dupont JY, Larrain M, et al: Lateral discoid menisci in children. Arthroscopy 5:52–56, 1989.
8. Belzer JP, Cannon WD Jr: Meniscus tears: Treatment in the stable and unstable knee. J Am Acad Orthop Surg 1:41–47, 1993.
9. Bertin KC, Goble EM: Ligament injuries associated with physeal fractures about the knee. Clin Orthop 177:188–195, 1983.
10. Bhaduri T, Glass A: Meniscectomy in children. Injury 3:176–178, 1972.
11. Bianchi M: Acute tears of the posterior cruciate ligament: Clinical study and results of operative treatment in 27 cases. Am J Sports Med 11:308–314, 1983.
12. Boden SD, Davis DO, Dina TS, et al: A prospective and blinded investigation of magnetic resonance imaging of the knee. Abnormal findings in asymptomatic subjects. Clin Orthop 282:177–185, 1992.
13. Bright RW: Physeal injuries. In Rockwood CA Jr, Wilkins KE, King RE (eds): Fractures in Children. Philadelphia, JB Lippincott, 1991, pp 87–146.
14. Burkhart SS, Peterson HA: Fractures of the proximal tibial epiphysis. J Bone Joint Surg Am 61:996–1002, 1979.
15. Burks RT: Gross anatomy. In Daniel DM (ed): Knee Ligaments: Structure, Function, Injury, and Repair. New York, Raven Press, 1990, pp 59–76.
16. Cannon WD Jr, Morgan CD: Meniscal repair: Arthroscopic repair techniques. Instr Course Lect 43:77–96, 1994.
17. Clancy WG Jr, et al: Treatment of knee joint instability secondary to rupture of the posterior cruciate ligament. Report of a new procedure. J Bone Joint Surg Am 65:310–322, 1983.
18. Colson J, Armour W: Sports Injuries and Their Treatment. Philadelphia, JB Lippincott, 1961.
19. Cook PC, Leit ME: Issues in the pediatric athlete. Orthop Clin North Am 26:453–464, 1995.
20. Arnoczky SP, Grewe SR, Paulos LE, et al: Instability of the anterior and posterior cruciate ligaments. Instr Course Lect 40:199–270, 1991.
21. Daniel DM, Stone ML, Barnett P, Sachs R: Use of the quadriceps active test to diagnose posterior cruciate-ligament disruption and measure posterior laxity of the knee. J Bone Joint Surg Am 70:386–391, 1988.
22. DeLee JC, Riley MB, Rockwood CA Jr: Acute posterolateral rotatory instability of the knee. Am J Sports Med 11:199–207, 1983.
23. Dickhaut SC, DeLee JC: The discoid lateral-meniscus syndrome. J Bone Joint Surg Am 64:1068–1073, 1982.
24. Dimakopoulos P, Patel D: Partial excision of discoid meniscus. Arthroscopic operation of 10 patients. Acta Orthop Scand 61:40–41, 1990.
25. Fairbank TJ: Knee joint changes after meniscectomy. J Bone Joint Surg Br 30:664–670, 1948.
26. Fischer SP, Fox JM, Del Pizzo W, et al: Accuracy of diagnoses from magnetic resonance imaging of the knee. A multi-center analysis of one thousand and fourteen patients. J Bone Joint Surg Am 73:2–10, 1991.
27. Fleissner PR, Eilert RE: Discoid lateral meniscus. Am J Knee Surg 12:125–131, 1999.
28. Frank C, Strother R: Isolated posterior cruciate ligament injury in a child: Literature review and a case report. Can J Surg 32:373–374, 1989.
29. Fujikawa K, Iseki F, Mikura Y: Partial resection of the discoid meniscus in the child's knee. J Bone Joint Surg Br 63:391–395, 1981.
30. Girgis FG, Marshall JL, Monajem A: The cruciate ligaments of the knee joint. Anatomical functional and experimental analysis. Clin Orthop 106:216–231, 1975.
31. Gollehon DL, Torzilli PA, Warren RF: The role of the posterolateral and cruciate ligaments in the stability of the human knee. A biomechanical study. J Bone Joint Surg Am 69:233–242, 1987.
32. Goodrich A, Ballard A: Posterior cruciate ligament avulsion associated with ipsilateral femur fracture in a 10-year-old child. J Trauma 28:1393–1396, 1988.
33. Gray DJ, Gardner E: Prenatal development of the human knee and superior tibiofibular joints. Am J Anat 86:235, 1950.
34. Grood ES, Stowers SF, Noyes FR: Limits of movement in the human knee. Effect of sectioning the posterior cruciate ligament and posterolateral structures. J Bone Joint Surg Am 70:88–97, 1988.
35. Hall FM: Arthrography of the discoid lateral meniscus. AJR Am J Roentgenol 128:993–1002, 1977.
36. Harvell JC Jr, Fu FH, Stanitski CL: Diagnostic arthroscopy of the knee in children and adolescents. Orthopedics 12:1555–1560, 1989.
37. Hayashi LK, Yamaga H, Ida K, Miura T: Arthroscopic meniscectomy for discoid lateral meniscus in children. J Bone Joint Surg Am 70:1495–1500, 1988.
38. Hede A, Larsen E, Sandberg H: The long term outcome of open total and partial meniscectomy related to the quantity and site of the meniscus removed. Int Orthop 16:122–125, 1992.
39. Heller L, Langman J: The menisco-femoral ligaments of the human knee. J Bone Joint Surg Br 46:307–313, 1964.
40. Holmes JC, Pruitt AL, Whalen NJ: Iliotibial band syndrome in cyclists. Am J Sports Med 21:419–424, 1993.

41. Hosen: Gray's Anatomy. Philadelphia, Lea & Febiger, 1950, pp 3–13.

42. Hughston JC: The importance of the posterior oblique ligament in repairs of acute tears of the medial ligaments in knees with and without an associated rupture of the anterior cruciate ligament. J Bone Joint Surg Am 76:1328–1344, 1994.

43. Hughston JC: The absent posterior drawer test in some acute posterior cruciate ligament tears of the knee. Am J Sports Med 16:39–43, 1988.

44. Hughston JC, Bowden JA, Andrews JR, Norwood LA: Acute tears of the posterior cruciate ligament. Results of operative treatment. J Bone Joint Surg Am 62:438–450, 1980.

45. Hughston JC, Degenhardt TC: Reconstruction of the posterior cruciate ligament. Clin Orthop 164:59–77, 1982.

46. Hughston JC, Jacobson KE: Chronic posterolateral rotary instability of the knee. J Bone Joint Surg Am 67:351–359, 1985.

47. Hughston JC, Norwood LA: The posterolateral drawer test and external rotational recurvatum test for posterolateral rotatory instability of the knee. Clin Orthop 147:82–87, 1980.

48. Ikeuchi H: Arthroscopic treatment of the discoid lateral meniscus. Technique and long-term results. Clin Orthop 167:19–28, 1982.

49. Imhoff A, Buess E, Hodler J, Fellmann J: Comparison between magnetic resonance imaging and arthroscopy for the diagnosis of knee meniscal lesions [in French]. Rev Chir Orthop Reparatrice Appar Mot 83:229–236, 1997.

50. Insall JN, Hood RW: Bone-block transfer of the medial head of the gastrocnemius for posterior cruciate insufficiency. J Bone Joint Surg Am 64:691–699, 1982.

51. Jacobsen K: Stress radiographical measurements of post-traumatic knee instability. A clinical study. Acta Orthop Scand 48:301–310, 1977.

52. Jerosch J, Lahm A, Castro WH, Assheuer J: Nuclear magnetic resonance and computerized tomography in meniscus injuries of the knee joint. Unfallchirurg 94:53–58, 1991.

53. Joyce MJ, Mankin HJ: Caveat arthroscopos: Extra-articular lesions of bone simulating intra-articular pathology. J Bone Joint Surg Am 65:289–292, 1983.

54. Kannus P, Jarvinen M: Knee ligament injuries in adolescents. Eight-year follow-up of conservative management. J Bone Joint Surg Br 70:772–776, 1988.

55. Kaplan EB: Discoid lateral meniscus of the knee joint. J Bone Joint Surg Am 39:77–87, 1957.

56. Kelly MA, Flock TJ, Kimmel JA, et al: MR imaging of the knee: Clarification of its role. Arthroscopy 7:78–85, 1991.

57. Kim SJ, Shin SJ, Kim HK, et al: Comparison of 1- and 2-incision posterior cruciate ligament reconstructions. Arthroscopy 16:268–78, 2000.

58. Kim SJ, Min BH, Han DY: Paradoxical phenomena of the McMurray test: An arthroscopic investigation. Am J Sports Med 24:83–87, 1996.

59. Kim SJ, Kim HK, Kim HJ: Arthroscopic posterior cruciate ligament reconstruction using a one-incision technique. Clin Orthop 359:156–166, 1999.

60. Kim SJ, Kim DW, Min B: Discoid lateral meniscus associated with anomolous insertion of the medial meniscus. Clin Orthop 315:234–237, 1995.

61. King A: Meniscal lesions in children and adolescents: A review of the pathology and clinical presentation. Injury 15:105–108, 1983.

62. King SJ, Carty ML, Brady O: Magnetic resonance imaging of knee injuries in children. Pediatr Radiol 26:287–290, 1996.

63. Kirk KL, Kuklo T, Klemme W: Iliotibial band friction syndrome. Orthopedics 23:1209–1214, 2000.

64. Kornick J, Trefelner E, McCarthy S, et al: Meniscal abnormalities in the asymptomatic population at MR imaging. Radiology 177:463–465, 1990.

65. LaPrade RF, Burnett QM, Veenstra MA, et al: The prevalence of abnormal magnetic resonance imaging findings in asymptomatic knees. With correlation of magnetic resonance imaging to arthroscopic findings in symptomatic knees. Am J Sports Med 22:739–745, 1994.

66. LaPrade RF, Terry GC: Injuries to the posterolateral aspect of the knee. Am J Sports Med 25:433–438, 1997.

67. Lewis MM, Reilly JF: Sports tumors. Am J Sports Med 15:362–365, 1987.

68. Makris CA, Georgoulis AD, Papageorgiou CD, et al: Posterior cruciate ligament architecture: Evaluation under microsurgical dissection. Arthroscopy 16:627–632, 2000.

69. Mandelbaum BR, Finerman GA, Reicher MA, et al: Magnetic resonance imaging as a tool for evaluation of traumatic knee injuries. Anatomical and pathoanatomical correlations. Am J Sports Med 14:361–370, 1986.

70. Manzione M, Pizzutillo PD, Peoples AB, et al: Meniscectomy in children: A long-term follow-up study. Am J Sports Med 11:111–115, 1983.

71. Martens M, Libbrecht P, Burssens A: Surgical treatment of the iliotibial band friction syndrome. Am J Sports Med 17:651–654, 1989.

72. McGinty JB, Geuss LF, Marvin RA: Partial or total meniscectomy; a comparative analysis. J Bone Joint Surg Am 59:763–766, 1977.

73. McMaster WC: Isolated posterior cruciate ligament injury: Literature review and case reports. J Trauma 15:1025–1029, 1975.

74. Meyers MH: Isolated avulsion of the tibial attachment of the posterior cruciate ligament of the knee. J Bone Joint Surg Am 57:669–672, 1975.

75. Mintzer CM, Richmond RC, Taylor JT: Meniscal repair in the young athlete. Am J Sports Med 26:630–633, 1998.

76. Morrissy R, Eubanks R, Park JP: Arthroscopy of the knee in children. Clin Orthop 162:103–107, 1982.

77. Muellner T, Weinstabl R, Schabus R, et al: The diagnosis of meniscal tears in athletes: A comparison of clinical and magnetic resonance imaging investigations. Am J Sports Med 25:7–12, 1997.

78. Neuschwander DC, Drez D, Finney T: Lateral meniscal variant with absence of the posterior coronary ligament. J Bone Joint Surg Am 74:1186–1190, 1992.

79. Noble CA: The treatment of iliotibial band friction syndrome. Br J Sports Med 13:51–54, 1979.

80. Noyes FR, Barber-Westin SD: Treatment of complex injuries involving the posterior cruciate and posterolateral ligaments of the knee. Am J Knee Surg 9:200–214, 1996.

81. Pellacci F, Montanari G, Prosperi P, et al: Lateral discoid meniscus: Treatment and results. Arthroscopy 8:526–530, 1992.

82. Raber DA, Freiderich NF, Hefti F: Discoid lateral meniscus n children: Long-term follow-up after total meniscectomy. J Bone Joint Surg Am 80:1579–1586, 1998.

83. Rang M: Children's Fractures. Philadelphia, JB Lippincott, 1974.

84. Raunest J, Oberle K, Loehnert J, et al: The clinical value of magnetic resonance imaging in the evaluation of meniscal disorders. J Bone Joint Surg Am 73:11–16, 1991.

85. Renne JW: The iliotibial band friction syndrome. J Bone Joint Surg Am 57:1110–1111, 1975.

86. Riseborough EJ, Barrett IR, Shapiro F: Growth disturbances following distal femoral physeal fracture-separations. J Bone Joint Surg Am 65:885–893, 1983.

87. Ritchie DM: Meniscectomy in children. Aust N Z J Surg 35:239–241, 1966.

88. Robert M, Khouri N, Carlioz H, et al: Fractures of the proximal tibial metaphysis in children: Review of a series of 25 cases. J Pediatr Orthop 7:444–449, 1987.

89. Ross AC, Chesterman PJ: Isolated avulsion of the tibial attachment of the posterior cruciate ligament in childhood. J Bone Joint Surg Br 68:747, 1986.

90. Rubman MH, Noyes FR, Barber-Westin SD: Arthroscopic repair of meniscal tears that extend into the avascular zone. Am J Sports Med 26:87–95, 1998.

91. Safran MR, Fu FH: Uncommon causes of knee pain in the athlete. Orthop Clin North Am 26:547–559, 1995.

92. Salter RB, Harris WR: Injuries involving the epiphyseal plate. J Bone Joint Surg Am 45:587–622, 1963.

93. Sanders W, Wilkins K, Neidre A: Acute insufficiency of the posterior cruciate ligament in children. J Bone Joint Surg Am 62:129–131, 1980.

94. Schlonsky J, Eyring EJ: Lateral meniscus tears in young children. Clin Orthop 97:117–118, 1973.

95. Seebacher JR, Inglis AE, Marshall JL, Warren RF: The structure of the posterolateral aspect of the knee. J Bone Joint Surg Am 64:536–541, 1982.

96. Shelbourne KD, Davis TJ, Patel DV: The natural history of acute, isolated, nonoperatively treated posterior cruciate ligament injuries. A prospective study. Am J Sports Med 27:276–283, 1999.

97. Shino K, Horibe S, Nakata K, et al: Conservative treatment of

isolated injuries to the posterior cruciate ligament in athletes. J Bone Joint Surg Br 77:895–900, 1995.

98. Silverman JM, Mink JH, Deutsch AL: Discoid menisci of the knee: MR imaging appearance. Radiology 173:351–354, 1989.

99. Smith CF, Van Dyk GE, Jurgutis J, Vangsness CT Jr: Cautious surgery for discoid menisci. Am J Knee Surg 12:25–28, 1999.

100. Speer KP, Spritzer CE, Goldner JL, et al: Magnetic resonance imaging of traumatic knee articular cartilage injuries. Am J Sports Med 19:396–402, 1991.

101. Stanitski CL: Correlation of arthroscopic and clinical examinations with magnetic resonance imaging findings of injured knees in children and adolescents. Am J Sports Med 26:743–744, 1998.

102. Stanitski C, Harvell JC, Fu F: Observations on acute knee hemarthrosis in children and adolescents. J Pediatr Orthop 13:506–510, 1993.

103. Sullivan JA: Ligamentous injuries of the knee in children. Clin Orthop 255:44–50, 1990.

104. Sutker A, Jackson D, Pagliano J: Iliotibial band syndrome in distance runners. Physician Sportsmed 9:69, 1981.

105. Takeda Y, Ikata T, Yoshida S, et al: MRI high-signal intensity in the menisci of asymptomatic children. J Bone Joint Surg Br 80:463–466, 1998.

106. Terry GC, LaPrade RF: The posterolateral aspect of the knee anatomy and surgical approach. Am J Sports Med 24:732–739, 1996.

107. Tria A: Ligaments of the Knee. New York, Churchill Livingstone, 1995.

108. Torg JS, et al: Natural history of the posterior cruciate ligament-deficient knee. Clin Orthop 246:209–216, 1989.

109. Torg JS, Conrad W, Kalen V: Clinical diagnosis of anterior cruciate ligament instability in the athlete. Am J Sports Med 4:84–93, 1976.

110. Torisu T: Avulsion fracture of the tibial attachment of the posterior cruciate ligament. Indications and results of delayed repair. Clin Orthop 143:107–114, 1979.

111. Torisu T: Isolated avulsion fracture of the tibial attachment of the posterior cruciate ligament. J Bone Joint Surg Am 59:68–72, 1977.

112. Trickey EL: Injuries to the posterior cruciate ligament: Diagnosis and treatment of early injuries and reconstruction of late instability. Clin Orthop 147:76–81, 1980.

113. Vahvanen V, Aalto K: Meniscectomy in children. Acta Orthop Scand 50:791–795, 1979.

114. Vandermeer RD, Cunningham FK: Arthroscopic treatment of the discoid lateral meniscus: Results of long-term follow-up. Arthroscopy 5:101–109, 1989.

115. Veltri DM, Deng XH, Torzilli PA, et al: The role of the cruciate and posterolateral ligaments in stability of the knee. A biomechanical study. Am J Sports Med 23:436–443, 1995.

116. Veltri DM, Warren RF: Isolated and combined posterior cruciate ligament injuries. J Am Acad Orthop Surg 1:67–75, 1993.

117. Warren RF: Meniscectomy and repair in the anterior cruciate ligament-deficient patient. Clin Orthop 252:55–63, 1990.

118. Washington ER, Root L, Liener UC: Discoid lateral meniscus in children. J Bone Joint Surg Am 77:1357–1360, 1995.

119. Watanabe M: Arthroscopy of the knee joint. In Helfet AJ (ed): Disorders of the Knee. Philadelphia, JB Lippincott, 1974, p 145.

120. Williams JS, Abate JA, Fadale PD, et al: Meniscal and nonosseus ACL injuries in children and adolescents. Am J Knee Surg 9:22–26, 1996.

121. Woods GW, Whelan JM: Discoid meniscus. Clin Sports Med 9:695–706, 1990.

122. Wroble RR, Henderson RC, Campion ER, et al: Meniscectomy in children and adolescents. Clin Orthop 279:180–189, 1992.

123. Zaman M, Leonard MA: Meniscectomy in children: A study of fifty-nine knees. J Bone Joint Surg Br 60:436–437, 1978.

124. Zionts LE, MacEwen GD: Spontaneous improvement of post-traumatic tibia valga. J Bone Joint Surg Am 68:680–687, 1986.

125. Zobel MS, Borrello JA, Siegel MJ, Stewart NR: Pediatric knee MR imaging: Pattern of injuries in the immature skeleton. Radiology 190:397–401, 1994.

Section J

Anterior Cruciate Ligament Injuries

1. ANTERIOR CRUCIATE LIGAMENT RECONSTRUCTION IN THE ADULT

Michael J. D'Amato, MD ■ Bernard R. Bach, Jr., MD

Basic Science

Anatomy

On the ultrastructural level, the anterior cruciate ligament (ACL) is composed of longitudinally oriented fibrils of collagen tissue ranging from 20 to 170 μm in diameter.[24] The mean diameter of these fibrils and the cross-sectional area increase from proximal to distal. Throughout the ligament, the percentage of total cross-sectional area occupied by collagen remains nearly constant.[24] Bundles of collagen fibrils make up subfascicular units, which are surrounded by a thin band of loose connective tissue called the endotenon. Several subfasciculi are grouped together to make up a collagen fasciculus. The fasciculus is surrounded by an epitenon, which is much denser than the endotenon. Surrounding the entire ligament is paratenon, which blends with the epitenon (Fig. 28J1–1).[11, 86] On histologic evaluation, the ligament is composed of fibroblasts surrounded by a matrix consisting primarily of type I collagen with a small amount of type III and type VI collagen near the insertion sites.[6, 24]

The cruciate ligaments are covered by a synovial fold that originates at the posterior inlet of the intercondylar notch and extends to the anterior tibial attachment of the ACL. Thus, the cruciate ligaments, although intra-articular, are extrasynovial.[11] The predominant blood supply of the cruciate ligaments is the middle genicular artery, which leaves the popliteal artery and directly pierces the posterior capsule.[12] Branches of the artery form a periligamentous plexus within the synovial sheath surrounding the ligament. This plexus, in addition to providing the nutritional requirements of the ACL, is the source of the hemarthrosis typically seen after an ACL injury. The osseous attachments of the ACL contribute little to its vascularity.[13] There is also a contributing blood supply from the fat pad through the inferior medial and lateral genicular arteries that may play a more important role when the ligament is injured.[13]

Innervation of the ACL is provided by a branch of the tibial nerve, the posterior articular nerve.[167] It arises from the tibial nerve in the popliteal fossa, wraps around the popliteal artery and vein, penetrates the posterior capsule, and forms the popliteal plexus. Branches of this plexus course through the synovial lining of the cruciate liga-

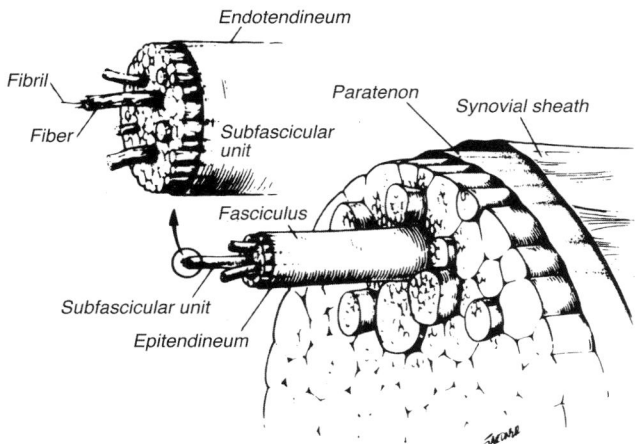

Figure 28J1–1. Microstructure of the anterior cruciate ligament. (From Nogalski MP, Bach BR Jr: Acute anterior cruciate ligament injuries. In Fu FH, Harner CD, Vince KG [eds]: Knee Surgery. Baltimore, Williams & Wilkins, 1994, pp 679–730.)

ments, following the course of the blood vessels, and extend as far anterior as the infrapatellar fat pad. Nerve fibers similar in size to pain fibers are readily visualized in the intrafascicular spaces of the ligaments.[165] Mechanoreceptors have been identified on the surface of the ligament amid fibrous fatty and vascular tissue, well beneath the external synovial sheath.[268, 269] The long axes of the receptor organs are parallel to the ligament, and the receptors are found primarily at the insertions of the ligament, usually at the femoral attachment.[268] The exact role of these mechanoreceptors has yet to be fully understood, but they most likely serve to enhance knee stability through sensory feedback loops controlling proprioception and muscle tone around the knee.[178, 252]

The insertion sites of the ACL are marked by a transition of ligament tissue merging into bone. Electron micro-

scopic evaluation of this region by Cooper and Mishol has demonstrated four zones.[76] Zone 1 is made up of ligament tissue, primarily collagen; zone 2 consists of a mix of collagen blending with fibrocartilage; zone 3 contains mineralized fibrocartilage; and zone 4 represents the subchondral bone. This transition reduces stress at the attachment site by dissipating the longitudinal and shear forces through a gradual change in the stiffness of the tissues from ligament to bone.

The ACL has attachments on the femur and tibia. Descriptions of the exact location, shape, and dimensions of these insertion points are similar but variable on examination of the literature.[116, 127, 232] The femoral attachment originates from the posteromedial aspect of the intercondylar notch on the lateral femoral condyle. The tibial attachment inserts about 15 mm behind the anterior border of the tibial articular surface, just medial to the attachment of the anterior horn of the lateral meniscus (Fig. 28J1–2).[107] The tibial and femoral insertion sites are broad expansions of the ligament, approximately three times the cross-sectional area of the ligament midsubstance.[127] The femoral insertion, as described by Harner and coworkers,[127] is circular, encompassing an average area of 113 mm²; the tibial insertion is more oval, with an average area of 136 mm². The midsubstance cross-sectional area of the ACL averaged just below 40 mm². Markolf and coworkers[189] demonstrated that for the ligament as a whole, the distance between insertion points lengthens approximately 3 mm during the terminal 30 degrees of extension. There is a twist of the fibers in the coronal plane of approximately 90 degrees with external rotation of the fibers.[232, 263] If all ligaments except the ACL are cut and the tibia is allowed to rotate freely, internal rotation of the tibia will result.[55, 263]

The ACL has been described as consisting of two discrete bundles, the anteromedial and posterolateral, named for their anatomic location at the tibial insertion site. The divisions are based on the fiber orientation and tensioning characteristics during flexion and extension.[110, 116, 127] The

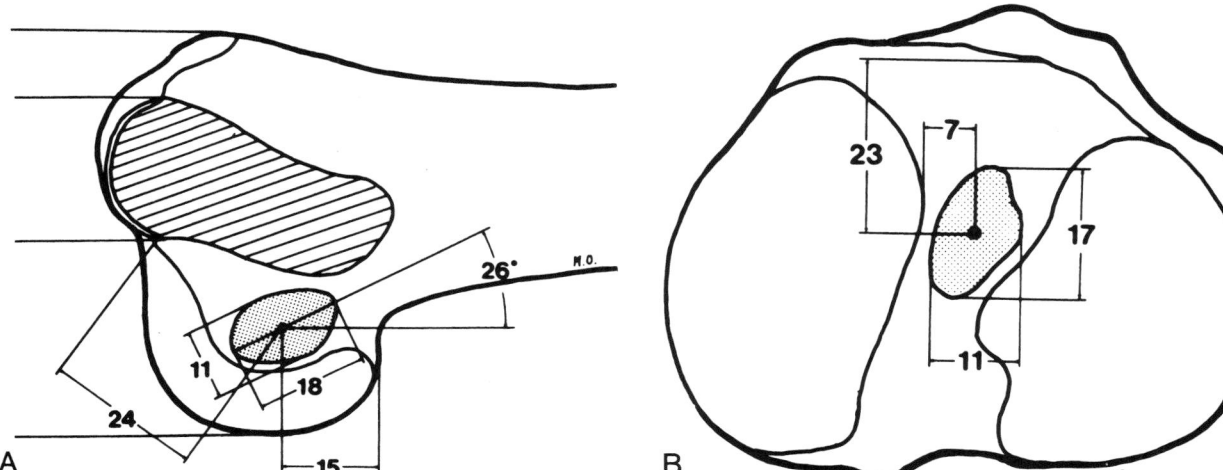

Figure 28J1–2. *A*, Femoral attachment of the anterior cruciate ligament with measurements in millimeters. *B*, Tibial attachment of the anterior cruciate ligament with measurements in millimeters. (*A* and *B*, From Odensten M, Gillquist J: Functional anatomy of the anterior cruciate ligament and a rationale for reconstruction. J Bone Joint Surg Am 67:257–262, 1985.)

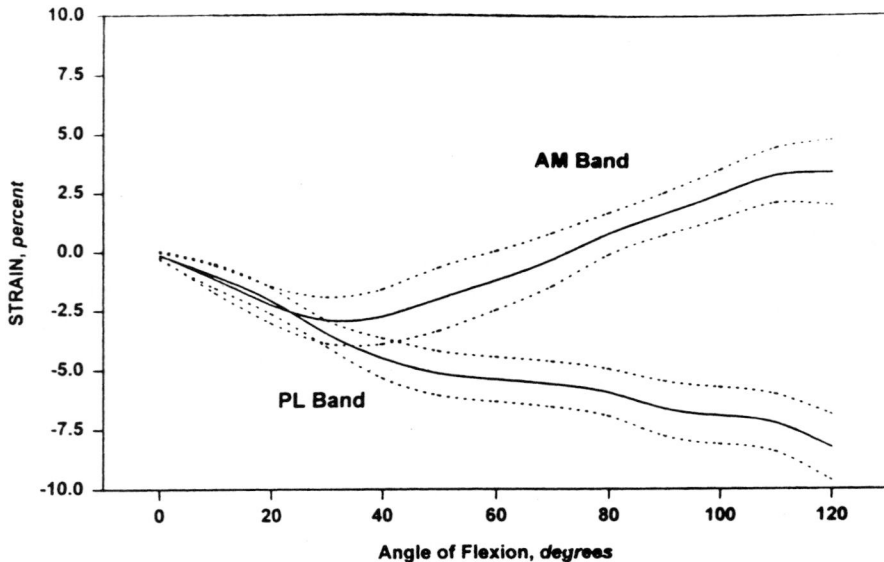

Figure 28J1–3. Strain patterns in the anteromedial (AM) and posterolateral (PL) bands of the anterior cruciate ligament as a function of knee flexion angle. (From Edwards TB, Guanche CA, Petrie SG, Thomas KA: In vitro comparison of elongation of the anterior cruciate ligament and single- and dual-tunnel anterior cruciate ligament reconstructions. Orthopedics 22:577–584, 1999.)

presence of a third, intermediate, bundle has been promoted by Amis and Dawkins,[7] whereas whether there exists a distinct anatomic division of the ligament at all has been questioned by others.[232, 318] The relative size attributed to each bundle has varied across studies, with Harner and coworkers finding a nearly equal division between the two bundles.[116, 127] Despite these discrepancies in anatomic description, it is clear that from a functional standpoint, the ACL demonstrates varying tensile properties across its width. Edwards and associates[92] demonstrated the elongation behavior of the ACL using differential variable reluctance transducers placed directly in each bundle (Fig. 28J1–3). The anteromedial bundle shortens from 0 to 30 degrees of knee flexion followed by progressive lengthening from 30 to 120 degrees of flexion. From 30 to 70 degrees, the ligament is returning to its baseline length, and only with flexion greater than 70 degrees does the ligament undergo actual lengthening beyond its baseline, reaching maximal strain at 120 degrees. The posterolateral bundle is longest with the knee in full extension and undergoes progressive shortening with diminished strain as the knee flexes, reaching minimal strain at 120 degrees. It is unlikely that any truly isometric fibers are present.

Biomechanics of the Normal Anterior Cruciate Ligament

The ACL functions as the primary restraint to anterior translation of the tibia.[62, 109] It serves as a secondary restraint to tibial rotation and to varus or valgus stress.[191] The ACL has an average cross-sectional area of 44 mm², with ultimate tensile load measured up to 2160 N and a stiffness of 242 N/mm, and can tolerate strain of about 20% before failing.[61, 105, 227, 326] Age is a factor in the strength of the ACL; older ACLs fail under lower loads than do younger ACLs.[199, 227] The forces in the intact ACL range from about 100 N during passive knee extension to about 400 N with walking and reach, and up to 1700 N with

cutting and acceleration-deceleration activities.[60, 190, 221] As such, the ACL experiences loads exceeding its failure capacity only with unusual combinations of loading patterns on the knee.[105]

Beynnon and Fleming[40] presented a comprehensive review of in vivo strain patterns in the intact ACL during a variety of activities and exercises (Table 28J1–1). The most important variables influencing ACL strain were the position of the knee and the dynamic interaction of muscle activity. Increased strain was seen with increasing knee extension. This differs from the findings found in vitro and points out the importance of the dynamic effects of muscle tone and contraction. Activities that produced isolated quadriceps activity led to the highest ACL strains, whereas those that generated isolated hamstring activity produced the lowest levels of ACL strain. Co-contraction of the hamstrings during closed chain extension activities provided a dampening effect to the strain produced by isolated quadriceps activity seen in open chain activities. A more thorough analysis of open versus closed chain exercises and of the implications on ACL rehabilitation is presented later.

Biologic Response to Anterior Cruciate Ligament Injury

Unlike the medial collateral ligament (MCL), which has an excellent healing potential after injury, the injured ACL fails to demonstrate the ability to regain a functional state after conservative treatment measures. A number of distinct biologic differences between the extra-articular MCL and the intra-articular ACL exist to explain this discrepancy in healing potential. These differences can be categorized as intrinsic or extrinsic to the ligament tissue itself.

Extrinsic differences between the MCL and ACL exist with regard to their external environment. It is important to understand how these environments may play a role in their healing capacity. Injuries to extra-articular ligaments like the MCL lead to a localized collection of bleeding and

TABLE 28J1–1
Rank Comparison of Peak Anterior Cruciate Ligament Strain Values During Commonly Prescribed Rehabilitation Activities

Rehabilitation Activity	Peak Strain (%)	No. of Subjects
Isometric quadriceps contraction at 15° (30 Nm of extension torque)	4.4	8
Squatting with sport cord	4.0	8
Active flexion-extension of the knee with 45-N weight boot	3.8	9
Lachman's test (150 N of anterior shear load)	3.7	10
Squatting	3.6	8
Active flexion-extension (no weight boot) of the knee	2.8	18
Simultaneous quadriceps and hamstrings contraction at 15°	2.8	8
Isometric quadriceps contraction at 30° (30 Nm of extension torque)	2.7	18
Anterior drawer (150 N of anterior shear load)	1.8	10
Stationary bicycling	1.7	8
Isometric hamstrings contraction at 15° (to −10 Nm of flexion torque)	0.6	8
Simultaneous quadriceps and hamstrings contraction at 30°	0.4	8
Passive flexion-extension of the knee	0.1	10
Isometric quadriceps contraction at 60° (30 Nm of extension torque)	0.0	8
Isometric quadriceps contraction at 90° (30 Nm of extension torque)	0.0	18
Simultaneous quadriceps and hamstrings contraction at 60°	0.0	8
Simultaneous quadriceps and hamstrings contraction at 90°	0.0	8
Isometric hamstrings contraction at 30°, 60°, and 90° (to −10 Nm of flexion torque)	0.0	8

From Beynnon BD, Fleming BC: Anterior cruciate ligament strain in-vivo: A review of previous work. J Biomech 31:519–525, 1998. © 1998, with permission from Elsevier Science.

the formation of a hematoma at the site of injury. As the hematoma organizes, inflammatory cells migrate into the region, adhering to the fibrinogen matrix that develops. These cells produce the chemical mediators, in the form of cytokines and growth factors, that attract fibroblasts and stem cells. The fibroblasts and stem cells lead to the formation of granulation tissue in the area of injury, and the granulation tissue matures over time into fibrous scar tissue, restoring function to the injured ligament.[107] The ACL, however, is intra-articular and enveloped by synovial tissue. When the ACL is injured and this synovial tissue is disrupted, a local hematoma fails to develop as the blood is eluted into the joint fluid. The remainder of the healing cascade is thus interrupted, and the ligament fails to regain any functional integrity. It is the injury to the synovial lining that has been demonstrated through ligament transection studies to be the key factor in determining the healing capacity of an injured ACL.[107, 131]

Intrinsic differences between the ACL and MCL may also affect the healing potential of each. Variations exist in the characteristics of fibroblast cell populations in each ligament.[107] The production of extracellular matrix and collagen is greater in the ACL fibroblast cell, which should give the ACL an advantage toward an improved healing response; however, it has also been demonstrated that the ACL fibroblast exhibits less mobility, slower migration, and lower proliferation rates than those of the MCL fibroblast, factors that inhibit the ability of the ACL to respond to injury.[218, 266, 297, 323]

In addition, Cameron and associates[68] demonstrated a significant alteration in the cytokine profile of synovial fluid in response to ACL injury. These alterations may have implications for the ability of the ACL to generate a healing response as well as for the long-term development of osteoarthritic changes. The role of nitric oxide as a mediator of these effects has been suggested, and in fact, it has been shown that both articular cartilage and cruciate ligament collagen and proteoglycan synthesis are inhibited by nitric oxide, whereas the MCL is unaffected.[70]

The healing response of ligament tissues is clearly complex and currently not fully understood. Further research into the interactions of cellular, chemical, and environmental mediators is needed to define the healing process clearly. How this will affect the future treatment of ACL injuries is unknown, but currently, the fact remains that the ACL does not demonstrate a functional ability to heal itself after injury, and our only active intervention remains reconstructive surgery.

Biologic Response of Anterior Cruciate Ligament Graft Reconstruction

After implantation, ACL grafts undergo a sequential process of incorporation into the host knee.[14] This process was first studied in animal models, both canine and rabbit, but more recently, evaluation of human specimens has provided sufficient data to confirm the findings of the animal studies.[14, 25, 97, 155]

The first phase consists of an inflammatory response during which the graft undergoes avascular necrosis. Donor fibroblasts undergo cell death, and the remaining tissue structure serves as a scaffold for future cell migration and matrix production. The second phase consists of a period of revascularization and migration of host fibroblasts into the graft tissue. Revascularization begins within 20 days after implantation and is complete between 3 and 6 months.[97, 155] The material properties of the graft change as this process of "ligamentization" proceeds. While the graft is revascularizing, the ultimate load to failure and stiffness in a patellar tendon autograft are significantly decreased. The graft strength can drop to as low as 11% of normal ACL strength, and the graft stiffness can fall to as low as 13% of normal ACL stiffness during graft maturation.[25, 41] The implications for graft protection and the potential for injury with a return to stressful activities during this period are obvious. In the final phase, the healing graft undergoes remodeling of its collagen structure into a more organized and structurally functional pattern. The collagen fibers align themselves along the longitudinal axis of the graft and develop a crimp pattern resembling that of the native ACL.[97] The graft continues to exhibit differences in the size of the collagen fibers and the content of the extracellular matrix, however, and it may never completely resemble the ultrastructural architecture of the native ACL.[107, 291]

Epidemiology

Injury to the ACL is common, particularly in the athletic population. Isolated ACL injuries account for nearly half of all ligamentous knee injuries. In the general population, an estimated 1 of every 3000 people will suffer an ACL injury in any given year[137, 205]; 70% of these injuries will occur during a sporting activity (Table 28J1–2).[137] Skiing is a particularly high-risk activity for ACL injury. Deibert and coworkers,[88] tracking injuries at a Vermont ski resort, found an ACL injury in almost 1 of every 2000 adult skier visits. Even more alarming is that despite advances in skiing equipment that have reduced the overall rate of injury to skiers, the incidence of ACL injury rose 280% between the 1972–1973 and 1993–1994 ski seasons.[88]

Women are at a greater risk for suffering an ACL injury than are men. Messina and colleagues,[202] looking at high-school basketball players in Texas, noted the ACL injury rate to be approximately four times greater for women than for men. This trend continues when other sports, such as soccer and volleyball, are evaluated. Lindenfeld and associates[180] reported a sixfold increase in the ACL injury rate for female soccer players compared with their male counterparts, and Ferretti and coworkers[100] reported a four times greater incidence of serious knee injuries in women volleyball players than in men.

In the past, these injuries would often prevent the return to meaningful sports activities. Now, with current surgical techniques, an injured person can predictably return to strenuous activities in more than 90% of all cases, usually within 6 months. This underscores the importance of maintaining an awareness of these injuries so that prompt treatment is initiated, time lost to injury is minimized, and additional injury is minimized. The alarmingly high injury rate, particularly in women, points out the need to focus on better understanding of the mechanisms of injury and to find more effective preventive measures.

Presentation of the Patient

The first step in diagnosis and treatment of an injured patient is obtaining a complete and thorough history. Useful information can be gleaned from an understanding of the mechanism of injury, the initial symptoms, the time since the initial injury, and any late sequelae, including reinjuries. These items will guide the clinician toward a focused clinical examination, which will ensure a proper diagnosis not only of any ACL injury but also of any associated injuries. The need for any additional testing is determined by the results of the history and physical examination. Therefore, a thorough understanding of each segment is crucial in leading to an accurate and complete diagnosis of all injuries present. Only then can the prompt initiation of proper treatment be carried out, with the best chance of a maximal functional recovery.

Understanding the mechanism of injury helps lead to a proper diagnosis. One quarter to one third of the time, the patient is unable to give a clear account of the mechanism of injury.[123, 226] In these cases, it may be helpful to gather accounts from any coaches, trainers, or teammates who may have witnessed the injuring event. If video replay is available, that can also be helpful in understanding the mechanism of injury.

Injuries to the ACL may occur with a variety of mechanisms, but there are a few common and predictable patterns. A low-energy injury occurring during an athletic activity is the most common mechanism. The injuries may be direct, contact injuries, or they may be secondary to indirect, noncontact mechanisms. Common noncontact mechanisms of injury are sudden deceleration and rotational maneuvers as seen during cutting-type running or jumping activities.[226] Hyperextension or valgus stress to

TABLE 28J1–2
Acute Knee Ligament Injuries with Pathologic Motion: Activity at Time of Injury*

Ligament Injury	Activity at Time of Injury								
	Football	*Baseball*	*Basketball*	*Soccer*	*Skiing*	*Other Sports*	*Vehicle*	*Miscellaneous*	**Total**
ACL single-ligament injury	27 (11%)	25 (11%)	19 (8%)	33 (14%)	23 (10%)	38 (16%)	15 (6%)	58 (24%)	238
MCL single-ligament injury	14 (10%)	16 (11%)	6 (4%)	10 (7%)	19 (13%)	13 (9%)	14 (10%)	52 (36%)	144
MCL-ACL combined injury	6 (9%)	1 (2%)	3 (5%)	9 (14%)	12 (19%)	8 (13%)	9 (14%)	16 (25%)	64
PCL injury (18 isolated, 19 combined)	1 (3%)	5 (14%)	2 (5%)	0	1 (3%)	6 (16%)	14 (38%)	8 (21%)	37
LCL injury (10 isolated, 7 combined)	0	3 (18%)	0	1 (6%)	1 (6%)	2 (12%)	1 (6%)	9 (53%)	17
Total	48 (10%)	50 (10%)	30 (6%)	53 (11%)	56 (11%)	67 (13%)	53 (10%)	143 (29%)	500

*Study performed at San Diego Kaiser; N = 500.
ACL, anterior cruciate ligament; LCL, lateral collateral ligament; MCL, medial collateral ligament; PCL, posterior cruciate ligament.
From Hirshman HP, Daniel DM, Miyasaka K: The fate of unoperated knee ligament injury. In Daniel DM, Akeson WH, O'Connor JJ (eds): Knee Ligaments: Structure, Function, Injury, and Repair. New York, Raven Press, 1990, pp 481–503.

the knee can also result in ACL injury; this is often secondary to a direct blow. Only about one third of all patients describe a contact mechanism of injury.[226]

Another subset of ACL injuries occurs after a high-energy event, such as a motor vehicle accident. These patients will commonly have sustained associated injuries, both musculoskeletal and systemic. A high degree of suspicion must be maintained to evaluate and diagnose these associated injuries.

The patient's subjective complaints from the time of injury and the period just after can be helpful toward making the diagnosis of an ACL injury. Patients may recall a "popping" or "tearing" sensation at the time of injury. Anywhere from 33% to 90% of patients with an ACL tear experience these sensations.[101, 226] Although indicative of an ACL rupture, these sensations may also occur with patellofemoral subluxation-dislocation events, MCL injury, and meniscal tears. Patients will have difficulty bearing weight after an ACL injury, and many experience the sensation of instability or have frank episodes of the knee's "giving out."[226] It is unlikely that an athlete will be able to continue to participate in competition after an acute ACL injury.[221]

The rapid onset of a knee effusion is common after an ACL injury. The swelling represents the development of a hemarthrosis and typically occurs within the first 4 to 12 hours in the setting of an ACL injury.[87, 226] The presence of a traumatic hemarthrosis is highly suggestive of an ACL tear. DeHaven[87] and Noyes and colleagues,[226] in separate studies, confirmed an ACL tear arthroscopically in almost three quarters of all patients presenting with an acute traumatic hemarthrosis. Other causes of an acute hemarthrosis in the knee may be patellar instability, posterior cruciate ligament (PCL) injuries, meniscal tears, fractures, osteochondral injuries, popliteus avulsion, and combinations of each. The absence or delayed onset of a hemarthrosis does not preclude an ACL injury.

Previous injury or surgery and the time interval from the initial injury are also important in considering patients with ACL injuries. Associated injuries, such as meniscal tears, osteochondral injuries, and other ligament injuries, as well as knee arthrosis may be present in the setting of an acute ACL injury, but they are more common after the repeated subluxation events that can occur in the presence of a chronically ACL-deficient knee.[156]

In taking the history, it is also important to gather information about the patient's job requirements, activity level, and goals for continued activities. These issues may influence the decision for surgery, the timing of surgery, and the ability to carry out postoperative rehabilitation and may have an impact on the selection of graft material. The physician must remember that the patient is not just an injured ACL but a complete person, with many complex psychological, social, and economic stresses, all of which need to be addressed in forming an appropriate treatment plan.

Physical Examination

In combination with the history, the physical examination should provide an accurate diagnosis of an ACL injury in nearly all cases. Radiography, magnetic resonance imaging (MRI), examination under anesthesia, and arthroscopy are necessary only for the diagnosis of associated injuries or in the rare instance in which the differentiation of a partial or complete ACL injury cannot be made through the clinical examination alone. It is therefore crucial for the clinician to become familiar with the typical examination findings in an ACL-deficient knee and to become proficient with the testing techniques used to measure anterior knee translation.

In the acute setting, the examination is most accurately performed immediately after the injury, before swelling, pain, and reflex muscle splinting occur. If the injury occurs in an athlete during participation, the examination may be performed at the time of initial evaluation on the field or immediately after the player is brought to the sidelines. If the time to presentation is delayed, the examination in the acute setting may be difficult, and a repeated examination after a few days have passed is often more revealing.

The examination begins with an inspection of the knee. The overall alignment of the knee should be observed. Severe distortion of the normal alignment may represent a fracture of the distal femur or proximal tibia or indicate knee dislocation, both of which require urgent treatment. An effusion will most commonly be present within a few hours after an ACL injury. Absence of an effusion does not mean that an ACL injury has not occurred; in fact, with more severe injuries that include the surrounding capsule and soft tissues, the hemarthrosis may be able to escape from the knee, and the degree of swelling may paradoxically be diminished. In addition, the presence of an effusion does not guarantee that an ACL injury has occurred. Meniscal injuries, PCL injuries, osteochondral injuries, and intra-articular fractures may present with a hemarthrosis, either alone or in combination with an ACL injury.

Palpation follows inspection and should begin with the uninvolved extremity. This provides the examiner with a baseline for reference against the examination findings of the injured knee. It also serves to familiarize the patient with the examination procedures in the hope that the patient will be more relaxed during manipulation of the involved knee. Palpation confirms the presence and degree of effusion. Subtle effusions missed during inspection should be picked up by a careful manual examination. Periarticular tenderness should be evaluated next. Although the ACL cannot be palpated, palpation of the medial and lateral joint lines may elicit pain in the presence of concomitant meniscal disease. Palpation should continue along the collateral ligaments and include assessment of both proximal and distal insertion sites. Tenderness along the patellar border may be an indication of injury to the retinacular structures, and patellar mobility, tracking, and apprehension should be examined.

Active and passive range of motion should be checked. Loss of motion may be secondary to pain, large effusions, an incompetent extensor mechanism, or a mechanical block. Sources of a mechanical block are displaced meniscal tears, loose osteochondral fragments, and the stump of a torn ACL. Aspiration of a large effusion may be beneficial in alleviating pain, improving motion, confirming the presence of a hemarthrosis, and allowing a more accurate

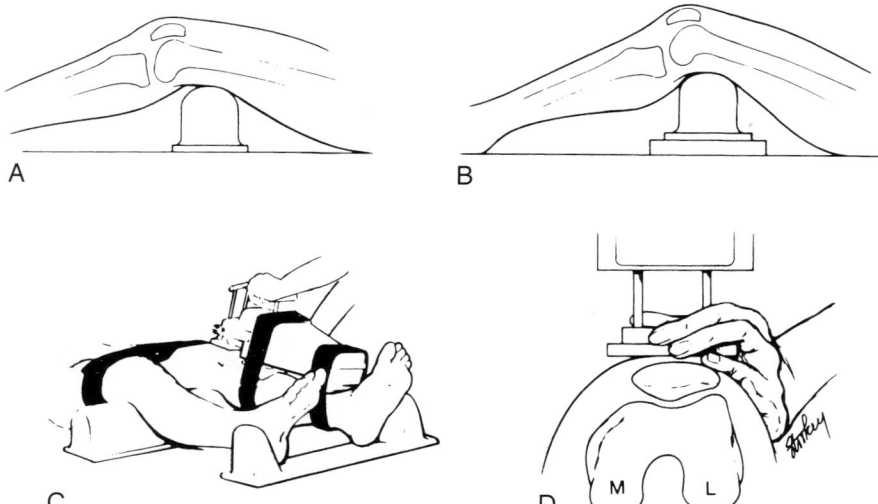

Figure 28J1–7. The knee is supported in a flexed position to engage the patella in the femoral trochlea (*A*). In some patients, the thigh support must be raised an additional 3 to 6 cm to provide sufficient knee flexion to engage the patella in the femoral trochlea. This may be done by placing a board under the thigh support (*B*). The thigh should be supported so that the patella is facing up. Occasionally, a thigh strap is used to accomplish this task (*C*). The foot support is not used to rotate the limb internally but simply supports the feet. The examiner stabilizes the patellar sensor with manual pressure. Before establishing the testing reference position, sufficient pressure should be applied to the patella to press it firmly into the femoral trochlea (2 to 6 pounds) so that the increase in pressure on the patellar pad that will inevitably occur while stabilizing the instrument and limb during testing will not change the position of the patella and the patellar sensor. The hand stabilizing the patellar sensor should rest against the lateral thigh to help stabilize the testing instrument and to prevent rotation of the instrument during testing (*D*). L, lateral; M, medial. (*A–D* from Daniel DM, Stone ML: KT1000 anterior-posterior displacement measurement. In Daniel DM, Akeson WH, O'Connor JJ [eds]: Knee Ligaments: Structure, Function, Injury, and Repair. New York, Raven Press, 1990, pp 427–447.)

Radiographic Imaging Studies

In most cases, the diagnosis of an ACL injury can be made after obtaining a careful history and performing a thorough physical examination. The role of radiographic imaging is primarily to exclude any associated injuries that may have an impact on the treatment plan. Plain radiographs are mandatory for all traumatic injuries. Although the ACL itself cannot be visualized with standard radio-

graphs, secondary signs of ACL injury may be seen in the form of lateral capsular avulsions known as Segond's fractures.[328] In younger patients, or in middle-aged patients with osteopenia, tibial eminence avulsion fractures can occur in the presence of an ACL injury. Plain radiographs will also reveal proximal tibia or distal femur fractures, may reveal osteochondral injuries or loose bodies, and will establish a baseline for the degree of joint degeneration at the time of presentation as well as the overall alignment of the knee. Warren and coworkers[315] described the lateral notch sign as an indication of ACL insufficiency, particularly in the chronic condition. An expansion of the normal indentation of the lateral condyle to a depth of 2 mm or more was correlated with an ACL-deficient knee (Fig.

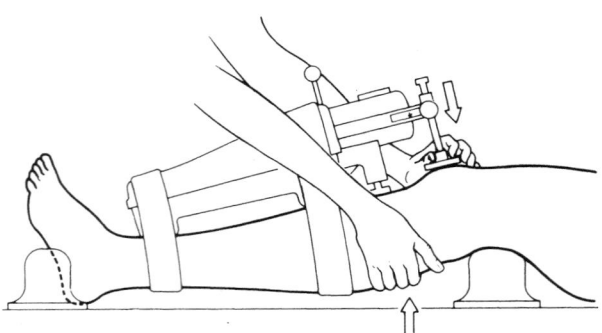

Figure 28J1–8. The manual maximum test. The limbs are positioned with the support system, the arthrometer is applied, and the testing reference position is obtained in the standard way. While the examiner stabilizes the patellar sensor pad with one hand, the other hand applies a strong anterior displacement force directly to the proximal calf to produce the maximum anterior displacement. Care is taken that the knee is not extended. The tibial displacement is read off the dial. (From Daniel DM, Stone ML: KT1000 anterior-posterior displacement measurements. In Daniel DM, Akeson WH, O'Connor JJ [eds]: Knee Ligaments: Structure, Function, Injury, and Repair. New York, Raven Press, 1990, pp 427–447.)

TABLE 28J1–3

Data on the Knees of Normal Subjects and the Knees of Patients Who Had an Acute or Chronic Tear of the Anterior Cruciate Ligament

	Test Results (mm)*		
	89 N and 30 Degrees of Flexion	*Maximum Manual Force*	*Compliance Index*
Normal	6.3 ± 1.84 (2–12)	7.0 (4–11)	1.1 ± 0.4 (0.5–2.0)
Acute tear	9.6 ± 3.1 (4.5–19)	13.0 (5–22)	2.2 ± 0.96 (0.5–4.0)
Chronic tear	11.4 ± 3.7 (3–21)	13.5 (7–22)	2.1 ± 1.05 (0.5–6.0)

*Ranges are give in parentheses.
Modified from Bach BR Jr, Warren RF, Flynn WM, et al: Arthrometric evaluation of knees that have a torn anterior cruciate ligament. J Bone Joint Surg Am 72: 1299–1306, 1990.

NORMAL KNEE ACL DEFICIENT KNEE

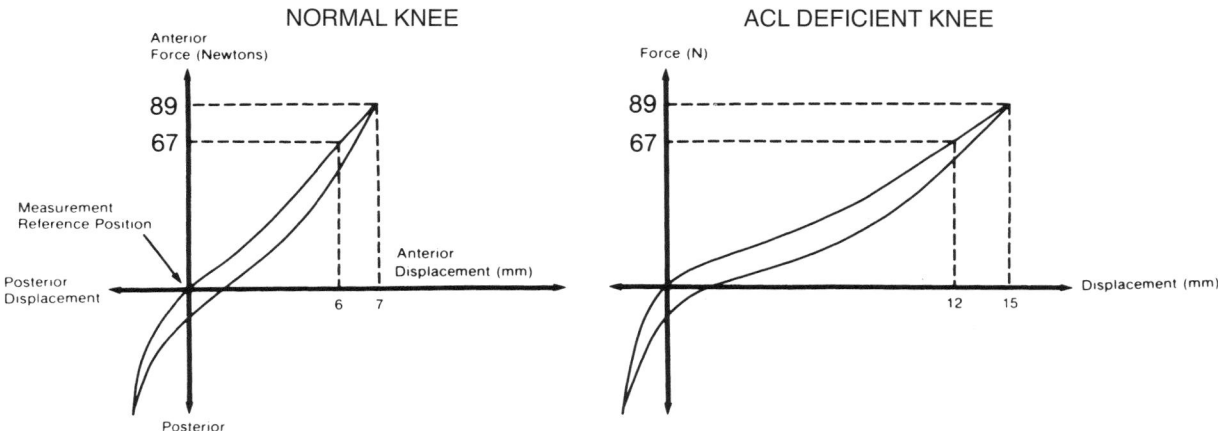

Figure 28J1–9. Compliance index. Force-displacement curves for normal knees (*left*) and for anterior cruciate ligament–deficient knees (*right*). The compliance index is obtained by measuring the difference in displacement that occurs between the 67-N and 89-N anterior force levels. On this curve, the compliance index for the normal knee is 1 mm; for the knee with an anterior cruciate ligament disruption, it is 3 mm. (From Daniel DM, Stone ML: KT1000 anterior-posterior displacement measurements. In Daniel DM, Akeson WH, O'Connor JJ [eds]: Knee Ligaments: Structure, Function, Injury, and Repair. New York, Raven Press, 1990, pp 427–447.)

28J1–10). Jacobsen[150] further described the radiographic changes observed in the chronic ACL-deficient knee. Before 2 years of ACL deficiency, only 2 of 21 knees demonstrated marginal osteophyte formation, whereas the remaining 19 knees showed no radiographic abnormalities. From 2 to 3 years, 7 of 12 knees demonstrated osteophytes, and one knee had developed structural changes in the form of joint space narrowing, subchondral cyst formation, and sclerosis. After 3 years of ACL deficiency, 80% of the knees had formed osteophytes; 20% had gone on to develop structural changes. Sherman and colleagues[289] found similar results in their series of 127 patients with ACL-deficient knees. They noted the development of osteophytes at the medial and lateral joint margins, spurring of the patella and tibial spines, tibial sclerosis, joint space narrowing, and cyst formation. These findings increased in severity in direct correlation to time from injury. They also noted a relationship between the presence of meniscal injury or meniscectomy and the development of osteoarthritis.

The need for further imaging studies is debatable. Historically, arthrography or computed tomography was used for diagnosis of ACL injuries. These modalities have been supplanted by the development of MRI. MRI has the advantage of providing a clearly defined image of all the anatomic structures of the knee. The normal ACL is seen as a well-defined band of low signal intensity on sagittal images through the intercondylar notch (Fig. 28J1–11).[308] With an acute injury to the ACL, the continuity of the

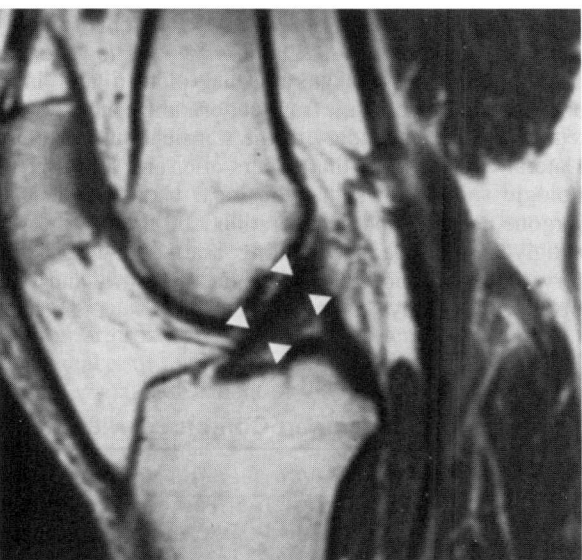

Figure 28J1–11. Normal anatomy of the anterior cruciate ligament, demonstrated by magnetic resonance imaging. Sagittal T$_1$-weighted image demonstrates the anterior cruciate ligament as a smooth low-signal-intensity structure (*arrowheads*). (From Daniel DM, Stone ML: KT1000 anterior-posterior displacement measurements. In Daniel DM, Akeson WH, O'Connor JJ [eds]: Knee Ligaments: Structure, Function, Injury, and Repair. New York, Raven Press, 1990, pp 427–447.)

Figure 28J1–10. Lateral notch sign. To measure the depth of the notch, a perpendicular line (A) is drawn tangent to the articular surface, and the depth of the notch (B) is measured from this line. (From Warren RF, Kaplan N, Bach BR Jr: The lateral notch sign of anterior cruciate ligament insufficiency. Am J Knee Surg 1:119–124, 1988.)

and will avoid the need to estimate the percentage of ACL fibers involved visually. A positive pivot shift test result under anesthesia establishes the diagnosis of ACL deficiency, regardless of the findings at surgery.

Critical review of the natural history of partial tears is complicated by the many different criteria used to establish the diagnosis. As such, it is difficult, if not impossible, to make a sound comparison from one study to the next. Noyes and colleagues[229] noted a 50% chance of instability and 75% chance of further knee injury for patients with a 50% disruption of ACL tissue at the time of arthroscopy. They also noted a poor prognosis for patients with more than 5 mm of side-to-side laxity during instrumented testing under anesthesia. In contrast, Buckley and associates[52] found no correlation of the percentage of tear to clinical outcome. Messner and Maletius[203] presented their 18- to 25-year follow-up on patients with partial ACL injuries. They defined a partial tear as less than 50% involvement of the ACL at arthroscopy and a maximum of 1+ instability on examination under anesthesia. No patient treated conservatively for the partial ACL injury went on to require an ACL reconstruction. Of 21 patients, 18 had no or slight limitation with sports activities, and 20 had no or slight limitations during work; 20 of 21 patients had grade 2 or less evidence of radiographic osteoarthrosis, and only 3 of 12 showed radiographic progression from the 12-year evaluation to the latest follow-up.

Partial ACL injuries are a treatment dilemma. The demands of the patient must be considered along with the symptoms and physical examination findings. Again, we believe that a positive pivot shift test result under anesthesia is pathognomonic of an ACL-deficient knee and treat this as a complete injury. For the patient who has sustained a true partial injury, treatment must be customized to the individual patient. Patients with symptoms of instability or patients in a high-risk, high-demand category should preferably be treated with reconstruction. Patients with a low-demand lifestyle and no symptoms can be treated conservatively and watched closely for any signs of progressive instability. In our experience of 65 conservatively treated partial ACL tears, less than 10% went on to require subsequent reconstruction.

Associated Injuries

The association of ACL tears with injuries to other structures of the knee has long been recognized.[67, 234, 235] O'Donoghue[234, 235] coined the phrase "the unhappy triad" in referring to the association of ACL injury with MCL and medial meniscal tears. More recently, it has been noted that lateral meniscal tears are more commonly seen in association with combined ACL-MCL injuries.[27, 281] Barber[27] reported an 80% incidence of lateral meniscal tears with combined ACL-MCL injury. Medial meniscal tears occurred only 25% to 29% of the time and always in association with a lateral meniscal injury. Bellabarba and coworkers[37] performed an extensive review of meniscal injuries associated with acute and chronic ACL insufficiency (Tables 28J1–5 and 28J1–6). They found a 41% to 81% incidence of meniscal tears in acute ACL injuries; 56% were lateral tears, and 44% were medial tears. In chronic ACL-deficient knees, the rate of associated meniscal injury ranged from 58% to 100%. In this population, medial meniscal tears were more common, representing 70% of all meniscal injuries.

Treatment of meniscal tears should focus on preserva-

TABLE 28J1–5
Mediolateral Distribution of Meniscal Tears in the Acutely Injured Anterior Cruciate Ligament (ACL)

Author	Incidence of Meniscal Tears in Acute ACL Injuries (%)	Medial vs. Lateral Distribution		
		No. of Injured Menisci	Medial (%)	Lateral (%)
DeHaven	65	56	37	63
McDaniel	82	10	50	50
Noyes	72	40	37	63
Woods	50	64	53	47
Indelicato	77	40	65	35
Cerabona	46	50	56	44
McCarroll	75	18	67	33
Henning	NA	76	55	45
Warren	65	—	50	50
Hirshman	53	127	39	61
Sgaglione	60	43	44	56
Shelbourne	NA	32	13	87
Shelbourne	67	286	42	58
Sherman	45	27	70	30
Paletta (skiers)	41	33	24	76
Paletta (nonskiers)	63	54	52	48
Keene	81	57	40	60
Sgaglione	73	24	46	54
Spindler	68	50	40	60
Ihara	NA	40	25	75
Overall		1127 (total)	44	56

From Bellabarba C, Bush-Joseph CA, Bach BR Jr: Patterns of meniscal injury in the anterior cruciate–deficient knee: A review of the literature. Am J Orthop 26: 18–23, 1997.

TABLE 28J1–6
Mediolateral Distribution of Meniscal Tears in Chronic Anterior Cruciate Ligament (ACL) Insufficiency

Author	Incidence of Meniscal Tears in Chronic ACL Injuries (%)	Medial vs. Lateral Distribution		
		No. of Injured Menisci	*Medial (%)*	*Lateral (%)*
Warren	98	107	87	13
McDaniel	86	27	81	19
Noyes	92	17	59	41
Woods	88	135	64	36
Indelicato	91	65	69	31
Fowleer	73	38	50	50
Warren	—	34	76	24
Aglietti	—	110	84	16
Kornblatt	82	36	75	25
McCarroll	100	6	67	33
Finsterbush	65	23	74	26
Henning	—	111	71	29
Hirshman	76	119	90	10
Irvine	86	127	44	56
Keene*	—	54	59	41
Keene†	89	02	58	42
Sgaglione	100	22	59	41
Satku	58	61	74	26
Overall		1184 (total)	70	30

*Less than 12 months after injury.
†More than 12 months after injury.
From Bellabarba C, Bush-Joseph CA, Bach BR Jr: Patterns of meniscal injury in the anterior cruciate–deficient knee: A review of the literature. Am J Orthop 26: 18–23, 1997.

tion of the meniscus. Our better understanding of the healing potential of meniscal injuries and the long-term deleterious effects of meniscectomy mandate repair of meniscal tears, if possible.[26, 54, 96, 98] Repair in the setting of an ACL reconstruction has been considered the ideal situation for healing of the meniscal tear; success rates approach 100% for lateral tears and 90% for medial tears.[37, 58, 69] Small longitudinal tears of less than 10 mm or partial-thickness tears of the lateral meniscus have been shown to have a high rate of healing and a low propensity for development of symptoms, and they may be treated conservatively.[102, 304, 317] The same has not been true of the medial meniscus tears, which have been shown to have a high propensity for progression with conservative treatment. Therefore, even small tears of the medial meniscus are best managed with meniscal repair.[102, 304]

Concurrent MCL injury has been shown to occur in about 21% of all ACL injuries.[137, 205] The MCL has been shown to have an excellent healing potential. Repair of the MCL in association with ACL reconstruction has led to increased risk for motion loss.[4, 128] Shelbourne and Porter[284] demonstrated excellent results with nonoperative treatment of MCL injuries combined with ACL reconstruction. They found a reduction in motion loss, improved recovery time, and no difference in valgus stability. We treat all MCL injures nonoperatively, and reconstruction of the ACL is delayed until the acute inflammatory phase has resolved and full range of motion of the knee is established.

We currently do not alter our rehabilitation protocol after ACL reconstruction for either MCL injuries or meniscal repairs.

Natural History

Before any treatment decisions can be made with regard to ACL injuries, an understanding of the natural history of the disorder is mandatory. Only then can one have a baseline against which to reference the results of any operative or nonoperative intervention. There are many variables to be considered in studying the natural history of ACL insufficiency. Both objective and subjective criteria have been evaluated, often with use of different rating scales or testing methods, making comparison of the many clinical reports difficult. Despite some reports to the contrary, most studies evaluating the conservative treatment of ACL injuries have demonstrated poor results.

Instability after nonoperative treatment is a frequent complaint. Noyes and colleagues[228] found a 65% incidence of giving way during strenuous activities. These episodes resulted in significant pain, swelling, and disability that lasted for days after the instability event. In a series from Hawkins and coworkers,[130] 86% of patients had similar episodes of instability. Seitz and associates[271] reported a 56% incidence of subjective instability. An identical number demonstrated objective instability in the form of a positive pivot shift test result, and 85% had either a grade 2 or grade 3 Lachman test result. Likewise, Odensten and coworkers[233] noted an 89% incidence of instability, as determined by a positive pivot shift test result, in their series of conservatively treated ACL injuries.

The inability to return successfully to strenuous sporting activities is well documented. Those who do return rarely do so at the same level as before their ACL injury. In Hawkins' series, only 14% returned to full athletic activity.[130] Seitz and associates[271] noted a 22% return to unrestricted activities. Similarly, Noyes and colleagues[228] reported that only 19% of their patients could perform turning or twisting activities.

ACL insufficiency predisposes the patient to injury to other knee structures. Another concern is the development of osteoarthritic changes in the knee after ACL injury.

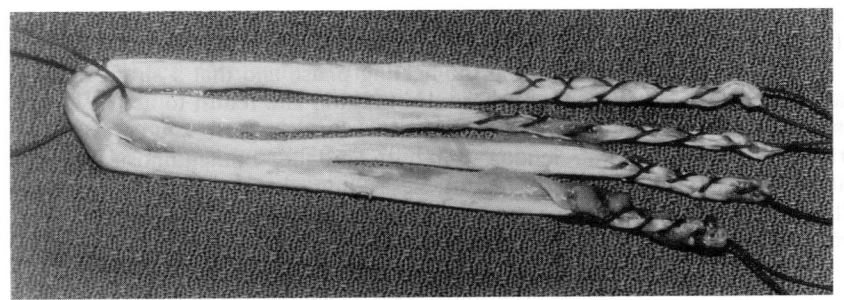

Figure 28J1–13. Quadrupled semitendinosus-gracilis autograft. (From Brown CH Jr, Sklar JH: Endoscopic anterior cruciate ligament reconstruction using doubled gracilis and semitendinosus tendons and endobutton femoral fixation. Operative Tech Sports Med 7:201–213, 1999.)

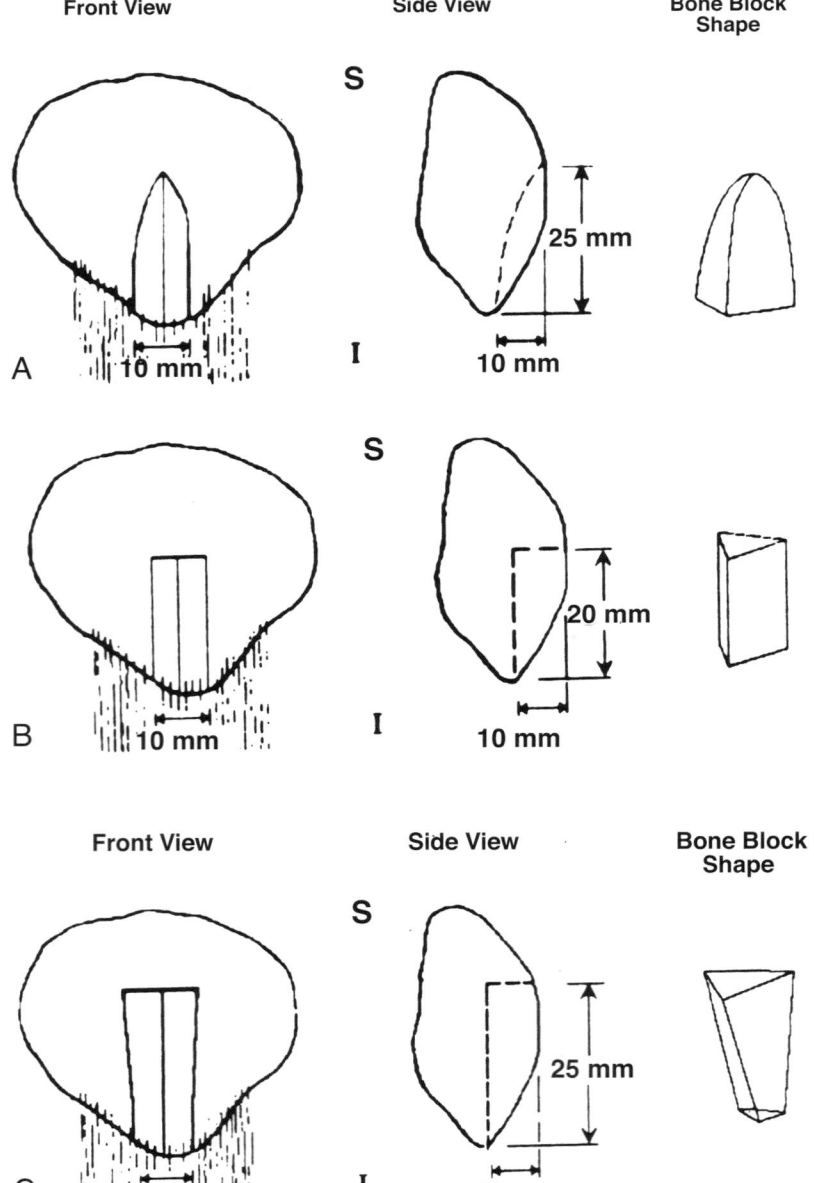

Figure 28J1–14. Size and shape of various patellar bone blocks. *A*, Tapered bone block with hull-shaped trough. *B*, Square bone block with triangular trough. *C*, Trapezoid bone block with triangular trough. (*A–C* from Friis EA, Cooke FW, McQueen DA, Henning CE: Effect of bone block removal and patellar prosthesis on stresses in the human patella. Am J Sports Med 22:696–701, 1994.)

other alternative graft choice. The average cross-sectional area is up to 64 mm^2.[299] The load to failure has been estimated to be as high as 2352 N.[265] Although not currently a popular choice for primary ACL reconstructions, the central-third quadriceps tendon–bone graft may be useful in revision surgery or in multiple ligament reconstructions.

The use of allografts is growing in popularity. The fear of disease transmission has largely been eliminated with the development of modern donor screening and testing procedures. In the past, sterilization by high-dose radiation resulted in weakened structural properties in the graft tissue.[114, 294] The alternative use of ethylene oxide sterilization resulted in adverse surgical reactions, particularly chronic knee effusions.[149] The current technique of cryopreservation has been shown to have no effect on the structural properties of the frozen tissue.[147, 327] One concern that does remain is the delayed incorporation and maturation of allograft tissue after implantation.[148] Advantages of allografts are the absence of donor site morbidity, larger graft constructs, faster initial recovery time, and improved cosmesis. The use of patellar tendon allografts also provides the advantage of bone-to-bone fixation and healing. They are valuable graft sources for revision and multiple ligament reconstructions and are a useful primary graft source for older or lower demand patients and for patients who require a faster surgical recovery time.

Graft Harvest

The goal of any graft harvest technique is not only to obtain an adequate graft specimen but also to minimize the chance of incurring a donor site complication. Each graft option presents a unique set of technical challenges and potential pitfalls. A firm understanding of these differences is vital for avoidance of the many hazards that can occur.

Harvest of the central third of the patellar tendon is performed with the patellar and tibial insertion sites attached as bone plugs at either end of the graft construct. In general, the recommended dimensions are a width of 10 mm and a length of 25 mm. Removal of the patellar bone block has been shown to increase the stress across the remaining patella.[106] Square or tapered blocks have been shown to result in lower stress increases than trapezoidal cuts (Fig. 28J1–14).[106] The trough should be angled in a triangular or trapezoidal fashion to minimize the amount of bone stock removed. Oversized bone blocks taken from the patella predispose the patella to fracture or to tendon rupture.[47, 81] Bone grafting the patellar defect has been suggested as a way of reducing the risk for complication.[81, 106] The significance of bone grafting in altering the natural history of the defect has been questioned, however.[49] In some cases, it has even been implicated as a source of patellar pain secondary to the development of bone spurring in the region of the graft.[108]

Fracture has not been a significant problem associated with harvest of the tibial bone block. Rupture of the remaining patellar tendon is a rare reported complication, however.[47, 174] To minimize the risk of tendon rupture, care must be taken to define the central third of the tendon accurately. The patellar tendon narrows from proximal to distal, and one must be certain to keep the longitudinal

incisions in line with the orientation of the graft fibers. We also recommend angling the block cut to leave a triangular trough. This will maximize the bone stock that is left under the remaining tendon attachments (Fig. 28J1–15). This should leave a stronger insertion site, which theoretically reduces the likelihood of tendon rupture.

Closure of the tendon defect is controversial. It has been suggested that direct closure of the tendon gap will result in shortening of the tendon by as much as 10% of its length.[50, 85] Others have demonstrated no difference in tendon length after patellar tendon or hamstring reconstructions, however.[201] A proposed alternative is closure of the paratenon without closure of the tendon.[39] Regeneration of a load-bearing tendon-like scar tissue within the defect is seen by 6 to 12 months after closure of the paratenon alone, and this tissue continues to remodel over time.[39, 163] Others have noted that even if the defect is left open, it will fill in with scar tissue.[105] These scar tissues differ histologically and on MRI examination from the normal tendon tissue.[163] We believe that a loose approximation of the tendon edges with the knee flexed approximately 70 degrees should have a minimal effect on overall tendon length and helps orient the direction of the healing scar tissue. In addition, we close the paratenon to minimize the scarring of the tendon to the overlying skin.

Patellar pain after patellar tendon graft harvest has been a big concern. Some studies report the incidence of anterior knee pain in excess of 50% after patellar tendon reconstructions.[19, 168, 187] Fortunately, the majority of these complaints decrease over time.[49, 187, 261] It has been suggested that rather than being due to graft harvest, patellar pain may be related to loss of motion and poor rehabilitation techniques after surgery.[49, 128, 260] This theory is supported by the finding that implementation of aggressive rehabilitation techniques and the elimination of open chain exercises have lowered the incidence of patellar symptoms after patellar tendon reconstructions.[260, 285] In a meta-analysis of 21 studies of patellar tendon autograft ACL reconstruction using an unaug-

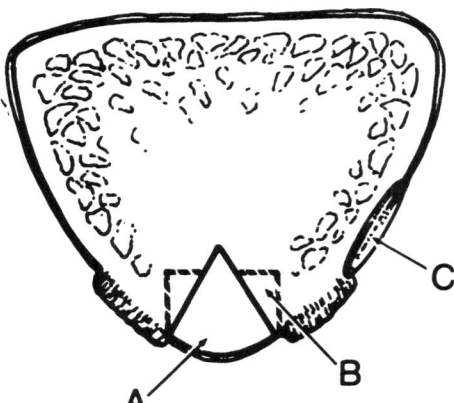

Figure 28J1–15. Triangular versus square tibial bone blocks. A triangular bone block (A) leaves more bone stock to protect the attachment of the remaining patellar tendon than does a square bone block (B). Placement of the tibial tunnel (C) should not violate the tibial bone block or the remaining patellar tendon. (From Nogalski MP, Bach BR Jr: Acute anterior cruciate ligament injuries. In Fu FH, Harner CD, Vince KG [eds]: Knee Surgery. Baltimore, Williams & Wilkins, 1994, pp 679–730.)

TABLE 28J1–8
Failure Strength of Various Techniques of Graft Fixation

Fixation	Ultimate Failure Load (N)	Reference
Patellar Tendon		
Interference screw		
Metal	558	66
Bioabsorbable	552	66
Soft Tissue		
Femoral		
Interference screw		
Metal	242	65
Bioabsorbable	341	65
EndoButton	430	306
Bone anchor	312	306
Cross-pin	1126	306
Tibial		
Interference screw	350	185
Tandem washer	1159	185
WasherLoc	905	185

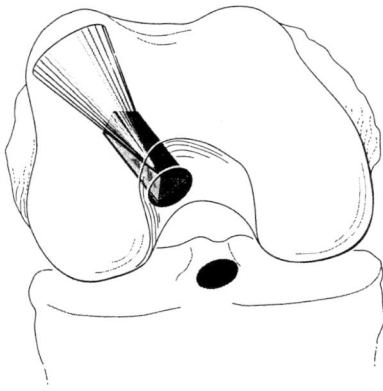

Figure 28J1–17. Demonstration of the wedge effect. With endoscopic interference screw placement (inside-out technique), the apex of fixation lies closer to the tunnel entrance. Therefore, for the graft to pull out of the tunnel, it must pull past the most secure (least divergent) point of fixation. The opposite would be the case using an outside-in technique, where the graft would be pulled away from the apex of fixation and toward the more divergent, and less secure, fixation points. (From Dworsky BD, Jewell BF, Bach BR Jr: Interference screw divergence in endoscopic anterior cruciate ligament reconstruction. Arthroscopy 12:45–49, 1996.)

block ranging from 423 N to 558 N (Table 28J1–8).[66, 172, 300] Combined with a proven clinical track record, interference screw fixation has become the standard for bone block fixation. Factors that may affect fixation strength of interference screws are screw diameter and divergence of the screw placement relative to the bone block. Screw diameter, typically 7 mm or 9 mm, has been shown to have an effect on pullout strength only when the gap between the bone block and tunnel wall exceeds 2 mm.[63] Under these circumstances, the 9-mm screw should be used. Screw placement with a divergence angle greater than 30 degrees has been shown to fail under lower loads than more parallel screw placement does.[91, 176] It has been shown that screw divergence has a more significant role during outside-in techniques, as occurs with tibial fixation or femoral fixation in the two-incision technique, as opposed to inside-out techniques, such as endoscopic femoral fixation.[91] We believe the reason for this phenomenon is the wedge effect that is created with endoscopic inside-out fixation. The bone block, to fail, must pull past the distal aspect of the screw. The bone block is being pulled toward the apex of fixation, which demonstrates the least divergence and greatest strength. With outside-in techniques, the distal aspect of the screw is the most divergent. As fixation fails, the bone block is pulled away from the apex of fixation and away from the screw (Fig. 28J1–17). Fortunately, outside-in techniques typically allow more accurate placement of the screws, with a lower incidence of screw divergence.[175] In addition, we recommend the use of a 9-mm screw on the tibial side to further protect against fixation failure. No difference has been noted in comparison of metal interference screws with bioabsorbable screws.[66]

Fixation strengths of soft tissue grafts have varied greatly, depending on the fixation method used (see Table 28J1–8). Different fixation methods are available for the tibial and femoral sides. Commonly used femoral fixation methods include buttons, suture posts, suture anchors, screw and washer constructs, cross-pins, and interference screws. Options for the tibial side include suture posts, staples, screw and washer constructs, and interference screws. Magen and colleagues[185] looked at six methods for tibial fixation of soft tissue grafts. They noted superior fixation strength (905 to 1159 N) and stiffness (414 to 516 N/mm) of the tandem soft tissue screw and washer construct and the WasherLoc (Arthrotek, Warsaw, Ind). To and coworkers[306] examined femoral fixation devices and found significantly improved strength and stiffness with cross-pin fixation (1126 N and 575 N/mm) compared with suture buttons or anchors (312 to 430 N and 24 to 26 N/mm). Interference screw fixation for soft tissue grafts has not been as successful as it has been for bone block fixation. Failure strengths for soft tissue interference screws range from 244 to 350 N.[65, 185, 293]

Fixation devices can be categorized as direct, meaning they achieve fixation through direct contact with the graft tissue and host bone, or indirect, meaning they secure the graft through the fixation of an intermediary material, such as a suture loop. Examples of direct fixation devices include interference screws, staples, screw and washer constructs, and cross-pins. Examples of indirect fixation devices include various buttons and suture posts. Direct fixation methods are superior to indirect methods. A large factor in the superiority of direct over indirect fixation methods is the relative weakness in the material properties of the bridging material compared with the graft tissue. Becker and associates[35] tested the strength and stiffness of No. 6 Ethibond, Mersilene, and polylene. They found strengths ranging from 338 N for Ethibond to 474 N for polylene, with the corresponding stiffness ranging from 37.1 N/mm for Ethibond to 47 N/mm for polylene. All three materials demonstrated significant reductions in their material properties when fashioned into suture loops by use of knots, as would be their use in clinical practice. They failed at the site of the knots and underwent elongation of about 1 cm before failure. Additional support for this concept was provided by Magen and coworkers,[185] who noted a significant decrease in the mechanical properties of their tandem washer construct when the length of the graft required the use of bridging sutures and did not allow direct fixation of the soft tissue to the washer.

The location of fixation is another factor to be considered. Fixation at the intra-articular tunnel entrance sites has been termed anatomic fixation. Theoretical advantages of anatomic graft fixation include improved stability and reduced graft tunnel motion. Morgan and associates[209] found improved isometricity with fixation of the graft closer to the joint surfaces. Ishibashi and colleagues[144] demonstrated increased stability to anterior translation with anatomic fixation in a cadaver model. In a clinical setting, however, Aglietti and coworkers[5] failed to find any difference in joint laxity between anatomic and nonanatomic fixation methods. They did note a lower incidence of tunnel widening with anatomic fixation but also found an increase in anterior knee pain. They did not think that the reduction in tunnel expansion justified the increased knee pain and greater technical difficulty associated with anatomic graft fixation.

The clinical significance of graft tunnel motion and tunnel expansion has not yet been determined. Graft tunnel motion is related not only to the fixation site but also to the stiffness of the graft construct.[107] Graft motion can occur in a longitudinal direction, known as the bungee effect, or in the sagittal plane, also known as windshield wiping. Longitudinal motion appears to be more of a problem with soft tissue constructs because of the more distal fixation methods typically employed and the reduced stiffness of the graft materials. Methods involving long segments of suture material, such as button fixation, result in a greater bungee effect. Increased longitudinal tunnel motion may compromise graft healing within the bone tunnel.[107] Sagittal graft motion is directly related to the distance of fixation relative to the joint line. Again, the effect is typically more pronounced in soft tissue grafts. Adverse effects of windshield wiping theoretically include increased bone tunnel expansion and damage to the graft related to wear on the bone tunnel edges.[117, 138, 267] The clinical significance of bone tunnel widening is unknown at this time.

Because patellar tendon grafts are typically fixed anatomically on the femoral side during endoscopic techniques and little clinical significance has been demonstrated with alterations in tibial fixation sites, we have not altered our standard technique of tibial fixation using an interference screw at the distal tunnel entrance. Because of the potential for greater reduction of graft motion in soft tissue grafts, however, we do support the use of supplemental interference screw fixation placed close to the anatomic insertion points for soft tissue grafts when distal fixation methods are used.

Graft Rotation

Many surgeons recommend rotation of patellar tendon grafts before tibial fixation. The normal ACL has been shown to have an external rotation within its fibers of approximately 90 degrees.[263] Re-creating this external graft rotation can be beneficial for a number of reasons. First, it re-creates the normal ACL morphologic characteristics. Second, rotation may help clear the lateral wall, reducing the chance of graft impingement. Third, rotation of 90 degrees has been shown to increase the tensile strength of patellar tendon grafts.[74, 75] Fourth, graft rotation effectively shortens the overall construct length.[17, 44] This can be beneficial in situations of graft mismatch, or in revision situations, to allow interference screw fixation when the graft would otherwise be too long. We have used rotation up to 540 degrees without any noticeable effect on clinical outcome. Auge and Yifan[17] have recommended up to 620 degrees of graft rotation without any detrimental outcome on clinical results. It is unclear at this time whether graft rotation greater than 180 degrees has any significant effect on graft strength. Finally, rotation of the graft typically places the cortical surface against the anterior tunnel wall. Placement of the screw on the cortical surface is more secure, and by moving the screw anterior on the tibia, the chance of graft abrasion against the screw during knee range of motion is minimized.

Graft Tension

The amount of tension created in the graft at the time of its fixation has a direct effect on the kinematics of the knee after ACL reconstruction. Factors that influence the tension in the graft are the position of the knee at the time of fixation, the tension applied to the graft, the position of the graft tunnels, and the mechanical properties of the graft tissue being used. Failure to generate enough tension results in graft laxity and an unstable knee, whereas excessive tensioning may lead to increased forces transmitted in the graft, leading to a failure of graft fixation or of the graft tissue itself.[43, 189, 190, 217] High graft forces may overconstrain the knee. This can theoretically lead to a limited range of motion in the knee or early degenerative changes in the knee secondary to the increased forces across the knee. The degree of tension has also been shown to influence the biologic healing of the graft.[332] Few surgeons control the amount of tension applied at the time of surgery, choosing instead to manually gauge the tension being applied. This leads to a wide variation in the range of tension placed on the graft.[84]

We know from kinematic studies that the forces generated in the graft as well as in the intact ACL are greatest at full extension and lowest at about 30 degrees of knee flexion.[43, 64, 190] Therefore, the tension applied to the graft with the knee positioned in full extension represents the highest force that will be generated in the graft throughout the entire range of motion of the knee. This is the safest position for the graft to be tensioned because it is unlikely that excessive tension in the graft will occur. There is a risk that the graft may become lax as the knee moves into flexion, however. With proper tunnel placement, this should not occur. When the graft is fixed with the knee positioned in 30 degrees of flexion, the result is an increase of tension in the graft as the knee is extended. This degree of increase is unpredictable, and concern exists that tensioning with the knee in flexion may lead to the generation of excessive loads within the graft.[64, 113] Tensioning the graft at 30 degrees of flexion results in an initially more stable knee,

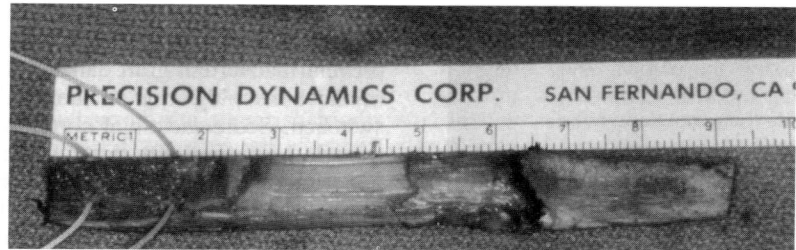

Figure 28J1–20. Prepared patellar tendon graft. Two No. 5 sutures are placed in the tibial bone block. The distal cortical surface on the tibial bone block and the tendo-osseous junction of the femoral bone block are marked with ink for visual identification. (From Ferrari JD, Bush-Joseph CA, Bach BR Jr: Anterior cruciate ligament reconstruction using bone–patellar tendon–bone grafts: Autograft and allograft endoscopic techniques and two-incision autograft technique. Operative Tech Sports Med 7:156–171, 1999.)

vested 10- × 25-mm bone plugs. If one bone plug is longer, use it on the femoral side to decrease length construct mismatch between the tibial tunnel and the graft. A small rongeur can be used to contour the bone plugs, and the excess bone removed should be saved for subsequent patellar defect bone grafting. A small spur of bone is often present proximal to the tendon insertion into the tibial bone plug and should be removed so that the bone edge is flush with the tendinous insertion. If one bone block is 11-mm wide, it can be used for the tibial tunnel side. Use a 0.062-inch K-wire to make two drill holes in the tibial bone plug, placed parallel to the cortical surface through the cancellous portion of the graft. Place a No. 5 Ti-Cron suture in each hole (Fig. 28J1–20). We have not had any occurrence of suture cutout through the cancellous bone with use of this technique in more than 900 cases of ACL reconstruction. Because we place our interference screw on the cortical surface of the bone plug, we avoid passing the suture holes through the cortex to minimize the risk of lacerating the sutures at the time of fixation. Alternatively, a 22-gauge wire can be placed, rather than suture, to preclude the potential for suture laceration. Because we use a "push-up" rather than "pull-through" technique in placing our graft intra-articularly, we do not place sutures in the femoral bone plug. If a pull-through technique with a passing pin is used, sutures may be placed in the femoral plug in an identical manner. After the graft is prepared, wrap it in a moist lap pad and place it in a kidney basin in the middle of the main instrument table. It is not immersed in water because this will cause the graft to become edematous.

Notch Preparation and Notchplasty

Intercondylar notch preparation is performed while the graft is being prepared at the back table. While evaluating the notch configuration, note the presence of tibial eminence and notch wall osteophytes. Although significant notch width variability may be encountered, 20 to 22 mm is required to avoid graft impingement. Removal of the ligamentum mucosum from the notch apex facilitates visualization, and it is occasionally necessary to débride some fat pad. Remove the remaining ACL tissue with the combination of arthroscopic scissors, arthroscopic osteotome, and motorized 5.5-mm full-radius resector. All soft tissue should be removed from the lateral wall of the notch.

Synovium overlying the PCL laterally may be removed to help visualize the posterior notch. This may create bleeding that requires electrocauterization.

The notchplasty is performed for two purposes. First, it promotes visualization of the over-the-top position and accurate placement of the femoral tunnel. Second, it helps prevent impingement of the graft with the knee in full extension. We initiate the notchplasty with a quarter-inch osteotome placed through the inferomedial portal (Fig. 28J1–21). This allows a more expeditious notchplasty, and the osteocartilaginous fragments can be removed with a grasper, the cartilaginous portion removed, and the remaining bone used to graft the patellar and tibial defects. Complete the notchplasty with a motorized 5.5-mm round bur, moving from anterior to posterior and from apex to inferior; pay careful attention to avoid misinterpreting a vertical ridge located two thirds of the way back in the notch ("resident's ridge") as the true posterior outlet (Fig. 28J1–22). When the ridge is identified, place the bur posterior to the ridge and move it from a posterior to an anterior direction to smooth the ridge. Use a curet to remove soft tissue from the posterior outlet, and then hook a probe over the posterior edge to confirm proper over-the-top positioning (Figs. 28J1–23 and 28J1–24). Minimal bone should be removed from the femoral ACL insertion to avoid lateralizing the isometric point. Proper perpendicular

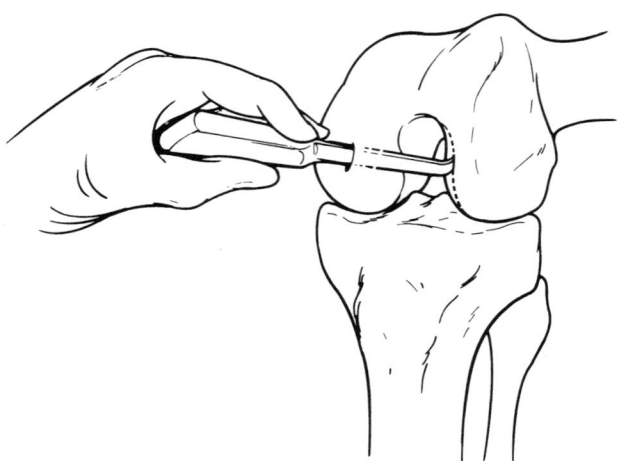

Figure 28J1–21. The notch may need to be widened to visualize the intercondylar notch adequately. The line of bone resection is marked with a ¼″ osteotome.

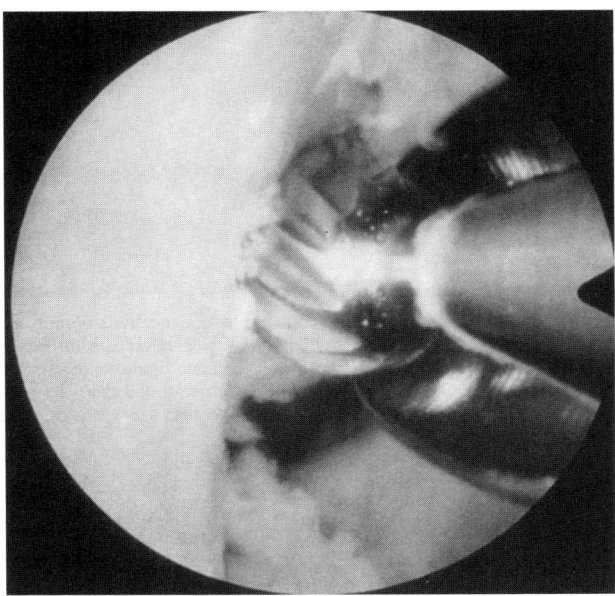

Figure 28J1–22. Arthroscopic view of a right knee. A 5.5-mm round bur is used to complete the notchplasty. Note the ridge of bone just anterior to the bur ("resident's ridge"). This bone must be removed to provide adequate visualization of the posterior notch before femoral tunnel placement. (From Ferrari JD, Bush-Joseph CA, Bach BR Jr: Anterior cruciate ligament reconstruction using bone–patellar tendon–bone grafts: Autograft and allograft endoscopic techniques and two-incision autograft technique. Operative Tech Sports Med 7:156–171, 1999.)

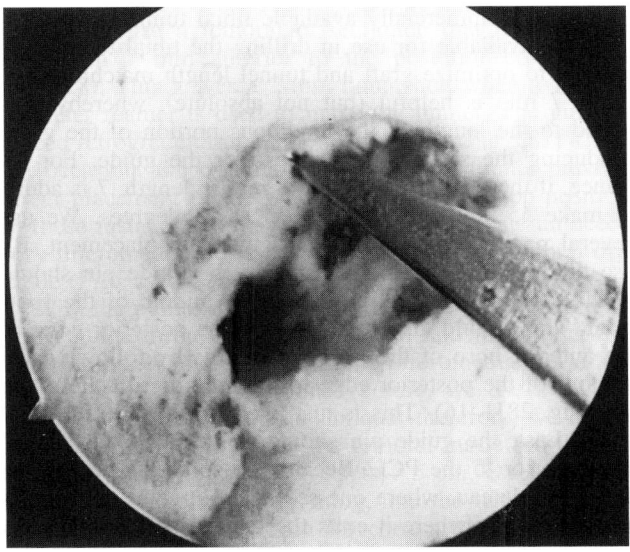

Figure 28J1–24. Arthroscopic view of a right knee. A probe is placed over the posterior edge of the femur, confirming adequate visualization of the over-the-top position. (From Ferrari JD, Bush-Joseph CA, Bach BR Jr: Anterior cruciate ligament reconstruction using bone–patellar tendon–bone grafts: Autograft and allograft endoscopic techniques and two-incision autograft technique. Operative Tech Sports Med 7:156–171, 1999.)

camera orientation is crucial in avoiding excessive removal of lateral femoral condyle bone in the midportion of the notch and insufficient bone from the inferior portion of the notch.

Tibial Tunnel Placement

After completion of the notchplasty, prepare the tibial tunnel. Make a medially based rectangular periosteal flap just medial to the tibial tubercle graft harvest site. The tibial tunnel entrance is generally 1.5 cm medial to the

tubercle and 1 cm proximal to the pes anserine tendons. Care must be taken to avoid injuring the superficial MCL, the pes anserine tendons, and the medial aspect of the patellar tendon. A more posteromedial starting point is desirable in the endoscopic technique to allow straighter access to the correct femoral tunnel position. The tibial tunnel's position will dictate the position of the femoral tunnel to a certain extent because the femoral tunnel guide is placed through the tibial tunnel, unlike in the two-incision technique (Fig. 28J1–25).

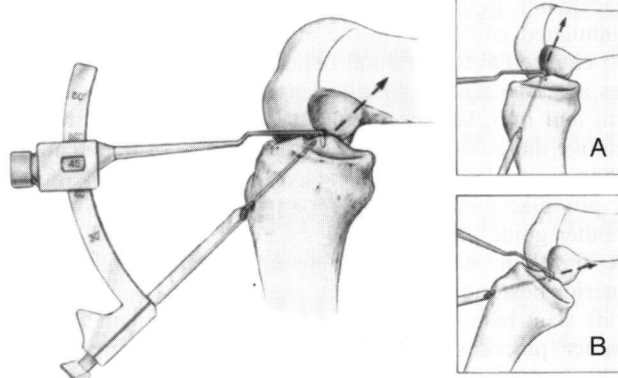

Figure 28J1–25. Placement of the tibial tunnel. A well-placed tibial tunnel will allow for direct placement of the femoral tunnel. A tibial tunnel that is too steep (*inset A*) will displace the femoral tunnel in an anterior direction. A tibial tunnel that is too flat (*inset B*) will displace the femoral tunnel in a posterior direction and will risk violation of the posterior cortex. (From Ferrari JD, Bush-Joseph CA, Bach BR Jr: Anterior cruciate ligament reconstruction using bone–patellar tendon–bone grafts: Autograft and allograft endoscopic techniques and two-incision autograft technique. Operative Tech Sports Med 7:156–171, 1999.)

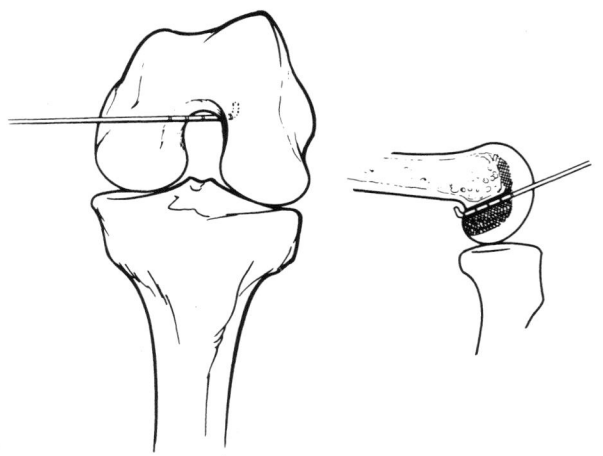

Figure 28J1–23. A probe is used to identify the over-the-top position.

After the reamer is removed, flush loose bone from the knee with the aid of the pump and collect these reamings with gauze placed at the exit of the tibial tunnel. Femoral tunnel integrity can be checked by placing the arthroscope retrograde through the tibial tunnel into the femoral tunnel (Fig. 28J1–30). During the process of femoral tunnel reaming, if the reamer engages the lateral wall, we use this observation to assist us in fine-tuning the amount of lateral wall expansion. The femoral tunnel entrance should appear circular. If there is an oval appearance laterally, we abrade the opening to produce a circular configuration. We then "ellipticize" (i.e., eccentrically abrade) the anterolateral quadrant to aid in screw placement and chamfer the anterior ridge with a shaver to facilitate guide pin placement and to protect the graft from abrasion along the tunnel edge.

Graft Placement and Fixation

After removing the graft from its gauze, we place a two-pronged pusher at the base of the femoral bone plug (Fig. 28J1–31) and position a curved hemostat through the inferomedial portal with its tips pointed up. We then push the graft up through the tibial tunnel, where it is then grasped by the hemostat at the junction of the proximal and middle thirds of the bone plug (Fig. 28J1–32A). Remove the pusher, and guide the graft up into the femoral socket (Fig. 28J1–32B). Orient the cortical surface of the femoral plug posteriorly and in the coronal plane.

Before fully seating the femoral plug into its socket, place the Nitenol hyperflex guide pin (Linvatec Corporation, Largo, Fla) into the femoral socket at the 11-o'clock position of the graft. The 11-o'clock position is used for

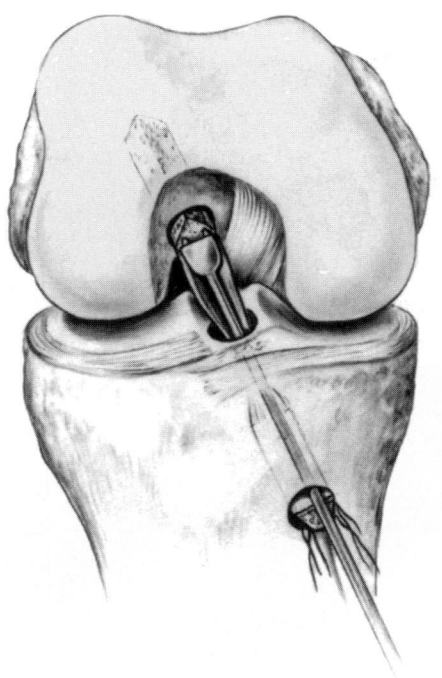

Figure 28J1–31. Right knee. A two-pronged pushing device is used to guide the femoral bone block through the tibial tunnel and into the knee joint. Unlike in this diagram, we grasp the femoral bone plug with a hemostat as it enters the knee joint, and we remove the pushing device before engaging the tibial bone plug in the tibial tunnel. This allows for the easy removal of the pushing device. (From Ferrari JD, Bush-Joseph CA, Bach BR Jr: Anterior cruciate ligament reconstruction using bone–patellar tendon–bone grafts: Autograft and allograft endoscopic techniques and two-incision autograft technique. Operative Tech Sports Med 7: 156–171, 1999.)

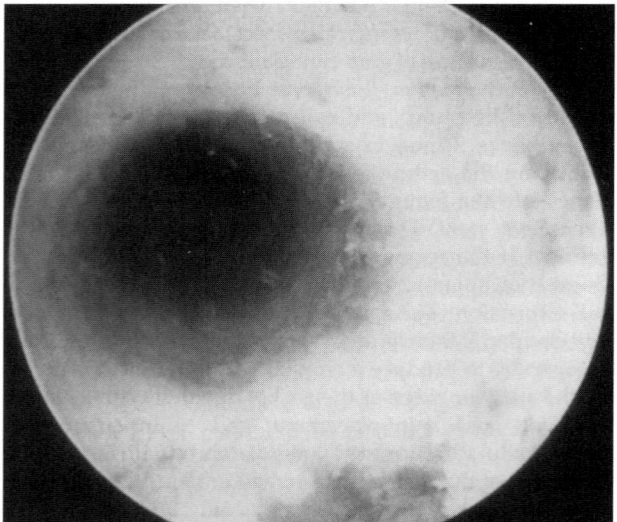

Figure 28J1–30. Arthroscopic view of the femoral tunnel with the arthroscope placed through the tibial tunnel. This view allows evaluation of the integrity of the femoral tunnel, particularly the posterior wall. (From Ferrari JD, Bush-Joseph CA, Bach BR Jr: Anterior cruciate ligament reconstruction using bone–patellar tendon–bone grafts: Autograft and allograft endoscopic techniques and two-incision autograft technique. Operative Tech Sports Med 7:156–171, 1999.)

both right and left knees to account for the clockwise rotation of the screw threads as the screw is advanced. If difficulty is encountered in placing the guide pin in the tunnel, a hemostat may be used to create a small opening to facilitate passage of the guide pin. Once the pin is initially positioned within the tunnel, the knee is flexed approximately 110 degrees, and the guide pin is fully seated within the tunnel (Fig. 28J1–32C). The pin should not be forced and should slide easily. If forced, the pin could potentially be placed through the bone plug or posterior femoral cortex. If the guide pin appears too divergent from the graft, as can often be seen if patella alta is present, the accessory inferomedial portal is helpful in placing the guide pin more parallel with the graft and reducing screw divergence. As the knee is flexed, the camera can be adjusted to visualize the "gap space interval" anteriorly between the femoral socket and bone plug. We then use a pushing device to fully seat the bone plug in its socket (Fig. 28J1–32D). The tibial plug should be checked to make sure it is not protruding excessively from its tunnel. If there is marked graft-tunnel mismatch at this time, the graft can be removed and the femoral socket deepened.

We use a 7- × 25-mm titanium fully threaded cannulated interference screw on the femoral side. We prefer interference screw fixation with nonheaded Kurosaka screws (Linvatec Corporation, Largo, Fla), and we generally use a screw that matches the length of our graft. Apply

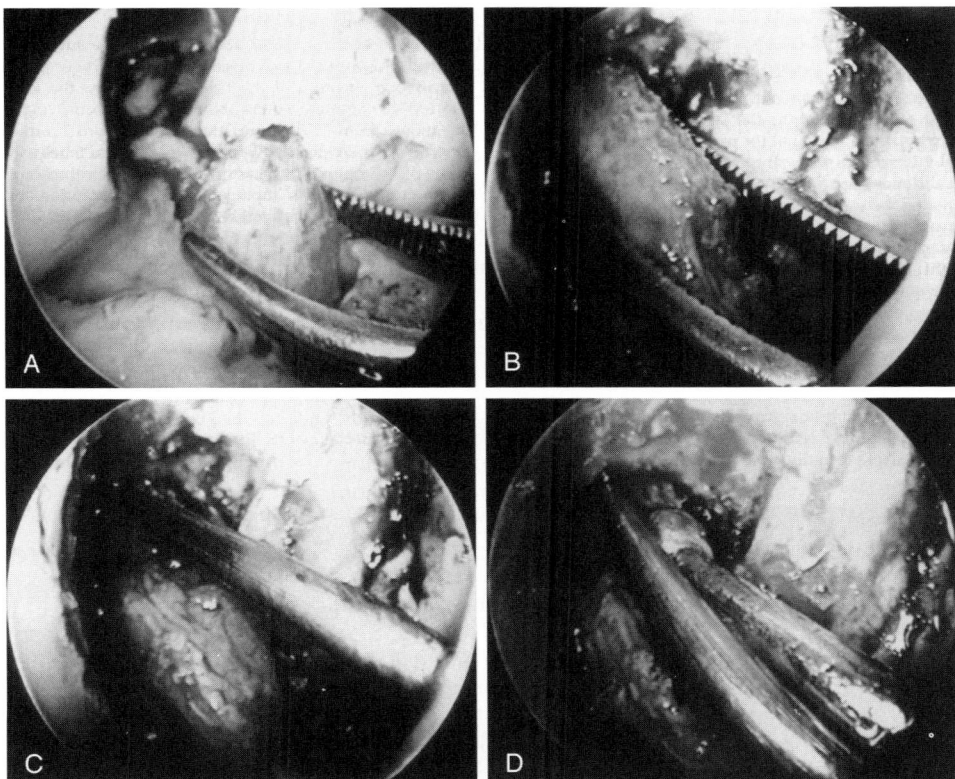

Figure 28J1–32. Arthroscopic view of the right knee. *A,* The femoral bone block is grasped with a curved hemostat placed through the inferomedial portal. *B,* The hemostat is used to guide the bone block into the femoral tunnel. *C,* When the bone block is seated up to the final 3 mm, a flexible guidewire is placed at the 11-o'clock position, the knee is hyperflexed, and the guide pin is seated in the base of the femoral tunnel. *D,* The bone block is seated the final 3 mm using a broad-faced tamp. (*A–D* from Ferrari JD, Bush-Joseph CA, Bach BR Jr: Anterior cruciate ligament reconstruction using bone–patellar tendon–bone grafts: Autograft and allograft endoscopic techniques and two-incision autograft technique. Operative Tech Sports Med 7:156–171, 1999.)

maximal tension to the sutures as the screws are placed to avoid graft advancement. We place the femoral screw against the cancellous surface, thus reducing the potential for soft tissue injury or laceration, whereas the tibial screw is placed against the cortical surface. Cannulated screws are used to help prevent divergence. Place the screw over the guidewire and push it into the joint (Fig. 28J1–33). To maximize the potential for parallel placement of the femoral interference screw, hyperflex the knee to 110 degrees. This additional knee flexion compensates for the difference between the tibial tunnel angle and the angle created by the flexible Nitenol pin placed through the inferomedial portal. As the screw is being placed, apply light tension to the tibial plug's sutures, which helps prevent the graft from

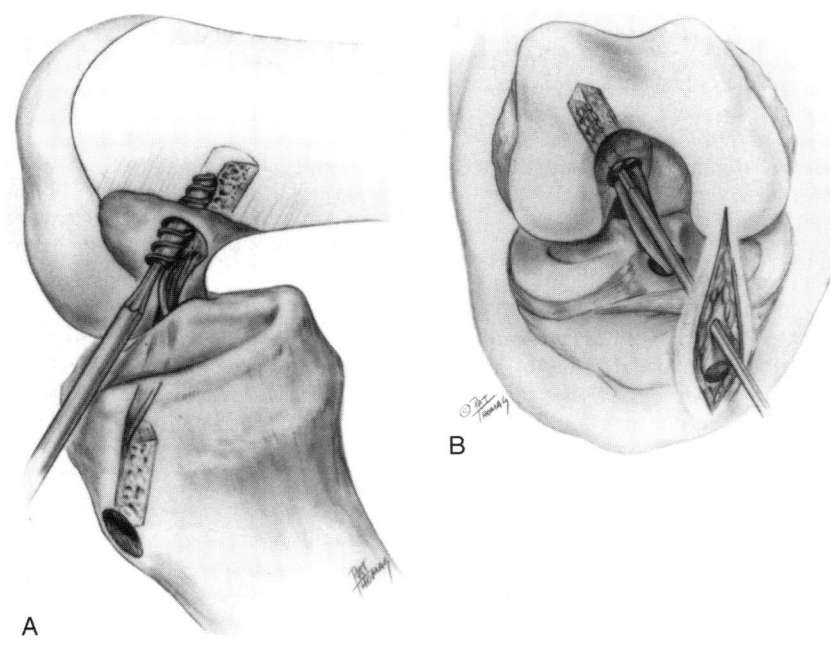

Figure 28J1–33. Right knee. Lateral (*A*) and coronal (*B*) views of interference screw placement. Note the placement of the screw at the 11-o'clock position relative to the femoral tunnel. (*A* and *B,* From Ferrari JD, Bush-Joseph CA, Bach BR Jr: Anterior cruciate ligament reconstruction using bone–patellar tendon–bone grafts: Autograft and allograft endoscopic techniques and two-incision autograft technique. Operative Tech Sports Med 7:156–171, 1999.)

being lacerated by the screw. The tendinous portion of the graft just inferior to the femoral plug is carefully observed. If this tissue begins to rotate, the screw may be wrapping up or lacerating the tendon. When the screw is halfway positioned, remove the guide pin, or it may be difficult to remove the wire when the screw is fully seated. The screw is fully seated when its base is flush with or slightly above the base of the femoral plug, or fraying and subsequent graft disruption can occur with motion. Commercially available graft protection sleeves are available to reduce the potential for soft tissue laceration. If we decide to recess the femoral bone plug more than 5 mm, we routinely use a protection sleeve.

Check the graft for gross isometry. Hold the sutures in the tibial plug tightly and place an index finger at the extraosseous entrance of the tibial tunnel. Flex the knee from 100 degrees to complete extension or hyperextension. As the knee moves from 30 degrees to complete extension, 1 to 2 mm of motion is generally noted. Cycle the knee several times with tension placed on the graft. Last, view the graft arthroscopically to ensure that it is impingement free in extension and does not abrade along the lateral wall with knee motion.

An alternative means of graft passage is the use of a passing pin that has an open slot at its base for placing suture. When using this technique, place two No. 5 Ti-Cron sutures through both bone plugs. Place the pin through the over-the-top guide and drill through the femur. Tap the pin with a mallet through the anterolateral thigh and out the skin. Overdrill with the 10-mm reamer, and pass the sutures through the bottom slot of the pin. Pull the pin out of the anterolateral thigh and securely grasp the sutures protruding out the pinhole. With a hand on each group of sutures, bring the graft into the knee joint. A probe in the inferomedial portal can facilitate placement of the femoral bone plug into its socket. After placing the femoral interference screw, remove the two No. 5 Ti-Cron sutures from the anterolateral thigh. We prefer the push-in technique to the pull-through method because it avoids placing a pin through the thigh and the possible complications, such as break in sterility, pin breakage, and creation of a stress riser in the femur. The phase II notchplasty and visualization of the femoral socket are also easier because the passing pin is not present, and no sutures need be placed through the femoral bone plug.

Before tibial fixation, we externally rotate the graft. This allows an anatomic rotation of the graft, can reduce graft-tunnel mismatch by shortening the graft construct, and allows the tibial screw to be placed against the cortical surface of the tibial plug, anterior to the graft. We do this for four reasons. First, with the screw placed anteriorly, when the knee flexes, there is no abrasion of the screw against the graft. If the screw is placed posteriorly and the screw tip extends beyond the tendo-osseous interval, knee flexion may result in abrasion of the graft. Second, the screw is more likely to diverge if it is placed posteriorly along the cancellous portion of the graft. Third, a screw placed posteriorly will anteriorize the graft and adversely affect isometricity and possibly create impingement of the graft. Last, fixation is greater when it is placed along the cortical surface.

One must ensure that the tibial plug is moving freely within the tibial tunnel before distal fixation. On occasion, the distal tip of the plug can get caught inside the tunnel on the inferior edge. If the plug is fixed in this position, graft tension will be lax. For fixation on the tibial side, position the knee in full extension and firmly tension the tibial plug sutures. Place a Nitenol hyperflex pin anterior to the tibial plug and secure the graft with a 9- × 20-mm cannulated interference screw. Recess the head of the screw just below the cortical surface of the tibia so that it is less likely to become symptomatic but not difficult to remove should the situation arise. If the tibial plug has been recessed in its tunnel because of mismatch, choose a longer screw.

Place the arthroscope back inside the knee for a final check of graft orientation and to ensure that proper tension is present at 20 to 30 degrees of knee flexion. A Lachman test and pivot shift examination can be done at this time.

Methods of Addressing Graft Construct Mismatch

As with most surgical problems, prevention is the best cure. By following the N + 7 rule, most but not all graft construct mismatches can be avoided. Our largest mismatches currently occur in use of bone-tendon-bone allografts when the allografts are derived from a cadaver of significantly larger size than the patient. Several methods are available to address mismatch problems. Small mismatches may be reduced by recessing the femoral bone plug deeper within its socket. If one is going to recess the femoral bone block, parallel placement of the interference screw is essential because the potential for graft injury increases. Commercially available graft protectors can be used to further protect the soft tissue component of the graft. An accessory inferomedial portal should also be considered for screw placement.

Externally rotating the graft 180 degrees or even 540 degrees will reduce mismatch as well. If 15 mm of tibial bone is within the tibial tunnel, our choice is to use an interference screw. An alternative to interference screw fixation is tying the sutures over a bicortical screw and washer or recessing the tibial tunnel bed so that the tibial plug can be placed within it and be fixed with either two 7/16-inch barbed staples or a bicortical 3.5-mm screw placed in a lag fashion. Last, should the entire bone plug be protruding, we remove the tibial bone block, place two No. 5 Ti-Cron sutures in the tendon perpendicular to one another in a Krackow fashion for traction, and then place the free tibial bone block into the tunnel. We secure this entire construct with a 9- × 20-mm interference screw placed over a guidewire. This construct has been found to be significantly stronger and stiffer than fixation with the bone block sutures tied over a post.

Closure

Loosely reapproximate the patellar tendon defect with three or four interrupted No. 1 Vicryl sutures while the knee is flexed, avoiding excessive shortening of the tendon.

The osteoperiosteal flap overlying the tibial drill hole is also closed with No. 1 Vicryl. We graft the patellar bone defect with the collected bone reamings, and any remaining bone is used to graft the tibial donor site. We close the peritenon with a running 2–0 Vicryl suture, the subcutaneous layer with interrupted 2–0 Vicryl, and the skin with a running 3–0 Prolene. We inject 0.5% bupivacaine (Marcaine) with epinephrine into the periosteal region, deep surgical wound region, portals, and skin and intra-articularly. We do not use HemoVac drains. Apply Steri-Strips to the wounds, then apply dry sterile gauze, Kerlex roll, cryotherapy pad, and ACE wrap. The cryotherapy pad must not contact the skin, or a superficial frostbite can occur. Last, place the leg in a hinged knee brace, which is locked in extension.

Rehabilitation

Rehabilitation after ACL surgery continues to evolve. The goal remains to return the patient to a normal and complete level of function in as short a time as possible without compromising the integrity of the surgically reconstructed knee. During the past 30 years, advancements in surgical techniques, graft selection, and fixation methods as well as an improved understanding of the biology and biomechanics of the knee have fueled a radical change in the way we rehabilitate a patient after ACL reconstruction. We now stress early motion and weight-bearing, focus on closed chain exercises, and return athletes to the playing field earlier than ever before. As we move into the new millennium, further research into the biology of graft healing, the appropriate limits of graft strain, and the effects of activity on graft stability will guide the continued evolution of rehabilitation after ACL reconstruction.

Open and Closed Kinetic Chain Exercise

Considerable debate has occurred in recent years about the use of closed kinetic chain activity versus open kinetic chain activity after ACL reconstruction. Open kinetic chain movement refers to isolated joint movement during which the distal component is free to move in space with a single rotational axis that is relatively stable. Thus, one segment of the limb is stabilized while the other segment moves freely. An example of open kinetic chain exercise is the leg extension machine (Fig. 28J1–34). Closed kinetic chain movement refers to multijoint movement around several joint axes. Multiple segments of the extremity are moving while the distal segment is fixed to a surface or object that can be moving or fixed. An example of closed kinetic chain exercise is the leg press machine (Fig. 28J1–35). Other examples are squatting exercises, stationary bicycle, and StairMaster. In theory, closed kinetic chain exercises provide a more significant compression force across the knee while activating co-contraction of the hamstring muscles. It has been suggested that these two factors help to decrease the anterior shear forces in the knee that would otherwise be taken up by the ACL graft. As a result, closed

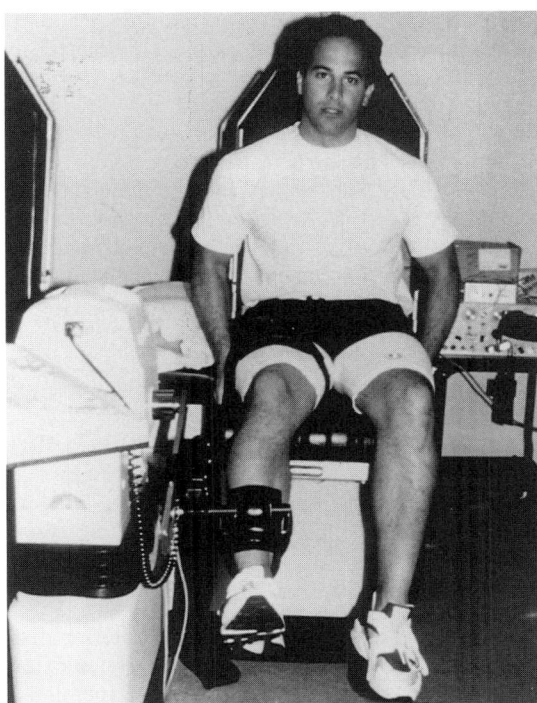

Figure 28J1–34. Leg extension machine. Patient is doing an open kinetic chain exercise.

kinetic chain exercises are favored over open kinetic chain exercises during rehabilitation after ACL reconstruction. The literature supporting this theory is not so definitive, however.

One of the confusing issues is that many common activities cannot be clearly classified as open or closed kinetic chain. Walking, running, stair climbing, and jumping have a combination of open and closed kinetic chain components to them. Regardless, a review of our current knowledge about the mechanics of activities is important to establish guidelines for safe activities after reconstructive ACL surgery. Understanding the relationship between a given activity and the resulting tibial translation, force generation in an intact ACL or ACL graft, and strain production in the ACL or ACL graft has been the primary focus of research efforts.

Jenkins and coworkers[152] measured side-to-side difference in anterior displacement of the tibia in subjects with unilateral ACL-deficient knees during open kinetic chain exercise (knee extension) and closed kinetic chain exercises (leg press) at 30 degrees and 60 degrees of knee flexion. The displacement for open kinetic chain exercise at 30 degrees was 4.7 mm greater in the involved extremity compared with 1.3 mm for closed kinetic chain exercise. The displacement for open kinetic chain exercise at 60 degrees was 1.2 mm compared with −0.1 mm for closed kinetic chain exercise. Side-to-side differences of 3 to 5 mm are commonly cited as abnormal, whereas more than 5 mm is usually defined as an arthrometric failure. Thus, open chain exercises at low flexion angles may place the graft at risk for development of laxity approaching a level considered a failure.

These findings were supported by the work of Yack and

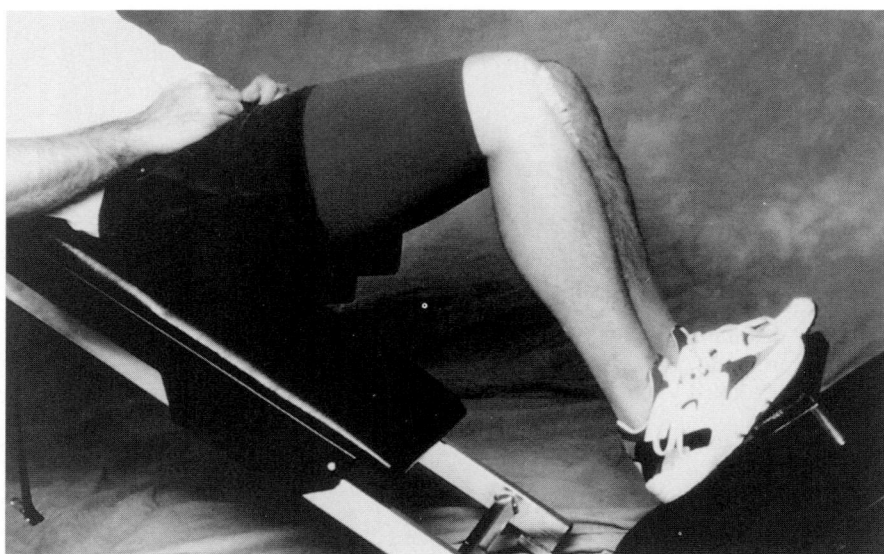

Figure 28J1–35. Leg press machine. Patient is doing a closed kinetic chain exercise.

associates,[329] who also found increased anterior displacements during open kinetic chain exercise (knee extension) compared with closed kinetic chain exercise (parallel squat) through a flexion range of 0 to 64 degrees. Kvist and Gillquist[173] have demonstrated that these displacements occur with even low levels of muscle activity. Generation of the first 10% of the peak quadriceps torque produced 80% of the total tibial translation seen with maximal quadriceps torque. Escamilla and coworkers[94] have developed a mathematical model to study forces in the knee during open and closed kinetic chain activities. Their model predicts that shear forces generating tension in the ACL are negligible during closed kinetic chain activities but are increased with open kinetic chain activities in a range from 0 to 30 degrees.[94, 250] Using a different model, Lutz and colleagues[183] also predicted an absence of anterior directed shear force during closed kinetic chain activities but predicted an increased force directed toward the ACL during open kinetic chain activities below 60 degrees of flexion. Jurist and Otis,[159] Zavetsky and colleagues,[333] and Wilk and Andrews[319] noted that changing the position of the resistance pad on isokinetic open kinetic chain devices could modify anterior shear force and anterior tibial displacement. In addition, Wilk and Andrews[319] also found greater anterior tibial displacements at slower isokinetic speeds.

Extensive work has been done by Beynnon and Fleming[40] using implanted transducers to measure the strain in the intact ACL during various exercises (see Table 28J1–1). Regardless of the exercise, maximal strain values were less than 5%. Strain values in the ACL were found to be higher during isometric quadriceps contraction at 15 degrees and 30 degrees of knee flexion and were minimal or absent with isometric quadriceps contraction at flexion angles of 60 degrees or greater or with simultaneous quadriceps and hamstring contractions at flexion angles of 30 degrees or greater. They did not find a consistent distinction between closed kinetic chain and open kinetic chain activities, however. Similar strain characteristics comparing active knee extension, an open kinetic chain exercise, with squatting, a closed kinetic chain exercise, were noted. Both exercises

resulted in increased strain values in the ACL, with squatting showing slightly higher strain values than knee extension. This finding contradicts the previous studies and indicates that certain closed chain activities, such as squatting, may not be as safe as the mathematical force models would predict, particularly at low flexion angles. One must question whether the apparent advantage of closed kinetic chain exercise over open kinetic chain exercise is real and whether it can be generalized to all methods of these exercises. One advantage they did find for closed kinetic chain exercises was that increasing resistance did not lead to an increased strain in the ACL during closed kinetic chain exercises, whereas it did during open kinetic chain exercises.

A protective effect of the hamstrings has been proposed on the basis of the findings of minimal or absent strain in the ACL with isolated hamstring contracture or when the hamstrings were simultaneously contracted along with the quadriceps.[40] Co-contraction of the quadriceps and hamstrings occurs in closed kinetic chain exercises, with a progressive decrease in hamstring activity as flexion angle of the knee increases. Not all closed kinetic chain activities produce the same degree of co-contraction, however. Co-contraction does not occur to any significant degree during open kinetic chain exercise.[94, 183, 250]

Closed kinetic chain exercises generate greater activity in the vasti musculature; open kinetic chain exercises generate more rectus femoris activity. Open chain activities generate more isolated muscle activity and thus allow more specific muscle strengthening. With fatigue, however, any stabilizing effect of these isolated muscles may be lost and can put the ACL at greater risk. Closed chain exercises, by allowing agonist muscle activity, may not provide focused muscle strengthening, but they may provide a safer environment for the ACL in the setting of fatigue.[94, 250]

An important consideration in comparing open and closed kinetic chain exercises for use during ACL rehabilitation is the effect of each on the patellofemoral joint. Closed chain exercises place low stress on the patellofemoral joint at low knee flexion angles, whereas open chain

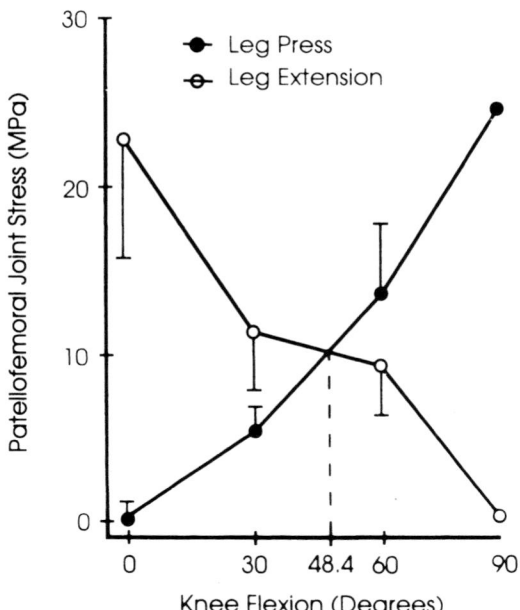

Figure 28J1–36. Contact stress in the patella as a function of knee flexion angle in open and closed kinetic chain exercises. (From Steinkamp LA, Dillingham MF, Markel MD, et al: Biomechanical considerations in patellofemoral joint rehabilitation. Am J Sports Med 21:438–444, 1993.)

exercises place a high stress on the patellofemoral joint at low flexion angles (Fig. 28J1–36).[301] From this, we can conclude that closed chain exercises are favorable in the functional ranges of motion and that open chain exercises should be avoided to reduce the likelihood of development of patellofemoral symptoms, which can interfere with the progression of therapy. An exception is the straight leg raise; although technically an open chain exercise, it places little stress on the patellofemoral joint because the patella is not in contact with the trochlea at this position of extension or slight hyperextension of the knee.[118]

To summarize, closed chain exercises can be used safely during rehabilitation of the ACL. Closed chain activities appear to generate low anterior shear force and tibial displacement through most of the flexion range, although some evidence now exists that low flexion angles during certain closed kinetic chain activities may strain the graft as much as open chain activities do. At what level strain becomes detrimental and whether some degree of strain is beneficial during the graft healing phase are currently unknown. Until these answers are realized, current trends have been to recommend activities that minimize graft strain to put the ACL at the lowest risk for development of laxity. Open chain flexion, dominated by hamstring activity, appears to pose little risk to the ACL throughout the entire flexion arc, but open chain extension places significant strain on the ACL as well as on the patellofemoral joint and should be avoided.

Rehabilitation Considerations
Pain and Effusion

Pain and swelling are common after any surgical procedure. Both act to cause reflex inhibition of muscle activity.

Therefore, it is important to control these problems to facilitate early range of motion and strengthening activities.

Standard therapeutic modalities to reduce pain and swelling include cryotherapy, compression, and elevation. Narcotic and anti-inflammatory pain medications should also be used judiciously in the acute postoperative setting. Muscle activity, in the form of quad setting and ankle pumps, helps to reduce swelling by improving venous return. Electrical muscle stimulation of the quadriceps may be used to promote muscle activity before the return of volitional control.

Cryotherapy

Cryotherapy is commonly used to reduce pain, inflammation, and effusion after ACL reconstruction surgery. Cryotherapy acts through a variety of local effects.[237] It lowers tissue metabolism, limiting the effects of hypoxia. This prevents cell death, which limits the release of the chemical mediators of pain, inflammation, and edema. It induces vasoconstriction, which reduces fluid extravasation and minimizes blood loss. Cryotherapy also inhibits afferent nerve conduction, which decreases pain and muscle spasm.[321] Decreased subjective pain scores and reduced analgesic use have been demonstrated in patients using cryotherapy after surgery.[72, 237]

The many forms of cryotherapy include ice packs, ice baths, and more recently, continuous flow cooling devices. Complications such as superficial frostbite and neurapraxia can be prevented by avoiding prolonged placement of the cold source directly on the skin. Contraindications to cryotherapy include hypersensitivity to cold (such as Raynaud's phenomenon), lupus erythematosus, periarteritis nodosa, and rheumatoid arthritis.[321]

Motion

Loss of motion is among the most common complications after ACL reconstruction. Loss of extension is more common than loss of flexion and is less tolerated.[162] Symptoms resulting from a loss of motion include anterior knee pain, quadriceps weakness, gait abnormalities, and early articular degenerative changes.[162, 231, 282] There are a number of causes of loss of motion after ACL reconstruction (Table 28J1–9). As our understanding of the causes has increased, and with the implementation of aggressive postoperative rehabilitation protocols, the incidence of postoperative motion problems has been reduced.[125]

Prevention is the first and most effective method for treatment of loss of motion after ACL reconstruction. Many of the factors leading to loss of motion can be prevented with proper surgical timing and technique. After surgery, rehabilitative measures to regain motion are started immediately. Early passive range of motion and active range of motion are begun and may be augmented with the use of a continuous passive motion machine. Postoperative immobilization has been shown to lead to a higher incidence of the need for later manipulation to regain motion.[241] Control of pain and swelling, early reactivation of the

TABLE 28J1–9
Factors That Can Cause Limitation of Knee Motion after Anterior Cruciate Ligament Reconstruction

Arthrofibrosis, infrapatellar contracture syndrome, and patella infera
Inappropriate graft placement or tensioning
"Cyclops" syndrome
Acute surgery on a swollen knee
Concomitant medial collateral ligament repair
Poorly supervised or poorly designed rehabilitation program, prolonged immobilization
Reflex sympathetic dystrophy

From Shelbourne KD, Patel DV: Treatment of limited motion after anterior cruciate ligament reconstruction. Knee Surg Sports Traumatol Arthrosc 7:85–92, 1999. © 1999, Springer-Verlag.

quadriceps musculature, and early return to weight-bearing will enhance the return of motion. Patellar mobilization techniques should be started to prevent patellar tendon shortening or retinacular contracture, both of which can lead to motion loss.

Our current goals include achieving and maintaining full knee extension immediately after surgery. Knee flexion to 90 degrees should be achieved by 7 to 10 days postoperatively. Failure to achieve these goals prompts the early initiation of countermeasures to prevent a chronic problem from occurring. These techniques are discussed in detail in the complications section to follow.

Continuous Passive Motion

The efficacy of continuous passive motion after ACL reconstruction is controversial (Fig. 28J1–37). Historically, its use was advocated to improve cartilage nutrition and limit motion loss when immobilization was common after surgery.[262] With the advancement of arthroscopic reconstruction techniques and the growing popularity of accelerated rehabilitation with use of early motion and weight-bearing, the benefits of continuous passive motion machines have waned. Few studies now demonstrate a significant benefit of continuous passive motion over a supervised motion program.[255] We currently do not believe that the added cost is justified and have not used continuous passive motion since 1993. There may still be a role for continuous passive motion after manipulation and arthroscopic surgery for patients who have arthrofibrosis, however.

Weight-bearing

Historically, patients were kept from bearing weight after ACL surgery. Concerns existed about graft fixation failure and the development of graft laxity. With the institution of more aggressive rehabilitation, brought on in part by observations of noncompliant patients, along with the advent of improved fixation methods, a trend toward immediate weight-bearing in the postoperative setting has evolved.[280] Theoretical advantages of weight-bearing include improved cartilage nutrition, decreased disuse osteopenia, reduced peripatellar fibrosis, and quicker quadriceps recovery.[309]

In a study by Tyler and coworkers,[309] immediate weight-bearing was shown to reduce muscle inhibition at the knee joint in the early postoperative period, as demonstrated by an increased return of electromyographic activity in the vastus medialis oblique muscle within the first 2 weeks after surgery. The same study also demonstrated a reduction in the subsequent development of anterior knee pain after surgery in patients who began immediate weight-bearing. No differences were noted between weight-bearing and non–weight-bearing groups with regard to knee laxity, range of motion, or functional scores.

One theoretical concern with weight-bearing in the first 4 to 6 weeks is donor site morbidity in patients with a bone–patellar tendon–bone autograft.[124] The risk for proximal tibia fracture, patellar fracture, or patellar tendon rupture in association with weight-bearing is unknown at this

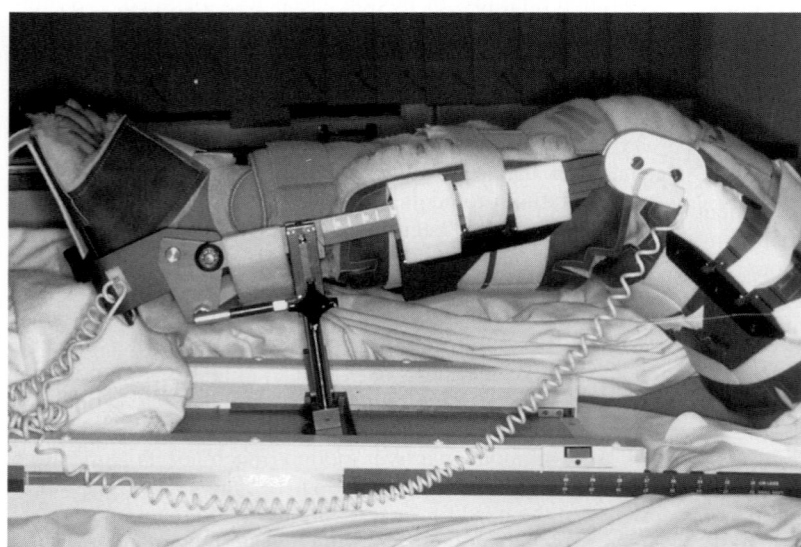

Figure 28J1–37. Continuous passive motion device.

time, but it is certainly less than 1%. Although rare, these complications can be difficult to treat and can lead to poor results. We currently recommend maintaining the knee in a brace locked in full extension during the first 4 to 6 weeks after surgery to limit the forces transmitted through the extensor mechanism and to protect the extensor mechanism in the event of a patient's slip or fall.

Properly initiated, immediate weight-bearing is safe and beneficial. It is part of a well-designed rehabilitation program.

Muscle Training Issues

The early initiation of muscle training is crucial for prevention of muscle atrophy and weakness. In fact, muscle activation and strengthening should begin shortly after injury, before surgery. Once surgery takes place, muscle retraining should begin immediately. Factors leading to muscle inhibition, such as pain and swelling, should be dealt with promptly. Electrical muscle stimulation may help initiate muscle activation in patients who are unable to overcome reflex inhibition voluntarily. Biofeedback may be used to enhance the force of muscle contraction. Weight-bearing has also been shown to be beneficial in promoting muscle reactivation.

Muscle balance is an important consideration. Achieving the appropriate hamstring-to-quadriceps ratio provides an improved dynamic protection for the ACL. Barratta and colleagues[32] pointed out the increased risk for injury with reduced hamstring antagonist activity and demonstrated improved coactivation ratios in response to exercise.

Fatigue has been shown significantly to affect not only the strength of muscle contraction but also the electromechanical response time and rate of muscle force generation.[314, 320] These factors are critical elements of dynamic stabilization of the knee, and deficits reduce the ability of the individual to protect the knee during activity. Endurance training should be included in the rehabilitation program.

Electrical Muscle Stimulation and Biofeedback

Electrical muscle stimulation (Fig. 28J1–38) and biofeedback are modalities that may be useful adjuncts to conventional muscle training techniques. The literature investigating the use of electrical muscle stimulation after ACL reconstruction varies in regard to its benefit. There is no convincing evidence that electrical muscle stimulation alone is superior to voluntary muscle contraction alone in promoting muscle strength after surgery.[179] It may certainly be of benefit in the early postoperative period, however, when reflex inhibition of the quadriceps due to pain and swelling prevents the initiation of voluntary muscle activity. Anderson and Lipscomb[8] did note a positive effect of electrical muscle stimulation in limiting quadriceps strength loss and patellofemoral crepitus after ACL reconstruction. The most appropriate use of electrical muscle stimulation seems to be in combination with volitional muscle activity in the early postoperative period.[295]

Biofeedback may be useful for reeducation of the muscles. With electromyographic monitoring, a visual or auditory signal is provided to the patient when a preset threshold of muscle activity is achieved. The threshold limits can be modified as the patient progresses. Through the use of positive "rewards," biofeedback encourages increased muscle contraction, which is beneficial during strength training. It can also improve the timing of muscle activation, which in turn benefits dynamic stabilization of the knee.

Proprioception

The role of the ACL in proprioception of the knee is still under investigation. It has been suggested that altered proprioception may reduce the effectiveness of the individual to protect the knee and may predispose the ACL to repetitive microtrauma and ultimately failure.[178] Patients

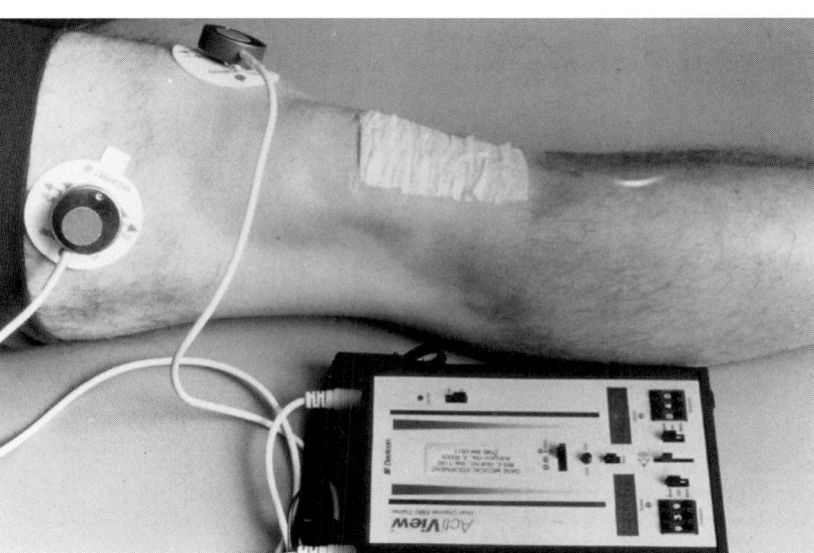

Figure 28J1–38. Electrical muscle stimulation.

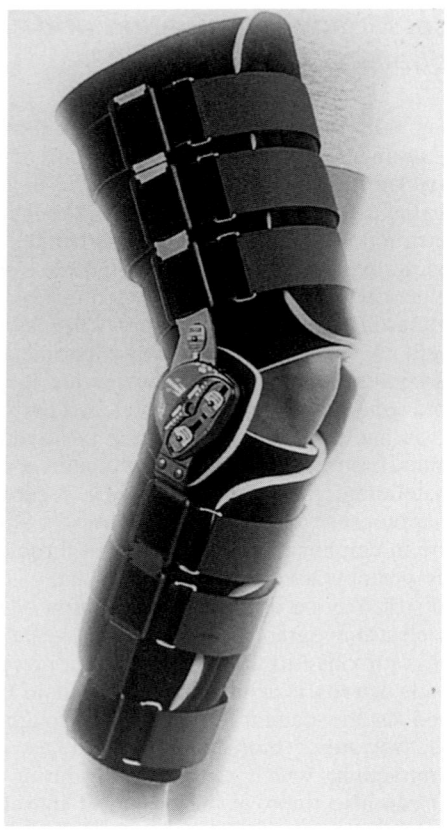

Figure 28J1–39. Rehabilitation knee brace.

with ACL-deficient knees have been shown to have decreased proprioceptive abilities, which in turn has a detrimental effect on the dynamic hamstring stabilization reflex.[31, 34, 252] Differences in proprioception between asymptomatic and symptomatic patients after ACL injury have been demonstrated.[252] A relationship between proprioception and outcome after ACL reconstruction has been noted.[33] The mechanism by which rehabilitation after ACL reconstruction has a beneficial effect on improving proprioception is not clear at this time. Improvement has been shown in patients with both ACL-reconstructed and ACL-deficient knees after proprioceptive training programs, however.[33, 177, 247]

Lephart and associates[178] recommended a program designed to assess all three levels of neuromuscular control. Higher brain center control is developed through conscious, repetitive positioning activities. The conscious repetition maximizes sensory input to reinforce proper joint stabilization activity. The patient then makes the transition to unconscious control by incorporating distraction techniques into the exercises, such as the addition of ball throwing or catching a ball while performing the required task.

The brain stem is involved in the maintenance of balance and equilibrium. To improve brain stem control, balance and postural maintenance activities should be implemented. The patient should start with visual activities, when the eyes are open, and progress to performing the exercises with the eyes closed, removing the visual input. The rehabilitation program should also use a progression

of activities from stable to unstable surfaces and from bilateral to unilateral stance.

To enhance proprioceptive control at the spinal level, activities involving sudden changes in joint position should be used. Plyometric activities and rapid movement exercises on unstable surfaces enhance the reflex dynamic stabilization arc.

Bracing

The effectiveness of and need for bracing after ACL reconstruction are controversial. Two forms of brace are currently in use, rehabilitation braces (Fig. 28J1–39) and functional braces (Fig. 28J1–40). Rehabilitation braces are used in the early postoperative period to protect the donor site while range of motion, weight-bearing, and muscle activity are initiated. Functional braces are used when the patient returns to strenuous activity or athletics in an attempt to provide increased stability to the knee and to protect the reconstructed ligament while it matures. The efficacy of functional braces in a prophylactic mode to prevent reinjury after graft maturation has not been supported in the literature and is not recommended.

The biomechanical effects of bracing have been studied. Beynnon and colleagues[40, 42] demonstrated a protective effect for the ACL of a brace under low-level loading condi-

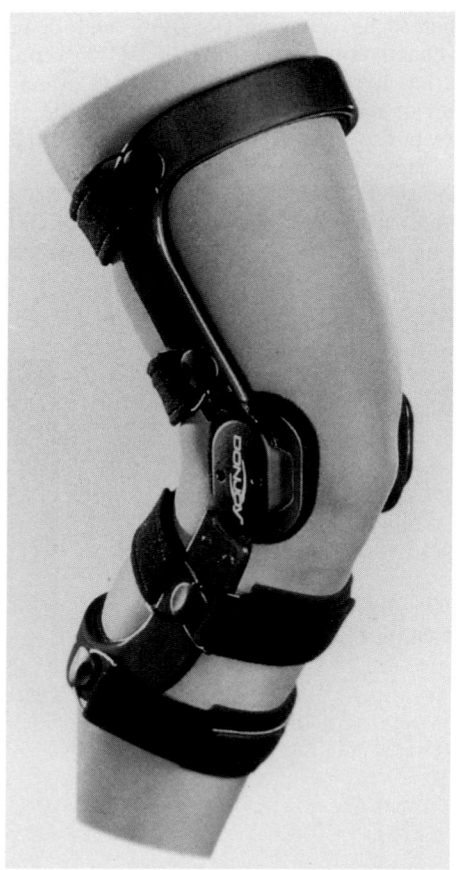

Figure 28J1–40. Functional knee brace.

TABLE 28J1–10
Jump Training Program

Exercise*	Duration or Repetitions by Week	
Phase I: Technique	*Week 1*	*Week 2*
Wall jumps	20 sec	25 sec
Tuck jumps†	20 sec	25 sec
Broad jumps, stick (hold) landing	5 reps	10 reps
Squat jumps†	10 sec	15 sec
Double-legged cone jumps†	30 sec/30 sec	30 sec/30 sec (side-to-side and back-to-front)
180-degree jumps	20 sec	25 sec
Bounding in place	20 sec	25 sec
Phase II: Fundamentals	*Week 3*	*Week 4*
Wall jumps	30 sec	30 sec
Tuck jumps†	30 sec	30 sec
Jump, jump, jump, vertical jump	5 reps	8 reps
Squat jumps†	20 sec	20 sec
Bounding for distance	1 run	2 runs
Double-legged cone jumps†	30 sec/30 sec	30 sec/30 sec (side-to-side and back-to-front)
Scissor jump	30 sec	30 sec
Hop, hop, stick landing†	5 reps/leg	5 reps/leg
Phase III: Performance	*Week 5*	*Week 6*
Wall jumps	30 sec	30 sec
Step, jump up, down, vertical	5 reps	20 reps
Mattress jumps	30 sec/30 sec	30 sec/30 sec (side-to-side and back-to-front)
Single-legged jumps, distance†	5 reps/leg	5 reps/leg
Squat jumps†	25 sec	25 sec
Jump into bounding†	3 runs	4 runs
Hop, hop, stick landing	5 reps/leg	5 reps/leg

*Before jumping exercises: stretching (15 to 20 minutes), skipping (two laps), side shuffle (two laps). After training: cool-down walk (2 minutes), stretching (5 minutes), weight training (after 15-minute rest). Note: Each jump exercise is followed by a 30-second rest period.

†These jumps performed on mat.

From Hewett TE, Lindenfeld TN, Riccobene JV, Noyes FR: The effect of neuromuscular training on the incidence of knee injury in female athletes. Am J Sports Med 27:699–706, 1999.

tions, but this effect was diminished with progressively increasing loads. DeVita and coworkers[90] found that functional bracing after ACL reconstruction promoted neuromuscular adaptations during the gait cycle that reduced the extensor moment at the knee produced by the quadriceps. This theoretically reduces the strain placed on the ACL during walking.

No long-term benefits of bracing have been demonstrated with regard to knee laxity, range of motion, or function. Bracing has been shown to increase quadriceps atrophy and inhibit the return of quadriceps strength after surgery, however.[251] This effect appears to resolve once use of the brace is discontinued.

Despite this, we currently recommend use of a drop-lock rehabilitation brace for the first 4 to 6 weeks after surgery. The brace is locked in extension when the patient is sleeping to prevent potential loss of extension range of motion, and for patients with bone–patellar tendon–bone autografts, it is locked in extension during weight-bearing to protect the extensor mechanism. The brace is removed or unlocked during range of motion and non–weight-bearing exercises. It is our belief that the risk for postoperative patellar fracture or patellar tendon rupture, although rare, outweighs the cost and inconvenience of brace use.

Gender Issues

Hewitt and colleagues[135, 136] have developed a prophylactic training program designed specifically for women to try to reduce the risk of knee injury (Tables 28J1–10 to 28J1–12). They demonstrated that they could reduce landing forces, increase muscle power, and improve the hamstring-to-quadriceps ratio in a 6-week training program.[136] They also observed that the program, when it is performed before a sports season, significantly reduces the number of knee injuries sustained by a trained population compared with an untrained population of women athletes.[135]

Wilk and associates[320] have proposed eight key factors that should be considered in rehabilitation after reconstruction of the ACL is performed in women (Table 28J1–13).

TABLE 28J1–11
Glossary of Jump Training Exercises

180-degree jumps	Two-footed jump. Rotate 180 degrees in midair. Hold landing for 2 seconds and then repeat in reverse direction.
Bounding for distance	Start bounding in place and slowly increase distance with each step, keeping knees high.
Bounding in place	Jump from one leg to the other straight up and down, progressively increasing rhythm and height.
Broad jumps–stick (hold) landing	Two-footed jump as far as possible. Hold landing for 5 seconds.
Cone jumps	Double-legged jump with feet together. Jump side-to-side over cones quickly. Repeat forward and backward.
Hop, hop, stick	Single-legged hop. Stick second landing for 5 seconds. Increase distance of hop as technique improves.
Jump into bounding	Two-footed broad jump. Land on single leg, then progress into bounding for distance.
Jump, jump, jump, vertical	Three broad jumps with vertical jump immediately after landing the third broad jump.
Mattress jump	Two-footed jump on mattress, trampoline, or other easily compressed device. Perform side-to-side and back-to-front.
Scissors jump	Start in stride position with one foot well in front of other.
Single-legged jumps, distance	Single-legged hop for distance. Hold landing (knees bent) for 5 seconds.
Squat jumps	Standing jump raising both arms overhead, land in squatting position touching both hands to floor.
Step, jump up, down, vertical	Two-footed jump onto 6- to 8-inch step. Jump off step with two feet, then vertical jump.
Tuck jumps	From standing position, jump, and bring both knees up to chest as high as possible. Repeat quickly.
Wall jumps (ankle bounces)	With knees slightly bent and arms raised overhead, bounce up and down off toes.

From Hewett TE, Lindenfeld TN, Riccobene JV, Noyes FR: The effect of neuromuscular training on the incidence of knee injury in female athletes. Am J Sports Med 27:699–706, 1999.

TABLE 28J1–15
Guidelines for Rehabilitation after Reconstruction of the Anterior Cruciate Ligament

Phase I

Begins immediately after surgery through approximately 2 weeks

Goals

Protect graft fixation
Minimize effects of immobilization
Control inflammation
No continuous passive motion
Full extension range of motion, 90 degrees of knee flexion
Achieve quadriceps control
Educate patient about rehabilitation progression

Brace

Locked in extension for ambulation and sleeping

Weight-bearing Status

Weight-bearing as tolerated with two crutches
Discontinue crutches as tolerated after 7 days

Therapeutic Exercises

Heel slides/wall slides
Quad sets, hamstring sets (electrical stimulation as needed)
Patellar mobilization
Non–weight-bearing gastrocnemius/soleus, hamstring stretches
Sitting assisted flexion hangs
Prone leg hangs (extension)
  Straight leg raise, all planes, with brace in full extension until quadriceps strength is sufficient to prevent extension lag
Phase I functional training
  Aerobic conditioning
    Upper extremity ergometry
    Well-leg bicycling
  Proprioception
    Active and passive joint positioning
    Balancing activities
      Stable platform, eyes open
      Stable platform, eyes closed
      Seated ball throwing and catching

Phase II

Begins approximately 2 weeks postoperatively and extends to approximately 6 weeks

Criteria

Good quad set, straight leg raise without extension lag
Approximately 90 degrees of flexion
Full extension
No signs of active inflammation

Goals

Restore normal gait
Restore full range of motion
Protect graft fixation
  Improve strength, endurance, and proprioception of the lower extremity to prepare for functional activities

Brace/Weight-bearing Status

Patellar tendon graft: continue ambulation with brace locked in extension; may unlock brace for sitting and sleeping, may remove brace for range of
  motion exercises
Hamstring and allograft: may discontinue brace use when normal gait pattern and quad control achieved

Therapeutic Exercises

Mini-squats 0–45 degrees
4-way hip exercises
Stationary bike (begin with high seat, low tension)
Closed chain extension (leg press: 0–45 degrees)
Toe raises
Continue hamstring stretches, progress to weight-bearing gastrocnemius/soleus stretches
Continue prone leg hangs with progressive ankle weights until extension is achieved

TABLE 28J1–15 *Continued*
Guidelines for Rehabilitation after Reconstruction of the Anterior Cruciate Ligament

Phase II functional training
  Aerobic conditioning
    Advance to two-leg bicycling
    Continue upper extremity ergometry
  Aquatherapy
    Pool walking/jogging
  Plyometrics/eccentric muscle training
    Stair walking
    Up/down, forward/backward
  Proprioception
    Balancing activities
      Unstable platform (KAT or BAPS), eyes open/closed
      Mini-tramp standing
    Standing ball throwing and catching

Phase III

Begins at approximately 6 weeks and extends through approximately 4 months

Criteria

Normal gait
Full range of motion
Sufficient strength and proprioception to initiate functional activities

Goals

Improve confidence in the knee
Avoid overstressing the graft fixation
Protect the patellofemoral joint
Progress strength, power, proprioception to prepare for return to functional activities

Therapeutic Exercises

Continue flexibility exercises as appropriate for patient
Advance closed kinetic chain strengthening (one-leg squats, leg press 0–60 degrees)
StairStepper/elliptical stepper
Cross-country skiing machine
Phase III functional training (6–12 weeks)
  Aerobic conditioning
    Continue bicyling and upper extremity ergometry
    Pool running/swimming
    StairStepper/elliptical stepper
    Cross-country skiing machine
  Running
    Straight-ahead jogging progressing to running
    Figure-of-eight pattern
    Large circles, walking or slow jogging
  Plyometrics
    Stair jogging
    Box jumps
    6- to 12-inch heights
  Proprioception
    Mini-tramp bouncing
    Pogo ball balancing
    Lateral slide board
    Ball throwing and catching on unstable surface
Phase IV functional training (12 + weeks)
  Aerobic conditioning
    Continue as above
  Running
    Figure-of-eight pattern
    Small circles, running
  Agility
    Start at slow speed, advance slowly
    Shuttle run
    Lateral slides
    Carioca crossovers
  Plyometrics
    Stair running
    Box jumps
    1- to 2-foot heights
  Proprioception
    Continue as above
    Add sport-specific activities ($\frac{1}{4}$- to $\frac{1}{2}$-speed)

Table continued on following page

TABLE 28J1–17
Patellar Tendon versus Hamstring Autografts for Arthroscopic Anterior Cruciate Ligament Reconstruction: Results of Literature Search of Studies with a Minimum 24-Month Follow-up

Patellar Tendon Studies	Hamstring Studies
Engebretsen 1990	Marder 1991
Marder 1991	Sgaglione 1992
Aglietti 1992	Sgaglione 1993
Buss 1993	Otero 1993
Otero 1993	Karlson 1994
Bach 1994	Howell 1996
Arciero 1996	Maeda 1996
Grontvedt 1996	Aglietti 1996
O'Neill 1996	O'Neill 1996
Aglietti 1997	Yasuda 1997
Heier 1997	Nebelung 1998
Sgaglione 1997	Corry 1999
Shelton 1997	Muneta 1999
Bach 1998 (endoscopic)	
Bach 1998 (two-incision)	
Kleipool 1998	
Otto 1998	
Webb 1998	
Jomha 1999	
Corry 1999	
Patel 2000	

chronic ACL-deficient knee do not fare as well as reconstructions performed in the acute setting once the initial inflammatory response has resolved.

Patellar Tendon versus Hamstring Autografts

We sought to perform a comprehensive analysis of the results of ACL reconstruction comparing patellar tendon and hamstring autografts. To accomplish this, we performed a thorough search of the literature to find all published series of arthroscopic ACL reconstruction using either patellar tendon or hamstring autografts with a minimum of 24 months of follow-up. We excluded those studies that performed arthrotomy or miniarthrotomy or used intra-articular or extra-articular augmentation. We discovered 21 studies representing 1348 patients using patellar tendon grafts and 13 studies representing 628 patients using hamstring grafts that fit these criteria. The results of the search are presented in Table 28J1–17. In Appendices A and B, we present the data gathered from the individual studies separated by graft source.

A meta-analysis of the data was then performed to

TABLE 28J1–18
KT1000 Laxity Testing*

	<3 mm	3–5 mm	>5 mm
Patellar tendon	79%	15%	6%
Hamstrings	74%	19%	7%

*$P = .02$

TABLE 28J1–19
Pivot Shift Test*

	Grade 0	Grade I	Grade II+
Patellar tendon	82%	15%	3%
Hamstrings	82%	14%	5%

*Not significant.

compare the patellar tendon group with the hamstring group. With regard to knee stability (Table 28J1–18), we found that side-to-side laxity, as measured by KT1000, was less than 3 mm in 79% and less than 5 mm in 94% in the patellar tendon group compared with 74% and 93% in the hamstring group, respectively. These differences were statistically significant. Elimination of the pivot shift was achieved in 82% of the patellar tendon group and in 82% of the hamstring group (Table 28J1–19). Only 3% and 5%, respectively, had a pivot shift of grade 2 or greater. These differences were not statistically significant.

A major goal of ACL surgery is not just to provide stability to the knee but also to allow the patient to return to unrestricted activities at the previous level of ability. There was no difference between the two groups; 68% of the patellar tendon patients and 66% of the hamstring patients were able to return to their previous activity level. Overall, the patient's subjective satisfaction is good for both; however, it was significantly greater in the patellar tendon group (95%) than in the hamstring group (87%).

Subsequent surgery was required in both groups (Table 28J1–20), but differences in the type of surgery required were noted. Lysis of adhesions or a manipulation under anesthesia was required to regain motion after patellar tendon reconstructions significantly more often than after hamstring reconstruction. Hardware removal was performed after 3% of the patellar tendon reconstructions, significantly less than after hamstring reconstructions, which required hardware removal in 6% of all cases. There was no difference in the need for subsequent meniscal repair or meniscectomy between the two groups.

A difference between the two groups can be seen in the type and frequency of complications that occurred (Table 28J1–21). Looking at graft failure or graft rupture, we found only a 2% failure rate for patellar tendon grafts, whereas hamstring grafts had a 5% failure rate. The incidence of anterior knee pain was higher in the patellar tendon group (17%) than in the hamstring group (12%). Both groups had similar infection rates, below 1%.

To summarize, both patellar tendon and hamstring autografts can be used to achieve excellent results in the major-

TABLE 28J1–20
Subsequent Surgery

	Patellar Tendon	Hamstrings	P Value
Meniscectomy or meniscal repair	3%	4%	NS
Lysis of adhesions or manipulation under anesthesia	6%	3%	.01
Hardware removal	3%	6%	.02

TABLE 28J1–21
Complications

	Patellar Tendon	Hamstrings	P Value
Graft failure	2%	5%	.001
Anterior knee pain	17%	12%	.01
Infection	0.5%	0.4%	NS

ity of cases. Patellar tendon grafts tend to be more stable; a greater percentage demonstrate less than 3 mm of side-to-side laxity, and a greater number of hamstring grafts fall in the 3- to 5-mm laxity range. Both grafts eliminate the pivot shift with equal efficacy. Hamstring grafts have a greater tendency to fail but cause less anterior knee pain. Both provide excellent satisfaction to the patient. Despite these results, however, about one third of the patients in each group failed to return to their previous level of activity. It is this last statistic that should be an incentive for further advancement of surgical techniques, rehabilitation protocols, and basic science understanding. Although we have come a long way with regard to ACL reconstruction, there is clearly still room for improvement.

Allograft versus Autograft

The results of patellar tendon allograft reconstructions have improved with the elimination of graft irradiation and ethylene oxide sterilization techniques. With use of nonirradiated, fresh frozen patellar tendon allografts, nearly identical results of ACL reconstruction have been found compared with autograft patellar tendon techniques.[168, 129, 287] Shelton and coworkers[287] compared autograft and allograft patellar tendon ACL reconstructions at 2 years of follow-up and found no statistically significant differences between the two groups. Similarly, Kleipool and associates[168] also found no statistically significant differences between allograft and autograft patellar tendon ACL reconstruction at an average follow-up of 4 years. Harner and colleagues[129] compared the results of ACL reconstruction with use of allograft and autograft tissue at 3- to 5-year follow-up. The only difference between the two groups was a small increase in extension loss in the autograft group. From these studies, it is apparent that nonirradiated, fresh frozen allograft patellar tendon tissue presents a viable alternative to autograft tissue for use in ACL reconstruction.

Chronic versus Acute Reconstruction

Concerns exist about the results of ACL reconstruction in the setting of chronic ACL insufficiency. A number of factors put this group at risk for poor outcomes. These include an increased risk for meniscal injury and the long-term effects of ACL deficiency on the stability of the secondary soft tissue restraints.

Comparing acute and chronic reconstructions with use of a patellar tendon autograft, Noyes and Barber-Westin[225] found no significant differences in laxity, although there was a trend for improved stability in the acute group. In addition, the acute group had a higher overall knee score (96 points) compared with the chronic group (90 points), and significantly more patients returned to strenuous activity after an acute reconstruction than in the chronic group. Not surprisingly, the number of operations preceding the reconstruction numbered 94 for the 57 patients in the chronic group, compared with only 2 for the 30 patients in the acute group.

Sgaglione and coworkers[273] evaluated the effect of injury chronicity on the results after ACL reconstruction with use of hamstring autografts. They found significantly improved results for those patients undergoing reconstruction in the acute setting compared with those with chronic ACL insufficiency. They also concluded that meniscal injury seems to be the most significant factor contributing to the inferior results in the chronic setting.

Clearly, there is a benefit to addressing ACL insufficiency in the early postinjury setting, before secondary injury can occur that may compromise the result of a future reconstruction.

Complications

Loss of Motion

Loss of motion is often cited as the most common complication after ACL reconstruction. The causes of motion loss are listed in Table 28J1–9. The definition of loss of motion varies in the literature. Harner and colleagues[128] use a loss of knee extension of 10 degrees or of knee flexion less than 125 degrees to define loss of motion, whereas Shelbourne and Patel[282] define loss of motion as any symptomatic deficit of extension or flexion compared with the opposite knee. The term *arthrofibrosis* has been used when the limitation of motion is symptomatic and resistant to rehabilitative measures.[282] It is often used synonymously with loss of motion in the literature.

Shelbourne and Patel[282] have developed a classification system for arthrofibrosis or loss of motion (Table 28J1–22). Type 1 arthrofibrosis is characterized by a flexible loss, less than 10 degrees, of extension only, which can be

TABLE 28J1–22
Classification of Arthrofibrosis

Type	Description
1	≤10° extension loss and normal flexion
2	>10° extension loss and normal flexion
3	>10° extension loss and >25° flexion loss with decreased medial and lateral movement of the patella (patellar tightness)
4	>10° extension loss and ≥30° flexion loss and patella infera with marked patellar tightness

From Shelbourne KD, Patel DV: Treatment of limited motion after anterior cruciate ligament reconstruction. Knee Surg Sports Traumatol Arthosc 7:85–92, 1999.

pens during a shift change or a staff break, must be informed of the location of the graft so that a similar error is not made.

Should the graft become contaminated for any reason, there are a few salvage options. The graft can be sterilized, a similar graft can be harvested from the contralateral knee, an alternative graft can be harvested from the ipsilateral or contralateral knee, or an allograft can be used if it is available. For sterilization of the graft once it has been contaminated, studies have found chlorhexidine to be the most effective agent.[53, 206] Burd and associates[53] discovered a 100% disinfection rate of contaminated bone-tendon allografts by use of a 3-L power irrigation with chlorhexidine solution. A 2% solution was as effective as the standard 4% solution. Molina and colleagues[206] noted a similar sterilization rate with use of a 4% chlorhexidine solution. These studies and others have found incomplete sterilization of contaminated graft tissue with irrigation solutions consisting of mixed antibiotic solutions, povidone-iodine, benzalkonium chloride, or Castile soap.[53, 206, 298] When chlorhexidine is used to decontaminate the graft, it is important to wash the tissue thoroughly in a saline bath to remove all of the chlorhexidine before the graft is introduced into the knee. Van Huyssteen and Bracey[310] demonstrated severe chondrolysis of articular cartilage in the knee after irrigation with a dilute 0.02% chlorhexidine solution.

Other Complications

A number of other rare complications that follow ACL reconstruction occur in less than 1% of all cases. After central-third patellar tendon autograft reconstructions, extensor mechanism problems, such as patellar fracture, patellar tendon rupture, and even quadriceps rupture, have been noted to occur infrequently.[47, 48, 89, 124, 196] Although rare, they occur when proper surgical techniques and rehabilitation methods are not employed. In our series of more than 900 patellar tendon reconstructions, we have had one distal rupture of the patellar tendon and no episodes of patellar fracture. This low rate most likely reflects the care taken to maintain proper graft harvesting techniques as well as the postoperative bracing protocol used.

Infection is another potentially devastating but fortunately rare complication. In a survey of 61 sports medicine fellowship directors, Matava and colleagues[193] found an average infection rate of 0.2% after ACL reconstruction. There was no relationship between infection rate and graft choice, reconstruction method, or duration of prophylactic antibiotic use. There was a significantly greater risk of infection, however, among those surgeons who routinely used a drain after surgery compared with those who did not. Williams and coworkers[322] noted that the majority of their infections occurred during those reconstructions performed in association with secondary procedures, such as a meniscal repair. If an infection does occur, the current recommended treatment regimen consists of culture-specific antibiotics, irrigation and débridement of the joint, and graft retention. Débridement of the graft and removal of hardware are reserved for resistant infections only. Outcomes after infection are less predictable than those of uncomplicated reconstructions.[193, 195, 313, 322]

Other rare complications include fixation failure, deep venous thrombosis, and reflex sympathetic dystrophy. Awareness of the signs and symptoms of these conditions will allow prompt diagnosis and initiation of early treatment. Maintaining a continuous dialogue with the physical therapist during the course of rehabilitation can help as well.

References

1. Aglietti P, Buzzi R, D'Andria S, Zaccherotti G: Arthroscopic anterior cruciate ligament reconstruction with patellar tendon. Arthroscopy 8:510–516, 1992.
2. Aglietti P, Buzzi R, Giron F, et al: Arthroscopic-assisted anterior cruciate ligament reconstruction with the central third patellar tendon. Knee Surg Sports Traumatol Arthrosc 5:138–144, 1997.
3. Aglietti P, Buzzi R, Menchetti PPM, Giron F: Arthroscopically assisted semitendinosus and gracilis graft in reconstruction for acute anterior cruciate ligament injuries in athletes. Am J Sports Med 24:726–731, 1996.
4. Aglietti P, Buzzi R, Zaccherotti G, D'Andria S: Operative treatment of acute complete lesions of the anterior cruciate and medial collateral ligaments. Am J Knee Surg 4:186–194, 1991.
5. Aglietti P, Zaccherotti G, Simeone AJ, Buzzi R: Anatomic versus non-anatomic tibial fixation in anterior cruciate ligament reconstruction with bone–patellar tendon–bone graft. Knee Surg Sports Traumatol Arthrosc 6(suppl 1):S43–S48, 1998.
6. Amiel D, Frank C, Harwood F, et al: Tendons and ligaments: A morphological and biochemical comparison. J Orthop Res 1:257–265, 1984.
7. Amis M, Dawkins GPC: Functional anatomy of the anterior cruciate ligament: Fibre bundle actions related to ligament replacements and injuries. J Bone Joint Surg Br 73:260–267, 1991.
8. Anderson AF, Lipscomb AB: Analysis of rehabilitation techniques after anterior cruciate reconstruction. Am J Sports Med 17:154–160, 1989.
9. Andersson C, Odensten M, Gillquist J: Knee function after surgical or non-surgical treatment of acute ACL. Clin Orthop 264:255–263, 1991.
10. Arciero RA, Scoville CR, Snyder RJ, et al: Single versus two-incision arthroscopic anterior cruciate ligament reconstruction. Arthroscopy 12:462–469, 1996.
11. Arnoczky SP: Anatomy of the anterior cruciate ligament. Clin Orthop 172:19–25, 1983.
12. Arnoczky SP: Blood supply to the anterior cruciate ligament and supporting structures. Orthop Clin North Am 16:15–28, 1985.
13. Arnoczky SP, Rubin RM, Marshall JL: Microvasculature of the cruciate ligaments and its response to injury. J Bone Joint Surg Am 61:1221–1229, 1979.
14. Arnoczky SP, Tarvin GB, Marshall JL: Anterior cruciate ligament replacement using patellar tendon: An evaluation of graft revascularization in the dog. J Bone Joint Surg Am 64:217–224, 1982.
15. Asahina S, Muneta T, Ezura Y: Notchplasty in anterior cruciate ligament reconstruction: An experimental animal study. Arthroscopy 16:165–172, 2000.
16. Asahina S, Yamamoto H, Muneta T, et al: Evaluation of anterior cruciate reconstruction reinforced by the Kennedy ligament augmentation device. Int Orthop 19:229–233, 1995.
17. Auge WK II, Yifan K: A technique for resolution of graft-tunnel length mismatch in central third bone–patellar tendon–bone anterior cruciate ligament reconstruction. Arthroscopy 15:877–881, 1999.
18. Bach BR Jr, Jones GT, Sweet FA, Hager CA: Arthroscopy-assisted anterior cruciate ligament reconstruction using patellar tendon substitute: Two- to four-year follow-up results. Am J Sports Med 22:758–767, 1994.
19. Bach BR Jr, Levy ME, Bojchuk J, et al: Single-incision endoscopic anterior cruciate ligament reconstruction using patellar tendon autograft. Minimum two-year follow-up evaluation. Am J Sports Med 26:30–40, 1998.
20. Bach BR Jr, Tradonsky S, Bojchuk J, et al: Arthroscopically assisted anterior cruciate ligament reconstruction using patellar tendon autograft. Am J Sports Med 26:20–29, 1998.

21. Bach BR Jr, Warren RF: "Empty wall" and "vertical strut" signs of ACL insufficiency. Arthroscopy 5:137–140, 1989.
22. Bach BR Jr, Warren RF, Flynn WM, et al: Arthrometric evaluation of knees that have a torn anterior cruciate ligament. J Bone Joint Surg Am 72:1299–1306, 1990.
23. Bach BR Jr, Warren RF, Wickiewicz TL: The pivot-shift phenomenon: Results and description of a modified clinical test for anterior cruciate ligament insufficiency. Am J Sports Med 16:571–576, 1988.
24. Baek GH, Carlin GJ, Vogrin TM, et al: Quantitative analysis of collagen fibrils of human cruciate and meniscofemoral ligaments. Clin Orthop 357:205–211, 1998.
25. Ballock RT, Woo SL-Y, Lyon RM, et al: Use of patellar tendon autograft for anterior cruciate ligament reconstruction in the rabbit: A long-term histological and biomechanical study. J Orthop Res 7:474–485, 1989.
26. Barantz ME, Fu FH, Mengato R: Meniscal tears: The effect of meniscectomy and repair on intra-articular contact areas and stress in the human knee. Am J Sports Med 14:270–276, 1986.
27. Barber FA: What is the terrible triad? Arthroscopy 8:19–22, 1992.
28. Barber FA, Click SD: Meniscus repair rehabilitation with concurrent anterior cruciate reconstruction. Arthroscopy 13:433–437, 1997.
29. Barber FA, Elrod BF, McGuire DA, Paulos LE: Is an anterior cruciate ligament reconstruction outcome age dependent? Arthroscopy 12:720–725, 1996.
30. Barber-Westin SD, Noyes FR, Heckmann TP, Shaffer BL: The effect of exercise and rehabilitation on anterior-posterior knee displacements after anterior cruciate ligament autograft reconstruction. Am J Sports Med 27:84–93, 1999.
31. Barrack RL, Skinner HB, Buckley SL: Proprioception in the anterior cruciate deficient knee. Am J Sports Med 17:1–6, 1989.
32. Barratta R, Solomonow M, Zhou BH, et al: Muscular coactivation: The role of the antagonist musculature in maintaining knee stability. Am J Sports Med 16:113–122, 1988.
33. Barrett DS: Proprioception and function after anterior cruciate ligament reconstruction. J Bone Joint Surg Br 73:833–837, 1991.
34. Beard DJ, Kyberd PJ, Ferguson CM, Dodd CAF: Proprioception after rupture of the anterior cruciate ligament. J Bone Joint Surg Br 75:311–315, 1993.
35. Becker R, Schroder M, Ropke M, et al: Structural properties of sutures used in anchoring multistranded hamstrings in anterior cruciate ligament reconstruction: A biomechanical study. Arthroscopy 15:297–300, 1999.
36. Bell DG, Jacobs I: Electro-mechanical response times and rate of force development in males and females. Med Sci Sports Exerc 18:31–36, 1986.
37. Bellabarba C, Bush-Joseph CA, Bach BR Jr: Patterns of meniscal injury in the anterior cruciate–deficient knee: A review of the literature. Am J Orthop 26:18–23, 1997.
38. Bents RT, Jones RC, May DA, Snearly WS: Intercondylar notch encroachment following anterior cruciate ligament reconstruction. Am J Knee Surg 11:81–88, 1998.
39. Berg EE: Intrinsic healing of a patellar tendon donor site defect after anterior cruciate ligament reconstruction. Clin Orthop 278:160–163, 1992.
40. Beynnon BD, Fleming BC: Anterior cruciate ligament strain in-vivo: A review of previous work. J Biomech 31:519–525, 1998.
41. Beynnon BD, Johnson RJ: Anterior cruciate ligament injury rehabilitation in athletes: Biomechanical considerations. Sports Med 22:54–64, 1996.
42. Beynnon BD, Johnson RJ, Fleming BC, et al: The effect of functional knee bracing on the anterior cruciate ligament in the weight-bearing and nonweightbearing knee. Am J Sports Med 25:353–359, 1997.
43. Beynnon BD, Johnson RJ, Fleming BC, et al: The measurement of elongation of anterior cruciate–ligament grafts in vivo. J Bone Joint Surg Am 76:520–531, 1994.
44. Blum MF, Garth WP, Lemons JE: The effects of graft rotation on attachment site separation distances in anterior cruciate ligament reconstruction. Am J Sports Med 23:282–287, 1995.
45. Bolgla LA, Keskula DR: Reliability of lower extremity functional performance tests. J Orthop Sports Phys Ther 26:138–142, 1997.
46. Bolton WC, Bruchman WC: The Gore-Tex expanded polytetrafluoroethylene prosthetic ligament. Clin Orthop 196:202–213, 1985.
47. Bonatus TJ, Alexander AH: Patellar fracture and avulsion of the patellar ligament complicating arthroscopic anterior cruciate ligament reconstruction. Orthop Rev 20:770–774, 1991.
48. Bonomo J, Krinick RM, Sporn AA: Rupture of the patellar ligament after use of its central third for anterior cruciate reconstruction. J Bone Joint Surg Am 66:1294–1297, 1984.
49. Boszotta H, Prunner K: Refilling of removal defects: Impact on extensor mechanism complaints after use of a bone-tendon-bone graft for anterior cruciate ligament reconstruction. Arthroscopy 16:160–164, 2000.
50. Breitfuss H, Frohlich R, Provacz P, et al: The tendon defect after anterior cruciate ligament reconstruction using the midthird patellar tendon—a problem for the patellofemoral joint? Knee Surg Sports Traumatol Arthrosc 3:194–198, 1996.
51. Brown CH, Hecker AT, Hipp JA, et al: The biomechanics of interference screw fixation of patellar tendon anterior cruciate ligament grafts. Am J Sports Med 21:880–886, 1993.
52. Buckley SL, Barrack RL, Alexander AH: The natural history of conservatively treated partial anterior cruciate ligament tears. Am J Sports Med 17:221–225, 1989.
53. Burd T, Conroy BP, Meyer SC, Allen WC: The effects of chlorhexidine irrigation solution on contaminated bone-tendon allografts. Am J Sports Med 28:241–244, 2000.
54. Burke DL, Ahmed AM, Miller J: A biomechanical study of partial and total medial meniscectomy. Trans Orthop Res Soc 3:91–96, 1978.
55. Burks RT: Gross anatomy. In Daniel DM, Akeson WH, O'Connor JJ (eds): Knee Ligaments: Structure, Function, Injury, and Repair. New York, Raven Press, 1990, pp 59–76.
56. Burks RT, Haut RC, Lancaster RL: Biomechanical and histological observations of the dog patellar tendon after removal of its central one-third. Am J Sports Med 18:146–153, 1990.
57. Burks RT, Leland R: Determination of graft tension before fixation in anterior cruciate ligament reconstruction. Arthroscopy 4:260–266, 1988.
58. Buseck MS, Noyes FR: Arthroscopic evaluations of meniscal repairs after anterior cruciate ligament reconstruction and immediate motion. Am J Sports Med 19:489–494, 1991.
59. Buss DD, Warren RF, Wickiewicz TL, et al: Arthroscopically assisted reconstruction of the anterior cruciate ligament with use of autogenous patellar-ligament grafts. J Bone Joint Surg Am 75:1346–1355, 1993.
60. Butler DL, Grood ES, Noyes FR, Sodd AN: On the interpretation of our ACL data. Clin Orthop 196:26–34, 1985.
61. Butler DL, Guan Y, Kay MD, et al: Location-dependent variations in the material properties of the anterior cruciate ligament. J Biomech 25:511–518, 1992.
62. Butler DL, Noyes FR, Grood ES: Ligamentous restraints to anterior-posterior drawer in the human knee. J Bone Joint Surg Am 62:259–270, 1980.
63. Butler JC, Branch TP, Hutton WC: Optimal graft fixation—the effect of gap size and screw size on bone plug fixation in ACL reconstruction. Arthroscopy 10:524–529, 1994.
64. Bylski-Austrow DI, Grood ES, Hefzy MS, et al: Anterior cruciate ligament replacements: A mechanical study of femoral attachment location, flexion angle at tensioning, and initial tension. J Orthop Res 8:522–531, 1990.
65. Caborn DNM, Coen M, Neef R, et al: Quadrupled semitendinosus-gracilis autograft fixation in the femoral tunnel: A comparison between a metal and a bioabsorbable interference screw. Arthroscopy 14:241–245, 1998.
66. Caborn DNM, Urban WP Jr, Johnson DL, et al: Biomechanical comparison between bioscrew and titanium alloy interference screws for bone–patellar tendon–bone graft fixation in anterior cruciate ligament reconstruction. Arthroscopy 13:229–232, 1997.
67. Campbell WC: Reconstruction of the ligaments of the knee. Am J Surg 43:473–480, 1939.
68. Cameron M, Buchgraber A, Passler H, et al: The natural history of the anterior cruciate ligament–deficient knee: Changes in synovial fluid cytokine and keratan sulfate concentrations. Am J Sports Med 25:751–754, 1997.
69. Cannon WD, Vittori JM: The incidence of healing in arthroscopic meniscal repair in anterior cruciate ligament reconstructed knees versus stable knees. Am J Sports Med 20:176–181, 1992.
70. Cao M, Stefanovic-Racic M, Georgescu HI, et al: Does nitric oxide help explain the differential healing capacity of the anterior cruciate, posterior cruciate, and medial collateral ligaments? Am J Sports Med 28:176–182, 2000.

isokinetic quadriceps work in healthy subjects. Scand J Med Sci Sports 9:189–194, 1999.

174. Langan P, Fontanetta AP: Rupture of the patellar tendon after use of its central third. Orthop Rev 16:317–321, 1987.

175. Lemos MJ, Albert J, Simon T, Jackson DW: Radiographic analysis of femoral interference screw placement during ACL reconstruction: Endoscopic versus open technique. Arthroscopy 9:154–158, 1993.

176. Lemos MJ, Jackson DW, Lee TQ, Simon TM: Assessment of initial fixation of endoscopic interference femoral screws with divergent and parallel placement. Arthroscopy 11:37–41, 1995.

177. Lephart SM, Kocher MS, Fu FH, et al: Proprioception following anterior cruciate ligament reconstruction. J Sports Rehabil 1:188–196, 1992.

178. Lephart SM, Pincivero DM, Rozzi SL: Proprioception of the ankle and knee. Sports Med 25:149–155, 1998.

179. Lieber RL, Silva PD, Daniel DM: Equal effectiveness of electrical and volitional strength training for quadriceps femoris muscles after anterior cruciate ligament surgery. J Orthop Res 14:131–138, 1996.

180. Lindenfeld TN, Schmitt DJ, Hendy MD, et al: Incidence of injury in indoor soccer. Am J Sports Med 22:364–371, 1994.

181. Liu SH, Al-Shaikh R, Panossian V, et al: Primary immunolocalization of estrogen and progesterone target cells in the human anterior cruciate ligament. J Orthop Res 14:526–533, 1996.

182. Lund-Hanssen H, Gannon J, Engebretsen L, et al: Intercondylar notch width and the risk for anterior cruciate ligament rupture: A case-control study in 46 female handball players. Acta Orthop Scand 65:529–532, 1994.

183. Lutz GE, Palmitier RA, An KN, Chao EYS: Comparison of tibiofemoral joint forces during open-kinetic-chain and closed-kinetic-chain exercises. J Bone Joint Surg Am 75:732–739, 1993.

184. Maeda A, Shino K, Horibe S, et al: Anterior cruciate ligament reconstruction with multistranded autogenous semitendinosus tendon. Am J Sports Med 24:504–508, 1996.

185. Magen HE, Howell SM, Hull ML: Structural properties of six tibial fixation methods for anterior cruciate ligament soft tissue grafts. Am J Sports Med 27:35–43, 1999.

186. Mann TA, Black KP, Zanotti DJ, et al: The natural history of the intercondylar notch after notchplasty. Am J Sports Med 27:181–188, 1999.

187. Marder RA, Raskind JR, Carrol M: Prospective evaluation of arthroscopically assisted anterior cruciate ligament reconstruction: Patellar tendon versus semitendinosus and gracilis tendons. Am J Sports Med 19:478–484, 1991.

188. Mariani PP, Santori N, Adriani E, Mastantuono M: Accelerated rehabilitation after arthroscopic meniscal repair: A clinical and magnetic resonance imaging evaluation. Arthroscopy 12:680–686, 1996.

189. Markolf KL, Burchfield DM, Shapiro MM, et al: Biomechanical consequences of replacement of the anterior cruciate ligament with a patellar ligament allograft. Part I: Insertion of the graft and anterior-posterior testing. J Bone Joint Surg Am 78:1720–1727, 1996.

190. Markolf KL, Burchfield DM, Shapiro MM, et al: Biomechanical consequences of replacement of the anterior cruciate ligament with a patellar ligament allograft. Part II: Forces in the graft compared with forces in the intact ligament. J Bone Joint Surg Am 78:1728–1734, 1996.

191. Markolf KL, Mensch JS, Amstutz HC: Stiffness and laxity of the knee: The contributions of the supporting structures. J Bone Joint Surg Am 58:583–593, 1976.

192. Marzo JM, Warren RF: Results of treatment of anterior cruciate ligament injury: Changing perspectives. Adv Orthop Surg 15:59–69, 1991.

193. Matava MJ, Evans TA, Wright RW, Shively RA: Septic arthritis of the knee following anterior cruciate ligament reconstruction: Results of a survey of sports medicine fellowship directors. Arthroscopy 14:717–725, 1998.

194. May DV, Snearly WN, Bents R, Jones R: MR imaging findings in anterior cruciate ligament reconstruction: Evaluation of notchplasty. AJR Am J Roentgenol 169:317–222, 1997.

195. McAllister DR, Parker RD, Cooper AE, et al: Outcomes of postoperative septic arthritis after anterior cruciate ligament reconstruction. Am J Sports Med 27:562–570, 1999.

196. McCarrol JR: Fracture of the patella during a golf swing following reconstruction of the anterior cruciate ligament. Am J Sports Med 1:26–27, 1983.

197. McDaniel WJ, Dameron TB: The untreated anterior cruciate ligament rupture. Clin Orthop 172:158–163, 1983.

198. McDaniel WJ, Dameron TB: Untreated ruptures of the anterior cruciate ligament. J Bone Joint Surg Am 62:696–705, 1980.

199. McKernan DJ, Paulos LE: Graft selection. In Fu FH, Harner CD, Vince KG (eds): Knee Surgery. Baltimore, Williams & Wilkins, 1994, pp 667–678.

200. McPherson GK, Mendenhall HV, Gibbons DF, et al: Experimental, mechanical, and histological evaluation of the Kennedy ligament augmentation device. Clin Orthop 196:186–195, 1985.

201. Meisterling RC, Wadsworth T, Ardill R, et al: Morphologic changes in the human patellar tendon after bone-tendon-bone anterior cruciate ligament reconstruction. Clin Orthop 289:208–212, 1993.

202. Messina DF, Farney WC, DeLee JC: The incidence of injury in Texas high school basketball. Am J Sports Med 27:294–299, 1999.

203. Messner K, Maletius W: Eighteen- to twenty-five-year follow-up after acute partial anterior cruciate ligament rupture. Am J Sports Med 27:455–459, 1999.

204. Miller MD, Hinkin DT: The "N + 7 rule" for tibial tunnel placement in endoscopic anterior cruciate ligament reconstruction. Arthroscopy 12:124–126, 1996.

205. Miyasaka KC, Daniel DM, Stone ML, Hirshman HP: The incidence of knee ligament injuries in the general population. Am J Knee Surg 4:3–8, 1991.

206. Molina ME, Nonweiller DE, Evans JA, DeLee JC: Contaminated anterior cruciate ligament grafts: The efficacy of 3 sterilization agents. Arthroscopy 16:373–378, 2000.

207. More RC, Markolf KL: Measurement of stability of the knee and ligament force after implantation of a synthetic anterior cruciate ligament. J Bone Joint Surg Am 70:1020–1031, 1988.

208. Morgan C, Kalmam V, Grawl D: Definitive landmarks for reproducible tibial tunnel placement in anterior cruciate ligament reconstruction. Arthroscopy 11:275–288, 1995.

209. Morgan C, Kalmam V, Grawl D: Isometry testing for anterior cruciate ligament reconstruction revisited. Arthroscopy 11:647–659, 1995.

210. Morgan EA, McElroy JJ, DesJardins JD, et al: The effect of intercondylar notchplasty on the patellofemoral articulation. Am J Sports Med 24:843–846, 1996.

211. Mueller W: The Knee: Form, Function, and Ligament Reconstruction. New York, Springer-Verlag, 1983, pp 8–75.

212. Muneta T, Sekiya I, Ogiuchi T, et al: Effects of aggressive early rehabilitation on the outcome of anterior cruciate ligament reconstruction with multi-strand semitendinosus tendon. Int Orthop 22:352–356, 1998.

213. Muneta T, Sekiya I, Yagishita K, et al: Two-bundle reconstruction of the anterior cruciate ligament using semitendinosus tendon with endobuttons: Operative technique and preliminary results. Arthroscopy 15:618–624, 1999.

214. Muneta T, Yamamoto H, Ishibashi T, et al: The effects of tibial tunnel placement and roofplasty on reconstructed anterior cruciate ligament knees. Arthroscopy 11:57–62, 1995.

215. Muren O, Dahlstedt L, Dalen N: Reconstruction of old anterior cruciate ligament injuries. Acta Orthop Scand 66:118–122, 1995.

216. Myer JW, Schulthies SS, Fellingham GW: Relative and absolute reliability of the KT-2000 arthrometer for uninjured knees. Am J Sports Med 24:104–108, 1996.

217. Nabors ED, Richmond JC, Vannah WM, McConville OR: Anterior cruciate ligament graft tensioning in full extension. Am J Sports Med 23:488–492, 1995.

218. Nagineni CN, Amiel D, Green MH, et al: Characterization of the intrinsic properties of the anterior cruciate and medial collateral ligament cells. J Orthop Res 10:465–475, 1992.

219. Nebelung W, Becker R, Merkel M, Ropke M: Bone tunnel enlargement after anterior cruciate ligament reconstruction with semitendinosus tendon using endobutton fixation on the femoral side. Arthroscopy 14:810–815, 1998.

220. Neeb TB, Aufdemkampe G, Wagener JH, Mastenbroek L: Assessing anterior cruciate ligament injuries: The association and differential value of questionnaires, clinical tests, and functional tests. J Orthop Sports Phys Ther 26:324–331, 1997.

221. Nogalski MP, Bach BR Jr: Acute anterior cruciate ligament injuries. In Fu FH, Harner CD, Vince KG (eds): Knee Surgery. Baltimore, Williams & Wilkins, 1994, pp 679–730.

222. Novak PJ, Bach BR Jr, Hager CA: Clinical and functional outcome of anterior cruciate ligament reconstruction in the recreational athlete over the age of 35. Am J Knee Surg 9:111–116, 1996.

223. Novak PJ, Wexler GM, Williams JS, et al: Comparison of screw post fixation and free bone block interference fixation for anterior cruciate ligament soft tissue grafts: Biomechanical considerations. Arthroscopy 12:470–473, 1996.
224. Noyes FR, Barber SD, Mangine RE: Abnormal lower limb symmetry determined by function hop tests after anterior cruciate ligament rupture. Am J Sports Med 19:513–518, 1991.
225. Noyes FR, Barber-Westin SD: A comparison of results in acute and chronic anterior cruciate ligament ruptures of arthroscopically assisted autogenous patellar tendon reconstruction. Am J Sports Med 25:460–471, 1997.
226. Noyes FR, Basset RW, Grood ES, Butler DL: Arthroscopy in acute traumatic hemarthrosis of the knee. J Bone Joint Surg Am 62:687–695, 1980.
227. Noyes FR, Butler DL, Grood ES, et al: Biomechanical analysis of human ligament grafts used in knee-ligament repairs and replacements. J Bone Joint Surg Am 66:344–352, 1984.
228. Noyes FR, Mooar PA, Matthews DS, Butler DL: The symptomatic anterior cruciate–deficient knee. Part I: The long-term functional disability in athletically active individuals. J Bone Joint Surg Am 65:154–162, 1983.
229. Noyes FR, Mooar PA, Moorman CT, McGinniss GH: Partial tears of the anterior cruciate ligament. Progression to complete ligament deficiency. J Bone Joint Surg Br 71:825–833, 1989.
230. Noyes FR, Wojyts EM, Marshall MT: The early diagnosis and treatment of developmental patella infera syndrome. Clin Orthop 265:241–252, 1991.
231. Nyland J: Rehabilitation complications following knee surgery. Clin Sports Med 18:905–925, 1999.
232. Odensten M, Gillquist J: Functional anatomy of the anterior cruciate ligament and a rationale for reconstruction. J Bone Joint Surg Am 67:257–262, 1985.
233. Odensten M, Hamberg P, Nordin M, et al: Surgical or conservative treatment of the acutely torn anterior cruciate ligament. Clin Orthop 198:87–93, 1985.
234. O'Donoghue DH: An analysis of end results of surgical treatment of major injuries to the ligaments of the knee. J Bone Joint Surg Am 37:1–13, 1955.
235. O'Donoghue DH: Surgical treatment of fresh injuries to the major ligaments of the knee. J Bone Joint Surg Am 32:721–738, 1950.
236. O'Donoghue DH: Surgical treatment of injuries to the knee. Clin Orthop 18:11–36, 1960.
237. Ohkoshi Y, Ohkoshi M, Nagasaki S, et al: The effect of cryotherapy on intraarticular temperature and postoperative care after anterior cruciate ligament reconstruction. Am J Sports Med 27:357–362, 1999.
238. O'Neill DB: Arthroscopically assisted reconstruction of the anterior cruciate ligament: A prospective randomized analysis of three techniques. J Bone Joint Surg Am 78:803–812, 1996.
239. Ostenberg A, Roos E, Ekdahl C, Roos H: Isokinetic knee extensor strength and functional performance in healthy female soccer players. Scand J Med Sci Sports 8:257–264, 1998.
240. Osteras H, Augestad LB, Tondel S: Isokinetic muscle strength after anterior cruciate ligament reconstruction. Scand J Med Sci Sports 8:279–282, 1998.
241. Otero AL, Hutcheson L: A comparison of the doubled semitendinosus/gracilis and central third of the patellar tendon autografts in arthroscopic anterior cruciate ligament reconstruction. Arthroscopy 9:143–148, 1993.
242. Otto D, Pinczewski LA, Clingeleffer A, Odell R: Five-year results of single-incision arthroscopic anterior cruciate ligament reconstruction with patellar tendon autograft. Am J Sports Med 26:181–188, 1998.
243. Palmer I: On the injuries to the ligaments of the knee joint. Acta Chir Scand 53(suppl):1–21, 1938.
244. Patel JV, Church JS, Hall AJ: Central third bone–patellar tendon–bone anterior cruciate ligament reconstruction: A 5-year follow-up. Arthroscopy 16:67–70, 2000.
245. Paulos LE, Rosenberg TD, Drawbert J, et al: Infrapatellar contracture syndrome: An unrecognized cause of knee stiffness with patella entrapment and patella infera. Am J Sports Med 15:331–341, 1987.
246. Pinar H, Gillquist J: Dacron augmentation of a free patellar tendon graft: A biomechanical study. Arthroscopy 5:328–330, 1989.
247. Pincivero DM, Lephart SM, Henry TJ: The effects of kinesthetic training on balance and proprioception in anterior cruciate ligament injured knee. J Athletic Training 31(suppl 2):S52, 1996.
248. Pomeroy G, Baltz M, Pierz K, et al: The effects of bone plug length and screw diameter on the holding strength of bone-tendon-bone grafts. Arthroscopy 14:148–152, 1998.
249. Puddu G, Cipolla M, Cerullo G, et al: Anterior cruciate ligament reconstruction and augmentation with PDS graft. Clin Sports Med 12:13–24, 1993.
250. Reinold MM, Fleisig GS, Wilk KE: Research supports both OKC and CKC activities. Biomechanics Nov(suppl):27–32, 1999.
251. Risberg MA, Holm I, Steen H, et al: The effect of knee bracing after anterior cruciate ligament reconstruction. Am J Sports Med 27:76–83, 1999.
252. Roberts D, Friden T, Zatterstrom R, et al: Proprioception in people with anterior cruciate ligament–deficient knees: Comparison of symptomatic and asymptomatic patients. J Orthop Sports Phys Ther 29:587–594, 1999.
253. Robson AWM: Ruptured crucial ligaments and their repair by operation. Ann Surg 37:716–718, 1903.
254. Rodeo SA, Arnoczky SP, Torzilli PA, et al: Tendon healing in a bone tunnel: A biomechanical and histological study in the dog. J Bone Joint Surg Am 75:1795–1803, 1993.
255. Rosen MA, Jackson DW, Atwell EA: The efficacy of continuous passive motion in the rehabilitation of anterior cruciate ligament reconstructions. Am J Sports Med 20:122–127, 1992.
256. Rosen MA, Jackson DW, Berger PE: Occult osseous lesions documented by magnetic resonance imaging associated with anterior cruciate ligament ruptures. Arthroscopy 7:45–51, 1991.
257. Roth JH, Kennedy JC, Lockstadt H, et al: Polypropylene braid augmented and nonaugmented intra-articular anterior cruciate ligament reconstruction. Am J Sports Med 13:321–336, 1985.
258. Roth JH, Shkrum MJ, Bray RC: Synovial reaction associated with disruption of polypropylene braid augmented intraarticular anterior cruciate ligament reconstruction. A case report. Am J Sports Med 16:301–305, 1988.
259. Rozzi SL, Lephart SM, Gear WS, et al: Knee joint laxity and neuromuscular characteristics of male and female soccer and basketball players. Am J Sports Med 27:312–319, 1999.
260. Rubinstein RA, Shelbourne KD, Van Meter CD: Isolated autologous bone–patellar tendon–bone graft site morbidity. Am J Sports Med 22:324–327, 1994.
261. Sachs RA, Daniel DM, Stone ML, Garfein RF: Patellofemoral problems after anterior cruciate ligament reconstruction. Am J Sports Med 17:760–765, 1989.
262. Salter RB, Simmonds DF, Malcolm BW, et al: The biological effect of continuous passive motion on the healing of full-thickness defects in articular cartilage. J Bone Joint Surg Am 62:1232–1251, 1980.
263. Samuelson TS, Drez D Jr, Maletis GB: Anterior cruciate ligament graft rotation: Reproduction of normal graft rotation. Am J Sports Med 24:67–71, 1996.
264. Santi MD, Richardson AB: The ligament augmentation device in hamstring grafts for reconstruction of the anterior cruciate ligament. Am J Sports Med 22:524–530, 1994.
265. Schatzmann L, Brunner P, Staubli HU: Effect of cyclic preconditioning on the tensile properties of human quadriceps tendons and patellar ligaments. Knee Surg Sports Traumatol Arthrosc 6:S56–S61, 1998.
266. Schreck PJ, Kitabayashi LR, Amiel D, et al: Integrin display increases in the wounded rabbit medial collateral ligament but not the wounded anterior cruciate ligament. J Orthop Res 13:174–183, 1995.
267. Schulte K, Majewski M, Irrgang J, et al: Radiographic tunnel changes following arthroscopic anterior cruciate ligament reconstruction. Am J Sports Med 23:372–373, 1995.
268. Schultz RA, Miller DC, Kerr CS, Micheli L: Mechanoreceptors in human cruciate ligaments. J Bone Joint Surg Am 66:1072–1076, 1984.
269. Schutte MJ, Dabezies EJ, Zimny ML, Happel LT: Neural anatomy of the human anterior cruciate ligament. J Bone Joint Surg Am 69:243–247, 1987.
270. Sciore P, Frank CB, Hart DA: Identification of sex hormone receptors in human and rabbit ligaments of the knee by reverse transcription–polymerase chain reaction: Evidence that receptors are present. J Orthop Res 16:604–612, 1998.
271. Seitz H, Schlenz I, Muller E, Vecsei V: Anterior instability of the knee despite an intensive rehabilitation program. Clin Orthop 328:159–164, 1996.
272. Sernert N, Kartus J, Kohler K, et al: Analysis of subjective, objec-

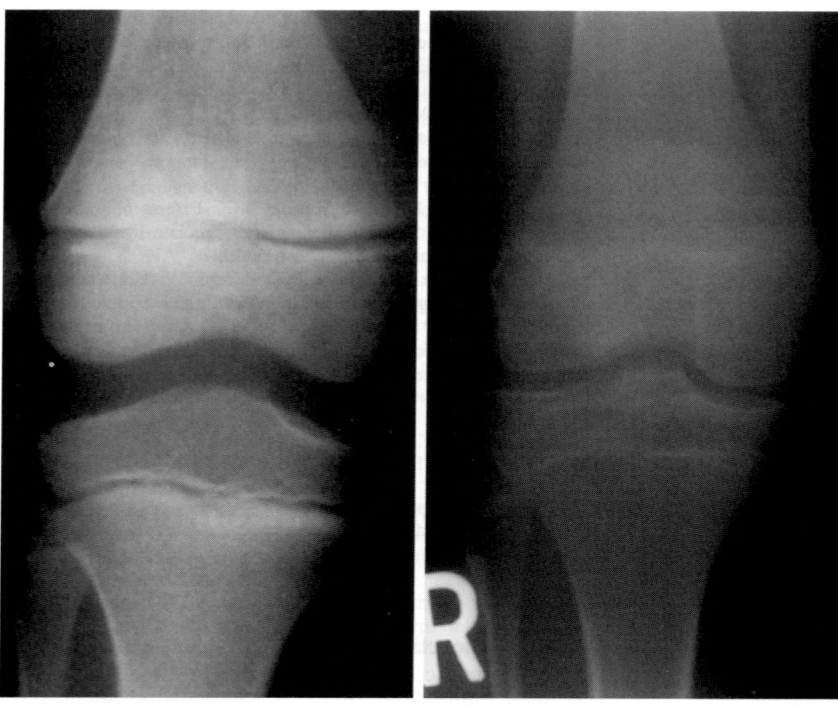

Figure 28J2–1. *Left,* Anteroposterior radiograph of a patient with *wide open* physis. *Right,* Radiograph of an adolescent with little growth remaining.

patterns, such as *capping* of the metaphysis by the epiphysis, which precedes physiologic physeal fusion.

Tibial Eminence Fractures

Tibial eminence fractures represent a unique variant of ACL disruption in which the bony insertion of the ligament on the intercondylar tibial eminence is avulsed. Rinaldi and Mazzarella[37] noted that in the skeletally immature patient, the tibial spine offers less resistance than the ACL substance to traction forces. An injury that could cause a midsubstance tear in an adult can cause an avulsion of the tibial spine in a child.

Meyers and McKeever[26] reported that the most common mechanism of injury is a fall from a bicycle or motorcycle and stated that a child with a swollen knee after such an injury should be considered to have a fracture of the intercondylar eminence until proved otherwise. Other mechanisms include sports injuries and pedestrian–motor vehicle trauma.[48] Many authors have reported collateral ligament and meniscal injuries with tibial spine avulsions.[10, 26, 28, 50]

Meyers and McKeever[26] classified tibial spine avulsions into three types: Type I has minimal or no displacement; type II is anterior hinging of one third to one half of the tibial eminence; type III is completely displaced from the fracture bed. Type III+ fractures are characterized by rotational malalignment. Zaricznyj[50] further documented a type IV fracture, in which the displaced fragment is comminuted.

Treatment

Type II and III fractures generally are treated successfully with closed reduction and immobilization. Aspiration of a tense hemarthrosis is necessary to allow the knee to be brought closer to full extension. Many authors recommend immobilization in approximately 20 degrees of flexion in a long leg cast for 4 to 6 weeks. Micheli and colleagues[25, 27] stated that the fracture fragment is subject to the least tension at 15 to 30 degrees of flexion and that further extension to 0 degrees results in its displacement. This empirical observation has been supported by biomechanical studies, which show in vitro that the lowest strain occurs at 35 degrees of flexion.[25, 34, 41, 45] Others have recommended immobilization in full extension to allow the femoral condyles to compress the fragment into the fracture bed.[36, 47–49] Roberts[38] stated that the terminal 5 degrees of extension mechanically reduces the tibial eminence fracture by producing direct contact with the lateral femoral condyle. The reduction must be confirmed fluoroscopically or under direct vision, by either arthroscopic or open methods, to determine what knee position would optimize the reduction.

If reduction with closed manipulation is unsatisfactory, open or arthroscopic reduction is necessary.[4, 20, 26, 48, 49] The fracture fragment and bed are débrided of interposed soft tissue, including meniscus or cartilage, that may be preventing proper seating of the fracture fragment. Arthroscopic fixation of the fracture fragment may employ sutures or wire.[18, 36, 39, 47] When the fracture fragment is larger than it appears radiographically, fixation may be achieved with a 3.5-mm cannulated screw or smooth pin fixation placed in retrograde fashion from the anterior epiphysis.[39, 50] Transepiphyseal fixation is not recommended because of the risk of anterior growth arrest and hyperextension deformity.[31] Some authors have recommended suturing the anterior horn of the lateral meniscus or the medial meniscus to the fragment.[39, 48]

The overall results after adequate reduction of the tibial

spine are good to excellent.[4, 26, 30] Sequelae following tibial spine fracture may include residual ACL laxity and loss of terminal knee extension.[4, 48] Residual ACL laxity may be secondary to many factors, including secondary hypertrophy and lengthening of the tibial spine, functional ACL lengthening, and associated ACL injury. In a primate study, Noyes and associates[33] showed disruption of normal collagen architecture of ACL fibers in which failure of the ACL had occurred at the tibial spine. At long-term follow-up of 45 patients with open reduction of tibial eminence fracture, Wiley and Baxter[48] found minimal side-to-side difference in anterior laxity in type I injuries with a mean difference of 1 mm, but more significant side-to-side differences in type II (3 mm) and type III (4 mm) injuries. Greater laxity (5 mm) was noted in patients who suffered pedestrian–motor vehicle trauma. Willis and associates[49] found mean side-to-side differences of 1 mm, 3.5 mm, and 4.5 mm in 56 patients with type I, II, and III tibial spine avulsions at 2- to 8-year evaluations. Two of these patients were treated by cast in 20 degrees of flexion; 36, with aspiration or arthroscopy and closed reduction in extension; and 18, with open reduction and internal fixation. Functional results were good, with 84% returning to the same level of sports activity and 98% having no complaints of giving way.

Loss of terminal knee extension may result after tibial spine fractures.[4, 26] Lengthening and hypertrophy of the tibial spine can occur secondary to hyperemia or residual displacement and can provide a bony block to extension. In Wiley and Baxter's[48] series of 45 patients, all patients had some decrease in extension (range, 4 to 15 degrees), and 64% were symptomatic. Willis and associates[49] reported no significant (>10 degrees) loss of extension.

Author's Recommendations

The most important goal of either closed (type II and III) or open (type IV) technique is anatomic reduction. Anatomic reduction should be confirmed arthroscopically or fluoroscopically. Displacement of the anterior cartilaginous component, usually elevation of the anterior segment,

can occur regardless of which method of reduction or fixation is used. A period of immobilization in extension prevents this. In cases in which internal fixation is necessary, placement of a posteriorly angled cannulated screw keeps the fragment reduced and allows earlier range of motion (Fig. 28J2–2). Care must be taken to ensure that the screw does not cross the tibial physes.

Midsubstance Anterior Cruciate Ligament Tears

Nonsurgical Treatment

The risk of physeal damage with surgical treatment has been the primary rationale for nonsurgical management of midsubstance ACL injuries in the skeletally immature patient.[27, 28] Rehabilitation and bracing to defer surgical treatment until skeletal maturity have been advocated by some. Most reports indicate, however, that these patients have a poor prognosis with respect to return to sports and long-term sequalae.[5, 7, 8, 17] Angel and Hall[2] reviewed 22 ACL-deficient, skeletally immature patients at an average follow-up of 51 months. No patient with a complete ACL tear was able to return to sports at a preinjury level. McCarroll and associates[23] treated 16 patients with quadriceps and hamstring rehabilitation and bracing. Nine were unable to return to sports, and all 16 patients had giving-way episodes.

Many long-term consequences have been reported in ACL-deficient, skeletally immature patients, including repeated giving-way episodes, meniscal damage, and early arthrosis. Graf and associates[14] treated eight patients with rehabilitation and bracing. At a follow-up of only 2 years, all had symptoms of giving way, and seven patients had developed new meniscal tears. Mizuta and associates[29] treated 18 patients with rehabilitation and bracing. At a minimum follow-up of 36 months, all patients were symptomatic. Of these patients, 17 had giving-way episodes, 9 had evidence of secondary meniscal tears, and 11 had evidence of early degenerative arthritis.

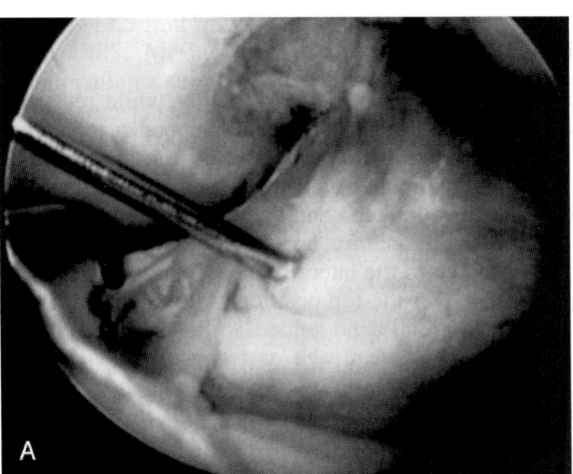 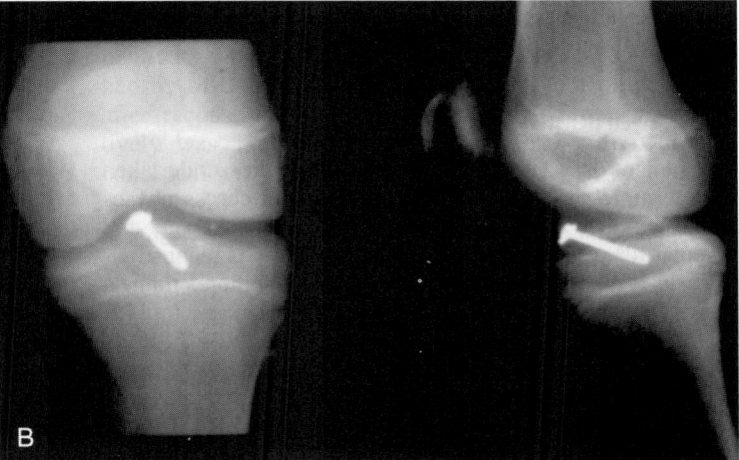

Figure 28J2–2. *A,* A guide pin is inserted into the reduced avulsed fragment, followed by a 3.5-mm cannulated screw (*B*). The screw is angled posteriorly, which prevents elevation of the anterior segment.

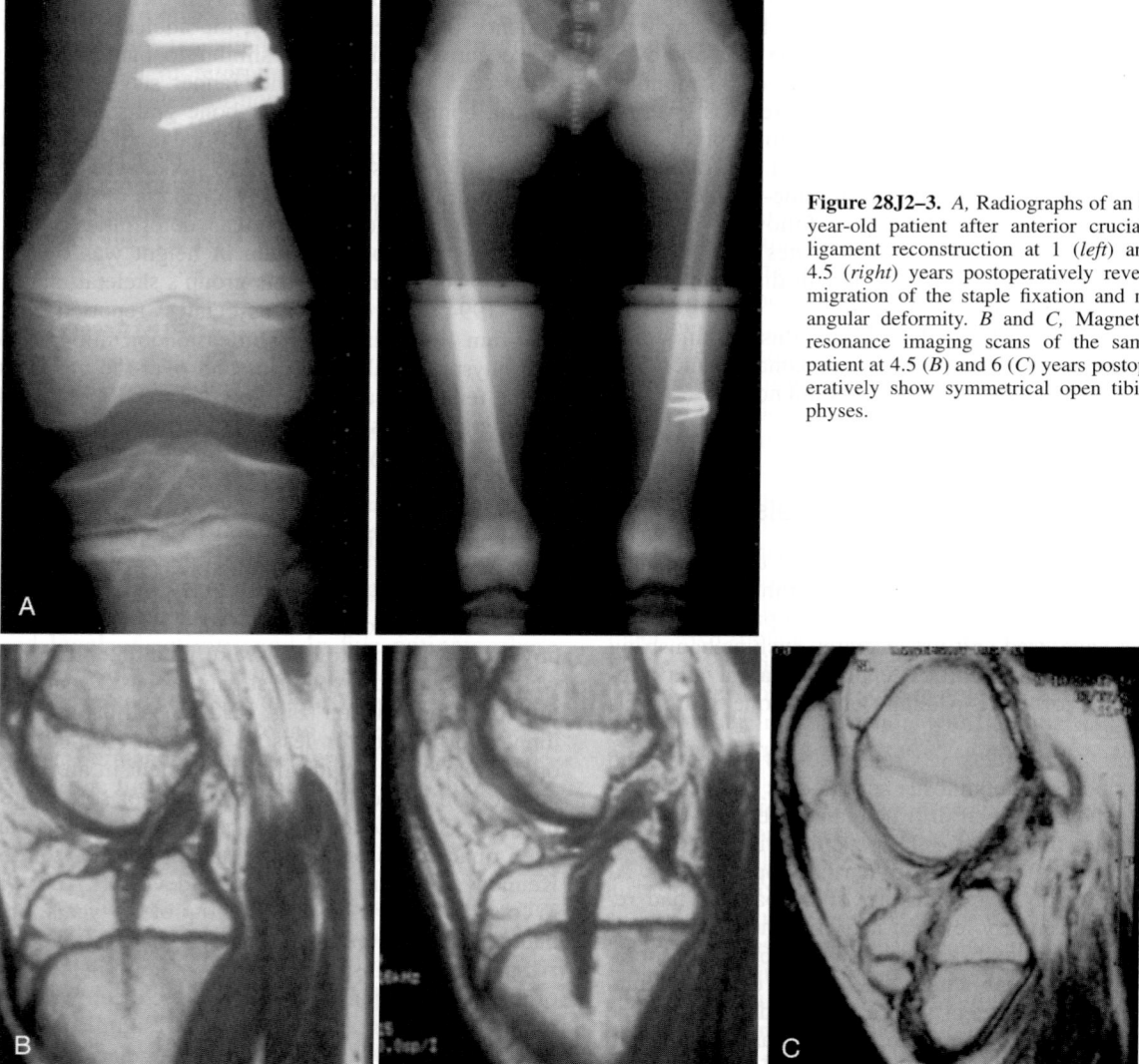

Figure 28J2–3. *A,* Radiographs of an 8-year-old patient after anterior cruciate ligament reconstruction at 1 (*left*) and 4.5 (*right*) years postoperatively reveal migration of the staple fixation and no angular deformity. *B* and *C,* Magnetic resonance imaging scans of the same patient at 4.5 (*B*) and 6 (*C*) years postoperatively show symmetrical open tibial physes.

reported, these are contraindicated when there is significant growth remaining.

Author's Preferred Treatment

It has been the practice at this center to manage the young ACL-injured patient with *wide open* physes with intra-articular hamstring ACL reconstruction. In our experience, growth disturbance and subsequent angular deformity have not occurred with this technique. We use small (6 mm), vertically placed tunnels; ensure that they are filled completely with graft tissue; and use over-the-top femoral placement. In Figure 28J2–4, MRI shows a hamstring tendon graft in the over-the-top position. The anatomic femoral origin of the ACL is closely reproduced. We take care not to overconstrain the knee by tensioning the graft at 20 pounds or less and to keep femoral and tibial graft fixation well away from the physes (Fig. 28J2–5). Meticulous attention to detail averts situations with potential for increasing the risk of growth arrest (Fig. 28J2–6). The rehabilitation

protocol for this group of patients is the standard for functional and progressive post-ACL reconstruction.

Summary

ACL injury in skeletally immature patients increasingly is recognized and reported. The functional results of non-surgical treatment of ACL injury, either as an attempt at definitive treatment or as a temporizing plan until skeletal maturity occurs, are poor, and the risks of reinjury and further meniscal and cartilage damage are significant. Primary ACL repair or extra-articular reconstruction alone is not efficacious. In an adolescent patient who is approaching skeletal maturity, risk of physeal injury is low, and intra-articular reconstruction can be performed as in an adult patient. Results with respect to decreased laxity and return to athletic activities mirror those described in adults. In truly skeletally immature patients, intra-articular reconstruction using a soft tissue graft through a transphyseal

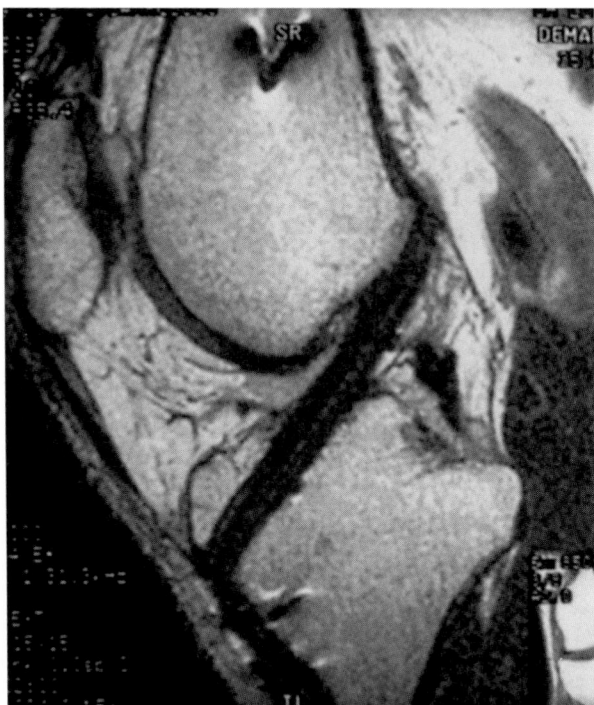

Figure 28J2–4. Magnetic resonance imaging shows a hamstring tendon graft in the over-the-top position. The anatomic femoral origin of the anterior cruciate ligament has been closely reproduced.

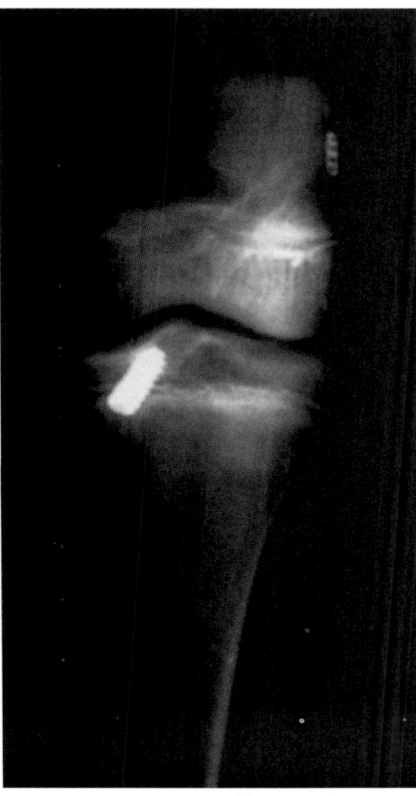

Figure 28J2–6. The tibial interference screw has been placed across the open physis, with a potential increased risk of growth arrest in the area.

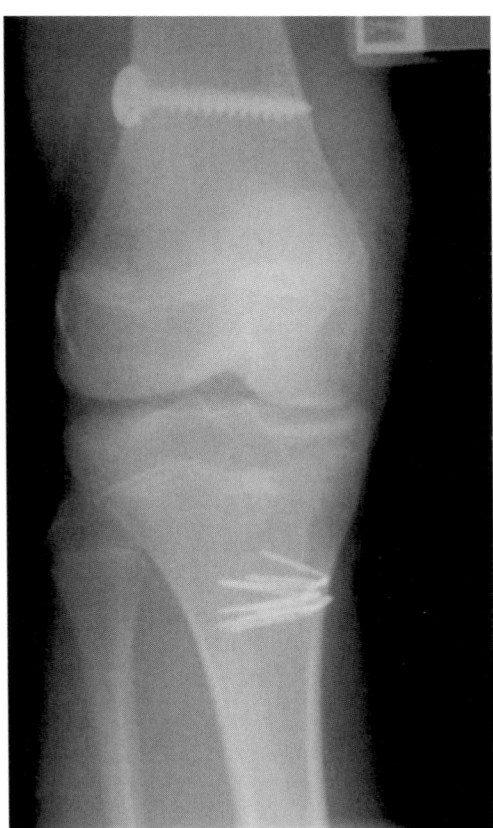

Figure 28J2–5. Anteroposterior radiograph of a 13-year-old girl 6 months after hamstring over-the-top anterior cruciate ligament reconstruction. Tibial fixation and femoral fixation are well away from the physes.

tibial tunnel of small diameter and the over-the-top position on the femur has not been shown to cause early physeal closure, limb-length discrepancy, or angular deformity.

References

1. Andrews M, Noyes F, Barber-Westin S: Anterior cruciate ligament allograft reconstruction in the skeletally immature athlete. Am J Sports Med 22:48–54, 1994.
2. Angel KR, Hall DJ: Anterior cruciate ligament injury in children and adolescents. Arthroscopy 5:197–200, 1989.
3. Arnowitz ER, Ganley TJ, Goode JR, et al: Anterior cruciate ligament reconstruction in adolescents with open physes. Am J Sports Med 28:168–175, 2000.
4. Baxter MP, Wiley JJ: Fractures of the tibial spine in children. J Bone Joint Surg Br 70:228–230, 1988.
5. Bradley GW, Shives TC, Samuelson KM: Ligament injuries of the knees of children. J Bone Joint Surg Am 61:588–591, 1979.
6. Brief LP: Anterior cruciate ligament reconstruction without drill holes. Arthroscopy 7:350–357, 1991.
7. Chick RR, Jackson DW: Tears of the anterior cruciate ligament in young athletes. J Bone Joint Surg Am 60:970–973, 1978.
8. Clanton T, DeLee JC, Sanders B, et al: Knee ligament injuries in children. J Bone Joint Surg Am 61:1195–1201, 1979.
9. Degenhardt TC, Hughston JC: Chronic posterior cruciate instability: Non-operative management. Orthop Trans 5:486–487, 1981.
10. DeLee JC: Ligamentous injury of the knee. In Stanitski C, DeLee JC, Drez D Jr (eds): Pediatric and Adolescent Sports Medicine. Philadelphia, WB Saunders, 1994, pp 406–432.
11. DeLee JC, Curtis RJ: Anterior cruciate ligament insufficiency in children. Clin Orthop 172:112–112, 1983.
12. Edwards TB, Greene CC, Baratta RV, Drez D: The effect of transphyseal anterior cruciate ligament reconstruction in an immature canine

model [abstract]. Paper presented at the 26th Annual Meeting of the American Orthopaedic Society for Sports Medicine, June 18–21, 2000, Sun Valley, Idaho.

13. Engebretsen L, Svenningsen S, Benum P: Poor results of anterior cruciate ligament repair in adolescence. Acta Orthop Scand 59:684–686, 1988.

14. Graf BK, Lange RH, Fujisaki CK, et al: Anterior cruciate ligament tears in skeletally immature patients: Meniscal pathology at presentation and after attempted conservative treatment. Arthroscopy 8:229–233, 1992.

15. Grontvedt T, Engebretsen L, Benum P, et al: A prospective, randomized study of three operations for acute rupture of the anterior cruciate ligament: Five-year follow-up of one hundred and thirty-one patients. J Bone Joint Surg Am 78:159–168, 1996.

16. Guzzanti V, Falciglia F, Gigante A, et al: The effect of intra-articular reconstruction on the growth plates of rabbits. J Bone Joint Surg Br 76:960–963, 1994.

17. Kannus P, Jarvinen M: Knee ligament injuries in adolescents. J Bone Joint Surg Br 70:772–776, 1988.

18. Kogan M, Amendola A: Arthroscopic suture fixation of displaced tibial intercondylar eminence fractures. Arthroscopy 13:306, 1997.

19. Letts RM, Yang J, Houle J-B: The effect of creating a bone tunnel across the physis [abstract]. Presented the 51st Annual Meeting of The Canadian Orthopaedic Association, Quebec City, 1996.

20. Lipscomb B, Anderson A: Tears of the anterior cruciate ligament in adolescents. J Bone Joint Surg Am 68:19–28, 1986.

21. Lo YPC, Kirkley A, Miniaci A, Fowler PJ: The outcome of operatively treated anterior cruciate ligament disruptions in the skeletally immature child. Arthroscopy 13:627–634, 1997.

22. Matz SO, Jackson DW: Anterior cruciate ligament injury in children. Am J Knee Surg 1:59–65, 1988.

23. McCarroll JR, Rettig AC, Shelbourne KD: Anterior cruciate ligament injuries in the young athlete with open physes. Am J Sports Med 16:44–47, 1988.

24. McCarroll JR, Shelbourne KD, Porter DA, et al: Patellar tendon graft reconstruction for mid-substance anterior cruciate ligament rupture in junior high school athletes. Am J Sports Med 22:478–484, 1994.

25. Meglan D, Zueler B, Buck W, et al: The effects of quadriceps force upon strain in the anterior cruciate ligament [abstract]. Trans Orthop Res Soc 11:55, 1986.

26. Meyers MH, McKeever FM: Fracture of the intercondylar eminence of the tibia. J Bone Joint Surg Am 52:1677–1684, 1970.

27. Micheli LJ: Pediatric and adolescent sports injuries: Recent trends. Exerc Sport Sci Rev 14:359–374, 1986.

28. Micheli LJ, Foster TE: Acute knee injuries in the immature athlete. Instr Course Lect 42:473–481, 1993.

29. Mizuta H, Kubota K, Shiraishi M, et al: The conservative treatment of complete tears of the anterior cruciate ligament in skeletally immature patients. J Bone Joint Surg Br 77:890–894, 1995.

30. Molander ML, Watkin G, Wikstad I: Fracture of the intercondylar eminence of the tibia: A review of 35 patients. J Bone Joint Surg Br 63:89–91, 1981.

31. Mylle J, Reynders P, Broos P: Transepiphyseal fixation of anterior cruciate avulsion in a child: Report of a complication and review of the literature. Arch Orthop Trauma Surg 112:101–103, 1993.

32. Nottage W, Matsuura P: Management of complete anterior cruciate ligament tears in the skeletally immature patient. Arthroscopy 10:569–573, 1994.

33. Noyes FR, DeLucas JL, Torvik PJ: Biomechanics of anterior cruciate ligament failure: An analysis of strain-rate sensitivity and mechanism of failure in primates. J Bone Joint Surg Am 56:253, 1974.

34. Noyes FR, Grood ES, Butler DL, et al: Clinical laxity tests and functional stability of the knee. Clin Orthop 146:84–89, 1980.

35. Parker AW, Drez D, Cooper JL: Anterior cruciate ligament injuries in patients with open physes. Am J Sports Med 22:44–47, 1994.

36. Rask BP, Micheli LJ: Knee ligament injuries and associated internal derangements in children and adolescents. In Fu FH, Harner CD, Vince KG (eds): Knee Surgery. Baltimore, Williams & Wilkins, 1995, pp 365–381.

37. Rinaldi E, Mazzarella F: Isolated fracture-avulsion of the tibial insertions of the cruciate ligaments of the knee. Ital J Orthop Traumatol 6:77–83, 1980.

38. Roberts JM: Avulsion fractures of the proximal tibial epiphysis. In Fowler PJ, Kennedy JC (eds): The Injured Adolescent Knee. Baltimore, Williams & Wilkins, 1979.

39. Roberts JM: Operative treatment of fractures about the knee. Orthop Clin North Am 21:365–679, 1990.

40. Roche AF, Wainer H, Thissen D: Skeletal Maturity: The Knee Joint as a Biological Indicator. New York, Plenum Medical, 1975.

41. Smith BA, Livesay GA, Woo SL: Biology and biomechanics of the anterior cruciate ligament. Clin Sports Med 12:637–670, 1993.

42. Stadlemaier DN, Arnozcky SP, Dodds H, et al: The effect of drilling and soft tissue grafting across open growth plates. Am J Sports Med 23:435, 1995.

43. Stanitski C: Anterior cruciate ligament injury in the skeletally immature patient: Diagnosis and treatment. J Am Acad Orthop Surg 3:146–158, 1995.

44. Stanitski C, Harvell J, Fu F: Observations on acute knee haemarthrosis in children and adolescents. J Pediatr Orthop 13:506–510, 1993.

45. Takeda Y, Xerogeanes JW, Livesay GA, et al: Biomechanical function of the human anterior cruciate ligament. Arthroscopy 13:361–364, 1994.

46. Tanner JM, Davies PS: Clinical longitudinal standards for height and height velocity for North American children. J Pediatr 107:317–329, 1985.

47. Warner JP, Micheli LJ: Pediatric and adolescent musculoskeletal injuries. In Grana AW, Kalenak A (eds): Clinical Sports Medicine. Philadelphia, WB Saunders, 1991, pp 490–498.

48. Wiley JJ, Baxter MP: Tibial spine fractures in children. Clin Orthop 225:54–60, 1990.

49. Willis RB, Blokker C, Stoll TM, et al: Long-term follow-up of anterior eminence tibial fractures. J Pediatr Orthop 13:361–364, 1993.

50. Zaricznyj B: Avulsion fracture of the tibial eminence: Treatment by open reduction and pinning. J Bone Joint Surg Am 59:1111–1114, 1977.

Patellar Tendon Autograft Reconstruction Minimum 2-Year Follow-up Studies

APPENDIX A–1
Demographics

Author and Year Published	Total No. of Patients	No. of Patients Evaluated	Follow-up (%)	Mean Age at Surgery (yr)	Mean Follow-up Interval (mo)	Gender (% male)
Engebretsen 1990	50	50	100	29	24	58
Marder 1991	40	37	93	22	29	65
Aglietti 1992	73	69	95	23	96	77
Buss 1993	69	67	97	24	32	66
Otero 1993	N/A	55	N/A	26	36	76
Bach 1994	75	62	83	27	37	71
Arciero 1996	82	82	100	20	31	88
Grondveldt 1996	51	47	92	26	24	45
O'Neill 1996	87	85	98	27	44	64
Aglietti 1997	101	89	88	23	84	81
Heier 1997	53	45	85	45	37	38
Sgaglione 1997	90	86	96	25	36	73
Shelton 1997	30	30	100	25	24	53
Bach (ENDO) 1998	128	103	81	25	26	63
Bach (DI) 1998	147	97	66	26	79	74
Kleipool 1998	29	26	90	28	52	35
Otto 1998	80	68	85	27	60	72
Webb 1998	90	82	91	25	24	53
Johma 1999	80	59	74	26	84	73
Corry 1999	90	82	91	25	24	53
Patel 2000	44	32	73	33	70	75

DI, double incision; ENDO, endoscopic; N/A, data not available.

APPENDIX A–2
Previous Surgery

Author and Year Published	Patients with Previous Surgery (%)	PMM (%)	PLM (%)	Previous ACLR (%)	Misc. Surgery (%)
Engebretsen 1990	N/A	N/A	N/A	0	0
Marder 1991	24	N/A	N/A	5	0
Aglietti 1992	26	17	4	3	2
Buss 1993	51	28	6	0	19
Otero 1993	N/A	N/A	N/A	0	N/A
Bach 1994	42	N/A	N/A	0	N/A
Arciero 1996	0	0	0	0	0
Grondveldt 1996	43	N/A	N/A	N/A	N/A
O'Neill 1996	34	N/A	N/A	11	8
Aglietti 1997	25	15	10	0	0
Heier 1997	9	7	2	0	N/A
Sgaglione 1997	26	8	3	0	15
Shelton 1997	N/A	N/A	N/A	N/A	N/A
Bach (ENDO) 1998	44	N/A	N/A	0	N/A
Bach (DI) 1998	47	N/A	N/A	0	N/A
Kleipool 1998	84	31	15	0	13
Otto 1998	22	9	4	0	9
Webb 1998	N/A	0	0	0	N/A

ACLR, anterior cruciate ligament reconstruction; DI, double incision; ENDO, endoscopic; N/A, data not available; PMM, partial medial meniscectomy; PLM, partial lateral meniscectomy.

APPENDIX A–3
Surgical Protocol

Author and Year Published	Technique	Femoral Graft Fixation	Tibial Graft Fixation
Engebretsen 1990	ENDO	IS and S/W	Staples or IS and S/W
Marder 1991	DI	S/W	S/W
Aglietti 1992	DI	Lig. button	IS and lig. button
Buss 1993	DI	Lig. button	IS and lig. button
Otero 1993	ENDO	IS	IS
Bach 1994	DI	IS	IS
Arciero 1996	Both	IS	IS
Grondveldt 1996	DI	IS	IS
O'Neill 1996	Both	IS	IS
Aglietti 1997	DI	Lig. button	IS and lig. button
Heier 1997	DI	S/W	S/W
Sgaglione 1997	Both	IS	IS
Shelton 1997	ENDO	IS	IS
Bach (ENDO) 1998	ENDO	IS	IS
Bach (DI) 1998	DI	IS	IS
Kleipool 1998	ENDO	IS	IS
Otto 1998	ENDO	IS	IS
Webb 1998	ENDO	IS	IS
Jomha 1999	ENDO	IS	IS
Corry 1999	ENDO	IS	IS
Patel 2000	ENDO	IS	IS

DI, double incision; ENDO, endoscopic; IS, interference screw; lig. button, ligament button; S/W, screw/washer.

APPENDIX A–4
Rehabilitation Protocol

Author and Year Published	Postoperative Weight-bearing	Postoperative CPM	Return to Full Sports (mo)
Engebretsen 1990	NWB × 8 wk	Not used	12
Marder 1991	TDWB × 6 wk	Not used	10–12
Aglietti 1992	NWB × 3 wk	Not used	N/A
Buss 1993	NWB × 6 wk	+	6
Otero 1993	NWB × 6 wk	+	N/A
Bach 1994	NWB × 2 wk	+	8
Arciero 1996	Progressive WB	Not used	N/A
Grondveldt 1996	WBAT	Not used	6
O'Neill 1996	WBAT	Not used	6
Aglietti 1997	NWB × 3 wk	Not used	6
Heier 1997	WBAT	Not used	6
Sgaglione 1997	NWB × 4 wk	Not used	9
Shelton 1997	WBAT	Not used	6
Bach (ENDO) 1998	WBAT	+	4–6
Bach (DI) 1998	NWB × 2 wk	+	6
Kleipool 1998	PWB × 4 wk	+	12
Otto 1998	NWB × 4 wk	+	9
Webb 1998	Progressive WB	Not used	9
Jomha 1999	NWB × 4 wk	+	9
Corry 1999	WBAT	Not used	9
Patel 2000	N/A	N/A	N/A

CPM; continuous passive motion; DI, double incision; ENDO, endoscopic; N/A, data not available; NWB, non–weight-bearing; PWB, partial weight-bearing; TDWB, touchdown weight-bearing; WBAT, weight-bearing as tolerated.

APPENDIX A–5
Meniscal Disease at Reconstruction

Author and Year Published	Patients with Meniscal Tears (%)	Meniscal Tears Treated by PMM (%)	Meniscal Tears Treated by MMR (%)	Meniscal Tears Treated by PLM (%)	Meniscal Tears Treated by LMR (%)
Engebretsen 1990	N/A	N/A	N/A	N/A	N/A
Marder 1991	32	50	25	25	0
Aglietti 1992	N/A	28	27	42	3
Buss 1993	51	40	34	17	9
Otero 1993	58	N/A	N/A	N/A	N/A
Bach 1994	63	21	47	24	8
Arciero 1996	49	8	43	30	20
Grondveldt 1996	43	N/A	N/A	N/A	N/A
O'Neill 1996	69	27	19	39	14
Aglietti 1997	94	30	26	37	2
Heier 1997	40	N/A	0	N/A	0
Sgaglione 1997	56	27	29	35	8
Shelton 1997	83	N/A	N/A	N/A	N/A
Bach (ENDO) 1998	52	34	17	42	9
Bach (DI) 1998	52	36	36	34	14
Kleipool 1998	45	29	50	7	14
Otto 1998	71	46	6	35	13
Webb 1998	28	0	10	12	4
Jomha 1999	N/A	31	5	25	8
Corry 1999	N/A	N/A	N/A	N/A	N/A
Patel 2000	40	77	0	23	0

DI, double incision; ENDO, endoscopic; LMR, lateral meniscal repair; MMR, medical meniscus repair; N/A, data not available; PLM, partial lateral meniscectomy; PMM, partial medial meniscectomy.

APPENDIX A–6
KT1000 Side-to-Side Differences

Author and Year Published	Preoperative			Postoperative		
Engebretsen 1990	N/A	N/A	N/A	<3 mm 79%	3–5 mm 21%	>5 mm 0%
Marder 1991	N/A	N/A	N/A	<3 mm 86%	3–5 mm 14%	>5 mm 0%
Aglietti 1992	<3 mm 2%	3–5 mm 6%	>5 mm 92%	<3 mm 56%	3–5 mm 32%	>5 mm 12%
Buss 1993	N/A	N/A	N/A	0–3 mm 84%	>3 mm 16%	>5 mm 0%
Otero 1993	N/A	N/A	N/A	N/A*	N/A*	N/A*
Bach 1994	<3 mm 12%	≥3 mm 88%	>5 mm N/A	≤3 mm 92%	3–5 mm 4%	≥5 mm 4%
Arciero 1996	N/A	N/A	N/A	<3 mm 70%	3–5 mm 22%	<5 mm 8%
Grondveldt 1996	<4 mm 18%	4–5 mm 41%	>5 mm 41%	<4 mm 98%	4–5 mm 2%	>5 mm 0%
O'Neill 1996	N/A	N/A	N/A	≤3 mm 89%	3–5 mm 7%	>5 mm 4%
Aglietti 1997	<5 mm 19%	—	>5 mm 81%	<3 mm 48%	3–5 mm 38%	>5 mm 13%
Heier 1997	<3 mm 35%	3–5 mm 15%	>5 mm 50%	<3 mm 78%	3–5 mm 10%	>5 mm 12%
Sgaglione 1997	N/A	N/A	N/A	≤3 mm 77%	3–5 mm 16%	>5 mm 7%
Shelton 1997	<3 mm 8%	3–5 mm 18%	>5 mm 74%	<3 mm 72%	3–5 mm 23%	>5 mm 5%
Bach (ENDO) 1998	≤3 mm 12%	3–5 mm 18%	≥5 mm 70%	≤3 mm 83%	3–5 mm 14%	≥5 mm 3%
Bach (DI) 1998	≤3 mm 9%	3–5 mm 13%	≥5 mm 78%	≥3 mm 70%	3–5 mm 26%	≥5 mm 4%
Kleipool 1998	≤3 mm 2%	3–5 mm 23%	>5 mm 75%	<3 mm 73%	3–5 mm 21%	>5 mm 6%
Otto 1998	N/A	N/A	N/A	N/A	N/A	N/A
Webb 1998	N/A	N/A	N/A	<3 mm 90%	3–5 mm 7%	>5 mm 3%
Jomha 1999	N/A	N/A	N/A	65%	33%	2%
Corry 1999	N/A	N/A	N/A	91%	1%	8%
Patel 2000	N/A	N/A	N/A	88%	12%	0%

*The authors reported their postoperative KT1000 mean difference of 1.5 mm.
DI, double incision; ENDO, endoscopic; N/A, data not available.

APPENDIX A–7
Pivot Shift Examination

Author and Year Published	Preoperative Grade (%)				Postoperative Grade (%)			
	0	*1 +*	*2 +*	*3 + or 4 +*	*0*	*1 +*	*2 +*	*3 + or 4 +*
Engebretsen 1990	0	22	70	8	89	11	0	0
Marder 1991	0	N/A*	N/A	N/A	78	16	6	2
Aglietti 1992	0	10	70	20	87	10	3	0
Buss 1993	0	N/A*	N/A	N/A	89	3	8	0
Otero 1993	N/A	N/A	N/A	N/A	N/A	N/A	N/A	N/A
Bach 1994	29†	26	40	5	92	5	3	0
Arciero 1996	N/A	N/A	N/A	N/A	74	22	4	0
Grondveldt 1996	0	0	8	92	68	32	0	0
O'Neill 1996	N/A	N/A	N/A	N/A	N/A	N/A	N/A	N/A
Aglietti 1997	0	7	73	20	70	19	11	0
Heier 1997	N/A	N/A	N/A	N/A	36	47	15	2
Sgaglione 1997	N/A	N/A	N/A	N/A	91	6	3	0
Shelton 1997	N/A	N/A	N/A	N/A	87	13	0	0
Bach (ENDO) 1998	34†	33	27	6	91	9	0	0
Bach (DI) 1998	1	18	60	20	84	16	0	0
Kleipool 1998	0	5	29	66	76	18	6	0
Otto 1998	0	7	74	19	65	34	1	0
Webb 1998	0	N/A*	N/A	N/A	91	9	0	0
Jomha 1999	N/A	N/A†	N/A	N/A	76	22	2	0
Corry 1999	N/A	N/A*	N/A	N/A	91	9	0	0
Patel 2000	N/A	N/A†	N/A	N/A	91	N/A§	N/A	N/A

*Remarked only that all patients had a positive pivot shift result (except patients with locked knees).
†All of these patients had positive pivot shift results under anesthesia.
‡A normal or 1 + examination finding was reported in 92% of the autograft and 89% of the allograft patients.
§Results were reported as positive in 9% of patients tested.
DI, double incision; ENDO, endoscopic; N/A, data not available.

APPENDIX A–8
Knee Scores

Author and Year Published	Tegner*	Lysholm (mean)	Noyes (mean)	HSS (mean)	IKDC† (%)	Zarins (mean)	NR
Engebretsen 1990		94					
Marder 1991						39	
Aglietti 1992							NR
Buss 1993				88			
Otero 1993		85					
Bach (DI 1994)	7.6/2.1/6.3	88	86	88			
Arciero 1996		90			85		
Grondveldt 1996		96					
O'Neill 1996		92% > 90			92		
Aglietti 1997					77		
Heier 1997		91			64		
Sgaglione 1997					94		
Shelton 1997							NR
Bach (ENDO 1998)	7.3/3.5/6.5	90	88	90			
Bach (DI 1998)	7.1/3.5/6.3	87	87	89			
Kleipool 1998	8/3/6	95			70		
Otto 1998		91			80		
Webb 1998		93			86		
Jomha 1999		94			76		
Corry 1999					80		
Patel 2000	6.3/3.1/5.1	89					

*Tegner results reported as mean preinjury/pre-reconstruction/post-reconstruction.
†Normal, nearly normal.
DI, double incision; ENDO, endoscopic; HSS, Hospital for Special Surgery; IKDC, International Knee Documentation Committee; NR, data not recorded.

APPENDIX A–9
Outcome

Author and Year Published	Subjective Satisfaction (%)	Return to Previous Level of Sports (%)
Engebretsen 1990	NR	64
Marder 1991	NR	65
Aglietti 1992	NR	78
Buss 1993	98	68
Otero 1993	NR	NR
Bach (DI 2–4) 1994	95	NR
Arciero 1996	NR	NR
Grondveldt 1996	NR	NR
O'Neill 1996	NR	92
Aglietti 1997	91	62
Heier 1997	98	76
Sgaglione 1997	97	80
Shelton 1997	NR	NR
Bach (ENDO) 1998	95	41
Bach (DI 5–9) 1998	94	46
Kleipool 1998	NR	NR
Otto 1998	NR	53
Webb 1998	NR	84
Jomha 1999	95	93
Corry 1999	95	88
Patel 2000	94	41

DI, double incision; NR, not recorded.

APPENDIX A–10
Complications*

Author and Year Published	Reoperation Rate	LOA or MUA	PM or MR	Graft Failure	Deep Infection	HWR	Patellar Trauma	Patellar Pain	Misc.
Engebretsen 1990	8	8	0	0	4	0	0	N/R	0
Marder 1991	N/A	N/A	N/A	3	0	N/A	0	32	0
Aglietti 1992	4	3	1	0	0	0	0	4	0
Buss 1993	6	3	0	0	0	1	0	26	0
Otero 1993	31	31	N/A	0	0	0	0	5	0
Bach 1994	11	5	3	0	0	0	0	18	0
Arciero 1996	7	4	0	0	0	4	0	N/R	4
Grondveldt 1996	2	2	0	0	0	0	0	9	0
O'Neill 1996	15	4	5	2	0	4	0	N/R	1
Aglietti 1997	8	1	7	0	0	0	0	3	0
Heier 1997	9	4	0	4	0	0	0	N/R	4
Sgaglione 1997	16	5	1	3	1	8	1	13	1
Shelton 1997	N/A	N/A	N/A	N/A	N/A	N/A	N/A	10	N/A
Bach (ENDO) 1998	15	5	7	0	0	0	0	14	0
Bach (DI) 1998	26	12	7	0	0	6	1	13	1
Kleipool 1998	31	12	8	0	0	31	0	50	0
Otto 1998	16	6	3	4	0	6	0	17	0
Webb 1998	4	4	0	3	2	0	0	N/R	1
Jomha 1999	N/A	8	5	10	2	12	0	44	7
Corry 1999	N/A	4	0	4	0	0	0	31	2
Patel 2000	N/A	6	6	9	0	0	N/A	N/A	N/A

*Complication results in percent.
DI, double incision; ENDO, endoscopic; HWR, hardware removal; LOA, lysis of adhesions; Misc., miscellaneous; MR, meniscal repair; MUA, manipulation under anesthesia; N/A, data not available; N/R, not reported; PM, partial meniscectomy.

Hamstring Anterior Cruciate Ligament Reconstruction
Minimum 2-Year Follow-up Studies

APPENDIX B–1
Demographics

Author and Year Published	Total No. of Patients	No. of Patients Evaluated	Follow-up (%)	Mean Age at Surgery (yr)	Follow-up Mean (mo)	Gender (% male)
Marder 1991	40	35	88	24	32	74
Sgaglione 1992	29	28	97	25	34	71
Sgaglione 1993	51	50	98	24	37	74
Otero 1993	N/A	36	N/A	25	36	81
Karlson 1994	87	64	74	28	34	66
Howell 1996	49	41	84	33	26	68
Maeda 1996	42	41	98	24	27	54
Aglietti 1996	77	69	90	23	60	63
O'Neill 1996	40	40	100	27	38	68
Yasuda 1997	70	64	91	24	30	52
Nebelung 1998	34	29	85	N/A	N/A	76
Corry 1999	90	85	94	25	24	52
Muneta 1999	62	54	87	24	27	39

N/A, data not available.

APPENDIX B–2
Previous Surgery

Author and Year Published	Patients with Previous Surgery (%)	PMM (%)	MMR (%)	PLM (%)	LMR (%)	Previous ACLR (%)	Misc. Surgery (%)
Marder 1991	10	N/A	N/A	N/A	N/A	0	N/A
Sgaglione 1992	71	36	N/A	18	N/A	0	39
Sgaglione 1993	40	20	N/A	10	N/A	0	39
Otero 1993	N/A	N/A	N/A	N/A	N/A	0	N/A
Karlson 1994	27	N/A	N/A	N/A	N/A	N/A	N/A
Howell 1996	17	12	N/A	2	N/A	0	5
Maeda 1996	68	12	24	20	20	0	N/A
Aglietti 1996	N/A	N/A	N/A	N/A	N/A	N/A	N/A
O'Neill 1996	28	N/A	N/A	N/A	N/A	5	N/A
Yasuda 1997	N/A	N/A	N/A	N/A	N/A	0	N/A
Nebelung 1998	N/A	N/A	N/A	N/A	N/A	N/A	N/A
Corry 1999	0	0	0	0	0	0	0
Muneta 1999	N/A	N/A	N/A	N/A	N/A	N/A	N/A

ACLR, anterior cruciate ligament reconstruction; LMR, lateral meniscal repair; N/A, data not available; MMR, medial meniscal repair; PLM, partial lateral meniscectomy; PMM, partial medial meniscectomy.

APPENDIX B–3
Surgical Protocol

Author and Year Published	Technique	Graft Construct	Femoral Graft Fixation	Tibial Graft Fixation
Marder 1991	DI	Doubled ST/G	S/W	S/W
Sgaglione 1992	N/A	Doubled ST or single ST/G	Staples ×2 or S/W	Staples ×2 or S/W
Sgaglione 1993	N/A	Doubled ST or single ST/G	N/A	N/A
Otero 1993	N/A	Doubled ST/G	Suture post	S/W
Karlson 1994	N/A	Single ST/G	S/W ×2	S/W
Howell 1996	DI	Doubled ST/G	S/W or staples	S/W or staples
Maeda 1996	DI	Multiple combinations of ST/G	Buttons or suture post	Buttons or suture post
Aglietti 1996	N/A	Single ST/G	Spiked staples ×2	N/A
O'Neill 1996	DI	Single ST/G	Spiked staples ×2	Spiked staples ×2
Yasuda 1997	DI	Doubled ST/G	Spiked staples ×2	Spiked staples ×2
Nebelung 1998	N/A	Doubled ST	EndoButton	Staples ×2
Corry 1999	DI	Doubled ST/G	Interference screw	Interference screw
Muneta 1999	N/A	Multistrand ST or multistrand ST/G	Acufex button or EndoButton	Suture post

DI, double incision; G, gracilis; N/A, data not available; ST, semitendinosus; S/W, screw and washer.

APPENDIX B–4
Postoperative Protocol

Author and Year Published	Postoperative Weight-bearing	Immobilization	Postoperative CPM	Return to Sports (mo)
Marder 1991	TDWB×6 wk	Hinged brace, 40° flexion	Not used	10–12
Sgaglione 1992	PWB×4–6 wk	Hinged brace 10°–60° flexion	Used in 82%	9
Sgaglione 1993	PWB×4–6 wk	Hinged brace 10°–60° flexion	Not used	9
Otero 1993	WBAT at 6 wk	Cast brace×4 wk	Not used	N/A
Karlson 1994	PWB×6 wk	Hinged brace 10°–30° flexion×6 wk	Not used	6
Howell 1996	TDWB×3 wk	None	Used in 100%	4
Maeda 1996	NWB×3 wk	Cast at 30°–50° flexion 5–10 days	Not used	9–10
Aglietti 1996	PWB×6 wk	Hinged brace×4 wk	Not used	6–8
O'Neill 1996	WBAT	None	Not used	6
Yasuda 1997	PWB at 2 wk FWB at 4 wk	Hinged brace	Not used	12
Nebelung 1998	FWB at 1–2 wk	Brace limited to 90° flexion	Not used	N/A
Corry 1999	Immediate	None	Not used	9
Muneta 1999	WBAT 3–4 days postoperatively	Knee brace in extension	Not used	6

CPM, continuous passive motion; N/A, data not available; NWB, non–weight-bearing; TDWB, touchdown weight-bearing; PWB, partial weight-bearing; WBAT, weight-bearing as tolerated.

APPENDIX B–5
Meniscal Disease at Reconstruction

Author and Year Published	Medial Meniscal Disease			Lateral Meniscal Disease		
	Patients with MM Tears (%)	MM Tears Treated by PMM (%)	MM Tears Treated by MMR (%)	Patients with LM Tears (%)	LM Tears Treated by PLM (%)	LM Tears Treated by LMR (%)
Marder 1991	9	N/A	N/A	9	N/A	N/A
Sgaglione 1992	46	54	46	32	100	0
Sgaglione 1993	48	33	50	44	95	5
Otero 1993	N/A	N/A	N/A	N/A	N/A	N/A
Karlson 1994	N/A	N/A	N/A	N/A	N/A	N/A
Howell 1996	47	53	29	28	73	0
Maeda 1996	N/A	N/A	N/A	N/A	N/A	N/A
Aglietti 1996	16	55	45	28	84	0
O'Neill 1996	35	50	50	35	79	21
Yasuda 1997	17	45	55	19	58	42
Nebelung 1998	N/A	N/A	N/A	N/A	N/A	N/A
Corry 1999	0	0	0	0	0	0
Muneta 1999	33	N/A	N/A	33	N/A	N/A

LM, lateral meniscus; LMR, lateral meniscal repair; MM, medial meniscus; MMR, medial meniscal repair; N/A, data not available; PLM, partial lateral meniscectomy; PMM, partial medial meniscectomy.

mately 3% of all knee injuries in the general population and as much as 37% in the trauma patients with acute hemarthroses.[30, 31, 87] Furthermore, the setting in which the injury occurred has diagnostic and therapeutic implications because 95% of PCL injuries in the trauma setting have associated ligamentous injuries as well.[31] In contrast, athletes suffer mainly isolated PCL injuries,[35, 98] although the overall incidence in this population remains unknown. Depending on the severity of the injury, the disability resulting from isolated PCL injuries and combined ligamentous injuries can range from minimal functional alterations to profound limitations in daily activities. This chapter reviews the current evaluation and management of isolated and combined PCL injuries.

Anatomy

Ligament Morphology

Although the PCL lies within the joint capsule of the knee and is easily visualized arthroscopically, it is technically an extra-articular structure because its own synovial sheath covers it. The PCL has a broad femoral origin at the posterolateral aspect of the medial condyle and inserts centrally on the posterior aspect of the tibia in a fovea, 1 to 1.5 cm below the joint line. The PCL has an average length and width of 38 mm and 13 mm, respectively, although its diameter is highly variable along its course.[40, 54] A study by Miller and Olszewski[86] found its intra-articular length to be 30.7 + 2.6 mm, which may have implications in the choice of graft used for reconstruction. The PCL is narrowest in its midportion (11 mm) and fans out at its origin (32 mm) and insertion (13 mm) (Figs. 28K1–1 and 28K1–2). The fibers of the PCL attach in a lateral to medial direction on the tibia and in an anteroposterior direction on the femur (Fig. 28K1–3). Its complex semicircular origin, which lies 1 cm posterior to the medial articular cartilage, has made past attempts at isometric reconstruction of this ligament difficult.[40]

Investigators have divided the PCL into various compo-

nents or bundles on the basis of their tensioning patterns.[54, 108] The ligament consists of three main components: the anterolateral bundle, the posteromedial bundle, and the meniscofemoral ligaments (ligaments of Humphry and Wrisberg). The components have been shown to possess unique anatomic and biomechanical properties as well as specific sites of bone insertion (Fig. 28K1–4).[54, 89] The nomenclature of the separate bundles refers to their anatomic position; the femoral insertion is specified first, followed by the tibial insertion.[40] The anterolateral and posteromedial bundles have different tensioning patterns, depending on the degree of knee flexion, and thus functionally behave differently (Fig. 28K1–5). The larger anterolateral bundle demonstrates increasing tension with knee flexion; the posteromedial bundle has a reciprocal pattern, becoming taut as the knee moves into extension.[40, 49, 54] Furthermore, the cross-sectional area of the anterolateral component is two times larger than the posteromedial bun-

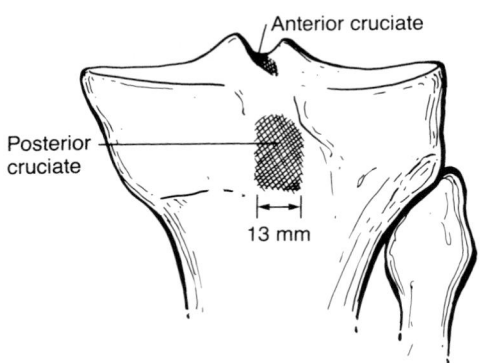

Figure 28K1–2. The posterior cruciate ligament inserts in a central fovea on the tibia approximately 1.5 cm below the joint line.

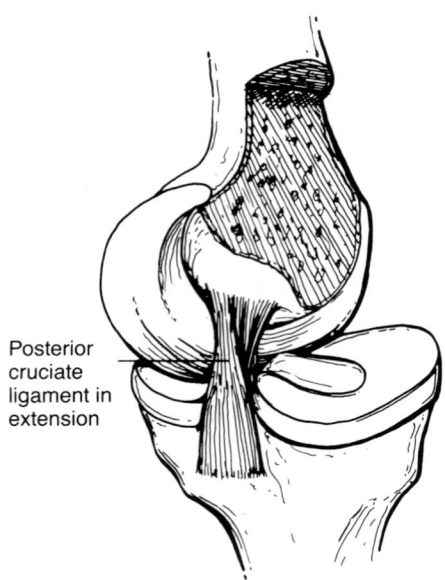

Figure 28K1–3. The fibers of the posterior cruciate ligament attach in an anterior-to-posterior direction on the femur and a medial-to-lateral direction on the tibia. (Redrawn from Girgis FG, Marshall JL, Monajem A: The cruciate ligaments of the knee joint. Anatomical, functional and experimental analysis. Clin Orthop 106:216–231, 1975.)

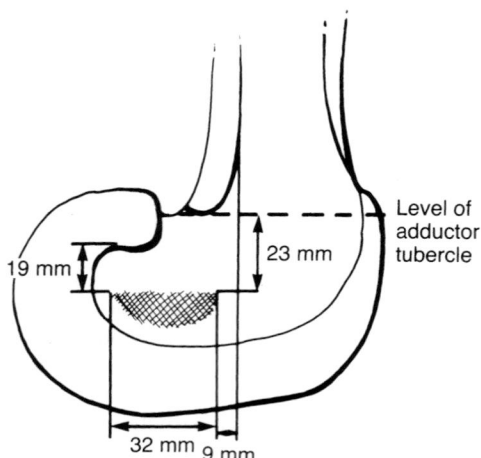

Figure 28K1–1. The broad complex origin of the posterior cruciate ligament is in the form of a semicircle on the medial femoral condyle.

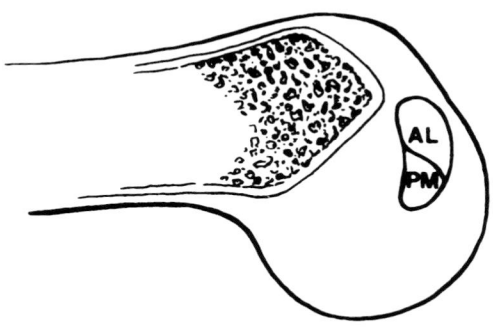

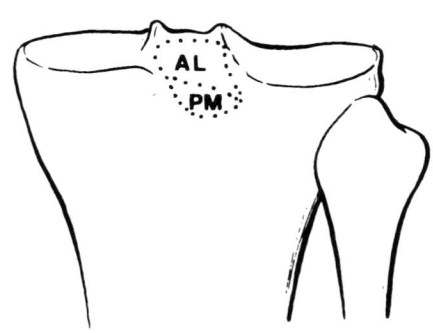

Figure 28K1–4. The anatomic position of the anterolateral (AL) and posteromedial bundles (PM) of the posterior cruciate ligament. (From Harner CD, Höher J: Current concepts: Evaluation and treatment of the posterior cruciate ligament injuries. Am J Sports Med 26:471–482, 1998.)

dle, whereas its structural properties (stiffness, ultimate strength) are approximately 150% of the posteromedial component.[54, 108]

The anterior and posterior meniscofemoral ligaments of Humphry and Wrisberg, respectively, are the third component of the PCL complex. Although reported to be variable

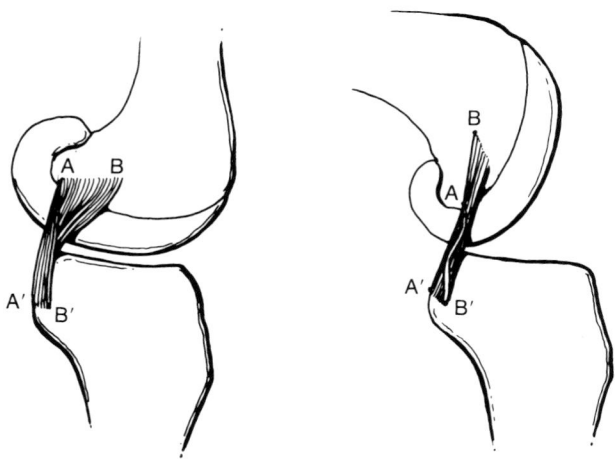

Figure 28K1–5. The posteromedial bundle of the posterior cruciate ligament (A–A′) is taut in extension and lax in flexion. The anterolateral bundle (B–B′) is tight in flexion and lax in extension. (Redrawn from Girgis FG, Marshall JL, Monajem A: The cruciate ligaments of the knee joint. Anatomical, functional and experimental analysis. Clin Orthop 106: 216–231, 1975.)

in their presence,[55] these ligaments arise from the posterior horn of the lateral meniscus and insert on the posterolateral aspect of the medial femoral condyle (Fig. 28K1–6). Despite their small size (22% of PCL cross-sectional area), the meniscofemoral ligaments have been shown to have significant mechanical strength. Their stiffness and ultimate load to failure are slightly greater than for the entire posteromedial bundle.[54, 71] Although the precise role of the meniscofemoral ligaments in knee kinematics has yet to be determined, their mechanical strength suggests that they contribute to knee stability.[49, 54]

Blood Supply and Innervation

The vascular supply of the knee and the cruciate ligaments has been well described.[3, 115] The popliteal artery gives rise to five branches that supply blood to the knee joint: the superior and inferior geniculate arteries (both with medial and lateral branches) and the middle geniculate artery (Fig. 28K1–7). The middle geniculate artery penetrates the posterior capsule of the knee, providing the major blood supply to the cruciate ligaments, synovial membrane, and posterior capsule itself. Furthermore, the synovial sleeve covering the PCL is well vascularized and is a major contributor to the blood supply of the ligament.[3, 115] The distal portion of the PCL also receives a portion of its blood supply from capsular vessels originating from the inferior geniculate and popliteal arteries.

The PCL and its synovial sleeve are supplied by nerve fibers from the popliteal plexus. This plexus receives contributions from the posterior articular nerve (prominent branch of posterior tibial nerve) and from the terminal portions of the obturator nerve.[67] Golgi tendon organ–like structures have been observed near ligament origins beneath the synovial sheath and are thought to have a proprioceptive function in the knee.[67, 117] Katonis and associates[65] have identified Ruffini's corpuscles (pressure receptors), Vater-Pacini corpuscles (velocity receptors), and free nerve endings (pain receptors) in a histologic study of mechanoreceptors in the PCL. These studies indicate that disruption of the PCL alters not only the knee kinematics but also the afferent signals to the central nervous system.[113]

Ligament Biomechanics

Biomechanical studies have shown that the PCL is the primary restraint to posterior translation and a secondary restraint to external rotation of the tibia.[13, 41, 44, 136, 137] Although the tensile strength of the PCL was once thought to be twice that of the anterior cruciate ligament (ACL),[68] tensile testing has shown that the load to failure of the PCL is only marginally stronger than that of the ACL.[105] The biomechanical properties of the PCL (i.e., stiffness, ultimate load, and modulus of elasticity) have been shown to be highly dependent on the portion of the ligament tested, however, with the anterolateral component exhibiting superior structural properties.[54, 108] It is critical that the orthopaedic surgeon attempting to reconstruct the PCL

Bone Scanning

A bone scan may prove helpful in the evaluation and management of chronic PCL injuries. Patients with these injuries are predisposed to early medial and patellofemoral compartment chondrosis.[17, 26, 66] In the setting of an isolated PCL-deficient knee with medial or patellofemoral compartment pain and normal radiographs, a bone scan to assess these compartments may be helpful. If there is increased uptake, surgical intervention may be beneficial.[131] If there is no increased uptake, a continued nonoperative approach is our treatment of choice.

Natural History

The natural history of the PCL-injured knee continues to be debated among experts in sports medicine. Unfortunately, the controversy will continue to exist until better prospective outcome studies are published in the literature. To date, the majority of papers that are available for review consist of retrospective studies with mixed populations combining both acute and chronic[66, 98] as well as isolated and combined ligament injuries.[24, 25, 131] Despite these short-comings, numerous investigators have shown that isolated acute PCL injuries (grade I to grade III) do relatively well with conservative treatment.[35, 66, 98, 118] The majority of patients in these studies, however, had grade II PCL laxity or less. The relatively benign course of these injuries is most likely due to the integrity of the secondary restraints and various portions of the PCL remaining intact.[49] Furthermore, satisfactory outcomes have also been reported for isolated PCL injuries in athletes, most of whom were able to return to full activity without surgery.[35, 66] Patients with combined ligament knee injuries and injuries resulting from high-energy trauma have not fared as well, however.[131] In these difficult cases, surgical repair or reconstruction within the first 3 weeks has shown results superior to those of conservative management.[49]

There is a general consensus that PCL injuries (especially grade III) are not as benign as previously thought in the long term.[83] Patients with chronic PCL injuries will have a variable progression of articular degeneration and symptoms over time (Fig. 28K1–15). A high incidence of

2) Tibiofemoral contact shifts anteriorly

- **Posterior horn medial menisci unloaded**
- **Increase wear of articular cartilage**

3) Force in the PLS

1) Posterior tibial translation

Figure 28K1–15. Pathomechanics of articular wear secondary to altered tibiofemoral contact forces in the chronically posterior cruciate ligament–deficient knee. PLS, posterior lateral structures.

late chondrosis[17, 26, 66] (involving the medial femoral condyle and patellofemoral joint) and meniscal tears[39] has been noted in patients treated nonoperatively. These findings are likely to be the result of increased contact pressure that occurs after PCL disruption.[76, 123] The problem is that investigators have been unable consistently to identify prognostic factors to help predict outcomes of patients. Although it has not been found universally, a positive correlation between isokinetic quadriceps strength and functional outcome has been found in several studies.[26, 98] Surprisingly, objective instability and time from injury have correlated poorly with final outcome and radiographic degenerative changes in most studies.[10, 26, 98, 121] A prospective study by Shelbourne and colleagues[118] provides further support for these findings. Patients in their series, with isolated grade I or grade II PCL injuries, had good subjective results for the most part, but only a limited number achieved good functional results. Thus, degenerative changes are probably inevitable in the PCL-deficient knee over time. The question remains, however, whether current surgical techniques of reconstruction can change or forestall this course of history.

Treatment

Controversy still exists with respect to the indications for nonoperative and surgical intervention, techniques of reconstruction, and methods of rehabilitation for the PCL-injured knee. The relatively infrequent occurrence of this injury has unfortunately led to clinical studies with small sample sizes and short-term follow-up. The limited understanding of the PCL and associated injuries has additionally resulted in studies that are frequently a collection of differing patterns of PCL injury—acute, chronic, isolated, combined, partial, and complete—and also lack well-defined indications for surgical management. Most series do not include control groups, combine primary repair and multiple reconstructive techniques, and use different outcome measures. Because of this, it has been difficult to compare results of different operative techniques and approaches.

This section focuses on a review of the pertinent literature followed by a discussion of current treatment recommendations. We conclude with a presentation of our approach to the management of the PCL-injured knee.

Review of the Literature on Nonoperative Treatment

Treatment of the isolated PCL injury is probably the most controversial. Recommendations have ranged from nonoperative management to various reconstructive techniques. Many have suggested a conservative approach. Dandy and Pusey[25] treated 20 patients with persistent knee symptoms due to unrecognized, isolated PCL injury. At 7.2 years of follow-up, 18 of the 20 had a good functional result. The authors thought that the subjective results, objective evaluation findings, and functional capacity without operative intervention were adequate and did not warrant surgical reconstruction or repair. Tietjens[130] likewise recommended that patients with isolated PCL injuries be treated nonoperatively after reporting 80% good or excellent functional results in 50 patients. The remaining 20%, however, had either disabling instability or meniscal tears. Similar success was reported by Cross and Powell.[24] They treated 67 of 116 PCL injuries nonoperatively and noted 54 good or excellent results. This study, like that of Dandy and Pusey,[25] lacked radiographic evaluation and additionally did not separate isolated from combined injury patterns. Parolie and Bergfeld[98] observed 25 patients with isolated PCL tears resulting from sporting injuries. At a minimum of 2 years of follow-up, 80% were satisfied with their knee function, and 68% returned to their previous level of activity. They also noted that those with unsatisfactory results tended to have diminished quadriceps strength compared with those with successful results. Torg and colleagues[131] observed 14 patients with isolated PCL injuries and 29 patients with combined PCL injuries for more than 6 years and concluded that the patients with isolated injuries remained without symptoms and did not require subsequent reconstruction. Medial compartment changes were noted in 60% of those with isolated injuries who underwent radiographic evaluation. Fowler and Messieh[35] also had good results with nonoperative management. They observed 13 patients with isolated PCL injuries for an average of 2.6 years and found that all achieved good subjective results and were able to return to their previous level of participation. The objective assessment of stability did not correlate with the good functional results. They concluded that functional stability was not dependent on objective stability, therefore, and that in light of the good functional results, nonoperative treatment is a viable option in those with isolated PCL injuries. In a later study, Shelbourne and associates[118] examined the results of patients with acute, isolated, nonoperatively treated PCL injuries. The study population consisted of 133 patients, all of whom returned subjective evaluations, and 68 who were available for long-term follow-up evaluation. All the patients had the equivalent of partial PCL tears (grade I or grade II) and were observed for an average of 5.4 years after the injury. The majority of patients had good subjective results that did not correlate with the degree of laxity, and 63 of 68 patients evaluated had the same or less laxity on physical examination. In addition, regardless of the amount of laxity, half of the patients returned to the same sport at the same or higher level, one third returned to the same sport at a lower level, and one sixth did not return to the same sport. From these results, they thought that patients with acute, isolated PCL injuries achieved a good result both objectively and subjectively with a nonoperative approach independent of the degree of laxity.

Whereas these studies varied with respect to injury mechanism, extent of the PCL or other ligament injury, physical therapy protocol, and evaluation of outcome and time of follow-up, they do suggest that most patients with PCL-injured knees will do well with conservative care. Even though nonoperative treatment seems to give relatively good results, these patients do not have a normal outcome in all series reported. The pathomechanics of the PCL-injured knee is different from that involving other ligamentous knee injuries (see Fig. 28K1–15). As a result

of the excessive posterior tibial translation, abnormal wear occurs, and pain rather than instability becomes the major symptomatic issue. In addition, the symptoms may take time to develop, so it is important that the patients be aware of this potential problem. We, like Shelbourne and associates, believe that in essence, this injury is analogous to a medial meniscus tear in its outcome.[118]

Review of the Literature on Operative Treatment

Avulsion Fractures Involving the Posterior Cruciate Ligament

Avulsion fractures of the PCL are relatively rare injuries. When isolated and nondisplaced, these fractures have been effectively managed with a brief period of immobilization. Most would agree, however, that displaced avulsions should undergo operative management.[73, 80, 132–134] Whereas several reports do not differentiate between isolated and combined injury patterns, surgical management of tibial avulsion fractures has been fairly successful. In independent studies, both Lee[73] and McMaster[80] were the first to report good results with this type of treatment. After treating 13 avulsion fractures, Trickey[134] noted better results in the surgical compared with the nonsurgical group. Torisu[133] treated 21 patients with tibial avulsion fractures with cast immobilization for nondisplaced fractures and early internal fixation for displaced fractures. At an average of 4 years of follow-up, all of the patients had good or excellent results.

Isolated Posterior Cruciate Ligament Injuries

Although many still favor the nonoperative approach to the PCL-injured knee, studies have suggested that the long-term outcome may not be without its detriments. Many of the patients treated conservatively had good functional results, but a significant percentage suffered from persistent objective instability and progressive post-traumatic arthritis. Dejour and associates[26] reported the long-term follow-up of PCL-deficient knees and noted that at an average of 15 years after injury, 89% had persistent pain and approximately 50% had chronic effusions. In addition, after 25 years of follow-up, progressive degenerative changes inevitably developed. Keller and colleagues[66] observed 40 patients with isolated PCL injuries for an average of 6 years. In this shorter interval, 90% still complained of pain, 65% stated that the knee limited their activity, and 43% reported difficulty with walking. Radiographic changes were directly related to the time elapsed from the injury, and the subjective complaints were related to the degree of remaining objective laxity.

Boynton and Tietjens[10] observed 38 patients with isolated PCL-deficient knees for an average of 13.4 years and found that the prognosis varies. Eight (21%) had surgery for subsequent meniscal tears. Among the 30 patients with isolated PCL-deficient knees with normal menisci, 24 (81%) had at least occasional pain, and 17 (56%) had at

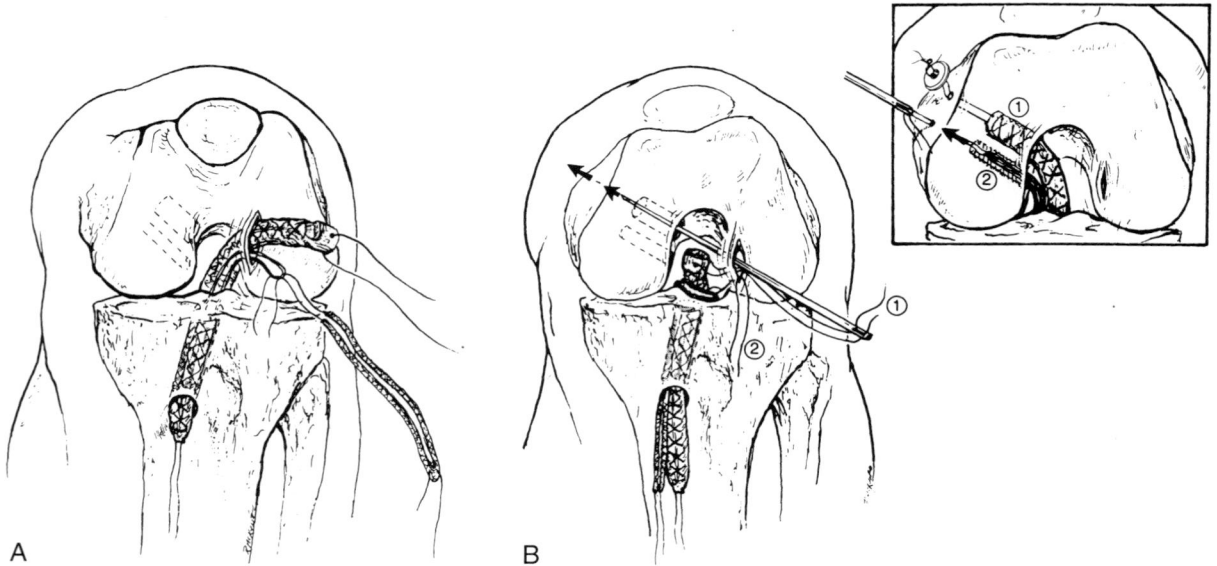

Figure 28K1–19. Graft placement. *A*, The Achilles tendon allograft (1) and the semitendinosus autograft (2) are passed in anterograde fashion through the tibial tunnel. *B*, Grafts are then fixed to corresponding femoral tunnels. (From Petrie RS, Harner CD: Double bundle posterior cruciate ligament reconstruction technique: University of Pittsburgh approach. Op Tech Sports Med 7:118–126, 1999.)

femoral side and then cycled. The Achilles graft, representing the reconstructed anterolateral bundle, is tensioned at 90 degrees and then fixed with a screw and pegged washer on the tibia. Subsequently, the hamstring tendon, or reconstructed posteromedial bundle, is tensioned at 30 degrees of flexion and then secured in a similar fashion or tied over a post (Fig. 28K1–20).

Although the tibial inlay procedure is favored by some surgeons, we think this approach is technically demanding and requires a prone or lateral decubitus position, adding operative time and becoming particularly burdensome in attempting repair of a combined ligament injury.[7, 8, 62, 82] At this time, tibial fixation variation has not been shown to affect the behavior of the graft significantly, and so the theoretical benefits may not outweigh the technical demands of this technique.[7, 8, 62, 82]

Combined PCL-PLS injury is one of the most complex treatment problems encountered in the management of knee ligament injuries. When both the PCL and PLS are ruptured, substantial posterior translation, external rotation, and varus opening can be present at differing angles of knee flexion.[21] This combination creates a complex surgical dilemma.[20] With several patterns of injury possible, it is difficult to have one surgical plan. It is essential that this injury be appropriately identified because if it is mistaken for an isolated PCL injury and treated nonsurgically, posterior and posterolateral instability will invariably persist.[30, 31, 49, 52, 53, 90, 125] Treatment of the acute PLS injury is generally more successful than that of the chronic injury; therefore, acute surgical intervention is recommended for combined PCL-PLS injury.[5, 21, 28, 49, 59, 83, 138] The timing for surgical treatment of the injured PLS is critical; acute repairs consistently give more favorable results than does reconstruction of chronic injuries.[21, 72, 83, 138] Attempts at surgical repair beyond this time frame are frequently disappointing both in localizing discrete anatomic structures and in finding any sturdy tissue to repair. Accordingly, surgical

options for chronic injuries are reconstructions rather than repairs. Many reconstructive techniques have been described, but none has consistently shown better results than acute repair.

Treatment of PLS injuries is therefore centered on recognizing the acute injury and following with the immediate, direct anatomic repair of all ligamentous injuries, preferably within the first 2 weeks. Depending on the quality of the tissue or type of injury, repair or reconstructive techniques may be used. Our approach begins with a lateral "hockey-stick" incision paralleling the posterior edge of the iliotibial band, which is then split, exposing the deep structures of the LCL anteriorly and the lateral head of the gastrocnemius muscle and underlying popliteus complex more posteriorly. Special attention is given to identifying the injured structures. In cases in which the posterolateral capsular structures are avulsed off their femoral attachments with preservation of the popliteus tendon, direct repair of these structures by use of suture anchors is recommended. The LCL should also be assessed, and if an avulsion injury is present, it should be similarly repaired with suture anchors. On occasion, there is interstitial tearing of this structure, mandating concomitant reconstruction (Fig. 28K1–21).[18] For this, an Achilles tendon allograft is used. The LCL can be detached and elevated from its distal insertion, and the allograft bone block is then fixed vertically into the fibular head by interference screw fixation. The native LCL can then be tensioned proximal and distal to the graft. Suture anchors are then placed into the lateral epicondyle, with passage of the suture arms through the Achilles tendon and proximal LCL to reinforce the repair.

The extent of injury to the popliteus and, more important, its attachments to the fibula through the popliteofibular ligament must then be visualized. The popliteofibular ligament is now recognized as a significant component of the popliteus complex, particularly as a static stabi-

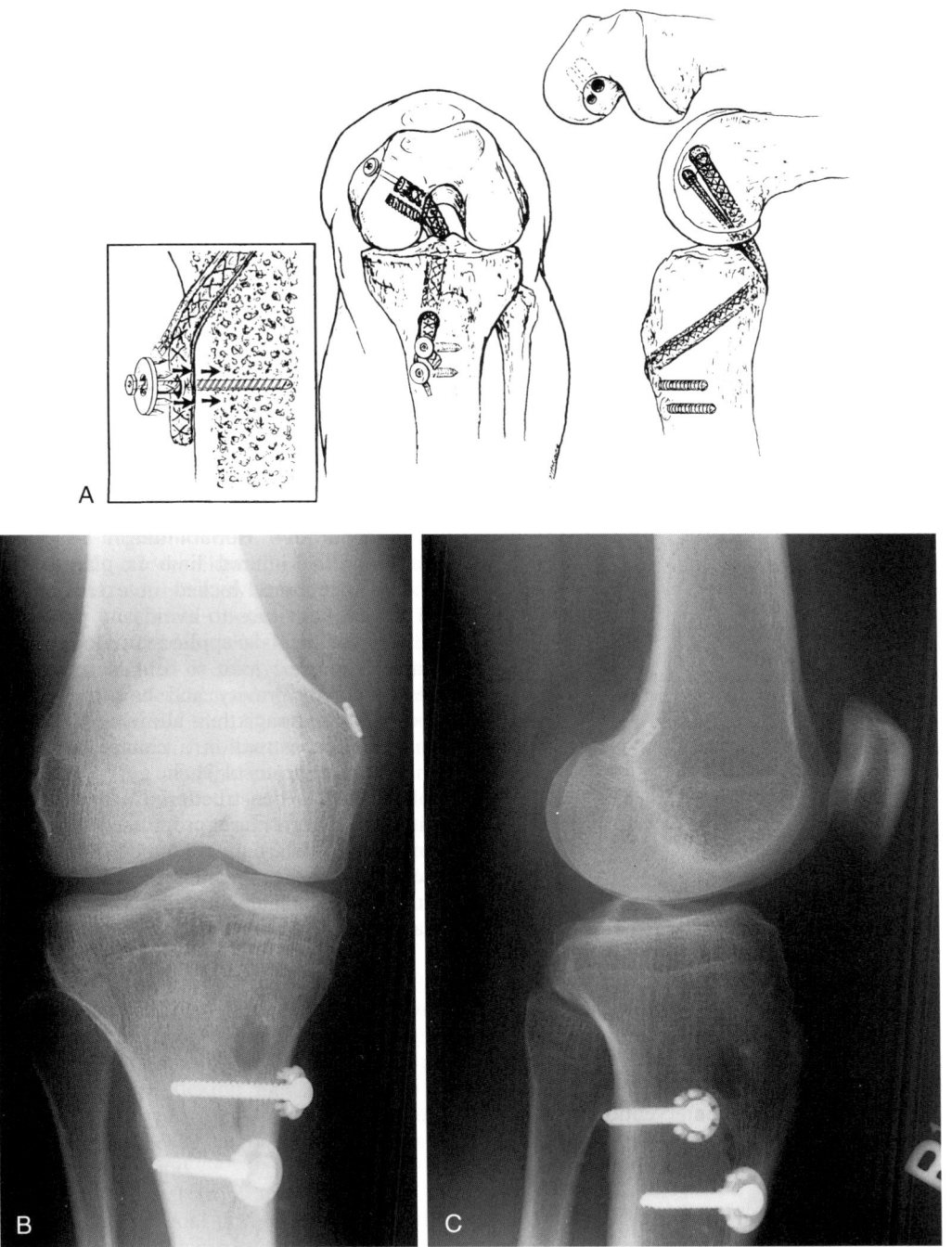

Figure 28K1–20. Tibial fixation of the posterior cruciate ligament graft. *A,* Individual graft fixation. Tibial fixation is achieved with a 4.5-mm screw and a spiked soft tissue washer *(inset).* Separate screws and washers are used for each graft. *B* and *C,* Anteroposterior and lateral radiographs with fixation in place. (From Petrie RS, Harner CD: Double bundle posterior cruciate ligament reconstruction technique: University of Pittsburgh approach. Op Tech Sports Med 7:118–126, 1999.)

lizer.[138] We therefore believe that this step is the most crucial to the overall success or failure of the procedure. In cases in which this tendon is avulsed off its tibial or femoral insertion, tension with anatomic restoration of the popliteofibular ligament is created through the use of sutures in combination with femoral or fibular fixation by means of a blind tunnel and one of several possible fixation devices. Tension is applied with the knee in 20 to 30 degrees of flexion during the final fixation. If the popliteus tendon tissue cannot be repaired by this approach, reconstruction is indicated as described next for the chronic injury.

Chronic injuries still present a therapeutic challenge. The initial evaluation of limb alignment and gait is essential for this problem. If varus malalignment or a lateral thrust exists, a proximal tibial osteotomy may be necessary

31. Fanelli GC, Edson CJ: Posterior cruciate ligament injuries in trauma patients. Part II. Arthroscopy 11:526–529, 1995.

32. Fanelli GC, Giannotti BF, Edson CJ: Arthroscopically assisted combined posterior cruciate ligament/posterolateral complex reconstruction. Arthroscopy 12:521–529, 1996.

33. Fanelli GC, Giannotti BF, Edson CJ: Current concepts review. The posterior cruciate ligament arthroscopic evaluation and treatment. Arthroscopy 10:673–688, 1994.

34. Fleming RE, Blatz DJ, McCarroll JR: Posterior problems in the knee: Posterior cruciate insufficiency and posterolateral rotatory insufficiency. Am J Sports Med 9:107–113, 1981.

35. Fowler PJ, Messieh SS: Isolated posterior cruciate ligament injuries in athletes. Am J Sports Med 15:553–557, 1987.

36. Fox RJ, Harner CD, Sakane M, et al: Determination of in situ forces in the human posterior cruciate ligament using robotic technology: A cadaveric study. Am J Sports Med 26:395–401, 1998.

37. Fukubayashi T, Torzilli PA, Sherman ME: An in vitro biomechanical evaluation of anteroposterior motion of the knee. J Bone Joint Surg Am 64:258–262, 1982.

38. Galloway MT, Grood ES, Mehalik JN, et al: Posterior cruciate ligament reconstruction. An in vitro study of femoral and tibial graft placement. Am J Sports Med 24:437–445, 1996.

39. Geissler WB, Whipple TL: Intraarticular abnormalities in association with posterior cruciate ligament injuries. Am J Sports Med 21: 846–849, 1993.

40. Girgis FG, Marshall JL, Al Monajem ARS: The cruciate ligaments of the knee joint: Anatomical, functional and experimental analysis. Clin Orthop 106:216–231, 1975.

41. Gollehon DL, Torzilli PA, Warren RF: The role of the posterolateral and cruciate ligaments in the stability of the human knee. A biomechanical study. J Bone Joint Surg Am 69:233–242, 1987.

42. Green NE, Allen BL: Vascular injuries associated with dislocation of the knee. J Bone Joint Surg Am 59:236–239, 1977.

43. Grood ES, Hefzy MS, Lindenfield TN: Factors affecting the region of most isometric femoral attachments. Part I: The posterior cruciate ligament. Am J Sports Med 17:197–207, 1989.

44. Grood ES, Stowers SF, Noyes FR: Limits of movement in the human knee. Effect of sectioning the posterior cruciate ligament and posterolateral structures. J Bone Joint Surg Am 70:88–97, 1988.

45. Gross M, Glover JS, Bassett LW, et al: Magnetic resonance imaging of the PCL: Clinical use to improve diagnostic accuracy. Am J Sports Med 20:732–737, 1992.

46. Grover JS, Bassett LW, Gross ML, et al: Posterior cruciate ligament: MR imaging. Radiology 174:527–530, 1990.

47. Hall FM, Hochman MG: Medial Segond-type fracture: Cortical avulsion off the medial tibial plateau associated with tears of the posterior cruciate ligament and medial meniscus. Skeletal Radiol 26:553–555, 1997.

48. Harner CD, Baek GH, Vogrin TM, et al: Quantitative analysis of human cruciate ligament insertions. Arthroscopy 15:741–749, 1999.

49. Harner CD, Höher J: Current concepts: Evaluation and treatment of posterior cruciate ligament injuries. Am J Sports Med 26:471–482, 1998.

50. Harner CD, Höher J, Vogrin TM, et al: The effects of a popliteus load on in situ forces in the posterior cruciate ligament on knee kinematics. Am J Sports Med 26:669–673, 1998.

51. Harner CD, Janaushek MA, Kanamori A, et al: Biomechanical analysis of a double bundle posterior cruciate ligament reconstruction. Am J Sports Med 28:144–151, 2000.

52. Harner CD, Janaushek MA, Ma B, et al: The effect of knee flexion angle and application of an anterior tibial load at the time of graft fixation on the biomechanics of a posterior cruciate ligament–reconstructed knee. Am J Sports Med 28:460–465, 2000.

53. Harner CD, Vogrin TM, Höher J, et al: Biomechanical analysis of a posterior cruciate ligament reconstruction: Deficiency of the posterolateral structures as a cause of graft failure. Am J Sports Med 28: 32–39, 2000.

54. Harner CD, Xerogeanes JW, Livesay GA, et al: The human posterior cruciate ligament complex: An interdisciplinary study. Ligament morphology and biomechanical evaluation. Am J Sports Med 23: 736–745, 1995.

55. Heller L, Langman J: The meniscofemoral ligaments of the human knee. J Bone Joint Surg Br 46:307–313, 1964.

56. Hewett TE, Noyes FR, Lee MD: Diagnosis of complete and partial posterior cruciate ligament ruptures: Stress radiography compared with KT-1000 arthrometer and posterior drawer testing. Am J Sports Med 25:648–655, 1997.

57. Höher J, Harner CD, Vogrin TM, et al: Hamstring loading increases in situ forces in the PCL. Trans Orthop Res Soc 23:48, 1998.

58. Höher J, Harner CD, Vogrin TM, et al: In situ forces in the posterolateral structures in the knee under posterior tibial loading in the intact and posterior cruciate ligament–deficient knee. J Orthop Res 16:675–681, 1998.

59. Hughston JC, Degenhardt TC: Reconstruction of the posterior cruciate ligament. Clin Orthop 164:59–77, 1982.

60. Hughston JC, Jacobson KE: Chronic posterolateral rotatory instability of the knee. J Bone Joint Surg Am 67:351–359, 1985.

61. Jackson DF: Posterior cruciate and associated ligament instabilities. Instructional Course Lecture, AAOS Annual Meeting, Washington, DC, 1992.

62. Jakob RP, Edwards JC: Posterior cruciate ligament reconstruction: Anterior-posterior two stage technique. Sports Med Arthrosc Rev 2: 137–145, 1994.

63. Jakob RP, Hassler H, Staeubli HU: Observations on rotatory instability of the lateral compartment of the knee: Experimental studies on the functional anatomy and the pathomechanism of the true and reversed pivot shift sign. Acta Orthop Scand Suppl 191:1–32, 1982.

64. Johnson JC, Bach BR: Current concepts review: Posterior cruciate ligament. Am J Knee Surg 3:145–153, 1990.

65. Katonis PG, Assimakopoulos AP, Agapitos MV, et al: Mechanoreceptors in the posterior cruciate ligament: Histologic study on cadaver knees. Acta Orthop Scand 62:176–178, 1991.

66. Keller PM, Shelbourne KD, McCarroll JR, et al: Nonoperatively treated isolated posterior cruciate ligament injuries. Am J Sports Med 21:132–136, 1993.

67. Kennedy JC, Alexander IJ, Hayes KC: Nerve supply of the human knee and its functional importance. Am J Sports Med 10:329–335, 1982.

68. Kennedy JC, Grainger RW: The posterior cruciate ligament. J Trauma 7:367–377, 1976.

69. Kim S-J, Kim H-K, Kim H-J: Arthroscopic posterior cruciate ligament reconstruction using a one-incision technique. Clin Orthop 359:156–166, 1999.

70. Klimkiewicz JJ, Harner CD, Fu FH: Single bundle posterior cruciate ligament reconstruction: University of Pittsburgh approach. Operative Tech Sports Med 7:105–109, 1999.

71. Kusayama T, Harner CD: Anatomical and biomechanical characteristics of the human meniscofemoral ligaments. Knee Surg Sports Traumatol Arthrosc 2:234–237, 1994.

72. LaPrade RF: The medial collateral ligament complex and the posterolateral aspect of the knee. In Arendt EA (ed): Orthopaedic Knowledge Update: Sports Medicine 2. Rosemont, Ill, American Academy of Orthopaedic Surgeons, 1999, pp 317–326.

73. Lee HG: Avulsion fracture of the tibial attachment of the cruciate ligaments. Treatment by operative reduction. J Bone Joint Surg Am 29:460, 1937.

74. Lipscomb AB Jr, Anderson AF, Norwig ED, et al: Isolated posterior cruciate ligament reconstruction. Long-term results. Am J Sports Med 21:490–496, 1993.

75. Loos WC, Fox JM, Blazina ME, et al: Acute posterior cruciate ligament injuries. Am J Sports Med 9:86–92, 1981.

76. MacDonald P, Miniaci A, Fowler P, et al: A biomechanical analysis of joint contact forces in the posterior cruciate deficient knee. Knee Surg Sports Traumatol Arthrosc 4:252–255, 1996.

77. Mariani PP, Adriani E, Santori N: Arthroscopic posterior cruciate ligament reconstruction with bone-tendon-bone patellar graft. Knee Surg Sports Traumatol Arthrosc 5:239–244, 1997.

78. Markolf KL, Wascher DC, Finerman GA: Direct in vitro measurement of forces in the cruciate ligaments. Part II: The effect of section of the posterolateral structures. J Bone Joint Surg Am 75: 387–394, 1993.

79. McCormick WC, Bagg RJ, Kennedy CW Jr, et al: Reconstruction of the posterior cruciate ligament. Preliminary report of a new procedure. Clin Orthop 118:30–31, 1976.

80. McMaster WC: Isolated posterior cruciate ligament injury: Literature review and case reports. J Trauma 15:1025–1029, 1975.

81. Meyers MH: Isolated avulsion of the tibial attachment of the posterior cruciate ligament of the knee. J Bone Joint Surg Am 57: 669–672, 1975.

82. Miller MD: Posterior cruciate ligament reconstruction: Tibial inlay technique. Sports Med Arthrosc Rev 7:225–234, 1999.

83. Miller MD, Bergfeld JA, Fowler PJ, et al: The posterior cruciate ligament injured knee: Principles of evaluation and treatment. Instr Course Lect 48:199–207, 1999.
84. Miller MD, Harner CD: The anatomic and surgical considerations for posterior cruciate ligament reconstruction. Instr Course Lect 44: 431–441, 1995.
85. Miller MD, Harner CD, Koshiwaguchi S: Acute posterior cruciate ligament injuries. In Fu FH, Harner CD, Vince KG (eds): Knee Surgery. Baltimore, Williams & Wilkins, 1994, pp 749–767.
86. Miller MD, Olszewski AD: Posterior cruciate ligament injuries: New treatment options. Am J Knee Surg 8:351–355, 1995.
87. Miyasaka KC, Daniel DM: The incidence of knee ligament injuries in the general population. Am J Knee Surg 4:3–8, 1991.
88. Moore HA, Larson RL: Posterior cruciate ligament injuries. Results of early surgical repair. Am J Sports Med 8:68–78, 1980.
89. Morgan CD, Kalman VR, Grawl DM: The anatomic origin of the posterior cruciate ligament: Where is it? Reference marks for PCL reconstruction. Arthroscopy 13:325–331, 1997.
90. Müller W: The Knee: Form, Function and Ligament Reconstruction. Berlin, Springer-Verlag, 1983.
91. Noyes FR, Barber-Westin SD: Posterior cruciate ligament allograft reconstruction with and without a ligament augmentation device. Arthroscopy 10:371–382, 1994.
92. Noyes FR, Barber-Westin SD: Surgical reconstruction of severe chronic posterolateral complex injuries of the knee using allograft tissues. Am J Sports Med 23:2–12, 1995.
93. Noyes FR, Barber-Westin SD: Surgical restoration to treat chronic deficiency of the posterolateral complex and cruciate ligaments of the knee joint. Am J Sports Med 24:415–426, 1996.
94. Noyes FR, Barber-Westin SD: Treatment of complex injuries involving the posterior cruciate and posterolateral ligaments of the knee. Am J Knee Surg 9:200–214, 1996.
95. Noyes FR, Stowers SF, Grood ES, et al: Posterior subluxations of the medial and lateral tibiofemoral compartments. An in vivo ligament sectioning study in cadaveric knees. Am J Sports Med 21:407–414, 1993.
96. O'Donoghue DH: An analysis of end results of surgical treatment of major injuries of the ligaments of the knee. J Bone Joint Surg Am 37:1–13, 1955.
97. Ogata K, McCarthy JA: Measurements of length and tension patterns during reconstruction of the posterior cruciate ligament. Am J Sports Med 20:351–355, 1992.
98. Parolie JM, Bergfeld JA: Long-term results of nonoperative treatment of isolated posterior cruciate ligament injuries in the athlete. Am J Sports Med 14:35–38, 1986.
99. Pearsall AW, Pyevich M, Draganich LF, et al: In vitro study of knee stability after posterior cruciate ligament reconstruction. Clin Orthop 327:264–271, 1996.
100. Petrie RS, Harner CD: Double bundle posterior cruciate ligament reconstruction technique: University of Pittsburgh approach. Operative Tech Sports Med 7:118–126, 1999.
101. Petrie RS, Harner CD: Evaluation and management of the posterior cruciate injured knee. Operative Tech Sports Med 7:93–103, 1999.
102. Plancher KD, Siliski JM, Ribbans W: Traumatic dislocation of the knee: Complications and results of operative and nonoperative treatment. Proceedings of the American Academy of Orthopaedic Surgeons 56th Annual Meeting, Las Vegas, Nev. Park Ridge, Ill, American Academy of Orthopaedic Surgeons, 1989, p 85.
103. Polly DW, Callaghan JJ, Sikes RA, et al: The accuracy of selective magnetic resonance imaging compared with the findings of arthroscopy of the knee. J Bone Joint Surg Am 70:192–198, 1988.
104. Pournaras J, Symeonides P: The results of surgical repair of acute tears of the posterior cruciate ligament. Clin Orthop 267:103–107, 1991.
105. Prietto MP, Bain JR, Stonebrook SN, et al: Tensile strength of the human posterior cruciate ligament (PCL). Trans Orthop Res Soc 13: 195, 1988.
106. Race A, Amis AA: PCL reconstruction: In-vitro biomechanical comparison of "isometric" versus single and double-bundled "anatomic" grafts. J Bone Joint Surg Br 80:173–179, 1998.
107. Race A, Amis AA: Are anatomic PCL reconstructions superior to isometric? An in-vitro biomechanical analysis. Trans Orthop Res Soc 43:874, 1997.
108. Race A, Amis AA: The mechanical properties of the two bundles of the human posterior cruciate ligament. J Biomech 27:13–24, 1994.
109. Renstrom P, Arms SW, Stanwyk TS, et al: Strain within the anterior cruciate ligament during hamstring and quadriceps activity. Am J Sports Med 14:83–87, 1986.
110. Richter M, Kiefer H, Hehl G, et al: Primary repair for posterior cruciate ligament injuries: An eight-year follow up of fifty-three patients. Am J Sports Med 24:298–305, 1996.
111. Roman PD, Hopson CN, Zenni EJ Jr: Traumatic dislocation of the knee: A report of 30 cases and literature review. Orthop Rev 16: 917–924, 1987.
112. Roth JH, Bray RC, Best TM, et al: Posterior cruciate ligament reconstruction by transfer of the medial gastrocnemius tendon. Am J Sports Med 16:21–28, 1988.
113. Safran MR, Allen AA, Lephart SM, et al: Proprioception in the posterior cruciate ligament deficient knee. Knee Surg Sports Traumatol Arthrosc 7:310–317, 1999.
114. Satku K, Chew CN, Seow H: Posterior cruciate ligament injuries. Acta Orthop Scand 55:26–29, 1984.
115. Scapinelli R: Studies on the vasculature on the human knee joint. Acta Anat 70:305–331, 1968.
116. Schulte KR, Chew CN, Fu FH: Arthroscopic posterior cruciate ligament reconstruction. Clin Sports Med 16:145–156, 1997.
117. Schultz RA, Miller DC, Kerr CS, et al: Mechanoreceptors in human cruciate ligaments. J Bone Joint Surg Am 66:1072–1076, 1984.
118. Shelbourne KD, Davis TJ, Patel DV: The natural history of acute, isolated, nonoperatively treated posterior cruciate ligament injuries. A prospective study. Am J Sports Med 27:276–283, 1999.
119. Shelbourne KD, Nitz P: Accelerated rehabilitation after anterior ligament reconstruction. Am J Sports Med 18:292–299, 1990.
120. Shields L, Mital M, Cave E: Complete dislocation of the knee: Experience at the Massachusetts General Hospital. J Trauma 9: 192–215, 1969.
121. Shino K, Horibe S, Nakata K, et al: Conservative treatment of isolated injuries to the posterior cruciate ligament in athletes. J Bone Joint Surg Br 77:895–900, 1995.
122. Sisto DJ, Warren RF: Complete knee dislocation: A follow-up study of operative treatment. Clin Orthop 198:94–101, 1985.
123. Skyhar MJ, Warren RF, Ortiz GJ, et al: The effects of sectioning of the posterior cruciate ligament and posterolateral complex on the articular contact pressures within the knee. J Bone Joint Surg Am 75:694–699, 1993.
124. Southmayd WW, Rubin BD: Posterior cruciate ligament using the semimembranosus tendon. Clin Orthop 150:196–197, 1980.
125. Stäubli HU: Posteromedial and posterolateral capsular injuries associated with posterior cruciate ligament insufficiency. Sports Med Arthrosc Rev 2:146–164, 1994.
126. Stäubli HU, Birrer S: The popliteus tendon and its fascicles at the popliteal hiatus: Gross anatomy and functional arthroscopic evaluation with and without anterior cruciate ligament deficiency. Arthroscopy 6:209–220, 1990.
127. Taft T, Almekinders L: The dislocated knee. In Fu FH, Harner CD, Vince K (eds): Knee Surgery. Baltimore, Williams & Wilkins, 1994, pp 837–858.
128. Terry GC, LaPrade RF: The biceps femoris muscle complex at the knee: Its anatomy and injury patterns associated with acute anterolateral-anteromedial rotatory instability. Am J Sports Med 24: 2–8, 1996.
129. Terry GC, LaPrade RF: The posterolateral aspect of the knee: Anatomy and surgical approach. Am J Sports Med 24:732–739, 1996.
130. Tietjens BR: Posterior cruciate ligament injuries. J Bone Joint Surg Br 67:674, 1985.
131. Torg JS, Barton TM, Pavlov H, et al: Natural history of posterior cruciate deficient knee. Clin Orthop 164:59–77, 1982.
132. Torisu T: Avulsion fracture of the tibial attachment of the posterior cruciate ligament. Indications and results of delayed repair. Clin Orthop 143:107–114, 1979.
133. Torisu T: Isolated avulsion fracture of the tibial attachment of the posterior cruciate ligament. J Bone Joint Surg Am 59:68–72, 1977.
134. Trickey EL: Injuries to the posterior cruciate ligament. Diagnosis and treatment of early injuries and reconstruction of late instability. Clin Orthop 147:76–81, 1980.
135. Turner DA, Prodromos CC, Petasnick JP, et al: Acute injuries of the ligaments of the knee: Magnetic resonance evaluation. Radiology 154:717–722, 1985.
136. Veltri DM, Deng X-H, Torzilli PA, et al: The role of the popliteofibular ligament in the stability of the human knee. A biomechanical study. Am J Sports Med 24:19–27, 1996.

137. Veltri DM, Deng X-H, Torzilli PA, et al: The role of the cruciate and posterolateral ligaments in stability of the knee. A biomechanical study. Am J Sports Med 23:436–443, 1995.
138. Veltri DM, Warren RF: Posterolateral instability of the knee. Instr Course Lect 44:441–453, 1995.
139. Vogrin TM, Höher J, Harner CD, et al: Effects of sectioning of the posterolateral structures on knee kinematics and in situ forces in the posterior cruciate ligament. Knee Surg Sports Traumatol Arthrosc 8:93–98, 2000.
140. Wascher DC, Dvimak PC, DeCoster TA: Knee dislocation: Initial assessment and implications for treatment. J Orthop Trauma 11: 525–529, 1997.
141. Watanabe Y, Moriya H, Takahashi K, et al: Functional anatomy of the posterolateral structures of the knee. Arthroscopy 9:57–62, 1993.

2. POSTERIOR CRUCIATE LIGAMENT INJURIES IN THE CHILD

J. Robert Giffin, MD, FRCSC ■ Christopher C. Annunziata, MD ■ Christopher D. Harner, MD

The knee is the most frequent site of injury in childhood sports.[2] It has been estimated that more than 30 million children and adolescents in the United States now participate in organized athletics.[28] Greater participation in cutting sports such as soccer, football, and basketball has increased the potential for acute traumatic as well as overuse knee injuries.[41] Acute ligamentous injury to the knee and, in particular, to the cruciate ligaments in children is being diagnosed more frequently.[21, 29, 34] This observation has been attributed to a better understanding of and greater clinical suspicion for ligamentous tears as well as to our ability to diagnose these injuries with improved imaging and arthroscopic techniques.[26, 29, 44] Furthermore, the increased intensity and participation of elite or highly skilled preadolescent athletes in competitive sporting programs have also been implicated in the growing frequency of knee injuries.[32] The level of commitment and the intensity of training required to reach this level of athletic prowess put the skeletally immature knee at considerable risk.

In addition to these elite young athletes, growing numbers of children and adolescents are now participating in recreational and competitive sports at a variety of skill levels.[32] Despite the participation of these young athletes in organized sports, there exists a definite overall trend toward more sedentary indoor activities, with fewer hours spent outdoors in free play during growth and development. It has been hypothesized that the decline in activity has resulted in a decrease in the level of fitness and strength in today's youth, which may increase their susceptibility to injury when they suddenly participate in a rigorous sporting activity.[34]

Young Athlete's Knee

The anatomic structures of the young athlete's knee resemble those of an adult, but there are important physiologic and biomechanical differences. The presence of open cartilaginous growth plates, increased bone porosity and pliability, unique musculotendinous apophyseal insertions, and growing articular cartilage lead to a different spectrum of injuries in children and adolescents than in adults. In addition, the child is lighter and has a lower center of gravity, shorter lever arms, and decreased muscle strength, thereby considerably reducing the magnitude of forces generated across the lower extremities. These factors, combined with the relatively greater strength of the ligaments compared with the physis, generally protect the pediatric knee from ligamentous injury. Unfortunately, however, growing articular cartilage has been shown to be more susceptible to injury, in both clinical and biomechanical studies, than mature cartilage.[34]

Knee injuries in children may involve the ligaments, the extensor mechanism, the menisci, the articular cartilage and subchondral bone, the epiphysis, and adjacent structures. The age of the athlete and the anatomic insertion of the ligament (i.e., metaphyseal versus epiphyseal) will determine whether physeal or ligamentous injury occurs (Fig. 28K2–1). Physeal and ligamentous injuries occur with relatively equal frequency in children between 7 and 11 years of age, whereas younger children are more likely to sustain metaphyseal fractures.[45] Teenagers sustain ligament injuries with low-energy trauma and physeal fractures with high-energy trauma.[39, 45] In general, the physis is more likely to be injured during times of rapid growth (i.e., peak height velocity during puberty). In some circumstances, even in young children, the ligament may fail before the physis.

Posterior Cruciate Ligament Injury

The posterior cruciate ligament (PCL) is widely recognized as the primary restraint to posterior tibial translation

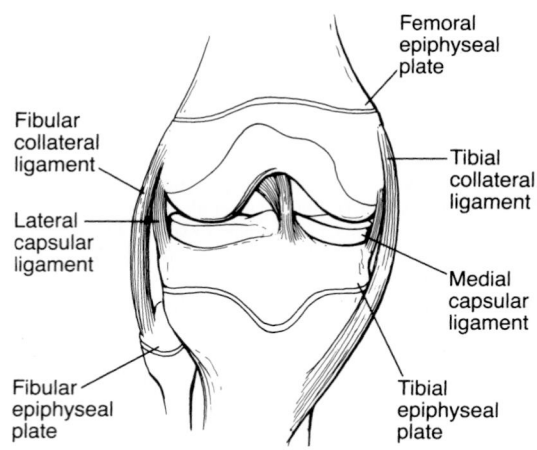

Figure 28K2–1. The attachment of the cruciate ligaments occurs within the epiphysis of the femur and the tibia. The medial collateral ligament is the only ligament to cross the tibial physeal plate. Because of the ligaments' relationship to the physeal plates and their relative strength, stress concentrates at the growth plates, producing physeal injury rather than ligament failure.

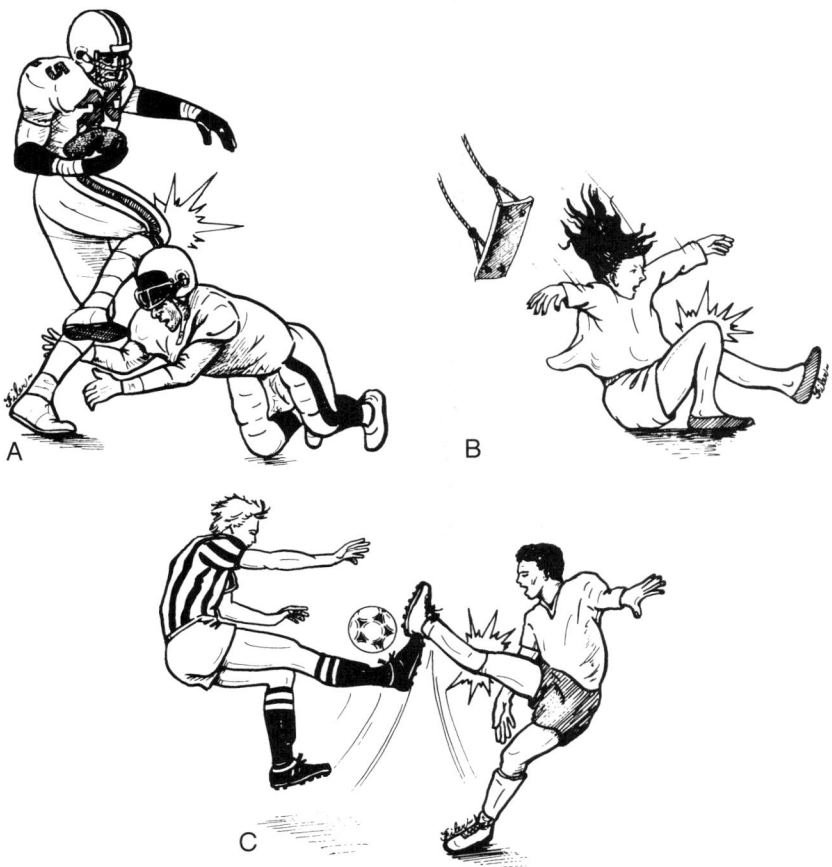

Figure 28K2–2. Three mechanisms of posterior cruciate ligament injury. *A*, Direct pretibial trauma. *B*, Forced hyperflexion. *C*, Hyperextension. (From Miller MD, Harner CD, Koshiwaguchi S: Acute posterior cruciate ligament injuries. In Fu FH, Harner CD, Vince KG [eds]: Knee Surgery, vol 1. Baltimore, Williams & Wilkins, 1994.)

and is a secondary restraint to external rotation. Although ligamentous disruptions of the anterior cruciate ligament (ACL) are being reported with increasing frequency in the pediatric population, PCL injuries in this age group are extremely uncommon. A thorough review of the literature reveals only sporadic case reports of PCL injuries in the skeletally immature knee.* Most of the reports of PCL injuries in children involve avulsions from either the tibial or the femoral attachments, with femoral avulsions being more common. The femoral attachment of the PCL has been reported to be the weakest at the chondro-osseous junction.[25, 46] Because this attachment site has not yet ossified, avulsion from the femur may not be appreciated on plain radiographs. This has important ramifications for treatment because the physician must be aware of this pattern of avulsion injury (with adjacent periosteum or perichondrium), which is amenable to a successful primary repair if recognized early.

Mechanism of Injury

Three mechanisms have been proposed for ligamentous disruption of the PCL: (1) direct pretibial trauma, (2) hyperflexion, and (3) hyperextension (Fig. 28K2–2). Pretibial trauma (i.e., a posteriorly directed blow on the anterior

aspect of the proximal tibia) is a commonly cited cause of PCL injury. For example, an athlete falling on a flexed knee with the foot in plantar flexion is at risk of tearing the PCL. If the foot is dorsiflexed, however, the force is transmitted proximally through the patella and the distal femur, thereby protecting the PCL from injury.[4] Noncontact injuries, such as forced hyperflexion, have been reported to be the most common isolated PCL injuries in athletes.[7] These injuries often result in only partial tearing of the PCL, with the posteromedial fibers remaining intact. Hyperextension injuries are often combined with varus or valgus forces to result in multiligament disruptions, which have a much more guarded prognosis.

Classification

Posterior cruciate ligament injuries in both children and adults can be classified according to severity (grades I to III), timing (acute versus chronic), and presence of associated injuries (isolated versus combined).[14] These variables have significant implications for patient outcome and thus are important to consider when making treatment decisions. Isolated injuries to the PCL can be classified as partial (grades I or II) or complete (grade III) tears. In the majority of cases, this is done clinically and corresponds to the laxity in the PCL, as measured by the step-off between the medial tibial plateau and the medial femoral condyle. Iso-

*See references 5, 8, 10, 15, 19, 22, 25, 27, 33, 35–37, and 46–48.

lated grade III injuries or complete PCL tears can occur, but they are frequently associated with other ligament injuries, in particular injury to the posterolateral structures. Distinguishing between isolated and combined PCL injuries is critical, because the prognosis and the treatment for these injuries are vastly different.[14]

Evaluation

An accurate and detailed history and physical examination are essential to arriving at the correct diagnosis and formulating an appropriate treatment plan. The acutely injured child is notoriously a poor historian, and the symptoms are frequently vague and generalized. Children younger than 6 to 7 years of age are usually unable to localize pain reliably. Their manifestation of a knee disorder may be a limp or refusal to walk.[34] Coaches or parents may provide helpful information, but often the injury occurs when the child is unsupervised. This makes a good physical examination even more important, which can be difficult if the child is frightened or in pain. It is very important to gain the child's trust before proceeding with the examination and to remember that pain from hip injuries may be referred to the medial aspect of the knee as a result of the common sensory supply by the obturator nerve.

Evaluation of the injured knee begins with obtaining a detailed history, trying to delineate the mechanism of injury, its severity, and possible associated injuries. Patients with PCL injuries may present for evaluation in a variety of different scenarios. Injuries may range from a seemingly benign fall on the athletic field to severe trauma caused by a motor vehicle accident. The more acutely traumatized the knee, the more difficult it will be to examine it. Unlike patients with isolated ACL injuries, those with acute isolated PCL injuries do not typically report hearing or feeling a "pop." Although many suspect a knee injury, patients do not typically relate a sense of instability. They may note mild to moderate swelling, accompanying stiffness, and occasionally mild knee pain.

The examination of the acutely injured knee begins with evaluation of the neurovascular status, followed by observation of the knee for its resting position and the presence and location of any ecchymosis. The examiner must differentiate between intra-articular effusion and extra-articular swelling. Acute hemarthrosis after trauma to the skeletally immature knee alerts the clinician to a significant intra-articular injury. Arthroscopic examination of the knee for acute hemarthrosis in children has shown ACL or meniscal injury to be present in the majority of patients[1, 6, 44]; however, hemophilia must be considered in the differential diagnosis of a child presenting with hemarthrosis and a history of no or minimal trauma.[12]

All important anatomic structures of the knee should be palpated sequentially, leaving those areas most likely to be tender (according to the suspected diagnosis) until last. Stress maneuvers to test ligament integrity in the mediolateral and anteroposterior planes may be performed gently. Comparison with the noninjured extremity is crucial because of the physiologic laxity present in many children.

If there is significant tenderness over a growth plate, it may be prudent to obtain radiographs before stressing the knee, which might displace a fracture. Finally, range of motion of both the knee *and the hip* (to rule out primary hip disease) is checked near the end of the examination once the patient's trust has been gained and the rest of the examination has been completed.

Extremely rare cases of congenital absence of the cruciate ligaments should be suspected when the adolescent presents with marked knee instability in the absence of pain, swelling, or history of trauma.[16] Although this condition may present as an isolated finding, it is usually associated with other lower limb abnormalities. Radiographs show a shallow intercondylar notch and hypoplasia or total aplasia of the tibial spines. This allows for the differentiation between this rare condition and naturally symmetrical and physiologic knee ligament laxity.

Imaging

Imaging studies play an important role in the diagnosis of PCL injuries in children. Plain radiographs may detect avulsion fractures of the femoral and tibial attachments of the PCL. As previously mentioned, the attachment site may not yet have ossified; thus, avulsion of the PCL (especially from the femur) may not be appreciated on plain films. The only clue may be a slight irregularity at the femoral or tibial attachment, which could easily be missed unless the radiographs are carefully scrutinized.[36, 43] Stress films may be helpful on occasion to rule out an occult physeal plate injury due to ligamentous disruption (Fig. 28K2–3). Magnetic resonance imaging is extremely useful for evaluating PCL injuries in the skeletally immature knee. It can accurately differentiate between in-substance and "peel-off" injuries and can determine if there is any associated chondral or meniscal disease.[14] Magnetic resonance imaging should not be considered a substitute for a thorough history and physical examination, however.

Natural History

Owing to the rarity of PCL injury in children and the limited short-term follow-up that has been reported in the literature, the consequences of PCL deficiency in the skeletally immature knee (with or without treatment) remain unknown. Unfortunately, the literature regarding adult PCL injuries is not extremely helpful because most of the studies are retrospective, combining both isolated and multiligamentous injuries, and do not stratify the outcome according to the degree of instability. There is a general consensus that PCL injuries (especially grade III) are not as benign as previously thought over the long term.[14, 30] Patients with chronic PCL injuries will experience a variable progression of articular degeneration and symptoms over time. A high incidence of late chondrosis[4, 18] (involving the medial femoral condyle and the patellofemoral joint) and meniscal tears[9] has been noted in adult patients treated nonoperatively. These findings are likely the result of the increased contact pressure that occurs in these compartments after

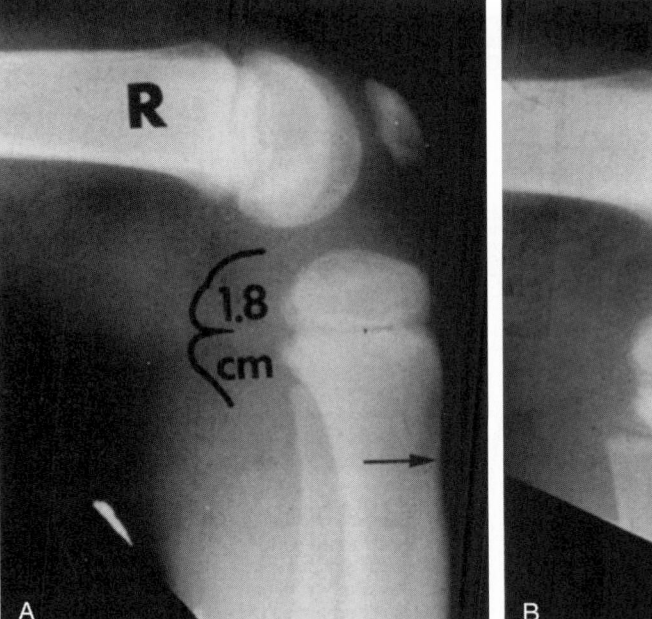

Figure 28K2–3. *A* and *B*, Posterior drawer stress view indicating injury to the posterior cruciate ligament and not the physeal plate.

PCL disruption.[23, 40] The fact that growing articular cartilage is more susceptible to injury than mature articular cartilage is particularly worrisome.[34] The problem to date has been that investigators have been unable to identify prognostic factors consistently to help predict patient outcome after PCL injury.

It should also be noted that the long-term outcome after nonsurgical treatment of ACL injuries in the skeletally immature has been poor with respect to return to sports and long-term sequelae.[3, 5, 11, 17, 21, 31]

Treatment

Rationale

The treatment of acute PCL injuries in children is dependent on both the pattern of ligamentous injury and whether there is any associated meniscal or chondral disease. The full extent of the injury must be determined before formulation of a treatment plan, because the site of injury (avulsion or midsubstance), its grade (partial or complete), and the presence of associated injuries will greatly influence the treatment algorithm. Furthermore, both the child and the parents must be actively involved in the decision-making process. The expectations of both the patient and the family, as well as the maturity of the patient and his or her commitment to rehabilitation, must be taken into consideration before embarking on any surgical intervention.

Avulsion Injuries

Posterior cruciate ligament avulsions (soft tissue or bony) from the femur or the tibia should be repaired primarily. If the child suffered a hyperflexion injury, an avulsion should be suspected; this can be confirmed with

magnetic resonance imaging of the knee. Arthroscopy and examination with the patient under anesthesia remain the most accurate means of determining the extent of the child's injury, however, because partial ligament tears can be difficult to distinguish, even with magnetic resonance imaging, in the skeletally immature knee.[34] Furthermore, arthroscopy will confirm the location of PCL disruption and the feasibility of repair as well as assist in evaluating the menisci and the chondral surfaces for injury. Meniscal repair should be attempted whenever possible, and PCL avulsions from the femur or the tibia should be repaired primarily with transosseous (intraepiphyseal) sutures through drill holes or, for bony avulsions, with either screw or transosseous suture fixation (Fig. 28K2–4).

Midsubstance Injuries

Isolated midsubstance cruciate tears are generally not repaired in children because the outcome has not been proven to be any better than in adults.[5] Permanent plastic deformation and early degeneration of the ligament may contribute to failure of the repair. Although transphyseal ACL reconstructions with soft tissue grafts (i.e., hamstring) are currently being performed at some centers,[20, 21] PCL reconstruction in the skeletally immature knee may be contraindicated. Animal studies have shown that the tibial physis can be very sensitive to transphyseal drilling.[13, 24, 42] The tibial tunnel in PCL reconstruction crosses the physis peripherally, in comparison to the more central location of an ACL tunnel, thereby theoretically posing a greater risk to physeal injury or closure.

Conservative treatment is currently recommended for skeletally immature patients with an isolated grade III midsubstance PCL tear. A recent study has suggested that interstitial tears of the PCL may have some propensity to heal with closed management, although there is some resid-

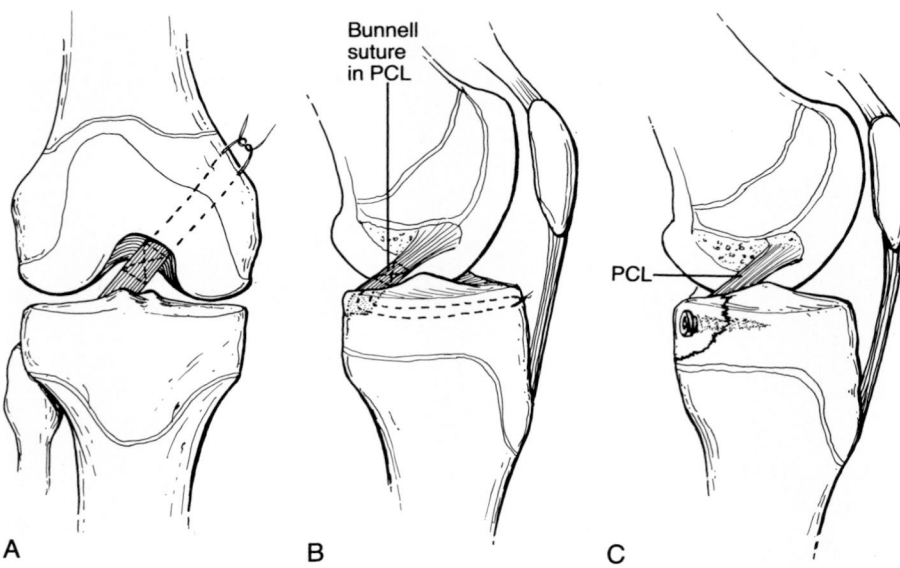

A   **B**   **C**

Figure 28K2–4. *A*, Posterior cruciate ligament (PCL) avulsion from the femur repaired with a Bunnell-type stitch through the femoral epiphysis. *B*, PCL avulsion from the tibia repaired with a Bunnell-type stitch through the tibial epiphysis. *C*, PCL bony avulsion repaired with an intraepiphyseal screw.

ual laxity.[38] Initial treatment should include immobilization of the knee in extension with anterior translation to reduce posterior sag. Restoration of range of motion and quadriceps/hamstring strength starts at 4 to 6 weeks. The patients must be followed annually. If functional instability or pain develops, or if radiographs or bone scans are notable for early signs of arthrosis, then reconstruction of the PCL can be performed after growth is completed.

Multiligament Injuries

In the presence of multiligament injuries, the collateral ligaments are repaired surgically along with any associated meniscal disease. In this scenario, attempting to repair a midsubstance tear of the PCL with suturing may be indicated if there is significant growth remaining. If the resultant posterior laxity is clinically significant, a PCL reconstruction can be performed in the future. In cases in which physeal growth is limited (<1 cm), an acute reconstruction can be performed to stabilize the knee.

If a nonoperative approach is preferred by the treating surgeon, the knee can be immobilized in a cast in full extension to reduce posterior sag. It is critical to obtain radiographs immediately after immobilization and at regular intervals to ensure that the knee remains reduced. Restoration of range of motion and quadriceps/hamstring strength will begin at 4 to 6 weeks. Late reconstruction can be performed in the future after physeal closure if the patient is symptomatic.

References

1. Angel KR, Hall DJ: The role of arthroscopy in children and adolescents. Arthroscopy 5:192–196, 1989.
2. Backx JG, Beijer HJM, Bol E, et al: Injuries in high-risk persons and high-risk sports: A longitudinal study of 1818 school children. Am J Sports Med 19:124–130, 1991.
3. Bradley GW, Shives TC, Samuelson KM: Ligament injuries in the knees of children. J Bone Joint Surg Am 61:588–591, 1979.
4. Clancy WG Jr, Shelbourne KD, Zoellner GB, et al: Treatment of knee joint instability secondary to rupture of the posterior cruciate ligament. Report of a new procedure. J Bone Joint Surg Am 65: 310–322, 1983.
5. Clanton TO, DeLee JC, Sanders B, et al: Knee ligament in children. J Bone Joint Surg Am 61:1195–1201, 1979.
6. Eiskjaer S, Larsen ST, Schmidt MB: The significance of hemarthrosis of the knee in children. Arch Orthop Trauma Surg 107:96–98, 1988.
7. Fowler PJ, Messiah SS: Isolated posterior cruciate ligament injuries in athletes. Am J Sports Med 15:553–557, 1987.
8. Frank C, Strother R: Isolated posterior cruciate ligament injury in a child: Literature review and a case report. Can J Surg 32:373–374, 1989.
9. Geissler WB, Whipple TL: Intraarticular abnormalities in association with posterior cruciate ligament injuries. Am J Sports Med 21:846–849, 1993.
10. Goodrich A, Ballard A: Posterior cruciate ligament avulsion associated with ipsilateral femur fracture in a 10-year-old child. J Trauma 28:1393–1396, 1988.
11. Graf BK, Lange RH, Fujisaki CK, et al: Anterior cruciate ligament tears in skeletally immature patients: Meniscal pathology at presentation and after attempted conservative treatment. Arthroscopy 8:229–233, 1992.
12. Gregosiewicz A, Wösko I, Kandzierski G: Intra-articular bleeding in children with hemophilia: The prevention of arthropathy. J Pediatr Orthop 9:182–185, 1989.
13. Guzzanti V, Falciglia F, Gigante A, Fabbriciani C: The effect of intra-articular ACL reconstruction on the growth plates of rabbits. J Bone Joint Surg Br 76:960–963, 1994.
14. Harner CD, Höher J: Current concepts: Evaluation and treatment of posterior cruciate ligament injuries. Am J Sports Med 26:471–482, 1998.
15. Itokazu M, Yamane T, Shoen S: Incomplete avulsion of the femoral attachment of the posterior cruciate ligament with an osteochondral fragment in a twelve-year-old boy. Arch Orthop Trauma Surg 110: 55–57, 1990.
16. Johansson E, Aparisi T: Congenital absence of the cruciate ligaments: A case report and review of the literature. Clin Orthop 162:108–111, 1982.
17. Kannus P, Järvinen M: Knee ligament injuries in adolescents: Eight-year follow-up of conservative management. J Bone Joint Surg Br 70:772–776, 1988.
18. Keller PM, Shelbourne KD, McCarroll JR, et al: Nonoperatively treated isolated posterior cruciate ligament injuries. Am J Sports Med 21:132–136, 1993.
19. Kunz M: Injuries of the cruciate ligament in children caused by sports accidents [in German]. Sportverletz Sportschaden 6:2–5, 1992.
20. Lipscomb AB, Anderson AF: Tears of the anterior cruciate ligament in adolescents. J Bone Joint Surg Am 68:19–28, 1986.

21. Lo IKY, Bell DM, Fowler PJ: Anterior cruciate ligament injuries in the skeletally immature patient. Instr Course Lect 47:351–359, 1998.

22. Lobenhoffer P, Wünsch L, Bosch U, et al: Arthroscopic repair of the posterior cruciate ligament in a 3-year-old child. Arthroscopy 13:248–253, 1997.

23. MacDonald P, Miniaci A, Fowler P, et al: A biomechanical analysis of joint contact forces in the posterior cruciate deficient knee. Knee Surg Sports Traumatol Arthrosc 4:252–255, 1996.

24. Makela EA, Vainionpaa S, Vihtonen K, et al: The effect of trauma to the lower femoral epiphyseal plate: An experimental study in rabbits. J Bone Joint Surg Br 70:187–191, 1988.

25. Mayer PJ, Micheli LJ: Avulsion of the femoral attachment of the posterior cruciate ligament in an eleven-year-old boy. J Bone Joint Surg Am 61:431–432, 1979.

26. McCarroll JR, Rettig AC, Shelbourne KD: Anterior cruciate ligament injuries in the young athlete with open physis. Am J Sports Med 16:44–47, 1988.

27. McMaster WC: Isolated posterior cruciate ligament injury: Literature review and case reports. J Trauma 15:1025–1029, 1975.

28. Micheli LJ: Preface. Clin Sport Med 14:xi, 1995.

29. Micheli LJ, Foster TE: Acute knee injuries in the immature athlete. Instr Course Lect 42:473–481, 1993.

30. Miller MD, Bergfeld JA, Fowler PJ, et al: The posterior cruciate ligament injured knee: Principles of evaluation and treatment. Instr Course Lect 48:199–207, 1999.

31. Nottage WM, Matsuura PA: Management of complete traumatic anterior cruciate ligament tears in the skeletally immature patient: Current concepts and review of the literature. Arthroscopy 10:569–573, 1994.

32. Outerbridge AR, Micheli LJ: Overuse injuries in the young athlete. Clin Sport Med 14:503–516, 1995.

33. Quintart C, Elbaum R: A case of isolated fracture of the posterior cruciate ligament in a child [in French]. Rev Chir Orthop Reparatrice Appar Mot 85:617–620, 1999.

34. Rask BP, Micheli LJ: Knee ligament injuries and associated derangements in children and adolescents. In Fu FH, Harner CD, Vince KG (eds): Knee Surgery. Baltimore, Williams & Wilkins, 1994, pp 365–381.

35. Ross AC, Chesterman PJ: Isolated avulsion of the tibial attachment of the posterior cruciate ligament in childhood. J Bone Joint Surg Br 68:747, 1986.

36. Rungu JL, Fay MJ: Acute posterior cruciate ligament insufficiency in children. Am J Knee Surg 3:192–203, 1990.

37. Sanders WE, Wilkins KE, Neidre A: Acute insufficiency of the posterior cruciate ligament in children. J Bone Joint Surg Am 62:129–130, 1980.

38. Shelbourne KD, Jennings RW, Vahey TN: Magnetic resonance imaging of posterior cruciate ligament injuries: Assessment of healing. Am J Knee Surg 12:209–213, 1999.

39. Skak SV, Jensen TT, Poulsen TD, et al: Epidemiology of knee injuries in children. Acta Orthop Scand 58:78–81, 1984.

40. Skyhar MJ, Warren RF, Ortiz GJ, et al: The effects of sectioning of the posterior cruciate ligament and posterolateral complex on the articular contact pressures within the knee. J Bone Joint Surg Am 75:694–699, 1993.

41. Smith AD, Tao SS: Knee injuries in young athletes. Clin Sports Med 14:629–650, 1995.

42. Stadlemaier DN, Arnocsky SP, Dodds H, et al: The effect of drilling and soft tissue grafting across open growth plates: A histologic study. Am J Sports Med 23:431–435, 1995.

43. Stanitski CL: Ligamentous injury of the knee. In Stanitski CL, DeLee JC, Drez DJ (eds): Pediatric and Adolescent Sports Medicine, vol 3. Philadelphia, WB Saunders, 1994, pp 422–432.

44. Stanitski CL, Harvell JC, Fu FH: Observations on acute hemarthrosis in children and adolescents. J Pediatr Orthop 13:506–510, 1993.

45. Sullivan JA: Ligamentous injuries of the knee in children. Clin Orthop 225:44–50, 1990.

46. Suprock MD, Rogers VP: Posterior cruciate avulsion in a 4-year-old boy. Orthopaedics 13:659–662, 1990.

47. Torisu T: Isolated avulsion of the tibial attachment of the posterior cruciate ligament. J Bone Joint Surg Am 59:68–72, 1977.

48. Wening JV, Mathiak G, Mathiak M, et al: Diagnosis and therapy of cruciate ligament injuries in childhood: Clinical results [in German]. Unfallchirurgie 21:285–291, 1995.

Section L

The Multiple Ligament–Injured Knee

Gregory C. Fanelli, MD ▪ Daniel D. Feldmann, MD
Craig J. Edson, MS, PT/ATC ▪ David Maish, MD

The dislocated knee is a severe injury resulting from violent trauma. It results in disruption of at least three of the four major ligaments of the knee and leads to significant functional instability. Vascular and nerve damage, as well as associated fractures, may contribute to the challenge of caring for this injury. Historical treatment was primarily limited to immobilization. With the advent of better surgical instrumentation and technique, however, the management of combined anterior and posterior cruciate ligament (ACL/PCL) tears associated with medial or lateral collateral ligament (MCL/LCL) disruption has become primarily surgical.

This chapter presents basic knee anatomy, mechanisms and classifications of injury, evaluation, treatment, postoperative rehabilitation, and the authors' experience with treating the dislocated knee.

Anatomy

Stability of the knee is due to several anatomic structures. The articulation of the femorotibial joint is maintained in part by the bony anatomy of the femoral condyles and the tibial plateau. The menisci serve to increase the contact area between femur and tibia and thus increase stability of the joint. The four major ligaments (ACL, PCL, MCL, LCL) and the posteromedial and posterolateral corners are the most significant ligamentous stabilizers of the knee. In addition to these static anatomic structures, dynamic anatomic structures, such as the musculature that crosses the knee joint, also play a role in stabilization. In any knee injury, examination must include evaluation of all these anatomic structures.

When evaluating a dislocated knee, it is imperative to evaluate the structural integrity of any remaining ligamentous structure; consequently, the functions of these structures must be well understood. The ACL primarily prevents anterior translation of the tibia relative to the femur and accounts for about 86% of the total resistance to anterior tibial translation.[4] It is also involved in limiting internal and external rotation of the tibia relative to the femur when the knee is in extension.[45] The ACL will also limit varus and valgus stress in the face of either an LCL or an MCL injury.

The PCL may be considered the primary static stabilizer

of the knee given its location near the center of rotation of the knee and its relative strength.[41] The PCL has been shown to provide 95% of the total restraint to posterior tibial displacement forces acting on the tibia.[4] The PCL works in concert with structures of the posterolateral corner, and injury to both structures is required to increase posterior translation significantly.[16]

The MCL and the LCL act alone to resist valgus and varus stresses, respectively, at 30 degrees of knee flexion. Together, they act in a secondary fashion to limit anterior and posterior translation as well as rotation of the tibia on the femur. The anatomy of the posterolateral corner of the knee is complex; its major structures consists of (1) the LCL, (2) the arcuate complex, (3) the popliteal tendon, and (4) the popliteal-fibular ligament.[5] The posterolateral corner primarily resists posterolateral rotation of the tibia relative to the femur but also contributes to resisting posterior tibial translation. The posteromedial corner of the knee consists primarily of the posterior oblique portion of the MCL and the associated joint capsule. These structures provide resistance to valgus stress and posteromedial tibial translation. Evaluation of traumatic knee dislocation must include these anatomic structures; typically, three areas or more are injured in knee dislocation. Failure to recognize and treat capsular and ligamentous injury, besides the obvious ACL/PCL injury, will produce less than optimal results.[6–8]

Neurovascular structures are also at risk of injury. The popliteal fossa is defined by the tendons of the pes anserinus and semimembranosus medially and the biceps femoris tendon laterally. The space is closed distally by the medial and lateral heads of the gastrocnemius and proximally by the hamstrings. Within this space, the popliteal artery and vein and the tibial and peroneal branches of the sciatic nerve are located. The popliteal artery may be most at risk of injury in knee dislocations. The popliteal artery is tethered proximally at the adductor hiatus as it exits from Hunter's canal and distally as it passes under the soleus arch, making it vulnerable to injury in these areas. This artery is considered to be an "end artery" of the lower limb; if it is injured, the surrounding geniculate arteries are not sufficient to maintain collateral blood flow to the lower extremity. The popliteal vein is in close association with the artery but seems to be less at risk during injury than the popliteal artery. From a surgical standpoint, the popliteal vessels are located directly posterior to the posterior horns of the medial and lateral menisci, and dissection in this area may put these structures at risk if they are not adequately protected. The sciatic nerve divides into its peroneal and tibial divisions within the popliteal space. These nerves are less likely to be injured with knee dislocation, probably because they are not tethered, as the popliteal artery is. The peroneal nerve does seem to be at higher risk, because its course around the fibular head functionally decreases its potential excursion and violent varus injuries may result in traction injury to this nerve. Its location must be identified during dissection to reconstruct the posterolateral corner.

Classification of Injury

Classification of knee dislocation is primarily based on the direction in which the tibia dislocates in relation to the femur.[14, 17] This results in five different categories: anterior, posterior, lateral, medial, and rotatory. The anteromedial, anterolateral, posteromedial, and posterolateral dislocations are classified as rotary dislocations. Other factors to be considered include whether (1) the injury is open or closed, (2) the injury is due to "high-energy" or "low-energy" trauma, (3) the knee is completely dislocated or subluxed, and (4) there is neurovascular involvement. Furthermore, one should be acutely conscious of the fact that a complete dislocation may reduce spontaneously, and any triple-ligament knee injury constitutes a frank dislocation.[7, 36, 43]

Reports vary, but anterior and posterior dislocations appear to be the most common directions of dislocation. Frassica and coworkers[13] found a 70% incidence of posterior dislocation, 25% incidence of anterior dislocation, and 5% incidence of rotatory dislocation in their series. Green and Allen[18] reported incidences of 31% for anterior, 25% for posterior, and 3% for rotatory dislocations in their series. Rotatory dislocations occur less frequently; however, the posterolateral dislocation seems to be the most common combination. This particular pattern may be irreducible secondary to the medial femoral condyle becoming "buttonholed" through the anteromedial joint capsule. In addition, the MCL invaginates into the joint space, blocking reduction. This buttonholing results in a skin furrow along the medial joint line where the subcutaneous tissue attachments to the joint capsule drag the skin into the joint.[42] Attempts at reduction in this scenario make the skin furrow more pronounced.

The actual incidence of different directional dislocations is not as important as the correct diagnosis of the direction of injury and how it relates to potential neurovascular injury. Hyperextension injuries (or posterior dislocations), because of the tethered popliteal artery and vein, may have the highest incidence of associated vascular injury; however, any dislocation, if initial displacement is severe enough, will result in injury to the popliteal artery. The common peroneal nerve is less at risk because it has a greater excursion than the popliteal vessels, but it is still susceptible when a varus force is applied to the knee. Posterolateral dislocation is associated with a high incidence of injury to the common peroneal nerve.[21, 37]

Open knee dislocations are not uncommon. Reported incidence is between 19% and 35% of all dislocations.[24, 37] An open knee dislocation, in general, carries a worse prognosis secondary to severe injury to the soft tissue envelope. Furthermore, an open injury may require an open ligament reconstruction, or staged reconstruction, because arthroscopically assisted techniques cannot be performed in the acute setting with these open injuries.

Distinguishing between low-energy and high-energy injuries is important. Low-energy or low-velocity injuries, usually associated with sports, have a decreased incidence of associated vascular injury. High-energy or high-velocity injuries, secondary to motor vehicle accidents or falls from a height, tend to have an increased incidence of vascular compromise. With decreased pulses in an injured limb and a history of a high-energy injury, one should obtain vascular studies on an urgent basis.

Mechanism of Injury

The mechanisms of injury for the two most common knee dislocation patterns, anterior and posterior, are reasonably well described. Kennedy[21] was able to reproduce anterior dislocation by using a hyperextension force acting on the knee. At 30 degrees of hyperextension, Kennedy found that the posterior capsule failed. When extended further, to about 50 degrees, the ACL, the PCL, and the popliteal artery fail. There is some question about whether the ACL or the PCL fails first with hyperextension[15, 21]; however, in our clinical experience, both the ACL and the PCL fail with dislocation.[7] Other series[13, 32, 38] demonstrated both ACL and PCL tears with complete knee dislocation.

A posteriorly directed force applied to the proximal tibia when the knee is flexed to 90 degrees is thought to produce a posterior dislocation, the so-called dashboard injury.[32] Medial and lateral dislocations result from varus/valgus stresses applied to the knee. A combination of varus/valgus stress with hyperextension and a blow to the proximal tibia will likely produce one of the rotatory dislocations.

Associated Injuries

Several anatomic structures are at risk in the dislocated knee. The four major ligaments of the knee as well as the posteromedial and posterolateral corners can be compromised. Vascular and nerve injuries are common. There may also be associated bony lesions, avulsion fractures of the ACL or the PCL, tibial plateau fractures, distal femur condylar fractures, or ipsilateral tibial or femoral shaft fractures.

There is evidence in the literature that a frank dislocation may not result in complete rupture of three of the four major ligaments[21, 25, 37]; however, this seems to be the exception rather than the rule. Several authors have found that a frank dislocation of the knee invariably results in rupture of at least three of the four major ligaments. Sisto and Warren[38] found that all knees in their series had three or more ligaments compromised. Frassica and colleagues found that all 13 patients treated operatively were found to have ACL, PCL, and MCL disruptions.[13] Fanelli and associates found that 19 of 20 were found to have a third component (posterolateral corner or MCL) in addition to complete ACL and PCL disruption.[7] With a frank dislocation of the knee, careful ligament examination is necessary to diagnose fully the extent of the injury.

The incidence of vascular compromise in knee dislocations has been estimated to be about 32%.[18] When limited to anterior or posterior dislocation, the incidence may be as high as 50%.[44] Recent studies confirm the significant incidence of arterial injury,[1, 13, 35, 38] reaffirming the need for careful vascular evaluation. The popliteal artery is an end-artery to the leg, with minimal collateral circulation through the genicular arteries. Furthermore, the popliteal vein is responsible for the majority of venous outflow from the knee. If either structure is compromised to the point of prolonged obstruction, ischemia and eventual amputation are often the result.[3, 30]

Two mechanisms have been described for injury to the popliteal artery. One is a stretching mechanism, seen with hyperextension, until the vessel ruptures. This may occur secondary to the tethered nature of the artery at the adductor hiatus and the entrance through the gastrocnemius-soleus complex. This type of injury should be suspected with an anterior dislocation. Posterior dislocation, the second mechanism, may cause direct contusion of the vessel by the posterior plateau, resulting in intimal damage. Under no circumstance should compromised vascular status be attributed to arterial spasm; in this situation, there is often intimal damage and impending thrombus formation. Cone[5] points out that initial examination may be normal; however, thrombus formation can occur hours to days later,[5, 19, 29, 33] and recent series have demonstrated delayed thrombus formation.[13, 38] Furthermore, a bicruciate ligament rupture presenting as a "reduced" dislocated knee may have as high an incidence of arterial injury as a frank dislocation.[43]

Popliteal vein injury occurs much less frequently; at least historically, this injury had not been reported. Nevertheless, venous occlusion must also be recognized and appropriately treated. Whether to repair venous injury seemed controversial in the past. Ligating the popliteal vein, a common practice during the Vietnam conflict, led to severe edema, phlebitis, and chronic venous stasis changes. Venous repair was thought to lead to thrombophlebitis and pulmonary embolism. Currently, if obstruction to outflow is recognized, surgical repair of the popliteal vein is warranted.[31]

Injury to either the peroneal nerve or the tibial nerve has been documented,[1, 21, 25, 35, 37, 38, 44, 46] with an incidence of about 20% to 30%. The nervous structures about the knee are not as tightly anchored as the popliteal vessels; this probably accounts for the lower incidence of injury compared with neighboring vascular structures. The mechanism of injury is usually stretch. The peroneal nerve seems to be more frequently involved than the tibial nerve, probably because of its anatomic location. With any varus loading of the knee, the peroneal nerve is placed under tension. In Shields' series,[37] posterior dislocation caused the majority of the nerve injuries.

Given the fact that knee dislocation is usually secondary to violent trauma, associated fractures are common; the incidence may be as high as 60%.[25] Tibial plateau fractures and avulsion fractures from the proximal tibia or the distal femur are common.[13, 22, 24, 25, 38, 46] Recognition of these injuries is also important, because additional bony involvement has implications for definitive treatment. Associated distal femur fractures and proximal tibial fractures treated with intramedullary nailing make bone tunnel placement for ACL and PCL reconstruction difficult. With violent trauma, any conceivable fracture or avulsion may occur with a dislocated knee; however, it is suggested that medial and lateral dislocations are associated with an increased frequency of minor bony lesions.[23]

Fracture-dislocations represent a separate entity in the spectrum from pure knee dislocation to tibial plateau fractures. Pure knee dislocation requires only soft tissue reconstruction to gain stability; tibial plateau fractures require purely bony stabilization. Fracture-dislocations of the knee often involve both bony and ligamentous repair or reconstruction, adding an element of complexity to their treatment.[17, 26] Long-term outcome for fracture-dislocation injuries to the knee joint falls somewhere between the outcomes for tibial plateau fractures and pure dislocations, with tibial plateau fractures doing the best and dislocations the worst.[26]

anterior to posterior translation in 10 of the 11 knees; at 70 degrees; there were 9 knees that had less than 3 mm side to side difference in anteroposterior translation. These authors concluded that simultaneous bicruciate ligament reconstruction is warranted to restore function to the knee.

Fanelli Sports Injury Clinic Experience

The authors' practice is at a tertiary care regional trauma center. There is a 38% incidence of PCL tears in acute knee injuries, with 45% of these being combined ACL/PCL tears.[10, 11] Careful assessment, evaluation, and treatment of vascular injuries are essential in these acute multiple ligament–injured knees. There is an 11% incidence of vascular injury associated with these acute multiple ligament–injured knees at our center.[9]

Our preferred approach to combined ACL/PCL injuries is an arthroscopic ACL/PCL reconstruction using the transtibial technique, with collateral/capsular ligament surgery as indicated. Not all cases are amenable to the arthroscopic approach, and the operating surgeon must assess each case individually. Surgical timing is dependent on vascular status, reduction stability, skin condition, systemic injuries, open versus closed knee injury, meniscus and articular surface injuries, other orthopaedic injuries, and the collateral/capsular ligaments involved.

Surgical Timing

Most ACL/PCL/MCL injuries can be treated with brace treatment of the medial collateral ligament followed by arthroscopic combined ACL/PCL reconstruction in 4 to 6 weeks after healing of the MCL. Certain cases may require repair or reconstruction of the medial structures and must be assessed on an individual basis. Our preferred surgical treatment is primary repair augmented with an Achilles tendon MCL reconstruction.

Combined ACL/PCL/posterolateral injuries should be addressed as early as is safely possible. ACL/PCL/posterolateral repair and reconstruction performed 2 to 3 weeks after injury allow sealing of capsular tissues to permit an arthroscopic approach and still permit primary repair of injured posterolateral structures. We have reported excellent results reconstructing these knees 6 to 8 weeks after injury.[6]

Open multiple-ligament knee injuries and dislocations may require staged procedures. The collateral/capsular structures are repaired after thorough irrigation and débridement, and the combined ACL/PCL reconstruction is performed at a later date after wound healing has occurred. Care must be taken in all cases of delayed reconstruction to ensure that the tibiofemoral joint is reduced on the AP and lateral radiographs in full extension.

The preceding surgical timing guidelines should be considered in the context of the individual patient. Many patients with multiple ligament injuries of the knee are severely injured multiple trauma patients with multisystem injuries. Modifiers of the ideal timing protocols outlined here include the vascular status of the involved extremity, reduction stability, skin condition, open or closed injury, and other orthopaedic and systemic injuries. These additional considerations may cause the knee ligament surgery to be performed earlier or later than desired. We have previously reported excellent results with delayed reconstruction in the multiple ligament–injured knee.[6, 7]

Graft Selection

The ideal graft material should be strong, provide secure fixation, be easy to pass, be readily available, and have low donor site morbidity. The available options in the United States are autograft and allograft sources. Our preferred graft for the PCL is the Achilles tendon allograft because of its large cross-sectional area and strength, absence of donor site morbidity, and easy passage with secure fixation. We prefer Achilles tendon allograft or bone–patellar tendon–bone allograft for ACL reconstruction. The preferred graft material for the posterolateral corner is a split biceps femoris tendon transfer, a biceps femoris tendon transfer, or free autograft (semitendinosus) or allograft (Achilles tendon) tissue when the biceps tendon is not available.[12] Cases requiring MCL and posteromedial corner surgery may have primary repair, reconstruction, or a combination of both. Our preferred method for MCL and posteromedial corner instability is a reconstruction with allograft tissue.

Surgical Approach

Our preferred surgical approach is a single-stage arthroscopic combined ACL/PCL reconstruction using the transtibial technique, with collateral/capsular ligament surgery as indicated. The posterolateral corner is repaired and is then augmented with a split biceps tendon transfer, a biceps tendon transfer, a semitendinosus free graft, or allograft tissue. Acute medial injuries not amenable to brace treatment undergo primary repair and allograft reconstruction as indicated. The operating surgeon must be prepared to convert to a dry arthroscopic procedure or to an open procedure if fluid extravasation becomes a problem.

Surgical Technique

The principle of reconstruction in the multiply injured knee is to identify and treat all disorders using accurate tunnel placement, anatomic graft insertion sites, strong graft material, secure graft fixation, and a well-defined postoperative rehabilitation program.

The patient is positioned supine on the operating table. The surgical leg hangs over the side of the operating table, and the well leg is supported by the fully extended table. A lateral post is used for control of the surgical leg. We do not use a leg holder. The surgery is done under tourniquet control unless previous arterial or venous repair contraindicates the use of a tourniquet. Fluid inflow is by gravity. We do not use an arthroscopic fluid pump.

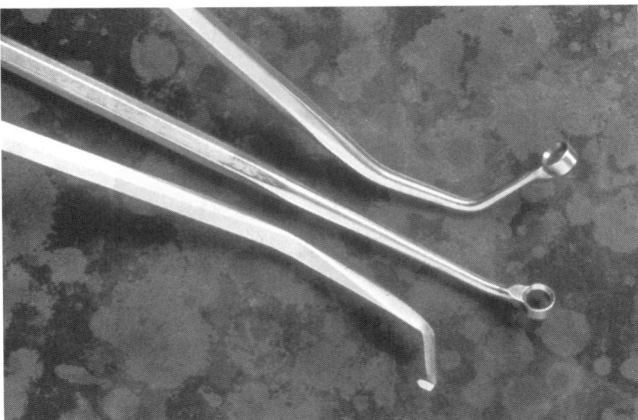

Figure 28L–2. Specially designed, curved over-the-back posterior cruciate ligament instruments are used to elevate the posterior capsule in preparation for tibial tunnel creation. (Courtesy of Arthrotek Inc., Warsaw, Ind.)

Allograft tissue is prepared before bringing the patient into the operating room. Arthroscopic instruments are placed with the inflow in the superolateral portal, the arthroscope in the inferolateral patellar portal, and instruments in the inferomedial patellar portal. An accessory extracapsular extra-articular posteromedial safety incision is used to protect the neurovascular structures and to confirm the accuracy of tibial tunnel placement.

The notchplasty, which is performed first, consists of ACL and PCL stump débridement, bone removal, and contouring of the medial wall of the lateral femoral condyle and the intercondylar roof. This allows visualization of the over-the-top position and prevents ACL graft impingement throughout the full range of motion. Specially curved PCL instruments are used to elevate the capsule from the posterior aspect of the tibia (Fig. 28L–2).

The PCL tibial and femoral tunnels are created with the help of a PCL/ACL drill guide (Fig. 28L–3). The transtibial PCL tunnel goes from the anteromedial aspect of the proximal tibia 1 cm below the tibial tubercle to exit in the inferolateral aspect of the PCL anatomic insertion site. The PCL femoral tunnel originates externally between the medial femoral epicondyle and the medial femoral condylar articular surface to emerge through the center of the stump of the anterolateral bundle of the PCL. The PCL graft is positioned and anchored on the femoral or the tibial side, and it is left free on the opposite side.

The ACL tunnels are created using the single-incision technique. The tibial tunnel begins externally at a point 1 cm proximal to the tibial tubercle on the anteromedial surface of the proximal tibia to emerge through the center of the stump of the ACL tibial footprint. The femoral tunnel is positioned next to the over-the-top position on the medial wall of the lateral femoral condyle near the ACL anatomic insertion site. The tunnel is created to leave a 1 to 2-mm posterior cortical wall so that interference fixation can be used. The ACL graft is positioned and is anchored on the femoral side, with the tibial side left free (Fig. 28L–4). Attention is then turned to the posterolateral corner.

Our preferred technique for posterolateral reconstruction is the split biceps tendon transfer to the lateral femoral epicondyle. The requirements for this procedure are the following: The proximal tibiofibular joint should be intact; the posterolateral capsular attachments to the common biceps tendon should be intact; and the biceps femoris tendon insertion into the fibular head must be intact. This technique restores the function of the popliteofibular ligament and the lateral collateral ligament, tightens the posterolateral capsule, and provides a post of strong autogenous tissue to reinforce the posterolateral corner.

A lateral hockey-stick incision is made. The peroneal nerve is dissected free and is protected throughout the procedure. The long head and common biceps femoris tendon is isolated, and the anterior two thirds is separated from the short-head muscle. The tendon is detached proximally and is left attached distally to its anatomic insertion

Figure 28L–3. Fanelli PCL/ACL drill guide. (Courtesy of Arthrotek Inc., Warsaw, Ind.)

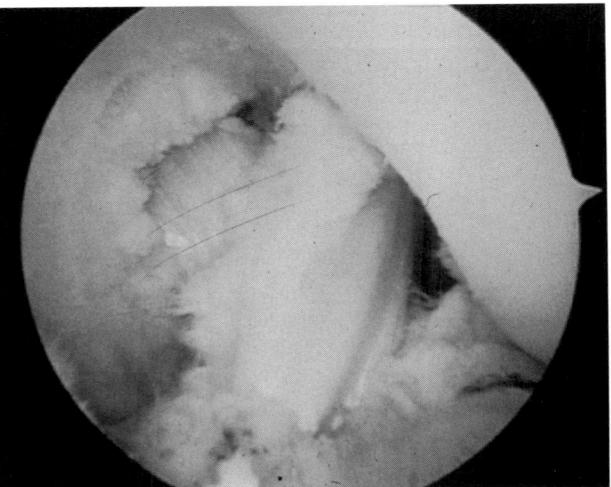

Figure 28L–4. Arthroscopically assisted combined anterior and posterior cruciate ligament reconstruction in a multiple ligament–injured knee using Achilles tendon allografts. Tunnels are anatomically placed to re-create the anterolateral bundle of the posterior cruciate ligament and the anatomic insertion sites of the anterior cruciate ligament.

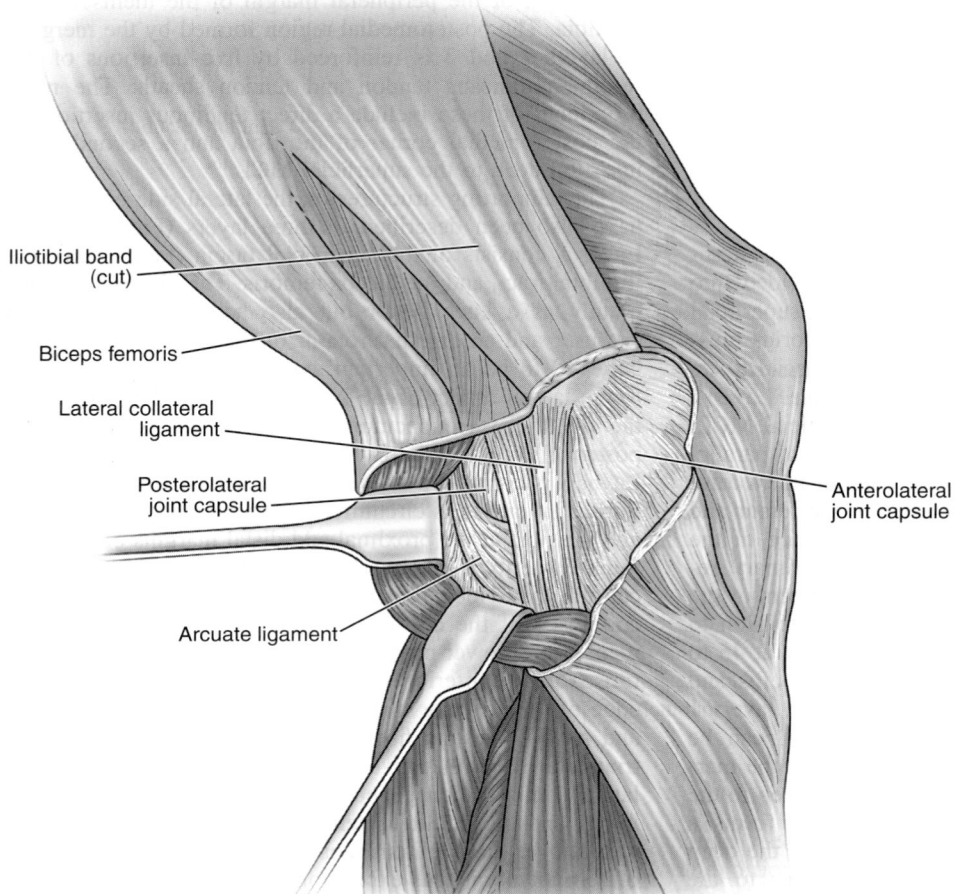

Iliotibial band
(cut)

Biceps femoris

Lateral collateral
ligament

Posterolateral
joint capsule

Arcuate ligament

Anterolateral
joint capsule

Figure 28N–7. Anatomic layers of the lateral knee. The iliotibial band and the superficial fascia (layer 1) have been removed, exposing the lateral collateral ligament and the arcuate ligament (layer 3). Layer 2 is incomplete at this location. (From Insall JN, Scott WN: Surgery of the Knee, 3rd ed. Philadelphia, WB Saunders, 2000.)

The superficial lamina represents the original capsule and consists of the LCL and the fabellofibular ligament. The LCL originates on the lateral epicondyle of the femur anterior to the origin of the gastrocnemius and inserts into the head of the fibula, blending with the insertion of the biceps femoris. The fabellofibular ligament is a condensation of fibers lying between the LCL and the arcuate ligaments and runs from the fabella, a sesamoid bone found in the lateral head of the gastrocnemius, to the fibular styloid.[53] The popliteus muscle arises as a tendon about 2.5 cm long from a depression at the anterior part of the groove on the lateral condyle of the femur. The tendon passes beneath the medial limb of the arcuate ligament and forms a thin, triangular muscle that inserts into the medial two thirds of the triangular surface proximal to the popliteal line on the posterior surface of the tibia. The primary role of the popliteus appears to be to unlock the knee to allow flexion by producing external rotation of the femur in the loaded position.[8, 68, 75] The LCL, the PCL, and the popliteus-arcuate complex act in concert to stabilize the posterolateral corner of the knee against varus stress, external tibial rotation, and posterior flexion.[4, 44, 45]

Anteriorly, the quadriceps muscle group consists of four distinct parts that share a common tendon of insertion. The rectus femoris arises as two heads (direct and indirect) from the ilium, which unite and narrow to a tendon 5 to 8 cm proximal to the superior pole of the patella.[87] The vastus lateralis arises from a broad linear strip, beginning at the proximal end of the trochanteric line and extending halfway down the linea aspera. It also arises from the lateral intermuscular septum. The vastus medialis originates from the distal part of the trochanteric line and follows the spiral line to the medial lip of the linea aspera. The most distal fibers of the muscle arise from the tendon of the adductor magnus and pass almost horizontally anterior to the insertion into the common tendon and the medial border of the patella. This part of the muscle is sometimes described as the vastus medialis obliquus. Like the vastus lateralis, the vastus medialis has a distal fibrous expansion that blends with the medial patellar retinaculum. The vastus intermedius arises from the anterior and lateral aspects of the shaft of the femur; medially, it partly blends with the vastus medialis.

The four muscles become confluent distally and form the quadriceps tendon, which extends anteriorly about the patella to become the patellar tendon. The quadriceps tendon is often depicted as a trilaminar structure, with the anterior layer being formed by the rectus femoris, the intermediate layer by the vastus medialis and lateralis, and the deep layer by the tendon of the vastus intermedius.[67, 87] In reality, the organization is more complex and variable.[87] The patellar tendon runs from the lower border of the patella to the tibial tubercle. Because there is an inclination toward the shaft of the femur, the quadriceps muscle does not pull in a direct line with the patellar tendon. The angle formed is always valgus; the average is 14 degrees in men and 17 degrees in women.[1] The resulting vector toward lateral patellar displacement is resisted by the lateral lip of the femoral trochlea, the horizontal fibers of the vastus medialis obliquus, and the medial patellar retinaculum. The posterior surface of the patellar tendon is separated from the synovial membrane of the joint by a large infrapatellar pad of fat and from the tibia by a bursa. The fat pad fills the space between the femoral condyles and the patellar tendon and adjusts its shape as the size of this potential cavity varies with movement.

The popliteal fossa is bounded laterally by the biceps femoris and medially by the semimembranosus and by the tendons of the pes anserinus. Distally, the space is closed by the two heads of the gastrocnemius (Fig. 28N–8). The roof of the fossa is formed by the deep fascia; the floor consists of the popliteal surface of the femur, the posterior capsule of the knee joint, and the popliteus muscle with its fascial covering. The popliteal artery exits from Hunter's canal and enters the popliteal fossa at the junction of the middle and lower thirds of the femur. Proximally, it is separated from the femur by a thick pad of fat, but in the region of the posterior joint line, it lies in direct contact

with the posterior capsule. Further distally, the artery runs superficial to the popliteus fascia and ends at the lower border of the popliteus by dividing into the anterior and posterior tibial arteries. The tibial nerve arises from the sciatic nerve halfway down the thigh. It runs distally through the popliteal fossa close to the popliteal vessels. The common peroneal nerve enters the popliteal fossa on the lateral side of the tibial nerve and runs distally along the medial side of the biceps tendon. It then passes between the biceps femoris tendon and the lateral head of the gastrocnemius and runs distally posterior to the fibula head. Next, it crosses superficial to the neck of the fibula before piercing the peroneus longus.

In addition to the comprehensive understanding of normal anatomy that is required to perform successful knee replacement, specific knowledge of the anatomic changes that result from the arthritic processes is important. Specific disease processes affect the anatomy of the knee differently. Post-traumatic arthritis may be associated with ligamentous incompetence and bony defects that are dependent on the initial injury. Old lateral plateau fractures with depression or malunited splits may result in bony deficiencies of the tibia, whereas extra-articular fractures may result in malalignment. These abnormalities may require the use of modular augmentations, bone grafting, or modifications in surgical technique. In degenerative arthritis, in addition to

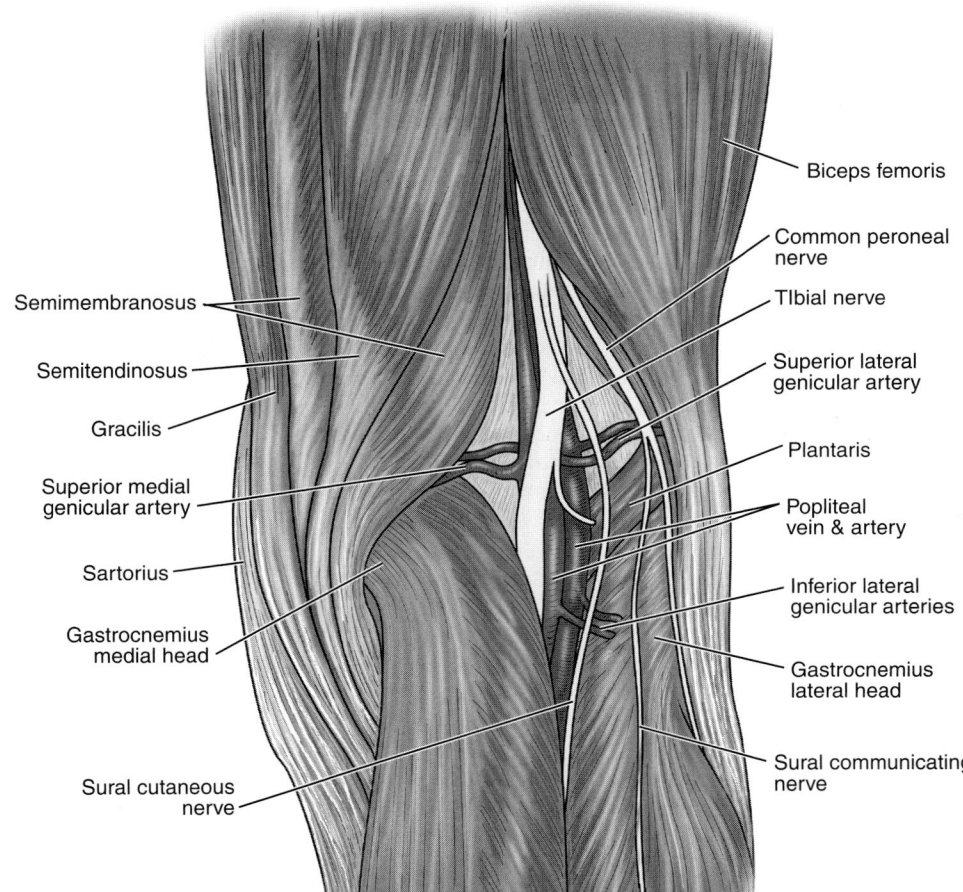

Figure 28N–8. The popliteal fossa. (From Insall JN, Scott WN: Surgery of the Knee, 3rd ed. Philadelphia, WB Saunders, 2000.)

Semimembranosus

Semitendinosus

Gracilis

Superior medial genicular artery

Sartorius

Gastrocnemius medial head

Sural cutaneous nerve

Biceps femoris

Common peroneal nerve

Tibial nerve

Superior lateral genicular artery

Plantaris

Popliteal vein & artery

Inferior lateral genicular arteries

Gastrocnemius lateral head

Sural communicating nerve

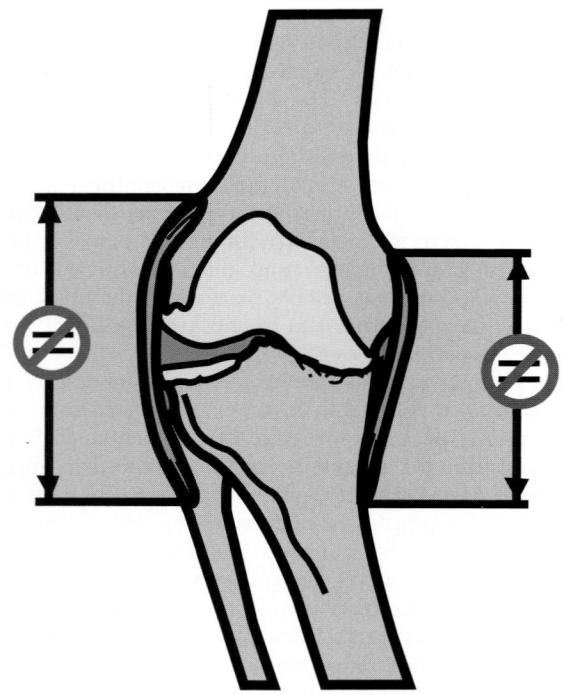

Figure 28N–9. Varus deformity of the knee associated with medial compartment osteoarthritis. The medial ligaments have contracted and the lateral structures are lax, producing a soft tissue imbalance.

bone erosion, the development of deformity is associated with contractures of the soft tissue structures on the concave side of the deformity and stretching of the structures on the convex side. For example, in the varus knee, the medial structures shorten and the lateral structures become attenuated in severe cases (Fig. 28N–9). In the latter, the contracted anatomic structures on the medial side of the knee include the pes anserinus tendons; the superficial MCL; the posteromedial corner, including the semimembranosus insertion; the medial capsule; and the deep MCL. In distinction, the contracted anatomic structures in the valgus knee include the ITB, the LCL, the popliteus tendon, and the arcuate ligament–posterolateral capsular complex. These commonly encountered abnormalities dictate the specific surgical techniques that are required to create a balanced knee after prosthetic replacement. These techniques are described in subsequent sections.

Clinical Evaluation

History

The primary indication for knee replacement is chronic disabling knee pain due to arthritis. In most circumstances, this pain is exacerbated by weight-bearing activity, is relieved by rest, and occurs in association with varying degrees of swelling. Other symptoms may include buckling, catching, and stiffness. Isolated unicompartmental arthritis may present as pain predominantly on the medial or the lateral side, whereas patellofemoral arthritis may present as isolated anterior knee pain, particularly with stair

climbing. Diffuse pain is more likely a result of involvement of more than one compartment. Other causes should always be considered, especially if the pain is not clearly activity related; radiates to the hip, the back, or the foot; or is inconsistent with the associated physical examination or radiographic studies. In these circumstances, arthritis of the hip, radiculopathy, and inflammatory or autoimmune diseases should be excluded. Also, especially in the young athletic population, any previous injuries to the ipsilateral knee should be detailed owing to the potential for possible ligamentous deficiencies. It is also important to elicit a history of failed nonoperative and operative treatment, including steroid injections, oral anti-inflammatory medication, physical therapy, bracing, arthroscopic débridement, and osteotomy. It is sometimes difficult to determine whether a patient's pain is disabling; this is partially dependent on the individual patient's expectations and goals. Older or less active patients may be content if ambulation is limited to a few blocks so long as they have little discomfort with activity about the house. In distinction, younger patients may find it severely disabling to be limited to the same activity levels. In patients with high expectations, a frank discussion of the goals of knee replacement is necessary. The indications for unicompartmental arthroplasty versus TKR are reviewed in subsequent sections.

Physical Examination

Important findings include incisions about the knee, joint-line and peripatellar tenderness, crepitus, overall alignment of the knee, and varus and valgus deformities, for which it must be determined whether they are passively correctable to neutral. In addition, the passive range of motion, fixed flexion contractures, and extension lags should be noted. Distal pulses, strength, and sensation in the extremity should also be evaluated.

Diagnostic Aids

In most cases, plain radiographs of the affected knee are adequate for preoperative counseling. Our standard radiography series includes a weight-bearing anteroposterior view in full extension, a standing posteroanterior view in 45 degrees of flexion, a lateral view, and a merchant view (Fig. 28N–10A and B). These standard radiographic images allow comprehensive evaluation of the involved compartments. If joint-space narrowing is less remarkable, magnetic resonance imaging of the knee may identify meniscal disease or other intra-articular disease. In patients with pain out of proportion to the radiographic changes noted, magnetic resonance imaging may also be used to identify other, more rare pathologic processes such as avascular necrosis, stress fractures, and bone lesions. In the recreational athlete, serologic screening for rheumatologic diseases is rarely required, but this should be performed if any concerns are raised by the patient's history. Before knee replacement, we also routinely obtain a full-length three-joint view of the lower extremity; however, this is

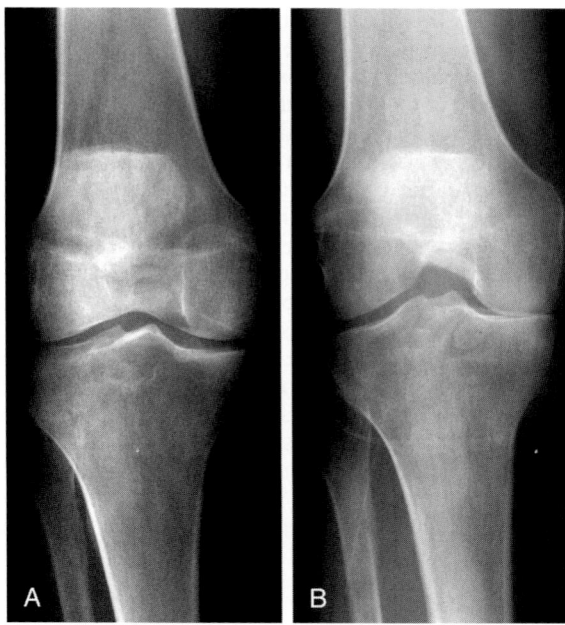

Figure 28N–10. *A*, Weight-bearing anteroposterior radiograph demonstrating medial compartment narrowing. *B*, Forty-five-degree weight-bearing posteroanterior flexion view in the same patient accentuates degenerative changes.

probably mandatory only if there is a history of fractures of the ipsilateral extremity or if the physical examination suggests unusual extra-articular deformities.

Treatment Options

Unicompartmental Arthroplasty

Because early reports on the long-term follow-up of unicondylar arthroplasty documented high revision rates, there was a significant decline in the use of this procedure during the early 1980s.[49] The use of these devices in selected patients who met specific criteria was continued, however, and has been associated with survival rates of approximately 80% to 85% at approximately 10 years.[32, 62, 93, 101] Unicompartmental replacement is currently undergoing a resurgence in popularity for unicompartmental arthritis both in the elderly population, in whom it may be considered a definitive procedure, and in younger patients, in whom some have reported that it is a superior temporizing procedure (compared with tibial osteotomy) before TKR.[16, 32, 91, 112] Although unicondylar replacement has a higher revision rate than does TKR at approximately 10 years, uncomplicated revision of unicondylar replacement to TKR has been used to justify this recent trend.[32] The development of minimally invasive surgical techniques has also contributed to the renewed interest in unicondylar arthroplasty because this procedure can be performed on an outpatient basis with a faster recovery than TKR. In a comparison study in which patients with either a unicondylar prosthesis or a total knee prosthesis were interviewed postoperatively, the unicondylar arthroplasty was associated with better range of motion and greater patient satisfaction.[69] Improved motion may be beneficial in the younger, more athletic population with symptomatic osteoarthritis. Despite these proposed benefits, there is no specific information documenting superior results versus TKR in the active, athletic population. Therefore, based on the excellent results that have been obtained at our institution with total knee prostheses, we continue to perform tricompartmental arthroplasty in the majority of young, active patients rather than osteotomy or unicompartmental replacement.[25, 80]

Total Knee Arthroplasty

By the 1980s, TKR had become accepted as the gold standard for salvage of the painful, arthritic knee. During the 1970s and 1980s, the development of the early condylar knee-resurfacing prosthesis occurred rapidly along two distinct evolutionary pathways, based on the management of the PCL. Early PCL-sacrificing prostheses evolved into PCL-substituting designs, which are distinct from the cruciate-retaining designs that spare the native PCL. A philosophical debate regarding the superiority of these design principles has been ongoing for years. Changes in the geometry of many cruciate-retaining designs during the 1990s to create more conforming articular surfaces have reduced some of the differences between these devices. In clinical practice, highly successful results have been documented at long-term follow-up with both cruciate-retaining and PCL-substituting designs. Good and excellent outcomes have been reported from independent centers at long-term follow-up in greater than 90% of patients.[22, 23, 82] Prosthesis survivorship free from revision also exceeds 90% at long-term follow-up.[22, 23, 82] Causes of failure include aseptic loosening, instability, infection, patellofemoral complications, periprosthetic fracture, and malalignment.[19, 34, 37, 41, 78, 79]

We have supported the use of posteriorly stabilized prostheses since their initial development and continue to use them in all patients. Despite the clinical success achieved with some designs of cruciate-retaining prostheses, we believe that certain features of the PCL-substituting designs are especially important in young, active patients. Recent studies have clarified many of the major points of contention in the debate about cruciate-retaining versus PCL-substituting knee replacement. These issues are reviewed in the context of the active patient in the following section. Additional factors that may influence prosthesis survival in athletes (e.g., limb alignment, fixation, and joint load) are also discussed within the framework of this debate.

Posterior Cruciate Ligament Retention versus Substitution

Surgical Exposure

Release of the cruciate ligaments facilitates surgical exposure, especially in tight knees, which makes the procedure less demanding. Also, it is technically easier to cut straight across the tibia than around the cruciate insertions.

These factors make it easier to make the correct bone cuts and to obtain accurate placement of the prosthesis. The importance of achieving tibiofemoral alignment close to 7 degrees of valgus to maximize long-term survival emphasizes the need for adequate exposure.[89, 103]

Correction of Deformity

Knees with significant preoperative fixed varus, valgus, or flexion deformities can be successfully managed with the use of PCL-retaining prostheses; however, the PCL is a deforming factor in these cases. Therefore, careful balancing of the PCL with release or recession may be required to achieve flexion- and extension-gap symmetry.[33, 88, 94] Balancing of the PCL may be difficult and seems to be experience dependent. In most circumstances, we believe that use of a posteriorly stabilized prosthesis is technically less difficult and allows more reliable correction of deformity. Failure to balance the PCL appropriately may lead to either reduced flexion or flexion instability.[82, 111, 115] Laskin has documented that in patients with fixed varus deformities exceeding 15 degrees in whom PCL-retaining rather than PCL-substituting prostheses were used, the results of knee replacement were inferior.[66] Finally, removal of the PCL and clearance of the intercondylar notch allow better visualization of the posterior knee. This facilitates capsular release and posterior osteophyte excision during correction of flexion deformities.

Kinematics

In the natural knee, tightening of the PCL during flexion produces femoral rollback. This rollback moves the tibiofemoral contact point posteriorly during flexion, which increases the quadriceps efficiency and range of motion. These effects were felt to be critical in activities such as stair climbing. Retention of the PCL was initially believed to allow preservation of normal knee kinematics after TKR.

In performing this function, the native PCL was initially perceived to be superior to the cam-and-post mechanism of posteriorly stabilized knee prostheses. Fluoroscopic studies, however, have demonstrated that PCL-retaining prostheses do not replicate the kinematics of the normal knee.[23, 99] Instead, in many cases, a paradoxical roll forward of the femur with anterior translation of the tibiofemoral contact area occurs. This motion is the direct opposite of normal knee kinematics and likely results from improper tension in the PCL. Adverse consequences may include decreased flexion and posterior tibial polyethylene wear. Although Dennis and coauthors demonstrated that posteriorly stabilized prostheses also do not completely reproduce normal knee kinematics, reliable femoral rollback occurred (Fig. 28N–11A and B).[23] Techniques for balancing the PCL have been described, but the success of these methods in restoring normal knee kinematics with cruciate-retaining prostheses has not yet been proven.[88, 94] The more reliable kinematics of the PCL-substituting designs is crucial to optimal function in the active patient.

Range of Motion

Experience with the use of the early cruciate-sacrificing total condylar prosthesis produced flexion of about 90 to 95 degrees. Improved flexion with both posteriorly stabilized and PCL-retaining prostheses has been reported. Averaged data from numerous studies document mean flexion of approximately 100 to 115 degrees with both types of prosthesis.[9, 82] With careful surgical technique, reliable passive flexion of 110 to 115 degrees should be obtainable with either type of prosthesis. Owing to the experience required to tension the PCL correctly, however, we believe that the posteriorly stabilized prosthesis produces more reproducible results. An improperly tensioned PCL that is left too tight can limit flexion. Arthroscopic release of the

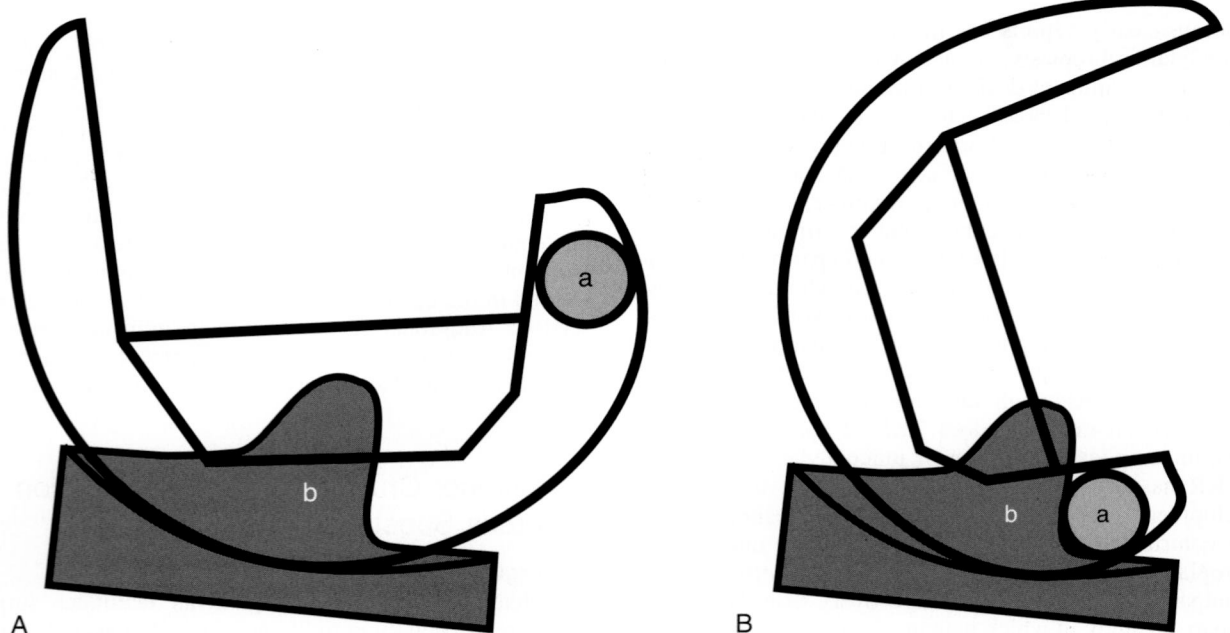

Figure 28N–11. *A,* The cam (a) and post (b) mechanisms of a posterior stabilized knee prosthesis. *B,* The interaction of the cam and the post as the prosthesis flexes results in femoral rollback and posterior translation of the femorotibial contact point.

tight PCL may improve flexion in selected patients with PCL-retaining prostheses.[115] Dennis and coauthors have also documented that maximum flexion of the knee under weight-bearing conditions is different from flexion measured passively.[24] Although neither cruciate-retaining nor PCL-substituting prostheses replicated normal knee flexion under weight-bearing conditions, the PCL-substituting design achieved significantly better results.

Evolution in the cam-and-post mechanism of posteriorly stabilized prostheses has made extreme flexion safer. In the latest design that we use, the cam engages the post at approximately 70 degrees and then rides down the post before eventually moving up the post with extreme flexion. This effectively increases the "jump distance" that must be exceeded before dislocation, which allows for a greater safety margin in positions of high flexion. In conjunction with slight changes in the sagittal radius of curvature of the posterior femoral condyles and more emphasis on removing the posterior osteophytes intraoperatively to reduce posterior impingement, this modification has helped increase the attainable flexion (Fig. 28N–12).

These concepts, in addition to further subtle modifications, are being incorporated into a new generation of "high flexion" posteriorly stabilized prostheses. With these designs, additional bone is resected from the posterior condyles, which allows augmentation of the posterior condyles of the prosthesis. This modification creates an enhanced bearing surface in deep flexion that eliminates the edge loading on the posterior polyethylene. Although good preoperative motion is probably the best predictor of postoperative motion, surgical technique and prosthesis design also play important roles. Therefore, in the athletic population, in whom range of motion under weight-bearing conditions is important, we believe that posteriorly stabilized prostheses are desirable.

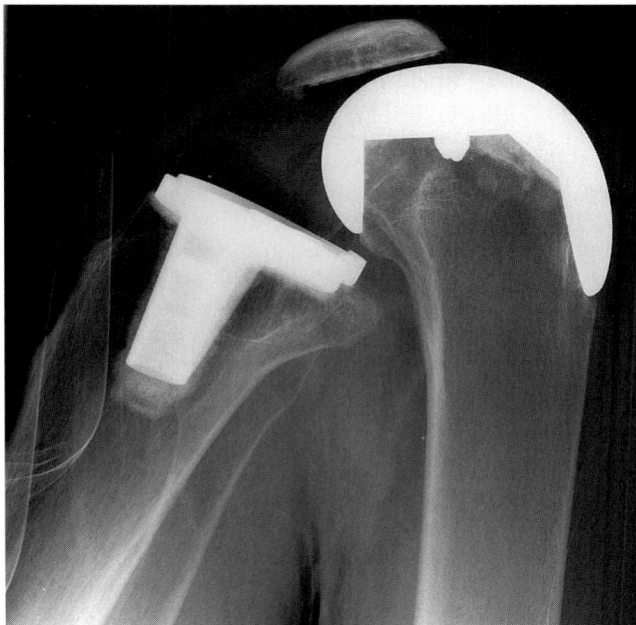

Figure 28N–12. Lateral radiograph of a posterior stabilized knee prosthesis in a highly flexed position, demonstrating rollback.

Proprioception

The cruciate ligaments contain mechanoreceptors; therefore, advocates of PCL retention have proposed that preserving the natural ligament would lead to superior proprioception after TKR. Recent reports have not demonstrated a clear advantage, however.[96, 110] Warren and coauthors have reported that although the improvement was greater in patients with a cruciate-retaining prosthesis, all patients had improved proprioception after TKR, regardless of whether a PCL-retaining or a PCL-substituting prosthesis was used.[110] This was speculated to be due to the elimination of pain and retensioning of the collateral ligaments and soft tissues. The inconclusive results may be due to the inherent qualities of the PCL in patients with arthritic knees. Significant degenerative changes in the PCLs of patients with arthritic knees exceeding those found in age-matched controls have been reported.[61] Therefore, the preserved PCL in a patient with a PCL-retaining prosthesis should not be expected to function in a normal manner, from either a biomechanical or a proprioceptive standpoint.

Gait Analysis

Early work suggested that the mechanics of walking and stair climbing were different in patients with PCL-retaining versus PCL-substituting prostheses.[3, 55] Andriacchi and associates described a characteristic forward lean of the trunk with less knee flexion in patients with PCL-substituting prostheses during stair climbing than in patients with PCL-retaining prostheses.[3] Recent gait analysis disputes these findings. Bolanos and coauthors were unable to identify any significant differences in spatiotemporal gait parameters or knee range of motion during level walking or stair climbing in either patients with PCL-retaining or those with PCL-substituting prostheses.[12]

Stability

Neither PCL-retaining nor PCL-substituting designs compensate for instability in the medial-lateral plane. Therefore, both require intact collateral ligaments for stability. In the anterior and posterior planes, the characteristics of the two designs are different. This results in different problems when adequate flexion-extension balance is not achieved. A less conforming tibial polyethylene insert should be used in PCL-retaining prostheses because kinematic conflict results during femoral rollback in flexion if a more conforming insert is used. If the PCL is improperly tensioned, anteroposterior instability may occur as the less conforming insert does little to prevent posterior translation of the femur. The phenomenon of symptomatic flexion instability in patients with PCL-retaining prostheses has recently gained widespread recognition.[82, 111] The consequences of a tight PCL have been previously discussed. Recent biomechanical studies have suggested that it is difficult to obtain the appropriate tension in the PCL.[48, 70] Although posteriorly stabilized prostheses eliminate the PCL as a factor in preventing adequate flexion-extension balancing, anterior and posterior instability can still occur. In some patients with significant flexion instability, the jump distance of the cam-and-post mechanism may be exceeded during extreme flexion, which results in acute dislocation. In previous series, a dislocation rate of 2% to 3% has been reported.[25, 86] Changes in the design of the cam-and-post mechanism have been successful in reducing dislocations.[86]

Polyethylene Wear

Polyethylene wear in posteriorly stabilized designs, which have moderately conforming articular surfaces, has not presented as a major clinical problem in older patients.[22, 86] These moderately conforming surfaces reduce the contact stresses in the polyethylene significantly (Fig. 28N–13).[6, 7] In contrast, the higher contact stresses encountered in the unconstrained, flat-on-flat articulations of PCL-retaining prostheses used during the 1980s in conjunction with thin, heat-pressed polyethylene inserts led to rapid wear in some cases.[11, 31, 59, 104] A trend toward more conforming polyethylene inserts in cruciate-retaining designs, in conjunction with PCL balancing, has reduced the differences in contact areas between these and cruciate-substituting designs; however, failure to balance the PCL may result in severe posteromedial polyethylene wear. The more conforming surfaces of the posteriorly stabilized implants seem better suited to optimizing long-term wear in active patients who are theoretically at risk for this problem.

Schmalzried and coauthors have documented that younger, male patients subject total joint replacements to significantly greater use.[92] Based on electronic pedometer measurements, the average patient took 4988 steps per day, which extrapolated to approximately 0.9 million cycles per year. The range was 395 to 17,718 steps per day, which represented approximately a 45-fold difference; in particular, men younger than 60 years of age walked 40% more than the average patient. Biomechanical analysis has also shown that high loads caused by high activity levels and increased patient weight routinely subject the polyethylene to stresses above the yield point.[65] In addition, polyethylene thickness and quality have been shown to be important factors in the rapid failure that occurred in cruciate-retaining prostheses in the 1980s.[6, 59] In view of these theoretical concerns, it seems desirable to use moderately conforming posteriorly stabilized prostheses, which provide larger contact areas, with polyethylene thickness greater than 10 mm in active patients.

Loosening

The increased constraint imposed by the moderately conforming articular surfaces of posteriorly stabilized prostheses was initially thought to be detrimental to long-term fixation at the cement-bone-prosthesis interface, owing to increased stress transmission. In distinction, a separate see-saw mechanism in cruciate-retaining devices, which resulted from the anteroposterior sliding of the femoral component on the less conforming tibial surface, was prob-

lematic. Despite these theoretical concerns, clinical studies have not shown aseptic loosening to be a significant problem in TKR, even in the young active patient. Survival rates free from aseptic loosening have been reported to be more than 90% at 10 years with both types of prostheses.[22, 71] Although clinical results have been favorable, the potential for an increased rate of failure in active patients should be considered because these devices may be subjected to 10 to 20 years of further use. Also, after total hip replacement, the rate of aseptic loosening in very active patients was twice that found in less active patients at 10 years.[58] The higher joint loads caused by obesity have also not been proven to produce higher clinical failure rates.[40]

During the 1980s, a trend toward cementless fixation was advocated in younger, more active patients for whom theoretical long-term advantages were anticipated.[47] This trend toward cementless fixation was intimately associated with the use of cruciate-retaining devices. The theoretical advantages of cementless fixation have not translated into clinical practice, however. Loosening rates at up to 10 years of follow-up have, at best, been equal to those in reported series of cemented posteriorly stabilized TKRs.[26, 90, 114] Currently, we continue to recommend cemented posteriorly stabilized prostheses in all patients.

Patellar Resurfacing

The role of patellar resurfacing in TKR has been another area of vigorous debate since the 1980s and is independent of the debate about cruciate retention or substitution. In North America, despite a recent trend toward selective resurfacing, the majority of surgeons continue to resurface the patella routinely; however, this is certainly not the standard of care around the world. Recent studies continue to support patellar resurfacing in most patients. Klebish and coauthors prospectively followed patients with bilateral TKAs in whom the patella was resurfaced on one side and not on the other.[60] The incidence of anterior knee pain was the same (10%) whether or not the patella was resurfaced, and both functional and subjective results were equivalent. Similar results have also been documented by Barrack and colleagues in another prospective study.[5] Again, function and pain scores were not statistically different, with approximately a 10% incidence of anterior knee pain. Patients in whom the patella had not been resurfaced had a significantly higher reoperation rate of 10%. This significantly higher complication rate has been confirmed by Boyd and associates.[13] These studies have failed to demonstrate any advantage to retaining the natural patella, and reoperation and complication rates were higher in patients in whom the patella was not resurfaced. Currently, patellar resurfacing remains the gold standard in TKR; therefore, we resurface the majority of the patellae with an all-polyethylene dome. In specific circumstances, we consider leaving the native patella intact. It may be advisable to omit patellar resurfacing in younger and more active patients if the articular surface has minimal degenerative changes. Also, Stern and Insall have documented that pain and complication rates are higher in obese patients who undergo resurfacing; therefore, this is another group in whom patellar resurfac-

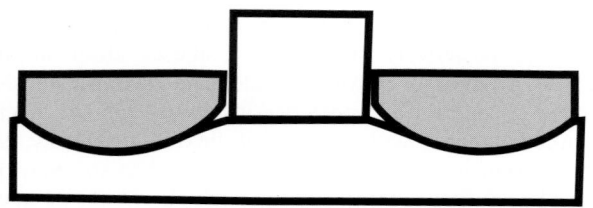

Figure 28N–13. Conforming femoral and tibial articular surfaces of a posterior stabilized prosthesis in the coronal plane.

ing may need to be avoided.[98] If patellar resurfacing is omitted, it seems desirable to use a femoral component that accommodates the natural patella. Therefore, the latest generation of posteriorly stabilized prostheses that we use has a side-specific femoral component and an extended trochlea with a more gradual transition with the distal condyles.

Future Developments in Knee Replacement

Conventional fixed-bearing knee prostheses have proven clinically successful with very favorable results at 10 to 15 years.[22] With only a few exceptions, these results have been obtained in older, less active patient populations.[25, 27] Despite the success achieved with posteriorly stabilized total knee prostheses, these devices have limitations. Concerns exist regarding the long-term durability of current prostheses in younger, more demanding patients. Polyethylene wear may be reduced by radical improvements in the inherent qualities of the material itself, which have not yet been realized, or by decreasing the contact stresses at the articular surfaces. Reduction in contact stresses can be achieved by increasing the conformity of the femoral component and the polyethylene insert. Owing to the inherent tradeoff that exists in fixed-bearing prostheses between conformity and freedom of motion, however, significant improvements in contact stresses are not feasible. Therefore, at present, a mobile-bearing prosthesis seems to represent the only plausible solution to this problem.

Mobile-Bearing Prostheses

A mobile-bearing prosthesis eliminates the relationship between articular conformity and freedom of rotation that exists in a fixed-bearing prosthesis. In a mobile-bearing prosthesis, rotation occurs at the interface between the superior surface of the tibial baseplate and the inferior surface of the polyethylene insert. In distinction, articular conformity is a property of the femoral component and the superior surface of the tibial polyethylene insert. In a mobile-bearing prosthesis, articular conformity can be maximized, thereby reducing contact stresses and wear on the superior surface of the polyethylene. Simultaneously, rotation can still occur at the undersurface. Although modern condylar prostheses have contact areas of approximately 100 to 300 mm², mobile-bearing designs provide contact areas in the range of 1000 mm². This increase in contact area reduces contact stresses from levels that routinely exceed the yield stress of polyethylene to safe levels.[51] At the same time that conformity is increased on the articular surface, rotation can also occur at the undersurface. With a fixed-bearing prosthesis, it is not possible to increase conformity and to allow rotation.

In addition to reducing wear on the articular surface, mobile-bearing designs may offer a solution to undersurface polyethylene wear. Undersurface wear has been recognized as a serious problem in fixed-bearing designs that have modular metal-backed tibial components.[51, 84] Debris is generated by undersurface motion between the tibial

baseplate and the polyethylene insert and may contribute to osteolysis. Although a number of different locking mechanisms have been designed, undersurface motion is ubiquitous in modern modular fixed-bearing designs.[84] Also, owing to manufacturing limitations, most tibial baseplates are made of unpolished titanium, which has poor bearing characteristics. Mobile-bearing prostheses paradoxically may offer a solution to undersurface debris generation and may allow the benefits of modular components, such as intraoperative sizing flexibility, to be retained. Because undersurface motion is intended in mobile-bearing designs, the interface can be optimized. In addition, because a locking mechanism is no longer required, the baseplate can be manufactured from highly polished cobalt chrome.

Many questions still remain about mobile-bearing prosthesis design. These issues include whether both rotation and translation should occur at the undersurface; whether the pivot point should be medialized, centralized, or anteriorized; whether stops to prevent bearing spinout are necessary; and whether the articular surface should be fully conforming or should have a decreasing contact area in flexion to optimize rollback. Many modern mobile-bearing designs are currently undergoing clinical evaluation, and further investigation will likely reveal the optimal in vivo characteristics. Despite the lack of long-term follow-up of new designs, the published long-term results for the original designs have been very favorable, with outcomes equal to those for the best fixed-bearing designs.[17, 52, 97] It seems likely that this class of knee prosthesis will offer significant advantages for the active, younger patient, including reduced polyethylene wear, better kinematics, and improved motion.

Authors' Preferred Method of Treatment

Technique of Total Knee Arthroplasty

Although prosthesis design certainly affects the outcome of TKR, this variable is largely beyond the control of most orthopaedic surgeons. In distinction, surgical technique is at least as important for successful results and is highly surgeon dependent, despite the instrumentation and the guides that have been developed to help make surgery easier and more reproducible. Regardless of the specific instrument system that is used, the surgical concepts remain the same. Crucial principles include adequate exposure, preparation of the bone surfaces, restoration of limb alignment, soft tissue balancing, selection of the correct component position, and closure. Before the incision, examination with the patient under anesthesia is performed to evaluate maximum flexion, the presence of flexion contractures, the integrity of the collateral soft tissue restraints, and whether the varus or valgus deformity can be passively corrected to neutral. Each of these factors must be considered and may require modifications in the basic surgical technique. For example, in patients with significant flexion contractures, we may elect to resect an additional 2 mm of distal femur. Furthermore, in these circumstances, we also elevate the capsule subperiosteally from the posterior femur. If the ligaments appear incompetent, a prosthesis with increased femoral-tibial constraint should be available for use. Finally, if the varus or valgus deformity can be corrected to neutral, a less aggressive soft tissue release should be anticipated than in a knee with a fixed deformity.

We favor an anterior midline skin incision. If a previous skin incision is present, we attempt to incorporate it unless large flaps would be created. Without extensive dissection, the quadriceps tendon is exposed, and a standard medial parapatellar arthrotomy is performed. The arthrotomy is begun at the superior aspect of the quadriceps tendon. The incision runs distally approximately 0.5 cm from the medial border of the tendon, curves around the patella, and continues along the medial border of the patellar tendon. The anterior horn of the medial meniscus is transected, and the medial capsule and the periosteum are elevated from the proximal 3 to 4 cm of the medial tibia. The infrapatellar fat pad is resected, and the patella is everted. If this is impossible, after the arthrotomy incision has been extended superiorly, a quadriceps snip is performed by continuing the incision from the apex of the arthrotomy into the fibers of the vastus lateralis at an angle of 45 degrees.[36]

Once it can be safely everted in extension, we like to prepare the patella. Remnants of the fat pad are excised from the patellar tendon, and any synovium is débrided from the quadriceps tendon. The patellar thickness is then measured at the high point, and marginal osteophytes are trimmed to allow accurate placement of the patellar reamer. We attempt to recreate the thickness of the patella or to reduce the composite thickness by 1 to 2 mm.

Once the patella has been prepared, the exposure about the tibia is continued. The varus knee and the valgus knee require different considerations. In the varus knee, the contracted anatomic structures on the medial side of the knee include the pes anserinus tendons, the superficial MCL, the posteromedial corner (including the semimembranosus insertion and the medial capsule), and the deep MCL. In this situation, the initial exposure of the medial tibia is extended distally and posteriorly to include subperiosteal elevation of the entire medial capsule and the superficial MCL. Next, the deep MCL is released from its attachment on the tibial plateau. The knee is then flexed, and both cruciate ligaments are released from the femur. The tibia is progressively externally rotated, and the subperiosteal elevation is continued sharply around the proximal tibia to include the insertion of the semimembranosus tendon at the posteromedial border. In distinction, in the valgus knee, the medial release should be limited. In this case, a ½ osteotome is used at the medial joint line to release the capsule from the margin of the tibial plateau. The superficial MCL is not elevated distally, however. In the flexed position, the cruciates are cut, and, if required for exposure, the semimembranosus insertion can be released from the posteromedial corner of the tibia.

Once adequate exposure has been obtained, preparation of the femur and the tibia is performed. Because they are independent, either the tibia or the femur may be cut first. Resection of the distal femur and the proximal tibia should achieve a desirable axis of 5 to 8 degrees of valgus alignment at the knee, with the components oriented perpendicular to the mechanical axis of the femur and the tibia. Both intramedullary and extramedullary referencing instrumentation has been developed. Currently, in primary knee replacement, we use an intramedullary referencing guide for the femur and an extramedullary guide for the tibia. In revision surgery, however, we also use an intramedullary guide for the tibia in many cases.

Although the tibia may be cut first, we begin with preparation of the femur. A starter hole is made in the distal femur slightly medial to the midline of the trochlea and just above the PCL origin. Before the intramedullary guide is inserted, the canal is suctioned to reduce the risk of fat embolism. The femoral intramedullary guide is set to produce a distal cut that is at 6 degrees of valgus angulation relative to the anatomic axis of the femur in the varus knee, and 4 to 5 degrees in the valgus knee. Although the exact sequence of events is system specific, the next important step is to perform anterior and posterior femoral cuts. Based on the dimensions of the distal femur, the appropriately sized anterior-posterior cutting guide is selected. We aim to resect the same thickness of bone from the posterior condyles as will be replaced by our femoral component without notching the anterior femur. If the dimensions of the femur are between sizes, we tend to select the larger size to avoid over-resection of the posterior condyles, which can make balancing flexion and extension gaps difficult. Once the appropriate size has been chosen, the anterior-posterior cutting guide is oriented parallel to the transepicondylar axis. This axis is defined by the center of the sulcus of the medial epicondyle and the high point of the lateral epicondyle, as described earlier in the anatomy section. These two points can be readily identified intraoperatively, and a line drawn between them on the distal femur is useful as a reference for positioning the cutting guide. The epicondylar axis has been shown to be the most reliable landmark for determining accurate femoral component rotation.[81] If the anterior-posterior guide is not oriented along this axis, the posterior condylar cuts will be rotated, which makes it difficult to produce a symmetric flexion space. In most circumstances, more bone will be resected from the posterior medial condyle, because in the varus knee the posterior condylar line is internally rotated by approximately 3 degrees relative to the epicondylar axis.[39] Once the guide has been correctly positioned, the anterior cut and the posterior condylar resections are performed.

On the tibial side, the extramedullary cutting guide is positioned to provide a cut perpendicular to the mechanical axis in the coronal plane and at approximately 7 degrees of posterior slope in the sagittal plane. After the bony cuts have been completed, the remnants of both cruciate ligaments and menisci should be excised. During excision of the medial meniscus—a potentially dangerous time—the fibers of the deep MCL that attach to the peripheral margin of the meniscus must be protected. In addition, posterior condylar osteophytes should be removed with an osteotome. Use of laminar spreaders can help provide the distraction that facilitates these steps. If there is a significant preoperative flexion contracture, a blunt periosteal elevator can be passed posteriorly through the notch to elevate the posterior capsule, which may act as a limiting force in restoring full extension.

Next, the largest spacer block that will fit in the flexion

gap is inserted, and stability is assessed. The orientation of the tibial cut is also evaluated. The knee is then brought into extension, and the overall alignment is assessed. We use an extramedullary guide rod to ensure that optimal overall limb alignment has been achieved from the hip to the center of the ankle. If the bone cuts fail to achieve the desired limb alignment, soft tissue balancing of the medial and lateral structures may be difficult to achieve. Furthermore, the abnormal mechanical stresses associated with chronic malalignment can lead to progressive laxity and instability. If appropriate femoral and tibial cuts have been made and the overall alignment is acceptable, the next crucial intraoperative step is to restore medial and lateral soft tissue balance. In addition to bone erosion, the development of deformity associated with degenerative arthritis involves contracture of the soft tissue structures on the concave side of the deformity and stretching of the structures on the convex side, as previously described.

The goal of soft tissue balancing is to release the tight structures to create a symmetric rectangular space in both flexion and extension. Failure to restore this soft tissue balance has the potential to lead to instability.[30] Although mild degrees of soft tissue imbalance appear to be clinically insignificant, it seems best to strive for optimal balance.[30] The techniques that we use to restore soft tissue balance adhere to the principles described by Insall, which require the release of the tight structures on the contracted side.[50] Other alternative techniques to tighten or imbricate the relatively elongated structures, such as the MCL in a valgus knee, have been also described.[63, 64]

The principles of soft tissue balancing described here are equally applicable to both primary and revision TKR. In the revision setting, however, preoperative ligament insufficiency, bone defects, and a higher risk of iatrogenic injury can complicate the balancing process; this discussion is beyond the scope of this chapter. Techniques for balancing the soft tissues in the varus and valgus knee are described subsequently.

In the varus knee, if the medial structures are still tight, an incremental release is performed to correct the imbalance. A ¾-inch straight osteotome is used to extend the subperiosteal elevation of the distal superficial MCL insertion and the deep fascia along the posteromedial border of the tibia (Fig. 28N–14). This release is extended to approximately the level of the middle third of the tibia. In addition, the pes tendons may or may not be released. In some cases, the popliteus tendon may impinge on the posterolateral aspect of the prosthesis; in these cases of varus deformity, it may be released. Next, the spacer is reinserted, and the efficacy of the release is evaluated. In many cases, once the extension space symmetry has been restored by the release, the next-thicker spacer block is required. If an imbalance persists, additional subperiosteal releases of any palpable tight bands should be performed distally.

In the valgus knee, the contracted anatomic structures

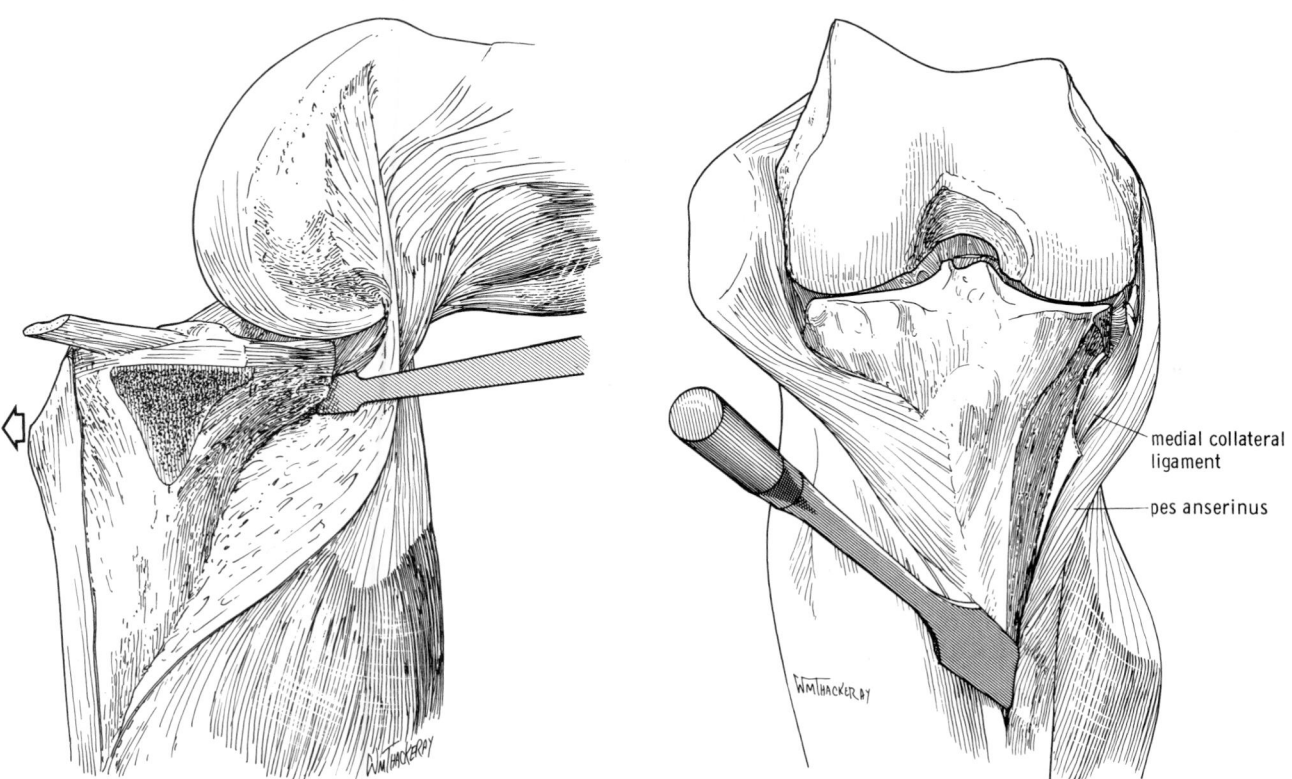

Figure 28N–14. Medial soft tissue releases in a knee with a fixed varus deformity. Subperiosteal release of the deep and superficial medial collateral ligament, the capsule, and the semimembranosus insertion about the proximal tibia (*left*). Complete release with subperiosteal elevation of the distal pes and the superficial medial collateral ligament insertions to the midtibia (*right*). (From Insall JN, Scott WN: Surgery of the Knee, 3rd ed. Philadelphia, WB Saunders, 2000.)

include the ITB, the LCL, the popliteus tendon, and the arcuate ligament–posterolateral capsular complex. If alignment is acceptable when the knee is brought into extension with the spacer block but the lateral side is tight, the spacer is removed and the laminar spreaders are inserted and gently opened. The lateral soft tissue structures are then released in a graduated fashion using an inside-out technique with the popliteus tendon as a landmark. The arcuate and the posterolateral capsular complexes are incised horizontally with a No. 15 blade at the level of the tibial bone cut. Next, multiple "pie crusting" puncture incisions are made through the ITB and the capsule, both at the level of the extension gap and proximal to the joint. Although no specific attempt is made to divide the LCL, it is likely that it is partially cut.

Once the extension gap appears to be rectangular, the spacer block is reinserted, and balance is re-evaluated. If at this stage the lateral side is still tight, further pie crusting is performed. In certain cases, the ITB may need to be totally released from Gerdy's tubercle. In the valgus knee, we avoid releasing the popliteus tendon if possible because this may provide stability in flexion and help prevent rotatory instability. In knees with severe valgus deformities, the lateral side may be tight despite maximal release. In these cases, it may be necessary to strip the lateral femoral condyle, including the insertion of the popliteus tendon. This can be done either sharply or by elevating a wafer of bone from the lateral epicondyle. In these situations, a prosthesis with increased femoral-tibial constraint may be required to provide medial and lateral stability. Use of a constrained prosthesis in elderly patients with significant valgus deformities has been associated with good long-term results despite theoretical concerns regarding loosening.[28]

Once a balanced extension space has been created in either the varus or the valgus knee, the knee is assessed to ensure that full extension is achieved without any tendency toward hyperextension. Finally, the flexion space must be re-evaluated to ensure that it is symmetric with the extension gap (Fig. 28N–15A and B). If flexion and extension gaps are not equal, further adjustments to the bone resection may be required. If the knee is balanced in flexion but tight in extension with a persistent flexion contracture, an additional 2 mm of femur must be removed, because femoral resection selectively changes only the extension gap. If the knee is so tight in both flexion and extension that the smallest 10-mm spacer cannot be inserted, then additional tibia must be cut, because tibial resection changes both flexion and extension gaps. In the primary setting, it is uncommon to find the knee balanced in extension and too tight in flexion. In this rare circumstance, over-resection of the posterior femoral condyles owing to the use of anterior referencing cutting guides or undersizing of the femoral component may be responsible. It may be necessary to resect an additional portion of distal femur and to use a larger polyethylene insert.

Once appropriate extension and flexion gap symmetry has been obtained, the bone surfaces can be prepared for final component positioning. On the femoral side, Chamfer cuts and a box cut for the posteriorly stabilized component must be made. The guide for these cuts should be positioned so that the component is lateralized to optimize patellar tracking without creating overhang. Next, tibial

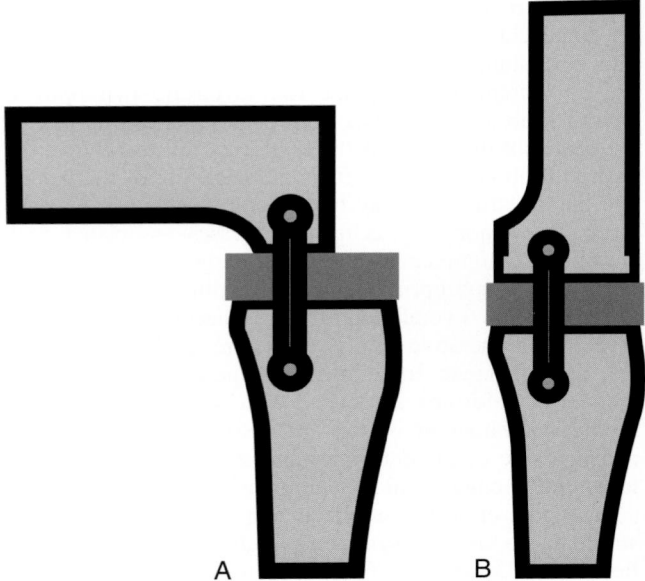

Figure 28N–15. Symmetric flexion (*A*) and extension (*B*) gaps.

rotation is set so that the center of the component is oriented in line with the junction of the medial and middle thirds of the tibial tubercle. Internal rotation may result in patellar subluxation. Finally, the patellar component is positioned slightly medially and superiorly on the prepared surface, which helps prevent patellar maltracking.

Once these steps have been completed, a trial using temporary components is performed to ensure that appropriate soft tissue balance has been achieved without flexion contracture or hyperextension. If imperfections exist, adjustments are made. A no-thumbs technique is used to evaluate patellar tracking. If femoral and tibial rotation has been correctly set, the thickness of the patella has been reproduced, and the other techniques for optimizing patellar tracking have been used, patellar subluxation is uncommon in the varus knee. If no technical errors can be identified and maltracking is present, we do not hesitate to perform a lateral patellar release. Once the result with the trial components is acceptable, the surfaces are cleaned and dried, and the real components are cemented in place. After the cement has hardened, we routinely drop the tourniquet and cauterize any significant bleeding vessels. The joint is irrigated, and a deep drain is placed before arthrotomy closure, which is performed in extension. After skin closure, a light sterile dressing is used, which permits immediate passive motion.

Postoperative Management and Rehabilitation

Perioperative Rehabilitation

In the immediate postoperative period, we use patient-controlled analgesia for pain control and continuous passive motion beginning in the recovery room. Passive flexion is advanced as tolerated, and the importance of active extension is emphasized to the patient. Ambulation with weight-bearing as tolerated is begun on postoperative day 1 without limitation. Early goals include independent transfers, walking as tolerated, and active motion from full extension to 90 degrees of flexion.

Criteria for Return to Sports Participation

By 3 weeks, most patients are walking with a cane and have gained active motion from full extension to greater than 90 degrees of flexion. Quadriceps strengthening, stationary biking, motion, and independent ambulation are advanced as tolerated. Swimming is encouraged once the staples are removed if the incision is well healed. If the patient can walk without a limp, activity is advanced; activity is somewhat patient specific depending on rate of recovery and goals. Putting and a gentle game of golf may be possible by 6 weeks, but a return to full activity is usually not practical until 3 months postoperatively. At 3 months, return to more vigorous activities such as golf, cross-country skiing, and doubles tennis may be possible. Interest in other activities is rare, and a return to other sports is based on individual progress. Factors such as persistence of swelling, equal return of quadriceps strength, absence of limp, achievement of required motion, and previous expertise are all considered.

Guidelines for Sports after Total Knee Replacement

Few reports have been published that specifically address the impact of sports on TKR.[14, 72–74] Although overall activity levels seem to increase after TKR owing to decreased pain and better function, it appears that it is relatively uncommon for patients to take up new sports.[14, 22] In view of the limited published information, recommendations for patient participation in sports after TKR are based on consensus. Theoretical concerns about sports after joint replacement include the risk of increased wear, loosening, and periprosthetic fractures related to falls.[20, 58] Mallon and coauthors surveyed members of the Knee Society about golf and found that 93% of the respondents did not limit participation after knee replacement; however, 66% recommended use of a cart.[72–74] Concern about the effects of the torque associated with the terminal swing led some members to warn against golf.[74]

Twenty-eight orthopaedic surgeons at the Mayo Clinic were surveyed to delineate activities that were recommended after TKR.[77] Responses from the attending surgeons were not significantly different from those of the house staff, except that residents and fellows were less likely to recommend participation in cross-country skiing. Sports recommended by more than 85% of respondents included swimming, cycling, golfing, bowling, sailing, and scuba diving; in distinction, sports recommended by fewer than 30% of the surgeons included jogging, baseball, bas-

ketball, football, hockey, handball, karate, soccer, racquetball, and water-skiing.[77] General principles for participation in sports were also discussed. Among the suggestions were the following:

1. Expectations about return to sports should be discussed preoperatively.
2. The benefits of exercise should be reviewed.
3. Patients should be informed about the theoretical concerns affecting prosthesis survival.
4. Return to low-impact sports should be encouraged.
5. High-impact sports should be discouraged.
6. Patient-specific factors should be considered.[77]

We agree with these general recommendations and base individual participation on similar principles.

Effect of Sports after Total Knee Replacement

Few reports have evaluated knee replacements in athletes. Mallon and coauthors have reported extensively on participation in golf after joint replacement.[72–74] After TKR, active golfers experienced a significant increase in their handicap (mean +4.6 strokes) and a decrease in the length of their drives. Also, the game caused discomfort in some golfers, with 15.7% experiencing a mild ache while playing and 34.9% experiencing mild ache after playing.[73] In addition, right-handed golfers with a left TKR were more likely to experience pain. This was speculated to be due to the increased torque experienced by the left knee at the end of the drive.[73] Based on these limited studies, it is difficult to draw specific conclusions about the impact of sports participation after knee replacement on prosthesis survival. Therefore, the best guidelines remain the reports on TKR in young, active patients reviewed previously.[25, 27]

Summary

In the young, active population, TKR has proven durable at intermediate- to long-term follow-up. Future modifications of prosthesis design to allow improved motion and to reduce polyethylene wear (e.g., mobile bearings) may further improve function and prosthesis survival. These changes remain unproven, however. Advances in unicondylar replacement have led to a resurgence of interest in this device. It is likely that increased use of this prosthesis as a less invasive temporary patch will occur in younger, active patients who are reluctant to undergo total joint replacement. Despite the advances in prosthesis design, the importance of optimal surgical technique in maximizing long-term survival must not be ignored. Unlike prosthesis design, which largely falls outside the control of most surgeons, surgical technique is highly dependent on the skill of the individual. Technical factors (e.g., restoration of limb alignment and soft tissue balance) that have been shown to enhance prosthesis survival should be emphasized. Although a well-designed prosthesis that is implanted in an optimal manner seems to be capable of withstanding the significant stresses associated with low-impact sports (e.g., walking, bicycling, swimming, and golf), persistent concerns exist regarding prosthesis survival under high-activity conditions. Therefore, research into all elements of materials development, prosthesis design, surgical technique, and alternative treatment solutions should be continued.

References

1. Aglietti P, Insall JN, Cerulli G, et al: Patella pain and incongruence. I: Measurements of incongruence. Clin Orthop 176:217–224, 1983.
2. Aglietti P, Insall JN, Walker PS, et al: A new patella prosthesis: Design and application. Clin Orthop 107:175–187, 1975.
3. Andriacchi TP, Galante JO, Fermier RW: The influence of total knee-replacement design on walking and stair-climbing. J Bone Joint Surg Am 64:1328–1335, 1982.
4. Baker CL, Norwood LA, Hughston JC: Acute posterolateral rotatory instability of the knee. J Bone Joint Surg Am 65:614–618, 1983.
5. Barrack RL, Wolfe MW, Waldman DA, et al: Resurfacing of the patella in total knee arthroplasty: A prospective, randomized, double-blind study. J Bone Joint Surg Am 79:1121–1131, 1997.
6. Bartel DL, Bicknell VL, Wright TM: The effect of conformity, thickness, and material on stresses in ultra-high molecular weight components for total joint replacement. J Bone Joint Surg Am 68:1041–1051, 1986.
7. Bartel DL, Rawlinson JJ, Burstein AH, et al: Stresses in polyethylene components of contemporary total knee replacements. Clin Orthop 317:76–82, 1995.
8. Basmajian JV, Lovejoy JF Jr: Functions of the popliteus muscle in man: A multifactorial electromyographic study. J Bone Joint Surg Am 53:557–562, 1971.
9. Becker MW, Insall JN, Farris PM: Bilateral total knee arthroplasty: One cruciate retaining and one cruciate substituting. Clin Orthop 271:122–124, 1991.
10. Berger RA, Rubash HE, Seel MJ, et al: Determining the rotational alignment of the femoral component in total knee arthroplasty using the epicondylar axis. Clin Orthop 286:40–47, 1993.
11. Bloebaum RD, Nelson K, Dorr LD, et al: Investigation of early surface delamination observed in retrieved heat-pressed tibial inserts. Clin Orthop 269:120–127, 1991.
12. Bolanos AA, Colizza WA, McCann PD, et al: A comparison of isokinetic strength testing and gait analysis in patients with posterior cruciate-retaining and substituting knee arthroplasties. J Arthroplasty 13:906–915, 1998.
13. Boyd AD, Ewald FC, Thomas WH, et al: Long-term complications after total knee arthroplasty with or without resurfacing of the patella. J Bone Joint Surg Am 75:674–681, 1993.
14. Bradbury N, Borton D, Spoo G, et al: Participation in sports after total knee replacement. Am J Sports Med 26:530–535, 1998.
15. Brantigan OC, Voshell AF: The tibial collateral ligament: Its function, its bursae, and its relation to the medial meniscus. J Bone Joint Surg 25:121–131, 1943.
16. Broughton NS, Newman JH, Baily RA: Unicompartmental replacement and high tibial osteotomy for osteoarthritis of the knee. A comparative study after 5–10 years' follow-up. J Bone Joint Surg Br 68:447–452, 1986.
17. Buechel FF, Pappas MJ: Long-term survivorship analysis of cruciate-sparing versus cruciate-sacrificing knee prostheses using meniscal bearings. Clin Orthop 260:162–169, 1990.
18. Butler DL, Noyes FR, Grood ES: Ligamentous restraints to anterior-posterior drawer in the human knee: A biomechanical study. J Bone Joint Surg Am 62:259–270, 1980.
19. Cameron HU, Hunter GA: Failure in total knee arthroplasty: Mechanisms, revisions, and results. Clin Orthop 170:141–146, 1982.
20. Cirincione RJ: Sports after total joint replacement. Md Med J 45:644–647, 1996.
21. Clancy WG, Shelbourne KD, Zoellner GB, et al: Treatment of knee joint instability secondary to rupture of the posterior cruciate ligament: Report of a new procedure. J Bone Joint Surg Am 65:310–322, 1983.
22. Colizza WA, Insall JN, Scuderi GR: The posterior stabilized total knee prosthesis: Assessment of polyethylene damage and osteolysis after a ten-year-minimum follow-up. J Bone Joint Surg Am 77:1713–1720, 1995.
23. Dennis DA, Komistek RD, Hoff WA, et al: In vivo knee kinematics derived using an inverse perspective technique. Clin Orthop 331:107–117, 1996.
24. Dennis DA, Komistek RD, Stiehl JB, et al: Range of motion after total knee arthroplasty: The effect of implant design and weight-bearing conditions. J Arthroplasty 13:748–752, 1998.
25. Diduch DR, Insall JN, Scott WN, et al: Total knee replacement in young active patients: Long-term follow-up and functional outcome. J Bone Joint Surg Am 79:575–582, 1997.
26. Duffy GP, Berry DJ, Rand JA: Cement versus cementless fixation in total knee arthroplasty. Clin Orthop 356:66–72, 1998.
27. Duffy GP, Trousdale RT, Stuart MJ: Total knee arthroplasty in patients 55 years old or younger. 10- to 17-year results. Clin Orthop 356:22–27, 1998.
28. Easley ME, Scuderi GR, Insall JN: Results of primary constrained condylar knee arthroplasty for knee arthritis associated with valgus deformity. Paper presented at the 67th Annual Meeting of the American Academy of Orthopaedic Surgeons, Orlando, Fla, March 15–19, 2000.
29. Eckhoff DG, Burke BJ, Dwyer TF, et al: Sulcus morphology of the distal femur. Clin Orthop 331:23–28, 1996.
30. Edwards E, Millar J, Chan C: An assessment of the effect of collateral ligament instability on results following total knee replacement. J Bone Joint Surg Br 71:338–339, 1989.
31. Engh GA: Failure of the polyethylene bearing surface of a total knee replacement within four years. A case report. J Bone Joint Surg Am 70:1093–1096, 1988.
32. Engh GA, McAuley JP: Unicondylar arthroplasty: An option for high-demand patients with gonarthrosis. Instr Course Lect 48:143–148, 1999.
33. Firestone TP, Krackow KA, Davis JD IV, et al: The management of fixed flexion contractures during total knee arthroplasty. Clin Orthop 284:221–227, 1992.
34. Friedman RJ, Hirst P, Poss R, et al: Results of revision total knee arthroplasty performed for aseptic loosening. Clin Orthop 255:235–241, 1990.
35. Furman W, Marshall JL, Girgis FG: The anterior cruciate ligament: A functional analysis based on postmortem studies. J Bone Joint Surg Am 58:179–185, 1976.
36. Garvin KL, Scuderi G, Insall JN: Evolution of the quadriceps snip. Clin Orthop 321:131–137, 1995.
37. Goldberg VM, Figgie MP, Figgie HE III, et al: The results of revision total knee arthroplasty. Clin Orthop 226:86–92, 1988.
38. Goodfellow J, Hungerford DS, Zindel M: Patello-femoral mechanics and pathology. I. Functional anatomy of the patello-femoral joint. J Bone Joint Surg Br 58:287–290, 1976.
39. Griffin FM, Insall JN, Scuderi GR: The posterior condylar angle in osteoarthritic knees. J Arthroplasty 13:812–815, 1998.
40. Griffin FM, Scuderi GR, Insall JN, et al: Total knee arthroplasty in patients who were obese with 10 years followup. Clin Orthop 356:28–33, 1998.
41. Haas SB, Insall JN, Montgomery W III, et al: Revision total knee arthroplasty with use of modular components with stems inserted without cement. J Bone Joint Surg Am 77:1700–1707, 1995.
42. Hsieh HH, Walker PS: Stabilizing mechanisms of the loaded and unloaded knee joint. J Bone Joint Surg Am 58:87–93, 1976.
43. Hughston JC, Andrews JR, Cross MJ, et al: Classification of knee ligament instabilities. Part I. The medial compartment and cruciate ligaments. J Bone Joint Surg Am 58:159–172, 1976.
44. Hughston JC, Andrews JR, Cross MJ, et al: Classification of knee ligament instabilities. Part II. The lateral compartment. J Bone Joint Surg Am 58:173–179, 1976.
45. Hughston JC, Norwood LA Jr: The posterolateral drawer test and external rotational recurvatum test for posterolateral rotatory instability of the knee. Clin Orthop 147:82–87, 1980.
46. Hungerford DS, Barry M: Biomechanics of the patellofemoral joint. Clin Orthop 144:9–15, 1979.
47. Hungerford DS, Krackow KA, Kenna RV: Cementless total knee replacement in patients 50 years old and under. Orthop Clin North Am 20:131–145, 1989.
48. Incavo SJ, Johnson CC, Beynnon BD, Howe JG: Posterior cruciate ligament strain biomechanics in total knee arthroplasty. Clin Orthop 309:88–93, 1994.

49. Insall J, Aglietti P: A five- to seven-year follow-up of unicondylar arthroplasty. J Bone Joint Surg Am 62:1329–1337, 1980.
50. Insall JN: Surgical techniques and instrumentation in total knee arthroplasty. In Insall JN (ed): Surgery of the Knee, 2nd ed. New York, Churchill Livingstone, 1993, pp 739–780.
51. Insall JN: Adventures in mobile-bearing knee design: A midlife crisis. Orthopedics 21:1021–1023, 1998.
52. Jordan LR, Olivo JL, Voorhorst PE: Survivorship analysis of cementless meniscal bearing total knee arthroplasty. Clin Orthop 338:119–123, 1997.
53. Kaplan EB: The fabellofibular and short lateral ligaments of the knee joint. J Bone Joint Surg Am 43:169–179, 1961.
54. Kaufer H: Mechanical function of the patella. J Bone Joint Surg Am 53:1551–1560, 1971.
55. Kelman GJ, Biden EN, Wyatt MP, et al: Gait laboratory analysis of a posterior cruciate-sparing total knee arthroplasty in stair ascent and descent. Clin Orthop 248:21–25, 1989.
56. Kennedy JC, Fowler PJ: Medial and anterior instability of the knee: An anatomical and clinical study using stress machines. J Bone Joint Surg Am 53:1257–1270, 1971.
57. Kennedy JC, Hawkins RJ, Willis RB, et al: Tension studies of human knee ligaments: Yield point, ultimate failure, and disruption of the cruciate and tibial collateral ligaments. J Bone Joint Surg Am 58:350–355, 1976.
58. Kilgus DJ, Dorey FJ, Finerman GA, et al: Patient activity, sports participation, and impact loading on the durability of cemented total hip replacements. Clin Orthop 269:25–31, 1991.
59. Kilgus DJ, Moreland JR, Finerman GA, et al: Catastrophic wear of tibial polyethylene inserts. Clin Orthop 273:223–231, 1991.
60. Klebish PA, Varma AK, Greenwald AS: Patellar resurfacing or retention in total knee arthroplasty. J Bone Joint Surg Br 76:930–937, 1994.
61. Kleinbart FA, Bryk E, Evangelista J, et al: Histologic comparison of posterior cruciate ligaments from arthritic and age-matched knee specimens. J Arthroplasty 11:726–731, 1996.
62. Kozinn SC, Scott R: Unicondylar knee arthroplasty. J Bone Joint Surg Am 71:145–150, 1989.
63. Krackow KA, Holtgrewe JL: Experience with a new technique for managing severely overcorrected valgus high tibial osteotomy at total knee arthroplasty. Clin Orthop 258:213–224, 1990.
64. Krackow KA, Jones MM, Teeny SM, et al: Primary total knee arthroplasty in patients with fixed valgus deformity. Clin Orthop 273:9–18, 1991.
65. Kuster MS, Wood GA, Stachowiak GW, et al: Joint load considerations in total knee replacement. J Bone Joint Surg Br 79:109–113, 1997.
66. Laskin RS: Total knee replacement with posterior cruciate ligament retention in patients with a fixed varus deformity. Clin Orthop 331:29–34, 1996.
67. Last RJ: Some anatomical details of the knee joint. J Bone Joint Surg Br 30:683–688, 1948.
68. Last RJ: The popliteus muscle and the lateral meniscus. J Bone Joint Surg Br 32:93–99, 1950.
69. Laurencin CT, Zelicof SB, Scott RD, et al: Unicompartmental versus total knee arthroplasty in the same patient. A comparative study. Clin Orthop 273:151–156, 1992.
70. Mahoney OM, Noble PC, Rhoads DD, et al: Posterior cruciate function following total knee arthroplasty: A biomechanical study. J. Arthroplasty 9:569–578, 1994.
71. Malkani AL, Rand JA, Bryan RS, Wallrichs SL: Total knee arthroplasty with the kinematic condylar prosthesis. A ten-year follow-up study. J Bone Joint Surg Am 77:423–431, 1995.
72. Mallon WJ, Callaghan JJ: Total knee arthroplasty in active golfers. J Arthroplasty 8:299–306, 1993.
73. Mallon WJ, Callaghan JJ: Total joint replacement in active golfers. J South Orthop Assoc 3:295–298, 1994.
74. Mallon WJ, Liebelt RA, Mason JB: Total joint replacement and golf. Clin Sports Med 15:179–190, 1996.
75. Mann RA, Hagy JL: The popliteus muscle. J Bone Joint Surg Am 59:924–927, 1977.
76. Marshall JL, Girgis FG, Zelko RR: The biceps femoris tendon and its functional significance. J Bone Joint Surg Am 54:1444–1450, 1972.
77. McGrory BJ, Stuart MJ, Sim FH: Participation in sports after hip and knee arthroplasty: Review of literature and survey of surgeon preferences. Mayo Clin Proc 70:342–348, 1995.
78. Moreland JR: Mechanisms of failure in total knee arthroplasty. Clin Orthop 226:49–64, 1988.
79. Murray PB, Rand JA, Hanssen AD: Cemented long-stem revision total knee arthroplasty. Clin Orthop 309:116–123, 1994.
80. Nagel A, Insall JN, Scuderi GR: Proximal tibial osteotomy. A subjective outcome study. J Bone Joint Surg Am 78:1353–1358, 1996.
81. Olcott CW, Scott RD: A comparison of 4 intraoperative methods to determine femoral component rotation during total knee arthroplasty. J Arthroplasty 15:22–26, 2000.
82. Pagnano MW, Cushner FD, Scott WN: Role of the posterior cruciate ligament in total knee arthroplasty. J Am Acad Orthop Surg 6:176–187, 1998.
83. Pagnano MW, Hanssen AD, Lewallen DG, Stuart MJ: Flexion instability after primary posterior cruciate retaining total knee arthroplasty. Clin Orthop 356:39–46, 1998.
84. Parks NL, Engh GA, Topoleski LD, et al: The Coventry Award. Modular tibial insert micromotion. A concern with contemporary knee implants. Clin Orthop 356:10–15, 1998.
85. Poilvache PL, Insall JN, Scuderi GR, et al: Rotational landmarks and sizing of the distal femur in total knee arthroplasty. Clin Orthop 331:35–46, 1996.
86. Ranawat CS, Luessenhop CP, Rodriguez JS: The press-fit condylar modular total knee system: Four-to-six-year results with a posterior-cruciate-substituting design. J Bone Joint Surg Am 79:342–348, 1997.
87. Reider B, Marshall JL, Koslin B, et al: The anterior aspect of the knee joint: An anatomical study. J Bone Joint Surg Am 63:351–356, 1981.
88. Ritter MA, Faris PM, Keating EM: Posterior cruciate ligament balancing during total knee arthroplasty. J Arthroplasty 3:323–326, 1988.
89. Ritter MA, Faris PM, Keating EM, et al: Postoperative alignment of total knee replacement: Its effect on survival. Clin Orthop 299:153–156, 1994.
90. Rosenberg AG, Barden RM, Galante JO: Cemented and ingrowth fixation of the Miller-Galante prosthesis. Clinical and roentgenographic comparison after three- to six-year follow-up studies. Clin Orthop 260:71–79, 1990.
91. Schai PA, Suh JT, Thornhill TS, et al: Unicompartmental knee arthroplasty in middle-aged patients: A 2- to 6-year follow-up evaluation. J Arthroplasty 13:365–372, 1998.
92. Schmalzried TP, Szuszczewicz ES, Northfield MR, et al: Quantitative assessment of walking activity after total hip or knee replacement. J Bone Joint Surg Am 80:54–59, 1998.
93. Scott RD, Cobb AG, McQueary FG, et al: Unicompartmental knee arthroplasty. Eight- to 12-year follow-up evaluation with survivorship analysis. Clin Orthop 271:96–100, 1991.
94. Scott RD, Thornhill TS: Posterior cruciate supplementing total knee replacements using conforming inserts and cruciate recession: Effect on range of motion and radiolucent lines. Clin Orthop 309:146–149, 1994.
95. Seebacher JR, Inglis AE, Marshall JL, et al: The structure of the posterolateral aspect of the knee. J Bone Joint Surg Am 64:536–541, 1982.
96. Simmons S, Lephart S, Rubash H, et al: Proprioception after unicondylar knee arthroplasty versus total knee arthroplasty. Clin Orthop 331:179–184, 1996.
97. Sorrells RB: The rotating platform mobile bearing TKA. Orthopedics 19:793–796, 1996.
98. Stern SH, Insall JN: Total knee arthroplasty in obese patients. J Bone Joint Surg Am 72:1400–1404, 1990.
99. Stiehl JB, Komistek RD, Dennis DA, et al: Fluoroscopic analysis of kinematics after posterior-cruciate-retaining knee arthroplasty. J Bone Joint Surg Br 77:884–889, 1995.
100. Sullivan D, Levy IM, Sheskier S, et al: Medial restraints to anterior-posterior motion of the knee. J Bone Joint Surg Am 66:930–936, 1984.
101. Tabor OB Jr, Tabor OB: Unicompartmental arthroplasty: A long-term follow-up study. J Arthroplasty 13:373–379, 1998.
102. Terry GC, LaPrade RF: The biceps femoris muscle complex at the knee: Its anatomy and injury patterns associated with acute anterolateral-anteromedial rotatory instability. Am J Sports Med 24:2–8, 1996.
103. Tew M, Waugh W: Tibiofemoral alignment and the results of knee replacement. J Bone Joint Surg Br 67:551–556, 1985.

104. Tsao A, Mintz L, McRae CR, et al: Failure of the porous-coated anatomic prosthesis in total knee arthroplasty due to severe polyethylene wear. J Bone Joint Surg Am 75:19–26, 1993.

105. United States Bureau of the Census: Current population reports, series P23-194, population profile of the United States: 1997. Washington, DC, U.S. Government Printing Office, 1998, pp 50–51.

106. Van Dommelen BA, Fowler PJ: Anatomy of the posterior cruciate ligament: A review. Am J Sports Med 17:24–29, 1989.

107. Vince KG: Evolution of total knee arthroplasty. In Scott WN (ed): The Knee. St. Louis, Mosby-Year Book, 1994, pp 1045–1049.

108. Warren LF, Marshall JL: The supporting structures and layers on the medial side of the knee: An anatomical analysis. J Bone Joint Surg Am 61:56–62, 1979.

109. Warren LF, Marshall JL, Girgis FG: The prime static stabilizer of the medial side of the knee. J Bone Joint Surg Am 56:665–674, 1974.

110. Warren PJ, Olanlokun TK, Cobb AG, Bentley G: Proprioception after total knee arthroplasty: The influence of prosthetic design. Clin Orthop 297:182–187, 1993.

111. Waslewski GL, Marson BM, Benjamin JB: Early, incapacitating instability of posterior cruciate ligament-retaining total knee arthroplasty. J Arthroplasty 13:763–767, 1998.

112. Weale AE, Newman JH: Unicompartmental arthroplasty and high tibial osteotomy for osteoarthrosis of the knee. A comparative study with a 12- to 17-year follow-up period. Clin Orthop 302:134–137, 1994.

113. Welsh PR: Knee joint structure and function. Clin Orthop 147:7–14, 1980.

114. Whiteside LA: Cementless total knee replacement. Nine- to 11-year results and 10-year survivorship analysis. Clin Orthop 309:185–192, 1994.

115. Williams RJ III, Westrich GH, Siegel J, Windsor RE: Arthroscopic release of the posterior cruciate ligament for stiff total knee arthroplasty. Clin Orthop 331:185–191, 1996.

CHAPTER TWENTY-NINE

The Leg

Jack T. Andrish, MD

This chapter deals with an interesting spectrum of injuries to the leg. Although divergent in their underlying pathoanatomy, the clinical presentations may overlap considerably. The literature supports an incidence of leg injury presenting to a sports medicine clinic ranging from 4.07% to 30%.[35, 74, 84, 124, 130] These figures, of course, are highly influenced by the practice profile of the particular clinic reporting and of the attending doctor. As we will see, confusion and controversy exist in the literature for many of these conditions. On the other hand, clear statements can be made about most of them regarding clinical presentation, underlying pathoanatomy, and treatment recommendations.

The Shin Splint Syndrome

Although the term *shin splint syndrome* is outdated and should probably be abandoned, the sheer magnitude of its common usage ensures its survival. Over the years, it has been applied to virtually any pain occurring in the lower leg as a result of overuse, usually from running or marching. In 1966, the American Medical Association, Subcommittee on Classification of Sports Injuries, issued a definition stating that the term *shin splints* refers to a condition that produces pain and discomfort in the leg owing to repetitive running or hiking.[4] Further, the condition should be limited to musculotendinous inflammations and should exclude stress fractures and ischemic disorders. Followed closely, this definition eliminates not only stress fractures but also acute and chronic compartment syndromes. In a general sense, however, these two entities will always figure prominently in the differential diagnosis of leg pains in the running athlete.

Shin splints account for about 13% of injuries in runners.[23, 74] In a prospective study of shin splints at the United States Naval Academy, the incidence of this disorder during "plebe summer" was found to be 4.07%.[7]

The exact nature of shin splints has been described in various ways in the literature. Because pain is most commonly located over the posteromedial border of the tibia in the middle and distal thirds of the leg, the condition has been felt to arise from an overload on the posterior tibial tendon.[104, 164] As we will see, this is probably an incorrect assumption, and the term *medial tibial stress syndrome,* proposed by Drez, is more appropriate.[110] Indeed, in this chapter we consider these terms to be interchangeable but refer to the syndrome as more precisely one of medial tibial stress.

Patients with medial tibial stress syndrome present with pain. The pain is initially felt on exertion and then may be relieved with continued running. The pain may recur toward the end of the workout or after running. At times, the pain is described as a dull ache or soreness. As the condition advances, the pain may be perceived as sharp, penetrating, and severe. As it becomes more severe, the pain can extend throughout the time of exertion and can impair, if not prohibit, performance. With time and continued abuse, the leg pain may be present with activities of daily living.

As with most overuse syndromes, shin splints seem to occur when there has been a significant change in activity. The unconditioned individual who decides to become a jogger and pursues this goal with unrealistic intensity is prone to develop shin splints. In fact, the experience described at the Naval Academy demonstrated that twice as many of the midshipmen who developed shin splints had no previous training before entering the Academy's rigorous physical education program as their counterparts who did not develop shin splints.[7] On the other hand, the shin splint syndrome is certainly not restricted to the unconditioned or ill-prepared athlete. Changes in footwear, running surface, and terrain as well as increased intensity of training have all been related at one time or another to the development of this problem.[66, 71, 74, 84, 116] Females may be at higher risk than males.[137]

Clinical Evaluation

The physical examination is invariably consistent. There is tenderness along the posteromedial border of the tibia, usually beginning at a location about 4 cm proximal to the medial malleolus and extending proximally for a variable distance up to 12 cm.[29, 110] Typically, up to a third of the posteromedial border of the tibia may be tender, and this area is usually centered around the junction of the distal and middle thirds of the leg. Slight swelling may be apparent as well. In the typical case, percussion elsewhere about the tibia does not elicit pain or tenderness. Passive and active flexion and extension and inversion and eversion of the foot or ankle are also usually pain free. Active resisted plantar flexion and toe raises, however, may elicit the characteristic pain.[101]

Routine plain radiographs of the leg are usually interpreted as normal. Not infrequently, however, there may be hypertrophy of the posterior cortex of the tibia. This is felt to be the result of bone remodeling as the bone adapts to the increased repetitive stress applied. Another finding variably described on plain radiographs is subperiosteal lucency and scalloping on the anterior or medial aspect of the tibia.[101] A faint periosteal reaction may also be seen at times. Although this may be attributed to periostitis, the association with tibial stress fracture must be kept in mind and ruled out by serial plain radiographs or bone scintigraphy.

Traditionally, the bone scan has been most helpful in

the evaluation of the shin splint syndrome. Numerous studies have documented the characteristic scintigraphic features.[19, 70, 86, 101, 107, 147, 161] Rupani and colleagues, in a retrospective study using three-phase radionuclide bone imaging in sports injuries, described the differences seen between the tibial stress fracture and the medial tibial stress syndrome.[149] Typically, in the medial tibial stress syndrome, there is a moderate increase of radionuclide activity along the posteromedial border of the tibia on delayed images. This extends for about a third of the length of the tibia. The ratio of the length of the lesion to the bone length, in their experience, ranged from 1:3 to 3:4. Phase one and phase two (radionuclide angiograms and blood pool images) were always normal. On the other hand, tibial stress fractures are characterized by a more focal and intense reaction (see Fig. 29–5). Uptake is typically fusiform, although sometimes it is transverse. The maximum ratio of the length of the stress fracture to the length of the long bone in the experience of these investigators was 1:5. When bone scans are used to evaluate the shin splint syndrome, both lateral and medial views should be obtained because they localize the precise focus of uptake better and indeed can correlate this uptake with the site of insertion of the soleus muscle.

More recently, magnetic resonance imaging (MRI) has been used for the detection of stress reactions of bone as a spectrum of injury that can result in stress fracture.[6, 10] MRI has been found to be highly sensitive and specific.[32] As with other conditions, MRI provides additional information about the soft tissues in the leg that may also be involved in the differential diagnosis of exercise-induced leg pain in the athlete. It has become our preferred imaging tool for this purpose.

Pertinent Anatomy

Although often described as the result of overuse of the tibialis posterior, stress fracture has also been perceived as the result of microstress fractures of the tibia as well as a deep posterior compartment syndrome.[14, 19, 129] Stress fractures can be ruled out nicely, however, by the presence or absence of a typical scintigraphic appearance. Further, Mubarak and associates have investigated compartment pressures in patients with the medial tibial stress syndrome, including pressures within the deep posterior compartment of the leg, and have found them normal.[110] Perhaps the most pertinent investigation into the anatomy of the medial tibial stress syndrome was done by Michael and Holder.[101] In this study, the authors investigated anatomic dissections of human cadavers and correlated clinical findings with electromyographic and bone scanning results. Their laboratory dissections clearly demonstrated that the site of increased activity on bone scans and the site of tenderness to direct palpation over the posteromedial border of the tibia do not correspond to the posterior tibialis muscle but rather to the medial origin of the soleus muscle. The soleus with its investing fascia forms the tough soleus bridge overlying the deep compartment of the leg (Fig. 29–1).

Relevant Biomechanics

Numerous authors have described the association of excessive foot pronation with the development of shin splints.[77, 101, 104, 185] Others have performed critical reviews and have found that the literature does not support clinical beliefs that lower extremity morphology and alignment are risk factors for overuse injury.[72] Messier and Pittala studied 17 subjects with shin splints and compared them with 19 normal controls.[100] Selected anthropometric measurements were investigated, including leg lengths, Q angles, and hamstring and ankle flexibility. Biomechanical evaluations using high-speed cinematography were studied. Two significant variables correlated significantly with the occurrence of shin splints: maximum pronation velocity and maximum pronation. Additionally, heel cord flexibility was less evident in patients with shin splints.

McKenzie and colleagues have also stressed the relationship between forefoot pronation and the development

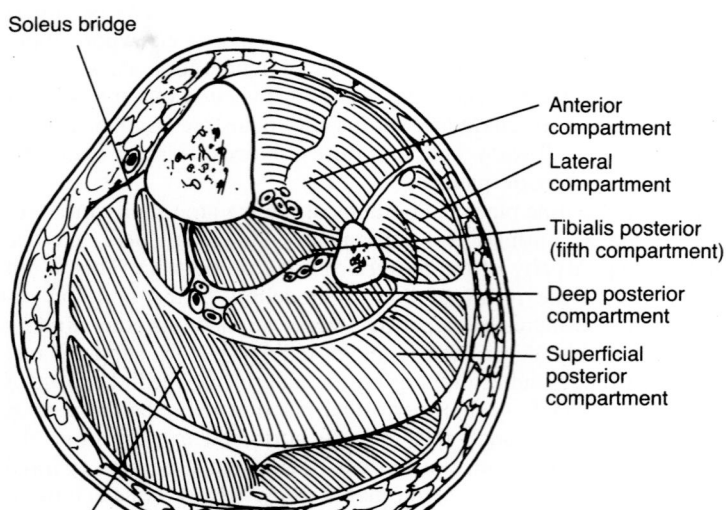

Soleus bridge

- Anterior compartment
- Lateral compartment
- Tibialis posterior (fifth compartment)
- Deep posterior compartment
- Superficial posterior compartment

Soleus muscle

Figure 29–1. The soleus bridge includes the tough superficial investing fascia of the soleus, which inserts along the posteromedial border of the tibia.

of overuse syndromes in the lower extremity.[97] They point out that in normal running, the initial contact is made at foot strike with the lateral aspect of the foot. The tibia is externally rotated, and, as stance phase progresses, the body is carried over the foot and the tibia rotates internally. To compensate for this internal tibial rotation, a simultaneous eversion of the subtalar joint is required, resulting in pronation of the foot. Thus, foot pronation is a normal occurrence that not only helps dissipate the initial forces of foot contact but also provides a smooth transition and adaptation to varying terrain and running surfaces. The medial soleus has been shown to effect inversion of the calcaneus. Thus, with normal running and foot pronation, an eccentric contracture is required of the soleus. Excessive pronation or excessive velocity of pronation can therefore apply increased stress and strain to the supporting musculature, including the medial soleus. It may be that the velocity of pronation is of greater importance in the development of an overuse syndrome in the lower extremity than the actual degree of eversion or pronation that occurs. Viitasalo and Kvist analyzed 35 male athletes with shin splints.[180] In particular, these authors used gait analysis methodology to investigate and describe subtalar mobility as well as the lower leg and heel position and angular displacements that occur during treadmill running. They found that during running, the Achilles tendon angle was significantly greater at heel strike in patients with shin splints than in a group of 13 normal long-distance runners and volunteers who had no foot problems. More recently, investigators are using gait analysis to create new methods of looking at old problems in an effort to understand better the significance of coupled motions of the lower extremity as well as the role of gait variability in the normal and the injured state.[68]

Treatment Options

A great deal of myth as well as methodology has been applied to the treatment of shin splints and medial tibial stress syndrome. A study performed at the United States Naval Academy is consistent with most authors' experience.[7] In this study, midshipmen diagnosed as having shin splints were managed with one of a number of treatments including rest, anti-inflammatory medication, heel cord stretching, heel pads, and casting. No treatment combination worked better than rest alone. We should remember that in managing overuse syndromes, rest implies "relative" rest. That is, the patient's activities are restricted to those that can be performed comfortably. This may mean abstaining from running and jumping activities, or it may require cutting back only on the intensity of running. A careful discussion with the patient is needed to assess what degree of rest will be required.

James and others have pointed out the importance of evaluating the runner's lower limb alignment as well as the mechanics of gait.[74] For example, the varus heel may do well with a medial heel wedge, and the varus foot may require a medial post beneath the forefoot. The runner inclined toward excessive foot pronation may do better with an orthotic device. If hindfoot valgus is a prominent feature of gait, a heel cup by itself or incorporated into the orthotic may prevent excessive foot translation. Trainers experienced in the care of athletes also have their favorite methods of taping (Fig. 29–2).

We should not forget to look at the running shoe. A wide heel can lead to increased velocity of foot pronation on heel strike.[175] This produces increased eccentric stress on the supporting musculature, including the medial soleus as well as the bony framework of the foot and leg. Although the addition of heel pads did not seem to help in one statistical study,[7] others have shown clinical efficacy of cushion insoles in preventing overuse injury of the leg.[42, 59] They do absorb impact forces at heel strike and thus dissipate stress.

Tight heel cords have been implicated in the development of shin splints. Garrett and others have shown that tight muscle-tendon groups are more susceptible to strain.[48, 151, 165] Therefore, heel cord stretching in the management of the medial tibial stress (soleus) syndrome has some merit.

Because biopsy studies have demonstrated periostitis

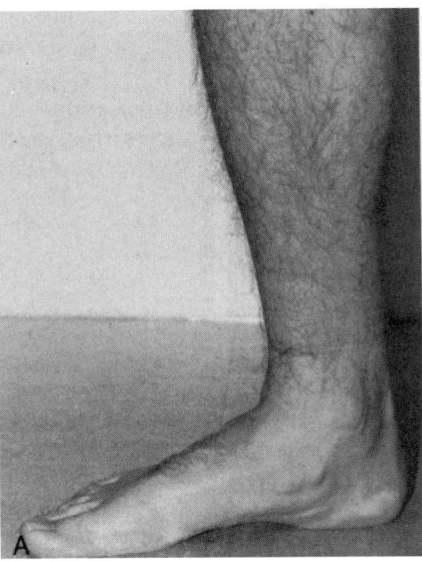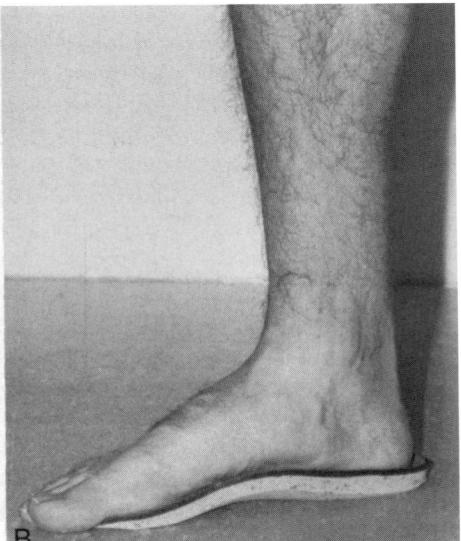

Figure 29–2. *A* and *B,* Custom-molded stress inlay orthotics can be useful in preventing hyperpronation of the foot during gait, thus relieving excess stress on the medial soleus and secondary foot flexors.

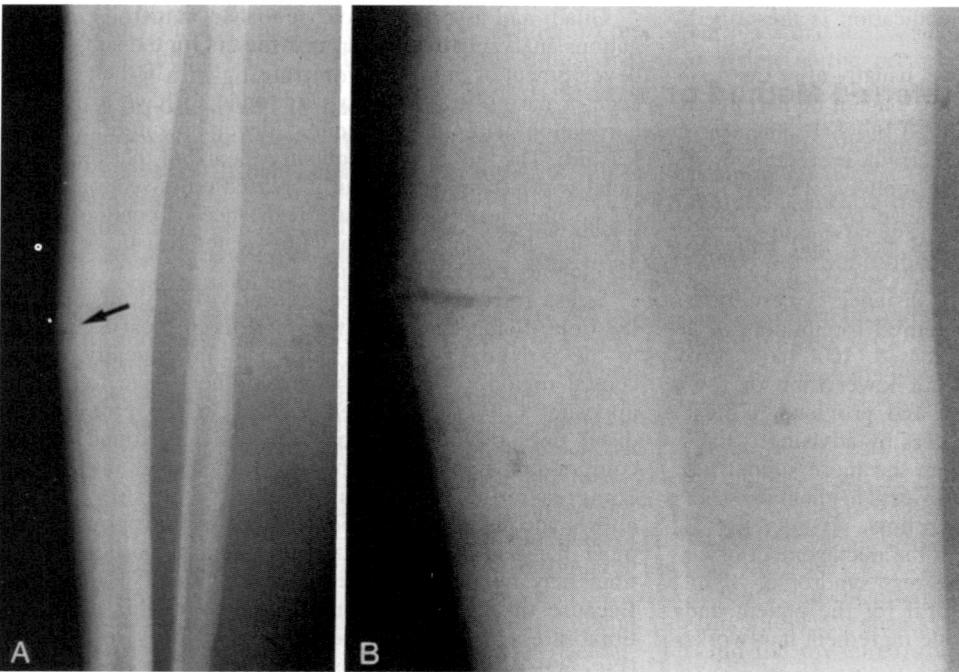

Figure 29–4. *A* and *B,* The "dreaded black line" of the anterior tibial cortex is notorious for its prolonged and unpredictable healing.

running is the most frequent offender. Other factors associated with stress fractures include running on hard surfaces, inadequate footwear with poor impact-absorbing qualities, and lower limb malalignment. As with the medial tibial stress syndrome, forefoot varus, hyperpronation, and tibia vara have all been shown to predispose the athlete to stress fractures.[92, 170]

Stress fractures are uncommon in prepubertal children, but case reports do exist in the literature.[38, 73, 124] On the other hand, in adolescence and afterward, the susceptibility appears to be about the same as in the adult population.

Pathoanatomy

Johnson in 1963 described the histopathology of stress fractures.[76] Li and his coworkers described the histopathologic processes that occur during the genesis of a tibial stress fracture in a rabbit model.[85] Their findings agree with the commonly held belief that the development of a stress fracture results from a continuum of bone resorption and remodeling in response to repetitive stress. They have demonstrated that the earliest stage of bone stress represents a vascular phenomenon. Increased numbers of erythrocytes are found within bone, resulting in vascular congestion and thrombosis. Subsequently, osteoclastic resorption takes place. Periosteal reaction is initiated as osteoclastic resorption progresses, and periosteal new bone proliferation results from the increase in osteoblasts. Within the cortical bone, development of resorption cavities as well as resorption of small cracks that form within cement lines is followed by bone remodeling. Periosteal callus forms, apparently as an attempt to stabilize the bone while the underlying remodeling process is carried out. The usual end result of this type of bone remodeling occurring in

response to repetitive bone stress is cortical hypertrophy. Further studies have shown that repetitive stress to bone leads to increased mineralization. Ideally, the bone hypertrophy and remodeling take place in sufficient time to prevent the subsequent development of a cortical stress fracture. If repetitive stress continues and overloads an already weakened cortex that is still undergoing remodeling, however, cortical fracture may result. More recently, Nattiv and Armsey have described the spectrum of stress injury of bone in the female as related to the context of their hormonal, nutritional, and environmental milieu.[115]

Relevant Biomechanics

Two theories about the pathomechanics of tibial and fibular stress fractures exist. The first, proposed by Clement, alleges that muscle fatigue and weakness reduce the relative shock-absorbing capabilities of muscle in the lower extremities.[24] This ultimately results first in higher stress being applied to the bone itself and then in fatigue fracture. Stanitski and colleagues proposed just the opposite.[164] They believe that highly concentrated muscle forces acting across a specific bone lead to a rhythmic, repetitive muscle action that causes subthreshold mechanical insults, ultimately resulting in fatigue fracture.

As noted, other intrinsic factors have been found to alter the biomechanics of running, ultimately predisposing to the development of stress fractures. These include excessive pronation of the foot, forefoot varus, subtalar varus, tibia vara, leg length inequalities, and pes cavus.[126] Excessive pronation probably contributes by producing an overload on the flexor musculature of the leg, primarily the medial half of the soleus muscle but also the other supporting flexors such as the tibialis posterior. Depending on which theory one subscribes to, either the repetitive overactivity of these muscle groups leads to tibial or fibular stress fracture or the resulting fatigue and subsequent weakness of the musculature predispose the underlying bone to fatigue failure. Forefoot varus and tibia vara contribute to risk by their association with compensatory increased foot pronation. Pes cavus results in a lack of normal foot pronation, which lessens the ability to smooth out the shock of heel strike and foot flat during gait. The resulting heightened forces are then transmitted proximally up the leg. Novacheck has summarized a biomechanical approach to running injuries and has emphasized the important energy absorption performed by the eccentric loading action of the muscles of the lower extremity.[119]

The atypical stress fracture of the anterior cortex of the midtibia occurs almost exclusively in athletes performing repetitive jumping and leaping activities. It is thought that the repetitive forceful contractions of the flexor musculature of the leg act like a bowstring against the tibia, producing repetitive increased tensile forces across the anterior cortex.[25, 132, 141] Ultimately, this can lead to fatigue fracture. The histopathologic findings in biopsies performed on this atypical stress fracture have been consistent with nonunion.[61] Surrounding cortical hypertrophy and sclerosis exist with a fracture line filled with granulation tissue.

Medial Malleolar Stress Fractures

Another variety of atypical tibial stress fracture occurs in the medial malleolus. The fracture extends from the tibial plafonds proximally in an oblique manner. Inherently unstable, this fracture may require an extensive period of casting to allow satisfactory healing (see Fig. 29–7), Shelbourne and his coworkers described their experience with this injury and advocated early internal fixation to achieve an earlier recovery and return to athletics.[157]

Although less common, fibular fractures do occur.[92, 125, 126, 130] The usual location of fibular stress fractures is just proximal to the distal tibiofibular syndesmoses. Biomechanical studies have demonstrated the amount of bending that occurs within the fibula during muscle contraction.[17, 172] Tethered to the tibia distally by the tibiofibular ligaments, stress is concentrated just proximal to this level. Although less common, stress fractures have been described at virtually every level of the fibula, including the fibular neck.[17, 172]

Clinical Evaluation

In the early stage of development, tibial and fibular stress fractures may be confused with the shin splint syndrome. The pain is experienced after activity, but as the condition advances, the pain begins to occur during activity as well. With time, it may be present with activities of daily living. Tenderness is usually well localized to bone, and periosteal thickening or even callus formation may be palpable. Usually, however, by the time callus formation

(about the tibia) can be palpated, the symptoms are resolving.

Findings on plain radiographs are variable.[34] Usually 2 to 3 weeks are required for changes to occur. Changes may include a very slight periosteal reaction and may be associated with scalloping or subperiosteal resorption. As the process matures, periosteal new bone formation occurs. Endosteal thickening may also be appreciated as well as cortical hypertrophy. The actual presence of a visible cortical fracture line on plain radiographs is variable. Rosen and colleagues demonstrated that 28% of stress fractures diagnosed by bone scan have associated plain roentgenographic abnormalities as well.[147]

Traditionally, the most reliable and sensitive means of detecting a stress fracture is the use of the technetium bone scan.[62, 103, 118, 120, 147, 149, 186] Although there are a few case reports of symptomatic individuals with negative bone scans who subsequently developed stress fractures, most studies show a virtual 100% sensitivity with the use of this technique. The characteristic focal fusiform appearance is readily distinguished from the linear activity seen with the tibial stress syndrome[149] (Fig. 29–5). Studies utilizing bone scans for the detection of stress fractures have also pointed out that approximately 40% of these lesions are asymptomatic.[147, 186] Many of these lesions subsequently become symptomatic if stress is not interrupted. Further, the use of the three-phase bone scan can provide an estimate of the age of the lesion.[149] When a stress fracture is 2 to 4 weeks old, all phases of the bone scan will be abnormal. As

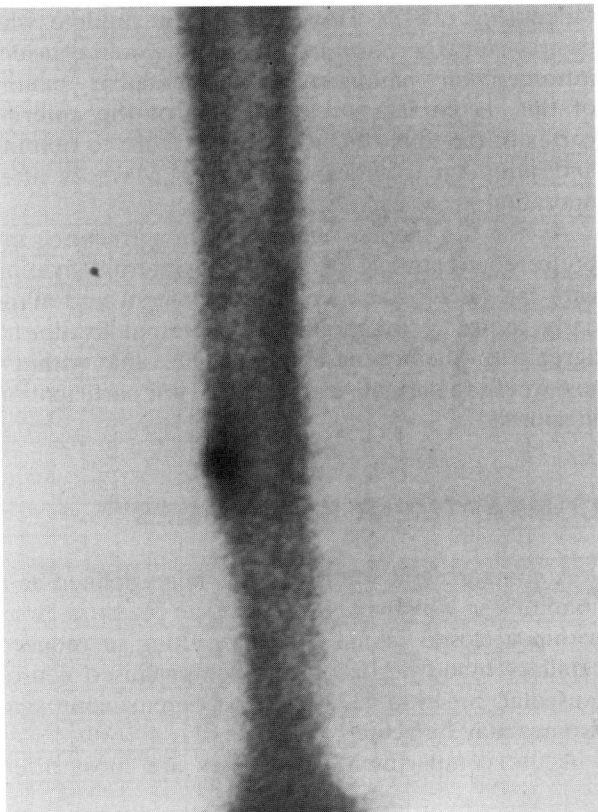

Figure 29–5. A focal, fusiform uptake is more consistent with tibial stress fracture than with the more diffuse linear pattern of tibial stress syndrome.

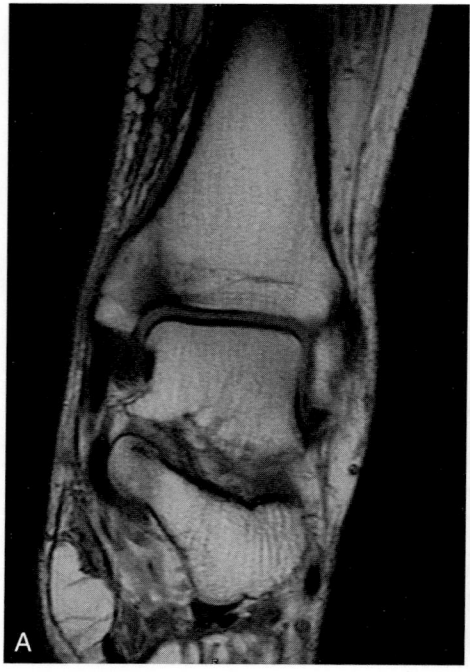 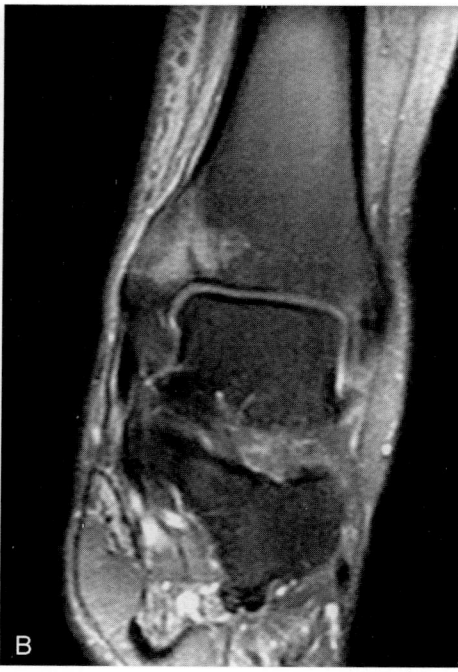

Figure 29–6. Magnetic resonance imaging is sensitive and accurate for detection of stress fracture. Here the T₁-weighted image reveals bone edema (low signal) about a medial malleolar stress fracture *(A),* and the fat-suppressed proton density image shows the edema (high signal) and the fracture line *(B).*

healing progresses, radionuclide angiograms (first phase) and subsequently the blood pool images no longer reveal abnormalities. The delayed images, however, remain positive for at least 3 to 6 months and usually longer.

Other modalities used to aid in the diagnosis have not been as helpful. Ultrasound and thermography have been used in an effort to obtain an inexpensive and safe screening modality, but they are not nearly as accurate as the bone scan.[36, 57, 92] Computed tomography can be disappointing and misleading, particularly when one is trying to differentiate between a stress fracture and a primary bone tumor.[57, 160, 185]

MRI has now become the preferred imaging technique for the detection of stress fracture when plain radiographs are not conclusive (Fig. 29–6). MRI has the ability to provide a biologic assessment of the state of the stress reaction in bone in addition to making the initial diagnosis.[10, 20, 32] Although initially felt to be an expensive test that was certainly no better than the bone scan and probably generally inferior to it,[82, 163] both statements are presently inaccurate. MRI has proven to be a sensitive tool for the detection of stress fracture. Furthermore, it avoids the use of radiation altogether at a comparable expense.

Treatment Options

The great majority (93%) of tibial and fibular stress fractures heal with conservative treatment.[126] That is, simply restricting running activities until the individual is pain free should suffice. Indeed, management of these fractures is quite similar to that of the medial tibial stress syndrome. The average length of time of rest for the tibia is 4 to 6 weeks; however, the average time until return to full athletic competition may be 3 months. Reports exist on the

use of functional bracing for tibial stress fractures, allowing the most immediate return to activity.[37] Clement has advocated a two-phase protocol.[24] Phase one includes pain control through local physiotherapy, nonsteroidal anti-inflammatory medication, and ice massage. Weight-bearing is allowed for normal activities, but running is stopped. Cycling, swimming, and water running are offered as alternative forms of conditioning. Physical therapy emphasizing flexibility exercises as well as isometric and other muscle strengthening exercises is encouraged. Phase two begins when the athlete has been pain free for 10 to 14 days and includes a graduated return to sport. This graded return is probably of most importance in preventing a recurrence. It should be remembered that recurrence rates of stress fractures in athletes, although not necessarily at the same site, approach 10%.[57, 104, 126]

There are two problem stress fractures of the tibia that deserve special mention with regard to treatment. The first is the "dreaded black line," the transverse cortical striation of the anterior tibial cortex (see Fig. 29–4A and B). These may be single or multiple. As already described, they represent stress fractures on the tension side of the bone and are thus prone to delayed union, nonunion, and even complete fracture. Although closed treatment has been advocated by most, excision and bone grafting remain as alternative treatments to be tried after 3 to 6 months of failed closed management.[61] More recently, intramedullary nailing has gained favor by its ability to allow a quicker return to athletic activity.[21]

The other special case is the medial malleolar tibial stress fracture, which has a potential for delayed union (Fig. 29–7). Although closed treatment can be successful, Shelbourne and colleagues advocate internal fixation with screws to prevent subsequent displacement and allow early return to functional activities.[157]

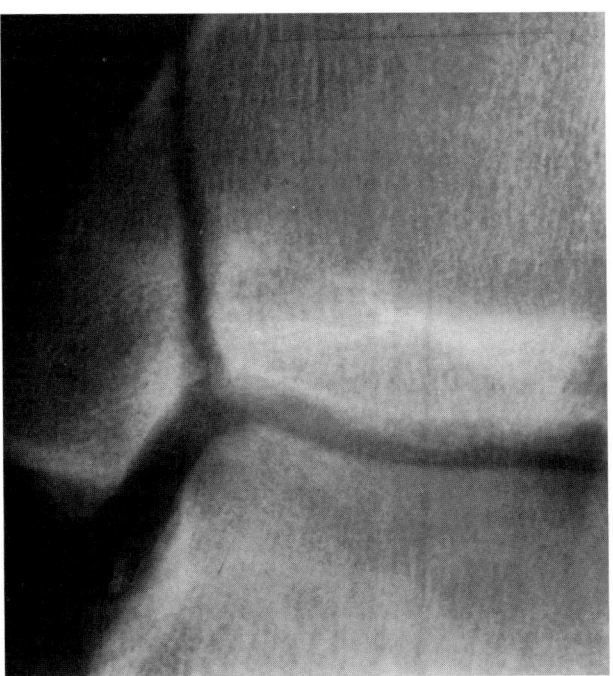

Figure 29–7. Excessive shear stress makes this medial malleolar stress fracture prone to delayed union. Bone scan is helpful in detecting this fracture, and a computed tomography scan can demonstrate the anatomic configuration and the extent of involvement.

Author's Preferred Method of Treatment

For the typical tibial stress fracture on the compression side of bone, I follow the guidelines recommended by Clement.[24] For fibular stress fractures, I prefer similar symptomatic treatment. I also have had success with functional braces such as the Aircast type of pneumatic tibial brace, which allows an earlier return to pain-free running.

For the anterior tibial midshaft stress fracture, my initial preference is a non–weight-bearing short-leg cast applied for 6 to 8 weeks. Although I have had healing occur within this amount of time, my experience is similar to that reported in the literature, which suggests that several months are needed to allow complete healing. I have had variable success with drilling alone as well as with bone grafting, but these are my secondary procedures, to be used at this point in patients in whom closed treatment has failed (Fig. 29–8). For the athlete who desires an early return to function, however, I consider intramedullary nailing (Fig. 29–9). After intramedullary nailing of this incomplete stress fracture of the anterior cortex of the tibia, the athlete can return to running and jumping activities as early as 6 weeks after operation.

As for the medial malleolar stress fracture, my preferred treatment for the skeletally mature athlete is immediate internal fixation with lag screws to prevent displacement and allow early return to function. I agree with Shelbourne and colleagues that after internal fixation, the athlete may return to full participation in sports within 4 to 6 weeks. For the skeletally immature patient, I provide a 6-week period in a non–weight-bearing cast followed by a walking cast or brace until radiographically healed.

Compartment Syndromes

A compartment syndrome has been defined as a condition in which an elevated tissue pressure exists within a closed fascial space, resulting in reduced capillary blood perfusion and compromised neuromuscular function.[144, 148] Compartment syndromes may be acute or chronic.

Acute compartment syndromes are most often located in the leg as the result of tibial fractures, but they can also result from a variety of other forms of trauma such as muscle rupture, crush injuries, and circumferential burns.[9, 60, 111] Studies have documented the influence of the external environment on intracompartmental pressures.[146] Direct pressure, circumferential dressings, and casts all significantly increase intracompartmental pressures. In the case of a cast, an 85% reduction in intracompartmental pressure can be achieved simply by bivalving the cast, releasing the underlying padding and removing half of the cast.[47]

Although acute compartment syndromes are fortunately uncommon in athletic participation, the condition must be recognized and treated (by fasciotomy) immediately. In sports, the two situations that are most likely to produce an acute compartment syndrome of the leg are tibial fracture and muscle rupture.

The acute compartment syndrome has been well defined clinically.[114] With the advent of improved methods of measuring intracompartmental tissue pressures, more precise and accurate objective criteria have been added. The needle manometer technique was first described in 1884.[79] More recently, the use of this technique has been advocated by Reneman and by Whitesides and colleagues.[138, 182] Matsen and his associates developed a needle technique that incorporates continuous infusion of saline into the compartment. This allows measurement of intracompartmental pressures over time by preventing catheter tip plugging.[94] Scholander and colleagues developed the wick catheter technique.[154] Its principal advantage is the absence of the need for continuous infusion of saline in an already compromised compartment. The wick catheter was also found to be appropriate for continuous monitoring of intracompartmental pressures during exercise. Rorabeck[146] designed the slit catheter, which remains a popular method and is also advocated by Mubarak and Horgens.[112] This device consists of five 3-mm long slits cut into the tip of a polyethylene tube and provides continuity between the tissue fluids and the saline within the catheter without requiring continuous saline injection. Finally, McDermott and associates described the use of the solid-state transducer intracompartmental catheter for the dynamic measurement of intracompartmental pressures.[96] With the use of either the wick or the slit catheter technique, it is now generally accepted that resting intracompartmental pressures of greater than 30 mm Hg represent a level that can be associated with interruption of the capillary circulation and thus can lead to muscle and nerve ischemic changes.[65]

The chronic compartment syndrome has also been described as an exertional compartment syndrome or an exer-

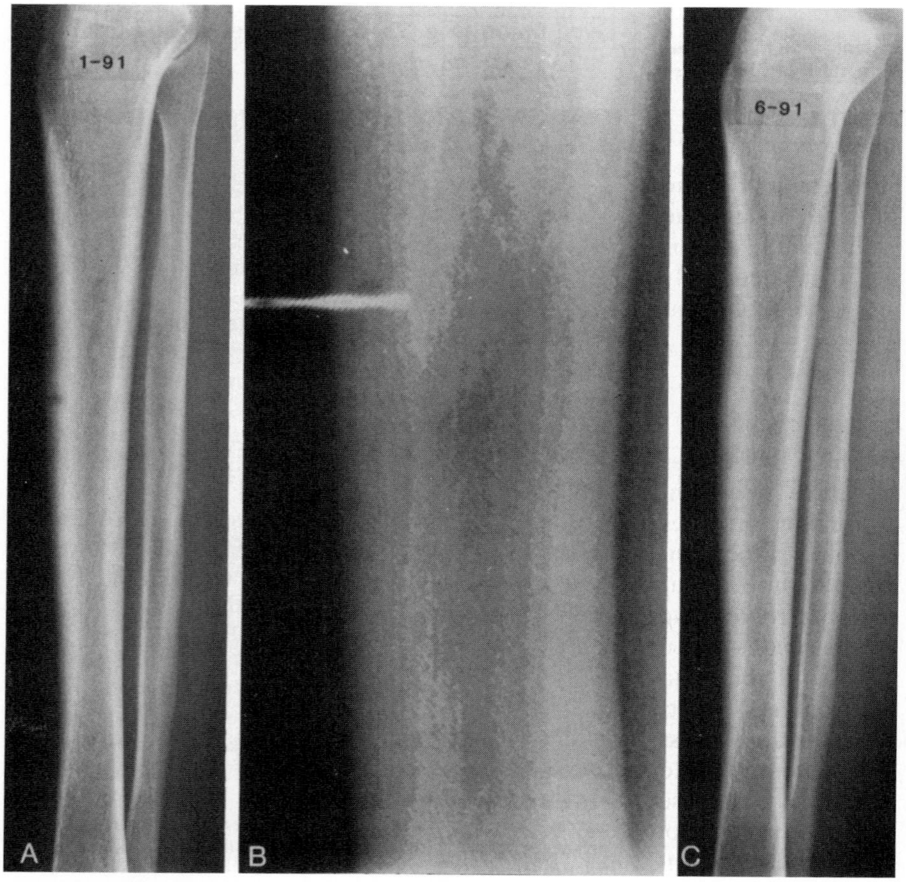

Figure 29–8. *A* to *C,* This recalcitrant anterior tibial stress fracture was drilled under fluoroscopic control and healed uneventfully by 3 months postoperatively.

cise-induced compartment syndrome. The exact underlying pathophysiology is not clear.[3, 69, 136] There are conflicting reports in the literature about the importance of ischemia in the generation of this symptom complex. What has been demonstrated, however, is that abnormal pressures are present with the chronic compartment syndrome (exercise induced).[133, 144] It has been demonstrated that with muscle contraction alone, significant elevations in intracompartmental pressures occur, up to 80 mm Hg and beyond.[87, 96, 98] The degree of pressure elevation is directly related to the extent of muscle contraction. Muscle weight can increase by as much as 20% owing to increased tissue perfusion with exercise. This increase in muscle size can lead to increased intracompartmental pressure if the surrounding fascial borders are unyielding. Sustained increase in this tissue pressure can lead to transudation of fluid into the interstitial space.[31, 45] As tissue pressures approach the level of the diastolic blood pressure, the microcirculation is impeded.[182]

Various authors have tried to establish objective guidelines for the diagnosis of chronic compartment syndrome by tissue pressure measurements. Most authors have observed elevated resting tissue pressure both before and immediately after exercise.[133, 144] In particular, there is a delayed return to normal tissue pressure after exercise. The criteria for chronic compartment syndrome developed by Rorabeck and colleagues include a resting intramuscular pressure above 10 mm Hg and an abnormally elevated tissue pressure in excess of 15 mm Hg measured 15 minutes after exercise.[144] Pedowitz and his coworkers devel-

oped criteria that include any one of the following: (1) a pre-exercise pressure greater than 15 mm Hg; (2) a 1-minute postexercise pressure of greater than 30 mm Hg; and (3) a 5-minute postexercise pressure in excess of 20 mm Hg.[133]

Pertinent Anatomy

There are at least four well-described fascial compartments within the leg: the anterior, lateral, superficial posterior, and deep posterior compartments.[94] Others have described subdivisions of these compartments resulting in at least five compartments.[30] The tibialis posterior functions as if it were within its own compartment and has been shown to be vulnerable itself to a chronic compartment syndrome.[28] Lying within the four major compartments are four major nerves with sensory components (Fig. 29–10). The sural nerve lies within the superficial posterior compartment. The tibial nerve is located in the deep posterior compartment. The deep peroneal nerve lies within the anterior compartment, and the superficial peroneal nerve is found within the lateral compartment. A thorough knowledge of the compartmental anatomy of the leg is important in making a precise clinical diagnosis of which compartment is involved.

Muscle hernias through fascial defects have been shown to exist in at least 40% of patients with chronic compart-

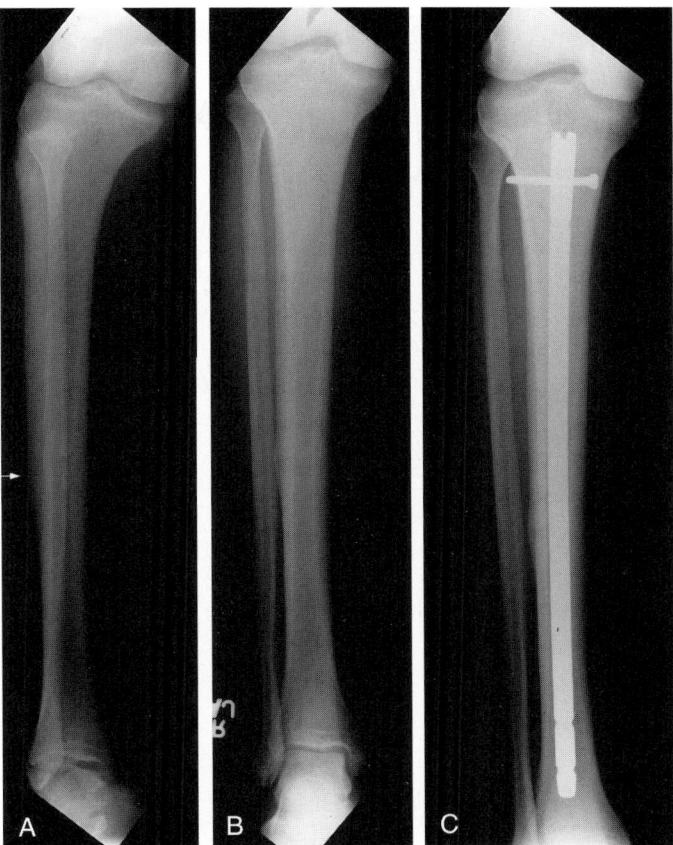

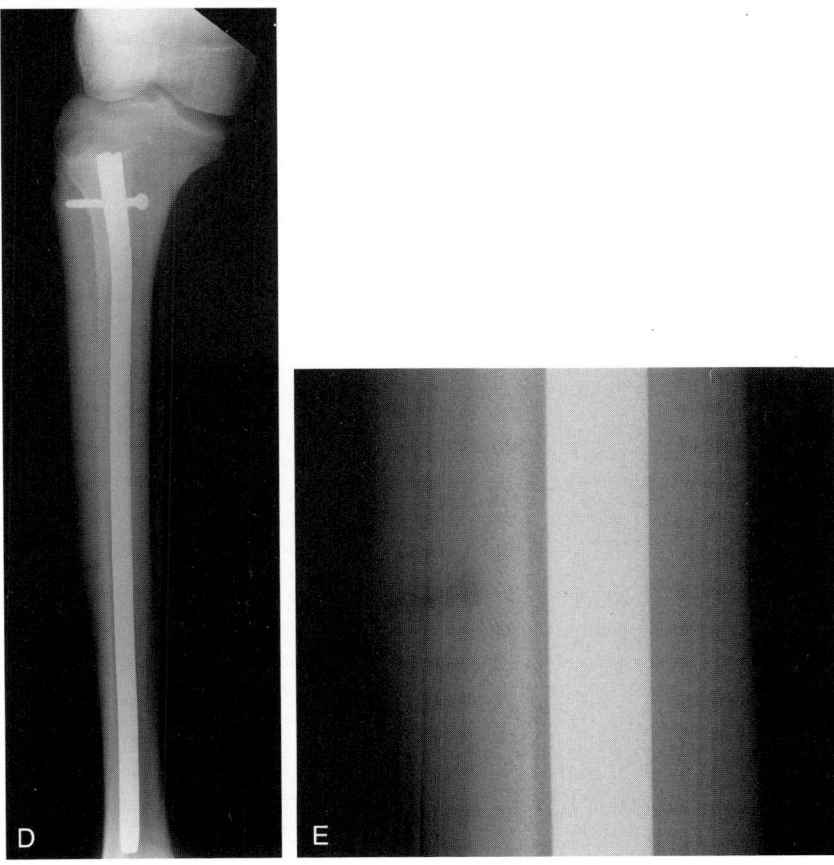

Figure 29–9. *A* and *B,* The highly competitive athlete, unwilling to accept prolonged protection and activity restrictions, may be better served by intramedullary nailing. The *arrow* in part *A* shows the stress fracture. *C* to *E,* This athlete returned to competitive basketball by 6 weeks after surgery and experienced uneventful healing.

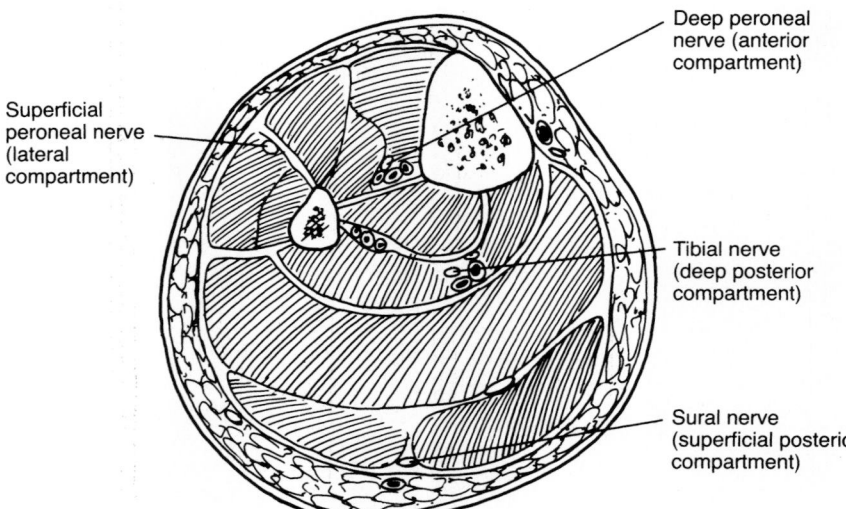

Superficial peroneal nerve (lateral compartment)

Deep peroneal nerve (anterior compartment)

Tibial nerve (deep posterior compartment)

Sural nerve (superficial posterior compartment)

Figure 29–10. Lying within the four major compartments of the leg are four major sensory nerves. The distribution of dysesthesias and hypesthesias can thus help identify the affected compartment.

ment syndromes.[133] This compares to the normal incidence of 5% among controls.

Relevant Biomechanics

Isolated reports in the literature have investigated the biomechanical factors that may lead to increased compartmental tissue pressures. Kirby and McDermott demonstrated that landing styles of rearfoot and forefoot during treadmill running can influence pressures within the anterior compartment of the leg.[78] They recommended that individuals whose pressures rise significantly during rearfoot landing should avoid this style, perhaps by shortening their stride. They also described footwear modifications that could be helpful. Gertsch and colleagues found that the Siitonen step, a new technique in cross-country ski racing, was related to development of an anterior compartment syndrome.[52]

Clinical Evaluation

Acute compartment syndrome is a clinical diagnosis.[146] It can be recognized by pain that is out of proportion to the clinical situation. There may also be palpable swelling or tenseness within the affected muscle compartment. Paresthesias frequently exist in the distribution of the nerve traveling through the affected compartment. The overlying skin may be tense, shiny, and warm. Passive stretch of the muscles involved produces severe pain. A sensory deficit such as decreased sensation to light touch, pinprick, or two-point discrimination in the distal sensory distribution of the affected nerve is a reliable indicator. Distal pedal pulses are routinely intact. A change in capillary refill of the toes is unreliable. In the presence of significant trauma known to be associated with compartment syndromes and with the clinical picture described, one can be confident enough of the diagnosis to proceed with definitive treatment (fasciotomy).

Differentiating acute compartment syndrome from cellulitis and deep vein thrombosis is usually possible. The differentiation of this condition from an arterial occlusion or a neurapraxia, however, can be more difficult.[94] At times, this differentiation can be impossible based on the clinical presentation alone. Compartmental pressure measurements in acute cases are most useful in the following situations: (1) evaluation of the unconscious patient; (2) continuous monitoring of compartmental pressures in an extremity that has been traumatized to such an extent that it is at risk for subsequent development of this condition; (3) further evaluation of a patient with a clinically suspicious but equivocal presentation.[93, 94, 111, 182]

Detmer and colleagues have very nicely outlined the typical history of a chronic compartment syndrome that they feel is virtually pathognomonic of the condition.[30] The problem occurs most often in runners who give a history of being completely asymptomatic in the off-season but gradually develop an aching in the lower leg with training. This pain is initially dull; it is located within the muscle mass and occurs following runs. As the symptoms progress, the pain may persist after the activity has ended and even into the next day. Paresthesias may develop in the plantar aspect of the foot in a patient with a deep posterior compartment syndrome, or similar paresthesias may be referred to the dorsum of the foot in a patient with an anterior compartment syndrome. The most frequent locations of a chronic compartment syndrome in the leg are the anterior compartment and the deep posterior compartment. These two compartments account for approximately 80% of all cases, the remainder being distributed among the lateral, superficial posterior, and the so-called fifth compartment about the tibialis posterior.[28, 133]

We should remember that in patients with chronic compartment syndromes, the average delay in treatment from the onset of symptoms is 22 months. The physical examination may be normal if the patient is presently asymptomatic. Most patients, however, can localize their pain to the particular muscle or compartment involved.

Still, in the clinical evaluation of a chronic compartment syndrome, the gold standard remains the demonstration of an elevated postexercise resting intracompartmental pressure. In the normal state, elevated intracompartmental pressures that occur with muscle contraction and with exercise will revert to normal within 2 minutes with rest.[11] The postexercise delay in normalization of pressure is prolonged in the patient with a chronic compartment syndrome. The wick catheter technique and the slit catheter technique are the most popular and reliable methods of assessment.

For evaluating the effects of exercise on intracompartmental pressures, the literature provides no standard protocol. Most authors have the patient exercise the muscle groups until either pain or fatigue limits further activity.[133, 144] Isokinetic equipment is used most commonly. It should be remembered that intracompartmental pressures are affected by knee and ankle positioning[50] (Fig. 29–11). Joint positions should be standardized when obtaining serial measurements of intracompartmental pressures.

Bone scan, plain radiography, and computed tomography scan are useful only in ruling out associated injuries. Ultrasound evaluation of compartmental width has been used and has indeed demonstrated differences between joggers and nonjoggers.[51] The relationship of these findings to intracompartmental pressures is not established, however. The use of MRI has been applied to the evaluation of chronic compartment syndromes. Amendola and colleagues published their experiences with MRI.[3] Nine of their patients had "classic symptoms," but only five had abnormal pressures. Of these five, four had prolonged relaxation constants for T_1- and T_2-weighted images, using hydrogen proton MRI rather than spectroscopy. Although their findings must be considered preliminary because of the small numbers, the use of MRI is attractive because it may eventually provide a noninvasive means of assessing intracompartmental pressures simultaneously in all compartments of the leg. More recently, others have demonstrated the efficacy of near-infrared spectroscopy as a noninvasive method of assessing extremities at risk for compartment syndrome.[54, 131]

Treatment Options

The treatment for acute compartment syndrome is fasciotomy. Nerve and muscle ischemia lasting for longer than 12 hours will result in severe and irreversible deterioration.[182] Ischemia lasting less than 4 hours is usually associated with no permanent sequelae. It thus is imperative to institute treatment for the acute compartment syndrome as soon as the diagnosis is established.

Treatment for chronic compartment syndrome is also surgical. Most reports in the literature have established that conservative measures such as exercise, orthotics, and nonsteroidal anti-inflammatory agents as well as activity modification will be uniformly unsuccessful in allowing the individual to return to the presymptom level of activity.[91] On the other hand, treatment by surgical decompression of the affected compartment should have at least a 90% probability of producing significant improvement, if not complete recovery.[45, 91, 145, 167] Many of the cases documented in the literature of "failure" of fasciotomy for chronic compartment syndrome ultimately proved to be the result of an inadequate fasciotomy or a missed diagnosis (i.e., failure to recognize the isolated tibialis posterior compartment syndrome and to institute adequate decompression of this compartment). Detmer and colleagues, in a review of 100 cases of chronic compartment syndrome including 233 compartments, reported a recurrence rate of only 3.4%.[30] More recent reports, however, suggest that long-

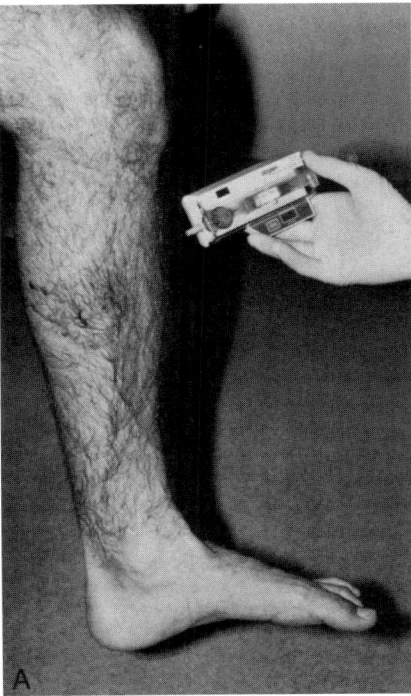
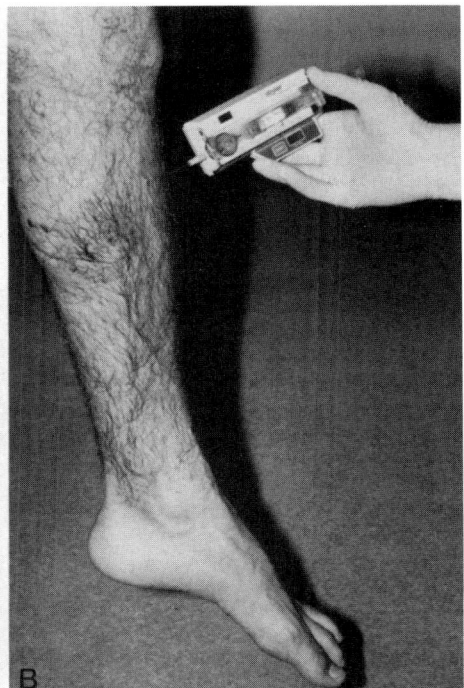

Figure 29–11. *A* and *B,* Remember that foot and ankle position can markedly affect intracompartmental pressures of the leg. For instance, active dorsiflexion or forced plantar flexion can elevate intracompartmental pressures of the anterior compartment. Standardization of the resting position of the limb should be maintained when measuring pre-exercise and postexercise compartment pressures.

term outcomes are better for the anterior and lateral compartments (80% satisfied) compared with those with deep posterior compartment involvement (50%) and that women athletes may be more often affected but less responsive to treatment.[71, 102]

It should be recognized that multiple compartments may be involved with elevated pressures. Most authors recommend assessing at least all four major compartments of the leg and decompressing those with persistently elevated postexercise pressures.

Several techniques exist for fasciotomy of the leg including (1) fibulectomy, (2) perifibular fasciotomy, and (3) double-incision fasciotomy. Fibulectomy has been popularized by Whitesides and colleagues and will adequately decompress all four major compartments of the leg as well as the posterior tibialis.[182] This is a rather extensive procedure, however, and there is conflict in the literature about subsequent disability. Fibulectomy is contraindicated in children and also in patients with compartment syndromes complicating tibial fractures.[146]

The perifibular fasciotomy through a single lateral incision has been popularized by Matsen and colleagues.[94] The incision is made from the fibular neck to the lateral malleolus. Cosmetically, this single-incision technique may be better than the double-incision technique proposed by Mubarak and associates,[113] but it is more difficult to obtain access to the deep posterior compartment. To gain entry, the interval between the peroneus longus and the soleus is followed down to the fibula, where the peroneal compartment is retracted anteriorly and the superficial posterior compartment is retracted posteriorly. Care must be taken to avoid injuring the peroneal nerve. In severely traumatized extremities, these landmarks may be less clearly defined, making this approach more difficult and hazardous.

The double-incision technique as proposed by Mubarak and Owen is relatively simple and safe.[113] The anterolateral incision is made midway between the tibia and the fibula. The underlying investing fascia is identified, and a short transverse incision is made just through the fascia to identify the anterolateral intermuscular septum. Then, approximately 1 cm anterior and 1 cm posterior to this septum, longitudinal fasciotomies are carried out, decompressing the anterior and lateral compartments. In performing this fasciotomy, care should be taken to identify and avoid the superficial peroneal nerve as it exits just lateral to the intermuscular septum. This nerve pierces the investing fascia over the lateral compartment immediately adjacent to the intermuscular septum at approximately the junction of the middle and distal thirds of the leg. The posteromedial skin incision is made about 1 cm medial to the tibia in the midportion of the leg. Investing fascia overlying the superficial compartment is divided longitudinally, and the musculature of the superficial compartment is retracted posteriorly to allow visualization of the fascia over the deep compartment. During this approach, care should be taken to avoid injuring the saphenous vein and nerve. Fasciotomy is then performed on the deep posterior compartment.

Exposure of the fascia over the tibialis posterior is more difficult. Two approaches have been recommended (Fig. 29–12). Davey and colleagues[28] recommend the single lateral incision for their fasciotomies and gain entry to the

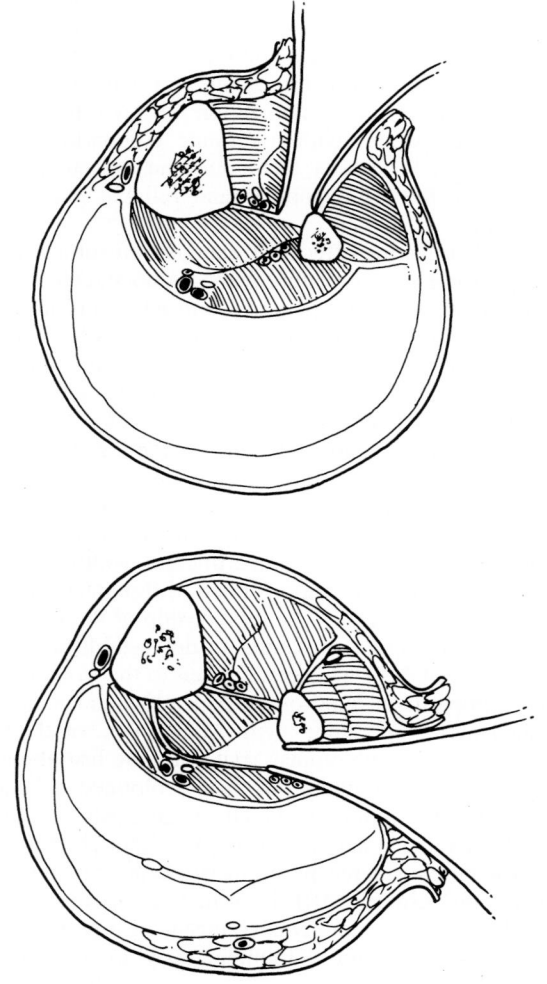

Figure 29–12. Entry and decompression of the "fifth compartment" of the leg may be obtained through either an anterolateral (*top*) or a posterolateral (*bottom*) approach.

fascia over the tibialis posterior by defining the interval between the superficial posterior and the lateral compartments, dissecting the flexor hallucis longus subperiosteally off the fibula, and retracting this muscle posteromedially.[29] The fascial attachment of the tibialis posterior muscle is then identified and incised. An alternative approach has been described by Nghiem and Boland, who gain entry to the fascia over the tibialis posterior through an anterolateral approach.[117] Dissection is carried along the anterolateral intermuscular septum to the fibula. The interosseous membrane is divided, thus decompressing the tibialis posterior as well as the deep posterior compartment of the leg. If one chooses the double-incision technique, the method described by Nghiem and Boland appears preferable.

For acute compartment syndromes, fasciotomies are performed as open procedures under direct vision. All wounds are left open throughout the length of the compartment and managed with sterile dressings. Rorabeck advocates the use of wet-to-dry dressings instituted on the third day, and on the seventh day performing either secondary wound closure or split-thickness skin grafting as appropriate.[146]

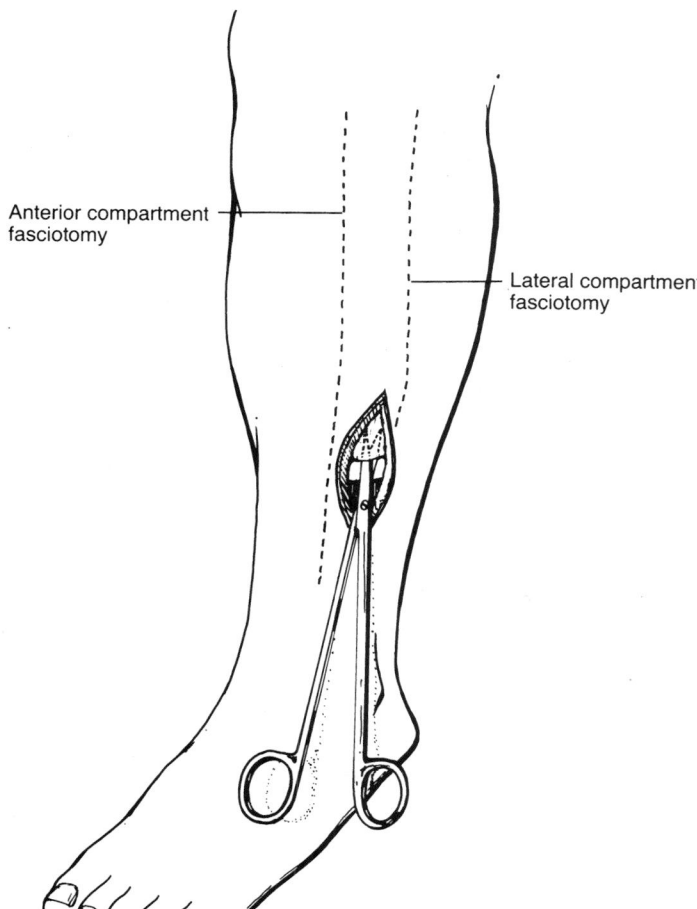

Anterior compartment
fasciotomy

Lateral compartment
fasciotomy

Figure 29–13. Because myofascial hernia is frequently present in patients with chronic compartment syndrome, it should be identified, and fasciotomy rather than fascial closure should be carried out. Perforating cutaneous nerves are frequently present at the site of a muscle hernia at these locations.

For chronic compartment syndrome, subcutaneous fasciotomies may do just as well, and the skin is closed primarily. These may be performed "arthroscopically assisted." Fronek and associates, however, emphasize the importance of a specially designed fasciotome.[45] A meniscotome is not deemed an adequate substitute. Because approximately 40% of patients with chronic compartment syndromes have an associated myofascial hernia, usually located at the site of penetration of the superficial peroneal nerve, fasciotomies should be instituted at this level (Fig. 29–13). These fascial defects should never be closed. It is well documented in the literature that increased intracompartmental pressures exist after fascial closure, and there are also reports of acute compartment syndromes being produced when these fascial defects are closed during the course of treatment for chronic compartment syndrome.[2, 45]

Postoperative Management and Rehabilitation

In a patient with a chronic compartment syndrome, subcutaneous fasciotomy may be performed on an outpatient basis under local anesthesia as recommended by Detmer and associates.[30] A supportive dressing is applied, and the patient is encouraged to elevate the extremity for the first 24 to 48 hours. Weight-bearing is allowed as tolerated. Crutches are discontinued by the seventh day. During the first week, gentle stretching exercises are instituted by the patient, and by the end of the second week, a more formal flexibility and strengthening program is instituted as well. Usually the level of comfort and the amount of healing are sufficient by 2 weeks to allow a return to running activities. Subsequent rehabilitation is much like that used for the medial tibial stress syndrome.

Criteria for Return to Sports Participation

As with most musculoskeletal injuries encountered in sports medicine, a return to full athletic participation is allowed when the following criteria have been met: absence of pain and tenderness in the leg, full return of strength and flexibility, and demonstration that the individual can run sufficiently well to allow participation in his or her particular sport.

Author's Preferred Method of Treatment

For the management of acute compartment syndromes, I follow the guidelines established by Rorabeck[146] (Table

TABLE 29–1
Indications for Surgical Decompression of Acute Compartment Syndrome

Absolute

1. Clinical signs of acute compartment syndrome with demonstrable motor or sensory loss
2. Elevated tissue pressure greater than 35 mm Hg
3. Interrupted arterial circulation to an extremity for more than 4 hours

Relative

4. Circumferential full-thickness burns
5. Muscle overuse syndrome
6. Limb compression syndrome

From Rorabeck C: A practical approach to compartmental syndromes—Part III. Instr Course Lect 32:102–113, 1983.

29–1). In patients with chronic compartment syndrome, I follow the guidelines suggested by Pedowitz and his associates[133] (Table 29–2). For the *chronic* exertional compartment syndrome, I release only those compartments with abnormal pressures or clinical symptoms, or both. We have continued to use the Stryker intracompartmental pressure monitor. This system is extremely portable and uses a disposable 18-gauge side-ported needle attached to an intracompartmental pressure monitor device. Less than 0.3 mL of saline is required for injection into the compartment, and multiple pressure measurements may be carried out quickly and easily. A disposable slit catheter may be used for continuous monitoring.[11]

Popliteal Artery Entrapment

Intermittent claudication of the leg is unusual in the young individual.[1] Even in the middle-aged athlete it remains an infrequent complaint among patients presenting to a sports medicine clinic. There are many reports in the literature, however, that document the existence of the popliteal artery entrapment syndrome and point to its frequency among runners and the confusion that may accompany this diagnosis.[27, 89, 142] The majority of individuals presenting with a popliteal artery entrapment syndrome are young males, 94% of whom are under the age of 40. First described by Love and Whelan[88] in 1965 and at times quite inappropriately labeled shin splints, this syndrome is more often confused with chronic posterior compartment syndrome.[15, 88, 89] The exact incidence of this condition is unknown, although it has been estimated to account for not more than 1% of all entities resulting in stenosis or occlu-

TABLE 29–2
Indications for Surgical Decompression of Chronic Compartment Syndrome

1. Pre-exercise compartmental pressure of >15 mm Hg
2. A 1-minute postexercise pressure of >30 mm Hg
3. A 5-minute postexercise pressure of >20 mm Hg

From Pedowitz R, Hargens A, Mubarak, S, et al: Modified criteria for the objective diagnosis of compartment syndrome of the leg. Am J Sports Med 18:35–40, 1990.

sion of the popliteal artery.[139] The condition is bilateral in 25% of cases.

Pertinent Anatomy

Although Rignault and colleagues attributed this syndrome to muscle hypertrophy, most reports describe various anatomic variations or congenital anomalies about the popliteal region of the leg.[40, 75, 88, 142, 173] Love and Whelan divided the popliteal artery entrapment syndrome into three types as follows[88, 173]:

Type 1—Medial deviation of the popliteal artery around and deep to the medial head of the gastrocnemius.

Type 2—Medial deviation of the popliteal artery about the medial head of the gastrocnemius, which arises abnormally from a more lateral position on the medial femoral condyle.

Type 3—Popliteal artery entrapment caused by an anomalous course of the artery deep to the popliteus muscle.

Represa and his coauthors classified the anomalies into three basic types:[139]

1. The popliteal artery passes deep to the medial head of the gastrocnemius, whose insertion may be normal or abnormal (63% of cases).
2. The popliteal artery cuts across the medial head of the gastrocnemius, occasionally dividing this structure into two tendons or origins (23% of cases).
3. The popliteal artery passes deep to the popliteus muscle (7% of cases).

In the remaining 7% of cases, the anatomic abnormality has not been categorized. Recently, Sammarco has described adductor canal compression of the superficial femoral artery presenting as ischemic pain of the leg.[152] Represa and colleagues further outlined the embryologic development of the popliteal artery system and recognized that our present knowledge of the ontogenic development in this region is incomplete.

Clinical Evaluation

Although the symptomatology may appear vague and may lead to a delay in diagnosis of months or even years, the syndrome should be suspected in any young athlete presenting with symptoms of intermittent claudication. This includes intermittent calf pain, cramping, coolness, and at times paresthesias into the foot. The condition is most often unilateral but may be bilateral. It is not unusual for symptoms to be present with walking and relieved with running, although the reverse may also be true.[88, 89] The syndrome may progress to the point where pain occurs with activities of daily living as well as recreation.

The physical examination may be entirely normal in the asymptomatic patient. In the mildly symptomatic patient, there may be mild calf tenderness. Provocative clinical tests for the syndrome include obliteration of pedal pulses by active plantar flexion or passive dorsiflexion of the ankle (Fig. 29–14). Doppler recordings at the ankle with

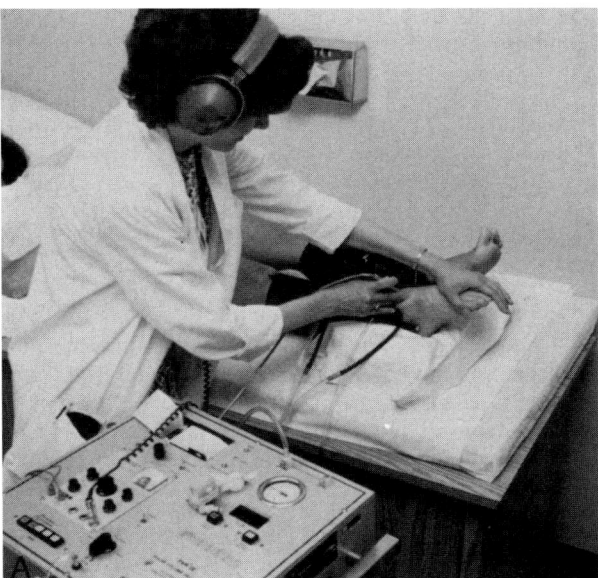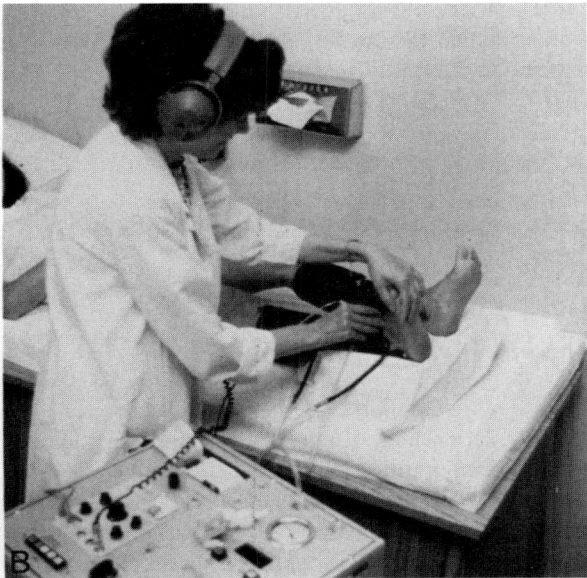

Figure 29–14. *A* and *B,* Provocative clinical tests for the syndrome of popliteal artery entrapment include obliteration of pedal pulses by active plantar flexion or passive dorsiflexion of the ankle as detected by Doppler recordings.

dorsiflexion and plantar flexion may be helpful. Rignault and associates, however, point out that noninvasive techniques are positive in as much as 50% of a normal control population.[142] Therefore, although these tests are suggestive of the syndrome, they are by no means diagnostic.

The definitive diagnosis of popliteal artery entrapment is provided by arteriography. Typically, a medial deviation of the popliteal artery is seen about the medial head of the gastrocnemius muscle. Most often, in the young athlete, the artery is patent, but active plantar flexion and passive dorsiflexion demonstrate stenosis and occlusion. Not uncommonly, a poststenotic dilatation of the artery is also present. Magnetic resonance arteriography is gaining favor as a noninvasive imaging modality that can provide information about the variations of the anatomic course of the popliteal artery that may be associated with this syndrome.

Treatment Options

The treatment of popliteal artery entrapment syndrome is surgical. Ideally, early diagnosis and treatment will prevent damage to the artery that might otherwise lead to progressive thrombosis. Limb ischemia has been reported and may be catastrophic.[89, 139]

Surgical treatment includes exploration of the popliteal artery and its relationship to the surrounding soft tissue structures. In the case of muscle hypertrophy with otherwise normal anatomic relationships, fasciotomy alone has been reported to provide a good result.[142] More typically, there is an anatomic variant or anomaly that requires release. With abnormal medial deviation of the popliteal artery, release and recession of the medial head of the gastrocnemius are advocated.[40, 75, 88] If abnormal fibrous bands, muscle bellies, or tendons constrict the popliteal artery, soft tissue release is performed. Assuming that sur-

gery is performed before permanent ischemic injury to the limb, the reported results are excellent.[134, 137, 142, 173]

Postoperative Management and Rehabilitation

In most instances, major arterial reconstruction or bypass is not required; however, in patients with chronic or severe disease, in whom permanent arterial damage has occurred, vascular reconstructive procedures may be required. Postoperative recovery and rehabilitation are therefore directed by the vascular surgeon. In patients with intermittent vascular compression without vessel damage, recovery is based on routine criteria of wound healing. Flexibility exercises for the leg as well as strengthening exercises are encouraged early. Duwelius and colleagues reported one case in which they documented Cybex isokinetic strength testing performed 1 year postoperatively in a high school athlete.[40] Strength deficits of 10%, 7%, and 11% were present at 60, 120, and 180 degrees per second. Plantar flexion total work and average power were 11% and 16% better in the involved extremity than in the noninvolved leg, a result that was attributed to the compliance of the patient with the rehabilitation program.

Criteria for Return to Sports Participation

Return to full athletic participation depends upon the return of strength and flexibility as well as adequate wound healing. Further, it should include documentation of adequate blood flow within the extremity, both in the normal state and in the stressed state (i.e., after walking or running). Provocative tests for pedal pulses in active plantar flexion and passive dorsiflexion should be normal. Repeat arteriography or magnetic resonance arteriography is not necessary unless a major reconstructive arterial procedure has been required or clinical signs and symptoms remain equivocal. In such a case, it should be remembered that "dynamic" arteriography done with active plantar flexion and passive dorsiflexion is an important component of this test.

Author's Preferred Method of Treatment

Because this syndrome can be confused with posterior compartment syndromes, I measure intracompartmental pressures before and after exercise and include fasciotomy as part of the treatment if necessary. Otherwise, my treatment protocol remains as described.

Effort-Induced Venous Thrombosis

Effort-induced venous thrombosis involving the upper extremity that occurs following repetitive muscular activity such as throwing has been well described in the literature.[184] In the lower extremity, the entity is less well recognized.[67, 176] The symptoms may even be confused with shin splints because the pain may be perceived as anterior. Physical examination, however, should demonstrate calf tenderness and a positive Homan's sign. Further diagnostic work-up including duplex ultrasound imaging or venography should confirm the diagnosis. Treatment includes anticoagulation regimens. With resolution of symptoms and completion of medical treatment, running may be resumed on a graduated basis.

Tennis Leg

This condition is well known and typically presents in the middle-aged or early middle-aged recreational athlete who makes a sudden move or jump while running. Sudden acute pain is felt in the calf; it often feels as if someone had kicked the athlete in the back of the leg. Significant pain and swelling usually develop during the ensuing 24 hours.

Although it is now recognized and documented that this condition is due to a tear of the medial head of the gastrocnemius muscle at the muscle-tendon junction, occasionally the condition is misinterpreted as a rupture of the plantaris tendon.[25, 81] Numerous authors, however, have put this myth to rest, and a review of the literature by Severance and Bassett failed to demonstrate any significant evidence to support rupture of the plantaris tendon as an occurrence.[156]

Pertinent Anatomy

Sutro and Sutro have analyzed the susceptibility of the gastrocnemius muscle to injury, particularly the medial

head at the musculotendinous junction.[171] The medial half of the muscle belly is larger than the lateral mass. Also, the muscle fibers of the gastrocnemius are fast twitch, as opposed to the underlying soleus muscle, which is primarily slow twitch. These authors imply, but do not prove, that there is an anatomic basis for the preference of medial gastrocnemius ruptures.

Relevant Biomechanics

Anouchi and associates have emphasized that the gastrocnemius muscle is particularly vulnerable to injury because it passes by two joints, the knee and the ankle.[8] The mechanism of injury often includes overstretching of this muscle unit by forced ankle dorsiflexion in combination with the extended knee. Froimson has noted that the gastrocnemius muscle is a "short action" muscle, making it particularly vulnerable to overstretch and injury.[44]

Clinical Evaluation

The history includes sudden onset of pain in the calf while running or making a sudden stop or cut. Usually a marked amount of calf swelling and pain develops over the next 24 hours. Tenderness is well localized to the musculotendinous junction of the medial head of the gastrocnemius. MRI can easily demonstrate hemorrhage within the gastrocnemius muscle and provide evidence of the tear.

The differential diagnosis must include thrombophlebitis as well as posterior compartment syndrome.[143] Thrombophlebitis can usually be differentiated on clinical grounds. The presence, however, of calf swelling, tenderness, and pain with dorsiflexion can make this differential diagnosis confusing. Duplex ultrasound imaging is helpful for detection and venography remains the definitive test to rule out thrombophlebitis. Sonographic study also has been shown to have efficacy for the demonstration of tears of the gastrocnemius muscle as well as the plantaris.[16, 83]

Acute posterior compartment syndrome has been described in conjunction with ruptures of the medial head of the gastrocnemius.[8, 165] Indeed, rupture of the gastrocnemius has been associated with anterior and lateral compartment syndromes as well.[165] Progressive pain out of proportion to the injury associated with paresthesias or weakness should alert the examining physician to the possibility of an associated compartment syndrome. As discussed earlier in this chapter, direct measurement of compartment pressures should be performed to rule out this diagnosis.

Treatment Options

Treatment for compartment syndrome is surgical (fasciotomy). Treatment for ruptures of the medial head of the gastrocnemius is nonsurgical. Many authors have outlined various nonoperative treatment regimens that provide consistently good long-term results.[49, 81, 108] Miller outlined an aggressive nonoperative management program in a study of 720 patients.[108] In his experience, treatment initiated within 48 hours of injury resulted in full rehabilitation of 85% of patients by 2 weeks.

Aggressive early management includes supportive wraps (Ace), ice applications three to five times a day, and crutches only if necessary. Early ankle motion is instituted along with nonsteroidal anti-inflammatory medications. As stretching exercises progress and pain subsides, calf strengthening exercises are initiated. Froimson recommends the use of a heel lift for 2 weeks and a return to full activity by 5 weeks.[44]

Criteria for Return to Sports Participation

When the patient has recovered normal pain-free motion and has demonstrated a return of calf strength of at least 90% of the contralateral normal leg, full return to athletic participation is allowed.

Author's Preferred Method of Treatment

For the athlete, I apply the principles of early control of swelling with the use of (1) elevation, (2) ice compresses, and (3) elastic supportive dressings (Ace or TED hose). Mobilization is begun early in the form of gentle active assisted and passive stretching exercises. These are carried out within the limits of pain three times daily. A heel lift is worn, and crutches may be required for the first 2 or 3 days; full weight-bearing is allowed as tolerated thereafter. Strengthening exercises are initiated as comfort allows, usually by 2 weeks. By 3 to 6 weeks, sufficient strength and motion have returned to allow a graduated return to sporting activities. Protective Achilles tendon taping may be used early when returning to sports. Full motion, absence of tenderness or pain, and a strength deficit of less than 10% are required for full athletic participation.

Proximal Tibiofibular Joint Disorders

Isolated dislocations and subluxations of the proximal tibiofibular joint are uncommon. In 1974, Ogden reviewed the existing literature and found a total of 108 cases.[122] Turco and Spinella, in 1985, reported 17 cases.[177] Numerous other case reports exist in the literature.[4, 41, 53, 158, 174, 179] Ogden classified these injuries into four types (Fig. 29–15). Type 1, subluxation, accounted for 23.3% of the 43 cases he presented. Type 2, anterolateral dislocation, was found most frequently and accounted for 67.4%. Type 3, posteromedial dislocation, accounted for only 7% of these injuries, and type 4, superior dislocation, accounted for 2.3% of proximal tibiofibular injuries. Type 4 injuries are usually associated with tibial fractures, fibular fractures, or diastasis of the ankle.

Pertinent Anatomy

As Thomason and Linson describe, the proximal tibiofibular joint is diarthrodial.[174] In approximately 10% of normal adults, the proximal tibiofibular joint space may communicate directly with the femoral tibial joint. The capsule is thicker and stronger anteriorly than posteriorly. There is a single posterior ligamentous band that passes upward obliquely from the fibula to the tibia and is reinforced by the popliteal tendon. The anterior tibiofibular ligament is formed by two or three bands, again passing obliquely and upward from the fibula to the tibia. The biceps femoris tendon passes anterior to this ligament, inserting into the lateral side of the fibula; a portion of it also extends anteriorly into the lateral condyle of the tibia.

Ogden described the inclination of this joint, dividing it into two types.[122] Type 1 is horizontal (with an inclination of less than 20 degrees), and type 2 is oblique (with an inclination of greater than 20 degrees). The surfaces of this joint consist of oval facets of articular cartilage. Type 2, an oblique joint, is the less stable of the two.

Relevant Biomechanics

The proximal tibiofibular joint glides as the talus spreads when the ankle comes into dorsiflexion.[5, 174, 177] Thomason and Linson note that this joint helps to relieve torsional stresses applied to the ankle as well as lateral tibial bending moments.[174] In addition to dissipating torsional loads, this joint allows normal distal motion of the fibula with weight-bearing secondary to contraction of those muscles attached to the fibula.

Clinical Evaluation

The mechanism of injury is distinct and reproducible.[5, 122, 174, 177] Inversion and plantar flexion of the foot causes tension on the peroneal muscles, extensor digitorum longus, and extensor hallucis longus. A violent contraction of these muscles will pull the fibula forward. Further, if the knee is in flexion, the biceps tendon and fibulocollateral ligaments are relaxed. Therefore, a fall on the adducted leg with the knee in flexion and the foot in plantar flexion and inversion is a typical example of the mechanism of injury. A slide tackle in soccer is a classic example of this mechanism (Fig. 29–16). Acutely, pain and tenderness are felt over the proximal tibiofibular joint. This sensation may be aggravated by flexion and extension of the ankle and by inversion and eversion of the foot. There may be a lack of full extension of the knee and transient paresthesia of the peroneal nerve.[179]

In chronic cases, patients may complain of knee instability, lateral knee pain (often poorly localized), and lack of full extension.

On physical examination, there may be an obvious lateral or anterolateral displacement of the fibular head. Tenderness is usually present. Especially in the type 1 injury (subluxation), gross instability may be found by manual

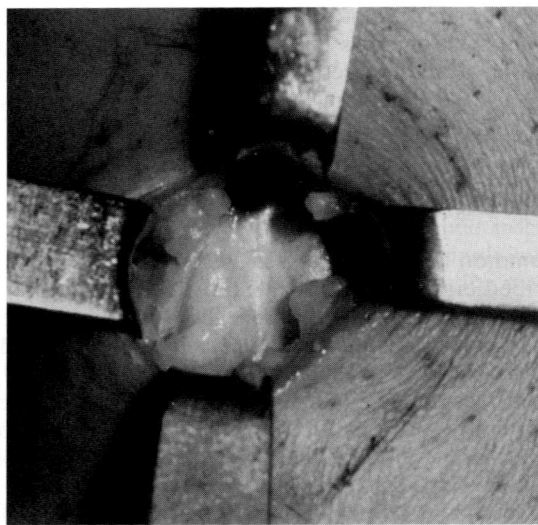

Figure 29–19. Superficial peroneal nerve entrapment is commonly associated with fascial defects and muscle hernia. Treatment should consist of fasciotomy, not fascial repair.

recognized that a pseudoradicular syndrome exists in the lower extremity among peripheral nerve entrapments. Saal and his coauthors point out that peripheral nerve entrapment may masquerade as a lumbar radiculopathy.[150] The distribution of sensory symptoms will allow recognition of the particular nerve involved. Tenderness is usually found over the area of entrapment and may be exacerbated by a simultaneous resistive muscle contraction of those muscles within the affected compartment. Motor weakness may be present, especially after exercise in patients with common peroneal or deep peroneal nerve entrapment.

For superficial peroneal nerve entrapment syndrome, three provocative diagnostic tests have been described: (1) tenderness to palpation may exist over the area of fascial exit, approximately 10 cm proximal to the lateral malleolus, with the patient providing active dorsiflexion and eversion of the ankle; (2) passive plantar flexion and inversion of the ankle may elicit pain or tenderness upon compression of the nerve; and (3) a positive Tinel's sign may be present with percussion over the nerve in the region of its exit from the deep fascia of the leg.[168] Electromyographic and nerve conduction studies may be helpful. Prolonged conduction velocity will be present on these studies. MRI may be used to detect muscle hernias that can be associated.[99]

Treatment Options

The treatment of peripheral nerve entrapment syndromes may be conservative if the symptoms are of recent onset. A tapered lateral sole wedge may be used to decrease repetitive inversion stress.[80] Peroneal muscle strengthening exercises and proprioceptive training have been thought to decrease the likelihood of repetitive injury. With an established entrapment syndrome, treatment is usually surgical and includes a careful fascial release and often a neurolysis.[169]

It should be emphasized again that at no time should

the treatment of a peripheral entrapment syndrome associated with a fascial defect include closure of the defect. An acute compartment syndrome with unfortunate consequences may result.[2]

Postoperative Management and Rehabilitation

After fascial release (fasciotomy) and neurolysis, weight-bearing is allowed as tolerated and return to full athletic participation is allowed according to the level of pain and tenderness experienced by the patient. Ten days to 5 weeks have been reported as the usual recovery time needed.[80]

References

1. Abraham P, Chevalier JM, Leftheriotis G, Saumet JL: Lower extremity arterial disease in sports. Am J Sports Med 25:581–584, 1997.
2. Almdahl S, Due J, Samdal F: Compartment syndrome with muscle necrosis following repair of hernia of tibialis anterior. Acta Chir Scand 153:695, 1987.
3. Amendola A, Rorabeck C, Vellett D, et al: The use of magnetic resonance imaging in exertional compartment syndromes. Am J Sports Med 18:29–34, 1990.
4. American Medical Association, Subcommittee on Classification of Sports Injuries: Standard Nomenclature of Athletic Injuries. Chicago, American Medical Association, 1966, pp 122–126.
5. Andersen K: Dislocation of the superior tibiofibular joint. Injury 16:494–498, 1985.
6. Anderson M, Ugalde V, Batt M, Gacayan J: Shin splints: MR appearance in a preliminary study. Radiology 204:177–180, 1997.
7. Andrish JT, Bergfeld JA, Walheim J: A prospective study on the management of shin splints. J Bone Joint Surg Am 56:1697–1700, 1974.
8. Anouchi Y, Parker R, Seitz W: Posterior compartment syndrome of the calf resulting from misdiagnosis of a rupture of the medial head of the gastrocnemius. J Trauma 27:678–680, 1987.
9. Arciero R, Shishido N, Parr T: Acute anterolateral compartment syndrome secondary to rupture of the peroneus longus muscle. Am J Sports Med 12:366–367, 1984.
10. Arendt E, Griffiths H: The use of MR imaging in the assessment and clinical management of stress reactions of bone in high-performance athletes. Clin Sports Med 16:291–306, 1997.
11. Awbrey B, Sienkiewicz P, Mankin H: Chronic exercise-induced compartment pressure elevation measured with a miniaturized fluid pressure monitor. Am J Sports Med 16:610–615, 1988.
12. Banerjee T, Koons D: Superficial peroneal nerve entrapment. J Neurosurg 55:991–992, 1981.
13. Barrow GW, Saha S: Menstrual irregularity and stress fractures in collegiate female distance runners. Am J Sports Med 16:209–216, 1988.
14. Bates P: Shin splints—a literature review. Br J Sports Med 19:132–137, 1985.
15. Bell S: Intracompartmental pressures on exertion in a patient with a popliteal artery entrapment syndrome. Am J Sports Med 13:365–366, 1985.
16. Bianchi S, Martinoli C, Abdelwahab I, et al: Sonographic evaluation of tears of the gastrocnemius medial head ("tennis leg"). J Ultrasound Med 17:157–162, 1998.
17. Blair WF, Hanley SR: Stress fracture of the proximal fibula. Am J Sports Med 8:212–213, 1980.
18. Blank S: Transverse tibial stress fractures. Am J Sports Med 15:597–602, 1987.
19. Brill DR: Sports nuclear medicine. Bone imaging for lower extremity pain in athletes. Clin Nucl Med 8:101–106, 1983.
20. Castillo M, Tehranzadeh J, Morillo G: Atypical healed stress fracture of the fibula masquerading as chronic osteomyelitis. Am J Sports Med 16:185–188, 1988.

21. Chang P, Harris R: Intramedullary nailing for chronic tibial stress fractures. Am J Sports Med 2495:688–692, 1996.

22. Christensen S: Dislocation of the upper end of the fibula. Acta Orthop Scand 37:107–109, 1966.

23. Clanton T, Solcher B: Chronic leg pain in the athlete. Clin Sports Med 13:743–759, 1994.

24. Clement DB: Tibial stress syndrome in athletes. J Sports Med 2: 81–85, 1974.

25. Daffner RH: Anterior tibial striations. AJR Am J Roentgenol 143: 651–653, 1984.

26. Darby RE: Stress fractures of the os calcis. JAMA 200:131–132, 1967.

27. Darling R, Buckley C, Abbott W, Raines J: Intermittent claudication in young athletes: Popliteal artery entrapment syndrome. J Trauma 14:543–552, 1974.

28. Davey J, Rorabeck C, Fowler P: The tibialis posterior muscle compartment. Am J Sports Med 12:391–397, 1984.

29. Detmer DE: Chronic shin splints. Classification and management of medial tibial stress syndrome. Sports Med 3:436–446, 1986.

30. Detmer D, Sharpe K, Sufit R, Girdley F: Chronic compartment syndrome: Diagnosis, management, and outcomes. Am J Sports Med 13:162–170, 1985.

31. Detmer D: Chronic leg pain. Am J Sports Med 8:141–144, 1980.

32. Deutsch A, Coel M, Mink J: Imaging of stress injuries to bone. Clin Sports Med 16:275–290, 1997.

33. Devas MB: Stress fractures in athletes. Proc R Soc Med 62:933–937, 1969.

34. Devas M: Stress Fractures. London, Churchill Livingstone, 1975, pp 56–91.

35. Devereaux MD, Lachmann SM: Athletes attending a sports injury clinic. A review. Br J Sports Med 17:137–142, 1983.

36. Devereaux M, Parr G, Lachmann S, et al: The diagnosis of stress fractures in athletes. JAMA 252:531–533, 1984.

37. Dickson T, Kichline P: Functional management of stress fractures in female athletes using a pneumatic leg brace. Am J Sports Med 15:86–89, 1987.

38. Donati R, Echo B, Powell C: Bilateral tibial stress fractures in a six year-old male: A case report. Am J Sports Med 18:323–325, 1990.

39. Drez D: Therapeutic Modalities for Sports Injuries. Chicago, Year Book, 1989.

40. Duwelius P, Kelbel M, Jardon O, Walsh W: Popliteal artery entrapment in a high school athlete. Am J Sports Med 15:371–373, 1987.

41. Falkenberg P, Nygaard H: Isolated anterior dislocation of the proximal tibiofibular joint. J Bone Joint Surg Br 65:310–311, 1983.

42. Fauno P, Kalund S, Andreason I, Jorgensen U: Soreness in lower extremities and back is reduced by use of shock absorbing heel inserts. Int J Sports Med 14:288–290, 1993.

43. Flandry F, Sanders R: Tibiofibular synostosis: An unusual cause of shin splintlike pain. Am J Sports Med 15:280–284, 1987.

44. Froimson A: Tennis leg. JAMA 209:415–416, 1969.

45. Fronek J, Mubarak S, Hargens A, et al: Management of chronic exertional anterior compartment syndrome of the lower extremity. Clin Orthop 220:217–227, 1987.

46. Gamble J: Proximal tibiofibular synostosis. J Pediatr Orthop 4: 243–245, 1984.

47. Garfin S, Mubarak S, Evans K, et al: Quantification of intracompartmental pressure and volume under plaster casts. J Bone Joint Surg Am 63:449, 1981.

48. Garrett WE Jr: Muscle strain injuries: Clinical and basic aspects. Med Sci Sports Exerc 22:436–443, 1990.

49. Gecha S, Torg E: Knee injuries in tennis. Clin Sports Med 7: 435–452, 1988.

50. Gershuni DH, Yaru NC, Hargens AR, et al: Ankle and knee position as a factor modifying intracompartmental pressure in the human leg. J Bone Joint Surg Am 66:1415–1420, 1989.

51. Gershuni D, Gosink B, Hargens A, et al: Ultrasound evaluation of the anterior musculofascial compartment of the leg following exercise. Clin Orthop 167:185–190, 1982.

52. Gertsch P, Borgeat A, Walli T: New crosscountry skiing technique and compartment syndrome. Am J Sports Med 15:612–613, 1987.

53. Giachino A: Recurrent dislocations of the proximal tibiofibular joint. J Bone Joint Surg Am 68:1104–1106, 1986.

54. Giannotti G, Cohn S, Brown M, et al: Utility of near-infared spectroscopy in the diagnosis of lower extremity compartment syndrome. J Trauma 48:396–401, 2000.

55. Giladi M, Milgrom C, Kashtan H, et al: Recurrent stress fractures in military recruits. J Bone Joint Surg Br 68:439–441, 1986.

56. Giladi M, Milgrom C, Simkin A, et al: Stress fractures and tibial bone width. J Bone Joint Surg Br 69:326–329, 1987.

57. Giladi M, Ziv Y, Aharonson Z, et al: Comparison between radiography, bone scan, and ultrasound in the diagnosis of stress fractures. Mil Med 149:459–461, 1984.

58. Gilbert RS, Johnson HA: Stress fractures in military recruits—a review of twelve years experience. Mil Med 131:716–721, 1966.

59. Gillespie WJ, Grant I: Interventions for preventing and treating stress reactions of bone of the lower limbs in young adults. The Cochrane Database of Systematic Reviews (1), 2001.

60. Goodman M: Isolated lateral-compartment syndrome. Report of a case. J Bone Joint Surg Am 62:834, 1980.

61. Green N, Rogers R, Lipscomb B: Nonunions of stress fractures of the tibia. Am J Sports Med 13:171–176, 1985.

62. Groshar D, Lam M, Even-Sapir E, et al: Stress fractures and bone pain: Are they closely associated? Injury 16:526–528, 1985.

63. Gross J, Hamilton W, Swift T: Isolated mechanical lesions of the sural nerve. Muscle Nerve 3:248–249, 1980.

64. Hamill J, van Emmerick R, Heiderscheit B: A dynamical systems approach to lower extremity running injuries. Clin Biomech 14: 297–308, 1999.

65. Hargens A, Akeson W, Mubarak S, et al: Tissue fluid pressures: From basic research tools to clinical applications. J Orthop Res 7: 902–909, 1989.

66. Harvey JS: Overuse syndromes in young athletes. Clin Sports Med 2:595–607, 1983.

67. Harvey J: Effort thrombosis in the lower extremity of a runner. Am J Sports Med 6:400–402, 1978.

68. Hoffman J, Chapnik L, Shamis A, et al: The effect of leg strength on the incidence of lower extremity overuse injuries during military training. Mil Med 164:153–156, 1999.

69. Hoffmeyer P, Cox J, Fritschy D: Ultrastructural modifications of muscle in three types of compartment syndrome. Int Orthop 11: 53–59, 1987.

70. Holder LE, Michael RH: The specific scintigraphic pattern of "shin splints in the lower leg": Concise communication. J Nucl Med 25: 865–869, 1984.

71. Howard J, Mohtadi N, Wiley J: Evaluation of outcomes in patient following surgical treatment of chronic exertional compartment syndrome in the leg. Clin J Sports Med 10:176–184, 2000.

72. Ilahi O, Kohl H: Lower extremity morphology and alignment and risk of overuse injury. Clin J Sport Med 8:38–42, 1998.

73. Israeli A, Ganel A, Blankstein A, Horoszowski H: Stress fractures of the tibial tuberosity in a high jumper: Case report. J Sports Med 5:299–300, 1984.

74. James SL, Bates BT, Osternig LR: Injuries to runners. Am J Sports Med 6:40–50, 1978.

75. Jiaju W, Cheng W, Guangsheng Z, Jingju Z: Popliteal artery entrapment syndrome. J Cardiovasc Surg 29:480–482, 1988.

76. Johnson LC, Stradford HT, Geis RW, et al: Histogenesis of stress fractures. J Bone Joint Surg Am 45:1542, 1963.

77. Kernohan J, Levack B, Wilson J: Entrapment of the superficial peroneal nerve. J Bone Joint Surg Br 67:60–61, 1985.

78. Kirby R, McDermott A: Anterior tibial compartment pressures during running with rearfoot and forefoot landing styles. Arch Phys Rehabil 64:296–299, 1983.

79. Landerer A: Die Gewebspannung in ihrem Einfluss und die ortiliche Blutbewegung und Lymphbewegung. Leipzig, Vogel, 1884.

80. Leach R, Purnell M, Saito A: Peroneal nerve entrapment in runners. Am J Sports Med 17:287–291, 1989.

81. Leach R: Leg and foot injuries in racquet sports. Clin Sports Med 7:359–370, 1988.

82. Lee JK, Yao L: Stress fractures: MR imaging. Radiology 169: 217–220, 1988.

83. Leekham R, Agur A, McKee N: Using sonography to diagnose injury of plantaris muscles and tendons. AJR Am J Roentgenol 172: 185–189, 1999.

84. Lehman WL Jr: Overuse syndromes in runners. Am Fam Physician 29:157–161, 1984.

85. Li G, Zhang S, Chen G, et al: Radiographic and histologic analyses of stress fracture in rabbit tibias. Am J Sports Med 13:285–294, 1985.

86. Lieberman CM, Hemingway DL: Scintigraphy of shin splints. Clin Nucl Med 5:31, 1980.

87. Logan J, Roabeck C, Castle G: The measurement of dynamic compartment pressure during exercise. Am J Sports Med 11:220–223, 1983.

88. Love J, Whelan T: Popliteal artery entrapment syndrome. Am J Surg 109:620–624, 1965.

89. Lysens R, Renson L, Ostyn M, Stalpaert G: Intermittent claudication in young athletes: Popliteal artery entrapment syndrome. Am J Sports Med 11:177–179, 1983.

90. Margulies J, Simkin A, Leichter I, et al: Effect of intense physical activity on the bone mineral content in the lower limbs of young adults. J Bone Joint Surg Am 68:1090–1093, 1986.

91. Martens M, Backaert M, Vermaut G, Mulier J: Chronic leg pain in athletes due to a recurrent compartment syndrome. Am J Sports Med 12:148–151, 1984.

92. Matheson GO, Clement DB, McKenzie DC, et al: Stress fractures in athletes: A study of 320 cases. Am J Sports Med 15:46–58, 1987.

93. Matsen F, Mayo K, Sheridan G, Krugmire R: Monitoring of intramuscular pressure. Surgery 79:702–709, 1976.

94. Matsen F, Winquist R, Krugmire R: Diagnosis and management of compartmental syndromes. J Bone Joint Surg Am 62:286–291, 1980.

95. McAuliffe T, Fiddian N, Browett J: Entrapment neuropathy of the superficial peroneal nerve. J Bone Joint Surg Br 67:62–63, 1985.

96. McDermott A, Marble A, Yabsley R, Phillips M: Monitoring dynamic anterior compartment pressures during exercise. Am J Sports Med 10:83–89, 1982.

97. McKenzie DC, Clement DB, Taunton JE: Running shoes, orthotics, and injuries. Sports Med 2:334–347, 1985.

98. Melberg P, Styf J: Posteromedial pain in the lower leg. Am J Sports Med 17:747–750, 1989.

99. Mellado J, Perez del Palomar L: Muscle hernias of the lower leg: MRI findings. Skeletal Radiol 28:465–469, 1999.

100. Messier SP, Pittala KA: Etiologic factors associated with selected running injuries. Med Sci Sports Exerc 20:501–505, 1988.

101. Michael RH, Holder LE: The soleus syndrome. A cause of medial tibial stress (shin splints). Am J Sports Med 13:87–94, 1985.

102. Micheli L, Solomon R, Solomon J, et al: Surgical treatment for chronic lower-leg compartment syndrome in young female athletes. Am J Sports Med 27:197–201, 1999.

103. Milgrom C, Chisin R, Giladi M, et al: Negative bone scans in impending tibial stress fractures. Am J Sports Med 12:488–491, 1984.

104. Milgrom C, Giladi M, Chisin R, Dizian R: The long-term followup of soldiers with stress fractures. Am J Sports Med 13:398–400, 1985.

105. Milgrom C, Giladi M, Simkin A, et al: An analysis of the biomechanical mechanism of tibial stress fractures among Israeli infantry recruits. Clin Orthop 231:216–221, 1988.

106. Milgrom C, Giladi M, Stein M, et al: Stress fractures in military recruits. J Bone Joint Surg Br 67:732–735, 1985.

107. Milgrom C, Giladi M, Stein M, et al: Medial tibial pain. Clin Orthop 213:167–171, 1986.

108. Miller W: Rupture of the musculotendinous juncture of the medial head of the gastrocnemius muscle. Am J Sports Med 5:191–193, 1977.

109. Moller B, Kadin S: Entrapment of the common peroneal nerve. Am J Sports Med 15:90–91, 1987.

110. Mubarak SJ, Gould RN, Lee YF, et al: R. The medial tibial stress syndrome. A cause of shin splints. Am J Sports Med 10:201–205, 1982.

111. Mubarak S, Owen C, Hargens A, et al: Acute compartment syndromes: Diagnosis and treatment with the aid of the Wick catheter. J Bone Joint Surg Am 60:1091–1095, 1978.

112. Mubarak S, Hargens A: Compartment Syndromes and Volkmann's Contractures. Philadelphia, WB Saunders, 1981.

113. Mubarak S, Owen C: Double incision fasciotomy of the leg for decompression in compartment syndromes. J Bone Joint Surg Am 59:184, 1977.

114. Mubarak S: A practical approach to compartmental syndromes. Part II. Instr Course Lect 32:92–102, 1983.

115. Nattiv A, Armsey T: Stress injury to bone in the female athlete. Clin Sports Med 16:197–224, 1997.

116. Neely F: Intrinsic risk factors for exercise-related lower limb injuries. Sports Med 26:253–263, 1998.

117. Nghiem D, Boland J: Four-compartment fasciotomy of the lower extremity without fibulectomy: A new approach. Am Surg 46:414–417, 1980.

118. Norfray J, Schlachter L, Kernahan W Jr, et al: Early confirmation of stress fractures in joggers. JAMA 243:1647–1649, 1980.

119. Novacheck T: Running injuries: A biomechanical approach. Instr Course Lect 47:397–406, 1998.

120. Nussbaum A, Treves S, Micheli L: Bone stress lesions in ballet dancers: Scintigraphic assessment. AJR Am J Roentgenol 150:851–855, 1988.

121. Ogden J: Subluxation of the proximal tibiofibular joint. Clin Orthop 101:192–197, 1974.

122. Ogden J: Subluxation and dislocation of the proximal tibiofibular joint. J Bone Joint Surg Am 56:145–154, 1974.

123. Orava S, Hulkko A, Jormakka E: Exertion injuries in female athletes. Br J Sports Med 15:229–233, 1981.

124. Orava S, Jormakka E, Hulkko A: Stress fractures in young athletes. Arch Orthop Trauma Surg 98:271–274, 1981.

125. Orava S, Puranen J, AlaKetola L: Stress fractures caused by physical exercise. Acta Orthop Scand 49:19–27, 1978.

126. Orava S, Hulkko A: Stress fractures in athletes. Int J Sports Med 8: 221–226, 1987.

127. Orava S, Hulkko A: Delayed unions and nonunions of stress fractures in athletes. Am J Sports Med 16:378–382, 1988.

128. Orava S, Hulkko A: Stress fractures of the midtibial shaft. Acta Orthop Scand 55:35–37, 1984.

129. Orava S, Puranen J: Athletes' leg pains. Br J Sports Med 13: 92–97, 1979.

130. Orava S: Stress fractures. Br J Sports Med 14:40–44, 1980.

131. Ota Y, Senda M, Hashizume H, Inoue H: Chronic compartment syndrome of the lower leg: A new diagnostic method using near-infared spectroscopy and a new technique of endoscopic fasciotomy. Arthroscopy 15:439–443, 1999.

132. Passa A, Rampoldi M: Fatigue fracture of the tibia in dancers (report of 3 cases). Ital J Orthop Traumatol 13:235–240, 1987.

133. Pedowitz R, Hargens A, Mubarak S, Gershuni D: Modified criteria for the objective diagnosis of chronic syndrome of the leg. Am J Sports Med 18:35–40, 1990.

134. Podore P: Popliteal entrapment syndromes: A report of tibial nerve entrapment. J Vasc Surg 2:335–336, 1985.

135. Pringle R, Protherol K, Mukherjee S: Entrapment neuropathy of the sural nerve. J Bone Joint Surg Br 56:465–468, 1974.

136. Qvarfordt P, Christenson J, Eklof B, et al: Intramuscular pressure, muscle blood flow, and skeletal muscle metabolism in chronic anterior tibial compartment syndrome. Clin Orthop 179:284–291, 1983.

137. Rauh M, Margherita A, Rice S, et al: High school cross country running injuries: A longitudinal study. J Clin Sports Med 10:110–116, 2000.

138. Reneman R: The Anterior and the Lateral Compartment Syndrome of the Leg. The Hague, Mouton, 1968.

139. Represa J, DeDiego J, Molina L, et al: Popliteal artery entrapment syndrome. J Cardiovasc Surg 27:426–430, 1986.

140. Resnick D, Newell J, Guerra J, et al: Proximal tibiofibular joint. Anatomic-pathologic-radiographic correlation. Am J Roentgenol 131:133–138, 1978.

141. Rettig A, Shelbourne D, McCarroll J, et al: The natural history and treatment of delayed union stress fractures of the anterior cortex of the tibia. Am J Sports Med 16:250–255, 1988.

142. Rignault D, Pailler J, Lunel F: The "functional" popliteal entrapment syndrome. Int Angiol 4:341–343, 1985.

143. Robinson N: Spontaneous rupture of the gastrocnemius muscle presenting as acute thrombophlebitis. Am Surg 38:385–388, 1972.

144. Rorabeck C, Bourne R, Fowler P, et al: The role of tissue pressure measurement in diagnosing chronic anterior compartment syndrome. Am J Sports Med 16:143–146, 1988.

145. Rorabeck C, Fowler P, Nott L: The results of fasciotomy in the management of chronic exertional compartment syndrome. Am J Sports Med 16:224–227, 1988.

146. Rorabeck C: A practical approach to compartmental syndromes. Part III. Instr Course Lect 32:102–113, 1983.

147. Rosen PR, Micheli LJ, Treves S: Early scintigraphic diagnosis of bone stress and fractures in athletic adolescents. Pediatrics 70: 11–15, 1982.

148. Roub L, Gumerman L, Hanley E, et al: Bone stress: A radionuclide imaging perspective. Radiology 132:431–438, 1979.

149. Rupani H, Holder L, Espinola D, Engin S: Three-phase radionuclide bone imaging in sports medicine. Radiology 156:187–196, 1985.

150. Saal J, Dillingham M, Gamburd R, Fanton G: The pseudoradicular syndrome. Spine 13:926–930, 1988.

151. Safran MR, Seaber A, Garrett WE Jr: Warmup and muscular injury prevention. An update. Sports Med 8:239–249, 1989.
152. Sammarco GJ, Russon-Alesi F, Munda R: Partial vascular occlusion causing pseudocompartment syndrome of the leg. Am J Sports Med 25:409–411, 1997.
153. Sanchez-Marquez A, Gil-Garcia M, Valls C, et al: Sports-related muscle injuries of the lower extremity: MR imaging appearances. Eur Radiol 9:1088–1093, 1999.
154. Scholander P, Hargens A, Miller S: Negative pressure in the interstitial fluid of animals. Science 161:321, 1968.
155. Scranton P, McMaster J, Kelly E: Dynamic fibular function: A new concept. Clin Orthop 118:76–81, 1976.
156. Severance H, Bassett FH III: Rupture of the plantaris—does it exist? J Bone Joint Surg Am 64:1387–1388, 1982.
157. Shelbourne K, Fisher D, Rettig A, McCarroll J: Stress fractures of the medial malleolus. Am J Sports Med 16:60–63, 1988.
158. Sijbrandij S: Instability of the proximal tibiofibular joint. Acta Orthop Scand 49:621–626, 1978.
159. Slocum DB: The shin splint syndrome. Am J Surg 114:875–881, 1967.
160. Somer K, Meurman KO: Computed tomography of stress fractures. J Comput Assist Tomogr 6:109–115, 1982.
161. Spencer R, Levinson E, Baldwin R, et al: Diverse bone scan abnormalities in "shin splints." J Nucl Med 20:1271–1272, 1979.
162. Sridhara C, Izzo K: Terminal sensory branches of the superficial peroneal nerve: An entrapment syndrome. Arch Phys Med Rehabil 66:789–791, 1985.
163. Stafford S, Rosenthal D, Gebhardt M, et al: MRI in stress fracture. AJR Am J Roentgenol 147:553–556, 1986.
164. Stanitski C, McMaster J, Scranton P: On the nature of stress fractures. Am J Sports Med 6:391–396, 1978.
165. Straehley D, Jones W: Acute compartment syndrome (anterior lateral, and superficial posterior) following tear of the medial head of the gastrocnemius muscle. Am J Sports Med 14:96–99, 1986.
166. Strickler T, Malone T, Garrett WE: The effects of passive warming on muscle injury. Am J Sports Med 18:141–145, 1990.
167. Styf J, Korner L: Chronic anterior compartment syndrome of the leg. J Bone Joint Surg Am 68:1338–1347, 1986.
168. Styf J: Diagnosis of exercise-induced pain in the anterior aspect of the lower leg. Am J Sports Med 16:165–169, 1988.
169. Styf J: Entrapment of the superficial peroneal nerve. J Bone Joint Surg Br 71:131–135, 1989.
170. Sullivan D, Warren RF, Pavlov H, Kelman G: Stress fractures in 51 runners. Clin Orthop 187:188–192, 1984.
171. Sutro C, Sutro W: The medial head of the gastrocnemius: A review of the basis for partial rupture and for intermittent claudication. Bull Hosp Jt Dis 45:150–157, 1985.
172. Symeonides PP: High stress fractures of the fibula. J Bone Joint Surg Br 62:192–193, 1980.
173. Taunton J, Maxwell T: Intermittent claudication in an athlete. Popliteal artery entrapment: A case report. Can J Appl Sport Sci 7:161–163, 1982.
174. Thomason P, Linson M: Isolated dislocation of the proximal tibiofibular joint. J Trauma 21:192–195, 1986.
175. Ting A, King W, Yocum L, et al: Stress fractures of the tarsal navicular in long-distance runners. Clin Sports Med 7:89–101, 1988.
176. Touliopolous S, Hershman E: Lower leg pain. Diagnosis and treatment of compartment syndromes and other pain syndromes of the leg. Sports Med 27:193–204, 1999.
177. Turco V, Spinella A: Anterolateral dislocation of the head of the fibula in sports. Am J Sports Med 13:209–215, 1985.
178. Veth R, Kingma L, Nielsen H: The abnormal proximal tibiofibular joint. Arch Orthop Trauma Surg 102:167–171, 1984.
179. Veth R, Klasen H, Kingma L: Traumatic instability of the proximal tibiofibular joint. Injury 13:159–164, 1981.
180. Viitasalo JT, Kvist M: Some biomechanical aspects of the foot and ankle in athletes with and without shin splints. Am J Sports Med 11:125–130, 1983.
181. Whiteside L, Reynolds F, Ellsasser J: Tibiofibular synostosis and recurrent ankle sprains in high performance athletes. J Sports Med 6:204–208, 1978.
182. Whitesides T, Haney T, Morimoto K, Harada H: Tissue pressure measurements as a determinant for the need of fasciotomy. Clin Orthop 113:43–51, 1975.
183. Wong K, Weiner D: Proximal tibiofibular synostosis. Clin Orthop 135:45–47, 1978.
184. Wright R, Lipscomb A: Acute occlusion of the subclavian vein in an athlete: Diagnosis, etiology and surgical management. J Sports Med 2:243, 1975.
185. Yousem D, Magid D, Fishman E, et al: Computed tomography of stress fractures. J Comput Assist Tomogr 10:92–95, 1986.
186. Zwas S, Elkanovitch R, Frank G: Interpretation and classification of bone scintigraphic findings in stress fractures. J Nucl Med 28:452–457, 1987.

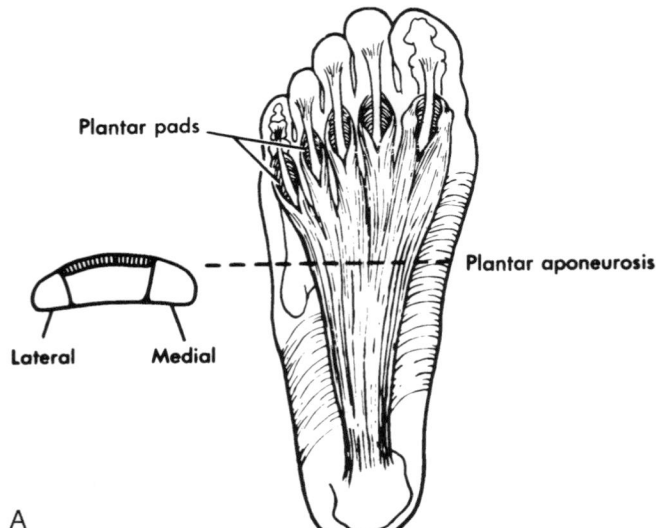

A

Figure 30A–1. *A,* Plantar aponeurosis. The plantar aponeurosis originates from the tubercle of the calcaneus and passes forward to insert into the base of the proximal phalanges. The aponeurosis divides, permitting the long flexor tendon to pass distally. *B,* The longitudinal arch at rest and the plantar aponeurosis nonfunctional. *C,* Dorsiflexion of the metatarsophalangeal joints results in the activation of the plantar aponeurosis, which results in depression of the metatarsal heads, elevation of the longitudinal arch, inversion of the calcaneus, and external rotation of the tibia. *(A–C* from Mann RA, Coughlin MJ: Biomechanics of walking in the foot and ankle. In Video Textbook of Foot and Ankle Surgery. St. Louis, Medical Video Productions, 1991.)

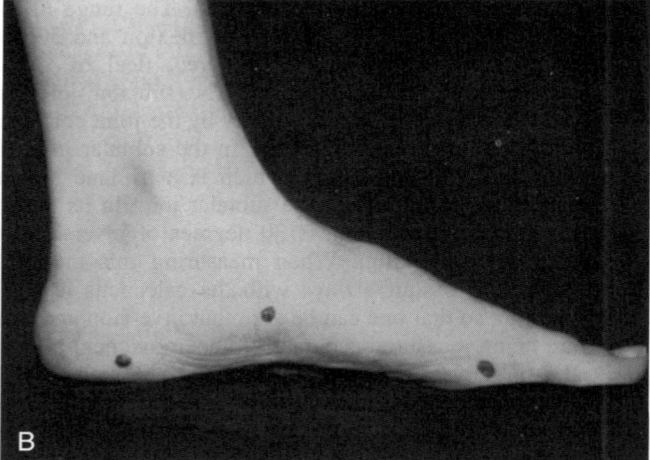

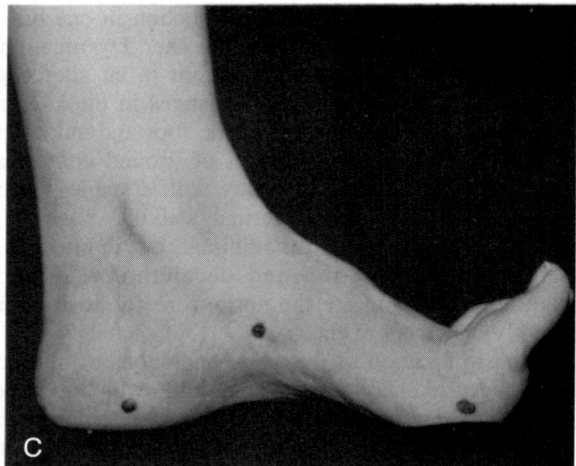

the foot. Dorsiflexion of the metatarsophalangeal joints is a passive motion that results in plantar flexion of the metatarsals, which elevates and stabilizes the longitudinal arch. Because of the configuration of the subtalar joint, this action also brings about inversion of the calcaneus, which imparts an external rotation torque to the lower extremity. The range of motion of the metatarsophalangeal joints is 60 degrees of dorsiflexion and 20 degrees of plantar flexion.

Ankle Joint

The ankle joint is not a simple hinge joint because the trochlear surface of the talus is a section from a cone whose apex is based medially (Fig. 30A–2).[4] The talus is stabilized within the ankle mortise by the medial and lateral malleoli. Medially, the deltoid ligament forms a dense supporting structure, whereas on the lateral aspect the ligament support is provided by three separate ligamentous bands—the anterior and posterior talofibular ligament and the calcaneofibular ligament.

The anterior talofibular ligament is taut with the ankle joint in plantar flexion, when it is in line with the fibula, and the calcaneofibular ligament is taut with the ankle joint in dorsiflexion, when the ligament is in line with the fibula (Fig. 30A–3).[4] It is well known that the anterior talofibular ligament is injured most frequently because most injuries occur with the ankle joint in plantar flexion, placing this ligament under tension. Isolated injuries to the calcaneofibular ligament are less frequent, and this injury occurs with the ankle joint in dorsiflexion.

Dorsiflexion and plantar flexion occur at the ankle joint. During walking, rapid plantar flexion occurs at heel strike and ends by foot flat, after which progressive dorsiflexion occurs. Dorsiflexion reaches a maximum at 40% of the walking cycle, when plantar flexion begins, and continues until toe-off, when dorsiflexion occurs again (Fig. 30A–4).

The force applied across the ankle joint during walking has been measured at approximately 4.5 times body weight.[6] This maximum stress occurs just before and just after the onset of plantar flexion of the ankle joint. If this force were extrapolated to running, in which the force is approximately 2 to 2.5 times greater than that of walking,

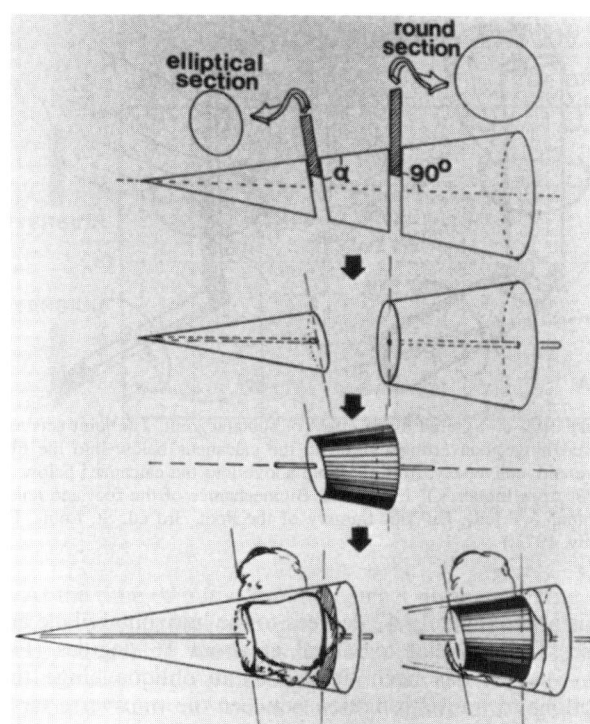

Figure 30A–2. The trochlear surface of the talus is a section from a cone. The apex of the cone is directed medially, and the open end is directed laterally. (From Inman VT: The Joints of the Ankle. Baltimore, Williams & Wilkins, 1976.)

we would see stress across the ankle joint that approaches 10 times body weight.

Muscle control of the ankle joint can be divided into the anterior and posterior compartments. The anterior compartment consists of the tibialis anterior, extensor hallucis longus, and extensor digitorum longus. The posterior compartment consists of the gastrocsoleus group, tibialis posterior, flexor digitorum longus, and flexor hallucis longus. The lateral compartment, consisting of the peroneus longus and brevis, functions with the posterior compartment.

During normal walking, the anterior compartment muscles become active late in stance phase to bring about dorsiflexion of the ankle joint by a concentric (shortening) contraction (see Fig. 30A–4). This muscle group remains

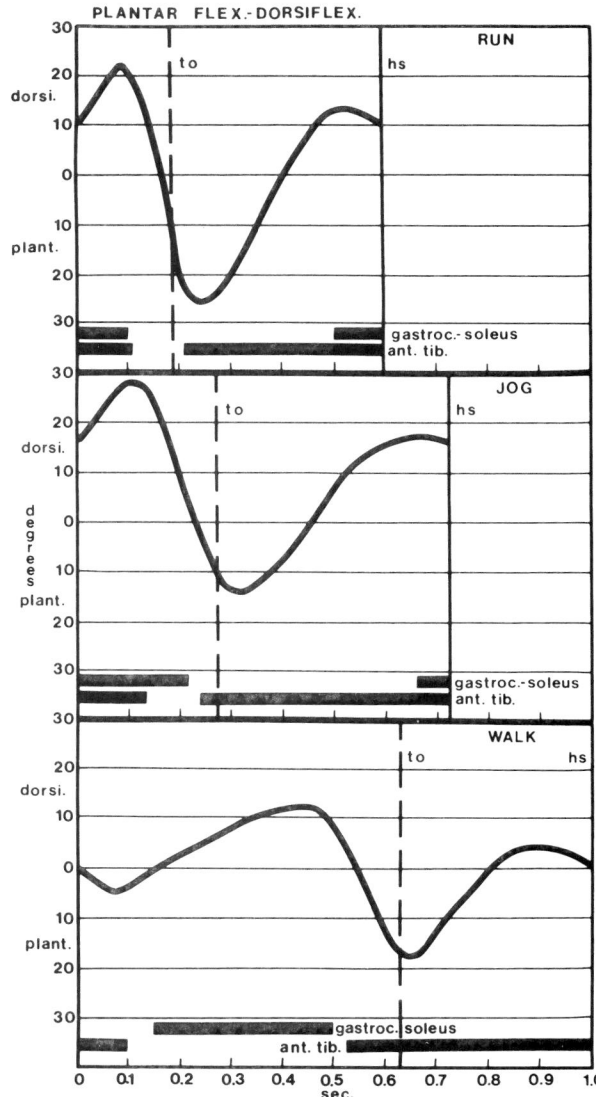

Figure 30A–4. Ankle joint range of motion for walking, jogging, and running. The muscle function of the anterior and posterior compartment is noted on the bottom of the graph. Ant. tib., anterior tibial; dorsi., dorsiflexion; flex., flexion; gastroc.-soleus, gastrocnemius-soleus; hs, heel strike; plant., plantar flexion; to, toe-off. (From Mann RA: Biomechanics of running. In American Academy of Orthopaedic Surgeons: Symposium on the Foot and Leg in Running Sports. St. Louis, CV Mosby, 1982.)

Figure 30A–3. Calcaneofibular (a) and anterior talofibular (b) ligaments. *A*, In plantar flexion, the anterior talofibular ligament is in line with the fibula, thereby providing most of the support to the lateral aspect of the ankle joint. *B*, When the ankle is in neutral position, both the anterior talofibular and the calcaneofibular ligaments support the joint. The obliquely placed structure depicts the axis of the subtalar joint. It should be noted that the calcaneofibular ligament parallels the axis. *C*, When the ankle joint is in dorsiflexion, the calcaneofibular ligament is in line with the fibula and supports the lateral aspect of the joint. (*A–C* from Inman VT: The Joints of the Ankle. Baltimore, Williams & Wilkins, 1976.)

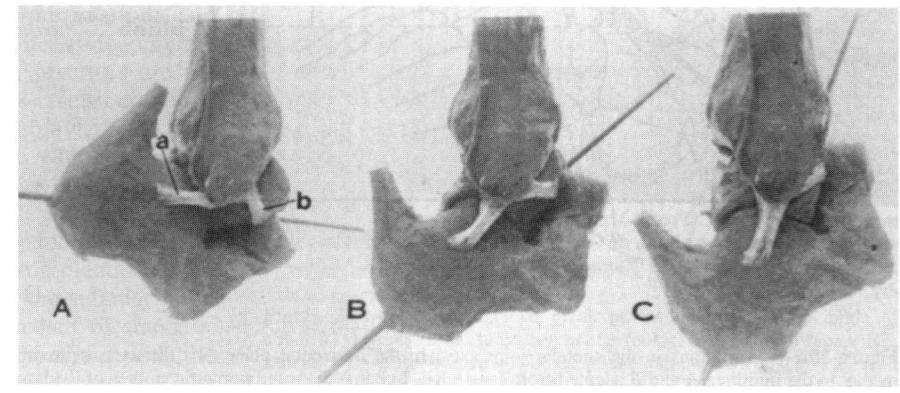

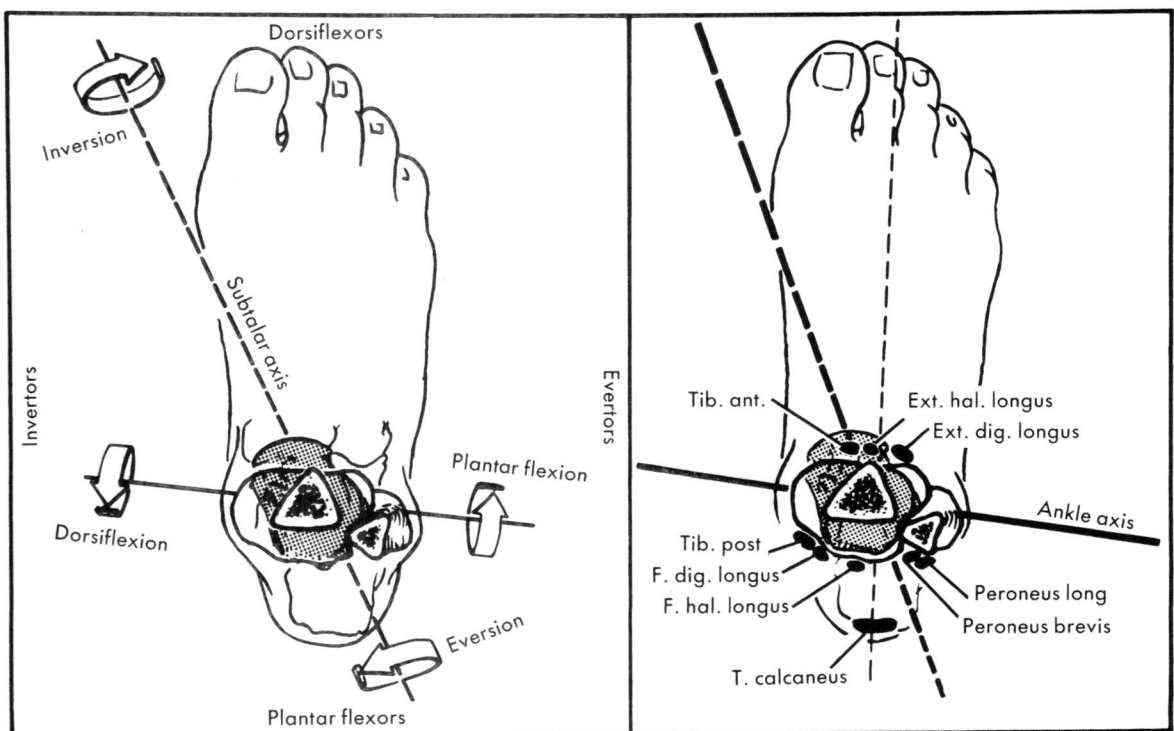

Figure 30A–9. *Left*, The location and the types of rotation that occur about the ankle and the subtalar axes. *Right*, The relationship of the various extrinsic muscles about the subtalar and ankle joint axes. (From Mann RA: Biomechanics of the foot. In American Academy of Orthopaedic Surgeons: Atlas of Orthotics. St. Louis, CV Mosby, 1975.)

Transverse Tarsal Joint

The transverse tarsal joint consists of the talonavicular and calcaneocuboid joints. As mentioned previously, motion at the transverse tarsal joint is that of adduction and abduction. The axes of the transverse tarsal joint are aligned so that when the calcaneus is in an everted position, the axes are parallel, permitting more motion to occur about this joint system. When the calcaneus is inverted, the axes are nonparallel, creating a stable joint system (Fig. 30A–10).[2]

It has been shown that when the subtalar joint is in an everted position, the transverse tarsal joint is unlocked, giving rise to a flexible forefoot. When the subtalar joint is in an inverted position, the transverse tarsal joint is locked, giving rise to a rigid forefoot. During normal walking, the foot is flexible at heel strike to absorb the impact, and this is due to the eversion of the calcaneus and the unlocked transverse tarsal joint. At toe-off, the calcaneus is inverted, and the transverse tarsal joint is locked, resulting in a rigid foot.

In the last half of stance phase, as pointed out earlier, the subtalar translates the external rotation that occurs in the lower extremity above and passes it distally to affect the stability of the transverse tarsal joint. At initial ground contact, it translates the eversion of the calcaneus to the talus, across the ankle joint, and into the lower extremity as internal rotation. The linkage mechanism can affect the transverse rotation of the lower extremity (Fig. 30A–11).

In a person with a flatfoot and increased eversion of the subtalar joint, an increased amount of internal rotation may occur, which in theory can affect even the knee, patellofemoral, or hip joint in some selected cases. An orthotic device that supports the longitudinal arch with

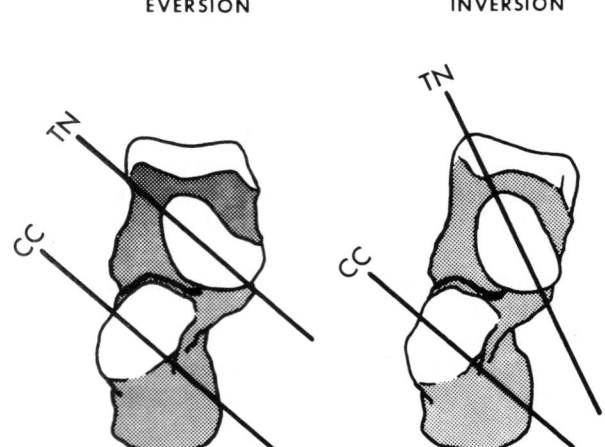

Figure 30A–10. The function of the transverse tarsal joint as described by Elftman. When the calcaneus is in eversion, the resultant axes of the talonavicular (TN) and calcaneocuboid (CC) joints are parallel or congruent. When the subtalar joint is in an inverted position, the axes are incongruent, giving increased stability to the midfoot. (From Mann RA, Coughlin MJ: Surgery of the Foot and Ankle. St. Louis, Mosby–Year Book, 1993, p 23.)

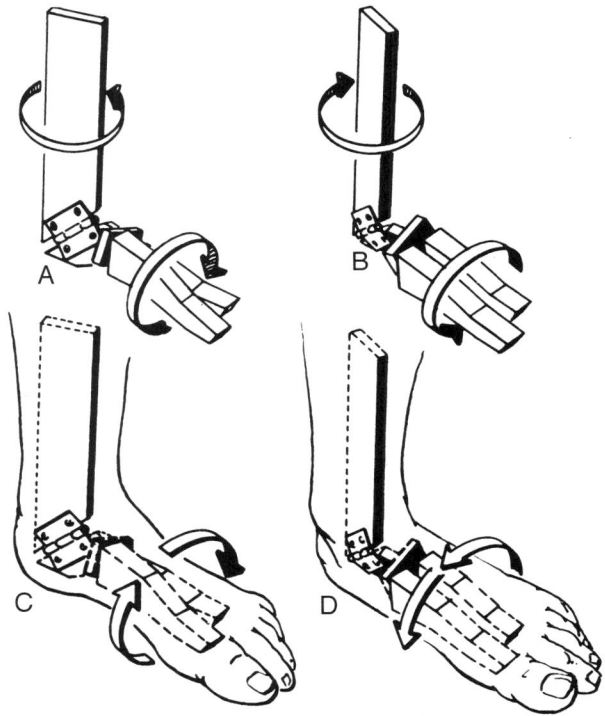

Figure 30A–11. Model demonstrating flattening and elevation of the longitudinal arch. *A* and *B*, Flattening of the longitudinal arch occurs at the time of heel strike with eversion of the calcaneus and internal rotation of the tibia. *C* and *D*, Elevation and stabilization of the longitudinal arch are associated with the outward rotation of the tibia, causing inversion of the calcaneus and locking of the transverse tarsal joint. (*A–D* from Inman VT, Mann RA: Biomechanics of the foot and ankle. In Inman VT [ed]: DuVries Surgery of the Foot, 3rd ed. St. Louis, CV Mosby, 1973.)

possibly medial heel posting may restrict subtalar joint rotation and decrease the internal rotation of the lower extremity, possibly resolving a clinical problem.

Linkage of the Foot and Ankle

The functions of the ankle joint, subtalar joint, transverse tarsal joint, and plantar aponeurosis have been examined and their interdependence pointed out. There exists, however, a certain linkage between these joints that should be emphasized further. Although the terms *inversion* and *eversion* pertain to pure subtalar joint motion, the terms *pronation* and *supination* describe a series of movements of the foot and ankle. Pronation is dorsiflexion of the ankle joint, eversion of the subtalar joint, and abduction of the transverse tarsal joint, whereas supination is plantar flexion of the ankle joint, inversion of the subtalar joint, and adduction of the transverse tarsal joint. It becomes immediately apparent that the pronated foot is a supple foot that can absorb impact, and the supinated foot is a rigid foot that serves as a platform for push-off. Although ankle joint motion during pronation is defined as dorsiflexion at the ankle joint, we initially observe plantar flexion during walking at heel strike. This plantar flexion also helps to absorb the initial ground contact. It is this linked series of movements that enables the athlete to absorb the impact, yet create a rigid platform from which to push off. We

have to consider, however, that these joint motions are enhanced further by the function of the plantar aponeurosis, the transverse metatarsal break, and the muscles of the leg and foot.

The joint linkage mentioned previously is essential for high-performance function of the lower extremity. If one of these linkages within the system fails to function in a satisfactory manner, stress is placed on the joints proximal and distal to it. Although we speak of ankle joint dorsiflexion and plantar flexion, only about half of this motion comes from the ankle joint; the remainder comes from the movement occurring within the subtalar and transverse tarsal joints.[1] If there is diminished motion of the ankle joint because of an anterior impingement or possibly degenerative changes within the joint, motion within the ankle is diminished, and the subtalar and transverse tarsal joints pick up the slack to compensate for the lost motion.

If there are changes within the subtalar and transverse tarsal joints, any loss of ankle joint motion is magnified. In the extreme case, such as in an ankle arthrodesis, there occurs during a long period of time increased motion within the subtalar and transverse tarsal joints, and at times degenerative changes occur.

Moving distally, if the motion in the subtalar joint is restricted, its ability to translate rotation proximally and distally is impaired, placing increased stress on the ankle and transverse tarsal joints. The degree of ankle joint dorsiflexion and plantar flexion also is affected because it contributes to this motion. Looking farther distally, impairment of the transverse tarsal joint impairs subtalar joint motion because for subtalar motion to occur, rotation must occur about the talonavicular joint as well as the calcaneocuboid joint.

If an isolated arthrodesis of the talonavicular or calcaneocuboid joint is carried out, most if not all subtalar joint motion is lost. For this reason, during performance of arthrodeses about the hindfoot, if the transverse tarsal joint motion can be maintained and only an isolated subtalar joint fusion carried out, patients usually have a more functional foot. The metatarsophalangeal joints also are affected by loss of motion.

When hallux rigidus, a degenerative arthritis of the first metatarsophalangeal joint, occurs, the metatarsophalangeal joint no longer dorsiflexes fully. This leads to compensation by placing the foot in more external rotation to relieve the stress across the involved area. This compensation in turn can affect the alignment of the lower extremity.

Because a linkage system exists within the lower extremity, questions should be raised about what effect an orthotic device will have, if any. As a general rule, a soft orthosis probably functions more to help absorb the impact of initial ground contact along with the shoe material. For individuals engaged in repetitive sports, such as long distance running, a material that helps to absorb some of this impact could be beneficial if the athlete is having problems related to impact, such as heel pain, metatarsalgia, or shin splints.

On a more sophisticated level, the use of a medial heel wedge, whether in the shoe or within an orthotic device, may have some influence on the rotation of the subtalar joint. Because at the time of initial ground contact rapid eversion of the subtalar joint and flattening of the longitudinal arch occur, a buildup of material along the medial arch that prevents some of this rotation from occurring in theory would decrease the amount of internal rotation being transmitted to the lower extremity. Reliable data to support this theory are lacking.

From a clinical standpoint, some patients seem to benefit from an orthotic device, although the benefit may be in part psychological. A runner with chronic knee pain may be helped by an orthotic device that limits eversion of the calcaneus, which in turn diminishes internal rotation of the tibia and affects the patellofemoral joint. Such use of orthoses remains based on trial and error rather than on firm scientific data.

References

1. Backer M, Kofoed H: Passive ankle mobility. J Bone Joint Surg Br 71:696, 1989.
2. Elftman H: The transverse tarsal joint and its control. Clin Orthop 16:41, 1960.
3. Hicks JH: The mechanics of the foot: II. The plantar aponeurosis and the arch. J Anat 88:25, 1954.
4. Inman VT: The Joints of the Ankle. Baltimore, Williams & Wilkins, 1976, pp 30–31, 70–71.
5. Inman VT, Mann RA: Biomechanics of the foot and ankle. In Inman VT (ed): DuVries Surgery of the Foot, 3rd ed. St. Louis, CV Mosby, 1973.
6. Isman RE, Inman VT: Anthropometric studies of the human foot and ankle. Bull Prosthet Res 10:97, 1969.
7. Mann RA: Biomechanics of the foot and ankle. In Mann RA (ed): Mann's Surgery of the Foot, 5th ed. St. Louis, CV Mosby, 1986, pp 7, 17.
8. Manter JT: Movements of the subtalar and transverse tarsal joints. Anat Rec 80:397, 1941.
9. Stauffer RN, Chao EY, Brewster RC: Force and motion analysis of the normal, diseased, and prosthetic ankle joint. Clin Orthop 127:189–196, 1977.
10. Wright DG, Desai ME, Henderson BS: Action of the subtalar and ankle joint complex during the stance phase of walking. J Bone Joint Surg Am 46:361, 1964.

Section B
Imaging of Sports Injuries of the Foot and Ankle

Douglas K. Smith, MD   ■   James S. Gilley, MD

The foot and ankle are frequently injured during sporting events, which may produce considerable disability in many athletes. Injuries of the foot and ankle may be acute or chronic problems. Cass and Morrey reported that acute foot and ankle injuries accounted for 10% of emergency room visits.[6] Garrick and Requa reported that foot and ankle injuries represented more than 25% of the 1600 athletic injuries in their series.[14] For most foot and ankle injuries, an accurate diagnosis can be made using the history, physical examination, and plain radiographs. Special imaging modalities are not required to make or to confirm the diagnosis in these cases. In other cases, the diagnosis may not be as clinically apparent, and special imaging (magnetic resonance imaging [MRI], computed tomography [CT], or bone scanning) may be useful for establishing or confirming a suspected diagnosis. This chapter presents the normal imaging appearances of the foot and ankle, as well as examples of common sports injuries viewed by special imaging modalities. The injuries of the foot and ankle are grouped by anatomic structure, that is, ligaments, tendons, osteochondral structures, and so forth.

Ligaments

The complex functions of the foot and ankle require that the osseous structures move in a controlled manner while supporting forces far exceeding body weight. The ligamentous structures of the foot and ankle bind the bones together and control the relative motion of the tarsal bones. Injury to these ligamentous structures can produce pain, instability, and disability. The ligamentous structures of the

ankle can be divided anatomically into the following: (1) distal tibial/fibular syndesmosis, (2) lateral ankle complex, (3) medial (deltoid) ankle complex, (4) posterior ankle complex, and (5) subtalar ligamentous complex.

The distal tibial/fibular syndesmosis is the fibrous synchondrosis between the distal fibula and the fibular notch of the distal tibia. The anterior and posterior tibial/fibular ligaments arise from the anterior and posterior rims of the distal tibia, respectively, and attach into the distal fibula (Fig. 30B–1A).[27] These ligaments help to maintain the stability of the distal tibial/fibular syndesmosis and prevent diastasis of the ankle mortise. Above the level of the syndesmosis, the vertically oriented tibial/fibular interosseous membrane attaches the tibia and fibula throughout the leg and ends just above the syndesmosis. The syndesmotic ligaments are located just above the tibiotalar joint. On axial images, the anterior tibial/fibular ligament (ATiFL) has a triangular shape, whereas the posterior tibial/fibular ligament has a more linear shape (see Fig. 30B–1A). The posterior cortex of the fibula has a convex shape at the level of the posterior tibial/fibular ligament insertion, whereas the posterior talofibular ligament arises lower from the lateral malleolus, where its posterior cortex has a concave shape.

Injuries to the distal tibial/fibular syndesmosis, or "high ankle sprains," usually tear the anterior tibial/fibular ligament before tearing the posterior tibial/fibular ligament. After an acute syndesmosis injury, edema typically develops adjacent to the anterior tibial/fibular ligament, which may have an ill-defined shape. Most acute syndesmotic injuries are treated as ankle sprains, and they are not commonly examined using MRI in the acute setting. MRI is typically obtained if the athlete complains of persistent

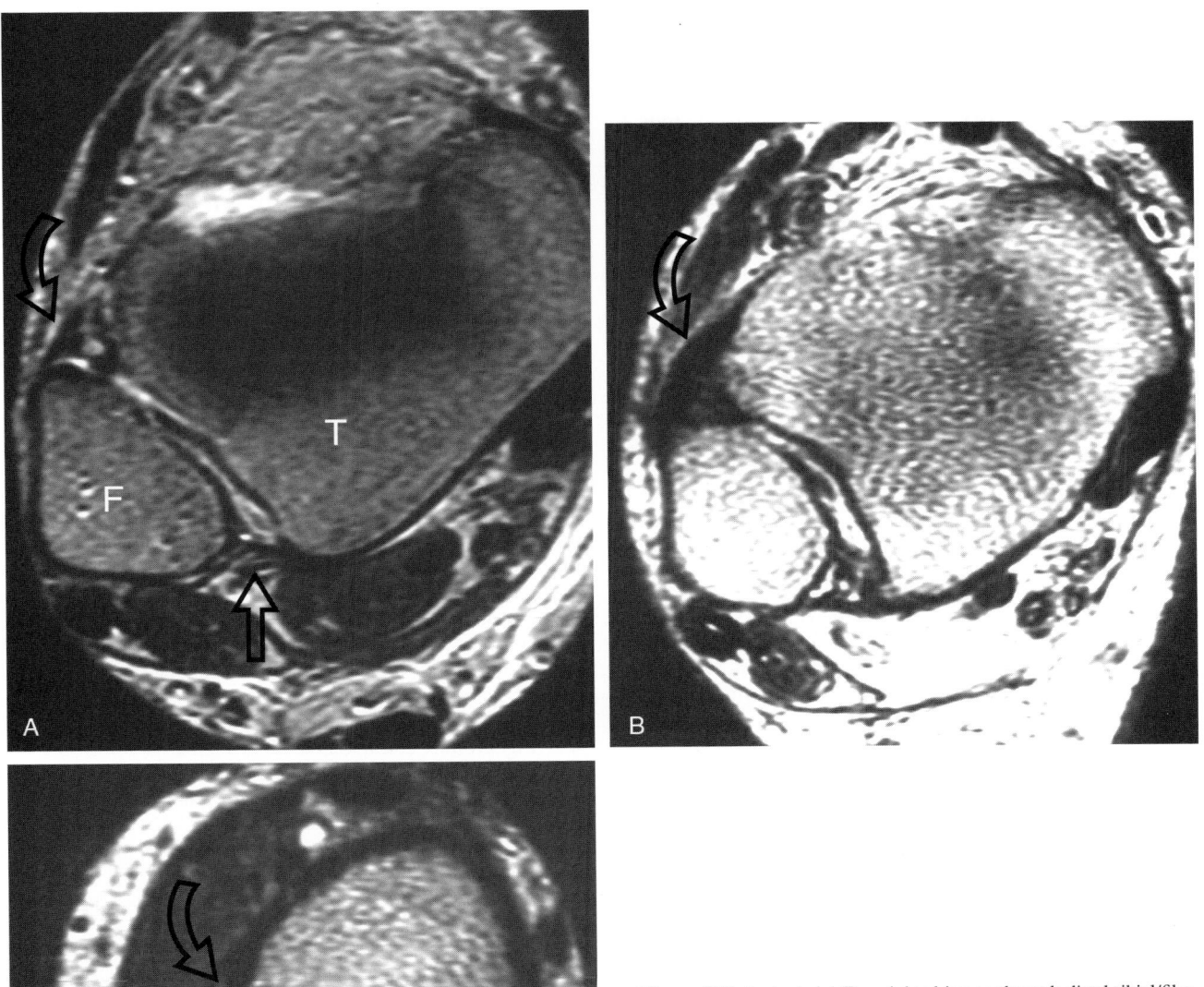

Figure 30B–1. *A,* Axial T_2-weighted image through distal tibial/fibular syndesmosis shows triangularly shaped anterior tibial/fibular ligament *(curved arrow)* and linearly shaped posterior tibial/fibular ligament *(straight arrow).* F, fibula; T, tibia. *B,* Axial T_2-weighted image shows marked thickening of the anterior tibial/fibular ligament *(curved arrow)* in a patient with an old syndesmosis injury. *C,* Axial T_2-weighted magnetic resonance image shows periosteal new bone at the site of the interosseous ligament avulsion *(curved arrow)* and thickening of the interosseous membrane *(straight arrow).*

pain after appropriate treatment has been provided for an ankle sprain. MRI typically shows a markedly thickened anterior tibial/fibular ligament with an ill-defined shape (see Fig. 30B–1*B*). If the injury extends above the syndesmosis into the leg, the tibial/fibular interosseous ligament may be torn or avulsed from the distal tibia. The resulting periosteal new bone or post-traumatic ossification of the interosseous membrane may be radiologically visible (see Fig. 30B–1*C*).

The lateral collateral ligament complex consists of the anterior and posterior talofibular (ATFL and PTFL) ligaments and the calcaneofibular ligament (CFL).[13] The ATFL and the PTFL are best seen on axial MRI at the level of the posterior concavity of the fibula. The normal ATFL extends from the anterior aspect of the lateral malleolus and attaches to the lateral margin of the talar neck (Fig. 30B–2). The ATFL is ribbon-shaped and approximately 2 to 3 mm thick. The ATFL is the most commonly injured ligament in the ankle. The PTFL arises from the posterior concavity of the lateral malleolus and inserts into the posterior process of the talus. The PTFL may be difficult to see on axial images because of the obliquity of its orientation. The calcaneofibular ligament is a vertically oriented, cord-like structure, extending from the tip of the lateral malleolus and traversing posteriorly and inferiorly to insert onto the lateral aspect of the calcaneus (Fig. 30B–3). The CFL lies deep to the peroneal tendons along the lateral aspect of the ankle.

Using MRI, ligament injuries are separated into three grades according to their anatomic appearance. A grade I tear or ligament sprain has surrounding soft tissue edema but no disruption or discrete tear of the ligament fibers. A grade II ligament tear is a partial tear. The ligament may be attenuated or may have a discrete tear (bright T_2 signal) extending through a portion of the ligament, but intact ligament fibers are present. In a grade III injury, the structural integrity and morphology of the ligament have been disrupted. The most frequently injured ligament in the ankle is the ATFL followed by the CFL. The posterior

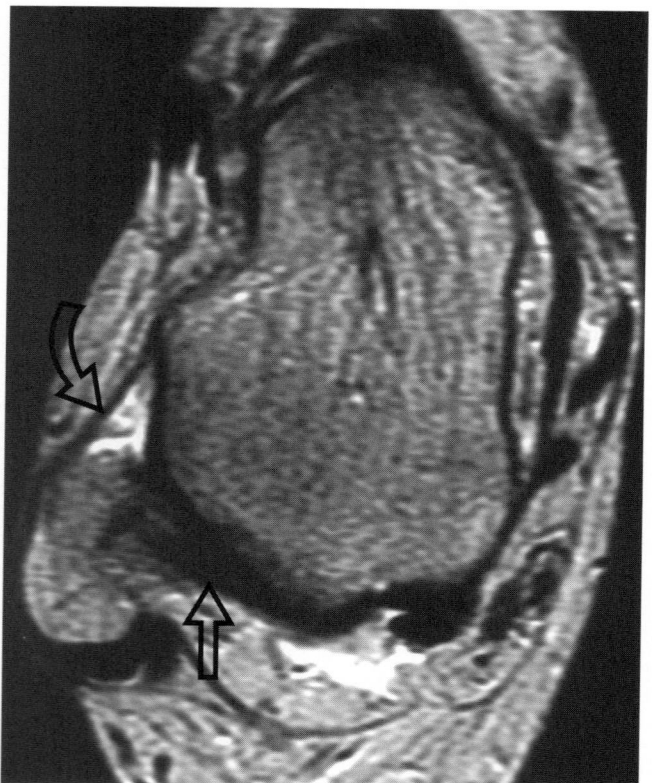

Figure 30B–2. Axial T_2-weighted magnetic resonance image just below the ankle mortise shows 2-mm-thick anterior talofibular ligament *(curved arrow)* arising from the anterior aspect of the lateral malleolus and inserting into the lateral aspect of the talar body. The posterior talofibular ligament *(straight arrow)* arises from the concavity of the posteromedial fibula and inserts into the posterolateral aspect of the talus.

talofibular ligament is rarely injured unless the ATFL and the CFL are also torn.

Lateral ankle sprains are common among athletes, who frequently injure the ATFL.[5] The MRI appearance of a grade I sprain is focal soft tissue swelling surrounding an intact ATFL. In a grade II injury, there is discontinuity of a portion of the ligament fibers or bright signal (hemorrhage) within the ATFL. In a grade III tear, a focal discontinuity of ligament fibers is noted. Chronic scarring of the ATFL produces a mass of low signal (black scar) in the expected location of the ATFL.

Following repetitive lateral ankle sprains, some individuals develop a focal soft tissue mass and focal pain in the interval between the anterior tibia and fibula (anterolateral gutter).[16] This clinicopathologic entity has become known as the "meniscoid syndrome."[25, 42] The anterolateral "gutter" of the ankle is located between the ATiFL and the ATFL; it is a potential space that may normally be filled with fat or joint fluid. Individuals with a meniscoid lesion have hyalinized scar tissue within the anterolateral ankle gutter that may cause impingement during ankle dorsiflexion. MRI of the meniscoid lesion shows abnormal tissue (low-signal soft tissue) filling the anterolateral ankle gutter between the talus and the fibula.

The CFL is a thick ligamentous band attaching the lateral malleolus to the lateral calcaneus (see Fig. 30B–3A). The CFL is rarely injured without a coexistent ATFL injury. Repetitive or chronic injury of the CFL can produce scarring around a thickened CFL (see Figs. 30B–3B and C). A complete tear (grade III) of the CFL involves a segmental defect or complete disruption of ligamentous fibers.

The medial collateral or deltoid ligament complex arises from the medial malleolus and is composed of superficial (tibiocalcaneal) and deep (tibiotalar) fascicles (Fig. 30B–4).[22, 35] The superficial fibers of the deltoid ligament complex can be separated into three groups of fascicles by the orientation and course of the ligament—the tibiocalcaneal, the tibiospring, and the tibionavicular ligaments. The deep layer is composed of the anterior and posterior tibiotalar ligaments. The posterior tibiotalar and tibiocalcaneal ligaments are most easily seen on conventional coronal plane imaging. The deltoid ligaments are usually torn during an ankle eversion injury and are less commonly torn than fibers of the lateral collateral ligaments (Fig. 30B–5A). Grade III injuries to the deltoid ligament are much less common than grade III injuries of the lateral complex and may occur as part of a more global ankle ligamentous injury (see Fig. 30B–5B). Scarring of the deltoid ligament following injury can produce pain in the medial gutter (see Fig. 30B–5C).[10] This scar is recognizable on MRI as poorly defined ligament fibers and surrounding ill-defined black signal in the medial gutter.

Tendons

The tendons of the ankle and foot serve important biomechanical functions, including supporting the bony arches and facilitating the complex motions of the foot and ankle by transmitting forces applied by the muscles of the leg

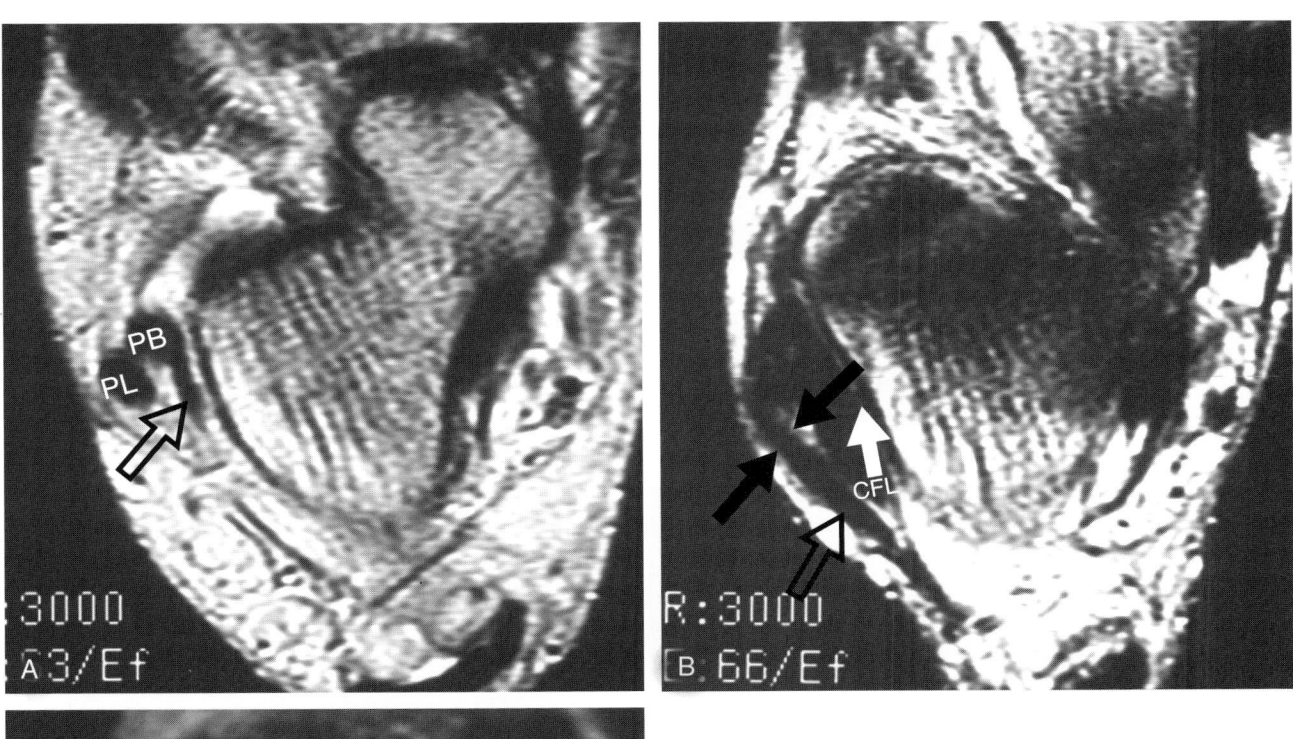

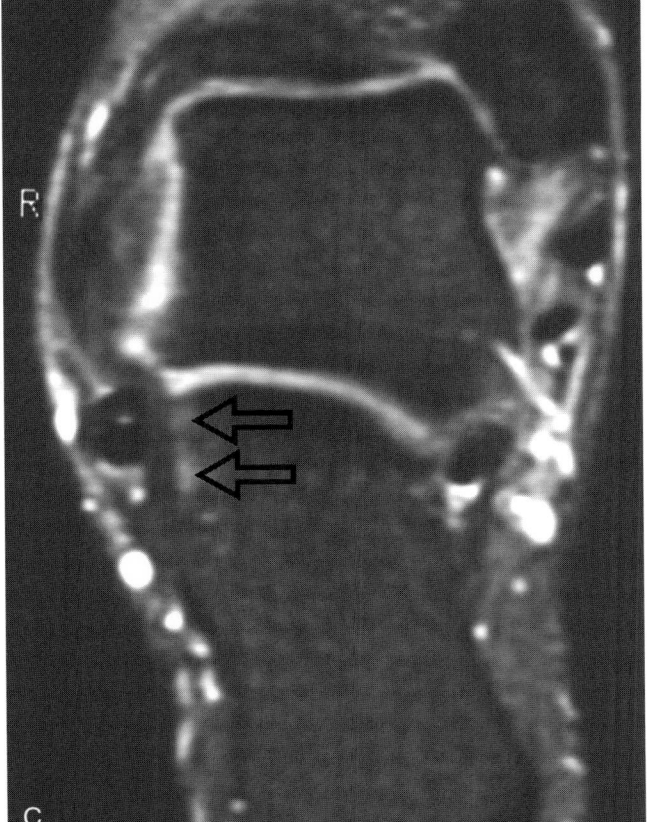

Figure 30B–3. *A,* Axial image through the midportion of a normal, 3-mm-thick, ribbon-shaped calcaneofibular ligament *(straight arrow).* Adjacent peroneus brevis (PB) and peroneus longus (PL) tendons. *B,* Axial image through a diffusely thickened, chronically torn calcaneofibular ligament (CFL) *(solid white arrow).* The peroneal retinaculum *(open arrow)* is also markedly thickened *(paired black arrows). C,* Coronal T_2-weighted image shows diffusely thickened and chronically injured CFL *(paired straight arrows).*

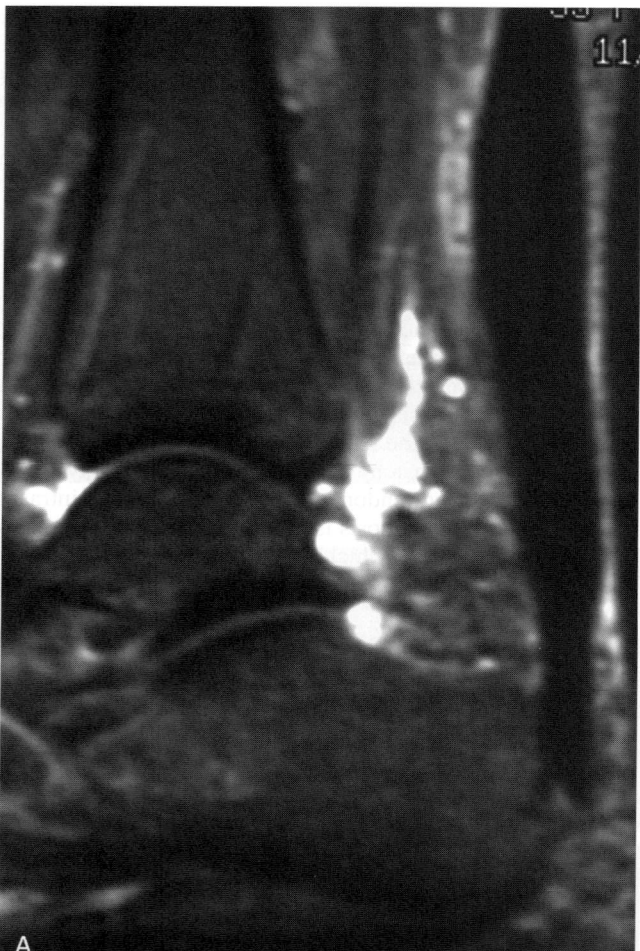

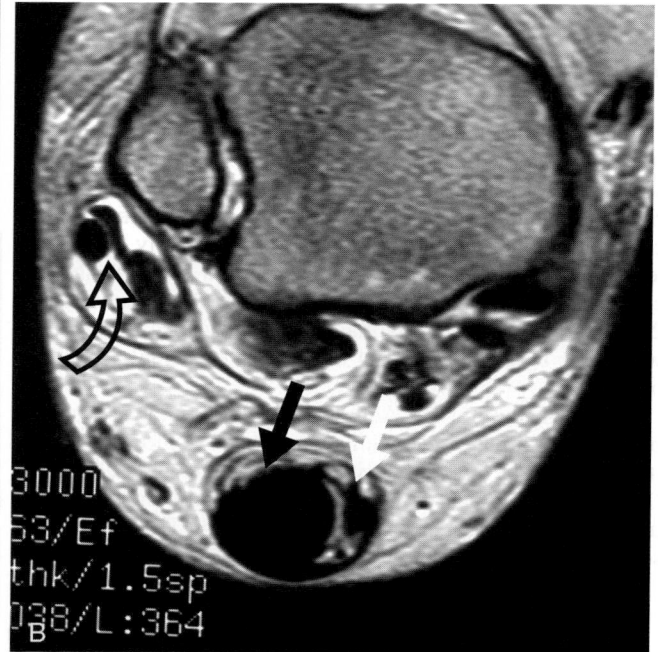

Figure 30B–7. *A,* Sagittal T$_2$-weighted image of diffusely thickened Achilles tendon shows that the intrasubstance signal of mucoid degeneration is not bright, as seen with hemorrhage from acute intrasubstance tearing. *B,* Axial T$_2$-weighted image shows enlarged Achilles tendon *(black arrow)* with rounded shape and internal intermediate (gray) signal within the tendon, consistent with mucoid degeneration. Thickened plantaris tendon *(white arrow)* and longitudinal peroneus tendon tear *(curved arrow)* are also seen.

becomes infiltrated with fluid or edema (Fig. 30B–8). In chronic peritendinitis, this fat pad may become fibrotic or infiltrated with low signal soft tissue on all MRI sequences. The retrocalcaneal bursa separates the calcaneus from the Achilles tendon. This bursa normally contains a small amount of fluid; however, the bursa may be distended in patients with Achilles peritendinitis.

Achilles tendon tears are divided into purely intrasubstance tears, partial-thickness tears, and full-thickness tears.[19] Intrasubstance tears have internal bright signal that is typically a combination of edema and hemorrhage (Fig. 30B–9).[2]

Complete, acute disruptions usually include a gap between the retracted proximal and distal ends of the Achilles tendon (Fig. 30B–10).[19] Hemorrhage and edema at the site of the tear are bright on T$_2$-weighted images and intermediate to low on T$_1$-weighted images. Acute partial tears do not have retracted ends and usually have bright signal at the site of the tear on T$_2$-weighted images (see Fig. 30B–10).[2] Partial tears may be linear intrasubstance tears or incomplete transverse tears. Partial intrasubstance tears have linear bands of bright signal on T$_2$-weighted sequences but relatively smooth surface contour of the tendon. A partial transverse tear is recognized by a segmental thinning or defect of the tendon substance, with hemor-

rhage and edema within the defect of the partial tear. An intact plantaris tendon can be misinterpreted as a remaining strand of Achilles tendon but can be recognized by its typical location and by its course on axial images (see Fig. 30B–6B).

Extensor Tendons

Three extensor tendons cross the ankle—the tibialis anterior, the extensor digitorum longus, and the extensor hallucis tendons. Repetitive ankle dorsiflexion can produce tenosynovitis or chronic tendinosis of the extensor tendons (Fig. 30B–11). The tibialis anterior tendon is the most commonly affected by tenosynovitis. The MRI appearance of tenosynovitis includes distention of the tendon sheath with bright signal fluid or thickened synovium. There may be nodular or diffuse thickening of the tendon with intrasubstance degeneration of the tendon or tendinosis. Traumatic injuries or ruptures of the extensor tendons are much less common than injuries of the flexor or peroneal tendons (see Fig. 30B–11). A full-thickness tear typically has a focal disruption of the tendon with retraction of the proximal tendon fragment. The tibialis anterior tendon is most commonly torn at the level of the extensor retinaculum.

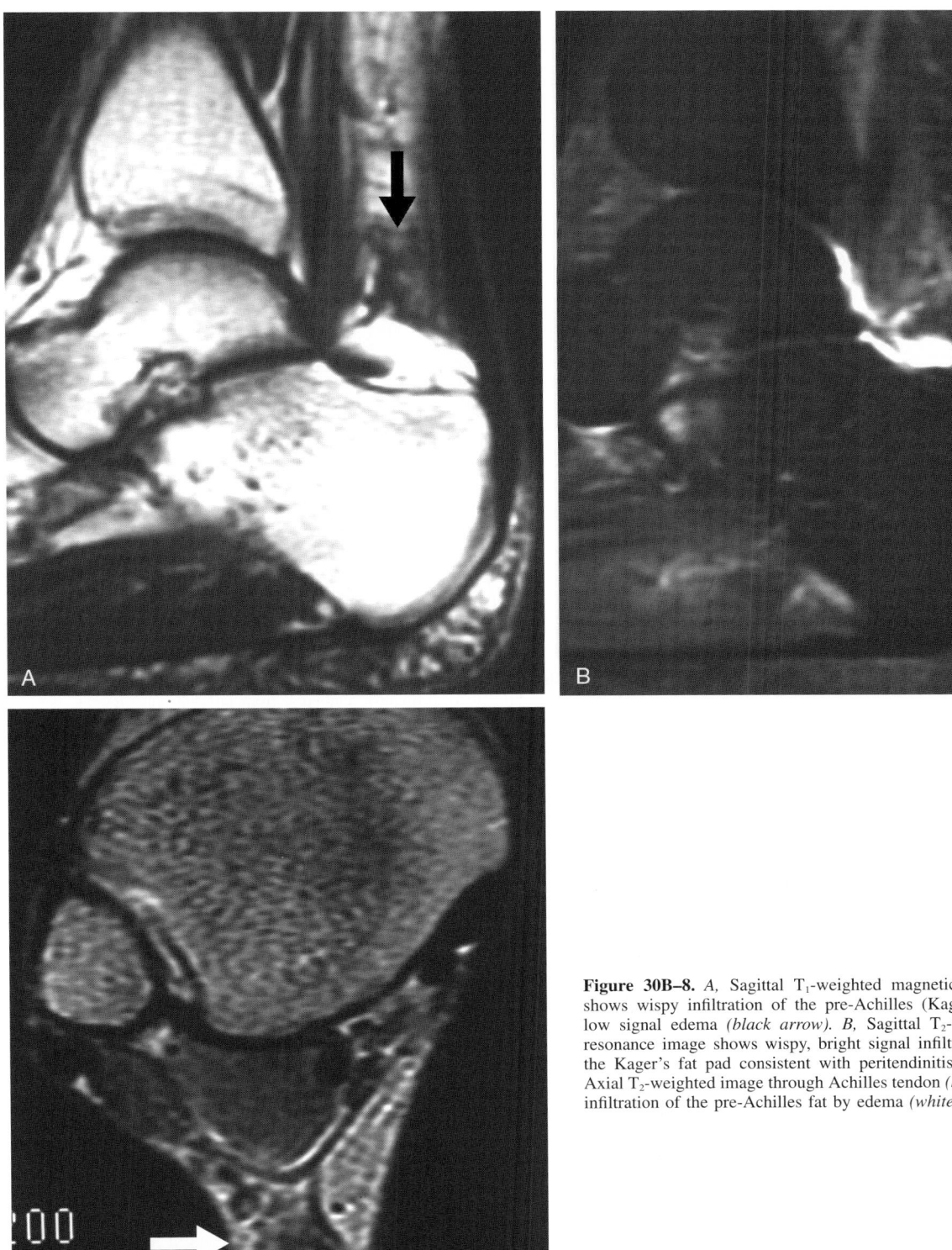

Figure 30B–8. *A,* Sagittal T_1-weighted magnetic resonance image shows wispy infiltration of the pre-Achilles (Kager's) fat pad with low signal edema *(black arrow). B,* Sagittal T_2-weighted magnetic resonance image shows wispy, bright signal infiltration or edema of the Kager's fat pad consistent with peritendinitis *(white arrow). C,* Axial T_2-weighted image through Achilles tendon *(black arrow)* shows infiltration of the pre-Achilles fat by edema *(white arrow).*

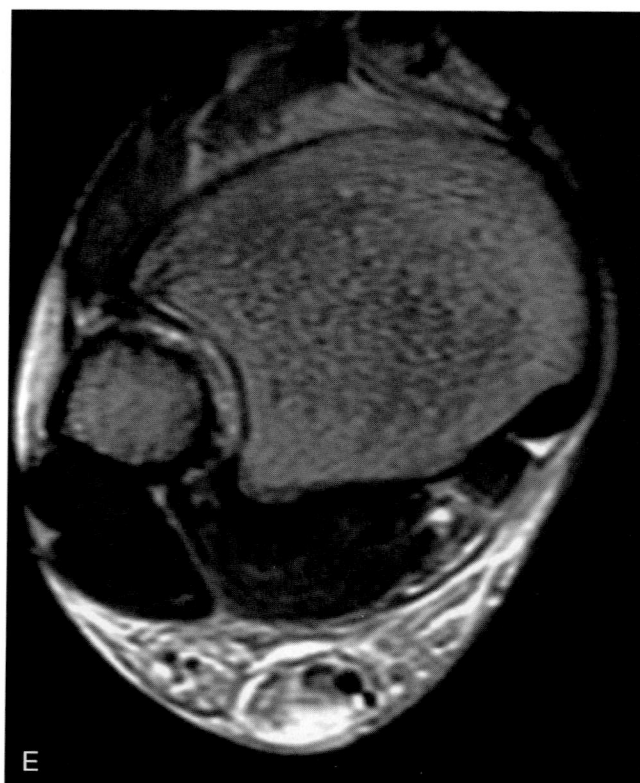

Figure 30B–10 *Continued. E,* Axial T$_2$-weighted image at the site of the full-thickness tear shows only ill-defined tissue. Contiguous images showed no continuous tendon fibers.

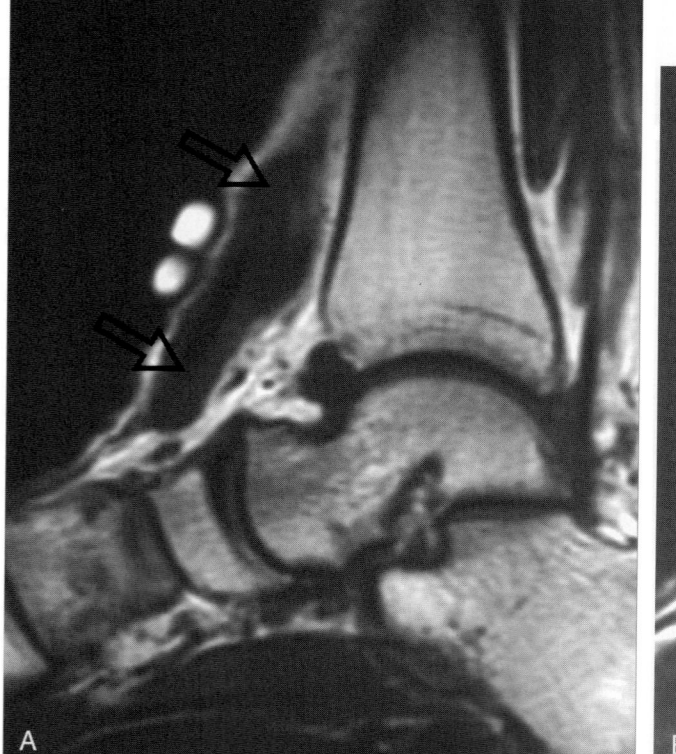

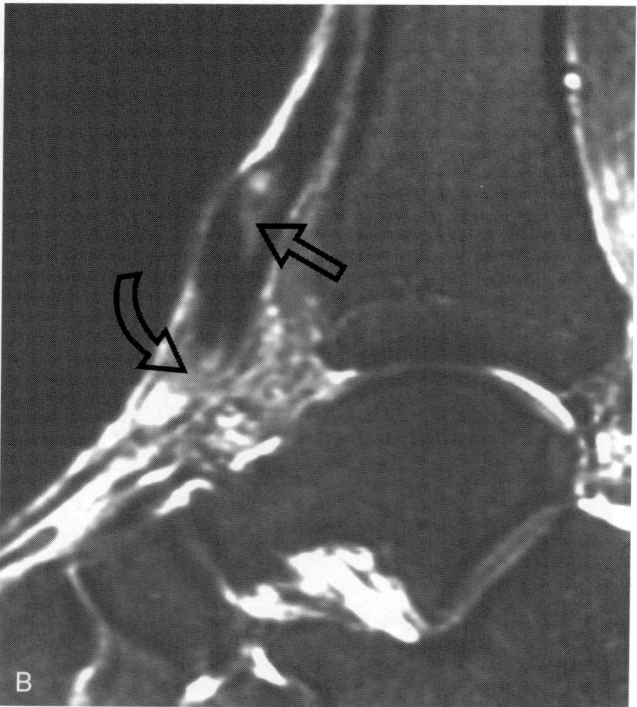

Figure 30B–11. *A,* Sagittal T$_1$-weighted image of a full-thickness tear of the tibialis anterior tendon. The tendon is markedly thickened with intrasubstance gray signal (*arrows:* tendinosis and intrasubstance tearing) above the level of the full-thickness tear, or ligament discontinuity at the level of the ankle joint. *B,* Sagittal T$_2$-weighted image of a full-thickness tear of the tibialis anterior tendon with discontinuity of the tendon *(curved arrow)* at the level of the ankle joint. Just above the site of the full-thickness tear is intrasubstance bright signal *(straight arrow),* reflecting intrasubstance, partial-thickness tearing.

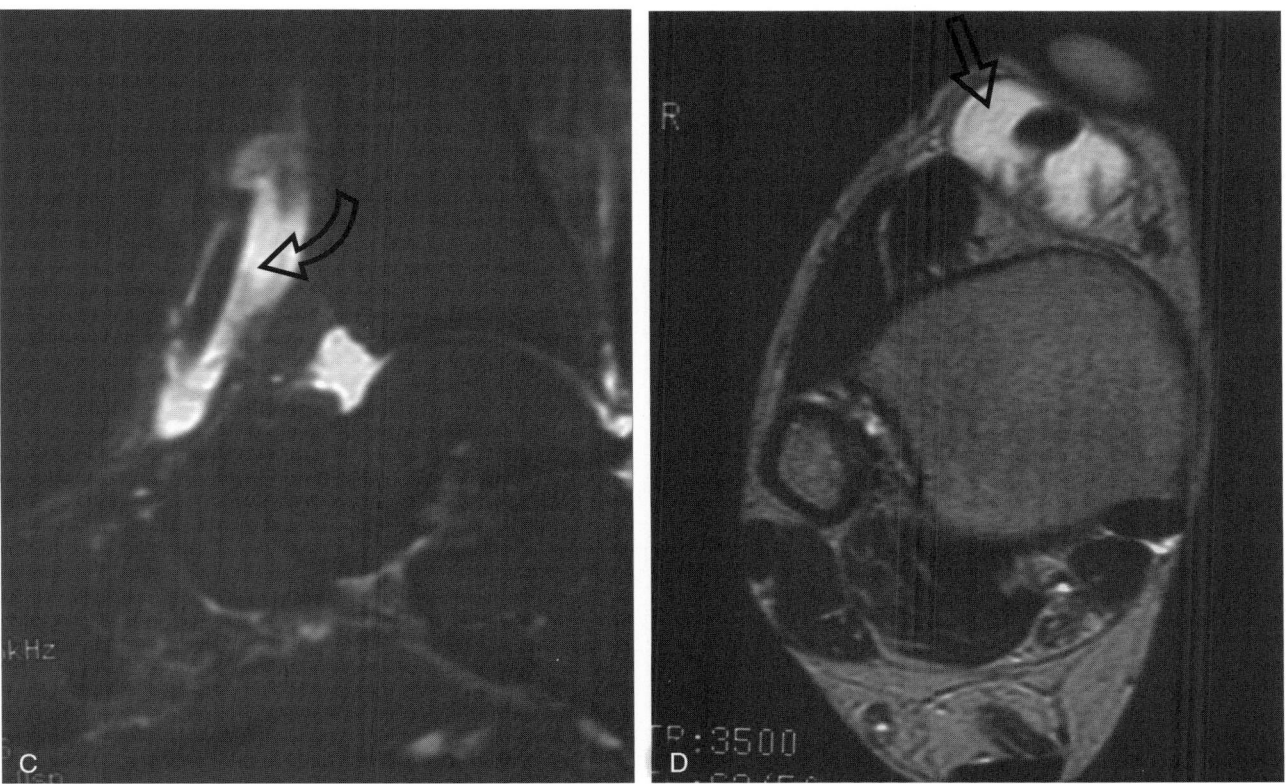

Figure 30B–11 *Continued. C,* Sagittal T$_2$-weighted magnetic resonance image shows marked tenosynovitis of the tibialis anterior tendon, with bright signal effusion and inflamed synovium *(curved arrow)* surrounding the tendon. *D,* Axial T$_2$-weighted image shows bright signal effusion and inflamed synovium *(arrow)* surrounding the tibialis anterior tendon.

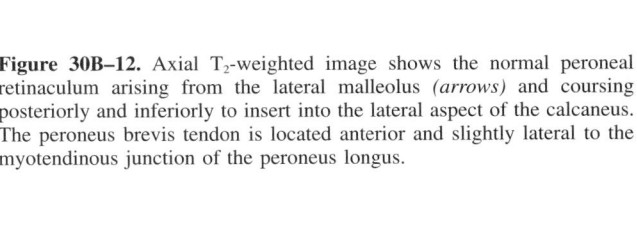

Figure 30B–12. Axial T$_2$-weighted image shows the normal peroneal retinaculum arising from the lateral malleolus *(arrows)* and coursing posteriorly and inferiorly to insert into the lateral aspect of the calcaneus. The peroneus brevis tendon is located anterior and slightly lateral to the myotendinous junction of the peroneus longus.

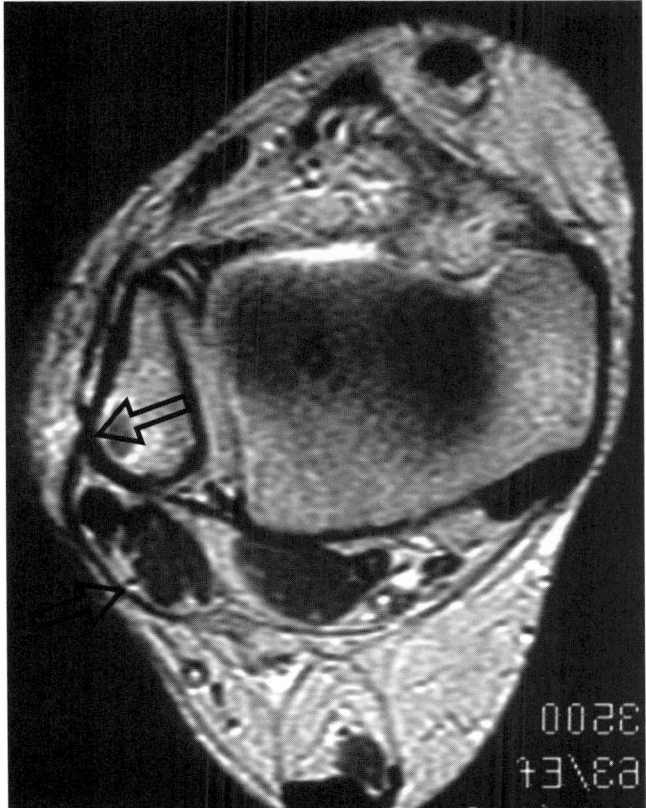

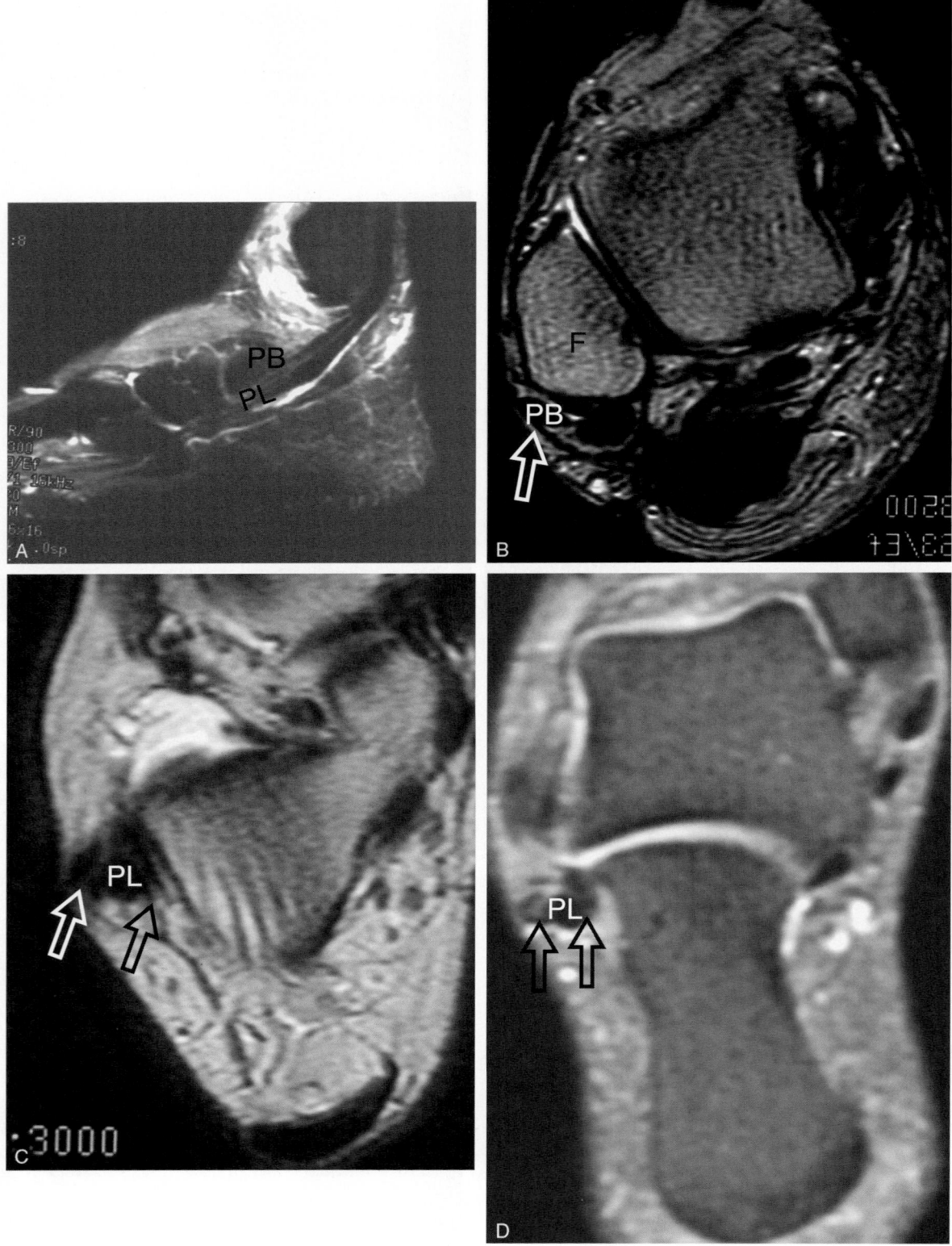

Figure 30B–13. *A,* Sagittal T$_2$-weighted magnetic resonance image shows diffuse attenuation of the peroneus brevis (PB) tendon (type 2 tear) and nodular thickening of the peroneus longus (PL) tendon in a patient with lateral ankle instability. *B,* Axial T$_2$-weighted image of the same ankle as in part *A* shows anterolateral dislocation of the peroneus brevis tendon (PB, *arrow*). Notice that the posterior aspect of the lateral malleolus (F) has a convex shape rather than the normal concave shape. *C,* Axial T$_2$-weighted image of a patient with a longitudinal split tear of the peroneus brevis tendon *(arrows).* The peroneus longus (PL) tendon is interposed between the two fragments of the peroneus brevis tendon. This type of tear can be seen in young individuals with peroneal tendon instability or lateral ankle ligament instability. *D,* Coronal T$_2$-weighted image of the same ankle as in part *C* shows two fragments of the split peroneus brevis tendon *(arrows)* and the peroneus longus tendon.

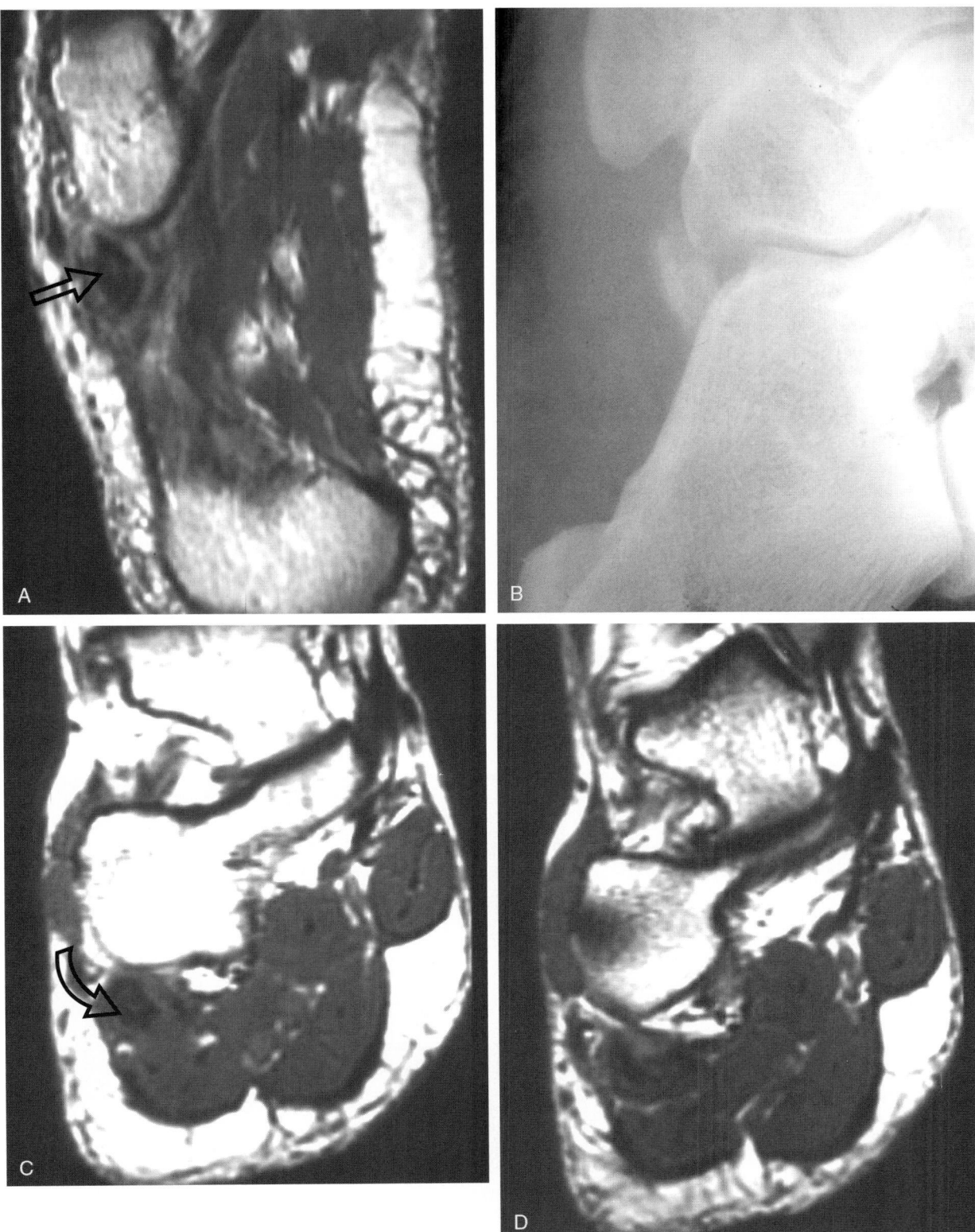

Figure 30B–14. *A,* T$_1$-weighted axial magnetic resonance image shows fracture of the os peroneum (linear gray signal, *arrow*) traversing the normally black signal of the os peroneum. *B,* Oblique radiograph of the foot shows elongation and a transversely oriented fracture of the os peroneum, suggesting a peroneus longus tendon tear. *C* and *D,* Coronal T$_1$-weighted images show flattening of the os peroneum with transversely oriented fracture *(curved arrow)* and attenuation of the peroneus longus tendon.

the tear and may have hemorrhage or edema (bright on T_2-weighted images) at the site of the tear. Partial-thickness tears may be recognized by focal increased size associated with internal increased signal or diffuse attenuation of the tendon (Fig. 30B–13A).[26, 36] The peroneus brevis tendon may develop a longitudinal tear that separates the tendon into two separate fascicles. These "longitudinal split" tears are associated with lateral ankle instability or calcaneal fracture (see Figs. 30B–13C and D).[3, 9, 32, 37] A tendon sheath effusion or tenosynovitis appears as bright signal within the tendon sheath on T_2-weighted images.

The peroneus longus tendon can be disrupted through a fracture of the os peroneum (normal variant of the intratendinous ossicle) (Fig. 30B–14).[26, 36] The two fracture fragments of the os peroneum may be distracted on plain radiographs.

Flexor Tendons

In most individuals, three flexor tendons pass posterior to the medial malleolus as they course to their insertion in the plantar aspect of the foot. The posterior tibial (PT) tendon is the most anterior of the three tendons and abuts the medial malleolus. The flexor digitorum longus (FDL) tendon is located just posterior to the PT and shares a common tendon sheath. The flexor hallucis longus (FHL) tendon is located several millimeters posterior to the PT and FDL tendons and passes beneath the sustentaculum talus on its route to the great toe (Fig. 30B–15). The posterior tibial artery and the tibial nerve course between the FDL and the FHL tendons at the level of the medial malleolus.

The posterior tibial tendon is the most frequently injured of the three flexor tendons.[17, 23, 33, 40] Overuse injuries of the PT can produce tenosynovitis of the common flexor tendon sheath. Tenosynovitis can be recognized on MRI as a tendon sheath distended with fluid or bright-signal tenosynovium. Posterior tibial tendon tears are thought to be the result of repeated microtrauma, leading to tendon degeneration, tendinitis, and eventually complete tears. Rosenberg and associates classified posterior tibial tendon tears into three types based on their morphologic appearances: type I—a partial-thickness tear with focal areas of fiber rupture, degeneration, and repair and characterized by focal tendon enlargement and increased signal on T_1-weighted MR images; type II—focal decreased width of the tendon representing partial tear with attenuation (usually at the level of the medial malleolus); and type III—discontinuity of the tendon consistent with complete rupture (Fig. 30B–16).[33] Tendon discontinuity, marked focal enlargement, and thinning of the PT tendon are still considered reliable signs of

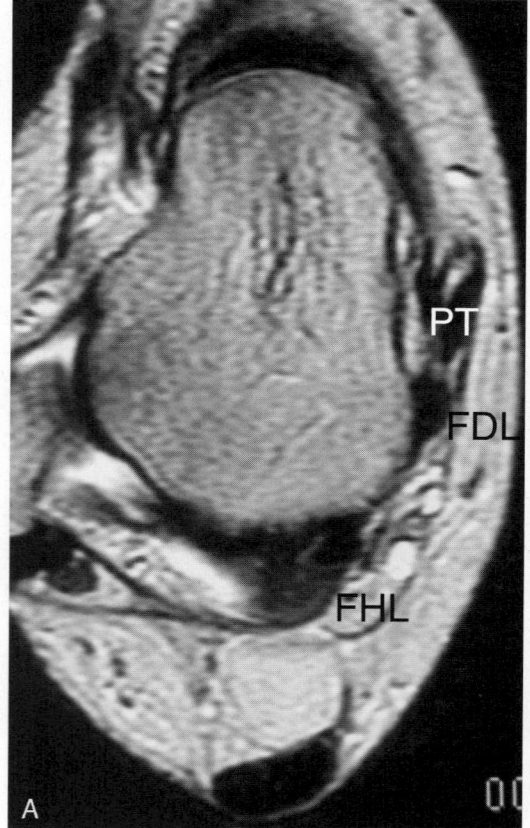
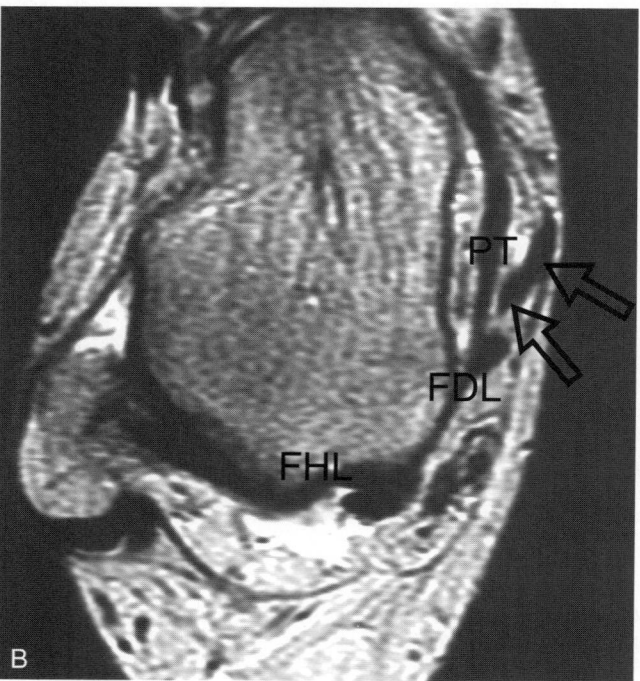

Figure 30B–15. *A,* Axial T_2-weighted magnetic resonance image shows normal morphology and position of the flexor tendons: PT, FDL, and FHL. *B,* Axial T_2-weighted magnetic resonance image shows two fascicles of the posterior tibial tendon *(arrows)* in a patient with a longitudinal split tear. The posterior tibial tendon fascicles are located anterior to the FDL tendon. FDL, flexor digitorum longus tendon; FHL, flexor hallucis longus tendon; PT, posterior tibial tendon.

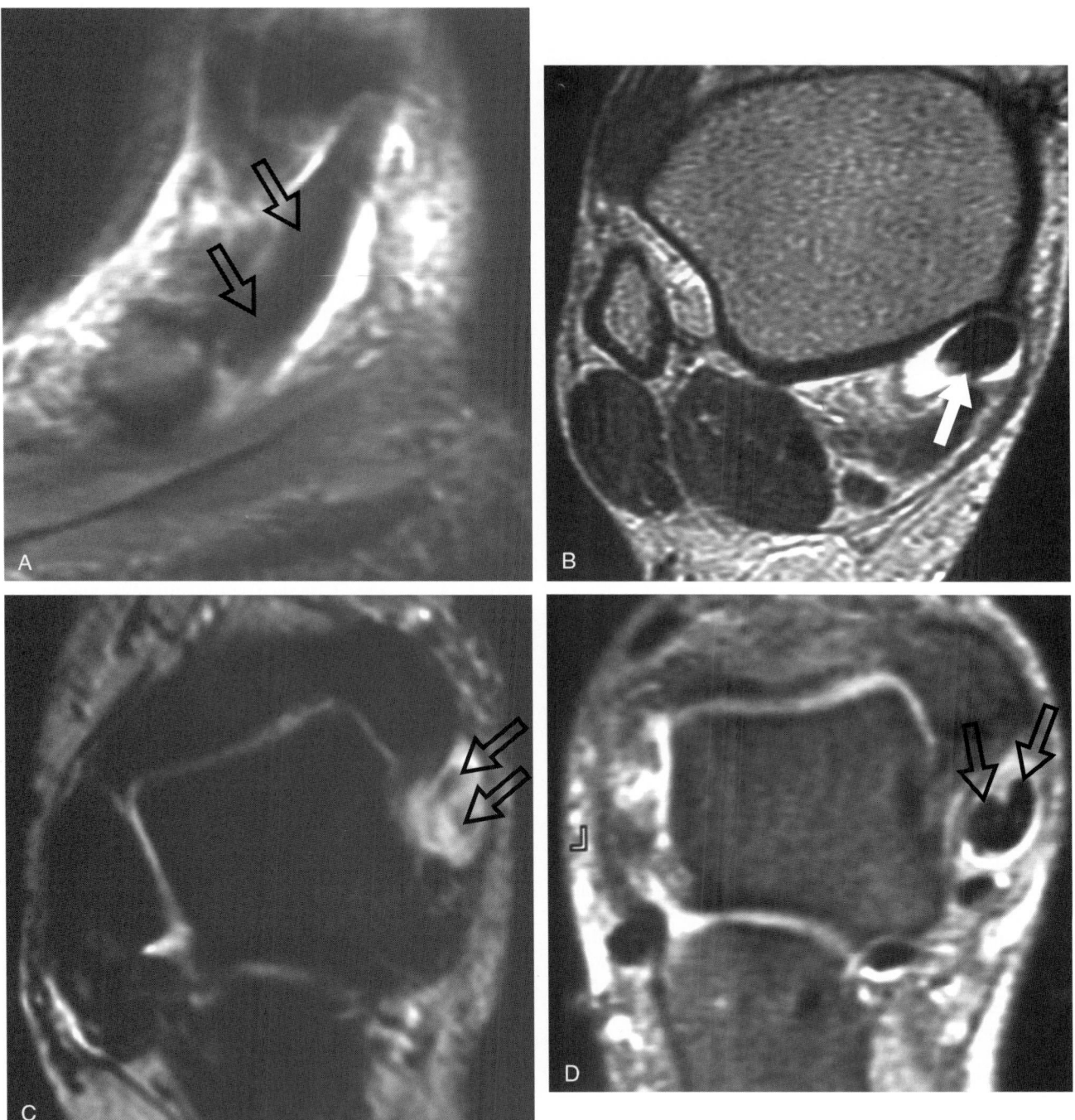

Figure 30B–16. *A,* Sagittal T$_2$-weighted magnetic resonance image shows diffuse enlargement of the torn posterior tibial tendon with a type I tear *(arrows)*. *B,* Axial T$_2$-weighted magnetic resonance image of the same ankle as in part *A* shows a type I tear with surface contour irregularity *(white arrow)*. *C,* Coronal T$_2$-weighted magnetic resonance image shows a comminuted, grade 3 tear of the posterior tibial tendon, with multiple separate fascicles of the torn tendon *(arrows)*. *D,* Coronal T$_2$-weighted image shows a longitudinal split tear of the posterior tibial tendon *(arrows)* surrounded by a tendon sheath effusion.

Illustration continued on following page

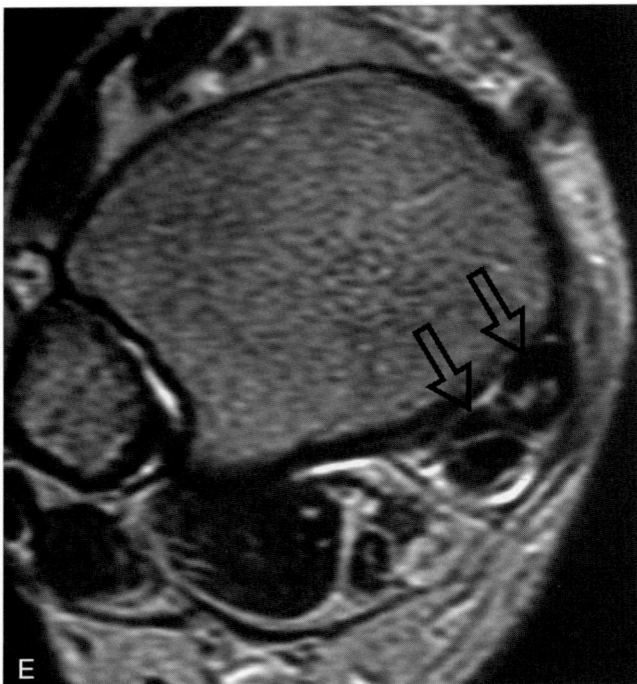

Figure 30B–16 *Continued. E,* Axial T$_2$-weighted image shows two separate fascicles *(arrows)* of the longitudinal split tear of the posterior tibial tendon.

PT tendon tears, but recent investigation of asymptomatic volunteers has shown a normal overlap in the width and signal characteristics of patients with tears of the PT tendon and asymptomatic volunteers.[40]

Plantar Fascia

The plantar fascia (deep fascia) of the plantar aspect of the foot comprises three distinct parts: A medial part covers the muscles of the great toe; a lateral part covers the flexor muscles of the small toe; and a central part is designated as the plantar aponeurosis (Figs. 30B–17*A* and *B*).[43, 44] The plantar aponeurosis supports the longitudinal arch of the foot with a similar function as the bowstring of a bow. All three components of the plantar fascia arise from the plantar tubercle of the calcaneus. This segment of the plantar fascia is prone to degeneration or discrete tear (Fig. 30B–18).[20, 28, 31, 43, 44] Plantar fasciitis is a chronic, recurrent, and frequently debilitating condition. The fascia may be thickened, with areas of nodularity in chronic cases. In acute fasciitis, there may be soft tissue edema adjacent to a normal-thickness plantar fascia.

Spring Ligament

The plantar calcaneonavicular or spring ligament runs from the anteromedial aspect of the calcaneus to the medial pole of the navicular. It serves as the major support for the medial arch and head of the talus. The spring ligament has

two major bands—a more elastic superomedial band and a more rigid plantar band. These two bands my be difficult to delineate with routine MRI scan planes; often 45-degree oblique coronal or sagittal scans are required for optimal visualization. The superomedial band is the one most often injured. On T$_2$-weighted MRI, a spring ligament tear presents as an area of high signal intensity and disruption of fibers in the distal portion of the superomedial band, just proximal to its navicular insertion (Fig. 30B–19*A*).[34] The spring ligament may be torn during severe ankle sprains with resulting loss of the medial arch height and persistent midfoot pain (see Fig. 30B–19*B* and *C*).[7, 35, 47]

Turf Toe

Traumatic hyperextension of the metatarsophalangeal (MTP) joint of the great toe can produce a sprain or tear of the plantar capsule–ligament complex. This is most commonly seen in football players who play on artificial turf and has been referred to as "turf toe." In a grade I injury or sprain, MRI shows only soft tissue edema adjacent to an intact plantar joint capsule. In a grade III injury or complete tear, there is typically disruption of the proximal aspect of the plantar plate, with an impaction-type bone contusion of the dorsal aspect of the metatarsal head. A chondral injury of the overlying cartilage of the metatarsal head or proximal phalanx may also occur (Fig. 30B–20).[46] T$_2$-weighted images show intraosseous marrow edema within the metatarsal head and joint effusion within the MTP joint. T$_1$-weighted MRI may show a trabecular impaction fracture or a discrete osteochondral fracture.

Hallux Sesamoid Bones

Sesamoid pain is common among long-distance runners. The tibial and fibular sesamoid bones lie in the medial and lateral slips of the flexor hallucis brevis. They serve to improve mechanical advantage at the first MTP joint, distribute weight, and protect the FHL tendon. The hallux sesamoid bones are subjected to significant stresses in athletes. A number of painful conditions can affect the sesamoid bones of the great toe, including avascular necrosis (osteochondrosis), inflammation (sesamoiditis), and fracture.

Osteochondrosis or avascular necrosis of the sesamoid bones may occur after a traumatic event and most commonly affects women during the second and third decades of life. Both sesamoid bones are affected with equal frequency. Plain radiographic findings include sclerosis and flattening of the involved sesamoid.[4, 18, 30] On MRI, the normally bright fatty marrow signal of the involved sesamoid is replaced by fibrous (dark) signal on all sequences.

Partite sesamoid bones are common and are more frequently found in the tibial compared with the fibular sesamoid (10 times more common). The synchondrosis of the sesamoid has sclerotic, smooth margins compared with the sharp margins seen in sesamoid fractures. Isolated fractures of the sesamoid bones are uncommon.

The term *sesamoiditis* refers to inflammation or an early

Text continued on page 2211

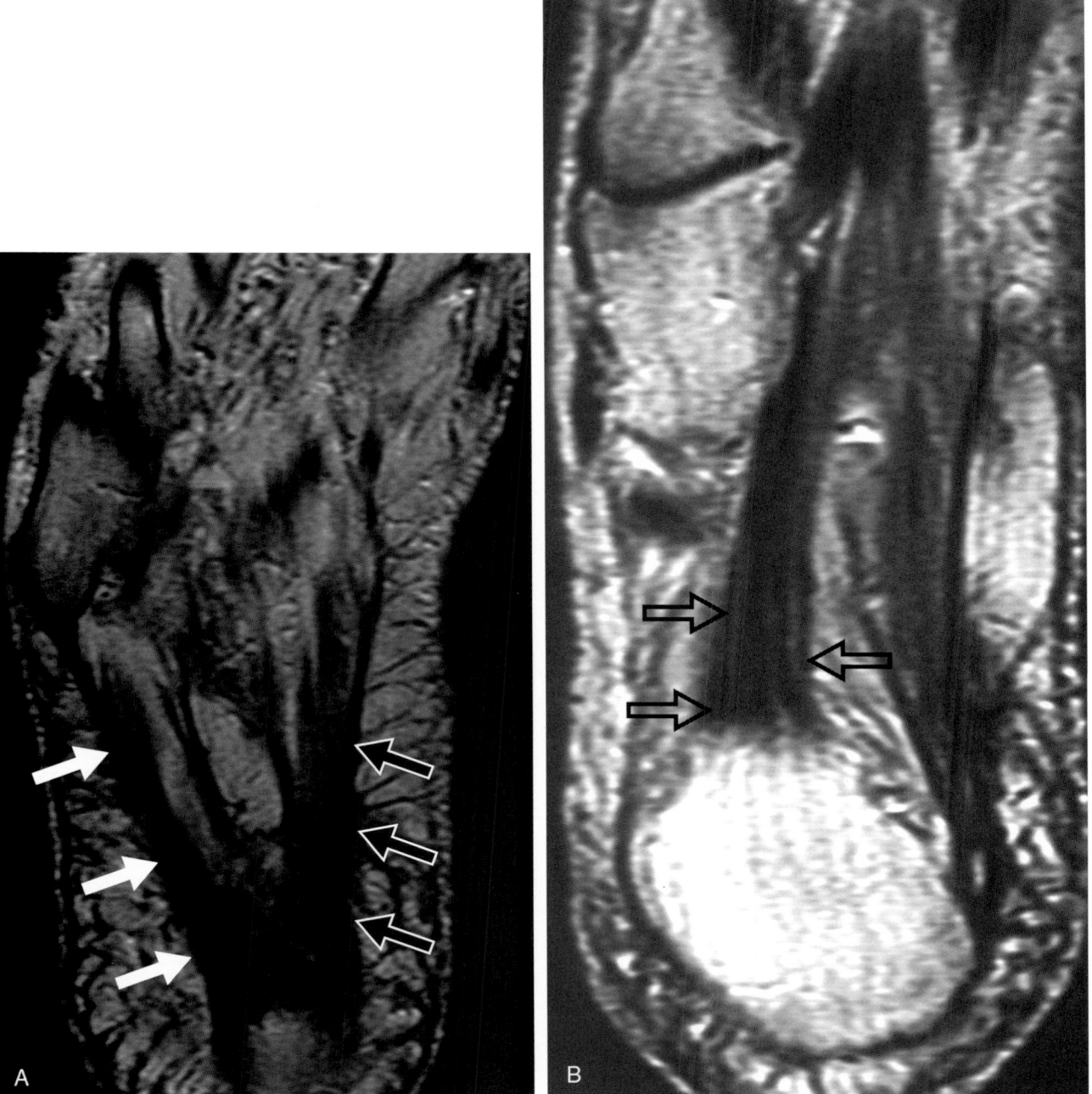

Figure 30B–17. *A,* Axial T$_1$-weighted image shows the lateral fascicle *(white arrows)* of the deep fascia covering muscles of the small toe, and the medial fascicle *(black arrows)* covering muscles of the great toe. *B,* Axial T$_1$-weighted image shows the central portion of the deep fascia, known as the plantar aponeurosis *(arrows)*.

Illustration continued on following page

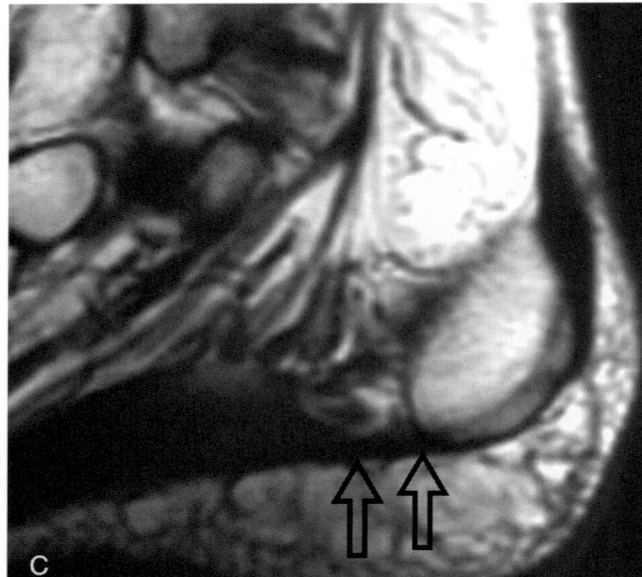

Figure 30B–17 *Continued. C,* Sagittal T$_1$-weighted image shows the insertion of the plantar aponeurosis into the plantar aspect of the calcaneus *(arrows).*

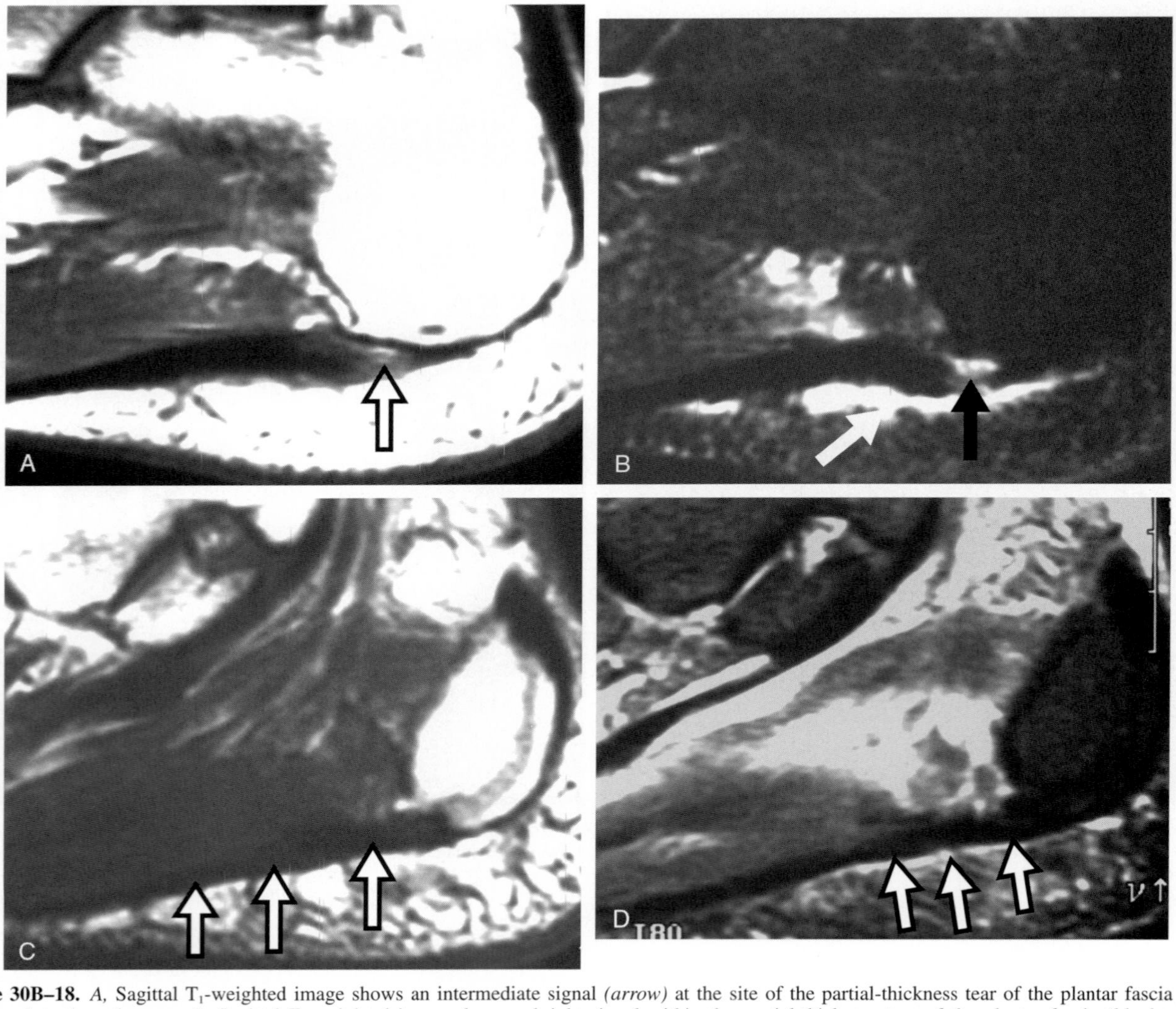

Figure 30B–18. *A,* Sagittal T$_1$-weighted image shows an intermediate signal *(arrow)* at the site of the partial-thickness tear of the plantar fascia at the insertion into the calcaneus. *B,* Sagittal T$_2$-weighted image shows a bright signal within the partial-thickness tear of the plantar fascia *(black arrow).* Bright signal, subcutaneous soft tissue edema is seen along the plantar aponeurosis *(white arrow). C,* Sagittal T$_1$-weighted image shows diffuse thickening *(arrows)* of the chronic plantar fasciitis. *D,* Sagittal T$_2$-weighted image shows diffuse thickening with an adjacent bright signal and subcutaneous soft tissue edema *(white arrows)* in chronic fasciitis.

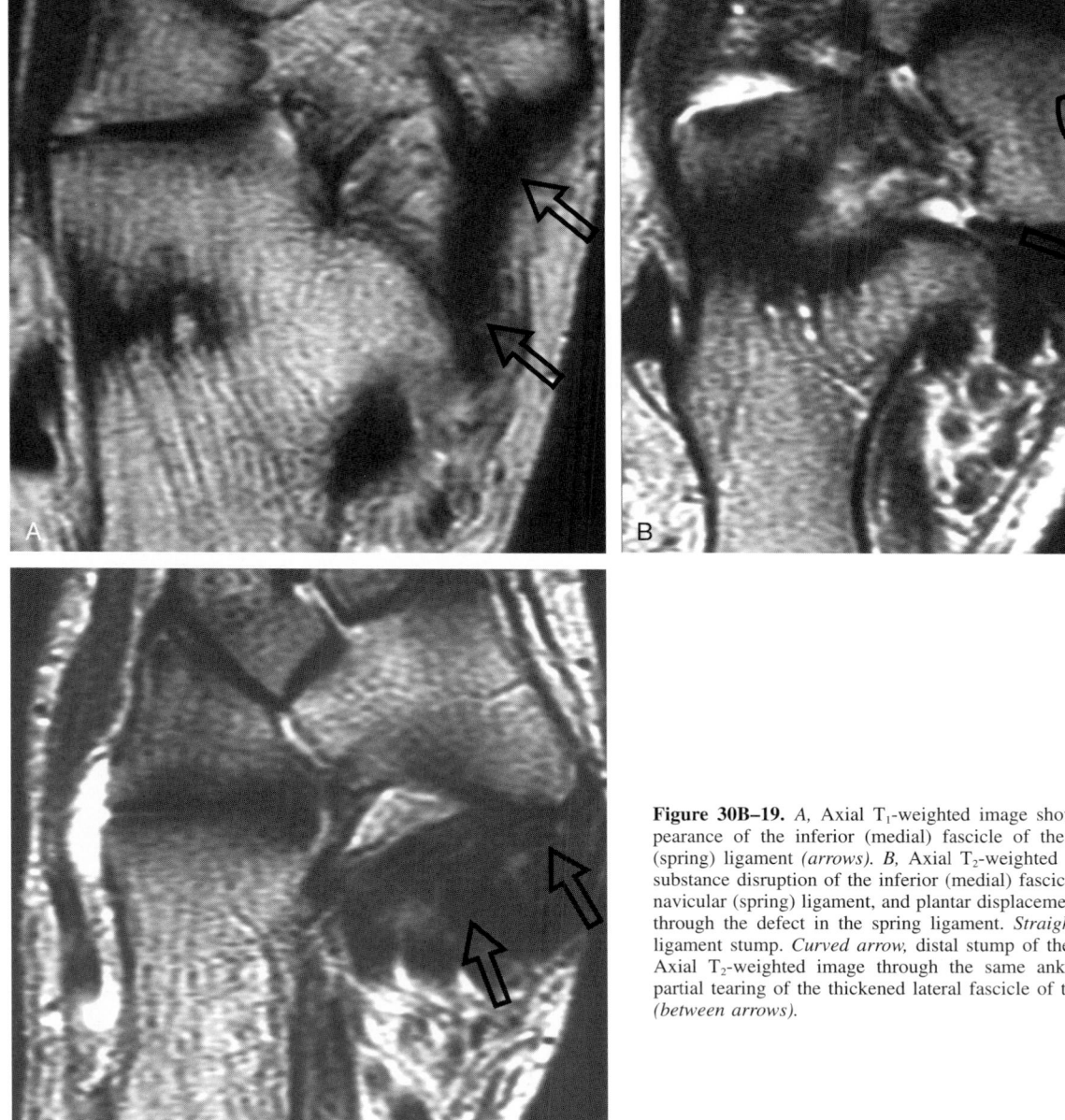

Figure 30B–19. *A,* Axial T$_1$-weighted image shows the normal appearance of the inferior (medial) fascicle of the calcaneonavicular (spring) ligament *(arrows). B,* Axial T$_2$-weighted image shows midsubstance disruption of the inferior (medial) fascicle of the calcaneonavicular (spring) ligament, and plantar displacement of the talar head through the defect in the spring ligament. *Straight arrow,* proximal ligament stump. *Curved arrow,* distal stump of the torn ligament. *C,* Axial T$_2$-weighted image through the same ankle as in *B* shows partial tearing of the thickened lateral fascicle of the spring ligament *(between arrows).*

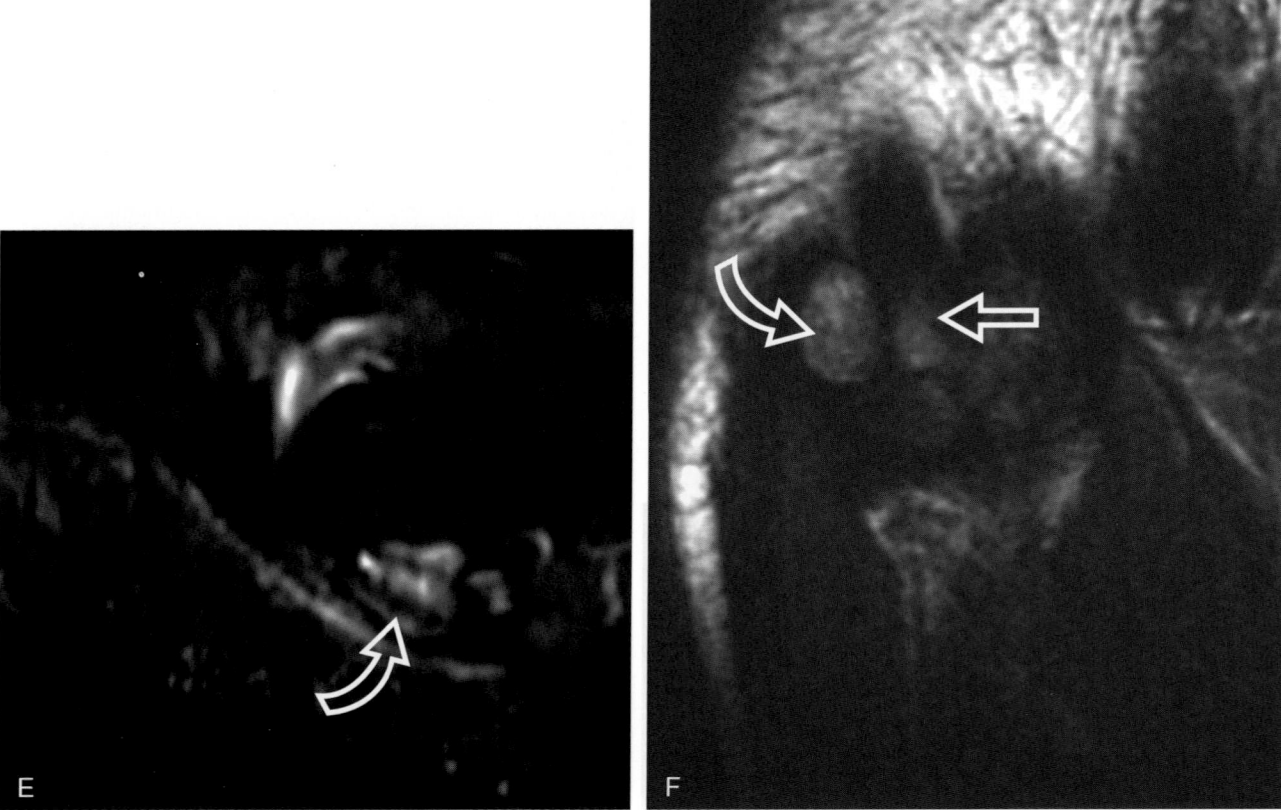

Figure 30B–21 *Continued. E*, Sagittal T₂-weighted image shows bright signal marrow edema *(curved arrow)* of the fibular sesamoid in sesamoiditis. *F*, Coronal T₁-weighted image shows dark signal (edema) in fibular sesamoid *(straight arrow)* and normal fatty marrow signal in tibial sesamoid *(curved arrow)*.

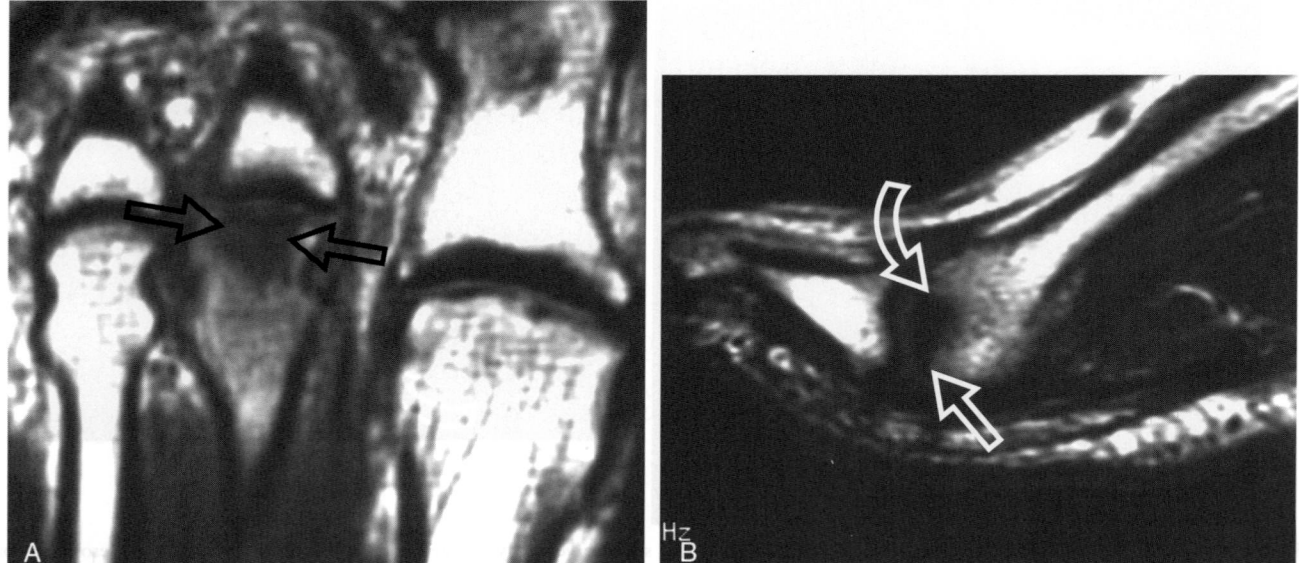

Figure 30B–22. *A*, Coronal T₁-weighted image shows crescent-shaped marrow infarction of the second metatarsal head *(between arrows)* in a patient with Freiberg's infarction. *B*, Sagittal T₁-weighted image of the same metatarsal head shows the black focus of the subchondral infarct *(arrows)* surrounded by gray marrow edema.

colleagues found that the tibia was involved in 49%, the tarsal bones in 25%, the metatarsals in 9%, the fibula in 7%, and the sesamoid bones in less than 1%.[24] Early stress fractures of the metatarsal bones may be difficult to identify on plain radiographs until they are healing and the periosteal new bone is visible. These fractures are common among long-distance runners and endurance athletes and may be identified earlier using bone scanning or MRI. MRI usually shows a transversely oriented black fracture line surrounded by bright signal marrow edema and adjacent soft tissue edema (Fig. 30B–23).

Calcaneal stress fractures are most frequently seen in endurance athletes or those participating in jumping sports. The fracture most often involves the dorsal tuberosity. Early fractures may be very difficult to identify on plain radiographs. Bone scanning usually shows a linear focus of intensely increased uptake. MRI shows a low-signal linear fracture line surrounded by marrow edema (Fig. 30B–24).

Stress fractures of the tarsal navicular are typically seen in jumping athletes such as basketball players or pole-vaulters and may be difficult to recognize on plain radio-

graphs because of the overlap of adjacent bones. Most navicular stress fractures are oriented in the sagittal plane and involve the dorsal/central aspect of the navicular. MRI shows a linear low-signal fracture line that usually extends to the talonavicular joint (Fig. 30B–25). Marrow edema and sclerosis usually surround the fracture line. Bone scanning may be useful to determine the chronicity of the fracture, and sequential CT scanning may be useful to evaluate healing after appropriate treatment has been provided. The sagittal plane fracture line of a navicular stress fracture could be mistaken for a bipartite navicular. The bipartite navicular typically has a dysmorphic shape with unequal size of the two fragments of the navicular (Fig. 30B–26).

Os Trigonum

The os trigonum is an accessory ossification center of the posterior process of the talus. The os trigonum can become painful in some athletes after repetitive ankle dorsi-

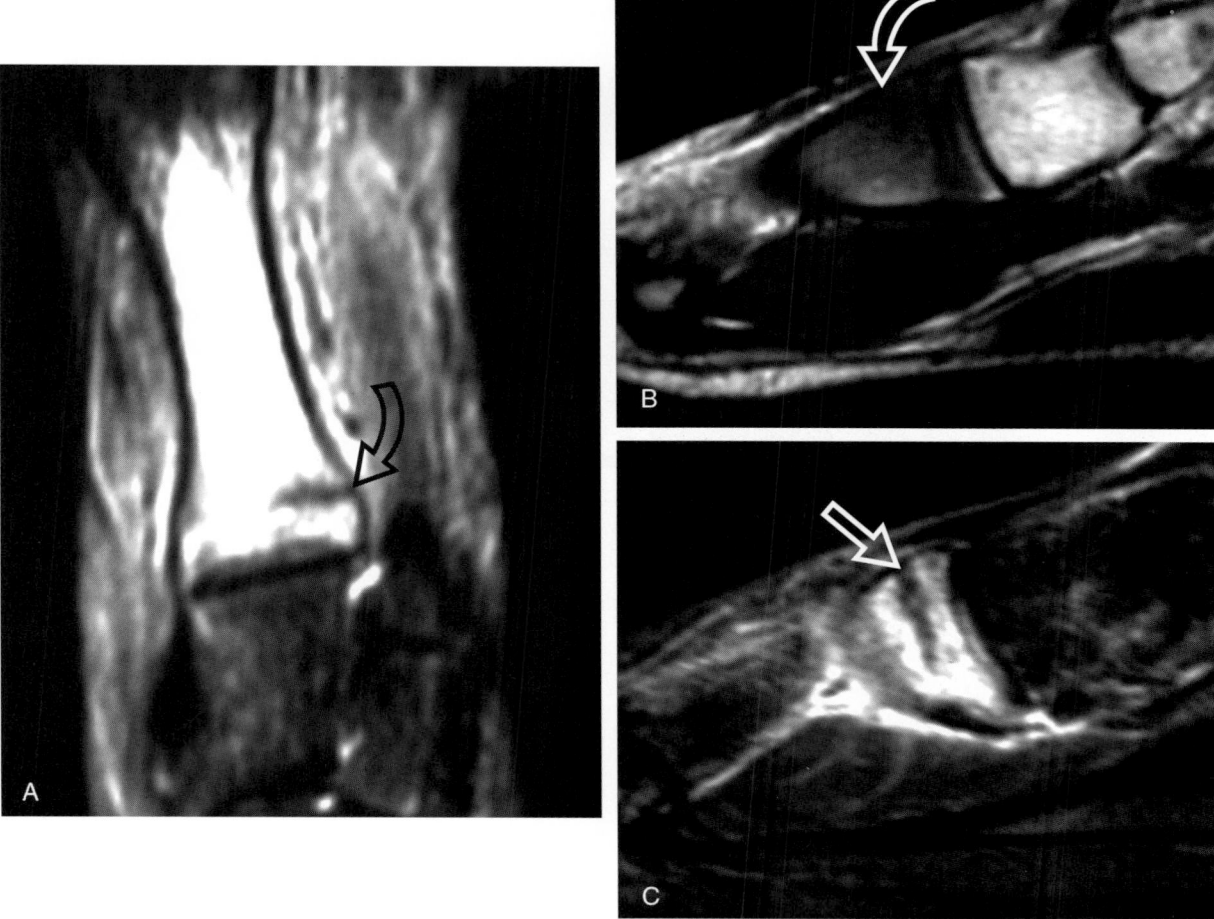

Figure 30B–23. *A,* Coronal T_2-weighted image shows bright signal marrow edema of the great toe metatarsal with transversely oriented black fracture line *(curved arrow)* through the lateral 40% of the metatarsal. *B,* Sagittal T_1-weighted image shows replacement of the normal bright signal fatty marrow with low signal marrow edema. Vertically oriented, black fracture line of stress fracture *(curved arrow)* is seen. *C,* Sagittal T_2-weighted image shows the vertically oriented black fracture line of the stress fracture *(arrow)* with surrounding bright signal marrow edema.

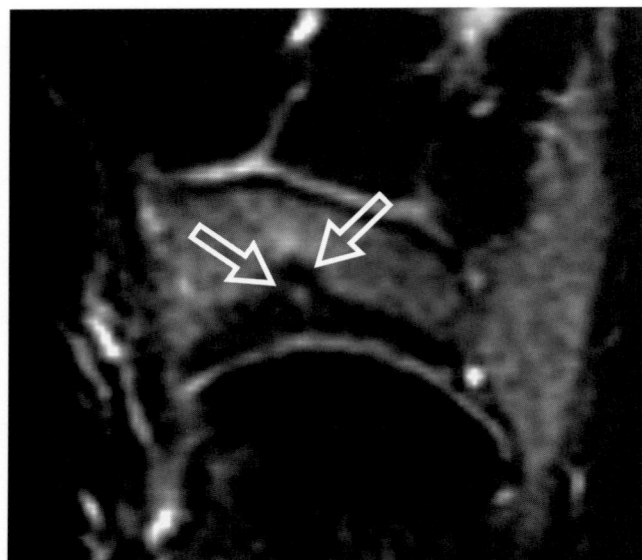

Figure 30B–24. Axial T₂-weighted magnetic resonance image shows a linear stress fracture *(arrows)* through the posterior aspect of the os calcis.

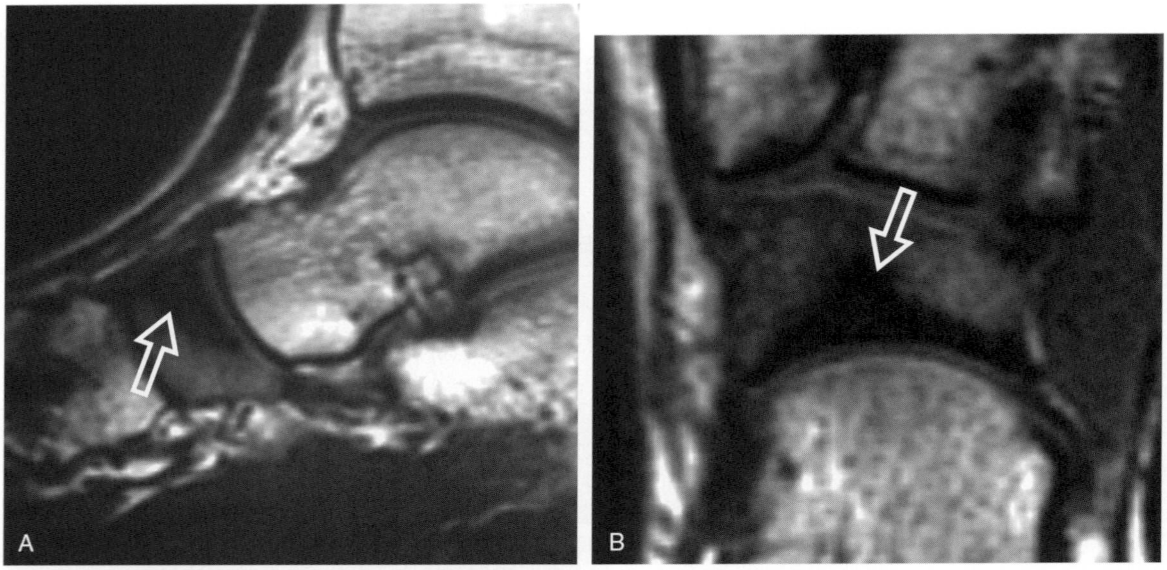

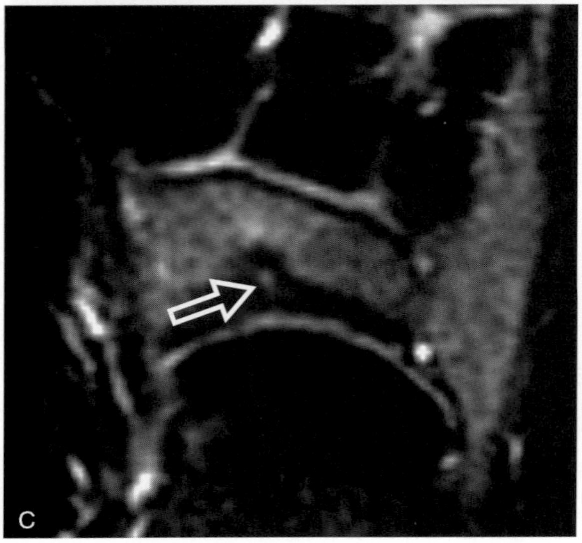

Figure 30B–25. *A,* Sagittal T₁-weighted image shows gray signal marrow edema in the dorsal aspect of the navicular adjacent to the site of a sagittal plane stress fracture *(arrow).* *B,* Coronal T₁-weighted image shows a linear black stress fracture line extending from the talonavicular articular surface in the dorsal aspect of the central navicular *(arrow).* *C,* Coronal T₂-weighted image shows bright signal marrow edema surrounding the fracture line *(arrow),* involving the proximal articular surface of the navicular.

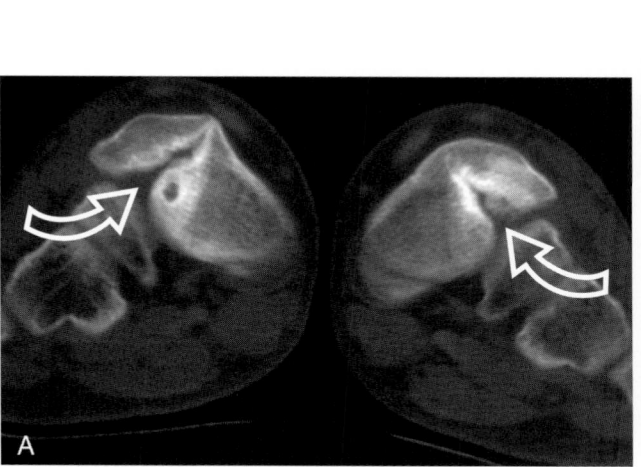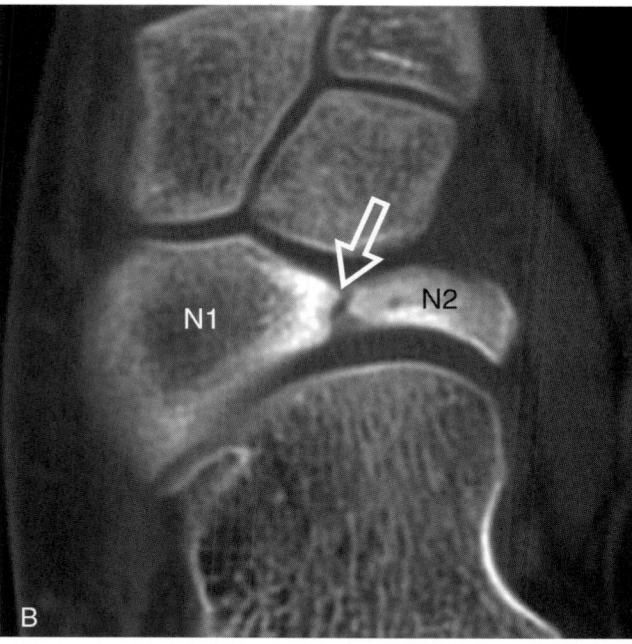

Figure 30B–26. *A,* Coronal plane computed tomographic (CT) images of both midfeet show obliquely oriented synchondrosis *(arrows)* of the bipartite navicular bones. The dysplasia or morphologic distortion of the navicular fragments distinguishes this from subacute stress fracture. *B,* Axial oblique CT of the right navicular shows a sagittal plane cleavage plane *(arrow)* between the two navicular fragments. The medial fragment (N2) is smaller than the lateral (N1), although the articular surfaces remain congruent. These findings are more consistent with a bipartite navicular than with a fracture deformity.

flexion (ballet dancers) or in jumping sports (basketball). The normal os trigonum has normal fatty marrow and smooth borders of the synchrondrosis that join it to the talus. Traumatic disruption or pseudarthrosis of the synchondrosis can produce pain. MRI of these injuries typically shows fluid signal traversing the synchondrosis with variable amounts of adjacent marrow edema (Fig. 30B–27). Inflammation of the os trigonum, or "trigonitis," is common among ballet dancers. In these individuals, the normal fatty marrow of the os trigonum is replaced by marrow edema (see Fig. 30B–27D). Trigonitis can usually be distinguished from a posterior process avulsion fracture by the absence of marrow edema within the talus. In posterior process fractures, marrow edema typically is noted in both the os trigonum and the adjacent talus and surrounding soft tissues (Fig. 30B–28).

Osteochondral Lesions of the Talar Dome

Osteochondritis dissecans is an acquired lesion in a diarthrodial joint that involves both the articular cartilage and subchondral bone. An osteochondral lesion is usually the result of either a single episode of trauma or multiple repetitive episodes, typically inversion injuries of the ankle in plantar flexion. The talar dome is most commonly involved, specifically the middle one third of the lateral dome and the posterior one third of the medial dome. Medial lesions tend to be deeper and cup-shaped, whereas lateral lesions are shallower and more wafer-like. The mechanism

of injury is believed to be a shearing impaction force between the talar dome and the tibial plafond at the time of an inversion sprain. Berndt and Harty[1a] described the sequencing and staging of these acute chondral or osteochondral fractures. Stage I represents a localized impaction and an area of bone bruising without violation of the cortex. These types of injuries may have sequelae with chondromalacia and subcortical cyst formation (Fig. 30B–29). Stage II lesions include an osteochondral fracture that is only partially detached. Stage III lesions are complete fractures that are nondisplaced. Stage IV lesions are displaced osteochondral fracture fragments. Stage I to III lesions may heal or partially heal, but they may also develop a nonunion.

The terms "stable," "loose-in-situ," and "loose" have been used to classify osteochondritis dissecans (OCD) lesions. A "stable" OCD lesion would indicate a healed osteochondral fracture with some residual radiographic lucency in the subchondral cortical bone. On MRI, these "stable" lesions have relatively normal marrow signal within the lesion and no marrow edema in the adjacent talus. "Loose-in-situ" refers to a lesion in which the overlying hyaline articular cartilage is intact but the subchondral bone fragment has not healed to the adjacent talus. This lesion has intact hyaline cartilage on MRI but has marrow edema at the interface between the OCD bone fragment and the adjacent talus. At surgery or arthroscopy, these lesions are usually ballotable. "Loose" OCD lesions are osteochondral fractures that have not healed but have not become displaced (Fig. 30B–30). A reliable but not invariable indicator of fragment instability with T_2-weighted MRI is a continuous line of fluid signal between

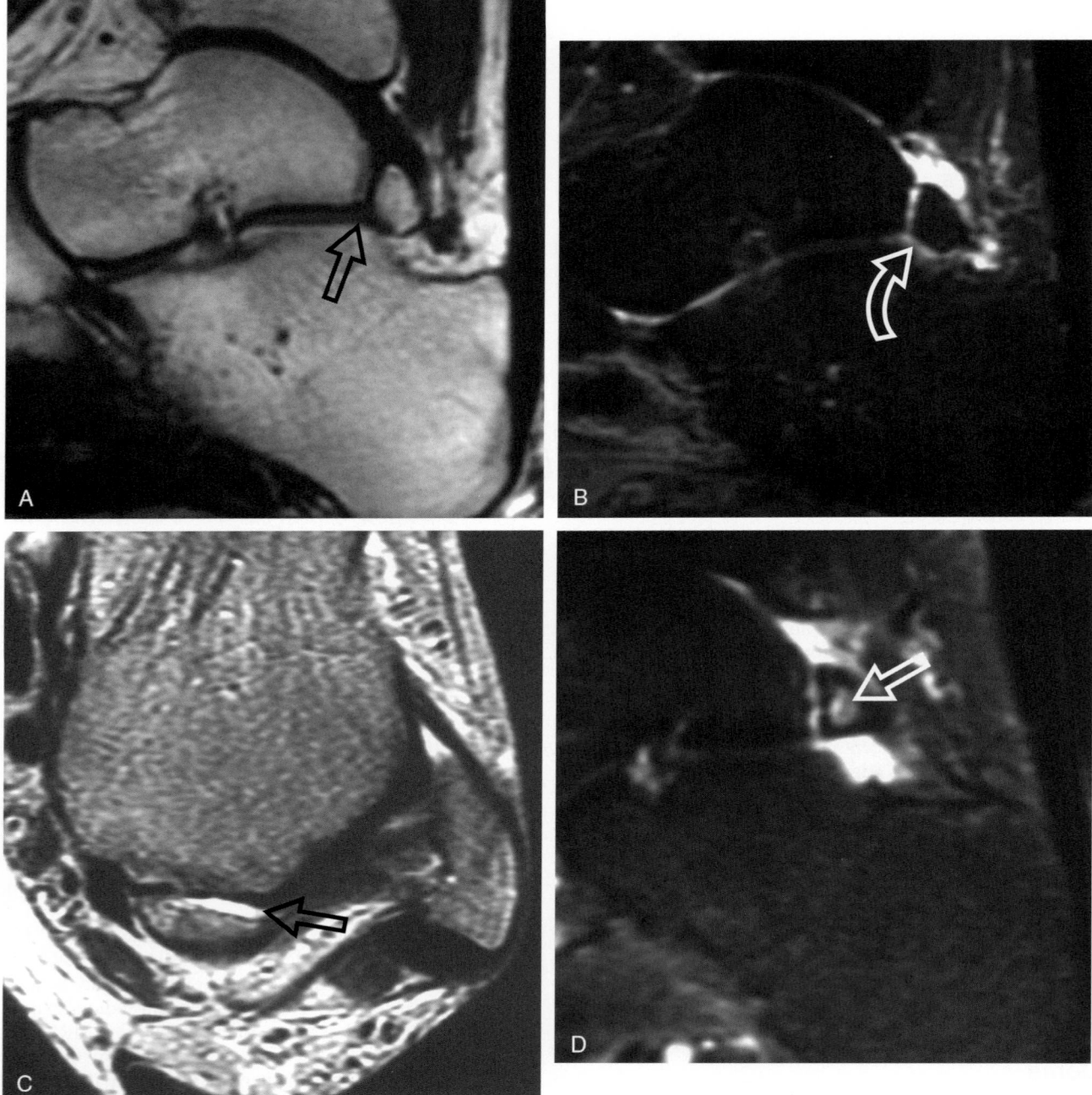

Figure 30B–27. *A*, Sagittal T$_1$-weighted magnetic resonance image shows a coronal plane pseudarthrosis *(arrow)* between the body of the talus and the os trigonum. *B*, Sagittal T$_2$-weighted image shows fluid signal within the pseudarthrosis *(curved arrow)*. No marrow edema within the os trigonum or the adjacent talus distinguishes this painful pseudarthrosis from a posterior process fracture or an os trigonitis. *C*, Axial T$_2$-weighted image shows fluid signal in the pseudarthrosis *(arrow)* between the body of the talus and the os trigonum. *D*, Sagittal T$_2$-weighted image of a patient with inflammation or osteitis of the os trigonum (also known as os trigonitis). There is marrow edema of the painful os trigonum *(arrow)* and normal marrow signal within the posterior talus, which distinguish trigonitis from a posterior process fracture.

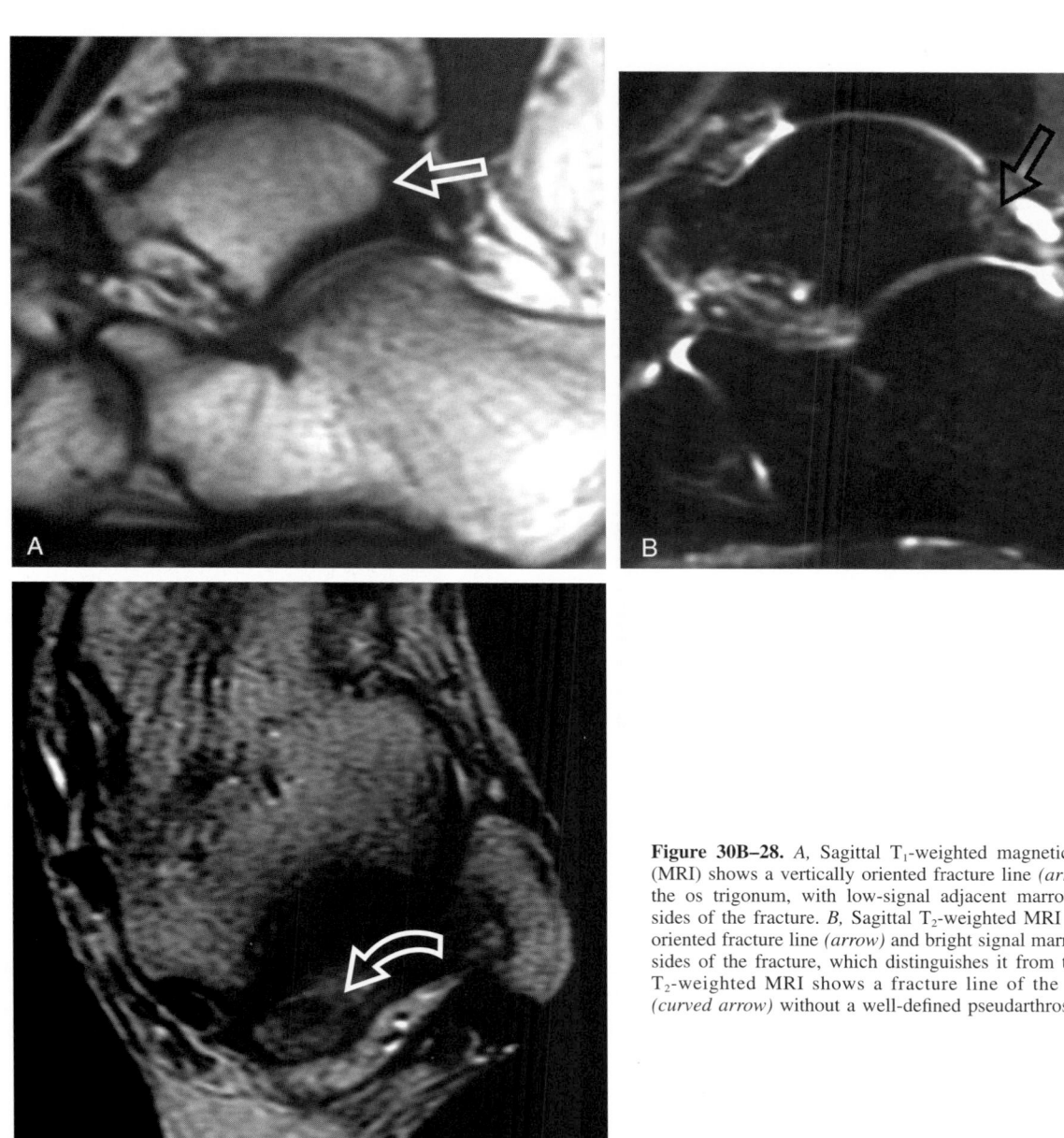

Figure 30B–28. *A,* Sagittal T$_1$-weighted magnetic resonance image (MRI) shows a vertically oriented fracture line *(arrow)* at the base of the os trigonum, with low-signal adjacent marrow edema on both sides of the fracture. *B,* Sagittal T$_2$-weighted MRI shows a vertically oriented fracture line *(arrow)* and bright signal marrow edema on both sides of the fracture, which distinguishes it from trigonitis. *C,* Axial T$_2$-weighted MRI shows a fracture line of the posterior process *(curved arrow)* without a well-defined pseudarthrosis.

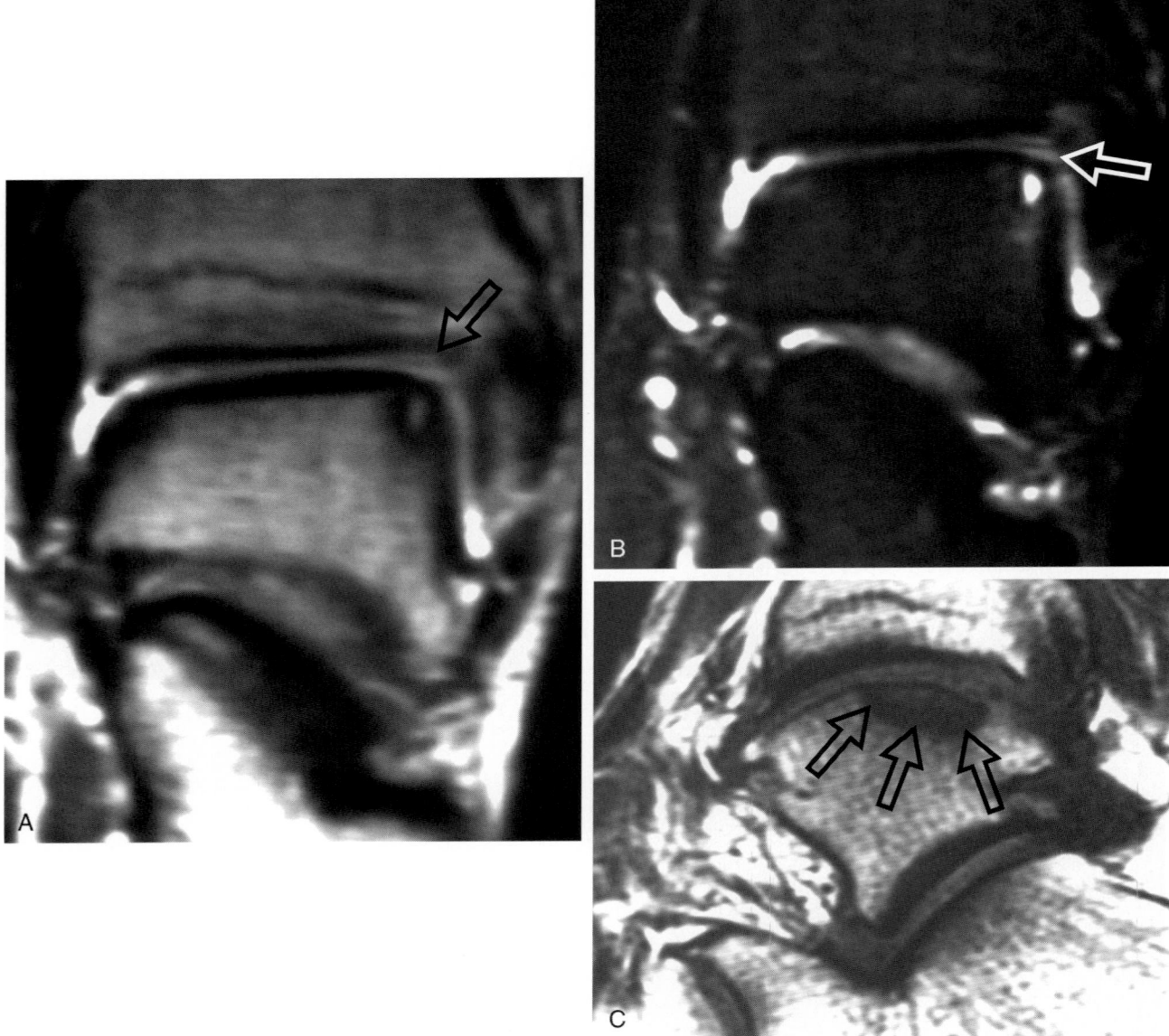

Figure 30B–29. *A,* Coronal T_2-weighted image of the Berndt and Harty stage I osteochondral lesion with a small focus of subchondral cyst formation surrounded by a peripheral rim of sclerosis. Chondromalacia of the overlying hyaline cartilage *(arrow)*. *B,* Coronal T_2-weighted image of the same lesion, showing a bright signal cyst in the subchondral bone, with chondromalacia of the overlying hyaline cartilage *(arrow)*. *C,* Sagittal T_1-weighted image shows crescent-shaped area of marrow signal abnormality *(arrows)* in the same ankle. No displacement of the subchondral cortex.

the fragment and the underlying subchondral bone. The difference between "loose-in-situ" and "loose" OCD fragments can be difficult to distinguish. Intra-articular injection of gadolinium and subsequent MRI may be useful for distinguishing these two entities in some cases.

Sinus Tarsi Syndrome

The sinus tarsi is a cone-shaped space located between the lateral margin of the talar neck and the anterior calcaneus.[1, 21] The apex of the cone is at the anterior margin of the posterior subtalar joint, and the base of the cone is at

the space between the talus and the calcaneus.[1, 21] This space is normally filled with fat and a few vessels. Infiltration of this space by edema, fibrosis, or a mass such as a ganglion cyst can produce severe pain in the area that may radiate into the foot (Figs. 30B–31 and 30B–32). This clinical entity is known as sinus tarsi syndrome.[1, 21]

Bone Contusions

Bone contusions, or trabecular microfractures, are common in sports-related injuries of the foot and ankle. Plain radiographs are usually normal, and individuals present

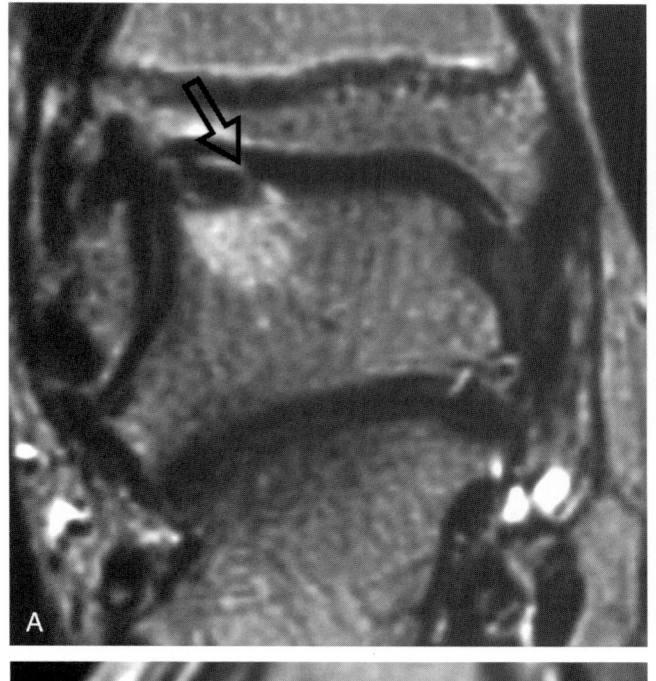

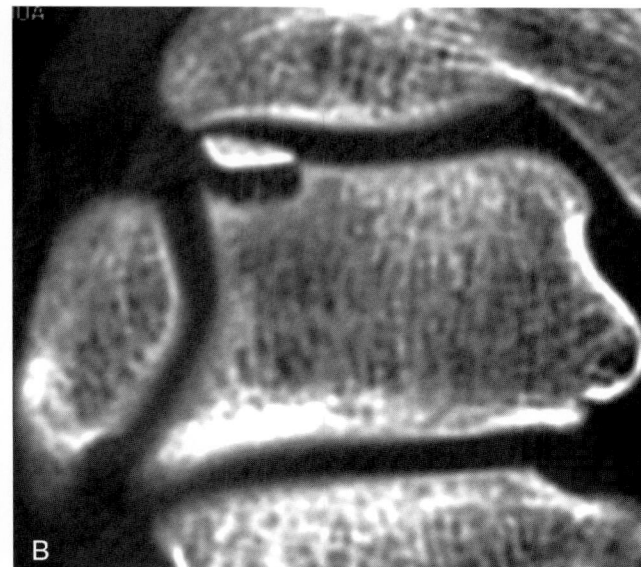

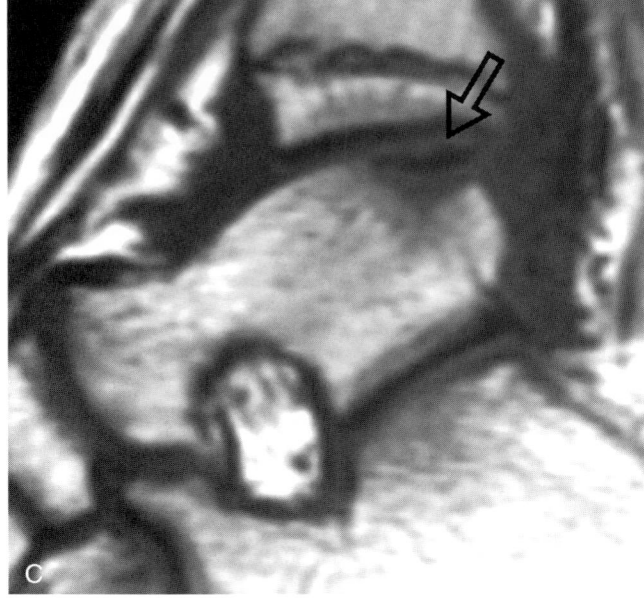

Figure 30B–30. *A,* Coronal T$_2$-weighted image of "loose" osteochondral lesion, with displacement of the osteochondral fragment *(arrow)* involving the lateral talar dome. *B,* Coronal plane computed tomographic image of the same ankle, showing displacement of the sclerotic osteochondral fragment. *C,* Sagittal plane magnetic resonance image shows sclerosis of the displaced osteochondral fragment *(arrow).*

with pain lasting longer than expected. The MRI appearance of bone contusions includes bone marrow edema beneath an articular surface or cortex of a bone. The location and distribution of bone contusions may help to identify the mechanism of injury and may suggest other occult injuries such as those noted in the patient with occult subtalar injury shown in Figure 30B–33.

Tarsal Tunnel Syndrome

The tarsal tunnel is a fibro-osseous canal through which the three flexor tendons, tibial nerve branches, and posterior tibial artery pass on their way to the foot. The roof of the tarsal tunnel is formed by the flexor retinaculum that arises from the anteromedial surface of the medial malleolus and inserts onto the medial tuberosity of the calcaneus and into the fascia overlying the abductor hallucis muscle. The tibial nerve gives off the medial calcaneal nerve and then divides into the medial and lateral plantar nerves. The medial calcaneal branch supplies sensory innervation to the medial aspect of the heel. The medial plantar nerve provides sensory innervation to most of the plantar aspect of the foot. The lateral plantar nerve provides sensory innervation to the lateral aspect of the foot and innervates many of the intrinsic muscles of the foot.

Tarsal tunnel syndrome is a clinical entity characterized by burning pain in the toes, sole of the foot, or medial heel that is aggravated by weight-bearing. Tarsal tunnel

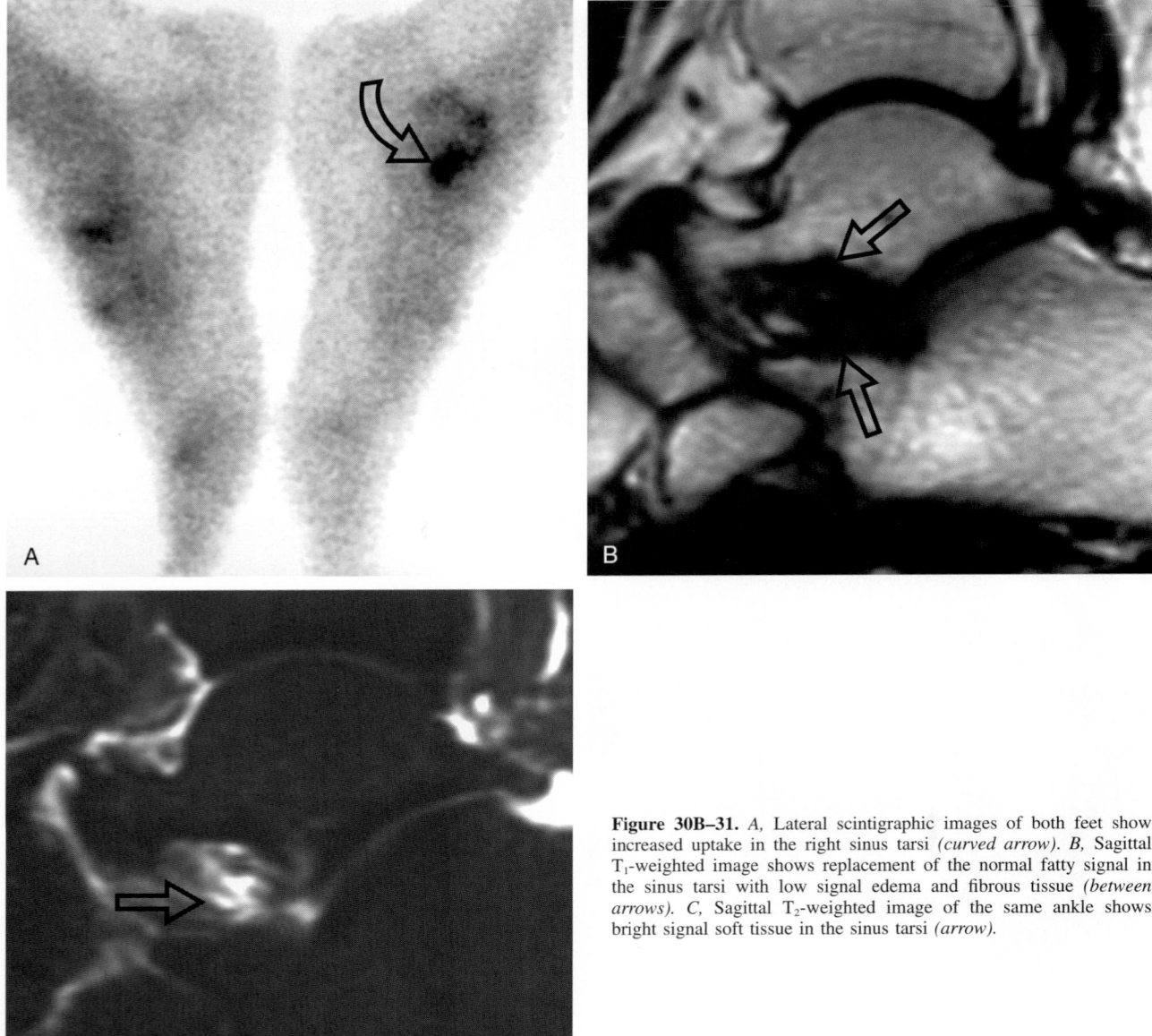

Figure 30B–31. *A,* Lateral scintigraphic images of both feet show increased uptake in the right sinus tarsi *(curved arrow). B,* Sagittal T₁-weighted image shows replacement of the normal fatty signal in the sinus tarsi with low signal edema and fibrous tissue *(between arrows). C,* Sagittal T₂-weighted image of the same ankle shows bright signal soft tissue in the sinus tarsi *(arrow).*

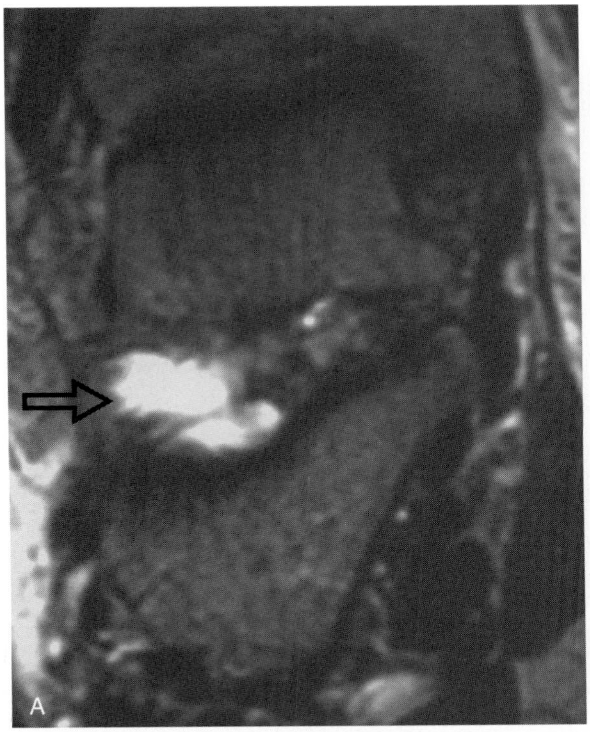

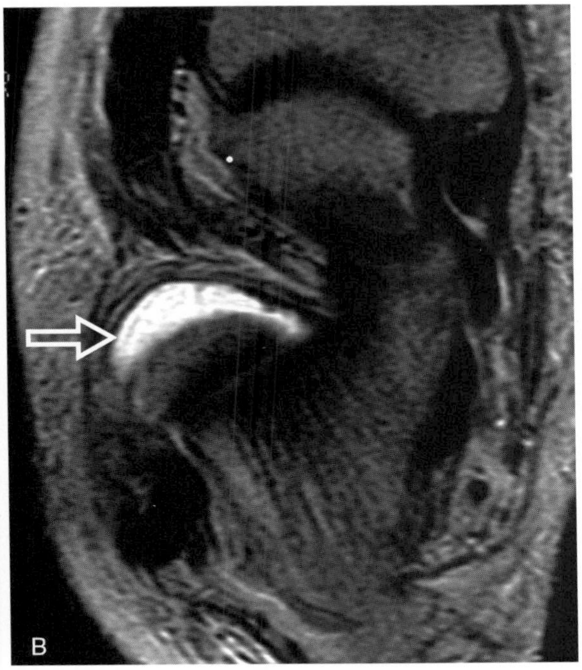

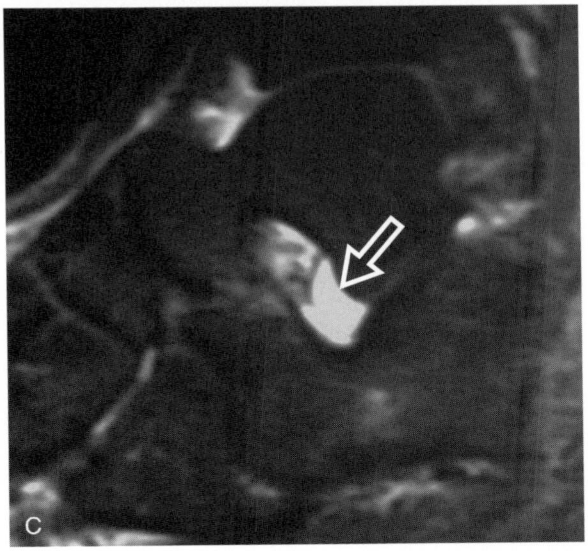

Figure 30B–32. *A,* Coronal T$_2$-weighted magnetic resonance image (MRI) shows a large ganglion cyst within the sinus tarsi *(arrow). B,* Axial T$_2$-weighted MRI shows a large ganglion cyst within the tarsal tunnel *(arrow). C,* Sagittal T$_2$-weighted MRI shows a large ganglion cyst within the sinus tarsi *(arrow).*

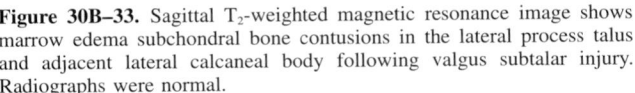

Figure 30B–33. Sagittal T$_2$-weighted magnetic resonance image shows marrow edema subchondral bone contusions in the lateral process talus and adjacent lateral calcaneal body following valgus subtalar injury. Radiographs were normal.

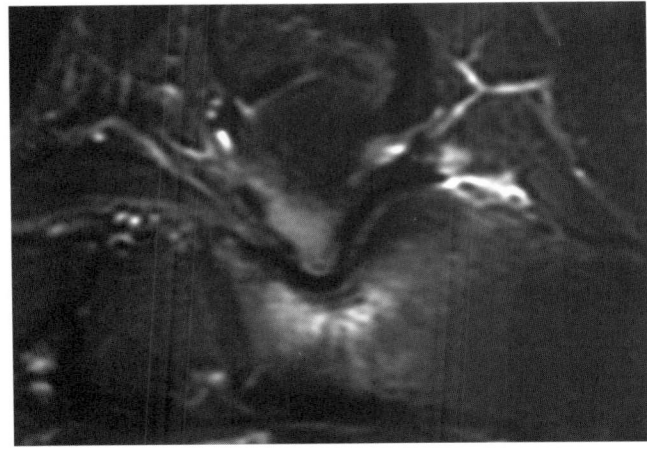

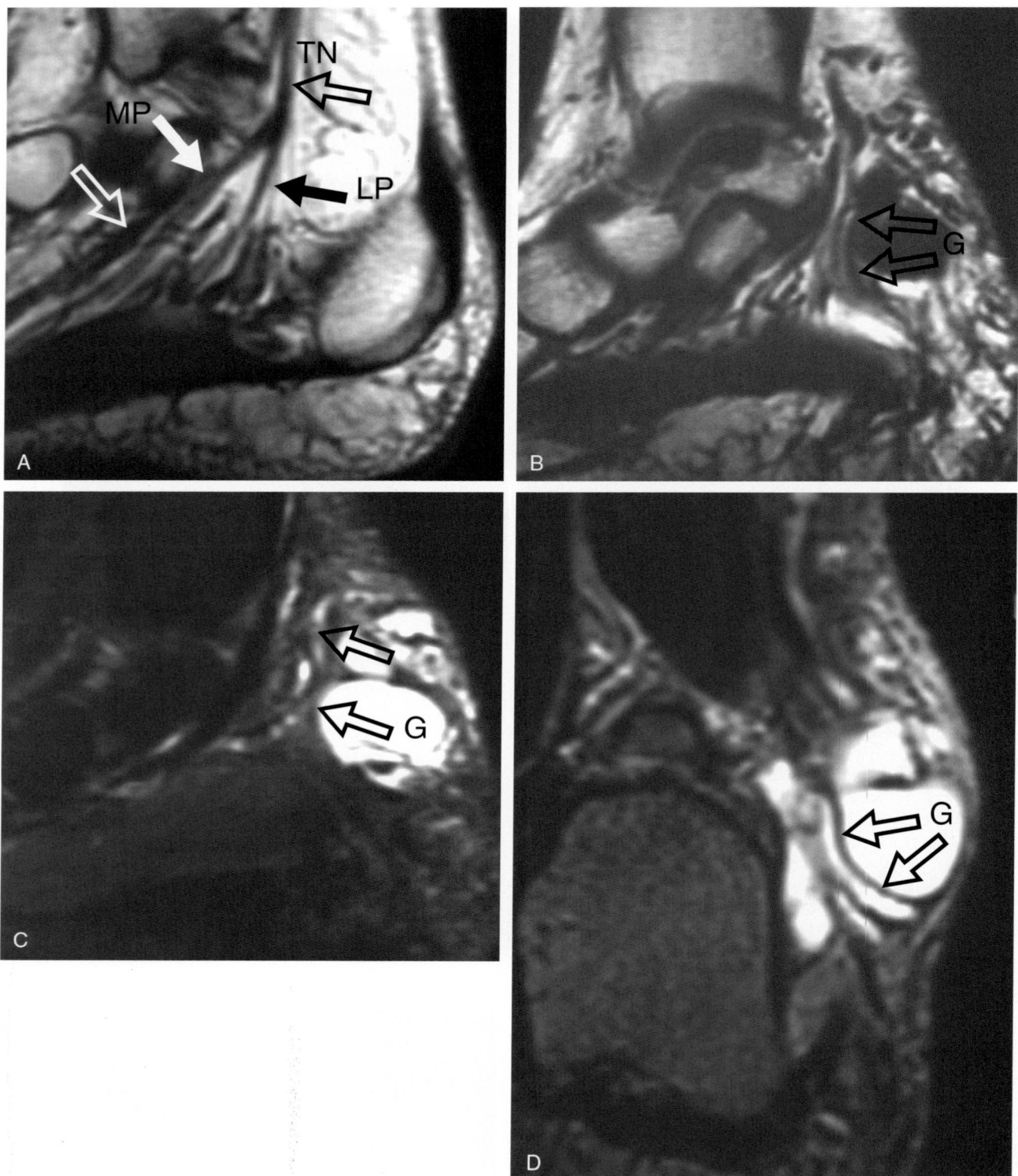

Figure 30B–34. *A,* Sagittal T$_1$-weighted magnetic resonance image of the tarsal tunnel shows a normal tibial nerve (TN, *open arrow*) branching into the medial plantar (MP) nerve *(white arrow)* and the lateral plantar (LP) nerve *(black arrow). B,* Sagittal T$_1$-weighted image in a patient with tarsal tunnel syndrome due to a multiloculated ganglion cyst (G) that displaces the plantar nerves *(arrows). C,* Sagittal T$_2$-weighted image through the same ankle shows a bright signal ganglion cyst in the tarsal tunnel, displacing the plantar nerves *(arrows). D,* Coronal T$_2$-weighted image shows medial displacement of the plantar nerves *(arrows)* by a ganglion cyst (G).

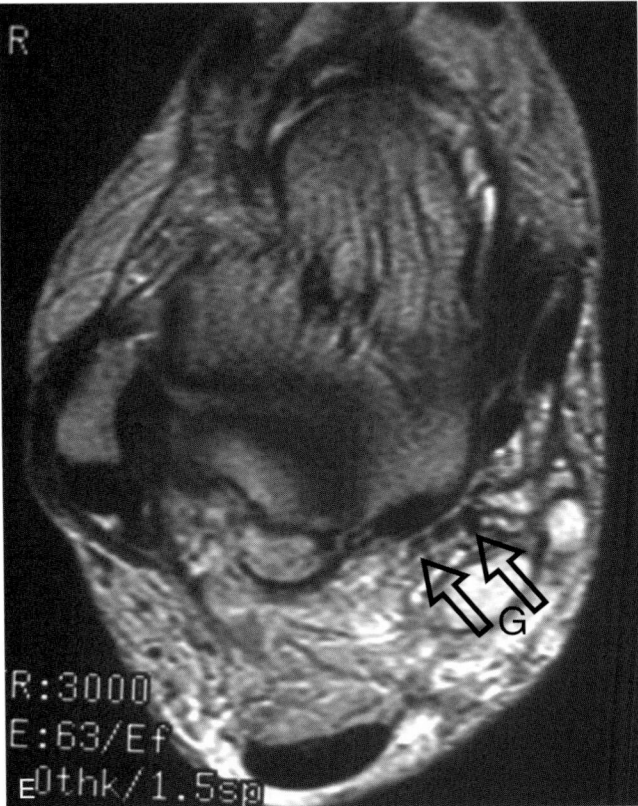

Figure 30B–34 *Continued. E,* Axial T_2-weighted magnetic resonance image shows medial displacement of the plantar nerves *(arrows)* by a ganglion cyst (G).

syndrome can be produced by any pathologic condition that produces extrinsic compression of the tibial nerve or its branches in the tarsal tunnel, including ganglion cysts (Fig. 30B–34), tenosynovitis or tendon sheath effusions of the flexor tendons, varicose veins, hindfoot valgus deformity with compression of the tibial nerve by the taut flexor retinaculum, or post-traumatic fibrosis.[12, 23]

Special imaging can be extremely helpful for the clinician in making the correct diagnosis of sports-related injuries. We cannot overemphasize the importance of communicating with the skeletal radiologist when referring patients for imaging. The optimal imaging modality for one entity may be very poor for another disease entity. If the history is known, the examination may be tailored to enable evaluation of the structures of greatest interest. We hope that this general overview is helpful and will stimulate the use of special imaging for diagnosing patients with problem cases as they arise.

References

1. Beltran J: Sinus tarsi syndrome. Magn Reson Imaging Clin North Am 2:59–65, 1994.
1a. Berndt AL, Harty M: Transchondral fractures (osteochondritis dissecans) of the talus. J Bone Joint Surg Am 41:988–1020, 1959.
2. Bonner A, Cloutier J, Econopouly J, Feitz D: Diagnosis of partial rupture of tendo Achillis with magnetic resonance imaging. J Foot Surg 29:212–217, 1990.
3. Bonnin M, Tavernier T, Bouysset M: Split lesions of the peroneus brevis tendon in chronic ankle laxity. Am J Sports Med 25:699–703, 1997.
4. Burton E, Amaker B: Stress fracture of the great toe sesamoid in a ballerina: MRI appearance. Pediatr Radiol 24:37–38, 1994.
5. Cardone BW, Erickson SJ, Den Hartog BD, Carrera GF: MRI of injury to the lateral collateral ligamentous complex of the ankle. J Comput Assist Tomogr 17:102–107, 1993.
6. Cass JR, Morrey BF: Ankle instability: Current concepts, diagnosis and treatment. Mayo Clin Proc 59:165–170, 1984.
7. Chen J, Allen A: MR diagnosis of traumatic tear of the spring ligament in a pole vaulter. Skeletal Radiol 26:310–312, 1997.
8. Cheung Y, Rosenberg Z, Ramsinghani R, et al: Peroneus quartus muscle: MR imaging features. Radiology 202:745–750, 1997.
9. Ebraheim N, Zeiss J, Skie M, Jackson W: Radiological evaluation of peroneal tendon pathology associated with calcaneal fractures. J Orthop Trauma 5:365–369, 1991.
10. Egol K, Parisien J: Impingement syndrome of the ankle caused by a medial meniscoid lesion. Arthroscopy 13:522–525, 1997.
11. Ekstrom J, Shuman W, Mack L: MR imaging of accessory soleus muscle. J Comput Assist Tomogr 14:239–242, 1990.
12. Erickson SJ, Quinn SF, Kneeland JB, et al: MR imaging of the tarsal tunnel and related spaces: Normal and abnormal findings with anatomic correlation. AJR Am J Roentgenol 155:323–328, 1990.
13. Erickson SJ, Smith JW, Ruiz ME, et al: MR imaging of the lateral collateral ligament of the ankle. AJR Am J Roentgenol 156:131–136, 1991.
14. Garrick JG, Requa RK: The epidemiology of foot and ankle injuries. Clin Sports Med 7:29–36, 1988.
15. Gray H: Muscles and fascia of the leg. In Goss CM (ed): Gray's Anatomy, 29th ed. Philadelphia, Lea and Febiger, 1973.
16. Hauger O, Moinard M, Lasalarie J, et al: Anterolateral compartment of the ankle in the lateral impingement syndrome: Appearance on CT arthrography. AJR Am J Roentgenol 173:685–690, 1999.
17. Hogan JF: Posterior tibial tendon dysfunction and MRI. J Foot Ankle Surg 32:467–472, 1993.
18. Karasick D, Schweitzer M: Disorders of the hallux sesamoid complex: MR features. Skeletal Radiol 27:411–418, 1998.
19. Keene J, Lash E, Fisher D, De SA: Magnetic resonance imaging of Achilles tendon ruptures. Am J Sports Med 17:333–337, 1989.
20. Kier R: Magnetic resonance imaging of plantar fasciitis and other causes of heel pain. Magn Reson Imaging Clin North Am 2:97–107, 1994.
21. Klein M, Spreitzer A: MR imaging of the tarsal sinus and canal: Normal anatomy, pathologic findings, and features of the sinus tarsi syndrome. Radiology 186:233–240, 1993.
22. Klein MA: MR imaging of the ankle: Normal and abnormal findings in the medial collateral ligament. AJR Am J Roentgenol 162:377–383, 1994.
23. Kneeland JB, Dalinka MK: Magnetic resonance imaging of the foot and ankle [review]. Magn Reson Q 8:97–115, 1992.
24. Matheson G, Clement D, McKenzie D, et al: Stress fractures in athletes. A study of 320 cases. Am J Sports Med 15:46–58, 1987.
25. McCarroll JR, Schrader JW, Shelbourne KD, et al: Meniscoid lesions of the ankle in soccer players. Am J Sports Med 15:255–257, 1987.
26. Mota J, Rosenberg Z: Magnetic resonance imaging of the peroneal tendons. Top Magn Reson Imaging 9:273–285, 1998.
27. Muhle C, Frank L, Rand T, et al: Tibiofibular syndesmosis: High-resolution MRI using a local gradient coil. J Comput Assist Tomogr 22:938–944, 1998.
28. Narvaez JA, Narvaez J, Ortega R, et al: Painful heel: MR imaging findings. Radiographics 20:333–352, 2000.
29. Neuhold A, Stiskal M, Kainberger F, Schwaighofer B: Degenerative Achilles tendon disease: Assessment by magnetic resonance imaging. Eur J Radiol 14:213–220, 1992.
30. Potter H, Pavlov H, Abrahams T: The hallux sesamoids revisited. Skeletal Radiol 21:437–444, 1992.
31. Rolf C, Guntner P, Ericsater J, Turan I: Plantar fascia rupture: Diagnosis and treatment. J Foot Ankle Surg 36:112–114, 1997.
32. Rosenberg Z, Beltran J, Cheung Y, et al: MR features of longitudinal tears of the peroneus brevis tendon. AJR Am J Roentgenol 168:141–147, 1997.
33. Rosenberg ZS, Cheung Y, Jahss MH, et al: Rupture of posterior tibial

tendon: CT and MR imaging with surgical correlation. Radiology 169:229–235, 1988.

34. Rule J, Yao L, Seeger LL: Spring ligament of the ankle: Normal MR anatomy. AJR Am J Roentgenol 161:1241–1244, 1993.

35. Schneck CD, Mesgarzadeh M, Bonakdarpour A, Ross GJ: MR imaging of the most commonly injured ankle ligaments. Part I. Normal anatomy. Radiology 184:499–506, 1992.

36. Schweitzer M: Magnetic resonance imaging of the foot and ankle. Magn Reson Q 9:214–234, 1993.

37. Schweitzer M, Eid M, Deely D, et al: Using MR imaging to differentiate peroneal splits from other peroneal disorders. AJR Am J Roentgenol 168:129–133, 1997.

38. Schweitzer M, Karasick D: MRI of the ankle and hindfoot. Semin Ultrasound CT MR 15:410–422, 1994.

39. Schweitzer ME: Magnetic resonance imaging of the foot and ankle [review]. Magn Reson Q 9:214–234, 1993.

40. Schweitzer ME, Caccese R, Karasick D, et al: Posterior tibial tendon tears: Utility of secondary signs for MR imaging diagnosis [see comments]. Radiology 188:655–659, 1993.

41. Shellock F, Feske W, Frey C, Terk M: Peroneal tendons: Use of kinematic MR imaging of the ankle to determine subluxation. J Magn Reson Imaging 7:451–454, 1997.

42. Stone J, Guhl J: Meniscoid lesions of the ankle. Clin Sports Med 10:661–676, 1991.

43. Theodorou D, Theodorou S, Farooki S, et al: Disorders of the plantar aponeurosis: A spectrum of MR imaging findings. AJR Am J Roentgenol 176:97–104, 2001.

44. Theodorou D, Theodorou S, Kakitsubata Y, et al: Plantar fasciitis and fascial rupture: MR imaging findings in 26 patients supplemented with anatomic data in cadavers. Radiographics 20:S181–S197, 2000.

45. Tjin AE, Schweitzer M, Karasick D: MR imaging of peroneal tendon disorders. AJR Am J Roentgenol 168:135–140, 1997.

46. Watson T, Anderson R, Davis W: Periarticular injuries to the hallux metatarsophalangeal joint in athletes. Foot Ankle Clin 5:687–713, 2000.

47. Yao L, Gentili A, Cracchiolo A: MR imaging findings in spring ligament insufficiency. Skeletal Radiol 28:245–250, 1999.

48. Yao L, Tong D, Cracchiolo A, Seeger L: MR findings in peroneal tendinopathy. J Comput Assist Tomogr 19:460–464, 1995.

Section C
Etiology of Injury to the Foot and Ankle

Thomas O. Clanton, MD ■ Robert M. Wood, MD, FRCS

The etiology of injury to the foot and ankle, as with other areas of the body, is a primary concern in sports medicine because prevention of injury requires the ability to recognize those conditions that are responsible for injury. Research has shown that when etiologic factors are addressed directly, it is possible to alter injury rates for a sport significantly.[128, 193] In studying etiology, it quickly becomes evident that multiple risk factors are interwoven to produce the common thread of excessive loading in either an acute or a chronic fashion.[290, 291, 301] In this chapter, we review predisposing conditions and the variables that may have a protective value. For the foot and ankle, the primary areas of attention are flexibility, shoe wear, and playing surfaces.

Injury variables can be divided into intrinsic and extrinsic factors.[237, 395] Intrinsic factors include the player's individual physical characteristics and personality traits. These physical characteristics include such things as age, sex, genotype, somatotype, strength, speed, agility, coordination, physical fitness, flexibility, malalignment, physical maturity level, rate of growth, muscle composition, anatomic variation, and previous injury with residual structural inadequacies or with inadequate rehabilitation.* Pure personality characteristics such as extroversion, anxiety level, conscientiousness, self-confidence, tough-mindedness, responsiveness to coaching, discipline, determination, tenacity, dependency, sensitivity, and others may play a role in whether an individual is injury prone.[52, 59, 153, 189, 204, 237, 286, 410, 411] The proportion of these factors and others left unmentioned constitutes the individual athlete's intrinsic risk of injury. Extrinsic factors, on the other hand, relate to the type of sports activity, the knowledge and skill of the coach or coaches, the practice or training methods, the level of competition, the environmental conditions, the playing surfaces, and the equipment.*

Sports activity can be separated further into high, medium, or low risk (Table 30C–1).[285, 386] Some sports pose different risks to certain body parts, whereas others carry a high risk or low risk to the body as a whole. For example, running carries a low risk of shoulder injury but a high risk of foot or knee injury. Conversely, swimming may pose a high risk of injury to the shoulders but a low risk of injury to the foot and ankle. One study found that football had 12 times more injuries than the next most common sport.[106] Another study suggested that football actually had a lower injury rate than soccer, wrestling, and women's gymnastics if the number of injuries per 1000 athlete exposures was taken into consideration.[448]

Although there may be disagreement about which sport produces the most injuries or has the highest percentage of injuries, it is clear that there is an inherent risk of injury connected with sports participation. Certain variables play a role in this, including playing time, position played, level of competition, movements required, equipment used, individual versus team play, enforcement of the rules and regulations, and level of physical fitness.[105, 146, 285] Practice methods (e.g., controlled versus uncontrolled contact drills) have a definite impact on injury statistics.[39, 105, 166] In competitive running, training techniques such as high-mileage workouts, excessive use of plyometrics, and interval work have been implicated in the incidence of overuse problems.[80, 81, 239] The environment affects injury risk in the sense that weather conditions can alter the playing surface, the shoes worn, the interface characteristics between shoe and surface, and the attitudes of players and coaches. Some

---

*See references 25, 34, 37, 39, 121, 139, 149, 152, 161, 172, 182, 189, 202, 214, 215, 236, 237, 254, 266, 276, 286, 290, 322, 367, 374, 375, 394, 395, 406, 414, and 427.

*See references 34, 37–39, 47, 64, 166, 178, 191, 192, 202, 203, 222, 223, 237, 254, 286, 290, 300, 306, 309, 322, 331, 373, 394, 395, and 425.

TABLE 30C–1
High-, Medium-, and Low-Risk Sports for Foot and Ankle Injury

High Risk	Medium Risk	Low Risk
Ballet	Aerobics	Archery
Basketball	Baseball	Boating
Dance	Football	Bowling
Ice skating	Gymnastics	Cycling
Mountaineering	Ice hockey	Equestrian
Running	Lacrosse	Fishing
Skateboarding	Racquetball/squash	Golf
Snowboarding	Roller skating	Parachuting
Soccer	Rugby	Rodeo
	Tennis	Skiing
	Volleyball	Weight training
	Water-skiing	Wrestling

Adapted from Sports Injuries. Accident Facts. Report of the National Safety Council, 1990, p 88; and from Table 26–1 in Clanton TO: Athletic injuries to the soft tissues of the foot and ankle. In Coughlin MJ, Mann RA (eds): Surgery of the Foot and Ankle, 7th ed. St Louis, Mosby, 1999.

of these factors are particularly crucial to the foot and ankle. The interaction between extrinsic and intrinsic elements makes statistical analysis difficult from a precise epidemiologic perspective. The reader must recognize that injury statistics are only as good as the integrity of the investigator, their statistical methods, and the research design.[87, 323, 434] George Bernard Shaw is credited with the phrase "There are lies, big lies, and statistics."[225] The earlier chapter on statistics provides more detailed analysis of this subject.

The coach is the main individual responsible for maximizing development and improving performance. Therefore, the coach's knowledge, experience, and ethics (along with these qualities in the physician and trainer) can be determinants of the athlete's health status.[39] Over the past decade, a controversial issue has been the use of performance-enhancing drugs and nutritional supplements.[97] Quite clearly, there are both positive and negative effects associated with their use. With respect to performance-enhancing drugs, one must deal with the fact that they are illegal, constitute an unfair advantage, and place on the athlete an unnecessary and potentially serious risk.[55, 98]

The same equilibrium between positive and negative effects shifts to the injury side with certain training techniques. Plyometric training is promoted to improve jumping ability and speed (Fig. 30C–1)[217]; however, such exercises as bench jumping and bounding can overload the system.[63] This is particularly true when stress accommodation is not allowed and when shoes and surfaces are inappropriate for these activities. Running programs that involve excessive mileage or, more commonly, "too much too soon" are responsible for stress fractures or other overuse syndromes.[34, 322]

Certain factors frequently lead to overstress: (1) when ill-suited or unprepared athletes are asked to train with long-distance running for such sports as swimming, basketball, or volleyball; (2) when athletes are out of shape because it is early in the season; and (3) when it is the transition period between seasons when a player shifts from one sport to another without recognizing the different stresses introduced by the variation in performance require-

ments, shoes, and playing surfaces. A lack of stress adaptation frequently results in overload problems such as tendinitis or stress fracture.

Stress tolerance varies widely from individual to individual. This must be recognized in the design of preseason, in-season, and off-season training programs. Unnecessary exposure to injury can be attributed to other coaching methods. Uncontrolled scrimmages and excessive contact work increase injury rates in football.[39] Gymnasts who perform complex maneuvers without adequate spotting or preparation have a higher risk of injury.[254] Baseball and softball players who practice sliding into fixed bases are unnecessarily exposed to foot and ankle trauma[191, 192] (Fig. 30C–2). Finally, the "no pain, no gain" coaching philosophy can pressure an athlete to return to play after an injury without adequate rehabilitation and increase the potential for injury. For example, an ankle syndesmosis injury treated functionally as a typical lateral ankle sprain can worsen considerably. In these times of astronomical salaries for professional athletes, there is increasing emphasis on players returning to sport after injury in the shortest amount of time possible. It is our job as physicians to act as educators for coaches, therapists, and athletic trainers so that they understand the benefit of returning an athlete to sport participation at the appropriate time after injury. Likewise, we should point out the risks involved when criteria for return to competition are ignored.

Injury risk is a natural and accepted part of sports participation. Different sports with different performance factors naturally provide varying degrees of exposure to injury.[285, 286] Three broad categories of analysis in the injury equation are neuromuscular, psychometric, and environmental factors.[286] These can be related to a classification of sports activities based on six basic motions: (1) stance, (2) walking, (3) running, (4) jumping, (5) throwing, and (6) kicking.[254, 256] Running, jumping, and kicking seemingly pose the greatest risk for injury to the foot and ankle. By using these types of categorization and classification combined with scientific analysis of biomechanical stresses, it may be possible to analyze injury potential more accurately and to design effective prevention strategies.

TABLE 30C–2
Injury Rates Calculated for the Foot and Ankle in Various Sports from a Review of the Literature

Sport/Study	Skill Level	Ankle Injury (%)	Foot Injury (%)
Aerobics			
Rothenberger[343]	Recreational	12	5
Garrick[143]	Recreational	11	18
Ballet			
Garrick[141]	Professional and nonprofessional	17	22
Sohl[389]	Review of literature	14	15
Baseball			
Garfinkel[140]	Professional	10	4
Basketball			
Zelisko[447]	Professional	19	4
Henry[173]	Professional	18	6
Moretz[277]	High school	31	8
Cycling			
Davis[107]	NA	F&A	8
Kiburz[207]	Club	F&A	14
Dance (general)			
Washington[435]	Various levels	17	15
Rovere[345]	Student	22	15
Equestrian			
Bernhang[30]	Top class	F&A	13
Bixby-Hammett[33]	Top class	F&A	6
Football			
Blyth[37]	High school	15	2
Culpepper[101]	High school	11	4
DeLee[112]	High school	18	2
Zemper[448]	College	16	4
		AE = 1	AE = 0.25
Canale[67]	College	11	2
Golf			
McCarroll[256]	Professional	2	3
McCarroll[257]	Amateur	3	2
Gymnastics			
Caine[65]	Club	21	3
Garrick[145]	High school	10	8
Ice hockey			
Sutherland[408]	Amateur	0	0
	High school	0	0
	College	7	10
	Professional	0	0
Park[313]	Junior	4	1
Lacrosse			
Muller[280]	College	15	4
Nelson[282]	College	14	4
Mountaineering			
McLennan[258]	NA	41	8
Tomczak[419]	NA	40	35
Parachuting			
Petras[315]	Military	7	0.3
Rodeo			
Meyers[265]	College	6	1
Roller skating			
Ferkel[132]	College	10	NA
Perlik[314]	NA	8	2
Rugby			
Micheli[267]	College/club	8	2
Running			
Gottlieb[154]	Recreational	19	11
Walter[433]	Recreational	15	16
Temple[416]	NA	26	26
Marti[249]	NA	30	10
Ice skating			
Brown	National males	8	8
Smith	Age 11–19 yr	29	8
Skiing			
Downhill			
Johnson[196]	Various	9	NA
Blitzer[36]	Youth	F&A	8
Freestyle			
Dowling[126]	USSA	8	NA

Table 30C–2
Injury Rates Calculated for the Foot and Ankle in Various Sports from a Review of the Literature *Continued*

Sport/Study	Skill Level	Ankle Injury (%)	Foot Injury (%)
Snowboarding			
Pino[319]	Recreational	26	3
Soccer			
Ekstrand[127]	Swedish senior male division	17	12
Nilson[289]	Various	36	8
Berger-Vachon[29]	Amateur leagues (France)	20	NA
Squash/raquetball			
Berson[31]	Recreational	21	2
Soderstrom[383]	NA	20	7
Tennis			
Winge[442]	Elite	11	9
Volleyball			
Schafle[357]	National amateur	18	6
Water skiing			
Humrnel[185]	NA	4	15
Weight training			
Kulund[216]	Elite/olympic	2	0
Wrestling			
Roy[347]	College	10	3
Lok[248]	Olympic	10	0
Snook[382]	College	4	0
Requa[332]	High school	3.8/100 wrestlers	

From Clanton TO: Athletic injuries to the soft tissues of the foot and ankle. In Coughlin MJ, Mann RA (eds): Surgery of the Foot and Ankle, 7th edition, St Louis, Mosby, 1999, pp 1093–1094.
AE, Number of injuries per athletic exposure; F&A, foot and ankle; NA, not available; USSA, United States Ski Association.

though this chapter encompasses only the foot and ankle, the factors responsible for injury in this region can also produce signs and symptoms outside the foot and ankle. Each individual has been endowed with certain unalienable anatomic characteristics that under the proper bionegative influences will result in an acute or chronic injury to the most vulnerable component in the system.

Flexibility is one of the components of physical fitness that has been judged to be critical for injury-free performance.[369] Its effect on injury to the foot and ankle has been discussed primarily in relation to (1) ankle joint stiffness affecting the incidence of ankle sprains and (2) flatfeet or hyperpronated feet as a source of injury or pain. For the foot and ankle, the concept of flexibility leads us into the area of hypermobility and joint laxity and includes such entities as the flatfoot, pronated foot, cavus foot, unstable ankle, unstable hindfoot, and hallux rigidus.

Definitions

Flexibility is the range of motion commonly present in a joint or group of joints that allows normal and unimpaired function.[5, 96] It can be subdivided into static and dynamic flexibility. The former does not consider the speed of the movement, whereas the latter implies immediate use of the full range of motion.[96, 369] Dynamic flexibility, therefore, is a key to athletic performance, particularly in sports such as diving, ballet, and gymnastics.[369] Beighton has pointed out that articular mobility is a graded trait where one end of the spectrum includes considerable joint laxity that may occur in normal individuals.[28] Nevertheless, when flexibility exceeds the normal range of movement in multiple joints, an individual is considered loose-jointed or hyper-

mobile. Hypermobility has been shown to have multiple inheritance patterns and can occur in both benign and pathologic forms.[27, 69, 181, 205, 438] Certain generalizations regarding joint mobility are summarized in Table 30C–3.

The loss of flexibility during rapid growth in children causes both muscle tendon imbalance and increased apophyseal traction. Resultant overuse injuries include traction apophysitis and tendinitis. Sever's disease is a common cause of heel pain in adolescents. Practitioners who treat athletes should emphasize the importance of maintaining good muscle flexibility in an attempt to reduce the incidence of overuse injury.

Hypermobility is often seen in athletes (Fig. 30C–3) and may be more frequently symptomatic than in the nonathletic population. This is likely due to the added stress of sports participation. According to Grahame, Hippocrates first mentioned hypermobility as a source of difficulty for athletes as early as the fourth century BC.[155] In the intervening years, little discussion in the medical literature centered

TABLE 30C–3
Flexibility Generalizations

1. Inherited characteristic
2. Individual variability
3. Joint-specific
4. Females more flexible then males
5. Decreases with age
6. Greater in certain ethnic groups (e.g., blacks and Native Americans)
7. Can be acquired through training
8. Strength training does not necessarily reduce flexibility
9. Little relationship with body proportion or limb length
10. Little relationship with injury rate

Data from references 4, 28, 96, 149, 155–157, and 224.

of maintaining flexibility and motion postoperatively in patients who have undergone musculoskeletal procedures. The benefits to the joints and to the surrounding musculo-tendinous and ligamentous structures are well established.[208, 352, 441]

Although the natural inclination and the accepted teaching for many years in the fields of sports medicine and exercise physiology has been that stretching is a preventive measure for athletic injury,[111, 330, 373] there is little conclusive epidemiologic evidence to support this idea.[166, 170] Two well-designed studies of running-related injuries failed to show a significant relationship between stretching or its absence and the frequency of injury.[223, 393] On the other hand, a study of military basic trainees showed a reduction in overuse injures with an effective hamstring flexibility program.[168] Research from Duke University has provided scientific groundwork on the preventive aspects of stretching and warm-up periods by showing that greater tension is required to rupture a muscle that has been stretched or preconditioned in the experimental situation.[350, 351] There is the possibility that a certain degree of tightness protects against injury by allowing load sharing when joints are stressed. This implies that stretching beyond a certain point may reduce the load-sharing ability of the musculotendi-nous units or the capsuloligamentous complex, which are responsible for joint stability.[170] If this is indeed the case, then excessive stretching or hypermobility could result in increased stress on the ligaments, bone, and cartilage at the joint, leading to injury or arthritis.[26, 327, 351] This may be the situation when ballet dancers force ankle plantar flexion to such an extent that it creates posterior impingement symptoms and reactive bone formation[209, 210] (Fig. 30C–6).

The balance between adequate and excessive stretching is further demonstrated in other areas. Research has shown that during level running a great deal of energy is stored in the muscle-tendon unit.[71] If the force-elongation curve of human skeletal muscle in vivo is examined, it can be shown that a stiffer muscle will have a greater potential for energy storage than a less stiff muscle when elongated to the same extent. In the submaximal range of motion of most joints involved in running, this would translate into a greater contribution from stored energy in a stiff muscle. Investigators have shown that clinical measures of flexibility that involve measurement of the end of the range of motion are inversely related to measures of muscle stiffness.[149] In other words, less flexible people have stiffer muscles throughout the range of motion. Perhaps it is for this reason that several laboratories have been able to show that less flexible individuals use less oxygen to cover the same distance while running at the same speed than more flexible individuals.[150] This interesting fact may explain why runners as a group are inflexible unless specific stretching exercises are pursued to prevent it. The importance of muscle stiffness in athletic injury remains an area for continued study because there is no scientifically based program for flexibility training with statistically reproducible results in lowering injury rates and/or improving performance.[149]

In summary, it is suggested that there is an optimal range of motion for each individual and for each of his or her joints. Warming up and stretching to obtain or maintain this range is conducive to the health of the tissues, but

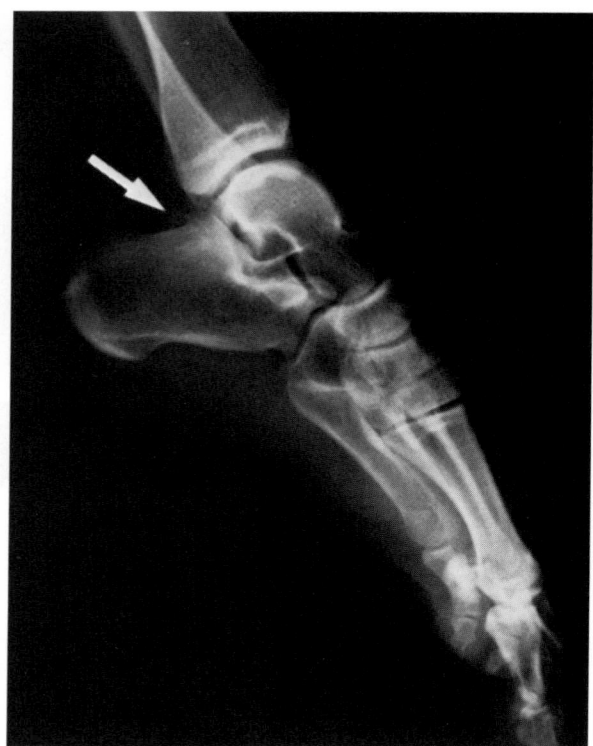

Figure 30C–6. Radiograph demonstrating reactive bone on the calcaneus resulting from posterior impingement in a ballet dancer. (Copyright by Thomas O. Clanton.)

stretching beyond this range is potentially harmful. Certain sports and certain movements within a sport require a particular range of motion. Athletic activity and the competitive process tend to select naturally those who can attain the movement criteria with the most efficiency and without a subsequent increase in injury rate.[77]

Joint Motion

In reviewing the literature for ankle, subtalar, and first metatarsophalangeal range of motion (Tables 30C–4 to 30C–6), it becomes obvious that there are different norms for range of motion in these joints. This is due to the degree of individual variability in anatomic constraints about these joints. A review of the literature shows that the average ankle range of motion is calculated as 53 degrees, with average dorsiflexion equaling 18 degrees and average plantar flexion equaling 35 degrees.[6, 45, 231, 354, 355] Variability in ankle motion measurements is introduced in a variety of ways including methodology (radiographic or clinical using flexometry, goniometry, or electrogoniometry), selection of landmarks, and measurement of specific tibiotalar movement or combined ankle-foot movement. Timing with regard to a warm-up period and geographic consideration may also be important.[2, 41, 440] Lundberg's study documents ankle motion and the ramifications involved in its measurement.[231]

As one moves distally, range of motion of the joints of the foot and ankle becomes increasingly difficult to mea-

TABLE 30C–4
Ankle Joint Motion*

Author	Method	Dorsiflexion (Extension) (degrees)	Plantar Flexion (degrees)	Total (degrees)
AAOS[6]	NS	20	50	70
Bonnin[43]	NS	10 to 20	25 to 35	35 to 55
Boone and Azen[45]	A	12.6 ± 4.4	56.2 ± 6.1	66.8 ± 5.5
Sammarco[353]				
WB	P	21 ± 7.21	23 ± 8	44 ± 7.6
NWB	P	23 ± 7.5	23 ± 9	46 ± 8.25
Weseley[437]	P	0 to 10 (max 23)	26 to 35 (min 10) (max 51)	26 to 45 (min 51) (max 84)
Lundberg[231]				
Review/summary	NS	13 to 33	23 to 56	36 to 89
Personal study	NS	24.9 ± 3.0	28.5 ± 7.5	53.4 ± 5.25
AMA[7]	A or P	20	40	60

* When a range is given, it signifies the range of greater concentration.
A, Active; NS, not specified; NWB, non–weight-bearing; P, passive; WB, weight-bearing.

sure objectively. This is particularly true of subtalar motion, for which numerous methods of measurement have been described. No consensus for normal motion has been reached (Fig. 30C–7; see Table 30C–5). This absence of a consensus creates considerable difficulty when one is trying to determine whether or not subtalar instability exists.[86] From personal experience and a review of the literature, it is clear that there is intersubject variability in subtalar motion. A more precise and standardized method of describing this joint's triplanar motion would be constructive. At the current state of knowledge, subtalar motion is generally described as movement in the frontal plane and averages 25 to 30 degrees. Of this total motion, 20 degrees is inversion and 5 to 10 degrees eversion.

Transverse tarsal joint motion is rarely discussed, but it plays an important role in lower extremity kinematics. Its instability has been described as medial swivel syndrome.[180, 242] There has even been one report of surgical treatment of patients with transverse tarsal joint instability.[449] This entity may have some relationship to cuboid syndrome—a painful condition of the hindfoot that has

TABLE 30C–6
First Metatarsophalangeal Joint Motion

Author		Dorsiflexion (degrees)		Plantar Flexion (degrees)
AAOS[6]		70		45
AMA[7]		50		30
Sammarco[353]		90		30
Joseph[198]	*Standing*	*Active*	*Total*	
	16	51 (40 to 100)	74	23 (3 to 43)
Clanton[85]		72.3 ± 12.4		35.0 ± 10.2

TABLE 30C–5
Subtalar Joint Motion

Author	Inversion (degrees)		Eversion (degrees)		Arc (degrees)
AAOS[6]	5		5		10
Inman[187]	–		–		44 ± 7
Sammarco[353]	20		5		25
DeLee[111]	–		–		35
McMaster[262]	25		5		30
Brantigan[54]	–		–		38 ± 6
James[190]	23 ± 6		8 ± 4		31 ± 7
Milgrom[270]					
Method	R	L	R	L	
AAOS	2.0 ± 7.4	31.2 ± 7.7	3.9 ± 4.1	4.0 ± 4.2	
Cailliet	21.4 ± 5.4	21.6 ± 5.5	3.4 ± 3.1	3.2 ± 3.3	
James	18.4 ± 5.2	18.4 ± 5.2	6.4 ± 3.7	6.7 ± 4.2	

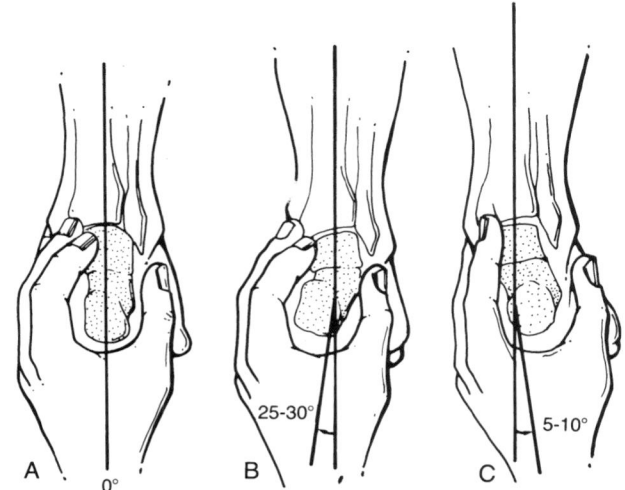

Figure 30C–7. Method of measuring subtalar motion with patient prone and knee flexed. *A*, Neutral position at 0 degrees on goniometer. *B*, Inversion. *C*, Eversion. (Redrawn from American Academy of Orthopaedic Surgeons: Joint Motion—Method of Measuring and Recording. Chicago, American Academy of Orthopaedic Surgeons, 1965; and Oatis C: Biomechanics of the foot and ankle under static conditions. Phys Ther 68:1815–1821, 1988.)

been described in the podiatric and dance literature.[167, 283] Average motion in the transverse tarsal joint depends on the position of the hindfoot, or subtalar joint, as described earlier in this chapter. As the subtalar joint undergoes eversion early in the gait cycle, the axes of the transverse tarsal joint are aligned so that they become parallel in this everted position of the heel, and this permits increased motion. According to Hicks, this is approximately 22 degrees.[175] Conversely, when the heel is inverted as occurs near the end of stance phase, the axes of the transverse tarsal joint become more divergent and less mobile, averaging 8 degrees of motion.[175] This fact is important when accessing range of motion about the tibiotalar joint. If range of motion of the tibiotalar joint is tested with the hindfoot in an everted position, one gets a falsely increased range of motion due to a combination of motion through the tibiotalar joint and transverse tarsal joint. With the heel inverted, a truer measure of tibiotalar joint motion can be obtained, due to the fact that a minimal amount of motion is taking place through the transverse tarsal joint. Large variations in motion exist in this region, and this makes the job of defining separate motions for the talonavicular and calcaneocuboid joints virtually impossible.[231]

Clearly, these descriptions portray motion in a single plane whether it is sagittal, frontal, or transverse. In discussing range of motion, it is important that standardized terminology is used. Beginning with the anatomic position, the aforementioned cardinal planes can be visualized together with their respective axes of motion (Fig. 30C–8). Using this as a framework, one can then use the appropriate terms to describe a movement, a position, or a deformity[308] (Table 30C–7). This system considers pronation and supination as triplane movements consisting of eversion, abduction, and dorsiflexion for pronation and inversion, adduction, and plantar flexion for supination.[248, 308] When analyzed carefully, it is apparent that motion in almost all joints and specifically in the ankle, subtalar, and transverse tarsal joints is actually triplane motion to one degree or another.[175, 187, 231, 248, 355] As an example, dorsiflexion of the ankle produces some degree of foot abduction as well as external rotation. Similarly, plantar flexion produces some adduction and internal rotation. As previously mentioned, motion in the transverse tarsal joint can occur in the sagittal plane and can thereby mimic motion of the tibiotalar joint. This transverse tarsal joint motion is particularly evident in patients who have undergone an ankle arthrodesis[188, 235, 253, 278, 399] (Fig. 30C–9). The literature indicates that 13 to 15 degrees of dorsiflexion or plantar flexion movement

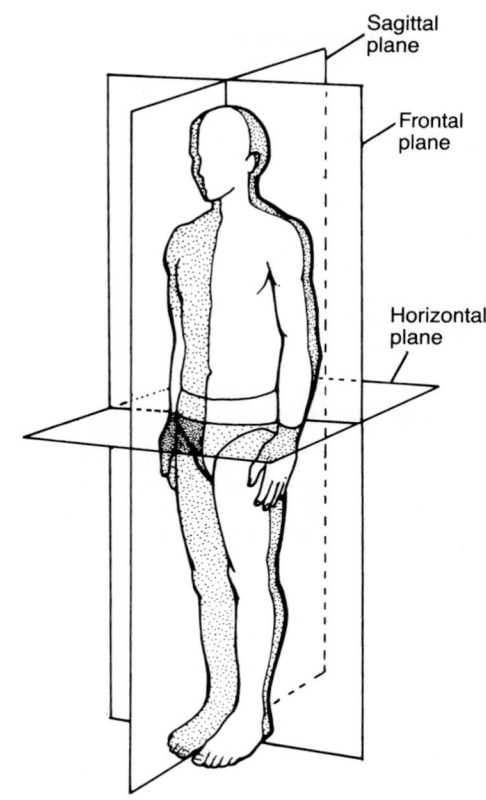

Figure 30C–8. The cardinal planes of motion. (Redrawn from Women in sports. Sport Research Review. Beaverton, Ore, Nike Sport Research Laboratory, Mar/Apr, 1990; and Oatis C: Biomechanics of the foot and ankle under static conditions. Phys Ther 68:1815–1821, 1988.)

occurs in the midfoot.[437] After an arthrodesis, an 8- to 11-degree increase in tarsal mobility has been noted, although this does not occur in all patients.[188, 278] Clinically, the triplane motion that occurs in joints is seldom described, but it becomes important in certain clinical situations and therefore should be recognized.

Motion in the tarsal-metatarsal joints is also a triplane motion occurring primarily in a single plane.[175, 355] This is most obvious in the first and fifth ray, where we describe dorsiflexion and plantar flexion movement. With dorsiflexion of the first ray, however, some degree of abduction and external rotation occurs, and with plantar flexion there is adduction and internal rotation.[342] Average dorsiflexion and plantar flexion in the first through fifth metatarsal joints

TABLE 30C–7
Terminology Used for Motion, Instability, and Deformity

Plane	Motion	Position	Deformity
Sagittal	Dorsiflexion	Dorsiflexed	Calcaneus
	Plantar flexion	Plantar flexed	Equinus
Frontal	Inversion	Inverted	Varus
	Eversion	Everted	Valgus
Transverse	Adduction	Adducted	Adductus
	Abduction	Abducted	Abductus
Triplane description	Pronation	Pronated	Pronatus
	Supination	Supinated	Supinatus

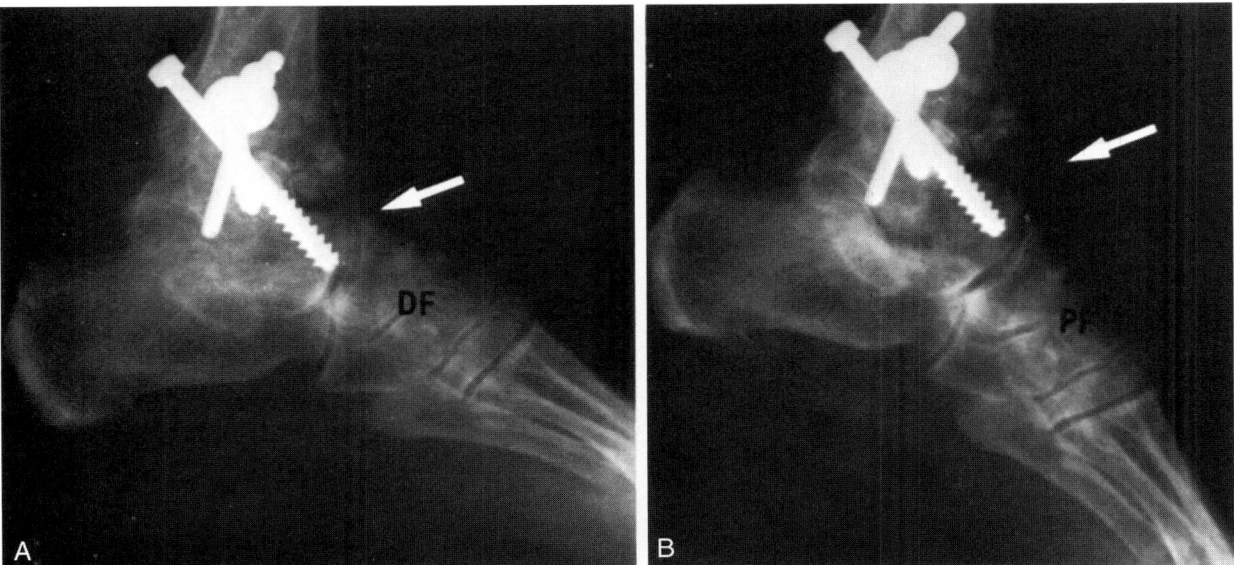

Figure 30C–9. Radiograph of patient with ankle fusion demonstrating increased transverse tarsal joint motion in the sagittal plane. *A,* Dorsiflexion. *B,* Plantar flexion. (Copyright Thomas O. Clanton.)

are 3.5, 0.6, 1.6, 9.6, and 10.2 degrees, respectively.[311] The triplane motion of supination and pronation was also described as 1.5, 1.2, 2.6, 11.1, and 9.0 degrees, respectively. This motion is used to advantage in the Lapidus procedure for treating hallux valgus and metatarsus primus varus in the hypermobile foot. Translational movements are abnormal in this area, and excessive forces are a cause of pathologic conditions ranging from stress fractures at the base of the second metatarsal (Fig. 30C–10) to mild diastasis between the first and second metatarsals (Fig. 30C–11) and on to the more severe forms of Lisfranc's fracture/dislocation.

The normal range of motion in the first metatarsophalangeal joint is quite variable (Fig. 30C–12). According to Joseph, the average range of motion is 51 degrees active dorsiflexion and 74 degrees total (active plus passive) using the axis of the first metatarsal as the neutral line[198] (Fig. 30C–13). The natural position for this joint in the standing posture is 16 degrees of dorsiflexion. In a study of range of motion in college football players, similar movement was documented, with total dorsiflexion averaging 72 ± 12 degrees.[85, 124] Active plantar flexion varies between 23 degrees and 45 degrees.[85, 124, 198] In performing these measurements, some variability occurs from the positioning of the ankle and subtalar joints. Motion is reduced when the ankle is in dorsiflexion and the subtalar joint is inverted. Furthermore, motion is reduced with advancing age.[198] When maximum dorsiflexion is reached in the first metatarsophalangeal joint, the normal gliding motion of proximal phalanx on the metatarsal head ceases and impingement can occur between the proximal phalangeal base and the first metatarsal head.[353] This may be a source of some of the problems seen in turf toe injury as well as hallux rigidus. First metatarsophalangeal joint dorsiflexion is important because of its relationship to gait and to stability of the skin of the metatarsal pad.[42]

Motion in the lesser metatarsophalangeal joints and in-

terphalangeal joints has been studied less thoroughly. Joseph's study included motion at the interphalangeal joint of the great toe. Average motion was 31 degrees of total extension and 46 degrees of active plantar flexion.[199] Recorded norms for lesser metatarsophalangeal joint motion range from 40 degrees to 90 degrees of dorsiflexion and

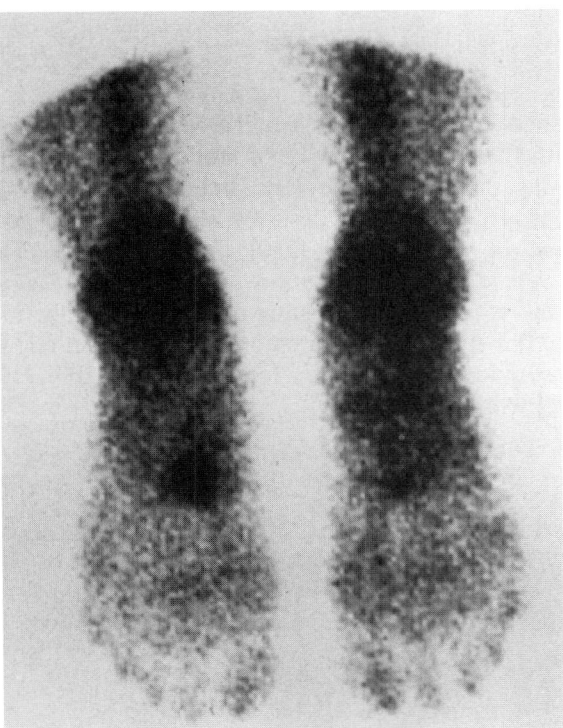

Figure 30C–10. Bone scan demonstrating a stress fracture at the second metatarsal base. (Copyright Thomas O. Clanton.)

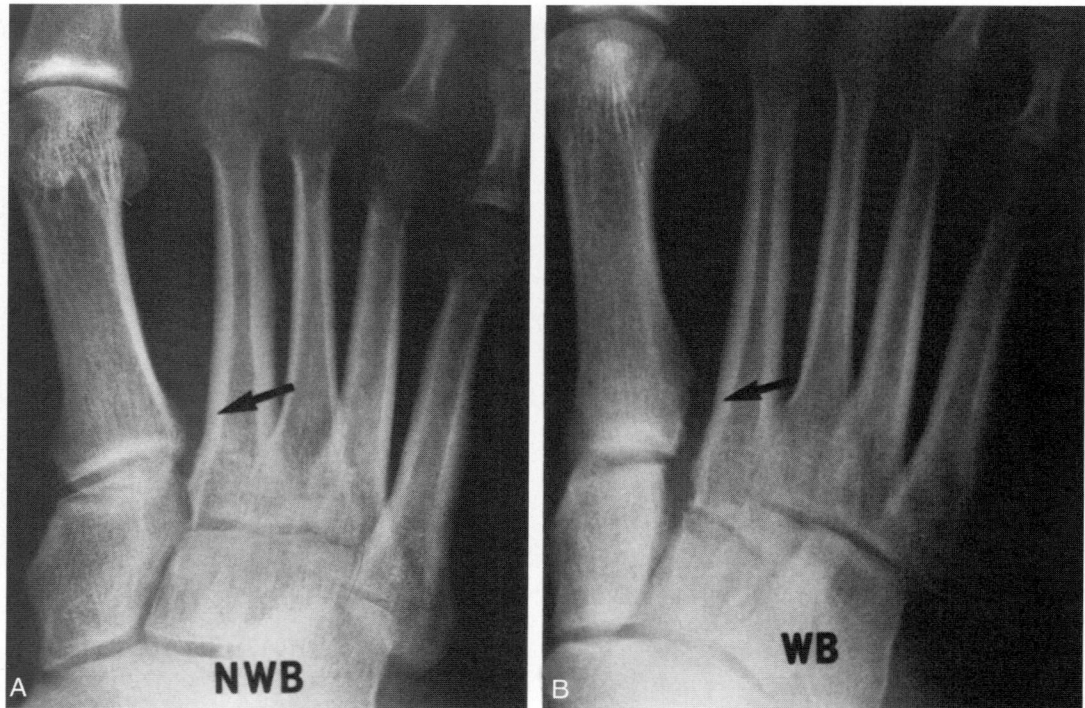

Figure 30C–11. Radiographs depicting subtle diastasis between the first and second metatarsal bases brought out by the weight-bearing radiograph. *A,* Non–weight-bearing. *B,* Weight-bearing. (Copyright Thomas O. Clanton.)

from 35 degrees to 50 degrees of plantar flexion.[6, 353] We have found 50 to 90 degrees of dorsiflexion and 40 to 65 degrees of plantar flexion in asymptomatic individuals, reflecting the wide range of movement that is normal for this area. Excessive movement or stress to the lesser metatarsophalangeal joints can be a rare source of disease. Isolated synovitis and instability of the lesser metatarsophalangeal joints, however, are becoming increasingly recognized as a source of forefoot pain in patients, including athletes[109, 274, 380] (Fig. 30C–14). Interphalangeal joint mo-

tion in the lesser toes is even less well defined, with 0 degrees being the standard for extension and 35 to 40 degrees for plantar flexion.[6] Loss of motion in these interphalangeal joints rarely creates symptomatology unless there is a fixed flexion deformity, such as a hammertoe or mallet toe. Knowledge of the normal range of motion allows one to determine the potential role of range of motion in the etiology of specific injuries to athletes, while being mindful that a considerable degree of variation exists that obscures a precise cause and effect relationship.

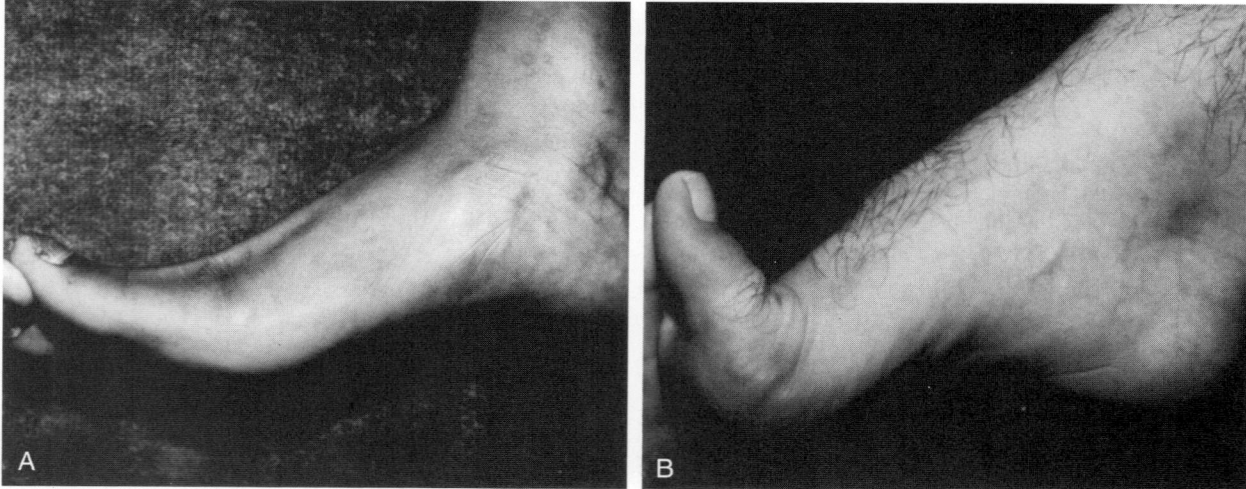

Figure 30C–12. Two asymptomatic athletes demonstrating variation in first metatarsophalangeal joint motion. *A,* Limited mobility. *B,* Hypermobility. (Photographs by Thomas O. Clanton.)

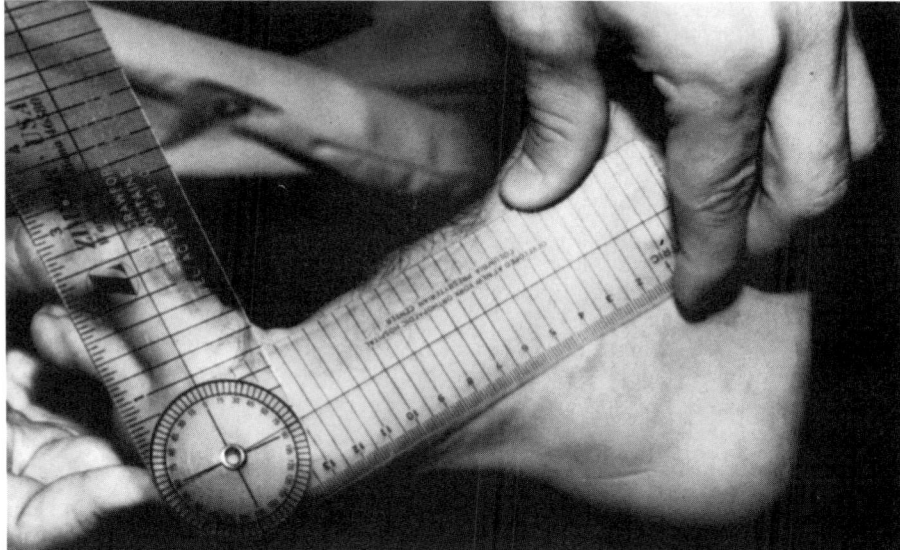

Figure 30C–13. Demonstration of goniometric method of measuring first metatarsophalangeal joint motion using the first metatarsal shaft as the neutral line. (Photograph by Thomas O. Clanton.)

Etiologic Role of Flexibility

With a more scientific understanding of joint motion and flexibility, it is appropriate to proceed to a more specific discussion of foot and ankle injuries related to flexibility or its absence. Beginning distally, the great toe provides one of the best examples of disease related to loss of flexibility. In hallux rigidus, a loss of motion occurs in the first metatarsophalangeal joint that produces pain.[246] This can cause significant disability when it affects an athlete. It was initially believed that turf toe was related to lack of flexibility in the first metatarsophalangeal joint.[84] Empiri-

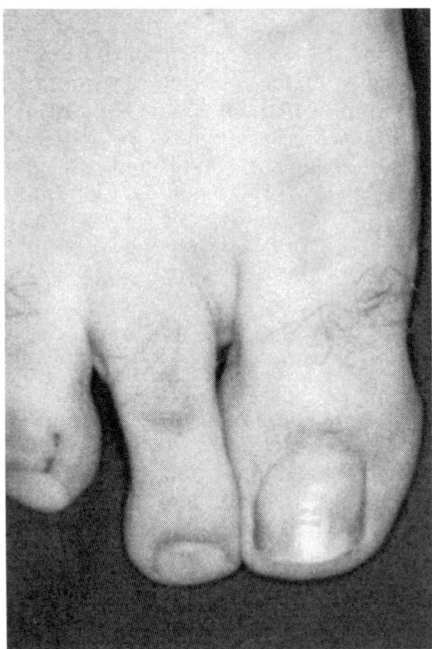

Figure 30C–14. Example of early second metatarsophalangeal joint instability in an athlete. (Photograph by Thomas O. Clanton.)

cally, one would expect a greater exposure to a hyperextension type of injury in athletes who have less natural dorsiflexion motion in the first metatarsophalangeal joint. Nevertheless, all the research to date in this area has failed to confirm an etiologic role for loss of dorsiflexion in turf toe injuries.[92, 341] This was specifically studied in a group of Rice University football players, and no definite relationship between restricted motion in the great toe and any predilection for turf toe injury could be found.[85, 124] One study purportedly found a role for lack of motion in the first metatarsophalangeal joint in another problem often seen in sports—plantar fasciitis. The study has some methodologic faults that cast doubt on the authors' conclusions and warrant repetition of the study.[98]

Lack of flexibility in the lesser metatarsophalangeal joints or interphalangeal joints is rarely linked with injuries or pathologic conditions in athletes. Certainly the loss of interphalangeal joint motion is a key component in mallet toes, hammer toes, and claw toes, and flexibility exercises are often advocated in the treatment of these conditions. A lack of flexibility in such toes can result in painful calluses at the tips of the toes and painful corns over the dorsum of the interphalangeal joints. A lack of dorsiflexion in a lesser metatarsophalangeal joint can be a source of pain and disability, particularly when this involves the second toe. There is usually an iatrogenic or post-traumatic cause. Conversely, increased motion seems to be a factor in variously named but seemingly interrelated conditions involving the second metatarsophalangeal joint, including transient synovitis, crossover second toe, and subluxation and dislocation of the second toe.[97, 109, 274, 380]

Hypermobility of the first ray has been implicated as a source of problems in the foot such as stress fractures, but confirmatory studies using accepted statistical techniques are lacking.[110, 255] Simkin and colleagues have suggested an association between low arches and metatarsal stress fractures.[371] Gross and Bunch measured stresses in 21 distance runners and found that the greatest force occurred under the first and second metatarsal heads.[162] Using the model of the metatarsals as proximally attached rigid cantilevers, the authors showed that the greatest bending strain and shear force occurred in the second metatarsal, where stress fractures are most common. These two studies provide circumstantial evidence that increased first ray flexibility is an anatomic factor in stress fractures of the second metatarsal shaft.

One would expect that the best source of a verifiable linkage between lack of flexibility and injury would come from the ankle. The tight Achilles tendon has been blamed for numerous conditions including bunions,[247] turf toe,[341] midfoot strain or plantar fasciitis,[206, 219, 385] ankle sprains,[432] Achilles tendinitis,[81] calf strains,[125, 272] and hyperpronation with its attendant problems.[57, 58, 245] With such a wide assortment of injuries, one would naturally conclude that the tight Achilles would be well defined by multiple studies as a major villain in the sports arena. Although there is no lack of accusers, the evidence remains scarce for a conviction. Walsh and Blackburn suggested heel cord stretching as a preventive maneuver to decrease the incidence of ankle sprains, but they reported no results from this program.[432] It seems somewhat paradoxical that on the one hand, the athletic trainer works hard to improve the athlete's flexibility at the ankle and on the other hand tapes or braces the ankle before practice or games to restrict motion. An even more considerable feat would be the unraveling of the mystery of midfoot-hindfoot flexibility and its relationship to sports injury. Is the runner with a hyperpronating foot truly more susceptible to injury? Does a rigid orthosis holding the foot in a subtalar neutral position reduce the likelihood of injury? What role do orthoses have in injury reduction or production? I will leave the last question to the following section on the etiology of foot and ankle injuries related to shoes and orthoses but will try to answer some of the other questions.

Hyperpronation has been blamed for almost every problem known to runners.[57, 58, 245] The prevalence of this complaint has reached such proportions that many runners come to their local orthopaedist, podiatrist, or running shoe salesperson with the self-made diagnosis of "pronated feet" and ask for a shoe or an orthotic device to cure their shin splints, knee pain, arch pain, and so on. Running shoes have been made and marketed specifically for this problem or its antithesis—the supinated, rigid, cavus foot.[129, 294, 390] By incorporating what we have learned about biomechanics and gait with an appreciation of the loads seen in long-distance running, we can see the potential for injury in this situation and recognize that anything that compromises the load-dissipating mechanism built into the lower extremity may contribute to injury.[291] In the cavus foot there is more rigidity in the joints of the foot in general.[233, 244] This means that loads are not dampened as effectively across the joints, and higher stress is applied at each level, which can frequently result in symptoms. So far, treatment has centered on the use of orthotic devices, but their success in the treatment of the athlete with a cavus foot is limited, and some form of stress reduction is often necessary to allow continued participation in sports.[232–234, 245]

An extreme example of the detrimental consequence of loss of motion is the iatrogenic rigidity created by an arthrodesis. In the example of a triple arthrodesis where the talonavicular, calcaneocuboid, and talocalcaneal joints are all fused, the elimination of motion in the hindfoot often results in progressive arthritic changes in the surrounding joints. The obvious inference is that loss of the load-dissipating capacity of the arthrodesed joints creates increased stress in the remaining joints, leading to subsequent arthritic changes. This is supported further by the effect of tarsal coalitions, which is lead to restricted hindfoot motion, and over time one sees the development of radiographic changes such as talar beaking and, eventually, arthritic changes.

The complex movements in the foot and ankle associated with pronation produce a more flexible foot at the time of weight transfer. This can produce problems in one of two ways. Whereas the normal foot (whatever that really is[360, 426]) goes through 6 to 10 degrees of subtalar eversion in the frontal plane during gait, the flat foot or pronated foot may have 12 to 15 degrees of motion.[90, 123, 307, 443] According to the linkage system detailed in the previous section on biomechanics, this increased motion will produce a corresponding increase in transverse plane motion affecting the lower extremity by imposing additional torsional stress on the soft tissue.[293] The second method by which pronation can produce problems is related to the speed with which the rearfoot angle changes.[244, 297] Researchers looking at the maximum velocity of pronation have claimed that this is as critical as the maximum angle of pronation.[73, 90] Because the foot goes through the available pronation range more quickly, less force is dissipated, resulting in a similar problem of increased load transmission. If that is the case, one can hypothesize that excessive stretching produces less passive constraint, allowing increased velocity to pronation or to ankle dorsiflexion during the early stance phase of the gait cycle. Both of these movements are important components of load absorption in running.

As exploration into the etiology of foot and ankle injuries related to flexibility continues, the questions seem to multiply. Because of the interrelationship of many factors and the extent of individual variability, it has been difficult, if not impossible, to impose the proper degree of control on in vivo studies of the pronated or cavus foot. Current studies have not provided a reliable prediction of the influence of the pronated or cavus foot on the risk of injury.[23, 76, 122, 123] Only a small number of epidemiologically valid clinical studies have looked at the relationship of flat and highly arched feet to injuries, and the majority of these have not shown a significant etiologic role for the hyperpronated foot.[240, 263, 322, 371] A recent study from the Mayo Clinic looked at the effect of foot structure and range of motion on musculoskeletal overuse injuries.[200] The study group was a well-defined cohort of 449 naval trainees. They were tracked prospectively for injuries throughout training. The risk factors that predisposed trainees to overuse injuries in this study were dynamic pes planus, pes cavus, restricted ankle dorsiflexion, and increased hindfoot inversion. In my experience, it is the cavus rather than the hyperpronated foot that gives athletes the greatest degree of difficulty and frustrates the clinician providing treatment.

Shoewear-Related Injury

Although the role of flexibility in sports injuries of the foot and ankle remains somewhat unclear, more evidence

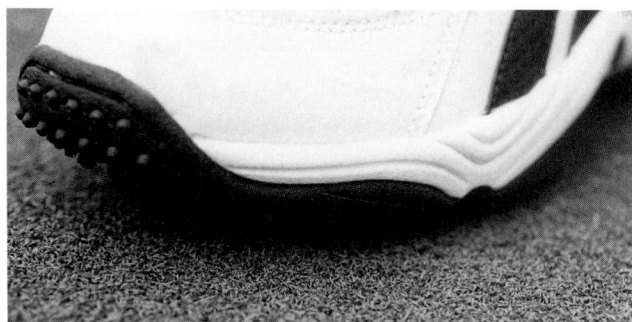

Figure 30C–15. The shoe-surface interface. (Photograph by Thomas O. Clanton.)

exists implicating shoewear and playing surfaces. The intimate relationship between these two makes separation into individual components difficult. Many studies of sports injuries look at these in a combined manner as the *shoe-surface interface*[9, 48, 50, 51, 405, 422–424, 429] (Fig. 30C–15). These studies are primarily concerned with shoes from the standpoint of foot fixation as an etiologic factor in ankle and knee injuries. The shoe can be a factor in athletic injuries in other ways, however, such as improper fit, lack of cushioning, inadequate support, and abnormal force generation. For this reason, shoewear and playing surfaces have been included as separate etiologic factors here, but the reader should maintain an awareness of their interdependency.

History

According to Stacoff and Luethi, shoewear has been recorded as a source of injury since the early Greeks.[393]

Because shoes can cause problems in so many ways, one has to wonder whether it might be better for athletes to participate without shoes. An advantage to barefoot play can be seen in young children who remove their shoes to race. One can speculate that there would be less tendency to sprain an ankle from landing on another player's foot if those feet were unshod. The symptom-free nature of primitive feet (regardless of their degree of pes planus or pes cavus) also makes one question the true value of modern shoewear.[179, 361, 400, 401] Barefoot participation in sports was the norm in ancient times. More recently, barefoot running received international attention with the successes of Zola Budd and Abebe Bikila, who each participated in Olympic competition sans shoes (Fig. 30C–16).

By ignoring scientific prejudices, one can make an empirical case for the advantages of the unshod condition. Numerous studies have demonstrated that the least amount of pronation occurs during barefoot running.[72, 90, 297, 392] This finding stimulates an inquiry into the role of pronation in injury versus the biomechanical alterations produced by the shoe and their promoted protective value. Robbins and colleagues championed the role of sensory feedback from the plantar surface of the foot in modifying load and protecting the runner from stress-related injury.[337–339] They suggested that this important system is impaired by modern footwear, creating a "pseudo-neuropathic" condition. In support of this heuristic approach, they point out that epidemiologic studies have shown no trend toward a reduction in injury from the use of modern athletic footwear. A recent study by DeWit and DeClercq looked at the stance phase during barefoot and shod running from a biomechanical standpoint.[118] They found that barefoot running is characterized by a significantly larger external loading rate and a flatter foot placement at touchdown. The flatter foot

Figure 30C–16. Barefoot runners. *A*, Zola Budd running in 1984 Olympic 3000-meter race against Mary Decker. (© 1991 David Madison.) *B*, Abebe Bikila of Ethiopia winning 1960 Olympic marathon in world record time. (© AP/Wide World Photos.)

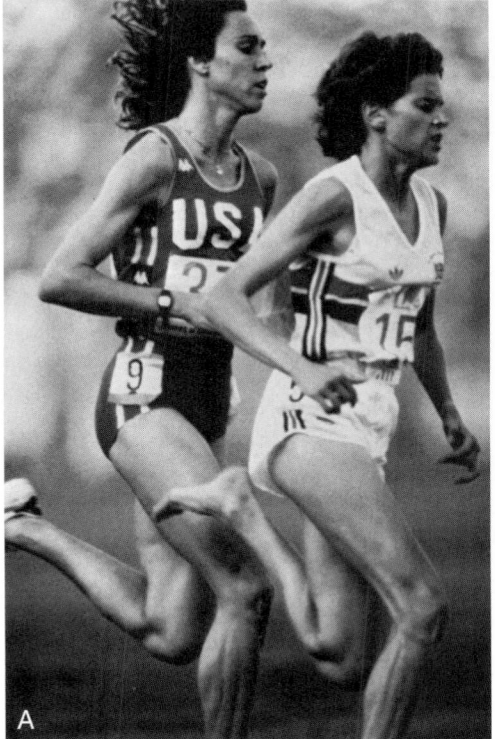

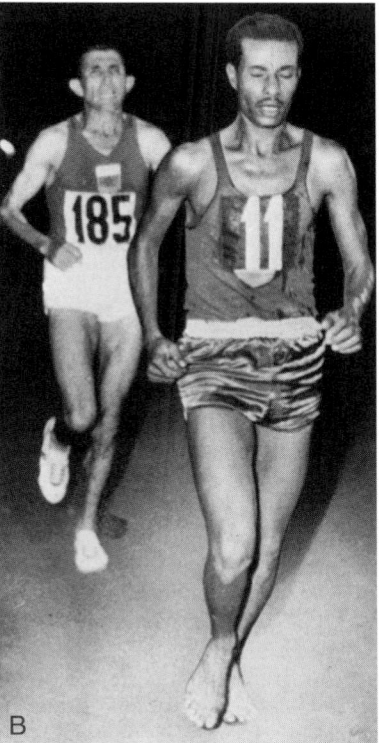

placement correlates with lower peak heel pressures. It was postulated that runners adopt this altered foot placement position in order to limit the local pressure beneath the heel. Barefoot running was also associated with significantly higher leg stiffness during the stance phase. Nostalgia aside, it is easily recognized that sports shoes are here to stay. Therefore, critical analysis of shoes is essential to discover how they fall short in their role as protective equipment for the sports participant.

Incidence

The exact incidence of injury attributable to athletes' shoes is a matter of conjecture, but several studies have included shoes as a separate factor in injury rates.[17] James and colleagues included shoes and surfaces as one of three categories under cause of injury in runners in addition to training errors and anatomic factors.[190] Nineteen percent of the 180 runners in their series were treated by a change or modification in shoewear. Lysholm and Wiklander studied 60 runners with 55 injuries during a 1-year period.[238] Surface or shoe problems were the primary sources of injury in three cases and one of multiple factors in ten others. Inferior footwear was the etiologic factor blamed in 34 of 318 injuries in soccer players.

Football has provided the best perspective on shoewear and its relationship to knee and ankle injuries. Torg and Quedenfeld published an extensive study in 1971 relating the incidence and severity of knee and ankle injuries to shoe type and cleat length in Philadelphia high school football players.[421] Rates of injury to the ankle were reduced from 0.08 per team per game to 0.01 per team per game by switching from conventional cleated football shoes to soccer style shoes with multiple shorter cleats. This result was substantiated by the work of Mueller and Blyth, who noted a reduction in knee and ankle injuries by resurfacing the playing field (30.5% reduction), changing from regular cleats to soccer shoes (22.3% reduction), or making both changes (46% reduction).[279] Using the data of Mueller and Blyth, one could estimate that 3.3% of knee and ankle injuries in high school football players in 1971 to 1972 were related specifically to the type of shoe worn. Although these studies do not consider such shoe-related problems as cleating-induced contusions or lacerations or turf toe, they do provide a framework for studying the role of shoes in sports injury.

Mechanical Factors

Shoe Fit

The most obvious problem with shoes is that which plagues the shod people of the world regardless of whether or not they are sports participants—proper fit. If the shoe does not fit the foot properly, all manner of problems can occur. Even the smallest problem with fit can prevent athletes from performing to the best of their capabilities. For example, a web corn can become so painful that each step is agony. The athlete with a congenital bunion may

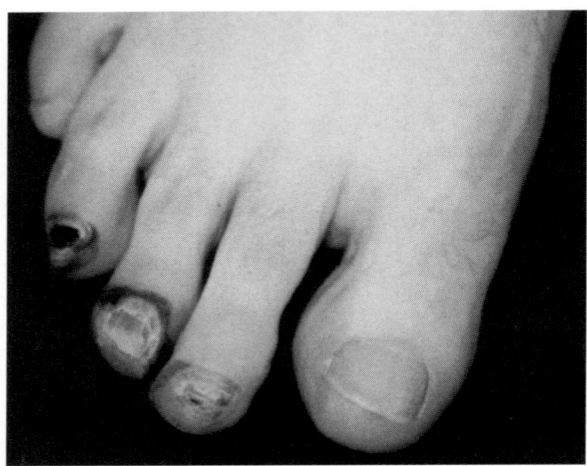

Figure 30C–17. The black toes of a marathon runner. (Photograph by Thomas O. Clanton.)

have few complaints until he is fitted with a narrow shoe or a shoe with a rigid vamp. Metatarsalgia can result from a shoe that is too tight across the forefoot. Similarly, a narrow shoe often aggravates a Morton's neuroma. The black toe of long-distance runners can be a sequela of improper shoe fit (Fig. 30C–17). Toe deformities such as hammer toes, claw toes, and overlapping fifth toes may become symptomatic in athletes whose shoes have toe boxes that are either too narrow or of insufficient depth.

Calluses and blisters are inherent in most sports participation (Fig. 30C–18). Improperly fitted shoes that rub the skin excessively or allow the foot to move or slide disproportionately in the shoe enhance their frequency. Other irritants include the insole edge, penetrating cleats, prominent seams, and orthotic device edges. Owing to variability in size characteristics of both feet and shoes, it is critical for the coach, trainer, equipment manager, or parent to direct individualized attention to the athlete and his or her shoes and be willing to make a change early when fitting problems become apparent. Important considerations in fitting shoes are described in more detail in Chapter 30D.

Cushioning

The importance of cushioning in protecting athletes from injury due to overload has been promoted largely by the running shoe industry and those whose research it supports.[13] The running literature (both lay and scientific) has seen a proliferation of articles addressing impact forces, shoe cushioning, shock absorption, and the effects of various alterations in shoe construction. The logical assumptions have been that load on the human body is directly attributable to impact forces at foot strike and that these forces are naturally altered by the cushioning properties of the shoe.[13, 72, 137, 292, 430] These assumptions foster the belief that changing the shoe's material properties (e.g., midsole thickness) can influence impact load, thereby affecting exposure to injury. For a detailed discussion of the biomechanics of running and the concept of load on the human body, the interested reader is referred to some of the numerous sources available.[13, 72, 75, 136, 291, 292, 295, 364, 397]

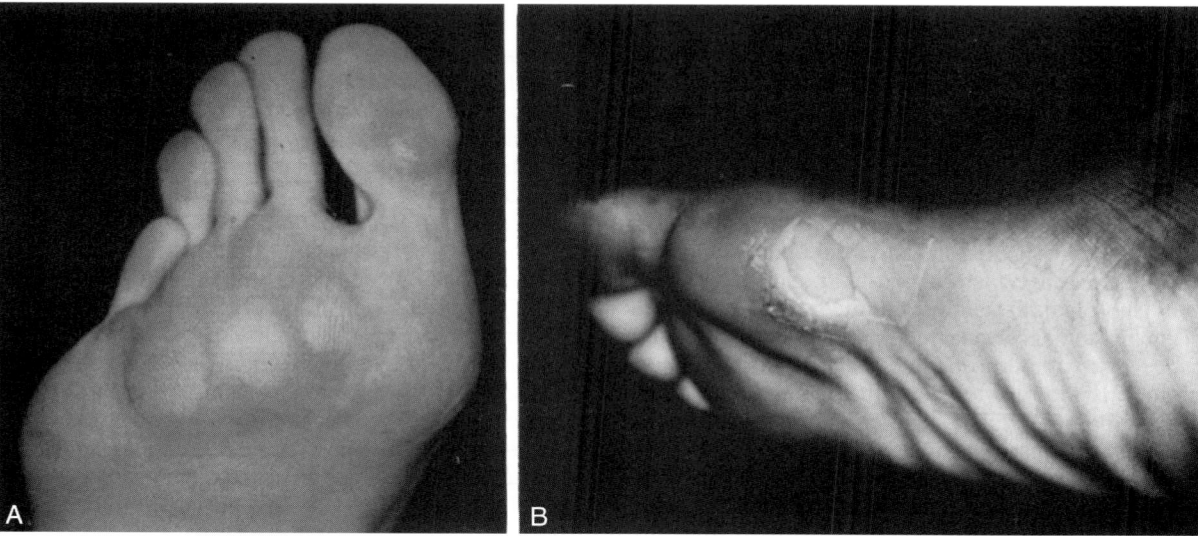

Figure 30C–18. Calluses and blisters are common in athletes. *A,* Diffuse pressure-related callus in female basketball player. *B,* Large blister in male basketball player. (Photographs by Thomas O. Clanton.)

Impact forces are a critical feature in the etiology of sports-related pain and injury whether acute or chronic[290] (Fig. 30C–19). The bionegative effects of impact loads are evident from the damage produced to articular cartilage by high-impact loads.[325, 326] Impact force transients and shock wave transmission play a role in the etiology of experimentally induced osteoarthritis.[226, 431] Radin and coworkers showed that deleterious changes occurred in the biochemical and biomechanical properties of articular cartilage of sheep walking constantly on concrete as opposed to those walking on wooden chips.[325, 326] Destruction of red blood cells as a result of mechanical stress in runners has been demonstrated, lending credence to the idea that heavy impact loads can have a bionegative effect.[130] Shock-absorbing insoles in the boots of South African military recruits produced a 9% reduction in their incidence of overuse injuries.[362] These studies support the belief that impact loads are an etiologic factor in certain injuries, but careful analysis leaves the impression that this load plays a much less consequential role than is often proposed.

Ground reaction forces are the primary external force acting on the human body during running.[74, 78, 273, 290, 402] These forces are increased as running velocity increases. Higher ground reaction forces are seen in the progression from walking to jogging to sprinting to jumping. Estimates vary from 1.2 times body weight (BW) for walking to 2.5 times BW for jogging. Sprinting increases load by three to six times BW, whereas jumping multiplies this force by six to eight times BW[290] (Table 30C–8). Impact force amplitude is reduced when soft materials are used in the shoe or running surface.[113] This reduction is achieved by increasing the deceleration distance of the foot (all else being equal). Calculations of impact peaks can be made from the equation

$$F_{max} = F_{xi} = v \, fm$$

where F_{max} is the maximum force or impact force occurring in the vertical direction (F_{xi}) and is related to velocity (v),

the mass of the body (m), and the spring constant for that body (f). From this equation it is apparent that impact velocity has the greatest influence on vertical load. It is also reduced by reducing the mass (e.g., shoe or body weight) or by reducing the spring constant (e.g., knee flexion angle). Other factors that influence impact loads include muscle reactivation, varying strategies used by the runner, and the geometry of the shoe or the surface. For a more in-depth study of these factors, refer to the later section of this chapter dealing with shoes and orthoses and books by Cavanagh, Frederick, Nigg, and Segesser and Pförringer.[75, 136, 292, 366]

Moving from theoretical to practical considerations has not been as easy as it might appear. As an etiologic factor in injury, lack of cushioning or shock absorption has not proved to be the critical factor that advertising would lead us to believe. Although changing from a new shoe with good cushioning properties to an old shoe lacking these properties can produce injury, an injury may come from changing to a newer shoe as well. It may be that change itself is the critical factor in an injury that occurs during a repetitive activity. One case example for the role of poor cushioning is that of a 26-year-old runner who sustained bilateral stress fractures of the fibulae associated with use of old tennis shoes for a 14-km race.[61] He borrowed some old tennis shoes after he lost one of his regular running shoes immediately before the race. Despite severe bilateral leg pain, he completed the race, only to discover 2 weeks later that he had radiographically documented, bilateral fibular stress fractures. Instrom testing of the remaining running shoe and the ipsilateral tennis shoe demonstrated that the running shoe had twice as much energy absorption and five times the deformation. Although lack of shock absorption is the postulated cause of injury in the aforementioned case, other factors might have played a role as well. These include the change itself, the altered muscle activity causing increased bending moments on the fibula, increased muscle activity resulting in muscle fatigue and loss of the protective function of the muscle, and variations in foot bly not to the degree to which some researchers and shoe manufacturers might lead us to believe.

Control

The control aspects of the sport shoe are the third consideration in the role of the shoe in causing athletic injuries. For the running shoe, control or support is primarily interpreted in the context of rearfoot control. This is defined as the shoe's ability to limit the amount or rate of pronation occurring through the subtalar joint at heel strike.[90] A less well-defined component of shoe support is its control of take-off supination, which is the falling-over movement that occurs at the lateral forefoot during toe-off.[297] Foot support also consists of the relative flexibility of the shoe, most often measured as forefoot flexibility.[72] This allows the shoe to bend at the metatarsal break. Greater flexibility has been considered desirable, but this shoe flexibility can be a major factor in certain injuries such as turf toe.[51, 84] Furthermore, stiffening the sole of the athletic shoe across the metatarsophalangeal joint may decrease the amount of energy loss and improve performance.[397] Control of movement in the sagittal plane by the shoe remains a subject for further investigation.

Support against medial and lateral shear is a concern in certain sports such as tennis and aerobic activities.[15, 230, 303, 391, 404] Design features emphasizing this parameter are relatively recent additions. The support provided for the ankle and hindfoot by high-top shoes has been an important consideration in preventing injury, particularly in basketball and football[144, 194, 195, 251, 316, 404] (Fig. 30C–21). Brizuela and associates recently performed a study on the influence of basketball shoes with increased support on shock attenuation and performance in running and jumping.[67] Two prototype shoes with identical soles but different uppers were used. The first was designed to provide greater ankle support, and the second was less supporting. The high support shoes resulted in higher forefoot impact forces and lower shock transmission to the tibia. The use of high support shoes resulted in lower ranges of eversion and higher ranges of inversion for the ankle on landing. In the motor performance tests, the high support shoes reduced the height jumped and increased the time to complete the running course relative to the low support shoes. This study underlines the importance of designing shoes that will maximize performance without compromising safety. Control characteristics are essential elements in modern sports shoes designed for prevention of injury, but not all features are beneficial.

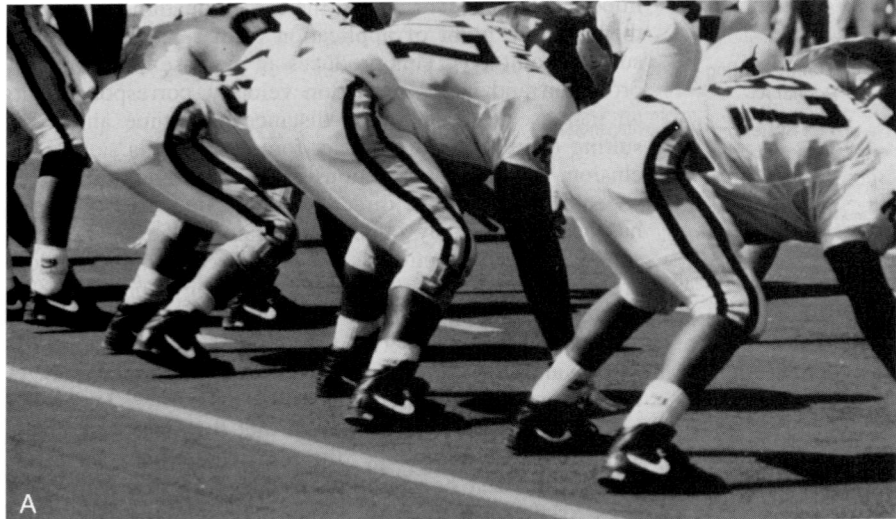

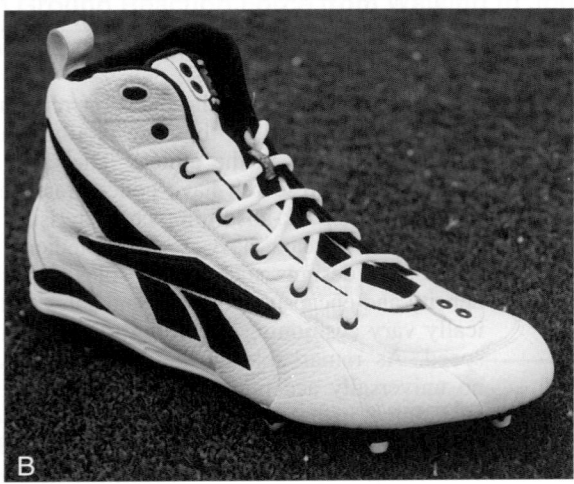

Figure 30C–21. High-top shoe support. *A*, Football linemen in their stance. *B*, High-top football shoe for grass field—2001 season. (Photographs by Thomas O. Clanton.)

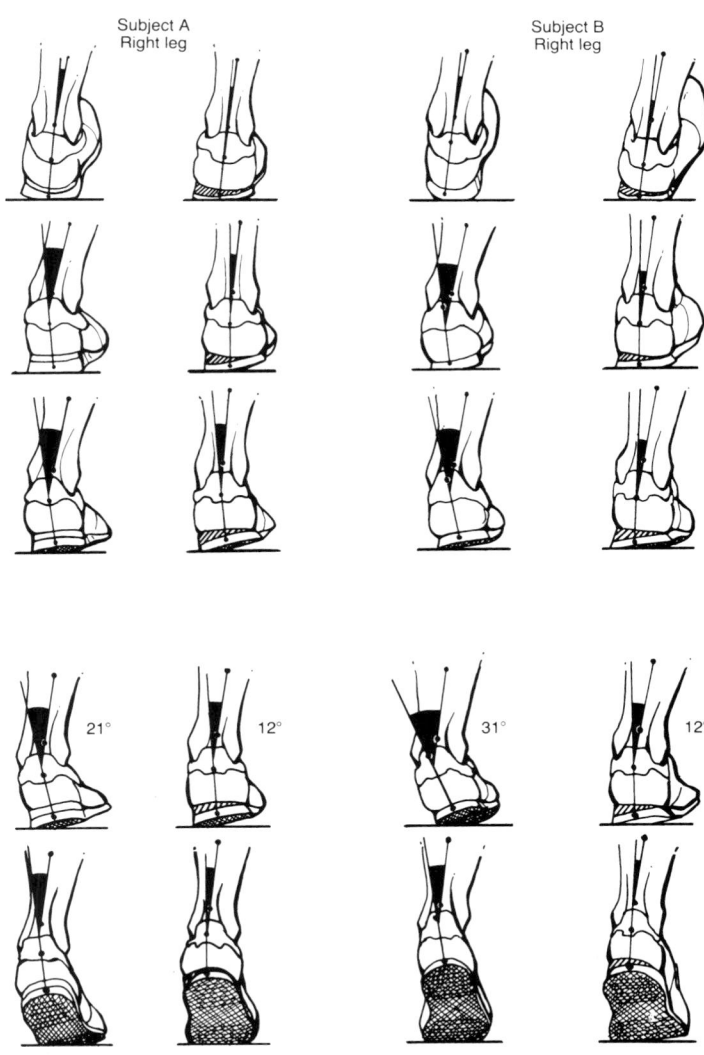

Figure 30C–22. Rearfoot stability provided by athletic shoewear. Illustration of two runners switching between their commonly used shoes without control features and shoes with special control features provided in the laboratory. (From Nigg BM, Bahlsen AH, Denoth J, et al: Factors influencing kinetic and kinematic variables in running. In Nigg BM [ed]: Biomechanics of Running Shoes. Champaign, Ill, Human Kinetics Publishers, 1986, p 157. © 1986 by Benno M. Nigg. Reprinted by permission.)

Rearfoot stability provided by the athletic shoe has become a critical ingredient in managing the overuse problems attributed to overpronation[89, 328] (Fig. 30C–22). Running shoes are marketed according to the innovative design features used to accomplish this control. Included are such creative concepts as cantilever soles with imbedded plastic stability devices, plastic torsion bars, materials of variable hardness in areas of the midsole, thermoplastic heel counters, heel flares, external stabilizers, and combination lasts. These aspects are reviewed in more detail in Chapter 30D. The importance attributed to rearfoot control is derived from the assumption that overpronation produces injuries in runners. This assumption has been extrapolated from studies of runners beginning with the classic study by James and colleagues, which analyzed 180 runners with 232 injuries. Fifty-eight percent of those injured were classified as pronators on biomechanical examination.[190] Clement and associates have confirmed the presence of biomechanical abnormalities in their own studies of runners with injuries.[91] The ability of the shoe or an orthosis to control

excessive pronation is supported by the work of Bates and associates, Cavanagh, Nigg and Morlock, and Smith and coworkers[22, 72, 304, 377] (Fig. 30C–23). Further evidence corroborating the effect of pronation control is provided by the results of treatment of injury by the use of orthoses, which led to improvement and resumption of training in 70% to 90% of those treated.[35, 106, 119, 190] Nigg and associates looked at the effect of shoe insert construction on foot and leg movement.[302] They found that the changes resulting from the use of all inserts in total shoe eversion, total foot eversion, and total internal tibial rotation were smaller than 1 degree when compared with the no-insert condition. Also, they found that the soft insert construction was more restrictive than the harder inserts. They concluded that it is important to match specific feet and shoe inserts optimally. In spite of the improvements in rearfoot control offered by current athletic shoewear, it has been difficult to relate this to any evidence for reduction in incidence of running injuries.

Take-off supination has been blamed for Achilles tendon

direct contact with the ground; therefore, durability is a prime consideration in the manufacturing process. The most frequently used materials are carbon rubber, styrene butadiene rubber, ethylene vinyl acetate, and polyurethane.[79, 93] In general, if the material is harder, its durability and weight are greater. Although carbon rubber is an ideal compound from the standpoint of its resistance to abrasion, it does not provide the traction characteristics necessary in a basketball or tennis shoe. Traction considerations must encompass the interaction of these materials with a variety of playing surfaces and conditions, including the artificial surfaces used indoors and outdoors as well as the amount of moisture or dust on the field or court.[333] Major differences occur in the coefficients of static and sliding friction for various shoe-surface combinations[299] (Table 30C–9).

Torque is another component of traction and can be measured as maximal torque exerted for a defined rotation. It correlates with the static coefficient of friction. Laboratory experiments have established large differences in torque between different shoe-surface combinations as illustrated in Figure 30C–27.[299] This example shows a variation in mean torque between approximately 20 Nm and 40 Nm. Rheinstein and colleagues performed similar experiments supporting this difference in torque as related to outsole material, outsole hardeners, player weight, and playing surface.[333] They found greater maximum torques with the softer outsoles combined with artificial and clean hardwood flooring in heavier players. Furthermore, rubber-soled shoes demonstrated much more sensitivity to dust than the polyurethane soles when analyzed for loss of traction. This research has considerable implications in sports medicine because higher torque means higher load transmission to the body and an increased potential for injury. Alternatively, lack of traction implies sliding, slip-

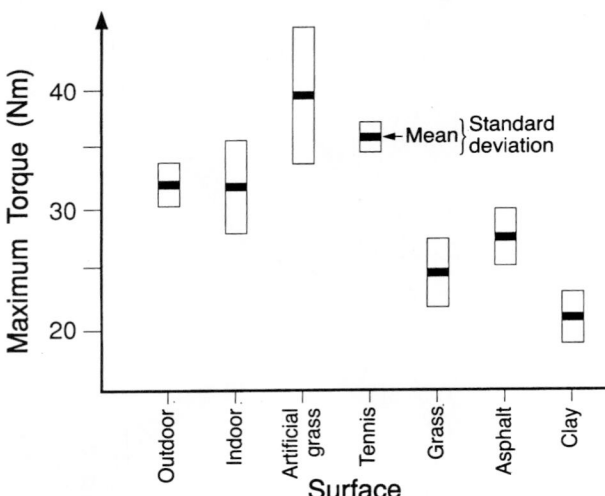

Figure 30C–27. Mean values and standard deviations for maximal torque for 12 subjects on seven surfaces in eight different shoes. (From Nigg BM, Denoth J, Keir B, et al: Load sport shoes and playing surfaces. In Frederick EC [ed]: Sport Shoes and Playing Surfaces. Champaign, Ill, Human Kinetics Publishers, 1984, p 12. © Nike, Inc. Reprinted by permission.)

ping, falling, and poor performance. Where is the proper balance? This question may be unanswerable but deserves attention.

Outersole tread design has developed from the flat rubber of the traditional canvas tennis shoe of yesteryear to the high-technology multiple-patterned sole we see in running shoes and court shoes today[40, 79] (Fig. 30C–28). These tread designs theoretically alter the mechanical properties of the

TABLE 30C–9
Friction Coefficients for Several Floor-Shoe Combinations Tested under Laboratory Conditions

Shoe	Surface				
	Carpet	*Synthetic Granular*	*PVC*	*Sand*	*Asphalt*
Sliding Friction Coefficients					
All-around shoe Little profile	1.05–1.15	0.95–1.05	1.00–1.20	0.40–0.60	0.70–0.80
Jogging shoe Treaded Profile	0.95–1.05	0.80–0.95	0.80–0.90	0.30–0.55	0.60–0.75
Tennis shoe Indoor No profile	0.50–0.60	0.75–0.90	0.40–0.50	0.30–0.50	0.65–0.75
Static Friction Coefficients					
All-around shoe Little profile	1.15–1.25	1.05–1.15	1.00–1.10	0.50–0.60	0.70–0.80
Jogging shoe Treaded Profile	1.05–1.15	0.95–1.05	0.80–0.90	0.40–0.60	0.70–0.80
Tennis shoe Indoor No profile	0.60–0.70	0.80–0.90	0.40–0.50	0.40–0.50	0.75–0.85

PVC, polyvinyl chloride.

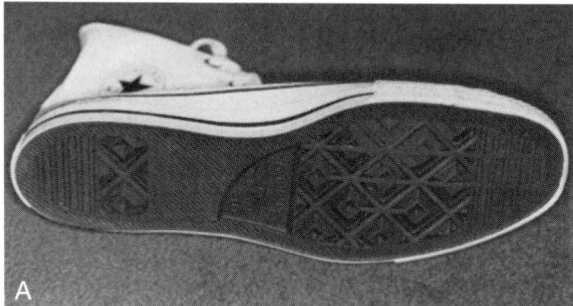

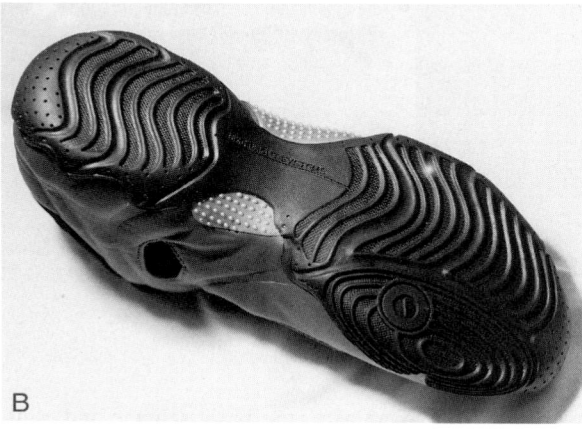

Figure 30C–28. *A,* Canvas sneaker outsole tread design. *B,* Modern court shoe outsole design. (Photograph by Thomas O. Clanton.)

shoe by enhancing performance or preventing injury by determining the flexion path for the shoe, the proper break point, and the pivot point, as well as by affecting traction and shock absorption.[93] The tread design has been used in marketing certain running shoes including the original Nike waffle sole and, more recently, Adidas' torsion sole. The

tread design can clearly alter the traction characteristics of the shoe, but its relationship to foot function and injury prevention remains unproven.

Efficiency of movement is an important factor in athletic performance, and proper traction ensures that internal forces generated by the body's muscles are efficiently converted into movement. A natural byproduct of this relationship was the introduction of appendages or cleats to the outsole of the shoe to improve traction. Introduced about 100 years ago for sports, they have been a source of controversy ever since they appeared. Rule changes in certain sports ensued that banned pointed cleats and placed size limits on cleats. The polemics continued with the concept that foot fixation was a leading cause of injury of the ankle and knee in sports.[66, 420] Dr. Daniel Hanley of Bowdoin College championed this attack on rigid cleating, particularly in the heel area, after he observed the incidence of significant noncontact injuries to the knee at Bowdoin.[79, 176, 420] Cleat modifications followed, including plastic heel disks,[424] lower profile oval cleats,[79] soccer cleats,[346] and cleats attached to a rotating turntable[66, 358] (Fig. 30C–29). This trend continued with the introduction in 1986 of the Tanel 360, which had a circular cleat design for artificial grass and a central forefoot cleat for natural grass[169, 413] (Fig. 30C–30). The design concept of a central cleat or circular cleating pattern theoretically allows pivoting with adequate traction but without the problem of foot fixation. This is an extension of the ideas incorporated in the aforementioned designs and the findings of Conrad that cleat arrangement affects injury in athletes.[93]

Research has documented the relationship between cleats and sports injuries. Rowe studied the effect of different shoes and cleats on knee and ankle injuries in the New York State Public High School Athletic Association during the 1967 and 1968 seasons.[346] He found a reduction in injuries with the use of a low-cut disk heel shoe compared with low- and hightop shoes with heel cleats and an even

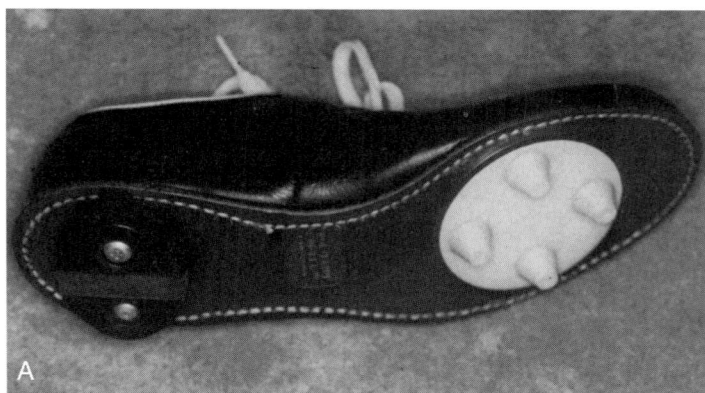

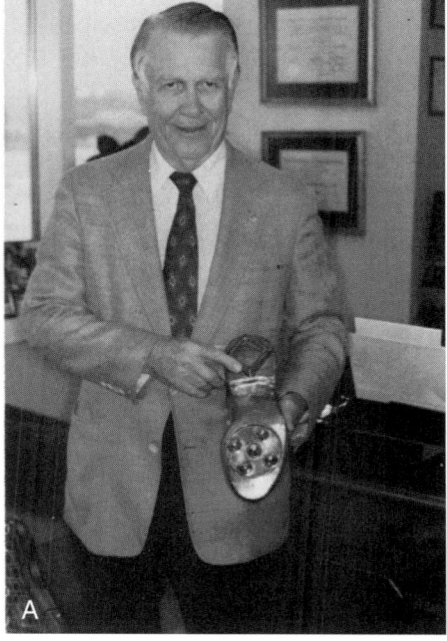

Figure 30C–29. *A,* Example of alternative cleat design used in the swivel shoe. *B,* Designer Bruce Cameron, MD, with the bronzed original of the swivel shoe. (Photographs by Thomas O. Clanton.)

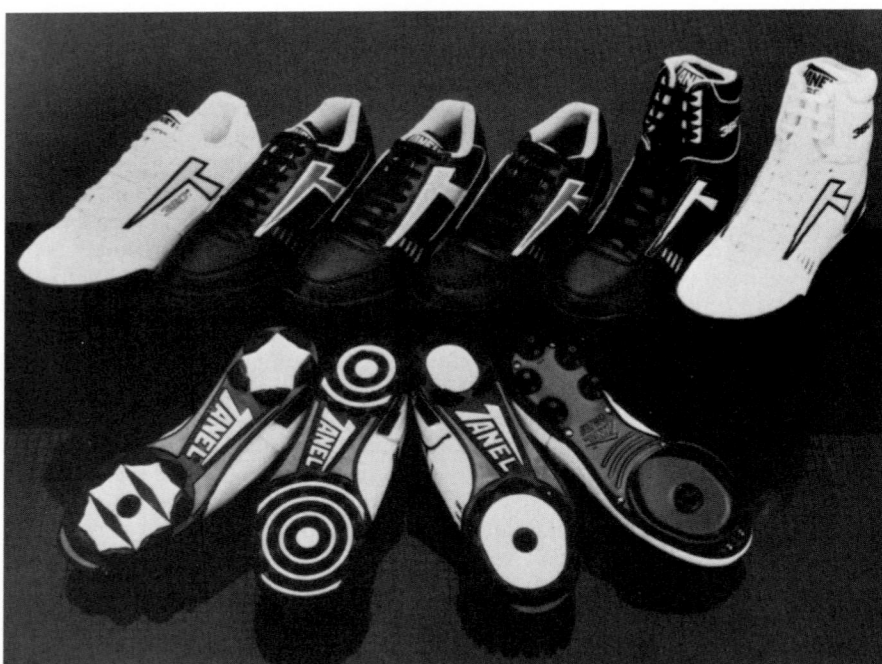

Figure 30C–30. Alternative cleating patterns in the Tanel 360 football shoe. (Photograph courtesy of Tanel Corporation.)

more substantial reduction with short soccer-type cleats used by athletes playing on natural grass. Because the effect of cleats on knee injuries has already been discussed, we will concentrate on the data compiled for the ankle. Although Rowe's findings were not subjected to statistical verification, ankle injuries were reduced from a high of 77 per 100,000 hours of participation to 34 per 100,000 by changing from the low-cut conventional heel to the soccer shoe. Rates of injury with the soccer shoe were lower than those seen with either type of high-top shoe. Torg and Quedenfeld found a similar reduction in ankle injuries from 0.45 per team per game with conventional cleats to 0.23 per team per game with a soccer-type shoe in their study of the Philadelphia Catholic High School Football League in 1969 and 1970.[421] Cameron and Davis found a progressive reduction in ankle injuries from 8.46% with a cleated shoe to 7.69% with a heel plate to 5.64% with a soccer shoe to 3.00% with their swivel shoe design.[66]

An exhaustive study of injuries in North Carolina high school football players by Mueller and Blyth emphasized the critical role of the playing surface in evaluating the role of cleats.[279] They reported a reduction in knee and ankle injuries from 14.8% to 11.5% by changing from traditional cleats to soccer-type shoes on properly maintained fields. Bonstingl and colleagues studied torque occurring with 11 shoe types on three artificial surfaces and natural grass at two player weights and two stance positions.[44] They concluded that there was a positive relationship between torque and injury and that the highest torque occurred with the conventional football shoe with seven ¾-inch cleats. A substantial reduction in torque occurs in circular pattern outsole design (e.g., the original Tanel 360 shoe) when compared with a traditional shoe or molded cleat soccer shoe.[220] Other studies have confirmed these differences in friction and torque between various outersoles, cleats, and playing surfaces.[9, 44, 50, 100, 212] This is one

of the most obvious areas where basic science and clinical research in the field of sports medicine have had an impact on sports equipment designed to prevent injury.

Playing Surfaces and Injury

Of all the etiologic factors involved in foot and ankle injury, the playing surface may be the most important and the least understood. If it is true that load on the human body is the common ground for discovering clues to the causes of athletic injury, then the influence of forces and moments intrinsic to the surface of play must be critically analyzed.[299, 305] As in other areas, both biopositive and bionegative effects are possible. Traditional sports surfaces have been composed of natural materials: wooden basketball courts, clay and grass tennis courts, cinder tracks, grass and dirt baseball diamonds, and natural grass football and soccer fields. With advancing technology, there was a move to replace these with more durable low-maintenance synthetic surfaces. Although such surfaces had some attractive advantages, they were not universally accepted and were subjected to quick criticism that followed their short-lived popularity.

Sports surfaces should accomplish three functions: (1) protection; (2) sports performance; and (3) maintenance.[211] The first is concerned with the protection of the athlete from excessive forces. The sports performance function relates to the optimization of the athletic experience through the qualities of the surface. Maintenance refers to the durability and conservation of the surface in preserving the former two qualities. The task of reviewing all sports surfaces is overwhelming, considering that wrestling mats, gymnastic beams, ice-skating rinks, and snow-packed slalom courses could all be included. To gain some understanding of this broad topic, we divide surfaces into indoor and outdoor surfaces and into natural and synthetic surfaces. For the outdoor surfaces used in football and soccer, grass and artificial grass are reviewed. Cinder, rubberized asphalt, and polyurethane tracks are also analyzed. Indoor surfaces used in basketball, volleyball, aerobic dance, and ballet are more diverse, and discussion is limited primarily to wooden floors and various types of synthetic floors. Tennis has become both an indoor and outdoor sport, and the spectrum of surfaces ranges from grass and clay to synthetic grass, concrete, carpets, and synthetic resins. There is some overlap between surfaces in sports, and multiple uses are the rule in most sports facilities. As the characteristics of a particular surface used in one sport are delineated, the reader is reminded that the surface characteristics are applicable in other sports, but protective, technical and performance characteristics may vary between sports, types of athletes, shoewear used, and environmental situations.

History

Since ancient times, humans have competed in running, jumping, and throwing. Participation occurred in a variety of locations, most commonly associated with some form of religious worship. The surface chosen was that which occurred naturally, most commonly grazed fields and dirt areas freed of rocks and other obstacles, not too unlike the sandlot fields of current times. As culture progressed, so did the playing fields, and stadiums were created for competition in ancient Greece. Improvements in these outdoor facilities were accomplished by maintaining the fields, using developments in soil and grass technology, crowning to improve drainage, and limiting play. It was not until 1964 that synthetic grass, produced by Monsanto, was introduced and installed on the playing field at Moses Brown School in Providence, Rhode Island.[197, 223, 330] Devel-

oped as a substitute for grass in a place where its natural growth was difficult, this artificial surface created little impact until 1966. On April 9, 1965, the "eighth wonder of the world," the Astrodome, was completed amid much hype in a city known for space age technology—Houston, Texas.[183] The Houston Astrodome was to house both baseball and football events as the first all-weather enclosed stadium (Fig. 30C–31). A special grass was developed to grow inside the Astrodome—Tifway 419 Bermuda.[183] Even the foundation soil required a unique design. Unfortunately when the clear Lucite roof panels were darkened to eliminate glare and lost fly balls, the grass withered, and management scrambled to find a suitable substitute. The following year the natural grass was replaced. Thus, Monsanto's synthetic grass became "AstroTurf," a name that is now almost as generic as Kleenex and Band-Aid.

Now, grass playing fields in natural and custom-installed varieties compete with synthetic surfaces that have undergone a technological revolution since they were first introduced. The field of sports turf management has become specialized enough that it now has its own association.[389] Entire publications advise facility managers in the most intricate detail of how to maintain playing fields.[388] Advertisements for different artificial turfs cover entire pages in the trade journals of athletic business managers.[11] The debate about which is the better surface has involved both the public and the scientific community, and more than 50 articles have appeared without a summary conclusion.* Perhaps the key deficiency in these studies is their poor control of other key factors in the turf equation such as the shoe, the field maintenance, weather, and the complicated nature of epidemiologic studies that include multiple individuals and teams and can involve intrinsic and extrinsic factors that can be overwhelming. A recent review of decision-making for installation of a grass versus an artificial turf field for a Texas high school stadium provides

---

*See references 1, 2, 68, 201, 223, 268, 305, 365, 373, 412, and 428.

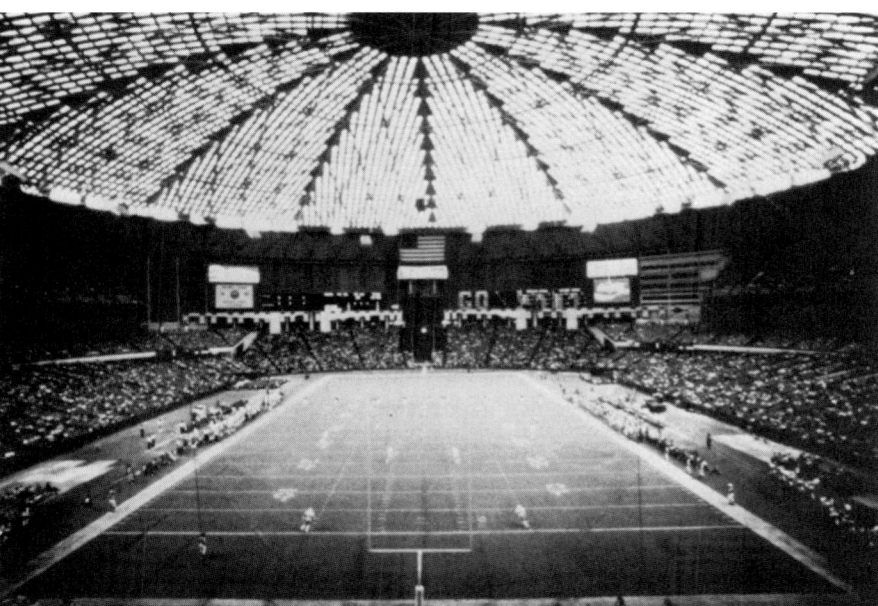

Figure 30C–31. The Houston Astrodome. (Photograph courtesy of Houston Hilights.)

one of the best overviews of this subject.[329] Because we encourage competition in other areas of society as a positive force, competition should be viewed in a similar light here. Not only have synthetic grass manufacturers been forced to make improvements in their fibers, mats, underpads, drainage, and so on, but advocates of natural grass have used modern methods to introduce advances of their own. As long as prevention of injury is a prime concern in these advances, both the individual athlete and society as a whole will benefit.

This same revolutionary process has occurred in other outdoor surface sports, such as tennis and track. Tennis originated from a French handball game called "jeu de paume" around the 13th century and was played in courtyards over a fringed or tasseled string or net.[417] Major Walter Wingfield of North Wales invented a game in 1873 from which modern outdoor tennis has more clearly evolved. Its popularity spread so rapidly that the All England Croquet Club added the name Lawn Tennis to its title and sponsored the first championship in 1877. As the name indicates, grass was the original surface used for play. As the popularity of tennis increased, other playing surfaces were needed to allow winter play and to bypass the problems inherent in growing a playing field. In 1909, Claude Brown used clay that he found too porous for brick making to introduce the hard or clay court. Although these surfaces remain popular, new court surfaces have flourished to such a degree that modern tennis has the widest choice of playing surface of any major sport (Table 30C–10). Only recently have the surface characteristics of these courts been subjected to laboratory and subject tests in an attempt to establish their safety.

Track and field is unquestionably the oldest form of organized sports activity, dating back 3500 years to ancient Greece. The religious festival at Olympia featuring this activity became an event of such proportions that the Greeks dated events with reference to the year of the Olympiad.[159, 310] Records dating back to 776 BC indicate that a race covering 192 meters (m) took place on a track about 32 m wide.[310] Other ancient Greek festivals include the Pythian games at Delphi, the Nemean Games at Nemea, and the Isthmian Games at Corinth. According to legend, the Irish Tailleann Games originated in the 19th century BC.[12] These early contests were held on grass, and later races took place on public thoroughfares.

Improvements in track design led to the use of cinders and a mixture of cinders and clay by the late 1800s. Synthetic surfaces began to appear in the 1960s with the production of a prototype track by the 3M Corporation for Macalester College in 1965.[197] The synthetic track gained wide appeal after its use in the 1968 Olympics in Mexico City, where numerous records were set, and the National Collegiate Athletic Association Track and Field Championship was held on a synthetic track the following year. Although athletes have long known the difference between "fast tracks" and "slow tracks," it remained for McMahon and Greene from Harvard to produce a track engineered to optimize running speed.[99, 259–261] Although this was an indoor track that theoretically and practically enhanced speed by about 2% (or 5 seconds per mile), the physics have since been incorporated into outdoor track surfacing technology. Although the cinder track has been virtually eliminated

from elite competition, its value in reducing injuries remains clear and some schools have preserved cinder tracks for use in training. Tracks for elite competition are generally made from rubber or synthetic materials such as polyurethane and are either poured or laid in place. Corporate research and development departments working in conjunction with bioengineers at universities in locations as far apart as Calgary, Zurich, Rome, and Boston design these surfaces to maximize performance and reduce injury potential.[324]

The origin of the movement of sports events from outdoors to inside can also be traced to ancient Greece. The name *gymnasium* is derived from the Greek word meaning "school for naked exercise," reflecting the all-male nature of this activity in that time period.[163] Exercise was an integral part of Greek society, but the gymnasium also served as a public facility for the training of male athletes to participate in the aforementioned public games. From its beginning as a room that served as a gathering place for exercise, the gymnasium grew in proportion to accommodate baths, dressing quarters, rooms for specialized purposes, and larger areas for contests and spectators.[163] Physical education including gymnastics and running centered around these facilities during the Hellenistic period and lasted until the fourth century, when literary interests suppressed the less cultured activity of bodily exercise. With the declining emphasis on physical education, the gymnasium disappeared until the reawakening of awareness of the link between body and mind in the 15th century. The first modern gymnasium opened in Copenhagen in 1799.[317] Educators such as Pestalozzi, Ling, and Spiess stimulated further development and groups such as the Young Men's Christian Association and the Young Men's Hebrew Association included physical exercise in their activities in the mid 1800s. The international Young Men's Christian Association training school in Springfield, Massachusetts, was the site where James Naismith introduced the new game of basketball to the world in 1891.[19] Wooden floors became the traditional gymnasium surface and continued to predominate for basketball courts as well as for other indoor courts and dance studios despite the influx of artificial surfaces. Contemporary surfaces have been said to have advantages ranging from improved durability to noise reduction to better space utilization, but seldom have their supporters argued for improved safety. In the study of sports surfaces, whether indoor or outdoor, it is quickly evident that many factors affect the safety value of the surface. These include not only the visible surface, but also and equally important, the under surface and the top finish.

Incidence

Although there is consensus that sports surfaces play a critical role in causing athletic injuries, it has been quite difficult to establish the incidence of injury in a sport or sports that can be attributed solely to the playing surface. Even in the area of traditional grass football fields, there have been studies that have suggested differences in incidence of injury from field to field, although the surface material is the same (Fig. 30C–32). The 1992 study by

TABLE 30C–10
Chart Comparing Various Tennis Court Surfaces

Court Type	Repairs May Be Costly	Glare	Initial Cost per Court including Base* (1992 prices)	Maintenance	Avg. Time before Resurfacing	Resurfacing Cost (1992 prices)	Surface Hardness	Ball Skid Length	Ball Spin Effective	Colors	Drying Time after Rain	Balls Discolored	Surface OK In & Out	Surface Cool on Hot Day	Slide Surface	Lines Affect Ball Bounce	Cushioned Surface	Durable	Court Speed Adjustable
Porous																			
Fast dry	no	no	14,000–18,000†	daily and yearly	annual	1000–3000	soft	short if damp court	yes	green red	fast	yes, slightly	yes	yes	yes	yes if tapes	no	no‡	yes
Clay (With subirrigation)	no	generally	24,000–26,000 / 9,000–11,000	daily and yearly	5 years	top dressing 1000–1500	soft	short if damp court	yes	varies	slow	yes	yes	yes	yes	yes if tapes	no	no‡	yes
Grass	no	no	15,000–17,000	daily and yearly	indefinite	varies	soft	moderately long	yes	green	slow	yes	out only	yes	yes	no	yes	hard objects can damage	no
Sand-filled synthetic turf‡	yes	no	25,000–30,000	daily and yearly	indefinite	N/A	soft	short	yes	green red	fast	no	yes	yes	yes	no	yes	hard objects can damage	yes
Porous concrete	yes	yes	27,000–31,000	minor	indefinite	N/A	hard	short	yes	concrete	fast	no	out only	no	no	no	no	yes	no
Nonporous Noncushioned																			
Concrete post-tensioned	yes	no (if colored)	22,000–25,000	very minor	5 years (if colored)	3000–3500	hard	controllable	yes	variety	fast	no	yes	no	no	no	no	yes	yes
Concrete reinforced	yes	no (if colored)	19,000–21,000	very minor	5 years (if colored)	3000–3500	hard	long if glossy finish, medium if gritty finish	no if glossy finish, yes if gritty finish	variety	fast	no	yes	no	no	no	no	yes	yes
Asphalt plant mix (colored)	no	no	16,000–18,000	very minor	5 years	2500–3000	hard	long if glossy finish, medium if gritty finish	no if glossy finish, yes if gritty finish	variety	fast	no	yes	no	no	no	no	yes	yes
Emulsified asphalt mix	no	no	19,000–21,000	very minor	5 years	2500–3500	hard	controllable	yes	variety	fast	no	yes	no	no	no	no	yes	yes
Combined hot plant and emulsified asphalt mix	no	no	19,000–21,000	very minor	5 years	2500–3500	hard	long if glossy finish, medium if gritty finish	yes if gritty finish	variety	fast	no	yes	no	no	no	no	yes	yes
Asphalt penetration macadam	no	no	15,000–17,000	very minor	5 years	3000–3500	hard	long if glossy finish, medium if gritty finish	yes if gritty finish	variety	fast	no	yes	no	no	no	no	yes	yes
Nonporous Cushioned																			
Asphalt bound system (colored)	no	no	19,000–23,000	very minor	5 years	2500–3500	soft	long if glossy finish, short if gritty finish	yes	variety	fast	no	yes	no	no	no	yes	yes	yes
Liquid applied synthetic	yes	possible	30,000–40,000	very minor	5–10 years	2500–3500	soft	varies shortest to longest	no if glossy finish, yes if gritty finish	variety	fast	no	yes	no	no	no	yes	yes	yes
Textile§	no	no	25,000–28,000	very minor	varies	varies	soft	short	yes	variety	fast	no	in only	N/A	no	no	yes	yes	no
Modular§	no	no	22,000–26,000	very minor	varies	varies	soft	medium to short	yes	green, red	fast	no	yes	yes	yes	no	yes	yes	yes
Removable§	no	no	25,000–30,000	very minor	varies	varies	soft	varies shortest to longest	yes	variety	fast	no	in only	N/A	no	no	minor	yes	no

* Prices vary regionally, do not include site preparation or fencing, and will be somewhat reduced when building or resurfacing batteries of courts.
† Including sprinkler system.
‡ Damaged areas may be readily repaired.
§ Including base construction and structurally sound surface.
Reprinted from Tennis Courts 1992–1993 with the permission of the United States Tennis Association, 707 Alexander Road, Princeton, NJ 08540.

2253

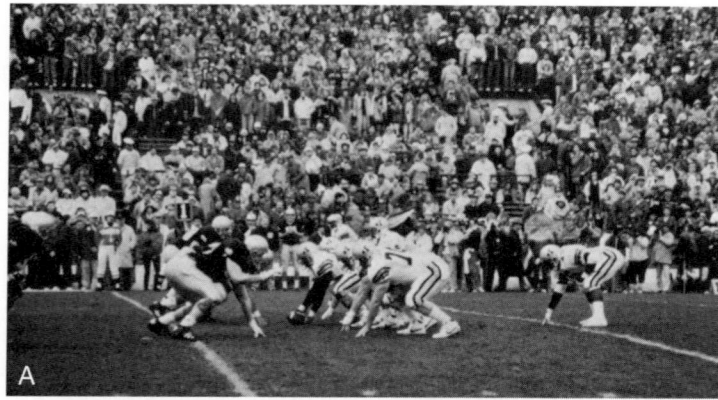

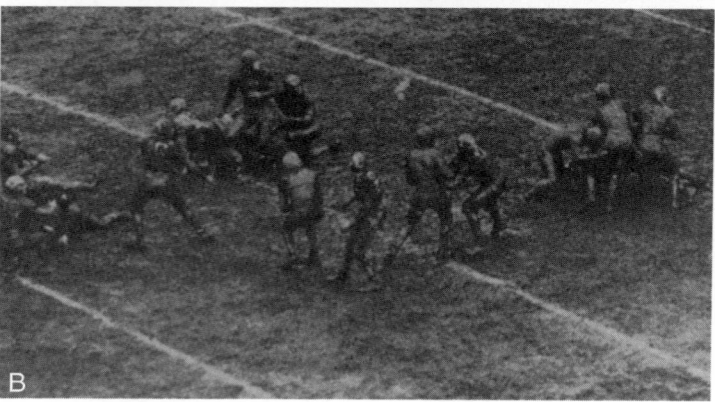

Figure 30C–32. Examples of differences between grass playing fields. *A*, Well-manicured college stadium grass field. (Photograph by Thomas O. Clanton.) *B*, Well-manicured college field destroyed in the rain. (Photograph courtesy of U.S. Naval Academy Athletic Association.)

Powell and Schootman is one of the best-controlled studies demonstrating that football players were at significantly higher risk of knee ligament injury when playing on AstroTurf as compared with natural grass.[321] Unfortunately, their study does not address injuries outside the knee. A study of North Carolina football players conducted by Mueller and Blyth[279] showed that a reduction in the injury rate resulted simply from resurfacing and maintaining the game and practice fields (Fig. 30C–33). Injury rates plum-meted from 29.3% and 21.3% on unresurfaced fields in 1969 to 1970 and 1971 to 1972, respectively, to a rate of 14.8% in 1971–1972 on resurfaced fields—about a 30% reduction. Poor field conditions were considered a factor in 8 of 34 soccer injuries in the paper by Sullivan,[407] 14 out of 18 outdoor soccer injuries in Hoff and Martin's series,[178] and 62 of 318 injuries in the Swedish study of Ekstrand and Gillquist.[126] These studies draw attention to the playing field and its importance and the need for further

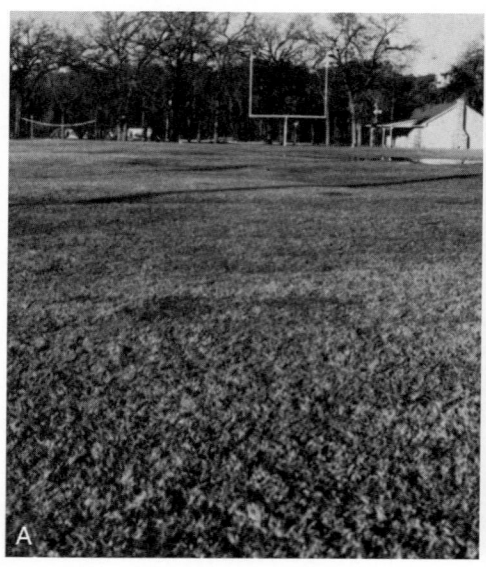
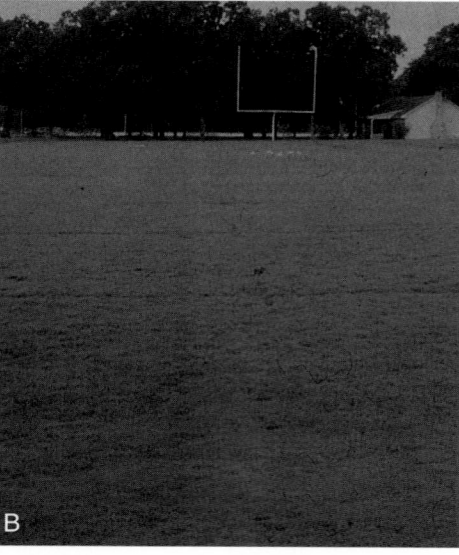

Figure 30C–33. *A*, Poorly maintained high school practice field. *B*, Same field 6 months later after maintenance. (Photograph by Thomas O. Clanton.)

work on proper playing surfaces and their maintenance to reduce injury rates in sports.

Studies of injuries and injury rates in sports ranging from dance[143, 167] to ice hockey[131, 370] have mentioned the sport's surface as a factor. Slipping on a wet tennis surface was a factor in 21% of the injuries cited in the retrospective analysis done by Biener and Calvori.[32] Although the surface is frequently named as a source of problems in runners, there have been no studies that have unequivocally confirmed this allegation.[322] The Ontario cohort study found no association between running surface and injury, whereas the companion study from South Carolina showed a statistically meaningful relationship only for females running on concrete.[240, 433] If the base is included as a part of the playing field surface, several studies can be cited indicating that this is the primary factor in ankle injuries in baseball and softball (Fig. 30C–34). Janda and coworkers found that 71% of the recreational softball injuries in their study were related to sliding, which has an obvious connection to the playing field and bases.[191] A follow-up to this study showed the implications of an injury-prevention method such as the use of a breakaway base on these surface-related injuries.[192] Janda and associates estimated that breakaway bases could reduce the incidence of serious injury in softball by 98% and result in a $2 billion per year savings in acute medical care costs. In the area of children's

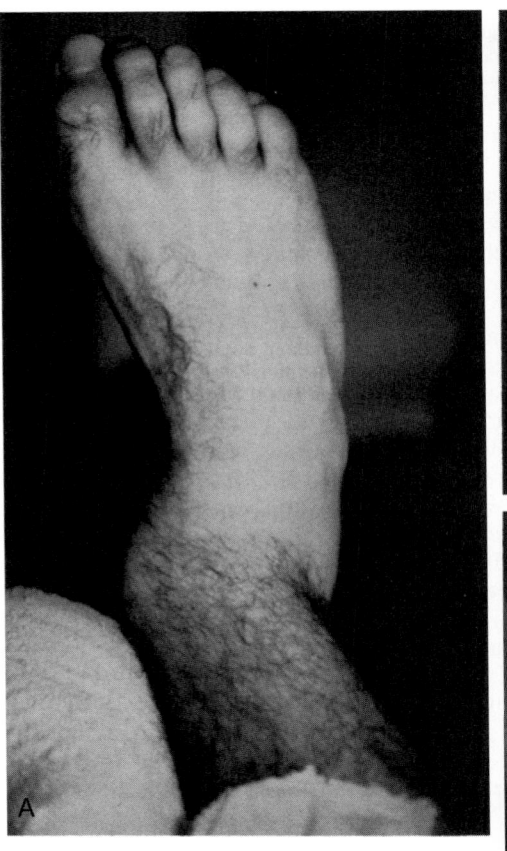
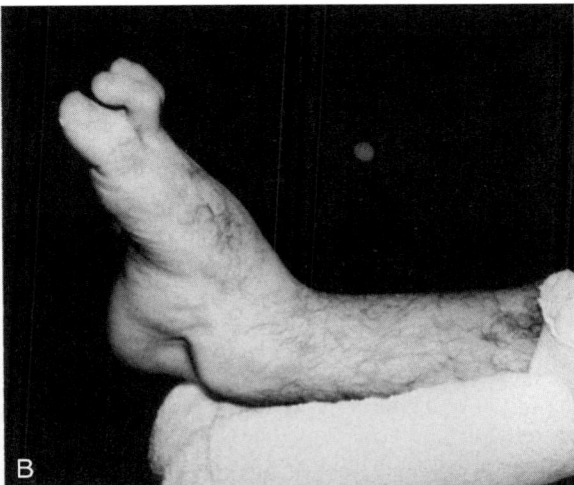
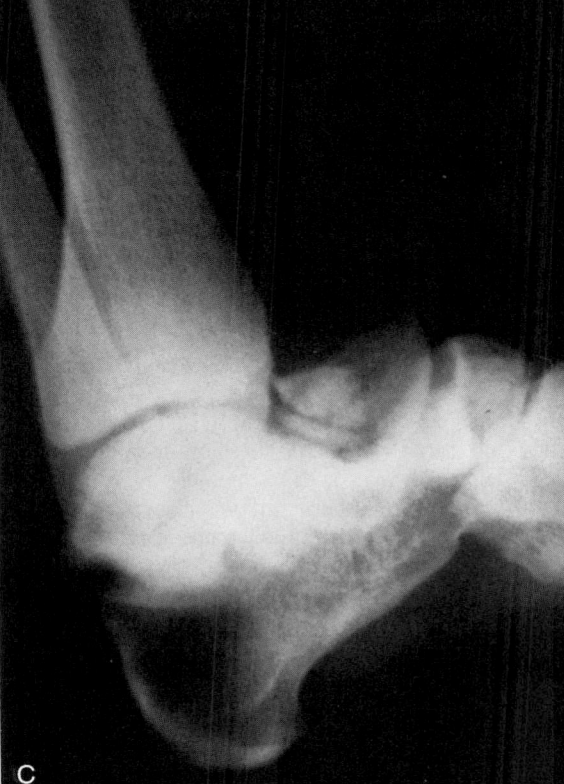

Figure 30C–34. Example of a fracture-dislocation in a baseball player resulting from stepping incorrectly on a base and another player's foot. *A* and *B*, Clinical photographs before reduction. (Photographs by Thomas O. Clanton.) *C*, Radiograph before reduction. (Copyright Thomas O. Clanton.)

playground injuries, statistics suggest that falls to the ground account for 60% of playground equipment injuries, yet barely half of daycare playground equipment is installed on impact-absorbing surfaces.[320] Certainly the playing surface is an important consideration in the prevention of injury.

Mechanical Factors

With the historical perspective and incidence of injury data in mind, the curious investigator must search for a unifying principle on which to base the study of sports surfaces and their relationship to injury. Regardless of the surface, the underlying question to be answered is how the surface affects load in the individual participant.[291, 299] For this purpose, attention has been focused on certain material properties of the sports surface such as hardness and friction together with performance properties such as energy loss or resilience. Nigg has reviewed the methods by which a playing surface may be characterized and specified some of the tests that are important in determining the aforementioned properties.[296]

Hardness

One of the most obvious differences between surfaces detected by casual observation as well as by sophisticated testing is the relative hardness or softness. Hardness is related to the ground reaction force, which was discussed earlier in the chapter in the section on biomechanics. In conformity with Newton's first law (for every action there is an equal and opposite reaction), the vertical reaction force responds to the vertical force component applied by the individual at foot strike. Its amplitude is affected by the shock-absorbing qualities of the surface to which the force is applied. The time needed for force absorption and reaction is the key to the amplitude of the reaction force and relates to the compliance of the surface material. Hard materials deform less than soft materials during identical impact testing conditions. For example, a well-maintained grass lawn is softer than a concrete sidewalk. When impact occurs between an object such as a leg and a surface such as grass or concrete, it is the surface hardness that limits the time of impact while increasing the amplitude of the reaction force (Fig. 30C–35). It takes little imagination to determine that sports participation on a soft surface such as a gymnastics mat carries less risk for certain impact-related injuries than a similar activity performed on a wooden floor. By the same token, athletes running on gymnastics mats compared with a tuned track would set few records.[261] From these mundane examples we can conclude that there are some opposing factors confronting us in this analysis. Although a harder surface may provide a better surface for performance needs in certain sports, it may create simultaneously an increased exposure to injury. This fact seems to be borne out most obviously by synthetic tracks.

Hardness is a variable that can be defined in terms of material science. Hardness is the resistance generated by a

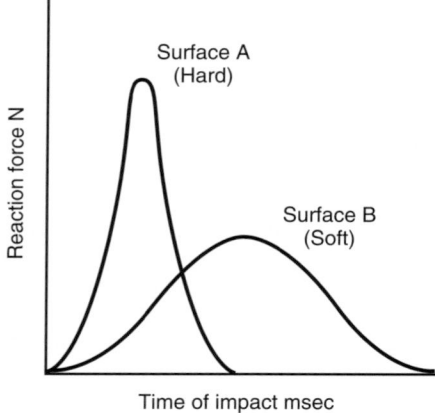

Figure 30C–35. Example of relationship between time of impact and type of surface. Hard surface A has a short time of impact but a high reaction force, whereas soft surface B has a longer time of impact and a lower reaction force.

material during deformation in response to an externally applied force.[114, 299] In the study of various materials, their behavior is described by means of a stress-strain curve or stress-deformation diagram. The elastic or plastic behavior of a material is determined by the remaining deformation once the acting force is removed. When the deformation persists, the material is described as plastic, and when the material returns to its original shape, it is elastic. A sports surface may be further characterized as being either area elastic or point elastic.[444] Owing to their high bending strength, area elastic surfaces distribute forces over a wide area. Point elastic surfaces have low bending strength and therefore deform only in a very confined area (Fig. 30C–36). This fact has implications for both performance and health.

From the clinical standpoint, there is a widespread belief that harder surfaces are associated with a higher incidence of injury for any given activity. This conclusion seems obvious, but it is more difficult to support scientifically.

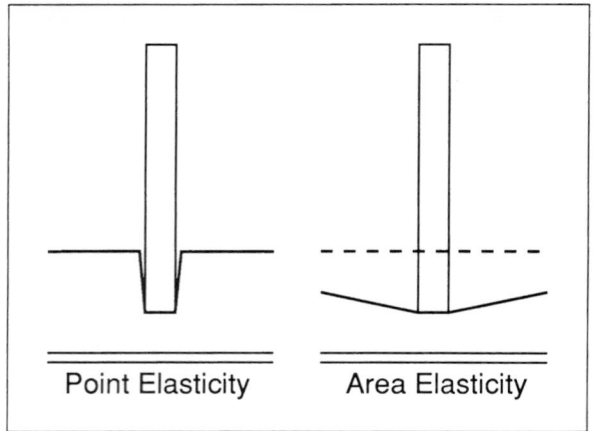

Figure 30C–36. Example of point elastic surface and area elastic surface. (From Denoth J: Indoor athletic playing surfaces—floor vs. shoe. In Segesser B, Pförringer W [eds]: The Shoe in Sport. Chicago, Year Book Medical Publishers, 1989, pp 65–69.)

Such conditions as shin splints, stress fractures, tibial stress syndrome, turf toe, bursitis, arthritis, and even acute fractures have been associated with the higher loads imparted by surfaces with limited compliance. Bowers and Martin demonstrated the existence of reduced shock-absorbing characteristics in 5-year-old AstroTurf compared with new AstroTurf, describing this as "clearly detrimental to player safety."[49] Unfortunately, they did not show a clear relationship between this lack of impact absorption and an increase in either acute or chronic injuries. Larson and Osternig[221] reported one of the few clinical studies implicating surface hardness as a source of specific athletic injury in 1974. In a survey of Pacific-8 Conference athletic trainers after the 1973 football season, they showed that the incidence of prepatellar and olecranon bursitis was increased on artificial grass compared with natural grass and attributed this increase to the hard underlying sub-base. Anecdotally, considerable evidence of problems with harder playing surfaces exists because players commonly complain of aching feet and legs after standing and practicing on older synthetic fields.

The injury most frequently associated with sports participation on artificial grass is turf toe.[51, 84, 341] This injury is a sprain of the first metatarsophalangeal joint that has been inextricably linked to the artificial playing surface. The nickname coined by Bowers and Martin has now become the diagnostic description and is recognized even by the artificial turf manufacturing companies. Turf toe is a distinct clinical entity related to the combination of a relatively flexible shoe and a hard artificial surface.[51] Despite the weight of clinical evidence pointing to the relationship between turf toe and the artificial surface, little statistical support exists implicating surface hardness as a major factor. The injury does indeed occur on natural grass and probably has more to do with the flexibility of the shoe and frictional characteristics of the surface than its hardness.

Impact forces, skeletal transient forces, and excess load produced by hard surfaces have been emphasized as etiologic factors in many other conditions ranging from osteoarthritis to shin splints to stress fractures. Statistical verification of this relationship, however, remains absent. An increased incidence of tibial periostitis, Achilles tendinitis, Achilles tendon rupture, and muscle rupture are postulated to be the result of hard surface synthetic tracks.[306] Haberl and Prokop have related these conditions to what they call "Tartan syndrome" and propose that surface hardness producing initial decelerations as high as 80 Gs is a primary etiologic factor.[164] The relationship between surface hardness and stress fractures has been mentioned in several studies. Other factors, such as repetitive and rhythmic activities, malalignment, and poorly cushioned shoewear, are also contributors to stress fractures.[63, 148, 158, 162, 229, 252, 356] With this as background, it is apparent that surface hardness is important in the study of athletic injury although its relative contribution among the interrelated factors is imprecise.

Friction

The frictional properties of the surface are the second critical mechanical factor of sport surfaces related to sports performance and injury. Whereas hardness is defined by a high vertical stiffness, friction relates to horizontal stiffness (Fig. 30C–37). Without friction, locomotion would be impossible. It is integral to acceleration and deceleration. The difficulties imposed by reduced friction are well known to the novice ice skater. High friction between the shoe and the surface translates into good traction for the athlete and improved performance. Unfortunately, this factor also means greater load on the body, which may exceed physiologic limits. Therefore, a trade-off exists between performance-enhancing qualities and safety considerations.

Friction can be viewed in several ways that are important to sports biomechanics. There are two types of friction to be considered: static and dynamic.[403] The former describes the resistance to movement between two bodies. It is a surface property of the contact surfaces. Dynamic friction, on the other hand, occurs only when relative movement between two objects is present and the force is opposing the horizontal movement and decelerating the object in motion. This type of friction is also related to the material properties of the surface, but in this relationship the dynamic force is less linear, particularly over large ranges in velocity. Friction can also be viewed in terms of horizontal or rotational friction.[296, 299, 403] Functionally, the former corresponds to the force resisting the foot sliding or moving sideways, whereas rotational friction relates to torque generated in activities such as turning or cutting. Torque is considered one of the primary etiologic factors in injuries to the knee and ankle.[9, 44]

Because the static coefficient of friction (μ) is a physical characteristic of a material surface, it can be calculated from the equation $\mu = F/W$ where W is the weight of the object being moved over a surface and F is the force required to move the object.[100, 396] This equation applies to smooth, uniform surfaces, but not to the shoe/turf interface. Therefore, a similar term has been described as the release coefficient (r). It is expressed as $r = F/W$ where W is the weight in the shoe and F is the force necessary to release the shoe/turf interface when engaged.[100] Torque is described in newton meters (Nm) or foot-pounds, whereas the release coefficient and the coefficient of friction are numerical descriptions without unit values.

Energy Loss

A separate but equally important property apart from hardness is the energy loss that occurs when a material is loaded. This property varies over a wide range from surface to surface and carries major implications in the field of sports biomechanics. As depicted in Figure 30C–38, materials can exhibit similar elastic behaviors on the stress/strain diagram yet have very different responses to the effects of loading and unloading. In this figure, material A shows no loss of mechanical energy, whereas material B depicts a loss of mechanical energy equivalent to the shaded area. This energy loss is not a true material property because it depends on the loading rate among other variables. When a material has the quality of variable deformation dependent upon velocity of deformation, it is described as viscoelastic. If energy applied to a surface is lost in the

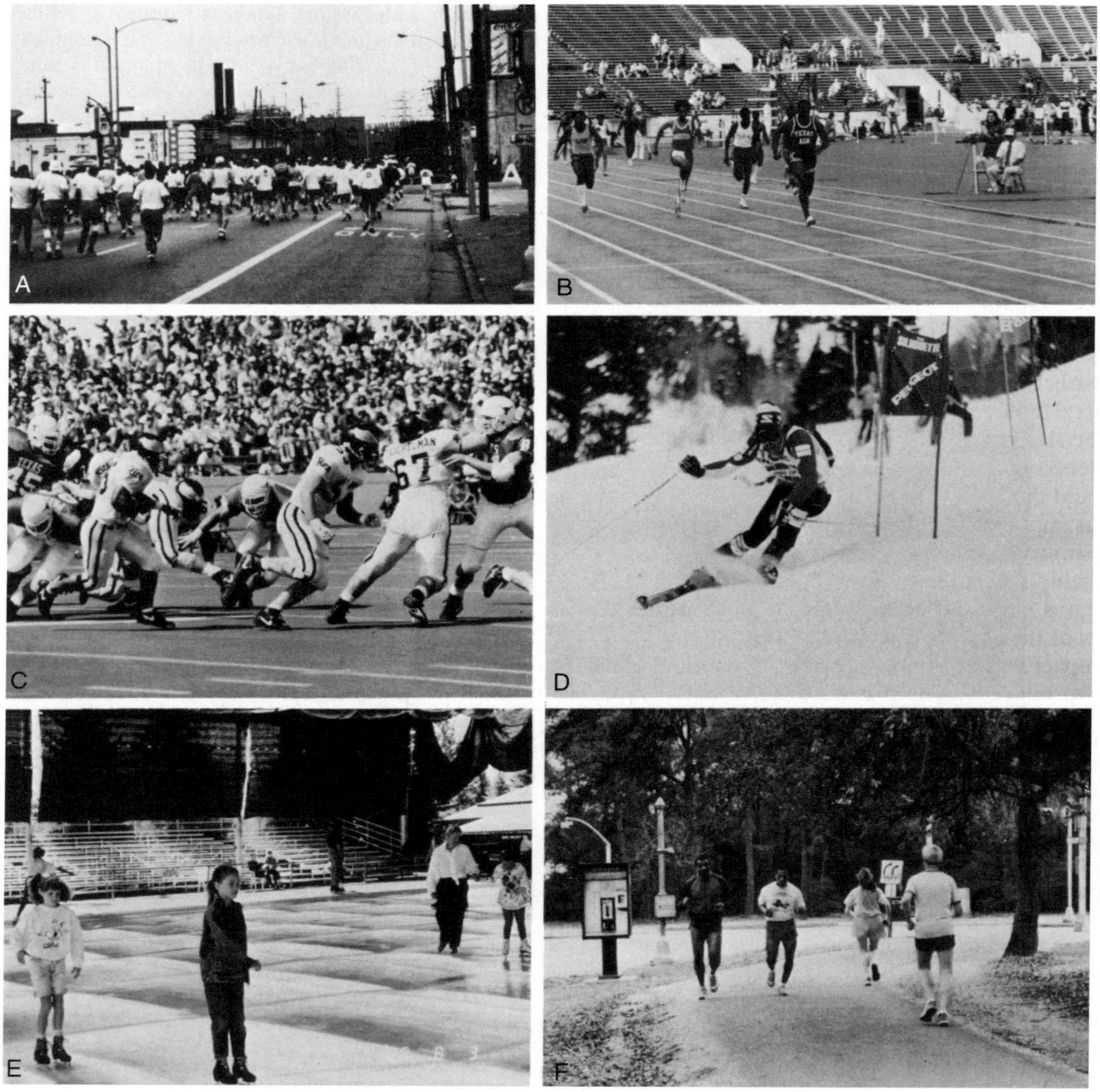

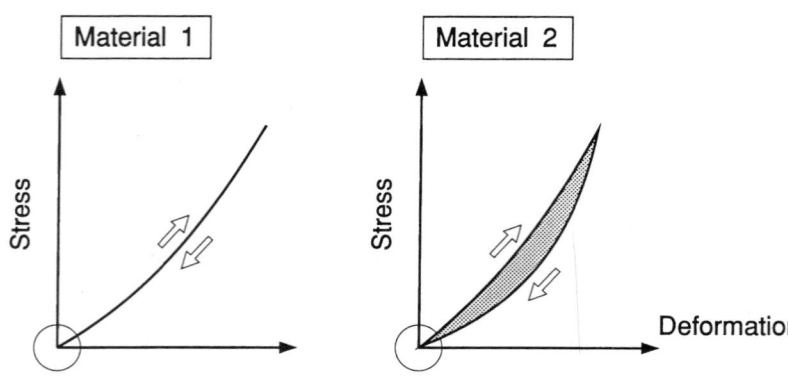

Figure 30C–37. Examples of vertical stiffness versus horizontal stiffness in surfaces. *A,* Concrete street with a high vertical and medium horizontal stiffness. *B,* Polyurethane track with high-medium vertical and high horizontal stiffness. *C,* Third-generation synthetic grass with low-medium vertical and high horizontal stiffness. *D,* Slalom course on snow with low vertical and horizontal stiffness. *E,* Ice-skating rink with high vertical and low horizontal stiffness. *F,* Cinder jogging path with medium vertical stiffness and low-medium horizontal stiffness. (Photographs by Thomas O. Clanton.)

Figure 30C–38. Differences in response of materials to loading and unloading despite similar elastic behavior. (From Denoth J: Load on the locomotor system and modelling. In Nigg BM [ed]: Biomechanics of Running Shoes. Champaign, Ill, Human Kinetics Publishers, 1986, p 96. © 1986 by Benno M. Nigg. Reprinted by permission.)

TABLE 30C–11
Results of Torque Testing in 12 Shoes for Nine Surface Conditions

	Release Coefficients							
Shoe	Grass	Grass Wet	AstroTurf	AstroTurf Wet	Tartan Turf	Tartan Turf Wet	PolyTurf	PolyTurf Wet
Group I	.55 ± .06		.35 ± .03		.34 ± .03		.29 ± 0.3	
Group II	.44 ± .04		.31 ± .03		.32 ± .02		.26 ± .02	
Group III	.37 ± .04		.26 ± .02		.26 ± .03		.20 ± .02	
Group IV	.36 ± .03	.32 ± .04	.41 ± .03	.26 ± .03	.34 ± .03	.23 ± .02	.33 ± .02	.23 ± .02
Group V	.28 ± .03	.27 ± .03	.29 ± .03	.29 ± .03	.27 ± .03	.24 ± .02	.26 ± .02	.23 ± .02
Group VI			.40 ± .01		.36 ± .01		.41 ± .02	
Group VII			.45 ± .04		.37 ± .02		.45 ± .02	

Shoes in groups I–V have plastic or polyurethane soles.
Shoes in groups VI–VII have rubber soles.

Group I: Conventional 7-posted football shoe, $^3/_4$-inch cleat length, $^3/_8$-inch tip diameter, plastic sole.
Group II: Conventional 7-posted football shoe, $^1/_2$-inch cleat length, $^3/_8$-inch tip diameter, polyurethane sole.
Group III: Conventional shoe with five $^3/_4$-inch cleats, $^3/_8$-inch tip diameter, Bowdoin heel, polyurethane sole.
Group IV: Soccer style, 15 cleats with $^3/_8$-inch tip diameter, polyurethane sole.
Group V: Soccer style, 15 cleats with $^1/_2$-inch tip diameter, polyurethane sole.
Group VI: Soccer style, 12 cleats (ten $^3/_8$-inch length and two $^1/_2$-inch length), $^1/_2$-inch tip diameter, rubber sole.
Group VII: Soccer style, 49 to 121 cleats ($^3/_8$-inch or $^5/_{16}$-inch length), $^3/_8$-inch tip diameter to pointed tips, rubber sole.

From Torg JS, Quedenfeld TC, Landau S: The shoe-surface interface and its relationship to football knee injuries. Am J Sports Med 2:261–269, 1974.

surface deformation, performance may suffer.[261] Surfaces that deform to greater degrees are called compliant and result in increased contact time. This is the means by which cushioning occurs. By increasing the time of collision, the force between the colliding bodies is decreased. The final property of importance in athletic performance on a given surface is its resilience. High resilience indicates that the energy stored in the surface owing to its stiffness and deformation is returned to the athlete—i.e., elastic behavior of the surface occurs quickly. This has implications for enhancing performance as well as lessening fatigue.[261, 444]

Experimental Work

Because of a presumed association with injuries, frictional properties of various sport surfaces and athletic shoes have been the subject of studies by several authors. To provide some historical perspective, these studies will be discussed in chronological sequence. Because there is a relationship between translational and rotational friction, studies of either or both forces are included. Furthermore, because friction involves the interaction between two surfaces, studies that have looked at the shoe or shoe cleat interface with the playing surface will be reviewed from the playing surface prospective.

Torg and Quedenfeld published pioneering work in the field of sports medicine in 1971 aimed at reducing injury rates by targeting the shoe-surface interface.[421] The study was done on grass and concentrated on the relationship between the number and size of shoe cleats and the incidence and severity of knee injuries in high school football players. As mentioned, this investigation was expanded to include ankle injuries in the Philadelphia Catholic Football League and showed a reduction in ankle injuries from 72 to 36 and in ankle fractures from 13 to 7 by changing from a traditional seven-cleated football shoe to a multi-cleated

soccer shoe. The study was continued through the 1971 season, and the trend remained, with only 39 ankle injuries and two fractures in the 1971 season. Continuing this study, Torg and colleagues performed laboratory studies to determine the torque necessary to release an engaged shoe-surface interface.[423, 424] Twelve shoes and nine surface conditions were tested for a total of 108 release coefficients. These are shown in Tables 30C–11 and 30C–12 for grass, AstroTurf, Tartan Turf, and PolyTurf under both wet and dry conditions. Coefficient differences of 0.05 were determined to be significant. The release coefficients ranged from a high of 0.55 ± 0.06, with a conventional seven-cleated football shoe on dry grass, to a low of 0.20 ± 0.02 with a conventional shoe that had an uncleated disk heel (Bowdoin modification) on dry PolyTurf. The use of wet versus dry conditions was based on the study by Bramwell and colleagues in 1972, which suggested that fewer injuries were sustained on wet synthetic fields than dry synthetic fields.[53] From their study, Torg and coworkers concluded that the release coefficient varies with (1) the number, length, and diameter of the cleats, (2) the type of surface—natural or artificial, (3) the condition of the

TABLE 30C–12
Relationship of Shoe-Turf Interface Release Coefficient to Incidence of Football Knee Injuries

Release Coefficient		
.60—	Not safe	
.50—		.49
	Probably safe	
.40—		
	Probably safe	
.30—		.31
	Safe	
.20—		
.10—		

From Torg JS, Quedenfeld TC, Landau S: The shoe-surface interface and its relationship to football knee injuries. Am J Sports Med 2:261–269, 1974.

TABLE 30C–13
Friction Coefficients for Various Surfaces and Shoes

Shoe	Coefficient of Sliding Friction Surface			
	PolyTurf	*AstroTurf*	*Tartan Turf*	*Grass*
A	1.49	1.34	1.42	1.23
B	1.54	1.31	1.16	1.21
C	1.33	1.23	1.13	1.07
D	1.38	1.16	0.92	0.92

From Stanitski CL, McMaster JH, Ferguson RJ: Synthetic turf and grass: A comparative study. Am J Sports Med 2:22–26, 1974.

surface—wet or dry, and (4) the outsole material of the shoe—polyurethane or soft rubber. They classified shoes as safe for a particular surface when the release coefficient was 0.31 or below.

Stanitski and associates in 1974 determined the static coefficient of 16 different shoe-surface combinations.[396] They used a drag test of a size 13 shoe with a 25-pound load pulled both with and against the grain, across various sections of football fields. Their results are shown in Table 30C–13. The coefficient of friction ranged from a high of 1.54 for a Riddell At-31 (standard last, leather upper, molded plastic sole, 20 ⅜-inch conical cleats) on Poly-

Turf to a low of 0.92 for the Puma 1430 ("soft last," molded rubber sole, 23 ⅜-inch cylindrical cleats with central indentations) on Tartan Turf and grass fields. These investigators found no grain effect and "essentially no change" when the surface was wet.

Bowers and Martin continued the study of cleat-surface friction, adding the new parameter of a new versus a worn synthetic surface.[50] The cleats from two different shoes were studied. One cleat was evaluated in both a slightly worn and very worn state. Three similar shoes were mounted in a triangular pattern on a platform weighted from two to fourteen pounds that was pulled across the new or worn turf. This study showed 16% more friction against the grain of a 5-year-old AstroTurf field when wet and 22% more friction when dry. This anisotropy in friction due to grain effect was minimal on new AstroTurf (Fig. 30C–39). From this study, the authors provided a formula for calculating coefficients of friction for individual shoes and surfaces that increased linearly with the number of cleats. They suggested that changes in friction altered player performance (e.g., smaller slip angles on wet turf) and that increasing friction could produce "foot lock" and result in increased injuries.

Bonstingl and coworkers expanded the study of shoes and surfaces by looking at dynamic torque for eleven shoe types on four dry turf samples at two different player weights.[44] They used the swivel shoe of Cameron's design, five styles of multicleated soccer shoes, four styles of

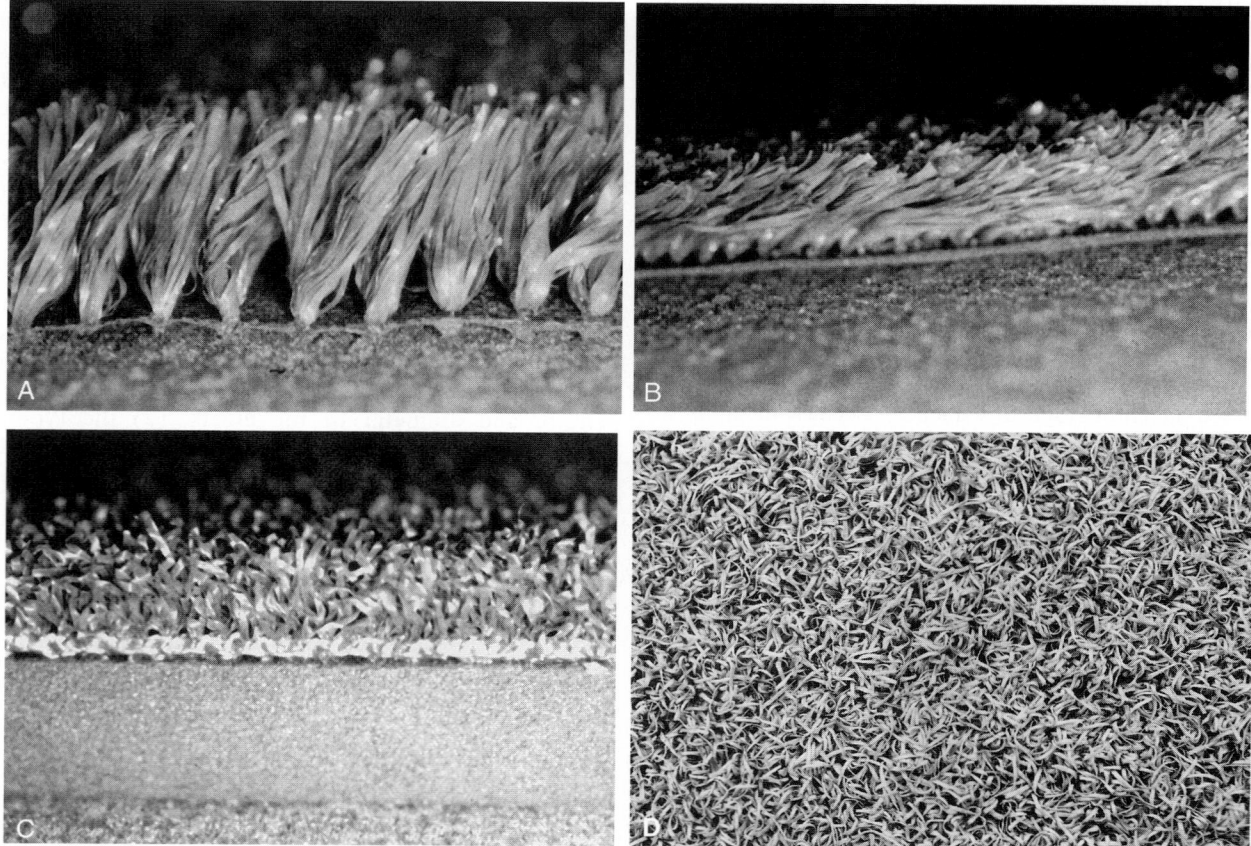

Figure 30C–39. AstroTurf evolution. *A,* Original AstroTurf (new) in its 1966 design with long nylon ribbon. *B,* Original AstroTurf showing its grain effect. *C,* Newer AstroTurf 8. *D,* Weave pattern of AstroTurf designed to prevent a grain effect. (Photographs by Thomas O. Clanton.)

noncleated basketball shoes, and a conventional football shoe for grass (seven ¾-inch plastic screw-on cleats with metal tips). The four surfaces were AstroTurf, Tartan Turf, PolyTurf, and grass. The two player weights used for the normal force were 170 pounds (77 kg) and 200 pounds (91 kg). All combinations were tested for both toe stance and foot stance positions. They found that all shoes except the swivel shoe developed about 70% more torque in foot stance than in toe stance and that the higher player weight resulted in more torque. There was no direct correlation between the torque for a given shoe type and all surface combinations except that the conventional shoe tested on grass had among the highest torque in both toe stance and foot stance. Although noncleated shoes generally had less torque for all playing surfaces, this was not absolutely true for all surfaces. Because this study proved that torque applied to an athlete's leg depends on (1) the type and outsole design of the shoe, (2) the playing surface, (3) the player weight being supported, and (4) the foot stance assumed, other studies must be considered in this light.

Culpepper and Niemann continued the study of the shoe/turf interface in 1983 by looking at the release coefficient for torque in several shoe-surface combinations.[100] They tested five different soccer style shoes of variable cleat number and configurations on old and new Poly-Turf and new AstroTurf under wet and dry conditions. Loads ranging from 10 to 90 pounds were transferred down a metal shaft to a prosthetic foot on which the different shoes were mounted (Fig. 30C–40). The release coefficient of torque was calculated for 30 different conditions (Table 30C–14). The range was from a low of 0.19 ± 0.01 to a high of 0.38 ± 0.03. The authors found that although a specific shoe did vary in its release coefficient ranking on different surfaces, *a shoe that had a low coefficient on one surface under one condition was generally lower on all three surfaces whether wet or dry, whereas a shoe that ranked higher did so for all conditions.* Using Torg's criteria for shoe safety, they rated all the shoes as either safe or probably safe.

Another study of both static friction and torque appeared in 1983, when Van Gheluwe and colleagues tested nine different shoes on three varieties of artificial turf in both the toe stance and foot stance positions.[429] The shoes were almost exclusively soccer style shoes with varying cleat number, height, and pattern; there was one conventional six-cleated natural turf shoe. The turfs used were AstroTurf (S90), Chevron Grass Sport 500, and Poligrass. The latter

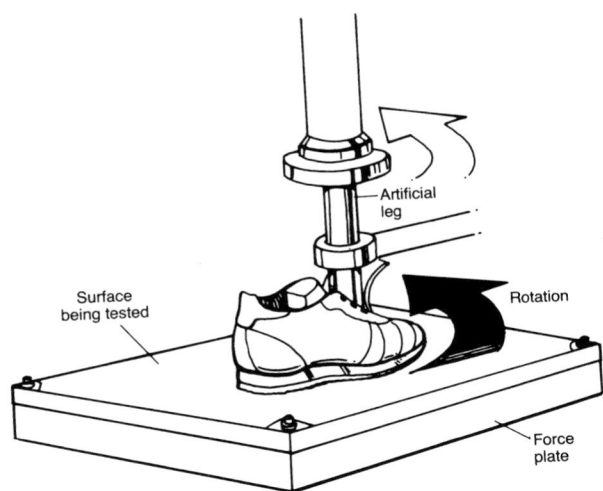

Figure 30C–40. Example of device for testing torque. (Redrawn from Physical tests. Sport Research Review. Beaverton, Ore, Nike Sport Research Laboratory, Jan/Feb, 1990; and Van Gheluwe B, Deporte E, Hebbelinck M: Frictional forces and torques of soccer shoes on artificial turf. In Nigg BM, Kerr BA [eds]: Biomechanical Aspects of Sport Shoes and Playing Surfaces. Calgary, University of Calgary Press, 1983, pp 161–168.)

was tested with and against the grain. The normal force applied to the test shoe was either 45 kg or 86.5 kg. In their analysis, the authors demonstrated higher values for friction and torque for AstroTurf compared with the other surfaces (AstroTurf scored highest in 22 of 36, or 61%, of the test conditions). They attributed this result to the nylon fiber of AstroTurf compared with the polypropylene fiber used in the other surfaces. The authors also pointed out a tendency toward increasing frictional torque with increasing values for total contact area of the cleats regardless of the type of artificial surface used. This confirmed the work of Bonstingl and colleagues; however, the results violate the law of physics for dry friction, which predicts the linear relationship for friction between two surfaces based on the normal load applied regardless of contact area. This contradiction is significant when interpreting the results of other studies that have assumed this linear relationship.

Andreasson and coworkers in Sweden published a more detailed study in 1986 evaluating torque and friction in a dynamic mode on an artificial surface.[9] This was the first study to specifically add dynamic torque (although Bowers

TABLE 30C–14
Release Coefficients of 30 Shoe-Surface Combinations

Shoe	New PolyTurf		Old PolyTurf		New AstroTurf	
	Dry	*Wet*	*Dry*	*Wet*	*Dry*	*Wet*
A	.27 ± .01	.21 ± .01	.24 ± .02	.24 ± .02	.19 ± .01	.24 ± .01
B	.35 ± .03	.29 ± .01	.33 ± .05	.31 ± .01	.38 ± .03	.35 ± .02
C	.21 ± .01	.23 ± .01	.29 ± .01	.22 ± .01	.19 ± .01	.22 ± .02
D	.32 ± .03	.24 ± .01	.32 ± .02	.31 ± .01	.34 ± .03	.26 ± .01
E	.28 ± .01	.29 ± .01	.30 ± .01	.25 ± .02	.26 ± .01	.28 ± .01

Data from Culpepper MI, Niemann KMW: An investigation of the shoe-turf interface using different types of shoes on Polyturf and Astro-turf: Torque and release coefficients. Alabama J Med Sci 20: 387–390, 1983.

and Martin measured dynamic friction) by using a rotating disk on which the surface was applied. The disk was rotated at a velocity varying between 1 and 5 m/sec in order to simulate speed from walking to running (but not sprinting). Twenty-five different shoes were tested including running shoes, tennis shoes, soccer shoes for artificial turf, and soccer shoes for natural turf. Values were obtained for toe stance for all shoes with and against the grain of the Poligrass test surface. Six shoes (four running and two soccer shoes for grass) were tested in a foot stance position. A single vertical load of 241 N was used for all tests. Torque in toe stance varied from a low of less than 10 Nm for one of the running shoes and one of the multicleated soccer shoes to a high of more than 50 Nm for another multicleated soccer shoe placed against the grain of the Poligrass test surface. Converting these figures to a value to allow comparison with a static release coefficient of others by dividing the torque by the normal force gives a range of less than 0.04 to 0.20. The authors showed that the frictional force is independent of speed between 1 and 5 m/sec. Unfortunately, this is below the 7 to 10 m/sec speeds that occur in modern football and soccer. Torques were generally lower for shoes with polypropylene outsoles compared with polyurethane and rubber-like soles. The ratio between torque (T) and friction (F) was calculated as a mean lever arm (L) by the equation $L = T/F$. This equation was proposed as a tool for predicting torque balance. The authors felt that a balanced shoe would reduce distortional forces on the knee and ankle by eliminating any torque when the shoe was sliding regardless of direction. The differences between this study and that of Bonstingl and colleagues were attributed to differences in the normal force used, although it seems clear that there are a number of other important differences.

Nigg and Segesser reported in 1988 on the variation in friction related to a change in normal force. They found when studying the six different surfaces considered for the

TABLE 30C–15
Variation in Static Coefficient of Friction for Translation with Variation in Vertical Load Using Football Shoes on Six Different Playing Surfaces (A through F)

Load (Vertical) (N)	Static Coefficient of Friction (Translational)					
	A	**B**	**C**	**D**	**E**	**F**
280	1.13	1.42	1.30	1.56	1.32	1.51
769	3.15	2.90	2.57	3.48	2.68	3.15

From Nigg BM, Segesser B: The influence of playing surfaces on the load on the locomotor system and on football and tennis injuries. Sports Med 5:375–385, 1988.

Toronto Skydome playing surface that the static coefficient of friction changed from lows of 1.13 to 1.56 for 280 N normal loads to highs of 2.57 to 3.48 for 769 N loads[305] (Table 30C–15). The tested surfaces ranked differently for the two load conditions. This result indicates the complexity of using material tests for choosing a playing surface because the individuals playing vary by a factor of 2 or more in weight and generate forces that may be well beyond those studied to date in laboratory tests.[164]

Just as there are differences between natural and artificial grass that affect the frictional properties of the playing surface and supposedly affect injury risk, similar differences have been known for other sport surfaces. Rheinstein and colleagues looked at static drag and dynamic torque characteristics of different shoes on two basketball surfaces.[333] The shoes were standard MK208-type basketball shoes with either synthetic rubber or polyurethane outsoles having a standard suction cup pattern. Sole hardness varied from 39 to 51 to 66 for elastomer and from 50 to 60 to 70 for the polyurethane as measured on the type A durometer scale (Fig. 30C–41). The three playing surfaces tested were

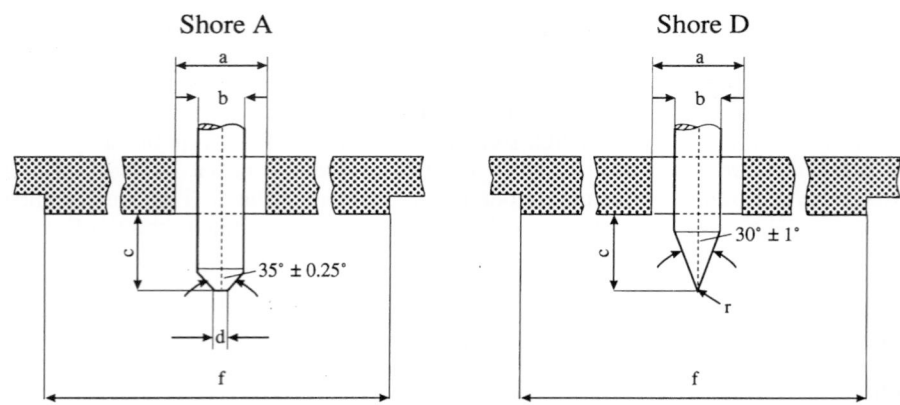

a	∅ (3.00 ±0.10) mm
b	∅ (1.25 ± 0.15) mm
c	$\left(2.50 \begin{smallmatrix} +0.04 \\ -0.01 \end{smallmatrix}\right)$ mm
d	∅(0.79 ± 0.01) mm
r	(0.10 ± 0.01) mm
f	∅ (16.0 ± 2.50) mm

Figure 30C–41. Methods for measuring shore hardness. (From Denoth J: Load on the locomotor system and modelling. In Nigg BM [ed]: Biomechanics of Running Shoes. Champaign, Ill, Human Kinetics Publishers, 1986, p 97. © 1986 by Benno M. Nigg. Reprinted by permission.)

clean hardwood, dusty hardwood, and clean artificial flooring (Tartan indoor surface manufactured by the 3M Corporation). Measurements were made at simulated player weights of 180 pounds (82 kg) and 150 pounds (68 kg). Torques ranged from a high of 42 foot-pounds for the soft elastomer shoe on the artificial floor at a 180-pound test load to a low of less than 20 foot-pounds for the softest polyurethane on dusty hardwood at a 150-pound test load. The results indicated a correlation between outsole material, outsole hardness, and player weight in the forces generated in friction and torque at the shoe-surface interface. Polyurethane soles produce less torque than the elastomer outsoles for all weight, floor, and surface condition parameters. Torque also decreased with increasing sole hardness for the elastomer outsoles on the clean hardwood and artificial surface, but varied for the polyurethane-soled shoes. As expected, greater player weight increased torque, and dust on the hardwood flooring cut torque almost in half. The polyurethane soles were considerably less affected by dust than the elastomer outsoles. The relationship of friction and torque to basketball-incurred injuries has not been studied, but it is clear that a certain minimum level of traction is necessary to prevent slipping, which affects both performance and injuries due to falling. Similarly, one would expect that high friction and torque could overload the athlete and result in injury. These findings have obvious implications for performance as well as prevention of injury in sports medicine.

Schlaepfer and colleagues studied the frictional characteristics of tennis shoes in 1983 for five different surface materials.[359] The five tennis shoes tested were similar except in their percentage of natural rubber versus synthetic rubber (shoe 1 = 100% natural rubber; shoe 3 = 50% each; shoe 5 = 100% synthetic rubber). The surfaces tested were porplastic grass (artificial grass), porplastic H (multipurpose hall flooring), porplastic F (porous SBR granules), porplastic SW (nonporous EPDM/SBR sandwich), and porplastic F covered with loose granulate (tennis surface "serde"). Three test situations were used. The first test varied the surface type and shoes with a constant velocity of 0.3 m/sec and a constant vertical load of 200 N. The second test varied the normal force (30 N, 100 N, 200 N, 400 N) applied to the shoe-surface interface. The third test varied the velocities using 0.14 m/sec, 0.3 m/sec, and 0.9 m/sec. The study showed a 25% decrease in the dynamic coefficient of friction from the artificial grass surface to the porplastic SW and an additional 30% decrease with the addition of the loose granulate. The shoes varied in their ranking depending on the surface tested except on the porplastic SW and the porplastic F with loose granulate, where outsole material had no influence. The normal force applied was linearly related to the friction coefficient for the porplastic H and F surfaces, but not for the artificial grass surface. The friction coefficient approached a linear relationship with increased weight applied to the shoe and was assumed to reach a linear relationship for normal forces above 200 N. The authors assumed the presence of Coulomb friction (i.e., linearly related) for all five shoes in the remainder of the test conditions. The frictional behavior of the tested shoes was concluded to be independent of velocity and weight (except

artificial grass at normal forces below 200 N) on these commonly used tennis surfaces.

Nigg and Denoth measured the coefficients of static and sliding friction in 1980 for five different surfaces and three styles of shoewear.[299] Results indicated that the sliding coefficient was slightly less than the static coefficient and the relationship remained constant for speeds up to 10 m/sec. The dynamic, or sliding, coefficient of friction ranged from a low of 0.3 on sand (clay) with an indoor tennis shoe or a treaded jogging shoe to a high of 1.20 on a polyvinylchloride floor with an all-around shoe (see Table 30C–9). Nigg expanded on this work in 1986 and has used these studies to emphasize the dominant role of the playing surface on the translational friction coefficient, although he acknowledged the open question of whether the structure, the material, or both are most responsible for the result.[293]

In a separate study, Nigg and Denoth measured torque for 12 subjects rotating 180 degrees on one leg on seven different sport surfaces and with eight different types of shoes.[303] Mean values for the different surfaces are shown in Figure 30C–27. The range varied from 20 Nm to 38 Nm, the highest torque being found on artificial grass. In an expanded study using average torque for five tested surfaces (10 Nm to 20 Nm) and average torque for ten tested shoes (13 Nm to 18 Nm), Nigg proposed that torque was shoe and surface codependent to a greater degree than translational friction.[293] In attempting to correlate the material tests for translational friction with the subject tests for rotational friction, Yeadon and Nigg found no relationship.[444] This study clarified the difficulty of combining material and subject tests, as occurs also in tests of impact load, in which the subject's response to a test condition may alter the result.[296]

In 1996, Heidt and associates examined the shoe-surface interaction of 15 different football shoes made by three manufacturers in both anterior translation and rotation using a specially designed pneumatic testing system.[171] The shoes tested included traditional cleated football shoes, court shoes, molded-cleat shoes, and turf shoes. All shoes were tested on synthetic turf under wet and dry conditions and on natural stadium grass. This study found that spatting, which is protective taping of the ankle and heel applied on the outside of the shoe, reduced both translational and rotational forces. There was no difference found between shoes on grass versus AstroTurf. There were, however, significant differences for cleated and turf shoes. They found that shoes tested in conditions for which they were not designed exhibited reproducible friction characteristics (either too high or too low) that could have safety implications. They recommended that shoe manufacturers display suggested playing surface conditions for which their shoes are recommended.

With the specialization that has occurred in the sports shoe manufacturing industry, there is no doubt that we will continue to see specific shoes designed for specific sports, specific surfaces, specific player positions and weight, and specific game or event conditions. When this is done with player safety in mind, it is a laudable venture, and this is even true when improved performance is the goal. It does, however, raise some interesting questions. Does this put schools that cannot afford multiple types of shoes at a measurable disadvantage? Does it put athletes at greater risk for injury when they are not afforded the best shoe for a given game condition? Does the use of a shoe on surfaces for which it is not designed carry liability exposure for the school? Does there exist a shoe or surface that is "the best" for a particular sport?

Clinical Relevance

In 1980, Nigg and Denoth reported the results of a retrospective study of tennis injuries using a questionnaire.[299] Although only 25% of the questionnaires were returned, they assumed that the ratio of impairments per type of court surface was unaffected by the poor response rate. Using one tennis player during one 6-month season as a single case, they analyzed 2481 cases to determine the relationship between injury and playing surface. The foot and ankle were the most commonly affected area when ankle joint, Achilles tendon, heel, and sole cases were combined (Fig. 30C–42). The authors factored in the variation and frequency of play for the different surfaces by determining the relative frequency of pain per hour per week[305] (Table 30C–16). Their data showed that the lowest frequency of injury occurred on clay and synthetic clay surfaces, and a lower frequency of pain occurred on asphalt or concrete than on carpet or synthetic grill. Using this information, Nigg and Segesser speculated that the compliance of a surface is less important in tennis injuries than its frictional properties.[305]

Studies of the frictional properties of track surfaces have also yielded interesting insight on performance and injury. Stucke and colleagues pointed out the importance of static friction coefficients for starting efficiency in running events.[403] When the static coefficient of friction is small, shorter steps and less body lean are used. The authors measured the static coefficient of friction for starting, stopping, and turning during 100 trials using five subjects wearing the same shoe type. They found that the cinder track had an intermediate value between 0.65 and 1.72, compared with the synthetic outdoor surfaces' values of

TABLE 30C–16
Frequency and Relative Frequency of Pain in Tennis Players Related to Six Different Playing Surfaces

Surface	Frequency of Pain (%)	Relative Frequency (%/hour/week)
Clay	2.2	0.5
Synthetic sand	3.0	1.6
Synthetic surface	10.7	3.0
Asphalt	14.5	3.9
Felt carpet	14.8	4.8
Synthetic grill	18.0	3.8

From Nigg BM, Segesser B: The influence of playing surfaces on the load on the locomotor system and on football and tennis injuries. Sports Med 5: 375–385, 1988.

0.8 to 2.22 and the synthetic indoor surface values of 0.54 to 1.47 (Fig. 30C–43).

This study emphasizes the variability between surfaces by pointing out that an artificial surface does not automatically indicate a surface with greater frictional stresses. Changes in movement technique are influenced by the variation in surface friction properties. These changes are connected with different muscle work, varying stress on the body, and changes in energy expenditure that may affect both injury rate and performance. The authors speculate that the use of surfaces of varying frictional properties during training and competition is disadvantageous because of the time necessary to perfect a repertoire of movement skills to meet the requirements of different sport surfaces. This conclusion begs the question of whether it is preferable to train on one surface (e.g., natural grass) to reduce injury exposure when contests will be held on a different surface (e.g., artificial grass), or to train on the same surface on which the contest will be conducted with scheduled training in a sequence of graduated stress to allow proper adaptation by the body.

When frictional properties of a surface are too low, slipping can occur and injuries may result.[305] When the

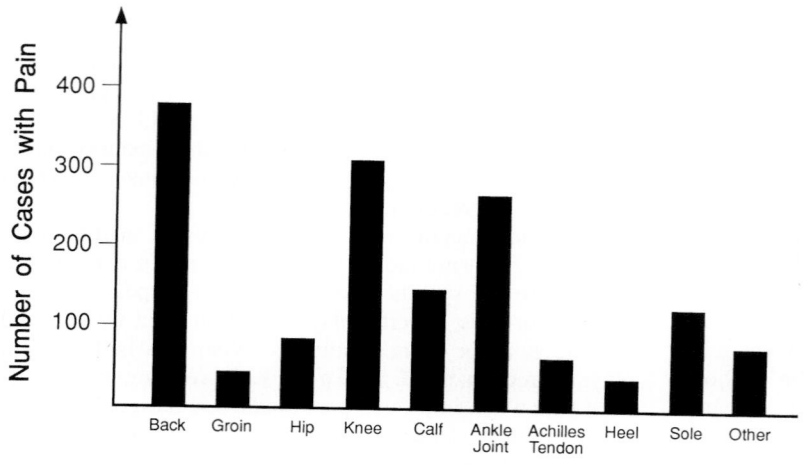

Figure 30C–42. Number of cases of tennis players with back and lower extremity pain by area of involvement. (From Nigg BM, Segesser B: The influence of playing surfaces on the load on the locomotor system and on football and tennis injuries. Sports Med 5:375–385, 1988.)

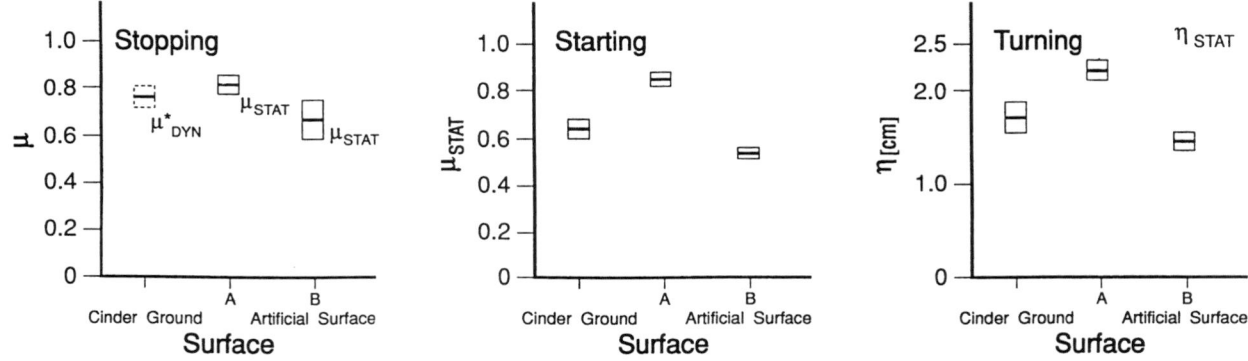

Figure 30C–43. Variation in coefficient of friction between three different track surfaces for starting, stopping, and turning. μ, coefficient of friction for translation; η, coefficient of friction for rotation; DYN, dynamic; STAT, static. (From Stucke H, Baudzus W, Baumann W: On friction characteristics of playing surfaces. In Frederick EC [ed]: Sport Shoes and Playing Surfaces. Champaign, Ill, Human Kinetics Publishers, 1984, pp 91–96. © Nike, Inc. Adapted and reprinted by permission.)

frictional resistance is too high, the load transference to the body may exceed its range of tolerance, resulting in injury. An optimal range in which both frictional overload and lack of traction are at acceptably low levels should exist. Ichii has suggested optimal ranges for the coefficient of translational friction for various sports.[305] He based his recommendations on both objective and subjective assessments, and the range was always between 0.5 and 0.7. Stussi and colleagues calculated the coefficients of static and sliding friction to be about 0.6 and 0.5, respectively, for clay; values on fabric courts approached 1.0.[404] Ankle strain is clearly reduced, according to Stussi and colleagues, during braking maneuvers on sandy surfaces as confirmed by both the force and electromyographic analysis. Stussi and associates acknowledged that greater performance demands might require increasing coefficients of friction and suggested that more stable shoe wear (e.g., with improved ankle support) might allow the player to tolerate the greater strain of the higher friction surfaces. They made no comment on the obvious question of how this would then affect the potentially increased strain on the knee (as occurred with the introduction of higher ski boots). Owing to the epidemiologic flaws in the study of tennis injuries by Nigg and coworkers, the final answer on the relationship between the frictional properties of playing surfaces and athletic injuries has not been determined, but the stage is certainly set for such a study.

Ice Sports

The sports of ice hockey and figure skating have enjoyed enormous growth in the United States and around the world over the past decade. These sports, with their unique footwear and playing surface, deserve special mention in any discussion of etiology of injury to the foot and ankle.

Ice hockey has evolved from a game traditionally played on frozen rivers and ponds to a game that today is played by more than a million people, from the frozen north of Canada to the sun and beaches of California and Florida. With its fast pace and aggressive action, hockey is a sport

in which participants are routinely exposed to the risk of injury. With increasing numbers of participants in hockey, those who care for athletes must be aware of the injuries that commonly occur in hockey, as well as their causes and prevention.

Similarly, figure skating has enjoyed an increase in popularity, owing mainly to the media exposure of the Olympic figure skating contest. With a significant portion of its participants being young females, figure skating poses many unique challenges to the physicians and trainers involved in the treatment of their injuries.[227] This section deals with the etiology of injuries in these two sports and includes a discussion of the recent literature regarding management and prevention of these injuries.

Ice Skates

Ice hockey and figure skating are unique sports because they require that their participants acquire a skill of locomotion unnatural to human beings. As such, skates are, arguably, the most important piece of equipment used by the hockey player or figure skater. The earliest skates, made of bone, were found in Sweden. Wooden skates with iron facings appeared in the 14th century, and skates made entirely of iron were introduced in the 17th century. Steel skates, with straps and clamps to fasten them to shoes, were sold in the 1850s and later became an integral part of the shoe. Skating has long been a means of travel in countries with long cold winters, such as Norway, Sweden, Finland, Russia, and especially Holland. There are references to skating in English books as early as the 12th century. By the early 18th century, skating was not only a means of travel but also a well-established sport.

Figure skates consist of three basic components: the boot, the blade, and the toe pick. As a rule of thumb, all boots have at least two thicknesses of leather—the outer skin and the lining. Higher end, more advanced boots have a three-piece construction, which consists of an extra layer of leather between the outer and inner layers. Boot manufacturers also use many different materials such as foam, plastic, and gel in order to vary the stiffness of their boots. Most competitive figure skaters use custom-fitted boots to ensure an exact fit. The type of boot and the boot's construction should correspond to the type of skating for which it is intended. In general, three-piece boots are recommended for freestyle figure skating, and two-piece boots are recommended for ice dancing.

Ice skating blades have three main design considerations: (1) rocker radius; (2) radius of hollow; and (3) toe pick design. The rocker radius of a blade is the actual curve of the blade from toe to heel and is expressed in feet. Generally, the rocker radius will vary from 6 to 8 feet or more depending on the blade and its intended application. A blade with a shorter radius will allow for easier turning; for this reason, short radius blades are a favorite choice of instructors for beginning freestylers. More advanced skaters who have developed a good feel for their edges will usually choose a blade of slightly larger radius, in the 7-foot range. The advantage of a larger radius is that the blade "runs" faster. That is to say, because there is a slightly larger section of the blade on the ice, the skater's body weight is being supported by a larger area of contact, thereby allowing the skate blade to glide over the ice faster.

The radius of hollow is the groove or the "U" on the blade. It is the depression between the inner and outer edges of the blade. The radius of hollow is expressed as a fraction—the smaller the fraction, the deeper the groove. Generally speaking, a beginning skater should start with a slightly flatter radius (e.g. ½ inch), and more advanced freestylers use 7/16 to 3/8 inch. Some dance skaters go even smaller, down to 5/16 inch.

Toe picks are unique to figure skates and are used both to initiate and terminate motion. Beginning level skaters should use less pronounced toe picks in order to avoid inadvertent digging into the ice. More advanced freestylers will typically have skates with larger toe picks in order to generate the enormous power needed for jumping and spinning. Dance blades still have toe picks of some size, but the lower picks are rounded off to prevent scratching the ice.[186]

Studies

As previously mentioned, both skates and the skating ice have changed significantly since humans first skated. Today's hockey players and skaters are skating on ice that is significantly softer, using skate blades that allow deeper penetration into the ice. Although this combination of softer ice and improved blade technology has improved the ability to stop, start, and turn more quickly and efficiently, it has theoretically exposed the skating athlete to a greater risk of injury. As with football and soccer players, in whom different cleat designs and patterns have been tested with respect to their interaction with the playing surface, it is important to determine the best combination of ice and skate blade so that performance can be maximized while minimizing the risk of injury.

Ice hockey is associated with many potential dangers because of the numerous contacts between players and collisions with sticks, pucks, and boards. One rarely thinks of foot and ankle injuries in such an aggressive sport as hockey where more serious injuries receive considerably more notoriety, but foot and ankle injuries do occur and can be season or career-ending, just as in other sports.

Molsa and Airaksinen performed a prospective epidemiologic study of ice hockey injuries in the two highest-level hockey programs in Finland in 1997.[275] The injuries were classified into three categories of severity: (1) minor, causing absence from practice or games for 0 to 7 days; (2) moderate, absence for 8 to 28 days; and (3) major, absence for more than 28 days. Injuries to the foot and ankle accounted for 12% of all sprain-type injuries in this study. More importantly, ankle injuries accounted for 10% of all major injuries in this study. This paper made several interesting and important observations. First, it was found that a greater number of injuries occurred at or near the end of the period or game. It was postulated that this might be due to an increase in intensity as the game progresses. Also, fatigue may influence a player's reaction time, thereby putting the player at increased risk for injury. Second, the majority of injuries occurred in areas of the body that were felt to have adequate protective equipment (58%). In only one case was there obviously defective equipment present at the injury site. This point emphasizes the need for continued research into improving protective equipment. Finally, foul play caused surprisingly few injuries in this study (9%). This point is contrary to the belief that foul play allowed by the referees is one of the most important reasons for injuries in ice hockey.

Smith and colleagues from the Mayo Clinic looked at the predictors of injury in ice hockey players from a multivariate, multidisciplinary point of view.[381] This prospective study of the incidence of injury in a season of high school ice hockey showed that high school hockey injuries were most strongly influenced by whether players experienced preseason perceived fatigue, were on the ice more during games than practices, were involved in collisions, and were in the high-playing-time group. Fatigue in this study was measured with a psychosocial screening test. Both preseason and midseason fatigue correlated with injuries, indicating that it was a very strong predictor of injuries. Fatigue is also a physical phenomenon. It was noted that after 20 seconds of "all out" skating, there is measurable decrease in stride efficiency. This may, in part, explain the increased injury rate experienced by players with the most playing time. Mair and associates studied the role of fatigue in susceptibility to acute muscle strain injuries.[243] They noted that fatigued muscles were less able to absorb energy before reaching the degree of stretch that causes injuries. This study underlines the importance of testing physical and psychosocial variables simultaneously in an integrated design in order to detect those at greatest risk for injury.

Ferrara and Schurr performed a study that looked at the relationship of position, mechanism of injury, type of injury, and body part injured to playing time lost due to an injury.[133] They did a causal analysis within a prospective cohort of seven schools from Hockey East and the Eastern Collegiate Athletic Conference for three consecutive competitive seasons. They found that the most important variable related to days lost was injury type. Fractures and dislocations resulted in an average of 22.22 days lost, and sprains resulted in an average of 13.61 days lost. In terms of mechanism of injury, direct impact with other players and the ice accounted for the greatest number of injuries. Also, impact with the puck, boards, and the goal resulted in a high number of days lost. The position played by the athlete had no statistical relationship to days lost owing to an injury. In this study, foot and ankle injuries accounted for 14% of the total number of injuries. Although other areas of the body were injured more frequently, injuries to the foot and ankle resulted in the largest number of mean days lost per injury.

Figure skating has an inherent risk of injury because of the high technical and physiologic demands on the young athletes involved. Muscular strength, flexibility, and explosive power are important requirements for successful figure skaters. Common causes of musculoskeletal injuries include inflexibility, asymmetrical or inadequate strength, inappropriate warm-up or cool-down, poor diet, fatigue, and overuse. The most common location of injuries for a figure skater is the foot; these injuries are often attributed to the boot. The United States Figure Skating Association is currently giving significant attention to injury prevention. A 4-year prospective study that began in 1991 found that approximately 50% of all injuries in ice dancers and pairs skaters could be prevented by early diagnosis of the injury and appropriate rehabilitation focusing on strength, flexibility, boot fitting, and decreased emotional stress.[227] Also, there are data showing that up to 78% of injuries may be prevented by comprehensive office conditioning programs. Data obtained from figure skating sports science camps have demonstrated that off-ice training programs can decrease stress fractures, overuse injuries, and ankle injuries, and increase ankle proprioception.

The boot and blade are the most important pieces of equipment of the figure skater. Unfortunately, they are often the cause of many injuries. Many clinicians believe that the boot, blade, and ice interface plays a crucial role in injury production. When new boots are stiff, they must be slowly and carefully broken in; if they are not, undue pressure points are created in the lower leg and foot, thereby putting the skater at risk for stress injury. The intrinsic stiffness of the boot transmits tremendous ground reaction forces when the skater lands a jump. Correct boot fit is of the utmost importance in injury prevention. The skater's boot should fit snugly around the heel and have a wide toe box. Orthotics, if required, can be built into a boot or created separately for insertion. When breaking in the boots, the skater should be sure that the tongue remains in a neutral position; often the tongue has a tendency to migrate laterally and cause increased pressure over the foot extensors. This can result in a troublesome tendinitis referred to as "skate-bite" or "lace-bite."

Studies in injury prevention in figure skaters have shown that it is useful to include a comprehensive foot and ankle program focusing on strength and proprioception in the skaters' overall training.[227] Some clinicians have suggested that young skaters wear less stiff boots in order to improve intrinsic ankle and foot strength and proprioception. In addition, this would force the skater to develop more precise technique because the boots would be less able to absorb the ground reaction forces.

Summary

This discussion of the etiologic factors involved in the foot and ankle injuries should introduce the concepts necessary to understand the injuries discussed in the remaining sections in this chapter. It is only after one understands the underlying causes of a problem that solutions are forthcoming. In the foot and ankle, as in no other area of the body, there is a direct interaction between anatomy and the environment—between flexibility or its lack as the anatomic constraint, between shoewear with its numerous effects as the immediate environment, and between the playing surface as the all-encompassing athletic milieu. As the reader investigates the specific injuries and pathologic conditions that beset athletes in sports, he or she should keep in mind the individual nature of these injuries and their potential risk factors. When causes are discovered, prevention is only a step behind.

References

1. Adkison JW, Requa RK, Garrick JG: Injury rates in high school football. A comparison of synthetic surfaces and grass fields. Clin Orthop 99:131–136, 1974.
2. Ahlberg A, Moussa M, Al-Nahdi M: On geographical variations in the normal range of joint motion. Clin Orthop 234:229–231, 1988.
3. Alles WF, Powell JW, Buckley W, Hunt EE: The national athletic injury/illness reporting system: 3-year findings of high school and college football injuries. J Orthop Sports Phys Ther 1:103–108, 1979.
4. Al-Rawi ZS, Al-Aszawi AJ, Al-Chalabi T: Joint mobility among university students in Iraq. Br J Rheum 24:326–331, 1985.
5. Alter MJ: The Science of Stretching. Champaign, Ill, Human Kinetics Books, 1988.
6. American Academy of Orthopaedic Surgeons: Joint Motion-Method of Measuring and Recording. Chicago, American Academy of Orthopaedic Surgeons, 1965, pp 68–71, 85.
7. American Medical Association: Guides to the Evaluation of Permanent Impairment, 3rd ed (revised). Chicago, American Medical Association, 1990, pp 58, 66.
8. Anderson LJ: Ligamentous laxity and athletics. JAMA 256:527, 1986.
9. Andréasson G, Lindenberger U, Renström P, Peterson L: Torque developed at simulated sliding between sport shoes and an artificial turf. Am J Sports Med 14:225–230, 1986.
10. Asken MJ, Schwartz RC: Heading the ball in soccer: What's the risk of brain injury? Physician Sportsmed 26, November 1998, http://www.physsportsmed.com/issues/1998/11nov/asken.htm.
11. Athletic Business. Madison, Wis, Athletic Business Publications, 1992.
12. Athletics. Encyclopaedia Britannica, Vol 1. Chicago, Encyclopaedia Britannica, 1987, pp 668–670.
13. Athletic shoe cushioning. Sport Research Review. Beaverton, Ore, Nike Sport Research Laboratory, Sept/Oct, 1988.
14. Backx FJG, Erich WBM, Kemper ABA, Verbeek ALM: Sports injuries in school-aged children. An epidemiologic study. Am J Sports Med 17:234–240, 1989.
15. Bahlsen HA, Nigg BM: Selection of a lateral test movement for tennis shoes. In Nigg BM, Kerr BA (eds): Biomechanical Aspects of Sport Shoes and Playing Surfaces. Calgary, University of Calgary Press, 1983, pp 169–176.
16. Baker J, Frankel VH, Burstein A: Fatigue fractures: Biomechanical considerations. J Bone Joint Surg Am 54:1345–1346, 1972.
17. Barnes RA, Smith PD: The role of footwear in minimizing lower limb injury. J Sports Sci 12:341–353, 1994.
18. Barrett JR, Tanji JL, Drake C, et al: High versus low-top shoes for the prevention of ankle sprains in basketball players: A prospective randomized study. Am J Sports Med 21:582–585, 1993.

19. Basketball. Encyclopaedia Britannica, Vol 28. Chicago, Encyclopaedia Britannica, 1987, pp 151–157.
20. Bates BT, DeVita P, Kinoshita H: The effect of intra-individual variability of sample size. In Nigg BM, Kerr BA (eds): Biomechanical Aspects of Sport Shoes and Playing Surfaces. Calgary, University of Calgary Press, 1983, pp 191–198.
21. Bates BT, Haven BH: Effects of fatigue on the mechanical characteristics of highly skilled female runners. In Nelson RC, Morehouse CA (eds): Biomechanics IV. Baltimore, University Park Press, 1974, pp 121–125.
22. Bates BT, Osternig LR, Mason B, James LS: Foot orthotic devices to modify selected aspects of lower extremity mechanics. Am J Sports Med 7:338–342, 1979.
23. Bates BT, Osternig LR, Sawhill JA: An assessment of subject variability, subject-shoe interaction, and the evaluation of running shoes using ground reaction force data. J Biomech 16:181–191, 1983.
24. Bates BT, Simpson KJ, Panzer VP: The evaluation of subject, shoe, and movement variability. In Jonsson B (ed): Biomechanics X-B. Champaign, Ill, Human Kinetics, 1987, pp 909–912.
25. Baylis WJ, Rzonca EC: Functional and structural limb length discrepancies: Evaluation and treatment. Clin Podiatr Med Surg 5:509–520, 1988.
26. Beaulieu JE: Developing a stretching program. Physician Sportsmed 9:59–69, 1981.
27. Beighton PH, Horan FT: Dominant inheritance in familial generalised articular hypermobility. J Bone Joint Surg Br 52:145–147, 1970.
28. Beighton P, Solomon L, Soskolne CL: Articular mobility in an African population. Ann Rheum Dis 32:413–418, 1973.
29. Berger-Vachon C, Gabard G, Moyen B: Soccer accidents in the French Rhone-Alps Soccer Association. Sports Med 3:69–77, 1986.
30. Bernhang AM, Winslett G: Equestrian injuries. Physician Sportsmed 11:90–97, 1983.
31. Berson BL, Passoff TL, Nagelberg S, et al: Injury patterns in squash players. Am J Sports Med 6:323–325, 1978.
32. Biener K, Calvori P: Tennissportunfulle [Sports accidents of tennis players]. Med Klin 72:754–757, 1977.
33. Bixby-Hammett DM: Youth accidents with horses. Physician Sportsmed 13:105–117, 1985.
34. Blair SN, Kohl HW, Goodyear NN: Rates and risks for running and exercise injuries: Studies in three populations. Res Q 58:221–228, 1987.
35. Blake RL, Denton JA: Functional foot orthoses for athletic injuries: A retrospective study. J Am Podiatr Med Assoc 75:359–362, 1985.
36. Blitzer CM, Johnson RJ, Ettlinger CF, et al: Downhill skiing injuries in children. Am J Sports Med 12:142–147, 1984.
37. Blyth CS, Mueller FO: Football injury survey: Part 1. When and where players get hurt. Physician Sportsmed 2:45–52, 1974.
38. Blyth CS, Mueller FO: Football injury survey: Part 2. Identifying the causes. Physician Sportsmed 2:71–78, 1974.
39. Blyth CS, Mueller FO: Football injury survey: Part 3. Injury rates vary with coaching. Physician Sportsmed 2:45–50, 1974.
40. Bodziak WJ: Manufacturing processes for athletic shoe outsoles and their significance in the examination of footwear impression evidence. J Forensic Sci 31:153–176, 1986.
41. Bohannon RW, Tiberio D, Zito M: Selected measures of ankle dorsiflexion range of motion: Differences and intercorrelations. Foot Ankle 10:99–103, 1989.
42. Bojsen-Møller F, Lamoreux L: Significance of free dorsiflexion of the toes in walking. Acta Orthop Scand 50:471–479, 1979.
43. Bonnin JG: Injuries to the Ankle. London, William Heinemann Medical Books, 1950, pp 47–48.
44. Bonstingl RW, Morehouse CA, Niebel BW: Torques developed by different types of shoes on various playing surfaces. Med Sci Sports Exerc 7:127–131, 1975.
45. Boone DC, Azen SP: Normal range of motion of joints in male subjects. J Bone Joint Surg Am 61:756–759, 1979.
46. Bot SDM, van Mechelen W: The effect of ankle bracing on athletic performance. Sports Med 27:171–178, 1999
47. Bouter LM, Knipschild PG, Volovics A: Personal and environmental factors in relation to injury risk in downhill skiing. Int J Sports Med 10:298–301, 1989.
48. Bowers KD Jr: Ankle and knee injuries at West Virginia University before and after Astro Turf. West Virginia Med J 69:1–3, 1973.
49. Bowers KD Jr, Martin RB: Impact absorption, new and old

AstroTurf at West Virginia University. Med Sci Sports 6:217–221, 1974.
50. Bowers KD Jr, Martin RB: Cleat-surface friction on new and old Astroturf. Med Sci Sports 7:132–135, 1975.
51. Bowers KD Jr, Martin RB: Turf-toe: A shoe-surface related football injury. Med Sci Sports 8:81–83, 1976.
52. Bramwell ST, Masuda M, Wagner NN, Holmes TH: Psychosocial factors in athletic injuries: Development and application of the Social and Athletic Readjustment Rating Scale (SARRS). J Human Stress 1:6–20, 1975.
53. Bramwell ST, Requa RK, Garrick JG: High school football injuries: A pilot comparison of playing surfaces. Med Sci Sports 4:166–169, 1972.
54. Brantigan JW, Pedegana LR, Lippert FG: Instability of the subtalar joint. Diagnosis by stress tomography in three cases. J Bone Joint Surg Am 59:321–324, 1977.
55. Breo DL: Of MDs and muscles—lessons from two "retired steroid doctors." JAMA 263:1697–1705, 1990.
56. Brizuela G, Llana S, Ferrandis R, Garcia-Belenguer AC: The influence of basketball shoes with increased ankle support on shock attenuation and performance in running and jumping. J Sports Sci 15:505–515, 1997
57. Brody DM: Running injuries. CIBA Clinical Symposia 32:1–36, 1980.
58. Brody DM: Running injuries—prevention and management. CIBA Clinical Symposia 39:1–36, 1987.
59. Brown RB: Personality characteristics related to injury in football. Res Q 42:133–138, 1971.
60. Brown EW, McKeag DB: Training, experience, and medical history of pairs skaters. Physician Sportsmed 15:101–114, 1987.
61. Burgess I, Ryan MD: Bilateral fatigue fractures of the distal fibulae caused by a change of running shoes. Med J Austral 143:304–305, 1985.
62. Burrows HJ: Fatigue fractures of the fibula. J Bone Joint Surg Br 30:266–279, 1948.
63. Butler JE, Brown SL, McConnell BG: Subtrochanteric stress fractures in runners. Am J Sports Med 10:228–232, 1982.
64. Cahill BR, Griffith EH: Effect of preseason conditioning on the incidence and severity of high school football knee injuries. Am J Sports Med 6:180–184, 1978.
65. Caine D, Cochrane B, Caine C, et al: An epidemiologic investigation of injuries affecting young competitive female gymnasts. Am J Sports Med 17:811–820, 1989.
66. Cameron BM, Davis O: The swivel football shoe: A controlled study. Am J Sports Med 1:16–27, 1973.
67. Canale ST, Cantler ED, Sisk TD, Freeman BL: A chronicle of injuries of an American intercollegiate football team. Am J Sports Med 9:384–389, 1981.
68. Caplan A, Carlson B, Faulkner J, et al: Skeletal muscle. In Woo SL-Y, Buckwalter JA (eds): Injury and Repair of the Musculoskeletal Soft Tissues. Park Ridge, Ill, American Academy of Orthopaedic Surgeons, 1988, pp 213–291.
69. Carter C, Sweetnam R: Recurrent dislocation of the patella and of the shoulder. Their association with familial joint laxity. J Bone Joint Surg 42:721–727, 1960.
70. Carter C, Wilkinson J: Persistent joint laxity and congenital dislocation of the hip. J Bone Joint Surg Br 46:40–45, 1964.
71. Cavagna GA: Storage and utilization of elastic energy in skeletal muscle. Exerc Sport Sci Rev 5:89–129, 1977.
72. Cavanagh PR: The Running Shoe Book. Mountain View, Calif, Anderson World, 1980.
73. Cavanagh PR: The biomechanics of lower extremity action in distance running. Foot Ankle 7:197–217, 1987.
74. Cavanagh PR: The biomechanics of running and running shoe problems. In Segesser B, Pförringer W (eds): The Shoe in Sport. Chicago, Year Book, 1989, pp 3–15.
75. Cavanagh PR: Biomechanics of Distance Running. Champaign, Ill, Human Kinetics, 1990.
76. Cavanagh PR, Kram R: Stride length in distance running: Velocity, body dimensions, and added mass effects. In Cavanagh PR (ed): Biomechanics of Distance Running. Champaign, Ill, Human Kinetics, 1990, pp 35–63.
77. Cavanagh PR, Kram R: The efficiency of human movement—a statement of the problem. Med Sci Sports Exerc 17:304–308, 1985.
78. Cavanagh PR, Lafortune MA: Ground reaction forces in distance running. J Biomech 13:397–406, 1980.

79. Cheskin MP: The Complete Handbook of Athletic Footwear. New York, Fairchild Publications, 1987.

80. Clancy WG Jr: Symposium: Runners' injuries. Part one. Am J Sports Med 8:137–138, 1980.

81. Clancy WG Jr: Specific rehabilitation for the injured recreational runner. Instr Course Lect 38:483–486, 1989.

82. Clancy WG Jr: Tendinitis and plantar fasciitis in runners. In D'Ambrosia RD, Drez D Jr (eds): Prevention and Treatment of Running Injuries, 2nd ed. Thorofare, NJ, Slack, 1989, pp 121–131.

83. Clanton TO: Athletic injuries to the soft tissues of the foot and ankle. In Coughlin MJ, Mann RA (eds): Surgery of the Foot and Ankle, 7th ed. St Louis, Mosby, 1999.

84. Clanton TO, Butler JE, Eggert A: Injuries to the metatarsophalangeal joints in athletes. Foot Ankle 7:162–176, 1986.

85. Clanton TO, Ford JJ: Turf toe injury. Clin Sports Med 13:731–741, 1994

86. Clanton TO, Schon LC, Baxter DE: An overview of subtalar instability and its treatment. Perspectives Orthop Surg 1:103–113, 1990.

87. Clarke KS: Premises and pitfalls of athletic injury surveillance. Am J Sports Med 3:292–295, 1976.

88. Clarke TE, Frederick EC, Cooper LB: Biomechanical measurement of running shoe cushioning properties. In Nigg BM, Kerr BA (eds): Biomechanical Aspects of Sport Shoes and Playing Surfaces. Calgary, The University of Calgary Press, 1983, pp 25–33.

89. Clarke TE, Frederick EC, Hamill C: The effects of shoe design parameters on rearfoot control in running. Med Sci Sports 15:376–381, 1983.

90. Clarke TE, Frederick EC, Hamill C: The study of rearfoot movement in running. In Frederick EC (ed): Sport Shoes and Playing Surfaces. Biomechanical Properties. Champaign, Ill, Human Kinetics, 1984, pp 166–189.

91. Clement DB, Taunton JE, Smart GW, McNicol KL: A survey of overuse running injuries. Physician Sportsmed 9:47–58, 1981.

92. Coker TP, Arnold JA, Weber DL: Traumatic lesions of the metatarsophalangeal joint of the great toe in athletes. Am J Sports Med 6:326–334, 1978.

93. Conrad NL: Cleated shoe problems. An observation. J Am Podiatr Assoc 72:352–353, 1982.

94. Cook SD, Kester MA, and Brunet ME: Shock absorption characteristics of running shoes. Am J Sports Med 13:248–253, 1985.

95. Cook SD, Kester MA, Brunet ME, Haddad RJ Jr: Biomechanics of running shoe performance. Clin Sports Med 4:619–626, 1985.

96. Corbin CB: Flexibility. Clin Sports Med 3:101–117, 1984.

97. Coughlin MJ: Subluxation and dislocation of the second metatarsophalangeal joint. Orthop Clin North Am 20:535–551, 1989.

98. Council on Scientific Affairs: Drug abuse in athletes. Anabolic steroids and human growth hormone. JAMA 259:1703–1705, 1988.

99. Cuin DE: Design and construction of a tuned track. In Frederick EC (ed): Sport Shoes and Playing Surfaces. Biomechanical Properties. Champaign, Ill, Human Kinetics, 1984, pp 163–165.

100. Culpepper MI, Niemann KMW: An investigation of the shoe-turf interface using different types of shoes on Poly-turf and Astro-turf: Torque and release coefficients. Alabama J Med Sci 20:387–390, 1983.

101. Culpepper MI, Niemann KMW: High school football injuries in Birmingham, Alabama. South Med J 76:873–875, 878, 1983.

102. Cureton TK: Flexibility as an aspect of physical fitness. Res Q 12:381–390, 1941.

103. Cureton TK Jr: Physical Fitness of Champion Athletes. Urbana, Ill, The University of Illinois Press, 1951.

104. Daffner RH, Martinez S, Gehweiler JA: Stress fractures in runners. JAMA 247:1039–1041, 1982.

105. Dagiau RF, Dillman CJ, Milner EK: Relationship between exposure time and injury in football. Am J Sports Med 8:257–260, 1980.

106. D'Ambrosia RD: Orthotic devices in running injuries. Clin Sports Med 4:611–618, 1985.

107. Davis MW, Litman T, Crenshaw RW: Bicycling injuries. Physician Sportsmed 8:88–96, 1980.

108. DeHaven KE, Lintner DM: Athletic injuries: Comparison by age, sport, and gender. Am J Sports Med 14:218–224, 1986.

109. Deland JT, Sung IH: The medial crossover toe: A cadaveric dissection. Foot Ankle Int 21:375–378, 2000.

110. DeLee JC: Fractures and dislocations of the foot. In Mann RA (ed): Surgery of the Foot, 5th ed. St Louis, CV Mosby, 1986, p 746.

111. DeLee JC, Curtis R: Subtalar dislocation of the foot. J Bone Joint Surg Am 64:433–437, 1982.

112. DeLee JC, Farney WC: Incidence of injury in Texas high school football. Am J Sports Med 20:575–580, 1992.

113. Denoth J: Load on the locomotor system and modelling. In Nigg BM (ed): Biomechanics of Running Shoes. Champaign, Ill, Human Kinetics, 1986, pp 63–116.

114. Denoth J: Indoor athletic playing surfaces—floor vs. shoe. In Segesser B, Pförringer W (eds): The Shoe in Sport. Chicago, Year Book, 1989, pp 65–69.

115. Devas MB, Sweetnam R: Stress fractures of the fibula. A review of fifty cases in athletes. J Bone Joint Surg Br 38:818–829, 1956.

116. DeVries HA: Evaluation of static stretching procedures for improvement of flexibility. Res Q 33:222–229, 1962.

117. DeVries HA: Physiology of Exercise for Physical Education and Athletics, 3rd ed. Dubuque, Iowa, Wm C Brown, 1980.

118. DeWit B, DeClerq D, Aerts P: Biomechanical analysis of the stance phase during barefoot and shoe running. J Biomech 33:269–278, 2000.

119. Donatelli R, Hurlbert C, Conaway D, St Pierre R: Biomechanical foot orthotics: A retrospective study. J Orthop Sports Phys Ther 10:205–212, 1988.

120. Dowling PA: Prospective study of injuries in United States Ski Association freestyle skiing: 1976–77 to 1979–80. Am J Sports Med 10:268–275, 1982.

121. Drinkwater BL, Bruemner B, Chesnut CH III: Menstrual history as a determinant of current bone density in young athletes. JAMA 263:545–548, 1990.

122. Dufek JS, Bates BT: The evaluation and prediction of impact forces during landings. Med Sci Sports 22:370–377, 1990.

123. Edington CJ, Frederick EC, Cavanagh PR: Rearfoot motion in distance running. In Cavanagh PR (ed): Biomechanics of Distance Running. Champaign, Ill, Human Kinetics, 1990, pp 135–164.

124. Eggert K: First metatarsophalangeal joint range of motion as a factor in turf toe injuries. Master's thesis, University of Houston, 1991.

125. Ekstrand J, Gillquist J: The frequency of muscle tightness and injuries in soccer players. Am J Sports Med 10:75–78, 1982.

126. Ekstrand J, Gillquist J: The avoidability of soccer injuries. Int J Sports Med 4:124–128, 1983.

127. Ekstrand J, Gillquist J: Soccer injuries and their mechanisms: A prospective study. Med Sci Sports Exerc 15:267–270, 1983.

128. Ekstrand J, Gillquist J, Liljedahl SO: Prevention of soccer injuries. Supervision by doctor and physiotherapist. Am J Sports Med 11:116–120, 1983.

129. Ellis J: The myth of oversupination. Runner's World 25:52–54, 1990.

130. Falsetti HL, Burke ER, Feld RD, et al: Hematological variations after endurance running with hard- and soft-soled running shoes. Physician Sportsmed 11:118–127, 1983.

131. Feriencik K: Trends in ice hockey injuries 1965–1977. Physician Sportsmed 7:81–84, 1979.

132. Ferkel RD, Mai LL, Ullis KC, et al: An analysis of roller skating injuries. Am J Sports Med 10:24–30, 1981.

133. Ferrera MS, Schurr KT: Intercollegiate ice hockey injuries: A causal analysis. Clin J Sports Med 9:30–33, 1999.

134. Finkelstein H: Joint hypotonia with congenital and familial manifestations. NY State Med J 104:942–944, 1916.

135. Fleishman EA: The Structure and Measurement of Physical Fitness. Englewood Cliffs, NJ, Prentice-Hall, 1964.

136. Frederick EC (ed): Sports Shoes and Playing Surfaces. Biomechanical Properties. Champaign, Ill, Human Kinetics, 1984.

137. Frederick EC, Clarke TE, Hamill CL: The effect of running shoe design on shock attenuation. In Frederick EC (ed): Sport Shoes and Playing Surfaces. Biomechanical Properties. Champaign, Ill, Human Kinetics, 1984, pp 190–198.

138. Freeman MAR, Dean MRE, Hanham IWF: The etiology and prevention of functional instability of the foot. J Bone Joint Surg Br 47:679–685, 1965.

139. Fyhrie DP, Milgrom C, Hoshaw SJ, et al: Effect of fatiguing exercise on longitudinal bone strain as related to stress fracture in humans. Ann Biomed Eng 26:660–665, 1998.

140. Garfinkel D, Talbot AA, Clarizio M, et al: Medical problems on a professional baseball team. Physician Sportsmed 9:85–93, 1981.

141. Garrick JG: Ballet injuries. Med Probl Perform Arts 1:123–127, 1986.

142. Garrick JG: Characterization of the patient population in a sports medicine facility. Physician Sportsmed 13:73–76, 1985.

143. Garrick JG, Gillien DM, Whiteside P: The epidemiology of aerobic dance injuries. Am J Sports Med 14:67–72, 1986.

144. Garrick JG, Requa RK: Role of external support in the prevention of ankle sprains. Med Sci Sports 5:200–203, 1972.

145. Garrick JG, Requa RK: Epidemiology of women's gymnastics injuries. Am J Sports Med 8:261–262, 1980.

146. Garrick JG, Requa R: Medical care and injury surveillance in the high school setting. Physician Sportsmed 9:115–120, 1981.

147. Garrick JG, Requa RK: The epidemiology of foot and ankle injuries in sports. Clin Sports Med 7:29–36, 1988.

148. Gilbert RS, Johnson HA: Stress fractures in military recruits—a review of twelve years' experience. Mil Med 131:716–721, 1966.

149. Gleim GW, McHugh MP: Flexibility and its effects on sports injury and performance. Sports Med 24:289–299, 1997.

150. Gleim GW, Stachenfeld NS, Nicholas JA: The influence of flexibility on the economy of walking and jogging. J Orthop Res 8:814–823, 1990.

151. Glick JM, Gordon RB, Nishimoto D: The prevention and treatment of ankle injuries. Am J Sports Med 4:136–141, 1976.

152. Godshall RW: Junior league football: Risks vs benefits. Am J Sports Med 3:139–144, 1975.

153. Godshall RW: The predictability of athletic injuries: An eight-year study. Am J Sports Med 3:50–54, 1975.

154. Gottlieb G, White JR: Responses of recreational runners to their injuries. Physician Sportsmed 8:145–149, 1980.

155. Grahame R: Joint hypermobility—clinical aspects. Proc R Soc Med 64:692–694, 1971.

156. Grahame R, Jenkins JM: Joint hypermobility—asset or liability? A study of joint mobility in ballet dancers. Ann Rheum Dis 31:109–111, 1972.

157. Grana WA, Moretz JA: Ligamentous laxity in secondary school athletes. JAMA 240:1975–1976, 1978.

158. Greaney RB, Gerber FH, Laughlin RL, et al: Distribution and natural history of stress fractures in U.S. marine recruits. Radiology 146:339–346, 1983.

159. Greece. Encyclopaedia Britannica, Vol 20. Chicago, Encyclopaedia Britannica, 1987, p 375.

160. Greene TA, Hillman SK: Comparison of support provided by a semirigid orthosis and adhesive ankle taping before, during, and after exercise, Am J Sports Med 18:498–506, 1990.

161. Gross RH: Leg length discrepancy in marathon runners. Am J Sports Med 11:121–124, 1983.

162. Gross TS, Bunch RP: A mechanical model of metatarsal stress fracture during distance running. Am J Sports Med 17:669–674, 1989.

163. Gymnasium. Encyclopaedia Britannica, Vol 5. Chicago, Encyclopaedia Britannica, 1987, pp 590–591.

164. Haberl R, Prokop L: Physiological aspects of synthetic tracks. Foot motions during support phase of various running types on different track materials. Biotelemetry 1:171–178, 1974.

165. Hale RW, Mitchell W: Football injuries in Hawaii 1979. Hawaii Med J 40:180–183, 1981.

166. Halpern B, Thompson N, Curl WW, et al: High school football injuries: Identifying the risk factors. Am J Sports Med 15:316–320, 1987.

167. Hamilton WG: Foot and ankle injuries in dancers. Clin Sports Med 7:143–173, 1988.

168. Hartig DE, Henderson JM: Increasing hamstring flexibility decreases lower extremity overuse injuries in military basic trainees. Am J Sports Med 27:173–176, 1999.

169. Harvey J: This cleat could be pivotal. Sports Illus 65:W4, 1987.

170. Hattori K, Ohta S: Ankle joint flexibility in college soccer players. J Human Ergol 15:85–89, 1986.

171. Heidt RS Jr, Dormer SG, Cawley PW, et al: Differences in friction and torsional resistance in athletic shoe-turf surface interfaces. Am J Sports Med 24:834–842, 1996.

172. Helzlsouer KJ, Hayden FG, Rogol AD: Severe metabolic complications in a cross-country runner with sickle cell trait. JAMA 249:777–779, 1983.

173. Henry JH, Lareau B, Neigut D: The injury rate in professional basketball. Am J Sports Med 10:16–18, 1982.

174. Hertel J: Functional instability following lateral ankle sprain. Sports Med 29:361–371, 2000.

175. Hicks JH: The mechanics of the foot. I. The joints. J Anat 87:345–357, 1953.

176. Hirata I Jr: The Hanley cleat and the Ivy League: A progress report. J Am Coll Health 17:369–370, 1969.

177. Hirata I Jr: Proper playing conditions. Am J Sports Med 2:228–234, 1974.

178. Hoff GL, Martin TA: Outdoor and indoor soccer: Injuries among youth players. Am J Sports Med 14:231–233, 1986.

179. Hoffman P: Conclusions drawn from a comparative study of the feet of barefooted and shoe-wearing peoples. Am J Orthop Surg 3:105–136, 1905.

180. Hooper G, McMaster MJ: Recurrent bilateral mid-tarsal subluxations. J Bone Joint Surg Am 61:617–619, 1979.

181. Horan FT, Beighton PH: Recessive inheritance of generalized joint hypermobility. Rheum Rehab 12:47–49, 1973.

182. Hosea TM, Carey CC, Harrer HF: The gender issue: Epidemiology of ankle injuries in athletes who participate in basketball. Clin Orthop 372:45–49, 2000.

183. Houston Sports Association: Inside the Astrodome. Houston, Houston Sports Association, 1965.

184. Hubley-Kozey CL, Stanish WD: Can stretching prevent athletic injuries? J Musculoskeletal Med 7:21–31, 1990.

185. Hummel G, Gainor BJ: Waterskiing-related injuries. Am J Sports Med 10:215–218, 1982.

186. Ice Skating Institute website www.skateisi.com, May, 2000.

187. Inman VT: The Joints of the Ankle. Baltimore, Williams & Wilkins, 1976.

188. Jackson A, Glasgow M: Tarsal hypermobility after ankle fusion—fact or fiction? J Bone Joint Surg Br 61:470–473, 1979.

189. Jackson DW, Jarrett H, Bailey D, et al: Injury prediction in the young athlete: A preliminary report. Am J Sports Med 6:6–14, 1978.

190. James SL, Bates BT, Osternig LR: Injuries to runners. Am J Sports Med 6:40–50, 1978.

191. Janda DH, Wojtys EM, Hankin FM, Benedict ME: Softball sliding injuries. A prospective study comparing standard and modified bases. JAMA 259:1848–1850, 1988.

192. Janda DH, Wojtys EM, Hankin FM, et al: A three-phase analysis of the prevention of recreational softball injuries. Am J Sports Med 18:632–635, 1990.

193. Jessee EF, Owen DS Jr, Sagar KB: The benign hypermobile joint syndrome. Arthritis Rheum 23:1053–1056, 1980.

194. Johnson GR, Dowson D, Wright V: A biomechanical approach to the design of football boots. J Biomech 9:581–585, 1976.

195. Johnson GR, Dowson D, Wright V: Ankle loading and football boots. Rheum Rehab 15:194–196, 1976.

196. Johnson RJ, Ettlinger CF, Campbell RJ, et al: Trends in skiing injuries: Analysis of a 6-year study (1972–1978). Am J Sports Med 8:106–113, 1980.

197. Johnson WO: The tyranny of phony fields. Sports Illus 63:34–42, 1985.

198. Joseph J: Range of movement of the great toe in men. J Bone Joint Surg Br 36:450–457, 1954.

199. Kannus P, Aho H, Jarvinen M, Nittymaki S: Computerized recording of visits to an outpatient sports clinic. Am J Sports Med 15:79–85, 1987.

200. Kaufman KR, Brodine SK, Shaffer RA, et al: The effect of foot structure and range of motion on musculoskeletal overuse injuries. Am J Sports Med 27:585–593, 1999.

201. Keene JS, Narechania RG, Sachtjen KM, Clancy WG: Tartan Turf on trial: A comparison of intercollegiate football injuries occurring on natural grass and Tartan Turf. Am J Sports Med 8:43–47, 1980.

202. Keller CS, Noyes FR, Buncher CR: The medical aspects of soccer injury epidemiology. Am J Sports Med 15:230–237, 1987.

203. Kelley EJ, Kalenak A: Knowledge obsolescence: The need for sports medicine education among physical educators and coaches. Am J Sports Med 3:277–281, 1975.

204. Kerr G, Fowler B: The relationship between psychological factors and sports injuries. Sports Med 6:127–134, 1988.

205. Key JA: Hypermobility of joints as a sex linked hereditary characteristic. JAMA 88:1710–1712, 1927.

206. Kibler WB, Goldberg C, Chandler TJ: Functional biomechanical deficits in running athletes with plantar fasciitis. Am J Sports Med 19:66–71, 1991.

207. Kiburz D, Jacobs R, Reckling F, et al: Bicycle accidents and injuries among adult cyclists. Am J Sports Med 14:416–419, 1986.

208. Kim HK, Kerr RG, Cruz TF, Salter RB: Effects of continuous passive motion and immobilization on synovitis and cartilage degradation in antigen induced arthritis. J Rheumatol 22:1714–1721, 1995.

209. Klemp P, Chalton D: Articular mobility in ballet dancers. A follow-up study after four years. Am J Sports Med 17:72–75, 1989.
210. Klemp P, Stevens JE, Isaacs S: A hypermobility study in ballet dancers. J Rheum 11:692–696, 1984.
211. Komi PV, Gollhofer A, Schmidtbleicher D, Frick U: Interaction between man and shoe in running: Considerations for a more comprehensive measurement approach. Int J Sports Med 8:196–202, 1987.
212. Krahenbuhl GS: Speed of movement with varying footwear conditions on synthetic turf and natural grass. Res Q 45:28–33, 1974.
213. Kraus H: Backache, Stress, and Tension. Their Cause, Prevention and Treatment. New York, Simon and Schuster, 1965.
214. Kreipe RE, Gewanter HL: Physical maturity screening for participation in sports. Pediatrics 75:1076–1080, 1985.
215. Krivickas LS: Anatomical factors associated with overuse sports injuries. Sports Med 24:132–146, 1997.
216. Kulund DN, Dewey JB, Brubaker CE, et al: Olympic weight lifting injuries. Physician Sportsmed 6:111–119, 1978.
217. Kuland DN, Tottossy M: Warm-up, strength, and power. Orthop Clin North Am 14:427–448, 1983.
218. Kvist M, Kujala UM, Heinonen OJ, et al: Sports-related injuries in children. Int J Sports Med 10:81–86, 1989.
219. Kwong PK, Kay D, Voner RT, White MW: Plantar fasciitis. Mechanics and pathomechanics of treatment. Clin Sports Med 7:119–126, 1988.
220. Laeuger MJ, Ryan RE, Deichmann JB: Final Report on Athletic Shoe Testing System. Report submitted to The Tanel Corporation. Milwaukee, Wis, The University of Wisconsin, 1985.
221. Larson RL, Osternig LR: Traumatic bursitis and artificial turf. Am J Sports Med 2:183–188, 1974.
222. Laws K: Physics and the potential for dance injury. Med Probl Perform Art 1:73–79, 1986.
223. Levy IM, Skovron ML, Agel J: Living with artificial grass: A knowledge update. Part 1: Basic science. Am J Sports Med 18:406–412, 1990.
224. Lichtor J: The loose-jointed young athlete: Recognition and treatment. Am J Sports Med 1:22–23, 1972.
225. Lieblich L: Statistics, lies and citations. N Engl J Med 296:178, 1977.
226. Light LH, McLellan GE, Klenerman L: Skeletal transients on heel strike in normal walking with different footwear. J Biomech 13:477–480, 1980.
227. Lipetz J, Kruse RJ: Injuries and special concerns of female figure skaters. Clin Sports Med 19:369–380, 2000.
228. Lok V, Yuceturk G: Injuries of wrestling. J Sports Med 2:324–328, 1975.
229. Lombardo SJ, Benson DW: Stress fractures of the femur in runners. Am J Sports Med 10:219–227, 1982.
230. Luethi SM, Frederick EC, Hawes MR, Nigg BM: Influence of shoe construction on lower extremity kinematics and load during lateral movements in tennis. Int J Sports Biomech 2:166–174, 1986.
231. Lundberg A: Kinematics of the ankle and foot. In vivo roentgen stereophotogrammetry. Acta Orthop Scand 60(Suppl 233):1–24, 1989.
232. Lutter LD: Orthopaedic management of runners. In Bateman JE, Trott AW (eds): The Foot and Ankle. New York, Thieme-Stratton, 1980, pp 155–158.
233. Lutter LD: Cavus foot in runners. Foot Ankle 1:225–228, 1981.
234. Lutter LD: Running athlete in office practice. Foot Ankle 3:53–59, 1982.
235. Lynch AF, Bourne RB, Rorabeck CH: The long-term results of ankle arthrodesis. J Bone Joint Surg Br 70:113–116, 1988.
236. Lysens RJ, Ostyn MS, Vanden Auweele Y, et al: The accident-prone and overuse-prone profiles of the young athlete. Am J Sports Med 17:612–619, 1989.
237. Lysens R, Steverlynck A, Vanden Auweele Y, et al: The predictability of sports injuries. Sports Med 1:6–10, 1984.
238. Lysholm J, Wiklander J: Injuries in runners. Am J Sports Med 15:168–171, 1987.
239. MacDougall D, Sale D: Continuous vs. interval training: A review for the athlete and the coach. Can J Appl Sport Sci 6:93–97, 1981.
240. Macera CA, Pate RR, Powell KE, et al: Predicting lower-extremity injuries among habitual runners. Arch Intern Med 149:2565–2568, 1989.
241. Macpherson K, Sitler M, Kimura I, et al: Effects of a semirigid and softshell prophylactic ankle stabilizer on selected performance tests among high school football players. J Orthop Sports Phys Ther 21:147–152, 1995.
242. Main BJ, Jowett RL: Injuries of the midtarsal joint. J Bone Joint Surg Br 57:89–97, 1975.
243. Mair SD, Seaber AV, Glisson RR, Garrett WE Jr: The role of fatigue in susceptibility to acute muscle strain injury. Am J Sports Med 24:137–143, 1996.
244. Mann RA: Biomechanics of running. In D'Ambrosia RD, Drez D Jr (eds): Prevention and Treatment of Running Injuries, 2nd ed. Thorofare, NJ, Slack, 1989, pp 1–20.
245. Mann RA, Baxter DE, Lutter LD: Running symposium. Foot Ankle 1:190–224, 1981.
246. Mann RA, Clanton TO: Hallux rigidus: Treatment by cheilectomy. J Bone Joint Surg Am 70:400–406, 1988.
247. Mann RA, Coughlin MJ: Hallux valgus and complications of hallux valgus. In Mann RA (ed): Surgery of the Foot, 5th ed. St Louis, CV Mosby, 1986, pp 70–71.
248. Manter JT: Movements of the subtalar and transverse tarsal joints. Anat Rec 80:397–410, 1941.
249. Marti B, Vader JP, Minder CE, et al: On the epidemiology of running injuries: The 1984 Bern Grand-Prix study. Am J Sports Med 16:285–294, 1988.
250. Martin RK, Yesalis CE, Foster D, Albright JP: Sports injuries at the 1988 Junior Olympics. An epidemiologic analysis. Am J Sport Med 15:603–608, 1987.
251. Masson M, Hess H: Typical soccer injuries—their effects on the design of the athletic shoe. In Segesser B, Pförringer W (eds): The Shoe in Sport. Chicago, Year Book, 1989, pp 89–95.
252. Matheson GO, Clement DB, McKenzie DC, et al: Stress fractures in athletes. A study of 320 cases. Am J Sports Med 15:46–58, 1987.
253. Mazur JM, Schwartz E, Simon SR: Ankle arthrodesis. Long-term follow-up with gait analysis. J Bone Joint Surg Am 61:964–975, 1979.
254. McAuley E, Hudash G, Shields K, et al: Injuries in women's gymnastics: The state of the art. Am J Sports Med 15:558–565, 1987.
255. McBryde AM Jr: Stress fracture in runners. In D'Ambrosia RD, Drez D Jr (eds): Prevention and Treatment of Running Injuries, 2nd ed. Thorofare, NJ, Slack, 1989, pp 43–82.
256. McCarroll JR, Gioe TJ: Professional golfers and the price they pay. Physician Sportsmed 10:64–70, 1982.
257. McCarroll JR, Rettig AC, Shelbourne KD: Injuries in the amateur golfer. Physician Sportsmed 18:122–126, 1990.
258. McLennan JG, Ungersma J: Mountaineering accidents in the Sierra Nevada. Am J Sports Med 11:160–163, 1983.
259. McMahon TA, Greene PR: The influence of track compliance on running. J Biomech 12:893–904, 1979.
260. McMahon TA, Greene PR: Fast running tracks. Sci Am 239:148–163, 1978.
261. McMahon TA, Greene PR: The influence of track compliance on running. In Frederick EC (ed): Sport Shoes and Playing Surfaces. Biomechanical Properties. Champaign, Ill, Human Kinetics, 1984, pp 138–162.
262. McMaster M: Disability of the hindfoot after fracture of the tibial shaft. J Bone Joint Surg Br 58:90–93, 1976.
263. McNeal AP, Watkins A, Clarkson PM, Tremblay I: Lower extremity alignment and injury in young, preprofessional, college and professional ballet dancers. Part II: Dancer-reported injuries. Med Probl Perform Art 5:83–88, 1990.
264. McNitt-Gray JL: Landing strategy adjustments made by female gymnasts in response to drop height and mat composition. J Appl Biomech 9:173–190, 1991.
265. Meyers MC, Elledge JR, Sterling JC, et al: Injuries in interscholastic rodeo athletes. Am J Sports Med 18:87–91, 1990.
266. Micheli LJ: Overuse injuries in children's sports: The growth factor. Orthop Clin North Am 14:337–360, 1983.
267. Micheli LJ, Riseborough EM: The incidence of injuries in rugby football. J Sports Med 2:93–98, 1974.
268. Milburn PD, Barry EB: Shoe-surface interaction and the reduction of injury in rugby union. Sports Med 25:319–327, 1998.
269. Milgrom C, Finestone A, Levi Y, et al: Do high impact exercises produce higher tibial strains than running? Br J Sports Med 34:195–199, 2000.
270. Milgrom C, Giladi M, Simkin A, et al: The normal range of subtalar

inversion and eversion in young males as measured by three different techniques. Foot Ankle 6:143–145, 1985.

271. Milgrom C, Shlamkovitch N, Finestone A, et al: Risk factors for the lateral ankle sprain: A prospective study among military recruits. Foot Ankle 12:26–30, 1991.

272. Millar AP: An early stretching routine for calf muscle strains. Med Sci Sports 8:39–42, 1976.

273. Miller DI: Ground reaction forces in distance running. In Cavanagh PR (ed): Biomechanics of Distance Running. Champaign, Ill, Human Kinetics, 1990, pp 203–224.

274. Mizel MS, Yodlowski ML: Disorders of the lesser metatarsophalangeal joints. J Am Acad Orthop Surg 3:166–173, 1995.

275. Molsa J, Airaksinen O, Nasman O, Torstila I: Ice hockey injuries in Finland. A prospective epidemiologic study. Am J Sports Med 25:495–499, 1997.

276. Montgomery LC, Nelson FRT, Norton JP, Deuster PA: Orthopedic history and examination in the etiology of overuse injuries. Med Sci Sports 21:237–243, 1989.

277. Moretz A III, Grana WA: High school injuries. Physician Sportsmed 6:92–95, 1978.

278. Morgan CD, Henke JA, Bailey RW, Kaufer H: Long-term results of tibiotalar arthrodesis. J Bone Joint Surg Am 67:546–550, 1985.

279. Mueller FO, Blyth CS: North Carolina high school football injury study: Equipment and prevention. Am J Sports Med 2:1–10, 1974.

280. Mueller FO, Blyth CS: A Survey of 1981 college lacrosse injuries. Physician Sportsmed 10:87–93, 1982.

281. 1982–00 NCAA Participation Statistics Report. URL http://www.ncaa.org/participation_rates/.

282. Nelson WE, DePalma B, Gieck JH, et al: Intercollegiate lacrosse injuries. Physician Sportsmed 10:86–92, 1981.

283. Newell SG, Woodle A: Cuboid syndrome. Physician Sportsmed 9:71–76, 1981.

284. Nicholas JA: Injuries to knee ligaments. Relationship of looseness and tightness in football players. JAMA 212:2236–2239, 1970.

285. Nicholas JA: Risk factors, sports medicine and the orthopedic system: An overview. Am J Sports Med 3:243–259, 1976.

286. Nicholas JA: Report of the Committee on Research and Education. Am J Sports Med 6:295–304, 1978.

287. Nicholas JA, Grossman RB, Hershman EB: The importance of a simplified classification of motion in sports in relation to performance. Orthop Clin North Am 8:499–532, 1977.

288. Nicholas JA, Rosenthal PP, Gleim GW: A historical perspective of injuries in professional football. Twenty-six years of game-related events. JAMA 260:939–944, 1988.

289. Nielson AB, Yde J: Epidemiology and traumatology of injuries in soccer. Am J Sports Med 17:803–807, 1989.

290. Nigg BM: Biomechanics, load analysis and sports injuries in the lower extremities. Sports Med 2:367–379, 1985.

291. Nigg BM: Biomechanical aspects of running. In Nigg BM (ed): Biomechanics of Running Shoes. Champaign, Ill, Human Kinetics, 1986, pp 1–25.

292. Nigg BM: Biomechanics of Running Shoes. Champaign, Ill, Human Kinetics, 1986.

293. Nigg BM: Experimental techniques used in running shoe research. In Nigg BM (ed): Biomechanics of Running Shoes. Champaign, Ill, Human Kinetics, 1986, pp 27–61.

294. Nigg BM: Some comments for runners. In Nigg BM (ed): Biomechanics of Running Shoes. Champaign, Ill, Human Kinetics, 1986, pp 161–165.

295. Nigg BM: The assessment of loads acting on the locomotor system in running and other sport activities. Semin Orthop 3:197–206, 1988.

296. Nigg BM: The validity and relevance of tests used for the assessment of sports surfaces. Med Sci Sports 22:131–139, 1990.

297. Nigg BM, Bahlsen AH, Denoth J, et al: Factors influencing kinetic and kinematic variables in running. In Nigg BM (ed): Biomechanics of Running Shoes. Champaign, Ill, Human Kinetics, 1986, pp 139–159.

298. Nigg BM, Bahlsen HA, Luethi SM, Stokes S: The influence of running velocity and midsole hardness on external impact forces in heel-toe running. J Biomech 20:951–959, 1987.

299. Nigg BM, Denoth J, Kerr B, et al: Load sport shoes and playing surfaces. In Frederick EC (ed): Sport Shoes and Playing Surfaces. Biomechanical Properties. Champaign, Ill, Human Kinetics, 1984, pp 1–23.

300. Nigg BM, Frederick EC, Hawes MR, Luethi SM: Factors influencing short-term pain and injuries in tennis. Int J Sports Biomech 2:156–165, 1986.

301. Nigg BM, Herzog W, Read LJ: Effect of viscoelastic shoe insoles on vertical impact forces in heel-toe running. Am J Sports Med 16:70–76, 1988.

302. Nigg BM, Khan A, Fisher V, Stefanyshyn D: Effect of shoe insert construction on foot and leg movement. Med Sci Sports Exerc 30:550–555, 1998.

303. Nigg BM, Luethi SM, Bahlsen HA: The tennis shoe—biomechanical design criteria. In Segesser B, Pförringer W (eds): The Shoe in Sport. Chicago, Year Book, 1989, pp 39–46.

304. Nigg BM, Morlock M: The influence of lateral heel flare of running shoes on pronation and impact forces. Med Sci Sports 19:294–302, 1987.

305. Nigg BM, Segesser B: The influence of playing surfaces on the load on the locomotor system and on football and tennis injuries. Sports Med 5:375–385, 1988.

306. Nigg BM, Yeadon MR: Biomechanical aspects of playing surfaces. J Sport Sci 5:117–145, 1987.

307. Nuber GW: Biomechanics of the foot and ankle during gait. Clin Sports Med 7:1–13, 1988.

308. Oatis C: Biomechanics of the foot and ankle under static conditions. Physical Ther 68:1815–1821, 1988.

309. Olson OC: The Spokane Study: High school football injuries. Physician Sportsmed 7:75–82, 1979.

310. Olympic Games. Encyclopaedia Britannica, Vol 25. Chicago, Encyclopaedia Britannica, 1987, pp 197–201.

311. Ouzounian TJ, Shereff MJ: In vitro determination of midfoot motion. Foot Ankle 10:140–146, 1989.

312. Pardon ET: Lower extremities are site of most soccer injuries. Physician Sportsmed 5:43–48, 1977.

313. Park RD, Castaldi CR: Injuries in junior ice hockey. Physician Sportsmed 8:81–90, 1980.

314. Perlik PC, Kalvoda DD, Wellman AS, et al: Roller-skating injuries. Physician Sportsmed 10:76–80, 1982.

315. Petras AF, Hoffman EP: Roentgenographic skeletal injury patterns in parachute jumping. Am J Sports Med 11:325–328, 1983.

316. Petrov O, Blocher K, Bradbury RL, et al: Footwear and ankle stability in the basketball player. Clin Podiatr Med Surg 5:275–290, 1988.

317. Physical Education. Encyclopaedia Britannica, Vol 9. Chicago, Encyclopaedia Britannica, 1987, pp 412–413.

318. Physical tests. Sport Research Review. Beaverton, Ore, Nike Sport Research Laboratory, Jan/Feb, 1990.

319. Pino EC, Colville MR: Snowboard injuries. Am J Sports Med 17:778–781, 1989.

320. Playground-related injuries in preschool-aged children—United States, 1983–1987. JAMA 260:2799–2800, 1988.

321. Powell JW, Schootman M: A multivariate risk analysis of selected playing surfaces in the National Football League: 1980 to 1989. An epidemiologic study of knee injuries. Am J Sports Med 20:686–694, 1992.

322. Powell KE, Kohl HW, Caspersen CJ, Blair SN: An epidemiological perspective on the causes of running injuries. Physician Sportsmed 14:100–114, 1986.

323. Prager BI, Fitton WL, Cahill BR, Olson GH: High school football injuries: A prospective study and pitfalls of data collection. Am J Sports Med 17:681–685, 1989.

324. R&D Advanced Manufacturing. Mondo home page. URL http://www.mondousa.com/

325. Radin EL, Eyre D, Kelman JL, Schiller AL: Effect of prolonged walking on concrete on the joints of sheep. Arthritis Rheum 22:649, 1980.

326. Radin EL, Orr RB, Kelman JL, et al: Effect of prolonged walking on concrete on the knees of sheep. J Biomech 15:487–492, 1982.

327. Read M: Overstretched. Br J Sports Med 23:257–258, 1989.

328. Rearfoot stability. Sport Research Review. Beaverton, Ore, Nike Sport Research Laboratory, Nov/Dec, 1989.

329. Reddin P: Internal Audit Review of Artificial Turf. Jan 7, 2000. URL http://www.roundrockisd.org/rrweb/bondturf.htm/

330. Reid J: The real mean green. Texas Monthly, Dec. 1979, pp 153–156, 259–266.

331. Renström P, Johnson RJ: Overuse injuries in sports: A review. Sports Med 2:316–333, 1985.

332. Requa R, Garrick JG: Injuries in interscholastic wrestling. Physician Sportsmed 9:44–51, 1981.

333. Rheinstein DJ, Morehouse CA, Niebel BW: Effects on traction of outsole composition and hardnesses of basketball shoes and three types of playing surfaces. Med Sci Sports 10:282–288, 1978.
334. Richmond DA, Shafar J: A case of bilateral fatigue fracture of the fibula. Br Med J 1:264–265, 1955.
335. Robbins S, Waked E: Factors associated with ankle injuries. Preventive measures. Sports Med 25:63–72, 1998
336. Robbins S, Waked EG: Humans amplify impact to compensate for instability caused by shoe sole materials. Arch Phys Med Rehabil 78:463–467, 1997.
337. Robbins SE, Gouw GJ: Athletic footwear and chronic overloading. A brief review. Sports Med 9:76–85, 1990.
338. Robbins SE, Gouw GJ: Athletic footwear: Unsafe due to perceptual illusions. Med Sci Sports 23:217–224, 1991.
339. Robbins SE, Hanna AM: Running-related injury prevention through barefoot adaptations. Med Sci Sports 19:148–156, 1987.
340. Robbins S, Waked E, Rappel R: Ankle taping improves proprioception before and after exercise in young men. Br J Sports Med 29:242–249, 1995.
341. Rodeo SA, O'Brien S, Warren RF, et al: Turf-toe: An analysis of metatarsophalangeal joint sprains in professional football players. Am J Sports Med 18:280–285, 1990.
342. Romash MM, Fugate D, Yanklowit B: Passive motion of the first metatarsal cuneiform joint: Preoperative assessment. Foot Ankle 10:293–298, 1990.
343. Rothenberger LA, Chang JI, Cable TA: Prevalence and types of injuries in aerobic dancers. Am J Sports Med 16:403–407, 1988.
344. Rovere GD, Clarke TJ, Yates CS, et al: Retrospective comparison of taping and ankle stabilizers in preventing ankle injuries. Am J Sports Med 16:228–233, 1988.
345. Rovere GD, Webb LX, Gristina AG, et al: Musculoskeletal injuries in theatrical dance students. Am J Sports Med 11:195–198, 1983.
346. Rowe ML: Varsity football. Knee and ankle injury. NY State J Med 69:3000–3003, 1969.
347. Roy SP: Intercollegiate wrestling injuries. Physician Sportsmed 7:83–91, 1979.
348. Ryan AJ: The concept of physical fitness. In Ryan AJ (ed): Sports Medicine. New York, Academic Press, 1974, pp 31–55.
349. Ryan AJ: The Physician and Sportsmedicine Guide to Running. New York, McGraw-Hill, 1980.
350. Safran MR, Garrett WE Jr, Seaber AV, et al: The role of warmup in muscular injury prevention. Am J Sports Med 16:123–129, 1988.
351. Safran MR, Seaber AV, Garrett WE Jr: Warm-up and muscular injury prevention. An update. Sports Med 8:239–249, 1989.
352. Salter RB: History of rest and motion and the scientific basis for early continuous passive. motion. Hand Clin 12:1–11, 1996.
353. Sammarco GJ: Biomechanics of the foot. In Frankel VH, Nordin M (eds): Basic Biomechanics of the Skeletal System. Philadelphia, Lea & Febiger, 1980, pp 193–219.
354. Sammarco GJ, Burstein AJ, Frankel VH: Biomechanics of the ankle: A kinematic study. Orthop Clin North Am 4:75–96, 1973.
355. Sarrafian SK: Anatomy of the Foot and Ankle. Philadelphia, JB Lippincott, 1983, pp 375–425.
356. Saunders AJS, El Sayed TF, Hilson AJW, et al: Stress lesions of the lower leg and foot. Clin Radiol 30:649–651, 1979.
357. Schafle MD, Requa RK, Patton WL, Garrick JG: Injuries in the 1987 National Amateur Volleyball Tournament. Am J Sports Med 18:624–631, 1990.
358. Schier MJ: Houston MD tackles football injuries. Texas Med 69:106–109, 1973.
359. Schlaepfer F, Unold E, Nigg BM: The frictional characteristics of tennis shoes. In Nigg BM, Kerr BA (eds): Biomechanical Aspects of Sport Shoes and Playing Surfaces. Calgary, The University of Calgary Press, 1983, pp 153–160.
360. Schwartz RP, Heath AL, Misiek W: The influence of the shoe on gait. J Bone Joint Surg 17:406–418, 1935.
361. Schwartz RP, Heath AL, Misiek W, Wright JN: Kinetics of human gait. The making and interpretation of electrobasographic records of gait. The influence of rate of walking and the height of shoe heel on duration of weight-bearing on the osseous tripod of the respective feet. J Bone Joint Surg 16:343–350, 1934.
362. Schwellnus MP, Jordaan G, Noakes TD: Prevention of common overuse injuries by the use of shock absorbing insoles. A prospective study. Am J Sports Med 18:636–641, 1990.
363. Scott D, Bird H, Wright V: Joint laxity leading to osteoarthrosis. Rheum Rehab 18:167–169, 1979.
364. Scott SH, Winter DA: Internal forces at chronic running injury sites. Med Sci Sports Exerc 22:357–369, 1990.
365. Scranton PE Jr, Whitesel JP, Powell JW, et al: A review of selected noncontact anterior cruciate ligament injuries in the National Football League. Foot Ankle Int 18:772–776, 1997.
366. Segesser B, Pförringer W: The Shoe in Sport. Chicago, Year Book, 1989.
367. Shangold M, Rebar RW, Wentz AC, Schigg I: Evaluation and management of menstrual dysfunction in athletes. JAMA 263:1665–1669, 1990.
368. Shapiro MS, Kabo JM, Mitchell PW, et al: Ankle sprain prophylaxis: An analysis of the stabilizing effects of braces and tape. Am J Sports Med 22:78–82, 1994.
369. Shellock FG, Prentice WE: Warming-up and stretching for improved physical performance and prevention of sports-related injuries. Sports Med 2:267–278, 1985.
370. Sim FH, Simonet WT, Melton LJ, Lehn TA: Ice hockey injuries. Am J Sports Med 15:30–40, 1987.
371. Simkin A, Leichter I, Giladi M, et al: Combined effect of foot arch structure and an orthotic device on stress fractures. Foot Ankle 10:25–29, 1989.
372. Sitler M, Ryan J, Wheeler B, et al: The efficacy of semirigid ankle stabilizer to reduce acute ankle injuries in basketball. A randomized clinical study at West Point. Am J Sports Med 22:454–461, 1994.
373. Skovron ML, Levy IM, Agel J: Living with artificial grass: A knowledge update. Part 2: Epidemiology. Am J Sports Med 18:510–513, 1990.
374. Slocum DB: Overuse syndromes of the lower leg and foot in athletes. Instr Course Lect 17:359–367, 1960.
375. Slocum DB, James SL: Biomechanics of running. JAMA 205:97–104, 1968.
376. Smith AM, Stuart MJ, Wiese-Bjornstal DM, Gunnon C: Predictors of injury in ice hockey players. A multivariate, multidisciplinary approach. Am J Sports Med 25:500–507, 1997.
377. Smith LS, Bunch R: Athletic footwear. Clin Podiatr Med Surg 3:637–647, 1986.
378. Smith AD, Micheli LJ: Injuries in competitive figure skaters. Physician Sportsmed 10:36–47, 1982.
379. Smith LS, Clarke TE, Hamill CL, Santopietro F: The effects of soft and semi-rigid orthoses upon rearfoot movement in running. J Am Podiatr Med Assoc 76:227–233, 1986.
380. Smith RW, Reischl SF: Treatment of ankle sprains in young athletes. Am J Sports Med 14:465–471, 1986.
381. Smith RW, Reischl SF: Metatarsophalangeal joint synovitis in athletes. Clin Sports Med 7:75–88, 1988.
382. Snook GA: Injuries in intercollegiate wrestling: A five year study. Am J Sports Med 10:142–144, 1982.
383. Soderstrom CA, Doxanas MT: Racquetball: A game with preventable injuries. Am J Sports Med 10:180–183, 1982.
384. Sohl P, Bowling A: Injuries to dancers. Sports Med 9:317–322, 1990.
385. Spiegl PV, Johnson KA: Heel pain syndrome: Which treatments to choose? J Musculoskeletal Med 1:66–71, 1984.
386. Sports Injuries. Accident Facts. Report of the National Safety Council, 1990, p 88.
387. Sports injuries and footwear. Sport Research Review. Beaverton, Ore, Nike Sport Research Laboratory, Nov/Dec, 1988.
388. SportsTURF. Chicago, Ill, Adams Business Media, 2001.
389. Sports Turf Managers Association. URL http://www.sports-turfmanager.com/
390. Stacoff A, Kaelin X: Pronation and sportshoe design. In Nigg BM, Kerr BA (eds): Biomechanical Aspects of Sport Shoes and Playing Surfaces. Calgary, The University of Calgary Press, 1983, pp 143–151.
391. Stacoff A, Kaelin X: Technological and biomechanical criteria of the court shoe. In Segesser B, Pförringer W (eds): The Shoe in Sport. Chicago, Year Book, 1989, pp 77–86.
392. Stacoff A, Kalin X, Stussi E: The effects of shoes on the torsion and rearfoot motion in running. Med Sci Sports 23:482–490, 1991.
393. Stacoff A, Luethi SM: Special aspects of shoe construction and foot anatomy. In Nigg BM (ed): Biomechanics of Running Shoes. Champaign, Ill, Human Kinetics, 1986, pp 117–137.
394. Stanitski CL: Common injuries in preadolescent and adolescent athletes. Recommendations for prevention. Sports Med 7:32–41, 1989.

395. Stanitski CL: Pediatric sports injuries. Adv Orthop Surg 9:53–57, 1985.

396. Stanitski CL, McMaster JH, Ferguson RJ: Synthetic turf and grass: A comparative study. Am J Sports Med 2:22–26, 1974.

397. Stefanyshyn DJ, Nigg BM: Influence of midsole bending stiffness on joint energy and jump height performance. Med Sci Sports Exerc 32:471–476, 2000.

398. Steiner ME: Hypermobility and knee injuries. Physician Sportsmed 15:159–165, 1987.

399. Stewart MJ, Beeler TC, McConnell JC: Compression arthrodesis of the ankle. Evaluation of a cosmetic modification. J Bone Joint Surg Am 65:219–225, 1983.

400. Stewart SF: Footgear—Its history, uses and abuses. Clin Orthop 88:119–130, 1972.

401. Stewart SF: Human gait and the human foot: An ethnological study of flatfoot. Clin Orthop 70:111–123, 1970.

402. Stott JRR, Hutton WC, Stokes IAF: Forces under the foot. J Bone Joint Surg Br 55:335–344, 1973.

403. Stucke H, Baudzus W, Baumann W: On friction characteristics of playing surfaces. In Frederick EC (ed): Sport Shoes and Playing Surfaces. Biomechanical Properties. Champaign, Ill, Human Kinetics, 1984, pp 87–97.

404. Stussi A, Stacoff A, Tiegermann V: Rapid sideward movements in tennis. In Segesser B, Pförringer W (eds): The Shoe in Sport. Chicago, Year Book, 1989, pp 53–62.

405. Stussi E, Denoth J, Muller R, Stacoff A: Sports medicine and rehabilitation. Surface and footwear. Orthopade 26:993–998, 1997.

406. Subotnick SI: The short-leg syndrome. Physician Sportsmed 3:61–63, 1975.

407. Sullivan JA: Outdoor and indoor soccer: Injuries among youth players. Am J Sports Med 14:231–233, 1986.

408. Sutherland GW: Fire on ice. Am J Sports Med 4:264–269, 1976.

409. Sutro CJ: Hypermobility of bones due to "overlengthened" capsular and ligamentous tissues. A cause for recurrent intra-articular effusions. Surgery 21:67–76, 1947.

410. Taerk GS: The injury-prone athlete: A psychosocial approach. J Sports Med 17:187–194, 1977.

411. Taimela S, Kujala UM, Osterman K: Intrinsic risk factors and athletic injuries. Sports Med 9:205–215, 1990.

412. Tancred WR, Barnett E: Injuries and different playing surfaces. Sheffield, UK, University of Sheffield, 1989.

413. Tanel Corporation. Personal communication, 1991.

414. Taunton JE, McKenzie DC, Clement DB: The role of biomechanics in the epidemiology of injuries. Sports Med 6:107–120, 1988.

415. Taylor DC, Dalton JD Jr, Seaber AV, Garrett WE Jr: Viscoelastic properties of muscle-tendon units. The biomechanical effects of stretching. Am J Sports Med 18:300–309, 1990.

416. Temple C: Hazards of jogging and marathon running. Br J Hosp Med 29:237–239, 1983.

417. Tennis. The New Encyclopaedia Britannica, Vol 28. Chicago, Encyclopaedia Britannica, 1987, pp 164–169.

418. Thompson N, Halpern B, Curl WW, et al: High school football injuries: Evaluation. Am J Sports Med 15:117–124, 1987.

419. Tomczak RL, Wilshire WM, Lane JW, et al: Injury patterns in rock climbers. J Osteopath Sports Med 3:11–16, 1989.

420. Torg JS: Athletic footwear and orthotic appliances. Clin Sports Med 1:157–175, 1982.

421. Torg JS, Quedenfeld T: Effect of shoe type and cleat length on incidence and severity of knee injuries among high school football players. Res Q 42:203–211, 1971.

422. Torg JS, Quedenfeld T: Knee and ankle injuries traced to shoes and cleats. Physician Sportsmed 1:39–43, 1973.

423. Torg JS, Quedenfeld TC, Landau S: Football shoes and playing surfaces: From safe to unsafe. Physician Sportsmed 1:51–54, 1973.

424. Torg JS, Quedenfeld TC, Landau S: The shoe-surface interface and its relationship to football knee injuries. Am J Sports Med 2:261–269, 1974.

425. Torg JS, Stilwell G, Rogers K: The effect of ambient temperature on the shoe-surface interface release coefficient. Am J Sports Med 24:79–82, 1996.

426. Trott AW: The normal human foot—what is it? In Bateman JE, Trott AW (eds): The Foot and Ankle. New York, Thieme-Stratton, 1980, pp 1–4.

427. Tursz A, Crost M: Sports-related injuries in children: A study of their characteristics, frequency, and severity, with comparison to other types of accidental injuries. Am J Sports Med 14:294–299, 1986.

428. Underwood J: Turf: Just an awful toll. Sports Illus 63:48–62, 1985.

429. Van Gheluwe B, Deporte E, Hebbelinck M: Frictional forces and torques of soccer shoes on artificial turf. In Nigg BM, Kerr BA (eds): Biomechanical Aspects of Sport Shoes and Playing Surfaces. Calgary, The University of Calgary Press, 1983, pp 161–168.

430. Voloshin AS: Shock absorption during running and walking. J Am Podiatr Assoc 78:295–299, 1988.

431. Voloshin A, Wosk J, Brull M: Force wave transmission through the human locomotor system. J Biomech Eng 103:48–50, 1981.

432. Walsh WM, Blackburn T: Prevention of ankle sprains. Am J Sports Med 5:243–245, 1977.

433. Walter SD, Hart LE, McIntosh JM, Sutton JR: The Ontario Cohort Study of running-related injuries. Arch Intern Med 149:2561–2564, 1989.

434. Walter SD, Sutton JR, McIntosh JM, Connolly C: The aetiology of sports injuries. A review of methodologies. Sports Med 2:47–58, 1985.

435. Washington EL: Musculoskeletal injuries in theatrical dancers: Site, frequency, and severity. Am J Sports Med 6:75–98, 1978.

436. Watson AWS: Sports injuries during one academic year in 6799 Irish school children. Am J Sports Med 12:65–71, 1984.

437. Weseley MS, Koval R, Kleiger B: Roentgen measurement of ankle flexion-extension motion. Clin Orthop 65:167–174, 1969.

438. Whitney LF: Inheritance of double-jointedness of thumb. J Hered 23:425–426, 1932.

439. Whittle MW: Generation and attenuation of transient impulsive forces beneath the foot: A review. Gait Posture 10:264–275, 1999.

440. Wiktorsson-Möller M, Oberg B, Ekstrand J, Gillquist J: Effects of warming up, massage, and stretching on range of motion and muscle strength in the lower extremity. Am J Sports Med 11:249–252, 1983.

441. Williams JM, Moran M, Thonar EJ, Salter RB: Continuous passive motion stimulates repair of rabbit knee articular cartilage after matrix proteoglycan loss. Clin Orthop 304:252–262, 1994.

442. Winge S, Jorgensen U, Nielsen AL: Epidemiology of injuries in Danish championship tennis. Int J Sports Med 10:368–371, 1989.

443. Wright DG, Desai SM, Henderson WH: Action of the subtalar and ankle-joint complex during the stance phase of walking. J Bone Joint Surg Am 46:361–382, 464, 1964.

444. Yeadon MR, Nigg BM: A method for the assessment of area-elastic surfaces. Med Sci Sports 20:403–407, 1988.

445. Year 2000 Participation—Ranked by Total Participation. The National Sporting Goods Association. URL http://www.nsga.org/public/articles/details.cfm?id=28

446. Zaricznyj B, Shattuck LJ, Mast TA, et al: Sports-related injuries in school-aged children. Am J Sports Med 8:318–324, 1980.

447. Zelisko JA, Noble HB, Porter M: A comparison of men's and women's professional basketball injuries. Am J Sports Med 10:297–299, 1982.

448. Zemper ED: Injury rates in a national sample of college football teams: A 2-year prospective study. Physician Sportsmed 17:100–113, 1989.

449. Zwipp H, Krettek C: Diagnostik und Therapie der akuten und chronischen Bandinstabilität des unteren Sprunggelenkes [Diagnosis and therapy of acute and chronic ligament instability of the transverse tarsal joint]. Orthopade 15:472–478, 1986.

Section D
Sports Shoes and Orthoses

Andrew H. Borom, MD ■ Thomas O. Clanton, MD

There should be little surprise that an entire section of one chapter would be devoted to a discussion of sports shoes. The athletic shoewear industry has grown to such an extent that it has reached one of the pinnacles of achievement in our society—the front cover of *Sports Illustrated* (Fig. 30D–1).[251] With this achievement, both increasing recognition from Wall Street investors and harsh criticism alleging consumer exploitation surfaced.[174, 185, 229] Sports shoes became "high-tech" and rode a wave of advertising to become a status symbol.[229, 264] Among today's youth, the "right" shoe may vary from week to week. Athletic shoe sales rose to approach $8 billion in 1998, with fully half of that total brought in by the top two athletic shoe manufacturers. Not surprisingly, the top retailer of athletic shoes spent more on promotions and advertisements (some $163.2 million) than the next nine producers combined.[112] Major shoewear manufacturers have paid six-figure salaries to high-profile athletes and coaches to endorse their products.[147, 229] Financial benefits from shoe contracts have become a major consideration for college athletic programs and their coaches.[147] In this distorted environment, it is often difficult to wade through the hype to discover the contributions of merit in shoewear

technology. This section attempts to do just that. A foundation of relatively stable information is provided to guide the reader through this subject despite the constant changes fueled by fashion trends and advertising gimmickry as well as scientific research. To understand where we are and where we are headed, some historical perspective is necessary.

History

The history of sports shoes parallels the history of shoewear itself. According to legend, shoes were originally designed after an Arab chief dismounted from his camel onto a thorn and declared that all the earth would be covered with leather. Seeing the error in this logic, the chief's main advisor decided to make something that would cover just the feet. Although this makes a good story, it has not been supported by the discovery of shoes in the Fertile Crescent.[19] Indeed, the earliest footwear was discovered in south central Oregon in 1932 by anthropologist Luther Cressman—a sandal made from sagebrush bark (Fig. 30D–2).[19, 31] This find dates back 10,000 years to pre-Columbian times, but design features indicate a much earlier origin. It supports the notion that the shoe's primary function is to protect the sole from the hazards of the environment.

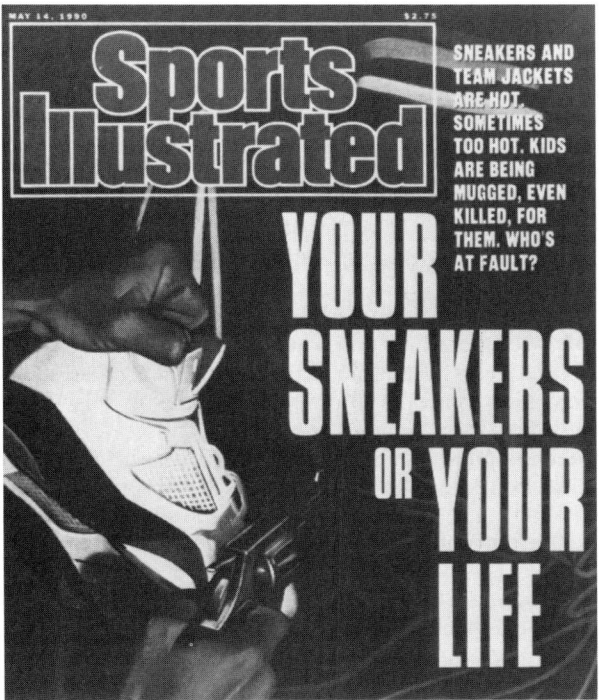

Figure 30D–1. *Sports Illustrated* cover indicating notoriety of sports shoes. (Illustration by Julian Allen. From *Sports Illustrated,* vol. 72, May 14, 1990.)

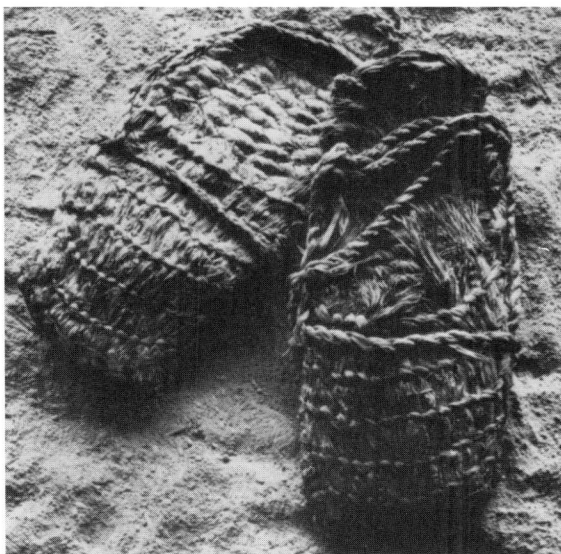

Figure 30D–2. Earliest existing footwear, dating back some 10,000 years. It is made from sagebrush bark and was found in south central Oregon by anthropologist Luther Cressman in 1932. (Photograph by Steve Bonini. Courtesy of University of Oregon Museum of Natural History and State Museum of Anthropology.)

A more ancient type of shoe was a hide shoe made by folding the skin or hide of a beast around the foot. This is the forerunner of what we call a moccasin, a term derived from the Algonquin Indians and introduced into English literature in 1612 by John Smith's "Map of Virginia."[90] Examples of this form of shoe come from excavations in Denmark of early Bronze Age oak-log coffins dating to around 1000 BC.[90] Although earlier examples do not seem to have been preserved, one can assume that the early hunters of the Stone and Ice Ages must have been capable of seeing the advantages of covering the foot for protection. What could be more logical than using the hide of their prey to provide a suitable foot covering?

Rock carvings have provided evidence that these hide shoes were secured to the foot by lashing them around the instep and arch.[90] Cave paintings found in Spain dating to 15,000 BC depict boots made of animal skin and fur.[133] More recent descriptions of shoemaking from animal hides are provided in the works of Xenophon, Carsten Niebuhr, and John Pinkerton.[154, 182, 267] Examples of the bear paw used as a shoe are seen in Figure 30D–3 from the Musée de l'Homme in Paris.[90] This bear paw with claws attached could be considered the first shoe with cleats.

A later development in shoewear and the second broad type of shoe is made of two components, an upper and a sole.[90] These are joined together at the lower edge of the foot. The appearance of this shoe occurs in Roman times, when a hide shoe reinforced by an extra piece of sole material was used.[133] Furthermore, during this time, the insole appears as a layer added for comfort and protection against chafing. These design features were a product of

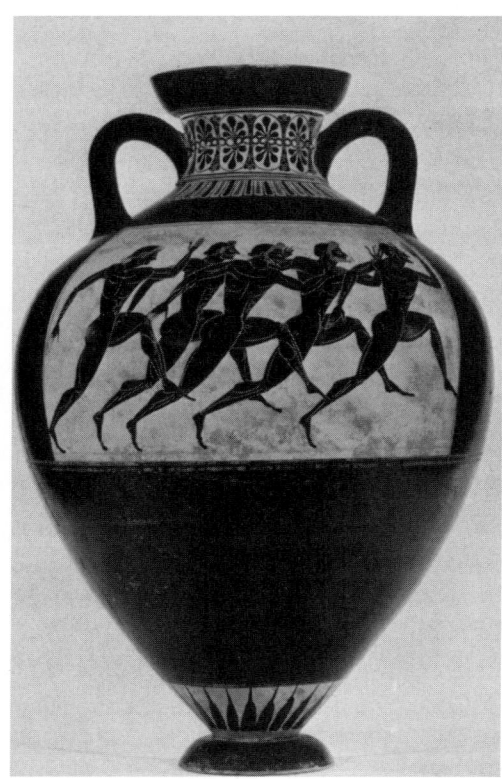

Figure 30D–4. Competitors in the early Greek games competed barefoot, according to early drawings found on vases from that period. (Courtesy of the Metropolitan Museum of Art, Rogers Fund, 1914.)

necessity owing to the abuse to which soldiers' feet were subjected. Similarly, modern design features were generated to protect the athletes' feet, particularly those involved in distance running.

Because early man was largely dependent on hunting, one can postulate that the earliest footwear was used in running. With civilization's advancement and socialization, shoes took on symbolic functions.[133] Papyrus sandals for religious ceremonies and jeweled sandals for high-fashion gatherings have been discovered in the burial holdings of Egyptian pharaohs.[239] Although these have little to do with sports shoes, they do foreshadow the current specialization, trendy colors, and designs incorporated into athletic shoewear construction. Competitors in the early Greek games competed barefoot according to early drawings found on vases of that period (Fig. 30D–4).[31] Inasmuch as shoemaking was a well-developed trade by this time, it seems that early athletes eschewed comfort for the presumed benefits of barefoot performance, that is, less weight, better feel for the surface, and improved traction.

Robbins and Hanna revived interest in barefoot running with their hypothesis that the excessive cushioning found in modern shoewear prevents appropriate sensory feedback and results in a "pseudoneurotrophic" effect.[201] The sensibility of the plantar foot is a key reason that gymnasts and dancers perform with bare or minimally shod feet. While an individual is running, plantar tactile reflexes and the intrinsic shock absorption system of the body complement one another and result in behavior modification to control load magnitude. Specifically, humans dramatically reduce

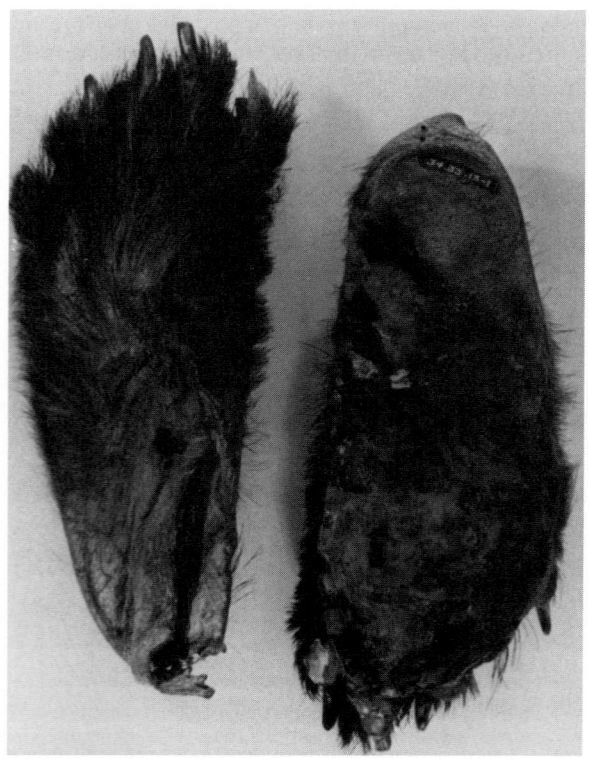

Figure 30D–3. Example of the bear paw shoe. (Courtesy of the Musée de l'Homme in Paris.)

impact force by altering knee and hip flexion at ground contact.[201] A series of studies by Robbins and coworkers have proposed that cushioned shoes lead to negligible decreases in load because subjects decrease flexion to accommodate the instability produced by softer surfaces.[139, 201] A recent study demonstrated that subjects presented with a "deceptive" advertisement of the ability of a surface to cushion impact led individuals to increase the ground reaction force of a barefoot footfall when compared with a "warning" and "neutral" message. This was despite the fact that the surface was covered with an identical thickness of ethyl-vinyl acetate surfacing material.[200]

Although the notion that "deceptive" advertising can lead to potentially harmful behavior associated with shoewear is intriguing in light of the enormous sums spent on advertisements by shoe companies, noted authorities on running and running shoes have not been impressed with this theory of the importance of sensory feedback.[189] They point out that biomechanical abnormalities such as excessive pronation, excessive Q angle at the knee, forefoot varus, and so on are the primary causes of running injuries, not a lack of sensory feedback. Furthermore, it is only with shoewear adaptations that these abnormalities can be corrected, according to these experts.[189] Ironically, one of the editors of *Runner's World* magazine recorded his shoewear experience over a 20-year period in a shoe diary and noted that a 5-year period of barefoot running was his healthiest period.[31] There is even a Web site now that promotes the benefits of shoeless running: www.running-barefoot.com.[213] Although it is clear that Western-style shoes have contributed to many of the foot ills of modern society such as bunions, corns, calluses, and neuromas,[71, 101] there is circumstantial evidence to suggest that improvements in running shoe construction have reduced the prevalence of Achilles tendinitis and allowed greater numbers of everyday citizens to participate in the sport of distance running.[31]

Tracing the history of the running shoe is an enlightening look at the shoe industry itself, at the role of sports in society, and at the international trade competition surrounding sport and its premier athletes. The most thorough sources of information in this area are *The Running Shoe Book*, written in 1980 by Peter Cavanagh, and *The Complete Book of Athletic Footwear*, written by Melvyn Cheskin in 1987.[31, 35] Both trace the evolution of running shoes through the footraces of 16th century fairs and the pedestrian races of the later 1800s to modern-day track and field competition. Important landmarks in this history can be picked out along the way. The turnshoe construction technique was firmly established by the 12th century. It allowed a shoe to be made with the seams on the outside and the smooth material inside next to the foot. The shoe was turned inside out to produce the finished product.[31, 35] By the 14th century, shoe construction had incorporated small strips of leather called welts to allow a replaceable outsole to be added to the upper.[134] Since the 14th century, shoemaking has been fairly standardized, with shoes consisting of the following:

1. Two parts, upper and lower.
2. Four processes: cutting, fitting, lasting, and bottoming.

3. Eight tools: knife, awl, needle, pinchers, last, hammer, lapstone, and stirrup.[80]

With the Industrial Revolution, the craft of shoemaking went from an in-home trade to a model of manufacturing method with the use of machines and mass production. Entire books have discussed the significance of this method to the development of industry in the United States.[52, 62] Leather was the mainstay of shoemaking throughout this period and continued as such into the 1900s. A change in shoemaking and the origin of the sneaker were presaged by the first patent, granted in 1832, for attaching rubber to the sole of the shoe. Unfortunately, the material was too unstable and lacked durability.[133] In 1839, Charles Goodyear's vulcanization process turned rubber into a usable material, but it was more than 100 years before rubber replaced leather as the most desirable outsole material for running shoes.[31]

Cavanagh cites the development of the Spencer shoe, a spiked shoe found in England's Northampton Museum, as the 1865 precursor of modern track shoes (Fig. 30D–5).[31] This shoe shows the separation of running shoes into a line separate from street shoes, although a spiked shoe used for cricket was patented in England in 1861. Spiked shoes were used in the short races popular in that day. Longer distances became popular in the latter part of the 19th century. Races around circular tracks for 144 straight hours became a spectator event imbued with international flavor. These pedestrians, as the participants were called, wore high-top leather boots and thick wool socks reminiscent of combat boots used in the military. Although pedestrian races faded in popularity, long-distance racing gained an audience, and the Olympics were reborn in Athens, Greece, in 1896. A marathon was included as a race of forty kilometers to commemorate the legend of Pheidippides. Cavanagh marks this Olympic race as the impetus for

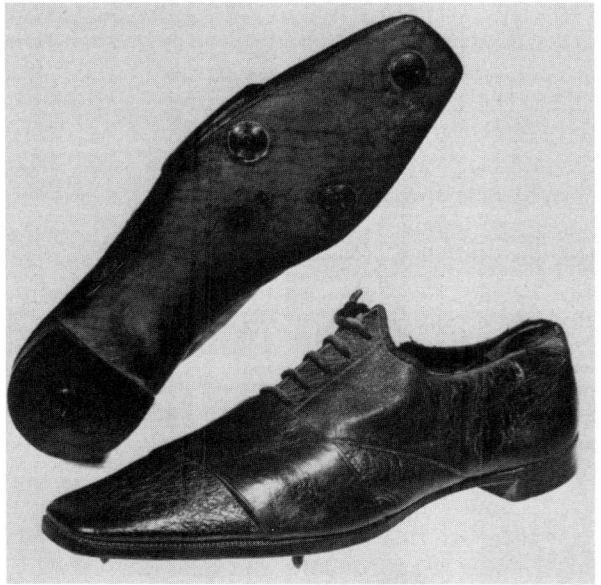

Figure 30D–5. The Spencer shoe, a spiked shoe found in England's Northampton Museum, was the 1865 precursor to modern track shoes. (Courtesy of the Northampton Museum, Northampton, England.)

development of the distance shoe, or training shoe, we use today.[31]

The popularity of the marathon prompted the Spalding Company to introduce a long-distance shoe for the general public in 1909.[31] Three shoes were advertised, two being high-tops (Fig. 30D–6). They had leather uppers and rubber soles and were priced at $5 to $8. A retired shoemaker named Richings began custom making a shoe for distance runners around the 1930s that predated the custom shoewear used by elite athletes of our day.[31] By the early 1900s, production of running shoes was in full swing, and the 1915 Spalding catalog advertised shoes for sprinting, middle-distance running, jumping, and pole-vaulting (Fig. 30D–7).[35] Competition entered the scene around the same time when Sears Roebuck entered the catalog shoe sales market and began the continuing controversy over who makes the best running shoe.[35] Endorsements by famous athletes were seen much earlier, but notable shoes were the Kiki Cuyler, Jr., basketball shoe and the Chuck Taylor All-Star shoe. We continue to see society's ongoing enchantment with famous athletes and their shoewear, as evidenced by the incredible popularity of the "Air Jordan" and "Bo Knows" campaigns of the Nike shoe company in the late 1980s and early 1990s. Despite recent cuts in advertising budgets for most of the major shoe manufacturers,[7] the fact that basketball shoe sales alone are responsible for as much as 25% of total athletic shoe revenue[26] ensures that certain

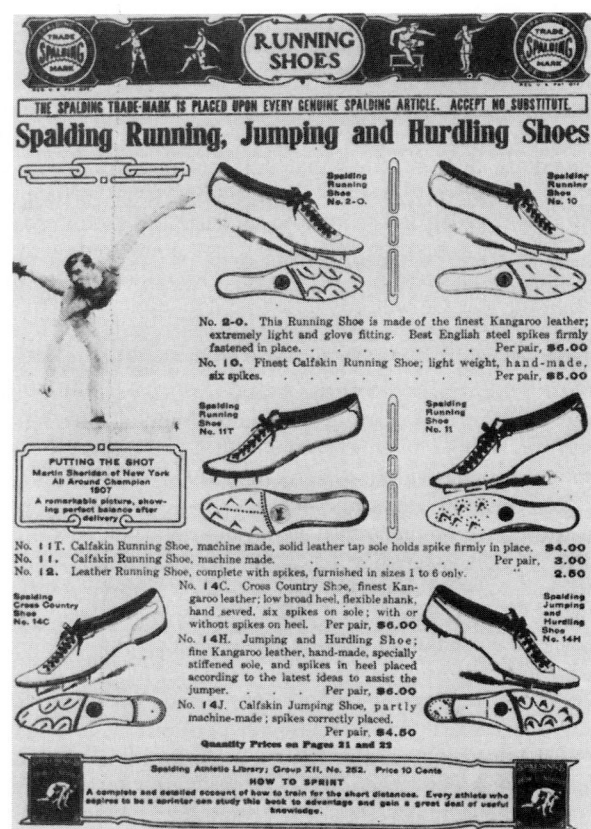

Figure 30D–7. Page from the 1915 Spalding catalog advertising shoes for sprinting, middle distance running, jumping, and pole-vaulting. (From Cheskin MP: The Complete Handbook of Athletic Footwear. New York, Fairchild Publications, 1987.)

National Basketball Association stars will expand their talent into marketing.

Beyond the running shoe, the history of other types of athletic shoes is rather scarce. The tennis shoe has been likened to the alcibiade, a low military boot with laces, which has been attributed to the Athenian general Alcibiades around the fourth century BC.[263] This foreshadows our modern tendency to associate a particular shoe with a famous individual—military then and sports now. The penchant of youth for shoes like those of their heroes has a precedent in Spartan times, when the red boots of Spartan soldiers were coveted by their youth.[263] The high cost of modern athletic shoes is nothing new, either. In Greco-Roman times, extravagant shoewear was the most costly item of dress, just as it is today for many in our society.[263] Concern about the cost of shoes has continued through the years. A report was submitted to the U.S. Congress on June 10, 1921, by the Federal Trade Commission explaining the reasons for the large increase in the price of shoes between 1918 and 1919.[193] The use of varying sole patterns and outsole spiking can also be traced to ancient times, when traction was critical for foot soldiers.[133] They placed nails through the soles of their sandals or boots, a practice known as hobnailing.[263] A Roman sandal with spikes was called the "caliga" and became associated with Gaius Caesar, Roman emperor from 37 to 41 AD, who was known as Caligula.[133]

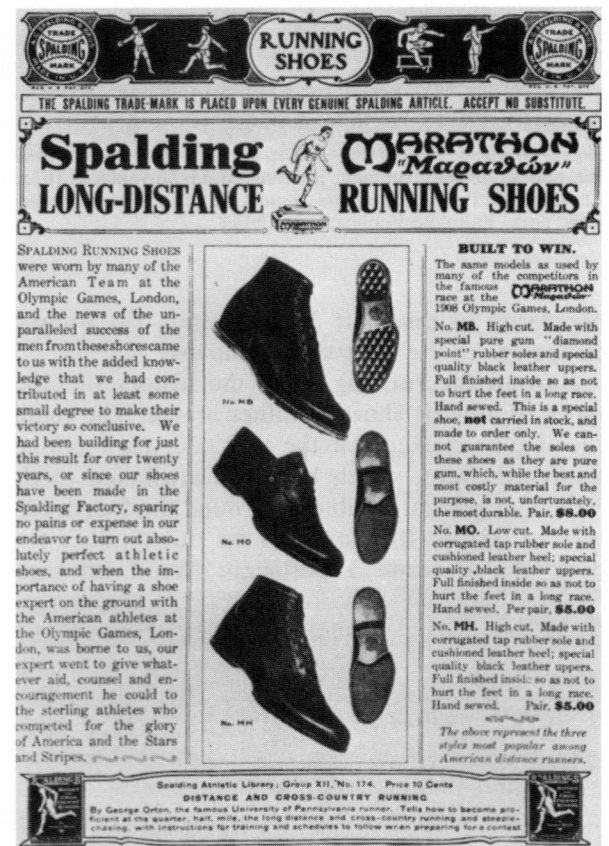

Figure 30D–6. Long-distance shoes introduced by the Spalding Company for the general public in 1909. (From Cheskin MP: The Complete Handbook of Athletic Footwear. New York, Fairchild Publications, 1987.)

A shoe designed for sports alone did not come into existence until the latter half of the 19th century. Croquet was a popular recreation during the Victorian period, and a croquet sandal appeared during this time.[133] Known as the "sneaker," it was in use by the 1860s and had a fabric upper, a rubber sole, and laces.[31, 133, 263] Further sports development in the late 1800s spawned the need for durable but lightweight shoes with variable traction requirements depending on the playing surface. Wilcox provides several illustrations of these specialized sports shoes of the late 1800s in his book, *The Mode in Footwear* (Fig. 30D–8).[263] From these developments, we can trace the roots of the multibillion-dollar sports shoe industry and can conclude that the protection of our feet and fashionable design have always been important concerns of mankind. From this foundation, an explosion occurred in sports-specific footwear that has provided us with today's shoes for basketball, rock climbing, tennis, snowboarding, soccer, gymnastics, fishing, rollerblading, skating, jumping, sprinting, and so forth (Fig. 30D–9).

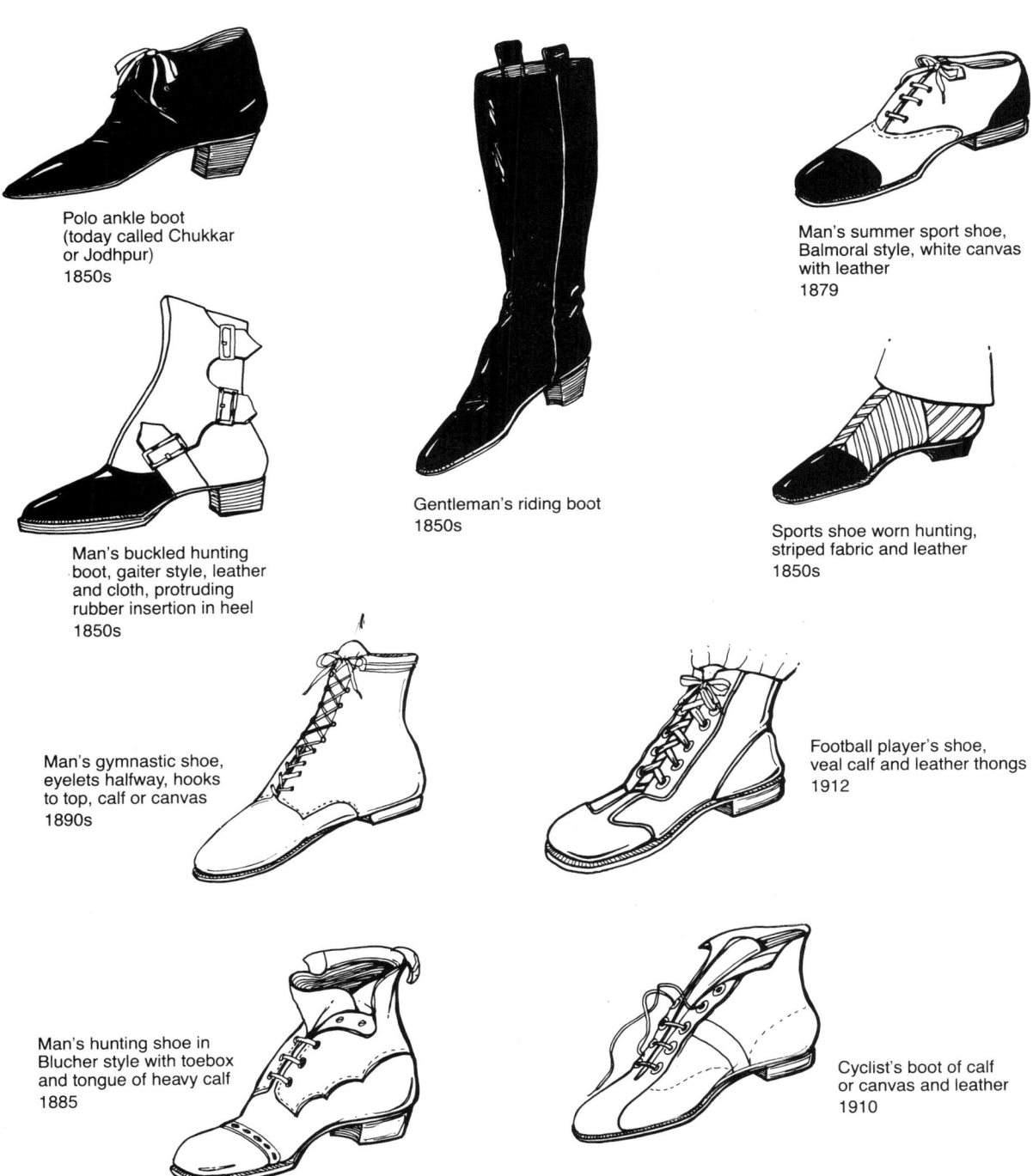

Polo ankle boot
(today called Chukkar
or Jodhpur)
1850s

Man's buckled hunting
boot, gaiter style, leather
and cloth, protruding
rubber insertion in heel
1850s

Gentleman's riding boot
1850s

Man's summer sport shoe,
Balmoral style, white canvas
with leather
1879

Sports shoe worn hunting,
striped fabric and leather
1850s

Man's gymnastic shoe,
eyelets halfway, hooks
to top, calf or canvas
1890s

Football player's shoe,
veal calf and leather thongs
1912

Man's hunting shoe in
Blucher style with toebox
and tongue of heavy calf
1885

Cyclist's boot of calf
or canvas and leather
1910

Figure 30D–8. Illustrations of specialized sports shoes of the late 1800s. (Adapted from Wilcox RT: The Mode in Footwear. New York, Charles Scribner and Sons, 1948.)

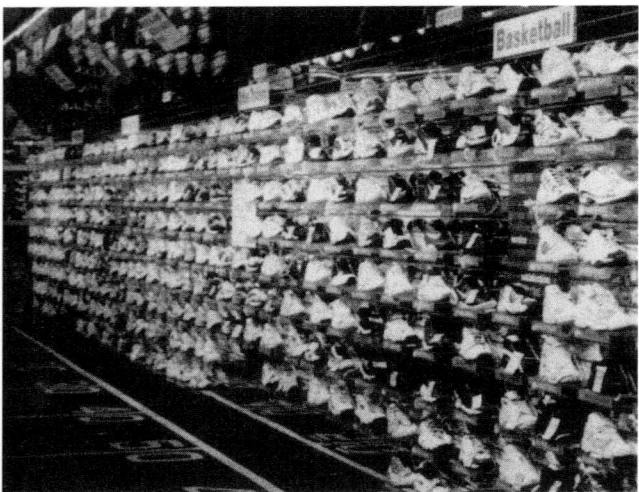

Figure 30D–9. Photograph from typical shoe store with wall of sport-specific shoes in all varieties. (Photograph by Andrew Borom.)

Anatomy of the Sports Shoe

Just as the anatomy of the human body is the basis upon which the surgeon's skill rests, the anatomy of the sports shoe is critical to those who must understand athletes and their injuries. Although the process of shoe manufacturing has evolved into a multibillion-dollar industry, the basic

shoe remains the same. This section first looks at the anatomy of the basic sports shoe and then discusses the shoe features unique to particular sports. The actual manufacturing process is discussed briefly.

Most of what has been written about athletic footwear has concentrated on shoes designed for the runner. Therefore, the prototype shoe for this section is the running shoe, and shoes for other sports are described in similar terms with specific modifications. The shoe pictured in Figure 30D–10 illustrates the components of the shoe.

For the sake of simplicity, the shoe can be broken down into two basic components: the upper and the bottom. The upper covers the foot, whereas the bottom cushions it and provides the interface between the foot and the surface. These two basic components are then subdivided into their various parts. The upper is composed of toe box, toe cap, vamp, quarter, saddle or arch bandage, eyelet stay, eyelets, throat, tongue, collar, Achilles tendon protector, heel counter, foxing, forefoot and rearfoot stabilizers, and lining. The bottom consists of sockliner or insole, insole board, midsole, wedge, and outer sole. Although some of these names differ from those used in traditional shoemaking, the actual construction of a sports shoe does not vary remarkably from the traditional shoe manufacturing process (see Glossary at the end of this chapter).

To understand the shoe itself, it is necessary to review the steps by which the shoe is made. Integral to this process is the last (from the Old English "laesk," meaning sole or footprint), which acts as an artificial foot form.[35, 114] This

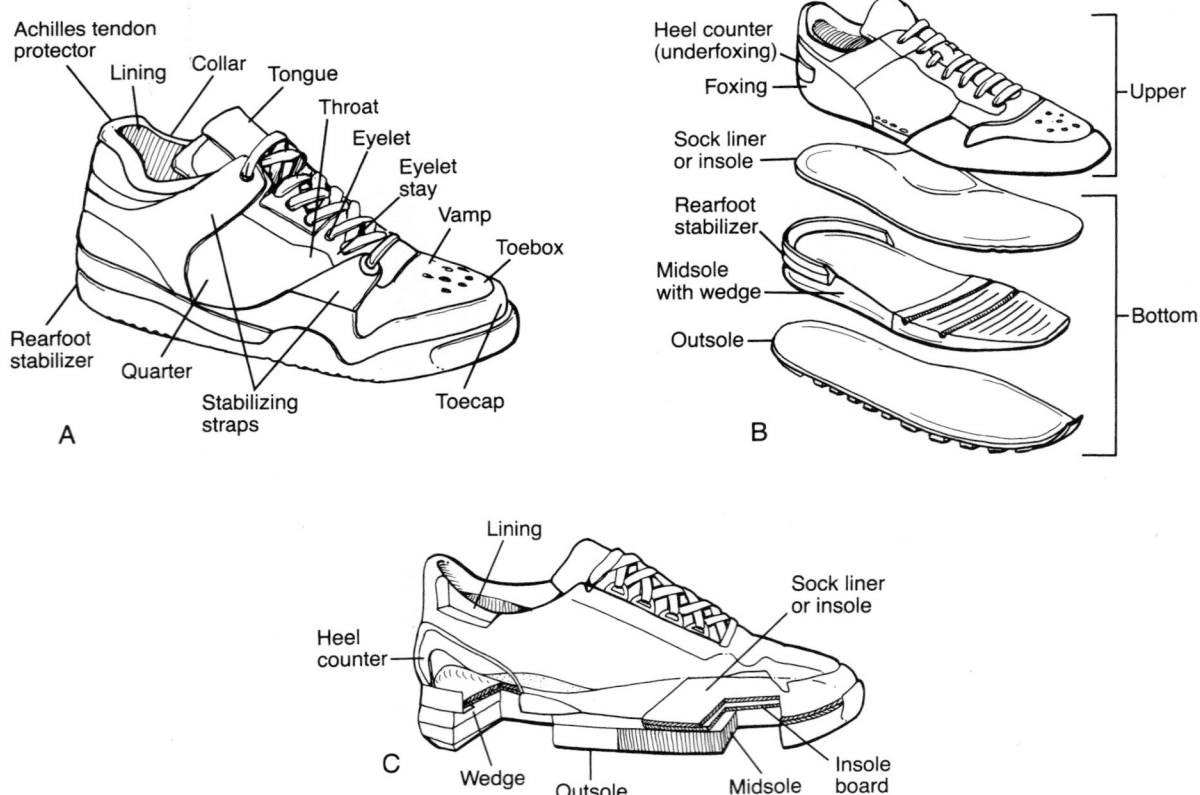

Figure 30D–10. Illustrations of athletic shoes. *A,* Overview of external appearance. *B,* Separation of shoe into component parts. *C,* Sectional view of interior of shoe.

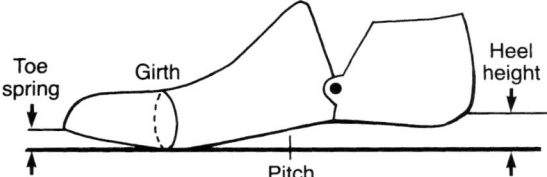

Figure 30D–11. Important measurements with respect to the last are toe pitch or toe spring, girth, and heel height or pitch. (Adapted from Cheskin MP: The Complete Handbook of Athletic Footwear. New York, Fairchild Publications, 1987; and Stacoff A, Luethi SM: Special aspects of shoe construction and foot anatomy. In Nigg BM: Biomechanics of Running Shoes. Champaign, Ill: Human Kinetics, 1986; Copyright 1986 by Benno M. Nigg. Reprinted by permission.)

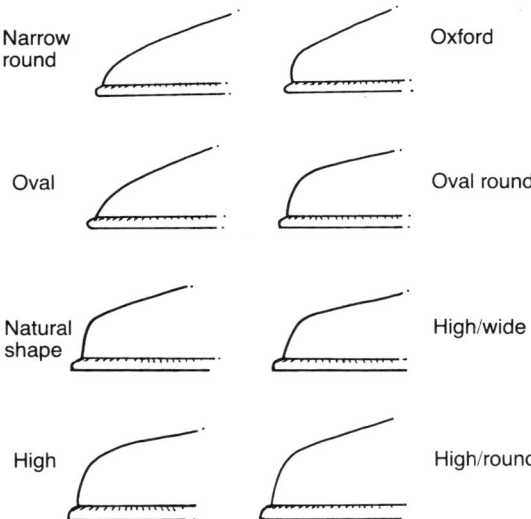

Figure 30D–13. Various alternatives for the shape of the toe box. (From Cheskin MP: The Complete Handbook of Athletic Footwear. New York, Fairchild Publications, 1987.)

allows the shoe upper to be created in the proper shape, size, and dimensions. Important measurements with respect to the last are the toe pitch or toe spring, the girth, and the heel height or pitch (Fig. 30D–11).[35, 236] The variation in toe spring and heel height can affect the movement of the foot by improving or impairing the rocker action of the foot during gait.[236]

Shape is also a critical consideration in analyzing the form for the last of a shoe. This shape can be either straight-lasted or curve-lasted depending on the amount of inward curve built into the last. Because most feet have a slight inward curve, the curved type of last provides better comfort and fit for most feet. The curved last allows the most shoe flexibility and is particularly well suited to the athlete with a highly arched or cavus foot. When the last is straighter, it translates into better medial support for the foot and is best suited to the flatter foot or to the person with an overpronated foot. Figure 30D–12 depicts the difference between straight and curved lasts. Sports shoe manufacturers use a curve of about 7 degrees in a curved last.[35] Variations exist now as slightly curved and semicurved lasts.

As we examine the last, the next consideration is the shape of the toe box. The various alternatives are depicted in Figure 30D–13.[35] It is clear that this feature has an important bearing on fit and comfort. The best example of this is the need for the athlete with clawing in the toes or

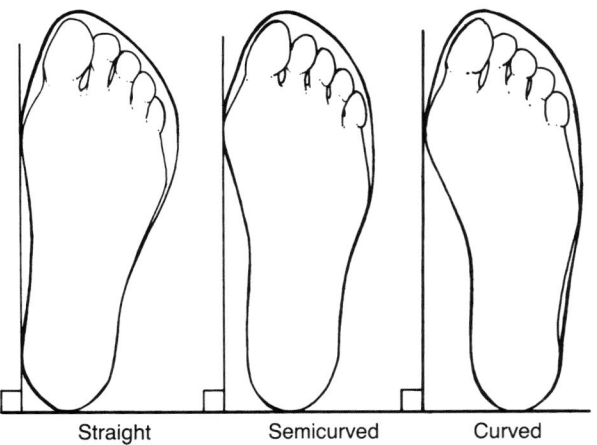

Figure 30D–12. Illustration of the difference between straight, semicurved, and curved last shoe.

even a single hammer toe to have a toe box of sufficient height to prevent chafing.

In the evolution of shoewear, the last was originally chiseled out of stone.[236] Later models were whittled from wood. A machine used in shaping gunstocks was converted to make lathes and led to the first lastmaking plant in Lynn, Massachusetts, in 1820.[236] Today the majority of lasts are made from plastic, a process developed by the Sterling Last Corporation in 1969.[236] Metal lasts are used when direct- or injection-molded soles are attached to the upper because the heat used in this process is poorly tolerated by wood or plastic.[35]

The dimensions of lasts are based on the average measurements of the segment of the population to whom the shoe will be marketed (e.g., men or women).[31, 35] In the past, women's shoes were based on scaled-down versions of lasts derived from the male foot anatomy. Recent investigations have noted several structural differences between the male and the female foot. Specifically, the female foot typically has a narrower Achilles tendon, a narrower heel in relation to the forefoot, and a foot that is narrower in general than its male counterpart.[69] In addition to these dimensional discrepancies, women have proportionately shorter leg length to total body height than do men, necessitating more foot strikes per distance covered. Because of their smaller feet, the heel-to-toe gait cycle is completed more quickly. Consequently, the cumulative ground reaction force is increased in the female runner, particularly in elite women runners, who tend to be midfoot strikers.[265] The repetitive nature of running causes these factors to be magnified tremendously over the life of a typical athletic or running shoe. Until recently, women's shoe manufacturers typically scaled down all key internal dimensions of a male athletic shoe in fixed proportion. This practice, termed scaling or grading, persists today. Fortunately, the majority of major athletic shoe companies now have divisions devoted to female athletic footwear, and many have developed lasts based on the anatomy of the female foot.[69] Now,

Throat

The topline of the vamp in front of the instep forms the throat. It is generally the narrowest part of the shoe at the base of the tongue and should be checked carefully for proper fit without excessive pressure.

Tongue

The portion of the upper that extends under the laces is called the tongue. It may be padded to reduce irritation to the dorsum of the foot. The tongue is often slit in a way that allows the laces to anchor the tongue and prevent it from sliding laterally.

Collar

The collar forms the uppermost part of the quarters and is the part through which the foot enters the shoe. When excessively stiff or high, the collar can irritate the hindfoot or ankle malleoli. It often has extra padding.

Achilles Tendon Protector

The extended area on the back of the shoe acts as a pull tab and protection for the Achilles tendon. It should be both molded and padded well to prevent irritation of this area. The high tab design that caused irritation of the Achilles tendon has been replaced by a "bunny-ear" design with a dip in the center.[82] The cutaway should be wide enough to prevent friction on the sides of the Achilles tendon.

Heel Counter

This reinforcement to the upper of the shoe is located in the heel area. It is a stiffened material of fiberboard or plastic that is molded to the heel and provides greater rearfoot control. The size of the heel counter and the quality of the material vary between shoes.

Foxing

Reinforcing material between the sole and the upper is called foxing and is usually composed of rubber or leather. Durability is improved by double stitching this material.

Forefoot and Rearfoot External Stabilizers (Footframe)

Material is used as a reinforcing component to cup the rearfoot or forefoot of the shoe for greater stability. This is a molded material that may or may not be an integral part of the midsole.

Lining

This is the material that acts as the inside backing for the material of the upper. It must be smooth and nonirritating because it is in direct contact with the foot.

Bottom

The bottom, or sole, of the shoe is important in protecting the foot from the environment. Therefore, it requires materials that are both comfortable and durable. In modern athletic footwear, these two features are accomplished by using multiple components.

Sockliner or Insole

This material cushions the foot and is the layer between the foot and the bottom of the shoe. Various materials have been used for this layer and are discussed in the next section. Most sports shoes come with removable sockliners to allow them to be replaced when they are worn out or when a corrective orthosis is necessary. The insole reduces friction and provides some degree of shock absorption. It also absorbs perspiration and can provide some canting or control of overpronation. The capability of this material to mold to the shape of the foot can be a source of additional comfort and control.

Insole Board

The cellulose fiberboard to which the upper is attached in the conventional lasting process is called the insole board; hence the term *board-lasted*. This process provides the greatest stability, as opposed to slip lasting, which has no insole board under the sockliner, and leads to improved comfort and flexibility. The intermediate option is combination lasting, in which there is an insole board in the hindfoot with stitching in the forefoot where it has been slip lasted (Fig. 30D–17).

Midsole

Known as the "heart" of the running shoe, the midsole is sandwiched between the upper and the outsole of the shoe and provides the bulk of shock absorption. With the wedge, this component also produces the desired heel lift, rocker action, and toe spring. Through the use of canting and variable hardness, the midsole can control foot motion. With the use of anatomic contouring, even greater stability and comfort can be achieved. Variations in the materials used add another dimension to what the midsole can do for the foot.

Many of the more significant and recent design advances have occurred through alteration of the midsole.[70] These modifications are seen as significant enough by the manufacturers that they are frequently incorporated in the name or advertising campaigns of the various shoe products (Table 30D–1). One particular midsole modification has even contributed to the most recognizable nickname of one of the greatest basketball players of all time—Michael "Air" Jordan.

Outsole

This is the bottom layer of the shoe that makes contact with the ground. The outsole can be constructed with

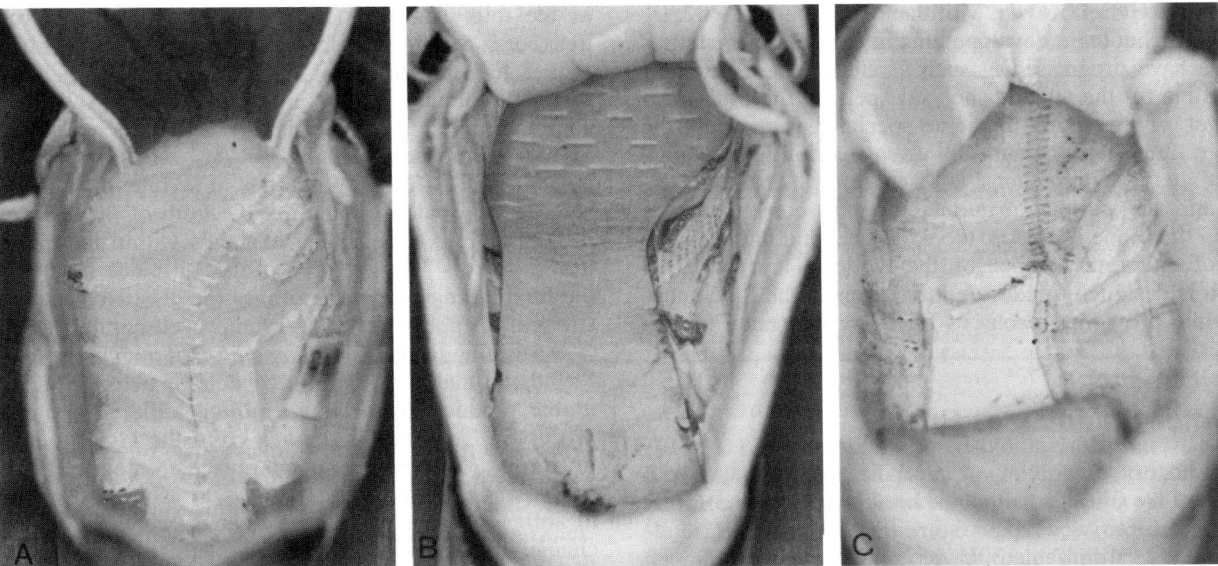

Figure 30D–17. Examples of different lasting methods for running shoes. *A*, Slip-last shoe. *B*, Board-last shoe. *C*, Combination-last shoe. (Photographs by Thomas O. Clanton.)

different materials, patterns, colors, and densities. These factors, excluding color variations, can be used to modify the shoe's stability, flexibility, comfort, and shock absorption. These features are discussed in greater detail later in this chapter.

Cleats or Traction Aids

The appendages or prominent patterning attached to, or incorporated into, the outsole of the shoe appears in innumerable designs, but its purpose is invariably the enhancement of friction between the athlete's foot and the playing surface. In track, this is accomplished with small metal spikes affixed to the outsole, whereas in football there may be plastic projections coming off an injection-molded outsole. From the viewpoint of sports medicine, cleats have the most direct influence on the performance characteristics of a shoe from the athlete's perspective and on the injury potential of a shoe. Optimization of the athlete/shoe/surface interface is critical in maximizing performance and reducing injury. This optimization continues to be elusive and is dependent on a number of variables, including turf (artificial vs. natural), environmental conditions (wet vs. dry), cleat spacing, cleat design, cleat length, outsole material, spatting, and others.[61, 81, 106] This complex subject is covered in more detail in Chapter 30C.

Materials Used in Shoes and Shoe Inserts

The petroleum industry has affected many areas of society, including shoe construction. Traditional materials such as leather, rubber, and cotton (canvas) still have their place, but the search for lighter, more durable, more shock-absorbing materials has led to the development of complex foams with high-tech names such as Elvalite, Hexalite,

TABLE 30D–1
Materials Encapsulated in Midsole Cushioning Designs

Shoe Manufacturer	Trade Name	Material/Design
Asics	Gel	Silicone resin in a pad
Avia	Arc	Dupont Hytrel in polyurethane
Brooks	Hydroflow	Silicone fluid in a two-chambered plastic bladder
Converse	He:01	Helium gas in polyurethane and nylon
Etonic	Soft Cell	Combined gel and ambient air
New Balance	N-ergy Cartridge	Hytrel in a blow-molded cartridge
New Balance	ENCAP	Ethylene vinyl acetate core in polyurethane shell
Nike	Air	Freon gas in polyurethane
Puma		Honeycomb pads
Reebok	Hexalite	Honeycomb pads
Reebok	DMX	Pods connected by tubing which allows air flow during stride

Compiled from Heil B: Running shoe design and selection related to lower limb biomechanics. Physiotherapy 78:406–412, 1992; Frey C: Footwear and stress fractures. Clin Sports Med 16:249–257, 1997; shoe product brochures and the Web sites of the named shoe manufacturers.

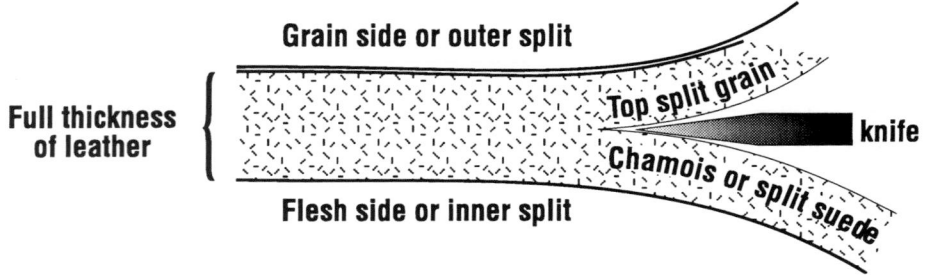

Full thickness of leather

Grain side or outer split

Top split grain

Chamois or split suede

knife

Flesh side or inner split

Figure 30D–18. Splitting of leather into two layers of skin for use in shoemaking. (Redrawn from Cheskin MP: The Complete Handbook of Athletic Footwear. New York, Fairchild Publications, 1987; and Philps JW: The Functional Foot Orthosis. New York, Churchill Livingstone, 1990.)

cability to footwear construction since ancient times. It has the ability to adapt to the shape of the foot and maintain the altered configuration. Leather transmits perspiration ("breathes") and can be treated to resist or repel water.[35, 220] Tensile strength is outstanding (up to 4 tons per square inch), flexibility is excellent, and puncture and abrasion resistance is superior.[35] The tanning process along with the finishing and dyeing of the leather can accentuate one or all of these properties. The disadvantages of leather are its deformability under stress, its tendency to crack when successively moistened and dried, its weight, and cost variations.

Nylon-weave uppers are made from polyamide resin fibers woven together into a taffeta and doubled or interfaced with a thin foam or tricot lining.[35] In the assembly process, these layers are "flamed," or heat-bonded. This bonds the laminates together, resulting in a material more flexible and absorbent than if the layers were glued.[82] The variables in this composition process are the exact material used in the thread, the size of the thread, the number of threads in the bundles, and the number and orientation of the bundles going lengthwise and widthwise (Fig. 30D–19).[31] The closeness of the weave affects the mechanical properties of the fabric. The nylon weave of a taffeta upper has good durability, softness, and flexibility and is lightweight, making it a superior replacement for leather in many athletic shoes.[31, 35]

Nylon mesh is made from the same nylon threads, but in a knitted rather than a woven process (Fig. 30D–20).[31]

This knitted process adds space within the strands without compromising strength. Thus, the breathability of the upper is improved. It can be used as a single-, double- or triple-mesh knit. Increasing the denier of the thread adds body and strength to the fabric. Whether used in mesh or woven form, the nylon upper is generally combined with a thin foam and a tricot lining for improved fit and comfort.[35]

Other synthetic materials are finding their way into athletic shoe uppers, including Gore-Tex (W. L. Gore and Associates, Elkton, Md).[114] Thermoplastic vinyl has uses in golf shoes in coated or laminated applications to leather or fabric. Slush- and dip-molded uppers of thermoplastic materials are used in recreational ice skates and certain waterproof footwear, whereas injection-molded thermoset plastic is the norm for ski boots.[35] Depending on the shoe's intended use, the shoewear manufacturer can provide a full range of breathability, extending from complete breathability up to complete insulation and waterproofing. The upper can be easily or barely deformable. Weight can be varied over a wide range, and the foot can be protected minimally or maximally.

Inlays, Inserts, Insoles, and Orthoses

Since ancient times, it has been known that the addition of leaves, moss, or animal skin to the inside of the shoe could provide cushioning for the foot and protection from

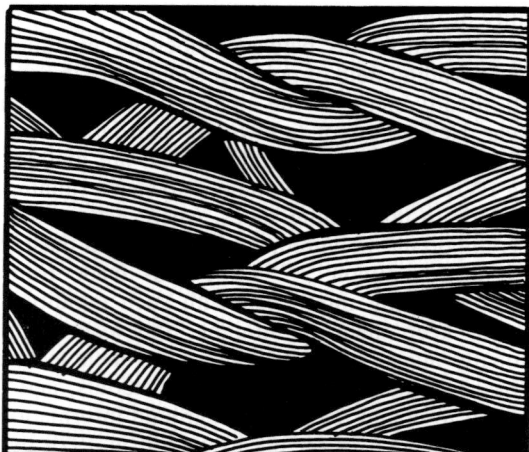

Figure 30D–19. Nylon-weave uppers made from fibers woven together into a taffeta. (Redrawn from Cavanagh PR: The Running Shoe Book. Mountain View, Calif, Anderson World, 1980.)

Figure 30D–20. Nylon mesh made from threads with a knitted rather than a woven process. (Redrawn from Cavanagh PR: The Running Shoe Book. Mountain View, Calif, Anderson World, 1980.)

environmental stresses.[90] For soldiers on long marches, this extra protection might mean the difference between life and death. For modern-day runners and athletes, this cushioning is intended to protect the most readily identifiable weak link in the kinetic chain. Many athletes would provide testimonial support for the merits of their orthotic devices or inserts in preventing injury or enhancing performance. Although it has been more difficult to document these beneficial effects objectively,[142, 236, 253] scientific evidence of the shock absorption properties of the various materials used in these devices does exist.[21, 219, 259, 266] This section provides some acceptable definitions to help make sense of this confusing area and then describes some of the materials used. The following section discusses their biomechanical properties.

Because of the confusion that surrounds this area, we have chosen to use the definitions of terms accepted by the Pedorthic Footwear Association.[96] The *insole* is the integral design component (layer) of the shoe that is the shoe's structural anchor to which is attached the upper, toe box, heel counter, linings, and/or welting. The *inlay* is a prefabricated removable material upon which the foot directly rests inside the shoe. In some shoes, the inlay is an integral design component. The *insert* is a type of orthosis, although the term has been used interchangeably with inlays and insoles in some circles to designate an off-the-shelf device placed inside the shoe. For the purpose of this chapter, we use the definition for an insert supplied by the Health Care Financing Agency: a total contact, multiple density, removable inlay that is directly molded to the patient's foot or a model of the patient's foot and that is made of a suitable material with regard to the patient's condition. An *orthosis* (or orthotic device) is a device that is used to protect, support, or improve function of parts of the body that move. A common error is to use the adjective orthotic(s) as a noun. A *pad* is a device placed inside a shoe to provide support or relieve pressure from a specific location such as a longitudinal arch pad or a metatarsal pad. Pads are made of various materials and come in a variety of shapes and sizes.

Inlays and inserts can be made from a single material or a composite of several materials. The most commonly used materials are leather, cork, foam, felt, and plastic.[115] Based on the previous definitions, inlays are "off-the-shelf," whereas inserts are "custom made." The latter can be subdivided into those made from a casting of the foot and those made from an impression of the foot (Fig. 30D–21).[18, 115, 181] These can be formulated in a weight-bearing, partial weight-bearing, or non–weight-bearing fashion. A recent trend in orthosis manufacture uses digital foot scanners, obviating the need for a negative mold of the foot. A topographic reading of the plantar foot is obtained using laser scanning, digitized force-plate gait and pressure analysis, or digital analysis of multiple air pegs. These manufacturing devices employ computer-assisted design in the final conversion of data to orthosis.[1, 13, 64, 248] The devices, which are at present quite expensive, largely rely on the subtalar neutral position as a starting point for data collection. The subtalar neutral position has been variously defined as the position from which there is equal inversion and eversion range of motion, the position from which there is twice as much inversion as eversion, or the position

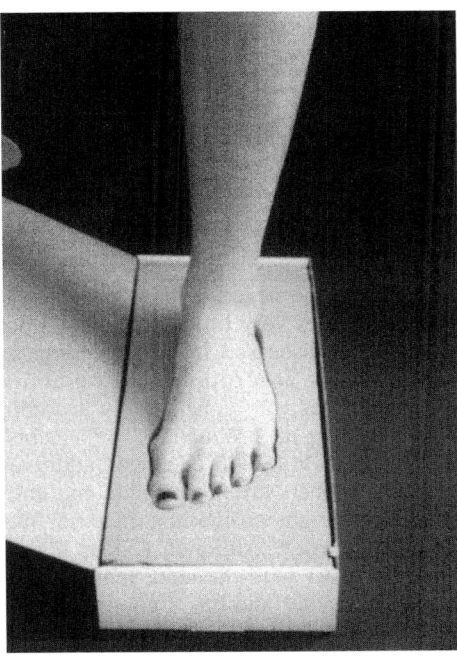

Figure 30D–21. Foam box used for taking an impression of a foot to make a custom-made orthosis. (Photograph by Andrew Borom.)

where the talar head is most fully covered by the tarsal navicular when palpating the foot. It is unclear how much a small variation in this point affects readings and ultimately function. Adequate data in the form of prospective, randomized, controlled studies comparing the use of orthoses manufactured with these systems and inserts made with traditional methods are lacking. There are no data confirming their superiority or justifying their cost.[14] Given the uncertainty surrounding the multitude of theories guiding orthotic prescriptions, it would be helpful to have some scientific support for the ability of foot orthoses to accomplish their stated objective.

For general classification purposes, inserts can be further divided into accommodative or functional varieties. *Accommodative* devices are those that are designed with a primary goal of conforming to the individual's anatomy, whereas *functional* devices are designed with the primary goal of controlling an individual's anatomic function, such as providing support or stability, or assisting ambulation.[4, 96, 181] Different materials can be used for these purposes, leading to an additional subdivision into rigid, semirigid, and soft, in which the material becomes the critical factor.

As discussed previously, the materials used in shoes, and now in orthotic devices, can be either natural or synthetic.[115] The most commonly used natural materials are leather, rubber, cork, metal, and felt. Synthetics include plastics and foams (both closed and open cell), which can be manufactured with varying qualities of hardness, density, durability, and moldability. The following paragraphs consider the advantages and disadvantages of these materials.

Natural Materials

Leather is extremely durable and conforms well to the contours of the foot. It is readily available, is tolerated well men—hence the interested reader is referred to their original works, the references from Mann's section on biomechanics, and the preceding section on the causes of injury to the foot and ankle. Without the contributions of these individuals, there would be no foundation on which we could base further research.

Whether one is talking about shoes or orthoses or a combination of these, from a biomechanical standpoint, one is primarily concentrating on (1) the effect of shoes or orthoses on reducing the forces present at foot strike, (2) their ability to improve functional motion within the foot, and (3) their efficacy in preventing or treating pathologic conditions in the lower extremity. Although it is known that certain other biomechanical parameters such as running economy and speed can be altered by shoes and orthoses, these factors will not be discussed in any depth in this section.

Nigg reviewed the available literature and combined this with nearly two decades of his own investigations in the field of shoewear research to formulate a new concept for inserts and orthoses. Although the interested reader is referred to this excellent review for details, the Human Performance Laboratory in Calgary proposes that the traditional view of the ability of orthoses or inserts to align the skeleton is not supported in the available literature. Rather, the concept that an orthosis or insert functions most effectively if it minimizes muscle work is advanced by these investigators.[170] The basics of this proposed concept are found in Table 30D–9. The situation-dependent variables can be influenced by the shoe, insert, orthosis or selection of the movement task, whereas the subject-dependent variables, by definition, vary from individual to individual. If this proposal is accepted, the authors suggest that it is possible to conclude the following regarding orthoses:

- The skeleton has a preferred path for a given movement task (e.g., running).
- If an intervention supports the preferred movement path, muscle activity is decreased. Interference with the preferred path increases muscle activity.
- An optimal insert or orthosis decreases muscle activity.
- An optimal insert feels comfortable owing to decreased muscle activity with resultant decreased fatigue.

TABLE 30D–9
Proposed Concept for Inserts and Orthoses

Situation-Dependent Variables	Subject-Dependent Variables
A force signal acts as an input variable on the shoe, based on the chosen movement.	The soft tissue and mechanoreceptors on the plantar surface of the foot act as a third filter.
The shoe acts as a first filter for the force input signal.	The filtered information is detected by the central nervous system, which provides a subject-specific dynamic response.
The insert or orthosis acts as a second filter for the force input signal.	The subject performs the movement task at hand.

From Nigg BM, Nurse MA, Stefanyshyn DJ: Shoe inserts and orthotics for sport and physical activities. Med Sci Sports Exerc 31(suppl 7):S421–S428, 1999.

- With an optimal insert, performance should increase in association with decreased muscle activity and fatigue.

This proposal is clearly innovative and controversial because it is unsupported by adequate experimental evidence. Further research matching subject and insert characteristics to identify the optimal solution for insert/orthosis fitting will, it is hoped, fill this evidence gap.[170]

As mentioned previously, the functional orthosis is fabricated based on a specific biomechanical theory. It usually uses the "subtalar neutral" position as the starting point. This theoretically aligns the hindfoot with the forefoot and allows the foot to function in its most biomechanically advantageous position. The functional orthosis changes the position of the foot with respect to the weight-bearing surface. The accommodative orthosis, on the other hand, brings the surface up to meet the foot in its steady-state position in an effort to improve weight distribution and alleviate symptoms. The accommodative device must be fabricated from a material that will mold easily to the surface of the foot because one of its primary purposes is to accommodate deformities. In contrast, the functional orthosis must be rigid enough to maintain the foot in the position chosen for maximum function. This makes it apparent why plastic is usually selected for the functional device, and a polyethylene or polyurethane foam is more commonly the choice if accommodation is the goal.

Shock Absorption

Loading of the athlete's body during sports activities has been implicated as a significant causal factor in pain and injury.[156, 157, 160, 167] The study of this relationship is an essential element in the field of sports biomechanics.[29, 30, 158] Numerous works have been published on the biomechanics of walking and running,[28, 94, 123, 124, 145, 158, 172, 226, 247] and a like number have documented the forces acting on the foot during various activities.[32, 55, 85, 146, 157, 159, 217, 240] Measurement of the pressure under the foot during gait dates back to 1882 with the work of Beely, who used crude manual methods. Since then, measurement of load has progressed to the use of force plates with the aid of piezoelectric transducers or strain gauge technology with computer analysis.[146, 240] The vertical force component produces skeletal transients beginning at heel strike or foot strike, and these have been theorized to produce injury through their resultant shock and shear waves.[79, 116, 141, 190, 255, 260] Experimental support for this analysis was provided by the finding that osteoarthritis developed in the joints of sheep housed on concrete.[187, 188] The association between chronic repetitive trauma, exercise, and arthritis has been the source of considerable controversy.[84, 151, 177, 230] Although controlled studies have failed to demonstrate a clear relationship between osteoarthritis and the loads generated in sports such as running (in otherwise healthy participants),[104, 107–109, 177, 230] this relationship has nevertheless served as an important catalyst for the athletic shoe industry to improve the shock absorption qualities of shoes.

Although increasing cushioning in shoewear seems intuitively appealing as a method to diminish shock transmission to the skeleton, Robbins and coworkers have produced a sizeable volume of work outlining the potentially detrimental effects of soft materials in shoes.[196–200, 202, 204, 205] Robbins and Hanna proposed that shoewear creates a "pseudo-neurotrophic" condition that eliminates the plantar tactile response from the human system designed to minimize impact loading through alteration of musculoskeletal response.[198] It has been demonstrated that whereas certain interface materials reduce vertical impact from inanimate objects dropped on them, human landing paradoxically increases these forces.[40] Gymnasts landing on a 10-cm thick mat demonstrated a 20% increase in vertical impact compared with a rigid surface.[199] Behavioral modifications that can either amplify or reduce vertical impact include variation in amplitude of hip and knee flexion.[139] Bending at these joints is decreased when landing on soft surfaces. This stiff-legged landing serves to heighten impact, whereas landing on hard surfaces results in increased hip and knee flexion to absorb energy.[199] Stability is part of this equation. When soft materials are placed beneath the plantar surface of individuals on a force platform, stability declines as measured by increased sway.[186] Human balance improves when placed on thin, stiff surfaces.[203, 206] To accommodate these factors, humans adopt landing strategies to deal with the landing surface. Decreased hip and knee flexion is used momentarily to increase stability by compressing the interface material.[199] Robbins and Waked examined ground reaction force in 12 men without disability using a 4.5-cm foot fall onto a force platform covered with one of four materials. Vertical impact was inversely related to surface stiffness, with the softest surface producing the greatest impact. They concluded that balance and vertical impact are closely related and hypothesized that landing on a soft surface is accompanied by an attempt to render it more stable by compressing the material, decreasing its thickness and increasing its stiffness. Although recognizing the impracticality of barefoot activity, they propose that currently available athletic shoes are too soft and thick, and recommend redesign.[199] In a further study by the same investigators, a "deceptive" advertising message associated with an EVA-covered platform was shown to produce higher vertical impact forces than the identical platform with a preceding "neutral" or "warning" message.[200] Although this theory has not been universally accepted, there is evidence that shoe manufacturers are incorporating thinner midsole shoes into their product lines, with the purported advantage of "more speed and stability."[66] Despite this opposing viewpoint, there is scientific data to support the incorporation of elements of cushioning for the reduction of certain overuse injuries.

Experimental Work

Available independent data on laboratory testing of various materials used in shoes and orthotic devices are somewhat limited compared with other areas of research in the fields of sports medicine, orthopaedics, and podiatry. In one of the earliest studies of this kind, Brodsky and co-workers studied the effects of repeated compression and the effects of repeated shear and compression on the behavior of five commonly used materials for shoe inserts.[21] They also determined the force-attenuation properties of the new and used materials. The materials tested were

Plastazote (Apex Foot Products, South Hackensack, NJ), Pelite (Durr-Fillauer Medical Inc., Chattanooga, Tenn), PPT (Langer Biomechanics Group, Inc., Deer Park, NY), Sorbothane (Sorbothane, Inc., Kent, Ohio), and Spenco (Spenco Medical Corp., Waco, Tex). To test compression, the authors used an Instrom testing machine and subjected the materials to cyclic loads. The greatest degree of compression was seen with the soft-grade Plastazote, which went from an original thickness of 6.6 mm to 4.55 mm after 5000 cycles. Lesser amounts of compression were seen with medium-grade Pelite, Spenco, and Sorbothane, and the least change was found with PPT.

In the same study the authors also looked at the resilience of the different materials. Resilience is a measure of a material's ability to resume its original shape after having been distorted. This is an important property in an insole or orthotic device. The resilience of the above materials was determined by remeasuring their thickness after a period of rest. Both Plastazote and Pelite showed good rebound in thickness after a 12-hour rest, which allowed a return to 6.0 mm for the Plastazote (a 70% return). Unfortunately, after rebound takes place, accelerated compression occurs when the material is again subjected to the same stress. Some of the results of this study are displayed in Table 30D–10.[21]

Foto and Birke recently investigated resilience for the most commonly prescribed multidensity material combinations used in manufacturing orthotic devices. Dynamic strain, or the material's percent deformation per cycle, as well as strain loss (or compression set), reflective of the material's permanent deformation, was measured for each of four combinations of materials. Cyclic loading to 10,000 and 100,000 cycles demonstrated marked differences in the temporary and permanent deformation of the various combinations. Although the materials tested are more commonly used in treatment of diabetic plantar pressure problems, the authors point out that an ideal pressure-relieving orthosis should demonstrate a dynamic strain of 50% or better at 350 kPa of pressure, and that compression set should be minimal. Excessive compression set corresponds to losses in posting, pressure relief and/or accommodation of deformity.[66] Furthermore, composite material performance is affected by the overall thickness, as well as the ratio of the individual materials.

TABLE 30D–10

Maximum Loss in Thickness Expressed as Percentage of Original Thickness after 10,000 Cycles

Material	Compression (%)	Shear Compression (%)
Plastazote (soft)	55	45
Pelite (medium)	15	16
Spenco	15	3.6
Sorbothane	3	10.2
PPT	0	0

From Brodsky JW, Kourosh S, Stills M, et al: Objective evaluation of insert material for diabetic and athletic footwear. Foot Ankle 9:111–116. © American Orthopaedic Foot and Ankle Society, 1988.

A

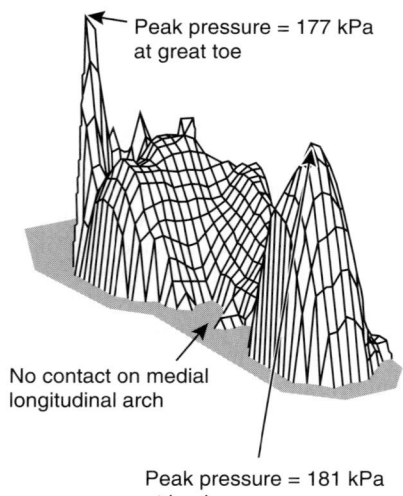

Peak pressure = 177 kPa
at great toe

No contact on medial
longitudinal arch

Peak pressure = 181 kPa
at heel

Contact area = 131 cm²

B

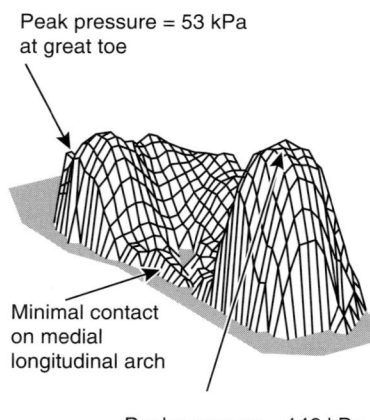

Peak pressure = 53 kPa
at great toe

Minimal contact
on medial
longitudinal arch

Peak pressure = 146 kPa
at heel

Contact area = 144 cm²

Figure 30D–23. Example of peak pressure measurements comparing different shoes. *A,* Shoe with limited cushioning properties. *B,* Shoe with improved cushioning properties. (Redrawn from Mueller MJ: Application of plantar pressure assessment in footwear and insert design. J Orthop Sports Phys Ther 29:747–755, 1999, by permission.)

knee pain,[22, 23, 95, 97, 110, 162, 210] iliotibial band syndrome,[22, 110, 136, 162, 171, 210] pes anserinus bursitis,[110] and popliteal tendinitis[22, 110, 132] (see Chapter 28C).

The problems attributed to excessive pronation have not been limited to the knee. In the leg, ankle, and foot, excessive pronation has been associated with posterior tibial tendinitis,[22, 37, 38, 95, 119, 162] overuse syndromes in runners,[8, 95] medial tibial stress syndrome,[119, 257] tarsal tunnel syndrome,[120, 215] cuboid syndrome,[127, 153] plantar fasciitis,[95, 105, 162] Achilles tendinitis,[22, 41, 95, 119] metatarsalgia,[119] and stress fractures.[131, 225] From this listing of virtually every known medical condition affecting the lower leg, it should become obvious to the astute reader that excessive pronation is a seemingly disastrous condition for the athlete. As such, it is natural to expect a plethora of laboratory and clinical studies offering scientific confirmation of the relationship between excessive pronation or rearfoot instability and these pathologic conditions. Unfortunately, the few studies that have addressed this question have failed to provide a conclusive answer.

Although the majority of studies that have been done on the use of rearfoot control features and orthotic devices have focused on the advantages of these features in the treatment of the pronated foot, shoe features and orthotic devices have also been used to treat the opposite foot condition—the cavus or highly arched foot. As discussed in Chapter 30A, the cavus foot type tends to be more rigid and has less available motion to dissipate the forces of weight-bearing. Consequently, it is the cavus foot that has been implicated in the production of plantar fasciitis,[22, 105, 117, 120, 125] stress fractures,[73, 131, 225] and medial tibial stress syndrome.[119] Because the cavus foot is generally more rigid and is commonly associated with a plantar flexed first ray and a varus hindfoot, orthotic support is designed to alleviate these problems. A less rigid orthosis is preferable to provide improved shock absorption and allow some degree

of flexibility. Whereas reports have found that up to 75% of patients who have pronation-related problems benefit from the use of an orthotic device, there has been a considerably less favorable response to the use of orthoses in the cavus foot population.[50, 76, 95, 118] Clinical experience has been the source of most of the evidence supporting the use of orthotic devices for the treatment of a variety of conditions that plague the athlete, particularly the runner.

Although much of the scientific and anatomic basis for the use of orthoses can be traced to the work of Manter,[60, 126] Elftman,[57–60] Hicks,[86, 87] Close,[44–46] and Inman,[33, 34, 92] it has primarily been orthotists and podiatrists who have experimented with various shapes and materials in an effort to develop a practical approach to the prescription of orthoses. The field of orthotic prescriptions has a pseudoscientific aura. This is created by many factors: erudite yet ambiguous terminology, seemingly contradictory theories, failure to establish what constitutes the normal foot (much less the abnormal), lack of recognition of normal anatomic variation, confusing concepts of what is compensated and what is not, and limited use of the scientific method in establishing the criteria for employment of orthoses and evaluation of their usefulness.[4, 56, 98, 236, 242–246] Faced with this conundrum, it is valuable to reflect on the former foundational work while viewing current shoe and orthotic research with a combination of skepticism and open-mindedness. One can then investigate the available experimental and clinical work, which either supports or refutes the scientific basis for prescribing orthoses or using particular modifications in athletic shoewear.

Experimental Work

Studies concerned with control of alignment and maintenance of rearfoot stability must begin by determining an acceptable indication of foot pronation.[42] Because pronation is a complicated triplane movement, it is difficult to quantify this movement with currently available techniques. Therefore, it has been generally agreed in the research community to use the degree of calcaneal eversion (valgus) as the indicator of pronation.[56, 191, 232] By using heel eversion alone, the associated abduction and dorsiflexion are discounted.[126] Nevertheless, this seems to be the most practical method and the one that has gained acceptance.

Measurement is done by observing the subject from a posterior viewpoint using reference markers on the lower leg to define its axis and a second set of markers on the calcaneus to denote its position (Fig. 30D–24). Gait analysis is then performed using high-speed film cinematography, video cameras, or optoelectronic systems to visualize the markers during each phase of gait.[252] The marker positions can then be plotted using anatomic landmarks and sent to a computer for analysis. This is the process of digitalization, from which are derived the specific angles exhibited at specific points in time in the gait cycle.

In the cinematographic system originally used, the manual plotting and calculations needed for each frame of film made this an incredibly time-consuming and laborious method subject to a certain degree of human error. Kinematic analysis provides information on a number of variables including initial Achilles tendon angle, maximal Achilles tendon angle, initial pronation, total pronation, initial pronation velocity, and so on.[159] By employing a video system, one can use a video processor to analyze the film and eliminate part of the tedious process of manual plotting. In the more sophisticated optoelectronic systems, the markers are actually infrared light–emitting diodes and are filmed by infrared-sensing cameras, thereby allowing further automation of the kinematic analysis.[191]

Regardless of the visualization method used, certain important factors must be taken into consideration. Sampling must be performed at a rate that is at least twice the frequency of the movement being analyzed, requiring a

minimal rate of 200 Hz for rearfoot movement.[252] The accuracy of the data collection system must be ensured both by the equipment manufacturer and by the on-site testing facility. Calibration, marker-to-marker distance testing, optimization of the collection environment, and meticulous attention to detail are just some of the factors necessary to ensure validity in kinematic testing.[252] For example, the markers can be placed using either a relative method, wherein four markers are arbitrarily placed on the posterior foot or shoe and the posterior calf, or an absolute method, which uses standard anatomic landmarks. Furthermore, it should be remembered that testing is done in a variety of conditions including different test subjects, different speeds from walking to sprinting, different surfaces ranging from treadmill to various over-ground conditions, in shoed and shoeless conditions, in varying types of shoewear, and in shoes with or without orthoses.[56]

This background is necessary to understand some of the information provided by the studies on rearfoot control. Although it is easy to see how a determination of rearfoot position could be performed in the barefoot runner, an obvious problem exists when the heel is hidden inside a shoe.[9] How does one determine the proper position for the markers? This question has been answered by studies that have used a window in the heel of the shoe to allow visualization of the calcaneus position.[42] One such study reported by Nigg analyzed measurements using one type of shoe in three test subjects with three trials per subject. A 2- to 3-degree shift was noted between the subject's heel and the shoe itself.[159] Because this shift was systematic, it was not believed to invalidate the test method. In a more recent study, Stacoff placed intracortical bone pins into volunteers to monitor movement coupling between shoe, calcaneus, and tibia. Apart from the difficulty of recruiting volunteers for this type of invasive monitoring, they observed considerable individual differences in coupling between these areas, and suggested that we have yet to unravel the details of this complex interaction.[237]

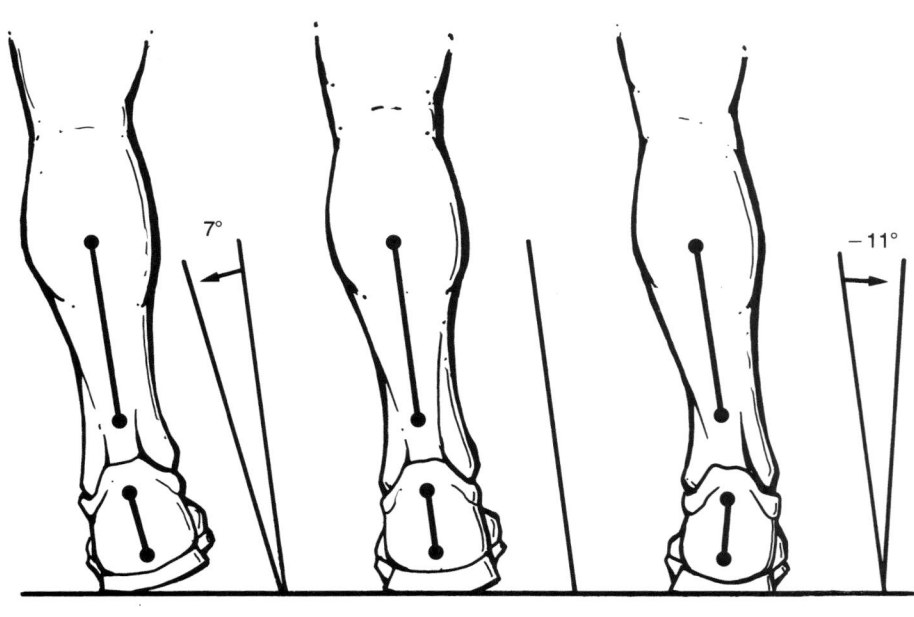

Figure 30D–24. Position of reference markers on the lower leg to define its axis and a second set of markers on the calcaneus to denote its position in kinematic analysis of gait. (Redrawn from Sport Research Review. Beaverton, Ore, Nike Sport Research Laboratory, Nov/Dec 1989.)

Supinated   Neutral   Pronated

Shoes and shoe design characteristics can have considerable effect on the kinematics of the foot in running and other sports activities including rearfoot control. Some of this effect is simply the result of displacement of the foot away from the contact surface by the shoe. It has been shown by several investigators that the Achilles tendon angle is decreased in the shoeless condition.[9, 56, 191] The total rearfoot movement and rate of pronation are also reduced in the barefoot runner.[9, 56, 159, 191, 235] This suggests that wearing shoes increases not only pronation but also other temporally related variables.[56, 191] This effect of shoewear is demonstrated in Figure 30D–25.

The shoe design variables that have been investigated most thoroughly with respect to kinematic effect include sole hardness, heel height, use of a heel flare, width of the midsole, and torsional flexibility.[56, 191] Sole hardness is measured in terms of durometer, a 25 shore A durometer sole being considerably softer than a 45 shore A durometer sole. Clarke and associates showed that the softer the sole, the greater the degree of maximum pronation and total rearfoot movement.[41] A similar study by Nigg found exactly the opposite result, the softer sole having less total pronation.[159] A later study by Nigg and colleagues confirmed their previous results, and further elaborated that the total foot eversion was roughly double for hard versus soft inserts. The harder inserts allowed for more individual variation of movement and did not force a preset movement pattern to the foot. Despite significant inter-individual variance, the subjects with a flexible foot were more likely to have diminished tibial rotation. This study concluded that individual variation must be taken into account when matching feet to inserts.[169] Because other factors such as overall shoe stiffness, shoe construction techniques, and variations in sole geometry can have significant effects on the kinematic function of the foot, it is easy to surmise how different results can be forthcoming from different laboratories when performing similar tests.[56]

Potential confusion in test results also occurs in the relationship of heel height to rearfoot control variables.

Bates and coworkers found that raising the heel height in relation to the forefoot could reduce both maximum pronation and the period of pronation.[9] Stacoff and Kaelin analyzed the effect of heel height over the range from 18 to 43 mm and found the same effect in the range from 23 to 33 mm but the opposite effect on pronation at the upper and lower ends of heel height.[234] To cap things off, Clarke and associates discovered no significant effect of varying heel heights between 10 and 30 mm. It is apparent that there are inconsistencies in the studies generating dissimilar results and adding to an already confusing picture.

With the introduction of the New Balance 305 Interval shoe in 1975, a new variable appeared in the shoe–foot control equation.[31] The flared heel, seen originally in this shoe, was added primarily to improve the stability of the shoe by widening the base of support when the foot was on the ground. Following the principle that "if a little bit is good, then more will be better," Nike introduced a shoe in the late 1970s that had a full 1-inch lateral heel flare. Unfortunately, a negative byproduct was quickly perceived in the increasing incidence of lateral knee pain that occurred with this shoe.[31] Nigg and Morlock discovered the underlying problem with the flared heel in a scientific study of 14 runners reported in 1987.[162] Using three shoes identical except in their degree of lateral heel flare, the authors noted increased initial pronation with wider flare but no difference in total pronation or impact forces at heel strike. Increasing the lateral heel flare increases the lever arm on the axis of motion across the subtalar joint, resulting in earlier initiation of a pronating movement, greater rearfoot angulatory velocity, and an increased initial Achilles tendon (touchdown) angle. A similar study by Nigg and Bahlsen confirmed this result but indicated that heel flare was less important when a softer midsole was used.[161] This study supported the earlier work of Cavanagh on a rounded heel design by demonstrating a reduction of more than 15% in the time of peak force with use of this modification.[56, 161]

Two shoe design characteristics that have been intro-

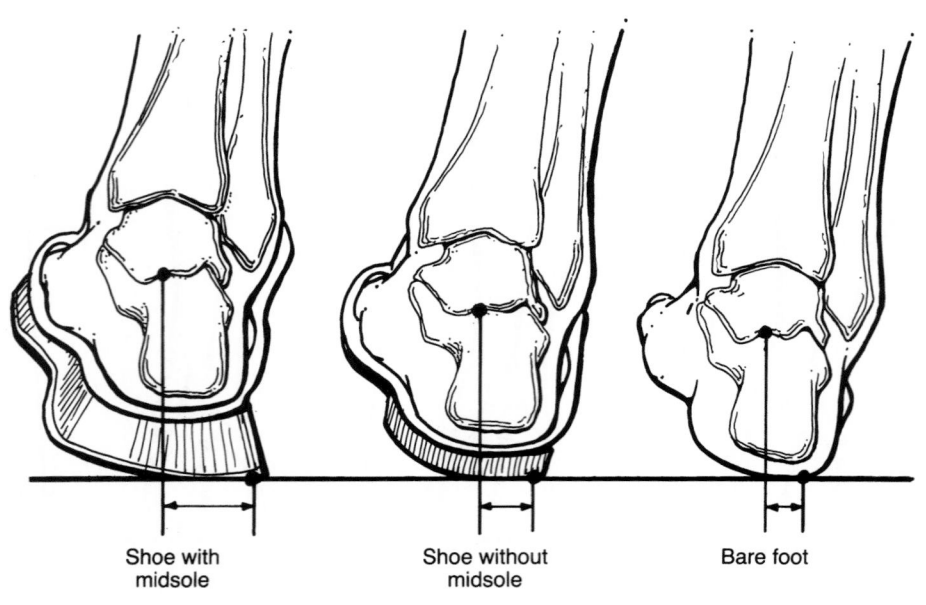

Shoe with midsole   Shoe without midsole   Bare foot

Figure 30D–25. Depiction of the effect of shoewear in increasing pronation from the barefoot condition. (Redrawn from Sport Research Review. Beaverton, Ore, Nike Sport Research Laboratory, Nov/Dec 1989.)

duced recently are related to midsole width and torsional flexibility. Both have been supported by shoe companies—Nike promoting the wider midsole and Adidas promoting running shoes with greater torsional flexibility.[3, 191, 223] According to the results provided by the Nike Sports Research Laboratory, reductions in maximum pronation and maximum pronation velocity can be obtained by increasing sole width to about 90 mm.[191] Torsional flexibility is a new concept related to evaluating the foot in three dimensions rather than by the traditional two-plane analysis of rearfoot inversion and eversion. Work by Stacoff and colleagues has demonstrated that large torsional movement occurs between the forefoot and hindfoot in the barefoot state.[235] This three-dimensional linkage between the forefoot and hindfoot is mediated through the tarsometatarsal (Lisfranc's) and transverse tarsal (Chopart's) joints and in a shoe can be influenced by shoe sole construction factors.

Shoe soles that are stiff in the longitudinal direction restrict the torsional movement normally produced when the forefoot adapts to the ground. Adidas has taken this concept and developed an entire line of running shoes with "a unique construction that controls the natural torsion, or twisting of the foot."[3] They also claim "the foot moves as nature intended it to. The natural twisting of the front part of the foot is controlled so that it no longer strains joints and tendons. Performance greatly improves, whereas injury and muscle strain are substantially diminished."[3] This seems to be an exaggerated claim for a shoe design feature that affects a foot movement that itself is not entirely understood, much less how it is changed by the shoe design and how that relates to other kinematic values. More time and research will be necessary to establish the importance of such factors as shoe width and torsional flexibility because they appear to be mutually exclusive based on examination of the shoes produced with this technology (Fig. 30D–26).

The fabrication of orthotic devices to control rearfoot stability, thereby treating various disorders of the lower extremity, has a rather short history. In 1962, Rose presented one of the earliest studies on the ability of a position-modifying device (the Schwartz meniscus) within the shoe to alter the rotation of the lower leg.[208] Sheehan, writing in the Preface to *The Foot Book* by Harry Hlavac, traced the origin of biomechanical therapy to the early 1970s and the development of sports podiatry.[88] He theorized that the increasing problem with anterior knee pain in runners was the key to the development of orthotic devices for the foot. The ability of a shoe insert to provide benefit when a surgical solution was not forthcoming led to "the ascendancy of orthopedic medicine."[88] And ascend it did, as orthoses for sports scaled new heights in cost, in numbers, and in varieties of conditions for which they were recommended. At present, many athletes and coaches think that the orthotic device is standard athletic equipment. Athletes come to the clinician with one sort of complaint or another and a self-made diagnosis requesting "orthotics." In this environment, it is critical that individuals involved in the field of sports medicine understand not only the biomechanical principles behind the use of orthotic devices but also the relevant literature from gait laboratory studies.

As in the evaluation of shoewear, kinematic analysis of

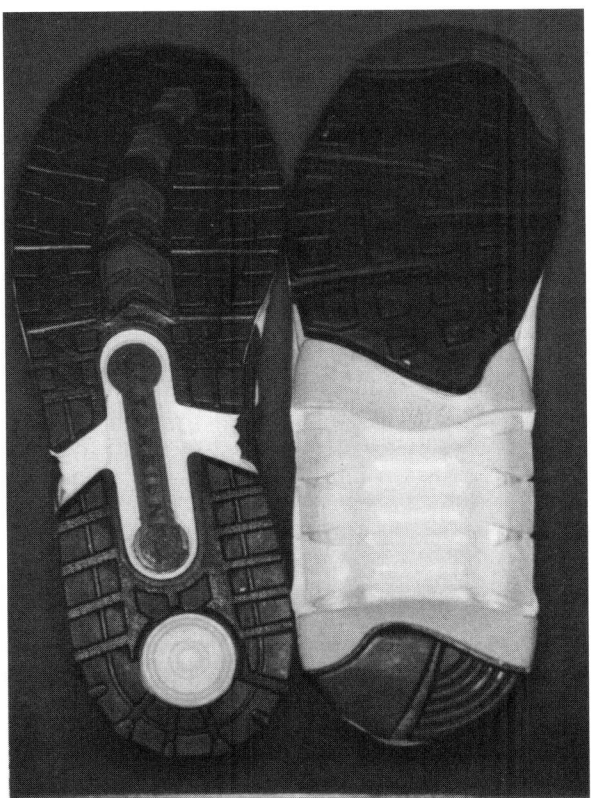

Figure 30D–26. Example of wide versus narrow midsole widths used in the Nike (*right*) and Adidas (*left*) running shoes. (Photograph by Thomas O. Clanton.)

various parameters is essential to the documentation of orthotic effects on gait. According to Stacoff and Luethi, it was Nigg who first determined the effect of shoe inserts on gait using film analysis.[236] Nigg's study concluded that a properly functioning insert should change gait characteristics toward values consistent with those of normal feet. Cavanagh and colleagues presented a paper at the 1978 meeting of the American Orthopaedic Society for Sports Medicine in Lake Placid, New York, that showed a reduction in maximum pronation and maximum velocity of pronation in runners who used a properly placed felt shoe pad as a medial support.[56] Nigg and associates reported in 1986 on the use of various conditions and positions (from no support to anterior to posterior positions) for medial supports within the shoe, demonstrating that placing the pad (elastic cork in this instance) more posterior reduced initial pronation and maximum pronation to a lesser extent (Fig. 30D–27).[165] Taunton and coworkers found a similar reduction in maximum pronation with the use of an orthosis.[250] These studies support the ability of an orthosis to affect kinematic parameters.

Further work in this area was provided by Smith and colleagues, who studied 11 well-trained runners using soft or semirigid orthoses while running on a treadmill at a 6- and 7-minute-mile pace.[227, 228] They found that calcaneal eversion was reduced in their subjects, who had an average rearfoot varus posting of 4.2 degrees. This reduced maximum pronation from a mean of 11.3 degrees in controls to 10.5 degrees for the soft orthosis to 10.1 degrees for the

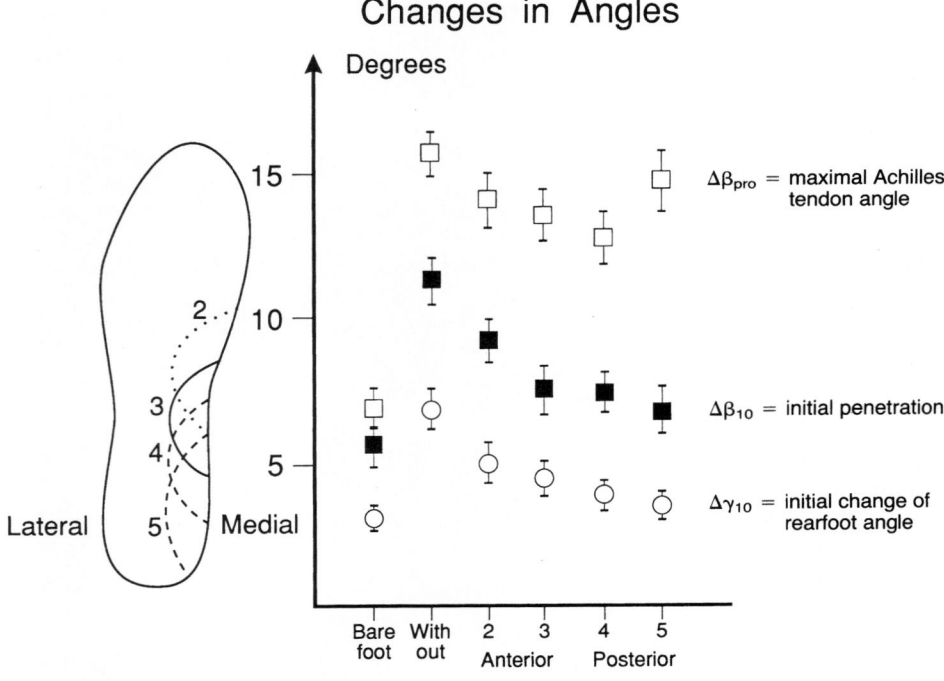

Changes in Angles

$\Delta\beta_{pro}$ = maximal Achilles tendon angle

$\Delta\beta_{10}$ = initial penetration

$\Delta\gamma_{10}$ = initial change of rearfoot angle

Figure 30D–27. Graphic demonstration that placing an insert more posteriorly reduces initial pronation and maximum pronation. (From Nigg BM: Biomechanics of Running Shoes. Champaign, Ill, Human Kinetics, 1986. Copyright 1986 by Benno M. Nigg. Reprinted by permission.)

semirigid device, only a 1% change. Maximum velocity of pronation was reduced from a mean of 540 degrees per second in controls to 430 degrees per second for the soft orthosis to 464 degrees per second for the semirigid group, an 11% change. Although the reduction in maximum pronation is quite small compared to the expected result for this amount of posting, the reduction in pronation velocity may play a larger role in symptomatic relief provided by orthoses—an effect that can be achieved as adequately by the less expensive soft orthosis as by the semirigid orthosis. Although these studies further augment the role of orthoses in adjusting kinematic variables, other authors have had results that are less supportive.

One of the most widely recognized studies of foot orthoses and their effect on gait is that done by Bates and associates in 1979.[8] This study failed to confirm a significant reduction in maximum pronation with a custom-molded orthotic device compared with shoes in six symptomatic runners. The study compared its results with control values obtained in a previous study of 10 asymptomatic runners.[9] Their results also suggested that an increased velocity of pronation occurred with the orthotic device in contrast to the findings of the previously mentioned studies. Rodgers and LeVeau produced a similar study using 29 runners fitted with custom-made semirigid orthoses made from polypropylene.[207] Subjects ran in their own shoes on an outdoor track and were filmed with 16-mm film at 120 frames per second. Runners completed three randomly sequenced runs in the following conditions: (1) barefoot, (2) shoe without orthosis, and (3) shoe with orthosis. Values obtained for maximum pronation, angulatory velocity of pronation, and time spent in pronation were not significantly different among the three conditions. There was, however, a trend toward decreased maximum pronation and time in pronation in the shoe with orthosis group. Smith and colleagues pointed out some of the flaws in the

various studies related to inadequate control of confounding variables such as type of shoe, type of orthosis, and physical measurements of test subjects.[228] Given the number of variables that are being analyzed in these gait studies of running, there should be little surprise that some discrepancies exist. More study will be necessary to determine which of the variables is important in relation to the clinical situation and the prevention or treatment of injuries. Progress in this field would proceed at a more rapid rate if there could be some universal agreement on terminology, methods of measurement, normal values, and sharing of information without commercial self-interest.

Clinical Work

Although there is a widespread belief in sports medicine circles that biomechanical abnormalities are a significant causal factor in lower extremity injuries, clinical studies have had paradoxical results. The military formerly believed that the pronated flat foot was more susceptible to injury, but recent work has disproved this belief. Devan and Carlton suggested as early as 1954 that stress fractures of the metatarsals were equally common among pronated, normal, and cavus foot types.[53] Gilbert and Johnson[12] and Bensel[74] reached the same conclusion from their research. Further confirmation of this conclusion has come from the Israeli Army study of 295 recruits, which indicated that the low-arched foot might even protect against the development of stress fractures.[73] The overall incidence of stress fractures in their study was 39.6% in recruits with a high arch, 31.3% in those with average arch height, and 10% in those with a low arch. It is important to note that in these studies, the criteria for defining arch height were subjective, and determinations were made in a non–weight-bearing position.

A continuation of the Israeli Army study was reported

in 1989 with a more quantitative determination of the longitudinal arch based on radiographic analysis.[225] This study reported a higher number of metatarsal stress fractures in recruits with low arches, whereas the incidence of femoral and tibial fractures in these recruits was less than that in those who had a higher arch. This result seemingly contradicts the findings of the previous studies. It should be noted that both of the Israeli Army studies excluded those with marked pes cavus or pes planus from the outset. A subsequent Israeli Army study examined the use of custom soft or semirigid functional orthoses and suggested a benefit in reducing stress fractures; however, fewer than half the recruits completed the study using their assigned orthoses (25% dropped out because of dissatisfaction with the orthosis). Nearly 50% of the arriving recruits were already using orthoses (30% custom-made).[266] All of this adds further confounding variables complicating interpretation of the various clinical studies and extrapolating an association between biomechanical parameters and symptomatology.

In dancing, a sport much different from running, dancers as well as their teachers and dance medicine specialists have related lower extremity injury to poor technique and malalignment.[77, 92, 127] Despite this, two independent studies failed to confirm such an association. McNeal and coworkers studied 350 dancers and found no significant relationship between alignment and injury rate for the knee, ankle, or foot.[138] Solomon and colleagues reported a similar lack of correlation between degree of hindfoot pronation and self-reported injuries in professional ballet and modern dancers.[231] Although faulty technique no doubt plays a role in exposing a dancer to potential injury, pronation has not been firmly established as the culprit.

Among runners it is evident that a number of risk factors have been implicated in the production of injuries (Table 30D–11).[121, 183, 261] Because so much emphasis is placed on the relationship between overpronation and injury, it is natural to expect confirmation of this in the epidemiologic surveys of running injuries. One of the first studies to focus attention on the role of pronation in runners was that of James and colleagues in 1978.[95] They reported a 58% incidence of pronation in 180 patients evaluated for a variety of complaints. It is important to note that one cannot draw the conclusion that the majority of injured runners have pronated feet because there is no way of determining the overall incidence of pronation in the running population. Despite this fact, it is our opinion that this study was instrumental in focusing the attention of sports medicine specialists on the role of alignment in sports injuries. Unfortunately (or perhaps fortunately for the overpronator), no such relationship has been clearly determined in epidemiologically valid studies.[183] One of the most comprehensive studies of running injuries is the Ontario cohort study, which included 1680 runners. Anthropometric measurements including femoral neck anteversion, pelvic obliquity, knee and patella alignment, rearfoot valgus, pes cavus and pes planus, somatotype, and running shoe wear pattern were made in 1000 of these runners. The study concluded that "none of the anthropometric variables measured was significantly related to risk."[261] The most consistent risk factor for a running-related injury is weekly training mileage, and this has been proven in study after study.[15, 121, 129, 183, 261] When weekly distance reaches 64 kilometers or 40 miles per week, the risk for injury increases by three times.[121, 261] Additionally, no correlation has been shown between shoe characteristics (e.g., varus wedge or waffle sole) or shoe expense and injury reduction in these studies.[72, 128, 261] Given all this information, what role does rearfoot stability provided by shoes or orthoses play in the prevention or treatment of athletic injury?

Although the scientific approach of systematically establishing a basis for the use of orthoses has failed, there does appear to be some practical basis for prescribing orthoses to injured athletes. Seventy-eight percent of the injured runners in the oft-quoted series of James and colleagues reported some benefit from the use of either rigid or flexible orthoses.[95] D'Ambrosia subdivided patients by diagnosis and analyzed the numbers who benefited from the use of an orthosis. The subgroup with pes planovalgus had the most benefit (90% of patients), whereas the subgroup with pes cavus had the least benefit (25% of patients) (Table 30D–12).[50] Another study from the Louisiana State University Medical Center Runner's Clinic reported a 72% im-

TABLE 30D–11
Risk Factors in Running Injuries

Characteristics of Runners	Characteristics of Running	Characteristics of Running Environment
Age	Distance	Terrain
Gender	Speed	Surface
Structural abnormalities	Stability of pattern	Climate
Body build	Form	Time of day
Experience	Stretching, weight training, warm-up/ cool-down	Shoes
Individual susceptibility		
Past injury		

From Powell KE, Kohl HW, Caspersen CJ, et al: An epidemiological perspective on the causes of running injuries. Physician Sportsmed 14:100–114, 1986.

TABLE 30D–12
Effectiveness of Orthoses

Diagnosis	N (%)	Percentage Improved with Orthosis
Posterior tibial syndrome	55 (27.5)	77
Pes planovalgum	23 (11.5)	90
Metatarsalgia	30 (15)	87
Plantar fasciitis	20 (10)	81
Calcaneal spur	18 (9)	81
Iliotibial band tendinitis	14 (7)	66
Cavus foot	13 (6.5)	25
Leg length inequality	10 (5)	NA
Chondromalacia patellae	6 (3)	NA
Achilles tendinitis	4 (2)	NA
Miscellaneous	7 (3.5)	NA
Total	200 (100)	

NA, not available.

From D'Ambrosia RD: Orthotic devices in running injuries. Clin Sports Med 4:611–618, 1985.

shoes were designed. Of 171 models of shoes, including spikes as well as running and general athletic shoes, 26% were purported to be for both pronators and supinators, 36% claimed an advantage for both the high-arched and flat-footed individual, and amazingly, two shoes in the survey claimed benefit for every distance, foot type, heel-strike pattern, and surface mentioned.[82]

The technologic gimmickry that has been introduced into the athletic shoewear industry in recent years has seldom met with commercial success unless the athlete has perceived a significant functional benefit. Examples of such less than successful innovations have included the swivel football shoe introduced by American Bilt-rite in the late 1960s,[27, 214] the Lotto running shoe with the safety tail light,[35] the Puma computerized shoe,[35] the Reebok "Pump," and the various component shoes introduced by several companies.[31, 35] Reebok introduced the Traxtar "smart shoe" for children. This shoe is equipped with a microprocessor and motion sensor, and it measures the child's performance in jumping and running. A light and sound display actually plays "Pomp and Circumstance" when specific performance levels are reached.[2] It remains to be seen whether the current gimmicks will follow the trend toward extinction or achieve the success of the "air sole" that has become the trademark of the Nike athletic shoes.[3, 6, 31, 78, 109, 130, 152, 221–223]

Summary

Knowledge of athletic shoes, pads, inlays, inserts, and orthoses has become important in the field of sports medicine for many reasons. This knowledge is essential not only from the standpoint of treating and preventing injuries but also to halt the propagation of misleading information and avoid unnecessary expense. Athletic shoewear is essential for the protection of the athlete's foot, but this protection must extend to the athlete as a whole. With a brief historical perspective and knowledge of the construction of shoes and orthoses, individuals can better understand the factors involved in this protection. These factors include shock absorption, stability, friction and torque, and proper fit. Their specific contributions to athletic performance, comfort, and injury risk remain incompletely elucidated despite numerous laboratory and clinical studies. It is hoped that this chapter will not only stimulate increased awareness of the role of athletic shoes and orthoses in the field of sports medicine but also point out the need for further research.

Glossary of Foot and Shoe Terminology*

Abduction: To move away from the midline of the body.

---

*This glossary has been compiled from: An A to Z guide to shoe terminology. Runner's World, 25:48–49, 1990; Cheskin MP: The Complete Handbook of Athletic Footwear. New York, Fairchild Publications, 1987, pp 163–245; Prescription Footwear Association/Board for Certification in Pedorthics: 1992/93 Desk Reference and Directory. Columbia, Md, Prescription Footwear Association, 1992, pp 65–78; and Janisse D (ed): Introduction to Pedorthics. Columbia, Md, Pedorthic Footwear Association, 1998.

Abrasion tester: A machine used to determine the quantity of material lost by friction (wear) under specified conditions.

Accelerometer: A device that measures acceleration or the rate of change of velocity as it relates to impact force.

Achilles notch: A depression cut into the back of the heel collar to provide a secure fit and prevent irritation of the Achilles tendon.

Acrylic resin: Synthetic resin prepared from acrylic acid.

Adduct: To move toward the midline of the body.

Adduction: Moving a part toward the midline of the body.

Adhesive (cement): Substance capable of holding materials together by surface attachment.

Aglet: Metal or plastic tip of lace.

Air: First introduced in 1979, Nike's cushioning concept of encapsulated air units in the midsole isn't actually air, it's freon. Depending on the model, the air units may be in the heel, forefoot, or both.

Air ball: An air-pressurized ball imbedded in the heel of Hi-Tec Badwater models for additional shock absorption.

Anatomical: Pertaining to the structure of the body.

Anatomical last: A stabilizing footbed contoured in such a way that the heel sits down in the midsole, rather than resting atop a flat platform. Developed and used extensively by Turntec.

Anatomy: The study of the structure of the body and the relationships between its parts.

Aniline: Leather tanning finish.

Anterior: Front portion.

Anterior heel: Type of metatarsal bar, also known as Denver bar or Denver heel; the apex coincides with the posterior edge under the posterior half of the metatarsal shafts.

Applique: Logo or other ornament in the form of a piece of leather or material sewn to the shoe.

Apron cut: Design of the toe cap.

ARC: Avia's stabilizing system, which is made of plastic in one of two configurations. Placed in the rearfoot, the "fingers" of the ARC spread out on impact to absorb shock and stabilize the foot.

Arch bandage: Reinforcing strips of fabric stitched inside the shoe on the medial and lateral quarters.

Arch cushion (cookie): Support pad for the medial arch of the foot.

Asymmetrical: In shoemaking this applies to lasts and patterns that have uneven shapes, the right side different from the left.

ATP (heel horn): Extended padding at the back heel collar to protect the Achilles tendon (Achilles tendon protector).

Autoclave: Vessel or oven in which chemical reaction or cooking takes place under pressure such as in the vulcanizing construction method.

Axis: A reference line for making measurements. Ground reaction forces are usually evaluated relative to a set of three orthogonal axes: vertical, longitudinal (direction of motion), and transverse (right angle to direction of motion).

Back cone: Portion of the cone surface between the "V" cut and the back end of the last.

Back cone height: The vertical distance between the heel featherline plane and the back cone top plane.

Backer: Lining material.

Backpart (rear foot): Portion of the last extending rearward from the break of the joint to the back of the last.

Backpart width: The width of the heel end measured parallel to the heel featherline plane at a specified distance from the heel point.

Back seam: Stitching line at the back of the heel joining quarters.

Bagged edge: Clean inside seam hiding stitching.

Bal (Balmoral): Front-laced shoe in which the meeting of the quarters and the vamp is stitched or continuous at the distal end of the throat. Bal is the abbreviation of Balmoral, the Scottish castle where this style was first introduced.

Balance: To support or arrange to equalize opposing forces.

Ball: Widest part of the sole, at the metatarsal head.

Ball girth: Circumference measure around the last encompassing the first to the fifth metatarsal area.

Banbury: Apparatus for mixing compounds.

Bar, comma: Comma-shaped bar wedged laterally and posteriorly, also known as Hauser.

Bar, Denver: See Anterior heel.

Bar, Jones: Metatarsal bar placed between the inner sole and outer sole.

Bar, Mayo: Metatarsal bar with the anterior edge curved to approximate the position of the metatarsal heads.

Bar, metatarsal: Rubber, leather, or synthetic bar applied transversely across the bottom of the sole, with the apex immediately posterior to the metatarsal heads.

Bar, rocker: Sole bar having its apex beneath the metatarsal shafts causing rocking instead of flexing action.

Bar, Thomas: Narrow metatarsal bar with abrupt anterior and posterior drop-offs.

Bar, transverse: See Bar, metatarsal.

Base plane: The plane to which the last in its proper attitude is referenced for the purpose of defining certain terms.

Bellows tongue: Outside attached tongue to prevent snow entry.

Benchmade: Shoes made entirely by hand at the shoemaker's workbench.

Bias cut: Cut away upswept heel.

Bicycle shoe: Low-quarter shoe laced to the toe.

Bilateral: Affecting both right and left sides.

Binding: Reinforcement for the edge of material used in upper.

Biomechanics: The study of the internal and external forces acting on the human body and the effects produced by these forces.

Bisect: Divide into two equal parts.

Blind eyelet: A metal or plastic eyelet concealed beneath the top surface of the shoe leaving only a small, rimless hole.

Blowing agent: Chemicals added to plastics or rubber that generate cellular structure.

Blown rubber: The lightest kind of rubber outsole material. As the outsoles are manufactured, air is injected into the rubber to lighten and soften the outsole. Few outsoles today are made with full blown rubber because it lacks durability, but many outsoles have blown rubber in the forefoot and midfoot for lightness and a harder carbon rubber in the high-wear area of the heel.

Blucher: Front-laced shoe in which the quarters are not attached distally to the vamp, giving more allowance at the throat and instep in fitting. Opposite of bal style. Front quarters or tabs are stitched over the vamp for a short distance at the throat.

Board last: One of three ways shoes are constructed. A fully board lasted shoe is constructed by gluing the upper to fiberboard before it is attached to the midsole. Board lasting promotes stability and provides a good platform for orthotics but lacks flexibility. Few new models are fully board lasted. (See combination last and slip last for information about the more common types of last.)

Boot, high top: High quarter shoe in which the quarters cover the malleoli.

Bottom: The sole up to the breast of the heel. On a wedge sole, the term covers the complete sole.

Bottom filler: Material that fills the cavity between the outer and inner soles.

Bottoming: The operation of attaching the completed sole to the upper.

Bottoming out: When the midsole material has worn out and is too soft relative to a runner's size, it compresses too quickly, which results in compromised shock absorption and support.

Box toe: Hardener used to maintain shape of front toe area.

Break: Flex point or path; creasing formed at the vamp when the shoe is dorsiflexed.

Breastline: An arbitrary line defining the forward boundary of the heel seat.

Breathability: The ability of a material to absorb and ventilate foot moisture; not to be confused with porous.

Buckskin: Leather or deerskin with suede finish.

Built-up: Construction used in vulcanized rubber process.

Bumper: Rubber toe strip attached over front toe area.

Butadiene: A gas obtained from petroleum, used to make plastics.

Calender sole: Sheet sole pressed between rollers.

Calfskin leather: Leather made from the skin of calves.

Cam: A projection on a wheel or shaft that changes a regular circular motion into an irregular rotary motion or a back and forth motion.

Cantilever: A concave outsole design in which the outer edges flare out on impact to dissipate shock. Used extensively by Avia.

Carbon black: Pigment added to outside rubber for better durability.

Carbon rubber: The most durable kind of rubber outsole material. It's a solid rubber with a carbon additive that makes the material stronger. If an outsole isn't full carbon rubber, it probably has a carbon-rubber heel pad.

C-cap: A term that New Balance uses for the process of heating and molding EVA to improve its durability and cushioning.

Celluloid: A thermoplastic material.

Cellulose: Natural polymeric.

Cement: See Adhesive.

Sagittal plane: The vertical plane that passes through the body from back to front dividing it into a left and right half.

Seam: Sewing that joins together pieces of the upper.

Semi cut: A design cut just on or over the ankle. (Also called three-quarter cut.)

Shank: The reinforcement under the arch between the heel and the sole; the bottom area of the last between the breastline and the joint break.

Shank piece: Rigid reinforcement of the shank.

Shank plug: A metal piece inserted in the shank in order to clinch metal shank fasting staple.

Shearing force: A force that causes or tends to cause two parts of a body to slide relative to each other.

Shell (dish) sole: A unit sole with foxing sides molded to the bottom. (Also called a cup sole.)

Shoe size:

Prewalkers: 3000–4
Big boys: 5½–11
Infants: 1–8
Growing girls: 3½–10
Children: 8½–12
Men: 6½–16
Misses: 12½–4
Ladies: 4–13
Youths: 12½–4
Boys: 3½–6

Shore hardness: The durometer hardness on a scale of 0–100.

Side leather: Leather made from the skin of cattle; commonly used leather in American footwear.

Silicone: A slippery polymeric material used in treating shoes for water repellency.

Skinfit: Nylon tricot lining.

Skive: The thinning down of edges of leather or poromeric material; to cut in thin layers or to a fine edge.

Slip last: The most flexible type of shoe construction. With a slip-lasted shoe, the upper is stitched together like a moccasin and glued to the midsole. Slip lasting allows for a better fit. Lasting method whereby a closed upper is formed before being stretched over the last.

Slip sole: A half-sole from toe to shank.

Slush molding: A PVC construction molding process.

Sneaker: The American name for vulcanized, canvas rubber shoe.

Socklining: The material (regularly called an insole) inserted between the foot and lasting insole next to the foot; material covering the dorsal surface of the inner sole.

Sole: Bottom or ground contact area of footwear.

Sole leather: Heavy leather, usually cattlehide that is dry-finished and used for outer soles.

Specific gravity: The density of any material.

Speed lacing: A lacing method that uses D-rings.

Spikes: Metal appendages protruding from the shoe sole.

Splint, Denis-Browne: Rigid bar between both shoes used to abduct the feet.

Splint, Friedman-counter: Flexible strip attached to both counters; used to limit internal rotation.

Split: The flesh or the underside of the leather hide after the grain side has been removed.

Split leather: See Sole leather.

Sprocket: A projection on the rim of a wheel or cylinder that engages the links of a chain.

Stability: The ability of the shoe to keep the foot moving in a forward direction, rather than allowing for excessive side-to-side movement.

Stabilizer: An ingredient used in formulating elastomers and synthetics.

StableAir: Etonic's new "air" system. StableAir is ambient, air-filled units placed in the heel or in the heel and forefoot for cushioning.

Standard deviation: A standard measure of dispersion of a frequency distribution about the average value. A distribution is typically made up of three standard deviations on either side of the average value.

Stick length: Overall length of a last measured with a last size stick.

Stitchdown: A method of sewing the uppers to the bottom.

Straight last: A last that is relatively straight on the medial side to add stability. The straighter the last, the greater the medial support. 1. Form for constructing a shoe that can be worn on either foot. 2. Form for constructing a shoe in which the medial border approximates a straight line.

Strain gauge: A device for measuring forces by monitoring the change in resistance to a small wire that has been deformed by the force.

Studs: Large knobs protruding from the sole.

Suction cups: Indentations on the outsole that provide traction on smooth surfaces.

Suede: The buffed reverse or flesh side of leather.

Supination: A triplane motion of the foot or part of the foot which consists of simultaneous movements: adduction, plantar flexion, and inversion; basically, a movement toward the midline of the body, down and in; elevation of the medial foot arch; the opposite of pronation. Oversupination occurs when the foot remains on its outside edge after heel strike instead of pronating. A true oversupinating foot underpronates or does not pronate at all so it doesn't absorb shock well. It is a rare condition, occurring in less than 1 per cent of the running population.

Symmetrical: In shoemaking, this applies to lasts or patterns that have even sides, the right side the same as the left side.

Synthetic: Something resulting from synthesis rather than occurring naturally; a product (as drug or plastic) of chemical synthesis.

Tack hole plug: A plastic insert in the bottom of the last for receiving insole tacks.

Tanning: Process of converting raw hides and skins into leather by a combination of chemical and mechanical means.

Tensile strength: The pulling force expressed in measuring leathers or fabrics; the resistance of a material to being pulled apart.

Terminal wear condition: A condition in which the outsole of a shoe is worn completely through to the midsole or underlying material.

Thermoplastic: Material capable of being repeatedly softened by heat and hardened by cooling; a type of rigid, durable plastic used for most heel counters.

Thimble: A metal sleeve inserted in the top heel end of last providing an opening for a mounting spindle or last pin.

Thomas bar: See Bar, Thomas.

Throat: Entrance of the shoe where normally the vamp and quarters meet; the topline of the vamp in front of the instep.

Throat opening: The distance in a straight line from the vamp point to the back seam tuck.

Toe box: Reinforcement used to retain the original contour of the toe and guard the foot against trauma or abrasion.

Toe cap: An additional protective device on the frontal toe area.

Toe profile: A side view profile of the toe end of the last.

Toe recede: The slope of the top surface of the last extending from the toe point to the point of full toe thickness.

Toe spring: The vertical distance between the base plane and the toe point of a last having the desired heel elevation; the vertical distance between the ground and the toe point giving the shoe frontal pitch.

Tongue: A layer of upper material that protects the top part of the foot from pressure from the laces. Some tongues on Asics shoes are now split to allow the foot to expand.

Tongue guide: The tag or slit in the tongue through which the laces are slotted to hold the tongue in place (lace keeper).

Toplift: Layer of material forming the plantar surface of the heel.

Top line: The open area of the shoe around the ankle.

Torque: A force that causes or tends to cause rotation of an object about an axis. The torque (also called moment) is the result of the magnitude of the force, its direction, and distance from the axis of rotation.

Torsion: The stress caused by twisting a material.

Torsional rigidity: The amount of stiffness in the shank and waist of a shoe.

Torsion rigidity bar: A motion-control device in some Saucony shoes. It consists of a bar (made of Kevlar and Hytrel) encapsulated in the midsole by EVA.

Torsion system: The flagship technology of Adidas. It's a system designed to allow the forefoot and rearfoot to move independently of each other to encourage freedom of movement. Shoes designed with the Torsion system have a groove cut into the midsole where the foot bends naturally during the running gait. The Torsion Bar is a Kevlar strip embedded lengthwise into the midsole to control excessive twisting of the foot.

TPR: Thermoplastic rubber.

Traction: The amount of friction or resistance to slip between a shoe outsole and the contact surface.

Transducer: A device that converts an applied load or force into an electrical signal.

Transverse arch: Curvature of metatarsal heads.

Transverse force: The force generated at a right angle to the direction of motion by a walker or runner during foot contact and most closely related to rearfoot stability. Also referred to as the mediolateral force.

Transverse plane: The horizontal plane that passes through the body from side to side and back to front dividing it into an upper and lower half.

Tread: The soling configuration of the outsole.

Treadmill: A rotary machine-driven belt that allows subjects to run in a confined space.

Treadpoint: Point of the bottom forepart of last or shoe in contact with the treading surface.

Tricot: Knitted fabric commonly used for linings in women's shoes.

Turnshoe: An early shoemaking technique; the reverse of the simple stitched shoe.

Unit sole: The bottom unit with sole and heel portions molded together as a single piece.

Universal last: A standard last used by sports shoemakers for all width fittings.

Upper: The material making up the "top" part of the shoe.

Upper leather: Any leather used for uppers.

Urethane: Plastic used for uppers, soles, top lifts, and other components; commonly known as polyurethane.

Urethane: A resin combination with polymers.

U-throat: A lacing eyestay pattern at the front of the shoe.

Vamp: Forepart of the upper. The top or front part of the upper over the toe and lacing area.

Vamp length or depth: The distance measured along the toe profile from the vamp tack to the toe point.

Vamp tack: An arbitrary point on top of a last forepart marked by a tack, measured from the toe.

V cut: The portion of the cone that is removed to permit "breaking" of the hinge.

Vegetable tanning: Tanning that uses plant or vegetable materials; uses materials derived from plant life such as oak, chestnut, quebracho, myrobalans, or divi-divi.

Velcro: Nylon hook and loop tape fastener that clings on contact.

Vertical force: The force perpendicular to a level surface. The dominant force generated by a walker or runner during foot contact and most closely related to the shock absorption characteristics of a shoe.

Vinyl: A PVC material that's available in expanding and nonexpanding types.

Vulcanize: A method of shoemaking in which the rubber sole and/or foxing is cured by heat after attaching to the upper; bonding of the outer sole to the upper from a sole mold in which the soft rubber molds to the shoe, then is allowed to cool and harden. Common in footwear such as sneakers.

Waffle: An outsole profile developed by former Oregon coach Bill Bowerman and used extensively by Nike.

Waist: Section of the last or shoe between the ball and instep.

Waist girth: The smallest dimension around a last between the joint girth and the instep girth.

Wall: Straight sides around the periphery of the forepart of certain style lasts.

Water repellent: Shoes treated so that they will shed water.

Waterproof: Shoes treated so that water cannot penetrate.

Wear tester: A piece of equipment used to evaluate the resistance of the outsole of a shoe to abrasion.

Wedge: Tapered leather, rubber, or other material used to elevate one side of the sole or heel; replaces the heel.

Wedge angle: The angle between the heel featherline

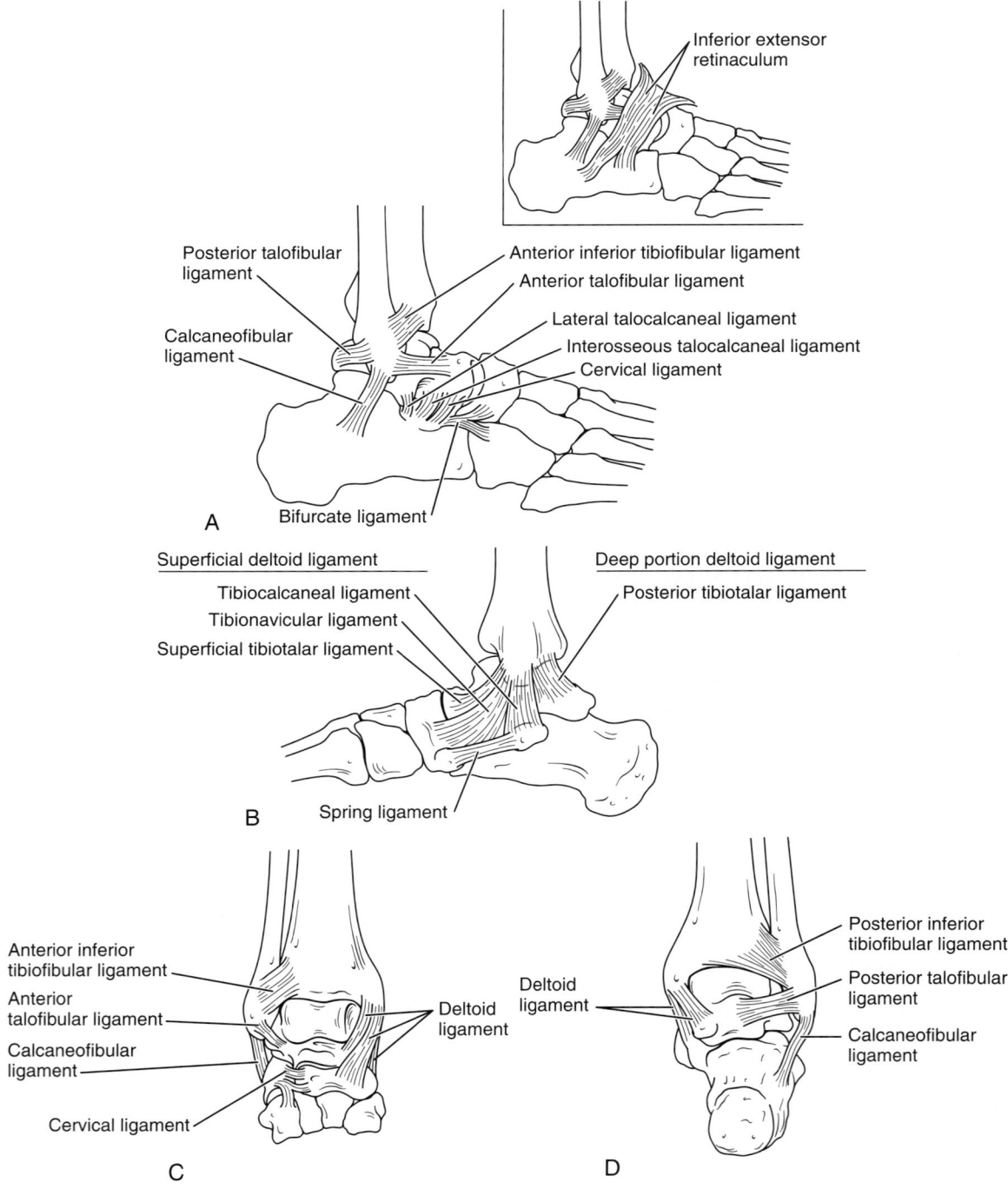

Figure 30E1–1. Compendium of the foot and ankle ligaments. *A,* Lateral view of the foot and ankle demonstrating the anterior talofibular ligament, calcaneofibular ligament, posterior talofibular ligament, anterior inferior tibiofibular ligament, lateral talocalcaneal ligament, inferior extensor retinaculum, interosseous talocalcaneal ligament, cervical ligament, and bifurcate ligament. *B,* Medial view of the foot and ankle demonstrating the superficial deltoid ligament, including the tibionavicular, spring ligament, tibiocalcaneal, and superficial tibiotalar components. *C,* An anterior view of the ankle and hindfoot demonstrating the deltoid ligament with its superficial and deep components, the anterior inferior tibiofibular ligament, the cervical ligament, the anterior talofibular ligament, and the calcaneofibular ligament. *D,* A posterior view of the ankle and hindfoot demonstrating the deltoid ligament with its superficial and deep components, the posterior inferior tibiofibular ligament, the posterior talofibular ligament, and the calcaneofibular ligament.

activity. Glick and colleagues reported that preexisting laxity of the lateral ankle ligaments, in the form of increased talar tilt on stress radiograph, is a significant risk factor.[87] Furthermore, Thacker and coworkers completed a review

of the literature and determined that a history of previous lateral ankle sprain is the most commonly cited risk factor for ankle sprain.[262]

Although hypermobility, generalized joint laxity, and

TABLE 30E1–1
Ankle Ligament Groups

Lateral ankle ligaments	Anterior talofibular ligament (ATFL)
	Calcaneofibular ligament (CFL)
	Posterior talofibular ligament (PTFL)
Medial ankle ligaments	Superficial deltoid (tibionavicular ligament,
	tibiospring ligament, tibiocalcaneal ligament,
	and superficial tibiotalar ligament)
	Deep deltoid (deep anterior tibiotalar ligament
	and deep posterior tibiotalar ligament)
Ankle syndesmosis	Anterior inferior tibiofibular ligament (AITFL)
	Posterior inferior tibiofibular ligament (PITFL)
	Distal interosseous ligament (IOL)

previous ligament injury should intuitively qualify as significant risk factors for lateral ankle injury, Baumhauer and associates published a contrary conclusion.[14] They completed a prospective study of joint laxity, foot and ankle alignment, ankle ligament stability, and isokinetic strength as risk factors for inversion ankle injuries. Among 145 college-age athletes, 15 injuries were reported during a single intercollegiate season (lacrosse, soccer, and field hockey). No significant differences were found between the injured and uninjured groups with regard to the stated risk factors.

Relevant Anatomy

Normal Anatomy. The talus articulates with the tibia and fibula to form the ankle joint (talocrural joint). The clinical range of motion is variable but includes 15 to 25 degrees of dorsiflexion and 40 to 55 degrees of plantar flexion. The empirical axis of the joint is somewhat oblique such that plantar flexion and dorsiflexion produce concomitant internal and external rotation of the foot relative to the leg. The rotational movements are translated through the subtalar joint and the remainder of the foot to produce supination and pronation during the gait cycle.

Inman noted that the anterior margin of the talar dome

is wider than the posterior margin by an average of 2.4 mm.[113] The obvious implication of this differential width is the stability imparted to the ankle joint during ankle dorsiflexion, along with the relative instability associated with ankle plantar flexion.

The functional stability of the ankle is the product of its soft tissue support. The ankle capsule is reinforced by several groups of ligamentous structures. The lateral ankle ligaments include the anterior talofibular ligament (ATFL), the calcaneofibular ligament (CFL), and the posterior talofibular ligament (PTFL) (Fig. 30E1–3).

The ATFL originates from the anterior aspect of the distal fibula, inserts on the lateral aspect of the talar neck, and measures 5 mm in width and 12 mm in length.[214] The CFL originates from the distal tip of the fibula, inserts at the lateral wall of the calcaneus, and is variable in dimension and orientation. Typically a cordlike structure 4 to 6 mm in diameter, the CFL is directed posteriorly 10 to 45 degrees from the tip of the fibula to the calcaneal insertion.[214] The PTFL originates from the posterior border of the fibula and inserts at the posterior lateral aspect of the talus; it is 6 mm in diameter and 9 mm in length.[214]

The position of the talus relative to the long axis of the leg is important for determination of the function of the lateral ankle ligaments (Fig. 30E1–4).[113] At a position of neutral dorsiflexion, the ATFL is perpendicular to the axis of the tibia and the CFL is oriented parallel to the tibia.[153] In this position, the CFL provides resistance to inversion stress or varus tilt of the talus. If, however, the talus is plantar flexed (the most common position for lateral ankle inversion injuries), then the ATFL is parallel and the CFL is perpendicular to the axis of the tibia. Therefore, with the foot in the most common position for lateral ankle ligament injury, the anatomy dictates an unfavorable ligamentous configuration in that the ATFL is placed in the precarious situation of providing resistance to inversion stress.[3]

Colville and colleagues used 10 cadaver ankles to measure strain in the lateral ankle ligaments with the ankle moving from dorsiflexion to plantar flexion.[53] The ATFL strain increased with increasing degrees of plantar flexion, internal rotation, and inversion. Conversely, the CFL strain increased with increasing degrees of dorsiflexion and internal rotation. The authors concluded that the ATFL and the

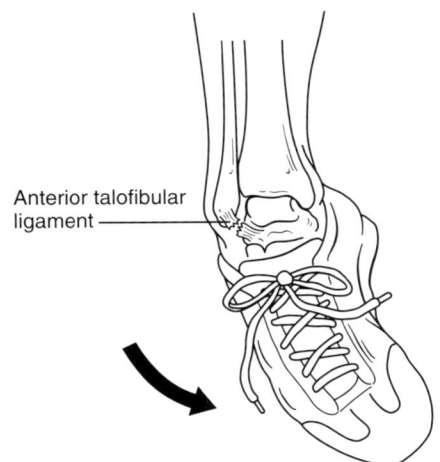

Figure 30E1–2. Inversion of the plantar flexed ankle is the mechanism of injury for lateral ankle sprain associated with a tear of the anterior talofibular ligament.

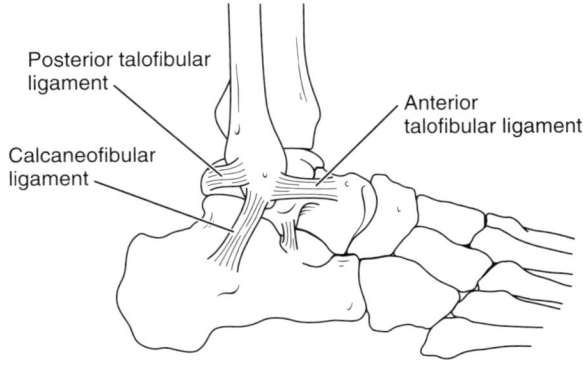

Figure 30E1–3. The lateral ligamentous complex of the ankle consists of the anterior talofibular ligament, calcaneofibular ligament, and posterior talofibular ligament.

with subtalar instability isolated or combined with lateral ankle ligament instability has been shown to occur in up to two thirds of patients[38]), subtalar coalition, bifurcate ligament sprain, peroneal tendon instability, peroneal tendon tear, lateral malleolus fracture, talar dome osteochondral injury, anterior process of the calcaneus fracture, and fracture of the base of the fifth metatarsal.

Examination of the patient includes evaluation of the entire extremity. Inspection of the leg, ankle, and foot may reveal swelling, ecchymosis, blister formation, or gross deformity. Palpation begins with a vascular and sensory assessment followed by a detailed assessment of the entire leg, ankle, and foot. Tenderness at the ATFL and the CFL is particularly important to note.

Motion about the foot and ankle is always assessed with the patient seated and relaxed. The knees are flexed and the feet allowed to fall into an equinus position. The leg is gently grasped while the heel is held in a neutral position and the ankle brought to a right angle or neutral dorsiflexion. From this position, maximal dorsiflexion and plantar flexion are observed in both passive and active modes.

Provocative maneuvers include resisted motor function to test specific motor units, in particular the peroneus brevis and longus; the squeeze test; and stability tests in varus, valgus, and external rotation.

Hopkinson and colleagues described a *squeeze test* used to identify syndesmosis ruptures at the time of initial presentation (Fig. 30E1–5).[110] The squeeze test was attributed to a former chief athletic trainer at the United States Military Academy. The test is performed by compression of the midleg from posterior lateral to anterior medial. Pain produced at the anterior inferior tibiofibular ligament (AITFL) suggests injury to the same, as long as fracture, contusion, and compartment syndrome are not present. The authors retrospectively reviewed eight patients with syndesmosis sprains; all were noted to have a positive squeeze test at initial evaluation. A separate biomechanical analysis of the squeeze test demonstrated that this test produced reproducible separation of the fibula and tibia.[261]

Stress testing is a useful clinical and radiographic tool that provides a portion of the diagnostic data needed for grading ankle sprains. Stress testing alone is not adequate for reproducible diagnosis of lateral ankle ligament injuries.[16, 213] Ankle stability is evaluated by means of three separate stress tests.

The *anterior drawer test* is used to demonstrate the integrity of the ATFL (Fig. 30E1–6). The patient is seated and the flexed leg secured with the examiner's open hand; the heel is then grasped from behind with the opposite hand, and an anterior force is placed in an effort to produce forward translation. The test is performed in both ankle neutral and plantar flexion positions. The results are compared with those of the contralateral ankle, and the test is repeated as required. A few millimeters of translation is normal. A portable ankle ligament arthrometer may be used in conjunction with manual testing to improve the accuracy and reliability of the test.[144]

Testing is occasionally uncomfortable, particularly in the acute setting. False-negative results may be caused by involuntary guarding or pain response. Local anesthesia increases the accuracy of the anterior drawer test (when performed with a mechanical testing device).[16]

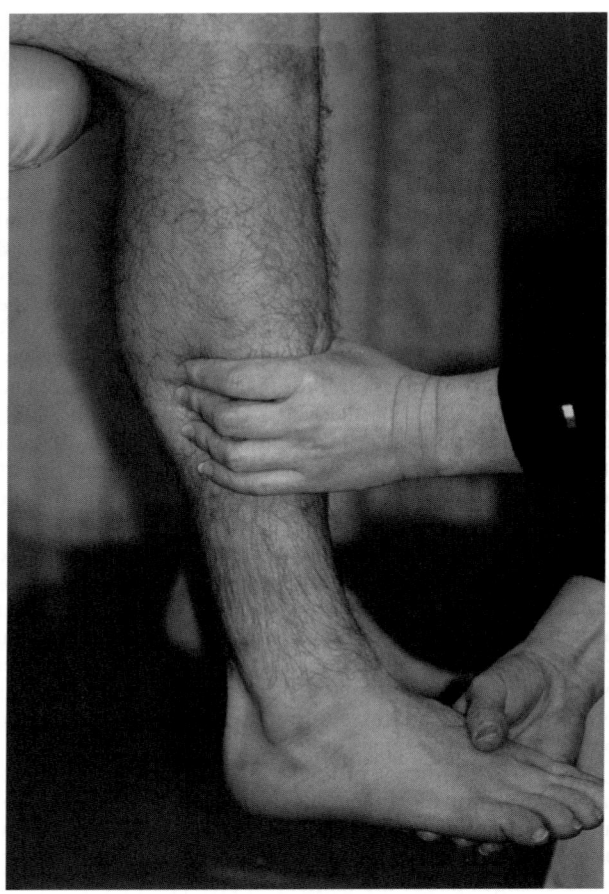

Figure 30E1–5. The squeeze test.[110] Syndesmosis injury is suspected when compression of the midleg produces pain at the ankle syndesmosis.

Broström noted that clinical instability was almost never present among arthrographically proven, acute, nonanesthetized ankle ligament ruptures.[32] After a spinal anesthesia was established, all ankles with a proven ATFL rupture demonstrated a positive anterior drawer sign. Broström went on to report in a separate publication that the anterior drawer test without any form of anesthesia was useful in diagnosing persistent (chronic) tears of the ATFL.[33] The results of the anterior drawer test are also influenced by the thickness of the fat pad at the posterior calcaneal tuberosity and by ligamentous laxity.[120]

The *talar tilt test* is performed with the patient seated (Fig. 30E1–7). The leg is secured with the examiner's open hand, the heel is grasped from behind with the opposite hand, and a varus or inversion force is placed in an effort to produce talar tilt. The results are compared with those of the contralateral ankle, and the test is repeated as required. The test is performed in both ankle neutral and plantar flexion positions. Varus stress against a neutral dorsiflexion talus differentially tests the function of the CFL; stressing a plantar flexed talus tests the ATFL.[153] Increased inversion of the calcaneus may represent talocrural (ankle) and/or talocalcaneal (subtalar) instability.[38] Varus tilt to a limited degree is probably normal.[19]

The chronic or recurrent lateral ankle sprain is associated with apprehension, discomfort, swelling, muscular

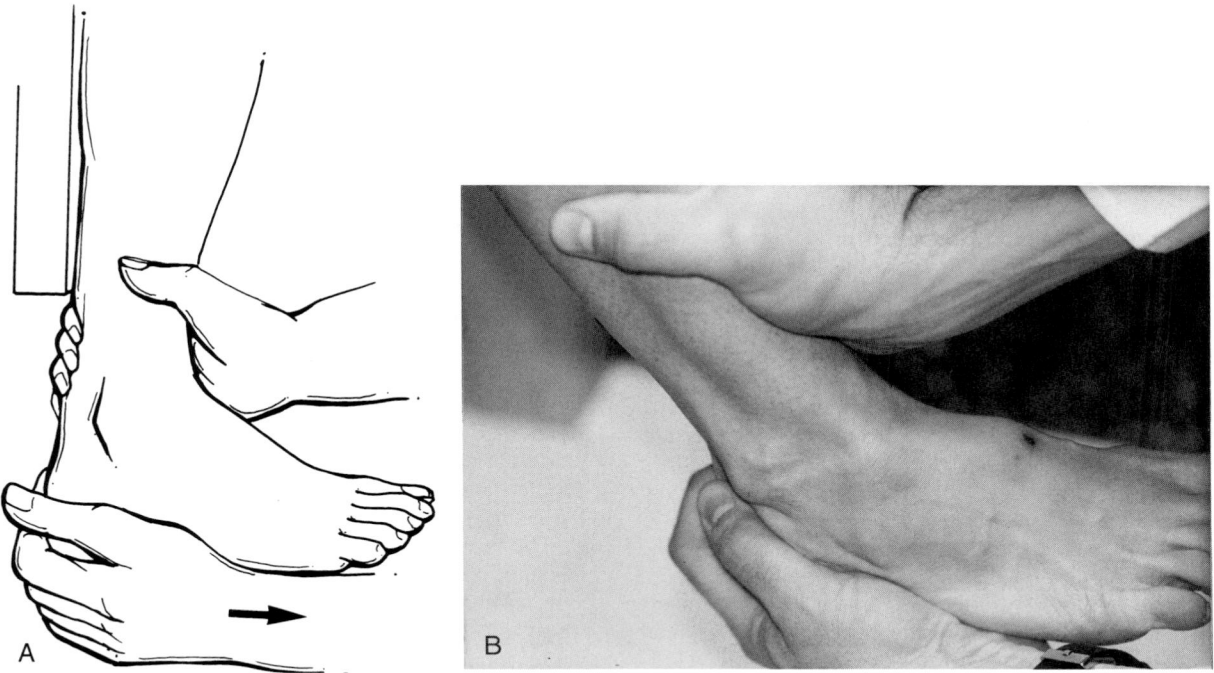

Figure 30E1–6. *A* and *B,* The anterior drawer test of the ankle.

Figure 30E1–7. *A* and *B,* The talar tilt (inversion stress) test of the ankle.

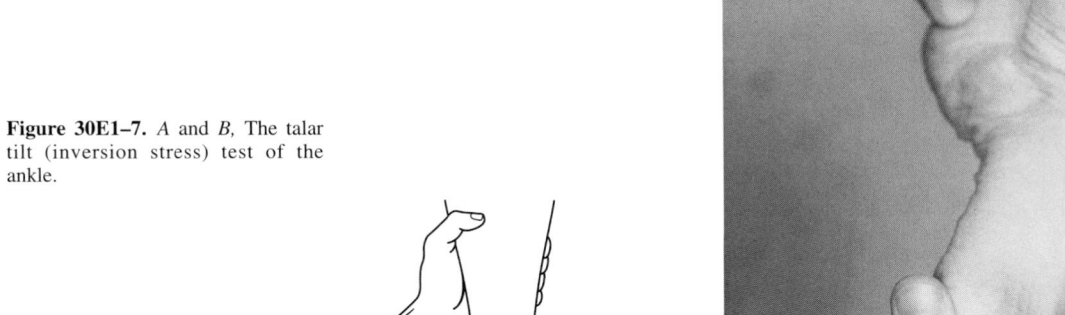

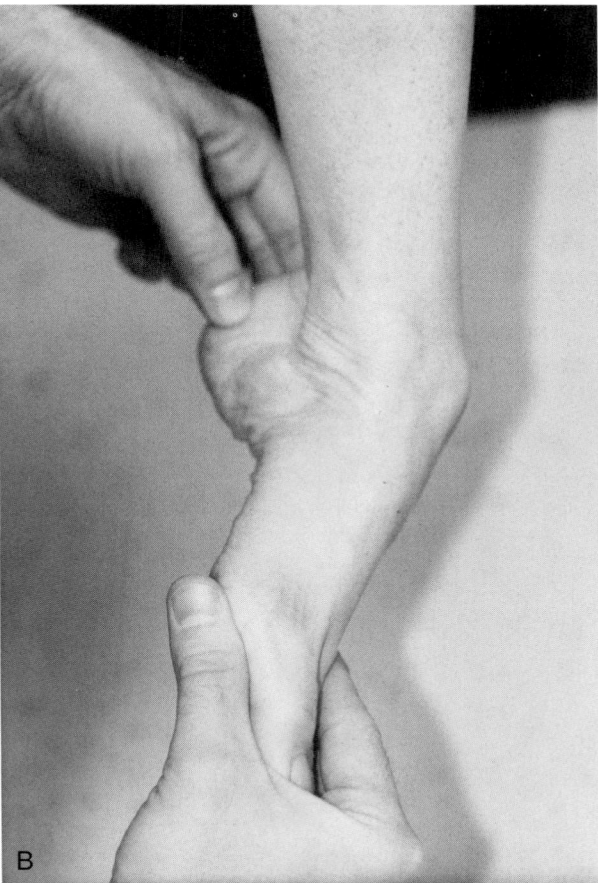

weakness, tenderness, and loss of coordination.[34, 78] Instability may be overt or subtle and has been described as a "giving way" of the ankle.[78] Significant disability is noted, particularly if the patient runs on uneven or loose surfaces. Broström noted a positive anterior drawer sign in 44 of 60 ankles with chronic instability.[34] He also noted that not all patients with persistent ruptures of the ATFL demonstrated a positive anterior drawer sign.

Boytim and coworkers described an *external rotation stress test*[25] (Fig. 30E1–8). The patient is seated and relaxed with the hip and knee flexed and the foot and ankle held in a neutral position. The knee is maintained in a forward-facing position while a gentle but firm external rotation force is applied to the foot. Pain reproduced at the anterior syndesmosis is diagnostic of a syndesmosis injury.

The high incidence of bifurcate ligament sprain warrants a brief discussion with regard to its presentation. Broström noted clinical evidence of bifurcate ligament injury in 18.6% of patients with acute ankle sprains and 3.7% of patients with confirmed lateral ankle ligament ruptures.[32] Bifurcate ligament injury is characterized by diffuse lateral hindfoot and midfoot swelling with associated ecchymosis. Tenderness tends to localize to the course of the bifurcate ligament, which is distinct from the course of the ATFL. The ankle and midfoot remain stable. Pain is easily reproduced with forced inversion of the plantar flexed foot.

Broström noted that the differentiation between lateral ankle ligament injury and bifurcate ligament injury was best achieved by eliciting indirect tenderness.[32] He suggested manipulation of the heel to produce lateral ankle pain and stabilization of the heel with simultaneous forced forefoot motion to produce bifurcate pain.

Imaging

A complete review of foot and ankle imaging is presented in a previous section (see Chapter 30B, Imaging of Sports Injuries of the Foot and Ankle).

Radiographs. Radiographs in the anteroposterior, mortise, and lateral projections are required for ankle evaluation after fracture. This may not apply to emergency department evaluations but it certainly applies to any physician in another setting who is asked to provide evaluation of an ankle sprain. Weight-bearing radiographs better reproduce physiologic loading, but they are not always obtainable in the acute phase owing to pain.

The radiographs are evaluated with regard to malleolar fracture, physeal fracture, osteochondral fracture, and avulsion fracture. Alignment and translation deformity are also inspected, particularly at the syndesmosis and the medial ankle joint space. (Please refer to the syndesmosis and deltoid sections for further review.)

During surgical exploration of 60 chronic ankle sprains,

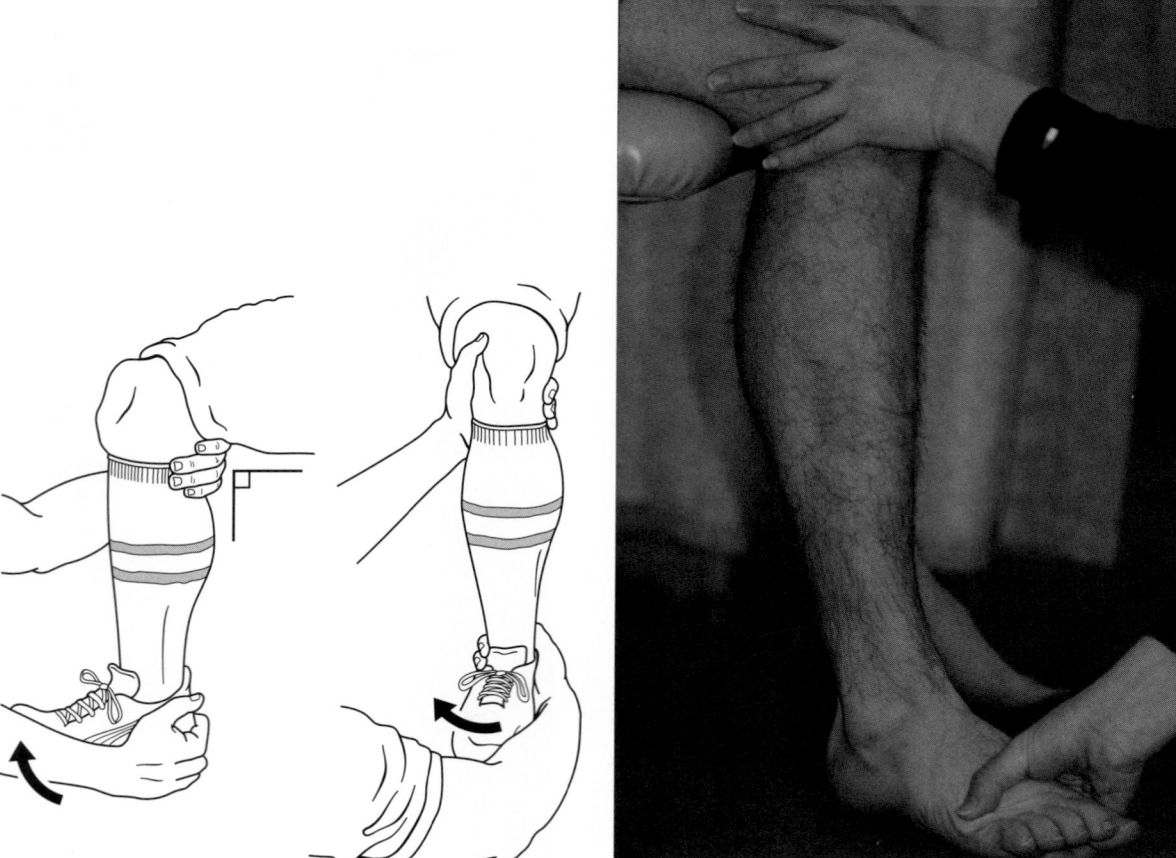

Figure 30E1–8. The external rotation stress test of the syndesmosis. (From Boytim MJ, Fischer DA, Neumann L: Syndesmotic ankle sprains. Am J Sports Med 19:294–298, 1991.)

Broström noted 5 cases (8%) with anterior lateral talar osteochondritis dissecans.[34] Anderson and Lecocq reported a 22% incidence of osteochondral lesions in a mixed series of 27 cases of single and recurrent lateral ankle injuries.[3] The lesions were located at the lateral talus in 5 patients and at the medial talus in 1 patient.

The presence of a subfibular ossicle may be indicative of acute or chronic injury to the ATFL,[17] or it may be a normal variant (os subfibulare). Broström noted that avulsion of bone fragments is an uncommon pathologic finding after an acute ankle sprain.[32] He further noted that patients who sustained an avulsion fracture were more likely to be older and female.

Stress Radiographs. The bilateral stress radiograph is used to quantify anterior talar translation and/or varus tilt of the talus. The external rotation stress radiograph is described in the syndesmosis section. Stress radiographs are not routinely necessary for the evaluation of acute lateral ankle ligament injury.[38, 115] Accuracy is compromised by pain response, peroneal spasm,[47] variable stress technique, and lack of control data in the case of a previously injured contralateral ankle. The literature offers no consensus with regard to normal and pathologic findings in radiographic stress tests.

The talar tilt stress test is similar to the clinical test but is performed during an anteroposterior radiograph. The degree of tilt is determined by measuring the angular divergence between the distal tibial articular surface and the talar dome (Fig. 30E1–9). Stress radiographs may provide additional data if the position of the talus is varied. Varus stress against a neutral dorsiflexion talus differentially tests the function of the CFL; stressing a plantar flexed talus tests the ATFL.[153]

Bonnin reported radiographic data demonstrating 4 degrees of varus tilt in 10% to 15% of noninjured ankles.[23] Hughes evaluated varus stress radiographs of both ankles in 90 injured and 90 noninjured patients and concluded

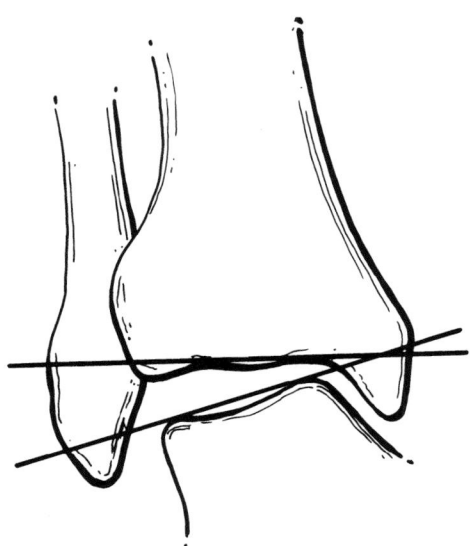

Figure 30E1–9. The talar tilt (inversion) stress radiograph. The talar tilt angle refers to the angle between two lines drawn to the tibial plafond and the talar dome.

that 6 degrees of increased talar tilt represents the transition from "normal to abnormal" talar tilt.[112]

Rubin and Whitten published data that suggest the presence of even more laxity in the normal ankle.[213] Approximately 56% of the noninjured ankles in their study had talar tilts of 3 to 23 degrees. Seligson and associates used mechanical devices to obtain controlled stress radiographs of 25 functionally normal ankles.[227] The talar tilt in these asymptomatic ankles varied from 0 to 18 degrees. The anterior translation as seen on the lateral stress radiograph never exceeded 3 mm.

Brand and colleagues reported symptomatic lateral ankle instability in 75% of Naval Academy cadets, with a difference in talar tilt angle of greater than 10 degrees.[26] In a separate report, Brand and coworkers noted, but did not substantiate, that preoperative, nonanesthetized talar tilt results were typically within 5 degrees of repeat, intraoperative, anesthetized values.[27]

Cox and Hewes performed stress radiographs on 404 ankles of patients with no history of previous ankle injury.[55] Manual stress was applied to the plantar flexed ankle for an anteroposterior radiograph. No talar tilt was detected in 365 (90.3%) of the ankles, 1 to 5 degrees of talar tilt was detected in 32 ankles (7.9%), and greater than 5 degrees of talar tilt was detected in only 7 ankles (1.7%).

Martin and associates used a mechanical stress device to produce stress radiographs with variable, reproducible inversion forces.[165] Because of a lack of correlation between symptoms, force, and talar tilt, the authors concluded that a single maximal force stress radiograph is more useful than multiple graded stress radiographs.

Glasgow and colleagues suggested the need for a lateral stress radiograph.[86] They cited the prevalence of ATFL ruptures and the associated anterior instability. The anterior drawer stress test is similar to the clinical test but is performed during a lateral radiograph. The degree of translation is determined by measuring the shortest distance between the talar dome and the posterior margin of the tibial articular surface[142] (Fig. 30E1–10).

Johanssen prospectively compared the talar tilt and anterior drawer stress radiographs of 244 recent lateral ankle sprains with the respective operative findings.[118] A positive anterior drawer/negative talar tilt was more often associated with an isolated ATFL disruption. The tests were not specific enough to differentiate isolated ATFL injuries from combined ATFL and CFL injuries.

Freeman reported "functional instability" (the tendency to give way) in 21 of 42 patients 1 year after initial lateral ankle ligament rupture.[76] Mechanical instability, defined by increased varus tilt on stress radiograph, was present in only 6 of these cases. Hansen and coworkers noted a similar lack of agreement between clinical symptoms and persistent talar tilt.[98]

Arthrography. The unpredictable effect of patient guarding during stress radiography is overcome by the use of ankle arthrography.[21, 22] This method is relatively simple. Contrast material is injected into the acutely injured ankle, preferably with fluoroscopic guidance, and radiographs are obtained in various projections with attention to areas of extravasation. A false-negative result from an early capsular seal is possible. The procedure has been made obsolete

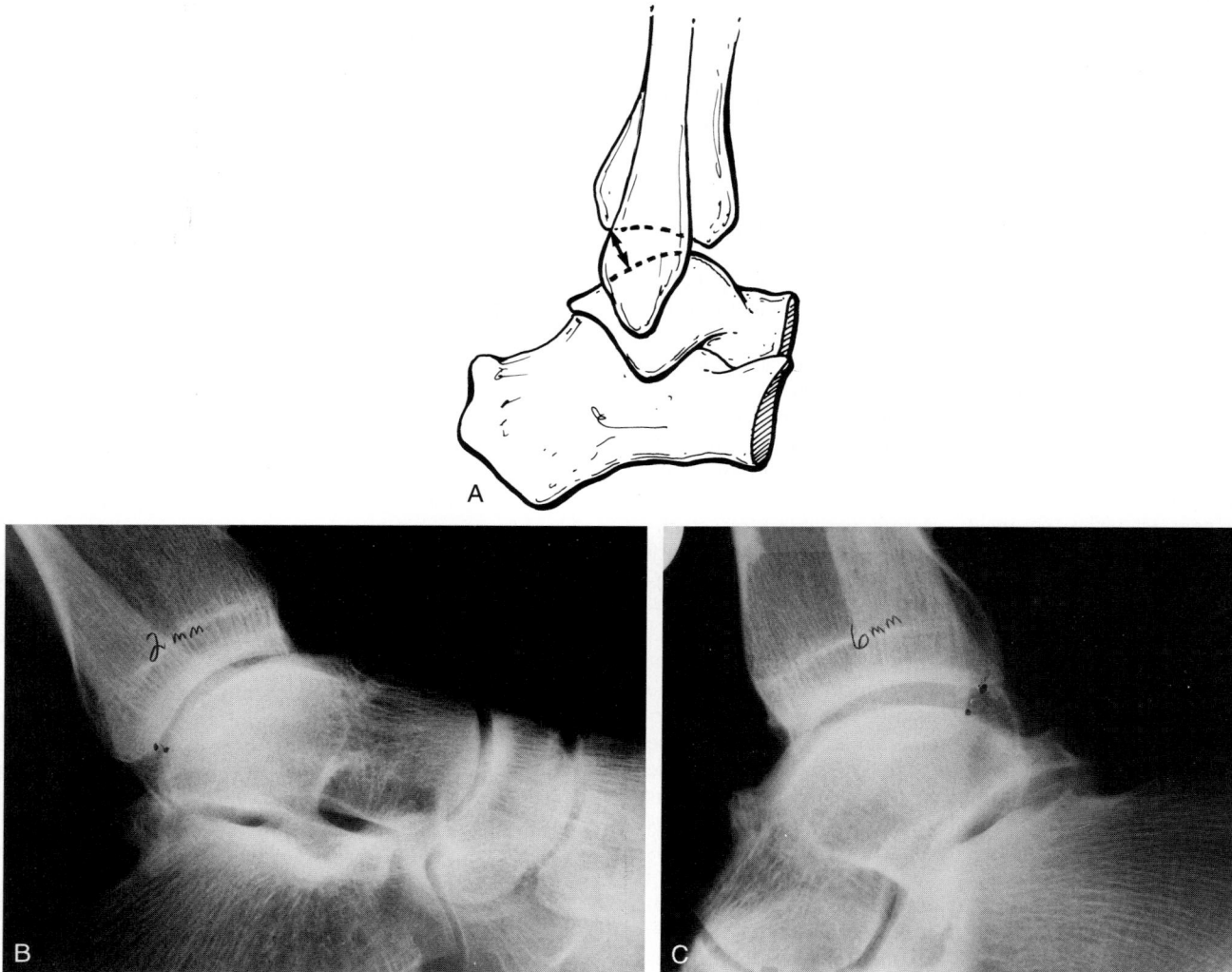

Figure 30E1–10. *A,* The anterior drawer stress radiograph. Anterior talar displacement (in millimeters) is recorded by measuring the shortest distance from the most posterior articular surface of the tibia to the talar dome. *B,* The anterior drawer stress radiograph with no anterior talar displacement, negative test. *C,* The anterior drawer stress radiograph with 6 mm anterior talar displacement, positive test.

by the use of MRI. The method is reviewed here for completeness and historical perspective.

In 1944, Berridge and Bonnin described the characteristics of a normal ankle arthrography.[19] These authors were able to diagnose ligament and capsular rupture, but they did not find the technique to be practical. Later, in 1957, Arner and associates used arthrography and surgical exploration and noted a correlation between extra-articular leakage of contrast and tear of the ATFL and CFL.[5]

Broström and colleagues performed arthrography of 321 fresh ankle sprains.[35] Extra-articular leakage occurred in 239 cases (74%). Surgical exploration was performed in 99 of these cases and in an additional 6 cases that did not demonstrate leakage. The authors concluded that arthrography was useful within the first 7 days of an acute ankle sprain. Leakage of contrast into the peroneal tendon sheath correlated with tear of the CFL. Leakage in front of the lateral malleolus correlated with ATFL rupture. Leakage in front of the syndesmosis correlated with complete rupture

of the syndesmosis. Leakage at the medial malleolus correlated with partial deltoid rupture. The presence of extra-articular contrast in the flexor hallucis longus (FHL) and flexor digitorum longus (FDL) tendon sheaths, as well as the posterior facet of the subtalar joint, was not diagnostic.

Raatikainen and coworkers compared arthrography, clinical examination, and stress radiography with surgical findings in 66 acute ankle sprains.[201] Arthrography predicted 100% of the ATFL disruptions and 77% of the CFL disruptions. Clinical examination and stress radiography failed to reliably predict lateral ankle ligament disruption.

Peroneal sheath injection (tenography), as described by Black and associates, is useful in discerning injury of the CFL.[22] Contrast leakage from the sheath or passage into the ankle joint suggests CFL disruption.

Magnetic Resonance Imaging. MRI is a useful method for evaluation of acute, subacute, and chronic lateral ankle ligament injuries[211] (Fig. 30E1–11). Associated injuries to the talar dome, subchondral bone, and peroneal tendons, as

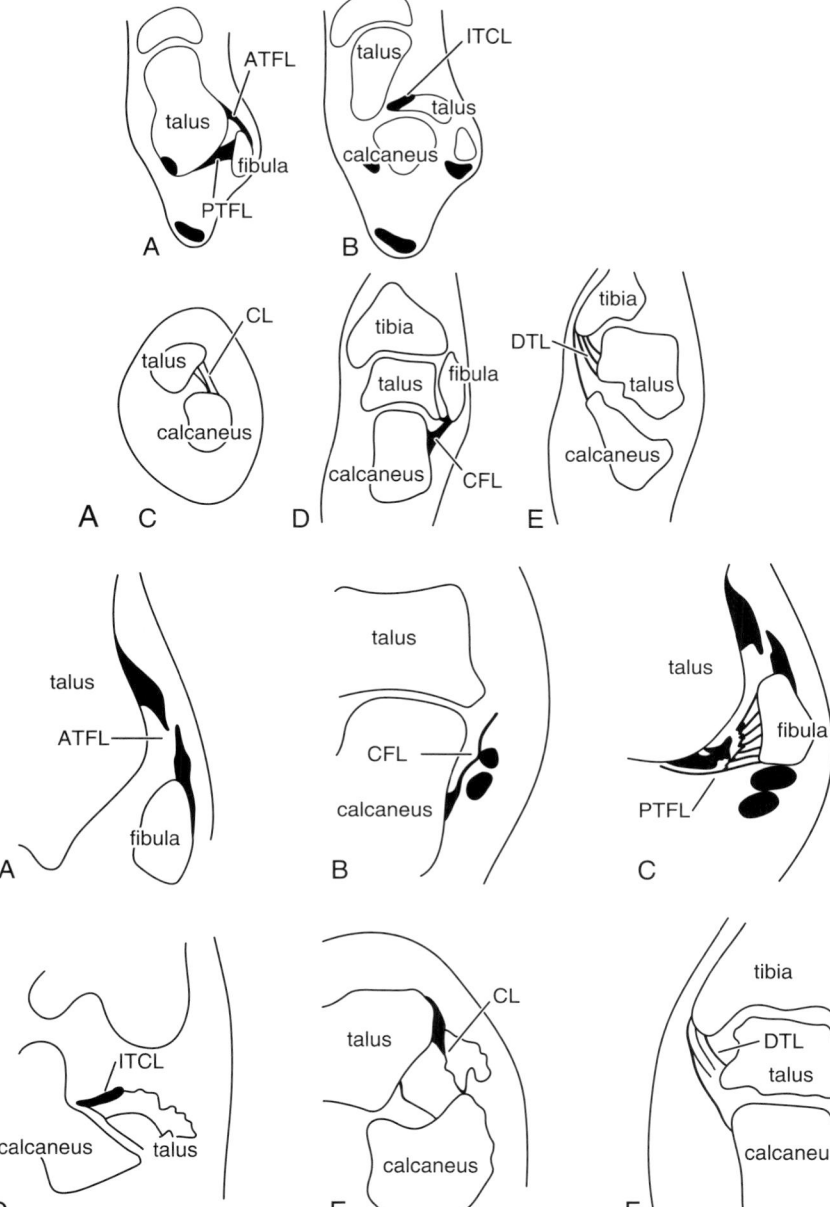

Figure 30E1–11. *A,* Magnetic resonance imaging key for the normal ankle. *B,* Magnetic resonance imaging key for the injured ankle. (*A* and *B,* From Tochigi Y, Yoshinaga K, Wada Y, Moriya H: Acute inversion injury of the ankle: Magnetic resonance imaging and clinical outcomes. Foot Ankle Int 19:730–734, 1998.)

well as the interosseous and cervical ligaments of the subtalar joint, are visualized.[266] MRI also reveals tarsal coalition.

Rijke and colleagues used a dedicated knee coil and axial images of the neutral and plantar flexed ankle to describe various ligament injuries.[211] Complete disruption, partial disruption, and laxity were all visualized. Additionally, hemorrhage and soft tissue swelling were indicative of an acute injury.

The high sensitivity associated with MRI mandates that images be carefully correlated with clinical findings. Its accuracy, lack of ionizing radiation, noninvasiveness, decreasing cost, and increasing availability suggest that MRI

is the imaging modality of choice for the ankle and subtalar joint.

Therapeutic Options

All acute injuries are treated with the RICE (*R*est, *I*ce, *C*ompression, *E*levation) method followed by gentle range of motion and protected weight-bearing. The amount of rest required after an acute ankle sprain is determined by the degree of pain.

Many studies have reviewed the effect of cold application to the injured extremity. Cold therapy is an effective, inexpensive, and easy-to-use modality for the treatment of

As was noted earlier, Ruth published a contrary conclusion based on the open treatment of 45 acute injuries; in fact, according to Ruth, the ruptured ligament ends were never in approximation, a finding that did not resolve with manipulation of the foot and ankle.[214]

Drez and coworkers used a more protracted immobilization method to treat 39 patients with first-time, combined ATFL and CFL injuries.[62] All cases were evaluated by stress radiography before and after treatment. The protocol included 7 to 10 days in an everted splint and 6 weeks in an everted walking cast, followed by ankle rehabilitation and a 1-month delay in return to athletic activity. A 79.5% success rate was obtained as determined by a repeat talar tilt stress radiograph with 5 degrees or less angulation compared with the uninjured ankle.

Eiff and associates used a prospective study to compare early mobilization and immobilization for the treatment of first-time lateral ankle sprains.[68] The early mobilization group was treated with an elastic wrap for 48 hours followed by application of a semirigid pneumatic brace and a common rehabilitation program. The immobilization group was treated with a non–weight-bearing plaster splint for 10 days followed by a common rehabilitation program. Both methods produced excellent results at 1-year follow-up with low rates for residual symptoms (5%) and re-injury (8%).

Surgical Repair

Surgical management of the acute lateral ankle sprain appears to produce good results on a routine basis. Kaikkonen and colleagues reported excellent and good results at a 6- to 8-year follow-up after primary repair of acute lateral ligament rupture.[123] No operative complications occurred. Others have reported favorable, reproducible results with primary repair of acute ruptures.[33, 214, 245]

Freeman compared strapping and early mobilization, immobilization with plaster for 6 weeks, and ligament repair with immobilization for the treatment of complete lateral ankle ligament ruptures.[75] The periods of disability were 12, 22, and 26 weeks for patients in the early mobilization, immobilization, and ligament repair groups, respectively. Ligament repair produced the greatest number of complaints at 1-year follow-up, including the only cases with residual loss of motion. Freeman suggested early mobilization as the treatment of choice for lateral ankle ligament ruptures.

Broström used a prospective study to compare the use of primary surgical repair followed by 3 weeks of plaster immobilization (95 cases), 3 weeks of plaster immobilization alone (82 cases), and strapping with early mobilization (104 cases).[33] Primary surgical repair provided the best results, including a low (3%) residual symptomatic instability rate. Broström went on to suggest that primary surgical repair should not be the routine treatment for acute ruptures. He cited the protracted postoperative recovery, the risk of infection, the risk of painful scar formation, and the success of late lateral ankle ligament reconstruction.

It is remarkable that early studies compared operative cases with nonoperative cases that used 3 to 8 weeks of plaster immobilization. Evans and coworkers recognized the discrepancy in immobilization periods and performed a prospective, randomized trial with 3 weeks of immobilization in a plaster cast with or without surgical repair of the acute lateral ankle ligament rupture.[73] An independent 2-year follow-up concluded that surgical repair yielded similar radiographic results (stress radiographs) and slightly worse functional results. Twice as many patients in the operative group were forced to give up athletic activity. Loss of subtalar inversion and surgical complications were also cited as disadvantages of primary repair of acute injury.

Cass and associates reviewed 25 consecutive primary repairs for grade III lateral ankle sprain and 40 delayed reconstructions for chronic lateral ankle instability at a mean follow-up of 9.5 years.[42] Subjective and objective results did not significantly differ. The authors concluded that chronic lateral ankle instability following conservative, nonoperative management is effectively treated with delayed reconstruction.

Repair of acute injury produces results similar to those associated with delayed reconstruction. Because most patients respond to nonsurgical management, primary repair offers few advantages. Today, operative repair of the complete, acute lateral ankle ligament injury is very infrequent.[18] Most authors favor nonsurgical treatment for acute ruptures.[33, 75, 124, 178]

Several authors recommend primary surgical repair for severe injury or injury in the high-demand athlete[33, 42, 54, 93, 96] (Fig. 30E1–13).

Technique: *Primary Lateral Ankle Ligament Repair*

1. The procedure is performed with the patient under general anesthetic. The patient is supine with a well-padded proximal tourniquet and a 3000-mL saline bag placed beneath the ipsilateral hemipelvis.

2. An image intensifier is used to obtain bilateral varus tilt and anterior drawer stress views. Broden's stress views are also obtained, if indicated.

3. Arthroscopy of the ankle is performed if clinical presentation or imaging suggests intra-articular disease.

4. The extremity is exsanguinated and the tourniquet is inflated. A bump is placed under the leg to prevent anterior translation of the talus.

5. A short oblique incision is made at the anterior margin of the distal fibula. This incision incorporates the lateral arthroscopy portal.

6. Blunt subcutaneous dissection is performed, with care taken to protect the superficial peroneal nerve and the sural nerve.

7. The anterior lateral capsule is exposed and the ATFL, the CFL, and capsular tears are identified. The ankle joint is inspected.

8. The tears are approximated and repaired with absorbable suture. Avulsion fractures are repaired directly to the fibula or talus.

9. The wound is closed in layers and a short leg splint is applied. At 10 days, the incision is inspected and a short leg non–weight-bearing cast is applied. Four to 6 weeks postoperatively, a rehabilitation program is instituted and monitored. A semirigid pneumatic ankle brace is used for 6 months postoperatively.

Chronic Lateral Ankle Ligament Instability

Chronic lateral ankle instability is defined as persistent mechanical instability of the talocrural joint. The condition

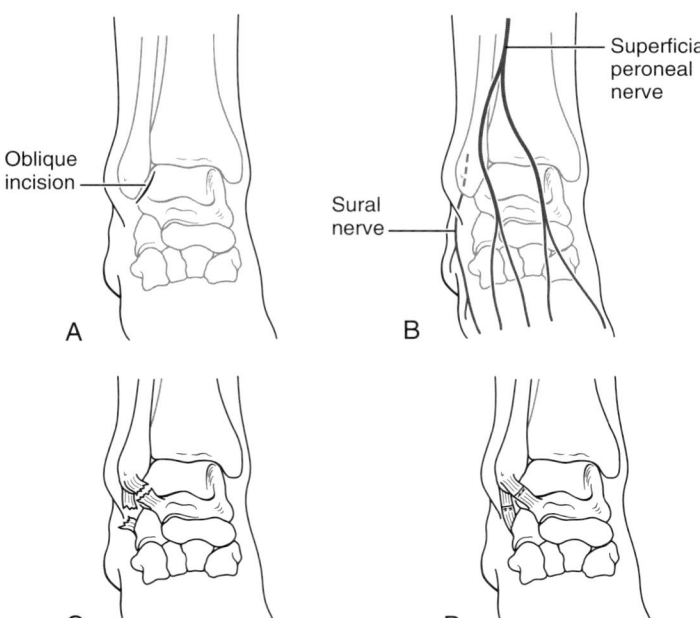

Figure 30E1–13. Surgical technique for primary lateral ankle ligament reconstruction. *A,* A short oblique incision is made at the anterior margin of the distal fibula. *B,* Blunt subcutaneous dissection is performed with care taken to protect the superficial peroneal nerve and the sural nerve. *C,* The anterior lateral capsule is exposed and the anterior talofibular ligament, calcaneofibular ligament, and capsular tears identified. *D,* The tears are approximated and repaired with absorbable suture.

develops after acute rupture and occurs in up to 20% of patients.[33, 124, 183]

A related condition is functional lateral ankle instability, defined by frequent sprains, difficulty running on uneven surfaces, and difficulty jumping and cutting. Brand and colleagues reported a 10% prevalence of functional lateral ankle instability among 1300 Naval Academy freshmen.[26] Functional instability may be related to previous ankle sprain, chronic lateral ankle instability, or peroneal weakness. The group was able to demonstrate a relationship between functional instability and comparative talar tilt angles. Seven percent of cadets had both a talar tilt of 10 degrees or greater and a difference between the talar tilts of both ankles in excess of 5 degrees. Within this subgroup, each cadet reported at least one previous severe ankle sprain, and 41% labeled themselves as having a "trick" ankle.

Rehabilitation without Surgery. Successful resolution of chronic lateral ankle instability is possible without surgical stabilization.[34, 247, 270] Patients with chronic, recurrent injuries are treated with a rehabilitation program and their activity levels are reduced. Functional ankle bracing is continued throughout the treatment period. The key points are motor strength (particularly of the peroneal muscles), proprioception, and coordination.

Surgical Treatment. Patients with chronic injuries that remain symptomatic after a supervised rehabilitation program are candidates for surgical management. A multitude of procedures have been used for lateral ankle ligament reconstruction, many with reasonable success.

In 1932, Nilsonne described a procedure for stabilization of the lateral ankle.[184] He repaired a chronic CFL rupture and reinforced the repair with a peroneus brevis tenodesis. Evans[20, 72, 145] and Watson-Jones[269, 270] modified the tenodesis. A further modification in the form of an augmentation procedure was proposed by Elmslie[70] and refined by Chrisman and Snook.[43]

The *Evans procedure* is a transposition of the entire peroneus brevis tendon through the distal fibula (Fig. 30E1–14). Evans recognized the occurrence of tenodesis and the loss of subtalar inversion associated with the procedure.[72]

The *Watson-Jones procedure* reconstructs the lateral ankle ligaments with a peroneus brevis tenodesis configured so as to replace the course of the ATFL (Fig. 30E1–15).[269, 270] The classical method uses the entire peroneus brevis tendon.[85] The procedure does not reproduce the anatomic orientation of the CFL. Because the tenodesis of the peroneus brevis lies at a right angle to the subtalar joint empirical axis, loss of subtalar motion is to be expected.[113]

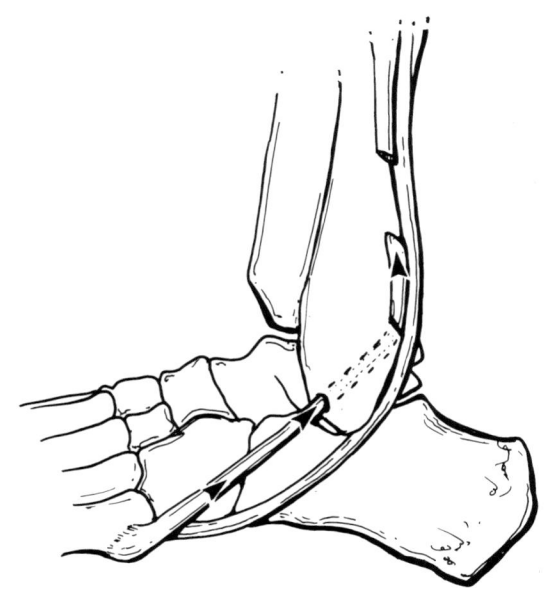

Figure 30E1–14. The Evans procedure.

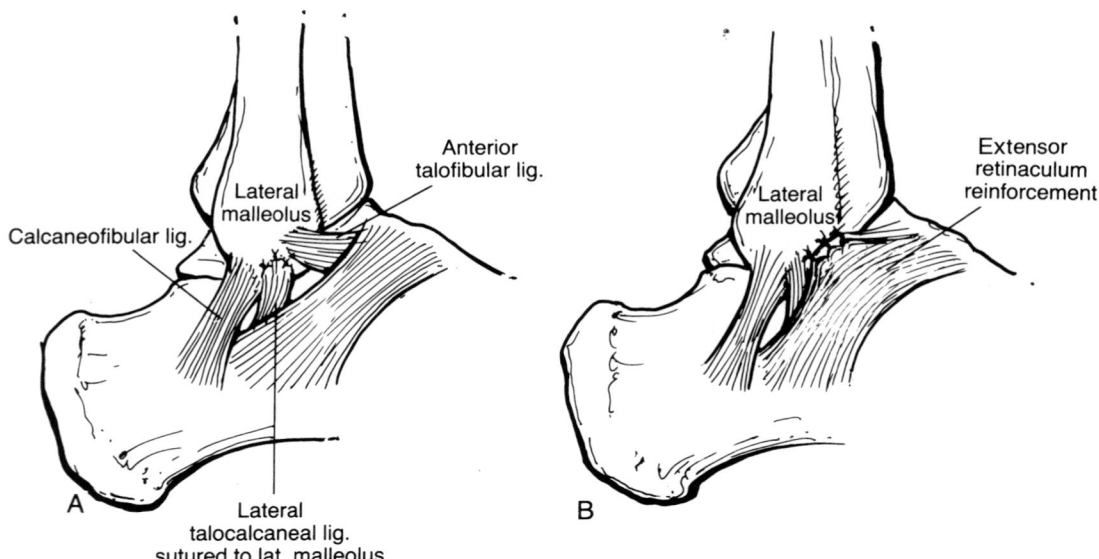

Figure 30E1–19. Gould modification of the Broström technique. After repair of the anterior talofibular or calcaneofibular ligament, reinforcements with the lateral talocalcaneal ligament *(A)* and extensor retinaculum *(B)* are made.

eral ankle instability, or a history of previous ankle reconstruction.

Karlsson and coworkers performed 60 lateral ankle ligament reconstructions with a modification of the Broström repair.[126] These authors advanced the ATFL and the CFL into a 4 × 4-mm bone trough at the anterior aspect of the distal fibula. The remaining periosteal flap was repaired over the ATFL. Good or excellent results were obtained in 53 (88%) of the patients. Unsatisfactory results were associated with generalized ligamentous laxity or longstanding instability.

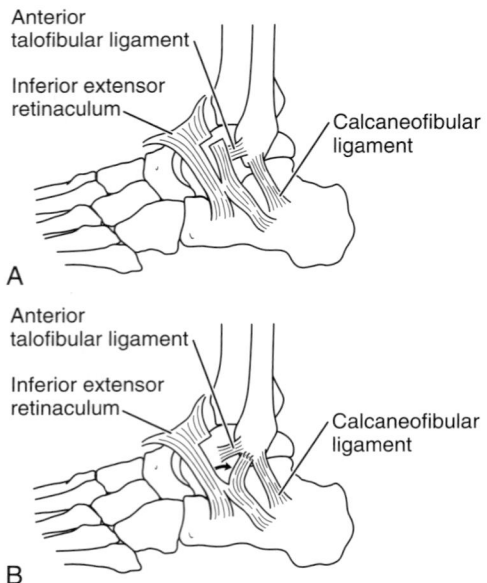

Figure 30E1–20. Harper modification of the Gould modification of the Broström technique. A flap from the inferior extensor retinaculum is mobilized and sutured to the lateral fibula. (From Harper MC: Modification of the Gould modification of the Broström ankle repair. Foot Ankle Int 19:788, 1998.)

Despite the many surgical options, ankle stabilization is effective and produces good or excellent results in more than 91% of chronic lateral ankle ligament instability cases.[216, 242] Radiographic stability does not always correlate with clinical outcome. Patients with early signs of osteoarthritis may experience progressive arthrosis despite stabilization. Persistent instability leads to osteoarthritis of the ankle joint.[50, 105, 131]

Ankle arthroscopy at the time of lateral ankle ligament reconstruction provides the surgeon with an opportunity for a more thorough evaluation of the ankle joint. Komenda and Ferkel suggest the use of ankle arthroscopy before lateral ankle ligament stabilization for treatment of loose bodies, osteochondral lesions of the talus, and ankle pain unrelated to instability.[140] They also suggest the procedure for evaluation of ATFL integrity and suitability of local tissue for reconstruction.

Patients with failed lateral ankle reconstruction due to re-rupture are placed into rehabilitation and fitted with an orthosis. Repair of the acute injury is a reasonable alternative to functional treatment. Persistent instability is treated with a Broström repair with the Gould modification, or an anatomic reconstruction with local tissue.[217] Sammarco and Idusuyi reconstructed four ankles after failed Broström procedures.[218] They used a split peroneus brevis technique that reconstructed the ATFL and the CFL with the facilitation of bone anchors. With the use of a tendon stripper, the incision was reduced to 4 cm. Ankle stability was achieved in each case, with one excellent and three good results (Fig. 30E1–21).

Technique: *Lateral Ankle Ligament Reconstruction with a Gould Modification of the Broström Repair*

1. The procedure is performed with the patient under general anesthetic. The patient is supine with a well-padded proximal tourniquet and a 3000-mL saline bag placed beneath the ipsilateral hemipelvis.

2. An image intensifier is used to obtain bilateral varus

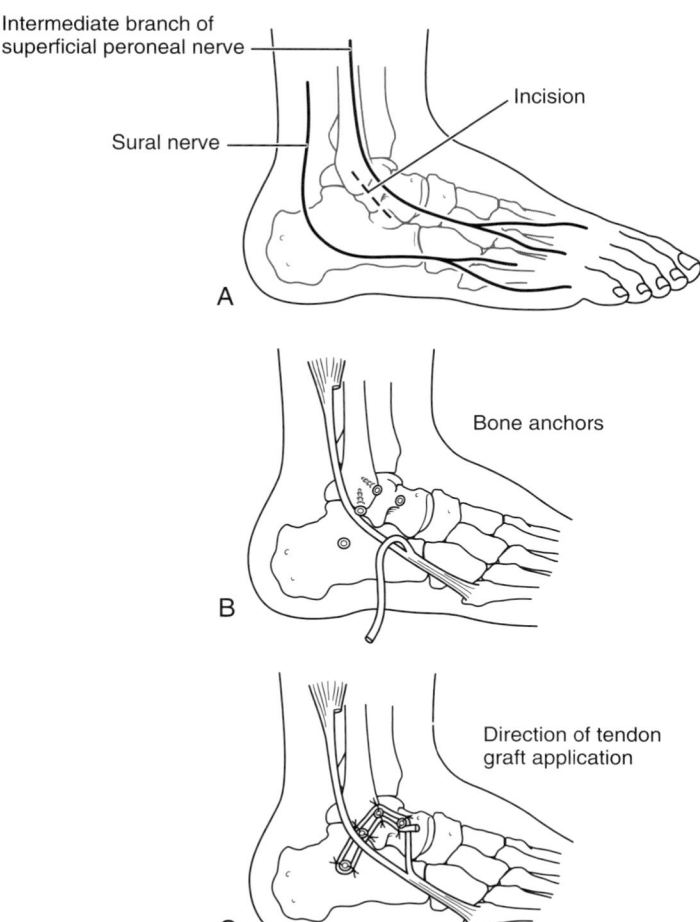

Figure 30E1–21. Lateral ankle reconstruction using a split peroneus brevis tendon graft and bone anchors. *A,* The tendon is harvested through a 4-cm incision. *B,* The bone anchors are positioned at the origin and insertion of the anterior talofibular ligament (ATFL) and calcaneofibular ligament (CFL). *C,* The ankle is held in a neutral position as the graft is positioned to reconstruct the ATFL and CFL. (From Sammarco GJ, Idusuyi OB: Reconstruction of the lateral ankle ligaments using a split peroneus brevis tendon graft. Foot Ankle Int 20:97–103, 1999.)

tilt and anterior drawer stress views. Brodén's stress views are also obtained, if indicated.

3. Arthroscopy of the ankle is performed if clinical presentation or imaging suggests intra-articular disease.

4. The extremity is exsanguinated and the tourniquet is inflated. A bump is placed under the leg to prevent anterior translation of the talus.

5. A short oblique incision is made at the anterior margin of the distal fibula. The incision incorporates the lateral arthroscopy portal.

6. Blunt subcutaneous dissection is performed, with care taken to protect the superficial peroneal nerve and the sural nerve. The extensor retinaculum is identified and tagged.

7. The anterior lateral capsule is exposed, and the ATFL and the CFL are identified. The capsule is incised just distal to the origin of the ATFL and the CFL, and the ankle joint is inspected.

8. The anterior margin of the fibula is exposed by subperiosteal elevation of the proximal capsule. The anterior fibula is decorticated, and three to five tunnels are produced with a small K-wire. The capsule with the ATFL and the CFL is secured with multiple nonabsorbable braided sutures. The sutures are passed through the tunnels and the capsule is advanced onto the decorticated margin

of the fibula. The lateral periosteal sleeve and the proximal capsule are repaired over the advanced ligament.

9. The superficial layer of the extensor retinaculum is secured with suture and advanced to the anterior fibula. This provides significant subtalar stability.

10. The wound is closed in layers, and a short leg splint is applied. At 10 days, the incision is inspected and a short leg weight-bearing cast is applied. At 4 weeks postoperatively, a rehabilitation program is instituted and monitored. A removable cast boot or a semirigid pneumatic ankle brace is used for an additional 4 to 6 weeks. The repair is further protected during subsequent athletic activity with a semirigid pneumatic ankle brace for 6 months postoperatively.

Rehabilitation after Surgery. Tissue injury initiates a predictable and sequential series of events known as the healing response. The response is typically divided into three phases with arbitrary and overlapping time lines.[208] The initial phase is the inflammatory phase, which includes the first through the third day following injury. The second phase is a proliferative phase of tissue repair that extends from day 3 to day 20. The final phase is a remodeling phase that proceeds after day 9.

To a certain degree, rehabilitation follows the phases of the healing response in an effort to reduce the undesirable

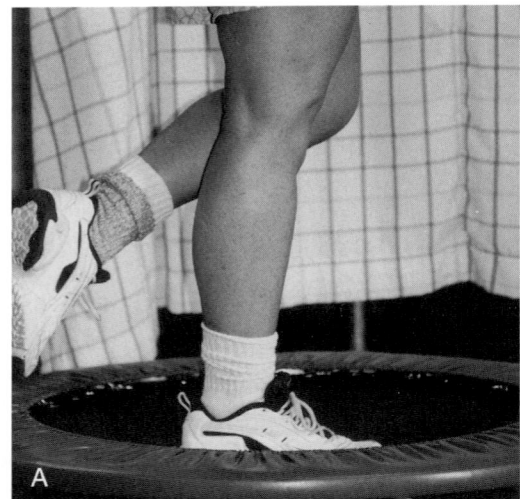
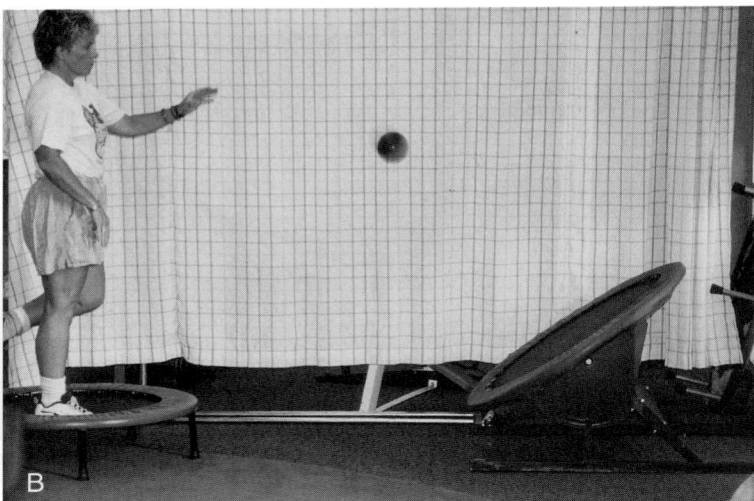

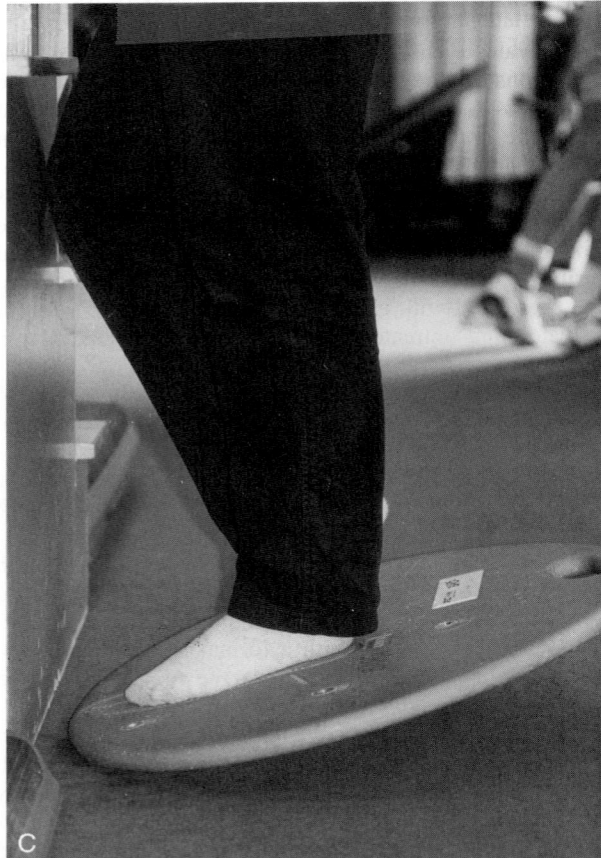

Figure 30E1–26. Closed chain activities. *A,* One-leg balance on a trampoline. *B,* Sports-specific activity (throwing) on a trampoline. *C,* Biomechanical ankle platform system.

ligamentous injury to the ankle and that the pattern and location of the lesion correlate with a specific mechanism of injury.[146, 185] Alanen and coworkers used a prospective study to establish a 27% incidence of bone bruise (i.e., microtrabecular fracture) after ankle inversion injury.[2] Ninety-five patients with otherwise normal radiographs were imaged. No clinical significance was related to the occurrence of the bone bruise.

Anterior Lateral Ankle Impingement. Chronic anterior lateral ankle pain after an inversion ankle injury is a well-

recognized entity. Bassett and associates described a distal fascicle of the anterior inferior tibiofibular ligament; the structure was found in 10 of 11 cadaver specimens[13] (Fig. 30E1–28). Impingement of the fascicle against the talar dome occurs with ankle dorsiflexion between 9 and 17 degrees. The clinical component of the study identified abrasion of the talar articular cartilage in five of the seven patients. Resection of the fascicle was curative and did not increase ankle instability.

A meniscoid lesion of the anterior lateral ankle has

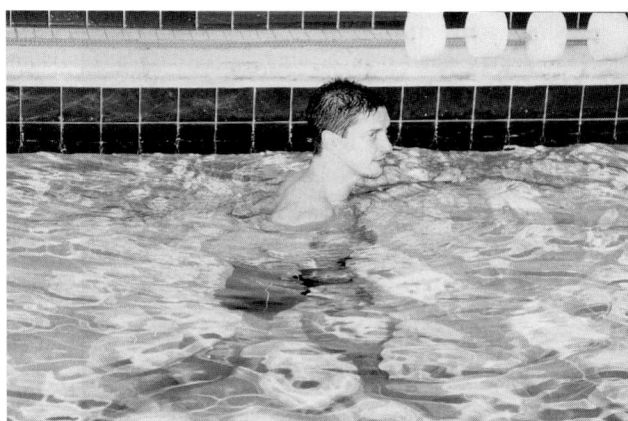

Figure 30E1–27. Water running for cross-training after foot or ankle injury.

also been described[278] (Fig. 30E1–29). Hamilton reported finding entrapment of the capsule between the talus and the lateral malleolus during the surgical management of two of three acute, high-grade, lateral ankle sprains.[96] He speculated that the capsular interposition might provide the substrate for the classical meniscoid lesion.

Chronic anterior lateral ankle pain is treated with an aggressive 6-week course of physical therapy and bracing to eliminate subtle instability. Oral anti-inflammatory and cortisone injection therapy may also be used. Patients who fail conservative management are treated with ankle arthroscopy and débridement of the anterolateral lesion (meniscoid lesion), if present.

Peroneal Tendon Instability. Peroneal tendon instability is a relatively common entity that may be associated with lateral ankle instability. The condition may be secondary to an inversion ankle injury,[3] or it may produce functional ankle instability caused by the dysfunction of the peroneal tendons. Chronic subluxation or frank dislocation of the peroneal tendons may also produce degenerative tears of the peroneus brevis tendon.

The peroneus brevis and longus muscles form individual tendons that pass behind the lateral malleolus to turn anteriorly toward their respective insertions at the base of the fifth metatarsal and the base of the first metatarsal. At the level of the lateral malleolus, the tendon of the peroneus brevis remains anterior to the peroneus longus. The tendons are retained within the peroneal groove by the superior peroneal retinaculum (SPR).[200] The SPR originates from the periosteum on the posterolateral ridge of the fibula.[58] The peroneal groove is a shallow bony groove[67] deepened by a fibrocartilaginous ridge.

The mechanism of injury is related to a sudden, forceful, passive dorsiflexion of the inverted foot combined with reflex contraction of the peroneal tendons.[65, 179, 251] As has been stated previously, the condition may also be related to chronic lateral instability.[83] The injury produces a variety of pathologic features, which include elevation of the SPR off the lateral border of the fibula with concomitant dissection of the tendons beneath the lateral fibular periosteum, tear of the SPR, or fracture of the posterolateral margin of the fibula. The anatomic classification of peroneal tendon instability, as described by Oden, is based on the location of SPR disruption.[188]

Chronic subluxation of the peroneus brevis tendon onto the posterolateral border of the fibula has been implicated in the development of longitudinal tears of the peroneus brevis tendon.[30, 238] Longitudinal tear of the peroneal tendons has also been described after acute and chronic lateral ankle inversion injury.[12, 215] Acute peroneal tendon dislocation produces pain over the course of the peroneal tendons as well as along the lateral border of the fibula. The patient may recall a "pop" at the time of injury. Oftentimes, the patient is capable of providing a vivid description of dislocation. The tendon may or may not spontaneously reduce.

A careful examination of the acute injury confirms swelling and tenderness posterior to the lateral malleolus.[7, 65, 71, 168, 179] Active dorsiflexion of the foot secured in a plantar flexed and everted position may produce apprehension, subluxation, or dislocation. Dislocation is not a neces-

Figure 30E1–28. The distal fascicle of the anterior inferior tibiofibular ligament is normally parallel and distal to the main ligament and separated from it by a fibrofatty septum. *Inset:* After an inversion sprain of the ankle, the distal fascicle may impinge on the anterolateral aspect of the talus. (From Bassett FH, Gates HS, Billys JB, et al: Talar impingement by the anteroinferior tibiofibular ligament. A cause of chronic pain in the ankle after inversion sprain. J Bone Joint Surg Am 72:55–59, 1990.)

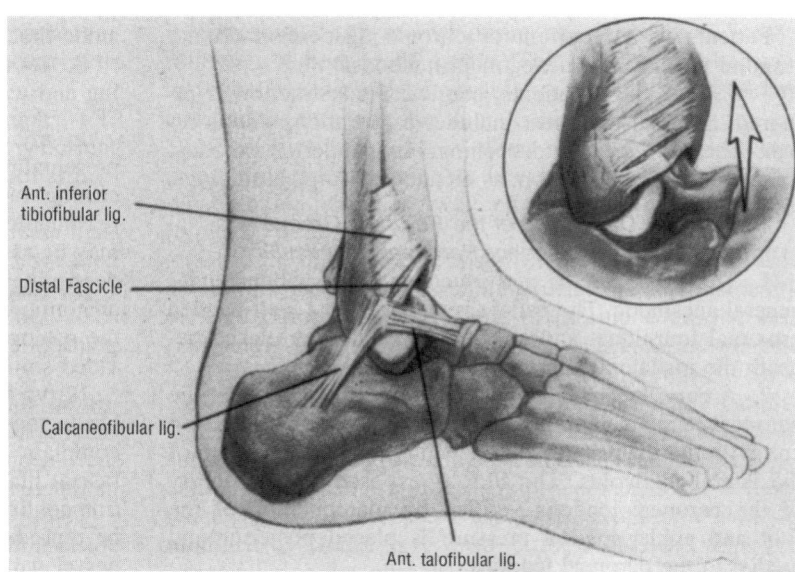

views of the ankles to document instability. Arthroscopy of the ankle is used before stabilization, if indicated by clinical examination (e.g., anterolateral tenderness, talar dome tenderness) or MRI findings (e.g., osteochondral lesion of the talus, loose body).

Return to Play Criteria

Recovery of function after a lateral ankle sprain follows a logical sequence of events. Once the initial pain and swelling subside, coordination and strengthening activities are emphasized. Gradually, the patient is able to return to walking, running, and cutting programs. I return patients to sport once they master sport-specific drills with minimal discomfort. A semirigid pneumatic ankle brace or taping accelerates the schedule, and these are used to prevent recurrent injury.

Prevention of recurrence and new injuries has received much attention in the literature. Conditioning, including strength, coordination, and proprioception; warm-up; comprehensive stretching; and external support are key components of prevention.

Taping of the ankle is perhaps the most widely used prophylactic method.[162] Rovere and colleagues published a retrospective analysis of taping and the laced ankle stabilizer that confirmed that taping is much less effective in the prevention of new and recurrent ankle injuries among collegiate football players.[212] Taping appears to be limited by time-related loosening.[94, 204] Glick and coworkers studied the effect of tape on six ankles with significant (>5 degrees) talar tilt.[87] Each subject performed 20 minutes of exercise. Only one of the six ankles remained firmly supported by the ankle tape.

Walsh and Blackburn acknowledge the time-related loosening associated with ankle taping.[268] They contend that the method continues to play a supportive role, perhaps limited to restricting the extremes of motion. They recommend taping against the skin and secondarily around the shoe (football). They emphasize that tape, in any amount or configuration, is not a substitute for rehabilitation. Although taping is inexpensive on a per-use basis, significant cost is associated with long-term application by trained personnel.[212]

Manfroy and associates studied resistance to maximal inversion in a weight-bearing, near–maximally inverted ankle, with and without supportive taping.[162] The method attempted to reproduce the conditions just before ankle injury. The taped ankle was capable of resisting inversion to a greater degree than the nontaped ankle; however, the protective effect was lost after 40 minutes of exercise.

Hamill and colleagues suggested the use of a semirigid pneumatic orthosis for the prevention of recurrent lateral ankle sprains; they cite a reduction in mediolateral excursion force and velocity in an experimental setting.[95] Decreased inversion, based on angular displacement, has also been demonstrated.[132]

Sitler and coworkers completed a prospective randomized study to evaluate the effectiveness of a semirigid pneumatic ankle brace in the prevention of ankle sprains.[232] The participants all competed in an intramural basketball program at the United States Military Academy. Over a 2-year period, 59 injuries were documented; 12 occurred in the braced group and 47 in the nonbraced control group. Although the frequency of injury was significantly reduced by bracing, the severity of the individual injuries remained similar.

Soccer players with and without a history of lateral ankle sprains were randomly assigned by Surve and associates to use a semirigid pneumatic ankle brace (Sport Stirrup, Aircast, Inc., Summit, NJ).[257] The orthosis reduced the incidence of lateral ankle sprains in the group with a history of previous ankle injury but not in the group without such a history.

Thacker and colleagues completed a review of 113 studies and concluded that supervised rehabilitation must be completed before resumption of running or practice.[262] Furthermore, these authors recommended the use of an orthosis for 6 months following a severe lateral ankle sprain.

On the question of peroneal rehabilitation, the importance of strong, coordinated activity appears obvious. The reality of the matter is not so self-evident. Konradsen and coworkers elegantly demonstrated that the time to development of reflex eversion mediated by the peroneal tendons is longer than the time required to incur injury of the lateral ligaments after exposure to a sudden inversion moment.[143]

A sobering study completed by Gerber and associates clearly illustrates the long-term disability associated with ankle sprain.[84] This prospective observational study of 104 West Point cadets confirmed that 95% of the cadets had returned to athletic activity by the 6-week follow-up. At the time of the 6-month follow-up, all cadets had returned to athletic activity, but 40% remained symptomatic. The persistent dysfunction was related neither to the grade of sprain nor to the presence of joint laxity.

In summary, I allow return to sport after recovery of pain-free ankle motion, strength, and protective reflexes. I expect the athlete to complete sport-specific drills with a high degree of confidence and comfort. Most importantly, the ankle is braced until functional and anatomic stability are achieved.

Medial Ankle Sprain

Isolated injury to the deltoid ligament is rare. Staples reviewed 110 cases of deltoid injury.[244] Deltoid rupture without associated ankle fracture was noted in only 10 cases. Of these 10 cases, five were isolated to the deltoid, three were associated with syndesmosis injury, and two were associated with anterior capsule injury.

Relevant Anatomy

The medial ligaments of the ankle, the deltoid ligaments, consist of superficial and deep components[48, 192] (Fig. 30E1–30). Close has demonstrated the importance of the medial ligaments in maintaining a normal medial clear space, that is, a normal intermalleolar distance.[48] He provided a detailed anatomic description but no data to support his conclusions.

Pankovich and Shivaram identified the superficial deltoid origin at the anterior colliculus of the medial malleo-

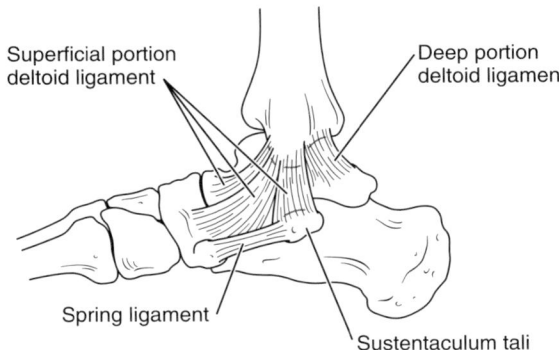

Superficial portion deltoid ligament

Deep portion deltoid ligament

Spring ligament

Sustentaculum tali

Figure 30E1–30. The superficial and deep layers of the deltoid ligament. (Redrawn from Close JR: Some applications of the functional anatomy of the ankle joint. J Bone Joint Surg Am 38:761–781, 1956.)

lus, and the deep deltoid origin at the posterior colliculus and the intercollicular groove.[192] The superficial deltoid includes four parts—the tibionavicular ligament, the tibiospring ligament, the tibiocalcaneal ligament, and the superficial tibiotalar ligament. The deep deltoid includes two parts—the deep anterior tibiotalar ligament and the deep posterior tibiotalar ligament.

The biomechanical characteristics of the ankle ligaments are such that failure (rupture) is due to increasing load as opposed to twisting or shearing.[8] Isolated testing of the individual ankle ligaments demonstrates that the ATFL is the first to fail and the deep deltoid ligament is the last to fail.[8]

Siegler and colleagues tested 20 fresh cadaver ankles.[231] Based on increasing ultimate load, components of the deltoid were ordered from weakest to strongest as follows: the tibiocalcaneal ligament, the tibionavicular ligament, the tibiospring ligament, and the posterior tibiotalar ligament.

Earll and coworkers conducted a cadaver study to assess the importance of the deltoid ligament relative to talocrural contact and pressure.[63] Division of the tibiocalcaneal fibers of the superficial deltoid resulted in significant decreased contact area (maximum 43%) and an associated increase in contact pressure (maximum 30%). Division of the other components of the deltoid resulted in insignificant changes in joint contact.

Most deltoid ruptures are associated with ankle fractures. Ankle fractures associated with a pure deltoid rupture typically involve the posterior deep tibiotalar ligament.[193]

Broström described the ligamentous lesions found during the surgical exploration of 105 recent ankle sprains.[31] The ATFL was the most commonly injured structure. The ATFL was completely torn as an isolated injury in 65 patients and as an associated injury in an additional 25 patients. The CFL was the second most commonly injured ligament. It was completely or partially torn as an associated injury in 23 patients. The deltoid ligament was partially torn in only 5 cases. No complete ruptures were noted. The torn ends of the ligament remained well opposed. The tears typically occurred at midsubstance close to the medial malleolus. Medial ankle instability was not found in any of these cases.

Kjærsgaard-Andersen and associates used a cadaver model to study the effect of isolated division of the tibiocal-

caneal ligament.[136] They reported a maximum median increase in tibiotalocalcaneal abduction of 6.1 degrees and a corresponding maximum median increase in talocalcaneal abduction of 3.6 degrees. The authors concluded that the tibiocalcaneal ligament is an important stabilizer of the medial hindfoot.

Rasmussen and colleagues used a cadaver model to study the effect of isolated division of the deltoid ligament with a device that allowed recording of rotatory movements in two planes.[206] The tibiocalcaneal ligament (superficial deltoid) and the intermediate tibiotalar ligament (deep deltoid) provided resistance to abduction of the talus. The deltoid also provided significant resistance to external rotation of the talus.

Reporting on a single case, Jackson and coworkers documented an eversion mechanism that produced rupture of the anterior aspect of the superficial and deep deltoid without other associated bony or ligamentous injury.[116] This injury occurred in a 23-year-old football player with a long-term history of medial ankle pain before the acute injury.

Clinical Evaluation

Evaluation of the medial ankle sprain is designed to elicit information that allows classification of the injury. As has been stated previously, I consider sprains from the simplistic perspective of graded ligament injury, as suggested by the American Medical Association[202] and by O'Donoghue.[189] Injuries are graded based on stretch (grade I), partial tear (grade II), or complete rupture of the ligament (grade III). Additional information with regard to associated ligamentous injuries is noted.

History. Information relevant to previous ankle injury, the mechanism of injury, the ability of the patient to continue to play or walk, and current complaints represent the salient historical points.

Physical Examination. It is imperative that the examination not be limited to the medial ankle ligaments. Inspection of the leg, ankle, and foot may reveal swelling, ecchymosis, blister formation, or gross deformity. Palpation begins with a vascular and sensory assessment followed by a detailed assessment of the entire leg, ankle, and foot. Tenderness at the deltoid and surrounding area is particularly important to note.

Motion about the foot and ankle is determined with the patient seated and relaxed. The knees are flexed and the feet allowed to fall into an equinus position. Ankle and subtalar range of motion is documented and motor function graded.

Stress testing is a useful clinical and radiographic tool that provides a portion of the diagnostic data required for grading ankle sprains. The *anterior drawer test* and the *varus talar tilt test* are used to demonstrate the integrity of the ATFL and the CFL. A *valgus talar tilt test* is used to evaluate the integrity of the deltoid. Testing is occasionally uncomfortable, particularly in the acute setting. False-negative results may be caused by involuntary guarding or pain response.

The test is performed in both ankle neutral and plantar flexion positions. Valgus stress is applied to the talus through the hindfoot, and a comparison is made between injured and noninjured ankles.

Ankle Syndesmosis Sprain

Injury to the ankle syndesmosis is most common in collision sports.[25] Boytim and colleagues reported 98 ankle injuries among the players of a professional football team over a 6-year period.[25] Twenty-eight significant lateral ankle sprains and 15 syndesmosis sprains were reported. The players with syndesmosis sprains missed more games and more practices and used more treatments than players with lateral ankle sprains.

Hopkinson and coworkers retrospectively reviewed 1344 ankle sprains that occurred over a 41-month period at the United States Military Academy.[110] Fifteen of these patients (1.1%) were diagnosed with syndesmosis sprain. A subsequent prospective study at the same institution revealed that syndesmosis sprains accounted for 17% of ankle sprains over a 2-month period.[84]

Relevant Anatomy

The ankle syndesmosis is composed of the anterior inferior tibiofibular ligament (AITFL), the posterior inferior tibiofibular ligament (PITFL), and the interosseous ligament (IOL) (Fig. 30E1–33). The syndesmosis, along with the deltoid, maintains the critical anatomic relationship between the tibia and the talus. Ramsey and Hamilton used a carbon black transference technique to clearly demonstrate that lateral displacement of the talus results in an incremental decrease in contact area with each millimeter of translation.[203] The first millimeter of lateral translation produced an average 42% reduction in contact area between the tibia and the talus. Failure to reduce the ankle syndesmosis and the associated lateral talar translation greatly increases the risk of post-traumatic ankle arthritis (Fig. 30E1–34).

Anatomic dissection by Close revealed that division of the syndesmosis and of the interosseous ligament produces minimal widening of the intermalleolar distance.[48] Only after the deltoid ligaments are divided does the syndesmosis separate. His conclusion is that significant trauma to the ankle must occur for the ankle mortise to appear wide.

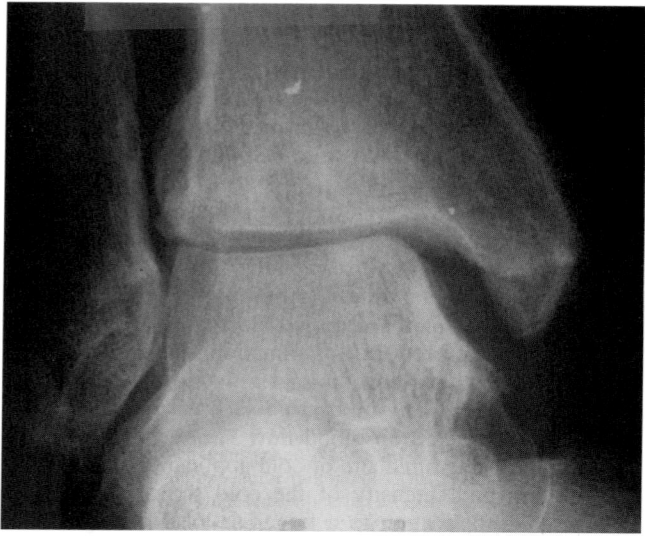

Figure 30E1–34. Post-traumatic ankle arthritis subsequent to an incompletely reduced ankle syndesmosis and lateral talar translation. Note the wide syndesmosis and medial joint space width, the narrow superior joint space, and the lateral subchondral cyst formation.

Broström described the ligamentous lesions found during the surgical exploration of 105 recent ankle sprains.[31] The ATFL was the most commonly injured structure. The ATFL was completely torn as an isolated injury in 65 cases and as an associated injury in an additional 25 patients. The CFL was the second most commonly injured ligament. It was completely or partially torn as an associated injury in 23 patients. The AITFL was completely torn in 6 cases. No incomplete ruptures were noted. Five of these injuries occurred at midsubstance and 1 involved an avulsion fracture off the anterior tibia. The torn ends of the ligament remained well opposed. External rotation of the talus produced up to 5 mm of diastasis in 5 cases and 1 to 2 mm in the sixth case.

The mechanism of injury is thought to be external rotation. In 1968, Lovell described the case of a 13-year-old tobogganner who sustained a forced external rotation

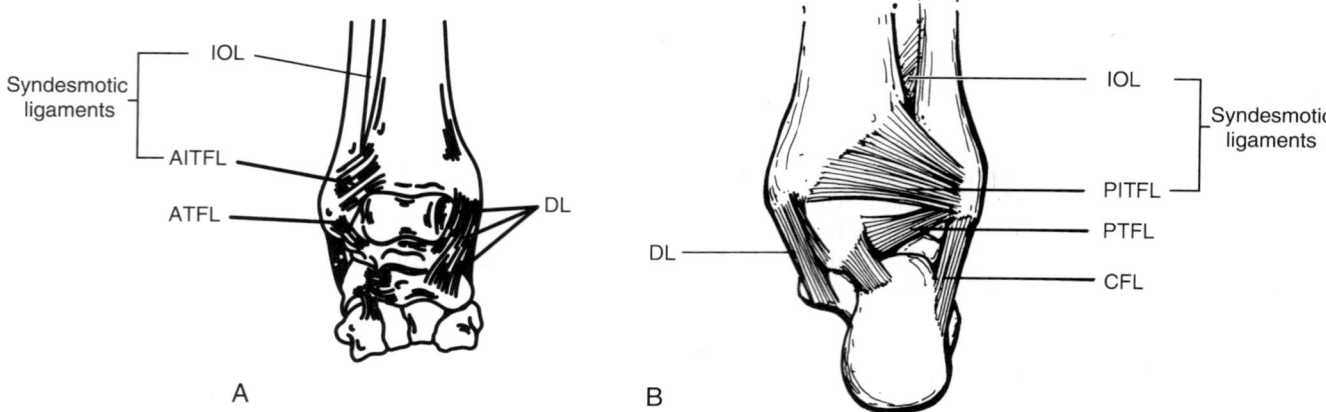

Figure 30E1–33. *A,* The tibiofibular syndesmosis from the front—anterior inferior tibiofibular ligament (AITFL), anterior talofibular ligament (ATFL), and deltoid ligament (DL). *B,* The tibiofibular syndesmosis from the back—posterior inferior tibiofibular ligament (PITFL), distal interosseous ligament (IOL), posterior talofibular ligament (PTFL), calcaneofibular ligament (CFL), deltoid ligament (DL).

injury to the ankle.[158] The patient presented with a fixed external rotation foot deformity that was associated with a posterior dislocation of the fibula perched behind the lateral tibia. Closed reduction and casting produced an excellent result.

Boytim and associates suggested two specific mechanisms of injury in the professional football player.[25] The first is direct force applied to the posterior leg of a downed player whose foot is in an externally rotated position. The second is an external rotation force at the knee while the foot is firmly planted.

Fritschy evaluated 10 world-class slalom skiers with syndesmosis injuries.[80] He speculated that a common mechanism of forced external rotation of the talus against the fibula produced all of their injuries. A retrospective review by Hopkinson and colleagues failed to establish a consistent mechanism of injury among eight patients with syndesmosis sprain.[110]

Clinical Evaluation

As has been stated previously, I consider sprains from the simplistic perspective of graded ligament injury, as suggested by the American Medical Association[202] and by O'Donoghue.[189] Injuries are graded based on stretch (grade I), partial tear (grade II), or complete rupture (grade III) of the AITFL. Additional information with regard to associated ligamentous injuries is noted.

Edwards and DeLee described a classification system for ankle diastasis without fracture (grade III sprain) based on the presence of radiographic diastasis with and without stress.[66] A *latent* syndesmosis injury appeared normal on an unstressed radiograph *and* abnormal or widened on external rotation stress mortise radiograph. A *frank* injury was seen as a widened syndesmosis on unstressed radiographs. The frank injuries were further divided into four types: type I, lateral fibular subluxation without plastic deformity of the fibula; type II, lateral fibular subluxation with plastic deformity of the fibula; type III, posterior subluxation of the fibula behind the lateral tibia; and type IV, superior dislocation of the talus with a wide diastasis.

History. Information relevant to previous ankle injury, the mechanism of injury, the ability of the patient to continue to play or walk, and current complaints represent the salient historical points. Syndesmosis injury is suggested by a mechanism of forced external rotation of the foot.

Physical Examination. The examination is systematic and includes careful palpation along the entire interosseous ligament and the fibula. Fracture of the fibula at all levels must be considered. Although dislocation of the proximal tibiofibular joint is rare,[224] it must also be considered when proximal leg symptoms are present. Local tenderness at the AITFL or along the interosseous ligament suggests a syndesmosis sprain.

Ankle range of motion is carefully assessed. Also, lateral ankle stability is determined with performance of the anterior drawer and talar tilt tests. One must never forget that pain out of proportion to the injury is a finding consistent with acute compartment syndrome.

Hopkinson and coworkers described a squeeze test used to identify syndesmosis ruptures at the time of initial presentation[110] (see Fig. 30E1–5). The squeeze test was attrib-

uted to a former chief athletic trainer at the United States Military Academy. The test is performed by compression of the midleg from posterior lateral to anterior medial. Pain produced at the AITFL suggests injury to the same, as long as fracture, contusion, and compartment syndrome are not present. The authors retrospectively reviewed eight patients with syndesmosis sprains; all were noted to have a positive squeeze test at initial evaluation. A separate biomechanical analysis of the squeeze test demonstrated that the squeeze test produced reproducible separation of the fibula and tibia.[261]

Boytim and associates described an external rotation stress test[25] (see Fig. 30E1–8). The patient is seated and relaxed with the hip and knee flexed and the foot and ankle held in a neutral position. The knee is maintained in a forward-facing position while a gentle but firm external rotation force is applied to the foot. Pain reproduced at the anterior syndesmosis is diagnostic of a syndesmosis injury.

A secondary test is the direct eversion maneuver[248] (Fig. 30E1–35). The maneuver is accomplished with the patient in a seated and relaxed position. The examiner gently secures the leg and foot as a direct eversion or abduction force is applied across the ankle. Increased translation as compared with the contralateral ankle is a positive result.

Imaging
Radiographs and Computed Tomography. The radiographic examination includes weight-bearing views of the

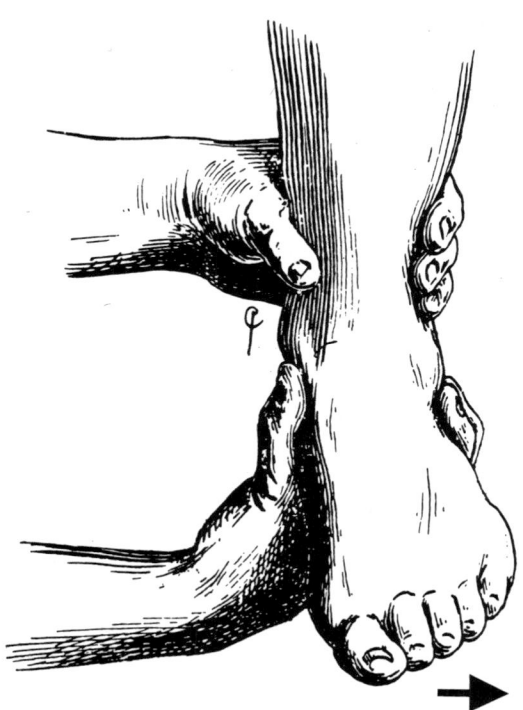

Figure 30E1–35. The direct eversion maneuver is accomplished with the patient in a seated and relaxed position. The examiner gently secures the leg and foot as a direct eversion or abduction force is applied across the ankle. Increased translation as compared with the contralateral ankle is a positive result. (From Stiehl JB: Complex ankle fracture dislocations with syndesmotic diastasis. Orthop Rev 19:499–507, 1990.)

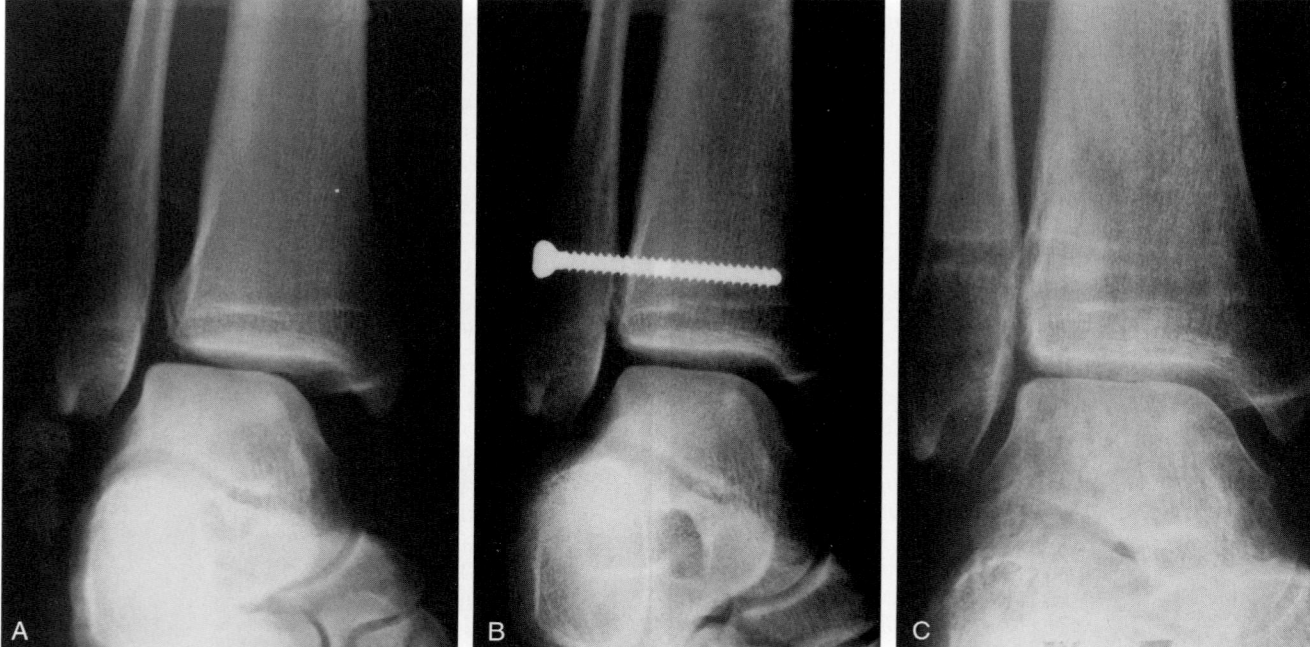

Figure 30E1–37. Syndesmosis rupture. *A,* Anteroposterior injury radiograph. *B,* Internal fixation with fully threaded 4.5-mm screw. *C,* Anteroposterior radiograph after screw removal.

Surgical Repair

Technique: *Closed or Open Reduction and Internal Fixation of the Ankle Syndesmosis*

1. The procedure is performed with the patient under general anesthesia. The patient is supine with a well-padded proximal tourniquet and a 3000-mL saline bag placed beneath the ipsilateral hemipelvis.

2. An image intensifier is used to attempt closed reduction of the syndesmosis. If reduction is not satisfactory, an open reduction is performed.

3. The extremity is exsanguinated and the tourniquet inflated. A linear incision is placed over the lateral border of the distal fibula. The syndesmosis is exposed and open reduction is accomplished by débridement of the distal tibiofibular articulation. If reduction of the medial joint space remains incomplete, then a medial ankle arthrotomy and a deltoid ligament repair are performed.

4. The tears of the AITFL are approximated and repaired with absorbable suture. Avulsion fractures are repaired directly to the fibula or tibia.

5. The syndesmosis repair is then protected by placement of one or two 3.5- or 4.0-mm screws. These screws are placed 2 cm[167] above the ankle joint line with the ankle in a neutral dorsiflexion position. The fixation is directed from the relatively posterior fibula into the more anterior tibia. Three or four cortices are captured with the screw. A nonlag technique is used in an effort to prevent overreduction of the mortise and subsequent loss of ankle dorsiflexion (see Fig. 30E1–37*B*).

6. The wound is closed in layers and a short leg splint applied. At 10 days, the incision is inspected and a short leg non–weight-bearing cast applied. Three to six weeks postoperatively, a rehabilitation program is instituted and

monitored. Weight-bearing is allowed after 10 to 12 weeks. The fixation is removed 3 months postoperatively before resumption of athletic activity is permitted.

Unusual Syndesmosis Injuries. Olerud reported a single case of posterior dislocation of the fibula (Edwards and DeLee type III) and subluxed talus associated with a violent supination and external rotation mechanism of injury.[190] This patient was successfully treated with primary open reduction and syndesmotic screw placement.

Edwards and DeLee used a fibular osteotomy to reduce lateral displacement of the fibula associated with plastic deformity of the fibula (Edwards and DeLee type II).[66] The procedure was successfully used on two patients with this unusual injury.

Chronic Syndesmosis Sprains. Katznelson, Lin, and Militiano used a distal tibiofibular arthrodesis to treat chronic syndesmosis ruptures.[128] All five injuries were the sequelae of injuries initially diagnosed as lateral ankle ligament sprains. All five patients obtained excellent results at the time of final follow-up. The report did not discuss return to athletic activity, nor was the time to follow-up noted.

Rehabilitation

Patients with low-grade syndesmosis sprains are placed in an aggressive rehabilitation program, as outlined in the lateral ankle sprain section. Rehabilitation for postoperative syndesmosis injuries is effectively delayed by 3 weeks. Non–weight-bearing status is maintained for 10 to 12 weeks.

Ankle and subtalar flexibility, motor function, and coordination[78] are emphasized throughout the protocol. The ankle is supported by a semirigid pneumatic ankle brace. In addition to the ankle brace, an elastic sock is available for mobilization of edema (see Fig. 30E1–22). Alternatively, the ankle is taped as described earlier.

Author's Preferred Method of Treatment

I treat acute syndesmosis injury *not* associated with fracture with the RICE (*R*est, *I*ce, *C*ompression, *E*levation) method and non–weight-bearing until the definitive diagnosis is established. Isolated grade I or grade II syndesmosis injuries are allowed to begin weight-bearing to tolerance after the acute pain and swelling remit. Treatment is symptomatic with an emphasis on recovery of range of motion, strength, and coordination. Taping is applied (as described earlier) for support of the syndesmosis and resistance to external rotation.

I use the Edwards and DeLee classification system for grade III sprains.[66] This system is based on the presence of radiographic diastasis with and without stress. A *latent* syndesmosis injury appears normal on an unstressed radiograph *and* abnormal or widened on external rotation stress mortise radiograph. A *frank* injury is seen as a widened syndesmosis on unstressed radiographs. Patients with latent grade III injuries are instructed to remain non–weight-bearing for at least 8 to 10 weeks. Sequential radiographs are used to monitor alignment. Frank injuries require closed or open reduction and screw fixation. A comprehensive rehabilitation program is instituted 3 to 6 weeks postoperatively. Screw fixation is removed 3 months postoperatively before resumption of full athletic activity is permitted.

Return to Play Criteria

Recovery follows a logical sequence of events. Once the initial pain and swelling subside, coordination and strengthening activities are emphasized. Gradually, the patient is able to return to walking, running, and cutting programs. Patients are returned to sport once they master sport-specific drills. A semirigid pneumatic ankle brace or syndesmosis taping accelerates the schedule. Conditioning, including strength, coordination, and proprioception; warm-up; comprehensive stretching; and external support are key components of prevention.

Fritschy evaluated 10 world-class slalom skiers with syndesmosis injuries.[80] The unexpected finding was that all skiers returned to their original level of competition but the time to return ranged between 18 months and 12 years.

Gerber and colleagues completed a prospective observational study of 96 West Point cadets with ankle sprains, including 16 syndesmosis sprains.[84] All patients were treated with a functional rehabilitation program. At the time of the 6-week and 6-month follow-up examinations, grade I syndesmosis sprains were associated with worse outcomes compared with all ankle sprains, including grade II and III syndesmosis sprains.

Ankle Dislocation without Fracture

Dislocation of the ankle joint is typically associated with major or minor bony injuries. Dislocation without associated fracture is rare.

Relevant Anatomy

The ankle joint ligamentous support is described in detail earlier. The stability of the ankle joint is such that talocrural dislocation without associated malleolar fracture is uncommon.

Wilson and coworkers reviewed the literature and found 14 cases of ankle dislocation without fracture.[276] Most of these injuries were associated with falls or direct trauma. The authors further described two cases. The first was a posterior dislocation of the ankle and the second an upward dislocation of the ankle associated with a wide diastasis of the distal tibiofibular joint.

Clinical Evaluation

History. Dislocation of the ankle joint with or without fracture produces dramatic pain and deformity. The patient may report spontaneous reduction, or reduction on the field may be noted by the patient or a trainer. Reduction produces significant relief of pain. Information relevant to previous ankle and subtalar injury, the mechanism of injury, and current complaints represent the salient historical points.

Physical Examination. Examination of the patient includes evaluation of the entire extremity. Inspection of the leg, ankle, and foot may reveal swelling, ecchymosis, blister formation, or gross deformity. Palpation begins with a vascular and sensory assessment followed by a detailed assessment of the entire leg, ankle, and foot.

Imaging

Radiographs. Radiographs of a dislocated ankle are typically dramatic (Fig. 30E1–38). Three standard views are reviewed and a lack of talocrural continuity is diagnostic for an ankle dislocation. Radiographs taken after a formal reduction or after spontaneous reduction are less dramatic but nonetheless must be obtained and carefully scrutinized for malleolar fractures, talar fractures, and osteochondral fractures (Fig. 30E1–39). Subsequent radiographs are obtained to ensure anatomic reduction and to monitor heterotopic ossification.

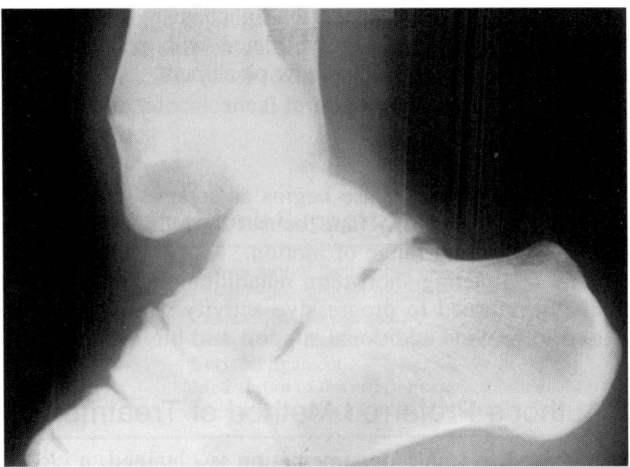

Figure 30E1–38. Ankle dislocation without fracture.

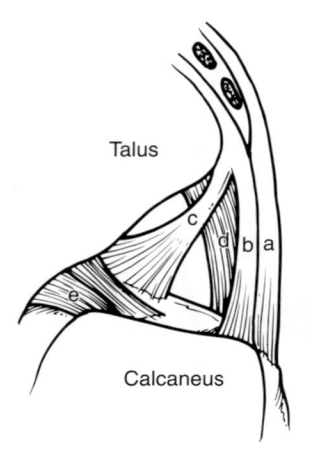

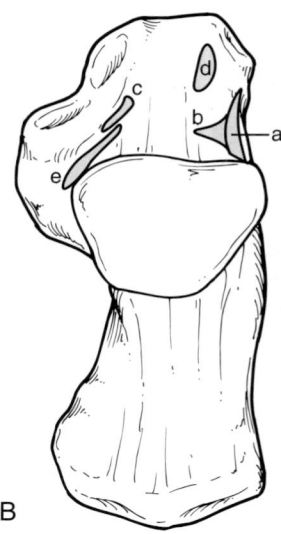

Figure 30E1–41. Ligaments of the sinus tarsi. *A,* Labels include: a, lateral retinacular root; b, intermediate retinacular root; c, medial retinacular root; d, cervical ligament; e, interosseous ligament. *B,* Calcaneal attachments of the ligaments of the sinus tarsi. (From Harper MC: Lateral ligamentous support of the subtalar joint. Foot Ankle 11:354–358, 1991.)

joint. This incremental difference was maximal at 5 degrees of ankle dorsiflexion. The clinical application, as suggested by the authors, is to place the ankle in slight dorsiflexion during stress testing of the ankle and subtalar joints.

A second cadaver study by Kjærsgaard-Andersen and associates revealed that the CFL provides significant rotatory stability to the talocalcaneal joint.[134] External rotation after isolated division of the CFL increased up to 5.4 degrees at the tibiotalocalcaneal complex and up to 2.9 degrees at the talocalcaneal complex. The authors concluded that the CFL is the primary restraint to hindfoot external rotation.

Heilman and colleagues used 10 fresh cadaver ankles to demonstrate that the CFL tightens with supination and dorsiflexion.[106] Selective division of the CFL produced 5 degrees of lateral opening across the posterior facet of the subtalar joint. Division of the lateral subtalar capsule added no further instability to the joint. Finally, division of the

interosseous ligament completely de-stabilized the joint, leading to dislocation (Fig. 30E1–42).

A third experimental study by Kjærsgaard-Andersen and coworkers demonstrated that isolated division of the cervical or interosseous ligaments resulted in relatively minor increases in three-plane joint motion.[135] These authors concluded that the resulting instability was significant despite the small angular changes. Furthermore, injury to either ligament may be related to the sinus tarsi syndrome or talocalcaneal instability.

Knudson and associates used a cadaver model to specifically study the effect of interosseous ligament division.[139] Measurements taken before and after interosseous ligament sectioning suggested that the interosseous ligament provides significant subtalar joint support, particularly in supination.

The study completed by Kato demonstrated a relationship between subtalar instability and generalized ligamen-

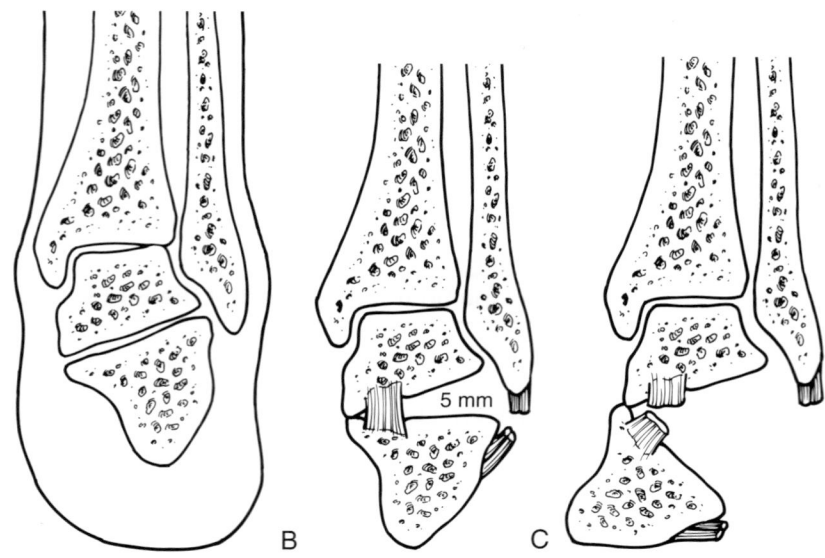

Figure 30E1–42. Stability of the subtalar joint after serial ligament sectioning. *A,* Brodén's view of the subtalar joint, intact ligaments. *B,* Brodén's view of the subtalar joint, after sectioning of the calcaneofibular ligament (CFL). *C,* Brodén's view of the subtalar joint, after sectioning of the CFL, capsule, and interosseous ligament. (From Heilmen AE, Braly G, Bishop JO, et al: An anatomic study of subtalar instability. Foot Ankle 10:224–228, 1990.)

tous laxity, a flattened posterior facet, chronic stress, and trauma.[127]

Clinical Evaluation

As has been stated previously, I consider sprains from the simplistic perspective of graded ligament injury, as suggested by the American Medical Association[202] and by O'Donoghue.[189] Acute injuries are graded based on stretch (grade I), partial tear (grade II), or complete rupture (grade III) of the subtalar capsule or supporting ligaments, including the CFL, the interosseus ligament, and the cervical ligament. A grade III tear is suggested by a clinical history of severe deformity or swelling, examination consistent with gross subtalar instability, or MRI demonstrating ligamentous disruption. The clinical evaluation provides additional information with regard to associated ligamentous injuries, especially at the lateral ankle.

History. Information relevant to previous ankle and subtalar injury, the mechanism of injury, the ability of the patient to continue to play or walk, and current complaints represent the salient historical points. Severe subtalar sprains are associated with a history of inversion injury with a characteristic "pop"; acute severe pain, swelling, or deformity; and inability of the patient to continue activity or to walk.

Physical Examination. An inversion foot or ankle injury is approached as a constellation of possible injuries, including ATFL sprain, CFL sprain, syndesmosis sprain, deltoid sprain, subtalar sprain (chronic insufficiency of the lateral hindfoot associated with subtalar instability isolated or combined with lateral ankle ligament instability has been shown to occur in up to two thirds of patients[38]), subtalar coalition, bifurcate ligament sprain, peroneal tendon instability, peroneal tendon tear, lateral malleolus fracture, talar dome osteochondral injury, anterior process fracture, and fracture of the base of the fifth metatarsal.

Examination of the patient includes evaluation of the entire extremity. Inspection of the leg, ankle, and foot may reveal swelling, ecchymosis, blister formation, or gross deformity. Palpation begins with a vascular and sensory assessment followed by a detailed assessment of the entire leg, ankle, and foot. Tenderness at the sinus tarsi, the ATFL, and the CFL is particularly important to note.

Clinical examination of the subtalar joint is difficult to complete owing to the complex nature of subtalar motion and its association with leg, ankle, and foot motion.[137] Evaluation of motion is determined by gently grasping the leg while the ankle is held at a right angle or a neutral dorsiflexion position. With the widest part of the talus engaged into the ankle mortise, adduction of the heel is more likely to represent motion through the talocalcaneal joint rather than the talocrural joint. From a neutral position (heel vertical), maximum passive inversion and eversion are measured. An alternative method is placement of the empirical subtalar joint axis horizontal with the ground by allowing the foot to fall into 45 degrees of equinus, or by examining the patient prone with the knee flexed 135 degrees[113] (Fig. 30E1–43). Gross clinical instability is consistent with a grade III sprain.

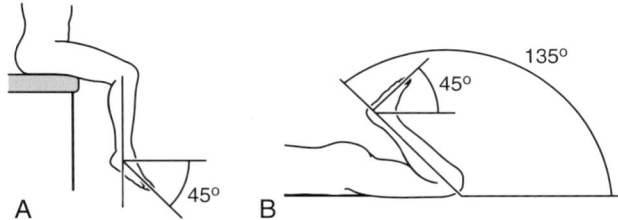

Figure 30E1–43. Clinical examination of the subtalar joint is facilitated by placement of the empirical subtalar joint axis horizontal with the ground. *A,* Place the foot in 45 degrees of equinus. *B,* Examine the patient prone with the knee flexed 135 degrees. (Redrawn from Inman VT: The Joints of the Ankle. Baltimore, Williams & Wilkins, 1976, p 108.)

Imaging

Radiographs. Radiographic demonstration of the subtalar joint is difficult.[230] Brodén described an oblique view of the foot designed to produce tangential images of the posterior facet of the subtalar joint[29] (Fig. 30E1–44). The view is obtained with the foot in 45 degrees of internal rotation and the beam centered on the sinus tarsi and angled posteriorly (by 10, 20, 30, or 40 degrees). The images are carefully inspected with attention to small fractures and nonconcentric joint alignment.

Stress Radiographs. Several methods for stress radiography of the subtalar joint have been described. Perhaps the most important method is stress radiography of the talocrural joint to quantify the extent of concomitant ankle instability.

The ankle *talar tilt test* is dependent on the contralateral ankle for control measurements. Varus tilt of the ankle, to a limited degree, is probably normal. Increased inversion of the calcaneus may represent talocrural (ankle) and/or talocalcaneal (subtalar) instability.[38] Radiographic data suggest that 4 degrees of varus tilt occurs in 10% to 15% of noninjured ankles.[23] Varus stress radiographs of both ankles in 90 injured and 90 normal ankles reveal that 6 degrees of increased tilt represents the transition from "normal to abnormal" tilt.[112]

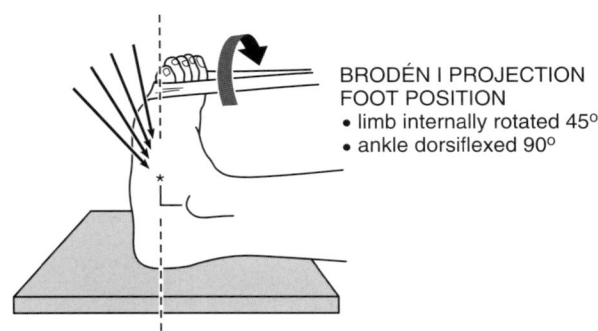

BRODÉN I PROJECTION FOOT POSITION
• limb internally rotated 45°
• ankle dorsiflexed 90°

CENTRAL RAY
• centered 2-3 cm distal and anterior to lateral malleolus
• four pictures, 10°, 20°, 30°, and 40° off the perpendicular

Figure 30E1–44. Brodén's oblique view of the foot designed to produce tangential images of the posterior facet of the subtalar joint. The view is obtained with the foot in 45 degrees of internal rotation and the beam centered on the sinus tarsi and angled posteriorly (10, 20, 30, or 40 degrees).

The *subtalar varus tilt test* is performed with the ankle in a neutral position.[133] A Brodén view of the posterior facet of the subtalar joint is obtained as a varus stress is applied to the subtalar joint. Angular divergence or lateral opening at the posterior facet is compared with the contralateral foot for quantification of instability.

Brantigan used a mechanical device to maintain simultaneous inversion force on both feet during tomography of the ankle and hindfoot.[28] Three patients with subtalar instability and one without instability were studied. The subtalar inversion angle was determined by calculating the tibiocalcaneal angle minus the talocrural tilt. The symptomatic group produced an average subtalar inversion angle of 57 degrees, and the asymptomatic group produced an average subtalar inversion angle of 38 degrees.

Harper completed a review of ankle and subtalar stress radiographs in 14 injured extremities, the contralateral non-injured extremities, and 18 additional asymptomatic extremities.[102] Lateral opening of the subtalar joint, as seen on the Brodén stress view, did *not* significantly differ between the injured and the uninjured contralateral extremity. Furthermore, results from the asymptomatic extremities revealed subtalar articular divergence between 0 and 20 degrees, with an average of 9 degrees. Similar findings using fluoroscopic methods have also been reported.[157]

An anterior stress view of the subtalar joint was used by Kato to assess instability[127] (Fig. 30E1–45). The anteroposterior view of the foot was taken with a constant anterior force applied to the heel while the leg remained stabilized. A line was drawn across the malleoli, and the perpendicular distance to the anterior edge of the talus and calcaneus was measured. Routine and stress views were compared, with attention to anterior calcaneal translation relative to the talus. Clinical data from 50 patients with subtalar instability revealed an average calcaneal displacement of 5 mm in the subtalar instability group and an average of 2 mm in the ankle instability group.

A relatively new method is the dorsiflexion-supination stress lateral radiograph described by Ishii and colleagues.[114] The true lateral radiograph is used to establish the position of the lateral talar process relative to the posterior facet of the calcaneus. Clinical and cadaver experiments indicate that this method is useful for detecting subtalar instability.

Arthrography. Subtalar arthrography for evaluation of acute injury to the CFL or the interosseous ligament remains a useful technique. Meyer and coworkers performed ankle stress radiographs and subtalar joint arthrography in 40 patients with acute inversion sprains.[173] They classified the injuries based on the extent of lateral ankle ligament and subtalar ligament injury. Thirty-two (80%) of the patients sustained injury to both the lateral ankle and the subtalar joint. Six patients with negative stress ankle radiographs had positive subtalar arthrograms.

Sugimoto and associates recommend using an image intensifier to obtain anteroposterior, lateral, and 45-degree oblique views of the subtalar joint.[256] Extravasation of contrast into the peroneal sheath or ankle joint suggests CFL rupture; leakage into the sinus tarsi suggests interosseous ligament or anterior capsule of the posterior facet joint rupture. The authors also noted that this method is not limited by the lack of availability and the cost associated with MRI.

Computed Tomography. The inability of the stress Brodén view to provide useful screening for subtalar instability was confirmed by van Hellemondt.[267] Using helical CT, the author demonstrated no significant difference in subtalar tilt between a group of patients with suspected subtalar instability and the contralateral asymptomatic extremities. The authors suspect that translation produces the tilt seen on routine stress radiographs, as opposed to true divergence of the talus and calcaneus. It is interesting to note that the CT did isolate four cases of fibrous middle facet coalition and a large calcaneal cyst. Finely cut CT is also useful in the evaluation of high-grade sprains to rule out associated fractures.

Magnetic Resonance Imaging. MRI is useful for the diagnosis of acute and chronic ankle and subtalar ligamentous injury[266] and their sequelae (see Fig. 30E1–11). MRI is also useful for identification of tarsal coalition.

High sensitivity mandates that images be carefully correlated with clinical findings. Its accuracy, lack of ionizing radiation, noninvasiveness, decreasing cost, and increasing availability suggest that MRI is the imaging modality of choice for the subtalar joint.

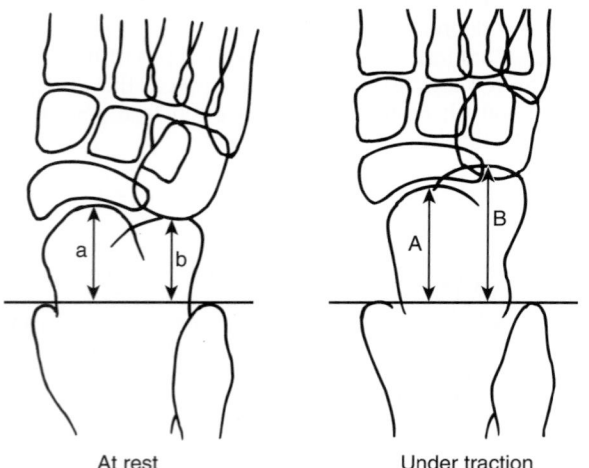

At rest   Under traction

a: Talomalleolar distance
b: Calcaneomalleolar distance

Displacement of the ankle: (A-a)
Displacement of the subtalar joint: (B-b)-(A-a)

Figure 30E1–45. Anterior stress view of the subtalar joint as described by Kato. Routine and stress anteroposterior views of the foot are compared, with attention to anterior calcaneal translation relative to the talus. (From Kato T: The diagnosis and treatment of instability of the subtalar joint. J Bone Joint Surg Br 77:400–406, 1995.)

Therapeutic Options

All acute injuries are treated with the RICE (*R*est, *I*ce, *C*ompression, *E*levation) method, as detailed in the ankle section. Patients with high-grade injuries are placed at non–weight-bearing status until finely cut CT scans are completed.

Many studies have reviewed the effect of cold application to the injured extremity. Cold therapy is an effective, inexpensive, and easy-to-use modality for the treatment of acute musculoskeletal injury. Appropriately applied cold therapy decreases pain perception, decreases the biochemical reactions that produce inflammation, and produces vasoconstriction with a concomitant reduction in soft tissue swelling and bleeding.

The effect of cold on blood flow varies and appears to depend on the anatomic site of cold application, along with the duration and intensity of the cold source.[46, 154, 155, 265] Intense cold application to a finger or toe for longer than 5 to 10 minutes produces a protective cycle of vasoconstriction and vasodilation, the so-called "hunting" response.[154] The ongoing intermittent vasodilation presumably is the digit's attempt to prevent tissue necrosis by hunting for a viable temperature. In the therapeutic setting, cold application to the degree that the "hunting" response is encountered is undesirable; this can be avoided by gradual, moderate, and limited cold application.

Hocutt and colleagues demonstrated the importance of using cold therapy (e.g., ice whirlpool or ice pack for 15 minutes one to three times a day) in the treatment of acute ankle sprains.[108] Furthermore, the group demonstrated a faster recovery associated with early cold therapy (i.e., within the initial 36 hours after an ankle sprain) as compared with delayed cold therapy or early heat therapy.

Grade I and Grade II Subtalar Sprains. Low-grade sprains are treated with early mobilization; weight-bearing to tolerance is encouraged and a rehabilitation program is instituted. Treatment is symptomatic, with an emphasis on recovery of foot and ankle range of motion, strength, and coordination. A cast boot is used during the initial recovery period followed by use of a semirigid pneumatic ankle brace.

Grade III Subtalar Sprains. High-grade injuries as determined by clinical findings are treated with a 2- to 3-week period of non–weight-bearing in a short leg cast. Once clinical stability is achieved, a comprehensive foot and ankle rehabilitation program is instituted. A cast boot is used during the second 3-week period followed by the use of a semirigid pneumatic ankle brace.

Chronic Subtalar Instability. Subtalar instability is surgically addressed by the Broström anatomic ligament reconstruction with the Gould modification. Imbrication of the extensor retinaculum to the lateral fibula effectively limits excessive subtalar motion. Furthermore, the lateral capsular imbrication or advancement is easily extended to include the CFL.

Kato demonstrated that conservative management designed to prevent anterior translation of the calcaneus relative to the talus was effective for most patients.[127] Fourteen patients underwent reconstruction of the interosseus ligament with an Achilles tendon graft augmented by an artificial ligament. Because the reconstruction was performed near the center of rotation, subtalar motion was not limited (the publication did not provide data to substantiate this finding). All patients reported excellent outcomes.

Schon and coworkers reviewed several tendon transfers used for lateral ankle stabilization that also have utility for subtalar stabilization.[222] Stabilization with a tendon transfer is suggested in cases of severe injury, generalized ligamentous laxity, and previous failed reconstruction.

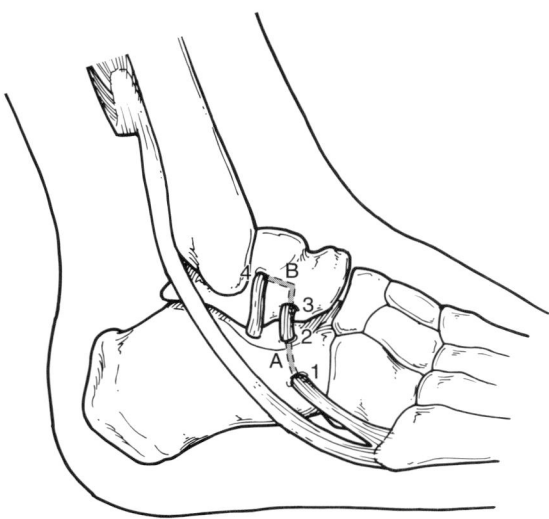

Figure 30E1–46. Interosseous ligament reconstruction as described by Schon has the advantage of an anatomic reconstruction. (From Schon LC, Clanton TO, Baxter DE: Reconstruction of subtalar instability: A review. Foot Ankle 11:324, 1991.)

Interosseous ligament reconstruction, as described by Schon, has the advantage of an anatomic reconstruction (Fig. 30E1–46). The anatomic configuration ensures preservation of ankle and subtalar motion. The authors recommend its use for cases limited to mild subtalar instability.

Rehabilitation

Tissue injury initiates a predictable and sequential series of events known as the healing response. This response is typically divided into three phases with arbitrary and overlapping time lines.[208] The initial phase is the inflammatory phase that includes the first through third days following injury. The second phase is a proliferative phase of tissue repair that extends from day 3 to day 20. The final phase is a remodeling phase that proceeds after day 9.

To a certain degree, rehabilitation follows the phases of the healing response in an effort to reduce the undesirable effects of inflammation (e.g., pain, swelling, loss of function) while simultaneously promoting tissue repair and functional recovery. For rehabilitation of the foot, emphasis throughout the protocol is placed on ankle, subtalar, midfoot, and forefoot flexibility, motor function, and coordination.[78] The hindfoot is supported by a functional ankle brace or various taping methods. An elastic sock is available for additional mobilization of edema (see Fig. 30E1–22).

Acute Phase. The pain and inflammation associated with the first few days following subtalar joint sprain are addressed with rest, cold therapy, and whirlpool. A trial of electrical stimulation may be considered for nonbony injuries. Foot and ankle passive and active range of motion are re-established. Isometrics may be initiated as pain allows.

Subacute Phase. Once the acute pain subsides, flexibility is addressed in all planes. An inclined board is a useful adjunct to gastrocsoleus and Achilles stretching (see

Fig. 30E1–23). Strengthening is initiated with towel scrunches (see Fig. 30E1–24), toe pick-up activities, manual resistive inversion and eversion, elastic bands (see Fig. 30E1–25), seated toe and ankle dorsiflexion with progression to standing, and seated supination-pronation with progression to standing.

Closed chain activities are gradually introduced, including one-leg balance, sports-specific activities on a trampoline, and the use of the BAPS (see Fig. 30E1–26). Aerobic fitness is maintained with cross-training activities such as water running (see Fig. 30E1–27) and cycling.

Heat therapy, such as the application of warm packs, is a useful modality before the therapy session. It reduces pain and spasms and thus facilitates increased range of motion. Cold therapy, compression, and elevation are used after each therapy session to reduce inflammation.

Return to Sport Phase. During this critical phase, walking and running activities are allowed to progress within the limits of a pain-free schedule. Once running activity is mastered, a monitored plyometric program is introduced with progression of difficulty. Schedules are carefully controlled to avoid re-injury.

Associated Injury

Sinus Tarsi Syndrome. O'Connor described a sinus tarsi syndrome as persistent pain at the sinus tarsi that follows a lateral ankle sprain.[187] Others have noted the syndrome to follow as a sequela of subtalar instability.[135] Taillard and associates noted that, in addition to pain over the sinus tarsi, patients with sinus tarsi syndrome complain of lateral ankle instability[259] (Table 30E1–6).

O'Connor speculated that the condition was related to fat pad scarring.[187] The diagnosis was made in 45 patients, 14 of whom were treated with sinus tarsi débridement, a procedure that included resection of the fat pad and the superficial ligaments at the floor of the sinus tarsi. Complete relief was noted in nine patients and partial relief in the remaining five.

Brown performed the O'Connor operation on 11 patients with sinus tarsi syndrome.[36] Ten patients reported significant relief. A single patient with early signs of talar osteoarthritis did not improve.

TABLE 30E1–6
Clinical Signs of Sinus Tarsi Syndrome[173, 187, 259]

History of foot or ankle inversion sprain	Yes
Subjective instability	Yes
Tenderness	Localized to the sinus tarsi
Ankle stability	Yes/no
Anesthetic injection to the sinus tarsi	Temporary symptomatic improvement
Radiographic findings	Normal
Arthrography (subtalar)	Loss of sinus tarsi filling
Magnetic resonance imaging	Rupture of interosseous ligament or cervical ligament; bone edema, soft tissue swelling, or fibrosis at sinus tarsi
Laboratory testing (rule out systemic inflammatory process)	Negative

Meyer and Lagier presented four cases of sinus tarsi syndrome, all successfully treated by curettage of the sinus tarsi contents.[171] Histologic findings from the small series indicated fibrous scar formation consistent with a traumatic cause. Two of the patients were treated with simultaneous subtalar arthrodesis, and one was treated with repair of a ruptured CFL.

Parisien and Vangsness described the use of subtalar joint arthroscopy for evaluation of the posterior facet and its anterior recess.[195] Parisien used this technique to rule out intra-articular disease, to biopsy synovium, and to release periarticular adhesions in three patients with post-traumatic hindfoot pain.[194]

Using 15 cadavers to evaluate subtalar joint arthroscopy portals, Frey and colleagues suggested that the technique may be useful for evaluation of subtalar joint instability and sinus tarsi syndrome.[79] A subsequent report, again led by Frey,[78a] addressed specifically subtalar arthroscopy for patients with sinus tarsi syndrome. Each of 14 patients was noted at the time of arthroscopy to a have a more specific diagnosis, including interosseous ligament rupture, arthrofibrosis, and osteoarthrosis, in 10, 2, and 2 cases, respectively.

A diagnostic approach to chronic sinus tarsi pain includes routine and stress radiographs to rule out ankle and subtalar instability, as well as MRI to rule out contiguous arthrosis and ganglion formation. Local injection of anesthetic and corticosteroid is most important for diagnosis and initial empirical treatment. Ankle bracing and foot and ankle rehabilitation are used as adjunctive treatments. Occasionally, sinus tarsi exploration and débridement are performed.

Author's Preferred Method of Treatment

I treat low-grade subtalar sprains with a semirigid pneumatic orthosis, weight-bearing to tolerance, and early rehabilitation of the foot. Most of these injuries are associated with a lateral ankle sprain, and treatment is dictated by the ankle injury. High-grade injuries, as suggested by a clinical history of severe deformity or swelling, examination consistent with gross subtalar instability, or MRI demonstrating ligamentous disruption, are placed in non–weight-bearing short leg casts for 2 to 3 weeks. This is followed by application of a removable cast boot for an additional 3 weeks of weight-bearing to tolerance. A comprehensive rehabilitation program is used, with an emphasis placed on reducing swelling and improving range of motion, strength, and proprioception.

Return to Play Criteria

Recovery follows a logical sequence of events. Once the initial pain and swelling subside, coordination and strengthening activities are emphasized. Gradually, the patient is able to return to walking, running, and cutting programs. A semirigid pneumatic brace (see Fig. 30E1–12) or taping accelerates the schedule. Patients are returned to sport once they have mastered sport-specific drills.

Subtalar Dislocation

Subtalar joint dislocation varies from isolated subtalar and talonavicular dislocation to dislocation associated with talar, calcaneal, or navicular fractures. The injury is unusual during athletic participation; it most commonly is associated with high-energy mechanisms.

Grantham reported five case of medial subtalar dislocation, all with an inversion mechanism of injury.[90] Four of these patients sustained the injury while playing basketball. Dendrinos and coworkers reported a single case of subtalar dislocation without fracture in a professional basketball player.[60] DeLee and Curtis identified 17 subtalar dislocations in a 7-year period.[59] The direction of the dislocation was anterior, lateral, and medial, for one, four, and twelve patients, respectively. Four of the medial dislocations were associated with an inversion mechanism of injury; each patient attained full subtalar range of motion and was asymptomatic at the last follow-up. Avascular necrosis did not occur.

Christiensen and associates noted arthrosis in each of 17 patients with a fracture dislocation of the subtalar joint and 6 of 13 patients with isolated dislocation of the subtalar joint.[44]

Relevant Anatomy

A review of hindfoot bony and ligamentous anatomy is presented in the preceding section (see "Subtalar Sprain"). The subtalar joint is stable in an everted position. This suggests that lateral dislocations are more likely to be associated with higher degrees of trauma, fractures, and less favorable outcomes.[44, 107, 137]

Clinical Evaluation

History. Patients with subtalar joint dislocation present with a history of acute and severe pain associated with obvious hindfoot deformity.

Physical Examination. After trauma protocols are followed, the extremity is carefully examined. Open injuries are documented, along with the neurologic and vascular status of the extremity.

Imaging

Radiographs. Routine radiographs of the foot and ankle in orthogonal views confirm the preliminary diagnosis. Repeat radiographs with anteroposterior, oblique, Brodén,[29] and lateral projections, as well as CT, are required before definitive and complete diagnosis is determined.

Therapeutic Options

Subtalar dislocation without fracture is treated expediently with closed reduction. Reduction is required for decompression of neurovascular structures and should not be delayed without appropriate reason. General anesthesia is probably more predictable and is less likely to produce associated injury to the foot. The knee is flexed in an effort to relax the gastrocnemius muscle.[137] Longitudinal traction is applied through the foot.

As has been noted earlier, repeat and complete radiographs and CT imaging are required for verification of subtalar joint reduction and assessment of associated fractures. After reduction of isolated subtalar joint dislocations is performed, immobilization for 3 to 8 weeks is indicated. DeLee and Curtis suggest 3 weeks of immobilization, immediate toe range of motion, and early subtalar range of motion.[59]

Dendrinos and colleagues reported a single case of subtalar dislocation without fracture in a professional basketball player.[60] The patient was treated with closed reduction. After 5 years of continued professional play, the same foot suffered an almost identical subtalar dislocation. The recurrence was attributed to coincidence.

Recurrent dislocation did not occur in any of the 17 subtalar dislocations in the series of DeLee and Curtis.[59]

Rehabilitation

A comprehensive foot and ankle rehabilitation program (as described earlier in the subtalar sprain section) is essential for maximum recovery of hindfoot function. Continued subtalar support is provided by a semirigid pneumatic orthosis.

Author's Preferred Method of Treatment

My experience with subtalar dislocations, both related and unrelated to athletic activity, suggests that the injury be given significant attention at the outset. Historical information to determine the mechanism of injury is paramount. Trauma protocols are followed as indicated. After radiographic documentation is obtained, a closed reduction is performed with the patient under conscious sedation or general anesthesia. The stability of the reduction is ideally simultaneously determined. Immobilization and complete radiographic studies, including CT imaging, are obtained after reduction. The length of immobilization is determined by postreduction stability. A non–weight-bearing cast is used for 3 weeks. This is followed by application of a removable cast boot for an additional 3 to 6 weeks of weight-bearing to tolerance and initial rehabilitation. Emphasis is placed on reducing swelling and improving range of motion, strength, and proprioception.

Return to Play Criteria

After completing short-term rehabilitation, the athlete is gradually returned to progressive activity. An ankle brace is used to provide additional support and biofeedback. Return to play is allowed only after local tenderness and swelling have resolved.

Bifurcate Sprain

Broström noted clinical evidence of bifurcate ligament injury in 18.6% of patients with acute ankle sprains and 3.7% of patients with confirmed lateral ankle ligament ruptures.[32] Backmann and Johnson considered bifurcate ligament rupture to be a common injury.[9] Søndergaard reported a 24% incidence of bifurcate and/or talonavicular sprain among patients presenting with an acute ankle/foot inversion sprain.[241] An additional 9% of patients were noted to have a combination of bifurcate /talonavicular ligament and lateral talocrural ligament injuries.

Relevant Anatomy

The bifurcate ligament is a short, stout ligament that originates from the anterior process of the calcaneus, divides into two arms, and inserts onto the navicular and cuboid[148] (see Figs. 30E1–1; Fig. 30E1–47). The origin is contiguous with the superior aspect of the calcaneal facet of the calcaneocuboid joint. The origin of the ligament is routinely visualized during the lateral approach to the sinus tarsi for triple arthrodesis. The ligament is distal and anterior to the inferior tip of the fibula, and superior and proximal to the base of the fifth metatarsal. The mechanism of injury is inversion, adduction, and forced plantar flexion of the foot.

Clinical Evaluation

As has been stated previously, I consider sprains from the simplistic perspective of graded ligament injury, as suggested by the American Medical Association[202] and by O'Donoghue.[189] Acute injuries are graded based on stretch (grade I), partial tear (grade II), or complete rupture (grade III) of the bifurcate ligament. Additional information with regard to associated ligamentous injuries, especially at the lateral ankle, is noted.

History. A bifurcate ligament sprain or an anterior process of the calcaneus avulsion fracture must be considered when one is presented with a suspected ankle sprain. The plantar flexion inversion mechanism associated with injury to the ATFL is the same mechanism as that responsible for the bifurcate ligament sprain. The patient often recalls a "pop" or "snap" followed by swelling and ecchymosis. The patient's ability to continue play after the acute injury is variable.

Physical Examination. Physical examination confirms diffuse lateral hindfoot and midfoot swelling with associated ecchymosis. Tenderness tends to localize to the course of the bifurcate ligament, an area that is distinct from the course of the ATFL. The ankle and midfoot remain stable. Pain is easily reproduced with forced inversion of the plantar flexed foot. Broström noted that the differentiation between lateral ankle ligament injury and bifurcate ligament injury was best achieved by eliciting indirect tenderness.[32] He suggested manipulation of the heel to produce lateral ankle pain and stabilization of the heel with simultaneous forced forefoot motion to produce bifurcate pain.

Imaging
Radiographs. Routine radiographs, including anteroposterior, lateral, and oblique views of the foot and ankle, are obtained. A pure bifurcate ligament sprain is not associated with bony injury; however, an avulsion fracture of the anterior process of the calcaneus is confirmed with the lateral radiograph (Fig. 30E1–48). The size of the fragment may vary from a fine calcified body to a significant portion of the anterior process and the contiguous calcaneocuboid facet.

Computed Tomography. Computed tomography is the preferred method for assessing avulsion fractures, but it is not particularly useful for evaluating an isolated bifurcate ligament sprain.

Magnetic Resonance Imaging. Isolated bifurcate ligament injury is not routinely imaged by MRI. A sprain is confirmed by edema within or adjacent to the ligament, as well as by increased marrow signal at the anterior process of the calcaneus.

Therapeutic Options

Acute bifurcate sprains are treated with the RICE (*R*est, *I*ce, *C*ompression, *E*levation) method followed by gentle range of motion and protected weight-bearing. The hindfoot is supported by the use of a variety of methods, including a splint, a removable walking cast, a functional ankle brace, and various taping methods.

Chronic bifurcate sprains are treated with a range of motion program and reduced activity levels. Intralesional and intra-articular (calcaneocuboid) steroids are placed, under fluoroscopic guidance, with the patient either in the sports medicine practitioner's office or in a radiology suite.

Operative treatment is rare for bifurcate ligament injuries. Large, displaced, intra-articular anterior process fractures are treated with open reduction internal fixation (ORIF) through a sinus tarsi approach. The extensor digitorum brevis muscle is elevated and the fragment reduced. Fixation is most easily accomplished with a small staple; alternatively, a percutaneous cannulated screw may be used. For symptomatic nonunions, the same approach is used, with the addition of local bone graft. Unfortunately, most bony nonunions are not amenable to ORIF owing to their small size. Excision is a reasonable option, but it does not yield the immediate relief that both patient and surgeon expect. Therefore, excision of a symptomatic nonunion is considered only after 6 to 12 months of aggressive rehabilitation.

Rehabilitation

Emphasis throughout the protocol is placed on rehabilitation of the foot and ankle and on subtalar flexibility,

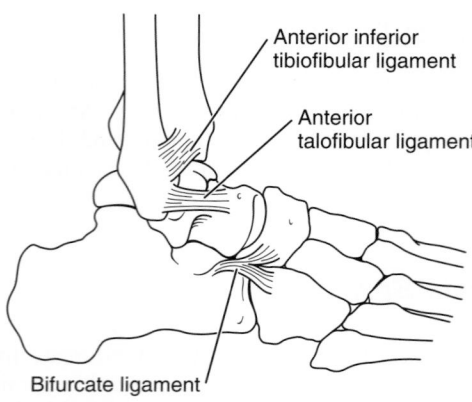

Anterior inferior tibiofibular ligament

Anterior talofibular ligament

Bifurcate ligament

Figure 30E1–47. Schematic drawing demonstrating the bifurcate ligament.

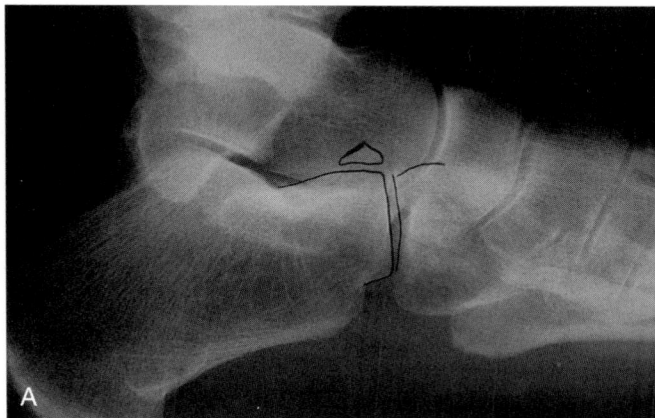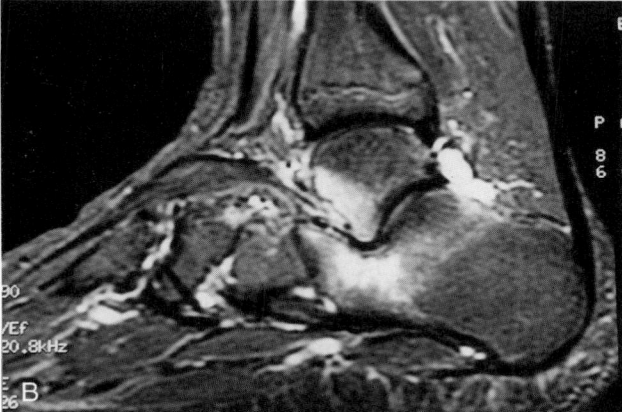

Figure 30E1–48. *A,* Avulsion fracture of the anterior process of the calcaneus. The triangular fragment is either intra-articular or extra-articular and varies in size. *B,* Magnetic resonance image demonstrating increased signal, with the bifurcate ligament consistent with sprain.

motor function, and coordination.[78] The foot is supported by a functional ankle brace or various taping methods. An elastic sock is available for additional mobilization of edema (see Fig. 30E1–22).

Acute Phase. The athlete's pain and inflammation are addressed with rest, cold therapy, and whirlpool. A trial of electrical stimulation may be considered for nonbony injuries.

Foot and ankle passive and active range of motion are re-established. Isometrics may be initiated as pain allows.

Subacute Phase. Once the acute pain subsides, flexibility is addressed in all planes. An inclined board is a useful adjunct to gastrocsoleus and Achilles stretching (see Fig. 30E1–23). Strengthening is initiated with towel scrunches (see Fig. 30E1–24), toe pick-up activities, manual resistive inversion and eversion, elastic bands (see Fig. 30E1–25), seated toe and ankle dorsiflexion with progression to standing, and seated supination-pronation with progression to standing.

Closed chain activities are gradually introduced (see Fig. 30E1–26), including one-leg balance, sports-specific activities on a trampoline, and the use of the BAPS.

Aerobic fitness is maintained with cross-training activities such as water running (see Fig. 30E1–27) and cycling.

Heat therapy, such as the application of warm packs, is a useful modality before the therapy session. It reduces pain and spasms and thus facilitates increased range of motion. Cold therapy, compression, and elevation are used after each therapy session to reduce inflammation.

Return to Sport Phase. During this critical phase, walking and running activities are allowed to progress within the limits of a pain-free schedule. Once running activity is mastered, a monitored, progressively difficult plyometric and cutting program is introduced. Schedules are carefully controlled to avoid re-injury.

Søndergaard and coworkers reviewed the results of treatment for 162 midtarsal sprains (bifurcate ligament and/or talonavicular ligament) and 161 talocrural sprains and concluded that the two injuries produce similar outcomes.[241] Both groups returned to pre-injury athletic activity at an average of 21 days.

Author's Preferred Method of Treatment

I treat bifurcate ligament sprains with a semirigid pneumatic orthosis, weight-bearing to tolerance, and early rehabilitation of the foot. Occasionally, I place a less athletic patient in a short leg walking cast in an effort to improve pain control and allow increased levels of independent activity.

Injuries associated with small anterior process fractures are treated as severe sprains. Delayed union or nonunion is unlikely and is even less likely to remain symptomatic. Large, intra-articular fractures are treated with a short leg cast and weight-bearing to tolerance. Displaced fractures are treated with ORIF.

Chronic pain related to nonunion or malunion is conservatively treated for a minimum of 6 to 12 months. In my experience, delayed excision is less effective than repair of nonunion with internal fixation.

Return to Play Criteria

Recovery follows a logical sequence of events. Once the initial pain and swelling subside, coordination and strengthening activities are emphasized. Gradually, the patient is able to return to walking, running, and cutting programs. A protective brace or taping accelerates the schedule. Patients are returned to sport once they master sport-specific drills.

Lisfranc Sprain

Injury to the Lisfranc joint complex is commonly associated with severe high-energy trauma. The poor outcome among these patients is well known by orthopaedic surgeons.

Lisfranc injury does occur during athletic activity. Curtis and associates described 19 such injuries associated with athletic activity.[56] The most common activity was basketball, followed by running. Meyer noted 24 midfoot sprains among university football players between 1987 and

1991.[174] The incidence was calculated at 4% of football players per year. Shapiro and colleagues identified nine injuries to the Lisfranc ligament associated with collegiate gymnastics (four), collegiate football (three), collegiate pole vault (one), and recreational tennis (one).[228]

Relevant Anatomy

The midfoot is a stable configuration of five bones (navicular, cuboid, medial cuneiform, middle cuneiform, and lateral cuneiform) joined together in a complex system of multifaceted, relatively immobile joints (Fig. 30E1–49). The articulation between the midfoot and the metatarsals is known as the Lisfranc joint (the tarsometatarsal joint or the metatarsal cuneiform joint). The second metatarsal cuneiform joint is significant in that it is the most stable of the entire complex. Two factors contributing to the second metatarsal cuneiform joint stability include a recessed bony configuration (keystone) and a strong plantar ligament connecting the base of the second metatarsal to the medial cuneiform.

A significant amount of force is required to produce fracture-dislocation. The mechanism of injury is either direct crushing or indirect loading of the fixed forefoot.[1] Wiley reviewed 20 cases of Lisfranc injury and identified direct and indirect mechanisms of injury.[272] The indirect mechanisms of injury were acute abduction of the forefoot (most common) and forced plantar flexion of the forefoot.

Forced dorsiflexion of the forefoot may occur as the result of landing from a jump, continued forward motion on a planted forefoot, a fall from a height, or a brake pedal injury. Curtis and coworkers described the mechanism of injury to include plantar flexion and rotation with or without abduction of the forefoot.[56] Meyer and associates determined a mechanism of injury from 16 football players with midfoot sprains.[174] Eight players reported an indirect twisting mechanism; six players reported contact to the heel of a plantar flexed forefoot; two players reported a crush injury to the dorsum of the foot. Shapiro and colleagues identified a consistent mechanism in nine athletes who sustained a Lisfranc injury.[228] Each athlete placed full weight onto the first ray with the foot in an externally rotated and pronated position.

The resulting injury includes tearing of relatively weak dorsal capsular structure, tearing of the strong plantar ligament between the medial cuneiform and the base of the second metatarsal, and to a varying degree, fracture of chondral and bony structures on both sides of the joint. Subsequent to the displacement that occurs at the time of injury, the joint complex either returns to a nondisplaced state or remains displaced owing to the interposition of the capsule and osteochondral fragments.

Clinical Evaluation

I consider sprains from the simplistic perspective of graded ligament injury, as suggested by the American Medical Association[202] and by O'Donoghue.[189] Acute injuries are graded based on stretch (grade I), partial tear (grade II), or complete rupture (grade III) of the Lisfranc capsule and supporting ligaments, including the Lisfranc ligament.

Stable injuries, including grade I and II sprains, are not associated with displacement or deformity. Unstable injuries, grade III sprains, vary between nondisplaced injuries and frank fracture-dislocations.

History. Typically, the athlete is able to recall a specific mechanism of injury. The injury is associated with a "pop" or "snap" followed by pain, swelling, and ecchymosis localized to the midfoot. The ability to continue play after the acute injury is variable for mild injury. Weight-bearing is very painful and unlikely after a severe injury. Occasionally, the patient describes sensing the midfoot collapse.

Physical Examination. Physical examination confirms diffuse midfoot swelling with associated ecchymosis. Sensory and vascular examination with particular attention to the deep peroneal nerve and the dorsalis pedis artery is documented.

Tenderness tends to localize to the course of the Lisfranc joint. Meyer and coworkers correlated prolonged recovery with medial and global midfoot tenderness, as opposed to injuries with lateral tenderness.[174] The remainder of the forefoot and hindfoot must also be carefully palpated.

Stability is tested in the midsagittal plane (dorsiflexion/plantar flexion) by securing the midfoot with one hand and grasping the individual metatarsal head with the other hand. A dorsiflexion force is applied; when compared with the opposite midfoot, pain and increased mobility are abnormal findings. Frontal plane stability is demonstrated by applying an adduction or abduction force across the Lisfranc joint. Myerson described a passive pronation-abduction test to evaluate the stability of the joint complex[141, 181, 182] (Fig. 30E1–50).

Imaging

Radiographs. The bilateral standing anteroposterior radiograph provides critical information used to help classify the injury. A diastasis between the bases of the first and second metatarsals suggests an unstable injury. A small fragment of bone representing an avulsion fracture of the Lisfranc ligament is often present (Fig. 30E1–51).

Faciszewski and associates reviewed 15 cases of subtle injury of the Lisfranc joint and determined that flattening of the longitudinal arch correlated with a poor outcome,

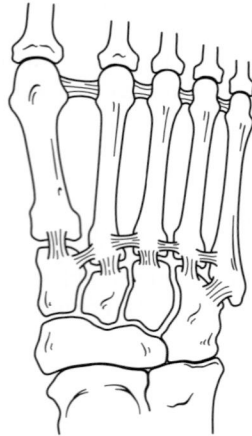

Figure 30E1–49. The Lisfranc articulation with its ligamentous attachments. Note the recessed second tarsometatarsal joint and the Lisfranc ligament in place of the first-second intermetatarsal ligament.

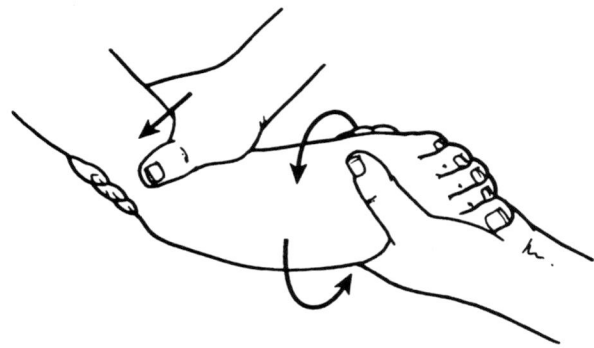

Figure 30E1–50. Frontal plane stability at the Lisfranc joint is demonstrated by application of a passive pronation-abduction. (From Komenda GA, Meyerson MS, Biddinger KR: Results of arthrodesis of the tarsometatarsal joints after traumatic injury. J Bone Joint Surg Am 78:1668, 1996.)

whereas persistent diastasis up to 5 mm did not correlate with a poor outcome.[74]. The authors also studied 20 normal volunteers. With the use of the standing lateral radiograph, the distance between the plantar aspect of the medial cuneiform was related to the plantar aspect of the fifth metatarsal base. In all cases, the medial cuneiform was higher than the fifth metatarsal base; furthermore, the difference between right and left feet averaged 1.5 mm.

Stress Radiographs. Goossens and De Stoop suggested stress films in cases with prominent clinical signs and normal radiographs.[88] The procedure is performed with the patient under general anesthesia with either an eversion and pronation or inversion and supination applied to the forefoot.

Computed Tomography. Further imaging with CT allows for a more detailed analysis. Alignment, displacement, and subtle osseous injury are best evaluated with fine-cut CT imaging (see Fig. 30E1–51B).

Magnetic Resonance Imaging. MRI is occasionally used to identify the hemorrhage and edema associated with acute ligamentous injury or to differentiate complete and partial tears.[198]

Therapeutic Options

All acute injuries are treated with the RICE (*R*est, *I*ce, *C*ompression, *E*levation) method, as described earlier. Patients are placed at non–weight-bearing status until definitive diagnosis is established and the initial pain and swelling remit. Subsequent treatment is predicated on the stability of the Lisfranc complex.

Grade I and Grade II Lisfranc Sprains. Upon verification of stability by clinical and radiographic examination, weight-bearing to tolerance is encouraged and a rehabilitation program instituted. Treatment is symptomatic, with an

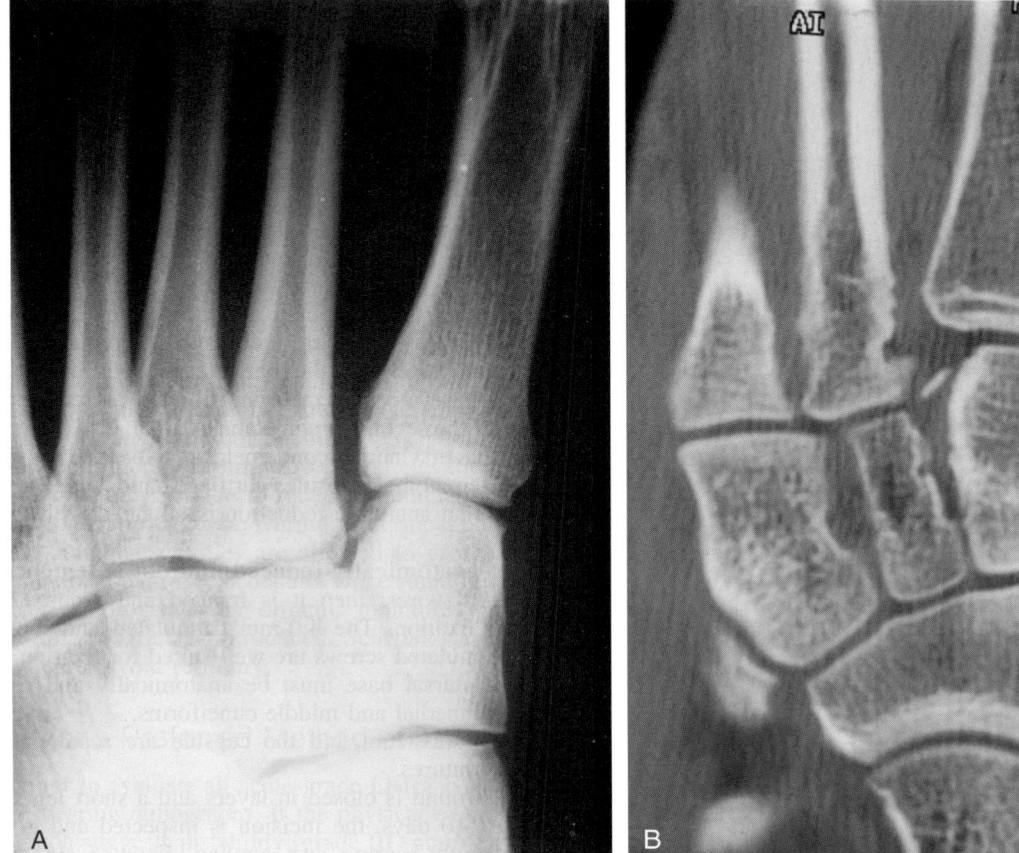
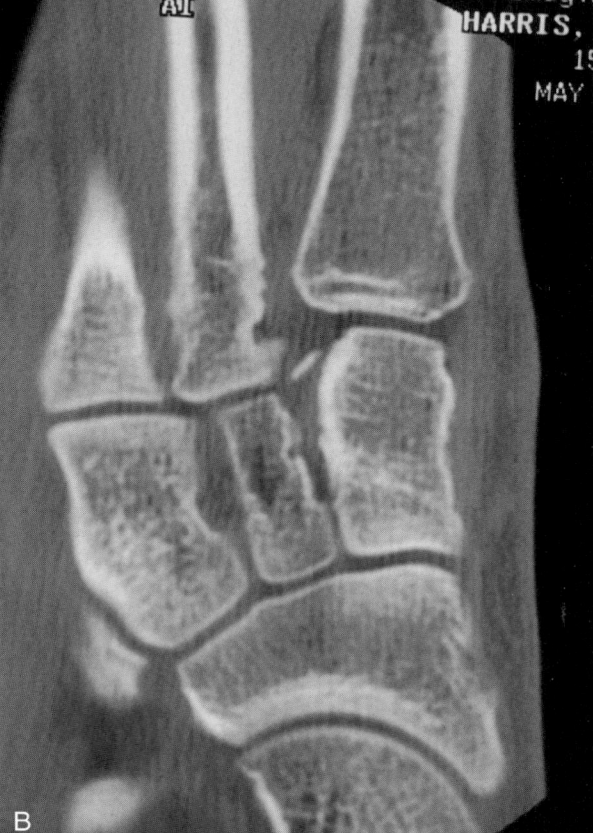

Figure 30E1–51. A diastasis and occasionally a bone fragment between the first and second metatarsal bases suggest injury to the Lisfranc joint. *A,* Lisfranc injury as seen on routine standing radiograph. *B,* Lisfranc injury as seen on computed tomography.

tous structures of the ankle with a modified Watson-Jones procedure. Foot Ankle Int 7:362–368, 1987.

12. Bassett F, Speer K: Longitudinal rupture of the peroneal tendon. Am J Sports Med 21:354–357, 1993.

13. Bassett FH, Gates HS, Billys JB, et al: Talar impingement by the anteroinferior tibiofibular ligament. A cause of chronic pain in the ankle after inversion sprain. Foot Ankle Int 72:55–59, 1990.

14. Baumhauer JF, Alosa DM, Renström AFH, et al: A prospective study of ankle injury risk factors. Am J Sports Med 23:564–570, 1995.

15. Beals TC, Manoli A: Late syndesmosis reconstruction: A case report. Foot Ankle Int 19:485–488, 1998.

16. Becker HP, Komischke A, Danz B, et al: Stress diagnostics of the sprained ankle: Evaluation of the anterior drawer test with and without anesthesia. Foot Ankle Int 14:459–464, 1993.

17. Berg EE: The symptomatic os subfibulare: Avulsion fracture of the fibula with recurrent instability of the ankle. J Bone Joint Surg Am 73:1251–1254, 1991.

18. Bergfeld JA, Cox JS, Drez D, et al: Symposium: Management of acute ankle sprains. Contemp Orthop 13:83–116, 1986.

19. Berridge FR, Bonnin JG: The radiographic examination of the ankle joint including arthrography. Surg Gynecol Obstet 79:383–389, 1944.

20. Björkenheim JM, Sandelin J, Santavirta S: Evans' procedure in the treatment of chronic instability of the ankle. Injury 19:70–72, 1988.

21. Black H: Roentgenographic considerations. Am J Sports Med 5:238–240, 1977.

22. Black H, Brand RL, Eichelberger M: An improved technique for the evaluation of ligamentous injury in severe ankle sprains. Am J Sports Med 6:276–282, 1978.

23. Bonnin JG: Radiologic diagnosis of recent lesions of the lateral ligament of the ankle. J Bone Joint Surg Br 31:478, 1949.

24. Bonnin JG: Injuries to the ligaments of the ankle. J Bone Joint Surg Br 47:609–611, 1965.

25. Boytim MJ, Fischer DA, Neumann L: Syndesmotic ankle sprains. Am J Sports Med 19:294–298, 1991.

26. Brand RL, Black HM, Cox JS: The natural history of inadequately treated ankle sprain. Am J Sports Med 5:248–249, 1977.

27. Brand RL, Collins MDF, Templeton T: Surgical repair of ruptured lateral ankle ligaments. Am J Sports Med 9:40–44, 1981.

28. Brantigan JW, Pedegana LR, Lippert FG: Instability of the subtalar joint. Diagnosis by stress tomography in three cases. J Bone Joint Surg Am 59:321–324, 1977.

29. Brodén G: Roentgen examination of the subtaloid joint in fractures of the calcaneus. Acta Radiol 31:85–91, 1949.

30. Brodsky J, Krause J: Peroneus brevis tendon tears: Pathophysiology, surgical reconstruction, and clinical results. Foot Ankle Int 19:271–279, 1998.

31. Broström L: Sprained ankles. I. Anatomic lesions in recent sprains. Acta Chir Scand 128:483–495, 1964.

32. Broström L: Sprained ankles: III. Clinical observations in recent ligament ruptures. Acta Chir Scand 130:560–569, 1965.

33. Broström L: Sprained ankles. V. Treatment and prognosis in recent ligament ruptures. Acta Chir Scand 132:537–550, 1966.

34. Broström L: Sprained ankles: VI. Surgical treatment of "chronic" ligament ruptures. Acta Chir Scand 132:551–565, 1966.

35. Broström L, Liljedahl SO, Lindvall N: Sprained ankles: II. Arthrographic diagnosis of recent ligament ruptures. Acta Chir Scand 129:485–499, 1965.

36. Brown JE: The sinus tarsi syndrome. Clin Orthop 18:231–233, 1960.

37. Brunet JA, Wiley JJ: The late results of tarsometatarsal joint injuries. J Bone Joint Surg Br 69:337–440, 1987.

38. Brunner R, Gaechter A: Repair of the fibular ligaments: Comparison of reconstructive techniques using plantaris and peroneal tendons. Foot Ankle Int 11:359–367, 1991.

39. Bulucu C, Thomas KA, Halvorson TL, et al: Biomechanical evaluation of the anterior drawer test: The contribution of the lateral ankle ligaments. Foot Ankle Int 11:389–393, 1991.

40. Cass JR, Settles H: Ankle instability: In vitro kinematics in response to axial load. Foot Ankle Int 15:134–140, 1994.

41. Cass JR, Morrey BF, Chao EYS: Three-dimensional kinematics of ankle instability following serial sectioning of lateral collateral ligaments. Foot Ankle Int 5:142–149, 1984.

42. Cass JR, Morrey BF, Katoh Y, et al: Ankle instability: Comparison of primary repair and delayed reconstruction after long-term follow-up study. Foot Ankle Int 5:142–149, 1984.

43. Chrisman OD, Snook GA: Reconstruction of lateral ligament tears of the ankle. An experimental study and clinical evaluation of seven patients treated by a new modification of the Elmslie procedure. J Bone Joint Surg Am 51:904–912, 1969.

44. Christiensen SB, Lorentzen JE, Krogsøe O, et al: Subtalar dislocations. Acta Orthop Scand 48:707–711, 1977.

45. Clanton TO: Instability of the subtalar joint. Orthop Clin North Am 20:583–592, 1989.

46. Clarke R, Hellon R, Lind A: Vascular reactions of the human forearm to cold. Clin Sci 17:165–179, 1958.

47. Clayton ML, Trott AW, Ulin R: Recurrent subluxations of the ankle. With special reference to peroneal nerve block as a diagnostic aid. J Bone Joint Surg Am 33:502–504, 1951.

48. Close JR: Some applications of the functional anatomy of the ankle joint. J Bone Joint Surg Am 38:761–781, 1956.

49. Close JR, Inman VT, Poor PM, et al: The function of the subtalar joint. Clin Orthop 50:159–179, 1967.

50. Coltart WD: Sprained ankle. BMJ ii:957–961, 1951.

51. Colville MR, Grondel J: Anatomic reconstruction of the lateral ankle ligaments using a split peroneus brevis tendon graft. Am J Sports Med 23:210–213, 1995.

52. Colville MR, Marder RA, Zarins B: Reconstruction of the lateral ankle ligaments. A biochemical analysis. Am J Sports Med 20:594–600, 1992.

53. Colville MR, Marder RA, Boyle JJ, et al: Strain measurement in lateral ankle ligaments. Am J Sports Med 18:196–200, 1990.

54. Cox JS: Surgical treatment of ankle sprains. Am J Sports Med 5:250–251, 1977.

55. Cox JS, Hewes TF: "Normal" talar tilt angle. Clin Orthop 140:37–41, 1979.

56. Curtis MJ, Myerson M, Szura B: Tarsometatarsal joint injuries in the athlete. Am J Sports Med 21:497–502, 1993.

57. Daseler EH, Anson BJ: The plantaris muscle. An anatomic study of 750 specimens. J Bone Joint Surg 25:822–827, 1943.

58. Davis W, Sobel M, Deland J, et al: The superior peroneal retinaculum: An anatomical study. Foot Ankle 15:271–275, 1994.

59. DeLee JC, Curtis R: Subtalar dislocation of the foot. J Bone Joint Surg Am 64:433, 1982.

60. Dendrinos G, Zisi G, Haralambos T: Recurrence of subtalar dislocation in a basketball player. Am J Sports Med 22:143–145, 1994.

61. Dias LS: The lateral ankle sprain: An experimental study. J Trauma 19:266–269, 1979.

62. Drez D, Yound JC, Waldman D, et al: Nonoperative treatment of double lateral ligament tears of the ankle. Am J Sports Med 10:197–200, 1982.

63. Earll M, Wayne J, Brodrick C, et al: Contribution of the deltoid ligament to ankle joint contact characteristics: A cadaver study. Foot Ankle Int 17:317–324, 1996.

64. Ebraheim NA, Lu J, Yang H, et al: Radiographic and CT evaluation of tibiofibular syndesmotic diastasis: A cadaver study. Foot Ankle Int 18:693–698, 1997.

65. Eckert W, Davis EJ: Acute rupture of the peroneal retinaculum. J Bone Joint Surg Am 58:670–673, 1976.

66. Edwards GS, DeLee JC: Ankle diastasis without fracture. Foot Ankle Int 4:305–312, 1984.

67. Edwards M: The relationship of the peroneal tendons to the fibula, calcaneus, and cuboideum. Am J Anat 42:213–253, 1928.

68. Eiff MP, Smith AT, Smith GE: Early mobilization versus immobilization in the treatment of lateral ankle sprains. Am J Sports Med 22:83–88, 1994.

69. Ekstrand J, Tropp H: The incidence of ankle sprains in soccer. Foot Ankle Int 11:41–44, 1990.

70. Elmslie RC: Recurrent subluxation of the ankle joint. Ann Surg 100:364–367, 1934.

71. Escalas F, Figueras J, Merino J: Dislocation of the peroneal tendons. Long-term results of surgical treatment. J Bone Joint Surg Am 62:451–453, 1980.

72. Evans DL: Recurrent instability of the ankle—a method of surgical treatment. Proc Roy Soc Med 46:343–344, 1953.

73. Evans GA, Hardcastle P, Frenyo AD: Acute rupture of the lateral ligament of the ankle. To suture or not to suture? J Bone Joint Surg Br 66:209–212, 1984.

74. Faciszewski T, Burks RT, Manaster BJ: Subtle injuries of the Lisfranc joint. J Bone Joint Surg Am 72:1519–1522, 1990.

75. Freeman MAR: Treatment of ruptures of the lateral ligament of the ankle. J Bone Joint Surg Br 47:661–668, 1965.

76. Freeman MAR: Instability of the foot after injuries to the lateral ligament of the ankle. J Bone Joint Surg Br 47:669–677, 1965.

77. Freeman MAR, Wyke BD: The innervation of the cat's knee joint. J Anat 98:299, 1964.

78. Freeman MAR, Dean MRE, Hanham IWF: The etiology and prevention of functional instability of the foot. J Bone Joint Surg Br 47: 678–685, 1965.

78a. Frey C, Feder KS, DiGiovanni C: Arthroscopic evaluation of the subtalar joint: Does sinus tarsi syndrome exist? Foot Ankle Int 20: 185–191, 1999.

79. Frey C, Gasser S, Feder K: Arthroscopy of the subtalar joint. Foot Ankle Int 15:424–428, 1994.

80. Fritschy D: An unusual ankle injury in top skiers. Am J Sports Med 17:282–286, 1989.

81. Fritschy D, Junet C, Bonivin JC: Functional treatment of severe ankle sprain. J Traumatol Sport 4:131–136, 1987.

82. Garrick JM: The frequency of injury, mechanism of injury, and epidemiology of ankle sprains. Am J Sports Med 5:241–242, 1977.

83. Geppert M, Sobel M, Bohne W: Lateral ankle instability as a cause of superior peroneal retinacular laxity: An anatomic and biomechanical study of cadaveric feet. Foot Ankle Int 14:330–334, 1993.

84. Gerber JP, Williams GN, Scoville CR, et al: Persistent disability associated with ankle sprains: A prospective examination of an athletic population. Foot Ankle Int 19:653–660, 1998.

85. Gillespie HS, Boucher P: Watson-Jones repair of lateral instability of the ankle. J Bone Joint Surg Am 53:920–924, 1971.

86. Glasgow M, Jackson A, Jamieson AM: Instability of the ankle after injury to the lateral ligament. J Bone Joint Surg Br 62:196–200, 1980.

87. Glick JM, Gordon RB, Nashimoto D: The prevention and treatment of ankle injuries. Am J Sports Med 4:136–141, 1976.

88. Goossens M, De Stoop N: Lisfranc's fracture-dislocation: Etiology, radiology, and results of treatment. Clin Orthop 176:154–162, 1983.

89. Gould N, Seligson D, Gassman J: Early and late repair of lateral ligament of the ankle. Foot Ankle Int 1:84–89, 1980.

90. Grantham SA: Medial subtalar dislocation: Five cases with a common etiology. J Trauma 4:845–849, 1964.

91. Grath GB: Widening of the ankle mortise. Acta Chir Scand 263: 72–77, 1960.

92. Greene TA, Hillman SK: Comparison of support provided by a semirigid orthosis and adhesive ankle taping before, during, and after exercise. Am J Sports Med 18:498–506, 1990.

93. Grønmark T, Johnsen O, Kogstad O: Rupture of the lateral ligaments of the ankle: A controlled clinical trial. Injury 11:215–218, 1980.

94. Gross MEA: Comparison of support by ankle taping and semirigid orthosis. J Orthop Sports Phys Ther 9:33–39, 1987.

95. Hamill J, Morin G, Clarkson P, et al: Exercise moderation of foot function during walking with a reusable semi-rigid ankle orthosis. Clin Biomech 3:153–158, 1988.

96. Hamilton WG: Sprained ankles in ballet dancers. Foot Ankle Int 3: 99–102, 1982.

97. Hamilton WG, Thompson FM, Snow SW: The modified Brostrom procedure for lateral ankle instability. Foot Ankle Int 14:1–7, 1993.

98. Hansen H, Damholt V, Termansen NB: Clinical and social status following injury to the lateral ligaments of the ankle. Acta Orthop Scand 50:699–704, 1979.

99. Hardcastle PH, Reschauer R, Kutsch-Lissberg E, et al: Injuries to the tarsometatarsal joint. Incidence, classification, treatment. J Bone Joint Surg Br 64:349–356, 1982.

100. Harper MC: The deltoid ligament. An evaluation of need for surgical repair. Clin Orthop 226:156–168, 1988.

101. Harper MC: The lateral ligamentous support of the subtalar joint. Foot Ankle Int 11:354–358, 1991.

102. Harper MC: Stress radiographs in the diagnosis of lateral instability of the ankle and hindfoot. Foot Ankle Int 13:435–438, 1992.

103. Harper MC: Modification of the Gould modification of the Brostrom ankle repair. Foot Ankle Int 19:788, 1998.

104. Harper MC, Keller TS: A radiographic evaluation of the tibiofibular syndesmosis. Foot Ankle Int 10:156–160, 1989.

105. Harrington KD: Degenerative arthritis of the ankle secondary to long-standing lateral ligament instability. J Bone Joint Surg Am 61: 354–361, 1979.

106. Heilman AE, Braly WG, Bishop JO, et al: An anatomic study of subtalar instability. Foot Ankle Int 10:224–228, 1990.

107. Heppenstall RB, Farahvar H, Balderston R, et al: Evaluation and management of subtalar dislocations. J Trauma 20:494–497, 1980.

108. Hocutt J, Jaffe R, Rylander C, et al: Cryotherapy in ankle sprains. Am J Sports Med 10:316–319, 1982.

109. Hollis JM, Blasier RD, Flahiff CM: Simulated lateral ankle ligamentous injury. Change in ankle stability. Am J Sports Med 23:672–677, 1995.

110. Hopkinson WJ, St. Pierre P, Ryan JB, et al: Syndesmosis sprains of the ankle. Foot Ankle Int 10:325–330, 1990.

111. Hortsman JK, Kantor GS, Samuelson KM: Investigation of lateral ankle ligament reconstruction. Foot Ankle Int 1:338–342, 1981.

112. Hughes JR: Radiologic diagnosis of recent lesions of the lateral ligament of the ankle. J Bone Joint Surg Br 31:478, 1949.

113. Inman VT: The Joints of the Ankle. Baltimore, Williams and Wilkins, 1976, pp 2, 37, 62–66, 74, 108.

114. Ishii T, Miyagawa S, Fukubayashi T, et al: Subtalar stress radiography using forced dorsiflexion and supination. J Bone Joint Surg Br 78:56–60, 1996.

115. Jackson DW, Ashley RD, Powell JW: Ankle sprains in young athletes: Relation of severity and disability. Clin Orthop 101:201–215, 1974.

116. Jackson R, Wills RE, Jackson R: Rupture of deltoid ligament without involvement of the lateral ligament. Am J Sports Med 16:541–543, 1988.

117. Javors JR, Violet JT: Correction of chronic lateral ligament instability of the ankle by use of the Brostrom procedure. A report of 15 cases. Clin Orthop 198:201–207, 1985.

118. Johanssen A: Radiological diagnosis of lateral ligament lesion of the ankle. Acta Orthop Scand 49:295–301, 1978.

119. Johnson D, Urban W, Caborn D, et al: Articular cartilage changes seen with magnetic resonance imaging–detected bone bruises associated with acute anterior cruciate ligament rupture. Am J Sports Med 26:409–414, 1998.

120. Johnson EE, Markolf KL: The contribution of the anterior talofibular ligament to ankle laxity. J Bone Joint Surg Am 65:81–88, 1983.

121. Johnston EC, Howell SJ: Tension neuropathy of the superficial peroneal nerve: Associated conditions and results of release. Foot Ankle Int 20:576–582, 1999.

122. Jones E: Operative treatment of chronic dislocations of the peroneal tendons. J Bone Joint Surg 14:574–576, 1932.

123. Kaikkonen A, Hyppanen E, Kannus P, et al: Long-term functional outcome after primary repair of the lateral ligaments of the ankle. Am J Sports Med 25:150–155, 1997.

124. Kannus P, Renström P: Current concepts review. Treatment for acute tears of the lateral ligaments of the ankle: Operation, cast, or early controlled mobilization. J Bone Joint Surg Am 73:305–312, 1991.

125. Karlsson J, Bergsten T, Lasinger O, et al: Reconstruction of the lateral ligaments of the ankle for chronic lateral instability. J Bone Joint Surg Am 70:581–588, 1988.

126. Karlsson J, Bergsten T, Lasinger O, et al: Surgical treatment of chronic lateral instability of the ankle joint. A new procedure. Am J Sports Med 17:268–274, 1989.

127. Kato T: The diagnosis and treatment of instability of the subtalar joint. J Bone Joint Surg Br 77:400–406, 1995.

128. Katznelson A, Lin E, Militiano J: Ruptures of the ligaments about the tibio-fibular syndesmosis. Injury 15:170–172, 1983.

129. Kaye RA: Stabilization of ankle syndesmosis injuries with a syndesmosis screw. Foot Ankle Int 9:290–293, 1989.

130. Kelikian H, Kelikian AS: Disorders of the Ankle. Philadelphia, WB Saunders, 1985, p 437.

131. Kelly JH, Janes JM: The chronic subluxing ankle. Arch Surg 72: 618–621, 1956.

132. Kimura IF, Nawoczenski DA, Epler M, et al: Effect of the air stirrup in controlling ankle inversion stress. J Orthop Sports Phys Ther 9: 190–193, 1987.

133. Kjærsgaard-Andersen P, Wethelund J, Nielsen S: Lateral talocalcaneal instability following section of the calcaneofibular ligament: A kinesiologic study. Foot Ankle Int 7:355–361, 1987.

134. Kjærsgaard-Andersen P, Wethelund JO, Helmig P, et al: Effect of the calcaneofibular ligament on hindfoot rotation in amputation specimens. Acta Orthop Scand 58:135–138, 1987.

135. Kjærsgaard-Andersen P, Wethelund JO, Hlemig P, et al: The stabilizing effect of the ligamentous structures in the sinus and canalis tarsi on movements of the hindfoot. An experimental study. Am J Sports Med 16:512–517, 1988.

136. Kjærsgaard-Andersen P, Wethelund JO, Helmig P, et al: Stabilizing effect of the tibiocalcaneal fascicle of the deltoid ligament on hind-

251. Stover C, Bryan D: Traumatic dislocation of the peroneal tendons. Am J Surg 103:180–186, 1962.

252. Stover CN: Air-stirrup management of ankle injuries in the athlete. Am J Sports Med 8:360–365, 1980.

253. Stover CN: Functional sprain management of the ankle. Ambulatory Care 6:25–28, 1986.

254. Stuart PR, Brumby C, Smith SR: Comparative study of functional bracing and plaster cast treatment of stable lateral malleolar fractures. Injury 20:317–320, 1989.

255. Stuessi E, Tiegermann V, Gerber H, et al: A biomechanical study of the stabilization effect of the Aircast ankle brace. Biomechanics X-A International Series on Biomechanics 6:159–164, 1987.

256. Sugimoto K, Samoto N, Takaoka T, et al: Subtalar arthrography in acute injuries of the calcaneofibular ligament. J Bone Joint Surg Br 80:785–790, 1998.

257. Surve I, Schwellnus MP, Noakes T, et al: A fivefold reduction in the incidence of recurrent ankle sprains in soccer players using the sport-stirrup orthosis. Am J Sports Med 22:601–606, 1994.

258. Taga I, Shino K, Inoue M, et al: Articular cartilage lesions in ankles with lateral ligament injury: An arthroscopic study. Am J Sports Med 21:120–127, 1993.

259. Taillard W, Meyer JM, Garcia J, et al: The sinus tarsi syndrome. Int Orthop 5:117–130, 1981.

260. Taylor DC, Englehardt DL, Bassett FH: Syndesmosis sprains of the ankle. The influence of heterotopic ossification. Am J Sports Med 20:146–150, 1992.

261. Teitz CC, Harrington RM: A biomechanical analysis of the squeeze test for sprains of the syndesmotic ligaments of the ankle. Foot Ankle Int 19:489–492, 1998.

262. Thacker SB, Stroup DF, Branche CM, et al: The prevention of ankle sprains in sports. A systematic review of the literature. Am J Sports Med 27:753–760, 1999.

263. Thordarson DB: Fixation of the ankle syndesmosis with bioabsorbable screws. Technique Orthop 13:187–191, 1998.

264. Thordarson DB, Hedman TP, Gross D, et al: Biomechanical evaluation of polylactide absorbable screws used for syndesmosis injury repair. Foot Ankle Int 18:622–627, 1997.

265. Thorsson O, Lilja B, Ahlgren L, et al: The effect of local cold application on intramuscular blood flow at rest and after running. Med Sci Sports Exerc 17:710–713, 1985.

266. Tochigi Y, Yoshinaga K, Wada Y, et al: Acute inversion injury of the ankle: Magnetic resonance imagining and clinical outcomes. Foot Ankle Int 19:730–734, 1998.

267. Van Hellemondt FJ, Louwerens JW, Sijbrandij ES, van Gils AP: Stress radiography and stress examination of the talocrural and subtalar joint on helical computed tomography. Foot Ankle Int 18:482–488, 1997.

268. Walsh WM, Blackburn T: Prevention of ankle sprains. Am J Sports Med 5:243–245, 1977.

269. Watson-Jones R: Recurrent forward dislocation of the ankle joint. J Bone Joint Surg Br 34:519, 1952.

270. Watson-Jones R: Fractures and Joint Injuries, 4th ed. Edinburgh, Livingstone, 1955, pp 821–823.

271. Whiteside LA, Reynolds FC, Ellsasser JC: Tibiofibular synostosis and recurrent ankle sprains in high performance athletes. Am J Sports Med 6:204–208, 1978.

272. Wiley JJ: The mechanism of tarso-metatarsal joint injuries. J Bone Joint Surg Br 53:474–482, 1971.

273. Wilkerson GB: Comparative biomechanical effects of the standard method of ankle taping and a taping method designed to enhance subtalar stability. Am J Sports Med 19:588–595, 1991.

274. Wilppula E: Tarsometatarsal fracture-dislocation. Acta Orthop Scand 44:335–345, 1973.

275. Wilson DW: Injuries of the tarso-metatarsal joints. Etiology, classification and results of treatment. J Bone Joint Surg Br 54:677–686, 1972.

276. Wilson MJ, Michele AA, Jakobson EW: Ankle dislocation without fracture. J Bone Joint Surg 21:198–204, 1939.

277. Windfeld P: Treatment of undue mobility of the ankle joint following severe sprains of the ankle with avulsion of the anterior and middle bands of the external ligament. Acta Chir Scand 105:299–304, 1953.

278. Wolin I, Glassman F, Sideman S, et al: Internal derangement of the talofibular component of the ankle. Surg Gynecol Obstet 91:193–200, 1950.

279. Wright R, Phaneuf M, Limbird T, et al: Clinical outcome of isolated subcortical trabecular fractures (bone bruise) detected on magnetic resonance imaging in knees. Am J Sports Med 28:663–667, 2000.

280. Xenos JS, Hopkinson WJ, Mulligan ME, et al: The tibiofibular syndesmosis. Evaluation of the ligamentous structures, methods of fixation, and radiographic assessment. J Bone Joint Surg Am 77:847–856, 1995.

281. Zenni EJ, Grefer M, Krieg JK, et al: Lateral ligamentous instability of the ankle: A method of surgical reconstruction by a modified Watson-Jones technique. Am J Sports Med 5:78–83, 1977.

282. Zoellner G, Clancy WJ: Recurrent dislocation of the peroneal tendon. J Bone Joint Surg Am 61:292–294, 1979.

2. LIGAMENT INJURIES OF THE FOOT/ANKLE IN THE PEDIATRIC ATHLETE

J. Andy Sullivan, MD

Most of the injuries that occur in the ankle and foot of the pediatric athlete are not unique to athletic participation but occur normally during childhood. Some, however, occur with greater frequency in the athlete. The conditions covered in this chapter occur in childhood and may present in the athlete, raising the question of whether he or she should be allowed to participate in sports activities.

Variations of Normal Anatomy

Tarsal Coalition

Tarsal coalition is a bony or fibrocartilaginous connection of two or more of the tarsal bones. The cause is unknown, but it has been established that the condition results from failure of differentiation and segmentation of the primitive mesenchyme.[17] The overall incidence is 1% to 3%.[11, 25] The most common coalitions are the calcaneo-navicular and talocalcaneal types. The first is bilateral in about 60% of cases, and the second is bilateral in about 50%.[11, 18, 25] More than one type of coalition can exist in one foot, and coalition may be more common than was previously appreciated, as is discussed later. The exact mode of inheritance is unknown, but it is postulated to be autosomal dominant with variable penetrance.[11]

Most patients seek medical care during early adolescence, at a time when the coalition is ossifying. The pain is vague in nature and insidious in onset. There may be a history of precipitating trauma. Sports participation or running over uneven ground may accentuate the pain. The pain is felt to be due to microfractures in the coalition.[23] Physical findings include pain on palpation over the subtalar joint, limited subtalar motion, and at times pes planus and ankle valgus. The peroneal muscles may be tight and resist inversion, but true muscle spasm occurs rarely (Fig. 30E2–1). Any condition that injures the subtalar joint can produce similar symptoms.

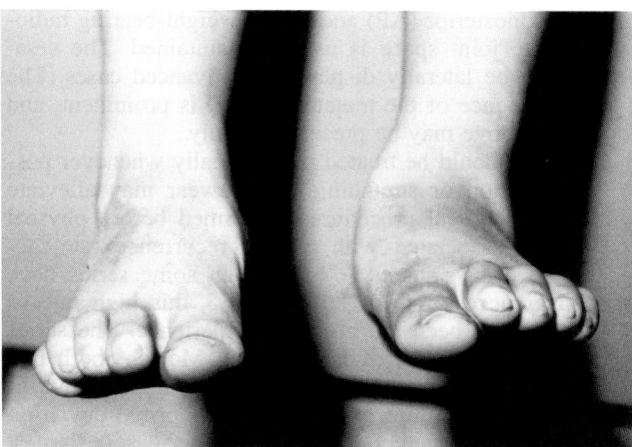

Figure 30E2–1. This patient had a tarsal coalition in the left foot. Note that the foot is held in an everted position. Attempted inversion caused pain and resistance.

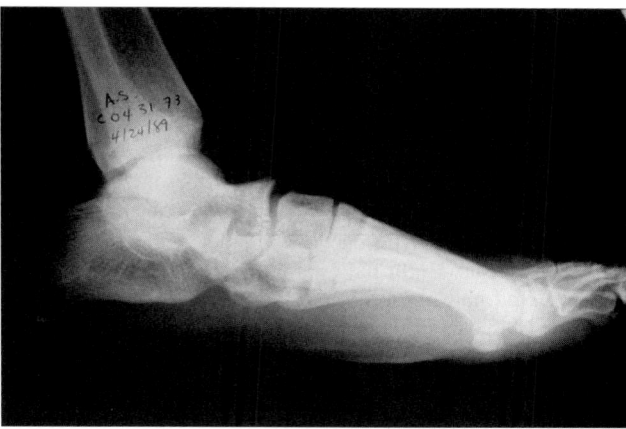

Figure 30E2–3. Lateral radiograph of the foot. Note the beaking of the talus and the widening of the talonavicular joint. The subtalar joint is narrowed.

The clinical diagnosis can be confirmed by radiographic imaging. Plain radiographs, especially the 45-degree oblique view (Fig. 30E2–2), usually demonstrate the calcaneonavicular coalition and other less common coalitions, such as the calcaneocuboid. The talocalcaneal coalition is difficult to visualize on plain radiographs, but secondary changes, which may suggest the need for other studies (Fig. 30E2–3), include beaking and shortening of the talar neck, a middle subtalar facet that cannot be seen, elongation of the lateral process of the calcaneus, and ball-and-socket ankle joint (see Fig. 30E2–3). Special views (e.g., Harris-Beath view), scintigraphy, plain tomography, and arthrography all have been used to demonstrate these coalitions. Computed tomography (CT), which is now the method of choice for the diagnosis of tarsal coalitions not identified on plain films,[16] is comparable in cost and radiation dosage to the other studies. It is technically simple to perform, noninvasive, and accurate. CT provides precise delineation of the anatomy if surgical resection is contem-

plated. It may also demonstrate the presence of more than one coalition, which is important for treatment planning (see Fig. 30E2–2). Magnetic resonance imaging (MRI), which also can be used, provides the advantage of demonstrating fibrous coalitions.[37] It is a more costly technique.

The initial treatment of these conditions should include conservative measures aimed at relieving the pain. These measures are empirical and include casting and the use of various shoe inserts and orthotics. The main indication for surgical resection is persistent pain. For calcaneonavicular coalition, resection of the bar with interposition of the extensor digitorum brevis is usually associated with good results. Studies by Cowell and by Cowell and Jayakuman have indicated that 23 of 26 feet treated in this manner became symptom-free.[11, 18]

Talocalcaneal coalition is more difficult to recognize, and its surgical management is less certain.[36] Before the advent of CT, the diagnosis was often confirmed at the time of surgery. Jayakuman and Cowell[18] reported that up to one third of their patients responded to conservative

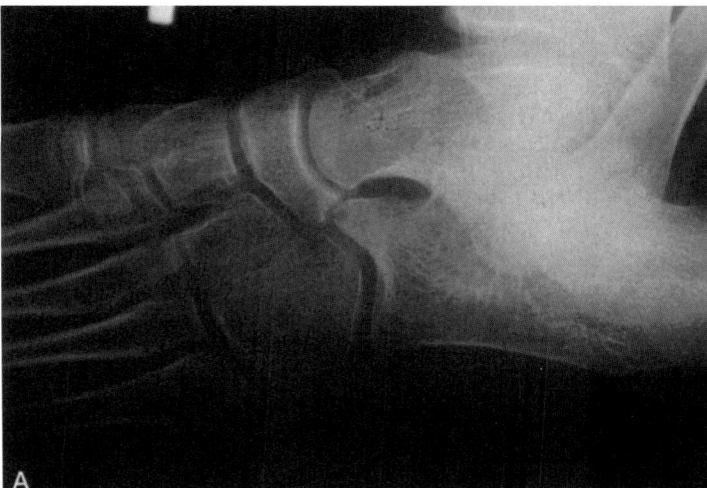
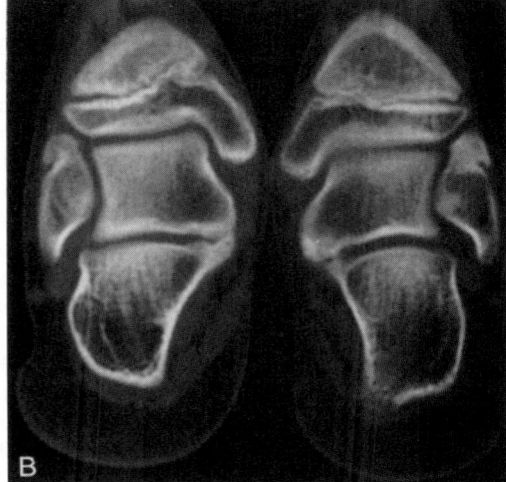

Figure 30E2–2. Plain radiography *(A)* and computed tomographic scan *(B)* showing calcaneonavicular and talocalcaneal coalitions, which occurred bilaterally in this patient. The patient presented with a painful, rigid foot and was having difficulty playing tennis.

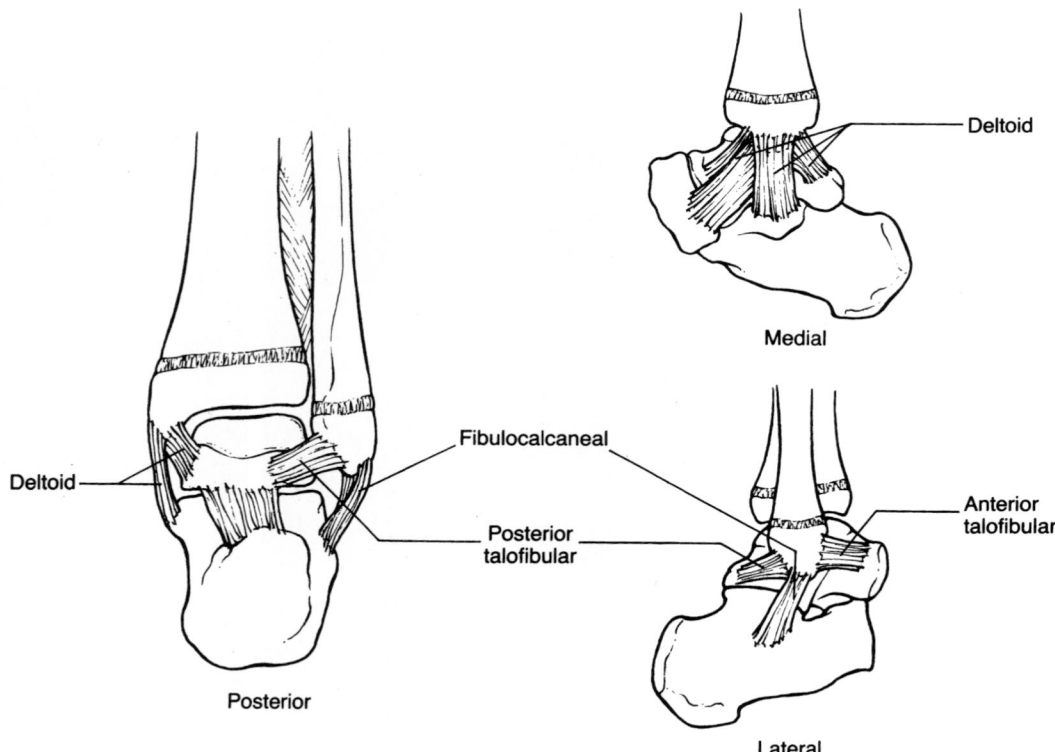

Figure 30E2–5. The ligaments of the ankle in posterior, medial, and lateral views.

rarely necessary but may be beneficial for the competitive athlete. Players should not return to play until the swelling has subsided and they have regained normal motion, are pain-free with normal strength, and are able to perform the maneuvers of the sport. Continued pain or disability should provoke a search for other, more serious injury.

Recurrent subluxation of peroneal tendons can occur in the adolescent athlete. Usually, a history of injury is followed by recurrent episodes of a snapping sensation and pain. The subluxation can be provoked by forceful dorsiflexion with the foot everted. In patients whose symptoms are sufficiently severe, surgical correction may be indicated. Surgical alternatives include deepening the groove on the fibula, creating a bony block, and reconstructing the superior peroneal retinaculum. The first two are rarely useful in treatment of the pediatric athlete because the physis is still open. Poll and Duijfjes[29] reviewed nine patients aged 15 to 45 (average age, 25) who underwent reconstruction with the posterior calcaneofibular ligament attached to a bone block. Results were said to be good.

Contusions on the foot are treated in the same way as those on any other area. Blisters are a frequent problem and require alleviation of the stress, which is usually provided by a new shoe, and protection until healing occurs. Tinea pedis (athlete's foot) usually responds to a regimen of antifungal medication, along with education about the need to change socks frequently and to use antifungal powders.

Fractures About the Ankle

Multiple systems have been proposed to classify ankle injuries. Dias and Giergerich[12] proposed using the systems that are applied to adult ankle fractures. All these classification systems take into account the position of the foot at the time of injury and the force applied. The Salter-Harris classification is based on the mechanism of injury and the pathoanatomy of the fracture pattern through the physis, as is interpreted on plain radiographs. Salter has described types I through V. Type V, a crush injury to the physis, is difficult to recognize on plain radiographs and is not discussed in this chapter (Fig. 30E2–6).

CT and MRI are valuable techniques in assessing some fractures because they allow more accurate evaluation of the fragments. Carey and associates[8] performed a study of plain films and MRI in 14 patients with acute injuries and reached the following conclusions. Direct visualization of cartilage afforded by MRI improved evaluation of growth plate injury in each case. MRI changed Salter-Harris classification or staging in 2 of 9 patients with fractures visualized on conventional radiographs, allowed the detection of radiographically occult fractures in 5 of 14 cases, and resulted in a physical change in management for 5 of the 14 patients studied. MRI has an important role in the evaluation of acute pediatric growth plate injury, particularly when diagnostic uncertainty persists following the evaluation of conventional radiographs. MRI allows detection of occult fractures, may alter Salter-Harris staging, and may lead to a change in patient management.[8]

Dias and Giergerich[12] proposed a modification of the Lauge-Hanson system by combining it with the Salter-Harris classification, suggesting that this is of benefit for planning the closed reduction of these injuries. Although these other systems may be important in the adult, the Salter-Harris classification is the most important system in

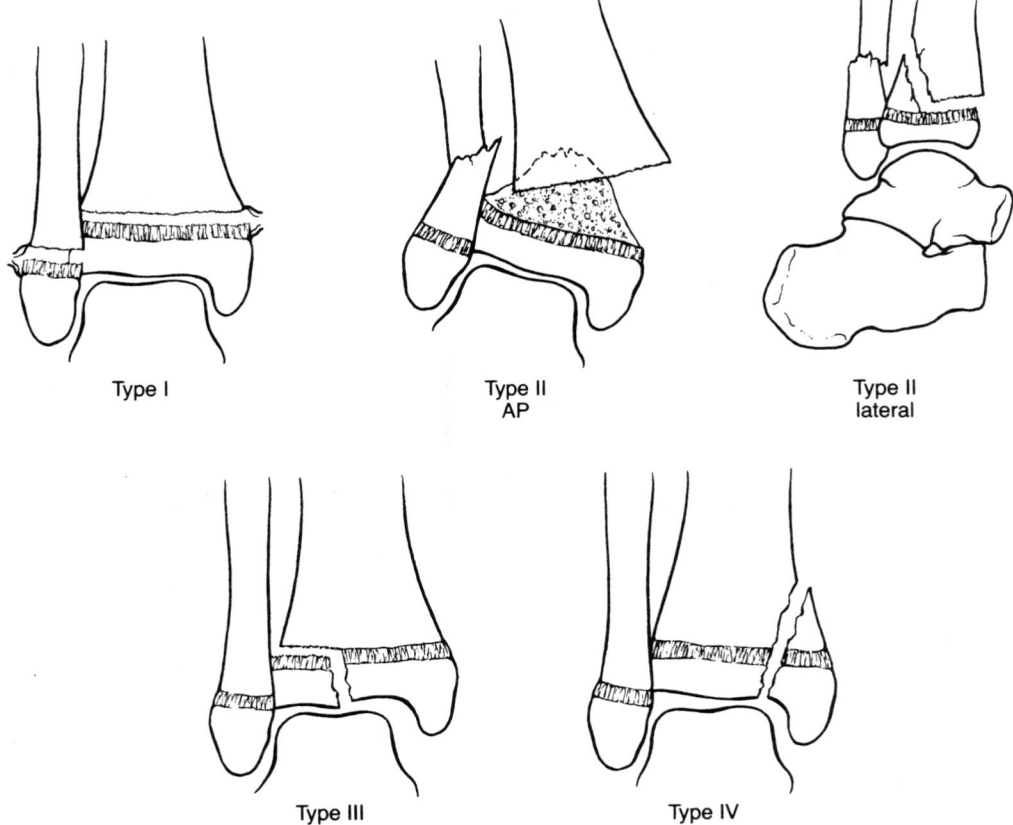

Figure 30E2–6. Fracture patterns of the distal tibial and fibular physes classified by the Salter-Harris system.

the child for planning treatment and predicting outcome. In the skeletally immature patient, the tibiotalar joint surface is rarely disturbed. The injury pattern changes in adolescence as the physis begins to close. The outcome of the injury depends on the type of physeal injury and its management. Tension injuries usually produce Salter-Harris type I and II injuries of the physis. Compression forces can produce Salter-Harris type III and IV injuries.

Salter-Harris type V injuries are severe crush injuries. A type VI injury in which the perichondrial ring is injured has been described.[30] These injuries rarely occur during usual sports activities.

Clinical Evaluation

The mechanism of injury and the time elapsed since the accident should be noted. The neurovascular status of the foot should be carefully documented. The amount of swelling and the status of the skin are important. Gentle examination should be carried out to seek areas of point tenderness, especially over the physis. This examination may be more useful than radiographs in the diagnosis of Salter-Harris type I injuries.

Radiographs should always include three views of the ankle. Only in this manner will the physician be able to see some fractures and determine if there is disruption of the ankle mortise. Plain tomography and CT may be indicated in the juvenile fracture of Tillaux and in triplane fractures, which are discussed later. Because treatment and prognosis depend on the Salter-Harris classification, the fractures are discussed according to fracture type.

Salter-Harris Type I

Salter-Harris type I injuries of the tibia occur in very young children and are not a consideration in the athlete. Salter-Harris type I fractures of the fibula are common and may be missed entirely or misdiagnosed as a sprain. The characteristic history of an external rotation force in a patient who presents with localized tenderness and swelling directly over the distal fibular physis is diagnostic. The radiograph shows only localized swelling and widening of the fibular physis. Many of these injuries probably go unrecognized and untreated. Gleeson has used ultrasound to identify these injuries and reports that they may be treated with tubular gauze and crutches or with a cast. They respond quite well to 2 to 3 weeks of immobilization in a short-leg walking cast.

Salter-Harris Type II

This injury is uncommon or is infrequently recognized in the fibula. Salter-Harris type II injury of the distal tibia combined with a fracture of the distal fibula is one of the most common injuries about the ankle, accounting for 47.3% of cases in the series compiled by Peterson and Cass.[27] In most instances, this injury can be reduced closed with the patient under sedation. Periosteum or other soft tissue, if it is inverted into the fracture site, can block the reduction. Traditional treatment consists of a long-leg bent-knee cast for 2 to 3 weeks followed by a short-leg walking cast for 4 weeks. Dugan and colleagues[13] reviewed 56 patients with this injury who were treated with a long-leg weight-bearing cast for 4 weeks. There were no nonunions and no angular deformities. There was one case of clinically insignificant premature closure of the growth plate. This seems to be the treatment of choice because it allows early healing, low morbidity, and rapid rehabilitation.

Salter-Harris Type III

This injury is also known as the juvenile fracture of Tillaux. The distal tibial physis closes first in the central region, and then from the medial side toward the fibula. An external rotation force applied to the partially closed physis applies traction on the physis through the anterior talofibular ligament. This avulses a fragment of the lateral physis, which remains attached to the ligament (Fig. 30E2–7). Closed reduction under anesthesia should be attempted. The injury can be treated closed if the fragment is not displaced more than 2 mm, or if it can be reduced closed and percutaneously fixed. Most of these injuries require open reduction and fixation of the fragment with a pin or cancellous screw.[37] Fractures of the medial malleolus can be either type III or IV injuries. If displaced less than 2 mm, they may be treated closed. This treatment should consist initially of a long-leg non–weight-bearing cast for 3 weeks followed by a short-leg walking cast for 3 weeks. These injuries are the most unpredictable of ankle epiphyseal injuries. Near-anatomic reduction must be obtained.[22]

Salter-Harris Type IV

This group includes some of the medial malleolar fractures and the triplane fractures. The triplane fracture, first described by Marmor, is so named because the fracture lines extend from the physis into the transverse, sagittal, and coronal planes (see Fig. 30E2–7).[9, 14, 33] This type of fracture may be mistaken for a Salter-Harris type II injury if the radiographs are not carefully scrutinized.

Many authors have described this fracture and have argued over the number of fragments involved.[9, 12, 14, 33] Cooperman and colleagues[9] studied 15 triplane fractures (average age, 13 years). This number represented 6% of 237 consecutive physeal fractures of the tibia and fibula. Average follow-up was 26 months. Thirteen fractures had been treated closed, and two had been treated by open reduction and internal fixation. In this series, plain tomographic studies supported the opinion that this was a two-part fracture. Dias and Giergerich[12] reviewed a series of fractures that included eight triplane fractures, which comprised both two-part and three-part fractures. Three patients were treated by open reduction, at which time it was

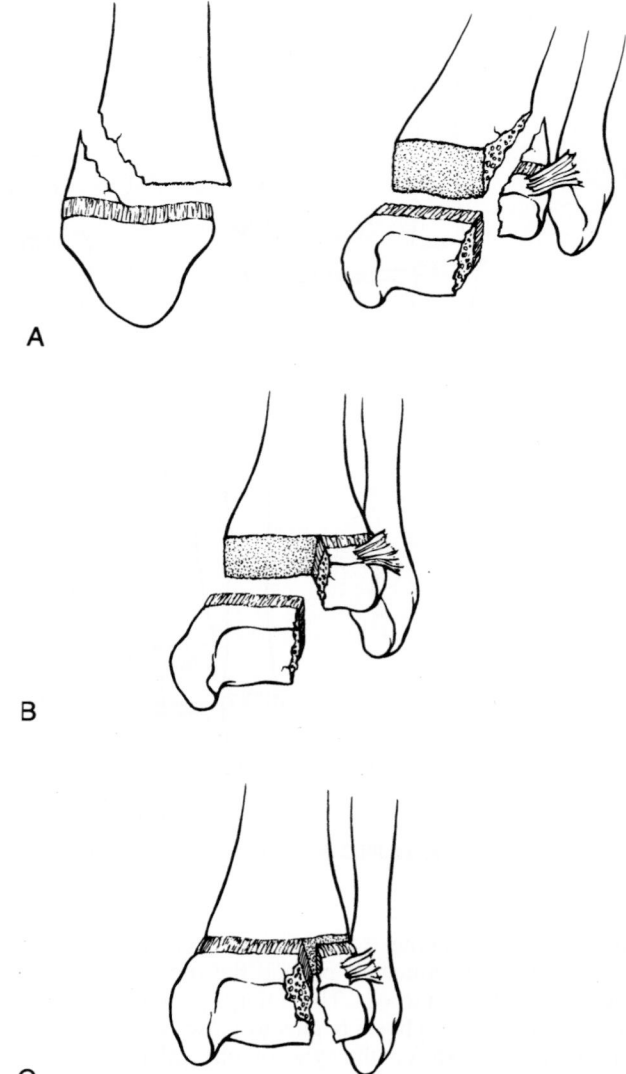

Figure 30E2–7. *A* and *B,* The triplane fracture can consist of two or more fragments. *C,* The juvenile fracture of Tillaux.

confirmed that these were three-part fractures. In two patients, studies confirmed that it was a two-part injury, and they were treated in a long-leg cast for 6 weeks. Ertl and associates[14] reviewed 23 patients with this injury. Eleven of fifteen had a three-part fracture. In these patients, plain radiographs did not accurately demonstrate the configuration of the fracture and were unreliable in distinguishing two-part from three-part fractures.

Figure 30E2–7 illustrates the possibilities. In the two-part fracture, the main fragment is the tibial shaft, including the medial malleolus and a portion of the medial epiphysis. The second fragment is the remaining epiphysis, which is attached to the fibula. In the three-part injury, the third fragment is usually an anterior free epiphyseal fragment.

Karrholm reviewed the literature on this injury.[19] Triplane fracture made up 7% of physeal injuries in girls and 15% in boys. Of the injuries, 35% were treated closed without manipulation, 30% by manipulation and casting, and 35% by open reduction and internal fixation.

If this injury can be reduced to within 2 mm, it may be treated closed. In Cooperman and colleagues' series,[9] 13 of 15 fractures were treated closed, and in the series of Dias and Giergerich,[12] 5 of 8 were treated in this way. In the series by Ertl and coworkers,[14] residual displacement of more than 2 mm was associated with a high incidence of late symptoms. Obtaining a reduction of less than 2 mm by either closed or open means did not ensure an excellent result. Poor results may be related to damage done to the articular surface, or to the amount of displacement. Fractures outside the weight-bearing area did not show this tendency toward poor results.

Evaluation of the adequacy of reduction in this injury is very difficult, and because most authors recommend manipulation under general anesthesia, the only radiographic means of diagnosis available is plain radiography. The author's preferred method is manipulation by internal rotation of the foot under sedation, which usually occurs in the emergency room. If there is any question about the adequacy of reduction on plain radiographs, CT or plain tomography is used to evaluate the articular surface and the reduction (Fig. 30E2–8) If displacement is greater than 2 mm, open reduction and internal fixation are carried out. This may require two incisions. The first is an anterolateral

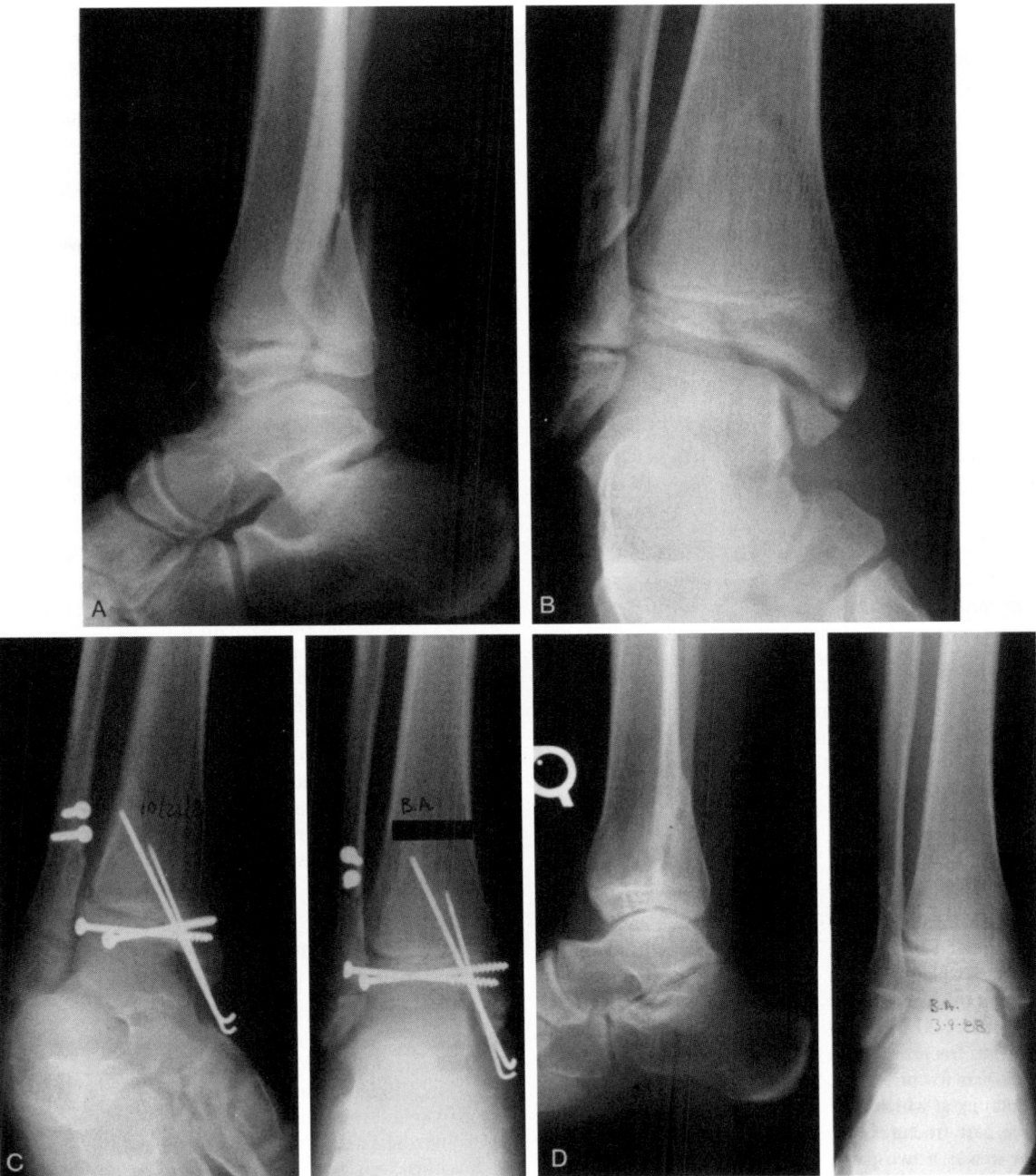

Figure 30E2–8. *A* and *B,* The position attained after manipulation of a severely displaced triplane fracture. The position was not acceptable, so further imaging was not necessary. *C,* The position achieved by open reduction. *D,* The position that is retained after hardware removal.

incision, which allows identification of the anterolateral fragment. Usually, it is first necessary to reduce and fix the posterior fragment. If this cannot be done closed or percutaneously, a second incision is required. These injuries require 6 weeks in a cast.

Prediction of Outcome

The prognosis for an ankle fracture in a skeletally immature patient depends on the following factors:

1. Salter-Harris classification
2. Quality of reduction
3. State of skeletal maturity
4. Amount of displacement
5. Miscellaneous modifiers (open fracture, vascular injury, infection, systemic illness, and so on)

Spiegel and colleagues[33] retrospectively studied a series of closed distal tibial physeal injuries. One hundred eighty-four patients (of 237) were followed for an average of 28 months. The authors looked specifically at the complications of angular deformity of greater than 5 degrees and shortening of more than 1 cm, joint incongruity, or asymmetrical closure of the physis. These complications seemed to correlate with the Salter-Harris grade, the amount of displacement or comminution, and the adequacy of reduction. The patients were divided into the groups shown in Table 30E2–1.

The overall complication rate was 14.1% for 184 patients. Salter-Harris type II injuries of the tibia seemed to be the least predictable because the incidence of complications remained approximately the same, regardless of the amount of displacement. Displacement is not always mentioned as one of the factors involved in prediction of outcome, but it is intuitive that greater displacement implies greater force, with more likely damage to the articular cartilage, the circulation, and the soft tissues important in healing. Karrholm[19] in his review felt the good results were based on the adequacy of the reduction.

Near-anatomic reduction of type II injuries of the tibia is desirable. These injuries are easy to reduce and often benign but must be followed until the patient attains skeletal maturity or a normal growth pattern is ensured because some will go on to premature closure and angular deformity.[22] The juvenile fracture of Tillaux and the triplane

fracture result from incomplete closure of the physis. Because growth is nearing an end, angular deformity and shortening are uncommon. In these patients, the tibiotalar joint surface is disturbed and must be restored to as near normal as possible to prevent incongruity and subsequent traumatic arthritis. In Cooperman and colleagues' series,[9] triplane fractures were reduced with the patient under general anesthesia by internally rotating the foot. The adequacy of reduction was determined by plain tomography. Dias and Giergerich[12] had nine Tillaux and triplane fractures that were followed for an average of 18 months, and all did well.

Peterson and Cass[27] reviewed all Salter-Harris type IV distal tibial injuries seen at the Mayo Clinic, paying particular attention to injuries of the medial malleolus. Nine of eighteen of these injuries went on to premature physeal closure sufficient to require additional surgery for physeal bar resection, angular deformity, or leg-length discrepancy. Thirteen of these patients received their care at the Mayo Clinic, and of these, 11 were closed injuries. Six patients were treated by closed reduction and a short-leg cast. Five had open reduction and internal fixation. Five additional patients in the study had been referred to the clinic because of complications of a closed injury that had been treated closed. Peterson and Cass concluded that oblique radiographs are necessary to ensure an accurate diagnosis. They are also necessary to confirm the adequacy of reduction. Some injuries that resemble type III injuries are actually type IV. The authors also found that partial arrest that results in angular deformity was more common than complete arrest. They concluded that there are three patterns of medial malleolar injury, and that type IV injuries constitute the most common and most dangerous pattern because they usually occur in a patient who has remaining growth potential (Fig. 30E2–9). They also concluded that the medial malleolus requires anatomic reduction, which often necessitates open reduction and internal fixation.

In any patient with an open physis, it is preferable to avoid crossing the physis with a fixation device. This goal can usually be achieved by placing smooth pins from metaphysis to metaphysis, or from epiphysis to epiphysis. At times, crossing the physis cannot be avoided. In these instances, smooth pins can be used, and care should be taken that they do not cross in the physis. Patients need to be followed to skeletal maturity, or until one is certain that a normal growth pattern is occurring. An asymmetrical Harris growth arrest line may be the earliest clue to an abnormal growth pattern (see Fig. 30E2–9).

TABLE 30E2–1
Complications of Ankle Fractures

Group	Complication Rate (%)	Salter-Harris Group and Bone Involved
Low risk (89 patients)	6.7	Type I and II of fibula, I of tibia, III and IV with displacement of less than 2 mm, epiphyseal avulsion injuries
High risk (28 patients)	32	Types III, IV, and V of tibia Tillaux and triplane
Unpredictable (66 patients)	16.7	Type II of the tibia

Fractures in the Foot

Fractures about the foot resulting from sports are unusual in children. Fractures of the metatarsals can result from direct trauma (Fig. 30E2–10). These can be treated by immobilization in a short-leg walking cast. The most controversial fracture about the foot may be an avulsion injury at the base of the fifth metatarsal.

Fractures of the fifth metatarsal in children can be divided into distal physeal fractures, fractures of the proximal diaphysis, and avulsion fractures of the apophysis. The

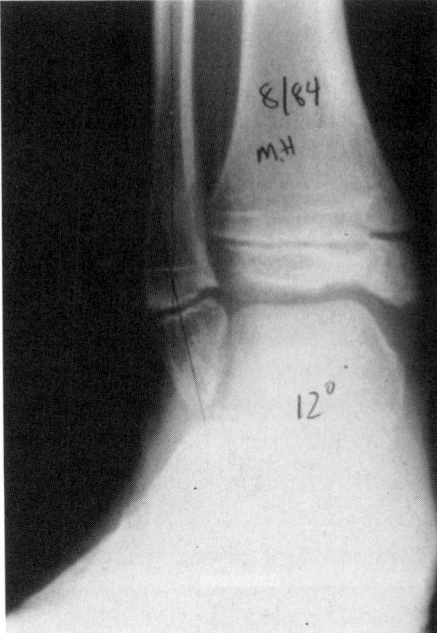
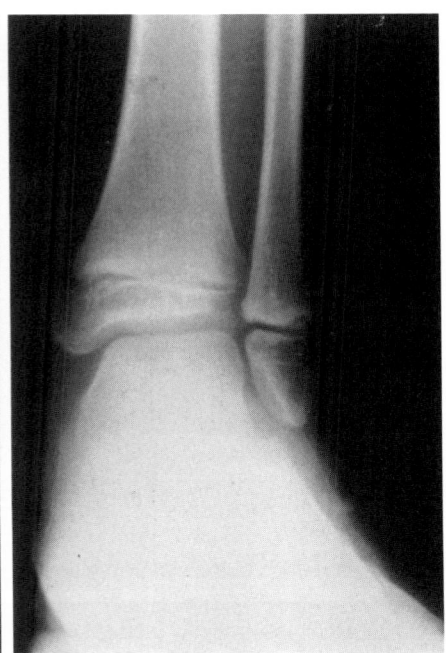

Figure 30E2–9. This patient sustained a Salter-Harris type IV medial malleolar fracture, which was treated closed. The patient was referred 6 months after injury, at which time she had trouble remembering which ankle had been injured. These radiographs were taken 18 months after the injury. Resection of a bony bridge and interposition were required. She resumed growth, and the fibular angular deformity had been corrected. Note the irregular Harris growth arrest lines.

fifth metatarsal has its epiphysis distally and an apophysis proximally. The tendon of the peroneus brevis is inserted into the apophysis. With inversion stress, the apophysis can be avulsed. Findings include tenderness at the base of the fifth metatarsal and radiographic confirmation of widening of the apophysis. Treatment should be symptomatic with compression and partial weight-bearing until the pain subsides. Crutches and an elastic bandage may be sufficient. Two to three weeks in a short-leg cast also yields good results.

Fracture of the proximal diaphysis of the fifth metatarsal (the Jones fracture) is less common in skeletally immature patients and usually occurs in the 15- to 20-year age range.[20] When such fractures do occur, a trial of immobilization in a short-leg walking cast is indicated because many acute fractures do heal. Even fractures with delayed union may heal if they are treated conservatively.[1] Early operative intervention in highly competitive athletes has been advocated by some, but others have shown that each patient needs to be treated individually because some of these fractures will heal if treated conservatively, allowing early return to athletics.[1, 20, 24] Early operative intervention in the pediatric athlete is rarely if ever indicated. Patients with established nonunion require operative treatment that includes reopening of the medullary canal, bone grafting, and internal fixation (Fig. 30E2–11).

Fractures of the toes are unusual in sports. Most phalangeal fractures can be treated by "buddy taping" them to the adjacent toe, wearing appropriate shoes for a few weeks, and avoiding sports until the toe is asymptomatic. Articular fractures are even more rare. The only one that may merit consideration of operative management is an intra-articular physeal fracture of the great toe. These should be reduced to as near-anatomic alignment as possible by whatever means necessary (Fig. 30E2–12).

Stress fractures are less common among children than in adults but cannot be entirely dismissed. Some children participate in marathons and other sporting events that can result in stress fractures. Basketball, soccer, and other team sports have tournaments that may require considerable running. The stress fracture shown in Figure 30E2–13 resulted from a tournament and was thought to be a sprain.

Yngve[39] found 131 pediatric stress fractures in 23 references in the literature. Two reports of the 131 documented metatarsal fractures—two of the tarsal navicular, and one of the medial sesamoid. The primary training error was too much too soon. Other factors that should be considered are a change in training surface or equipment (shoes) and a sudden change in intensity of training (tournaments). Diagnosis depends on an appropriate history, a high index of suspicion, and the presence of localized tenderness. The differential diagnosis includes contusion, tendinitis, and sprains.

The initial radiograph may be normal but should be diagnostic in half of cases. One should look for cortical thickening or a translucent fracture line. A bone scan may be diagnostic at this stage and may be particularly helpful if the diagnosis is in question and one wishes to avoid immobilization. A bone scan may be indicated when the diagnosis is in doubt and the athlete wishes to return to play. MRI has also been used to identify occult stress fractures. On the other hand, immobilization for 2 weeks in a cast is usually diagnostic in that pain is relieved; repeat radiographs are then positive, making a bone scan unnecessary. Although some of these fractures heal without a cast, the athlete should be immobilized for protection from himself or herself, as well as from well-meaning parents and coaches.

Osteochondral Lesions of the Talus

The term *osteochondritis dissecans* has been used to describe lesions in the dome of the talus. These lesions

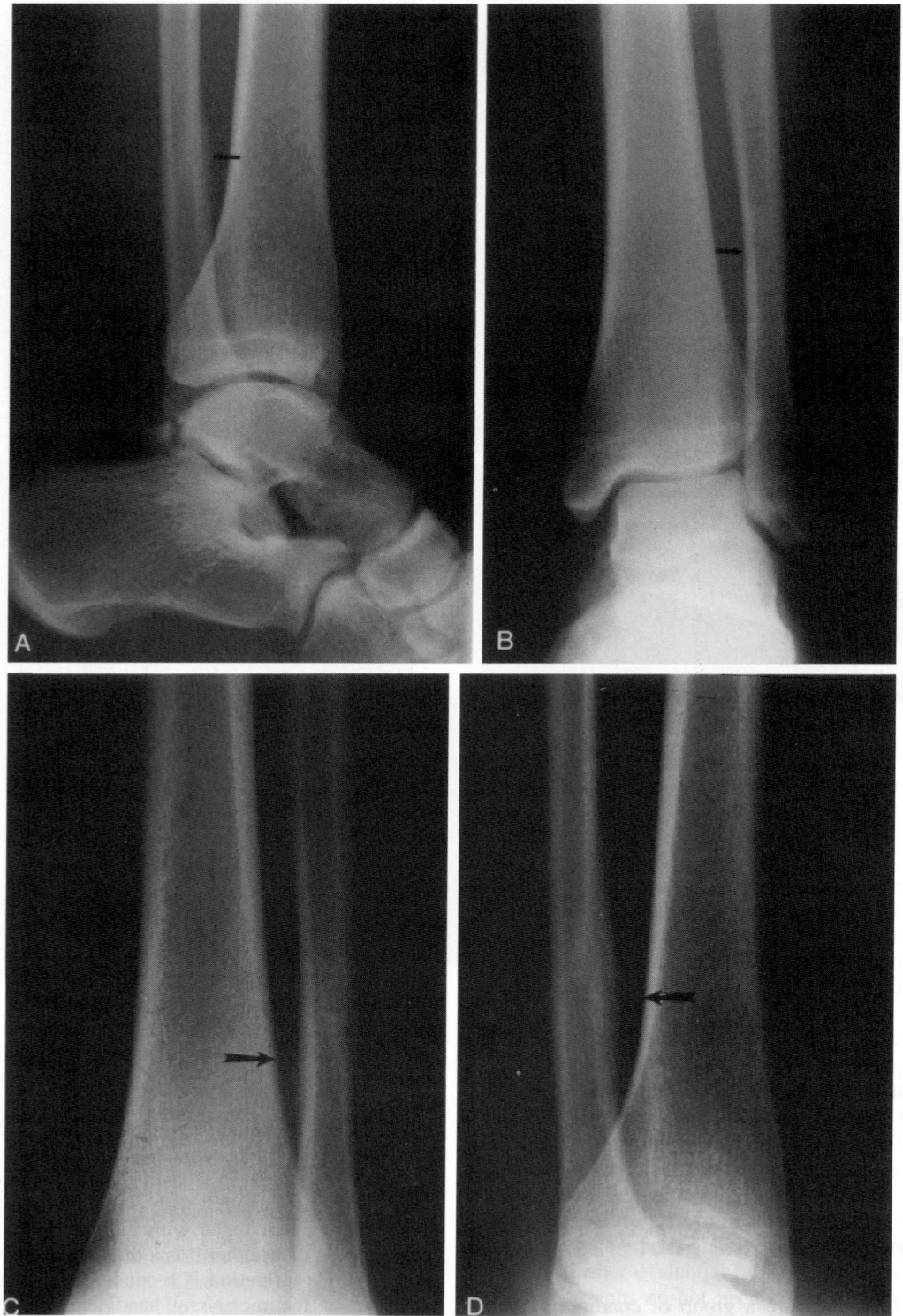

Figure 30E2–13. This patient presented with localized tenderness just above the ankle. After being injured in a basketball tournament, she continued to play with a presumptive diagnosis of a sprained ankle. The initial radiographs (*A* and *B*) showed periosteal elevation. Follow-up radiographs (*C* and *D*) taken after 2 weeks of short-leg walking cast treatment illustrate new bone formation.

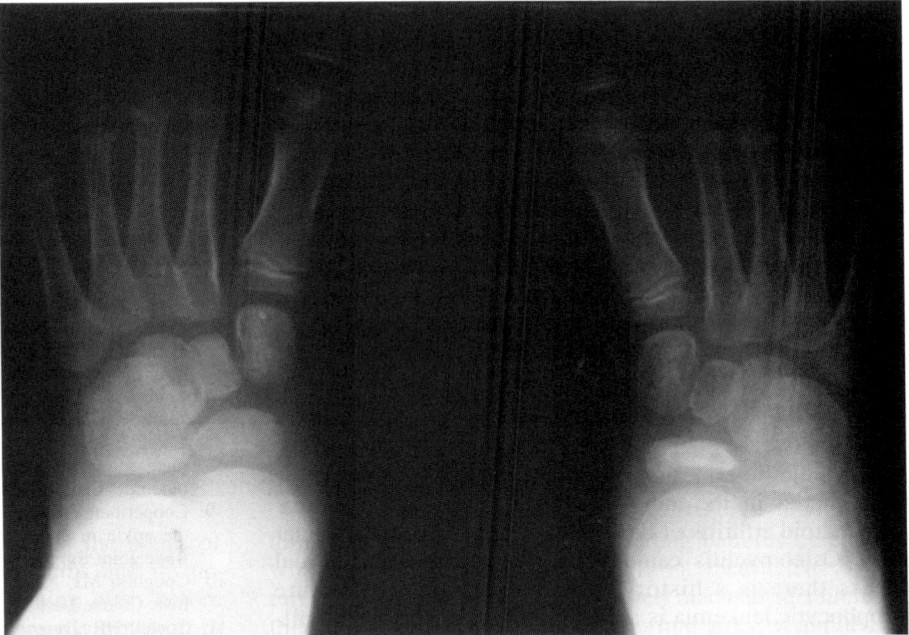

Figure 30E2–14. This patient presented with undisplaced fractures of the metatarsals. The condensed, narrowed appearance of the navicular is the same as that seen in patients with Kohler's syndrome, but it was an incidental finding in this patient.

on weight-bearing and has localized tenderness over the metatarsal head. Radiographs reveal collapse of the articular surface (see Fig. 30E2–15). Conservative treatment with a cast or orthotic device that minimizes weight-bearing over the involved head is often successful in relieving the pain. Surgical treatment consisting of removal of loose bodies or bone grafting has been reported for persistent symptoms. A dorsiflexion osteotomy to relieve weight-bearing has also been reported to work well. Removal of the metatarsal head should be avoided because this results in transfer of weight-bearing to the adjacent metatarsal heads. Prosthetic replacement has also been tried but is not indicated in children. In most instances, the disease runs its course, and the head re-ossifies within 2 to 3 years.

Sever's disease is a term used to refer to a nonarticular osteochondrosis or a traction apophysitis (Fig. 30E2–16). The real question is whether a distinct syndrome exists and, if it does, whether the apophysis has anything to do with it. The calcaneal apophysis appears and develops in the 5- to 12-year age range and is typically irregular. Often, a child with heel pain and an irregular apophysis has the same radiographic finding in the opposite asymptomatic heel. These children are usually in the 9- to 12-year age range and are active in sports. They may have a tight heel cord. The calcaneus serves as the insertion of the powerful gastrocnemius-soleus muscle and the origin of the plantar fascia. Traction or overuse can strain these structures, producing pain. Stretching may be beneficial. Symptomatic treatment by avoidance of the offending exercise is usually curative. Shock-absorbing inserts or a heel cup may be advantageous. A heel lift to relieve some of the pull of the

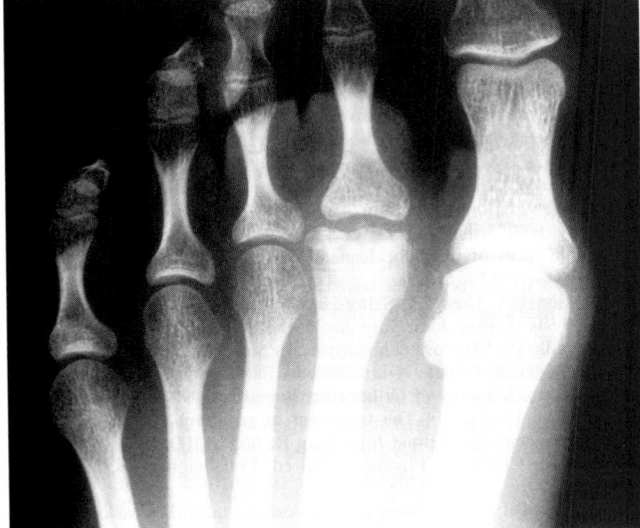

Figure 30E2–15. This anteroposterior radiograph of the foot shows irregularity and collapse of the second metatarsal head.

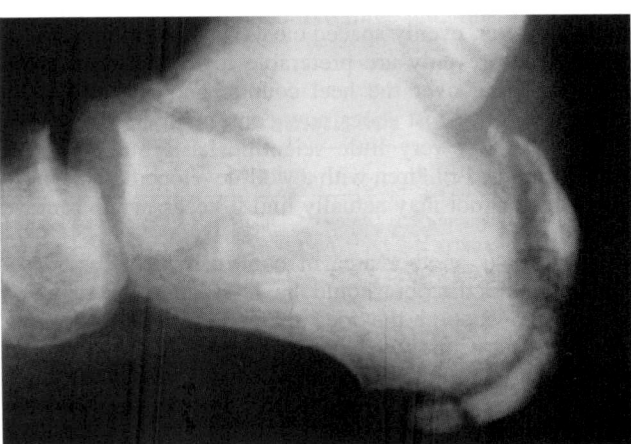

Figure 30E2–16. Lateral radiograph of the calcaneus. Note the irregularity, especially in the superior part of the apophysis. Fragmentation and increased density are common occurrences in the calcaneal apophysis.

"foot flat," and push-off. During the first interval, the foot is being loaded with the weight of the body while the ankle undergoes rapid plantar flexion under control of the anterior musculature. The foot is in pronation that originates at the subtalar joint, allowing absorption and dissipation of the forces generated by ground contact. The second interval begins with foot flat and forward transfer of the center of gravity over the foot. The ankle initially dorsiflexes, and the subtalar joint demonstrates progressive inversion brought on by multiple factors. The progressive inversion helps transform the flexible hindfoot and midfoot into a rigid lever. In the third interval, rapid plantar flexion of the ankle by concentric contraction of the posterior muscula-ture occurs with further inversion of the subtalar joint, reaching a maximum at toe-off. When the heel is elevated at the time of lift-off, the weight of the body is normally shared by all of the metatarsal heads. Because of the oblique nature of the metatarsophalangeal break, the foot must supinate to distribute the body weight evenly among the metatarsal heads.

Alterations and variations in anatomy and range of mo-tion may affect the loading of the foot during the stance phase of gait, which can lead to localized overloading and subsequent stress fracture. Patients with rigid foot deformities such as cavovarus foot or tarsal coalition are poorly able to absorb the forces during the first interval of the stance phase.[22, 35, 58] Stress is subsequently transferred to the midfoot (navicular, base of metatarsals), laterally (5th metatarsal), or distally to the forefoot. Inability to invert (supinate) the hindfoot during the second and third intervals leads to failure to distribute the body weight evenly among the metatarsals. Kaufman showed that pes planus increases the risk of stress fracture and does not protect the foot, as other studies have suggested.[22, 35] Clini-cally, overloading of the medial column of the foot occurs with sesamoid symptoms. Most authors accept that an abnormally short first metatarsal (congenital, traumatic, iat-rogenic) or abnormally long second or third metatarsals (Morton's foot) contribute to a stress fracture due to loss of the normal metatarsophalangeal break, which results in isolated overloading of specific metatarsals; Drez and associates,[17] however, showed that the lengths of the first and second metatarsals in their study of stress fracture patients did not differ significantly from those of randomly selected controls. Kaufman[35] was unable to demonstrate a relationship between loss of ankle or hindfoot motion and stress fracture.

Biomechanics

Bone is a dynamic organ that is capable of repair and reconfiguration. Wolff's law states that stresses applied to a bone stimulate remodeling of the bony architecture for optimal withstanding of the forces being applied. Rapid disuse osteopenia results when normal forces are with-drawn from a healthy bone. This phenomenon is clearly demonstrated in experimental models, as well as in humans experiencing weightlessness.[38] During steady state, daily stresses applied to bone stimulate development of a bony architecture that is optimally fit in terms of strength and density, according to Wolff's law. When activities and therefore stresses are increased, remodeling of the bone takes place. The exact mechanism that initiates this process is unknown. Several authors state that it is likely due to the creation of microfractures.[1] Microfractures stimulate osteoclastic resorption in initiation of the repair process. As osteoclasts resorb bone, osteoblasts fill in the voids with new osteons. If high levels of activity continue, micro-fractures and osteoclastic resorption exceed osteoblastic new bone formation, resulting in metabolic imbalance. If stresses continue to accumulate at a rate beyond that oc-curring in the repair process, fatigue fracture may result. Although microfractures of the bone are a physiologic process that responds to Wolff's law, disease is apparent when reparative processes cannot keep pace with the frac-ture process.

Stresses to bone result from both tension and compres-sion. Tensile forces occur on the convex sides of long bones; compressive forces occur on the concave border. Muscular activity and/or fatigue can attenuate these forces applied to bones. In normal, nonmaximal activity, muscular contractions tend to dampen the forces applied with weight-bearing. As activity level and duration increase, muscles fatigue, and the dampening effect of muscle diminishes. Microfractures begin to accumulate, thus shifting the bal-ance in favor of bone damage. Continued impact forces from weight-bearing lead to damage that exceeds repair capabilities, and eventually to fatigue fracture. Fatigue frac-ture is a function of the number of loading cycles and the amount of force applied. As the metabolic balance in nor-mal healthy bones relies on the ability of bone to heal, osseous vascularity plays an important role in this balance. As such, "watershed areas" of bone with relative hypovas-cularity (base of 5th metatarsal; midtarsal navicular; meta-tarsal necks; anterior tibia) are known to be predisposed to fatigue fractures.

Risk Factors

Various risk factors for development of a lower extrem-ity stress fracture have been identified. Clearly, running is responsible for the greatest number of stress fractures in the nonmilitary population.[1] Running is the athletic activity that produces the greatest number of repetitions of the same impact-loading activity. The force of each stride is a magnification of body weight, as has been shown in the gait studies of Mann.[39] Thus, a 70-kilogram individual dissipates 120 tons of force per foot per mile walked, and this increases to 210 tons of force per foot per mile in running.[39] It is not hard to see why runners and joggers develop stress injury after running multiple miles, several times a week, on concrete streets. In this context, it is hard to understand why the incidence of stress fractures is not higher still. Other predisposing factors may include poor training techniques, such as abruptly increasing the inten-sity, duration, or type of training. Alterations in warm-ups, running surface or grade, shoewear, and orthoses may be predisposing factors. Other impact activities such as jump-ing, sprinting, and hurdles can independently lead to stress fractures; they also increase the risk of stress injury in run-ners.

Anatomic factors play a role in stress-related injuries. The height of the arch has been shown by Simkin and colleagues[58] to correlate with an increased risk of stress fracture. A cavus foot deformity tends to be rigid and unable to absorb forces imparted during physical activities. Leg-length discrepancies overload the longer limb, resulting in the application of higher stresses. Hallux valgus deformities and long second metatarsals (Morton's foot) lead to second ray overload, with development of stress fractures. Excessive external rotation at the hip has been shown to increase the risk of stress fracture.[23]

Female gender as a risk factor has received increased attention in the recent literature on stress fractures. In their study of stress fractures in dancers, Kadel and coworkers[34] showed that excessive training and prolonged duration of amenorrhea contribute independently to the risk of fracture. Bone mineral density has been shown to be significantly decreased in amenorrheic athletes compared with eumenorrheic athletes and controls.[13, 47] Although estrogen supplementation has been shown to be clearly beneficial in preventing postmenopausal bone loss, the literature is contradictory as to whether estrogen supplementation decreases the incidence of stress fracture among amenorrheic athletes.[3, 13]

Previous surgical procedures to the lower extremities may expose the bones to new or varied forces. Metatarsal osteotomies, either for hallux valgus or for lesser ray problems, may lead to overloading of adjacent rays and increased risk for subsequent development of stress fractures.[20] Ankle and hindfoot procedures to fuse or realign the joint can lead to increased loading, especially if there is a malunion. Sammarco and Idusuyi[55] reported a case of a third metatarsal stress fracture following endoscopic plantar fascia release. They felt that excess strain was created owing to the loss of the stress-relieving function of the plantar fascia. Stress fractures following total joint replacement have been reported, presumably due to newly increased stresses in a poorly conditioned, previously underused extremity.[26]

Age has been shown to be a risk factor for stress fracture likely related to osteoporosis. Myburgh and associates[47] showed that athletes with stress fractures had lower bone mineral density in both the appendicular and the axial skeleton. They also showed that these same athletes had lower dietary calcium intake than did control subjects. Caucasian race has also been shown to be a risk factor.

Diagnosis

History

Whereas history and physical examination have classically been the standard for diagnosis of stress injuries, imaging studies have evolved to aid significantly in the diagnosis. Patients sustaining stress fractures of the foot and ankle generally present with a history of insidious onset of a vague, aching pain. The patient usually does not remember a specific traumatic event but may note a recent change in activity level or a change in type or duration of training. For the casual athlete, a new recreational sport or a diet-related exercise program may be the only change.

For more highly trained athletes, the change may be as simple as new athletic shoes, a different surface for running, or minor increases in speed or distance. Routine daily activities without a history of strenuous activity may produce insufficiency stress fractures in patients with osteoporosis or underlying diseased bone.[36] Dull, aching pain is characteristically present midway through or near the end of the activity; it usually resolves with cessation of the activity. The patient can usually localize the pain to a specific area. This pain progresses and eventually may develop into a sharp, severe pain that results from all weight-bearing activities, as the stress fracture becomes complete. Although a history of menstrual irregularities certainly aids in the diagnosis of stress fracture, a high index of suspicion is necessary early in the course, especially if a history of increased activity level is not forthcoming.

Physical Findings

The most reliable physical finding is a discrete, localized area of tenderness and swelling over the affected bone. Sixty-six percent of the athletes with stress fractures in Matheson's study had localized tenderness, and 25% had soft tissue swelling.[40] Erythema and warmth may be present but are much less likely. Patients may present with a limp but rarely with muscular atrophy. Joint range of motion is usually not affected. Percussion and vibratory and ultrasonic stimulation have been reported to aid in the diagnosis but are usually unnecessary.[16]

Physical examination should also include assessment of ankle and hindfoot position. Equinus contracture or hindfoot varus can predispose an athlete to high levels of forefoot or lateral foot stress. Cavus deformities are associated with hindfoot varus and neurologic disease. Alignment and range of motion of the knee and hip should be assessed as should leg lengths.

Imaging Studies

A patient's history of temporally related altered activity level, along with findings of localized tenderness, is often sufficient for the diagnosis of stress fracture to be made and treatment initiated. Plain radiographs, however, should still be obtained. Standard three-view studies of the ankle or foot are initially performed. Special oblique studies can be obtained as required by the particular case. Not uncommonly, in fact, more often than not, the initial radiographs are negative, with radiographic changes lagging behind clinical symptoms by at least 2 to 3 weeks.[36, 51] Cortical hypertrophy may be present, suggesting a condition of longstanding overload. Linear radiolucencies from osteoclastic resorption may eventually appear. More commonly, increased radiodensity as the body attempts a healing response can be present. Prather and colleagues[51] found radiographic assessment alone to be diagnostic only 64% of the time.

In many patients with nonarticular involvement, diagnosis of stress fracture by history and physical findings, despite negative plain radiographs, is sufficient (and reasonable) for treatment to be initiated. With higher-risk lesions or in high-caliber/elite athletes, further diagnostic studies are appropriate. Bone scintigraphy with radionuclide technetium[99m] diphosphonate is the study of choice owing to its ability to demonstrate early physiologic abnormality, thus increasing sensitivity.[59] Bone scans are routinely positive as early as 2 days following injury and may be so as early as 24 hours.[41] The isotope is incorporated into the bone by the activated osteoblasts. Even in subradiographic stress fractures, scintigraphic uptake is usually intense (Fig. 30F–1). Some fractures have a characteristic appearance on bone scan, and certain fractures (e.g., navicular, sesamoid, talar processes) often require further anatomic definition with computed tomography.

Magnetic resonance imaging (MRI) has emerged as a useful adjunct in the diagnosis of stress fractures (Fig. 30F–2). Stress fractures have a characteristic appearance on MRI, that is, low signal intensity on T_1-weighted images and high signal intensity on T_2-weighted images.[37] T_1 and short T_1 (tau) inversion recovery (STIR) sequence images demonstrate the lesion best when it is out of the acute phase.[56] MRI has the advantage of better accuracy in diagnosis than bone scan in terms of definition of the anatomy of the fracture site.[37] The benefits may be offset by the higher cost and, therefore, this approach should not be used indiscriminately in all patients.

Treatment Principles

The treatment of stress fractures of the foot and ankle may vary somewhat in duration, timing, and the election of aggressive intervention in comparison with the treatment of those fractures caused by acute, discrete traumatic incidents. These variations are discussed later according to the specific fractures. The basic principles of fracture care must still be followed, however, to achieve predictable healing. The two most basic of these principles are rest and immobilization of the injured limb. Rest takes on an additional (and negative) nuance of meaning for many athletes in sports-induced stress fractures because it is most often the highly repetitive motions and impacts of the sport itself that induce the injury. Rest, then, does not simply suggest the sensible alteration of everyday activity that comes to mind in the nonathlete; rather, it means that the athlete must severely modify or even suspend the previously intense pursuit of the sport. This can, and often is, met with howls of protest and anger, given the passion or payment associated with participation in amateur or professional sports, respectively. The physician or surgeon is in turn subjected to pressure from patient, parent, coach, trainer, or agent (sometimes subtle, and often overt) to violate these basic principles so that the athlete may return to the sport as quickly as possible. Sometimes the doctor feels that the demand is not just for a prognosis, nor even treatment, but for something just short of magic, as if the fracture will be healed if the doctor would only acquiesce to a quick return to the sport. In addition to the science discussed elsewhere in this chapter, successful treatment usually requires the skillful application of the art of medicine, encompassing that unique blend of rational decision-making, sympathetic coercion, and thoughtful compromise.

Rest, then, signifies decrease in, or cessation of, the sport, together with the judicious use of cross-training so that generalized deconditioning is minimized while the specific injury to the limb is protected from further microtrauma and repetitive stress.

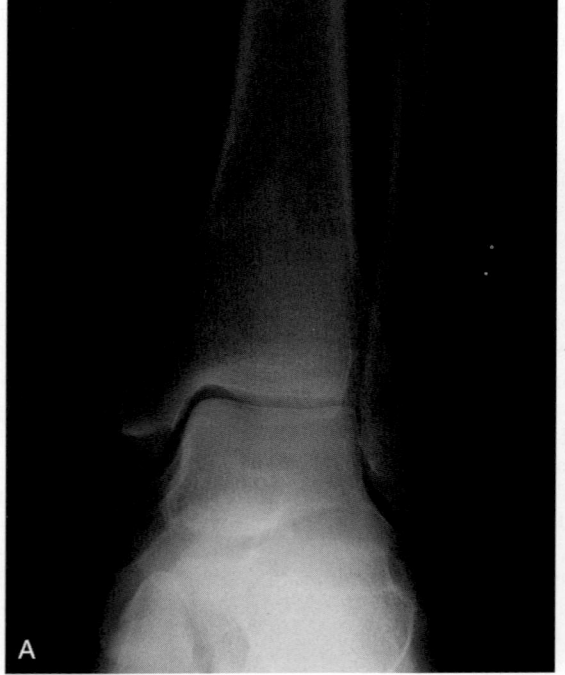
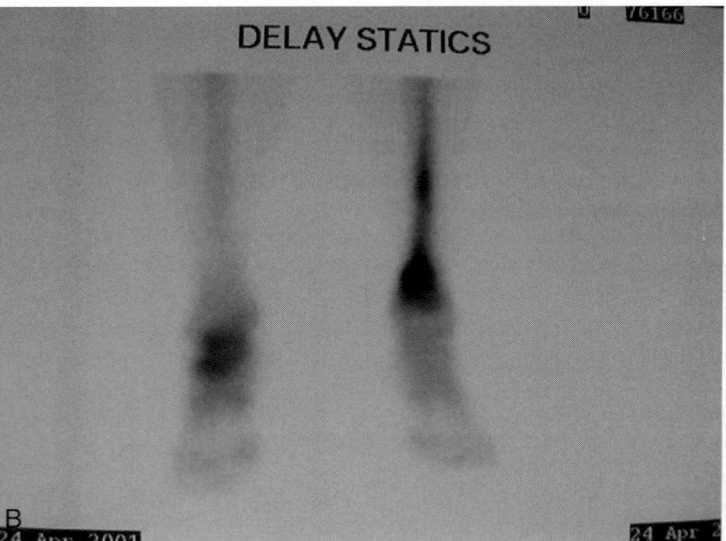

Figure 30F–1. *A,* Minimal radiographic findings with no cortical involvement. *B,* Diagnosis of tibial stress fracture confirmed by technetium[99m] bone scan. (Courtesy of James W. Brodsky, MD.)

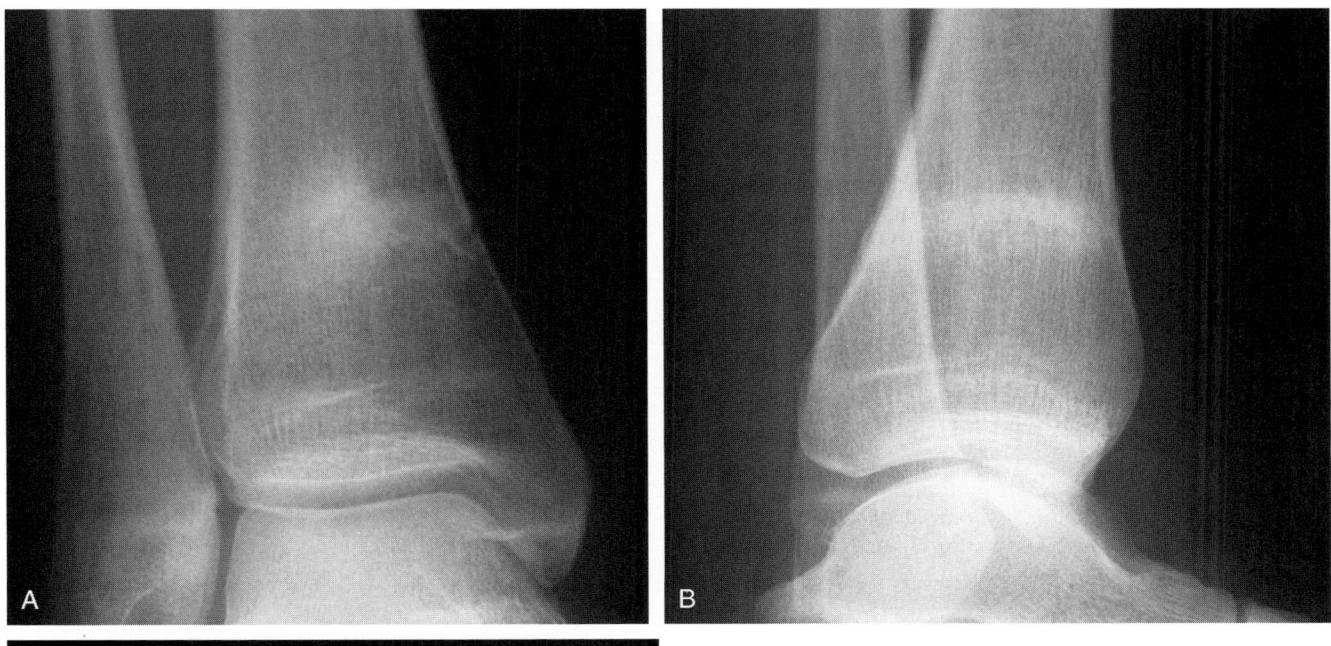

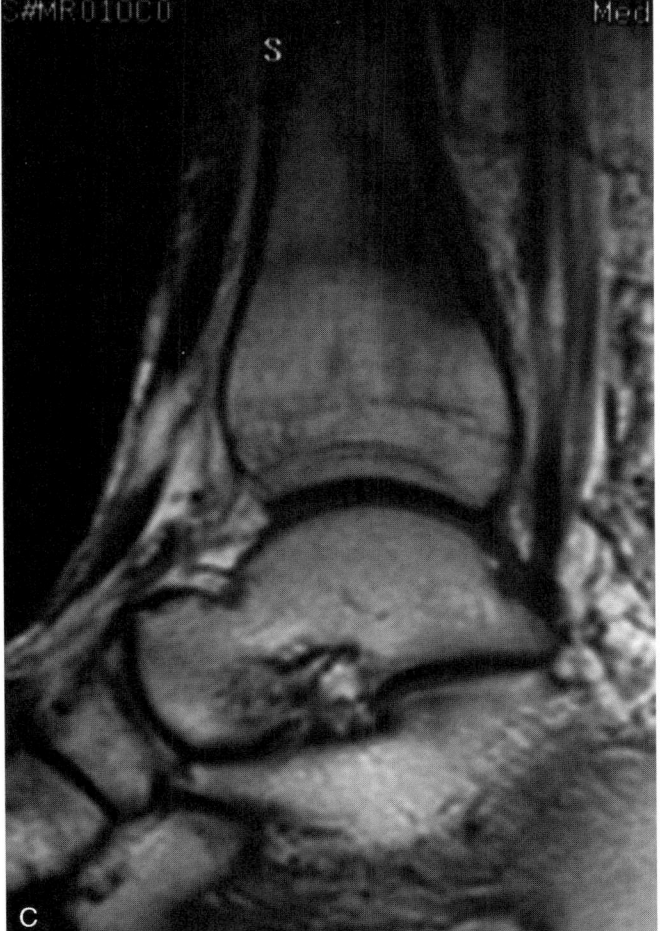

Figure 30F–2. *A* and *B,* Tibial stress fracture: Incomplete medial to lateral, but cortical portion facilitates diagnosis. *C,* Magnetic resonance imaging also demonstrates the lesion with high sensitivity. (Courtesy of James W. Brodsky, MD.)

Traditionally, immobilization has signified cast application. The advent of prefabricated braces, orthoses, and walking boots, as well as rigid-soled shoes, has made it easier to comply with immobilization. Although the use of casts has been supplanted in many cases, there are still many instances in which the superior immobilization provided by a cast is required in treatment of the fracture. The advantage of the removable devices is that even in fractures that require strict non–weight-bearing, the benefit of being able to remove the device for bathing is exceeded by the benefit of the patient being able to perform active range of motion exercises to maintain some muscle tone and bulk, and to reduce joint stiffness and the period of rehabilitation once the fracture is healed. The majority of stress fractures of the foot and ankle heal by the application of these two principal treatments alone.

Dietary change and metabolic treatment are important adjuncts to treatment of stress fracture in the patient with insufficiency fracture, less for the healing of the specific stress fracture than for the prevention of future stress fractures, because stabilization or reversal of the disease process is slow. Fractures in osteoporotic bone are not slower to heal than those in normal bone; however, they heal with the same porotic bone. Dietary and metabolic interventions are frequently supervised by an internal medicine or endocrine specialist. These include adequate intake of calcium with vitamin D in a diet that has sufficient calories and protein to ensure that the patient is not in a catabolic state. These interventions also frequently include hormone replacement therapy in postmenopausal women (unless there is a medical contraindication such as a history of estrogen-sensitive breast cancer) and occasionally the use of osteoblast-inhibiting medications such as nasal calcitonin (Miacalcin) or alendronate (Fosamax).

Although surgery is required in the minority of stress fractures of the foot and ankle, the need for surgery follows the same basic indications as for other fractures: Nonunion, malunion, or displacement that would lead to either of the two. In practical terms, there are several stress fractures of the foot and ankle for which surgery is more the rule than the exception, although the opposite is true for the rest. Those fractures that frequently require surgery are stress fractures of the tarsal navicular and the Jones fifth metatarsal fracture at the junction of the proximal metaphysis and diaphysis of the fifth metatarsal. Fractures that not infrequently require surgery are stress fractures of the base of the second metatarsal, disruption of the synchondrosis between the accessory and primary navicular bones, and stress fractures of the sesamoids of the hallux. Specific recommendations are discussed in the following sections.

It should be emphasized to all patients with fractures, injuries, or surgeries of the foot or ankle that it is typical to have a great deal of swelling, and for the swelling to be very persistent, often lasting 6 months or longer.

Specific Fractures and Their Treatment

Ankle Fractures

Stress fractures of the supramalleolar area are relatively uncommon. Fractures of the distal tibial metaphysis are most often associated with overuse, usually in the absence of deformity. Factors that increase the risk of a distal tibial stress fracture include previous prolonged immobilization, change in the modulus of elasticity of the bone caused by adjacent internal fixation, osteoporosis, and sudden increase in physical activity. Radiographic appearance often does not include a cortical component of the fracture. The initially negative radiographs later demonstrate condensation of new bone within the diaphysis (see Fig. 30F–2A and B), which seldom progresses to a complete fracture or to any discernible displacement (Fig. 30F–3). Treatment consists of immobilization and patience, as these tend to be slow to heal. An initial period of non–weight-bearing of 6 to 8 weeks is followed by weight-bearing immobilization until symptoms subside entirely. Weaning out of the removable walking brace is followed by participation in a rehabilitation program.

In contrast to distal tibial fractures, stress fractures of the distal fibular diaphysis and metaphysis are not infrequently associated with deformity. Typically, this would be a valgus hindfoot that increases biomechanical stress on the distal fibula (Fig. 30F–4). Otherwise, the same predisposing factors apply as those enumerated in the discussion of stress fractures of the distal tibia. As early as 1940, Burrows subclassified stress fractures of the distal fibula into two groups—young male athletes with fractures 5 to 6 cm proximal to the distal tip of the lateral malleolus; and middle-aged females with fractures 3 to 4 cm proximal to the malleolar tip (Fig. 30F–5).[11, 36, 45] Treatment for the two groups is substantially the same, that is, immobilization and/or activity modification. In the second subgroup, consideration should be given to metabolic status and appropriate diagnostic tests or referral should be considered. As with all stress fractures, clinical healing may precede completion of radiographic fracture healing. Surgery is seldom required.

Fractures of the medial malleolus, which are even less common than supramalleolar fractures of either the tibia or fibula, tend to be fatigue-type fractures due to overexertion in athletes or patients initiating a new exercise program.

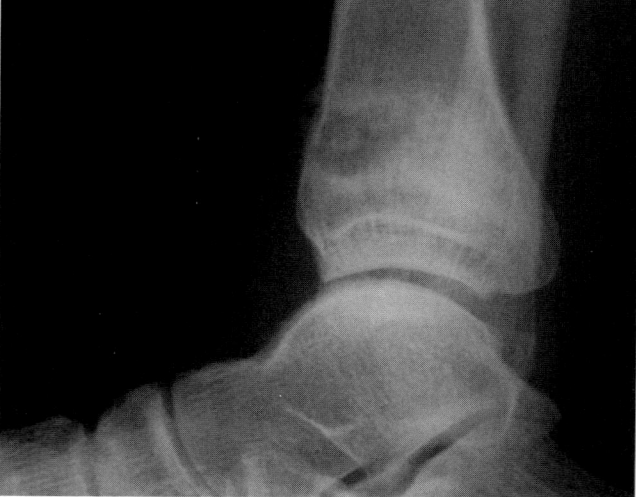

Figure 30F–3. Less typical finding of cystic resorption at tibial stress fracture site. (Courtesy of James W. Brodsky, MD.)

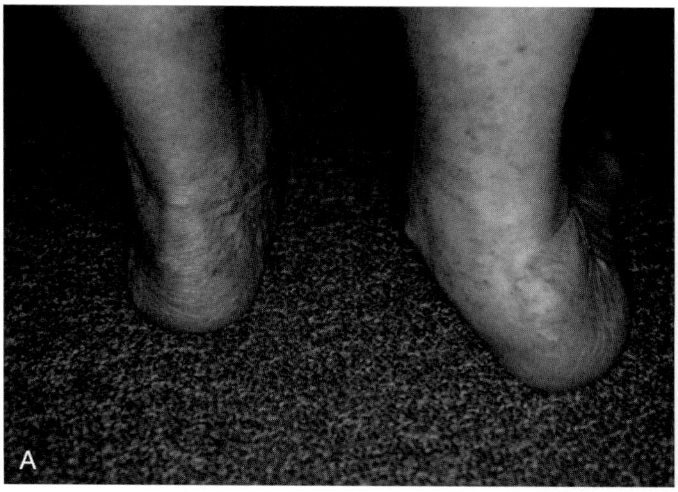

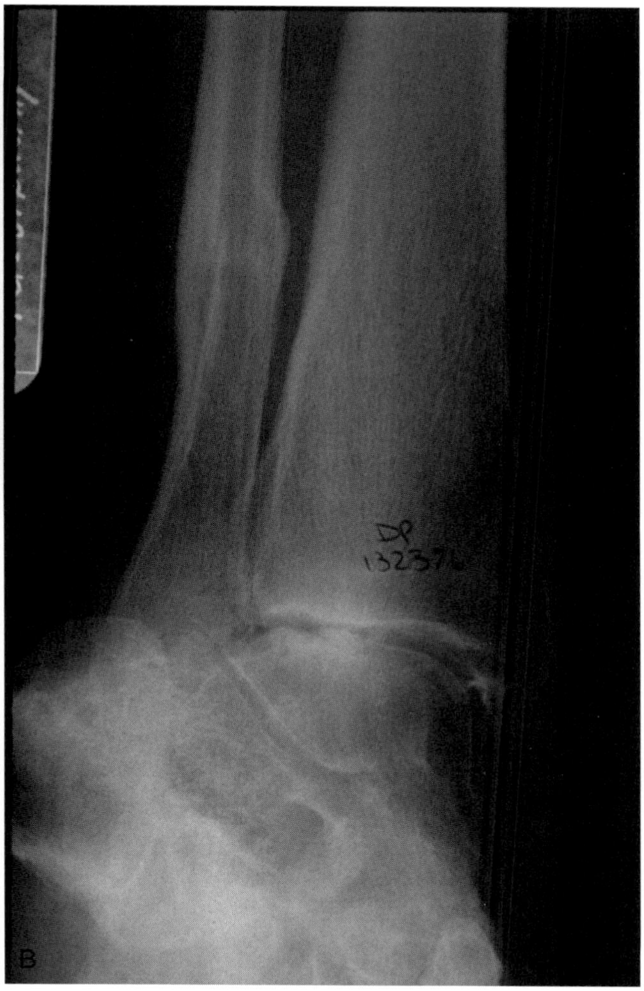

Figure 30F–4. Patient with valgus hindfoot *(A)* developed this fibular stress fracture *(B)* after initiation of a walking program. (Courtesy of James W. Brodsky, MD.)

Although general treatment principles should be followed, treatment is more likely to be surgical because of a greater proclivity for nonunion. Nonsurgical treatment with immobilization can and should be used initially in most patients. Exceptions include fractures that are fully intra-articular, displaced fractures, and fractures in selected professional or other serious athletes who require the fastest possible return to sport. Percutaneous screw fixation is an excellent choice unless the fracture has displaced or has developed a delayed union or nonunion. Bone grafting should be considered in cases of nonunion or delayed union. Illustrated in Figure 30F–6 is a professional basketball player with recurrent stress fractures of both medial malleoli. Neither pedobarographic analysis nor gait laboratory evaluation revealed an underlying biomechanical abnormality to explain the occurrence of the fractures. Treatment in this individual was variably successful, with failures and recurrences both after periods of immobilization and after internal fixation with and without bone grafting.

Fractures of the Hindfoot and Midfoot

Stress fractures of the talus are quite uncommon and are seen most often in runners and military recruits, but can occur in dancers and jumping athletes such as gymnasts. Fractures classically occur in the talar neck, but several reports describe talar process (i.e., lateral, posteromedial, posterolateral) stress fractures. Treatment is usually nonoperative, but the challenge is to make the diagnosis promptly. Plain radiographs are typically unrevealing, and an imaging study such as MRI or technetium scanning is required in most cases. Making the diagnosis can be difficult owing to the misleading, deep but vague localization of the patient's pain. Healing time varies, averaging between 2 and 4 months.

Fractures of the posterolateral process of the talus and disruption of the synchondrosis between an os trigonum and the posterior body of the talus are also uncommon injuries. They are most typically associated with classical ballet because of the hyperplantar flexion of the tibiotalar joint when the female dancer is dancing on toe *(en pointe)*.[8, 25] An important variation of stress fracture is the posterior impingement of the os trigonum against the posterior tibia, which causes direct mechanical pain (Fig. 30F–7). This often requires excision of the os trigonum through a posterior or posterolateral approach, usually with excellent results.[8, 25]

Stress injuries of the lateral process of the talus are very unusual. Cases of acute fracture, although uncommon, are

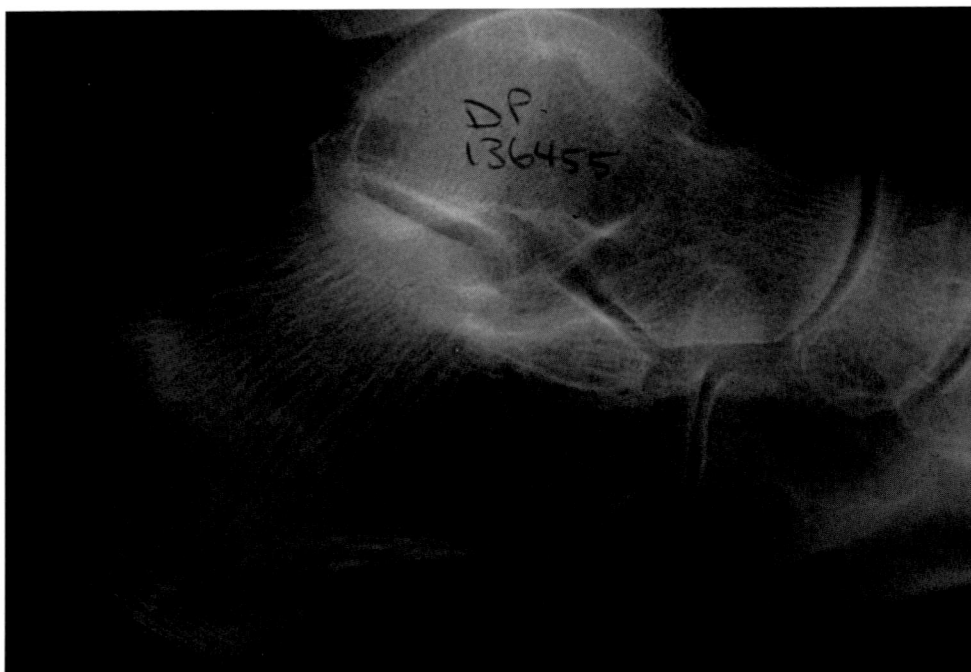

Figure 30F–9. Calcaneal stress fracture in a runner. The propagation of the fracture from the superior cortex of the tubercle is the most common pattern. (Courtesy of James W. Brodsky, MD.)

rarity in relation to other common heel pain diagnoses, stress fractures of the calcaneus are frequently overlooked because the initial radiographs are nearly always negative, and the pain is frequently quite diffuse and nonspecific. Although imaging studies such as MRI or technetium bone scan may be required to make the diagnosis, repeat radiographs after an interval of several weeks eventually show the typical, albeit often subtle, radiographic appearance. Calcaneal stress fractures are typically incomplete and manifest as a vertical condensation or radiodensity within the cancellous bone of the calcaneal tubercle. This usually occurs in the dorsal two thirds as can be seen on the lateral standing radiograph of the foot, and does not extend down to the plantar cortex (Fig. 30F–9). Rarely, the fracture might be posterior in the tubercle (Fig. 30F–10). Changes on the imaging studies correspond to the same anatomic distribution as that described for radiographs. Technetium bone scans that show increased uptake on the plantar surface of the calcaneus do not signify stress fracture, but rather are typical of plantar fasciitis. The inflammatory process at the insertion of the plantar fascia involves the periosteum and Sharpey's fibers, the latter of which produce the positive uptake on the scan.

On close physical examination, the distinguishing characteristic of calcaneal stress fracture is that the pain is dorsal and anterior on the calcaneal tubercle, and the patient will point to the medial and lateral sides of the heel anterior to the Achilles tendon as the center of the pain. Treatment consists of diminished activity with variable immobilization until symptoms subside, usually between 2 and 3 months.

Stress fractures of the tarsal navicular are the most difficult stress fractures of the foot and ankle to treat because of the typically slow and recalcitrant healing. Presentation is one of vague, poorly localized pain that is gradual in onset. On careful questioning, the patient will point to the dorsum of the hindfoot, but the examiner can easily be misled into thinking that the pain emanates from the adjacent tibiotalar joint. These relatively uncommon fractures occur primarily in running athletes. The largest series to date is that undertaken by Torg and associates.[60] They showed that all 21 of the fractures in their study were in the sagittal plane, in the central one third of the navicular. Microangiographic studies showed the central one third

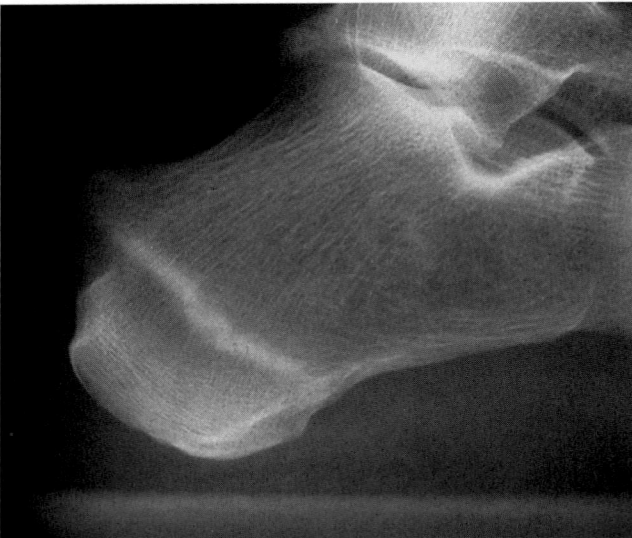

Figure 30F–10. Persistent heel pain in this 29-year-old woman was initially attributed to plantar fasciitis at another institution, where her radiographs were negative. After an interval of 4 weeks, the stress fracture of the calcaneal tubercle became apparent. (Courtesy of James W. Brodsky, MD.)

of the navicular to be relatively avascular.[60] Strict enforcement of non–weight-bearing has a markedly positive impact on healing of the fracture.

The routine, three-view foot radiographic evaluation is frequently unrevealing because the navicular is underpenetrated and the fracture is in the sagittal plane. Cone down views assist in diagnosis. Telltale radiographic signs include sclerosis in the subchondral bone adjacent to the talonavicular joint. Although bone scan or MRI adequately screens for the presence of a navicular stress fracture, the study of choice is computed tomography (CT). Sections in two planes are recommended. Images in the coronal plane should be parallel to the talonavicular joint and roughly parallel to the plantar surface of the foot. The typical appearance of the fracture on CT scan is a vertical fracture line (in the sagittal plane) that begins on the dorsum of the navicular, proceeds plantarward, and is almost always incomplete (Fig. 30F–11A to C). Although Torg and associates[60] described these as occurring in the central third, the location is usually more lateral than medial, and often at the junction of the medial two thirds and the lateral third. Sclerosis usually is noted on both sides of the fracture, which in the horizontal plane extends to and through the proximal subchondral bone of the navicular at the talonavicular joint. The location of the fracture line has been demonstrated to correspond to a zone of avascularity in the tarsal navicular. The intraosseous blood supply has been shown to enter from medial and lateral poles of the bone, and to diminish in the zone where the fracture occurs.

Tarsal navicular stress fractures frequently require surgical intervention because diagnosis is commonly delayed. If treatment is initiated early, an attempt at non–weight-bearing immobilization should be tried. Surgical treatment consists of bone grafting and internal fixation; the surgical procedure is technically challenging. The incision should be on the dorsolateral aspect of the hindfoot, corresponding to the lateral one third of the navicular bone. The fracture site is exposed and carefully débrided. The major pitfall is to lose the three-dimensional orientation of the navicular bone, so one must remember that the medial and lateral parts of the articular surface (and cartilage) are more proximal, and the articular surface is farther distal in the midportion of the bone. Thus, it is easy to penetrate the central portion of the proximal articular surface, damaging the talonavicular joint. Further risks to the joint are posed by the placement of the internal fixation screws, again attributable to the sharply curved proximal articular surface of the navicular. The screws are best and most easily placed from lateral to medial because the medial fragment is larger, thus affording a greater area for placement of the

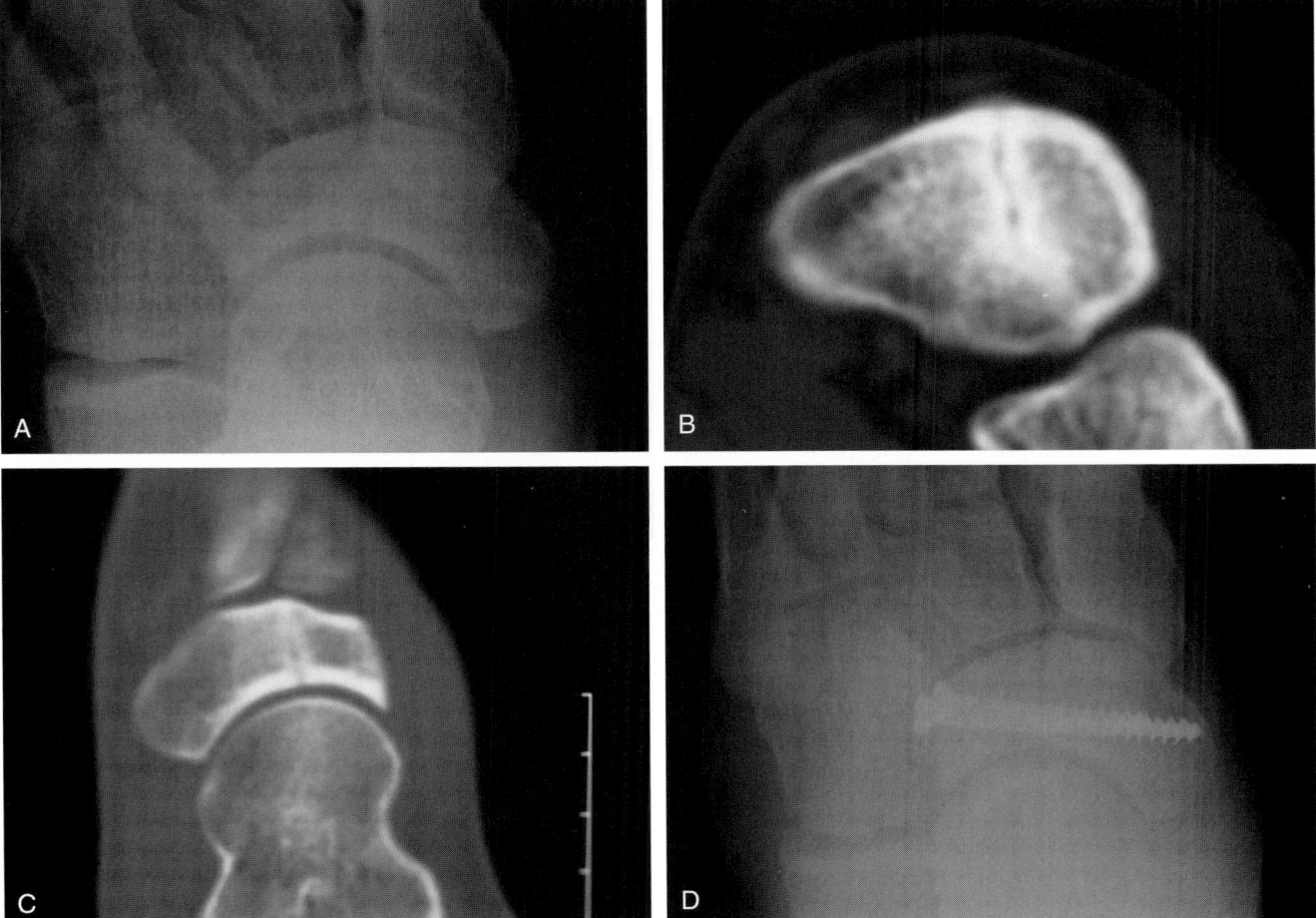

Figure 30F–11. *A,* Defensive lineman with vague, persistent hindfoot pain. Very subtle linear lucency in navicular on radiograph. *B* and *C,* Computed tomography confirmed the diagnosis. *D,* Patient was treated with internal fixation and bone grafting. (Courtesy of James W. Brodsky, MD.)

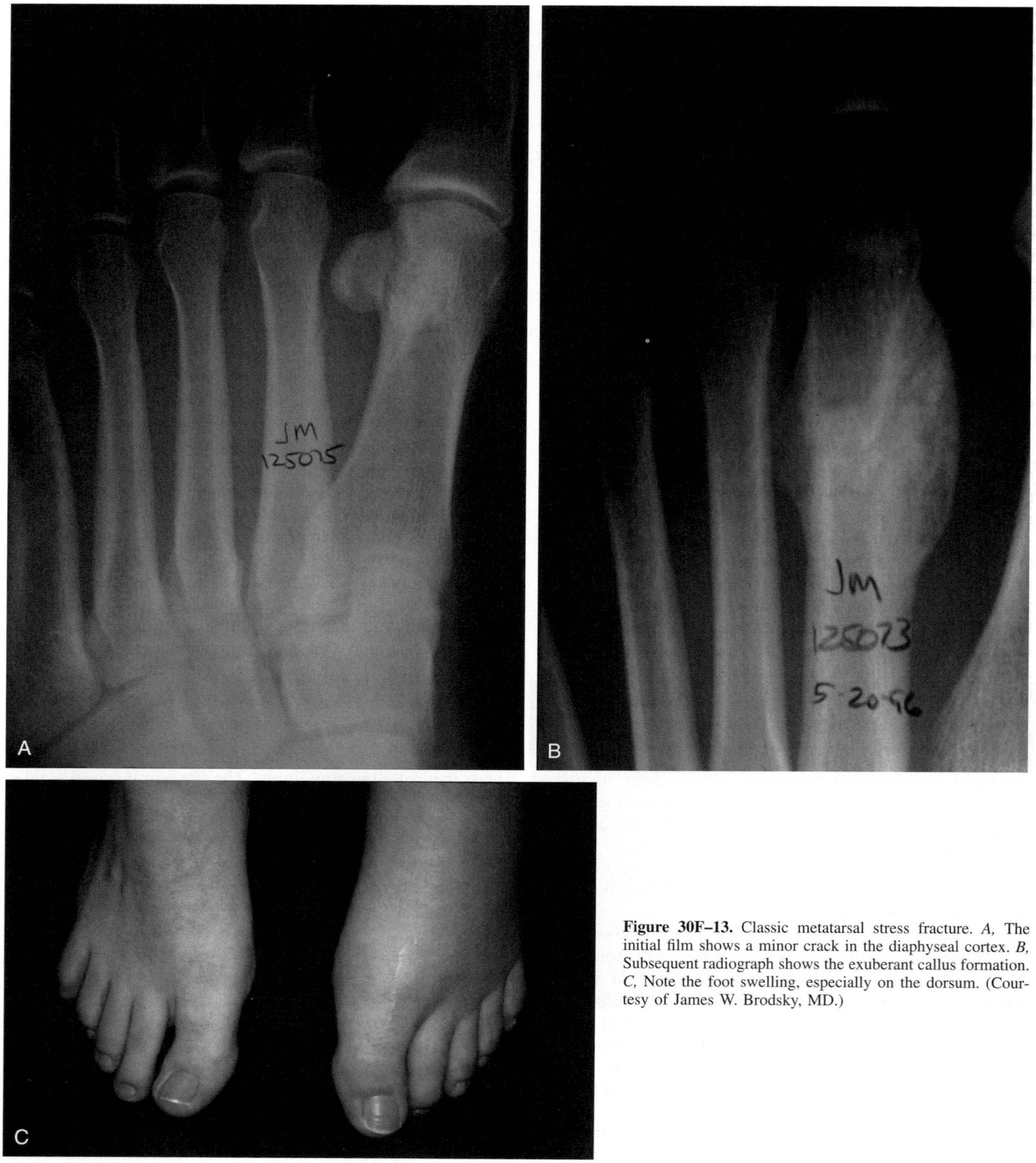

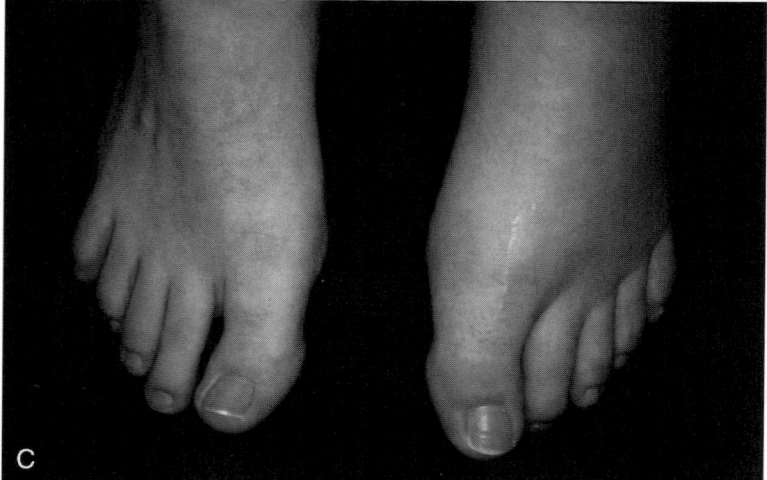

Figure 30F–13. Classic metatarsal stress fracture. *A,* The initial film shows a minor crack in the diaphyseal cortex. *B,* Subsequent radiograph shows the exuberant callus formation. *C,* Note the foot swelling, especially on the dorsum. (Courtesy of James W. Brodsky, MD.)

especially in cases with evidence of a hypertrophic non-union, or chronic stress injury. Six weeks of cast immobilization and non–weight-bearing is recommended after surgery, followed by appropriate progression, based on radiographic findings, to weight-bearing in a below-the-knee boot. In high-performance athletes, it is recommended that the screw be retained after healing, as long as the player continues to compete, because of the risk of recurrent fracture. Once the fracture is healed, strong consideration should be given to the use of a supportive athletic shoe and a custom-molded cushioning orthosis. A good example is a dual-density device made of a heat-molded polyethylene foam (e.g., medium-grade plastazote or Pelite) combined with a nondeforming open-cell foam (e.g.,

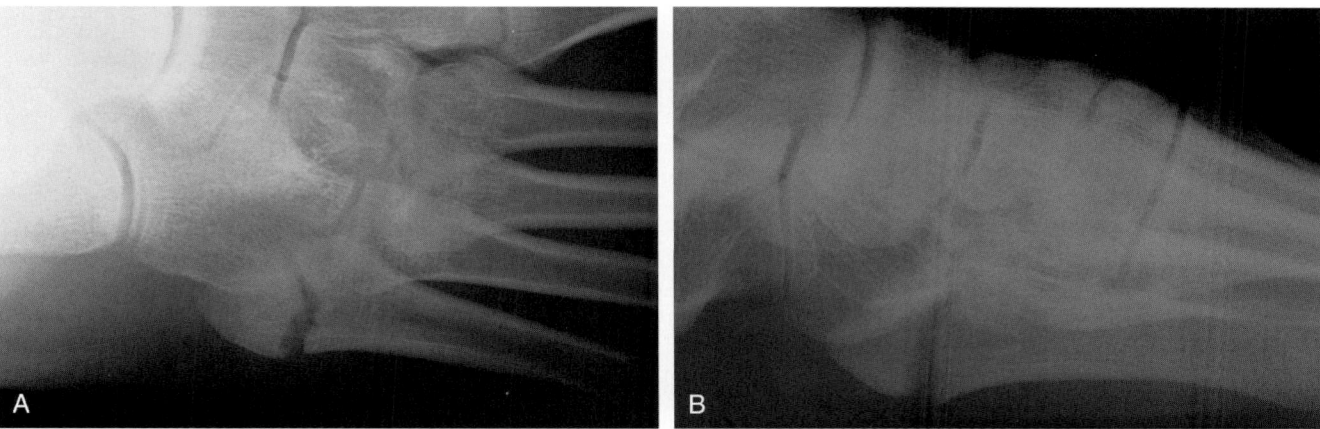

Figure 30F–14. A "dancer's fracture." This is the most common foot fracture, that is, avulsion fracture of the base of the fifth metatarsal associated with acute inversion injury. (Courtesy of James W. Brodsky, MD.)

Figure 30F–15. Acute Jones fracture at the diaphyseal-metaphyseal junction of the fifth metatarsal. (Courtesy of James W. Brodsky, MD.)

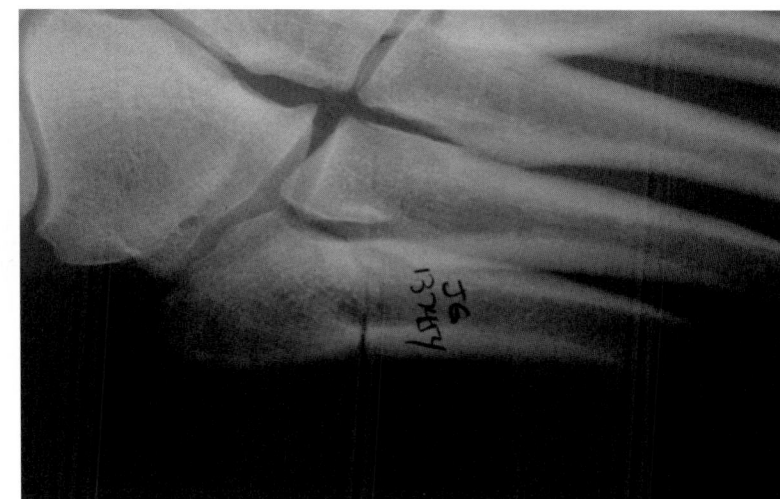

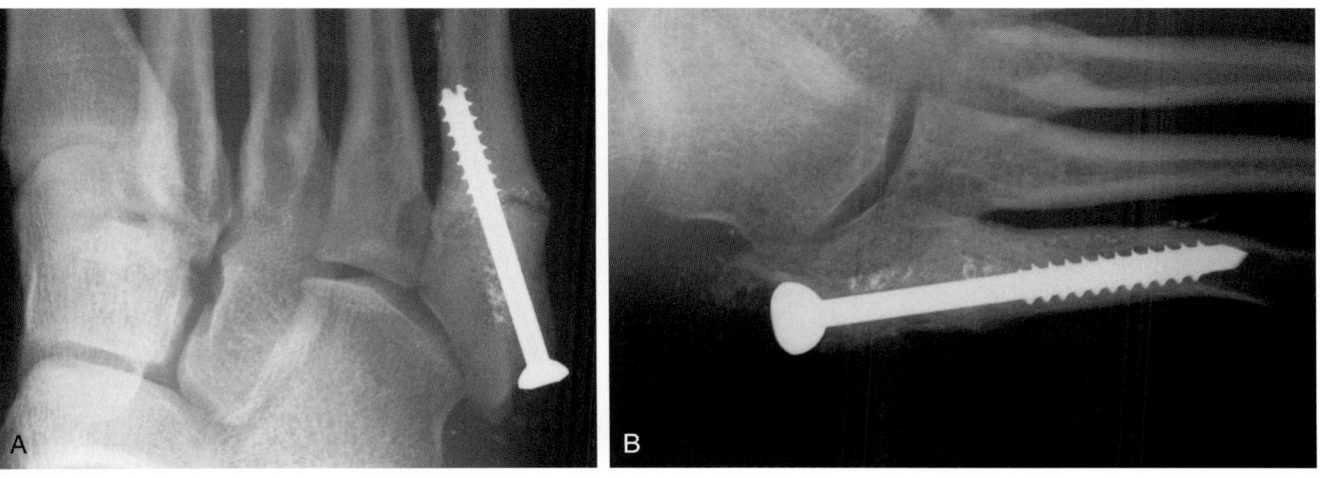

Figure 30F–16. Images of 18-year-old collegiate soccer player with recurrent pain and nonunion of Jones fracture after previous surgery. *A,* Note the hypertrophic beaking and sclerosis at the fracture site. *B,* Healing was achieved 10 weeks after revision intramedullary fixation and bone grafting. (Courtesy of James W. Brodsky, MD.)

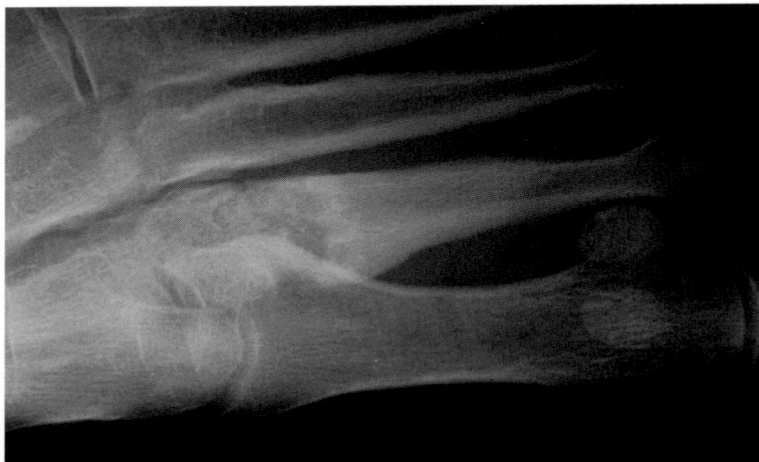

Figure 30F–17. A 66-year-old woman with large joint osteoarthritis developed this stress fracture of the proximal second metatarsal while participating in a walking program for knee rehabilitation. Note the chronic hypertrophy of the metatarsal. (Courtesy of James W. Brodsky, MD.)

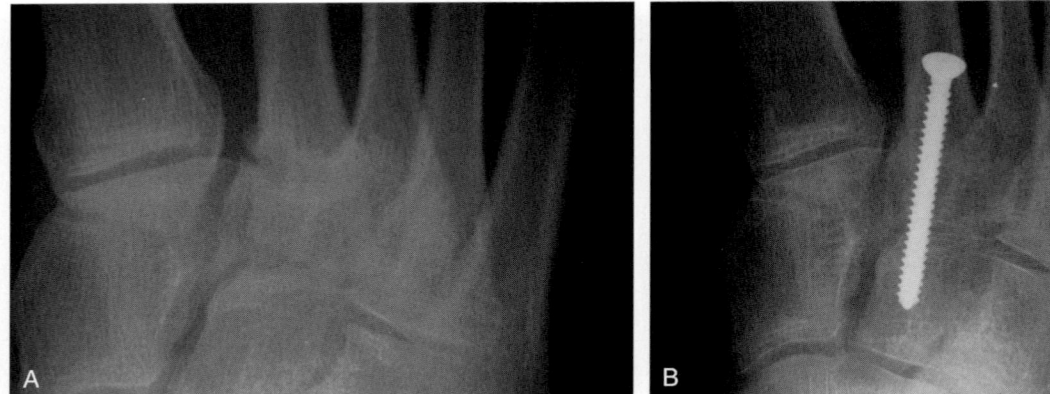

Figure 30F–18. Image of a 27-year-old woman with persistent dull midfoot pain. The correct diagnosis of stress fracture of the base of the second metatarsal was made after 1 year of multiple consultations. Operative treatment required bone grafting as well as arthrodesis of the metatarsal-cuneiform joint. (Courtesy of James W. Brodsky, MD.)

poron). To the plantar surface of the orthosis should be added a lateral wedge to counter the varus thrust of the hindfoot, and to facilitate the transfer of weight to the medial side of the midfoot.

Risk factors for the Jones fracture include a high level of activity in a running and/or jumping athlete. This fracture is typically seen in soccer and basketball players, although its occurrence is not exclusive of other sports and activities. Athletes with hindfoot varus of any cause have a predilection for this fracture because of lateral column overloading.

Basilar metatarsal stress fractures are less common among the general population but are the most common stress fracture seen in ballet dancers.[27, 48] The typical location is at the proximal metaphyseal-diaphyseal junction, with possible extension into the tarsometatarsal joint. Multiple theories exist as to the mechanism for a basilar metatarsal fracture; all of these theories center around the *en pointe* position.

Fractures of the bases of the metatarsals are less common than are those of the diaphysis and neck, but they are not rare.[48] Most typically, this fracture occurs at the base of the second metatarsal (Fig. 30F–17). By the time it is diagnosed, radiographs demonstrate sclerosis without

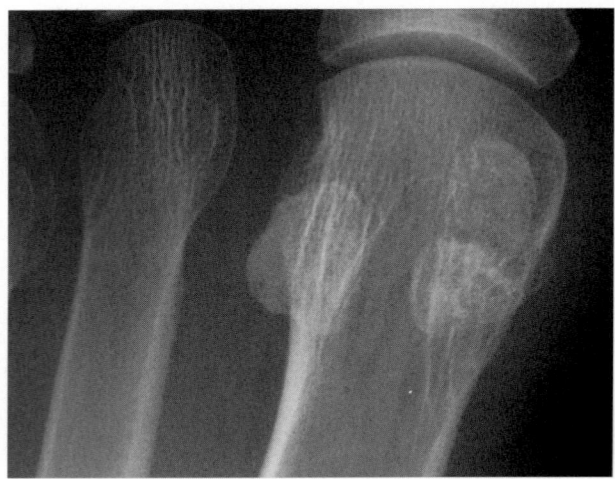

Figure 30F–19. Stress fracture of the medial sesamoids. Note the irregular edges, the elongation compared with the lateral sesamoids, and the difference in density of the proximal and distal portions. (Courtesy of James W. Brodsky, MD.)

displacement. The patient gives a history of chronic aching in the midfoot region, which must be distinguished from tarsometatarsal arthritis. Some of these fractures are chronically symptomatic but not so severe as to demand surgery, although they seldom heal with immobilization alone. Some patients elect to live with the pseudarthrosis untreated. Most require surgical intervention with bone grafting, with or without internal fixation. If the fracture is

very close to the second tarsometatarsal joint, it may be technically impossible to achieve fixation to the narrow proximal fragment. In these cases, it may be necessary to do an arthrodesis of the adjacent joint in order to gain stabilization and fixation (Fig. 30F–18).

Stress injury to the hallux sesamoids is relatively common in active populations. The hallux sesamoids are the points of weight transfer along the medial column of the

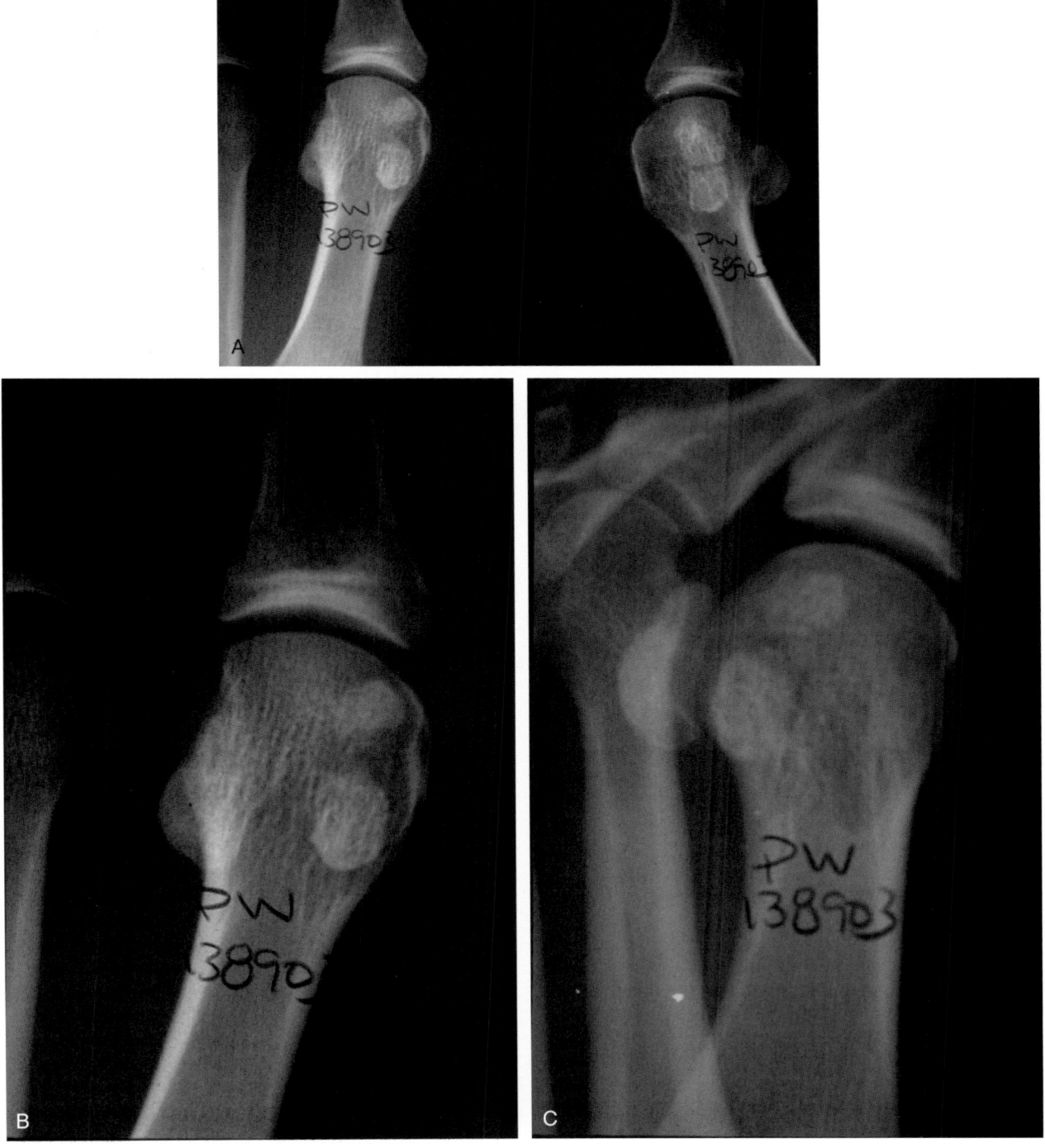

Figure 30F–20. Sesamoid fracture equivalent: There is disruption of the synchondrosis of this bipartite sesamoid. Note the separation between the two poles. (Courtesy of James W. Brodsky, MD.)

forefoot, and they are covered with very little soft tissue padding. Injuries to the sesamoids vary from acute fracture and stress fracture to sesamoiditis. Sesamoid stress fractures can occur in either the medial or the lateral sesamoid. The medial sesamoid is usually slightly larger than the lateral, and fracture of the medial sesamoid is somewhat more common.[62] The sesamoids are often difficult to visualize on radiographs because of the obscuring shadow of the first metatarsal head (Fig. 30F–19).

Patients with sesamoid stress fractures are generally active, although most give a history of a recent change in activity level. They present with insidious onset of medial forefoot pain, primarily with weight-bearing activities; this pain is exacerbated by running, jumping, and participating in toe-off activities. Physical examination reveals tenderness localized to the plantar first metatarsophalangeal joint (tenderness may localize to a specific sesamoid), which is worsened with passive dorsiflexion and plantar flexion of the hallux. Ecchymosis and swelling are unlikely. Radiographs may demonstrate a transverse fracture of the sesamoid, but differentiation from a bipartite sesamoid becomes problematic (Fig. 30F–20). If physical examination does not absolutely localize the pain to a specific sesamoid, anteroposterior (AP) and sesamoid views with a metallic marker are helpful. In most patients, treatment can be initiated without additional studies. If an absolute diagnosis is necessary, bone scan (from the plantar surface of the foot) is the modality of choice.[12]

Treatment is largely conservative, with activity modification and the use of off-loading orthoses being the mainstay of treatment. Protected weight-bearing in a cast or boot is used in recalcitrant cases and in those with a definite acute fracture line on plain films. Surgical treatment is reserved for cases that are recalcitrant to nonoperative treatment and symptomatic cases with radiographically documented distraction between the fragments. Sesamoid excision and reconstruction of the flexor hallucis brevis tendon and intersesamoid ligament is the appropriate surgical treatment. This approach has led to good results in the authors' hands, with little evidence of late hallux deformity. The soft tissue reconstruction is critical to obtaining a good result because the position of the remaining sesamoids must be maintained and late deviation of the great toe must be prevented. (The risk is that hallux valgus deformity may develop after medial sesamoid excision, and hallux varus after excision of the lateral sesamoids.) Other authors have suggested bone grafting of nondisplaced sesamoid nonunions, with satisfactory results. This approach has been reported in a small series of young, primarily collegiate athletes.[2]

Although partial excision of one of the poles of the fractured sesamoid has been suggested, this seldom is feasible unless one piece is very much smaller than the other. Leaving half-sesamoids usually results in a painful condition due to the poor tracking of the fragment under the metatarsal condyles.

References

1. Anderson MW, Greenspan A: Stress fractures. Radiology 199:1–12, 1996.
2. Anderson RB, McBryde AM Jr: Autogenous bone grafting of hallux sesamoid nonunions. Foot Ankle Int 18:293–296, 1997.
3. Barrow GW, Saha S: Menstrual irregularity and stress fractures in collegiate female distance runners. Am J Sports Med 16:209–216, 1988.
4. Belkin SC: Stress fractures in athletes. Orthop Clin North Am 11:735, 1980.
5. Bennell KL, Malcolm SA, Thomas SA, et al: Risk factors for stress fractures in female track-and-field athlete: A retrospective analysis. Clin J Sport Med 5:229, 1995.
6. Bennell KL, Malcolm SA, Thomas SA, et al: The incidence and distribution of stress fractures in competitive track and field athletes. Am J Sports Med 245:211, 1996.
7. Bradshaw C, Khan K, Brukner P: Stress fracture of the body of the talus in athletes demonstrated with computer tomography. Clin J Sport Med 6:48, 1996.
8. Brodsky AE, Kahlil MA: Talar compression syndrome. Foot Ankle 7:338, 1987.
9. Brudvig TJ, Gudger TD, Obermeyer L: Stress fracture in 295 trainees: A one year study as related to age, sex, and race. Mil Med 148:666, 1983.
10. Brukner P, Bradshaw C, Khan KM, et al: Stress fractures: A review of 180 cases. Clin J Sport Med 6:85–89, 1996.
11. Burrows HJ: Spontaneous fracture of the apparently normal fibula in its lowest third. J Bone Joint Surg 28:82, 1940.
12. Chisin R, Peyser A, Milgrom C: Bone scintigraphy in the assessment of the hallucal sesamoids. Foot Ankle Int 16:291, 1995.
13. Cook SD, Harding AF, Thomas KA, et al: Trabecular bone density and menstrual function in women runners. Am J Sports Med 15:503–507, 1987.
14. Creighton R, Sonoga A, Gordon G: Stress fracture of the tarsal middle cuneiform bone. J Am Podiatr Med Assoc 80:489, 1990.
15. Darby RE: Stress fractures of the os calcis. JAMA 200:131, 1967.
16. Delacerda FG: A case study: Application of ultrasound to determine a stress fracture of the fibula. J Orthop Sports Phys Ther 2:134, 1981.
17. Drez D, Young JC, Johnston RD, et al: Metatarsal stress fractures. Am J Sports Med 8:123–125, 1980.
18. Eisele SA, Sammarco GJ: Fatigue fractures of the foot and ankle in the athlete. J Bone Joint Surg Am 75:290, 1993.
19. Fishco WD, Stiles RG: Atypical heel pain, hyperparathyroidism-induced stress fracture of the calcaneus. J Am Podiatr Med Assoc 89:413–418, 1999.
20. Ford LT, Gilula LA: Stress fractures of the middle metatarsals following the Keller operation. J Bone Joint Surg Am 59:117–118, 1977.
21. Frusztajer NT, Dhuper S, Warren MP, et al: Nutrition and the incidence of stress fractures in ballet dancers. Am J Clin Nutr 51:779, 1990.
22. Giladi M, Milgrom C, Stein M, et al: The low arch, a protective factor in stress fractures. A prospective study of 295 military recruits. Orthop Rev 14:709–712, 1985.
23. Giladi M, Milgrom C, Simkin A, et al: Stress fractures, identifiable risk factors. Am J Sports Med 19:647–652, 1991.
24. Griffin LY: Common sports injuries of the foot and ankle seen in children and adolescents. Orthop Clin North Am 25:83, 1994.
25. Hamilton WG: Stenosing tenosynovitis of the flexor hallucis longus tendon and posterior impingement upon the os trigonum in ballet dancers. Foot Ankle 3:74, 1982.
26. Hardy DC, Delince PE, Yasik E, et al: Stress fracture of the hip: An unusual complication of total knee arthroplasty. Clin Orthop Rel Res 281:140–144, 1992.
27. Harrington T, Crichton KJ, Anderson IF: Overuse ballet injury of the base of the second metatarsal. Am J Sports Med 21:591, 1993.
28. Helstad PE, Ringstrom JB, Erdmann BB, et al: Bilateral stress fractures of the tarsal navicular with associated avascular necrosis in a pole vaulter. J Am Podiatr Med Assoc 86:551, 1996.
29. Hickey GJ, Fricker PA, McDonald WA: Injuries to young elite basketball players over a six-year period. Clin J Sport Med 7:252, 1997.
30. Hopson CN, Perry DR: Stress fractures of the calcaneus in women marine recruits. Clin Orthop 128:159, 1977.
31. Hulkko A, Orava S, Pellinen P: Stress fractures of the sesamoid bones of the first metatarsophalangeal joint in athletes. Arch Orthop Trauma Surg 104:113, 1985.
32. Hulkko A, Orava S, Peltokallio P, et al: Stress fracture of the navicular bone: Nine cases in athletes. Acta Orthop Scand 56:503, 1985.
33. Jones R: Fractures of the base of the fifth metatarsal by indirect violence. Ann Surg 35:697–700, 1902.

34. Kadel NJ, Teitz CC, Kronmal RA: Stress fractures in ballet dancers. Am J Sports Med 20:4465–4469, 1992.
35. Kaufman KR, Brodine SK, Shaffer RA, et al: The effect of foot structure and range of motion on musculoskeletal overuse injuries. Am J Sports Med 25:585–593, 1999.
36. Kaye R: Insufficiency stress fractures of the foot and ankle in post-menopausal women. Foot Ankle Int 19:221–224, 1998.
37. Lee JK, Yao L: Stress fractures: MR imaging. Radiology 169:217–220, 1998.
38. Li G, Zhang S, Chen C, et al: Radiographic and histologic analysis of stress fracture in rabbit tibias. Am J Sports Med 13:285–294, 1985.
39. Mann RA, Baxter DE, Lutter LD: Running symposium. Foot Ankle 1:190, 1981.
40. Matheson GO, Clement DB, McKenzie DC, et al: Stress fractures in athletes: A study of 320 cases. Am J Sports Med 15:46, 1987.
41. Matin P: The appearance of bone scans following fractures, including immediate and long-term studies. J Nucl Med 20:1227–1231, 1979.
42. Meurman KOA, Elfving S: Stress fractures of the cuneiform bones. Br J Radiol 53:157, 1980.
43. Milgrom C, Giladi M, Stein M, et al: Stress fracture in military recruits: A prospective study showing an unusually high incidence. J Bone Joint Surg Br 67:732, 1985.
44. Miller B, Markheim HR, Towbin MN: Multiple stress fractures in rheumatoid arthritis. J Bone Joint Surg Am 49:1408–1414, 1967.
45. Miller MD, Marks PH, Fu FH: Bilateral stress fractures of the distal fibula in a 35-year-old woman. Foot Ankle Int 15:450, 1994.
46. Motto SG: Stress fracture of the lateral process of the talus—A case report. Br J Sport Med 27:275, 1993.
47. Myburgh KH, Hutchins J, Fataar AB, et al: Low bone density is an etiologic factor for stress fracture in athletes. Ann Intern Med 113:754–759, 1990.
48. O'Malley MJ, Hamilton WG, Munyak J, et al: Stress fractures at the base of the second metatarsal in ballet dancers. Foot Ankle Int 17:89, 1996.
49. Okada K, Senma S, Abe E, et al: Stress fractures of the medial malleolus: A case report. Foot Ankle Int 16:49, 1995.
50. Orava S, Karpakka J, Teimela S, et al: Stress fracture of the medial malleolus. J Bone Joint Surg Am 77:362, 1995.
51. Prather JL, Nusynowitz ML, Snowdy HA, et al: Scintigraphic findings in stress fractures. J Bone Joint Surg Am 59:869–874, 1977.
52. Prozman RR, Griffis CG: Stress fractures in men and women undergoing military training. J Bone Joint Surg Am 59:825, 1977.
53. Reider B, Falconiero R, Yurkofsky J: Nonunion of a medial malleolus stress fracture. Am J Sports Med 21:478, 1993.
54. Rudzki SJ: Injuries in Australian army recruits. Part II: Location and cause of injuries seen in recruits. Mil Med 162:477, 1997.
55. Sammarco GJ, Idusuyi OB: Stress fracture of the base of the third metatarsal after an endoscopic plantar fasciotomy: A case report. Foot Ankle Int 19:157–159, 1998.
56. Schweitzer M: Magnetic resonance imaging of the foot and ankle. Magn Reson Q 9:214–234, 1993.
57. Shiraishi M, Mizuta H, Kubota K, et al: Stress fractures of the proximal phalanx of the great toe. Foot Ankle 14:28, 1993.
58. Simkin A, Leichter I, Giladi M, et al: Combined effect of foot arch structure and an orthotic device on stress fractures. Foot Ankle 10:25–29, 1989.
59. Steinbronn DJ, Bennett GL, Kay DB: The use of magnetic resonance imaging in the diagnosis of stress fractures of the foot and ankle: Four case reports. Foot Ankle 15:80–83, 1994.
60. Torg JS, Pavlov H, Cooley JH, et al: Stress fractures of the tarsal navicular. J Bone Joint Surg Am 64:700, 1982.
61. Umans H, Pavlov H: Stress fractures of the lower extremities. Semin Roentgenol 19:176–193, 1994.
62. Van Hal ME, Keene JS, Lange TA, et al: Stress fractures of the great toe sesamoids. Am J Sports Med 10:122, 1982.
63. Wei N: Stress fractures of the distal fibula presenting as monoarticular flares in patients with rheumatoid arthritis. Arthritis Rheum 37:1555–1556, 1994.
64. Weinstein SB, Haddad SL, Myerson MS: Metatarsal stress fractures. Clin Sport Med 2:319, 1997.

Section G
Tendon Injuries of the Foot and Ankle
James S. Keene, MD

Although the Achilles tendon has been the focus of most reports on tendon injuries of the foot and ankle, athletes sustain many disabling injuries that involve other tendons (e.g., anterior and posterior tibial, flexor hallucis longus) in this anatomic region. The frequency of tendon injuries about the foot and ankle has been recorded in only a limited number of studies.[6, 77, 134, 157, 159] In 1959, Anzel and colleagues reviewed 1014 cases of muscle and tendon disruptions treated at the Mayo Clinic and found that 143 (14%) of the injuries occurred in the lower extremity.[6] Of these 143 injuries, 34 (24%) involved the Achilles tendon or triceps surae, 10 (7%) the anterior tibial, 3 (2%) the posterior tibial, 3 (2%) the flexor hallucis longus (FHL), and 2 (1%) the peroneus longus or brevis tendon. Although earlier studies[70, 71, 81] do not provide specific numbers or percentages, they do state that muscles and tendons are torn in the following order of frequency: triceps surae, quadriceps, biceps, triceps, and rectus abdominis.

Most of these studies emphasize the rarity of injuries to the tendons of the foot and ankle, and several suggest that these injuries, if untreated, cause little functional impairment.[26, 63, 109, 133, 171] Other studies emphasize that disruptions of the tendons of the foot and ankle, particularly those that

occur in the fibro-osseous tunnels, are subject to the same complications characterizing tendon injuries in other anatomic regions.* These latter studies conclude that the same principles of treatment, well established in injuries of the wrist and hand, should be applied to tendon injuries of the foot and ankle if maximum function is to be regained.

In this chapter, the issues related to operative versus nonoperative treatment of injuries to the Achilles, anterior and posterior tibial, FHL, and peroneal tendons are addressed, and pertinent demographic data (age, sex, sport, and so forth) relative to an athlete's predisposition to injure the aforementioned structures are delineated.

Injuries Defined

Before beginning a discussion of specific tendon injuries, it seems germane to define the terms used to describe and classify these conditions. The dictionary definition of

---

*See references 39, 74, 77, 101, 134, 147, 149, 159, 166, and 182.

malleolus. The other had locking of the ankle and painful inversion and eversion of the foot.[126] Surgery was performed on all four athletes with this problem.[20, 111, 126] At surgery, the posterior tibial tendon either was found to be lying over the medial malleolus or was easily dislocatable. In all cases, the majority of the deltoid ligament was intact, and the flexor retinaculum, which was torn, was sutured to the periosteum of the posterior margin of the medial malleolus. All athletes had excellent results from surgery and returned to their competitive sport, symptom free, 10 to 14 weeks after surgery.

The frequency of closed disruptions has only recently been appreciated.[101, 147, 254] In 1983, Johnson reported the results of 11 surgical repairs of ruptured posterior tibial tendons that were performed over a 3-year period.[101] In 1985, Mann and Thompson,[148] reported on 17 cases that were treated over a 4-year period, and noted that the results of only 50 operatively treated disruptions had been previously reported.[74, 98, 101, 109, 219, 240, 255] In 1991, Woods and Leach reported on six athletic people, 20 to 50 years of age, who required surgery for partial (three cases) or complete ruptures of the posterior tibial tendon.[254] Holmes and Mann reported on 67 patients diagnosed with rupture of the posterior tibial tendon.[88] They divided their 67 patients into older (>50 years of age) and younger (<50 years of age) groups. The profile of the older group was significantly different in that 60% of the cases were associated with hypertension, diabetes, and obesity. Younger patients had no significant association with the aforementioned problems, but 5 of these 14 patients had significant trauma to the foot.[88]

All of the aforementioned studies stressed that closed disruptions often are not diagnosed because the signs and symptoms, although pathognomonic, are not recognized. In Mann and Thompson's series of patients, all had seen one or more physicians (in only two was the proper diagnosis made), and the average delay in diagnosis was 43 months (range, 1 month to 12 years). Average time to diagnosis in Johnson's series of patients was 19 months; he noted that 10 of his 11 patients had had previous medical evaluations, but in no instance was disruption of the posterior tibial tendon recognized.[101] Woods and Leach noted that the delay in diagnosis in five of their six athletes (range, 6 to 18 months) adversely affected the results of operative treatment.[254] They concluded that the key to successful treatment, particularly in athletic individuals, is to make the diagnosis early, before deformity occurs.

Pertinent Anatomy

The tibialis posterior (TP) tendon is formed in the distal third of the leg by the convergence of the large muscle units that arise more proximally from the posterior surfaces of the tibia and fibula and the adjacent interosseous membrane. At the level of the medial malleolus, the TP tendon is the most anterior structure, located immediately adjacent to the posterior surface of the malleolus. The other structures, in order from anterior to posterior, are the flexor digitorum, the posterior tibial artery, vein, and nerve, and the FHL (one mnemonic for remembering the order of

these structures is "Tom, Dick, and A Very Nervous Harry"). The posterior tibial tendon has numerous insertion sites on the plantar aspect of the foot. These include the inferior aspect of the navicular bone, all three cuneiform bones, and the bases of the second, third, and fourth metacarpals.[66, 233] The incidence of an accessory navicular or os tibial externum, a sesamoid bone invested in the TP near its insertion, is 10% to 20%.[33, 66, 233] If present, it may be a small accessory bone within the TP without attachment to the navicular (type I); an accessory navicular with a synchondrosis (type II); or a cornuate bony, navicular tuberosity (type III).[66] The TP is the main dynamic stabilizer of the hindfoot against valgus (eversion) forces owing to its multiple insertions, which are variously taut at different positions of foot function, and to the size and strength of its muscle. Disruption of the tendon, therefore, results in elongation of the ligaments of the hind and midfoot and a painful flatfoot deformity.

Variations in the vascular anatomy of the flexor tendons also may play a role in the frequency and location of injury. In a recent study, Frey and colleagues used injection techniques to examine the intrinsic vascularity of the posterior tibial and flexor digitorum longus tendons in 28 cadaveric limbs.[64] In all 28 specimens, they found that the posterior tibial tendon had a zone of hypovascularity in its midportion. The zone started approximately 4 cm from the tendon's insertion on the medial tubercle of the navicular bone and ran proximally for an average of 14 mm. Their dissections confirmed that there was no mesotenon present in this region and that the visceral layer of synovial tissue was present but hypovascular. Although this zone of hypovascularity may predispose the tendon to degenerative processes, it is proximal to the most common site of rupture of this tendon (1.0 to 1.5 cm from its insertion into the navicular) reported in the literature.[74, 101, 147] In contrast, the midportion of the flexor digitorum longus tendon has ample vascularity throughout its length owing to a longitudinal system of vessels arising from the proximal and distal arteries.[64]

Clinical Evaluation

The hallmark of a posterior tibial tendon disruption is the progressive deformity of the foot. Patients usually present with a painful flatfoot and note that they cannot walk "normally," have difficulty going up and down stairs, and have lost control of their foot. Disruptions most commonly occur in women older than 40 years of age, and many patients cannot recall any significant previous acute trauma.[101] The majority of patients do, however, have a history of antecedent tenosynovitis[254] and state that the problem began after twisting the foot, slipping off a curb, or stepping in a hole.[147] Most do not seek emergent care because their pain, located medially between the tip of the malleolus and the navicular bone, is not incapacitating.[101, 147, 254]

Salient physical findings include valgus of the hindfoot, adduction of the forefoot, a positive single heel rise test, a "too many toes" sign, and loss of function on manual testing of the tendon. The concurrent development of ab-

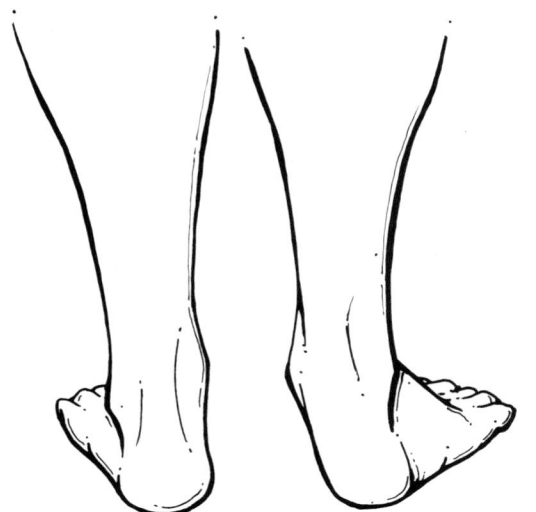

Figure 30G–1. The "too many toes" sign. More toes are visible lateral to the heel on the patient's right side.

normal hindfoot valgus and forefoot adduction produces the flatfoot deformity. These deformities are best evaluated by observing and comparing the posterior aspects of both feet with the patient standing. Patients with tendon ruptures have either a unilateral flatfoot or, in those who had previous flat feet, a relatively flatter foot on the involved side. Excessive forefoot abduction also can be suspected from posterior observation when more toes are visible lateral to the patient's heel on the involved side. This finding is called the "too many toes" sign (Fig. 30G–1).

The best method for evaluating loss of posterior tibial function is the single heel rise test.[101] In this test, the patient is instructed to stand on one leg with the knee extended and to rise onto the ball of the foot and the tips of the toes. The test is positive if the hindfoot (heel) on the involved side fails to invert and assume a stable (varus) position (Fig. 30G–2). The patient also will have great difficulty in raising the heel off the floor because gastrocnemius muscle

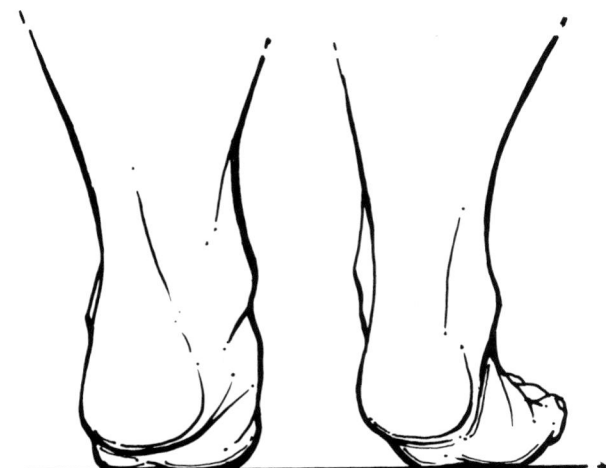

Figure 30G–2. Single heel rise test. The right heel does not assume a stable (varus) position (as seen on the left) when the patient attempts to stand on the toes.

function is compromised when there is no posterior tibialis to bring the heel into a locked, stable varus position.[101] Manual testing of the strength of the posterior tibial tendon can be misleading because of the inversion strength of the tibialis anterior. This latter muscle and its tendon effectively resist eversion of the foot when the foot is in full inversion. Thus, loss of posterior tibial function is best assessed by everting the heel and placing the forefoot in full abduction. The patient is then asked to invert the foot. The presence of tibialis posterior weakness will be apparent with this maneuver, particularly if one compares it with the strength of the opposite foot.

Standard weight-bearing AP and lateral radiographs show variable changes depending upon the time elapsed since the injury. Although several studies state that standard radiographs are not useful in making a diagnosis of posterior tibial tendon disruption,[109, 110, 147] Johnson concluded that standard films usually show pronounced changes.[101] Specifically, an increase in the talocalcaneal angle and inferior subluxation of the talus at the talonavicular articulation are evident on the lateral view. On the AP view, subluxation of the forefoot at the talonavicular articulation and an increased talocalcaneal angle are evident.[101] In Mann's study, the lateral talar–first metatarsal angle averaged 22 degrees.[147] This angle is 0 degrees in normal feet, 1 to 15 degrees in mild flatfoot deformities, and more than 15 degrees in severe flatfoot deformities.[22] Ancillary studies such as computed tomography and MRI are rarely indicated. Computed tomography scans should be obtained in feet with rigid deformities to rule out tarsal coalitions. Although MRI demonstrates the site or sites of tendon disease, it is not required to establish the diagnosis of posterior tibial tendon disruption.

Treatment Options

Nonoperative treatment of posterior tibial tendon disruption is appropriate in patients who have low activity levels, are in their sixties or seventies, have life-limiting medical problems, or have minimal discomfort from their acquired deformity. If the injury is diagnosed acutely, immobilization of 4 weeks' duration in a short-leg cast that is well molded along the longitudinal arch is recommended.[74, 101, 109, 133] In subacute cases, the use of an orthosis (a flexible leather arch support with a 3/16-inch heel wedge) is appropriate if the patient's only complaint is that he or she is wearing out the medial counter of his or her shoe because the results of later surgery will not be compromised if the foot is flexible.[74, 147] In the majority of patients, however, the prognosis for an unrepaired posterior tibial tendon is poor because of the inevitable development of a painful flatfoot. Thus, early surgical repair or reconstruction is the best treatment, particularly in athletic individuals.[254]

Appropriate surgical treatment of a posterior tibial tendon disruption is predicated upon the site and extent of the tear, the flexibility (duration) of the foot deformity, and the expectations of the patient. Based on these factors, there are four distinct surgical procedures: (1) end-to-end suture; (2) reattachment or advancement of the tendon to its primary site of insertion on the navicular bone; (3) reconstruction of the tendon; and (4) a triple or limited arthrodesis.

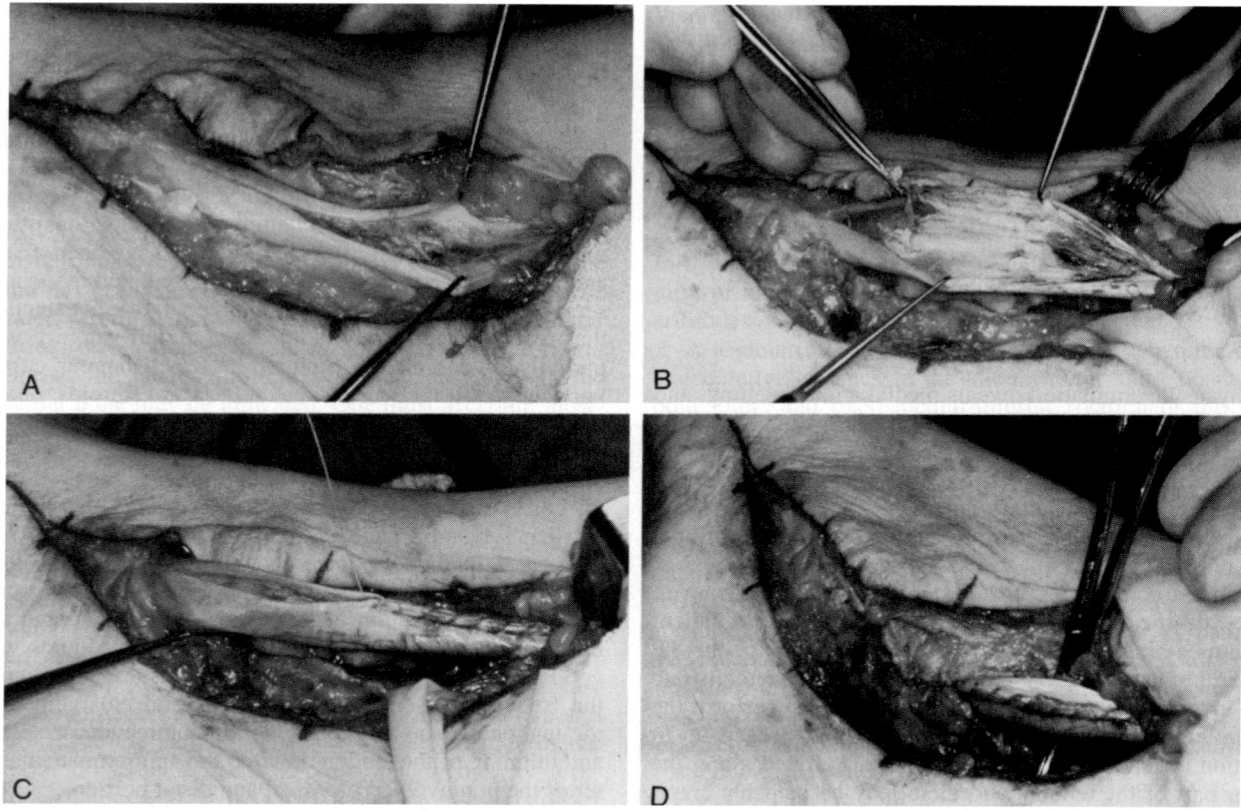

Figure 30G–3. Posterior tibial tendinitis. *A,* The surface of the tendon appears normal, but intrinsic degeneration is apparent when the tendon is opened. *B,* The degenerated central segment of tendon was excised, but the peripheral fibers were intact. *C,* The periphery of the tendon was closed with a running absorbable 2–0 suture. *D,* The retinaculum was closed at the medial malleolus to prevent subsequent subluxation of the tendon.

where MRI has demonstrated abnormalities because, as noted earlier (see Fig. 30G–3*A*), intrinsic degeneration may not be apparent on the surface. Subsequently, all degenerative tissue is removed with a curet or knife (Fig. 30G–3*B*), and after débridement, the tendon is closed with a running absorbable 2–0 suture (Fig. 30G–3*C*). Although several studies have concluded that releasing and not repairing the tendon sheath is appropriate,[124, 125, 252] subluxation of the posterior tibial tendon has been reported as a complication of tarsal tunnel decompressions.[123] Thus, I routinely preserve, restore, or reconstruct the posterior tibial tendon sheath at the medial malleolus to prevent this complication (Fig. 30G–3*D*). The wound is then closed with a running, subcuticular, nonabsorbable 3–0 Prolene suture, and the ankle is immobilized for 2 weeks to allow the incision to heal. At that juncture, immobilization is discontinued, the suture is removed, and the patient is instructed and supervised in gaining full range of motion, full strength, and full function. Relief of symptoms and return to full activity can be anticipated within 12 to 14 weeks of surgery.

Flexor Hallucis Longus Injuries

There are a limited number of published reports about complete disruptions of the FHL tendon.* Only seven cases

---

*See references 6, 38, 59, 63, 89, 94, 118, 196, 201, and 237.

of closed complete disruptions of the FHL tendon have been reported to date.[38, 89, 94, 118, 196, 201, 237] Six of the seven individuals were injured during the following sports activities: diving from a board; marathon running; walking; and playing soccer.[38, 89, 94, 118, 201, 237] The average age of the seven injured was 40 years (range 27 to 54 years), and the sites of tendon injury were in the groove of the posterior process of the talus (1); under the sustentaculum tali (2); mid-arch (1); at the metatarsal head (1); and 0.5 cm proximal to the tendon's insertion on the great toe (2). All seven FHL tendon ruptures were repaired because of functional disability due to loss of great toe push-off. Five were repaired acutely, and two late, at 4 months and at 2 years. Although only two of the seven patients regained active interphalangeal joint flexion, all of the six athletes regained their pre-injury level of performance.[38, 89, 94, 118, 201, 237] Postoperative stiffness of the interphalangeal joint did not cause any functional deficit.

The frequency and cause of FHL tendon lacerations are well chronicled in two studies.[59, 63] In 1977, Frenette and Jackson reported on 10 young athletes (median age 11 years) with FHL tendon lacerations. In 8 of their 10 patients, the laceration was caused when the athlete was running barefooted and stepped on a sharp object, usually broken glass. To find that number of cases, they surveyed 100 orthopaedic surgeons and did a 5-year review of the hospital records of four large hospitals. They found that four of the six primary repairs of this tendon resulted in no active plantar flexion of the interphalangeal joint of the great toe, and concluded that repair of the FHL tendon was not essential for good push-off or balance in running sports.[63] In contrast, Floyd and associates reported on 13 cases of open FHL tendon lacerations and found that of 12 tendons repaired (10 sutured primarily, 2 delayed), 9 retained active motion of the interphalangeal joint of the great toe.[59] The majority of the reports on open or closed disruptions of the FHL tendon have concluded that an intact tendon is essential for good push-off and balance in running sports.[38, 59, 89, 94, 118, 196, 201, 237]

Tendinitis of the FHL tendon is more common than complete disruption. Although cases of flexor hallucis tendinitis and tenosynovitis have been reported in tennis players and long distance runners,[167, 236, 239] it is much more prevalent, and is the most common site of lower extremity tendinitis, in classical ballet dancers.[41, 65, 82, 83, 116, 209, 210, 241] Washington's survey study of musculoskeletal injuries in dancers puts the incidence of this problem in perspective.[247] Of 414 injuries reported by individual dancers, 55 involved the ankle joint, and 3 of these 55 (5.5%) were diagnosed as tendinitis. Hamilton noted that tendinitis about the ankle is common in classical ballet dancers and that the tendon involved is almost always the FHL. He stated that in ballet the FHL is the Achilles tendon of the foot when a dancer is en pointe.[83, 84] FHL tendinitis is more often seen in the left foot than the right because choreography more often calls for the dancer to turn to the right (clockwise). This requires the dancer to be en pointe on the left foot.

Pertinent Anatomy

The FHL arises from the lower two thirds of the posterior surface of the shaft of the fibula, and the FHL tendon inserts into the base of the distal phalanx of the great toe. In the sole of the foot, the FHL tendon is connected by a fibrous slip to the flexor digitorum longus tendon. This slip (vide supra) tethers the FHL tendon and prevents excessive retraction of the proximal segment after the FHL tendon is severed. In the great toe, the FHL tendon lies superficial to and between the two heads of the flexor hallucis brevis. Thus, it is relatively easy to find the proximal end of the FHL tendon when it is severed in this location.[63] At the level of the ankle joint, the FHL, posterior tibial, and flexor digitorum longus tendons pass under the flexor retinaculum (lancinate ligament), and septa from this strong fibrous retinaculum convert a series of bony grooves into fibroosseous tunnels. The tendons also are enclosed in separate synovial sheaths, which are 8 cm long and extend proximal and distal to the aforementioned tunnels.

The constrictive nature of the fibro-osseous tunnels can cause "triggering" of a flexor tendon when partial tearing and healing of the tendon produce exuberant scar tissue. The most common tendon involved is the FHL, and the most common precipitating activity is classical ballet dancing.[41, 65, 82, 83, 116, 209, 210, 241] The FHL tendon is further constrained by bony grooves in the posterior surface of the tibia, the talus, and the sustentaculum tali.

Clinical Evaluation

Dancers with FHL tendinitis often note the insidious onset of pain at the posterior medial aspect of both ankles behind the malleolus, and often seek evaluation only when triggering of the FHL tendon produces so much pain that they are unable to dance en pointe.[41, 83, 209, 210, 241] Sammarco and Miller reported on four ballet dancers who had triggering of the FHL; in two of these dancers the hallux became locked in a flexed position.[210] They noted that the triggering becomes more severe over a period of several months, but pain is not an outstanding characteristic of this condition.[210] In Kolettis and associates' series of 13 female ballet dancers that had operative release because of isolated stenosing tendosynovitis, all had pain and tenderness over the medial aspect of the subtalar joint.[116] Their symptoms were exacerbated by jumping and attempts to perform en pointe work, and all 13 had lost the ability to stand en pointe. Crepitus was present in six patients, but triggering was present in only three. None of their dancers had pain or tenderness in the posterolateral aspect of the ankle with forced passive plantar flexion, which would have suggested involvement of an os trigonum.

In contrast, Hamilton and associates reported on 37 dancers that had 41 operations for posterior ankle pain. In their series, only 9 operations were performed for isolated tendinitis. Of the remaining 32 ankles, 26 were operated on for tendinitis and posterior impingement and 6 for isolated posterior impingement.[83]

Physical examination of patients with triggering of the FHL tendon reveals that the hallux can be flexed with ease when the foot is in a neutral position. When the foot is brought into plantar flexion, however, the patient is unable to flex the hallux. On forcible active contraction of the FHL, however, a snap or pop is noted in the posterior medial region of the ankle, and the patient is then unable to extend the interphalangeal or metatarsal phalangeal joints of the great toe. Subsequent passive extension of the interphalangeal joint produces a painless snap or pop posterior to the medial malleolus with subsequent freeing of motion in the great toe.

In dancers who have tendinitis without triggering, localized tenderness and swelling are present, occasionally with crepitus over the FHL tendon just posterior to the medial malleolus.[65] Hamilton stated that FHL tendinitis can be distinguished from tendinitis of other adjacent tendons by the following maneuver. The foot is placed in the pointe position, and the patient is asked to flex the great toe against mild resistance and then to flex toes two through five against resistance. Sequential palpation of the FHL and the flexor digitorum longus will reveal which tendon is locally tender and has the tendinitis.[82, 83]

Differential diagnosis of FHL tendinitis includes peroneal tendinitis, posterior impingement of the os trigonum, acute fracture of the lateral tubercle of the posterior process of the talus, Achilles tendinitis, bone spurs, and arthritic or osteochondritic lesions of the talus.[82, 83, 150] Posterior impingement can be tested for by forcibly plantar flexing the ankle. When impingement is present, this maneuver usually produces pain in a posterolateral location.[40, 83, 150] Achilles tendinitis can be differentiated from FHL tendinitained inversion injuries of the ankle,[45, 54] and two occurred in middle-aged woman (ages 48 and 58 years) who had twisted the ankle.[3, 163]

Disruption of the PLT due to a fracture of the os peroneum also has been reported.[141, 146, 184–186, 246] Most cases are the result of either repetitive inversion injuries or forced eversion of the ankle against resistance. Although PLT rupture with an associated os peroneum fracture is an uncommon occurrence, it should be included in the differential diagnosis of any patient with lateral ankle pain and instability, and either of the aforementioned mechanisms of injury.

Although longitudinal and interstitial tears of the peroneus brevis tendon (PBT) have been well described in the literature,[12, 16, 21, 27, 119, 207, 212, 224] only three cases of complete PBT rupture have been reported.[2, 143, 207] All three PBT tears occurred in combination with partial or complete PLT tears. Two were discovered at the time of surgical treatment of the PLT tears[143, 207] and the other when the PBT was going to be used for correction of chronic lateral ankle instability.[2]

Pertinent Anatomy

The PLT and PBT cross the ankle joint within a common fibro-osseous tunnel and synovial sheath. The tunnel is created laterally by the superior peroneal retinaculum; medially by the posterior talofibular, calcaneal fibular, and posterior inferior tibiofibular ligaments; and anteriorly by the posterior surface of the lateral malleolus. The superior peroneal retinaculum (SPR) is a strong fibrous band that blends with the periosteum of the lateral surface of the lateral malleolus and is rarely torn when subluxations or dislocations of the peroneal tendons occur.[50] Eckert and Davis, who described the retinaculum's origin from the periosteum of the posterior ridge of the fibula, found no actual tears of the SPR in their 73 repairs for subluxating peroneal tendons.[50] Davis and colleagues delineated the different patterns of insertions, and the relationship of the superior retinaculum to the peroneal tendons and the lateral ankle ligaments.[46] They observed that the SPR has at least one insertional band that parallels and inserts just lateral to the calcaneofibular ligament, and that these two structures are at maximum length in ankle dorsiflexion. They concluded that inversion ankle sprains that cause calcaneofibular ligament ruptures may often produce concomitant SPR injuries.[46] Numerous studies have documented the relationship between lateral ankle instability and peroneal tendon disease.[16, 21, 119, 141, 185, 207, 212, 224, 246]

The inferior peroneal retinaculum is continuous (anteriorly) with the fibers of the inferior extensor retinaculum and is attached posteriorly to the lateral surface of the calcaneus. Some retinacular fibers attach to the peroneal tubercle of the os calcis, forming a septum that creates separate compartments for the peroneus longus and brevis tendons. A thin vincula-like structure that runs between the PLT and PBT and is dorsally attached to the dorsolateral aspect of the fibula has also been described.[32] The peroneal tendons have a common synovial sheath until they separate under the inferior retinaculum. At that juncture, each tendon is enveloped by a distal progression of the common sheath. Proximal to the lateral malleolus, the PBT lies deep (medial) to that of the peroneus longus. Distal to the lateral malleolus, the PBT lies anterior to the peroneus longus. Knowledge of the changing spatial relationships of these tendons is important if one uses the PBT for lateral ankle reconstructions.

The PBT inserts into the tuberosity of the lateral aspect of the base of the fifth metatarsal. The PLT exits the posterior compartment of the inferior retinaculum, crosses the lateral surface of the cuboid bone, and traverses the plantar surface of the cuboid in a tunnel created by a groove in the bone and the lateral plantar ligament. The tendon inserts into the lateral side of the base of the first metatarsal and the medial cuneiform. There is an abrupt change in direction of the peroneus longus tendon at two points: first at the tip of the lateral malleolus, and second at the distal (lateral) edge of the cuboid bone. In both of these locations, the tendon is thickened, and at the point of contact with the smooth surface of the edge of the cuboid, there usually is a sesamoid within the tendon composed of fibrocartilage or bone. The blood supply of the peroneus longus and brevis tendons comes from the peroneal artery, and microvascular studies have documented that there are no critical zones of hypovascularity within these tendons that may be attributed to rupture.[222, 223]

Relevant Biomechanics

Several studies have noted the critical role that subluxation of the tendons over the posterolateral edge of the fibula plays in the development of peroneal tendon tears.[16, 21, 119, 224] Sobel and associates, in their study of 15 fresh-frozen specimens, demonstrated that PBT splits were uniformly located at the sharp posterior lateral edge of the fibula. They concluded that PBT tears were the result of either acute or repetitive mechanical trauma caused by subluxation of the tendon over the posterior corner of the lateral malleous.[224] Subsequent studies have supported this proposed mechanism of injury.[16, 119, 212]

Clinical Evaluation

Diagnosis of complete peroneal tendon disruptions is difficult and often is delayed.[3, 45, 54, 114, 163, 203] In one soccer player, the diagnosis was not suspected, and was discovered 10 hours after injury when an emergency fasciotomy was performed for an acute peroneal compartment syndrome.[45] The peroneus longus tendon was found to be avulsed from the muscle belly, and subsequently the entire muscle became necrotic and was excised. Seven months after the injury, function of the peroneus brevis and the anterior compartment muscles was normal, and the patient had returned to playing soccer. In the other case involving a soccer player, the individual sought treatment 8 months after his injury because of recurrent, painful swelling at the outer aspect of the heel.[54] At that time, he had full range of motion and full strength except for eversion, which was painful and weaker than normal. Ultimately, the tendon was explored because of his persistent tenosynovitis. At surgery, a bulbous enlargement and transverse tear of the tendon were discovered just below and behind the lateral malleolus. The enlarged portion of the tendon was excised, and the two ends of the peroneus longus were sutured to the adjacent tendon of the peroneus brevis. Two months after surgery, the patient had returned to full activity. The two runners with this injury were initially treated for lateral ankle sprains. The diagnosis of a complete PLT tear was made 4 weeks after injury when both sought a second opinion because of persistent pain and difficulty walking.[114, 203]

In the two middle-aged women with this injury, the diagnosis of a PLT disruption was made 1 or more years after the injury. One was treated successfully with 3 weeks of immobilization,[163] and the other was treated with end-to-end repair of both the peroneus longus and brevis tendons.[3]

It is apparent from the reports cited earlier that rupture of the PLT is an uncommon injury and diagnosis is delayed because the physical findings (pain and swelling about the lateral malleolus) usually imply a lateral ankle ligament injury. In addition, swelling often makes determination of point tenderness more difficult. Thus, one should look for increased hindfoot varus and test for pain with active eversion in all individuals with lateral ankle pain and tenderness proximally along the peroneal tendons.

Although fractures of the os peroneum without disruption of the tendon occur[78, 80] (and are the subject of a subsequent chapter), the association of this sesamoid fracture with PLT disruption warrants further emphasis. The os peroneum, which is present in 5% to 26% of individuals, is found within the PLT at the level of the plantar and lateral aspects of the cuboid.[246] One mechanism of injury, sudden forceful dorsiflexion of the foot and a violent reflex contraction of the peroneus muscles, is the same mechanism that produces a dislocation of the peroneal tendons.[146, 186] The other mechanism proposed (repetitive inversion injuries) is more subtle,[141, 184, 185] and thus recognition of this injury requires knowledge of its existence, careful examination of the lateral aspect of the foot, and standard radiographs that include AP, lateral, and calcaneal views.

The differential diagnosis for this combined injury includes lateral ankle ligament sprains, avulsion fractures at the insertion of the PBT, peroneal tendon subluxation, and tenosynovitis of the peroneal tendons. With a fracture of the os peroneum and disruption of the tendon, there is point-specific tenderness over the area of the sesamoid, and either wide separation of the fracture fragments or proximal migration of the sesamoid is evident on the standard radiographs.[184–186, 203, 246]

Peroneal Tendinitis

Far more common than complete disruption of one or both of the peroneal tendons are interstitial tears and chronic tendinitis. The evaluation and management of chronic tendinitis and tenosynovitis of the peroneal tendons have been addressed in only a limited number of studies.[3, 27, 28, 199, 213, 240] Scheller and colleagues postulated that peroneal tendinitis is due to the pulley action and abrupt change in direction of these tendons at the lateral malleolus. They suggest that the oblique stress placed on the tendon at the lateral malleolus produces an area of decreased vascularity that predisposes the tendon to injury.[213] Burman concluded that tenosynovitis of the peroneal tendons occurs in three specific locations: posterior to the lateral malleolus (peroneal sulcus), at the peroneal trochlea (a tunnel created by the attachment of the calcaneal fibular ligament to the peroneal tubercle of the os calcis), and at the plantar surface of the cuboid.[27] Burman also concluded that stenosing tenosynovitis of the peroneus longus and brevis occurs mainly in individuals with well-developed peroneal tubercles, and noted that anatomic studies have documented that 37% to 44% of humans have prominent peroneal tubercles. He operated on 6 of 25 patients that had chronic peroneal tenosynovitis at the level of the peroneal tubercle. In all six cases, the tendons were found to be intact, but the fibrous sheath and fibrous septum of the retinaculum were thickened. After resection of the stenotic sheath, the patients experienced relief from their peroneal pain.[27]

Trevino and coworkers reported on four cases of peroneal tenosynovitis that were treated surgically. They noted that the site of involvement was either the peroneal sulcus (two cases) or the peroneal trochlea.[240] Roggatz and Urban described three cases of peroneal tendinitis that were located distal to the peroneal trochlea at the lateral border or plantar surface of the cuboid bone.[199] Peroneal tendinitis also can be caused by congenital anomalies of the peroneal tendons.[84, 197, 208, 251] In the four cases reported to date, three had an anomalous bifurcation or trifurcation of the PBT,[84, 197, 251] and one had an accessory peroneal muscle and tendon.[208] In all cases, resection of the anomalous tendon and muscle produced good results.

The evaluation and management of interstitial tears (splits) of the peroneus longus and brevis tendons have been addressed in an increasing number of studies.[12, 16, 21, 27, 119, 207, 212, 224] Interstitial tears of the PLT can be classified as acute or chronic. Acute tears occur after a single event, after which symptoms develop. With chronic tears, there is no acute traumatic episode and symptoms are insidious in onset and develop over a long period of time.[207]

Acute tears may occur as primary injuries[40] or may occur in conjunction with other ankle injuries.[16] Bassett and Speer reported on eight athletes that sustained longitudinal ruptures of PLT (five patients) or PLB (three patients) as a result of a plantar flexion-inversion ankle injury.[16] Sammarco chronicled the evaluation and management of 14 cases of PLT tears, of which 8 had acute onset of symptoms.[207] In these two series of patients, delay in diagnoses was common, range 7 days to 6 months, and 7 to 48 months, respectively.[16, 207] In Bassett and Speer's study, all eight athletes noted persistent lateral ankle swelling, popping, and retrofibular pain after their initial sprain.[16] They all complained of a subjective feeling of ankle instability but were able to compete in their sport by taping the ankle. On physical examination, all ankles were stable and all had retrofibular tenderness, synovial sheath fullness, and palpable retrofibular popping with active foot rotation. None had evidence of clinical subluxation of the peroneal tendons. They and others[21] have concluded that splits in the PLT and PBT that go unrecognized may be the cause of residual pain after ligamentous repairs of lateral ankle injuries.

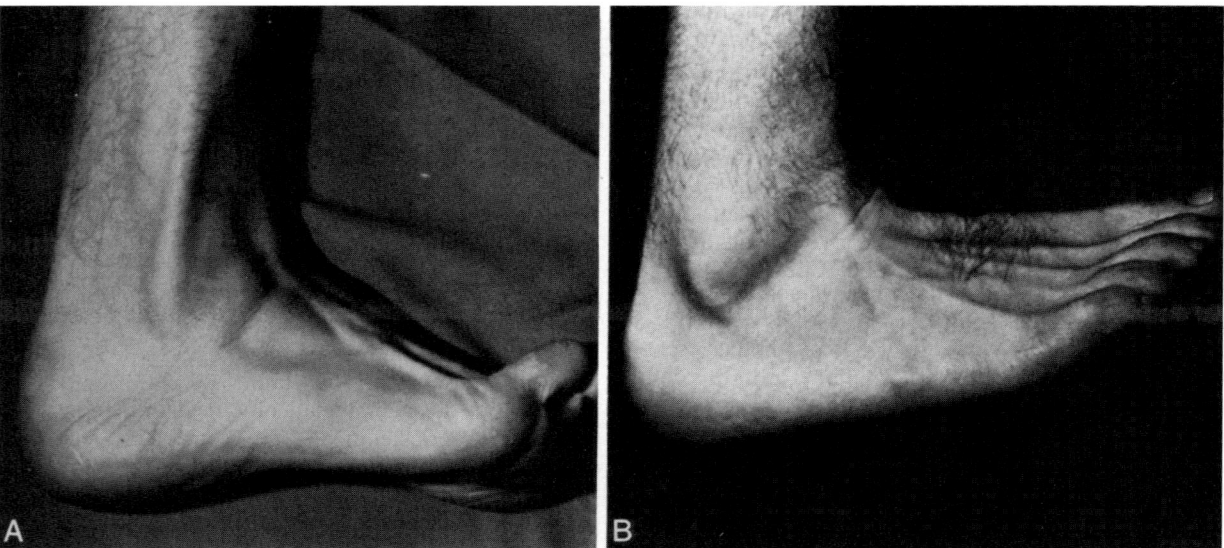

Figure 30G–5. Subluxation of the peroneal tendons. With dorsiflexion and eversion of the right foot *(A)*, the peroneal tendons dislocate anteriorly over the lateral malleolus. The dislocated tendons reduce when the foot is brought into plantar flexion and inversion *(B)*.

dorsiflexion causes a maximal change of direction of the tendons at the lateral malleolus and, in combination with eversion, also thrusts the tendons against the superior retinaculum. The key component of the injury, however, is the forceful reflex contraction of the peroneal muscles.

Clinical Evaluation

In acute injuries, the athlete usually notes a popping or snapping sound or sensation at the posterolateral aspect of the ankle, accompanied by intense localized pain behind the fibula and above the joint line.[50] There is usually diffuse lateral swelling and ecchymosis. The pain usually subsides rapidly and becomes relatively mild. If the individual is examined within hours of injury, one usually finds swelling localized over and just posterior to the lateral malleolus. If the swelling is not extensive, the peroneal tendons often can be palpated over the lateral malleolus, or their displacement can be appreciated when the ankle is dorsiflexed (Fig. 30G–5). When there is an associated fracture of the lateral malleolus, the bone fragment may be palpable in the deep tissues. In most cases, there are no signs of injury to the anterior talofibular, fibular calcaneal, or anterior tibiofibular ligaments as is commonly seen with lateral ligament injuries.

If the injury is evaluated 4 or more hours after the injury, the lateral aspect of the ankle often is markedly swollen, and palpation reveals only tenderness at the posterior lip of the lateral malleolus. At this juncture, the swelling may obscure frankly dislocated tendons and makes the diagnosis difficult. One must therefore attempt to stress the retinaculum by eliciting active eversion of the foot with the ankle held in dorsiflexion. In patients with an acute subluxation, this test may produce apprehension, severe pain, or show obvious dislocation, all of which are diagnostic of the problem. Safran and associates advocate that this provocative testing be done with the patient prone and the

knee flexed to 90 degrees.[205] They conclude that this position is a more comfortable position for the examiner and that dynamic instability is better visualized.

Because of the rapid resolution of symptoms and an initial diagnosis of an ankle sprain, most patients seek medical evaluation when chronic subluxation is established. Patients with recurrent subluxation complain of lateral ankle instability and pain. They also note a popping or snapping sensation in the ankle just before the ankle giving way.* The snapping or popping sensation is noted particularly during such activities as jogging or walking on uneven ground.

Chronic subluxation may tend to occur with increasing frequency owing to progressive stretching of the residual lateral soft tissue structures.[12] Many authors state that they can reproduce the tendon subluxation in all of their patients by having the patient contract the peroneal muscles with the foot in eversion.[53, 151, 190, 205, 213, 228, 258] Marti, however, stresses that one must examine the other ankle to identify those individuals with bilateral congenital subluxation of the peroneal tendon.[151] In addition, DeHaven reports that one can reproduce the dislocation in only about 50% of patients with chronic dislocation.[47]

The differential diagnosis of this injury includes longitudinal tears of the peroneal tendons, sprains of the lateral ligaments of the ankle, and in children, Salter I fractures of the lateral malleolus. Often a longitudinal tear of one of the tendons will result in internal snapping of one tendon over another, mimicking a subluxation.[85, 154] Patients with chronic dislocation of the peroneal tendons do not have instability of the ankle or subtalar joints. Specifically, they usually have a negative anterior drawer test and no increased lateral laxity in comparison with the opposite ankle. Salter I fractures can be documented by obtaining radiographs of the opposite ankle and noting the location of the pain. In patients with acute and chronic peroneal

---

*See references 85, 91, 117, 152, 161, 205, 211, 213, 228, and 258.

dislocations, the pain is located along the posterior lip of the lateral malleolus and not over the anterior tibial-talar area.

Radiographic evaluation of this injury should include AP, lateral, and mortise views of the ankle. Stress views, to assess increased talar tilt and lateral ankle instability, may be performed as indicated. Radiographs will be diagnostic only in patients with grade III injuries, those with an associated rim avulsion fracture of the lateral malleolus.[35, 168, 174, 231] The fragment, which is 1 to 1.5 cm in length, is best seen on the mortise view. This fracture occurs in 15% to 50% of individuals sustaining peroneal tendon dislocations,[174] and when this finding is present, it is pathognomonic of a dislocation of the peroneal tendons.* MRI will give further information regarding interstitial tendinopathy,[193, 202, 256] but MRI is not routinely necessary in cases of isolated peroneal instability.

Treatment Options

Nonoperative Treatment

Although most authorities agree that there is no place for nonoperative treatment of chronic dislocations, the treatment of acute injuries remains controversial. Stover and Bryan[231] stated that all acute cases should be treated conservatively with a well-molded cast and non–weight-bearing ambulation for 5 to 6 weeks. They reported on five patients treated in this manner, and all five had excellent results; however, two other patients in their series were immobilized for a shorter interval, and 6 of 10 patients treated by taping of the ankle in a neutral position for 4 to 6 weeks had recurrent dislocations. Thus, of a total of 17 acute peroneal dislocations treated nonoperatively, seven ultimately needed surgical repair.[231] In contrast, Scheller and colleagues treated seven patients with taping and a lateral felt pad over the fibula, and all seven had recurrent dislocations.[213] Similarly, Escalas and associates[53] reported that 28 of his 38 patients with acute dislocations, who were treated by immobilization and a compressive bandage for several weeks, had recurrent dislocations. Eckert and Davis[50] noted that only one of their seven patients who were treated with either adhesive strapping or casts for 4 weeks had a stable pain-free ankle, whereas four had recurrent dislocations.

McLennan reported on 16 athletes with subluxations or dislocations of the peroneal tendons.[156] Of the six acute injuries (diagnosis within 1 week), one had immediate surgery, and five had 3 weeks of taping of the ankle with a crescent-shaped, laterally placed pad. Three (60%) of these five athletes later had operative correction because of recurrent dislocations. Ten athletes with subacute and chronic injuries (diagnosis at 2 weeks to 2 years) also were treated with the aforementioned regimen of taping. Four (40%) of these athletes ultimately had surgery.[156] McLennan concluded that although nonoperative treatment gives satisfactory results in more than 50% of the cases, operative treatment of acute injuries is indicated in athletes seriously involved in sports, particularly those with rim fractures.[156]

*See references 17, 35, 53, 151, 168, 174, 190, 205, 211, 231, and 258.

All the aforementioned authors who have experienced failures with nonoperative treatment still recommend treating acute cases initially with a short-leg, non–weight-bearing cast for a minimum of 4 weeks.[53, 156, 213] They reserve surgical treatment for patients who have subsequent dislocations.

Operative Treatment

The results of operative treatment of acute dislocations have been reported in only a limited number of studies.[50, 151, 174] In Eckert and Davis's series of 73 patients, grade I (retinaculum and periosteum elevated from lateral malleolus) and grade II (fibrous ridge and periosteum elevated) lesions were repaired by suturing the retinaculum to the fibrous ridge or the ridge and retinaculum to the malleolus, respectively.[50] Grade III injuries (rim fractures) were treated with open reduction and K-wire fixation. At follow-up 6 or more months after surgery, the tendons had redislocated in three patients—all with grade II injuries. Twelve additional patients experienced mild pain after vigorous activity, but none of these felt that their symptoms warranted further treatment.[50]

Results of acute surgical repairs also have been reported by Marti[151] and Murr.[174] All three of Murr's patients had rim fractures of the lateral malleolus and were treated by open reduction and internal (suture) fixation. Within 1 year of surgery, all three patients had returned to skiing and were symptom-free.[174] Marti reported on five patients with acute injuries, one of whom had a rim fracture, and concluded that to achieve the best results, acute injuries should be treated operatively with primary repair of the torn peroneal retinaculum.[151] At an average follow-up of 3 1/2 years, all five patients were symptom-free and had normal ankle motion. In all of the aforementioned series of acute injuries, the patients were immobilized in a short-leg cast for 6 weeks after surgery.

Although over 18 surgical procedures have been proposed for treatment of recurrent dislocations, there are only five basic types of procedures. These are bone block procedures[17, 108, 151, 152, 160]; rerouting procedures[85, 190, 211]; reattachment of the retinaculum and reinforcement with local tissue[17, 44, 91, 205, 213, 248]; reconstruction of the superior peroneal retinaculum with tendon slings[53, 60, 102, 154, 161, 228]; and groove deepening procedures.[117, 234, 258]

The procedures that alter the osseous structure of the fibula are designed to contain the peroneal tendons either by deepening the peroneal groove or by augmenting the lateral osseous ridge of the fibula. Augmentation of the lateral border of the fibula usually is achieved with a bone block procedure. In the original procedure described by Kelly in 1920,[108] a "veneer-like graft, almost wholly composed of compact bone," was created by two saw cuts (one sagittal and one horizontal) in the distal 2 to 3 cm of the fibula. The graft was then rotated posteriorly so that it overlapped the posterior cortex of the fibula by 5 to 6 mm, and was fixed in its new position with two countersunk screws (Fig. 30G–6A). Kelly subsequently described a modification that eliminated screw fixation by dovetailing the graft so that it was wider anteriorly and was held tightly in its bed when it was displaced posteriorly (Fig. 30G–6B).

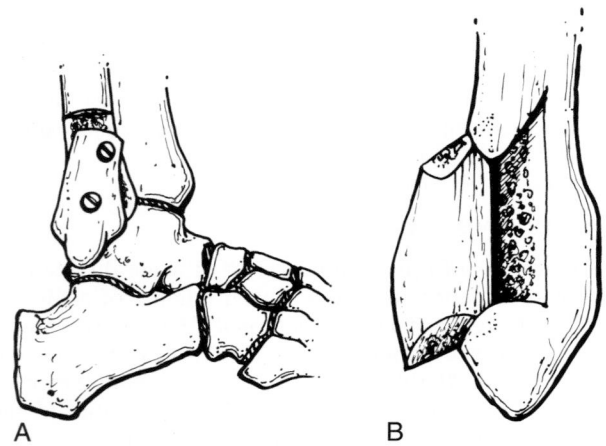

Figure 30G–6. Kelly's bone block procedures. The original technique *(A)* is shown on the left, and the modified procedure *(B)* is shown on the right.

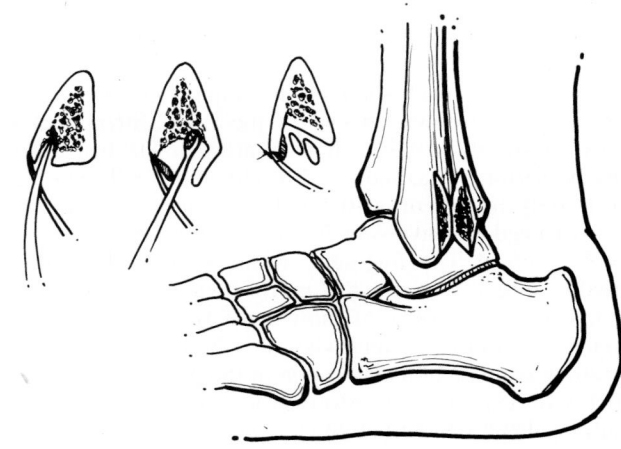

Figure 30G–8. Deepening of the peroneal groove via an osteoperiosteal flap.

DuVries modified Kelly's technique by using a wedge-shaped section of distal fibula that was 2 cm wide and half the depth of the lateral malleolus.[17] The wedge was displaced posteriorly 0.5 cm and held in place with a small screw or autogenous bone peg (Fig. 30G–7). Patients treated in this is manner were immobilized in a short-leg cast for 5 to 8 weeks.

The largest series of patients (11 to 12 cases) treated by the modified Kelly procedure were reported by Marti in 1977,[151] Micheli and colleagues in 1989,[160] and Mason and Henderson in 1996.[152] None of Marti's had redislocations 2 or more years after surgery, but two patients had crepitation of the tendons. He concluded that the crepitation was caused by insufficient posterior displacement of the bone block, which resulted in a shallow groove with a sharp inferior edge. In the more recent series of sliding,[160] or rotational[152] bone block procedures, similar results have been reported.

In patients with a shallow, flat, or convex peroneal

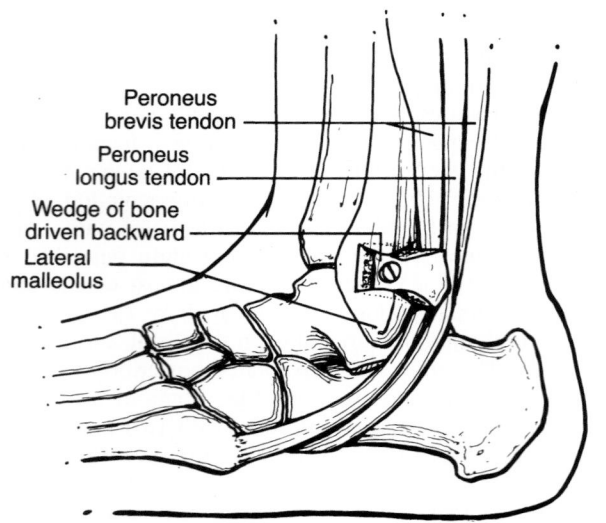

Peroneus brevis tendon
Peroneus longus tendon
Wedge of bone driven backward
Lateral malleolus

Figure 30G–7. The Du Vries modification of Kelly's bone block procedure.

groove, the groove-deepening procedure described by Zoellner and Clancy appears to be an effective method of correcting the basic deformity.[258] With this technique, a 1- × 3-cm osteoperiosteal flap is elevated from the posterior aspect of the distal part of the fibula and lateral malleolus. The posterior medial border of the cortical flap is left intact to act as a hinge. The flap is elevated and swung posteriorly, and the cancellous bone from the posterior aspect of the fibula is removed to a depth of 6 to 9 mm. The osteoperiosteal flap is then tapped back into place, and the peroneal groove is deepened over a length of 3 to 4 cm (Fig. 30G–8). Zoellner and Clancy used this technique in 10 patients and stated that the results were excellent at an average follow-up of 2 years (range 7 months to 3 years and 10 months).[258] In 6 of the 10 patients, however, the peroneal retinaculum was so tenuous that an additional (1- × 1-cm) periosteal flap was fashioned from the lateral surface of the malleolus and sutured to the medial part of the peroneal retinaculum. After surgery, the patients were immobilized in a short-leg cast for 3 weeks and then in a short-leg cast with an ankle hinge for an additional 3 weeks. Zoellner and Clancy recommended this technique because it (1) is technically easy to perform; (2) does not require metallic fixation; (3) corrects the basic deformity of a shallow peroneal groove; and (4) allows early motion because prolonged immobilization for union of bone or tendon is not needed.[258] Three subsequent studies have also reported excellent results with this technique in 17 additional patients.[12, 117, 234]

Results of the various soft tissue procedures (e.g., rerouting, periosteal flaps, and tendon slings) generally are very good. To date, however, there has not been a controlled study that compares the results of the different procedures to determine whether one is better than another.

Rerouting of the peroneal tendons has been advocated by Sarmiento and Wolf[211] and by Poll and Duijfjes.[190] Sarmiento and Wolf reported one case in which the tendons were divided, repositioned under the calcaneofibular ligament, and then repaired with a Bunnell stitch. At 3-year follow-up, the patient participated in athletic activities and had had no further dislocations.[211]

In 1984, Poll and Duijfjes reported on 10 patients in

whom the insertion of the calcaneofibular ligament was mobilized and lifted with a cancellous bone block from the calcaneus. The peroneal tendons were then brought under the ligament, and the bone block was replaced and fixed with a small cancellous screw. After surgery, the ankle was immobilized for 6 weeks in a short-leg plaster cast, but weight-bearing was allowed after 2 weeks. Poll and Duijfjes reported excellent results in all 10 patients and recommended the procedure because it precluded scarring and adhesions of the peroneal tendons to the surrounding structures.[190] They also described and critiqued similar procedures proposed by Platzgummer and by Leitz. Platzgummer divided the calcaneofibular ligament near the fibula, and Leitz osteotomized the lateral malleolus and refixed it with Kirschner wires.[190] Poll and Duijfjes stated that the disadvantage of the first technique was that the integrity of the ligament was disturbed, and a disadvantage of the second technique was that the osteotomy was near the articular surface of the fibula. Thus, these procedures increased the risk of adhesions forming between the tendons and the ligament or bone. Recently, Harper reported a good result in one patient that had transfer of both tendons under the calcaneofibular ligament after detachment of the ligament from the fibula.[85]

The use of a tendon sling to reconstruct the peroneal retinaculum was first described by Jones in 1932[102] (Fig. 30G–9). He reconstructed the retinaculum in a 22-year-old football player with a strip of tendon that was fashioned from the Achilles tendo at its calcaneal insertion. The tendon slip, which was 2 1/2 inches in length and approximately 1/4 inch in width, was passed through a transverse drill hole in the fibula, 1 inch above the tip of the lateral malleolus, looped posteriorly, and sutured to the periosteum of the fibula and to the tendon slip itself. Jones stressed that the tendon slip should be anchored with the foot held in full dorsiflexion and supination. After surgery, the athlete was placed in a short-leg cast for 6 weeks. At 6 weeks, he was permitted to return to full activity and subsequently returned to football without symptoms 3 months later.

The largest series of patients treated with the Jones

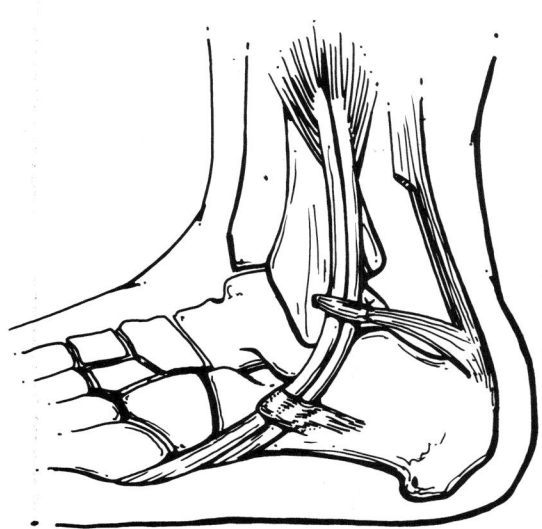

Figure 30G–9. The Jones (tendon-sling) procedure.

procedure was reported by Escalas and colleagues in 1980.[53] They performed the procedure in 28 patients, 15 of whom were followed for an average of 6.8 years (range 3 to 11 years). Fourteen of the 15 patients had excellent results and returned to sports activities after an average of 4.2 months. One patient reported instability of the ankle, but no instability could be demonstrated on physical examination. Three of the 15 patients had a moderate decrease in inversion of the hindfoot, and four lost up to 7 degrees of dorsiflexion. The authors noted that minor loss of motion occurred in spite of the fact that the tendon slip was sutured in all patients with the foot held in maximum dorsiflexion.[53]

Tendon slings have also been created from a portion of the PBT[228] and by transposition of the peroneus quartis tendon.[161] Stein used a free graft consisting of 50% of the diameter of the tendon of the peroneus brevis and anchored it through two drill holes to the fibula at a point 1.5 cm proximal to the inferior tip of the lateral malleolus.[228] The graft was passed through the distal drill hole in an anteroposterior direction, looped over the peroneal tendons, and passed through the proximal medially placed hole in a posterior to anterior direction. The free tendon was then sutured to itself with sufficient tension to restrain anterolateral subluxation of the tendons. Stein described the use of this technique in a 17-year-old quarterback who was placed in a short-leg cast for 6 weeks after the operation. The athlete was able to resume full sports-related activities 3 months after the operation and was asymptomatic when examined 3 years later. Stein felt that his procedure was superior to that of Jones[102] because the latter procedure had two disadvantages: (1) it weakened the Achilles tendon, and (2) restoring full ankle motion was a problem because the slip of tendon was left attached to the calcaneus.

Mick and Lynch[161] reported a case in which the peroneus quartis was used to reconstruct the superior and inferior peroneal retinaculum. The peroneus quartis, which is estimated to occur in 13% of the population, originates on the posterior surface of the fibula and inserts on the calcaneus. They rerouted this tendon anteriorly over the peroneus longus and brevis tendons and placed it in a 5-mm deep oblique groove created in the anterior aspect of the lateral malleolus. The periosteum and soft tissue on either side of the groove were sutured over the transferred peroneus quartis tendon. At follow-up 1 year later, their patient was performing all required duties as a firefighter and was asymptomatic.[161]

Reconstruction of the peroneal retinaculum with an osteoperiosteal flap was conceived and described by Watson-Jones in 1955.[248] With this technique, a flap of periosteum (1.0 × 1.35 cm) is elevated from the distal fibula. The posterior periosteum and soft tissue structures are left intact. The flap is reflected posteriorly and sutured to the remaining portion of the superior retinaculum and the fascia of the flexor muscles of the great toe. The tendon sheath of the peroneal muscles is not opened, and the groove is not deepened. After surgery, the patient is placed in a short-leg cast for 4 to 6 weeks and then rehabilitated until he or she has gained full range of motion and full strength.

The results of this procedure have been reported in only a limited number of studies. Scheller and colleagues performed this procedure in seven patients and subsequently described their follow-up at a minimum of 15 years. All seven patients had excellent results and returned to their pre-injury sporting activities.[213] In contrast, Das De and Balasubramaniam noted that two of three patients treated by them in this manner had recurrent dislocations and poor results.[44] They concluded that the failures were due to the fact that the procedure did not address the primary disease involved. They operated on seven subsequent patients with recurrent dislocations and noted that in all cases the periosteum was stripped from the lateral malleolus but remained in continuity with the superior retinaculum. The detached periosteum extended forward to the anterior margin of the lateral malleolus and down to its tip, creating a false pouch into which the peroneal tendons easily dislocated. They suggested that this injury was similar to that found in a Bankart's lesion in recurrent dislocations of the shoulder. They repaired the avulsed periosteum by scarifying the outer surface of the lateral malleolus and then suturing the periosteal flap to the lateral malleolus through the drill holes in the lateral edge of the peroneal groove. Their results in all seven cases were excellent at a minimum follow-up of 2 years.[44] In 1998, they published the results of 21 patients treated as outlined above. They reported that 18 had good results and had returned to their pre-injury level of activity. The three fair results were due to painful scars or neuromas.[113]

Subluxation of the peroneal tendons within the peroneal sheath has been described by McConkey and Favero[154] and Harper.[85] The former authors reported on a 28-year-old runner who, 5 years after a plantar flexion inversion injury, complained of intermittent pain and clicking in the area of the peroneal tendons during jumping and pivoting activities. There was no evidence of anterior subluxation of the peroneal tendons, but the patient was able to reproduce the painful clicking of the tendons with dorsiflexion and eversion of the foot. Direct compression over the tendons eliminated the clicking. When nonoperative treatment was unsuccessful, the peroneal tendons were surgically explored under a local anesthetic. At surgery, it was evident that dorsiflexion and eversion of the foot caused the peroneus brevis to rise out from under the peroneus longus and to displace posterolaterally. This maneuver produced the click that the patient had been experiencing. They corrected this problem by taking strips of the retinaculum and passing them under the peroneus longus but over the peroneus brevis. At follow-up 4 years later, the patient had returned to athletic participation, including basketball, without recurrence of the symptoms.[154]

Harper described two cases of subluxation of the tendons within the peroneal groove. One occurred insidiously in a 13-year-old girl, and the other developed in a 26-year-old man after several inversion injuries to the ankle.[85] Both were treated successfully, one with tenodesis of the brevis tendon to the longus after failure of a tendon-sling procedure, and the other with rerouting of the tendons.[85]

Author's Preferred Method of Treatment

My experience parallels that of Eckert and Davis and of Murr, who concluded that the results of closed methods of treatment are disappointing and doomed to failure.[50, 174] Thus, my preferred method of treatment for acute disloca-

tions is to reduce the tendons and tape the ankle with a felt pad over the perineal groove to allow the athlete to attempt to complete the current season. At the end of the season, a reconstruction of the retinaculum and deepening of the groove (as detailed later) are performed.

I have treated one athlete who presented with dislocated peroneal tendons that could not be reduced by closed methods. The injury had occurred 1 month before my evaluation of the athlete. During that interval, the individual had been examined by two physicians who, in spite of the mother's insistence that the tendon was dislocated, failed to recognize and diagnose the injury. This individual sought another opinion because he was unable to jog or participate in sports owing to pain, weakness, and lateral ankle instability. This athlete was surgically treated with the method outlined later for chronic dislocations.

My surgical treatment of chronic dislocations includes deepening the retromalleolar groove and reconstructing the superior peroneal retinaculum. Deepening of the peroneal groove is achieved using the method described by Zoellner and Clancy.[258] In this technique, a 5- to 7-mm J-shaped incision is made over the posterior aspect of the lateral malleolus along the course of the peroneal tendons. The superior and inferior retinaculi are incised, and the tendons are freed from their sheath and retracted anteriorly over the lateral malleolus. A small drill bit is then used to define the borders of an osteoperiosteal flap (4 cm in length and 1 cm in width) in the peroneal sulcus of the distal fibula and lateral malleolus. A small osteotome or an oscillating saw with a 3/8-inch blade is used to connect the drill holes along the superior, lateral, and inferior margins of the flap. The periosteum of the posterior medial border of the flap is left intact to act as a hinge. The flap is then raised and swung posteriorly to allow access to the cancellous bone beneath it. The cancellous bone from the posterior aspect of the fibula is removed to a depth of 8 to 10 mm. One should also remove the cancellous bone that remains on the posterior aspect of the flap and the cancellous bone under the intact medial edge of the sulcus to prevent the flap from springing open when it is tapped back into place. The flap will usually be held firmly when it is tapped back into position. If it is not, however, the flap can be held in its new bed with sutures that are passed through drill holes in the flap and the anterolateral cortex of the fibula.

The peroneal tendons are replaced in the new groove and the ankle is put through a full range of motion. If the tendons do not remain well seated and show a tendency to subluxate, the groove should be deepened by removing more cancellous bone. I also routinely reconstruct the superior retinaculum with a periosteal flap (1 cm^2) fashioned from the lateral surface of the malleolus, hinged on its posterolateral side, and sutured to the medial part of the peroneal retinaculum.

Although I have not found it necessary to perform additional procedures, I would not hesitate to augment the lateral edge of the fibula and further deepen the groove by using the modified bone block procedure described by Kelly.[108] The subcutaneous tissues are closed with a running 2–0 absorbable suture, and the skin is closed with a running subcuticular 3–0 nonabsorbable suture.

After surgery, the patient is placed in a short-leg boot for 2 weeks. At that juncture, the running subcuticular suture is removed, and the patient is allowed to bear full weight as wound healing and the patient's pain dictate. Three weeks after surgery, the patient is instructed to take off the boot and begin dorsiflexion and plantar flexion exercises three to four times per day. Immobilization is discontinued 6 weeks after surgery, and the patient begins further range of motion and strengthening exercises. The criteria for return to sports participation are the achievement of full range of motion and full strength, and completion of a running program.

The running program is initiated when the patient has a full range of motion and strength equal to 80% of that of the contralateral extremity. The athlete begins by jogging one quarter of a mile and then, if there is no pain or limp, progressing to 1 mile. At that time the athlete is instructed to perform six 40-yard "sprints" sequentially at half, three-quarters, and full speed. Athletes are allowed to increase their speed only when they have had no pain or limp at slower speeds. They subsequently repeat the same routine, alternately "cutting off" the injured and uninjured ankle every 10 yards. Most athletes are able to obtain a full range of motion and normal strength and to complete the running program within 12 to 16 weeks of surgery.

Achilles Tendon Injuries

Injuries of the Achilles tendon include peritendinitis, tendinosis, and partial or complete ruptures. Several authors report that peritendinitis of the Achilles is the most common overuse syndrome seen in sports medicine clinics.[37, 99, 121, 128, 177, 214] Although the true incidence of peritendinitis and tendinosis in athletes is not known, Achilles tendon pain accounted for 6.5% to 11% of the complaints of runners who were examined for lower extremity problems,[37, 99] and it has been reported in a variety of other sports such as soccer, football, tennis, volleyball, basketball, badminton, and handball.[62, 76, 177] Similarly, although there have been several studies of partial ruptures of the Achilles tendon, the true incidence of this phenomenon also has not been documented.[48, 57, 96, 135, 220] Reported estimates of the prevalence of Achilles tendinitis, however, are 11% in runners,[52] 9% in dancers,[204] 5% in gymnasts,[29] 2% in tennis players,[253] and less than 1% in football players.[257] In the various published reports to date, the mean age of patients with peritendinitis and tendinosis ranged from 24 to 30 years, and the youngest and oldest were 16 and 52 years, respectively.[29, 37, 48, 177, 204, 253, 257]

Basically, Achilles peritendinitis and tendinosis are overuse phenomena and are the result of accumulative impact loading and repetitive microtrauma to the tendon.[36, 37, 62, 76, 99, 214] In Clement and colleagues' series of 109 runners with Achilles tendinitis, the average distance run per week for males was 34 miles (range 12 to 70 miles) and for females it was 24 miles (range 10 to 50 miles).[37] There are, however, both intrinsic and extrinsic factors that predispose an athlete to these injuries. Intrinsic factors include areas of decreased vascularity,[86, 122] aging and degeneration of the tendon,[11, 36, 192] and anatomic deviations such as heel-leg or heel-forefoot malalignment,[99, 122, 221] and poor gastrocnemius-soleus flexibility.[37, 128, 214] Clement and

his colleagues proposed that a varus position of the heel or supination of the forefoot produced functional overpronation of the foot during running. He and others have concluded that this type of mechanical deformation may result in a whipping action in the tendon and increased friction between the tendon and the peritendinous tissues.[36, 37]

Extrinsic factors that predispose an athlete to tendinitis include a sudden increase in training intensity, interval training, change of surface (soft to hard), and inappropriate or worn-out footwear.[37, 177, 221] McCrory and coworkers did a discriminant analysis of significant variables to determine causal factors associated with Achilles tendinitis. Their study revealed that plantar flexion peak torque, touchdown angle, and years running were the strongest discriminators between runners afflicted with Achilles tendinitis and runners who had no history of overuse injury.[155] Although complete ruptures most often occur in middle-aged persons after a specific precipitating event, partial ruptures occur in younger individuals (20 to 30 years of age) who have reached their highest level of performance.[48, 62]

Anatomic Considerations

The tendo calcaneus (Achilles tendon), which is the thickest and strongest tendon in the body, is formed approximately 15 cm above the heel at the confluence of the soleus and the gastrocnemius muscles. Although the tendon begins where the muscle belly of the gastrocnemius ends, it continues to receive muscle fibers on its anterior surface from the soleus almost to the malleolar level. The soleus and gastrocnemius components of the tendon can be separated and identified almost to the tendon's insertion at the calcaneus, which is approximately 1.5 cm distal to the tip of the superior tuberosity. Between its origin and insertion, the tendon twists laterally (approximately 90 degrees) so that the tendinous fibers from the gastrocnemius insert into the posterolateral and those from the soleus insert into the posteromedial aspect of the calcaneus. Proximal to the site of insertion of the tendon, the retrocalcaneal bursa is interposed between the tendon and the upper part of the bony surface of the calcaneus. The narrowest part of the tendon is 4 cm proximal to its insertion, and throughout its length, the tendon is separated from the deep muscles by areolar and adipose tissue. The small saphenous vein and sural nerve are located along its lateral side. Lagergren demonstrated that the Achilles tendon has an avascular zone 2 to 6 cm above its insertion into the calcaneus.[122] Stein and colleagues confirmed these findings using a new method with injection of radioisotopes. They found that the intravascular volume of the middle part of the tendon (3 to 6 cm above the calcaneal insertion) was significantly lower than the proximal or distal parts of the tendon.[230] This area of avascularity is the most common site of peritendinitis, tendinosis, and rupture of the tendon.* Hastad and colleagues demonstrated through isotope clearance studies that there is deterioration in the nutrition of the tendon with advancing age.[86]

The pathologic changes in Achilles tendon injuries span

---

*See references 37, 62, 72, 92, 93, 97, 127, 129, 136, 148, 177, and 214.

a continuum of abnormalities but generally can be defined by three stages. In stage I, the tendon is normal, but there are inflammatory changes in the peritendinous tissue that include thickening and adherence of the sheath to the tendon and on occasion an exudative fluid around the tendon. This stage is most aptly described as peritendinitis.[76, 192] In two series of patients with Achilles tendinitis (a total of 188 tendons) in which the tendon was surgically explored, isolated peritendinitis was observed in 50% to 59% of the cases.[177, 214] The terms *tendinosis* and *peritendinitis with tendinosis* best describe the second stage, which is characterized either by degenerative and inflammatory changes within the tendon or by degenerative changes within the tendon and associated inflammation of the peritendinous tissue, respectively. Macroscopic examination of the tendon may reveal nodular thickening, areas of metaplastic calcification, or loss of the normal luster of the tendon at several locations.[11, 57, 62, 136, 177, 192] Microscopic examination reveals areas of mucoid degeneration, fibrinoid necrosis, and tearing of the tendon fibers.[11, 177, 192, 214] In general, tendinosis does not affect the whole tendon but may affect nonadjacent areas of the tendon. In the aforementioned series of Nelen and associates[177] and Schepsis and Leach,[214] tendinosis (intrinsic degeneration) without macroscopic ruptures was observed in 20% and 33% of the operated tendons, respectively.

In the final stage of injury, macroscopic, visible disruption of the tendon occurs. These macroscopic tears occur in both the peripheral and central areas of the tendon. In the studies cited above, macroscopic tears and partial disruption of the tendon were found in 21% of the cases.[177, 214]

Clinical Evaluation

The predominant symptom of Achilles tendinitis is pain, which is localized to the area of the tendon 2 to 6 cm above its insertion.[4, 5, 36, 37, 48, 62, 177, 183, 214] In Nelen and associates' series of 91 patients who were operated on for chronic Achilles tendinitis, the extrinsic factors that contributed to the onset of symptoms were sudden changes of training in 31% of the patients, inappropriate training surface in 15%, inappropriate shoes in 7%, and direct trauma in 10%. Clement and colleagues studied 109 runners and concluded that the three most prevalent causal factors were overtraining (75%), functional overpronation (56%), and poor gastrocnemius-soleus flexibility (38%).[37]

In the early stages of tendinitis, the athlete experiences pain only with prolonged running. The pain usually subsides rapidly with rest but may be exacerbated by climbing stairs. In the subacute stage, the pain is present at the start of a run and becomes worse with sprinting, sometimes forcing the athlete to stop or to cut down on sports activity. In the advanced stages, when there is tendinosis or a partial rupture, the athlete is unable to run and experiences pain at rest. The athlete may also complain of weakness and intermittent swelling.[220] Several authors think that the presence and severity of morning stiffness is a good standard by which to evaluate the seriousness of the condition.[128, 177] Nelen and associates found the following incidence of symptoms in the 91 patients that they explored surgically

for chronic Achilles tendinitis.[177] Thirty-five percent had pain only during sports activities, 65% had pain with daily activities, 86% had morning stiffness, 10% had pain at rest, and 35% had acute sharp pain, felt during a sprint or acceleration while running.[177] The aforementioned constellation of symptoms caused 54% of these athletes to decrease their sports activity and 46% to discontinue it.[177]

The physical findings in patients with Achilles peritendinitis and tendinosis include soft tissue swelling, local tenderness, and crepitus.[13, 128, 177, 183, 192, 215, 221] In the early stages, there is focal swelling and tenderness limited to a small area, usually no larger than the breadth of the palpating fingertips. The area of tenderness can be defined by squeezing the diseased tendon segment between the thumb and index finger. Crepitus, which is the result of an exudation around the tendon, is more commonly found in the acute stage and is accentuated by active dorsiflexion and plantar flexion of the foot. In all stages of tendinitis and tendinosis, including partial ruptures, Thompson's test is negative.

In chronic tendinitis, the area of tenderness is somewhat larger, and often the area is thickened and nodular. When one detects nodularity in the tendon, one should be suspicious of tendinosis or a partial rupture of the tendon.[177] In Denstad and Roass's series of 58 partial ruptures that were treated surgically, there was localized tenderness in 56 (97%), focal swelling in 53 (91%), but a palpable defect in the tendon in only 2 (3%).[48] In contrast, Skeoch examined 11 patients (16 tendons) with partial ruptures and concluded that palpation of the tendon generally reveals a partial defect.[220]

Differential diagnosis of patients with posterior heel pain includes retrocalcaneal bursitis and superficial tendo Achilles bursitis or "pump bumps."[36, 128] The superficial bursa of the Achilles tendon lies between the tendon and the skin and becomes inflamed as a result of friction from the heel counter of a shoe. The retrocalcaneal bursa lies anterior to the tendon, and inflammation of this structure usually is associated with prominence of the posterior superior tuberosity of the os calcis.

Standard AP and lateral radiographs of the ankle rarely show calcification of the soft tissues around the tendon or in the tendon itself; however, a prominent superior tuberosity of the os calcis will be evident on the lateral radiograph.[128] Lateral radiographs taken with a soft tissue technique may show localized swelling, particularly in the area of Kager's triangle,[121] which includes the retrocalcaneal bursa.[48, 121] The incidence of calcification within the Achilles tendon is not known because bone formation itself does not cause symptoms.[57] As noted in subsequent sections of this chapter, however, rupture of the Achilles tendon may occur through the ossified area[136] or in the tendon adjacent to the site of ossification.[57]

Studies on sonographic evaluation of athletes with chronic Achilles tendinosis have found that this modality accurately demonstrates both tendinitis and tendinosis (and associated microtears) of the tendon.[68, 69]

Treatment Options
Nonoperative Treatment

Most cases of Achilles peritendinitis and tendinosis are successfully managed nonoperatively. The basic modalities of nonoperative treatment are rest or a decrease in the runner's weekly mileage, use of a 1/4- to 3/8-inch heel lift, oral nonsteroidal anti-inflammatory medications, use of an orthotic to correct excessive pronation, ultrasound, and stretching exercises.[37, 128, 177, 214] Total rest usually is not required, but the athlete should be instructed to avoid hill work and interval training.[128, 214] Clement and colleagues suggest a form of modified rest in which the athlete is allowed to participate in swimming and cycling activities but is not allowed to resume running for 7 to 10 days after the symptoms have subsided.[37]

Although several authorities advise the use of a 1/4- to 3/8-inch heel lift to decrease tension on the Achilles tendon, a recent study did not substantiate the claimed benefit of these viscoelastic pads. In a blind observer, random prospective study of 33 subjects with Achilles tendinitis, Lowdon and associates found that subjects treated with ultrasound and exercises showed more profound improvement at both the 10-day and 2-month assessments than the two patient groups that received heel pads and exercises.[137]

The positive effects of ultrasound therapy on the repair of Achilles tendon injuries have been documented (in rats) by Jackson and coworkers.[96] They found that ultrasound increased the rate of collagen synthesis and the breaking strength of the Achilles tendon. The breaking strengths of treated tendons were significantly greater than those of untreated tendons at 5, 9, 15, and 21 days after injury.

Stretching exercises have been proposed by several authorities as a key to nonoperative treatment of Achilles tendinitis.[37, 128, 177, 214] Leach and associates stressed that the common finding in patients with posterior heel pain due to Achilles tendinitis is loss of passive dorsiflexion. There are two recommended methods of stretching, but with either method, the stretching should be slow and should be sustained for 20 to 30 seconds. With one method, the individual leans against a wall with the knees straight and the heel flat on the floor. With the other method, the involved foot is placed forward and both the knee and the ankle are flexed while the heel is held flat on the floor. It has been my experience that the former method of stretching affects the more proximal tendon and musculotendinous junction, whereas the latter method has a more profound effect on the insertion and distal aspect of the Achilles tendon.

Immobilization of the ankle for a period of 7 to 10 days may be indicated in individuals with severe acute symptoms.[128] Steroid injections, however, should be limited to the area of the retrocalcaneal bursa and should be employed only in patients with recalcitrant retrocalcaneal bursitis.[128, 214] There is a growing amount of evidence that steroid injections in and around the Achilles tendon may increase the risk of tendon rupture.[14, 15, 115, 128] Kleinman and Gross reported on three cases of Achilles tendon ruptures that occurred 2 to 6 weeks after the injection of steroids into the tendon. In all cases, the rupture was the result of minor trauma, and the tears were transverse.[115] They concluded that the tears were directly attributable to the steroid injection because rupture of the Achilles tendon usually is a sudden traumatic event, and in such patients, surgical exploration reveals that the tendon ends are shredded and interdigitated. In the three patients of Kleinman and Gross, however, the tears were transverse, and the tendon ends were rounded, with obvious preexisting degen-

erative changes. Astrom analyzed 342 cases of partial ruptures in 298 patients who were operated on for chronic painful Achilles tendinopathy.[13] A logistic regression analysis of age, gender, physical activity, and preoperative steroid injections found that only preoperative steroid injections and male gender predicted a partial rupture.[13]

A study by Balasubramaniam and Prathap[14] supports the conclusions reached by Kleinman and Gross,[115] and Astrom and Rausing.[13] They created central tears in the Achilles tendon of rabbits and then injected hydrocortisone acetate into one side and compared the effects of the injection with the rabbit's contralateral tendon. They subsequently sacrificed the animals at various intervals and observed the following changes on the injected side. Within 45 minutes there was separation of collagen bundles, and by 24 to 72 hours, areas of necrosis within the collagen were evident. At both 1 and 8 weeks after injection, they found that there was no evidence of repair of the Achilles tendon lesions, and in some animals, there was evidence of dystrophic calcification.[14]

Although most authors recommend nonoperative treatment of Achilles tendinitis, only Clement and colleagues have reported the results of a large series of patients (109 runners) treated in this manner.[37] Of these 109 athletes, 86 had complete follow-up and 85 had good or excellent results (e.g., they had achieved pre-injury training levels and either were symptom-free or had minor symptoms on occasion). Clement and colleagues and other authorities, however, stress that athletes will not remain symptom-free unless they understand the extrinsic factors that caused the injury.[4, 37, 128, 214] They should also be instructed in preventive measures, which include warming the Achilles tendon before running, applying ice for 10 to 15 minutes after running, and monitoring their shoe wear, particularly the posterolateral aspect of the shoe. The most important preventive measure is stretching the posterior structures to prevent contractures and loss of passive dorsiflexion.[37, 128, 214]

Recently, Alfredson and colleagues prospectively studied the effect of heavy-load eccentric training in 15 athletes who had chronic Achilles tendinosis.[4] All 15 experienced fast recovery in eccentric and concentric calf muscle and returned to previous running activity symptom-free. They concluded that there was little place for surgery in the treatment of chronic Achilles tendinosis located at the 2-cm to 6-cm level in the tendon.[4]

Operative Treatment

Operative treatment should be considered when a comprehensive nonoperative treatment program of several months' duration has failed and the athlete is not willing to alter or abandon the precipitating sports activity. Surgical treatment is required in about 25% of athletes with Achilles tendon overuse injuries.[120] Although the surgical procedure performed should depend entirely upon the disease found at the time of the operation, there are basically four distinct surgical procedures. These include release of the Achilles tendon sheath; excision of degenerated segments of tendon and side-to-side repair; excision of degenerated tissue and reconstruction of the tendon with fascial flaps from the gastrocnemius; and excision of the retrocalcaneal bursa and ostectomy of the superior tuberosity of the os calcis.[5, 13, 48, 76, 128, 177, 183, 214, 215, 221]

In cases of pure peritendinitis, it is recommended that the sheath of the Achilles tendon be released from the musculotendinous junction to the insertion of the tendon.[76, 128, 177, 214, 221] Adhesions between the tendon and the sheath should be released but only on the dorsal, medial, and lateral sides of the tendon. Circumferential dissection of the tendon will damage the anterior vascular supply of the tendon and cause excessive scarring.[37, 128, 177, 214] Several authors also make a number of vertical slits in the tendon to "vent" the tendon and encourage ingrowth of new blood vessels.[36, 76, 192]

In cases with focal tendinosis and partial rupture of the tendon, the diseased area of the tendon should be excised and the tendon repaired by side-to-side suture of the remaining normal tendinous fibers.[48, 177, 214] One must carefully inspect and palpate the tendon throughout its length because nonadjacent areas of tendinosis are common. The tendon should be opened in zones that have lost their normal luster and in areas of nodularity.

In cases where excision of the degenerated tissue disrupts the continuity of the tendon, one should reconstruct and reinforce the tendon with a turn-down flap of fascia from the gastrocnemius. In these cases, a modified Lindholm[132] repair, using only one flap of gastrocnemius fascia, will cover the defect.

When it is evident preoperatively that the patient has a retrocalcaneal bursitis, the bursa should be excised, and, if prominent, the posterior superior tuberosity of the os calcis should be removed.[128, 214] Ostectomy of the superior angle of the os calcis should begin just superior to the insertion of the Achilles fibers at an angle of 45 degrees to the long axis of the tendon. After excision of the fragment, any rough edges should be removed with a rasp or rongeur.[128, 214] The foot should then be put through a full range of motion to make sure that all areas of bony impingement have been excised.

Overall results of the aforementioned operative procedures were rated as good or excellent in 84% to 100% of the patients in the various series published to date.[13, 48, 128, 177, 183, 214, 215, 220, 221] In several studies, the results of specific procedures were reported.[177, 183, 214, 215] In Nelen and associates' series of 143 tendons that were surgically explored, release of the tendon sheath alone produced good or excellent results in 89% of the 93 tendons with peritendinitis. Excision of the degenerated tissues and side-to-side repair produced good or excellent results in 73% of the 26 tendons with tendinosis, and turned-down gastrocnemius flaps produced good or excellent results in 87% of the 24 tendons with more extensive tendinosis.[177] Complications from the aforementioned procedures included six cases of skin edge necrosis, two superficial wound infections, and one case of phlebitis.

Schepsis and Leach reported the results of 45 patients who underwent surgical exploration. In the 28 patients who had release of the sheath (15 cases), excision of areas of calcification (4 cases), or débridement of partial tears and repair of the tendon (nine cases), the results were good or excellent in 89%.[214] In the 11 patients who had excision of the retrocalcaneal bursa and a partial ostectomy of the os calcis, the results were good or excellent in 71% of the

cases. In the six remaining cases, a release of the tendon sheath, a retrocalcaneal bursectomy, and partial ostectomy of the os calcis were performed. All six patients had good or excellent results. They concluded that the higher percentage of unsatisfactory results in those treated for retrocalcaneal bursitis alone was due to technical errors. Specifically, either an inadequate amount of bone had been removed or concomitant adjacent Achilles tendinitis had not been appreciated at the time of the initial operation. In a subsequent long-term follow-up study that included an additional 21 patients (66 total), Schepsis and coworkers reported satisfactory results in 75% and 86% of the patients with retrocalcaneal bursitis, and insertional tendinitis, respectively.[216] They also reported that the highest percentage of satisfactory results (89%) were obtained in the paratendinitis group, and the lowest (67%) in the tendinosis group.[216]

In a recent study and the largest to date, Paavola and colleagues reported the results and complications of surgical treatment of Achilles tendon overuse injuries in 432 consecutive patients.[183] There was a total of 46 (11%) complications. Sixteen complications (35%) were classified as major: 14 skin edge necrosis; 1 new partial rupture; 1 deep vein thrombosis; and 30 (65%) were considered minor: 11 superficial wound infections; 5 seromas, 5 hematomas, 5 extensive scar/fibrotic reactions; and 4 sural nerve irritation. Fourteen (30%) of the 46 patients with complications had reoperations. They noted that every tenth patient treated surgically suffered a postoperative complication that clearly delayed recovery.[183] They suggested that these complications could be prevented through the meticulous adaptations in surgical techniques they describe.

Postoperative Management and Rehabilitation

In cases of peritendinitis in which only the sheath is divided, the postoperative protocols in the aforementioned series range from no immobilization[36, 183, 221] to cast immobilization for from 2 to 6 weeks.[128, 177, 214] A recent study found no advantages in recovery of muscle strength after surgery with a short immobilization time (2 weeks) versus a longer (6 weeks) period.[5] In those individuals with tendinosis and side-to-side repairs of the tendon, a non–weight-bearing splint is worn for 2 weeks and a short-leg walking cast is worn for an additional 2 weeks.[177, 183] Some authors, however, recommend no immobilization even after side-to-side repairs of the tendon.[48] When a flap of gastrocnemius has been used to reconstruct the Achilles tendon, most authorities recommend immobilization for a period of 5 to 7 weeks.[128, 177, 214, 215]

Stretching and strengthening of the Achilles tendon are initiated after immobilization has been discontinued. Patients then progressively increase their activity from walking and swimming to bicycling, jogging, and running. After a tendon reconstruction, they usually are able to jog within 8 to 12 weeks of surgery, but full recovery takes 5 to 6 months.[13, 128, 177, 183, 214]

Author's Preferred Method of Treatment

Initial treatment of Achilles peritendinitis and tendinosis always is conservative and focuses on control of pain and inflammation, correction of functional malalignment, and rehabilitation of the gastrocnemius–soleus muscle–tendon complex. In athletes who present within 1 to 2 weeks of the onset of symptoms, a short course (7 to 10 days) of oral, nonsteroidal anti-inflammatory medications and 2 weeks of rest usually will allow them to return to running, symptom-free. In addition, they are counseled about the extrinsic factors (e.g., errors in training) that may have caused their problem and about prophylactic measures (proper shoes, stretching) that can prevent Achilles tendinitis.

In most cases, however, the athlete seeks treatment only after he or she has attempted to "run through" the pain and has had to curtail or stop sports activities. In these cases, successful nonoperative treatment requires a more comprehensive program. First, the athlete must stop the precipitating activity (e.g., interval training, sprints, and so on), but is allowed to maintain aerobic fitness with alternative activities (such as swimming or cycling) if such activities can be performed without symptoms. This program of modified rest should be continued for 7 to 10 days after the Achilles tendon pain has subsided. Second, the athlete is started on a daily program of gastrocnemius-soleus stretching and strengthening exercises. Stretching is done in the manner outlined previously, and strengthening, initiated when pain has subsided, is achieved by performing toe raises with the heel hanging over the edge of a stair and moving the ankle through a full range of motion. Eccentric strengthening is accomplished with the toe raises by progressively increasing the speed of the heel drop. Third, functional components of malalignment are corrected with orthotics. Off-the-shelf flexible leather longitudinal arch supports (with or without a medial heel wedge) often are all that are needed to correct overpronation of the foot. Custom-made, rigid orthotics are obtained for patients with more severe or complex foot deformities.

Ten days to 2 weeks after symptoms subside, the athlete begins a gradual return to the pre-injury level of activity with a running program staged to include a progressive increase in intensity and duration. The rate at which an athlete is able to return to pre-injury training levels varies according to the severity and duration of each individual's symptoms. I use steroid injections only in athletes who have retrocalcaneal bursitis. In those individuals, the bursa (not the tendon) is injected with 1 mL of Xylocaine, 0.45% Marcaine, and 40 mg of dexamethasone. After the injection, the athlete is instructed to refrain from all physical activity for a minimum of 3 days. At that juncture, he or she begins the rehabilitation program outlined earlier for nonoperative treatment of Achilles tendinitis.

Operative treatment is offered to athletes who have Achilles pain after completing a 2- to 3-month program that includes "modified rest," oral anti-inflammatory medications, use of orthotics (arch supports and heel lifts), and physical therapy (stretching and ultrasound). The operation is performed with the patient prone on the operating table,

and the extent of the surgical procedure is dictated by the operative findings. In all patients, the tendon sheath is released throughout the length of the tendon, and the tendon is examined from its musculotendinous junction to its insertion on the calcaneus. In patients with peritendinitis and no macroscopic evidence of tendinosis, adhesions between the tendon and the tendon sheath are released, and vertical slits are made in the tendon in the area or areas that correspond with the patient's preoperative pain. If these vertical incisions reveal intrinsic degeneration of the tendon, the degenerated areas are excised, and a side-to-side repair of the tendon is performed.

In patients with partial ruptures or macroscopic evidence of tendinosis (nodularity, calcification, or loss of normal luster of the tendon), each area is opened through a longitudinal incision, and the abnormal segments of the tendon are excised. The method used to repair the tendon is predicated upon the amount of diseased tissue that is removed. A side-to-side repair is performed when 20% or less of the width of the tendon is excised. When wider segments are removed, an end-to-end repair and a turned-down flap of gastrocnemius fascia are used to reconstitute the integrity of the tendon. Details of the surgical technique and postoperative protocol for this procedure are provided in the following section on repair of Achilles tendon ruptures.

Patients who undergo a release of the tendon sheath or a side-to-side repair of the tendon are put in a short-leg, removable plastic boot for 2 weeks to facilitate wound healing. During that interval, they are allowed to bear weight on the extremity as tolerated. When the wound has healed, they begin the rehabilitation program outlined under the section on nonoperative treatment of Achilles tendinitis.

Achilles Tendon Ruptures

Spontaneous ruptures of the Achilles tendon generally occur in healthy, vigorous, "young" adults with no previous history of calf or heel pain.[18, 92, 103, 145, 178] Although the exact incidence of this injury is not known, Nistor reported that over a 4-year period, 107 people (0.02%) from a population of 500,000 were treated at his hospital (the only one in the area) for this injury.[178] In published series on this injury, the average age of the patients ranged from 37 to 43.5 years,[18, 23, 62, 92, 97, 127, 140, 145, 178] and 75% were between the ages of 20 and 49 years.[62, 93, 127, 140] In most series, the majority of individuals with this injury were men in their third to fifth decade of life who were participating in recreational sports activities.[18, 23, 92, 93, 129, 140, 145, 175, 178] The left Achilles is ruptured more frequently than the right,[228, 229] possibly because of the higher prevalence of individuals who are right-hand dominant and thus push off with their left foot. In many series, basketball and racket sports accounted for more than half of the injuries,[18, 93, 129, 178] and in one large study, 58 (52%) of 111 patients were playing badminton at the time of their Achilles tendon rupture.[31] One report noted a high (14.3%) incidence of gout in their patients compared with the normal prevalence in the general population of 0.2% to 0.3%.[18]

Although ruptures of the gastrocnemius musculotendinous junction (so-called tennis leg) occur, they are extremely rare injuries,[8] and the Achilles tendon most commonly ruptures 3 to 4 cm proximal to its insertion on the calcaneus, within the area of decreased vascularity.[122, 230] The pathogenesis of Achilles tendon rupture has been attributed to both degeneration of the tendon and excessive mechanical forces. Arner and Lindholm reported that all 92 ruptured tendons that they examined histologically had degenerative changes.[9] Kannus and Józsa found that 864 (97%) of the 891 spontaneously ruptured tendons they examined histologically had degenerative changes.[103] If tendon ischemia and secondary degeneration, however, were major factors, then patients older than 30 years of age would be expected to have a higher rate of rupture, which is not the case.[18, 62, 93, 97, 127, 140] In addition, pathologic specimens removed from acute ruptures often reveal the presence of hemorrhage and inflammation and no associated peritendinitis or tendinosis.[18, 93, 192] Thus, several authors have concluded that ruptures are due to a sudden overloading of the musculotendinous unit in a poorly conditioned individual rather than to underlying pathologic processes in the tendon.[92, 93]

The common precipitating event in 90% to 100% of individuals that sustain this injury is active forceful, sometimes unexpected plantar flexion of the foot.[18, 93] Arner and Lindholm classified the trauma that resulted in rupture in 92 patients into three categories.[9] The mechanism in the first category was pushing off with the weight-bearing foot while extending the knee. This type of movement, seen with sprint starts and in jumping sports, accounted for 53% of the ruptures in their series. The mechanism in the second category was sudden, unexpected dorsiflexion of the ankle. This mechanism, seen when an individual steps in a hole, accounted for 17% of the ruptures. The third category was violent dorsiflexion of a plantar flexed foot as occurs after a fall from a height. This mechanism was reported by 10% of the patients.[9]

The major current controversy regarding this injury is whether surgical repair or cast immobilization is the most appropriate method of treatment.

Clinical Evaluation

The great majority of patients who sustain spontaneous ruptures of the Achilles tendon note a sudden snap in the heel region at the time of injury and subsequent pain with flexion of the foot.[18, 62, 93, 103, 129, 144, 145] Kannus and Józsa reported that only 297 (33%) of the 891 patients in their study had symptoms before rupture of their Achilles tendon.[103] Many patients do not seek immediate treatment because they still are able to plantar flex their ankle, and approximately 70% of patients complain of pain in the ankle or heel only at the time of their initial medical evaluation. This presenting complaint along with a moderate limp and weakness in the ankle may suggest a mild sprain rather than a heel cord rupture. Thus, the correct diagnosis is missed at the time of initial evaluation in 25% of cases.[92, 93, 175, 177]

In acute cases, physical examination will reveal a palpable depression over the area of the tendon rupture, weakness of plantar flexion, and positive results on the calf squeeze or Thompson's test.[18, 62, 92, 93, 238] Thompson's test is performed with the patient prone on a table with the feet extending over the end of the table. The calf muscles are then squeezed between the examiner's thumb and forefingers in the middle third (the musculotendinous junction) below the place of widest girth. A "normal reaction" is shown by passive plantar movement of the foot. A "positive reaction" occurs when there is no plantar movement of the foot, indicating a rupture of the heel cord.[238] The test also can be performed with the patient kneeling on a chair.

The accuracy of Thompson's test for the diagnosis of fresh ruptures has been reported to be between 96% and 100%.[93, 179, 238] O'Brien, however, concluded that Thompson's test can be falsely positive.[179] He noted that with Thompson's test, tension in the Achilles tendon is produced by lifting and functionally shortening the gastrocnemius-soleus complex. When the gastrocnemius aponeurosis is torn and is no longer connected to that of the soleus, Thompson's test will indicate a complete rupture when in fact the Achilles tendon is intact.[179] Thus, he described and recommended a needle test for diagnosis of complete ruptures of the tendon.

The needle test is performed by inserting a 25-gauge needle into the calf just medial to the midline at a point 10 cm proximal to the superior border of the calcaneus. The foot is then passively dorsiflexed and plantar flexed, and the movement of the hub of the needle is noted. Movement of the needle in the direction opposite the direction of the foot indicates that the tendon is intact throughout its distal 10 cm.

O'Brien performed this test on 10 patients with suspected rupture of the Achilles tendon and found that two patients had a positive Thompson's test but a negative needle test. At surgery, both of these patients were found to have a partial rupture of the musculotendinous junction of the gastrocnemius, but the Achilles tendon was intact.[179] He further commented that false-positive results on Thompson's test may cause unwitting errors when the results of operative and nonoperative treatment of "complete" ruptures are compared.

A recent prospective study of 174 patients found that palpation of the gap was the least sensitive clinical test for an Achilles tendon rupture.[144] Although both the calf squeeze and O'Brien tests had a high positive predictive value, the calf squeeze test was significantly more sensitive (0.96 vs. 0.8) for diagnosis of an Achilles tendon tear.[144]

In chronic cases, defects in the tendon may not be evident or palpable owing to hematoma formation at the site of rupture and generalized swelling about the heel and ankle. Most patients do not have ecchymosis, swelling, or point tenderness as are usually found with acute ruptures,[148] and in one series, Thompson's test was positive in only 80% of the chronic cases.[18]

Standard radiographs usually are not diagnostic of an Achilles tendon rupture. Although Arner and colleagues reported that deformation of the contour of the distal stump was pathognomonic of an Achilles tendon rupture,[10] most authorities have concluded that standard radiographs are helpful only in confirming the diagnosis of rupture in patients with calcification of the tendon (Fig. 30G–10).[18, 148]

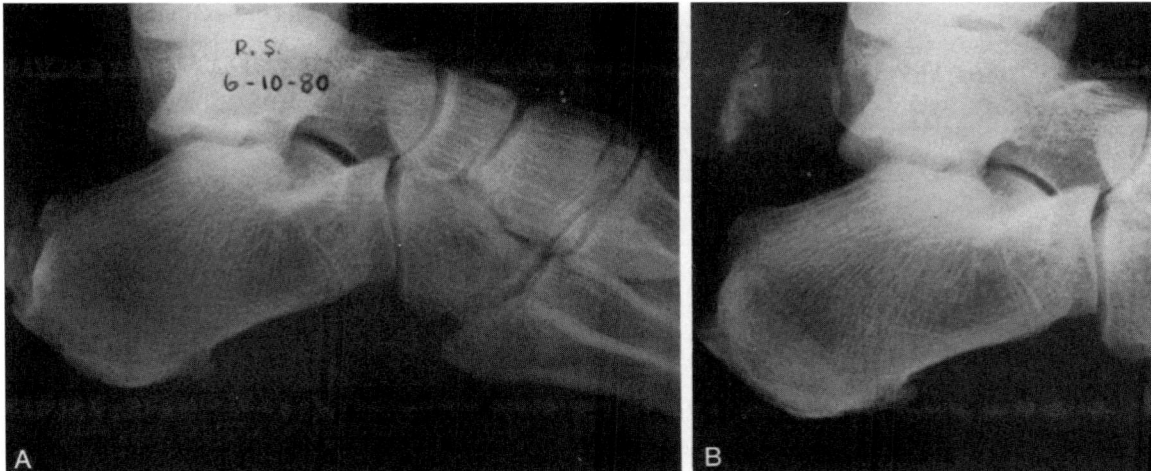

Figure 30G–10. Lateral radiographs of a 56-year-old patient with calcification of the Achilles tendon. The radiograph on the left *(A)* was obtained when the patient was evaluated for plantar fasciitis. Three years later *(B)*, the Achilles tendon was avulsed from the calcaneus.

With the advent of MRI, studies have been published that assess the diagnostic capabilities of this technique. One study found that MRI was extremely accurate for assessing the condition (e.g., shredded, uniform) and orientation (e.g., antegrade, retrograde) of the torn fibers and the width of the diastasis (with and without ankle flexion) between the ends of the tendon.[106] A second study identified four types of Achilles tendon lesions: type I, inflammatory reaction; type II, degenerative change; type III, incomplete rupture; and type IV, complete rupture.[250] I do not believe, however, that MRI is indicated for evaluation of Achilles tendon injuries because clinical tests are extremely reliable for diagnosis of complete ruptures, and treatment of lesser injuries should be predicated upon the results of nonoperative treatment.

Treatment Options

Controversy about Treatment Method

The best method of treatment for complete ruptures of the Achilles tendon remains controversial. A review of the literature reveals that there are comparable numbers of studies that advocate operative* and nonoperative[72, 127, 131, 153, 178, 229] methods of treatment. The advantages of nonoperative treatment are absence of wound complications, decreased patient cost, and lack of a scar. The disadvantages of nonoperative treatment are a re-rupture rate as high as 39% (Table 30G–1), a higher percentage of dissatisfied patients, and a significant loss of power, strength, and endurance compared with surgically treated patients.[18, 92, 93, 97] In addition, the results of surgical repair of re-rupture after nonsurgical treatment are not as good as those of primary repair.[216]

The advantages of surgical repair are a much lower rate of re-rupture, which ranges from 0 to 5% (Table 30G–2), a higher percentage of patients returning to sports, and a greater recovery of strength, power, and endurance.[18, 51, 93,]

*See references 18, 31, 51, 72, 92, 93, 97, 129, 130, 140, 187, 188, 225, and 249.

[97, 187, 188] The disadvantages of surgical repair are the cost of hospitalization and the major and minor complications of surgery (Table 30G–3). Complications such as deep venous thrombosis and pulmonary embolism have been reported with both methods of treatment.[9, 187, 188]

The limited number of studies (Table 30G–4) comparing operative and nonoperative methods of treatment have reached contradictory conclusions[72, 92, 97, 178] Nistor performed a prospective randomized study and found only minor differences in the results of the two methods of treatment.[178] He concluded that the treatment of choice is nonsurgical because in patients treated conservatively, there were fewer complications, fewer complaints, and no hospitalization. Gillies and Chalmers also concluded that owing to the complications of surgery, the results of operative repair of fresh ruptures were not significantly superior to those achieved with nonoperative management.[72] In both of these studies, the authors found no significant difference in the functional strength achieved by surgically and nonsurgically treated patients (see Table 30G–4).

TABLE 30G–1
Comparison of the Rate of Re-rupture in Reported Series of Nonoperatively Treated Achilles Tendon Ruptures

Authors	No. Cases	No. Re-ruptures	Percentage of Cases
Nistor[178]	60	5	8
Lea and Smith[127]	66	7	11
Lildholdt and Munch-Jorgensen[131]	14	2	12
Stein and Luekens[229]	8	1	13
Gillies and Chalmers[72]	7	1	14
Jacobs et al.[97]	32	7	22
Edna[51]	10	3	30
Persson and Wredmark[188]	20	7	35
Saleh et al.[206]	40	2	5
Inglis et al.[92]	23	9	39
Cetti et al.[31]	55	7	13
Totals	335	51	15.2

TABLE 30G–2
Comparison of the Rate of Re-rupture in Reported Series of "Open" Surgical Repairs of Achilles Tendon Ruptures

Authors	No. Cases	No. Re-ruptures	Percentage of Cases
Jacobs et al.[97]	26	0	0
Inglis and Sculco[93]	159	0	0
Lennox et al.[129]	20	0	0
Inglis et al.[92]	44	0	0
Percy and Conochie[187]	74	0	0
Shields et al.[217]	32	0	0
Gillies and Chalmers[72]	6	0	0
Ma and Griffith[140]	18	0	0
Beskin et al.[18]	42	0	0
Jessing and Hansen[100]	108	2	2
Arner and Lindholm[9]	92	4	4
Nistor[178]	44	2	5
Cetti et al.[31]	56	3	5
Soldatis et al.[225]	23	0	0
Mortensen et al.[169]	71	0	0
Speck and Klaue[227]	20	0	0
Aoki et al.[7]	22	0	0
Sölveborn and Moberg[226]	17	0	0
Totals	874	11	1.1%

In contrast, studies by Inglis and colleagues,[92] Jacobs and associates,[97] and Cetti and coworkers[31] not only documented a much higher rate of re-rupture with nonoperative treatment but also found that surgical repair resulted in significantly better restoration of strength, power, and endurance (see Table 30G–4). Both studies concluded that surgical treatment is the treatment of choice, particularly for active individuals. Two other relevant studies that examined the postoperative strength of patients found that surgical repair of re-rupture after failed conservative treat-

TABLE 30G–3
Comparison of the Rate of Postoperative Complications in Reported Series of Surgical Repairs of Achilles Tendon Ruptures

Authors	No. Cases	No. Major* Complications (%)	No. Minor† Complications (%)
Inglis and Sculco[93]	159	20 (13)	—
Jessing and Hansen[100]	108	7 (7)	18 (17)
Arner and Lindholm[9]	92	22 (24)	49 (53)
Percy and Conochie[187]	74	16 (22)	7 (10)
Inglis et al.[92]	44	2 (5)	—
Nistor[178]	44	4 (9)	29 (64)
Beskin et al.[18]	42	3 (7)	—
Shields et al.[217]	32	1 (3)	—
Jacobs et al.[97]	26	5 (19)	—
Lennox et al.[129]	20	8 (40)	1 (5)
Ma and Griffith[140]	18	0 (0)	2 (11)
Gillies and Chalmers[72]	6	1 (17)	—
Soldatis et al.[225]	23	0 (0)	2 (9)
Cetti et al.[31]	56	2 (4)	15 (27)
Totals	744	91 (12.2)	123 (16.5)

*Major complications include wound infection, delayed wound healing, skin slough, sinus tract formation, and re-rupture.

†Minor complications include adhesions of the tendon to the skin and sural nerve injury. (In several series, the number of minor complications was not reported.)

ment and early (less than 1 month of injury) surgical repair of acute ruptures produced better functional (strength) results than a second (8-week) period of casting and late surgical repair, respectively.[93, 188]

Nonoperative Treatment

The two largest series of patients treated nonoperatively were reported by Nistor[178] and by Lea and Smith.[127] Nonoperative treatment was popularized by Lea and Smith, who reported on 66 patients in 1972.[127] They immobilized their patients in a short-leg walking cast with the foot in a gravity equinus position for 8 weeks and allowed weight-bearing as soon as the cast was dry. The length (8 weeks) of immobilization was important because they documented a higher incidence of re-rupture with shorter periods of casting. After the cast was removed, the patient began active gastrocnemius strengthening exercises and used a 2.5-cm heel lift for 4 weeks.

In their series of patients, the average time to immobilization was 2.6 days (range, 1 to 42 days), and the majority (56%) of patients were placed in a cast within 24 hours of injury. At an average follow-up of 26 months (range, 5 months to 6.5 years), re-ruptures occurred in 7 (11%) of these 66 patients. All re-ruptures occurred within 1 to 4 weeks after the 8-week period of immobilization was completed. When a re-rupture occurred, they recommended a second full 8-week period of immobilization to ensure a good result.[127]

Nistor[178] modified this treatment protocol by using a below-knee gravity equinus cast for 4 weeks, a similar cast with less equinus for an additional 4 weeks, and a 2.5-cm heel lift for 4 subsequent weeks. In his series of 60 patients, there were five (8%) re-ruptures. All re-ruptures, which occurred between 9 and 16 weeks after the initial rupture, were treated with plaster casts for 7 to 9 weeks.

More recent studies have found that patients treated nonoperatively with splinting that allows controlled early mobilization are able to return to normal activities sooner.[153, 206] In 1997, McComis and colleagues reported on 15 patients who had nonoperative treatment of their Achilles tendon rupture with a functional bracing protocol.[153] The brace allowed immediate weight-bearing and active plantar flexion of the ankle, but limited dorsiflexion of the ankle. They graded their results (100-point scoring system) as Excellent in three patients, Good in nine, Fair in two, and Poor in one. Five patients had a positive result on the Thompson squeeze test at their 2-year follow-up.[153]

Operative Treatment

Surgical treatment of Achilles tendon ruptures initially recommended by Abrahamson in 1923 and by Queru and Stainovitch in 1929 has become increasingly popular since Arner and Lindholm published their results in 1959.[9] Open surgical procedures proposed for acute disruptions (less than 4 weeks after injury) include end-to-end repair with a Bunnell, modified Kessler, or pull-out wire suture[7, 18, 93, 97, 129, 169, 187, 226, 227]; end-to-end repair with the three-tissue bundle technique[18]; and direct repair and augmentation with tendon grafts,[18, 187] fascial flaps and grafts,[18, 93, 100, 129] or

TABLE 30G–4
Summary of Studies Comparing the Re-rupture Rate and Strength Achieved after Operative and Nonoperative Treatment of Achilles Tendon Ruptures

Authors	Operative				Nonoperative			
	No. Patients	No. Re-ruptures	Percentage of Cases	Strength* Achieved (%)	No. Patients	No. Re-ruptures	Percentage of Cases	Strength* Achieved (%)
Nistor[178]	44	2	5	83	60	5	8	79
Gillies & Chalmers[72]	6	0	0	84	7	1	14	80
Jacobs et al.[97]	26	0	0	75	32	7	22	65
Inglis et al.[92]	44	0	0	88	23	9	39	62
Totals	120	2	1.6		122	22	18	

*Strength of the normal leg was used to calculate the percentage of strength achieved after surgery.

synthetic (e.g., Dacron, Gore-Tex, and the like) grafts.[130] Closed surgical methods of repair include percutaneous suture[58, 75, 140, 249] and external fixation.[175]

In general, repairs are performed with the aid of a tourniquet and with the patient in the prone position. Although local anesthesia has been used successfully for repair of Achilles tendon ruptures,[7, 30, 107, 169] a general or regional anesthetic usually is administered to the patient for open repairs.[18, 93, 100, 187, 227] Many studies stress the importance of delaying surgery if there is substantial soft tissue swelling. They note that there is no difference in the functional result if the tendon is repaired within 30 days of rupture, and therefore optimizing local skin conditions is preferred over hasty surgical intervention.[18, 23, 93, 129]

For open repairs, an incision medial to the medial border of the Achilles tendon is recommended to minimize sural nerve injury. Inglis and colleagues recommend a darted incision, with darts created 1 inch apart at a 30-degree angle, to distribute skin pressure more evenly along the line of the incision and to increase the operating area of the incision.[93] The subcutaneous tissues are then opened to expose the deep (crural) fascia of the leg. The Achilles tendon is not a subcutaneous structure but lies beneath the deep crural fascia. The fascial layer is sharply dissected so that it can be closed carefully at the completion of the tendon repair. Closure of the deep fascia not only reduces tension on the skin closure but also acts as an interface between the subcutaneous tissue and the tendon repair and helps to prevent adherence of the tendon to the subcutaneous tissues and skin.

Although numerous surgical procedures have been proposed for repairing ruptures of the Achilles tendon, there is no single, uniformly superior technique. Analysis of the efficacy of one type of repair has been poorly documented because in most published series, several techniques were employed (Table 30G–5). It is evident from Table 30G–2, however, that all the techniques used in the different studies have been uniformly successful. In one study, Jessing and Hansen compared the results of end-to-end suture (54 patients) with those of direct repair augmented with a turndown graft of gastrocnemius fascia (48 patients). There was one re-rupture in each group, and they concluded that there were no significant differences in the functional results of these two operative procedures.[102] They did note, however, that although the rate of re-rupture with either technique was very low, the risk of sustaining a rupture of the contralateral tendon was quite high. Eight (26%) of the 31 patients in their series who resumed full sporting activities ruptured the other Achilles tendon within 2 to 14 years of their ipsilateral rupture. The basic concepts and principles of specific types of repairs are summarized in the following paragraphs.

TABLE 30G–5
Comparison of the Frequency of Various Procedures Performed for Open Repair of Acute Ruptures of the Achilles Tendon

Authors	No. Ruptures	Primary* Suture (%)	Local† Graft (%)	Three-Tissue Bundle (%)	Other‡ (%)
Inglis & Sculco[93]	162	79 (49)	81 (50)	—	2 (1)
Beskin et al.[18]	42	19 (45)	18 (43)	5 (12)	—
Lennox et al.[129]	20	16 (80)	4 (20)	—	—
Jacobs et al.[97]	25	16 (64)	9 (36)	—	—
Shields et al.[217]	32	—	26 (81)	—	6 (19)
Jessing & Hansen[100]	102	54 (53)	48 (47)	—	—
Totals	383	184 (48)	186 (49)	5 (1)	8 (2)

*In the primary suture group, direct repair with either a Bunnell or an amplified Kessler suture often was secured with a pullout wire.
†Local grafts included flaps of gastrocnemius fascia or augmentation with the plantaris or peroneus brevis tendon.
‡Includes reinsertion of the Achilles tendon into the os calcis via drill holes and os calcis bolt fixation.

pulled distally (1 to 1.5 cm) to approximate the ends of the tendon. The two K-wires are then maintained in their approximated position with an external fixator. The operation was performed under local anesthesia in 26 of the 33 patients.

Four weeks after the operation, the clamps and wires were removed, and the patients were placed in an equinus short-leg walking cast for an additional 4 to 5 weeks. After 8 weeks, immobilization was discontinued and the patients were given shoes with the heels built up 2.5 cm. Results at a mean follow-up of 2.4 years (range, 9 months to 4 years) were good or excellent in 30 of the 33 patients. Two patients had a fair result owing to sural nerve injuries, and one had a poor result owing to a Sudeck's atrophy. All except the patient with the poor result returned to their original level of activity, and there were no re-ruptures.

In the past decade, there have been additional studies to assess long-term results,[58] present new percutaneous techniques,[43, 75, 249] and compare the results of percutaneous and open surgical repair.[24] In 1990, Bradley and Tibone compared the results of 15 patients treated by open repair augmented with a gastrosoleus fascial graft, and 12 patients treated by percutaneous (Ma and Griffith type) repair.[24] They found that percutaneous repair resulted in strength levels similar to open repair, but had a re-rupture rate of 12%, significantly higher than the results of open repairs. They concluded that open repair should be performed in all high-caliber athletes who cannot afford any chance of re-rupture.[24]

Recently, new percutaneous surgical techniques have been developed to increase the strength of repairs[43] and decrease complications such as sural nerve injury.[249] Webb and Bannister reported results of 27 patients that had repairs through three midline stab incisions rather than Ma and Griffith's six (three lateral, three medial) skin incisions. They had no sural nerve injuries, compared with the 13% injury rate reported with the Ma and Griffith technique.[249]

In patients with neglected Achilles tendon ruptures, end-to-end repair often is not possible after excision of the intervening scar tissue. In these cases, grafts of fascia lata, local tendons (plantaris and peroneus brevis), or strips of Achilles tendon have been used to bridge the gap.[23, 194] Mann and colleagues oppose the use of free fascia and turn-down fascial grafts because they are avascular structures that must be revascularized to be incorporated into the repair.[148] They also note that transfer of the peroneus brevis carries the risk of changing the balance between the everters and inverters of the foot. Thus, they recommend transfer of the flexor digitorum longus and reported good and excellent results in six of the seven patients in which this procedure was performed.[148]

Abraham and Pankovich also found that results of repair of neglected rupture with strips of Achilles tendon and fascia lata were unsatisfactory.[1] They concluded that only an end-to-end repair of the chronic lesion would promote optimal functional recovery and restore muscle strength. Thus, they described a technique by which an end-to-end anastomosis was made possible by a proximal V-Y tendinous flap. With this technique, the tendon ends are appropriately trimmed and the length of the defect in the tendon is measured with the knee in 30 degrees of flexion and the ankle in 20 degrees of plantar flexion. An inverted V

incision, with arms that are 1½ times the length of the defect, is made over the central aponeurosis of the gastrocnemius. The incisions extend through the fascia and underlying muscle tissue of the gastrocnemius. The flap is then pulled distally and sutured to the distal stump of the ruptured tendon.

Postoperatively, the patient is placed in a long-leg cast for 6 to 8 weeks and then a short-leg, weight-bearing cast for an additional 4 to 6 weeks. The patient is subsequently placed in shoes with 3- to 5-cm heel lifts, which are worn for 1 month. Progressive resistive exercises are initiated immediately after the second cast is removed. In their series of four patients, there was only one surgical complication (a neuroma of the sural nerve), and three of the four patients regained full strength of the triceps surae muscle. The other patient had some residual weakness but was happy with the result.[1]

Author's Preferred Method of Treatment

Operative repair of Achilles tendon ruptures is my treatment of choice because the majority of my patients are intercollegiate or recreational athletes. Nonoperative treatment is always offered and discussed but usually is not recommended owing to the reported rate of re-rupture of 8% to 39% (see Table 30G–1) and the loss of strength after this method of treatment (see Table 30G–4). I have, however, treated acute ruptures with cast immobilization in patients who declined to have surgery, in elderly and chronically ill patients, and in middle-aged, sedentary, executive-type individuals who feel they cannot afford the time away from work required for operative treatment.

My preferred method of repair is shown in Figure 30G–13A to D. The procedure is performed on an outpatient basis, under a general or regional anesthetic. The patient is placed prone on the operating table, and the ruptured tendon is approached through a medial incision that parallels the medial border of the Achilles tendon. The skin and subcutaneous tissue are gently retracted with skin hooks and narrow retractors to expose the crural fascia. The fascia is incised along the medial border of the tendon so that its closure will be offset from that of the skin incision.

The ends of the tendon (see Fig. 30G–13A), which are not routinely débrided, are reapproximated with a modified Kessler stitch of No. 5 nonabsorbable suture. The peripheral fibers of each stump subsequently are sewn together with a running 2–0 absorbable suture (see Fig. 30G–13B). The repair is then reinforced with a strip of gastrocnemius fascia that is twisted 180 degrees on its distal pedicle and rotated distally to cover and extend 2 to 3 cm beyond the site of repair (see Fig. 30G–13C). A strip that is 10 to 12 cm long and 2 to 3 cm wide usually is sufficient because the fascia can easily be stretched to a width of 4 to 5 cm with tissue forceps. The fascial strip is secured to the distal stump and to the medial and lateral edges of the tendon with a running 2–0 absorbable suture (see Fig. 30G–13C). The ankle is then placed in a neutral position to assess the degree of tension on the repair. The defect in the gastrocnemius fascia and the sheath of the Achilles tendon are closed with interrupted and running 2–0 absorbable sutures, respectively (see Fig. 30G–13D). The skin is closed with a running subcuticular, 3–0 nonabsorbable su-

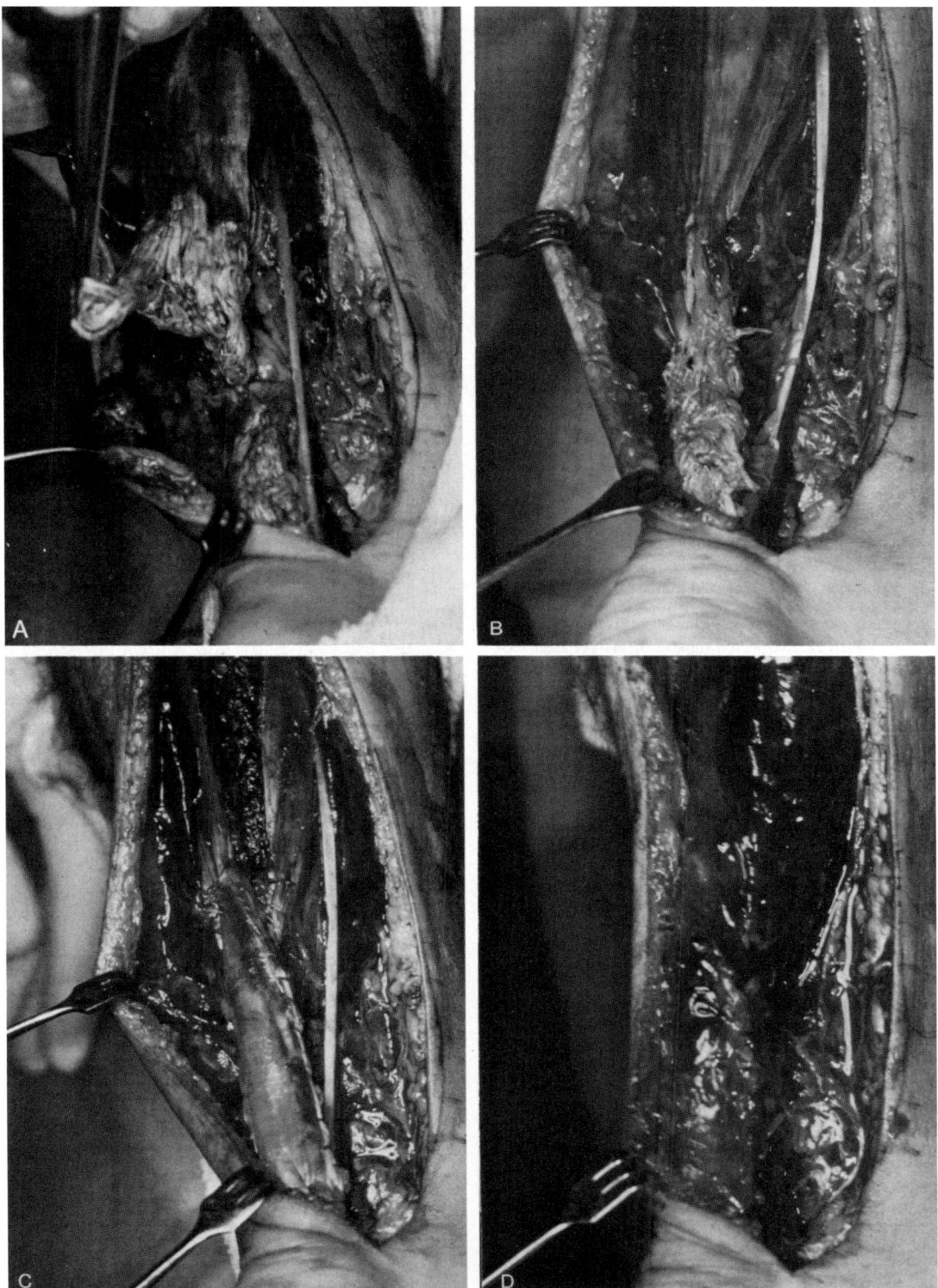

Figure 30G–13. The author's method for repair of Achilles tendon ruptures. The frayed ends of the tendon *(A)* are not routinely débrided. The ends of the tendon are reapproximated with a No. 5 nonabsorbable suture *(B)*, and the peripheral fibers are aligned and repaired with a running 2–0 absorbable suture. The repair is reinforced with a turned-down flap of gastrocnemius fascia *(C)*. The defect in the gastrocnemius fascia and the Achilles tendon sheath are repaired *(D)* before closure of the wound.

107. Keller J, Bak B: The use of anesthesia for surgical treatment of Achilles tendon rupture. Orthopedics 12:431–433, 1989.

108. Kelly RE: An operation for the chronic dislocation of the peroneal tendons. Br J Surg 7:502–504, 1920.

109. Kettelkamp DB, Alexander HH: Spontaneous rupture of the posterior tibial tendon. J Bone Joint Surg Am 51:759–764, 1969.

110. Key JA: Partial rupture of the tendon of the posterior tibial muscle. J Bone Joint Surg Am 35:1006–1008, 1953.

111. Khan KM, Gelber N, Slater K, Wark JD: Dislocated tibialis posterior tendon in a classical ballet dancer. J Dance Med Sci 1:160–162, 1997.

112. Khoury NJ, el Khoury GY, Saltzman CL, Brandser EA: MR imaging of posterior tibial tendon dysfunction. AJR Am J Roentgenol 167: 675–682, 1996.

113. Khoury NJ, el Khoury GY, Saltzman CL, Brandser EA: Rupture of the anterior tibial tendon: diagnosis by MR imaging. AJR Am J Roentgenol 167:351–354, 1996.

114. Kilkelly FX, McHale KA: Acute rupture of the peroneal longus tendon in a runner: A case report and review of the literature. Foot Ankle Int 15:567–569, 1994.

115. Kleinman M, Gross AE: Achilles tendon rupture following steroid injection. Report of three cases. J Bone Joint Surg Am 65:1345–1347, 1983.

116. Kolettis GJ, Micheli LJ, Klein JD: Release of the flexor hallucis longus tendon in ballet dancers. J Bone Joint Surg Am 78A:1386–1390, 1996.

117. Kollias SL, Ferkel RD: Fibular grooving for recurrent peroneal tendon subluxation. Am J Sports Med 25:329–335, 1997.

118. Krackow KA: Acute, traumatic rupture of a flexor hallucis longus tendon: A case report. Clin Orthop 150:261–262, 1980.

119. Krause JO, Brodsky JW: Peroneus brevis tendon tears: Pathophysiology, surgical reconstruction, and clinical results. Foot Ankle Int 19: 271–279, 1998.

120. Kvist M: Achilles tendon injuries in athletes. Sports Med 18:173–201, 1994.

121. Kvist MH, Lehto MU, Jozsa L, et al: Chronic Achilles paratenonitis. An immunohistologic study of fibronectin and fibrinogen. Am J Sports Med 16:616–623, 1988.

122. Lagergren C: Vascular distribution in the Achilles tendon. Acta Chir Scand 116:491–495, 1958.

123. Langan P, Weiss CA: Subluxation of the tibialis posterior, a complication of tarsal tunnel decompression: A case report. Clin Orthop 146:226–227, 1980.

124. Langenskiold A: Chronic non-specific tenosynovitis of the tibialis posterior tendon. Acta Orthop Scand 38:301–305, 1967.

125. Lapidus PW, Seidenstein H: Chronic non-specific tenosynovitis with effusion about the ankle: Report of three cases. J Bone Joint Surg Am 32:175–179, 1950.

126. Larsen E, Lauridsen F: Dislocation of the tibialis posterior tendon in two athletes. Am J Sports Med 12:429–430, 1984.

127. Lea RB, Smith L: Non-surgical treatment of tendo achillis rupture. J Bone Joint Surg Am 54:1398–1407, 1972.

128. Leach RE, James S, Wasilewski S: Achilles tendinitis. Am J Sports Med 9:93–98, 1981.

129. Lennox DW, Wang GJ, McCue FC, Stamp WG: The operative treatment of Achilles tendon injuries. Clin Orthop 148:152–155, 1980.

130. Levy M, Velkes S, Goldstein J, Rosner M: A method of repair for Achilles tendon ruptures without cast immobilization. Preliminary report. Clin Orthop 187:199–204, 1984.

131. Lildholdt T, Munch-Jorgensen T: Conservative treatment to Achilles tendon rupture. A follow-up study of 14 cases. Acta Orthop Scand 47:454–458, 1976.

132. Lindholm A: A new method of operation in subcutaneous rupture of the Achilles tendon. Acta Chir Scand 117:261–270, 1959.

133. Lipscomb PR: Nonsuppurative tenosynovitis and paratendinitis. American Academy of Orthopaedic Surgeons 7:254–261, 1950.

134. Lipscomb PR, Kelly PJ: Injuries of the extensor tendons in the distal part of the leg and in the ankle. J Bone Joint Surg Am 37:1206–1213, 1955.

135. Ljungqvist R: Subcutaneous partial rupture of the Achilles tendon. Acta Orthop Scand Suppl 113:1–86, 1967.

136. Lotke PA: Ossification of the Achilles tendon. Report of seven cases. J Bone Joint Surg Am 52:157–160, 1970.

137. Lowdon A, Bader DL, Mowat AG: The effect of heel pads on the treatment of Achilles tendinitis: A double blind trial. Am J Sports Med 12:431–435, 1984.

138. Lynn TA: Repair of the torn Achilles tendon, using the plantaris tendon as a reinforcing membrane. J Bone Joint Surg Am 48: 268–272, 1966.

139. Lysholm J, Wiklander J: Injuries in runners. Am J Sports Med 15: 168–171, 1987.

140. Ma GW, Griffith TG: Percutaneous repair of acute closed ruptured Achilles tendon: A new technique. Clin Orthop 128:247–255, 1977.

141. MacDonald BD, Wertheimer SJ: Bilateral os peroneum fractures: Comparison of conservative and surgical treatment and outcomes. J Foot Ankle Surg 36:220–225, 1997.

142. Macintyre JG, Taunton JE, Clement DB, et al: Running injuries: A clinical study of 4,173 cases. Clin J Sport Med 1:81–87, 1991.

143. Madsen BL, Noer HH: Simultaneous rupture of both peroneal tendons after corticosteroid injection: Operative treatment. Injury 30: 299–300, 1999.

144. Maffulli N: The clinical diagnosis of subcutaneous tear of the Achilles tendon: A prospective study in 174 patients. Am J Sports Med 26:266–270, 1998.

145. Maffulli N: Rupture of the Achilles tendon. J Bone Joint Surg Am 81:1019–1036, 1999.

146. Mains DB, Sullivan RC: Fracture of the os peroneum. A case report. J Bone Joint Surg Am 55:1529–1530, 1973.

147. Mann RA, Holmes GB Jr, Seale KS, Collins DN: Chronic rupture of the Achilles tendon: A new technique of repair. J Bone Joint Surg Am 73:214–219, 1991.

148. Mann RA, Thompson FM: Rupture of the posterior tibial tendon causing flat foot. Surgical treatment. J Bone Joint Surg Am 67: 556–561, 1985.

149. Markarian GG, Kelikian AS, Brage M, et al: Anterior tibialis tendon ruptures: An outcome analysis of operative versus nonoperative treatment. Foot Ankle Int 19:792–802, 1998.

150. Marotta JJ, Micheli LJ: Os trigonum impingement in dancers. Am J Sports Med 20:533–536, 1992.

151. Marti R: Dislocation of the peroneal tendons. Am J Sports Med 5: 19–22, 1977.

152. Mason RB, Henderson JP: Traumatic peroneal tendon instability. Am J Sports Med 24:652–658, 1996.

153. McComis GP, Nawoczenski DA, DeHaven KE: Functional bracing for rupture of the Achilles tendon. Clinical results and analysis of ground-reaction forces and temporal data. J Bone Joint Surg Am 79:1799–1808, 1997.

154. McConkey JP, Favero KJ: Subluxation of the peroneal tendons within the peroneal tendon sheath. A case report. Am J Sports Med 15:511–513, 1987.

155. McCrory JL, Martin DF, Lowery RB, et al: Etiologic factors associated with Achilles tendinitis in runners. Med Sci Sports Exerc 31: 1374–1381, 1999.

156. McLennan JG: Treatment of acute and chronic luxations of the peroneal tendons. Am J Sports Med 8:432–436, 1980.

157. McMaster PE: Tendon and muscle ruptures: Clinical and experimental studies on the causes and location of subcutaneous ruptures. J Bone Joint Surg Am 15:705–722, 1933.

158. Mensor MC, Ordway GL: Traumatic subcutaneous rupture of the tibialis anterior tendon. J Bone Joint Surg Am 35:675–680, 1953.

159. Meyn MA Jr: Closed rupture of the anterior tibial tendon. A case report and review of the literature. Clin Orthop 113:154–157, 1975.

160. Micheli LJ, Waters PM, Sanders DP: Sliding fibular graft repair for chronic dislocation of the peroneal tendons. Am J Sports Med 17: 68–71, 1989.

161. Mick CA, Lynch F: Reconstruction of the peroneal retinaculum using the peroneus quartus. A case report. J Bone Joint Surg Am 69:296–297, 1987.

162. Miki T, Kuzuoka K, Kotani H, Ikeda Y: Recurrent dislocation of tibialis posterior tendon. A report of two cases. Arch Orthop Trauma Surg 118:96–98, 1998.

163. Milgram JE: Muscle ruptures and avulsions with particular reference to the lower extremities. Instr Course Lect 10:233–243, 1953.

164. Miller RR, Mahan KT: Closed rupture of the anterior tibial tendon. A case report. J Am Podiatr Med Assoc 88:394–399, 1998.

165. Miller SD, Van Holsbeeck M, Boruta PM, et al: Ultrasound in the diagnosis of posterior tibial tendon pathology. Foot Ankle Int 17: 555–558, 1996.

166. Moberg E: Subcutaneous rupture of the tendon of the tibialis anterior muscle. Acta Chir Scand 95:455–460, 1947.

167. Moorman CT III, Monto RR, Bassett FH III: So-called trigger ankle due to an aberrant flexor hallucis longus muscle in a tennis player. A case report. J Bone Joint Surg Am 74:294–295, 1992.
168. Moritz JR: Ski injuries. Am J Surg 98:498–433, 1959.
169. Mortensen HM, Skov O, Jensen PE: Early motion of the ankle after operative treatment of a rupture of the Achilles tendon. A prospective, randomized clinical and radiographic study. J Bone Joint Surg Am 81:983–990, 1999.
170. Mosier SM, Lucas DR, Pomeroy G, Manoli A: Pathology of the posterior tibial tendon in posterior tibial tendon insufficiency. Foot Ankle Int 19:520–524, 1998.
171. Moskowitz E: Rupture of the tibialis anterior tendon simulating peroneal nerve palsy. Arch Phys Med Rehab 52:431–433, 1971.
172. Mota J, Rosenberg ZS: Magnetic resonance imaging of the peroneal tendons. Top Magn Reson Imaging 9:273–285, 1998.
173. Munk RL, Davis PH: Longitudinal rupture of the peroneus brevis tendon. J Trauma 16:803–806, 1976.
174. Murr S: Dislocation of the peroneal tendons with marginal fracture of the lateral malleolus. J Bone Joint Surg Br 43:563–565, 1961.
175. Nada A: Rupture of the calcaneal tendon. Treatment by external fixation. J Bone Joint Surg Br 67:449–453, 1985.
176. Nava BE: Traumatic dislocation of the tibialis posterior tendon at the ankle. Report of a case. J Bone Joint Surg Br 50:150–151, 1968.
177. Nelen G, Martens M, Burssens A: Surgical treatment of chronic Achilles tendinitis. Am J Sports Med 17:754–759, 1989.
178. Nistor L: Surgical and non-surgical treatment of Achilles tendon rupture. A prospective randomized study. J Bone Joint Surg Am 63:394–399, 1981.
179. O'Brien T: The needle test for complete rupture of the Achilles tendon. J Bone Joint Surg Am 66:1099–1101, 1984.
180. Oden RR: Tendon injuries about the ankle resulting from skiing. Clin Orthop 216:63–69, 1987.
181. Ouzounian TJ: Combined rupture of the anterior tibial and posterior tibial tendons: a new clinical entity. Foot Ankle Int 15:508–511, 1994.
182. Ouzounian TJ, Anderson R: Anterior tibial tendon rupture. Foot Ankle Int 16:406–410, 1995.
183. Paavola M, Orava S, Leppilahti J, et al: Chronic Achilles tendon overuse injury: Complications after surgical treatment—An analysis of 432 consecutive patients. Am J Sports Med 28:77–82, 2000.
184. Pai VS, Lawson D: Rupture of the peroneus longus tendon. J Foot Ankle Surg 34:475–477, 1995.
185. Patterson MJ, Cox WK: Peroneus longus tendon rupture as a cause of chronic lateral ankle pain. Clin Orthop 365:163–166, 1999.
186. Peacock KC, Resnick EJ, Thoder JJ: Fracture of the os peroneum with rupture of the peroneus longus tendon. A case report and review of the literature. Clin Orthop 202:223–226, 1986.
187. Percy EC, Conochie LB: The surgical treatment of ruptured tendo achillis. Am J Sports Med 6:132–136, 1978.
188. Persson A, Wredmark T: The treatment of total ruptures of the Achilles tendon by plaster immobilisation. Int Orthop 3:149–152, 1979.
189. Petersen W, Stein V, Tillmann B: Blood supply of the tibialis anterior tendon. Arch Orthop Trauma Surg 119:371–375, 1999.
190. Poll RG, Duijfjes F: The treatment of recurrent dislocation of the peroneal tendons. J Bone Joint Surg Br 66:98–100, 1984.
191. Porter DA, Baxter DE, Clanton TO, Klootwyk TE: Posterior tibial tendon tears in young competitive athletes: Two case reports. Foot Ankle Int 19:627–630, 1998.
192. Puddu G, Ippolito E, Postacchini F: A classification of Achilles tendon disease. Am J Sports Med 4:145–150, 1976.
193. Rademaker J, Rosenberg ZS, Delfaut EM, et al: Tear of the peroneus longus tendon: MR imaging features in nine patients. Radiology 214:700–704, 2000.
194. Ralston EL, Schmidt ER Jr: Repair of the ruptured Achilles tendon. J Trauma 11:15–21, 1971.
195. Rand T, Ahn JM, Muhle C, et al: Ligaments and tendons of the ankle—evaluation with low-field (0.2 T) MR imaging. Acta Radiol 40:303–308, 1999.
196. Rasmussen RB, Thyssen EP: Rupture of the flexor hallucis longus tendon: Case report. Foot Ankle 10:288–289, 1990.
197. Regan TP, Hughston JC: Chronic ankle "sprain" secondary to anomalous peroneal tendon. A case report. Clin Orthop 123:52–54, 1977.
198. Rockett MS, Waitches G, Sudakoff G, Brage M: Use of ultrasonography versus magnetic resonance imaging for tendon abnormalities around the ankle. Foot Ankle Int 19:604–612, 1998.
199. Roggatz J, Urban A: The calcareous peritendinitis of the long peroneal tendon. Arch Orthop Trauma Surg 96:161–164, 1980.
200. Rolf C, Guntner P, Ekenman I, Turan I: Dislocation of the tibialis posterior tendon: Diagnosis and treatment. J Foot Ankle Surg 36:63–65, 1997.
201. Romash MM: Closed rupture of the flexor hallucis longus tendon in a long distance runner: Report of a case and review of the literature. Foot Ankle Int 15:433–436, 1994.
202. Rosenberg ZS, Beltran J, Cheung YY, et al: MR features of longitudinal tears of the peroneus brevis tendon. AJR Am J Roentgenol 168:141–147, 1997.
203. Ross G, Regan KJ, McDevitt ER, Wilckens J: Rupture of the peroneus longus tendon in a military athlete. Am J Orthop 28:657–658, 1999.
204. Rovere GD, Webb LX, Gristina AG, Vogel JM: Musculoskeletal injuries in theatrical dance students. Am J Sports Med 11:195–198, 1983.
205. Safran MR, O'Malley D Jr, Fu FH: Peroneal tendon subluxation in athletes: New exam technique, case reports, and review. Med Sci Sports Exerc 31:S487–S492, 1999.
206. Saleh M, Marshall PD, Senior R, MacFarlane A: The Sheffield splint for controlled early mobilisation after rupture of the calcaneal tendon. A prospective, randomised comparison with plaster treatment. J Bone Joint Surg Br 74:206–209, 1992.
207. Sammarco GJ: Peroneus longus tendon tears: Acute and chronic. Foot Ankle Int 16:245–253, 1995.
208. Sammarco GJ, Brainard BJ: A symptomatic anomalous peroneus brevis in a high-jumper. A case report. J Bone Joint Surg Am 73:131–133, 1991.
209. Sammarco GJ, Cooper PS: Flexor hallucis longus tendon injury in dancers and nondancers. Foot Ankle Int 19:356–362, 1998.
210. Sammarco GJ, Miller EH: Partial rupture of the flexor hallucis longus tendon in classical ballet dancers: Two case reports. J Bone Joint Surg Am 61:149–150, 1979.
211. Sarmiento A, Wolf M: Subluxation of peroneal tendons. Case treated by rerouting tendons under calcaneofibular ligament. J Bone Joint Surg Am 57:115–116, 1975.
212. Saxena A, Pham B: Longitudinal peroneal tendon tears. J Foot Ankle Surg 36:173–179, 1997.
213. Scheller AD, Kasser JR, Quigley TB: Tendon injuries about the ankle. Orthop Clin North Am 11:801–811, 1980.
214. Schepsis AA, Leach RE: Surgical management of Achilles tendinitis. Am J Sports Med 15:308–315, 1987.
215. Schepsis AA, Wagner C, Leach RE: Surgical management of Achilles tendon overuse injuries. Am J Sports Med 22:611–619, 1994.
216. Scott WN, Inglis AE, Sculco TP: Surgical treatment of reruptures of the tendoachilles following nonsurgical treatment. Clin Orthop 140:175–177, 1979.
217. Shields CL, Kerlan RK, Jobe FW, et al: The Cybex II evaluation of surgically repaired Achilles tendon ruptures. Am J Sports Med 6:369–372, 1978.
218. Simonet WT, Sim L: Boot-top tendon lacerations in ice hockey. J Trauma 38:30–31, 1995.
219. Simpson RR, Gudas CJ: Posterior tibial tendon rupture in a world class runner. J Foot Surg 22:74–77, 1983.
220. Skeoch DU: Spontaneous partial subcutaneous ruptures of the tendo achillis. Review of the literature and evaluation of 16 involved tendons. Am J Sports Med 9:20–22, 1981.
221. Snook GA: Achilles tendon tenosynovitis in long-distance runners. Med Sci Sports 4:155–158, 1972.
222. Sobel M, DiCarlo EF, Bohne WH, Collins L: Longitudinal splitting of the peroneus brevis tendon: An anatomic and histologic study of cadaveric material. Foot Ankle 12:165–170, 1991.
223. Sobel M, Geppert MJ, Hannafin JA, et al: Microvascular anatomy of the peroneal tendons. Foot Ankle 13:469–472, 1992.
224. Sobel M, Geppert MJ, Olson EJ, et al: The dynamics of peroneus brevis tendon splits: A proposed mechanism, technique of diagnosis, and classification of injury. Foot Ankle 13:413–422, 1992.
225. Soldatis JJ, Goodfellow DB, Wilber JH: End-to-end operative repair of Achilles tendon rupture. Am J Sports Med 25:90–95, 1997.
226. Sölveborn SA, Moberg A: Immediate free ankle motion after surgical repair of acute Achilles tendon ruptures. Am J Sports Med 22:607–610, 1994.
227. Speck M, Klaue K: Early full weightbearing and functional treatment after surgical repair of acute Achilles tendon rupture. Am J Sports Med 26:789–793, 1998.

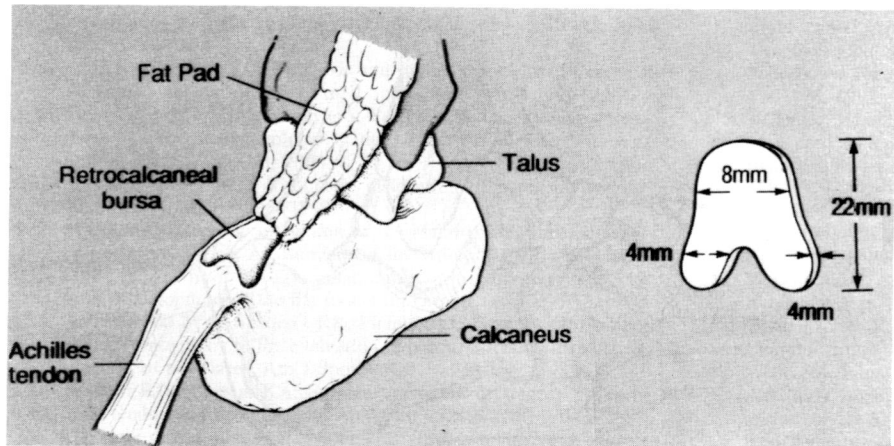

Figure 30H–3. Demonstration of the disk-shaped retrocalcaneal bursa. (From Frey C, Rosenberg Z, Shereff MJ: The retrocalcaneal bursa: Anatomy and bursography. Paper presented at the American Orthopaedic Foot and Ankle Society Specialty Day Meeting, February 1989, Las Vegas.)

hyaluronic acid, presumably secreted by its own lining. Because the Achilles tendon inserts in the middle third rather than in the more proximal upper portion of the posterior calcaneal surface, the plantar flexion lever is increased. The retrocalcaneal bursa, by accepting the fat pad, allows the necessary separation of tendon and bone that occurs in plantar flexion without creating excessive tissue tension.

Retrocalcaneal pain syndrome is commonly associated with the high-arched cavus foot and the varus heel.[7, 31] The combination of these factors tends to produce a foot that does not dorsiflex as readily as a normal foot. There is prominence of the heel, which is more susceptible to increased pressure from the tendons and the counter of the shoe. Ruch states that retrocalcaneal bursitis generally occurs in the circumstances of compensated rearfoot varus, compensated forefoot valgus, or plantar-flexed first ray because of the abnormal motion of the subtalar joint and the frontal and sagittal plane relationships.[31]

Clinical Evaluation

The history is generally that of slow onset of dull aching pain in the retrocalcaneal area aggravated by activity and certain shoewear. A common complaint is start-up pain after sitting or when arising in the morning. At times, there may be a history of acute onset of pain, sometimes associated with a traumatic incident. When this occurs, one must think of a tear or calcification of the Achilles tendon as perhaps the initiating factor.

Physical examination reveals swelling in the area of the retrocalcaneal bursa between the Achilles tendon and the calcaneus.[1] There is generally a prominence in the area of the superior portion of the heel. The swelling in the retrocalcaneal bursa will be found just anterior to the Achilles tendon. By palpating medially and laterally at the same time and with the aid of ballottement, one can sometimes feel fluid within the bursa (Fig. 30H–5). With careful and discrete palpation, one can generally differentiate between swelling in the Achilles tendon and swelling in the retrocalcaneal bursa. The swelling of the Achilles tendon associated with retrocalcaneal bursitis is usually at the level of the tendon at or just proximal to the insertion. Dorsiflexion of the foot usually increases the pain in the area. A great deal of swelling and inflammation on examination may indicate involvement of the retrocalcaneal bursa and involvement of the Achilles tendon. There may be redness and swelling between the Achilles tendon and the skin, usually owing to adventitious bursitis produced by pressure

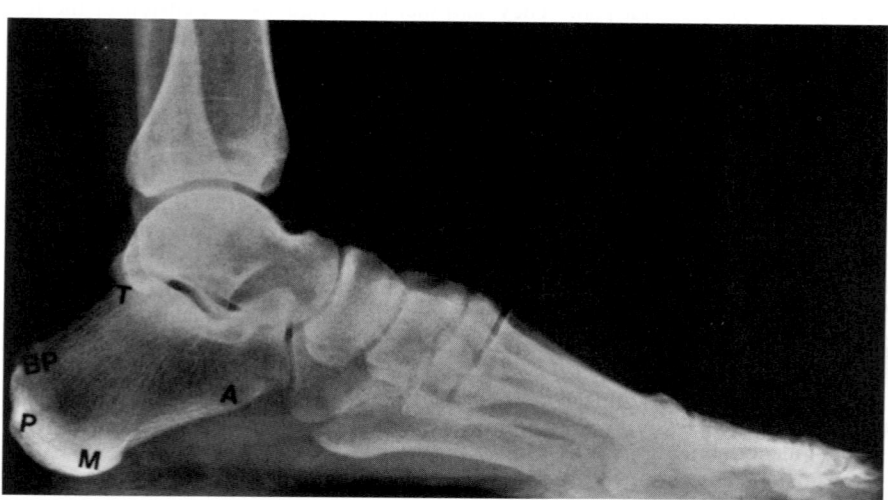

Figure 30H–4. Important radiographic landmarks of the os calcis. A, anterior tubercle; BP, bursal projection; M, medial tuberosity attachment of plantar aponeurosis; P, posterior tuberosity indicating attachment of Achilles tendon. T, superior aspect of talar articulation. (From Pavlov H, Heneghan MA, Hersh A, et al: The Haglund syndrome: Initial and differential diagnosis. Radiology 144:83–88, 1982.)

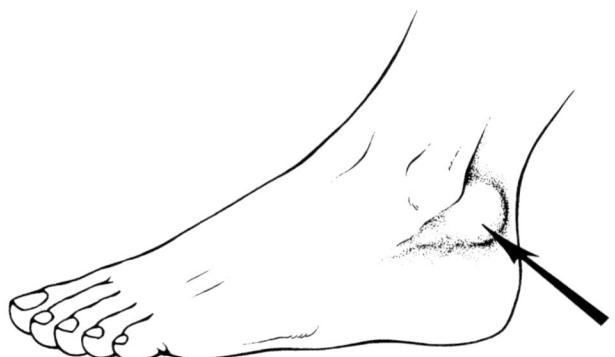

Figure 30H–5. Illustration demonstrating area of the swelling (*arrow*); retrocalcaneal bursitis with swelling is anterior to the Achilles tendon.

of the shoe counter against the Achilles tendon. There may be an area of periostitis, which is a discrete localized area of tenderness of the os calcis, usually on the lateral side of the posterior portion of the os calcis and produced by pressure of the shoe counter.

Diagnostic Studies

Radiographic Studies

A lateral view of the foot is taken with the patient standing. This allows biomechanical evaluation of the foot as well as evaluation of the specific points of the os calcis. The points of the os calcis are identified as the posterior margin of the posterior facet, the superior bursal projection, the tuberosity indicating the site of the Achilles tendon insertion, the medial tubercle, and the anterior tubercle.[29] The shape and appearance of the superior bursal prominence are noted. Radiographic evaluation of the lateral roentgenogram may be performed using the method of Fowler and Philip, which measures the posterior calcaneal angle (Fig. 30H–6).[9] Fowler and Philip consider the bursal projection prominent if the angle is greater than 75 degrees. Some authors have concluded that a combination of the Fowler angle and the angle of calcaneal inclination are more effective in correlating the radiographic appearance with symptomatology than the Fowler and Philip angle

alone,[31, 36] the combined angle being greater than 90 degrees in patients with symptomatic Haglund's disease.

Parallel pitch lines have been used by Heneghan and Pavlov[17] to determine the prominence of the bursal projection (Fig. 30H–7). The base line is constructed by placing a line along the medial tuberosity and the anterior tubercle and a parallel line from the posterior lip of the talar articular facet. The bursal prominence is considered abnormal if it extends above this line.

Pavlov and associates noted that the recessions seen on the lateral roentgenogram extend 2 mm inferior to the bursal projection, and with retrocalcaneal bursitis there is loss of the sharp interspace with the tendoachilles.[29] They also pointed out that the pre-Achilles fat pad outlines the anterior surface of the Achilles tendon, which normally measures 9 mm from anterior to posterior, 2 mm above the bursal projection.

Frey and colleagues described the retrocalcaneal bursa in a study of 12 fresh cadavers, 15 patients with signs and symptoms of retrocalcaneal bursitis, and 8 normal patients.[11] They found that in symptomatic patients, the amount of contrast material accepted averaged 0.92 mL and that the outline of the bursa was irregular in 100% of the patients in this group. The asymptomatic group accepted an average of 1.22 mL of contrast material, and 71% were noted to have a smooth bursal outline. The average area of the bursa on the lateral roentgenogram was 0.77 cm² in the normal patient and 1.18 cm² in the abnormal patient. Eighty-three percent of the patients noted significant (greater than 80%) improvement of their symptoms when 1% lidocaine was injected into the retrocalcaneal bursa.

Burhenne and Connell used xeroradiography to assess soft tissue and calcaneal detail in patients suffering from painful swelling localized in the heel.[3] They noted that neither a posterior calcaneal angle (of Philip and Fowler) of more than 75 degrees (see Fig. 30H–6) nor the parallel pitch line (see Fig. 30H–7) proved to be a reliable index. They evaluated four patients with heel pain and swelling in 100 control patients and found that the radiographic triad of retrocalcaneal bursitis, superficial tendoachilles bursitis, and Achilles tendon thickening, in the presence of an intact posterior superior calcaneal margin, was readily evaluated with xeroradiography.

Canoso and coworkers reported finding bursal fluid in

Figure 30H–6. Measurement of the Fowler and Philip angle. The normal angle is shown on the *left* and abnormal on the *right*. Upper level of normal is considered to be 69 degrees. Drawing at right indicates an abnormal angle of 75 degrees.

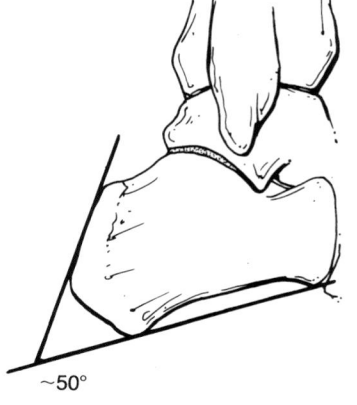

~50°

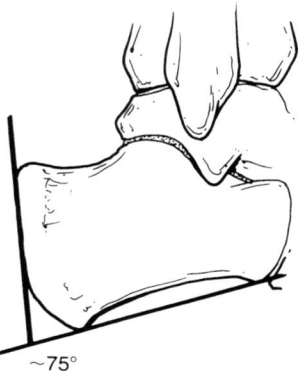

~75°

made into the retrocalcaneal area, not into the tendon. Even then, however, there is some contact with the Achilles tendon.[22]

Lagergren and Lindholm reported on the vascular supply of the Achilles tendon.[23] They found that ruptures of the Achilles tendon are usually limited to the segment of the tendon that lies between 2 and 6 cm proximal to its insertion in the os calcis and that this was an area of decreased vascularity and nutrition. This is an important finding relative to the retrocalcaneal bursal syndrome because this classic type of Achilles tendinosis is proximal to the area usually associated with the retrocalcaneal bursal syndrome. This may suggest that insertional tendinosis is brought on by impingement on the tendon rather than decreased circulation.

A soleus muscle anomaly associated with symptoms simulating retrocalcaneal bursitis has been reported.[27] In this entity, a soft bulge due to a large mass of anomalous soleus muscle in Kager's triangle was noted. The condition responded satisfactorily to excision.

Pavlov and colleagues reported the use of the parallel pitch line measurement in 10 symptomatic feet and 78 control feet.[29] They thought that the symptoms correlated statistically with a positive posterior pitch line but not with an abnormal posterior calcaneal angle. They concluded that radiographically the syndrome is characterized by (1) retrocalcaneal bursitis (loss of the lucent retrocalcaneal recess between the Achilles tendon and the bursal projection), (2) Achilles tendinitis (an Achilles tendon measuring more than 9 mm located 2 cm above the bursal projection), (3) superficial tendoachilles bursitis (a convexity of the soft tissues posterior to the Achilles tendon insertion), and (4) a cortically intact but prominent bursal projection with a positive parallel pitch line.

A series of 65 patients with Haglund's disease was reported by Ruch,[31] 17 were operated on by resection of the posterior superior portion of the os calcis, resecting the posterior superior aspect both medially and laterally and removing sufficient bone to render the previous palpable prominence entirely absent. They were evaluated 6 months to 5 years postoperatively. Fifteen demonstrated good to excellent results with elimination of symptoms. Three of the patients required a second procedure to obtain the desired result.

Vega and colleagues reported 20 cases of Haglund's deformity.[36] They noted that the combination of the Fowler and Philip angle and the calcaneal angle, when greater than 90 degrees, correlated with the manifestation of symptoms. This was similar to the findings of Ruch.[31] Vega and associates reported conservative treatment with pads, shoes, braces, and injections and resorted to surgical treatment only if conservative treatment was not successful. The surgical incision recommended was the lateral para-Achilles tendon approach.

Clancy stated that an articular-like surface lines the calcaneus in its superior surface where it comes in contact with the Achilles tendon.[7] He found that a bursa may form from constant overuse, enlargement of the bony prominence, or external pressure. He recommended steroid injection behind but not through or into the tendon. In patients who did not obtain relief with conservative measures, ostectomy has proved successful. Clancy noted that the ma-

jority of those who required surgery had significant cavus deformities.

Schepsis and Leach[32] reported that the majority of athletes, particularly runners, who presented with acute or chronic posterior heel pain were successfully managed nonoperatively using a combination of (1) a decrease in or cessation of the usual weekly mileage, (2) temporary termination of interval training and workouts on hills, (3) change from a harder bank surface to a softer surface, (4) a ¼- to ½-inch lift inside the shoe or added to the shoe, and (5) a program designed to stretch and strengthen the gastrocnemius-soleus complex. These measures were combined with oral anti-inflammatory medications and an occasional injection of corticosteroid into the retrocalcaneal bursa. Postural abnormalities were treated with orthotics. Schepsis and Leach studied retrospectively 45 cases of chronic posterior heel pain treated surgically in 37 patients. All but two of these patients were competitive long-distance runners who ran an average of 40 to 120 miles per week before the onset of symptoms. Their ages ranged from 19 to 56 years.

The surgical approach used by Schepsis and Leach was a longitudinal incision 1 cm medial to the Achilles tendon that was continued transversely to form a J-shaped incision if necessary (Fig. 30H–10). The patient was placed in a cast for 2 to 3 weeks with weight-bearing permitted after 1 week. When a disorder within the tendon existed requiring excision and repair, immobilization was continued for 1 to 2 weeks longer. Range of motion exercises were emphasized. A graduated program of swimming and stationary bicycling combined with isometric, isotonic, and isokinetic strengthening of the calf muscles was prescribed. Jogging was permitted after 8 to 12 weeks, rarely sooner. Full return to a competitive level of sports activity usually required 5 to 6 months.

The patients were divided into three groups—those with Achilles tenosynovitis-tendinitis, those with retrocalcaneal bursitis, and those with a combination of both. In a group of 24 patients with Achilles tendosynovitis-tendinitis, there were 15 (63%) excellent results, 7 (29%) good results, 1 (4%) fair result, and 1 (4%) poor result. In the 14 patients with retrocalcaneal bursitis, there were 7 (50%) excellent,

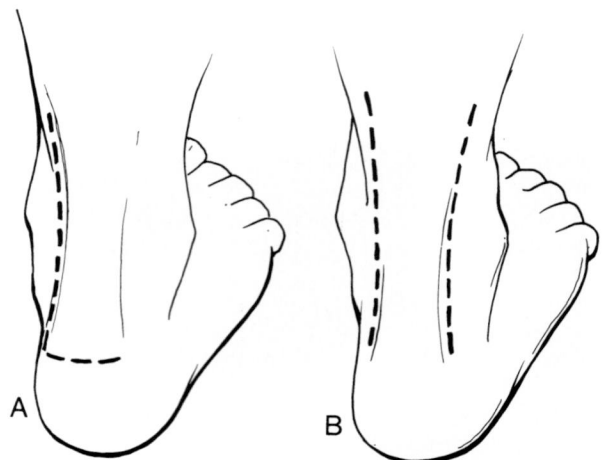

Figure 30H–10. Surgical incisions for retrocalcaneal bursitis. *Left,* medial approach with J extension, as described by Schepsis and Leach[32]; *right,* medial and lateral incisions, as described by Jones.[19]

3 (21%) good, and 4 (29%) fair results. In the group with a combination of both, there were 5 (71%) excellent and 2 (29%) good results. It was noted that four of the six unsatisfactory results occurred in the group with retrocalcaneal bursitis.

Jones and James[19] reported on 10 patients who underwent partial calcaneal exostosectomies for retrocalcaneal bursitis. They suggested that conservative measures should be attempted before considering surgical intervention. These included a decrease in the usual weekly mileage, elevation of the heel, instruction in Achilles tendon strengthening, removal of external pressure from the heel, use of oral anti-inflammatory medications, and evaluation and treatment of postural foot deformities. They also suggested immobilization of the leg in a short-leg walking cast for a brief period of time, thus allowing the athlete to continue cardiovascular maintenance on an exercise bicycle. Steroid injection was used as a last resort before surgery.

During an 8-year period, Jones and James operated on 10 patients with retrocalcaneal bursitis.[19] Six patients were competitive long-distance runners, and four were avid recreational runners. Their symptoms consisted of pain and tenderness in the retrocalcaneal area that developed either immediately or after running several miles. The patients ranged in age from 21 to 42 years. Surgery was performed through a longitudinal incision on both sides of the Achilles tendon (see Fig. 30H–10) and included exostosectomy and excision of the bursa. Jones and James emphasized that the ridge of bone at the insertion site must be carefully removed with a small curet and rongeur so that no prominence of bone is left beneath the Achilles tendon posteriorly. A short-leg walking cast was used for 8 weeks with partial weight-bearing allowed for the first 2 weeks and then full weight-bearing. After casting, a 1-inch heel elevation was used until the foot assumed the neutral position easily. General muscle conditioning was carried out until Cybex testing revealed symmetrical muscle strength. All of the patients went back to their desired level of activity within 6 months.

Sullivan,[35] addressing the problem of recurrent pain in the pediatric athlete, stated that heel pain may be due to osteochondrosis of the apophysis of the calcaneus (Sever's disease) or to Achilles tendinitis, which is characterized by pain on palpation of the tendon just above its insertion. In severe cases, there may be crepitation of the tendon. He recommended treatment comprising rest and aspirin or other mild anti-inflammatory agents. In differentiating these two entities, it may be helpful to note that the pain of osteochondrosis occurs on the inferior portion of the os calcis, and the pain associated with Achilles tendinitis is felt proximal to the insertion of the Achilles tendon on the os calcis.

Puddu and associates[30] proposed three stages of inflammation occurring at the insertion of the Achilles. Stage 1, peritendinitis, involves inflammation of the paratenon only. Peritendinitis with tendinosis, stage 2, is characterized by macroscopic thickening, nodularity, and microscopic focal degeneration of the Achilles tendon in addition to inflammation of the paratenon. Stage 3 is characterized by degenerative lesions of the substance of the tendon itself without associated peritendinitis.

Clain and Baxter[6] divided Achilles tendon disorders into insertional and noninsertional dysfunction. Insertional tendinosis occurs within and around the Achilles tendon at its insertion and may be associated with Haglund's deformity or spur formation within the tendon itself. In the presence of associated tendinosis, they advocated transfer of either the flexor digitorum longus as advocated by Mann[26] or the flexor hallucis longus as advocated by Wapner.[37, 38] Schepsis and associates[33] concurred that tendon transfer should be considered because it may enhance the blood supply and reinforce the Achilles tendon.

In summary, retrocalcaneal bursitis is a condition characterized by inflammation of the retrocalcaneal bursa, the Achilles tendon just above its insertion, and at times the tissue between the Achilles tendon and the skin. It is generally managed by conservative measures consisting of anti-inflammatory medication, decreased activity, padding to prevent pressure on the affected area, orthoses or heel lifts, and strengthening and stretching exercises. If it does not respond to these modalities, then surgical intervention may be considered. Surgery generally consists of excision of the exostosis and the retrocalcaneal bursa and at times the adventitious bursa, if it is present, and correction of the Achilles tendon disorder with tendon transfer if necessary. Although most series do report good results following surgery, in the athlete, this condition may present a serious threat to continued full activity even after surgical intervention.

Authors' Preferred Method of Treatment

The patient is first evaluated to ascertain the exact reason for the disorder. Adventitious bursitis is usually seen in women and does not seem to be a prominent problem in athletes. It is generally treated conservatively by softening the heel counter, using a small U-shaped pad (Fig. 30H–11) to relieve the pressure of the shoe or counter against the inflamed area, and anti-inflammatory medications. If the pain is refractory to these modalities, an injection of steroid directly into the inflamed area of the bursa, with care to avoid the tendon, may be tried once. Because of the risk of Achilles rupture following injections, the foot is immobilized in a removable cast walker for 2 weeks. Surgical intervention performed solely for adventitious bursitis is unusual.

Nonoperative management of insertional Achilles tendinitis is determined by the degree of inflammation and tendinosis present. When the degree is mild, a U-shaped heel pad, home stretching of the gastrocsoleus muscle, cross-training with bike riding, using a night splint to keep the foot in neutral, and avoiding activities such as running are generally successful. The addition of nonsteroidal anti-inflammatories can be considered.

In moderate to severe cases of tendinosis, a period of immobilization with a molded ankle foot orthosis can be used. This allows decreased load across the tendon but does not completely immobilize the tendon. The brace should have a relief molded into it to avoid direct contact on the posterior superior aspect of the calcaneus. The

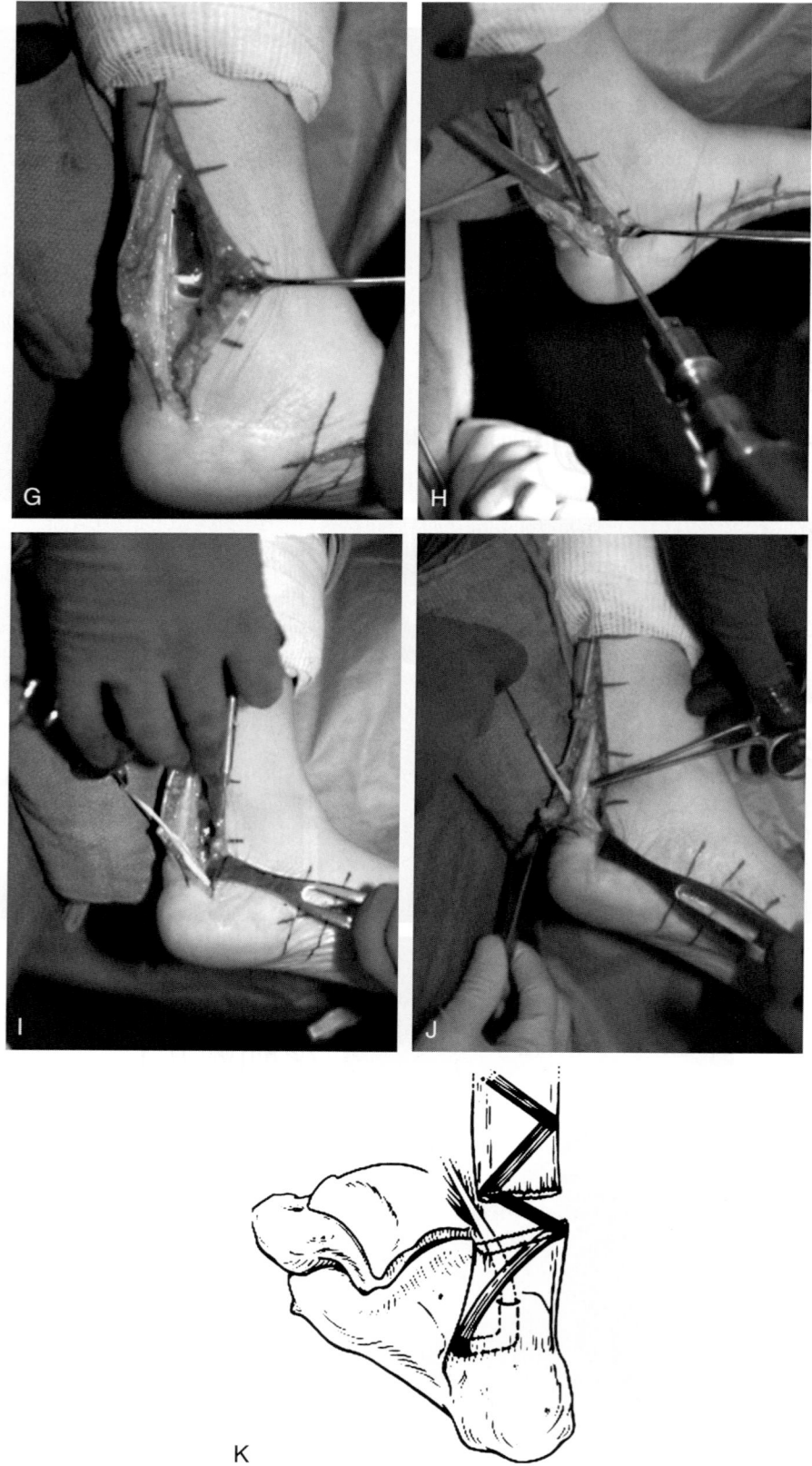

Figure 30H–13 *Continued. G,* A posterior incision is made, and the posterior fascia of the leg is opened to allow transfer of the FHL into the wound. *H,* Two drill holes are made, one superior and the other medial, to intersect in the posterior body of the calcaneus to create a tunnel for tendon transfer. *I,* The FHL tendon is passed through the superior hole and out the medial side of the tunnel. *J,* The FHL is woven through the Achilles tendon using a tendon weaver. *K,* Diagram of completed weaving of FHL through the Achilles demonstrating the orientation of the tunnel through the posterior calcaneus.

laner retractor is placed in the wound. The flexor hallucis brevis is then reflected plantarward, thus exposing the deep midfoot anatomy. In some instances, it is necessary to release the origin of the short flexors to assist visualization.

The FHL and flexor digitorum longus tendons are identified within the midfoot. They are generally covered by a layer of fatty tissue. Identification of the tendons is assisted by placing a finger over the lateral wall of the short flexor and manually plantar-flexing and dorsiflexing the first toe proximal interphalangeal joint. The motion of the tendon can be felt and dissection can be carried down to identify the tendons of the FHL medially and the flexor digitorum longus laterally. The FHL is divided as far distally as possible, but one must allow an adequate distal stump to be transferred to the flexor digitorum longus. The proximal portion is tagged with a suture. The distal limb of the FHL is then sewn into the flexor digitorum longus with all five toes in a neutral posture, providing flexion to all five toes via the flexor digitorum longus.

Attention is again turned to the posterior medial incision. The fascia overlying the posterior compartment of the leg is then incised longitudinally directly over the muscle belly of the FHL. The tendon is then retracted from the midfoot into the posterior incision.

A transverse drill hole is placed just distal to the insertion of the Achilles tendon halfway through the bone from medial to lateral. A second vertical drill hole is made just anterior to the level of resection of the posterior superior prominence to meet the first hole. A large towel clip is used to augment the tunnel created. A suture passer is placed through the tunnel from distal to proximal. The suture is then pulled through the tunnel, thus drawing the FHL tendon through the drill hole.

If the Achilles insertion has been detached, suture anchors can be used to reattach the tendon before securing the FHL transfer. The FHL is then woven from distal to proximal through the Achilles tendon using a tendon weaver. The tendon weaver is passed through the Achilles, creating a "tunnel" in the tendon. The tag suture on the flexor hallucis is then grasped and pulled back through the "tunnel," bringing the flexor tendon through the Achilles. This process is repeated to use the full length of tendon harvested. The tendon is secured with multiple sutures of number 1 cottony Dacron. After completion of the reconstruction, the paratenon is repaired. The subcutaneous tissue and skin are closed. Compressive dressings and plaster splints are applied to maintain 15 degrees of ankle plantar flexion.

The patient is placed in a short-leg non-weight-bearing cast at 15 degrees of equinus for 4 weeks. When the patient returns at 4 weeks, the dressing is removed and the forefoot is placed on a foot rest with the patient seated on an examining table with the hip flexed and allowed to stay in this position until the foot reaches neutral. The foot is then placed into a short-leg walking cast or removable cast walker with the ankle at neutral for an additional 4 weeks and weight-bearing is begun. A rehabilitation program for strengthening and range of motion is begun 8 weeks postoperatively. The patient is maintained in a removable cast walker for community ambulation until 10 degrees of dorsiflexion is obtained and grade 4/5 strength is demonstrated. In-home ambulation is allowed with a 7/16-inch heel lift

during this time. The patients are then advanced to regular shoe wear and continued on a home strengthening program with Thera-Band. Athletic activity is restricted for 6 months after surgery.

Criteria for Return to Sports Participation

The time needed for return to sports participation will depend upon the severity and perniciousness of the condition, the relationship of the pain component to the patient's sporting activity, and the extent of involvement of the Achilles tendon. Should the situation be severe enough to force the patient to stop the desired athletic activity, the following plan is used.

If retrocalcaneal bursitis is present with a normal Achilles tendon, conservative therapy is tried until the patient has been asymptomatic for 4 to 6 weeks. The patient may then return to sports participation, starting with limited activity and working up to full activity within 4 to 12 weeks, assuming that he or she has recovered full strength and mobility without pain. If retrocalcaneal bursitis is associated with degeneration of the Achilles tendon, nonoperative treatment should be used until the patient is asymptomatic. A gradual increase in activity is then allowed over a 6- to 12-week period. If surgery has been performed upon the tendon in combination with excision of the retrocalcaneal bursa and exostosectomy, immobilization is continued for 8 weeks but active range of motion is begun at 3 weeks. Strengthening and stretching exercises are started at 6 to 9 weeks. Increased activity according to tolerance can be started at 12 weeks, and return to strenuous activity is allowed at 4 to 6 months if local symptoms have resolved. When tendon transfer is used, the protocol is as described in the previous section.

Plantar Fasciitis Associated with Pain in Medial Tuberosity (Heel Spur, Subcalcaneal Pain Syndrome)

Pain in the region of the medial tuberosity of the heel associated with increased pain with activity and sometimes related to a spur of the os calcis has been described for many years. Initially, this condition was thought to be associated with gonococcus and was described as "gonorrheal spurs."[44, 51] Later it was thought that this entity was due to pull of the plantar fascia and musculature.[47–49, 92, 94, 98] More recently, Przylucki and Jones[110] and Baxter and Thigpen[44] have attributed this pain to entrapment of the nerve to the abductor digiti quinti arising from the lateral branch of the plantar nerve. Freeman[61] and others[47, 119] have attributed this pain to irritation of the medial calcaneal nerve. Other authors have attributed the pain to herniation or to compression of fat nodules.[62, 96] Bordelon[47, 48] described a clinical syndrome characterized by pain beneath the heel that is aggravated by ambulation and is not associated with any trauma. He proposed that this condition be considered in light of the structures that are present in the area.

Specific treatment should be directed toward the structures that are inflamed, the theory being that inflammation in one structure may produce inflammation in other structures.[47, 48] Reviewing the literature reveals that many different theories exist about the cause of subcalcaneal pain, and hence many different methods of treatment have been suggested for it.* It has been said that although this condition is familiar to all orthopaedic surgeons, it is probably fully understood by none.[48]

Snook and Chrisman[128] noted that there is conflicting literature on this subject on two salient points. The first is that there is no accepted explanation of the cause of the condition. Second, there is no generally approved method of treatment. They thought that perhaps the basic cause lay in the subcalcaneal pad, which in some unknown manner lost its compressibility, either by local loss of fat with thinning or by rupture of the fibrous tissue septa. Ali[42] stated that "the painful heel is due to a fibrotic response, similar to plantar fibromatosis and not to the spur of bone which is the end result of recurrent strain on the plantar fascia." Tanz[130] thought that "inferior heel pain is often due to irritation of a branch of the medial calcaneal nerve." Similarly, Baxter and Thigpen[44] and Przylucki and Jones[110] advanced the thought that the heel pain is due to an entrapment neuropathy that involves the branch of the lateral plantar nerve to the abductor digiti quinti. It has been noted that this branch passes more proximally than is shown in most anatomic studies and is in the area of the heel spur.

Mann[98] wrote that "in the early stages, fibrositis of low chronicity, with or without pain, anterior to the calcaneal tuberosity represents the pathological change. Continuation of the process leads to osteophytic changes and bone deposits on the sulcus just anterior to the tuberosity."

Kopell and Thompson[89] stated that calcaneodynia, or painful heel, "is usually ascribed to an inflammatory reaction based on mechanical stress at the common muscular and fascial origins on the anterior inferior surfaces of the calcaneus and in many cases, the inflamed structures are the calcaneal nerves which innervate the region of the common origin." Leach and coworkers[92, 94] also thought that the cause of plantar fasciitis appears to be repetitive trauma, which produces microtrauma in the plantar fascia near its attachments and leads to attempted repair and chronic inflammation.

Katoh and colleagues[83] reported on objective analysis of foot function during gait using vertical impulse distribution along the sole of the foot during the load-bearing period of gait. This was demonstrated to be reliable in distinguishing between patients with painful heel pads and those with plantar fasciitis.

Although there has been much discussion about the relationship of the calcaneal heel spur to subcalcaneal pain (Fig. 30H–14), the relationship has not been definitely established. Tanz[130] stated that a heel spur is located in the origin of the short toe flexors and not in the plantar fascia. He noted that 15% of normal asymptomatic adult feet have subcalcaneal plantar spurs, whereas about 50% of adult feet with plantar heel pain have spurs. He thought that heel spurs contributed to the plantar heel pain, although many

---

*See references 42–52, 54, 55, 59, 61, 62, 70, 71, 75, 76, 80, 84, 90, 92, 95–98, 100, 105, 110, 111, 113, 115, 119, 125, 127, 128, 130, and 133.

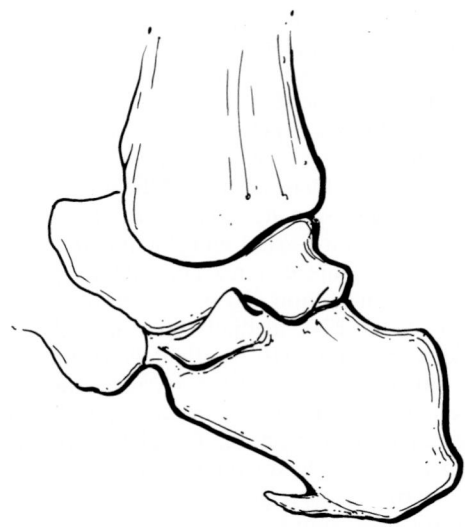

Figure 30H–14. Lateral view of foot demonstrating spur in the region of the medial tuberosity and the origin of the short flexors. Fifty percent of symptomatic patients have heel spurs.

patients with plantar heel pain did not have spurs. Snook and Chrisman[128] agreed with this. Their report on 27 patients with subcalcaneal pain noted that 13 had a calcaneal spur and 11 did not. Mann[98] stated that "over a long period of time, proliferative bony changes at the origin of the fascia may lead to the formation of a spur."

Shmokler and colleagues[126] reviewed 1000 patients at random with roentgenograms of the foot. There was a 13.2% incidence of heel spurs. Only 39% of those with heel spurs (5.2% of the total sample) reported any history of subcalcaneal heel pain. Shmokler and coworkers believed that these statistics tended to support the premise that the presence of a heel spur did not mandate pain.

Leach and colleagues[92, 94] stated that the spur is located in the short toe flexor origins as opposed to the plantar aponeurosis, casting doubt on the concept that the heel spur contributes to the pain in the plantar fascia. In evaluating 45 patients with 52 painful heels, Williams and associates[136] found that 75% of those with painful heels had a heel spur compared with 63% of the opposite nonpainful heels. Comparing 63 heels in 59 age- and sex-matched controls, the incidence of heel spur was 7.9%. Warren and Jones[134, 135] attempted to predict which factors would be associated with plantar fasciitis but found that a set of predictable variables was not present. Heel spurs may be present or absent and may or may not be the primary pathologic entity in heel pain. They have to be considered, however, in the context of the entire syndrome.

Pertinent Anatomy

The plantar aponeurosis arises from the os calcis and is composed of three segments (Fig. 30H–15).[69, 73, 74, 117] The central segment is the largest and arises from the plantar aspect of the posteromedial calcaneal tuberosity. It inserts into the toes. The lateral portion arises from the lateral process of the tuberosity of the os calcis and inserts into

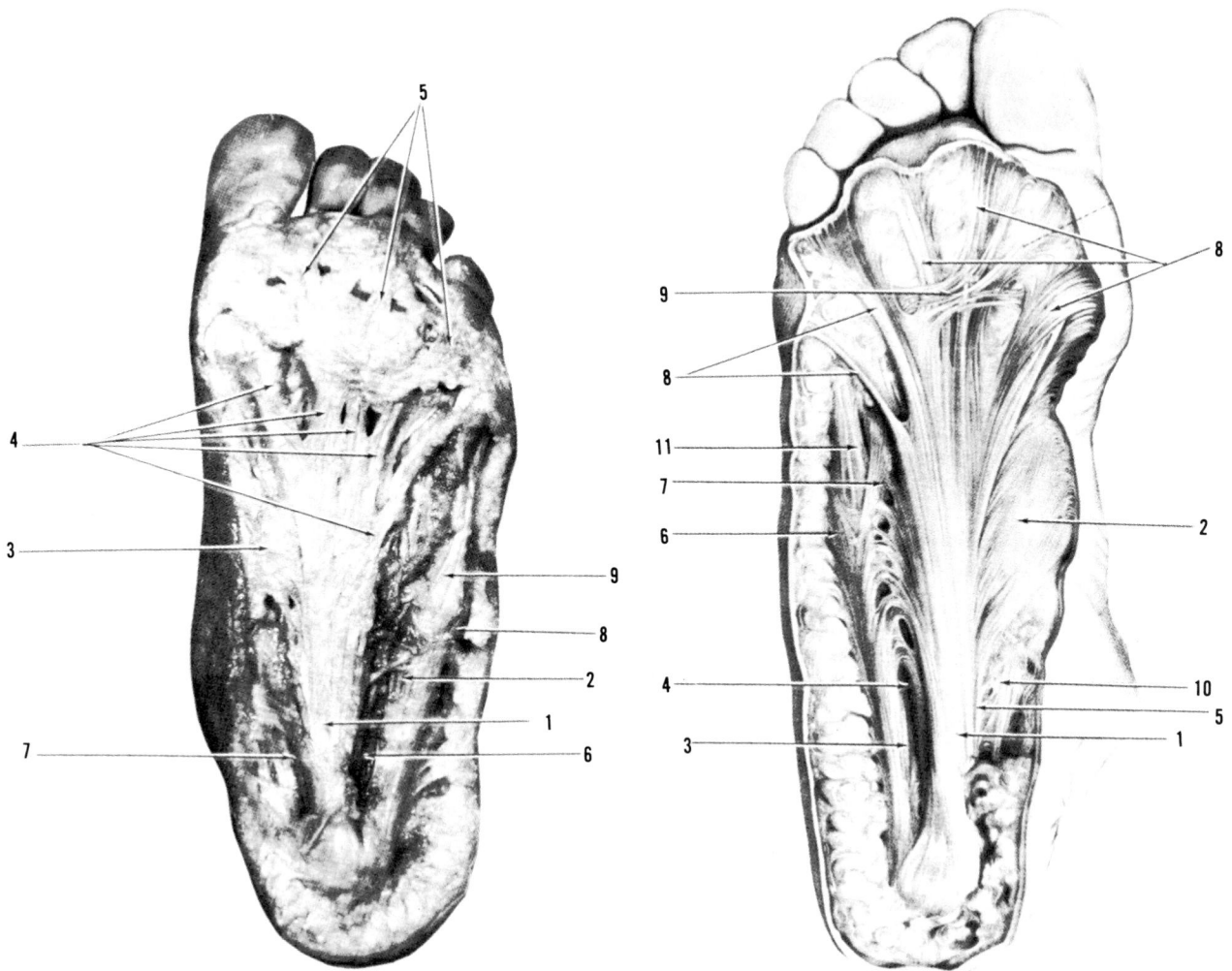

Figure 30H–15. The plantar aponeurosis is composed of three parts: central, medial, and lateral components. From the clinical standpoint, the central portion is considered to be in the plantar aponeurosis. 1, Central slip plantar fascia; 2, medial component plantar fascia; 3, lateral component plantar fascia; 4, lateral plantar sulcus; 5, medial plantar sulcus; 6, lateral crux; 7, medial crux; 8, superficial longitudinal tracts; 9, transverse superficial tract; 10, abductor hallucis muscle; 11, abductor digiti quinti muscle. (Redrawn from Rondhuis JJ, Hudson A: The first branch of the lateral plantar nerve and heel pain. Acta Morphol Neerland-Scand 24:269–279, 1986.)

the base of the fifth metatarsal. The medial portion is thin and covers the undersurface of the abductor hallucis.

Clinically, when considering the plantar aponeurosis, one is generally referring to the central portion, which extends from the medial tuberosity of the os calcis to the toes. It originates from the os calcis and passes to the proximal phalanges of the lesser toes through the longitudinal septa, to the big toe through the sesamoids, and into the skin of the ball of the foot through the vertical fibers.[70] Hyperextension of the toes and the metatarsophalangeal joints tenses the plantar aponeurosis, raises the longitudinal arch of the foot, inverts the hindfoot, and externally rotates the leg. This mechanism is passive and depends entirely on bony and ligamentous instability. This mechanism, whereby the arch is raised and supported with dorsiflexion of the toe, providing more stability to the foot, has been termed the *windlass mechanism* by Hicks.[77]

The posterior tibial nerve is located on the medial side of the foot behind the medial malleolus and beneath the flexor retinaculum (Fig. 30H–16). The medial calcaneal

nerve arises at the level of the medial malleolus or below and passes superficially to innervate the skin of the heel. It may consist of one or two branches. The important anatomic point is that this nerve passes in the subcutaneous tissue between the plantar fascia and the skin. The next nerve, which is the nerve to the abductor digiti quinti and which branches off the lateral plantar nerve, passes deeper, beneath the plantar ligament and underneath the spur, if present, to innervate the abductor digiti quinti (Fig. 30H–17). It is important to differentiate the medial calcaneal nerve from the nerve to the abductor digiti quinti.[47–49] They can be readily differentiated because the medial calcaneal nerve passes in the subcutaneous tissue and is superficial to the plantar aponeurosis, whereas the nerve to the abductor digiti quinti is deeper and passes beneath the plantar fascia.

Rondhuis and Hudson[114] noted that entrapment of the nerve to the abductor digiti quinti occurs between the abductor hallucis and the medial margin of the medial head of the quadratus plantae muscle. They did not find a

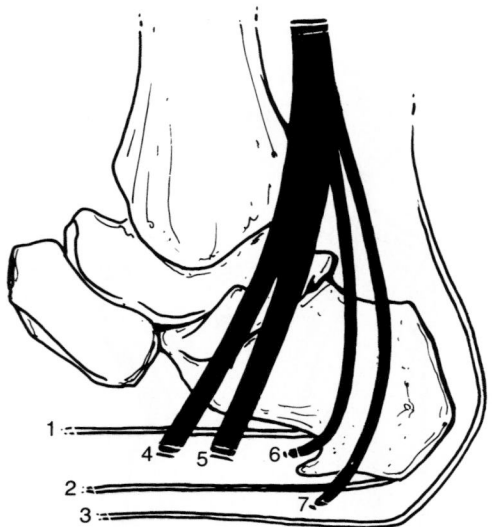

Figure 30H–16. Relationship of structures commonly associated with heel pain: (1) long plantar ligament; (2) plantar fascia; (3) skin; (4) medial plantar nerve; (5) lateral plantar nerve; (6) nerve to abductor digiti quinti; and (7) medial calcaneal nerve. Note that the medial calcaneal nerve supplying sensation to the heel passes superficial to the plantar fascia. The nerve to the abductor digiti quinti passes deep to the plantar fascia and beneath the spur.

perforation of the fascia as described by Baxter and Thigpen,[44] nor did they find any bursa in the origin of the plantar aponeurosis. They concluded that there are fibers that innervate the perichondrium, and sensory fibers are present and form free endings, producing pain sensation. They found motor branches to the flexor digitorum brevis and abductor digiti quinti muscles (Fig. 30H–18).

The medial and lateral plantar nerves continue to the foot and pass through prospective foramina of the abductor muscles. When considering entrapment of the posterior tibial nerve, it is important to note that this nerve may be entrapped either beneath the flexor retinaculum at the level of the medial malleolus or at the point where the medial

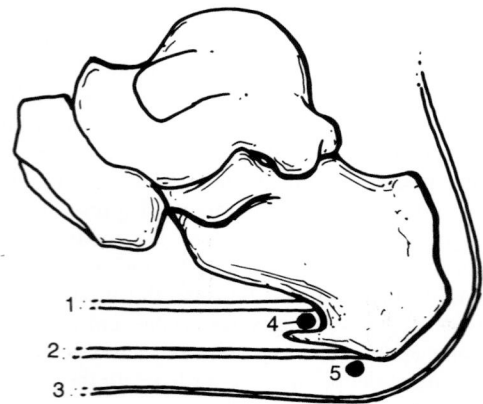

Figure 30H–17. Sagittal section of os calcis showing relationship of the nerves to the abductor digiti quinti and the medial calcaneal nerve as described by Baxter and Przylucki and Jones. (1) Long plantar ligament; (2) plantar fascia; (3) skin; (4) nerve to abductor digiti quinti; (5) medial calcaneal nerve.

and lateral plantar nerves exit through separate foramina in the abductor muscles (Fig. 30H–19).

Relevant Biomechanics

The foot must be evaluated to ascertain which specific type of foot and which biomechanical components are involved.[49] A supple foot with a tendency toward a flatfoot deformity will place increased strain on the origin of the plantar fascia on the calcaneus because the windlass mechanism will be under increased strain in maintaining a stable arch during the propulsive phase of gait. Biomechanically, in an effort to avoid this strain, one could consider an orthotic device to correct the biomechanical deformity and to increase the support of the foot during the stance phase. Strapping with tape may also be used to hold the forefoot in adduction and the heel in varus to relieve the pressure on the origin of the plantar aponeurosis during propulsion. When a cavus foot is present, there may be excessive strain on the heel area because the foot lacks the ability to evert to absorb the shock and adapt itself to the ground. With a cavus foot, a soft cushioning material may be used to decrease the shock component and increase the area of contact. The goals of these orthotic devices are to reduce the stress on the medial tuberosity and the plantar fascia (Fig. 30H–20).

Clinical Evaluation

History

The history usually reveals a slow but gradual onset of pain along the inside of the heel.[47–49] Occasionally, the pain may be associated with a twisting injury of the foot, producing an abrupt onset of pain.[74] The clinical course, however, is generally similar regardless of the onset. The location of the pain is generally described as along the medial side of the foot at the bottom of the heel. The pain is worse upon first arising in the morning and then decreases with increased activity. It may increase, however, after prolonged activity. Periods of inactivity are generally followed by an increase in pain as activity is started again. Numbness of the foot is not present. When severe pain is present, the patient is unable to bear weight on the heel and will bear weight on the forepart of the foot.

Physical Examination

Physical examination consists of evaluating the foot to determine what type of foot is present.[49] As with any examination of the foot, examination must include the entire lower extremity as well. Specific examination of the foot reveals acute tenderness along the medial tuberosity of the os calcis. This tenderness may be at the origin of the central slip of the plantar fascia, or it may be deep, in which case it probably represents a deep inflammation, perhaps with involvement of the nerve to the abductor digiti quinti. The medial calcaneal nerve is palpated and tapped to search for paresthesias of the medial calcaneal

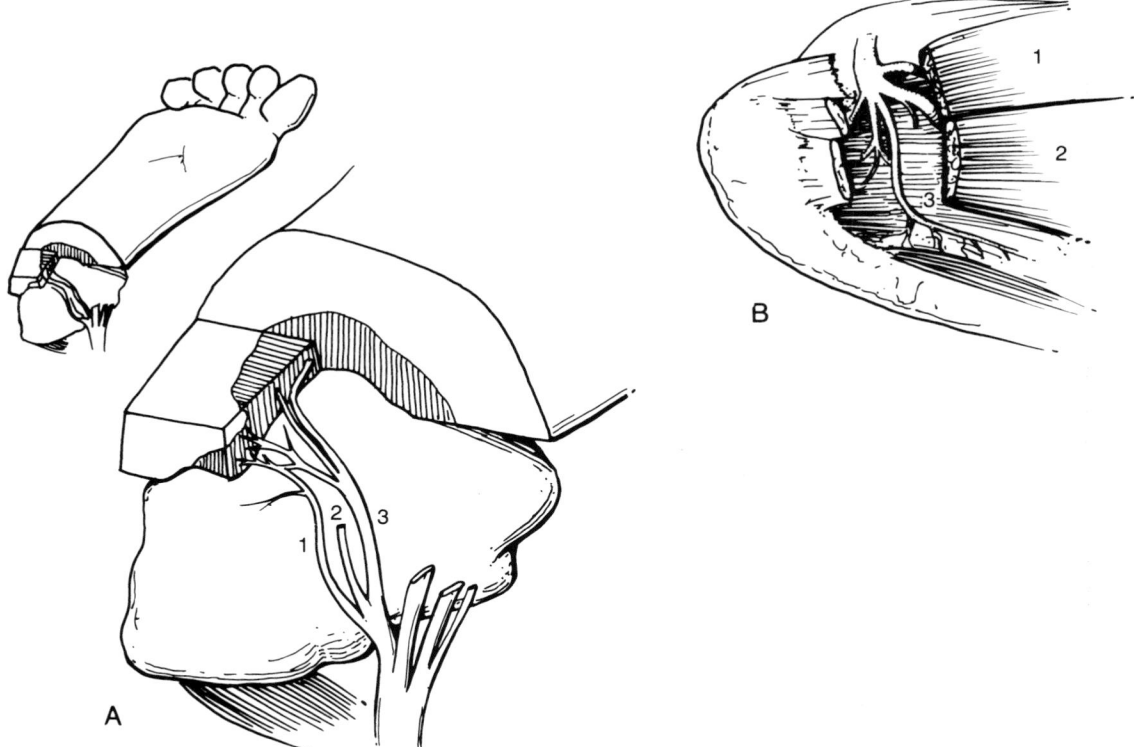

Figure 30H–18. *A,* Illustration of the nerve to the abductor digiti quinti. 1, Branch running to the medial process of the calcaneal tuberosity, bifurcating into a branch covering the perichondrium of the medial process and into another one running to a more lateral part of the calcaneal perichondrium. 2, Branch to the flexor digitorum muscle. 3, Branches to the abductor digiti minimi muscle.

B, Drawing of the nerve to the abductor digiti quinti as dissected in an adult foot showing parts of the abductor hallucis (1) and flexor digitorum (2) muscles, which have been removed; the nerve runs across the quadratus plantae muscle (3) in a plantar direction, then turns into a horizontal plane and proceeds laterally. (Redrawn from Rondhuis JJ, Hudson A: The first branch of the lateral plantar nerve and heel pain. Acta Morphol Neerland-Scand 24:269–279, 1986.)

nerve in the subcutaneous tissue; if found, this condition indicates inflammation and entrapment of the medial calcaneal nerve in this area. The plantar fascia is palpated to determine whether the plantar fascia is tender just at its origin or throughout its course. The plantar fascia is also palpated for nodules, the presence of which suggests plantar fibromatosis. The plantar fascia is palpated both with the toes flexed so that it is supple and with the toes extended, which places tension on the plantar fascia. The tarsal tunnel is palpated and percussed to elicit any tender-

Figure 30H–19. Site of entrapment of the posterior tibial nerve and its branches, demonstrating possible entrapment beneath the laciniate ligament and at the point where the nerve passes through the fascia of the abductor hallucis muscle. (Redrawn from Baxter DE, Thigpen CM: Heel pain—operative results. Foot Ankle 5:16–25, 1984. © American Orthopaedic Foot and Ankle Society, 1984.)

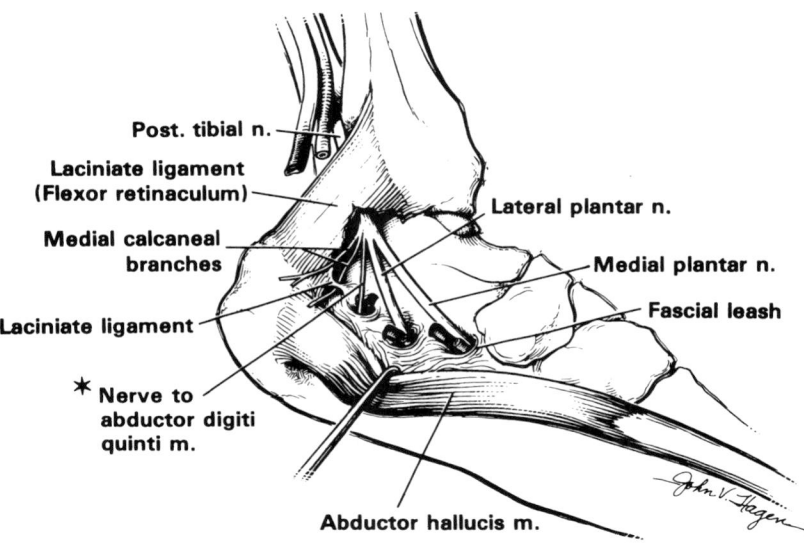

the calcaneal spur. This surgery failed, and Gerster and colleagues stated that surgery is contraindicated in patients with severe heel pain associated with seronegative spondyloarthritis.

Proximal neurologic causes of heel pain should also be considered. Tarsal tunnel syndrome may be present with referred pain to the heel and sole of the foot. A positive Tinel's sign may suggest this diagnosis. Electromyographic and nerve conduction studies should be used to rule out this condition.[49] Heel pain may also be referred from the lumbar spine. If a spinal or proximal cause appears to be a possibility, appropriate laboratory and radiographic studies should be performed as indicated.

MRI has shed light on the anatomic structures involved in subcalcaneal heel pain.[85] Heel pain can be caused by disorders of either the plantar fascia, calcaneus, tendons, or adjacent nerves. Because these conditions can lead to pain located in a small area of the heel, a precise clinical diagnosis may be difficult. This article describes some of these various causes of heel pain and how MRI helps to characterize them.

Grasel and colleagues[72] evaluated various MRI signs of plantar fasciitis to determine if a difference in these findings exists between clinically typical and atypical patients with chronic symptoms resistant to conservative treatment. They found signs on MRI that included occult marrow edema and fascial tears. Patients with these manifestations seemed to respond to treatment in a manner similar to that of patients in whom MRI revealed more benign findings.

Treatment Options

Management of subcalcaneal heel pain should initially begin with no operative treatment.[67] Plantar fasciitis is a common cause of heel pain, which frustrates patients and practitioners alike because of its resistance to treatment. Although normally managed with conservative treatment, plantar fasciitis is frequently resistant to the wide variety of treatments commonly used, such as nonsteroidal anti-inflammatory drugs, rest, pads, cups, splints, orthotics, corticosteroid injections, casts, physical therapy, ice, and heat. Although there is no consensus on the efficacy of any particular conservative treatment regimen, there is agreement that nonsurgical treatment is ultimately effective in approximately 90% of patients. Because the natural history of plantar fasciitis has not been established, it is unclear how much of symptom resolution is in fact due to the wide variety of commonly used treatments.

Gill and Kiebzak[68] studied 411 patients with a clinical diagnosis of plantar fasciitis and assessed them for predisposing factors. Each patient completed an outcomes assessment survey instrument that ranked effectiveness of various nonsurgical treatment modalities. Listed in descending order of effectiveness, the treatment modalities assessed were short-leg walking cast, steroid injection, rest, ice, runner's shoe, crepe-soled shoe, aspirin or nonsteroidal anti-inflammatory drug, heel cushion, low-profile plastic heel cup, heat, and Tuli's heel cup. Treatment with a cast ranked the best. The Tuli's heel cup ranked the poorest. Most of the treatments were found to be unpredictable or minimally effective. In their study, however, stretching and night splints were not included.

O'Brien and Martin[105] studied 58 painful heels in 41 patients who received conservative treatment. Seventy percent were classified as having excellent results (no remaining symptoms), 26% were classified as having good results (50% or less of the symptoms remained), and only 3.5% were symptomatic and classified as poor. Injection therapy was most successful when the preceding symptoms had been present for an average of 2.6 months. Orthotic therapy was most successful when the duration of the preceding symptoms was 2 ½ years.

Shikoff and coworkers[125] reported a retrospective study of 195 patients with heel pain. The typical patient was middle-aged and overweight—91% of the respondents were classified as having above normal weight for their sex and height. Approximately 50% of the patients continued to wear heel padding or to take oral medication or both for months after the initial visit. Thirty percent experienced only marginal relief from pain or had an unsatisfactory result.

Callison[50] reviewed 400 consecutive patients with heel pain who were seen in his office during a 40-month period from October 1985 to February 1989. Radiographs of all were obtained. Heel spurs were present in 45% and absent in 53%. The series consisted of 65% women and 35% men; 30% of the women were obese, but only 10% of the men were obese. Seven percent were involved in active sports. Patients were treated with steroid injections, orthoses, calf-stretching exercises, and nonsteroidal anti-inflammatory medications. Plaster immobilization was occasionally used. Results showed that 73% improved significantly within 6 months, 20% failed to improve, and 7% did not return and were lost to follow-up.

Davis and colleagues[57] studied 105 patients (70% female and 30% male; average age, 48 years) with 132 symptomatic heels who were treated according to a standard nonoperative protocol and then reviewed at an average follow-up of 29 months. The treatment protocol consisted of nonsteroidal anti-inflammatory medications, relative rest, viscoelastic polymer heel cushions, Achilles tendon stretching exercises, and, occasionally, injections. Obesity, lifestyle (athletic versus sedentary), sex, and presence or size of heel spur did not influence the treatment outcome. Ninety-four patients (89.5%) had resolution of heel pain within 10.9 months. Six patients (5.7%) continued to have significant pain, but did not elect to have operative treatment, and five patients (4.8%) elected to have surgical intervention. They concluded that despite attention to the outcome of surgical treatment for heel pain in the current literature, initial treatment for heel pain is nonoperative. The treatment protocol used in this study was successful for 89.5% of the patients.

Wolgin and coworkers[137] evaluated the long-term results of patients treated conservatively for plantar heel pain. After eliminating those patients with workers' compensation–related complaints and those with documented inflammatory arthritides, data on 100 patients (58 females and 42 males) were available for review. The average patient was 48 years old (range 20 to 85 years). The average follow-up was 47 months (24 to 132 months). Clinical results were classified as good (resolution of symptoms) for 82 patients, fair (continued symptoms but no limitation of activity or work) for 15 patients, and poor (continued symptoms limiting activity or changing work status) in 3 patients. The average duration of symptoms before medical attention was sought was 6.1, 18.9, and 10 months for the three groups, respectively. They conclude that although the treatment of heel pain can be frustrating owing to its indolent course, a given patient with plantar fasciitis has a very good chance of complete resolution of symptoms.

The use of steroid injection in the treatment of painful heel syndrome has been advocated but is controversial.[56, 91, 137] Few reports on the long-term efficacy of injection are available. Miller and coworkers[102] evaluated the results of a single injection of corticosteroids in patients with painful heel syndrome. Twenty-seven heels in 24 patients were injected with a combination of 1% lidocaine and 1 mL of betamethasone (6 mg). These patients had never previously received an injection to their heels and had continued symptoms of pain after a trial of other nonoperative treatment modalities. After the injection, patients were seen and surveyed periodically for a period of 5 months to 8 months. The amount of pain relief that they obtained, the length of time this lasted, and the amount of heel pain present at the final follow-up were recorded. At final follow-up, the pain had returned to its pre-injection level in 13 feet. Based on the results of our study, they believed that a steroid injection is a reasonable adjunct in the treatment of painful heel syndrome, but that it is unlikely to provide permanent pain relief.

Complications from steroid injection have been reported and can be severe. Rupture of the plantar fascia and irreversible fat pad atrophy[41, 58, 93, 121] have been reported. Loss of the plantar fad pad decreases the physiologic protection in the subcalcaneal region and increases the risk of the return of intractable symptoms. Injection should be used with caution in patients with a competent fat pad and not repeated more than once in any 3-month interval. If fat pad atrophy occurs, repeat injection should be avoided.

Pfeffer and associates[108] reviewed a 15-center prospective randomized trial to compare several nonoperative treatments for proximal plantar fasciitis (heel pain syndrome). Included were 236 patients with a duration of symptoms of 6 months or less. Patients with systemic disease, significant musculoskeletal complaints, sciatica, or local nerve entrapment were excluded. Patients were randomized prospectively into five different treatment groups. All groups performed Achilles tendon stretching and plantar fascia stretching in a similar manner. One group was treated with stretching only. The other four groups stretched and used one of four different shoe inserts, including a silicone heel pad, a felt pad, a rubber heel cup, or a custom-made polypropylene orthotic device. Patients were re-evaluated after 8 weeks of treatment. Combining all the patients who used a prefabricated insert, they found that their improvement rates were higher than those assigned to stretching only ($P = 0.022$) and those who stretched and used a custom orthosis ($P = 0.0074$). They concluded that when used in conjunction with a stretching program, a prefabricated shoe insert is more likely to produce improvement in symptoms as part of the initial treatment of proximal plantar fasciitis than a custom polypropylene orthotic device.

The use of night splints to prevent plantar flexion of the ankle, as an adjunct to the treatment of subcalcaneal pain, has received considerable interest in the last few years. Wapner and Sharkey[132] originally reported the results of the use of molded ankle foot orthosis night splints for the treatment of recalcitrant plantar fasciitis on 14 patients with a total of 18 symptomatic feet. All patients had symptoms for greater than 1 year and had previously undergone treatment with nonsteroidal anti-inflammatory medicines, cortisone injections, shoe modifications, and physical therapy without resolution. All patients were provided with custom-molded polypropylene ankle foot orthoses in 5 degrees of dorsiflexion because no commercially manufactured splints were yet available. With continued use of nonsteroidal anti-inflammatory medication, Tuli heel cups, Spenco liners, and general stretching exercises, successful resolution occurred in 11 patients in less than 4 months. There were three failures. It is felt that the use of night splints provides a useful, cost-effective adjunct to current therapeutic regimens for plantar fasciitis. Night splints appear to be useful in assisting to maintain the flexibility gained by stretching exercises and relieving morning start-up pain, and they reduce the time to resolution of symptoms. Multiple subsequent studies have demonstrated the usefulness of these devices and they are now readily commercially available.[46, 103, 104, 109, 112]

Martin and associates[99] reported on an outcome study of 400 patients with chronic plantar fasciitis treated nonoperatively and concluded that patients could expect a good outcome. Compliance with their protocols did not have a correlation with outcome with one exception. Patients with chronic conditions who are compliant with the use of the night splint had a better outcome. Patients' subjective perceptions were that stretching, night splints, and heel pads were of equal importance in their treatment. Their study suggests that within the first 12 months of onset, early, aggressive, nonsurgical treatment offers the best chance or a good outcome.

Alvarez[43] has reported on the OssaTron as another alternative for management heel pain syndrome after failure of nonoperative management and before surgical management. His study evaluated primarily the safety and early preliminary efficacy of the OssaTron in treatment of patients with plantar fasciitis unresponsive to nonoperative management. Twenty heels of 20 patients were treated with 1000 extracorporeal shock waves from the OssaTron to the affected heel after administration of a heel block. Each patient was evaluated by roentgenogram, KinCom, range of motion, and physical examination, including evaluation of point tenderness by means of a palpometer and according to a 10-cm visual analog scale. The control was the contralateral heel. Patients also performed self-evaluation by means of patient activities of daily living questionnaire and pain reported by a 10-cm visual analog scale. There were no complications or adverse effects attributed to the procedure of orthotripsy. Of the 20 patients treated, 17 were improved or pain free. Eighteen of the 20 subjects treated stated that they would undergo the procedure again instead of surgery. Based on these results, he concluded that orthotripsy is a safe and effective method of treating heel pain syndrome that has been unresponsive to nonoperative management.

the abductor, with release of the deep fascia of the abductor hallucis longus and removal of the heel spur if it impinged on or produced entrapment of the nerve. Among the 34 heels operated on, there were 32 good results and 2 poor results.

Clancy[51] treated patients with a medial heel wedge and flexible leather support, heel cord stretching, and rest for 6 to 12 weeks with a gradual return to running, wearing the orthotic and the medial heel wedge for 10 weeks. In patients who failed to respond, surgery consisting of release of the plantar fascia and the fascia over the abductor hallucis longus was recommended. The 15 patients in whom surgery was performed returned to running within 8 to 10 weeks. D'Ambrosia and colleagues[54, 55] had success using anti-inflammatory medication, physical therapy, orthotic devices, and shoe modifications. Orthotic devices seemed to be the most useful part of the treatment. These orthotic devices were made of Vitrathene, Plastazote II, or Plastazote III.

Henricson and Westlin[76] described 11 heels in 10 athletes with chronic heel pain that was unrelieved by conservative therapy. The pain was due to compression of the calcaneal branches of the tibial nerve. There was entrapment of the anterior calcaneal branch where the nerve passed between the tight and rigid edges of the deep fascia of the abductor hallucis and the medial edge of the os calcis. Surgery consisted of identifying and releasing the tibial nerve and both calcaneal branches and releasing the deep fascia of the abductor hallucis. Follow-up for 58 months after surgery revealed that 10 of the 11 heels were asymptomatic. The patients had resumed athletic participation after an average of 5 weeks. It seems to these authors that both the nerve to the abductor digiti quinti and the medial calcaneal nerve were released.

Jørgensen[82] described three athletes with unusually soft and fat heel pads who were heel strikers. These athletes were treated successfully with external heel shock absorption pads. Jørgensen reported a diagnostic method for evaluating the shock-absorbing ability of the heel pad by using a visual compressible index calculated on the basis of roentgenograms of the heel, loaded and unloaded by body weight.

According to Kwong and colleagues,[90] fasciitis is produced by an excessive amount or a prolonged duration of pronation. Temporary relief was obtained in their patients by the use of anti-inflammatory drugs and therapy. Long-term relief was obtained by achieving adequate control of pronation through the use of semirigid custom-molded orthotics that reduced plantar fascial strain by supporting the first metatarsal bone and controlling calcaneal position. These devices were used in conjunction with a firm posterior counter shoe.

Leach and coworkers[92] stated that most patients respond well to conservative therapy consisting of decreased activity, stretching, heel cups, and occasional local steroids. They described 15 competitive athletes in whom 16 operations were performed. Surgery consisted of release of the plantar fascia at the insertion of the os calcis, making the incision along the medial aspect of the heel. In one instance, the medial calcaneal nerve was involved in the inflammatory process. One patient returned to running at 6 weeks; the majority returned to running 9 weeks after

surgery. Most patients continued to improve up to 6 months after the surgical procedure. Of the 15 operations, 14 were entirely successful in that the athletes returned to their previous level of activity. One failure occurred in a marathon runner who improved but was unable to train at the level he desired. There were no complications.

In 1984, McBryde[100] reported that in his running clinic, plantar fasciitis comprised 9% of the total running disorders seen. The conservative (nonoperative) approach of McBryde and his group consisted of (1) ice massage for 2 minutes four to six times daily including before and after runs; (2) heel cord stretching for 3 to 5 minutes three to four times daily; (3) posterior tibial and peroneal strengthening; (4) heel cushioning and control; and (5) anti-inflammatory medication. This regimen was usually successful in treating runners with plantar fasciitis who were seen within the first 8 weeks. In runners with symptoms lasting longer than 6 weeks, a period of absolute rest with casting was usually required. Orthoses were used. Five percent of the patients in the series underwent surgery, consisting of plantar fascial release through a short 1-inch longitudinal incision in the medial arch. All re-embarked on a successful running program 6 to 12 weeks after surgery. Overall, among the 100 patients with plantar fasciitis, 82 recovered with a conservative approach, 11 stopped running, 5 underwent surgery (all of whom returned to running), and 2 refused surgery and continued to be symptomatic.

Rask[111] reported a medial plantar neurapraxia that he termed *jogger's foot*. Three cases were reported in which there was probable entrapment of the medial plantar nerve behind the navicular tuberosity in the fibromuscular tunnel formed by the abductor hallucis; the inciting factor was eversion of the foot. All three patients were treated successfully with conservative measures including change in running posture of the foot, anti-inflammatory medication, and proper footwear.

Sammarco[115] divided heel pain into three clinical classifications and provided a treatment algorithm for these conditions. First, calcaneodynia, produced by a stress fracture, was treated with a foot orthosis and decrease in running. Second, plantar fasciitis was treated with a foot orthosis, anti-inflammatory medication, and a flexibility program, plus occasional injections of corticosteroids. Recalcitrant plantar fasciitis (defined as symptoms lasting for more than 1 year) was considered for release of the plantar fascia and bone spur if one was present. Finally, calcaneodynia involving entrapment of the medial calcaneal nerve or the nerve to the abductor digiti quinti was diagnosed by a Tinel's sign and treated with an orthosis or release of the nerve.

Snider and colleagues[127] reported 11 operations for plantar fascial release for chronic fasciitis in nine distance runners who had had symptoms for an average of 20 months and had not responded to nonsurgical treatment. The results of the operations were excellent in 10 feet and good in one foot, with an average follow-up time of 25 months. Eight of nine patients returned to their desired level of full training at an average time of 4.5 months.

Treatment of Children

Calcaneal apophysitis (Sever's disease) is a common cause of heel pain in the young child. Micheli and Ireland[101] reported calcaneal apophysitis in 137 heels in 85 children, both heels being affected in 61% of the patients. Soft Plastazote orthotics or heel cups were used in 98% of the patients in combination with proper athletic footwear. Physical therapy consisted of lower extremity stretching and ankle dorsiflexion strengthening. All patients improved and were able to return to the sport of their choice 2 months after the diagnosis. Two patients had recurrent difficulty.

Sullivan[129] reported that radiographic irregularity of the calcaneal apophysis is the rule rather than the exception. He found no evidence that treatment altered the radiographic picture. Because there are a variety of conditions that cause pain in the heel, he believes that Sever's disease might not even be a true entity. This author notes that differentiation can be made on the basis of location of the pain, the pain of Achilles tendinitis being proximal to the medial bursa and the pain of calcaneal apophysitis being along the distal portion of the posterior part of the os calcis.

In summary, conservative treatment consisting of anti-inflammatory medications, orthoses, heel cups (Fig. 30H–24), injections, physical therapy, and decreased activity level is effective in 95% of cases of subcalcaneal pain syndrome. In patients who do not respond to an adequate trial of these conservative measures, surgery consisting of release of the plantar fascia or release of the nerve to the abductor digiti quinti or the sensory medial calcaneal nerve can be performed with an expectation of good results. Heel spur, if present, is removed. Problems with decreased sensation of the heel and persistent pain have been reported, however.

Authors' Preferred Method of Treatment

Plantar fasciitis arising at the medial tuberosity probably represents a traction periostitis with degeneration and tears of the plantar fascia and subsequent secondary involvement of the adjacent structures such as the medial calcaneal nerve and the nerve to the abductor digiti quinti. Occasionally, primary entrapment of the nerve of the abductor digiti quinti and the sensory branch of the medial calcaneal nerve may occur. A calcaneal spur is present in 50% of the cases and may be part of the inflammatory process. In longstanding cases, the chronic inflammation and traction on the insertion of the plantar fascia may result in a stress fracture of the os calcis, although this is more common in the older patient. An accurate diagnosis of the cause of the pain and any concomitant conditions such as chronic heel fat pad atrophy, cavus foot deformity, contraction of the Achilles tendon, or nerve entrapment must be determined because they will affect both the prognosis and treatment modalities employed.

At the first visit, we recommend a discussion with the patient to explain the nature of this condition. We tell them the good news is that it almost always gets better without the need for surgery. The bad news is that it usually does not get better quickly. In our initial consultation, we explain that we expect it to take at least 6 to 9 months to resolve completely and sometimes up to a year. It is important for both the physician and the patient to set this time frame early on to decrease the frustration often associated with this diagnosis.

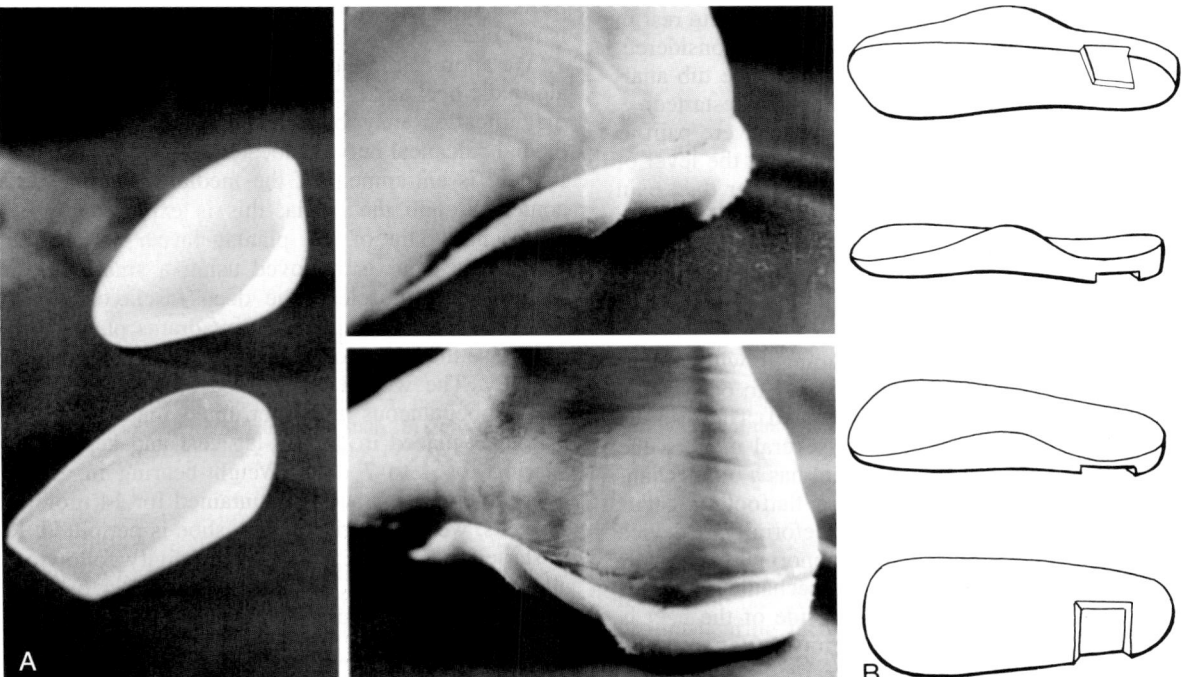

Figure 30H–24. *A*, Over-the-counter heel cups designed to compress the fat pad and cushion the heel. *B*, Custom orthoses used for treatment of subcalcaneal pain syndrome. These may be made of many types of material. Consistent features are support of the arch, presence of cushioning material, recess for area of pain beneath the heel, and slight medial elevation.

Criteria for Return to Sports Participation

Because plantar fasciitis associated with pain in the medial tuberosity in the athlete may be associated with a variety of presentations and degrees of severity and does not produce any significant structural effect other than alteration in form, activity may be allowed within the patient's symptomatic tolerance, although this varies greatly according to the pain component and the athlete's restriction. The exception to this is if the patient is developing a stress fracture. Once the pain has subsided with conservative treatment and no tenderness is present, gradually increasing activity is allowed using an orthotic within the shoe. If symptoms do not recur with the specific activity desired, full activity is allowed.

Following surgical intervention, the patient is allowed increased activity when the symptoms of pain with activity and acute tenderness have resolved. This usually occurs between 6 and 12 weeks postoperatively.

References

Retrocalcaneal Bursitis

1. Bordelon RL: Surgical and Conservative Foot Care. Thorofare, NJ, Slack, 1988.
2. Bottger BA, Schweitzer ME, El-Noueam KI, et al: MR imaging of the normal and abnormal retrocalcaneal AJR Am J Roentgenol 170:1239–1241, 1998.
3. Burhenne LJ, Connell DG: Xeroradiography in the diagnosis of the Haglund syndrome. J Can Assoc Radiol 37:157–160, 1986.
4. Canoso JJ, Liu N, Trail MR, Runge VM: Physiology of the retrocalcaneal bursa. Ann Rheum Dis 47:910–912, 1988.
5. Canoso JJ, Wohlgethan JR, Newberg AH, Goldsmith MR: Aspiration of the retrocalcaneal bursa. Ann Rheum Dis 43:308–312, 1984.
6. Clain MR, Baxter DE: Achilles tendinitis. Foot Ankle 13:482–487, 1992.
7. Clancy WG: Runners' injuries. Part II. Evaluation and treatment of specific injuries. Am J Sports Med 8:287–289, 1980.
8. Fiamengo SA, Warren RF, Marshall JL, et al: Posterior heel pain associated with a calcaneal step and Achilles tendon calcification. Clin Orthop 167:203–211, 1982.
9. Fowler A, Philip JF: Abnormality of the calcaneus as a cause of painful heel: Its diagnosis and operative treatment. Br J Surg 32:494–498, 1945.
10. Fox JM, Blazine ME, Jobe FW, et al: Degeneration and rupture of the Achilles tendon. Clin Orthop 107:221–224, 1975.
11. Frey C, Rosenberg Z, Shereff MJ: The retrocalcaneal bursa: Anatomy and bursography. Foot Ankle 13:203–207, 1992.
12. Gerster JC: Plantar fasciitis and Achilles tendinitis among 150 cases of seronegative spondarthritis. Rheumatol Rehabil 19:218–222, 1980.
13. Gerster JC, Piccinin P: Enthesopathy of the heels in juvenile onset seronegative B-27 positive spondyloarthropathy. J Rheumatol 12:310–314, 1985.
14. Gerster JC, Saudan Y, Fallet GH: Talalgia. A review of 30 severe cases. J Rheumatol 5:210–216, 1978.
15. Goss CM: Gray's Anatomy, 27th ed. Philadelphia, Lea & Febiger, 1959, pp 544–553.
16. Hartmann HO: The tendon sheaths and synovial bursae of the foot. Foot Ankle 1:247–296, 1981.
17. Heneghan JA, Pavlov H: The Haglund painful heel syndrome. Experimental investigation of cause and therapeutic implications. Clin Orthop 187:228–234, 1984.
18. Ippolito E, Ricciardi-Pollini PT: Invasive retrocalcaneal bursitis: A report on three cases. Foot Ankle 4:204–208, 1984.
19. Jones DC, James SL: Partial calcaneal osteotomy for retrocalcaneal bursitis. Am J Sports Med 12:72–73, 1984.
20. Karjalainen PT, Soila K, Aronen HJ, et al: MR imaging of overuse injuries of the Achilles tendon. AJR Am J Roentgenol 175:251–260, 2000.
21. Keck SW, Kelly PJ: Bursitis of the posterior part of the heel: Evaluation of surgical treatment of 18 patients. J Bone Joint Surg Am 47:267–273, 1965.
22. Kennedy JC, Willis RB: The effects of local steroid injections on tendons: A biomechanical and microscopic correlative study. Am J Sports Med 4:11–21, 1976.
23. Lagergren C, Lindholm A: Vascular distribution in the Achilles tendon: An angiographic and microangiographic study. Acta Chir Scand 116:491–495, 1958–1959.
24. Leach RE, James S, Wasilewski S: Achilles tendinitis. Am J Sports Med 9:93–98, 1981.
25. Mann RA: Surgery of the Foot, 5th ed. St. Louis, CV Mosby, 1986.
26. Mann RA, Holmes GB Jr, Seale KS, Collins DN: Chronic rupture of the Achilles tendon: A new technique of repair. J Bone Joint Surg Am 73:214–219, 1991.
27. Nelimarkka O, Lehto M, Jarvinen M: Soleus muscle anomaly in a patient with exertion pain in the ankle. A case report. Arch Orthop Traum Surg 107:120–121, 1988.
28. Olivieri I, Barozzi L, Padula A, et al: Retrocalcaneal bursitis in spondyloarthropathy: Assessment by ultrasonography and magnetic resonance imaging. J Rheumatol. 25:1352–1357, 1998.
29. Pavlov H, Heneghan MA, Hersh A, et al: The Haglund syndrome: Initial and differential diagnosis. Radiology 144:83–88, 1982.
30. Puddu G, Ippolito E, Postacchinni F: Classification of Achilles tendon disease. Am J Sports Med 4:145–150, 1976.
31. Ruch JA: Haglund's disease. J Am Podiatr Assoc 64:1000–1003, 1974.
32. Schepsis AA, Leach RE: Surgical management of Achilles tendinitis. Am J Sports Med 15:308–315, 1987.
33. Schepsis A, Wagner C, Leach RE: Surgical management of Achilles tendon overuse injuries. A long-term follow-up study. Am J Sports Med 22:611–619, 1994.
34. Schweitzer ME, Karasick D: MR imaging of disorders of the Achilles tendon. AJR Am J Roentgenol 175:613–254, 2000.
35. Sullivan JA: Recurring pain in the pediatric athlete. Pediatr Clin North Am 31:1097–1112, 1984.
36. Vega MR, Cavolo DJ, Green RM, Cohen RS: Haglund's deformity. J Am Podiatr Assoc 74:129–135, 1984.
37. Wapner KL, Hecht PJ, Mills RH Jr: Reconstruction of neglected Achilles tendon injury. Orthop Clin North Am 26:249–263, 2000.
38. Wapner KL, Pavlock GS, Hecht PJ, et al: Repair of chronic Achilles tendon rupture with FHL tendon transfer. Foot Ankle 14:443–449, 1993.
39. Watson AD, Anderson RB, Davis WH: Comparison of results of retrocalcaneal decompression for retrocalcaneal bursitis and insertional achilles tendinosis with calcific spur. Foot Ankle Int 21:638–642, 1993.
40. Zadek I: An operation for the cure of achillo-bursitis. Am J Surg 43:542–546, 1939.

Plantar Fasciitis

41. Acevedo JI, Beskin JL: Complications of plantar fascia rupture associated with corticosteroid injection. Foot Ankle Int 19:91–97, 1998.
42. Ali E: Calcaneal spur in Guyana. West Indian Med J 29:175–183, 1980.
43. Alvarez RG: Preliminary Results on the Safety and Efficacy of the OssaTron; for Treatment of Plantar Fasciitis. AOFAS Summer Meeting, July 1998, Boston.
44. Baxter DE, Thigpen CM: Heel pain—operative results. Foot Ankle 5:16–25, 1984.
45. Barrett SL, Day SV: Endoscopic plantar fasciotomy for chronic plantar fasciitis/heel spur syndrome: Surgical technique—early clinical results. J Foot Surg 30:568–70, 1991.
46. Batt ME, Tanji JL, Skattum N: Plantar fasciitis: A prospective randomized clinical trial of the tension night splint. Clin J Sport Med 6:158–162, 1996.
47. Bordelon RL: Subcalcaneal pain—a method of evaluation and plan for treatment. Clin Orthop 177:49–53, 1983.

48. Bordelon RL: Subcalcaneal pain: Present status, evaluation, and management. Instr Course Lect 33:283–287, 1984.
49. Bordelon RL: Surgical and Conservative Foot Care. Thorofare, NJ, Slack, 1988, pp 105–115.
50. Callison WJ: Heel pain: Analysis of results of treatment. Presented at meeting of the Orthopaedic Foot Club, Dallas, Texas, April 1989.
51. Clancy WG: Runners' injuries. Part II. Evaluation and treatment of specific injuries. Am J Sports Med 8:287–289, 1980.
52. Contompasis JP: Surgical treatment of calcaneal spurs: A three-year post-surgical study. J Am Podiatr Assoc 64:987–999, 1974.
53. Daly PJ, Kitaoka HB, Chao EY: Plantar fasciotomy for intractable plantar fasciitis: Clinical results and biomechanical evaluation. Foot Ankle 13:188–195, 1992.
54. D'Ambrosia RD: Conservative management of metatarsal and heel pain in the adult foot. Orthopedics 10:137–142, 1987.
55. D'Ambrosia RD, Richtor N, Douglas R: Orthotics. In D'Ambrosia RD, Drez D (eds): Prevention and Treatment of Running Injuries, 2nd ed. Thorofare, NJ, Slack, 1989, pp 245–258.
56. Dasgupta B, Bowles J: Scintigraphic localisation of steroid injection site in plantar fasciitis. Lancet 346:1400, 1995.
57. Davis PF, Severud E, Baxter DE: Painful heel syndrome: Results of nonoperative treatment Foot Ankle Int 15:531–535, 1994.
58. DeMaio M, Paine R, Mangine RE, Drez D Jr: Plantar fasciitis. Orthopedics 16:1153–1163, 1993.
59. DuVries HL: Heel spur (calcaneal spur). Arch Surg 74:536–542, 1957.
60. Eastmond CJ, Rajah SM, Tovey D, Wright V: Seronegative pauciarticular arthritis and HLA-B27. Ann Rheum Dis 39:231–234, 1980.
61. Freeman C: Heel pain. In Gould JS (ed): The Foot Book. Baltimore, Williams & Wilkins, 1988, pp 228–238.
62. Galinski AW: Calcaneodynia-herniation. J Am Podiatr Assoc 67:647–650, 1977.
63. Gentile AT, Zizzo CJ, Dahukey A, Berman SS: Traumatic pseudoaneurysm of the lateral plantar artery after endoscopic plantar fasciotomy. Foot Ankle Int 18:821–822, 1997.
64. Gerster JC: Plantar fasciitis and Achilles tendinitis among 150 cases of seronegative spondarthritis. Rheumatol Rehabil 19:218–222, 1980.
65. Gerster JC, Piccinin P: Enthesopathy of the heels in juvenile onset seronegative B-27 positive spondyloarthropathy. J Rheumatol 12:310–314, 1985.
66. Gerster JC, Saudan Y, Fallet GH: Talalgia. A review of 30 severe cases. J Rheumatol 5:210–216, 1978.
67. Gill LH: Plantar fasciitis: Diagnosis and conservative management. J Am Acad Orthop Surg 5:109–117, 1997.
68. Gill LH, Kiebzak GM: Outcome of nonsurgical treatment for plantar fasciitis. Foot Ankle Int 17:527–532, 1996.
69. Goss CM: Gray's Anatomy, 27th ed. Philadelphia, Lea & Febiger, 1959, pp 545–559.
70. Goulet MJ: Role of soft orthosis in treating plantar fasciitis. Suggestion from the field. Phys Ther 64:1544, 1984.
71. Graham CE: Painful heel syndrome: Rationale of diagnosis and treatment. Foot Ankle 3:261–267, 1983.
72. Grasel RP, Schweitzer ME, Kovalovich AM, et al: MR imaging of plantar fasciitis: Edema, tears, and occult marrow abnormalities correlated with outcomes AJR Am J Roentgenol 173:699–701, 1999.
73. Hamilton WG: Surgical anatomy of the foot and ankle. Clin Symp 37:2–32, 1985.
74. Hartmann HO: The tendon sheaths and synovial bursae of the foot. Foot Ankle 1:247–296, 1981.
75. Hassab HK, El-Sherif AS: Drilling of the os calcis for painful heel with calcanean spur. Acta Orthop Scand 45:152–157, 1974.
76. Henricson AS, Westlin NE: Chronic calcaneal pain in athletes: Entrapment of the calcaneal nerve? Am J Sports Med 12:152–154, 1984.
77. Hicks JH: The mechanics of the foot: The plantar aponeurosis and the arch. J Anat 88:25–31, 1954.
78. Hoffman SJ, Thul JR: Fractures of the calcaneus secondary to heel spur surgery. An analysis and case report. J Am Podiatr Med Assoc 75:267–271, 1985.
79. Intenzo CM, Wapner KL, Park CH, Kim SM: Evaluation of plantar fasciitis by three-phase bone scintigraphy. Clin Nucl Med 16:325–328, 1991.
80. Jay RM, Davis BA, Schoenhaus HD, Beckett D: Calcaneal decompression for chronic heel pain. J Am Podiatr Med Assoc 75:535–537, 1985.
81. Jerosch J: Endoscopic release of plantar fasciitis—a benign procedure? Foot Ankle Int 21:511–513, 2000.
82. Jørgensen U: Achillodynia and loss of heel pad shock absorbency. Am J Sports Med 13:128–132, 1985.
83. Katoh Y, Chao EY, Morrey BF, Laughman RK: Objective technique for evaluating painful heel syndrome and its treatment. Foot Ankle 3:227–237, 1983.
84. Kenzora JE: The painful heel syndrome: An entrapment neuropathy. Bull Hosp Joint Dis Orthop Inst 47:178–189, 1987.
85. Kier R: Magnetic resonance imaging of plantar fasciitis and other causes of heel pain. Magn Reson Imaging Clin N Am 2:97–107, 1994.
86. Kitaoka HB, Ahn TK, Luo ZP, An KN: Stability of the arch of the foot. Foot Ankle Int 18:644–648, 1997.
87. Kitaoka HB, Luo ZP, An KN: Mechanical behavior of the foot and ankle after plantar fascia release in the unstable foot. Foot Ankle Int 18:8–15, 1997.
88. Kitaoka HB, Luo ZP, An KN: Effect of plantar fasciotomy on stability of arch of foot. Clin Orthop 344:307–312, 1997.
89. Kopell HP, Thompson WAL: Peripheral Entrapment Neuropathies. Huntington, NY, Robert E. Krieger Publishing, 1986, pp 25–29.
90. Kwong PK, Kay D, Voner RT, White MW: Plantar fasciitis. Mechanics and pathomechanics of treatment. Clin Sports Med 7:119–126, 1988.
91. Lapidus PW, Guidotti FP: Painful heel: Report of 323 patients with 364 painful heels. Clin Orthop 39:178, 1965.
92. Leach RE, Dilorio E, Harney RA: Pathologic hindfoot conditions in the athlete. Clin Orthop 177:116–121, 1983.
93. Leach R, Jones R, Silva T: Rupture of the plantar fascia in athletes. J Bone Joint Surg Am 60:537–539, 1978.
94. Leach RE, Seavey MS, Salter DK: Results of surgery in athletes with plantar fasciitis. Foot Ankle 7:156–161, 1986.
95. Lester DK, Buchanan JR: Surgical treatment of plantar fasciitis. Clin Orthop 186:202–204, 1984.
96. Lin E, Ronen M, Stampler D, Suster S: Painful piezogenic heel papules. A case report. J Bone Joint Surg Am 67:601–604, 1985.
97. Lutter LD: Surgical decisions in athletes' subcalcaneal pain. Am J Sports Med 14:481–485, 1986.
98. Mann RA: Surgery of the Foot, 5th ed. St. Louis, CV Mosby, 1986, pp 244–247.
99. Martin RL, Irrgang JJ, Conti SF: Outcome study of subjects with insertional plantar fasciitis. Foot Ankle Int 19:803–811, 1998.
100. McBryde AM Jr: Plantar fasciitis. Instr Course Lect 33:278–282, 1984.
101. Micheli LJ, Ireland ML: Prevention and management of calcaneal apophysitis in children: An overuse syndrome. J Pediatr Orthop 7:34–38, 1987.
102. Miller RA, Torres J, McGuire M: Efficacy of first-time steroid injection for painful heel syndrome. Foot Ankle Int 16:610–612, 1995.
103. Mizel MS, Marymont JV, Trepman E: Treatment of plantar fasciitis with a night splint and shoe modification consisting of a steel shank and anterior rocker bottom. Foot Ankle Int 17:732–735, 1996.
104. Ng A: Treatment of plantar fasciitis with night splint and shoe modifications consisting of a steel shank and anterior rocker bottom. Foot Ankle Int 18:458, 1997.
105. O'Brien D, Martin WJ: A retrospective analysis of heel pain. J Am Podiatr Med Assoc 75:416–418, 1985.
106. O'Malley MJ, Page A, Cook R: Endoscopic plantar fasciotomy for chronic heel pain. Foot Ankle Int 21:505–510, 2000.
107. Paice EW, Hoffbrand BI: Nutritional osteomalacia presenting with plantar fasciitis. J Bone Joint Surg Br 69:38–40, 1987.
108. Pfeffer G, Bacchetti P, Deland J, et al: Comparison of custom and prefabricated orthoses in the initial treatment of proximal plantar fasciitis. Foot Ankle Int 20:214–221, 1999.
109. Powell M, Post WR, Keener J, Wearden S: Effective treatment of chronic plantar fasciitis with dorsiflexion night splints: A crossover prospective randomized outcome study. Foot Ankle Int 19:10, 1998.
110. Przylucki H, Jones CL: Entrapment neuropathy of muscle branch of lateral plantar nerve: A cause of heel pain. J Am Podiatr Assoc 71:119–124, 1981.
111. Rask MR: Medial plantar neurapraxia (jogger's foot): Report of 3 cases. Clin Orthop 134:193–195, 1978.
112. Ryan J: Use of posterior night splints in the treatment of plantar fasciitis. Am Fam Physician 52:891–898, 901–902, 1995.

If the problem is thought to be due to mechanical pressure on the nerve, usually conservative measures are not beneficial.

Surgical Management

Decompression of the posterior tibial nerve and its terminal branches should be undertaken through a longitudinal incision, which starts approximately 20 cm proximal to the medial malleolus and 2 cm behind the posterior border of the tibia and extends distally behind the medial malleolus and along the medial aspect of the foot. The direction of the incision below the malleolus depends on the area that needs to be explored. If most of the symptom complex involves the medial plantar nerve, the incision is brought along the dorsal margin of the abductor hallucis muscle, or if the symptoms seem to involve mainly the lateral plantar nerve, the incision is carried slightly more plantarward along the origin of the abductor hallucis muscle. The incision is deepened down to the fascial layer. Care is taken to identify and cauterize all bleeders.

The investing retinaculum is opened behind the posterior tibial tendon sheath, and usually the posterior tibial nerve lies just posterior to the flexor digitorum longus tendon. Occasionally, the flexor digitorum longus tendon is in its own tendon sheath; then one must open up the next tendon sheath posteriorly to identify the posterior tibial nerve. The nerve always is identified proximally, which makes the dissection easier as one proceeds distally toward the medial malleolus. As one reaches the area of the medial malleolus, the vascular leash, which accompanies the posterior tibial nerve, crosses over the nerve, making the dissection more difficult. At times, it is almost easier to identify the medial plantar nerve distal to the malleolus and work back retrograde, allowing identification of the medial plantar nerve along its entire course.

One follows the medial plantar nerve distally past the talonavicular joint, after which it passes through a fibroosseous tunnel onto the plantar aspect of the foot. It is important that a clamp be passed through this tunnel to be sure that no entrapment is present. If entrapment does appear to be present, the tunnel should be opened.

Returning proximally, the lateral plantar nerve carefully is identified posterior to the medial plantar nerve. Generally, the medial calcaneal branches come off the posterior aspect of the lateral plantar nerve at varying heights, usually starting at about the level of the medial malleolus, but at times they may branch off more proximally. Because of this, the dissection should be carried out along the anterior aspect of the lateral plantar nerve to avoid injury to the medial calcaneal branches.

The lateral plantar nerve is traced distally behind the vascular leash, after which it passes down beneath the origin of the abductor hallucis. At times, it is difficult to dissect out the lateral plantar nerve, but in patients in whom there is a positive Tinel's sign over the area of the nerve, it is imperative to take down the abductor origin sufficiently to allow the entire course of the lateral plantar nerve to be identified. Behind the abductor hallucis, the lateral plantar nerve passes through several firm fibroosseous tunnels, each of which needs to be identified by blunt dissection. If there is any evidence of entrapment, the tunnel needs to be released.

The medial calcaneal branch should be identified as it passes along the posterior aspect of the lateral plantar nerve, but it does not need to be dissected out unless the symptoms point to entrapment. As this dissection is carried out, if any ganglion or cystlike structure appears to be arising from a tendon sheath, it must be identified and excised. This structure could be the main cause of the patient's symptoms and should be looked for carefully, particularly if there is a localized Tinel's sign preoperatively over one of the terminal branches below the level of the malleolus.

After the nerve has been exposed completely, the vascular pattern of the nerve needs to be evaluated carefully. If the vascular pattern seems lacking in a localized area or along the course of the nerve, there may be some type of vascular constriction of the nerve that requires release of the epineurium to relieve it. After the dissection has been completed, the tourniquet is released, and all bleeding is brought under control. The wound is closed in a routine manner, and a compression dressing is applied. Postoperatively, the patient is kept non–weight bearing for 3 weeks, after which progressive weight bearing is begun as tolerated. Swelling should be controlled with an elastic stocking. I do not permit any impact-type activities for at least 2 months and then only as tolerated.

Clinical Results

The results after release of the tarsal tunnel are variable. The best results occur in patients who have a localized problem. In this group, a satisfaction rate of about 90% can be achieved. The remainder have about a 70% satisfaction rate. Many patients note that the pain or dysesthesias still are present but at a significantly reduced level. Patients who remain symptomatic may note no improvement at all or may feel slightly improved. In my experience, if an adequate release procedure appears to have been carried out, more than likely a second operation will not be successful either. Even after a successful release of the posterior tibial nerve and its terminal branches, tingling often occurs along the course of the nerve with percussion.

Entrapment of the Motor Branch to the Abductor Digiti Quinti

Entrapment of the nerve to the abductor digiti quinti has been identified as a source of heel pain.[2, 6, 16, 37, 40] Although it is not a common cause of heel pain, this nerve entrapment is something that should be sought carefully, particularly in the patient who presents with refractory pain about the heel.

Clinical Symptoms

Patients with this entrapment neuropathy complain of a vague burning pain about the heel pad area. The pain usually is poorly localized and rarely radiates out to the fore part of the foot or proximally in the heel. Generally, the symptoms are aggravated by activity and relieved by rest.

Etiology

The cause is believed to be the result of entrapment of the nerve to the abductor digiti quinti muscle (Fig. 30I–2), which arises from the lateral plantar nerve. The entrapment occurs as this nerve passes beneath the plantar aspect of the deep investing fascia of the abductor hallucis muscle as it courses laterally across the foot. The nerve, after passing the abductor hallucis, passes along the calcaneus, lying between the long plantar ligament, which is dorsal to it, and the plantar fascia, which is plantar to it. It lies adjacent to the plantar tuberosity of the calcaneus. Continuing laterally, the nerve terminates in the muscle mass of the abductor digiti quinti. The entrapment of the nerve usually occurs beneath the abductor fascia or, owing to its proximity to the calcaneal spur, secondary to inflammation, trauma, or healing of a stress fracture.

Diagnosis

Physical Examination

Pressure over the medial and slightly plantar aspect of the abductor hallucis muscle reproduces the patient's pain. Occasionally, a positive Tinel's sign can be elicited in the area. The patient with this condition usually needs to be evaluated on several occasions to be sure that the symptom complex is reproducible. Generally, electrodiagnostic studies are not useful in defining this problem.

Differential Diagnosis

The differential diagnosis in patients with this entrapment includes mainly other causes of heel pain, such as plantar fasciitis, a fasciitis or tendinitis of the origin of the abductor hallucis muscle, periostitis or stress fracture of the calcaneus, tarsal tunnel syndrome, systemic arthritides, or possibly a mechanical foot problem.

Treatment

Conservative Management

Conservative management consists of the use of nonsteroidal anti-inflammatory medications, local steroid injection, an orthotic device to attempt to keep the stress off the involved area and, occasionally, immobilization of the foot in a short-leg cast.

Surgical Treatment

In patients who fail to respond to conservative management, operative release can be considered.[2] The release is carried out through a 5-cm incision made along the upper border of the heel pad, care being taken to preserve the sensory branches to the calcaneus. The investing fascia over the abductor hallucis muscle is split, and the muscle is retracted dorsally. The deep layer of the investing fascia is released to observe the lateral plantar nerve. The branch to the abductor digiti quinti can be identified as it passes laterally. The nerve is traced laterally, and a hemostat is placed along the course of the nerve to ensure that an entrapment is not present as it passes adjacent to the calcaneal tuberosity. If there appears to be any evidence of pressure against the nerve from the medial half of the plantar fascia or the calcaneal tuberosity, the former is

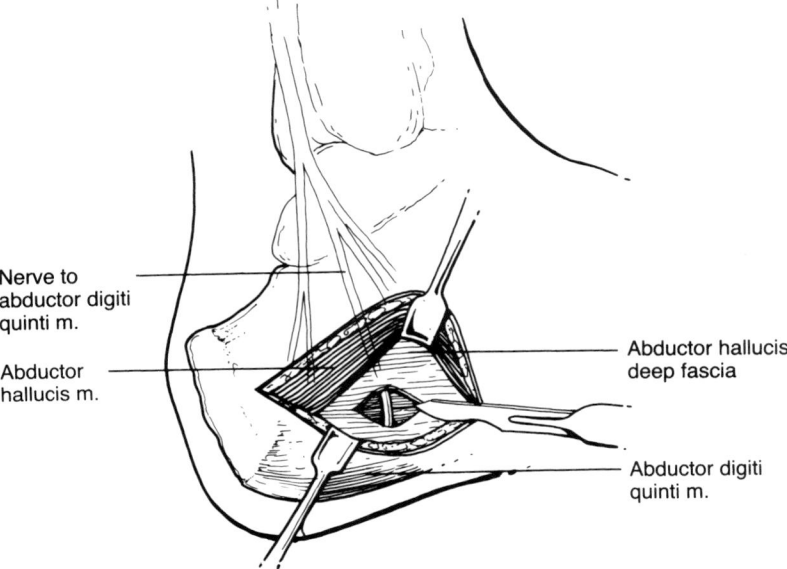

Figure 30I–2. Nerve to the abductor digiti quinti.

Nerve to abductor digiti quinti m.

Abductor hallucis m.

Abductor hallucis deep fascia

Abductor digiti quinti m.

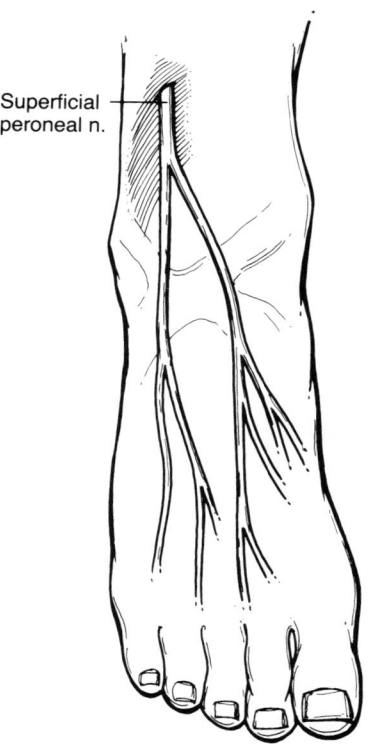

Figure 30I–5. Entrapment of the superficial peroneal nerve as it exits from the deep fascia of the leg.

which is innervated by the superficial portion of the deep peroneal nerve.

Clinical Symptoms

The patient usually complains of numbness and tingling over the dorsal aspect of the foot and ankle, but the first web space is not involved. The symptoms may be stimulated by sporting activities, but the condition occurs in the nonathlete as well. If the entrapment is due to a fascial defect with resultant muscle herniation, the patient may note a fullness or swelling over the anterolateral aspect of the leg where the nerve exits through the fascia.

Etiology

The cause frequently is undetermined, but sometimes the condition is secondary to a fascial defect with secondary muscle herniation, which results in tenting of the superficial peroneal nerve.[8] At times, compression from an external source, such as a lipoma or occasionally a bony callus resulting from a tibial fracture, may place pressure on the nerve.[1, 8, 39]

Diagnosis

Physical Findings

The physical examination usually brings out the cause of the problem. Tenderness or irritability of the nerve to percussion is evident where it exits through the fascial defect. A muscle herniation or an underlying lipoma or callus usually can be palpated. Frequently, there may be some sensory loss over the distribution of the nerve about the anterior aspect of the foot, sparing the first web space. Resisted dorsiflexion of the ankle joint may show the muscle herniation through the fascial defect.

Electromyographic Studies

A conduction study of the superficial peroneal nerve usually shows abnormal conduction velocities. Electromyography helps to rule out the presence of an L5 radiculopathy.

Differential Diagnosis

Superficial peroneal nerve entrapment may mimic a common peroneal nerve entrapment or possibly an L5 radiculopathy. The symptoms of a chronic ankle sprain or instability can mimic this condition, but with a careful history and examination, these usually can be differentiated.

Treatment

Conservative Management

Occasionally, a steroid injection or a diminished level of activity may be beneficial. If symptoms persist, however, and particularly if a muscle herniation or mass is present beneath the nerve, surgical release is indicated.

Surgical Treatment

The site of the entrapment is identified through a longitudinal incision, and the fascia over the anterior compartment is released. It is important to carry out an adequate release so that a muscle herniation does not result from the surgical decompression. If a mass is present, such as a lipoma or callus, this should be excised. Postoperatively, the patient is kept in a compression dressing until the soft tissues heal, at which time activities can be resumed as tolerated.

Clinical Results

Generally, surgical decompression of the nerve results in satisfactory relief for the patient. One must be cautious, however, not to damage the nerve inadvertently when the decompression is carried out.

Interdigital Neuroma

An interdigital neuroma (Fig. 30I–6) has been described as an entrapment-type phenomenon of the common digital

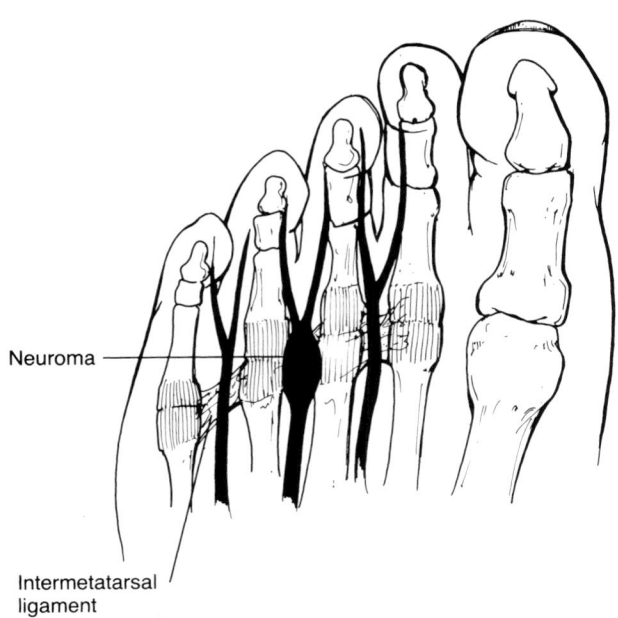

Figure 30I-6. Interdigital neuroma, plantar view.

Neuroma

Intermetatarsal ligament

nerve as it passes beneath the transverse metatarsal ligament to innervate the adjacent web space.[12, 13] For this reason, it is discussed in this section under entrapment neuropathies, although the precise cause of an interdigital neuroma in most cases still is not known. Other factors that may lead to the development of an interdigital neuroma include poor footwear,[5, 31] trauma,[30] and anatomic abnormalities.[19]

Clinical Symptoms

The patient with an interdigital neuroma usually is able to localize the pain precisely on the plantar aspect of the foot. The patient usually can point to the site of the pain with one finger. Frequently, the pain radiates out to the involved web space. The pain almost invariably is brought about by activities and is relieved by rest. Sometimes, removing a tight shoe brings about complete resolution of the symptoms. When walking barefoot, the symptoms are improved significantly in most patients. Occasionally, the patient notes a clicking sensation on the plantar aspect of the foot that may or may not exacerbate the pain. Localization of the pain in a patient with an interdigital neuroma is exactly opposite that noted in the tarsal tunnel syndrome, in which the pain is diffuse and poorly localized.

Etiology

Although multiple causes have been suggested, only rarely can the precise cause be found. When there is extrinsic pressure secondary to a ganglion or synovial cyst adjacent to the nerve, resulting in pressure, the cause is known precisely. Neuromas occur in women in 90% of cases, and this may be related to the position of the foot while wearing a high heel. Repetitive stress to this area could be the cause, but conversely, the incidence in runners and other individuals who are active on their feet is no greater than that observed in a more sedentary population. It has been hypothesized by some that the thickening of the nerve is due to an impingement of the nerve at the level of the transverse metatarsal ligament,[12] and some clinicians have proposed merely releasing the ligament without excising the nerve.[27] In my experience, however, this has not proved satisfactory.

As a rule, an interdigital neuroma involves the third interspace most frequently, followed closely by the second interspace.[5, 12, 31] In my experience, it is extremely unusual for a virgin neuroma to be found in the first or fourth web space.

Diagnosis

Physical Examination

Examination of the patient's foot should begin by careful palpation of the metatarsal heads, looking for evidence of pain and possible pathology in the metatarsophalangeal joint. After this, the web spaces should be palpated carefully. In the patient with an interdigital neuroma, the pain is elicited by firmly palpating the plantar aspect of the foot in the involved web space. When the area of pain has been identified, mediolateral compression of the foot usually is found to accentuate the pain. In most cases, the patient notes that the tingling radiates out toward the toes. Occasionally, an interdigital neuroma is associated with a mass in the web space, either a ganglion or a synovial cyst, which can be observed to move around, exacerbating the pain. Generally speaking, no sensory deficit is noted in these patients. Radiographs of the foot usually are negative.

At times, it is necessary to re-evaluate the patient with a neuroma on several occasions to be sure which web space is involved and to be sure that the symptom complex is present. Generally, if the patient has pain over the metatarsophalangeal joint as well as in the web space, one must be cautious about ascribing that pain wholly to the nerve because I believe it will be found more than likely to be due to a problem in the metatarsophalangeal joint rather than the common digital nerve.

Electromyographic Evaluation

To date, there does not appear to be a reliable electrodiagnostic study for the patient with a suspected interdigital neuroma.

Differential Diagnosis

An interdigital neuroma can be mimicked by many other conditions. These may be classified as follows:

1. Metatarsophalangeal joint pathology
   a. Degeneration of the plantar plate or capsule
   b. Synovitis of the metatarsophalangeal joint owing to nonspecific synovitis or rheumatoid arthritis

   c. Subluxation or dislocation of the metatarsophalangeal joint
   d. Freiberg's infraction
2. Pain of neuritic origin not related to an interdigital neuroma
   a. Degenerative disc disease
   b. Tarsal tunnel syndrome
   c. Lesion of the medial or lateral plantar nerve
   d. Peripheral neuropathy
3. Lesions on the plantar aspect of the foot
   a. Synovial cyst
   b. Soft tissue tumor not involving the metatarsophalangeal joint, such as a ganglion, lipoma, or soft tissue tumor
   c. Tumor of the metatarsal bone

Treatment

Conservative Management

Conservative management consists of prescribing a wide, soft shoe, preferably one with a low heel. A soft metatarsal support can be added to the shoe to remove the stress from the involved web space. This support spreads the distal portion of the foot, opening up the web spaces. Injection of a steroid preparation into the area of the nerve is practiced frequently, although I tend to avoid this, if possible. Occasionally, after a steroid injection, disruption of the capsule of the metatarsophalangeal joint may occur, resulting in deviation of the toes. If a steroid injection is carried out, it rarely should be done more than once for fear of doing more damage than good. If conservative management fails to bring about adequate relief of the problem, surgical excision of the neuroma is indicated.

Surgical Treatment

An interdigital neuroma should be excised through a dorsal approach. The incision is made in the web space and carried down between the two metatarsals. A Weitlander is used to spread the metatarsal heads apart, placing the transverse metatarsal ligament under tension. The transverse metatarsal ligament is cut. Using a small neurologic freer, the underlying web space is exposed, and the common digital nerve is identified. The nerve is traced proximal to the metatarsal head, at which point it is excised. The nerve is traced distally and excised just distal to its bifurcation. The skin is closed in a routine manner.

A compression dressing is used postoperatively for 3 weeks to permit the transverse metatarsal ligament to heal. Ambulation in a postoperative shoe with a firm sole is prescribed. The patient is allowed to resume activities as tolerated, although I prefer to restrict running for approximately 6 weeks.

If the patient has a recurrent neuroma, surgical exploration is carried out in the same manner as that described previously. I believe that incisions on the plantar aspect of the foot should be avoided if possible, especially in the athlete.

Clinical Results

After excision of an interdigital neuroma, approximately 80% of patients have satisfactory relief of symptoms. Careful review of our series of patients showed that 71% were asymptomatic, 9% were improved, 6% were marginally improved, and 14% were unchanged.[31] Results did not appear to differ whether the neuroma was removed from the second or third interspace. If a recurrent neuroma is present, as evident by well-localized pain and a positive Tinel's sign over the nerve, re-exploration produced satisfactory results in about 70% of our cases.

References

1. Banerjee T, Koons DD: Superficial peroneal nerve entrapment: Report of two cases. J Neurosurg 55:991, 1981.
2. Baxter DE, Thigpen CM: Heel pain: Operative results. Foot Ankle 5:16, 1984.
3. Byank RP, Clarke HJ, Bleecker ML: Standardized neurometric evaluation in tarsal tunnel syndrome. In: Advances in Orthopaedic Surgery. Baltimore, Williams & Wilkins, 1989.
4. Colbert, DS, Cunningham F, Mackey D: Sural nerve entrapment: Case report. J Irish Med Assoc 68:544, 1975.
5. Coughlin MJ: Soft tissue afflictions. In Chapman M (ed): Operative Orthopaedics. Philadelphia, JB Lippincott, 1988, pp 1819–1821.
6. Deese JM, Baxter DE: Compressive neuropathies of the lower extremity. J Musculoskel Med 5:68–91, 1988.
7. Docks GW, Salter, MS: Sural nerve entrapment: An unusual case report. J Foot Surg 18:42, 1979.
8. Garfin S, Mubarak SJ, Owen CA: Exertional anterolateral compartment syndrome: Case report with fascial defect, muscle herniation and superficial peroneal nerve entrapment. J Bone Joint Surg Am 59:404, 1977.
9. Gessini L, Jandolo B, Peitrangel A: The anterior tarsal tunnel syndrome: Report of four cases. J Bone Joint Surg Am 66:786, 1984.
10. Gould N, Alvarez R: Bilateral tarsal tunnel syndrome caused by varicosities. Foot Ankle 3:290–292, 1983.
11. Gould N, Trevina S: Sural nerve entrapment by avulsion fracture at the base of the fifth metatarsal bone. Foot Ankle 2:153, 1981.
12. Graham CE, Graham DM: Morton's neuroma: A microscopic evaluation. Foot Ankle 5:150, 1984.
13. Graham CE, Johnson KA, Ilstrup DM: The intermetatarsal nerve: A microscopic evaluation. Foot Ankle 2:150, 1981.
14. Gutmann L: Atypical deep peroneal neuropathy. J Neurol Neurosurg Psychiatry 33:453, 1970.
15. Hauser ED: Interdigital neuroma of the foot. Surg Gynecol Obstet 133:265, 1971.
16. Henricson AS, Westlin NE: Chronic calcaneal pain in athletes: Entrapment of the calcaneal nerve? Am J Sports Med 12:152, 1984.
17. Irani KD, Grabois M, Harvey SC: Standardized technique for diagnosis of tarsal tunnel syndrome. Am J Phys Med 61:26–31, 1982.
18. Johnson E, Ortiz P: Electrodiagnosis of tarsal tunnel syndrome. Arch Phys Med Rehabil 47:776–780, 1966.
19. Jones JR, Klenerman L: A study of the communicating branch between the medial and lateral plantar nerves. Foot Ankle 4:313, 1984.
20. Kaplan PE, Kernahan WT: Tarsal tunnel syndrome: An electrodiagnostic and surgical correlation. J Bone Joint Surg Am 63:96–99, 1981.
21. Keck C: The tarsal tunnel syndrome. J Bone Joint Surg Am 44:180–182, 1962.
22. Kenzora J, Lenet MD, Sherman M: Synovial cyst of the ankle joint as a cause of tarsal tunnel syndrome. Foot Ankle 3:181–183, 1982.
23. Kliman ME, Freiberg A: Ganglia of the foot and ankle. Foot Ankle 3:45–46, 1982.
24. Krause KH, Witt T, Ross A: The anterior tarsal tunnel syndrome. J Neurol 217:67, 1977.
25. Lam SJ: A tarsal tunnel syndrome. Lancet 2:1354–1355, 1962.
26. Lambert EH: The accessory deep peroneal nerve: A common variation in innervation of extensor digitorum brevis. Neurology 19:1169, 1969.

27. Lassman G: Morton's toe: Clinical, light and electron microscopic investigations in 133 cases. Clin Orthop 142:73, 1979.
28. Mackey D, Colbert DS, Chater EH: Musculocutaneous nerve entrapment. Irish J Med Sci 146:100, 1977.
29. Mann RA: The tarsal tunnel syndrome. Orthop Clin North Am 5: 109–115, 1974.
30. Mann RA: Diseases of the nerves of the foot. In Mann RA (ed): Surgery of the Foot, 5th ed. St. Louis, CV Mosby, 1985, pp 199–208.
31. Mann RA, Reynolds JC: Interdigital neuroma: A critical clinical analysis. Foot Ankle 3:238–243, 1983.
32. Menon J, Dorfman HD, Renbaum J, Friedler S: Tarsal tunnel syndrome secondary to neurilemoma of the medial plantar nerve. J Bone Joint Surg Am 62:301–303, 1980.
33. Mino DE, Hughes EC: Bony entrapment of the superficial peroneal nerve. Clin Orthop 185:203, 1984.
34. Oh SHJ, Kim HS, Ahmad BK: The near-nerve sensory nerve conduction in tarsal tunnel syndrome. J Neurol Neurosurg Psychiatry 48: 999–1003, 1985.
35. Pringle RM, Protheroe K, Mukherjee SK: Entrapment neuropathy of the sural nerve. J Bone Joint Surg Br 56:465, 1974.
36. Radin EL: The tarsal tunnel syndrome. Clin Orthop 181:167–170, 1983.
37. Rask MR: Medial plantar neurapraxia (jogger's foot): Report of three cases. Clin Orthop 134:193, 1978.
38. Sarrafian SK: Anatomy of the Foot and Ankle: Descriptive, Topographic, Functional. Philadelphia, JB Lippincott, 1983.
39. Srihara CR, Izzo KL: Terminal sensory branches of the superficial peroneal nerve: An entrapment syndrome. Arch Phys Med Rehabil 66:789, 1985.
40. Tranz SS: Heel pain. Clin Orthop 28:169, 1963.
41. Wilemon WK: Tarsal tunnel syndrome, a 50 year survey of the world literature and a report of two new cases. Orthop Rev 8:111–117, 1979.

Section J
Conditions of the Forefoot
Michael J. Coughlin, MD

HALLUX VALGUS

Hallux valgus is a static subluxation of the first metatarsophalangeal (MTP) joint.[14, 48] Hallux valgus is characterized by lateral or valgus deviation of the great toe and medial or varus deviation of the first metatarsal. Occasionally, pronation or rotation of the hallux occurs with severe deformity.

Hallux valgus is found almost exclusively in shoe-wearing societies,[12, 20] although it has been noted in primitive societies that do not wear shoes.[14, 48] Lam and Hodgson[40] conducted a study in China in which 30% of individuals wearing shoes were noted to have some elements of hallux valgus compared with 1.9% of individuals who did not wear shoes. In Japan before the 1970s and the introduction of high-fashion footwear, Kato and Watanabe[36] reported that the incidence of hallux valgus was relatively rare. The higher incidence of hallux valgus in women is thought to implicate constricting footwear as a major cause of hallux valgus.[20] Although shoes appear to be the major extrinsic cause of the development of hallux valgus, other intrinsic factors undoubtedly play a causative role because a small percentage of men develop hallux valgus despite the use of conservative footwear.[13] Many women do not develop hallux valgus despite wearing high-fashion footwear.

Pronation of the foot has been implicated in the development of hallux valgus.[48] Increased pressure on the medial border of the hallux leads to deformation of the medial capsular structures, which offer little resistance to pronation deformities of the foot. The repetitive activities required in sports coupled with pes planus may lead to progressive deformity. An increased first-second intermetatarsal (1–2 IM) angle often is associated with hallux valgus.[27] Mann and Coughlin[48] stated that metatarsus primus varus is often a primary deformity in juvenile or adolescent hallux valgus, whereas it is probably a secondary deformity in adult hallux valgus.

Miscellaneous causes, such as cystic degeneration of the medial capsule, Achilles tendon contracture, collagen-deficient diseases with hyperelasticity, neuromuscular disorders, poststroke syndrome, and cerebral palsy, all may predispose an individual to a hallux valgus deformity. Although such conditions are associated infrequently with athletes, the increased emphasis on health in all sectors of the population makes it necessary to consider these factors in evaluating a hallux valgus deformity.

A symptomatic hallux valgus deformity in a high-performance athlete presents a special problem for the treating physician. The increased stress manifested by running or jogging can affect the function of the foot significantly.[43] The increased force generated in the forefoot can approach 250% of body weight with running compared with 80% with walking. Lillich and Baxter[43] noted an increased range of motion of the joints of the lower extremity and an alteration in phasic activity of the muscles of the lower extremity with running activity. These factors must be considered when evaluating a hallux valgus deformity in an athlete.[44]

Anatomy

The MTP joint of the hallux is differentiated from the lesser toes by the sesamoid mechanism as well as by specific intrinsic muscles that stabilize the great toe and provide motor strength.[8] The first metatarsal head has a rounded cartilage-covered surface that articulates with the concave base of the proximal phalanx. There is significant variation in the joint surfaces of the first MTP articulation. A rounded MTP articulation (Fig. 30J–1) is more prone to the development of hallux valgus; a flattened or chevron-shaped MTP articulation is a stable configuration and is less prone to progressive development of hallux

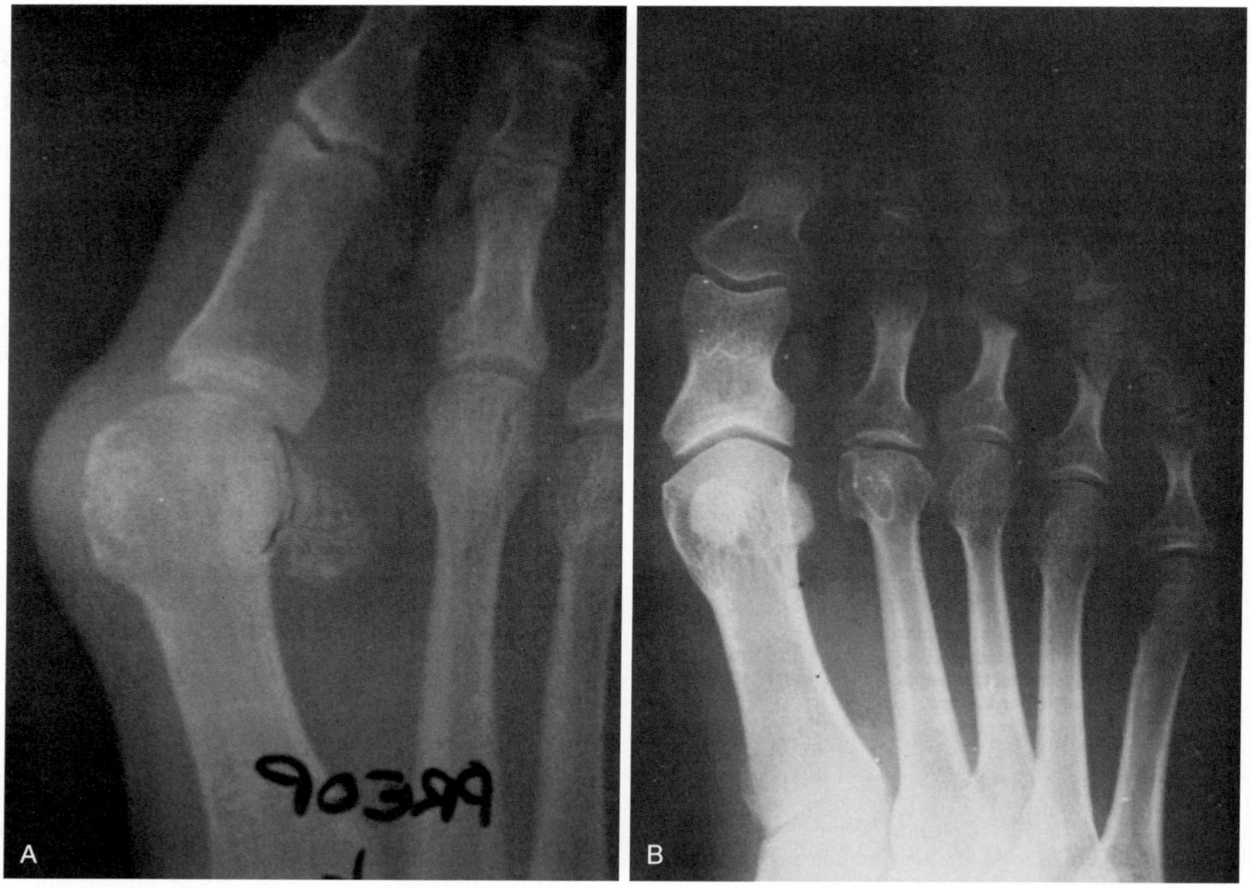

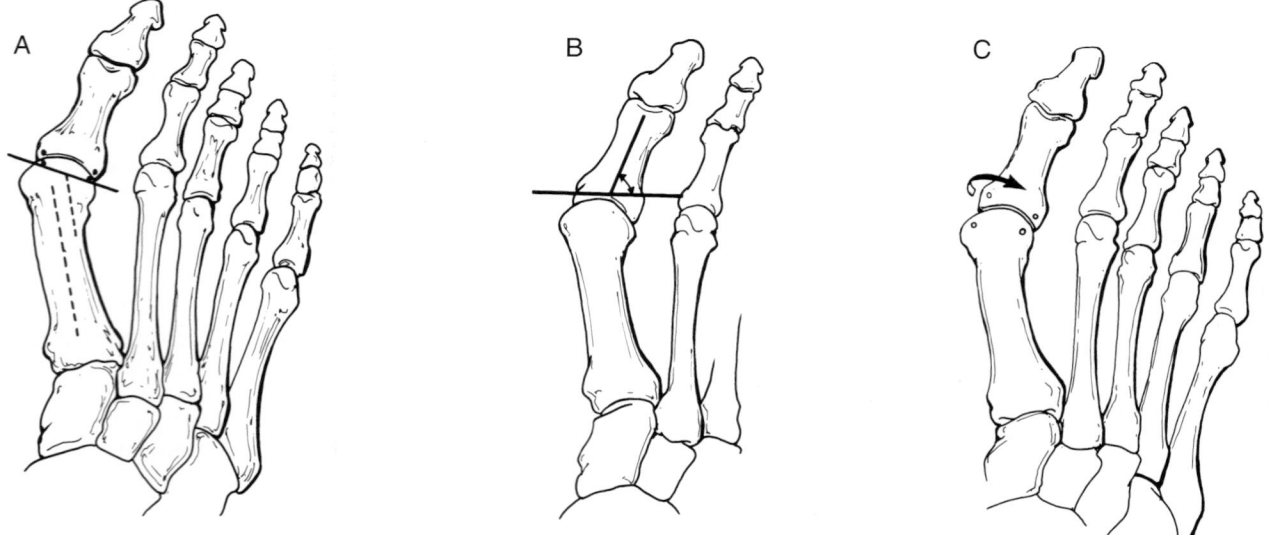

Figure 30J–1. *A,* A rounded metatarsal head is at risk for subluxation of the metatarsophalangeal joint. *B,* A flat metatarsophalangeal articulation is more resistant to subluxation. (© M. J. Coughlin. Used by permission.)

Figure 30J–2. *A,* The metatarsal articular orientation. The distal metatarsal articular angle is deviated in a lateral direction. *B,* When the articulation of the phalanx is deviated laterally (↑ proximal phalangeal articular angle), a hallux valgus interphalangeus deformity occurs. *C,* A subluxated metatarsophalangeal joint. In this noncongruent joint, the articular surface of the phalanx subluxates laterally on the metatarsal articular surface.

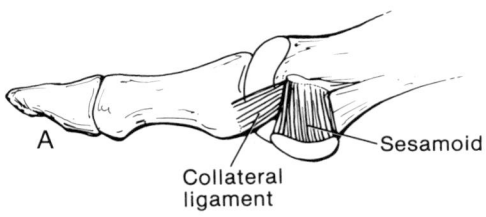

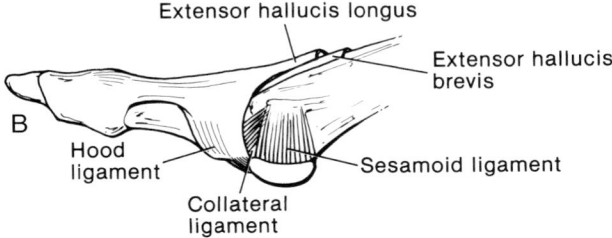

Figure 30J–3. *A,* The collateral ligaments and the sesamoid ligaments of the first metatarsophalangeal joint. *B,* The extensor hallucis longus inserts into the hood ligament.

valgus.[14, 48] The congruity of the joint surfaces describes the orientation of the articular surfaces of the proximal phalanx and the metatarsal head. The distal metatarsal articular angle (DMAA) (Fig. 30J–2*A*) describes the inclination of the distal metatarsal articular surface in relation

to the long axis of the first metatarsal.[14, 19] Although slight lateral deviation may be present, with a more oblique metatarsal orientation (10 to 15 degrees), the MTP joint may have a significant hallux valgus angle. The proximal phalangeal articular angle (Fig. 30J–2*B*) describes the inclination of the proximal phalangeal articular surface to the axis of the proximal phalanx. When a significant angulation is present here, a hallux valgus interphalangeus deformity exists.

Although the DMAA and proximal phalangeal articular angle define the orientation of the respective articular surfaces, in a congruent joint, the center of the metatarsal articular surface corresponds to the center of the articular surface of the proximal phalanx. In contrast, with an incongruent articulation, there is subluxation of the MTP joint (Fig. 30J–2*C*)—that is, the base of the proximal phalanx is deviated laterally in relation to the articular surface of the first metatarsal, resulting in an uncovering of the metatarsal head.[17] Piggott,[62] in a study of congruous and incongruous (subluxated) first MTP joints with hallux valgus, found that a congruous joint (with or without an increased DMAA) was a stable articulation. A hallux valgus deformity in this situation does not increase with time. With an incongruous or subluxated MTP joint, there is a significant risk of further progression of the deformity.

The first MTP joint is stabilized on the plantar-medial and plantar-lateral aspects by the collateral ligament and sesamoidal ligaments (Fig. 30J–3*A*). The fan-shaped collat-

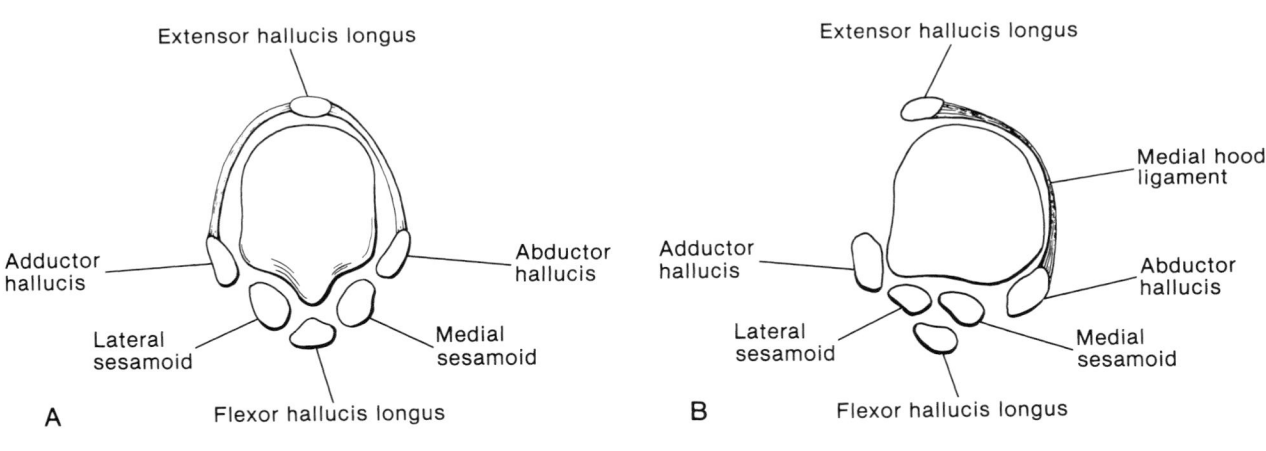

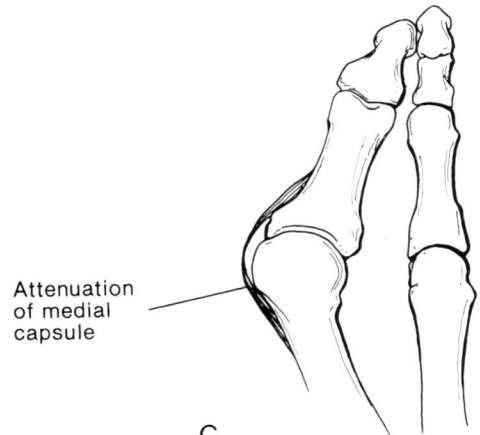

Figure 30J–4. *A–C,* With subluxation of the metatarsophalangeal joint, the dorsal capsule and the hood ligament become attenuated.

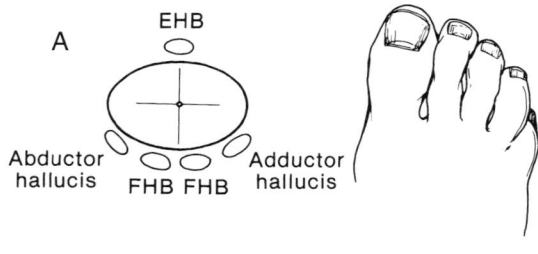

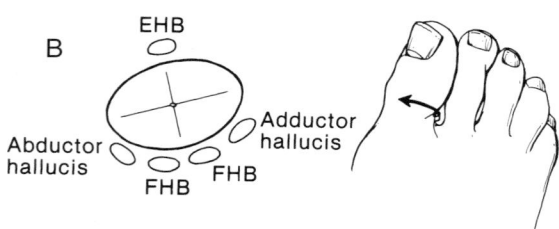

Figure 30J–9. *A,* Schematic representation of the intrinsic muscles surrounding the first metatarsal head. Normal articulation. *B,* With valgus deviation, the intrinsic muscles rotate. The abductor hallucis assumes a more plantar position, and the adductor hallucis assumes a more lateral orientation. EHB, extensor hallucis brevis; FHB, flexor hallucis brevis.

brevis, and the adductor hallucis) rotates (Fig. 30J–9) in relation to the metatarsal head, exposing the thin dorsal medial capsule to further deforming forces.

On the plantar aspect, the sesamoid complex displaces in relation to the first metatarsal head. The sesamoid mechanism, owing to the adductor hallucis insertion, retains its relationship to the lesser metatarsals, whereas the first metatarsal literally slides off the sesamoid complex. Although the term *sesamoid subluxation* is used to describe this progressive deformity, it is the first metatarsal that is displaced in relation to the sesamoids and lesser metatarsals. As this displacement occurs, the intersesamoidal ridge is smoothed out gradually (Fig. 30J–10) until it affords no resistance to further deformity. In severe hallux valgus deformities, as the first metatarsal displaces medially off the sesamoid mechanism, the extensor hallucis longus displaces into the first IM space. Dynamic contraction of the

Sesamoid Subluxation

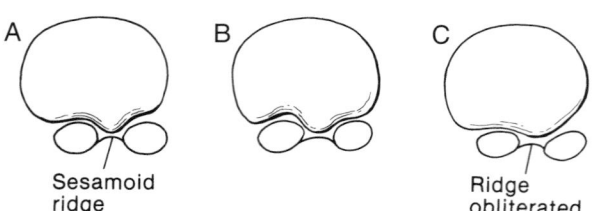

Figure 30J–10. *A,* Schematic representation shows sesamoid view with normal crista. *B,* Schematic representation of a patient with hallux valgus shows moderate obliteration of crista. *C,* Complete obliteration of crista with sesamoid subluxation.

extensor hallucis longus not only extends the toe but also adducts the toe. The abductor hallucis, having assumed a more plantar position in relation to the first metatarsal, loses its splinting effect on the first metatarsal head. The lateral sesamoid may come to lie on the lateral aspect of the first metatarsal head and on occasion lies vertically above the medial sesamoid. The medial sesamoid may articulate with the lateral facet of the first metatarsal.

The medial migration of the first metatarsal can be quantitated by measurement of the 1–2 IM angle (Fig. 30J–11), an angle subtended by lines drawn along the longitudinal axis of the first and second metatarsals. The lateral migration of the great toe can be quantitated by the measurements of the hallux valgus angle, the angle subtended by lines drawn along the longitudinal axis of the great toe and the first metatarsal.

Running places higher demands on the foot than walking.[3, 11, 43] Various athletic activities make varying demands on the foot and ankle. A sprinter may require extreme range of motion in dorsiflexion and plantar flexion at the first MTP joint, in contrast to a middle-distance or long-distance runner, in whom a large range of motion is important but not nearly so crucial.[43] Analysis of the particular sports avocation, training techniques, strength requirements of the first ray, and range of motion needed by the first MTP joint plays an important role in the assessment of the functional biomechanics of the forefoot. This careful evaluation helps the practitioner to develop a plan for the symptomatic athlete.

Although much attention has been paid to the bunion or medial eminence, it is most often the increased 1–2 IM

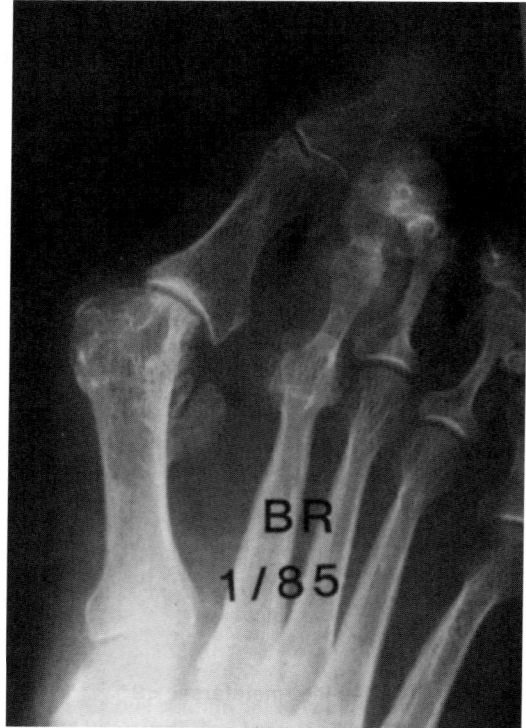

Figure 30J–11. Radiograph shows severe hallux valgus deformity with increased 1–2 intermetatarsal angle and increased hallux valgus deformity. (© M. J. Coughlin. Used by permission.)

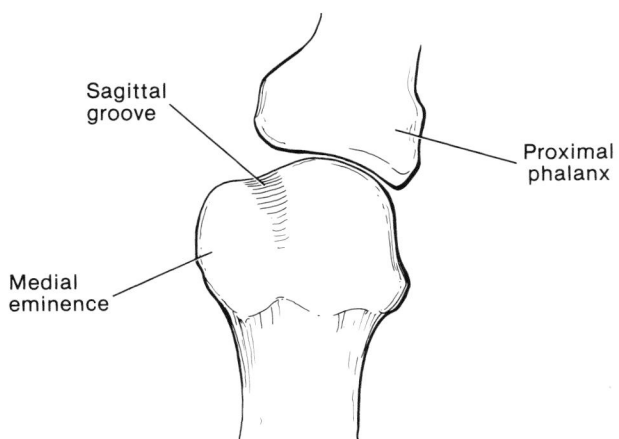

Figure 30J–12. The sagittal sulcus is created at the medial margin of the articular surface and is an osteophyte delineating the border of the medial eminence.

eminence. Although this anatomic landmark delineates the border of the metatarsal articular surface, its location is variable and depends on the severity of the deformity. Sometimes the sagittal sulcus is located in the center of the metatarsal head. It is important not to use the sagittal sulcus as a landmark for the medial eminence resection because in severe deformities an excessive amount of metatarsal head is removed. In mild and moderate cases of hallux valgus, attention must be directed to the location of the sagittal sulcus on the anteroposterior (AP) radiograph to determine whether resection of the medial eminence should be performed through the center of the sagittal sulcus or medial or lateral to the center of the sagittal sulcus.

Clinical Evaluation

The major subjective complaint of a patient with hallux valgus is pain over the medial eminence (Fig. 30J–13A). Typically, pain may be relieved by removing the shoes or exchanging a rigid, nonforgiving shoe for a soft, flexible one that yields to the bony prominence. At times, especially with repetitive athletic activities such as running, blistering of the skin or development of an inflamed bursa overlying the medial eminence may occur. Pressure from a shoe may cause compression of the dorsal medial sensory nerve to

angle coupled with lateral deviation of the great toe that creates a prominent and painful medial border of the first metatarsal head. At times, the medial eminence may become hypertrophied and symptomatic; however, this is uncommon. With progressive subluxation, a groove or sagittal sulcus (Fig. 30J–12) develops on the first metatarsal head, delineating the articular surface from the medial

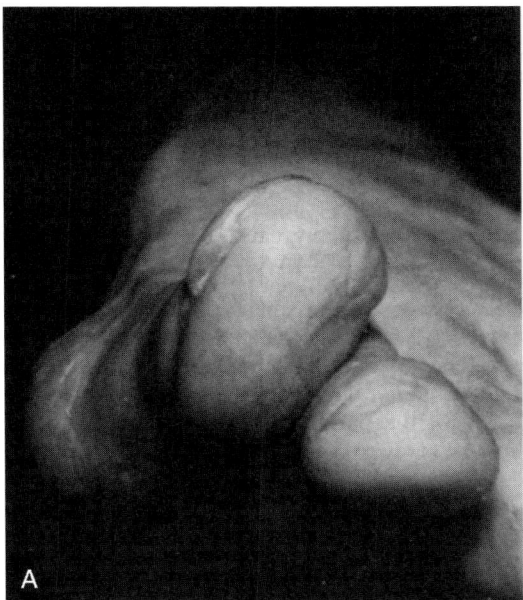

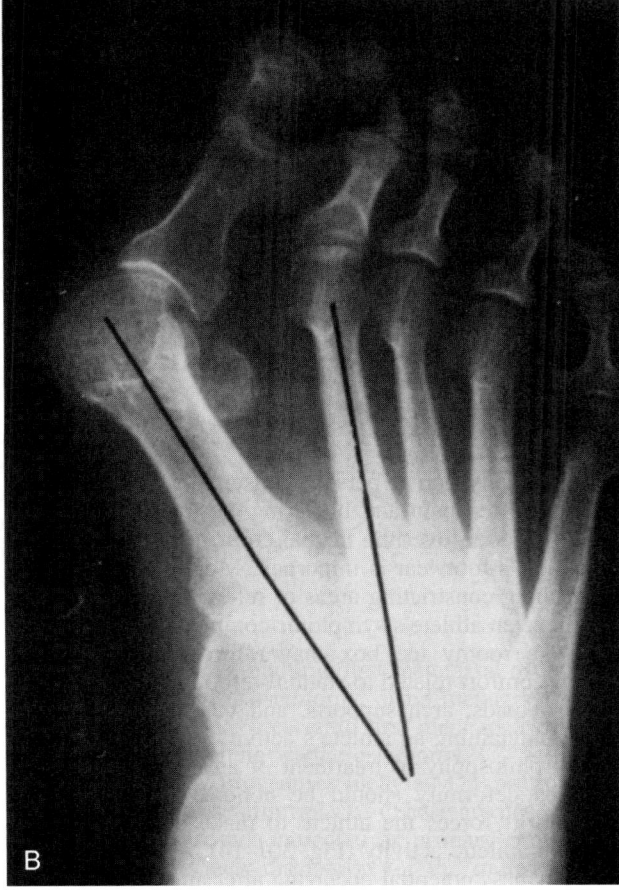

Figure 30J–13. *A,* The prominent medial eminence or bunion often is the most common complaint of the patient. *B,* Valgus deviation of the toe and medial deviation of the first metatarsal create a widened foot.

Akin Procedure

The Akin procedure[1, 70, 72, 77] involves a medial eminence resection and medial capsular reefing combined with a medial closing wedge osteotomy of the proximal phalanx. Although no correction of an increased 1–2 IM angle can be achieved with this procedure, indications for its use include hallux valgus interphalangeus, mild hallux valgus without significant metatarsus primus varus, and recurrent hallux valgus of a mild nature. In the presence of a congruent MTP joint, a proximal phalangeal osteotomy can be combined with a metatarsal osteotomy without significantly altering MTP joint congruity.

Technique. A medial longitudinal incision is made over the medial eminence, beginning at the interphalangeal joint and extending proximally. Care is taken to protect the dorsal and plantar digital nerves within the skin flap. An L-shaped capsular flap (Fig. 30J–15A) is developed by carefully dissecting the capsule off the medial eminence. The dorsal and proximal incisions are made in the capsule and are repaired later. The medial eminence is resected using an oscillating saw and starting at a point in the middle of or slightly toward the medial aspect of the sagittal sulcus. If any portion of the sagittal sulcus remains, it is resected with a rongeur.

The phalangeal osteotomy (Fig. 30J–15B) is made in the proximal metaphyseal region. Care is taken to protect the MTP capsular flap. A subperiosteal dissection is used to reflect tissue in the metaphyseal region on the dorsal, medial, and plantar surfaces. An oscillating saw is used to cut and remove a small, medially based wedge of bone. The lateral cortex is scored with the saw and cracked as the osteotomy site is closed. The osteotomy is stabilized with two 0.062 Kirschner wires placed in an oblique fashion to avoid the interphalangeal and MTP joints if possible.

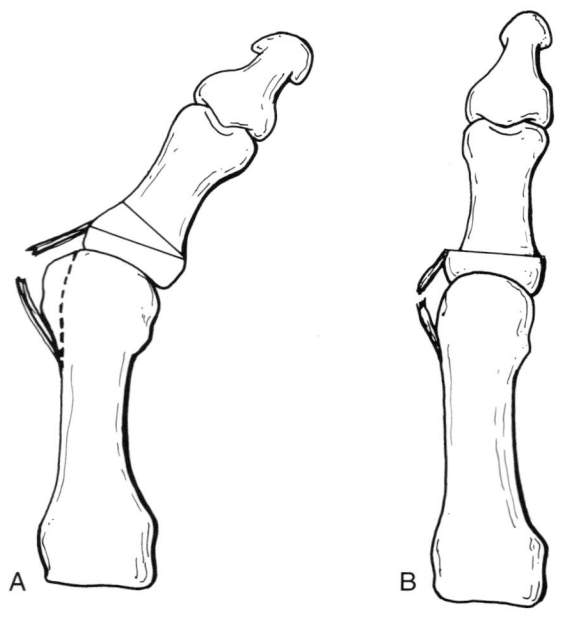

Akin procedure

Figure 30J–15. *A,* Location of osteotomy of proximal phalanx. *B,* After closure of osteotomy site.

Pronation of the toe may be corrected by derotating the toe at the osteotomy site. The medial capsule is repaired to the surrounding MTP capsule and periosteum. When insufficient tissue is present, a drill hole can be placed in the medial metaphyseal cortex, and the capsule flap can be sutured to the bone.

Postoperative Care. A soft compression dressing is applied at surgery, then changed weekly. The patient ambulates in a wooden-soled postoperative shoe. Kirschner wires are removed 4 to 6 weeks postoperatively. Range-of-motion exercises may be started 6 weeks after surgery. Aggressive walking activity can be started 6 weeks after surgery if the patient is progressing well. At 2 months after surgery, an athlete can start jogging in a shoe with a roomy toe box. A toe spacer is placed between the first and second toes to help maintain the correction. At 3 months, an athlete can progress to running if no problems are encountered.

Results and Complications. A phalangeal osteotomy as described by Akin[1] produces slight, if any, correction of the 1–2 IM angle.[24, 63] Plattner and Van Manen[63] reported on a series of 22 patients who had undergone an Akin procedure. An initial correction of the hallux valgus angle of 13 degrees decreased to a correction of only 6 degrees at an average 4.5 years of follow-up. Seelenfreund and Fried[70] reported a 16% recurrence (8 of 50 patients), and Goldberg and colleagues[24] reported a 21% recurrence (75 of 351 patients) (Fig. 30J–16).

Internal fixation to stabilize the osteotomy site is preferred. Nonunion of the phalangeal osteotomy is uncommon.[70] Although Colloff and Weitz[7] used a lateral MTP capsular release, this technique may devascularize the proximal phalangeal fragment and is not recommended. Other complications reported after the Akin procedure include a poor cosmetic appearance[24] and a high level of subjective postoperative patient dissatisfaction.[24, 63] Goldberg and associates[24] concluded that a phalangeal osteotomy as an isolated procedure in treatment of a hallux valgus deformity "does not have a sound biomechanical basis and should not be performed as an isolated procedure." Plattner and Van Manen[63] recommended this procedure for hallux valgus interphalangeus and not for a subluxated hallux valgus deformity (Fig. 30J–17). Mitchell and Baxter[59] and Colloff and Weitz[7] suggested that a phalangeal osteotomy may be used in combination with a proximal repair to gain increased correction.

Chevron Procedure

The chevron osteotomy as described by Johnson and colleagues[33] and others[2, 8] is indicated for a mild-to-moderate hallux valgus deformity with a hallux valgus angle of less than 30 degrees, an IM angle of less than 15 degrees, and no pronation of the hallux. Because the chevron osteotomy achieves an extra-articular correction, it may be used to correct a congruous deformity as well as a noncongruous or subluxated MTP joint.

Technique. A longitudinal medial incision is made over the medial eminence, progressing from the midportion of the proximal phalanx and extending proximally for about 5 cm. The incision is made directly down to the capsule. Care is taken to protect the dorsal and plantar cutaneous nerves in the skin flaps. The medial eminence is exposed

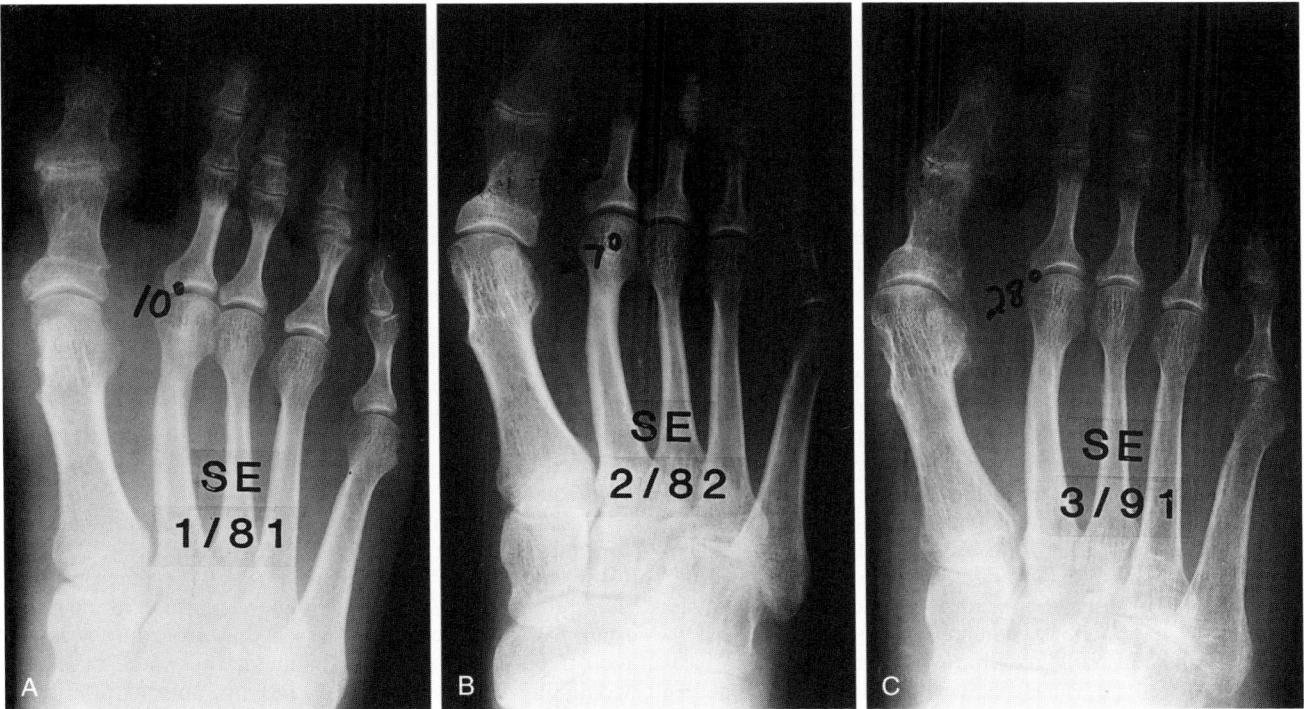

Figure 30J–16. *A*, Immediate postoperative radiograph shows correction with an Akin phalangeal osteotomy and medial eminence resection. *B*, One year after surgery, a recurrent deformity has developed with an increase in the hallux valgus angle. *C*, Ten years after surgery, further progression of deformity is noted.

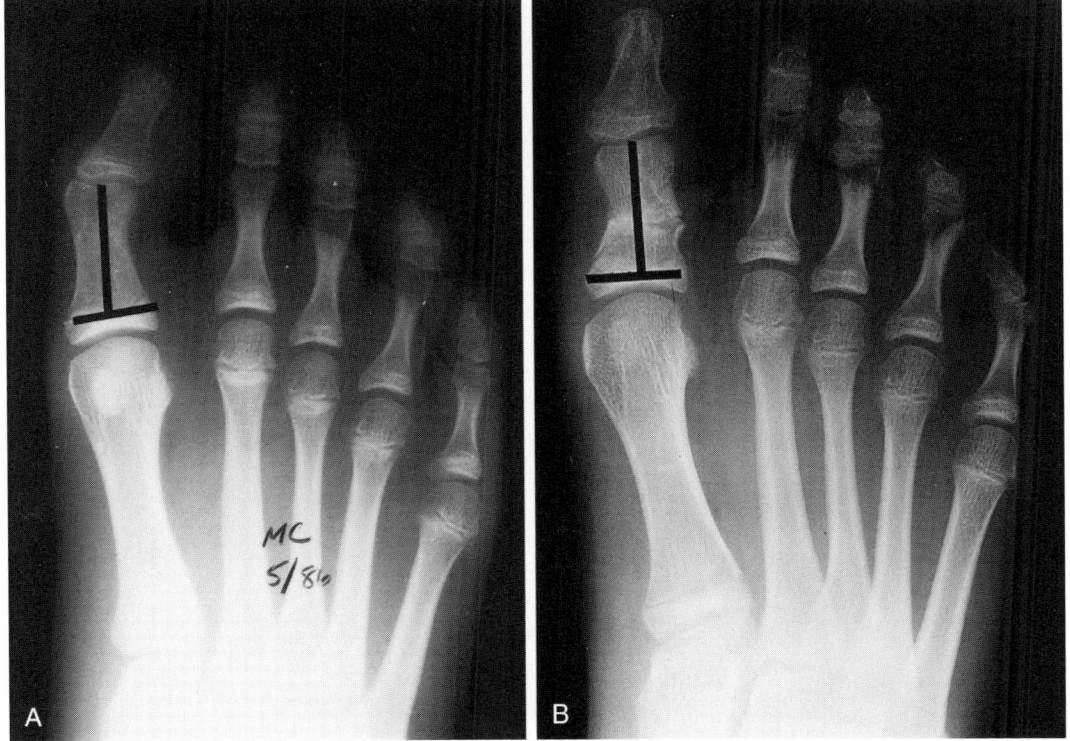

Figure 30J–17. *A*, Preoperative radiograph shows hallux valgus interphalangeus deformity. *B*, After Akin phalangeal osteotomy, adequate alignment is maintained.

by making an L-shaped, distally based capsular flap. The medial eminence is removed with an oscillating saw at a point just medial to or within the sagittal sulcus. Any ridge of bone that remains after the medial eminence is removed is smoothed with a rongeur. A horizontal drill hole is made in the center of the metatarsal head to mark the apex of the osteotomy. Then an oscillating saw with a fine blade is used to make a horizontal osteotomy (Fig. 30J–18) in a medial-to-lateral direction at an angle of approximately 60 degrees. The proximally based osteotomy is performed within the metaphyseal region, which provides a stable osteotomy site and a large surface for bony contact, which allows rapid healing.

Care is taken not to dissect the lateral aspect of the MTP joint because this may place a patient at greater risk for avascular necrosis of the first metatarsal head (Fig. 30J–19). The metatarsal head is displaced laterally (Fig. 30J–20) approximately one third the metaphyseal width, and the osteotomy site is impacted on itself, then fixed with a 0.062 Kirschner wire. Although the osteotomy is stable in a dorsal plantar direction, internal fixation decreases the possibility of medial displacement and loss of correction. The remaining metaphyseal flare is resected.

The medial capsule is repaired with interrupted absorbable sutures. If there is insufficient proximal capsule with which to secure the proximal capsular flap, small drill holes can be placed in the medial metaphyseal cortex to secure the proximal capsular flap.

Neither the lateral capsule nor the conjoined tendon is released. Although release of these structures may allow a greater correction,[2] Mann[45] and others[31, 57] have reported several cases of avascular necrosis of the metatarsal head after a chevron procedure. Although several authors have not found an increased incidence of avascular necrosis after a lateral MTP release,[2, 33, 39, 64] an extensive lateral release may place a patient at greater risk for avascular necrosis of the metatarsal head.[28, 71]

Postoperative Care. A soft compression dressing is applied at surgery and is changed weekly. The Kirschner wire is removed 3 weeks or more after surgery. Passive range-of-motion exercises may be started 3 to 4 weeks postoperatively. The patient ambulates initially in a wooden-soled postoperative shoe and later in an open-toed sandal.

Some authors have recommended the chevron procedure for mild-to-moderate hallux valgus deformities,[2, 8, 33] and Lillich and Baxter[43] reported the use of the chevron procedure in two elite female middle-distance and marathon runners. The rationale for using this procedure was that toe-off power could be maintained, and range of motion would not be altered significantly in this extra-articular type of repair. Lillich and Baxter[43] further stated that the

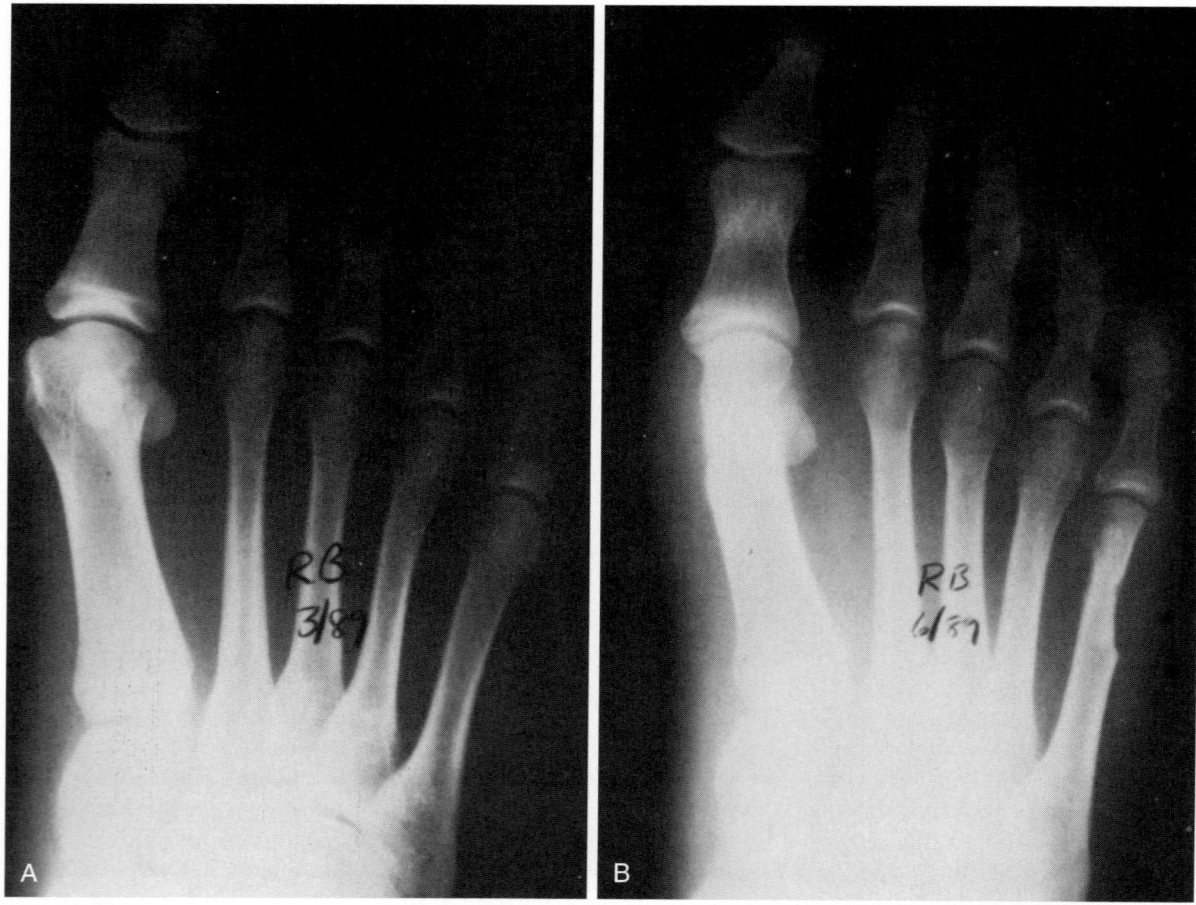

Figure 30J–18. *A* and *B*, Preoperative and postoperative radiographs of chevron osteotomy. (© M. J. Coughlin. Used by permission.)

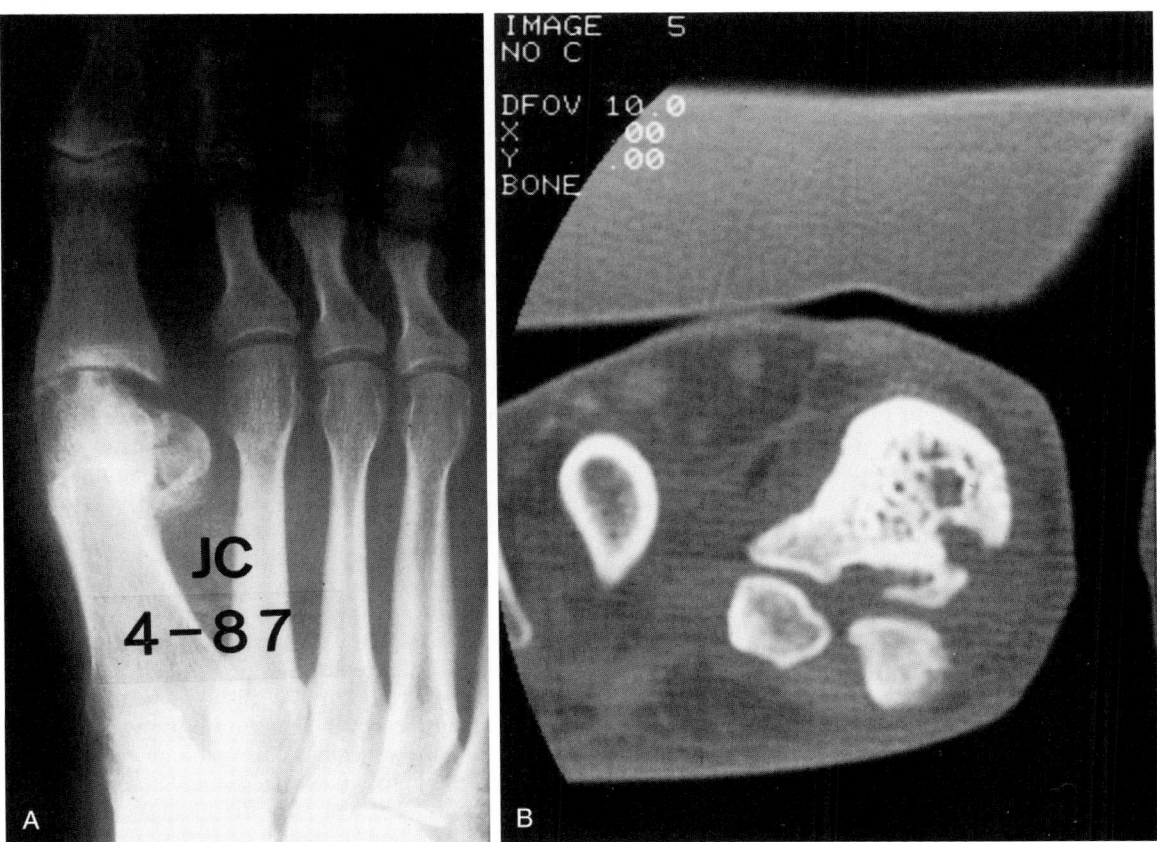

Figure 30J–19. *A,* Postoperative radiograph shows avascular necrosis after a distal metatarsal osteotomy. *B,* Computed tomography scan shows cystic degeneration consistent with avascular necrosis of the first metatarsal head.

stable nature of this osteotomy would make displacement unlikely, and the possibility of a transfer keratotic lesion is avoided. Lillich and Baxter[43] stressed the importance of a precise operative technique with a minimum of joint dissection. They allowed running 7 weeks postoperatively in a loose-fitting shoe with a toe spacer placed between the hallux and second toe. Running speed and duration were increased gradually, with a return to full activity achieved at 12 weeks after surgery.

Results and Complications. Johnson and colleagues[33] and others[2, 28, 29, 41, 42, 64] noted a high level of excellent results with this procedure, with a reported average correction of the hallux valgus angle of 12 to 13 degrees and an average correction of the 1–2 IM angle of 4 to 5 degrees. Because of the limited correction of the hallux valgus angle offered by the chevron procedure, it should be reserved for mild and low moderate deformities. Extension of the indications for this procedure to more severe deformities appears to increase the risk of recurrence, patient dissatisfaction, and complications. Meier and Kenzora[57] reported on 50 patients (72 feet) after a distal metatarsal osteotomy and noted a 74% satisfaction rate when the preoperative 1–2 IM angle was greater than 12 degrees and a 94% satisfaction rate when the 1–2 IM angle was 12 degrees or less.

The most frequent complication associated with the chevron procedure is undercorrection or recurrence, which varies from 10% to 14%.[2, 29, 42] Recurrent hallux valgus may develop when the indications for the chevron procedure are expanded to more severe deformities. Loss of correction can occur because of inadequate fixation or slippage at the osteotomy site. Shortening may occur as a result of excessive bone loss.[2, 29, 45, 57] Klosok and coworkers[39] reported postoperative transfer lesions in 12% of cases.

Distal Soft Tissue Repair

The modified McBride procedure has been used to correct mild-to-moderate hallux valgus deformities.[54, 55] Later, DuVries[22] used a technique that advocated (1) lateral capsular release, (2) adductor tendon release, (3) lateral sesamoid excision, (4) medial eminence resection, and (5) medial capsular reefing to achieve a bunion repair. Continuing modification of this procedure makes the use of the eponym *McBride* inappropriate. The description of this technique as a distal soft tissue repair is meant to clarify the fact that this is an intra-articular repair that does not use an osteotomy to achieve realignment. Although an osteotomy may be combined with this procedure to achieve an adequate repair, a distal soft tissue repair, when indicated, may be used by itself to correct a mild-to-moderate deformity.

Technique. A dorsal longitudinal incision is made in the first intermetatarsal web space approximately 2 to 3 cm in length. A Weitlaner retractor is used to spread the first and second metatarsals and to expose the tendon of the adductor hallucis. This tendon is dissected free from the

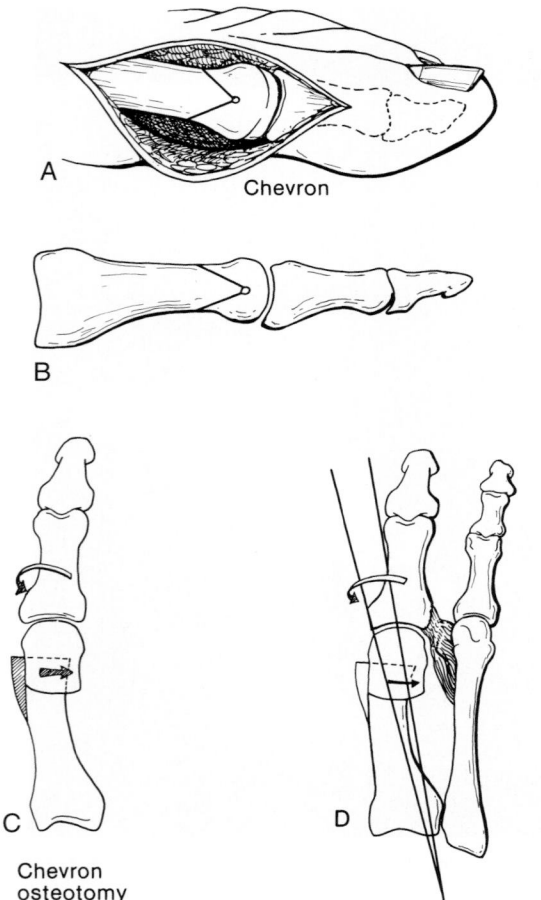

Figure 30J–20. *A,* Proposed chevron osteotomy of first metatarsal. *B,* A V-shaped osteotomy at approximately a 60-degree angle based proximally is centered in the metaphyseal region. *C* and *D,* The osteotomy is displaced laterally, and the remaining medial eminence is resected.

lateral sesamoid (Fig. 30J–21). The distal tendon insertion is left attached to the base of the proximal phalanx, and the tendon is severed about 1.5 cm proximal to this insertion at the musculotendinous junction. The distal stump of tendon is tagged with a 2–0 absorbable suture, which is used later to suture the tendon stump to the lateral metatarsal capsule. The remaining adductor hallucis muscle is allowed to retract. The lateral sesamoid is freed of any contracted tissue, and the transverse intermetatarsal ligament is incised. Care must be taken not to injure the common digital nerve directly beneath this ligament. The lateral sesamoid rarely is removed except in cases of severe deformity. Mann and Coughlin[49, 50] cautioned against performing a fibular sesamoid excision except in cases of severe deformity or severe degenerative arthritis of the sesamoid-metatarsal joint or in patients with severe sesamoid subluxation that prevented reduction of the MTP joint to reduce the risk of developing a postoperative hallux varus deformity (Fig. 30J–22).

The lateral capsule is perforated with several puncture incisions; then, with the toe angled into varus, the remaining capsule is torn. It is intended that by tearing the capsule, some scar tissue will form postoperatively, allowing the lateral capsular tissue to stabilize the lateral

aspect of the MTP joint. The stump of conjoined tendon is used later to reinforce the lateral capsule. A medial longitudinal incision directly over the medial eminence is made. The dissection is carried down to the capsule. The dorsal and plantar digital nerves are protected within the dorsal and plantar flaps. The capsule is released in an L-shaped fashion on the dorsal and proximal surfaces, leaving the distal and plantar capsular attachments in place (Fig. 30J–21*B*).

The medial eminence is resected using an oscillating saw (Fig. 30J–21*C*). Resection is performed in line with the medial diaphyseal cortex of the first metatarsal shaft. The cut is made without regard to the location of the sagittal sulcus, although in patients with a mild-to-moderate deformity, the osteotomy often is just medial to the sagittal sulcus. The area is rounded off with a rongeur if any part of the sagittal sulcus remains. (The sagittal sulcus is not used to define the medial eminence osteotomy because in patients with more severe deformities the sulcus may be oriented more laterally, and if this is used as a landmark, excessive resection of the medial eminence would result.)

When adequate reduction of the 1–2 IM angle deformity cannot be achieved with this distal realignment, a proximal first metatarsal osteotomy is performed. If adequate realignment is achieved with a distal soft tissue release and realignment, however, attention is directed to the first interspace incision. Three interrupted absorbable 2–0 sutures are used to approximate the first and second MTP capsules. These sutures are tied after the medial capsule plication is carried out. When the sutures are tied, the transverse metatarsal arch is compressed to approximate the first and second metatarsal heads. With the hallux held in appropriate alignment (varus-valgus and neutral rotation), several interrupted 2–0 absorbable sutures are used to reef the medial capsule (Fig. 30J–21*D* and *E*). Usually several sutures can be placed to repair the proximal and dorsal capsule. Occasionally, it is difficult to achieve an adequate repair of the dorsal medial capsule owing to a paucity of proximal capsular tissue. If this occurs, a small drill hole is placed in the medial metaphysis of the first metatarsal, and the dorsal medial capsule is secured with a suture placed through this drill hole.

Postoperative Care. A soft gauze and tape postoperative compression dressing (Fig. 30J–21*F*) is used to hold the toe in proper alignment. The dressing is changed on a weekly basis for 8 weeks. The patient is allowed to ambulate in a wooden-soled postoperative shoe. At 6 weeks after surgery, a stiff-soled sandal may be used. At this point, the patient may begin manipulating the toe in a dorsal-plantar flexion plane. Dressings are discontinued 8 weeks after surgery, and aggressive walking can be initiated at this time. A toe spacer is placed between the toes to protect the alignment of the great toe. Jogging may be initiated at 10 weeks after surgery if the postoperative course is uneventful, and running is introduced at 13 to 15 weeks postoperatively. An intra-articular repair requires a more lengthy recovery time than with previously described procedures. Premature athletic activity may impair the postoperative correction.

Results and Complications. Although Silver[73] recommended resection of the medial eminence and a lateral soft tissue release, he did not report on the results of this

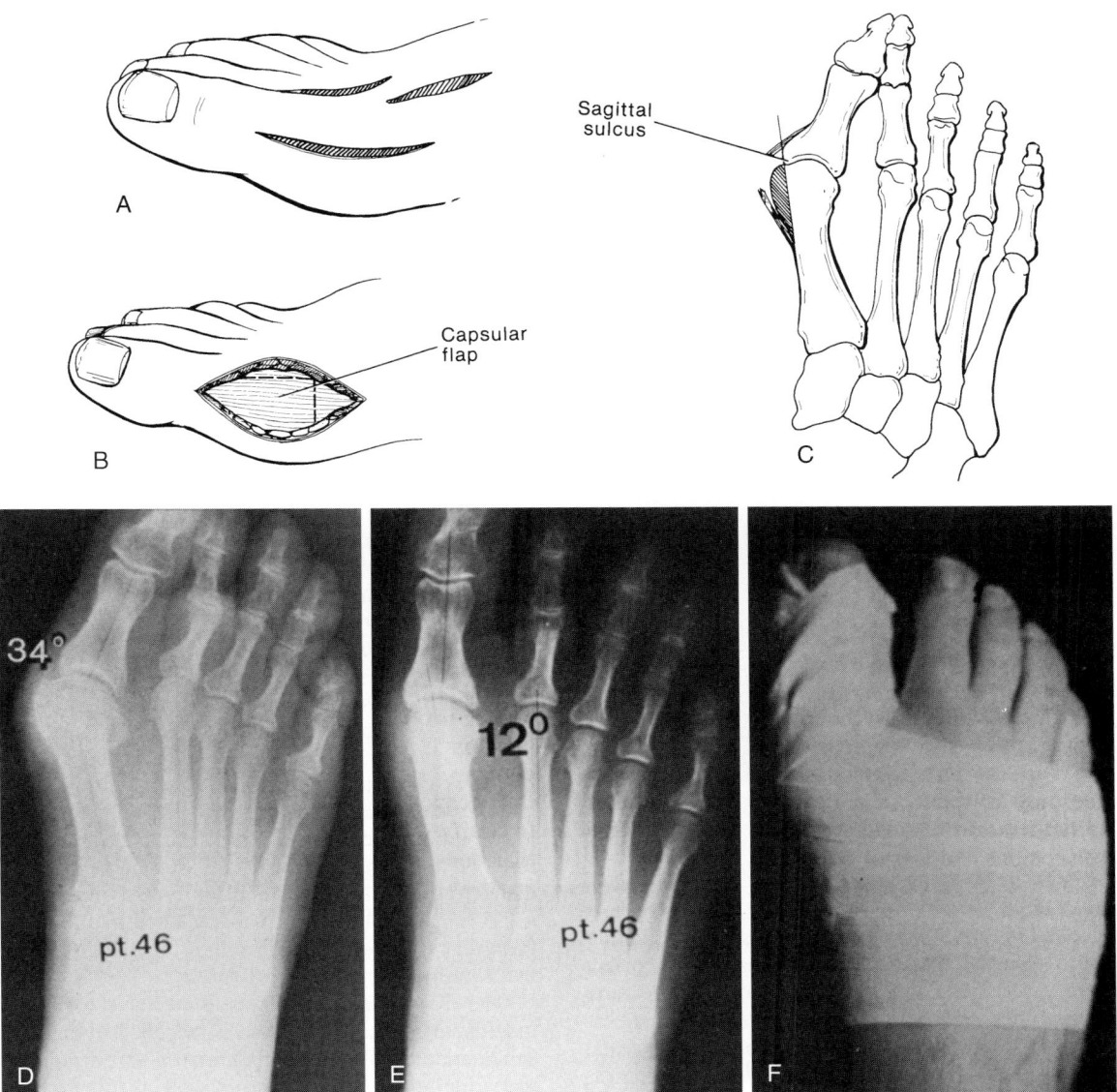

Figure 30J–21. *A,* Three incisions are used for surgical correction. *B,* A distally based, L-shaped capsular flap is used to expose the medial eminence. *C,* The medial eminence is resected along a line parallel with the long axis of the medial cortex of the first metatarsal. *D,* Preoperative radiograph. *E,* Postoperative radiograph after distal soft tissue realignment. *F,* A gauze and tape postoperative dressing is used. (*D–F,* © M. J. Coughlin. Used by permission.)

procedure. Later, Kitaoka and associates,[38] in reporting on the Mayo Clinic experience after simple bunionectomy and medial capsulorrhaphy with or without lateral capsulotomy, noted at an average 4.8-year follow-up that the hallux valgus angle had increased 4.8 degrees from the preoperative deformity, and the 1–2 IM angle had increased almost 2 degrees. Of the feet that had undergone a bunionectomy without a lateral capsulotomy, 29% underwent reoperation at 5 years. A failure rate of 24% for the entire group was reported.

Bonney and Macnab[4] reported generally poor results after simple exostectomy. Of their patients, 37% underwent additional treatment, and the authors concluded that the only indication for a simple bunionectomy is a large medial eminence that is the sole cause of symptoms in a patient whose general medical condition contraindicates an exten-

sive procedure and to whom the postoperative appearance is unimportant.

Meyer and colleagues[58] reported the results of the modified McBride procedure in 21 women joggers who had a symptomatic hallux valgus deformity. These authors reported a successful correction if the preoperative 1–2 IM angle was less than or equal to 14 degrees and the hallux valgus angle was less than 50 degrees. They reported an average overall hallux valgus correction of 20 degrees and an average correction of the 1–2 IM angle of 4.2 degrees. Of 21 patients, 19 (90%) reported significant improvement postoperatively. Two thirds of the patients resumed jogging 3 months after surgery, and 19 of 21 patients were involved in athletic activities 6 months after surgery.

Mann and Coughlin[50] in a review of the results of 100 McBride procedures reported an average correction of the

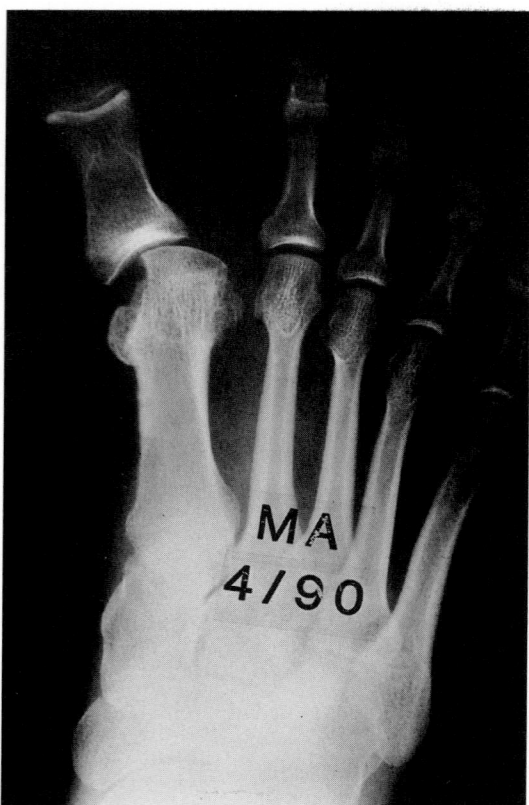

Figure 30J–22. Hallux valgus deformity (overcorrection) caused by excessive medial eminence resection.

hallux valgus angle of 14.8 degrees and an average correction of the 1–2 IM angle of 5.2 degrees. Mann and Coughlin[50] recommended that if more than 20 degrees of correction of the hallux valgus angle was indicated, the procedure should be combined with a first metatarsal osteotomy.

One of the most significant complications of the distal soft tissue procedure is a postoperative hallux varus deformity. Mann and Coughlin[50] reported hallux varus to occur in 11% of patients, although a severe deformity occurred in only 4%. Mann and Pfeffinger[52] reported a higher incidence of hallux varus deformities after attempted correction of severe deformities.

The limitations of a McBride or distal soft tissue reconstruction are substantial. Mann and Pfeffinger[52] observed that a severe hallux valgus deformity was not corrected adequately by a distal soft tissue reconstruction in half of the cases. The indication for this procedure is a subluxated hallux valgus deformity of less than 30 degrees with a 1–2 IM angle of less than 15 degrees.

Proximal First Metatarsal Osteotomy

A proximal metatarsal osteotomy that corrects an *increased* 1–2 IM angle can be combined with a distal soft tissue reconstruction that realigns the first MTP joint. As a rule, an osteotomy is indicated if the 1–2 IM angle is greater than or equal to 15 degrees, if the hallux valgus angle is greater than or equal to 30 to 40 degrees, or if after a distal soft tissue realignment an adequate correction

of the 1–2 IM angle cannot be obtained. Sometimes a more severe hallux valgus deformity (>40 degrees) with an increased 1–2 IM angle can be realigned adequately without an osteotomy; sometimes a moderate hallux valgus deformity (20 to 40 degrees) cannot be corrected adequately without a first metatarsal osteotomy. Although an opening or closing wedge osteotomy can be performed, significant lengthening or shortening of the first ray usually is not desirable. For this reason, a proximal crescentic osteotomy routinely is used.[16, 46, 48] This osteotomy is performed in the proximal first metatarsal metaphysis, an area that provides a broad, stable cancellous surface that allows fairly rapid healing.

Technique. A dorsal 3-cm longitudinal incision (Fig. 30J–23A) is made over the proximal first metatarsal. The dissection is carried down on the medial aspect of the extensor hallucis longus tendon, and a subperiosteal dissection is used to expose the proximal metatarsal shaft. The metatarsocuneiform joint is identified, and a crescentic osteotomy is performed using a curved saw blade (Zimmer, Inc, Warsaw, Ind, catalog no. 5053–176; Stryker, Kalamazoo, Mich, catalog no. 2296-31-4167 or 277-31-41651 Synthes 206 screw) (Fig. 30J–23B). The osteotomy, with the concave aspect based proximally, is performed approximately 1 cm distal to the metatarsocuneiform joint. The osteotomy is oriented in a dorsal plantar direction at about a 120-degree angle with the first metatarsal shaft. Occasionally, an osteotome is used to complete the cut. The distal fragment is rotated medially approximately 2 mm to ensure an adequate decrease in the 1–2 IM angle; however, care must be taken not to overcorrect the osteotomy. The osteotomy is fixed initially with a 0.062 Kirschner wire. The distal fragment is overdrilled with a 3.5-mm drill bit, then a 2.5-mm drill bit is used to create a fixation hole in the proximal fragment. The proximal drill hole is tapped and fixed with a small fragment screw.

The Kirschner wire is bent at the level of the first metatarsal shaft, and closure is begun, leaving the fixation subcutaneous. The dual fixation of screw and Kirschner wire provides compression as well as rotational stability. Intraoperative radiographs are taken to evaluate the correction of the 1–2 IM angle and the internal fixation. Often on the AP radiograph (Fig. 30J–23C to E), it appears that the fixation crosses the metatarsocuneiform joint, although this is unusual. Internal fixation can be removed easily under local anesthesia 6 weeks after surgery. The osteotomy is combined with a distal soft tissue realignment as previously described.

Postoperative Care. A soft gauze and tape compression dressing is used routinely for 8 weeks postoperatively. The patient is allowed to ambulate initially in a postoperative wooden-soled shoe; later at 6 weeks, the patient may use an open-toed, stiff-soled sandal. The patient can begin aggressive walking 7 to 8 weeks after surgery. Manipulation of the hallux in a dorsal-plantar plane should be initiated even with dressings in place to minimize restricted range of motion postoperatively. After discontinuance of the dressings, more aggressive manipulation is undertaken. Physical therapy may be used to increase motion and to improve the recovery rate. Jogging can be initiated 3 months postoperatively using a toe spacer between the first and second toes and wearing a roomy-toed running shoe.

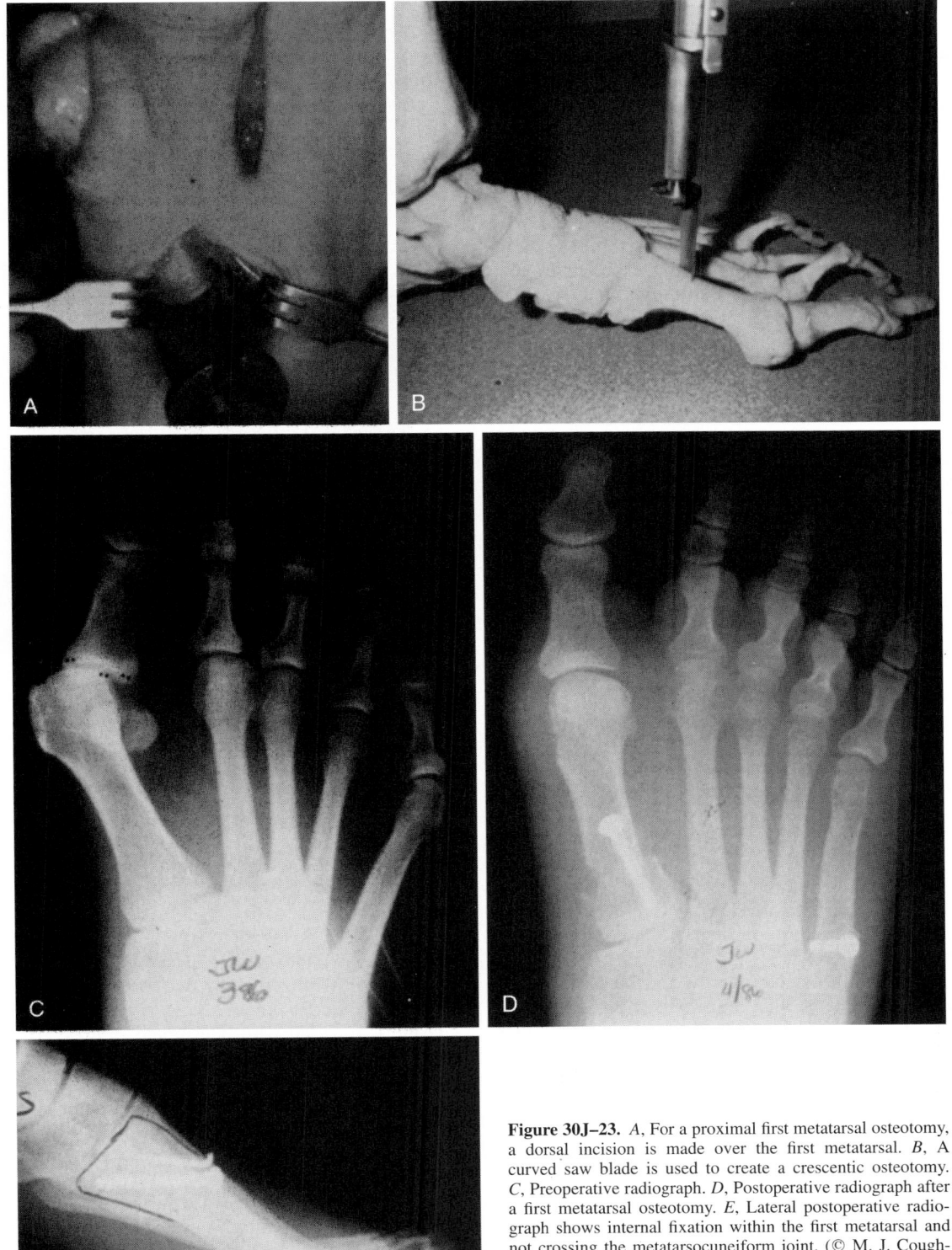

Figure 30J–23. *A*, For a proximal first metatarsal osteotomy, a dorsal incision is made over the first metatarsal. *B*, A curved saw blade is used to create a crescentic osteotomy. *C*, Preoperative radiograph. *D*, Postoperative radiograph after a first metatarsal osteotomy. *E*, Lateral postoperative radiograph shows internal fixation within the first metatarsal and not crossing the metatarsocuneiform joint. (© M. J. Coughlin. Used by permission.)

Aggressive running can be undertaken 4 months after surgery if there are no postoperative problems.

Results and Complications. A high satisfaction rate has been reported with the combined procedure of distal soft tissue reconstruction and proximal first metatarsal osteotomy (78% to 93%).[5, 53, 65, 69, 74, 75] The average correction of the hallux valgus angle has been reported consistently to be 23 to 24 degrees.[15, 20, 53, 75] The magnitude of improvement achieved is directly proportional to the severity of the preoperative hallux valgus deformity. A crescentic osteotomy is preferred[46, 48] because it results in minimal shortening of the first metatarsal. Lengthening of the first metatarsal with an opening wedge osteotomy may lead to instability at the osteotomy site, and a closing wedge osteotomy may lead to lateral metatarsalgia as a result of first ray shortening.

Complications associated with this procedure include overcorrection or hallux varus, undercorrection or recurrence, lateral metatarsalgia, and delayed union or malunion. Overcorrection often has been associated with lateral sesamoidectomy, and Simmonds and Menelaus[74] and Mann and Coughlin[48, 50] have recommended that a lateral sesamoidectomy should be avoided. Retention of the lateral sesamoid has decreased the prevalence of hallux varus in one series from 11%[50] to 8%.[52] Often hallux varus deformities less than 10 degrees are asymptomatic and are associated with a satisfactory result.

Combined Multiple First Metatarsal Osteotomies

In the presence of a congruent first MTP joint associated with a hallux valgus deformity, a distal soft tissue realignment is contraindicated because it would create an incongruent MTP joint (Fig. 30J–24).[14, 15, 17] An incongruent joint is at risk for later degenerative arthritis or recurrence of deformity. When a hallux valgus deformity occurs in a patient with a congruent first MTP joint, an extra-articular MTP joint correction with periarticular osteotomies (Akin, distal metatarsal, cuneiform) is indicated.

An Akin phalangeal osteotomy[1, 14, 15, 25] decreases phalangeal angulation associated with an increased proximal phalangeal articular angle; a first ray osteotomy (proximal first metatarsal osteotomy)[21, 61] or cuneiform osteotomy[15, 26] may correct an increased IM angle; occasionally, an increased DMAA may necessitate a medial closing wedge distal first metatarsal osteotomy.[23, 30, 60, 66] Mitchell and Baxter[59] recommended a combined chevron osteotomy and phalangeal osteotomy. The magnitude of the DMAA determines the necessity of multiple first ray osteotomies. Richardson and coworkers[67] stated that the average DMAA in normal feet was 6 degrees. As this angle increases, the magnitude of a congruent hallux valgus deformity increases.[15] Piggott[62] noted that 9% of adults with a hallux valgus deformity had a congruous MTP joint. Coughlin found this to occur in 46% of juveniles with hallux valgus and 37% of adult men with hallux valgus.[13] Coughlin and Carlson[17] reported a 2% incidence of congruent hallux valgus deformities in a large series of adults requiring hallux valgus surgery.

Technique. A medial longitudinal incision is centered

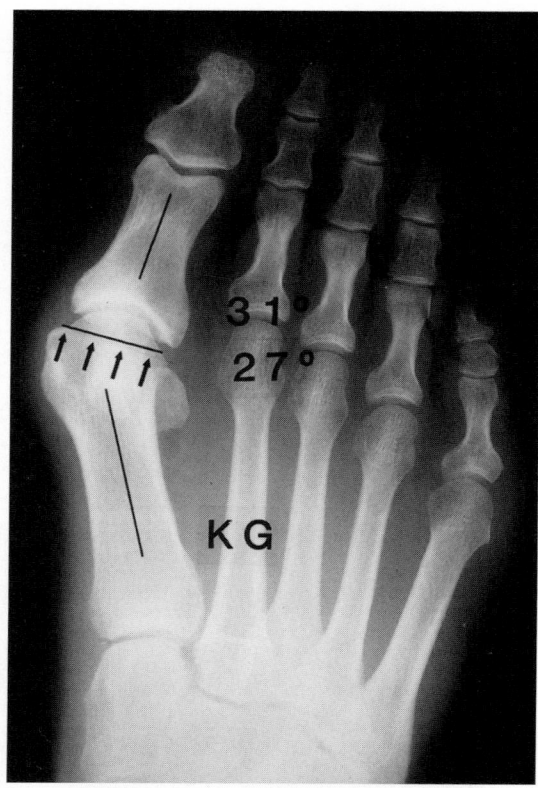

Figure 30J–24. Anteroposterior radiograph shows congruent hallux valgus deformity. The distal metatarsal articular angle is 27 degrees, and the hallux valgus angle is 31 degrees. The entire hallux valgus deformity is due to lateral sloping of the distal metatarsal articular surface.

over the first MTP joint. An L-shaped capsular release is used as previously described. A medial closing wedge osteotomy is performed 1.5 cm proximal to the metatarsal articular surface. The magnitude of the closing wedge depends on the magnitude of the DMAA. Usually, the size of this wedge is 6 to 10 mm at its medial base (Fig. 30J–25). Care is taken to avoid injury to the sesamoid mechanism on the plantar aspect. The osteotomy site is closed and stabilized with two oblique 0.062 Kirschner wires. The medial eminence is resected, and the medial capsule is repaired with interrupted sutures. After completion of the osteotomy, the hallux may appear to be in slight varus because the toe now closely parallels the longitudinal axis of the first metatarsal shaft. A proximal osteotomy of the first ray is necessary to diminish the 1–2 IM angle. A proximal first metatarsal osteotomy may be performed; however, care must be taken to avoid excessive soft tissue stripping, which may devascularize the first metatarsal. Alternatively, an opening wedge cuneiform osteotomy may be performed.[14] When a cuneiform osteotomy is performed, a medial longitudinal incision is centered over the first cuneiform. The naviculocuneiform and metatarsocuneiform joints are identified. A vertical osteotomy is centered in the first cuneiform, and the osteotomy site is opened medially. A triangular bicortical iliac crest bone graft is impacted into place and stabilized with two 0.062 Kirschner wires. (Bone removed from the metatarsal head or medial eminence usually is insufficient to serve as the graft.) The incision is approximated in a routine fashion (Fig. 30J–26).

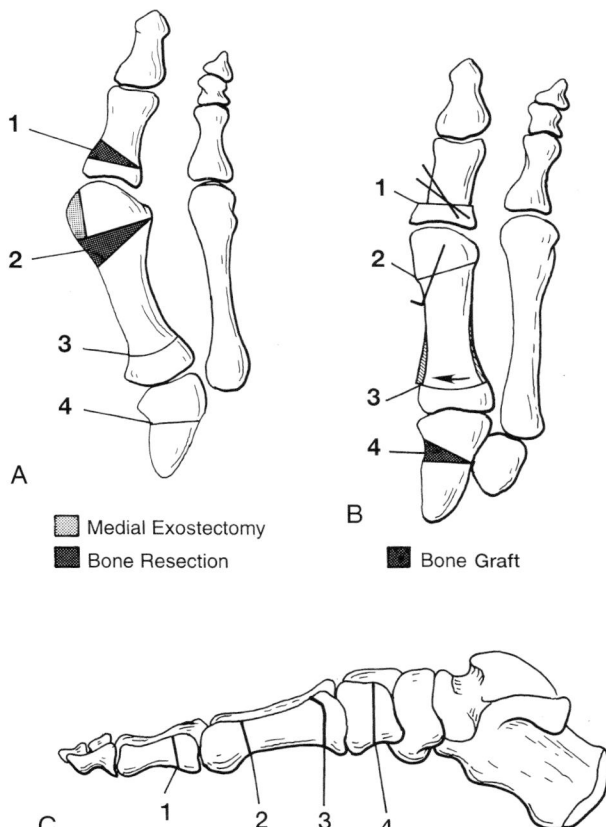

Figure 30J–25. Schematic diagram of double and triple first ray osteotomies. (*A* and *B* are anteroposterior views; *C* is a lateral view.) 1, Phalangeal osteotomy (closing wedge); 2, distal metatarsal osteotomies (closing wedge); 3, crescentic proximal first metatarsal osteotomy; 4, cuneiform osteotomy (opening wedge). (From Coughlin M, Carlson R: Treatment of hallux valgus with an increased distal metatarsal articular angle: Evaluation of double and triple first ray osteotomies. Foot Ankle Int 20:765, 1999.)

Postoperative Care. The foot is placed in a gauze and tape compression dressing, which is changed on an intermittent basis. A below-knee cast is applied. At 4 weeks, weight-bearing is allowed in the cast. The osteotomy sites typically are healed 6 to 8 weeks after surgery, and internal fixation routinely is removed. The cast is removed after radiographic confirmation of adequate healing, and range-of-motion exercises are initiated.

Results and Complications. Funk and Wells[23] and others[21, 25, 30, 60, 66] reported success with distal metatarsal osteotomies and double osteotomies. Funk and Wells[23] reported an average correction of the 1–2 IM angle of 7.2 degrees. Coughlin and Carlson[17] reported on the use of double and triple osteotomies in the treatment of adolescent hallux valgus deformities in 18 patients (21 feet) with a hallux valgus deformity characterized by an increased DMAA, who underwent either double or triple first ray periarticular osteotomies. The average hallux valgus correction measured 23 degrees, and the average 1–2 IM angle correction was 9 degrees. The DMAA averaged 23 degrees preoperatively and was corrected to an average of 9 degrees postoperatively. Peterson and Newman[61] reported a similar correction of the hallux valgus angle and the 1–2 IM angle.

Complications associated with multiple metatarsal osteotomies include loss of correction, loss of fixation, malunion, avascular necrosis, and degenerative arthritis of either the interphalangeal or MTP joint. These techniques are difficult and should be reserved for the occasional case of a hallux valgus deformity associated with a congruent joint with an increased DMAA of greater than 15 degrees (Fig. 30J–27).

Salvage Procedures

Excisional arthroplasty,[37] placement of MTP joint implants, and MTP arthrodesis all are techniques that must be considered salvage procedures. Although Cleveland and Winnant[6] and Jordan and Brodsky[34] found that the Keller procedure produced acceptable results, Rogers and Joplin[68] later remarked that "the operation does not restore the strength of the great toe essential to normal locomotion and it does not effect significantly a correction of the weakness that usually coexists in the foot as a whole. There is good evidence that the Keller reconstruction throws upon the rest of the foot a burden as great as, or greater than, that imposed by the deformity for which the operation was performed." Rogers and Joplin[68] reported weakened push-off in 55% of patients and noted, in regard to postoperative functional capacity, that 90% of their patients were employed in sedentary work, and 74% pursued sedentary leisure activities.

Turnbull and Grange[76] noted that the Keller procedure "so dysfunctions the great toe to cause more imbalance of load distribution." Hutton and Dhanendran[32] reported that excisional arthroplasty of the first MTP joint causes significant lateral transfer of weight-bearing capacity, which often increases the incidence of lateral metatarsalgia. Coughlin and Mann[18] noted a significant incidence of cock-up deformity in the hallux after the Keller procedure.

The decreased weight-bearing capacity of the first metatarsal,[32] the increased incidence of metatarsalgia and the cock-up deformity in the hallux, and the decreased strength and loss of stability created by disruption of the plantar aponeurosis and intrinsic musculature of the first ray make it unlikely that the Keller procedure would result in useful improvement for the symptomatic athlete with hallux valgus. As a salvage procedure in older patients, this procedure has merit, but in young and middle-aged athletes, strength and weight-bearing capacity of the first ray are functions that should be preserved if possible.

The use of a silicone hemiarthroplasty or double-stem total joint replacement is contraindicated in an athlete because the decreased weight-bearing capacity of the first ray after joint implantation may lead to lateral transfer metatarsalgia. The increased stress placed on the first MTP joint by a jogger or runner creates the potential for early failure of the implant.

Arthrodesis of the first MTP joint for severe hallux valgus and hallux rigidus is probably the best alternative of all these salvage procedures in an athlete. Arthrodesis leaves the athlete with increased rigidity of the forefoot, which leads to early lift-off[51] with walking and running and to potentially decreased function.

Although these salvage procedures should be part of the surgical armamentarium of an orthopaedic foot surgeon,

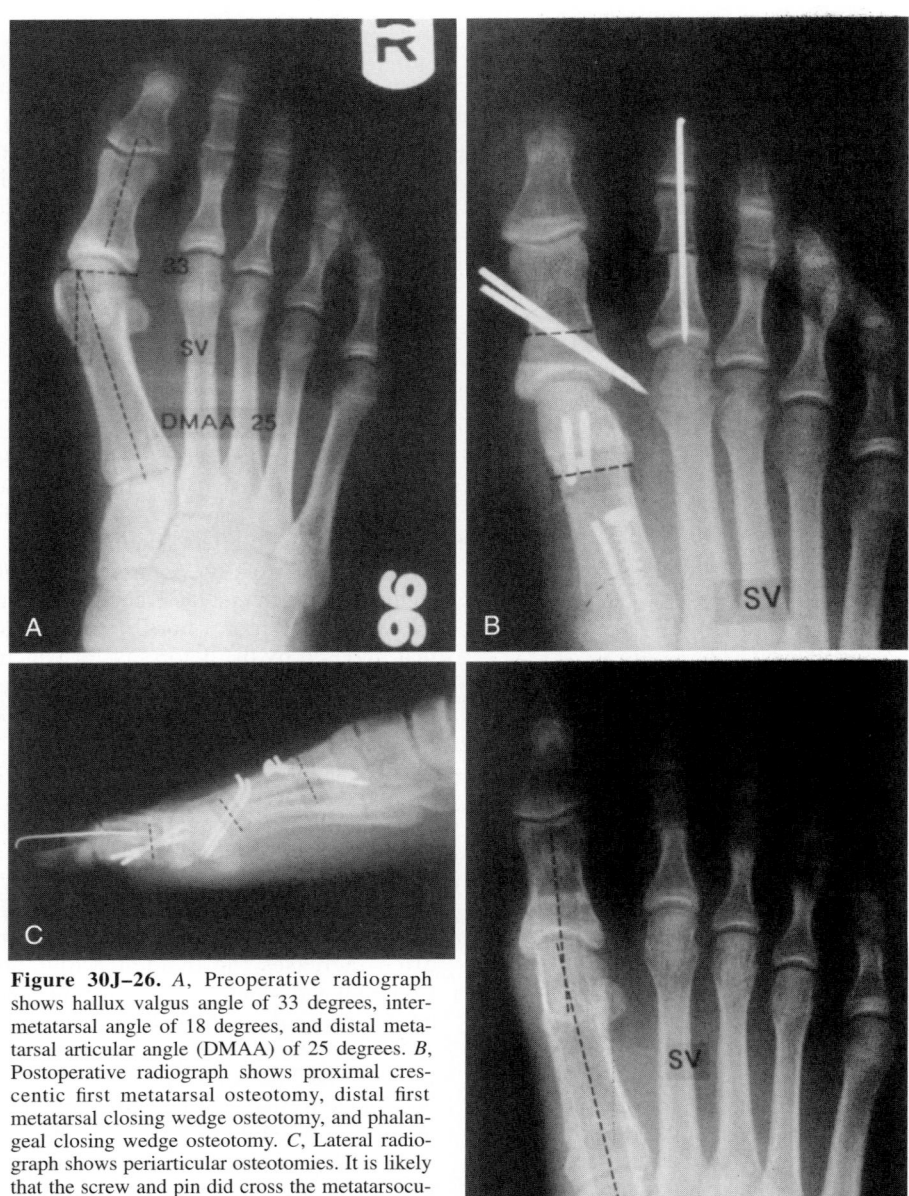

Figure 30J–26. *A*, Preoperative radiograph shows hallux valgus angle of 33 degrees, intermetatarsal angle of 18 degrees, and distal metatarsal articular angle (DMAA) of 25 degrees. *B*, Postoperative radiograph shows proximal crescentic first metatarsal osteotomy, distal first metatarsal closing wedge osteotomy, and phalangeal closing wedge osteotomy. *C*, Lateral radiograph shows periarticular osteotomies. It is likely that the screw and pin did cross the metatarsocuneiform joint. Hardware typically is removed 6 weeks after surgery, as shown in *D*. *D*, Radiograph at 3 years' follow-up shows hallux valgus angle of 16 degrees, intermetatarsal angle of 13 degrees, and DMAA of 11 degrees. (From Coughlin M, Carlson R: Treatment of hallux valgus with an increased distal metatarsal articular angle: Evaluation of double and triple first ray osteotomies. Foot Ankle Int 20:767, 1999.)

their applicability in an athletically active individual is limited. The primary procedures discussed earlier have lower postoperative morbidity than these salvage procedures and are preferable when surgery is indicated for an athlete with a symptomatic hallux valgus deformity.

Author's Preferred Method of Treatment

A symptomatic hallux valgus deformity presents a special problem to the treating physician. Although in general, conservative methods should be used in all athletes, a high-performance athlete requires more deliberate treatment. Hamilton (quoted by Lillich and Baxter[43]) stated that bunionectomies should be avoided in sprinters and ballet dancers. Restricted dorsiflexion and plantar flexion may interfere with a dancer's functional ability. Likewise, in sprinters, the need for dorsiflexion as well as strength in push-off makes them poor candidates for a hallux valgus repair. Middle- and long-distance runners appear to have less need for excessive dorsiflexion and push-off than sprinters. It is wise to treat most high-level athletes symptomatically until their desire for high-level competition

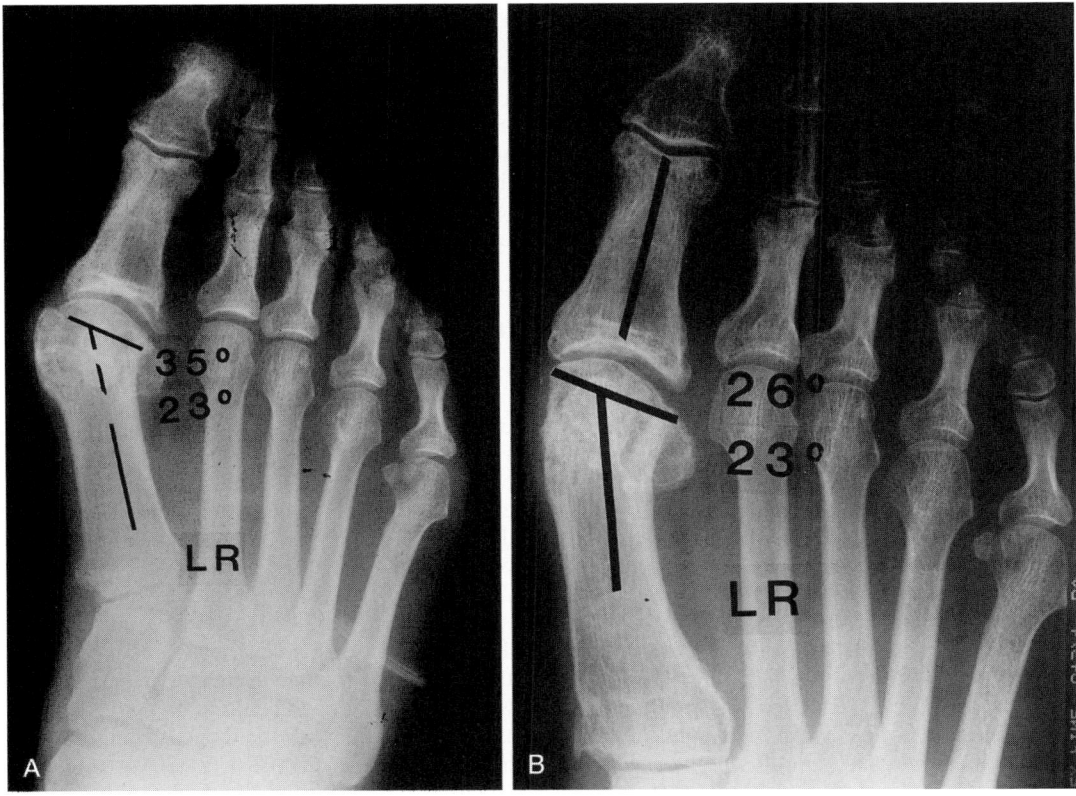

Figure 30J–27. *A,* Preoperative radiograph shows congruent hallux valgus deformity (hallux valgus angle, 35 degrees; distal metatarsal articular angle [DMAA], 23 degrees). *B,* Two years after distal soft tissue repair. Although the medial eminence has been resected, the DMAA is unchanged (DMAA, 23 degrees), and the hallux valgus is minimally corrected (hallux valgus angle, 26 degrees). The increased distal metatarsal articular angle prevented further realignment of the metatarsophalangeal joint.

wanes; if the hallux valgus deformity continues to be symptomatic, surgery can be performed at that time. When surgery is contemplated, careful analysis of the components of the hallux valgus deformity is essential in the decision-making process to ensure the appropriate choice of hallux valgus repair.

It is preferable to use a surgical procedure that (1) maintains a flexible MTP joint with as normal a range of motion as possible, (2) attempts to restore a normal weight-bearing pattern in the forefoot, (3) corrects the deformity without producing residual disability, and (4) allows a reasonable route of salvage if a complication develops. For a mild hallux deformity (0 to 20 degrees), usually conservative care suffices. An Akin procedure or a chevron repair is used when indicated. Because these two repairs are extra-articular, they can be carried out in a patient with a congruent (increased DMAA) or subluxated MTP joint. For a low moderate deformity (a hallux valgus angle of 20 to 30 degrees), a chevron procedure or a distal soft tissue realignment is the procedure of choice. The chevron procedure may be used to correct a congruent or subluxated MTP joint, but a distal soft tissue realignment can be used only in a patient with a noncongruent or subluxated joint.

For a high moderate deformity (a hallux valgus angle of 30 to 40 degrees), a distal soft tissue repair with or without a proximal first metatarsal osteotomy appears to offer the best chance for successful hallux valgus repair in the presence of a subluxated first MTP joint (Fig. 30J–28).

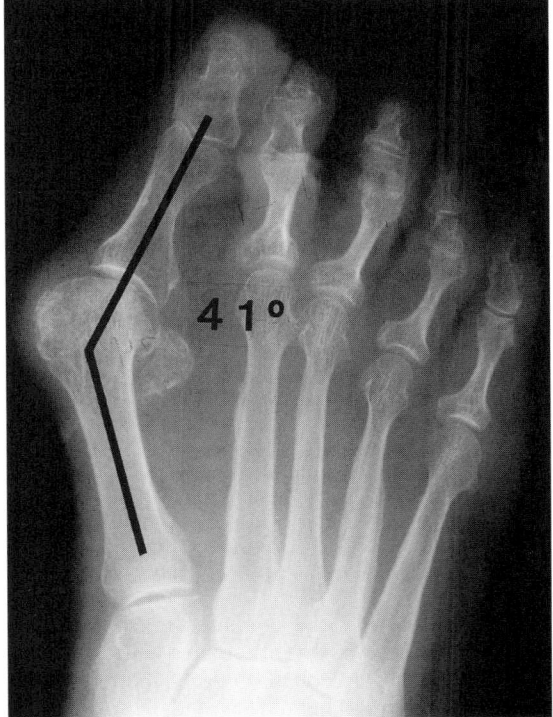

Figure 30J–28. Severe hallux valgus deformity with subluxation of first metatarsophalangeal joint.

For a congruent hallux valgus deformity, periarticular oste-otomies are indicated in the presence of an DMAA. An intra-articular correction of a congruent MTP joint with hallux valgus places the repair at high risk for recurrence, degenerative joint disease, or at least restricted range of motion. Adding an osteotomy undoubtedly increases the postoperative morbidity and recovery time in an athlete. When a more severe hallux valgus deformity is present, the magnitude of the surgical procedure increases, and postoperative swelling, reduced MTP joint range of motion, and reduced strength become more likely. For these reasons, patient counseling is especially advocated in this group. A change in athletic activity, substituting activities such as bicycling and other nonimpact activities for running, may reduce symptoms significantly in an athlete with hallux valgus.

TURF TOE

MTP joint injuries in competitive athletes have become an ever-increasing source of forefoot pain and dysfunction[80, 82, 94, 95, 97] and occasionally are characterized by a significant delay in return to sporting activities.[80] Bowers and Martin[78] initially reported on a syndrome in which "a sprain of the plantar capsuloligamentous complex of the great toe of the MTP joint" occurred. During a 4-year period, Bowers and Martin[78] reported on 27 such injuries of the foot in football players and coined the term *turf toe* because of the frequency with which the injury occurred on artificial playing surfaces as opposed to natural grass. Clanton and associates[80] reported on 62 MTP joint injuries in 53 collegiate football players, all of whom sustained injuries on artificial playing surfaces.

Although there are few documented studies of athletes with MTP joint injuries, Rodeo and colleagues[95] evaluated professional football players. Of players surveyed, 57% (38 players) reported symptoms of turf toe. Although this incidence was comparable to that seen in players from other teams whose home field was a natural grass surface, 84% of the players in this series reported that their initial injury occurred on artificial turf. Other factors that may predispose an individual to injury include increasing age of the player, number of years in professional football,[95] pes planus, decreased preinjury ankle range of motion, and decreased preinjury MTP range of motion.[80]

Severe trauma to the MTP joint of the hallux is relatively uncommon. Jahss,[88] Giannikas and coworkers,[87] DeLee,[85] and Rodeo and colleagues[93] reported on fracture-dislocations and dislocation of the first MTP joint after hyperextension injuries. Usually these injuries are associated with a significant dissipation of energy, and sesamoid fractures may be associated with these injuries. Hyperextension injuries[78, 80, 82, 83] to the hallux and lesser MTP joints[80] have been associated with flexible shoewear[86] and artificial playing surfaces[78, 82, 83, 99] and in certain cases may have long-term sequelae for the symptomatic athlete.

Anatomy

The first metatarsal head is characterized by a convex cartilage-covered surface that articulates with the congruent concave articular surface of the base of the proximal phalanx.[91] The medial and lateral sesamoids, contained within the tendon of the flexor hallucis brevis (Fig. 30J–29A), articulate on their dorsal surface with the medial and lateral facets on the plantar surface of the first metatarsal head (Fig. 30J–29B). Distally, the sesamoids are connected to the base of the proximal phalanx by the plantar plate. The tendon of the flexor hallucis longus is contained within a fibrous sheath located beneath the plantar surface of the two sesamoids. The tendons of the abductor hallucis and adductor hallucis insert on either border of the sesamoids as well as onto the plantar medial and plantar lateral bases of the proximal phalanx. These structures afford significant stability to the plantar aspect of the first metatarsal head. Dorsal to this, the MTP joint is stabilized by the medial and lateral collateral ligaments, which interdigitate with the sesamoid ligaments (Fig. 30J–30A). These capsular structures give significant stability to the medial and lateral aspects of the MTP joint. Centrally located on the dorsal aspect of the MTP joint are the tendons of the extensor hallucis longus and extensor hallucis brevis. The hood ligaments (Fig. 30J–30B) of the extensor expansion form the major capsular stabilizing structure dorsally; however, they are weak compared with the plantar supporting structures and afford less structural stability.

Biomechanics

In analyzing the MTP joint, Sammarco[96] noted that motion in this diarthrodial joint occurs by means of a sliding action along the joint surface. Joseph[89] reported that normal active extension of the MTP joint approximates 80 degrees (Fig. 30J–31) and that 25 degrees of additional motion can be achieved passively. With advancing age, joint excursion can be expected to diminish. Clanton and coworkers[79–81] and others[78] reported that an average of 60 degrees of dorsiflexion can be expected with normal gait. As the phalanx approaches the upper range of dorsiflexion excursion, this sliding action is replaced by axial compression forces onto the metatarsal and phalangeal articular surfaces, which can lead to joint injury.

The effectiveness of shoewear on MTP joint excursion can be dramatic. Shoes with soft flexible soles afford little restriction or protection (Fig. 30J–32), whereas shoes with a stiff sole may diminish MTP dorsiflexion by 30 degrees without causing any noticeable impairment of gait.

The classic mechanism of injury is a forced hyperextension injury to the first MTP joint.[78, 80, 81, 95] Coker and associates[82] described this as an axial loading of the foot with the MTP joint in hyperextension. Dorsiflexion in

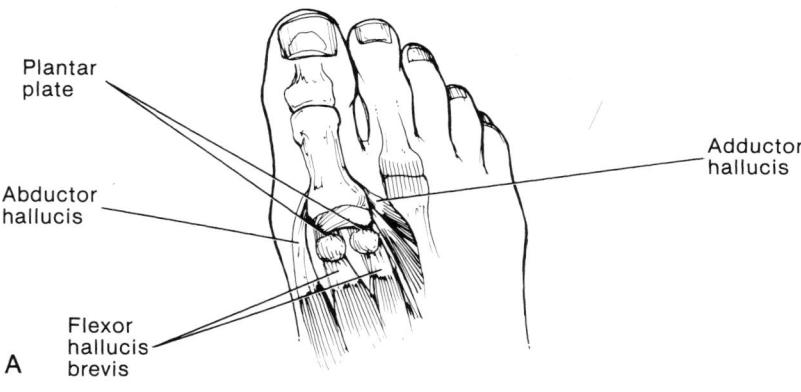

Figure 30J–29. *A,* The sesamoids are contained in the tendons of the flexor hallucis brevis. The abductor hallucis inserts onto the medial aspect of the medial sesamoid as well as the plantar medial base of the proximal phalanx, and the adductor hallucis inserts onto the lateral aspect of the lateral sesamoid as well as the plantar lateral base of the proximal phalanx. *B,* The sesamoid articulates with facets on the plantar aspect of the first metatarsal head.

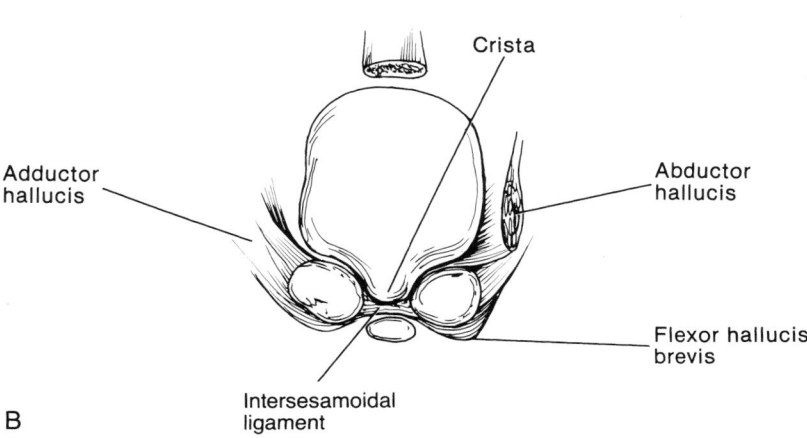

excess of a normal range of motion can lead to varying degrees of soft tissue capsular disruption, plantar plate rupture, or injury to the articular cartilage and subchondral bone. Only 35 of 51 patients in Clanton's series could recall the mechanism of injury[80]; however, 32 of the 35 patients (92%) could recall and describe a hyperextension injury. Rodeo and associates[95] reported that 85% of the football players in their series sustained a hyperextension injury. Coker and associates[82] reported that the mechanism of injury could be hyperextension, hyperflexion (which is

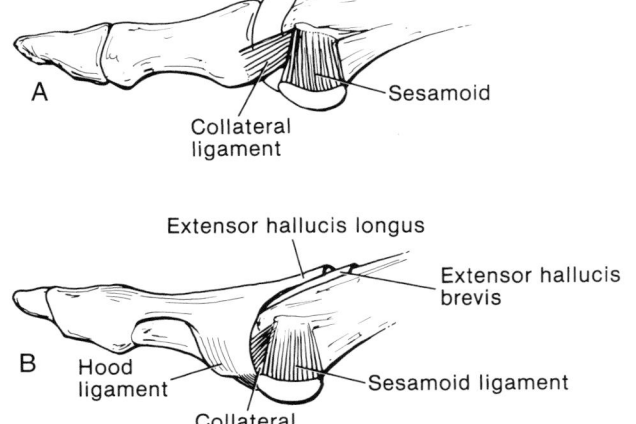

Figure 30J–30. *A,* The sesamoid and collateral ligaments stabilize the medial and lateral aspects of the first metatarsophalangeal joint. *B,* The hood ligament of the extensor expansion reinforces the dorsal aspect of the first metatarsophalangeal joint.

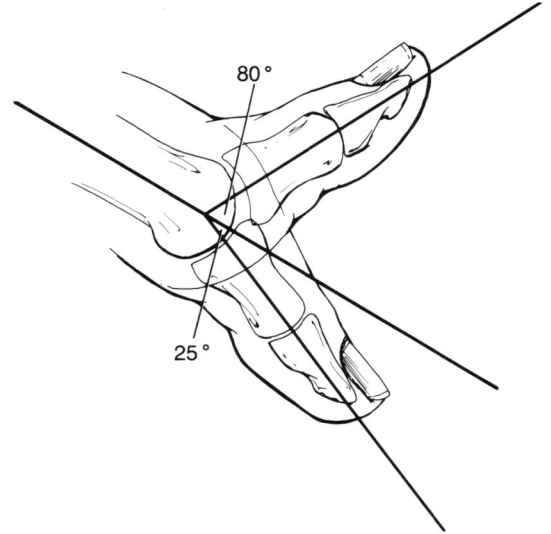

Figure 30J–31. Normal active extension of the first metatarsophalangeal joint averages 80 degrees. Active plantar flexion averages 20 to 25 degrees. This excursion may decrease with advancing age.

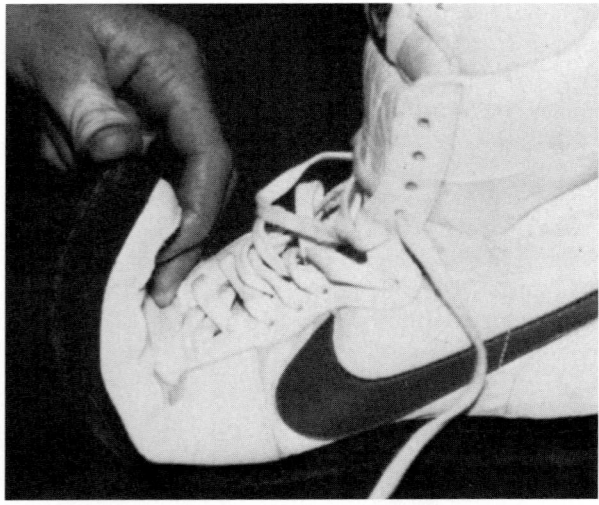

Figure 30J–32. A shoe with a flexible insole affords little protection for a hyperextension injury. (From Clanton TO, Butler JE, Eggert A: Injuries to the metatarsophalangeal joints in athletes. Foot Ankle 7:162–176, 1986. © American Orthopaedic Foot and Ankle Society, 1986.)

rare), or valgus, depending on the applied stress. Massari and coworkers[92] described a rare case of varus injury of the first MTP joint. Clanton and colleagues[80] hypothesized that more severe MTP joint injuries occur in players who have preexisting restricted motion of the first MTP joint. With continued forced dorsiflexion, capsular, ligamentous, or tendinous injury and axial compression of the joint surfaces may occur sooner than they would in a joint with more excursion.

Although Garrick[86] noted an increased injury rate in players playing on artificial surfaces, Bowers and Martin[78] found a correlation between flexible shoes and a relatively hard artificial playing surface. The use of relatively lightweight flexible shoes on artificial turf apparently predisposes the forefoot to injury.[82, 83, 99] In contrast, on grass surfaces, the use of a conventional cleated shoe, which is much stiffer (a steel plate is incorporated into the sole for attachment of the cleat), limits forefoot excursion.[80] Clanton and colleagues[80] observed that the rate of injury on artificial turf could be reduced markedly by inserting a steel forefoot insole inside the players' shoes.

Depending on the magnitude of force, the position of the MTP joint, and the direction of force, various injuries to the MTP joint can occur. Although most often a hyperextension injury leads to symptoms of turf toe, Coker and associates[82] and Clanton and colleagues[80] noted that occasionally a plantar flexion injury is associated with a turf toe injury. Valgus stress can occur as well, either alone or in combination with other forces, leading to different injury patterns.

First Metatarsophalangeal Joint Injury Classification

Rodeo and coworkers[93] proposed a classification of first MTP joint injury:

Grade 1: Acute sprain of the first MTP joint plantar capsule characterized by localized tenderness, pain with dorsiflexion, and swelling. Radiographs are normal. Treatment is conservative.
Grade 2: Acute sprain of the first MTP joint with significant plantar capsule disruption. There is extensive ecchymosis, painful dorsiflexion, and loss of motion. Radiographs may reveal a diastasis of a partite sesamoid or joint instability. No degenerative first MTP joint changes are present. Treatment may be conservative or surgical.
Grade 3: Chronic symptoms involving the first MTP joint resulting from previous injury. There is diminished motion and substantial radiographic changes of degenerative joint disease, hallux rigidus, or malalignment. Treatment is often surgical.

Clanton[79–81] proposed a classification for more acute injuries (Table 30J–1).

Clinical Evaluation

Attention to the range of motion of the MTP joint and the ankle joint in the preseason physical examination may be an important factor in selecting players who have a predisposition to turf toe injuries. Players with restricted motion may sustain an MTP joint injury with relatively less excursion of the hallux. Protection of the forefoot with an orthotic device may avoid more serious injury.[79–81] The history elicited from the athlete may give some indication of the mechanism of injury. It is important to ascertain the type of footwear used, the specific type of playing surface that the injury occurred on, and the location of maximal discomfort. After injury to the MTP joint, a player may complain of localized pain, swelling, discomfort, and pain with range of motion and ambulation. The magnitude of injury can vary from a mild MTP joint sprain to a complete capsular disruption.[79–81]

Physical Examination

On physical examination, obvious periarticular swelling is apparent. Ecchymosis often is noted adjacent to the area of capsular injury. Although plantar or plantar medial tenderness occurs with mild injuries, dorsal discomfort is associated with more severe capsular disruption. With severe injury, fracture-dislocation of the MTP joint may occur with obvious joint deformity. A palpable plantar defect may be noted indicating a partial or complete disruption of the plantar plate–sesamoid mechanism.[84]

An antalgic gait may be recognized as the athlete attempts to walk with the limb in external rotation or the foot in an everted position to minimize MTP joint excursion. With running, push-off is impaired, and it may be difficult to crouch with the MTP joint extended.[78] Passive manipulation of the MTP joint into dorsiflexion may cause significant discomfort,[78] and quantitation of the range of motion may show a corresponding decrease in dorsiflexion, plantar flexion, or both. Weakness of the MTP joint in plantar flexion may be observed.

TABLE 30J–1
Acute First Metatarsal Joint Injury

Grade	Objective Findings	Activity Level	Pathology	Treatment
1	Localized plantar or medial tenderness Minimal swelling No ecchymosis	Continued athletic participation	Stretching of capsuloligamentous complex	Symptomatic
2	More diffuse and intense tenderness Mild-to-moderate swelling Mild-to-moderate ecchymosis Painful and restricted range of motion	Loss of playing time for 3–14 days	Partial tear of capsuloligamentous complex	Walking boot and crutches as needed
3	Severe and diffuse tenderness Marked swelling Moderate-to-severe ecchymosis Range of motion painful and limited	Loss of playing time for 2–6 weeks	Tear of capsuloligamentous complex Articular cartilage and subchondral bone injury Possibility of sesamoid fracture or separation of bipartite sesamoid Possiblity of dislocated first MTP joint with spontaneous reduction	Long-term immobilization in boot or cast versus surgical repair

MTP, metatarsophalangeal.
Data from references 78–80.

Radiographic examination often fails to show bony abnormalities. Generalized soft tissue swelling frequently is shown.[78–80] Anteroposterior, lateral, and oblique radiographic views may be helpful in evaluating the MTP joint surface as well as the sesamoids. Occasionally, small periarticular flecks or chips of bone are noted (Fig. 30J–33A), probably indicating avulsion of the MTP capsule or ligamentous complex.

When a compression fracture of the metatarsal head has occurred, intra-articular loose bodies (Fig. 30J–33B) may be apparent. Chondrolysis of the joint space may occur with time, and Clanton and colleagues[80] have reported

cystic changes in the metatarsal head denoting progressive degenerative changes.[80] In patients with continued pain without obvious radiographic changes, Coker and associates[82] used MTP joint arthrograms to diagnose chronic capsular tears. Proximal migration of one or both of the sesamoids or migration of a bipartite sesamoid may indicate medial or lateral plantar plate disruption or sesamoid disruption.[93]

Use of high-resolution bone scans can be helpful in ascertaining whether sesamoid injury has occurred. The presence of a bipartite sesamoid may be difficult to differentiate from an acute fracture; a fracture shows increased

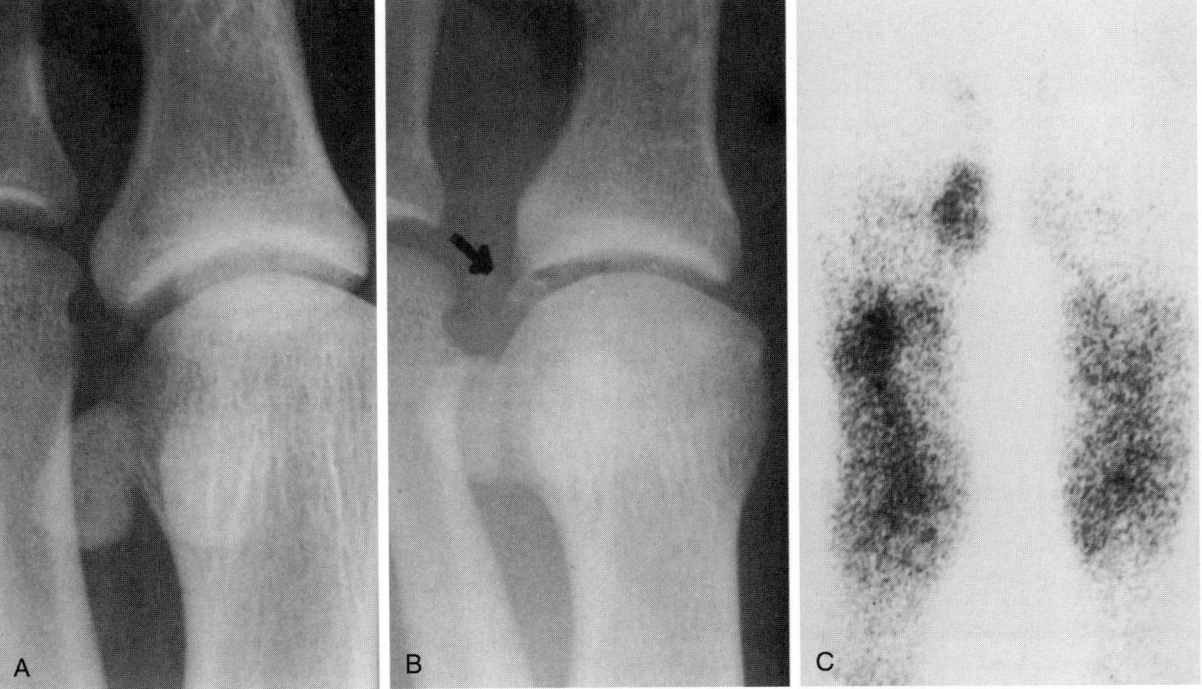

Figure 30J–33. *A*, A fleck of bone may indicate ligamentous or capsular disruption. *B*, Intra-articular loose bodies *(arrow)* may occur after turf toe injury. *C*, A bone scan may show increased uptake even when radiographs still appear normal. (From Clanton TO, Butler JE, Eggert A: Injuries to the metatarsophalangeal joint in athletes. Foot Ankle 7:162–176, 1986. © American Orthopaedic Foot and Ankle Society, 1986.)

uptake on a bone scan with time. Likewise, an impaction injury to the MTP articular surface may result in chondromalacia of the metatarsal head.[82] Radionuclear scanning (Fig. 30J–33C) may show increased uptake in the presence of normal radiographs. Magnetic resonance imaging (MRI) often is definitive in diagnosing capsular disruption and incomplete or complete plantar plate disruption.[90, 98]

Treatment Options and Rehabilitation

Depending on the magnitude of the injury, different options are available. For grade 1 injuries, which are characterized by localized tenderness, ice, compression, and nonsteroidal anti-inflammatory drugs (NSAIDs) may be used.[79–81] The patient may continue to participate in athletics if pain is minimal. Taping of the toe to reduce dorsiflexion excursion may be helpful. Inserting a rigid forefoot insole[79–81] to stiffen the shoe may decrease discomfort and help to reduce the incidence of recurrent injury.

In grade 2 injuries with diffuse tenderness, moderate swelling, ecchymosis, and significant restriction of motion, a moderate capsuloligamentous injury has occurred. Immersing the foot in ice three times a day until swelling has decreased[78] and protective taping often hasten recovery.[78–81] NSAIDs may be helpful as well.[79–81] Addition of a firm insole prevents dorsiflexion strain to the toe (Fig. 30J–34). Although it is unlikely that an articular joint injury has occurred, activity must be restricted until only minimal

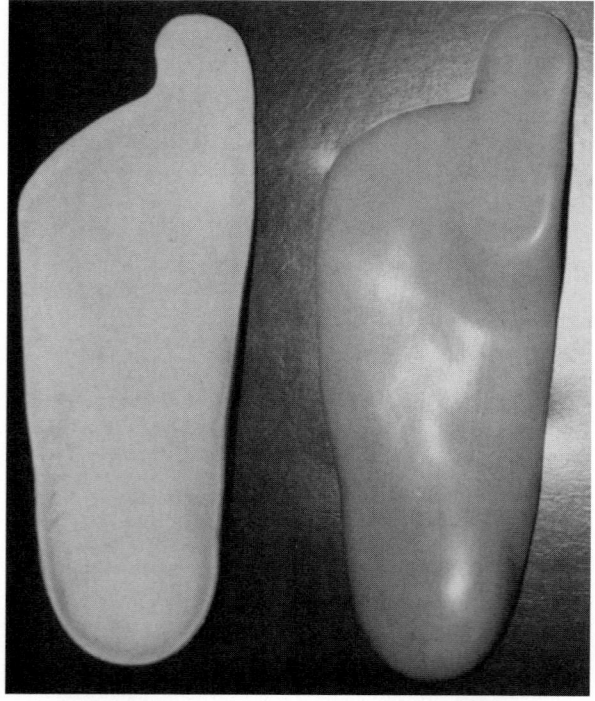

Figure 30J–34. Use of a firm insole that restricts forefoot motion may prevent injury and may diminish symptoms after injury. (From Clanton TO, Butler JE, Eggert A: Injuries to the metatarsophalangeal joints in athletes. Foot Ankle 7:162–176, 1986. © American Orthopaedic Foot and Ankle Society, 1986.)

discomfort exists.[78] Typically, refraining from athletic activity for 1 to 2 weeks allows significant improvement.

In grade 3 injuries, a significant capsuloligamentous injury has occurred. Dislocation of the MTP joint may occur in this situation (Fig. 30J–35). Spontaneous reduction may have occurred; when an unreduced dislocation is present, it should be reduced promptly by the trainer or team physician. The technique of hyperextension with concurrent longitudinal traction coupled with a plantar flexion push on the base of the proximal phalanx may achieve reduction. Follow-up radiographs are necessary to rule out the presence of fracture. Occasionally, an irreducible dislocation requires operative intervention.[85]

Clanton[79–81] stated that frequently a compression injury to the MTP articular cartilage and subchondral bone (Fig. 30J–36) occurs with this injury and may have long-term consequences. With a severe injury, ice, elevation, and compression are always helpful. Immobilization may be necessary after reduction of a frank dislocation. In patients without dislocation but with significant capsuloligamentous injury, crutches and reduced weight-bearing may be necessary initially. Weight-bearing may be initiated within the limits of pain.[82] Ultrasound and contrast baths may help to reduce swelling. As pain diminishes, a player may start walking with a weight-bearing configuration that allows comfortable gait. Joint mobilization assists in achieving more normal range of motion. NSAIDs may be employed, and taping to prevent excess dorsiflexion may decrease discomfort. As gait becomes less painful, the player is allowed to increase speed and to advance to a normal stride length until full speed is achieved. Last, cutting maneuvers can be initiated within the limits of pain. Shoe modification with a stiff forefoot insole may allow early return to athletic activity. Gradual return to sporting activities depends on the resolution of symptoms.[79–81] Intra-articular injections of steroids may disguise symptoms or give temporary relief only and are to be discouraged.[79–82]

Severe injuries may extend the recovery time from 2 to 6 weeks.[78–81] Clanton and coworkers[80] noted two patients with turf toe who developed progressive hallux valgus. Clanton and coworkers[80] noted several cases of hallux rigidus, which probably correlates with more severe articular injury.

Surgery is rarely necessary with an acute turf toe; management usually is centered on conservative methods. If there is a high clinical suspicion of major capsular or tendinous injury, an MRI scan should be obtained. After defining a capsular injury, an open repair occasionally is performed, especially in the presence of a partial or complete plantar plate injury.[82] The development of chronic pain, restricted motion, and discomfort with running may herald the end of an athletic career. Although MRI might be useful in defining the cause of chronic capsular pain, which may be a capsular ligamentous disruption, in the late phases of this disease, an MTP arthrodesis may be the sole means of eliminating pain. Often this procedure is incompatible with a return to high-level sports activities. Coker and associates[82] recommended operative repair for these injuries. When a sesamoid injury (fracture, osteonecrosis) occurred and did not heal successfully, Coughlin[84] believed that surgical excision may be warranted (see under Sesamoid Dysfunction, next).

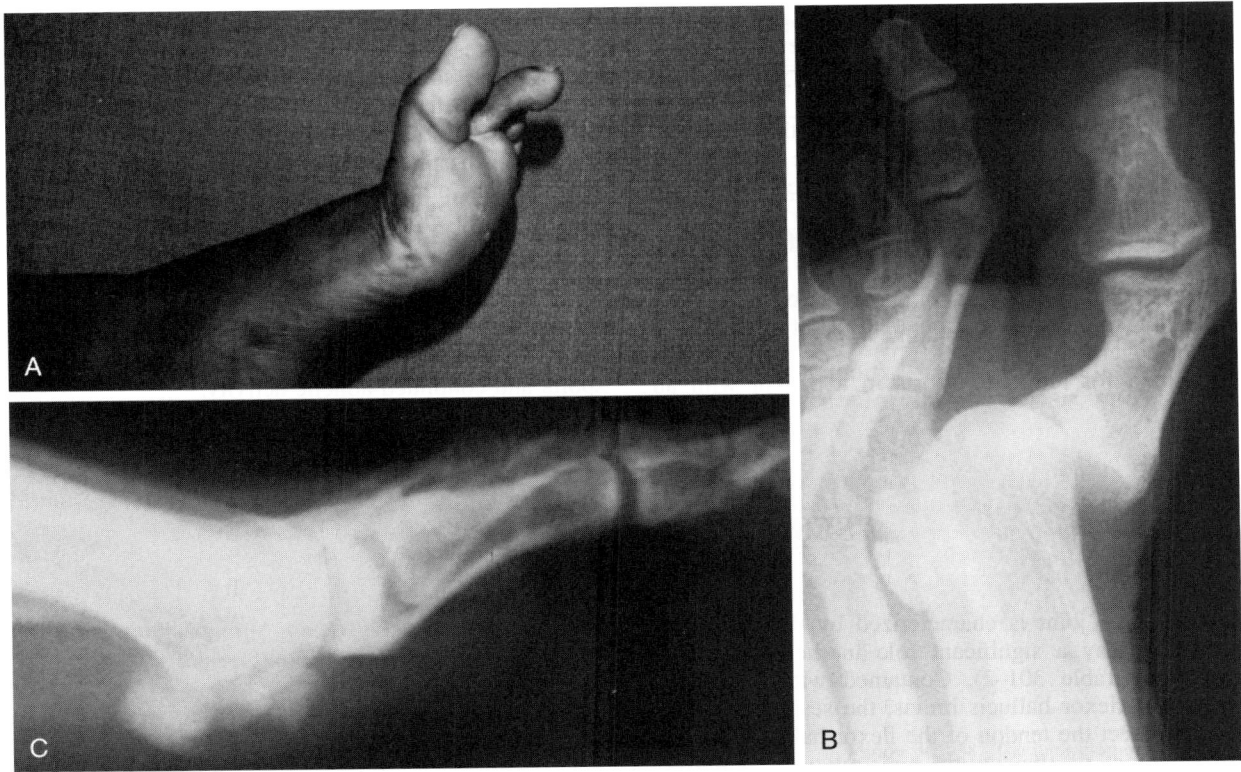

Figure 30J–35. *A–C*, Fracture-dislocation of the metatarsophalangeal-sesamoid joint (grade III injury). (From Clanton TO, Butler JE, Eggert A: Injuries to the metatarsophalangeal joints in athletes. Foot Ankle 7:162–176, 1986. © American Orthopaedic Foot and Ankle Society, 1986.)

With a progressive hallux valgus deformity, it is likely that disruption of the medial or plantar-medial capsule has occurred. Conservative treatment in the competitive athlete is warranted initially; however, with progression of pain and deformity, surgical repair is often necessary. Roomy footwear and the use of orthotic devices are preferred to surgical intervention if the progression of the deformity is insidious and asymptomatic. Operative treatment of hallux valgus in the competitive athlete may be associated with restricted range of motion, which may limit running activity significantly.

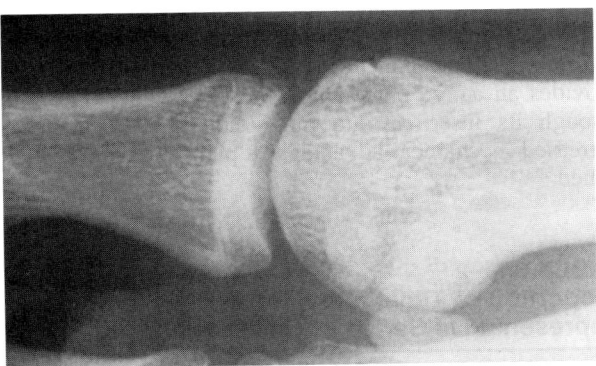

Figure 30J–36. A compression injury to the articular surface may be detected as a "divot" sign on the dorsal aspect of the first metatarsal head. (From Clanton TO, Butler JE, Eggert A: Injuries to the metatarsophalangeal joints in athletes. Foot Ankle 7:162–176, 1986. © American Orthopaedic Foot and Ankle Society, 1986.)

Author's Preferred Method of Treatment

The preference of athletes for lightweight flexible shoes that afford good traction but little structural support presents an increasing risk factor for competitive athletes. Coupled with a relatively hard playing surface, the chance of injury to the MTP joint increases significantly. Although a forced hyperextension injury is the most common mechanism of injury, plantar flexion or valgus stress can cause capsuloligamentous injury as well.

Preseason physical examination may help identify which players are at high risk for turf toe. Players with less than 60 degrees of dorsiflexion at the MTP joint or with significant reduction in dorsiflexion at the ankle joint should be protected with a stiff-soled shoe or a stiff insole. These modalities may prevent MTP joint injury or may reduce the magnitude of injury should it occur. An MRI scan should be obtained when there is suspicion of significant injury. In the high-performance athlete, open repair of partial and complete capsular, plantar plate, or sesamoid disruption may be indicated.

There are few better examples of injuries in which prophylactic intervention and the choice of footwear can help to reduce the incidence of athletic injury than turf toe. Although turf toe can be a disabling injury that can bring about the premature conclusion of an athletic career, prophylactic shoewear modification and counseling athletes at risk can reduce the frequency and magnitude of this injury.

In the athlete with an acute grade 1 turf toe injury, ice,

this may be the reason for the development of multipartite sesamoids.[128]

Biomechanics

The hallucal sesamoids function to absorb weight-bearing forces on the medial aspect of the forefoot, but most important, they appear to increase the mechanical advantage of the intrinsic musculature of the first ray. Just as the patella increases the mechanical advantage of the quadriceps mechanism in knee extension, the sesamoids increase the mechanical advantage of the intrinsic musculature in plantar flexing of the proximal phalanx.[128] The tendon of the flexor hallucis longus, which is protected in its tendon sheath by the medial and lateral sesamoids (Fig. 30J–40), provides a plantar flexion force to the interphalangeal joint of the great toe. Sesamoid dysfunction that restricts the range of motion of the MTP joint may lead to the development of a pathologic gait pattern. An athlete may tend to evert the forefoot to decrease dorsiflexion excursion in the latter part of gait or may tend to toe-off prematurely to minimize dorsiflexion excursion of the hallux. Pain with dorsiflexion or with direct pressure on the sesamoids may lead to a similar abnormal gait pattern. Although surgical excision may remove an abnormal sesamoid, it may leave a toe weakened with regard to plantar flexion force.[139] Disruption of the plantar aponeurosis after sesamoid excision may leave a weakened first ray, which may impair athletic function, such as jogging or running, significantly. Surgical repair of the intrinsic musculature and maintenance of either the abductor or the adductor hallucis when a sesamoid is excised are important factors to consider in maintaining the normal biomechanics of the first MTP joint.

Clinical Evaluation

In the history of a patient with a symptomatic sesamoid, the most frequent subjective symptoms are pain and discomfort in the toe-off phase of gait. The most common objective findings are as follows[139]:

1. Restricted range of motion
2. Pain on direct palpation
3. Pain with motion of the first MTP joint
4. Swelling in the first MTP joint
5. Diminished strength in plantar flexion or dorsiflexion

MTP joint synovitis may be noted on examination. A plantar keratosis beneath either the tibial or the fibular sesamoid occasionally may accompany a symptomatic sesamoid. The hallux must be inspected for either medial deviation (hallux varus) or lateral deviation (hallux valgus). Disruption of a sesamoid because of fracture or trauma may be associated with progressive insidious deviation of the great toe. A hallux valgus or hallux varus deformity may occur after previous sesamoid resection. It is important to examine the sensory nerves to the hallux because an adjacent digital nerve may be compressed[124] by the fibular or tibial sesamoid, resulting in neuritic symptoms or numbness. In this setting, a positive Tinel's sign may be elicited along the borders of the sesamoids.

Routine AP and lateral radiographs (Fig. 30J–41A and B) may not provide sufficient information with which to evaluate the sesamoids. On a lateral radiograph, the sesamoids often overlap each other; on the AP view, the metatarsal head obscures the medial and the lateral sesamoids. The tibial sesamoid is seen best on an oblique radiograph (Fig. 30J–41C)[146] with the MTP joint extended approximately 50 degrees; the x-ray beam is directed 15 degrees cephalad from a lateral position and is centered over the first metatarsal head. The fibular sesamoid is seen best on a lateral oblique radiograph (Fig. 30J–41D),[146] where it is shown in the first interspace between the first and second metatarsal heads. Often the most useful radiograph is the axial sesamoid view.

When radiographs appear normal despite subjective symptoms, a bone scan may be used.[129, 135] A bone scan may show increased uptake before any significant radiographic changes, such as fragmentation, disintegration, or sclerosis, appear. MRI[133] may be helpful in visualizing bone and soft tissue abnormalities of the sesamoid mechanism.

Diagnosis
Bipartite Sesamoids and Fracture

The incidence of bipartite sesamoids as well as their cause is a subject of significant controversy in the litera-

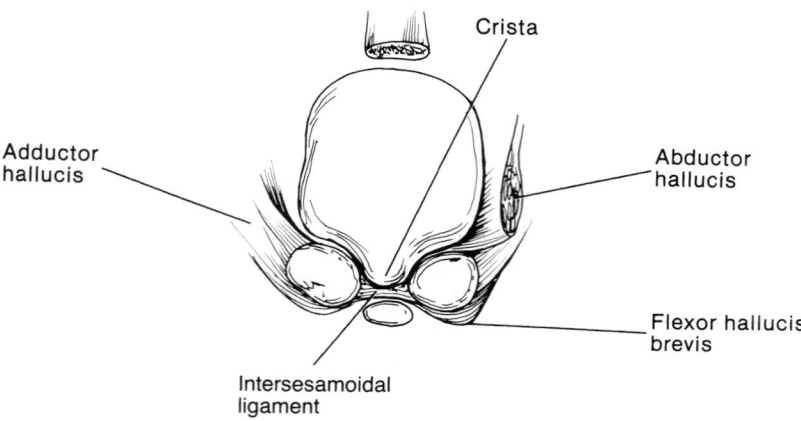

Figure 30J–40. A cross section through the first metatarsal head shows the flexor hallucis longus within a fibrous tendon sheath.

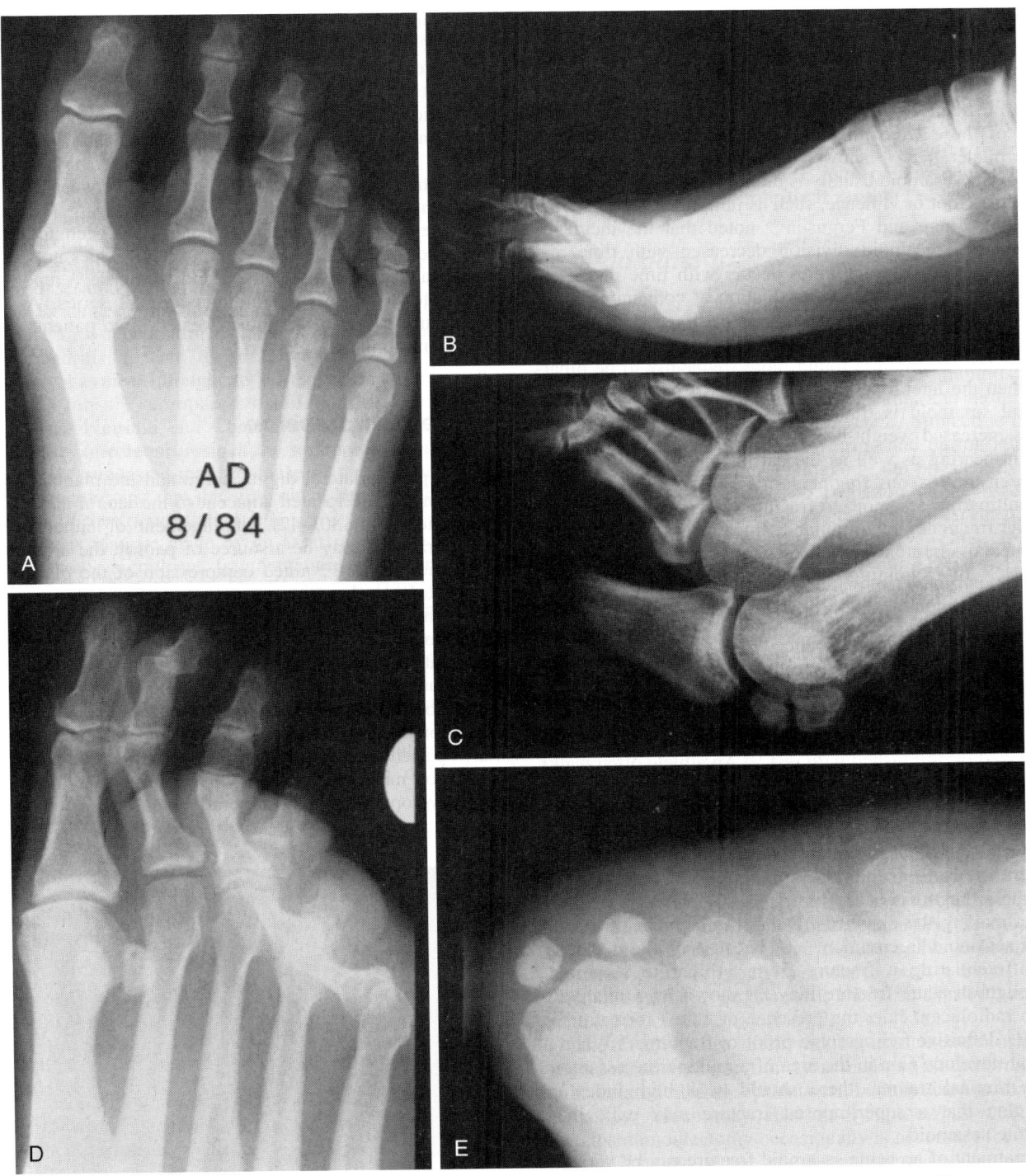

Figure 30J–41. *A,* Anteroposterior radiograph shows the sesamoids. *B,* Lateral radiograph shows sesamoids, although there is significant overlap that may conceal disease. *C,* An oblique radiograph shows the tibial sesamoid. *D,* A lateral oblique radiograph shows the fibular sesamoid. *E,* Axial view shows fracture of the lateral sesamoid. (*A,* from Coughlin MJ: Sesamoids and accessory bones of the foot. In Mann RA, Coughlin MJ [eds]: Surgery of the Foot and Ankle, 6th ed. St. Louis, Mosby, 1993; *B–E,* © M. J. Coughlin. Used by permission.)

ture.[159] Dobas and Silvers[113] found a 19% incidence of bipartite sesamoids, whereas Kewenter[134] found a 31% incidence. Rowe[148] reported a 6% to 8% frequency of bipartite sesamoids and noted that 90% of these were bilateral. Dobas and Silvers[113] noted that 87% of the bipartite sesamoids in their series involved the tibial or medial sesamoid.

Dobas and Silvers[113] noted that approximately 25% of the divided tibial sesamoids had an identical bipartite tibial sesamoid, and the remaining sesamoids were asymmetrical in regard to division. Jahss[129] reported that the medial sesamoid has a 10 times greater incidence of bipartitism. Although Giannestras[119] stated that bipartite sesamoids are

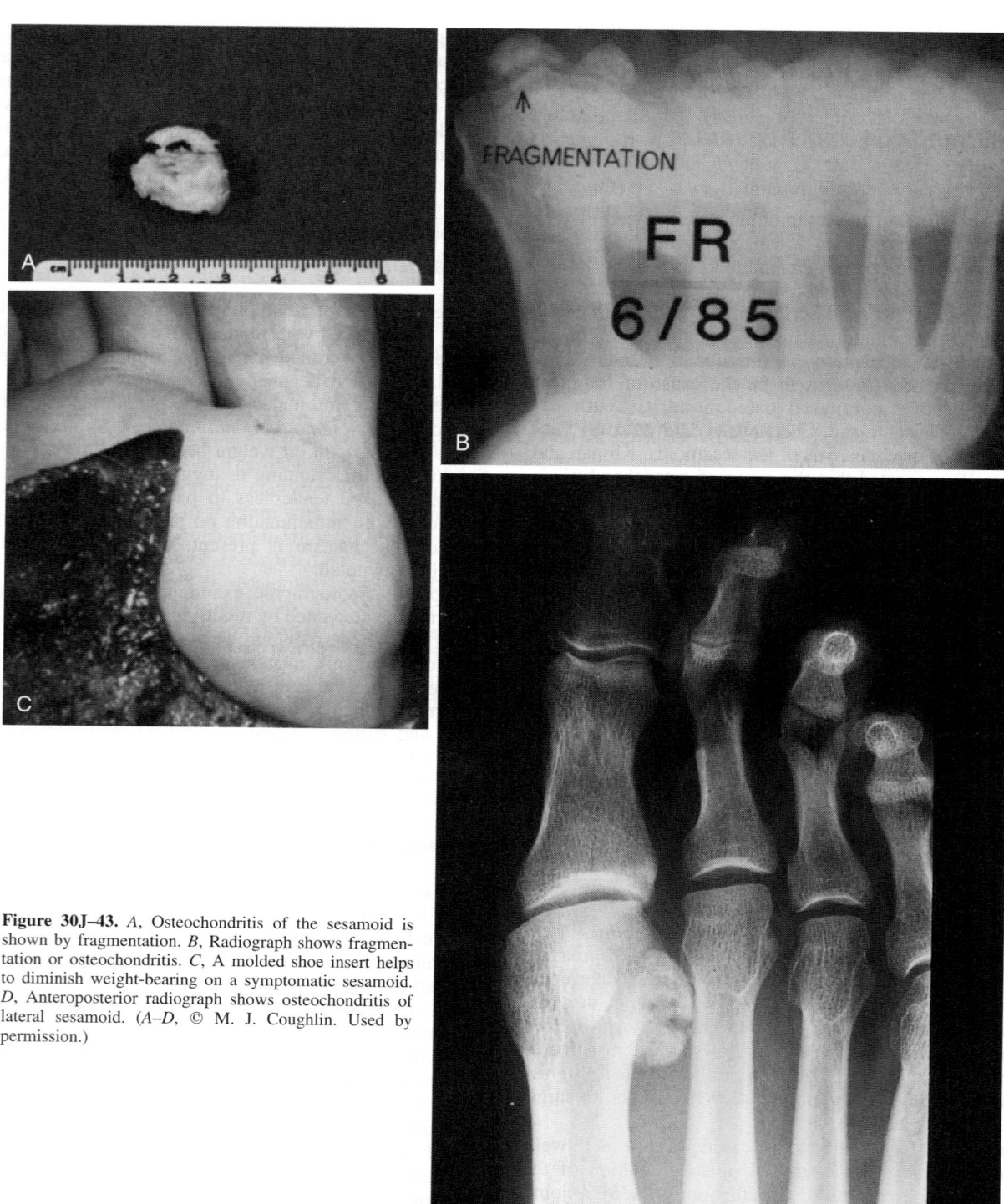

Figure 30J–43. *A*, Osteochondritis of the sesamoid is shown by fragmentation. *B*, Radiograph shows fragmentation or osteochondritis. *C*, A molded shoe insert helps to diminish weight-bearing on a symptomatic sesamoid. *D*, Anteroposterior radiograph shows osteochondritis of lateral sesamoid. (*A–D*, © M. J. Coughlin. Used by permission.)

running and implementing other aerobic activity may diminish symptoms. Decreasing the heel height of shoes may diminish pressure over the sesamoids. When a fracture has developed, a wooden-soled shoe, stiff sandal, or below-knee walking cast can be used. A molded insole or a metatarsal arch support is helpful in decreasing plantar

pressure in the sesamoid region for treatment of a fracture, sesamoiditis, or osteonecrosis. This type of support also may relieve the pressure of an IPK.

Taping the hallux into a neutral position may decrease MTP joint dorsiflexion and help to minimize discomfort (Fig. 30J–46). Although NSAIDs may be beneficial, the

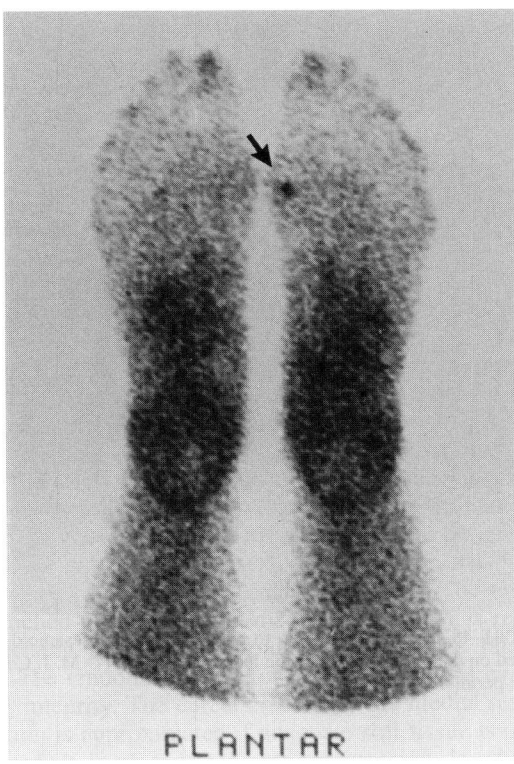

Figure 30J–44. The *arrow* marks increased uptake in the medial sesamoid consistent with osteochondritis.

use of intra-articular steroid injections should be infrequent. A steroid injection may help when there is localized inflammation or when sesamoiditis has occurred; however, in the presence of a fracture or osteonecrosis, intra-articular injection is contraindicated.

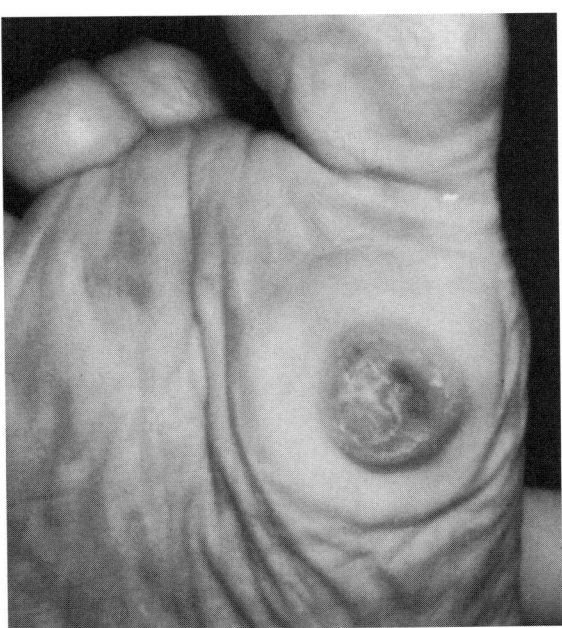

Figure 30J–45. An intractable plantar keratosis may develop beneath the tibial sesamoid. (© M. J. Coughlin. Used by permission.)

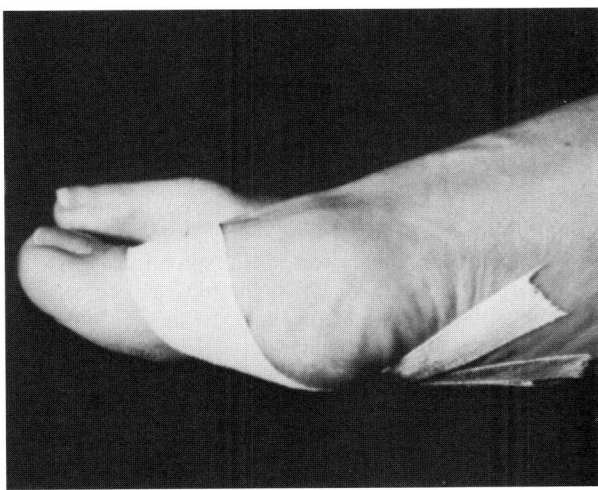

Figure 30J–46. Taping of the hallux minimizes dorsiflexion and may relieve symptoms. (© M. J. Coughlin. Used by permission.)

Surgical Excision

If conservative treatment has been unsuccessful, surgical excision of the chronically painful sesamoid is advocated.* Scranton and Rutkowski[152] and Speed[154] described excision of both sesamoids. Scranton[89] advised a reapproximation of the surgical defect to minimize postoperative disability. Helal[123] and Inge and Ferguson[128] cautioned against combined medial and lateral sesamoid excision because postoperative clawing of the hallux may occur with dual sesamoid excision. Jahss[129] recommended repair of the defect in the flexor hallucis brevis after dual sesamoid excision on the theory that it was comparable to repairing the quadriceps mechanism after patellectomy. Occasionally, dual sesamoidectomy may be necessary (i.e., with infection); elective dual sesamoidectomy should be avoided because a claw-toe deformity may occur.

Depending on which sesamoid is to be resected, various surgical approaches are available. The lateral or fibular sesamoid is approached through either a dorsal or a plantar approach. Mann and Coughlin[138] advocated a dorsal lateral approach to resect the fibular sesamoid in patients with hallux valgus; they recommended this approach for isolated fibular sesamoid excision also.[139] Inge and Ferguson[128] and others[135, 143] recommended a dorsal approach to avoid a painful plantar scar as well as injury to the plantar sensory nerve in the first interspace. Van Hal and colleagues,[156] Helal,[123] and Jahss[129] recommended a longitudinal plantar incision adjacent to the fibular sesamoid. Jahss[129] found a dorsal approach for a sesamoidectomy difficult. If one wishes to approximate the surgical defect, a plantar approach is necessary. The medial sesamoid may be resected by either a plantar medial incision[123, 156] or a direct medial incision.[128, 129, 135, 151] Kliman and associates[135] advocated a direct medial approach to avoid the plantar digital nerves, which may be in close proximity to the surgical dissection through a medial plantar approach. Mann and coworkers[139]

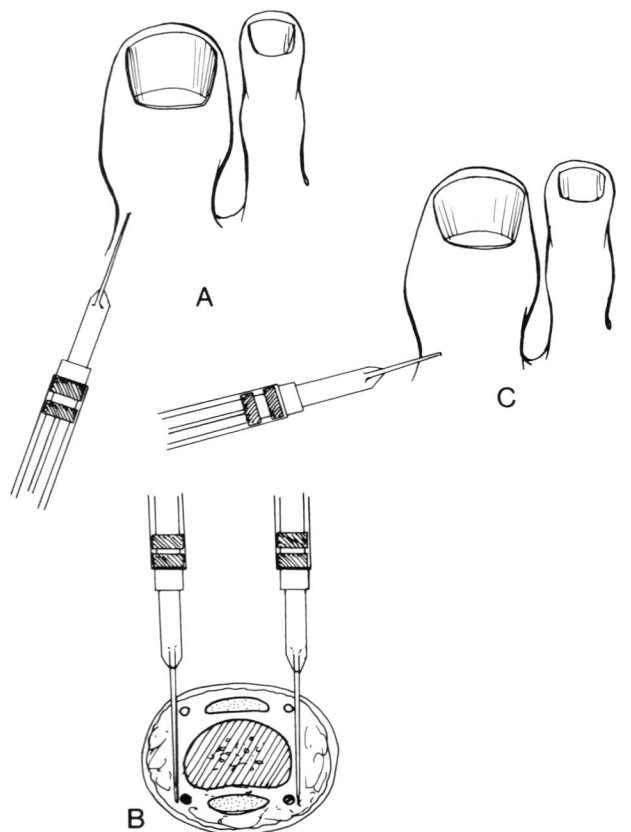

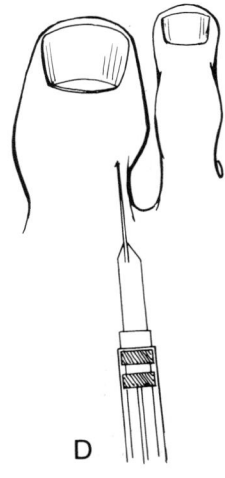

Figure 30J–54. Digital block of great toe. *A*, Injection of medial aspect of toe. *B*, Vertical injection techniques. *C*, The needle is turned in a horizontal direction. *D*, A final injection is used to anesthetize the lateral aspect of the toe.

dorsal medial aspect of the great toe at the base of the hallux, a small wheal (Fig. 30J–54A) is raised in the skin.[178] The needle is directed in a vertical fashion from the dorsal to the plantar surface (Fig. 30J–54B), anesthetizing the dorsal and plantar digital sensory nerves. Then the needle is turned horizontally (Fig. 30J–54C), and the dorsal aspect of the hallux is infiltrated. The needle is withdrawn and placed at the lateral base of the hallux (Fig. 30J–54D) for use in infiltration of the dorsolateral and dorsal plantar digital nerves.

Partial Nail Plate Avulsion. After an anesthetic block has been administered, the toe is prepared in a routine fashion. A ¼-inch Penrose drain may be used as a tourniquet if desired. The outer edge of the toenail plate is elevated proximally to the level of the cuticle (Fig. 30J–55A and B), then a scissors or small bone cutter is used to section the nail longitudinally (Fig. 30J–55C). Only the outer edge of the nail should be resected, taking care to remove as narrow a section of nail as possible (Fig. 30J–55D and E). The toe should be examined closely to ensure that no spike of the nail plate remains in the lateral nail fold because this would continue to incite a foreign body reaction. After removal of the nail edge, the acute or chronic infection often subsides. Antibiotics may be used depending on the severity of the infection.

Aftercare is important after a partial toenail avulsion. As the toenail regrows, the advancing edge is at risk for recurrent infection. A cotton wisp must be placed beneath the nail plate to elevate it as the edge grows distally. A digital block may be necessary to replace the initial pack-

ing. The patient is instructed in the packing procedure, and continues to perform the nail edge packing until the advancing nail edge has grown past the distal edge of the nail groove. Recurrence rate with subsequent infection after partial nail plate avulsion is 47% to 77%[174, 177] when further definitive care is deferred.

Complete Toenail Avulsion. When more extensive infection is present, a complete toenail avulsion may be necessary. A digital block is placed, and after the nail plate is elevated proximally (Fig. 30J–56A), the toenail is avulsed (Fig. 30J–56B and C). Although the procedure is associated with fairly brisk bleeding, a compression dressing usually can achieve rapid hemostasis. After 24 hours, the bandage is removed, and the foot is soaked in a tepid saltwater solution. The bandage is replaced and changed daily. Antibiotics may be prescribed depending on the severity of the infection. Re-epithelialization of the nail bed occurs in 2 to 3 weeks.[165] As the nail plate regrows, the advancing edges must be elevated, or an ingrown toenail can develop.[177] Murray[179] estimated that recurrent infection occurred in 64% of cases after the initial nail avulsion and in 86% of cases after the second toenail avulsion in the absence of definitive treatment. Although a toenail avulsion gives dramatic relief not only of an infection but also of symptoms, it has a poor long-term cure rate, and usually a second procedure is needed. Dixon[165] noted a much higher recurrence rate in patients in whom multiple avulsions of a single toenail have been performed. Lloyd-Davies and Brill[177] reported that within 6 months after nail avulsion, 31% of patients required further treat-

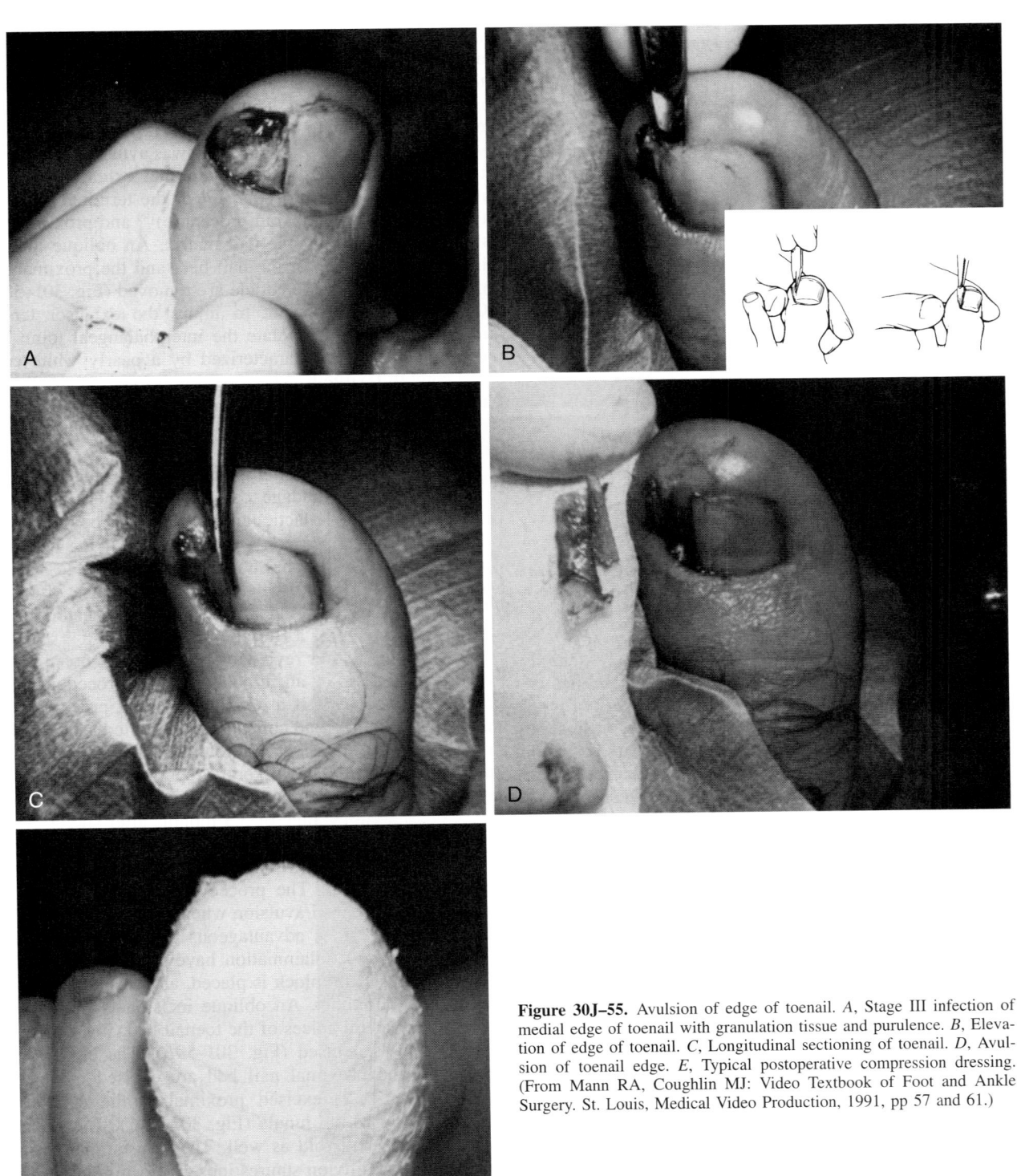

Figure 30J–55. Avulsion of edge of toenail. *A,* Stage III infection of medial edge of toenail with granulation tissue and purulence. *B,* Elevation of edge of toenail. *C,* Longitudinal sectioning of toenail. *D,* Avulsion of toenail edge. *E,* Typical postoperative compression dressing. (From Mann RA, Coughlin MJ: Video Textbook of Foot and Ankle Surgery. St. Louis, Medical Video Production, 1991, pp 57 and 61.)

ment. Palmer and Jones[181] reported a 70% recurrence rate after a nail plate avulsion.

Plastic Nail Wall Reduction. A plastic nail wall reduction is performed only after an acute infection has resolved following either successful conservative care or partial or complete toenail avulsion. This technique is used often in younger patients.[164, 165] After a digital anesthetic block, the toe is cleansed with an iodine solution. A Penrose drain is

Postoperative Management and Return to Sports Participation

Early mobilization of the foot after surgery limits postoperative stiffness and returns an athlete to activity sooner. Range-of-motion exercises of the toes and ankle should be carried out as soon as possible by the patient. Taping of the forefoot with a circumferential compression dressing protects the healing transverse metatarsal ligament, which is incised during surgery. The taping should be continued until adequate healing has occurred (this usually takes 3 to 6 weeks). Taping often can be performed by the patient. Sutures are removed 2 to 3 weeks after surgery, at which time physical therapy can be initiated. Whirlpool baths can be helpful in reducing edema. Range-of-motion exercises to the toes can be initiated early in the postoperative period.

Ambulation with full weight-bearing is allowed as soon as pain permits. Assistive devices such as crutches or a walker rarely are needed for younger patients. Instability with gait may necessitate temporary ambulatory aids in the older patient. Passive manipulation of the toes prevents restricted range of motion. General conditioning and aerobic exercises may be instituted as pain resolves and the wound heals.

Typically, a significant amount of fibrosis occurs at the site of surgery, and if this proves to be uncomfortable, aggressive massage may be used to relieve symptoms. A plantar metatarsal pad in the running shoe placed just proximal to the metatarsal head may provide comfort to the athlete during the postoperative period. Occasionally, an orthotic device may be needed; however, this is prescribed on an individual basis according to the patient's discomfort.

Author's Preferred Method of Treatment

When conservative methods fail to alleviate symptoms, surgical resection of a neuroma may be carried out. Injections of 1% lidocaine hydrochloride are helpful in identifying the location of the symptomatic neuroma. A dorsal approach is preferable for primary and secondary neuromas because (1) it avoids the possibility of a painful plantar scar, which may be the source of intractable postoperative pain, and (2) it can be extended should other web space pathology be identified.

Another source of web space pain may be second or third MTP joint capsular degeneration or disruption.[220, 221, 224, 225] Nonspecific synovitis can be a cause of ill-defined forefoot pain. A dorsal approach allows exploration of the dorsal aspect of the MTP joint should pathologic changes be shown. Likewise, when recurrent pain occurs after previous neurectomy, the possibility of MTP joint involvement makes a dorsal approach advantageous not only for exploring the intermetatarsal space but also for evaluating the adjacent MTP joint space.

INTRACTABLE PLANTAR KERATOSES

An IPK is a localized callosity occurring on the plantar aspect of the foot.[284] In contrast to diffuse callosities associated with systemic arthritides (e.g., rheumatoid arthritis or psoriatic arthritis), an isolated IPK typically develops beneath one or two metatarsal heads owing to increased pressure. The differential diagnosis of an isolated plantar keratotic lesion includes[286] (1) verrucae plantaris (Fig. 30J–73); (2) a small, well-circumscribed seed corn; (3) diffuse callus formation (Fig. 30J–74); (4) discrete, well-localized callus formation (Fig. 30J–75); (5) epidermal cysts; and (6) blistering or ulceration due to vascular insufficiency. Often a diagnosis of a plantar wart is made when in fact the cause may be one of the other disorders.[275] Because treatment of each lesion varies significantly, establishing a correct diagnosis is essential.

Plantar keratoses result from mechanical irritation, and it is normal for a moderate amount of callus to form, especially in individuals who are active in athletics. A callus indicates the presence of excess pressure. Typically, in these individuals, a broad, generalized callus develops in the forefoot region. In contrast, an IPK is a well-localized keratotic lesion. An IPK may occur as a small core (or seed corn) with a keratotic buildup around the periphery, as a well-circumscribed lesion (<1 cm in size), or as a broad diffuse lesion (>1 cm in size).

Plantar callus formation can result from many causes. High-fashion footwear can lead to increased pressure beneath symptomatic metatarsal heads. A hyperextension deformity of the MTP joint leads to buckling of the toe that can cause increased pressure beneath the metatarsal head.[266, 271, 273, 287, 288, 291]

Anatomy

Anatomic abnormalities can lead to callus formation. A plantar-flexed metatarsal (Fig. 30J–76),[281, 291] an elongated metatarsal in relation to adjacent metatarsals,[281, 284, 285] and a malunion of a metatarsal after fracture[281] all can lead to increased pressure beneath a metatarsal with subsequent callus formation. Positional deformities, such as forefoot equinus, a cavus midfoot deformity (Fig. 30J–77) coupled with a rigid forefoot, or a rotary deformity of the midfoot,[281] can lead to malalignment manifested by increased pressure beneath one or more metatarsal heads. Jahss[281] noted that fixed forefoot varus can lead to the development of callosities beneath the plantar aspect of the fifth ray. Jahss[281] noted that minor physiologic variations in the athlete can lead to development of IPKs as a result of the summation of repeated stresses that are involved with particular sporting activities. Varus or valgus malalignment of the forefoot or hindfoot can result in increased pressure

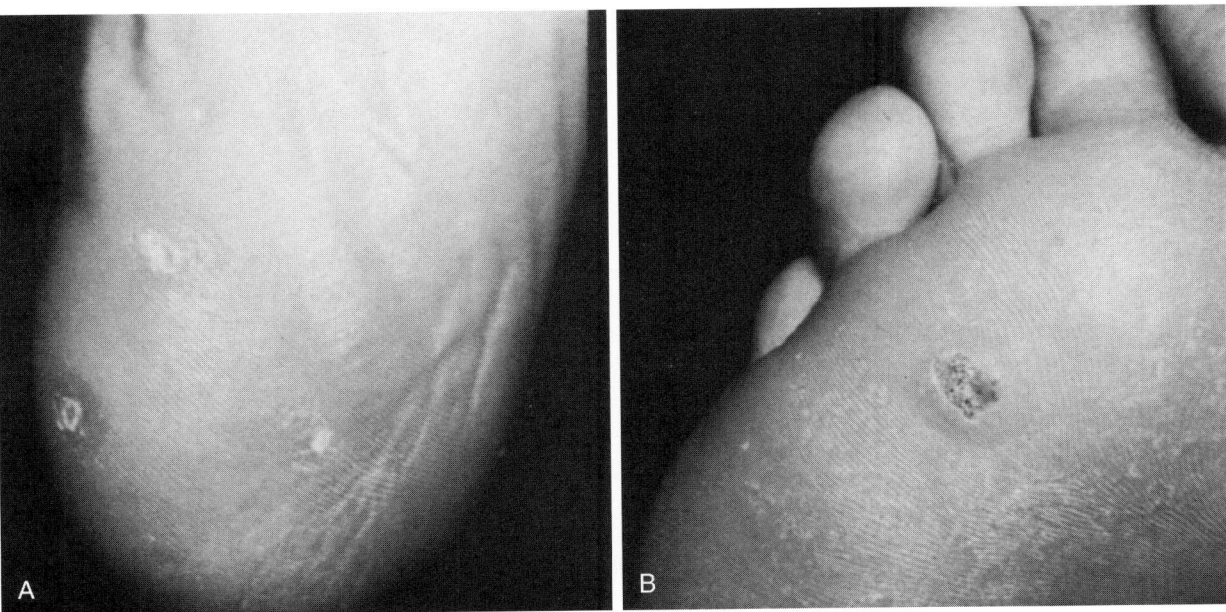

Figure 30J–73. *A,* Verruca plantaris, or wart. Warts usually are located in areas other than beneath the metatarsal head (e.g., heel region). *B,* Wart beneath the third metatarsal head. (*A,* © M. J. Coughlin. Used by permission; *B,* From Mann RA, Coughlin MJ: Video Textbook of Foot and Ankle Surgery. St. Louis, Medical Video Production, 1991, p 86.)

beneath specific metatarsals, leading to development of plantar keratoses. The repetitive stresses of athletic activity such as running, jogging, and walking may increase mechanical irritation to vulnerable areas, leading to increased symptoms.

Biomechanics

The first, fourth, and fifth metatarsal-tarsal articulations allow considerable flexibility compared with the second and third metatarsal-tarsal articulations, which are fairly rigid.[281] Reduced flexibility in the middle rays can increase

susceptibility to pressure buildup beneath the metatarsal heads. The length of individual metatarsals is variable, but in some situations an abnormally long second metatarsal (Fig. 30J–78) or second and third metatarsals subject a forefoot to increased weight-bearing, which may lead to symptoms of increased pressure.[265, 269, 273]

Midfoot flexibility and alignment can have a consider-

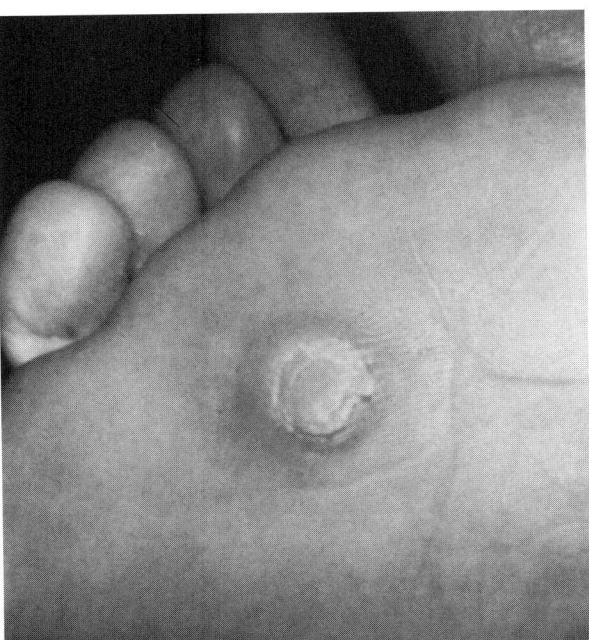

Figure 30J–75. A well-circumscribed intractable plantar keratosis resulting from a prominent fibular condyle. (From Mann RA, Coughlin MJ: Video Textbook of Foot and Ankle Surgery. St. Louis, Medical Video Production, 1991, p 86.)

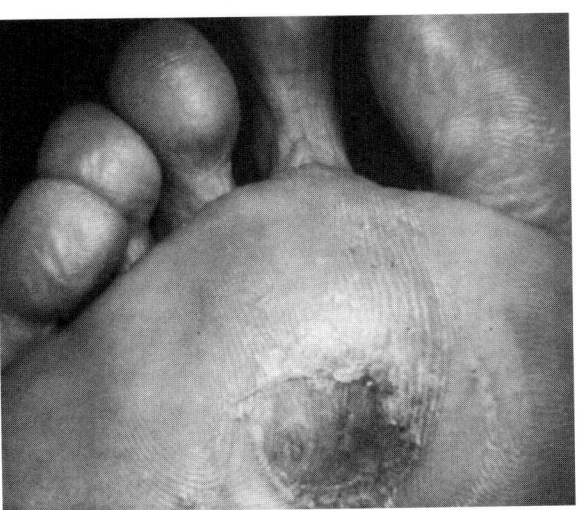

Figure 30J–74. Diffuse plantar keratosis. (© M. J. Coughlin. Used by permission.)

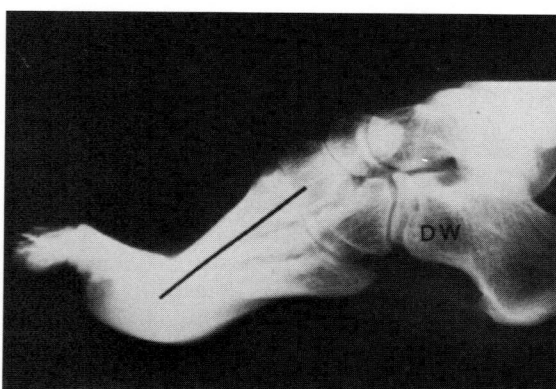

Figure 30J–76. Plantar-flexed first metatarsal. (© M. J. Coughlin. Used by permission.)

able effect on the distal metatarsals, whereas a pes planus configuration presents a flexible forefoot that rarely is associated with plantar keratoses. A cavus midfoot is characterized by decreased flexibility and is associated with a higher incidence of plantar keratoses.[281] A rotary midfoot deformity (Fig. 30J–79) can be characterized by either varus or valgus malalignment. A varus abnormality is characterized by increased pressure on the fifth ray, whereas a valgus malalignment is characterized by increased pressure beneath the first ray. Forefoot equinus can occur without a significant hindfoot deformity, presenting as a more rigid

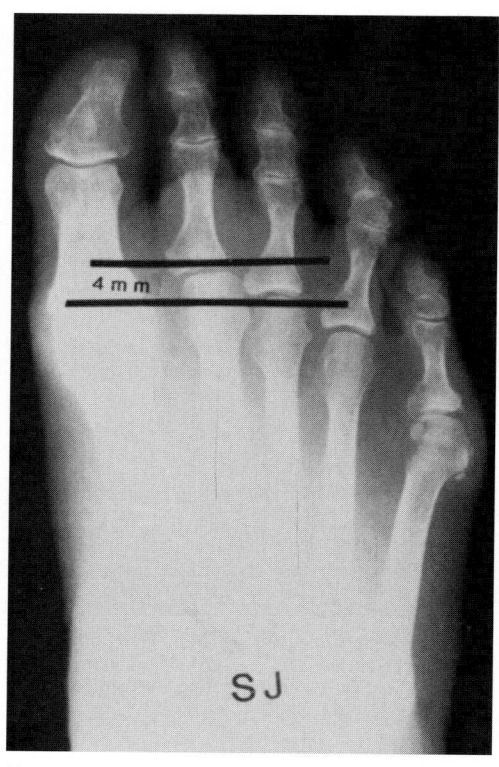

Figure 30J–78. A long second metatarsal may lead to increased callus formation. (© M. J. Coughlin. Used by permission.)

forefoot that is less resistant to pressure beneath the metatarsal heads.

In differentiating a true wart from an IPK, there are significant differences not only in the cutaneous presentation but also in location. Typically, an IPK is located under the weight-bearing part of the forefoot beneath the metatarsal heads.[275] A wart rarely is located under a meta-

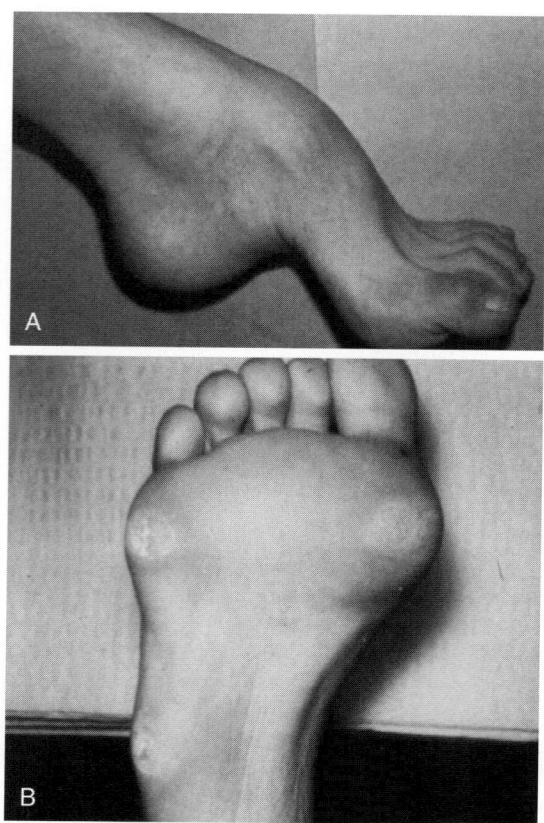

Figure 30J–77. *A* and *B*, A cavus deformity may lead to multiple areas of callus formation. (© M. J. Coughlin. Used by permission.)

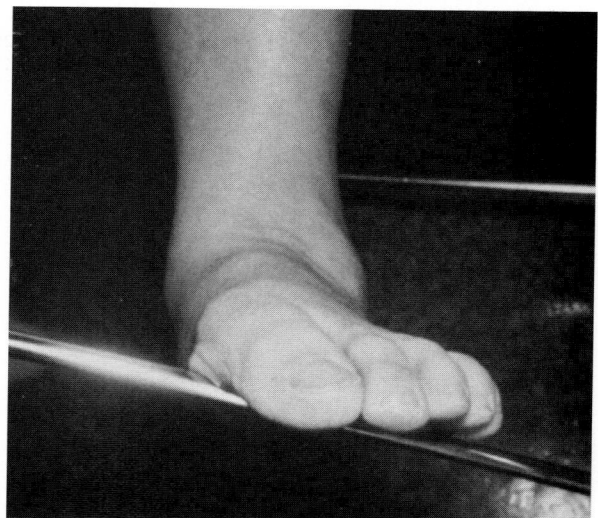

Figure 30J–79. A rotary midfoot deformity may subject the lateral border of the foot to callus formation. A varus deformity of the forefoot with a fixed hindfoot deformity is shown. (© M. J. Coughlin. Used by permission.)

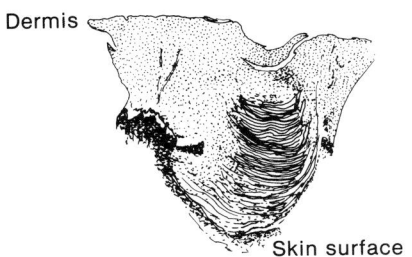

Microscopic section of callus
(compression of subdermal
lining epithelium)

Figure 30J–80. Cross section of intractable plantar keratosis.

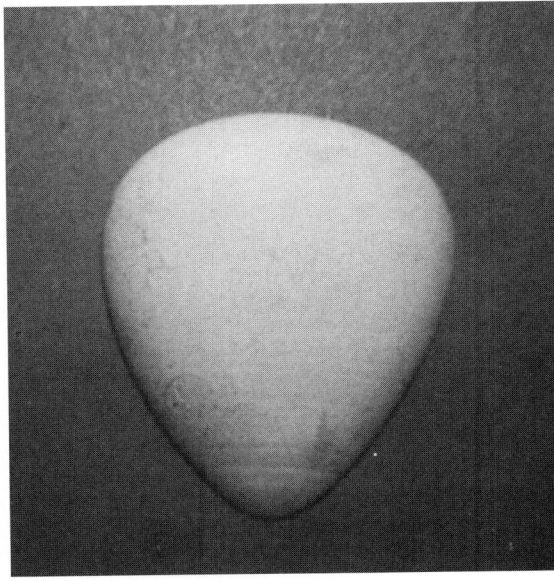

Figure 30J–82. A small metatarsal pad may be placed just proximal to the keratosis to redistribute the pressure. (© M. J. Coughlin. Used by permission.)

tarsal head and is more likely to be seen under other areas on the plantar aspect of the foot. When an IPK is trimmed, a small, pearl-gray avascular core is noted (Fig. 30J–80). This keratotic core is a buildup of the plantar callosity that invaginates owing to localized pressure beneath the metatarsal head. A wart is a well-localized lesion with sharp margins. When shaved, it bleeds vigorously because of the end arterioles that are present in the lesion (Fig. 30J–81).

Treatment Options

Conservative Treatment

The initial treatment of an IPK involves trimming the lesion to reduce the keratotic buildup. The keratotic center of a callus is delineated as it is shaved. This keratosis is a typical response to increased pressure; with time, the lesion invaginates slowly, and the keratosis increases in depth. As it deepens, it typically becomes more symptomatic. Frequently, it is not possible to trim a keratotic lesion completely in a single office visit; it may be necessary for a patient to return for subsequent visits to reduce the callus further.[284] As the keratotic core becomes more superficial, it typically becomes less symptomatic. A patient can be instructed in the technique of shaving a callosity and in time may be able to provide symptomatic care himself or herself. Trimming a callus may help in differentiating it from a wart. As the wart is shaved, small punctate arterioles characteristic of this lesion become apparent. An IPK has

an avascular central area, and further trimming does not uncover vascular structures. A seed corn has a well-differentiated keratotic core, usually 1 to 2 mm in size, and usually responds well to trimming or curettage.[284]

When the callus has been trimmed, a soft metatarsal pad (Fig. 30J–82) is placed proximal to the keratosis to redistribute the pressure more uniformly. Jahss[281] recommended relieving the pressure on areas of excess weight-bearing and increasing pressure on areas of too little weight-bearing. The use of a soft insole (Fig. 30J–83)[279] may alleviate the pressure further in athletes. Athletic

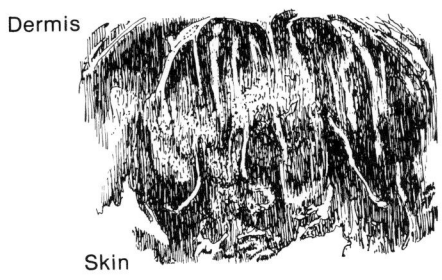

Microscopic section of wart—
mushrooming of entire epidermis

Figure 30J–81. Cross section of a wart.

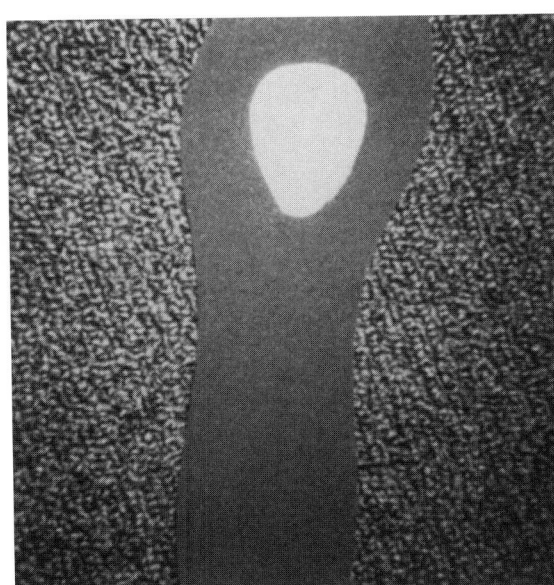

Figure 30J–83. A soft insole may be used to decrease the pressure in the forefoot region. (© M. J. Coughlin. Used by permission.)

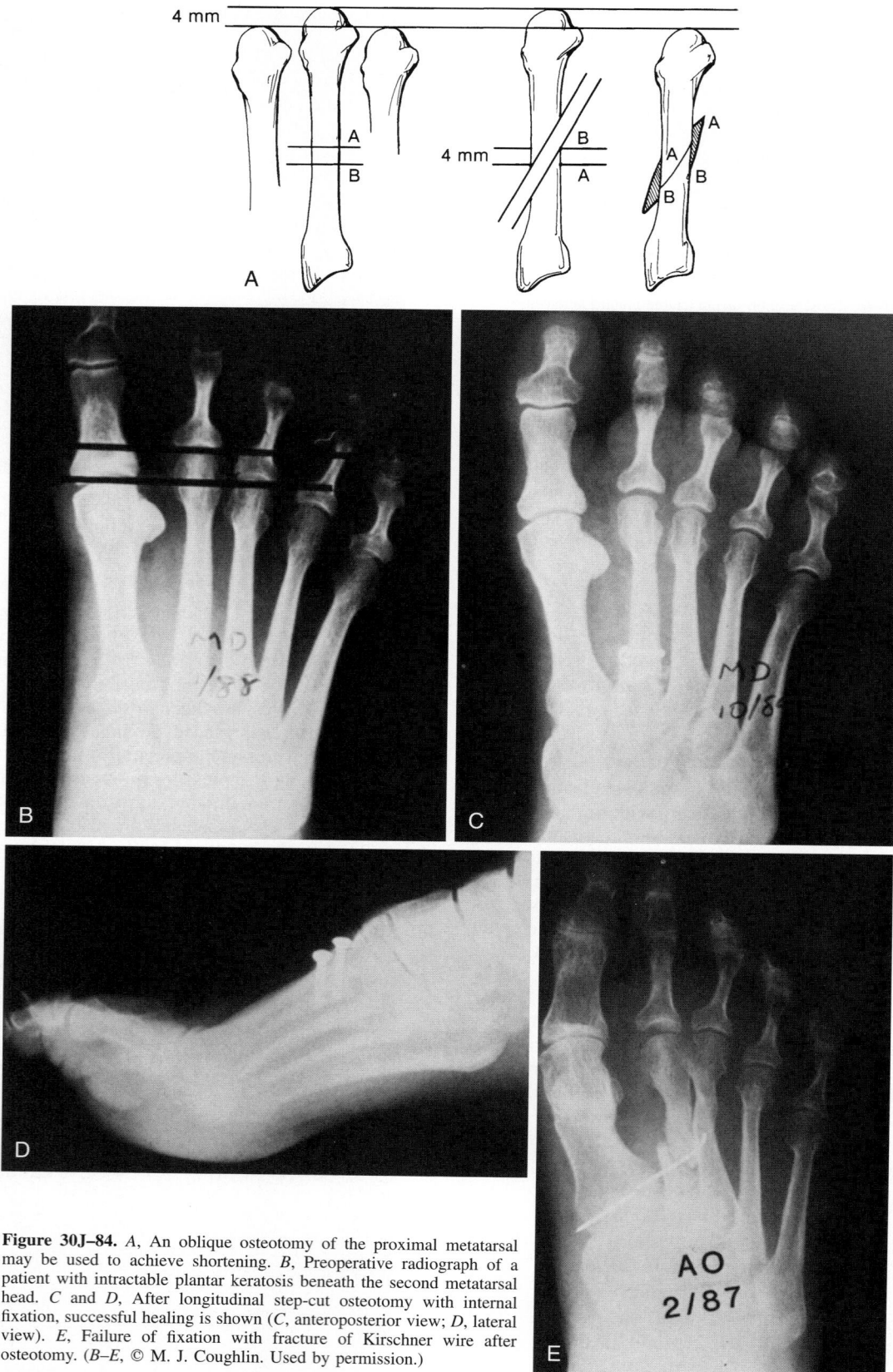

Figure 30J–84. *A,* An oblique osteotomy of the proximal metatarsal may be used to achieve shortening. *B,* Preoperative radiograph of a patient with intractable plantar keratosis beneath the second metatarsal head. *C* and *D,* After longitudinal step-cut osteotomy with internal fixation, successful healing is shown (*C,* anteroposterior view; *D,* lateral view). *E,* Failure of fixation with fracture of Kirschner wire after osteotomy. (*B–E,* © M. J. Coughlin. Used by permission.)

shoewear that provides a wide toe box and a soft sole to lessen impact when running should be selected.

When varus or valgus malalignment of the forefoot or hindfoot results in subsequent development of an IPK, appropriate orthotic devices may be selected to compensate for the malalignment and to redistribute weight-bearing forces beneath the metatarsal head. A Plastizote orthosis of medium or high density can be fabricated to relieve pressure beneath the IPK as well as to provide correction for a postural deformity.

If a keratotic lesion continues to be symptomatic and significantly impairs athletic function, surgical intervention may be contemplated. Because of the lengthy postoperative recovery time, the possibility of restricted MTP motion, and the possibility of recurrence of a lesion or development of a transfer lesion, a rigorous trial of trimming, padding, and orthotic management should be carried out before surgery is performed.

Surgical Treatment

IPKs beneath the second, third, and fourth metatarsal heads usually are classified as large, diffuse plantar keratoses or small, discrete keratoses. Differentiating between these two lesions is important to institute proper treatment.

Large, Diffuse Intractable Plantar Keratoses

A large, diffuse IPK often is associated with a long or plantar-flexed metatarsal. Although the second and third metatarsals are the most common sites of occurrence,[275] the other metatarsals occasionally are involved. Typically, these lesions are 1 to 2 cm in size and do not have an invaginated keratotic core. Giannestras[275] described a step-cut proximal metatarsal osteotomy that was used to decrease the length of a symptomatic metatarsal. Forty patients underwent metatarsal osteotomy to diminish the overall length. Giannestras[275] reported the occurrence of a transfer lesion in 10% of the patients in his series.

Mann[284, 286] suggested the use of an oblique longitudinal osteotomy (Fig. 30J–84A) rather than a step-cut osteotomy to shorten the elongated metatarsal. A longitudinal dorsal incision is used to expose the proximal metatarsal shaft. Care is taken to avoid the superficial sensory nerves. After a subperiosteal dissection, transverse marks are made on the proximal metatarsal diaphysis to indicate the amount of shortening desired. Preoperative radiographs are used to determine the appropriate amount of shortening (usually 4 to 8 mm is necessary). A longitudinal oblique osteotomy is carried out with a sagittal saw, and the metatarsal is allowed to shorten. The metatarsal is internally fixed with minifragment compression screws (Fig. 30J–84B and C), wire sutures, or Kirschner wires. Rigid internal fixation of the osteotomy helps to prevent angulation (Fig. 30J–84D) at the osteotomy site and promotes a more rapid union. Excess plantar flexion or dorsiflexion at the osteotomy site should be avoided. After routine skin closure, a compression dressing is applied. The patient is allowed to ambulate in a postoperative shoe until the osteotomy site has healed

(usually in 6 to 8 weeks). If a patient is unreliable, cast immobilization may be used.

Giannestras[275] reported development of transfer lesions in 10% of patients postoperatively. Mann[285] reported a 5% rate of transfer lesions. Delayed union occasionally occurs; however, with time, successful healing usually occurs.

A dorsal closing wedge osteotomy of the proximal metatarsal may be used to lessen the pressure beneath a metatarsal head. Through a similar dorsal longitudinal incision, the proximal metatarsal metaphysis is exposed. A small needle-nosed rongeur is used to remove a thin (approximately 2 mm) dorsal wedge. Alternatively, a power saw can be used to remove a thin dorsal wedge. Internal fixation with a wire suture, Kirschner wires, or a compression screw may be used. After routine skin closure, a compression dressing is applied. The patient is allowed to ambulate in a postoperative shoe, although a short-leg walking cast may be employed instead.

Small, Discrete Intractable Plantar Keratoses

A small, discrete IPK may develop. Mann and Du-Vries[288] proposed that this lesion is caused by a prominent fibular condyle on the plantar aspect of the metatarsal head. A discrete callus may develop after a metatarsal head fracture with a plantar flexion deformity, and it may be associated with a hyperextended MTP joint, leading to buckling of a toe with a plantar-flexed metatarsal. This type of lesion may be associated with an idiopathic plantar-flexed metatarsal. When conservative treatment has been unsuccessful, surgical intervention can be considered. DuVries[274] initially described a plantar condylectomy to correct this deformity. This procedure was later modified by Mann and DuVries,[288] who performed an MTP arthroplasty along with the plantar condylectomy (Fig. 30J–85).

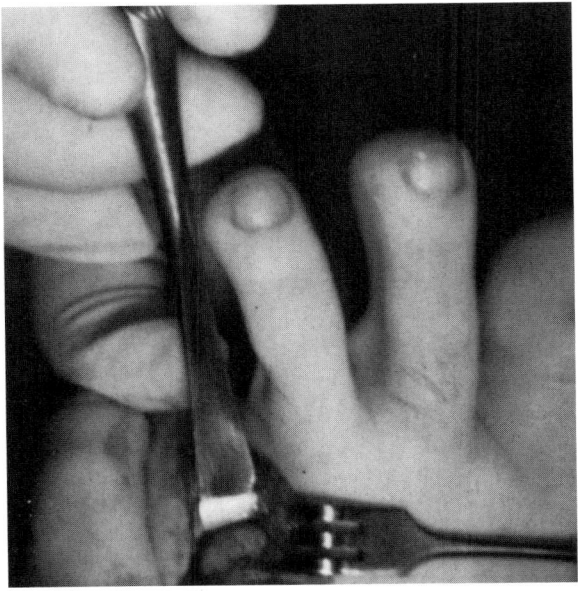

Figure 30J–85. Condylectomy for isolated intractable plantar keratosis. (© M. J. Coughlin. Used by permission.)

shortening. Based proximally, this metaphyseal osteotomy is oriented in a vertical direction. The osteotomy site is freed up, and the metatarsal head is elevated approximately 3 mm. It is believed that elevation of about 3 mm is necessary for adequate decrease of pressure beneath the symptomatic metatarsal head.[272] The osteotomy is fixed with a 0.045 Kirschner wire introduced through a separate puncture wound. The skin is closed in a routine fashion, and the patient is allowed to ambulate in a wooden-soled shoe. The Kirschner wire is removed 3 weeks after surgery, and the MTP joint is manipulated gently at this time.

Results and Complications

Helal,[277, 278] in describing the oblique distal metatarsal osteotomy, noted that the purpose was to elevate the metatarsal head and to reduce length (Fig. 30J–89). Although in his initial report, Helal[277] did not note specific complications, in a retrospective review of 310 patients (508 feet), 84% were noted to have no pain, and 8% recurrence of plantar callosities was noted (Fig. 30J–90).[278] Winson and coworkers[294] reported on 94 patients (124 feet) who underwent a similar procedure. In their report, 53% of the patients had significant postoperative symptoms, including transfer lesions in 32%, nonunion in 13%, and an overall recurrence of an IPK in 50% of patients. In 66 of the 124 feet, major complaints were noted postoperatively. Winson and coworkers[294] stressed that in either a cavus or a rigid foot, a distal oblique sliding osteotomy was contraindicated. Winson and coworkers[294] agreed with Giannestras[275] that the presence of a contracture at the MTP joint was a further contraindication to a metatarsal osteotomy (Fig. 30J–91). Pedowitz,[290] in a report on 69 distal oblique oste-

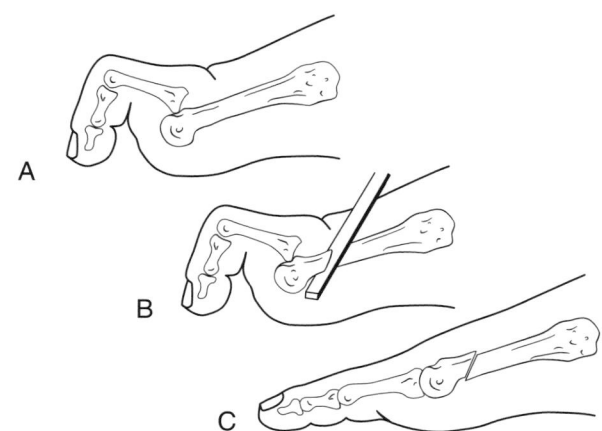

Figure 30J–90. Technique of Helal osteotomy. *A*, Dislocated metatarsophalangeal joint. *B*, Distal oblique osteotomy. *C*, The distal fragment has displaced dorsally and proximally. No internal fixation is used after the osteotomy.

otomies in 49 patients, reported good results in 83% of cases. Pedowitz[290] reported a 27% incidence of either residual callosity or transfer lesion. There were two nonunions in his series. Pedowitz[290] stressed that this procedure was contraindicated in patients who had a fixed MTP joint deformity. Idusuyi and associates,[280] in a report on 20 patients (23 feet) who had single osteotomies of the second, third, or fourth metatarsals without internal fixation, noted a 20% reoperation rate for recurrent plantar callosities. Of these patients, 65% were limited with footwear choices or required a shoe insert. Of 23 feet, 13 (56%) were rated as poor or fair, and the authors had significant reservations about recommending this procedure (Fig. 30J–92).

Trnka and colleagues,[292] in a comparison of the results

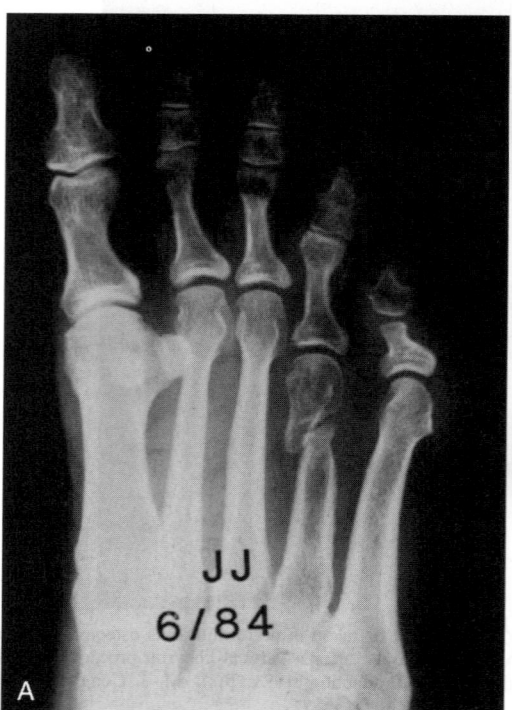

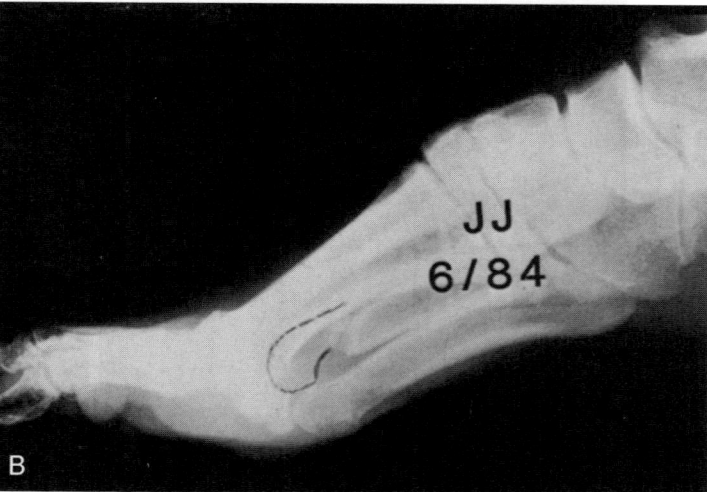

Figure 30J–89. *A* and *B*, Distal oblique osteotomy. Care must be taken to achieve a bony union. After a distal oblique osteotomy, this patient developed nonunion. (© M. J. Coughlin. Used by permission.)

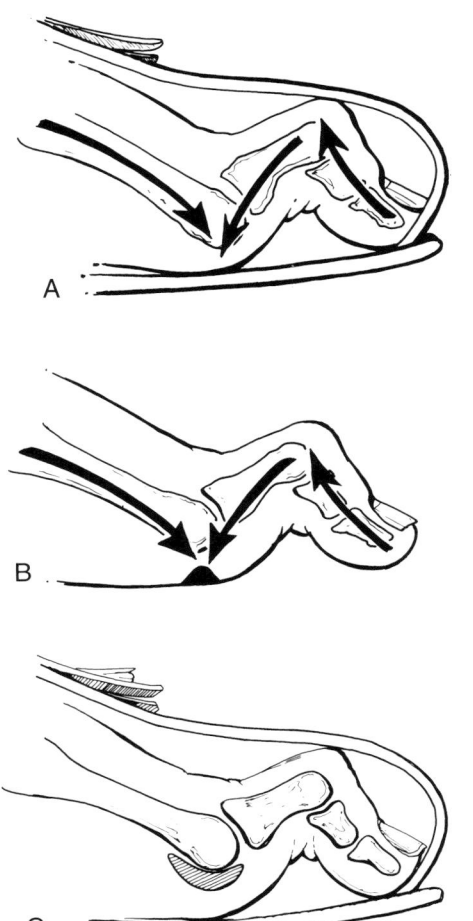

Figure 30J–91. *A–C,* A contracture of the metatarsophalangeal joint may lead to hammer toe formation and development of intractable plantar keratosis beneath the involved metatarsal head.

of an intra-articular capital oblique osteotomy (Weil type) and a distal oblique osteotomy (Helal type), reported a high level of satisfaction and a lower incidence of recurrent metatarsalgia in transfer lesions with the capital oblique osteotomy (Fig. 30J–93). No transfer lesions were noted with the capital oblique osteotomy, whereas 41 feet with an Helal-type osteotomy developed transfer lesions. Five

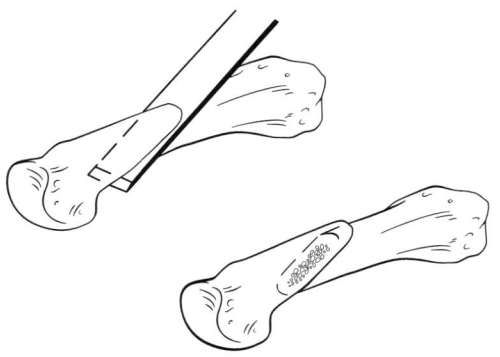

Figure 30J–92. Technique of oblique lesser metatarsal osteotomy showing dorsal displacement. *Top,* Preoperatively. *Bottom,* After osteotomy.

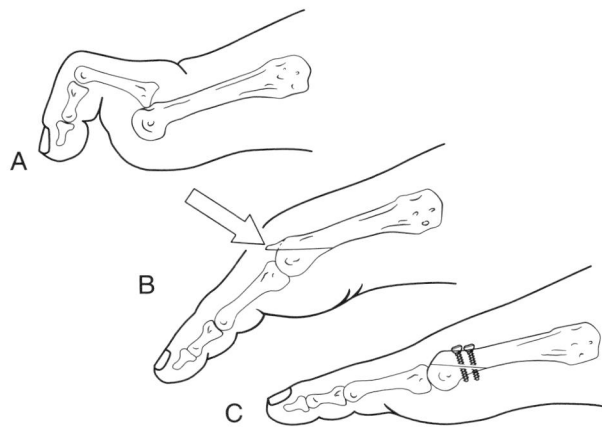

Figure 30J–93. *A,* Preoperative diagram shows dislocated lesser metatarsophalangeal joint. *B,* Technique of capital oblique osteotomy allows shortening but not plantar flexion. *C,* After internal fixation and resection of the dorsal flare, the lesser metatarsophalangeal joint has been reduced.

malunions and three pseudarthroses occurred in the 15 cases that underwent the Helal-type osteotomy compared with no malunions or pseudarthroses in the Weil-type group. Trnka and colleagues[292] concluded that the Weil-type osteotomy was a satisfactory method for treating metatarsalgia, but because of the high complication rate, the Helal-type osteotomy was not an acceptable procedure.

Metatarsal head resection should be avoided[281] because it tends to concentrate pressure beneath the remaining metatarsal head. Recurrence of callus formation in the form of a transfer lesion is inevitable.

Occasionally, an IPK may develop beneath a hallucal sesamoid.[289, 293] Mann and Wapner[289] reported on the results in 12 patients and noted 58% had excellent results with no recurrence, and 33% of patients had good results with slight recurrence of a plantar callosity. Van Enoo and Cane[293] reported on 17 tibial sesamoid shavings with an average 4-year follow-up. In two of the feet, a mild recurrent callosity developed postoperatively. A broad, diffuse callus may be associated with a plantar-flexed first metatarsal, whereas a discrete lesion is associated most commonly with a prominent sesamoid. When conservative treatment is unsuccessful, a plantar-flexed first metatarsal may be treated with a dorsal-based closing wedge osteotomy of the proximal first metatarsal. Discrete IPKs may be treated by sesamoid shaving or, more infrequently, with sesamoid excision (see earlier section on sesamoid dysfunction).

Although delayed union or nonunion is possible with the use of a proximal dorsal closing wedge osteotomy for an IPK, the location of this osteotomy in the metaphysis of the involved metatarsal usually allows fairly rapid healing. A transfer lesion may develop if an excess amount of bone is resected, and an IPK may recur if too little bone has been resected. Mann[285] reserved this osteotomy for recurrent lesions after failure of a longitudinal oblique osteotomy.

Although Hatcher and colleagues[276] advocated multiple metatarsal osteotomies as a method of reducing the occurrence of transfer lesions and the recurrence of plantar keratoses, Mann[285] and others[294] recommended an isolated osteotomy as a more reliable procedure. If two adjacent

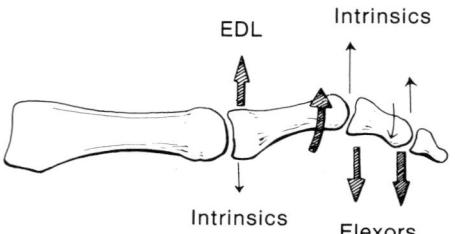

Figure 30J–96. At the various joints of the lesser toe, intrinsic and extrinsic muscles oppose each other. An obvious mismatch occurs between the larger intrinsic and the smaller intrinsic muscles, leaving two deformities. EDL, extensor digitorum longus.

and lumbricals. At the MTP joint and the interphalangeal joints, a mismatch occurs (Fig. 30J–96) in which the more powerful extrinsic muscles overpower the weaker intrinsic muscles.[303–305, 311] The position of the lesser toes is crucial in whether this mismatch leads to development of pathology. If the proximal phalanx is hyperextended, the extensor digitorum longus no longer assists in extending the proximal interphalangeal joint. If the MTP joint is in a relatively neutral position, the flexor digitorum longus helps to flex the MTP joint. As a chronic hyperextension deformity develops, the extensor digitorum longus loses its tenodesing effect on the interphalangeal joints, and the long and short flexors come under increased tension, increasing the flexion deformity at the interphalangeal joints. The weaker interossei and lumbricals are overpowered easily by the flexors of the interphalangeal joints, and the intrinsic muscles are overpowered at the MTP joint by the long and short extensor tendons.[303, 311, 333]

Hammer Toes

A hammer toe is a plantar flexion contracture of the proximal interphalangeal joint[303, 304, 310, 322] and frequently is associated with a hyperextension deformity of the MTP joint (Fig. 30J–97).[333] A hammer toe may vary from a fixed rigid deformity to a semiflexible or flexible deformity in which the toe can be corrected passively to a neutral position.[321] Hammer toes may occur in multiple toes, although most commonly they occur in the second toe.[310] A hammer toe is believed to be an acquired deformity. Although neuromuscular disease, degenerative disk disease, and connective tissue disorders may be associated with hammer toe development,[311, 312] the long-term use of fashionable footwear probably is the most common cause that leads to the development of progressive contractures of the lesser toes.[304, 305, 312, 321, 333]

Clinical Evaluation

The major complaint of a patient with a hammer toe deformity is discomfort over the dorsal aspect of the proximal interphalangeal joint where a callosity may develop as the toe buckles and strikes the top of the toe box (Fig. 30J–98).[321] On the plantar aspect of the foot, an IPK may

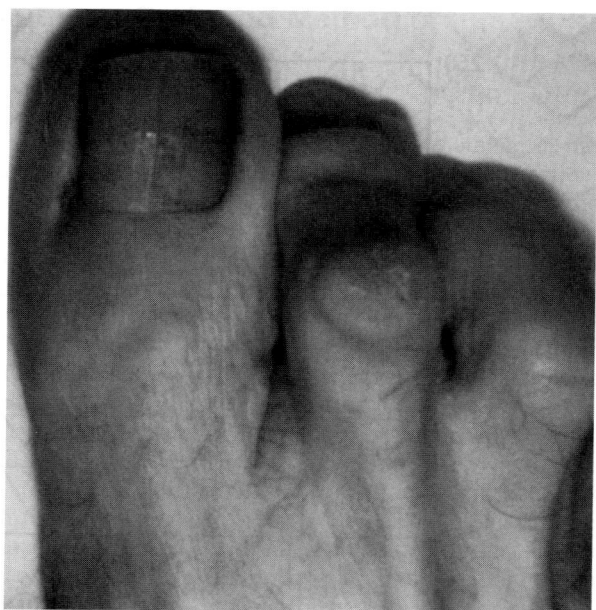

Figure 30J–97. Hammer toe deformity. (© M. J. Coughlin. Used by permission.)

develop beneath the metatarsal head owing to subluxation at the MTP joint.

The patient with a hammer toe deformity should be examined in a standing as well as a sitting position.[311, 321] The flexibility of the deformity is evaluated by passively manipulating the interphalangeal joint as well as the MTP joint. If a toe can be corrected passively to a neutral position, it is said to be a flexible hammer toe. If the toe cannot be corrected passively, it is defined as a rigid hammer toe deformity. The differentiation between these two entities is important in choosing the appropriate surgical treatment. With the patient in a standing position, the adjacent lesser toes are evaluated. If there is a contracture of the flexor digitorum longus, there also may be a flexion deformity of an adjacent toe. In this case, in addition to carrying out a hammer toe repair (Fig. 30J–99), a flexor tenotomy may be beneficial in the treatment of the hammer toe deformity.[304, 311]

It is important to evaluate the orientation of the MTP joint. The presence of subluxation or dislocation at this

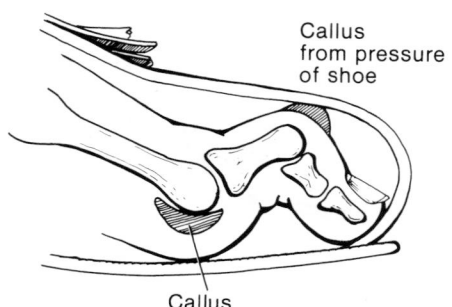

Figure 30J–98. Dorsal aspect of the proximal interphalangeal joint strikes the toe box, leading to callus formation. An intractable plantar keratosis may develop beneath the metatarsal head.

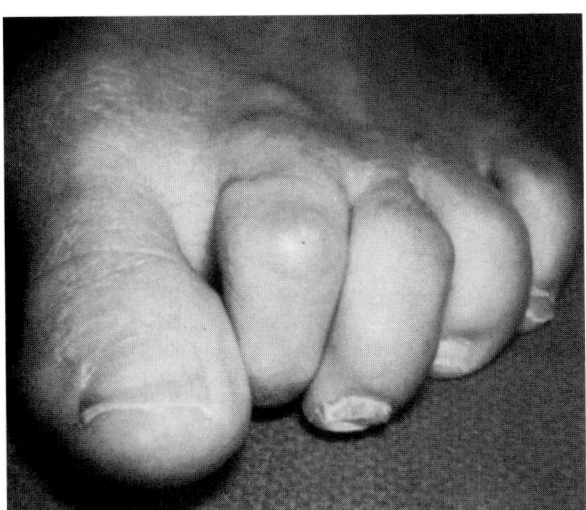

Figure 30J–99. Contracture of all the lesser toes may indicate a tightness of the flexor digitorum longus. (© M. J. Coughlin. Used by permission.)

joint may influence the treatment plan significantly. Subluxation and dislocation (Fig. 30J–100) may occur in a dorsal medial or lateral plane[301, 304, 307, 309]; the flexibility of any deformity of this joint must be assessed as well.

In the evaluation of lesser toe deformities, it is important to note the amount of space present between adjacent toes. Reduction of the interval between adjacent toes owing to deviation of adjacent lesser toes or to a concomitant hallux valgus deformity may diminish the space available for a lesser toe correction. This diminished space may require correction of an asymptomatic adjacent toe (i.e., hallux valgus or an adjacent lesser toe deformity).[311]

Radiographs of the forefoot are important in analyzing

a hammer toe deformity. The presence of subluxation or dislocation at the MTP joint is seen best on an AP radiograph, whereas evaluation of a hammer toe is carried out best with a lateral radiograph.

Treatment Options

Conservative Treatment

In the early stages of a hammer toe deformity, a flexible hammer toe may be treated with a roomy shoe with a low heel and an adequate toe box.[305, 321, 322] The deformity may be manipulated by the patient on a regular basis to maintain flexibility of the toe.[305, 311] An elevated toe box may eliminate dorsal pressure on the hammer toe at the level of the proximal interphalangeal joint.[311] When an IPK has developed, use of a soft insole or liner may decrease symptoms.[305, 311] Use of foam or viscoelastic padding over the hammer toe callosity or padding at the tip of a hammer toe where calluses have occurred (Fig. 30J–101) may relieve the pressure.[305] When a painful hammer toe does not respond to conservative care, surgical intervention may be considered. When a rigid deformity of the proximal interphalangeal joint is present, a proximal interphalangeal joint arthroplasty is carried out. When there is a flexible deformity of the proximal interphalangeal joint, a flexor tendon transfer is performed. An MTP joint abnormality[304] must be assessed in regard to the severity and rigidity of the deformity. Surgical correction must be performed at this level if a hammer toe repair is carried out, to prevent recurrence of deformity (Fig. 30J–102).[304]

Technique for a Rigid Hammer Toe Repair

An elliptical skin incision centered over the dorsal aspect of the proximal interphalangeal joint is used to excise

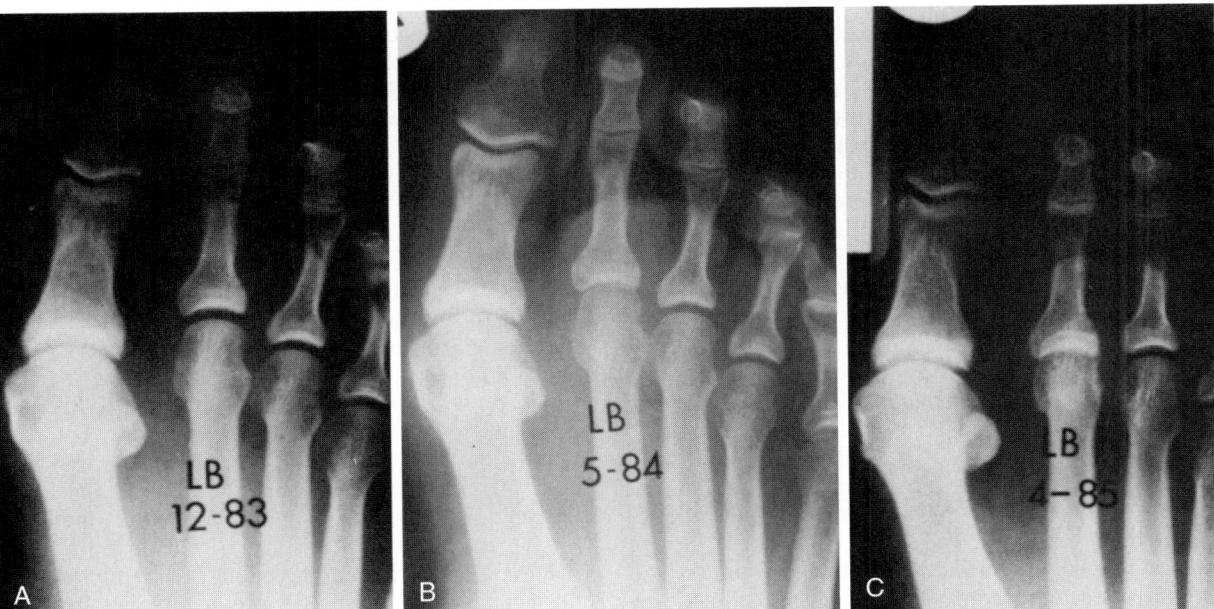

Figure 30J–100. *A–C*, Gradual subluxation of the metatarsophalangeal joint may occur. This tennis player developed subluxation and dislocation during a 5-year period. (*A*, From Coughlin MJ: Lesser toe deformities. Orthopaedics 10:65, 1987; *B*, from Coughlin MJ: Lesser toe deformities. In Mann RA, Coughlin MJ [eds]: Surgery of the Foot and Ankle, 6th ed. St. Louis, Mosby, 1993.)

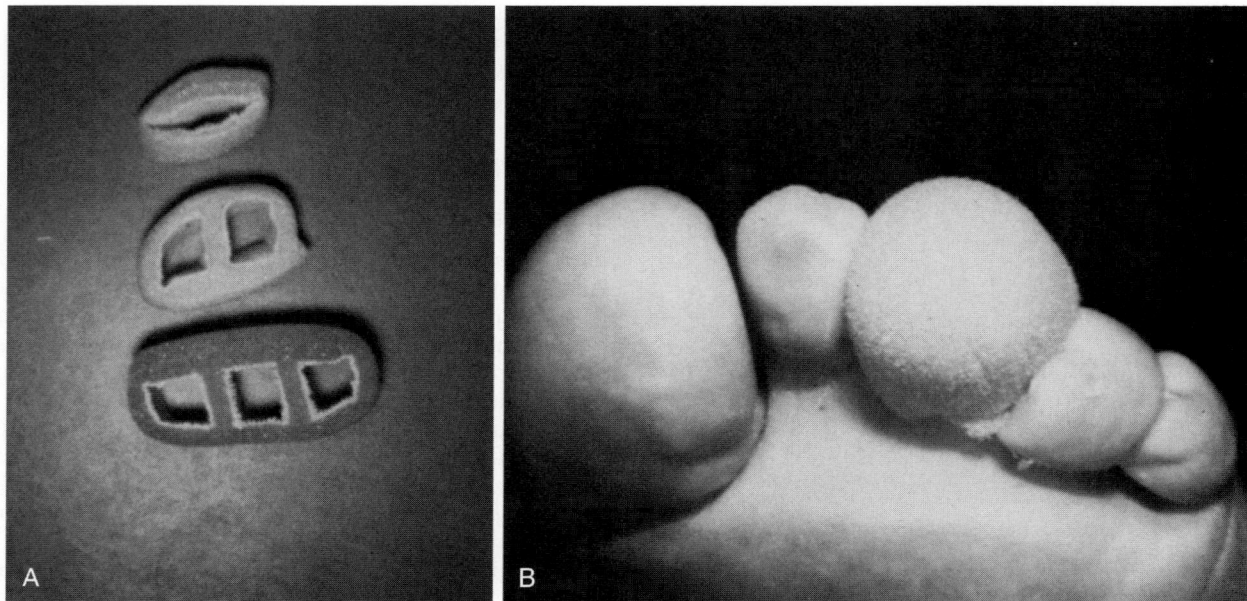

Figure 30J–101. *A,* Tube gauze may alleviate pain over a hammer toe. *B,* A toe cap may help to pad a callus at the tip of the toe. (*A,* From Coughlin MJ: Lesser toe deformities. In Mann RA, Coughlin MJ [eds]: Surgery of the Foot and Ankle, 6th ed. St. Louis, CV Mosby, 1993; *B,* from Mann RA, Coughlin MJ: Video Textbook of Foot and Ankle Surgery. St. Louis, Medical Video Production, 1991.)

the dorsal callus, the extensor tendon, and the joint capsule (Fig. 30J–103).[303, 304, 309–311, 321, 322] The scalpel is used to release the plantar capsule, and the collateral ligaments are severed carefully to deliver the head of the proximal phalanx. A bone cutter is used to resect the condyles of the proximal phalanx, and a rongeur is used to smooth any prominent edges. The amount of bone that is removed depends on the severity of the contracture. More bone must be removed if the deformity cannot be corrected completely after a condylectomy. If there is significant tightness of the long flexor tendon or if an adjacent lesser toe appears to be contracted, a flexor tenotomy is performed.[304, 311]

The articular cartilage of the base of the middle phalanx is removed. Whether an arthrodesis or an arthrofibrosis is obtained is not as important as the correction of the deformity and attaining stiffness at the proximal interphalangeal joint.[304] With a proximal interphalangeal joint arthroplasty, a fibrous arthroplasty may result with approximately 15 degrees of motion.[304, 311, 321, 322] After resection of the articular surfaces, the toe is fixed with a 0.045 intermedullary Kirschner wire.[311, 321] The wire is introduced at the proximal interphalangeal joint and driven through the middle and distal phalanges, exiting through the tip of the toe. The wire driver is placed on the Kirschner wire protruding from the tip of the toe, and the wire is pulled distally until only a small portion of its point remains in the joint. With the prepared surfaces aligned in a straight position in an AP and a medial-lateral plane, the Kirschner wire is driven in a proximal direction to stabilize the proximal interphalangeal joint. The Kirschner wire is bent at the tip of the toe to prevent proximal migration. The skin is closed with vertical mattress sutures, and a small compression dressing is applied. Sutures are removed 3 weeks after surgery, and the pin is removed 3 to 4 weeks postoperatively. The toe is taped in correct alignment for another 6 weeks. The patient is allowed to ambulate in a postoperative shoe.

Technique of Flexible Hammer Toe Repair

A dorsal longitudinal incision is centered over the proximal phalanx.[303, 304, 311, 317, 328, 329, 336, 337] The dissection is carried superficial to the extensor tendon, and a hemostat is used to dissect adjacent to the extensor hood on each side of the toe. This dissection is superficial to the extensor hood and deep to the neurovascular bundle.

A transverse incision is made at the plantar flexion crease of the MTP joint. The tendon sheath of the flexor tendons is identified and is incised longitudinally. The tendon of the flexor digitorum longus is characterized by a median raphe and is the largest and deepest of the three tendons in the sheath (Fig. 30J–104).[321, 322] After applying tension to the tendon through this proximal plantar incision, the tendon is detached distally through a percutaneous puncture incision at the level of the distal interphalangeal joint. The tendon is pulled into the proximal plantar incision and is split longitudinally along the median raphe. Each half of the tendon is passed on either side of the proximal phalanx in a dorsal direction. With the ankle held in a neutral position and the toe held in approximately 20 degrees of plantar flexion, the tendon is sutured to the extensor expansion or to the other limb of the tendon.[304] Either limb may be tightened until adequate alignment is achieved. A 0.045 Kirschner wire is used to stabilize the repair; the toe should be realigned adequately before placement of the Kirschner wire. The Kirschner wire should be used only to stabilize the repair because if the toe is not corrected completely, it may re-deform when the Kirschner wire is removed. The Kirschner wire is driven from the tip of the toe in a proximal direction. It may fail to penetrate the metatarsal head but still acts as a splint for the MTP joint. After a routine skin closure, a compressive dressing is used. Sutures are removed 3 weeks after surgery. The pin is removed 3 weeks postoperatively, then the toe is

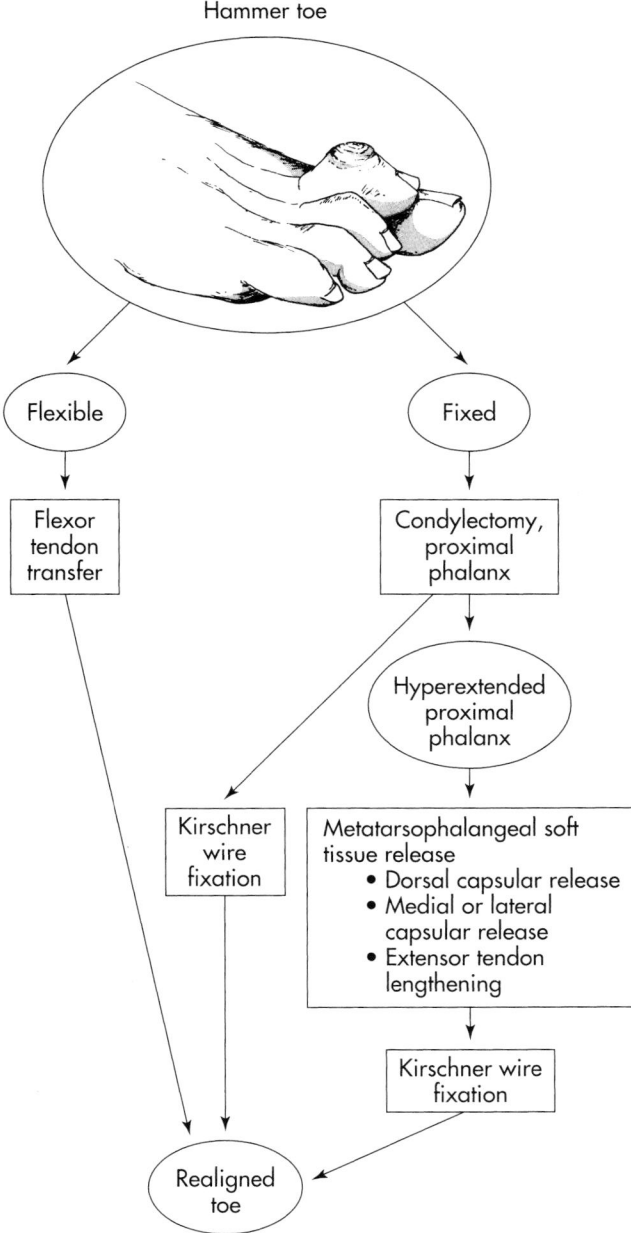

Hammer toe

Flexible → Flexor tendon transfer

Fixed → Condylectomy, proximal phalanx → Hyperextended proximal phalanx

Kirschner wire fixation

Metatarsophalangeal soft tissue release
• Dorsal capsular release
• Medial or lateral capsular release
• Extensor tendon lengthening

Kirschner wire fixation

Realigned toe

Figure 30J–102. Algorithm for treatment of hammer toe deformity. (From Coughlin MJ, Mann RA: Lesser toe deformities. In Coughlin MJ, Mann RA [eds]: Surgery of the Foot and Ankle, 7th edition. St. Louis, Mosby, 1999, p 331.)

taped in slight plantar flexion for approximately 6 weeks. The patient is allowed to ambulate in a wooden-soled shoe after surgery.

Results and Complications of Fixed and Flexible Hammer Toe Repairs

Ohm and colleagues[327] reported on 25 patients (62 hammer toe repairs) in whom a distal interphalangeal fusion was performed. A 100% fusion rate was achieved. An equal number of corrections were performed in the second, third, and fourth toes. Although many authors advocate attempted proximal interphalangeal arthrodesis,[295, 335, 341] ad-

equate resection with realignment that achieves a stable alignment of the toe is considered a successful result.[313, 318, 332] A fusion of the proximal interphalangeal joint or an arthrofibrosis succeeds by converting the flexor digitorum longus to a flexor of the entire digit. Coughlin and associates[310] reported on 63 patients (118 toes) with a fixed hammer toe deformity.

Involvement of the second toe was noted in 35%, the third toe in 21%, the fourth toe in 24%, and the fifth toe in 20%. After a resection arthroplasty technique with intramedullary Kirschner wire fixation, fusion of the proximal interphalangeal joint occurred in 81% of the involved toes. Subjective acceptable alignment was achieved in 86% of cases. Pain was relieved in 92%, and subjective satisfaction was noted by 84% of patients. Malalignment and numbness were the major factors reported to be associated with an unsuccessful result.

The rate of pseudarthrosis in some series approaches 50%, although a higher fusion rate has been achieved with peg-and-dowel type of technique.[295, 320, 334] Lehman and Smith[320] reported a 50% patient satisfaction rate with this technique, however. Major reasons for postoperative dissatisfaction included angulation of the lesser toe and incomplete relief of pain. McConnell[325, 326] reported on a large

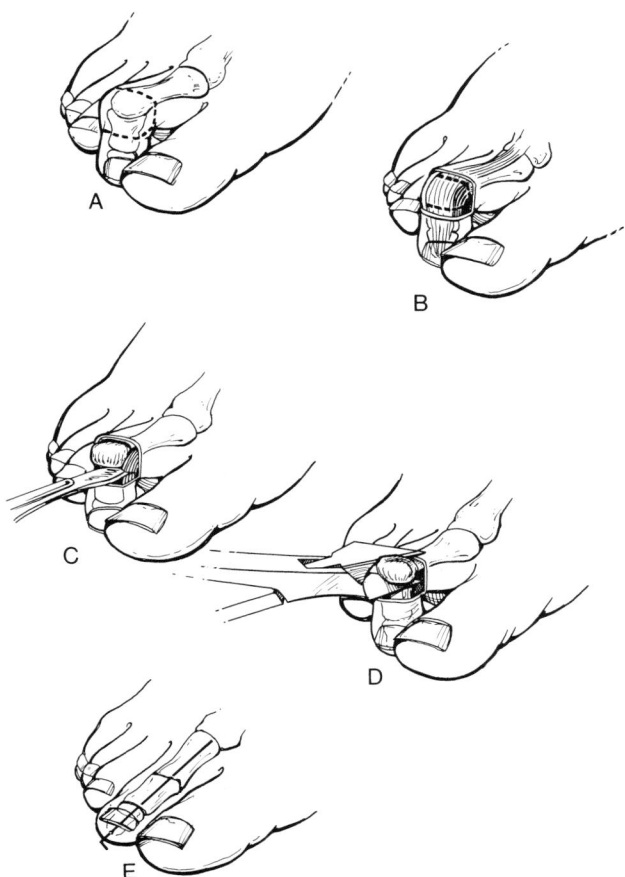

Figure 30J–103. A, Technique of fixed hammer toe repair. A dorsal elliptical incision excises skin, extensor tendon, and dorsal capsule. B, The collateral ligaments are released. C, The condyles of the proximal phalanx are delivered. D, The condyles are resected with a bone cutter. E, An intermedullary Kirschner wire is used for fixation.

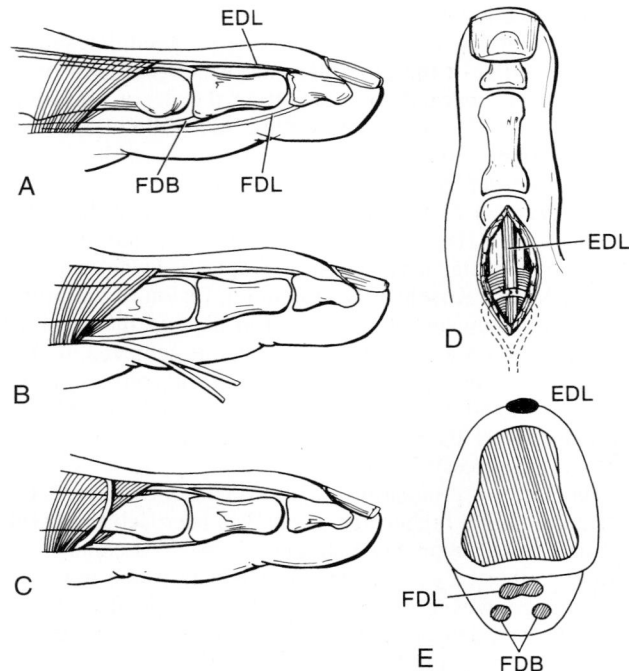

Figure 30J–104. *A*, Technique of flexor tendon transfer. Lateral view shows flexor digitorum longus (FDL), flexor digitorum brevis (FDB), and extensor digitorum longus (EDL). *B*, The flexor digitorum is detached through a distal puncture wound and is delivered through a transverse incision at the plantar metatarsophalangeal joint flexion crease. *C*, The tendon is split longitudinally, and each half is delivered on either side of the proximal phalanx and is sutured into either the extensor expansion or the corresponding limb of the flexor tendon. *D*, Dorsal view shows transferred flexor digitorum longus tendon. *E*, Cross-sectional view shows the characteristic position of the flexor digitorum longus tendon. It is deep to the flexor digitorum brevis and is characterized by a midline raphe.

series of patients treated with diaphysectomy. Although this technique was useful in treating a hammer toe deformity, it also may be used for shortening of a substantially long lesser toe. The actual postoperative alignment of the lesser toe and complication rate were not reported in either of McConnell's series. Daly and Johnson[314] reported on a large series of hammer toes treated with partial proximal phalangectomy. Although 75% patient satisfaction was noted, 43% of patients noted moderate footwear restrictions, 27% reported residual pain, 28% noted cosmetic dissatisfaction, and 18% reported recurrent cock-up deformity. Cahill and Connor[299] reported on 78 patients (84 feet). They noted 50% poor results after partial proximal phalangectomy. Conklin and Smith[300] noted 29% postoperative dissatisfaction after this procedure.

The results of fixed hammer toe repairs are in general gratifying, and few if any complications are reported routinely. Although swelling may be noted to persist for 1 to 6 months,[320, 327] it invariably subsides with time. Recurrence of a hammer toe deformity is a frustrating complication. Although excessive resection should be avoided because it leads to an unstable or floppy toe, an inadequate resection may lead to recurrence. In the face of recurrence, a flexor tenotomy may be performed to aid in correction. Postoperative malalignment can be a source of patient dissatisfaction.[310] Arthrodesis or arthrofibrosis gives an inherent sta-

bility to the digit and helps to resist the deforming forces of lesser toes. Complications associated with Kirschner wire fixations are uncommon, but migration or breakage or pin tract infection may develop.[343] Other uncommon complications include postoperative numbness, subsequent mallet-toe deformity, and decreased MTP range of motion. Uncommonly, patients may develop pain at the site of the pseudarthrosis. An injection of corticosteroid usually gives lasting relief. If a deformity of the MTP joint exists simultaneously, a hammer toe repair as well as correction of the MTP deformity must be considered.

Taylor,[336, 337] Pyper,[329] and others[314, 328] noted satisfactory results ranging from 51% to 89% after correction of a flexible hammer toe deformity. Thompson and Deland[338] reported excellent pain relief; however, only 54% of patients examined were noted to have complete correction of deformity. Kuwada[319] and Barbari and Brevig[296] reported greater than 90% satisfaction in patients after flexor tendon transfer.

After a tendon transfer, the ability to curl the toes is sacrificed. Frequently at long-term follow-up, stiffness develops at the proximal interphalangeal joint. A patient should be counseled preoperatively that dynamic function of the lesser toe is absent after flexor tendon transfer. Although this is not a cause of disability, a patient must be counseled about the tradeoff of function of the flexor digitorum longus for stability or realignment of the lesser toe.

Subluxation and Dislocation of the Metatarsophalangeal Joint

One of the most common forefoot deformities is subluxation or dislocation of a lesser MTP joint.[298, 301, 307, 308, 315] As a result of a constricting toe box or excessive length, the second toe may buckle.[311] Over a long period of time, the plantar aponeurosis and plantar capsule may become stretched, diminishing their stabilizing force over the MTP joint.[304, 311, 333] Concurrent contractures of the dorsal capsule and extensor tendons may add to the deformity. A hallux valgus deformity may destabilize the toe by exerting extrinsic pressure on the second toe.[311] With time, subluxation may progress to frank dislocation (Fig. 30J–105).

Although the most common deformity of the second MTP joint is dorsal dislocation, occasionally the second toe deviates medially.[301, 307, 311] A gap or space occurs between the second and third toes (Fig. 30J–106).[301, 307–309] This deformity may be associated with a hallux valgus deformity. Medial deviation of the toe may occur after trauma[301] as a result of degenerative or rheumatoid arthritis,[301, 311] nonspecific synovitis,[324] synovial cyst or ganglion formation,[301, 309] or erosion of the fibular collateral ligament or for no known reason at all.[301]

Clinical Evaluation

The main subjective complaints of patients with either a subluxated or dislocated toe are pain dorsally over the proximal interphalangeal joint, pain caused by the develop-

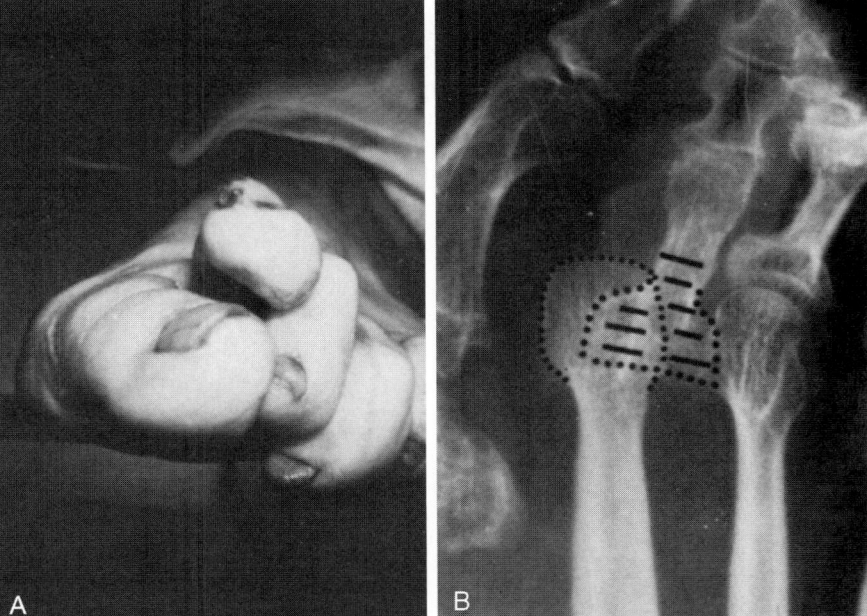

Figure 30J–105. A hallux valgus deformity may destabilize the second toe, leading to dislocation. *A,* Hallux valgus deformity causes medial pressure on the second toe with hammer toe formation. *B,* Radiograph shows dislocated second toe. (*A,* from Chapman, MW [ed]: Chapman's Operative Orthopaedics. Philadelphia, JB Lippincott, 1988; *B,* © M. J. Coughlin. Used by permission.)

ment of an IPK beneath the second metatarsal head, or capsular pain on the plantar aspect of the MTP joint at the insertion of the plantar capsule.[311] With the development of a deviated second toe, a patient may complain of vague pain in the second intermetatarsal space.[301, 304] This condition is often difficult to distinguish from an interdigital neuroma except that typically paresthesias or neuritic symptoms are not present in the toes.

On physical examination, deviation of the second toe either medially or dorsally is common. Pain may be noted with ambulation and may be elicited with palpation of the second intermetatarsal space.[301, 304] Manipulation of the toe

may cause discomfort as well. A dorsal plantar drawer test (Fig. 30J–107) is administered by thrusting the toe in a dorsal plantar direction. With capsulitis or MTP joint instability, pain is elicited. When a patient complains of presumable MTP pain, but no deformity is present, eliciting pain with a drawer test may assist in making the correct diagnosis.

Treatment Options

Conservative Treatment

The use of roomy footwear may alleviate discomfort in patients with a subluxated or dislocated second MTP

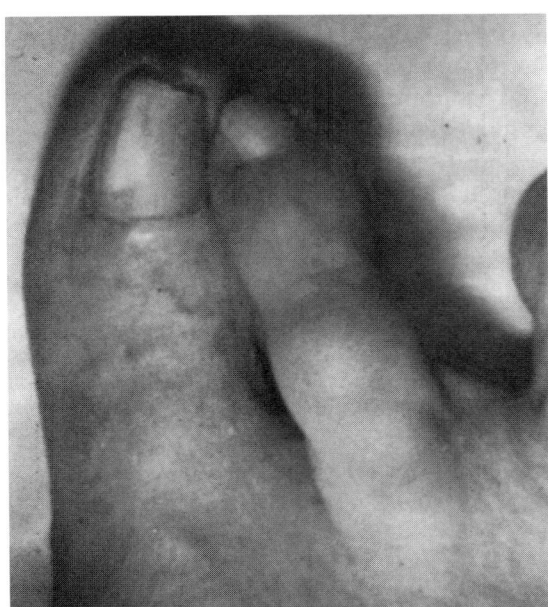

Figure 30J–106. Crossover second toe shows space between the second and third toes. (© M. J. Coughlin. Used by permission.)

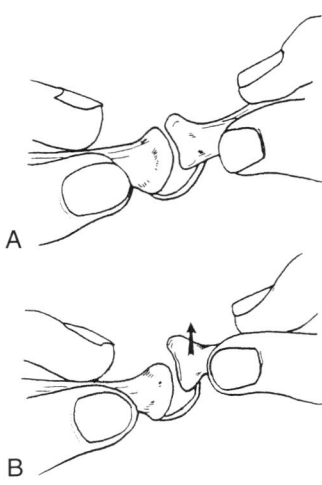

Figure 30J–107. Drawer test for metatarsophalangeal (MTP) joint instability. *A,* The toe is grasped between the thumb and the second finger. *B,* With a dorsal force, an attempt is made to subluxate the MTP joint. With instability of the MTP joint, pain is elicited with stress on the plantar structures. (From Coughlin MJ, Mann RA: Lesser toe deformities. In Coughlin MJ, Mann RA [eds]: Surgery of the Foot and Ankle, 7th ed. St. Louis, Mosby, 1999, p 354.)

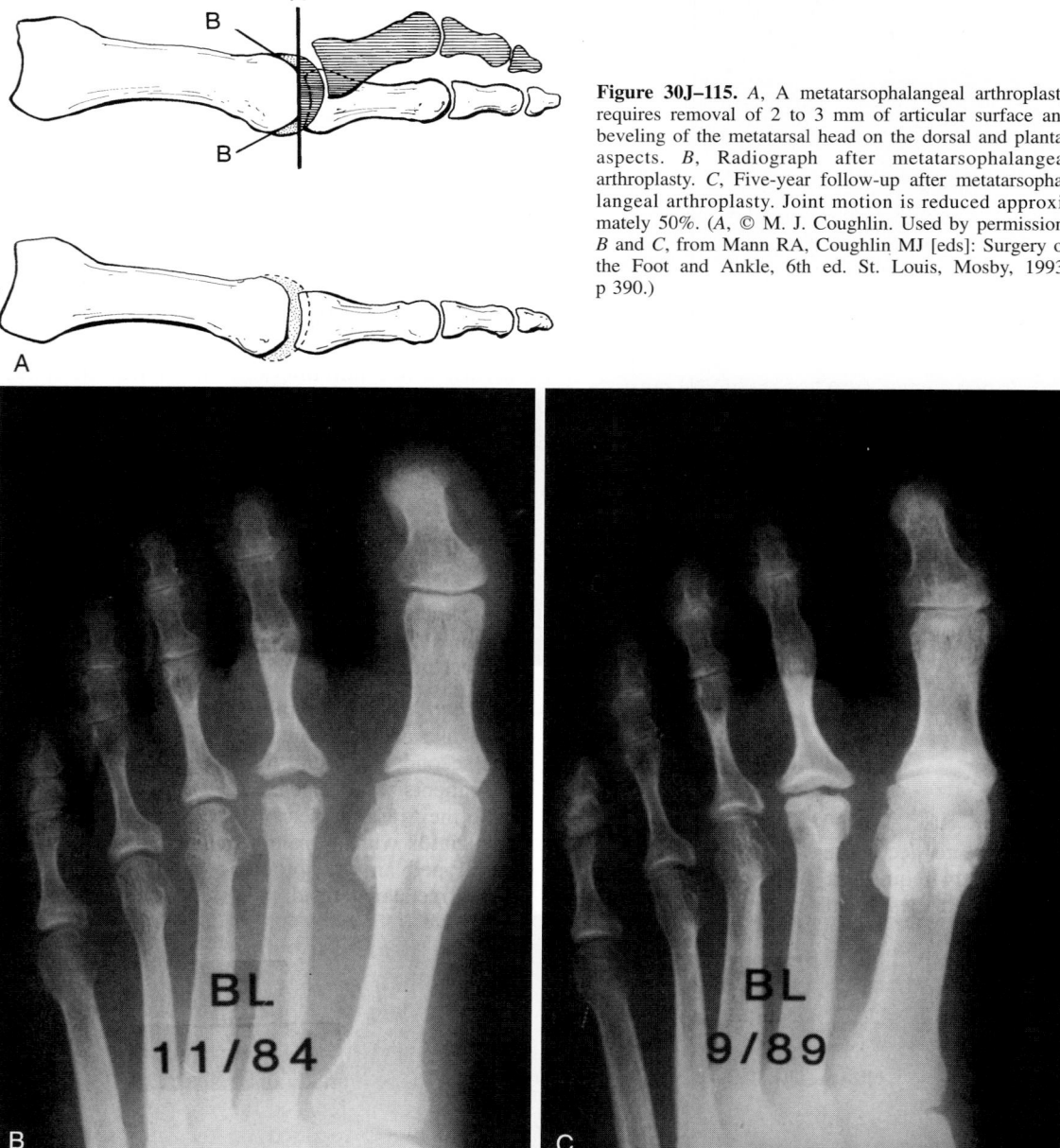

Figure 30J–115. *A*, A metatarsophalangeal arthroplasty requires removal of 2 to 3 mm of articular surface and beveling of the metatarsal head on the dorsal and plantar aspects. *B*, Radiograph after metatarsophalangeal arthroplasty. *C*, Five-year follow-up after metatarsophalangeal arthroplasty. Joint motion is reduced approximately 50%. (*A*, © M. J. Coughlin. Used by permission; *B* and *C*, from Mann RA, Coughlin MJ [eds]: Surgery of the Foot and Ankle, 6th ed. St. Louis, Mosby, 1993, p 390.)

realignment technique, good and excellent results were reported in 71%.

Mallet Toe

A mallet toe is characterized by a contracture or deformity of the distal interphalangeal joint (Fig. 30J–117).[306, 311] The distal phalanx is flexed at the distal interphalangeal joint, and most commonly the second toe is involved. The abnormality is believed to result from pressure of the toe box of a shoe against a long second toe.[302] In younger patients, contracture of the flexor digitorum longus may be the cause of this deformity. In younger patients, this is typically a flexible deformity, but in older patients, it is frequently a fixed contracture.[311]

Treatment Options

Conservative Treatment

Conservative treatment includes the use of shoes with a roomy toe box. Often, a toe cap or foam rubber pad can be used to protect the end of the second toe. When a fixed contracture is present, bony resection may be necessary. In a younger patient who has a contracture of the flexor digitorum longus, a flexor tenotomy may allow correction of the digit (Fig. 30J–118).[311]

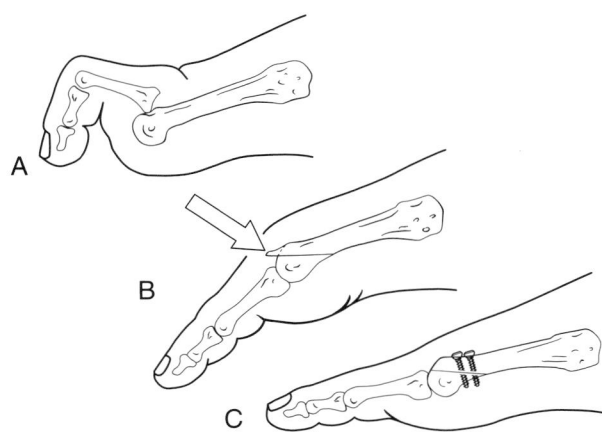

Figure 30J–116. *A–C*, Diagram of capital oblique osteotomy.

Technique of Mallet Toe Repair

An elliptical incision is performed over the dorsal aspect of the distal interphalangeal joint.[303–306, 311, 312, 321, 322] The extensor tendon, skin, and joint capsule are resected (Figs. 30J–119 and 30J–120). The collateral ligaments and plantar capsule are released, allowing the head of the middle phalanx to be delivered. A bone cutter is used to resect the condyles of the middle phalanx, and the flexor digitorum longus is released through the same incision. The articular surface of the distal phalanx is resected. A 0.045 Kirschner wire is driven through the distal phalanx, exiting through the tip of the toe. Then the Kirschner wire is driven in a retrograde fashion into the middle phalanx. The Kirschner wire is bent at the tip of the toe to prevent proximal migration. The toe is wrapped in a compressive dressing, and the patient is allowed to ambulate in a wooden-soled shoe. The sutures and pin are removed 3 weeks after surgery, and the toe is taped in alignment for approximately 6 weeks.

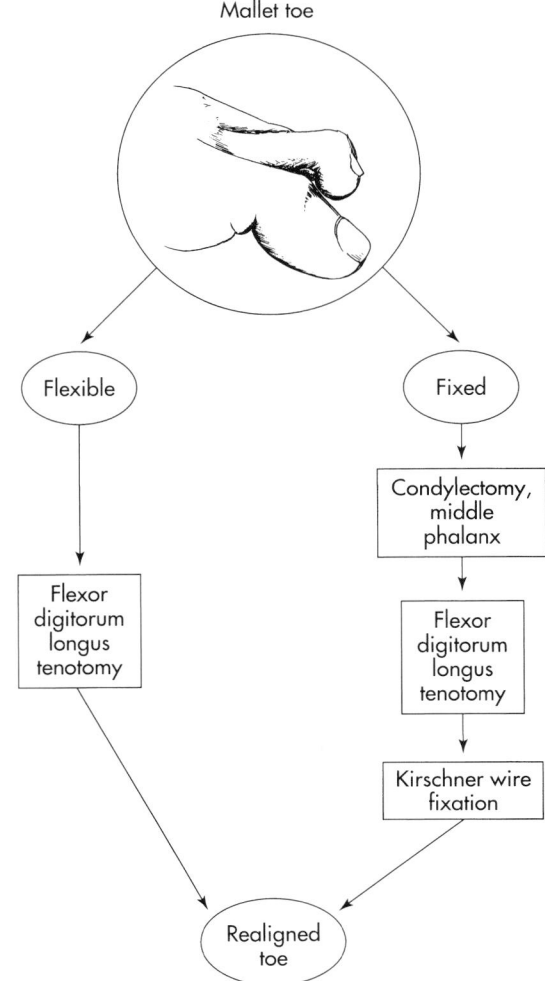

Figure 30J–118. Algorithm for mallet toe repair. (From Coughlin MJ, Mann RA: Lesser toe deformities. In Coughlin MJ, Mann RA [eds]: Surgery of the Foot and Ankle, 7th ed. St. Louis, Mosby, 1999, p 343.)

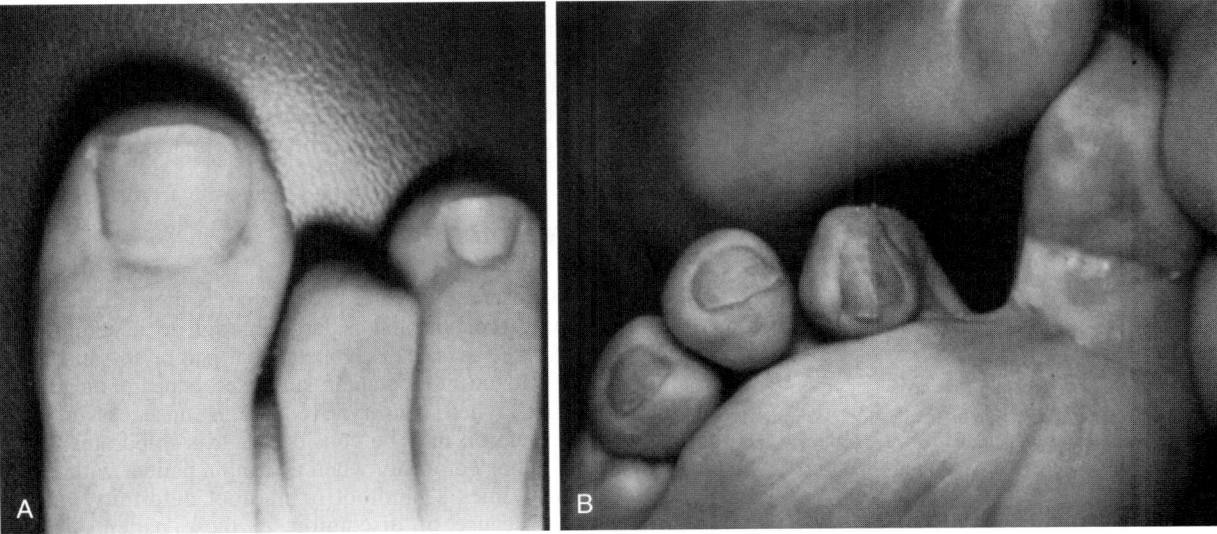

Figure 30J–117. *A* and *B*, Mallet toe deformity. (From Mann RA, Coughlin MJ: Video Textbook of Foot and Ankle Surgery. St. Louis, Medical Video Production, 1991, p 48.)

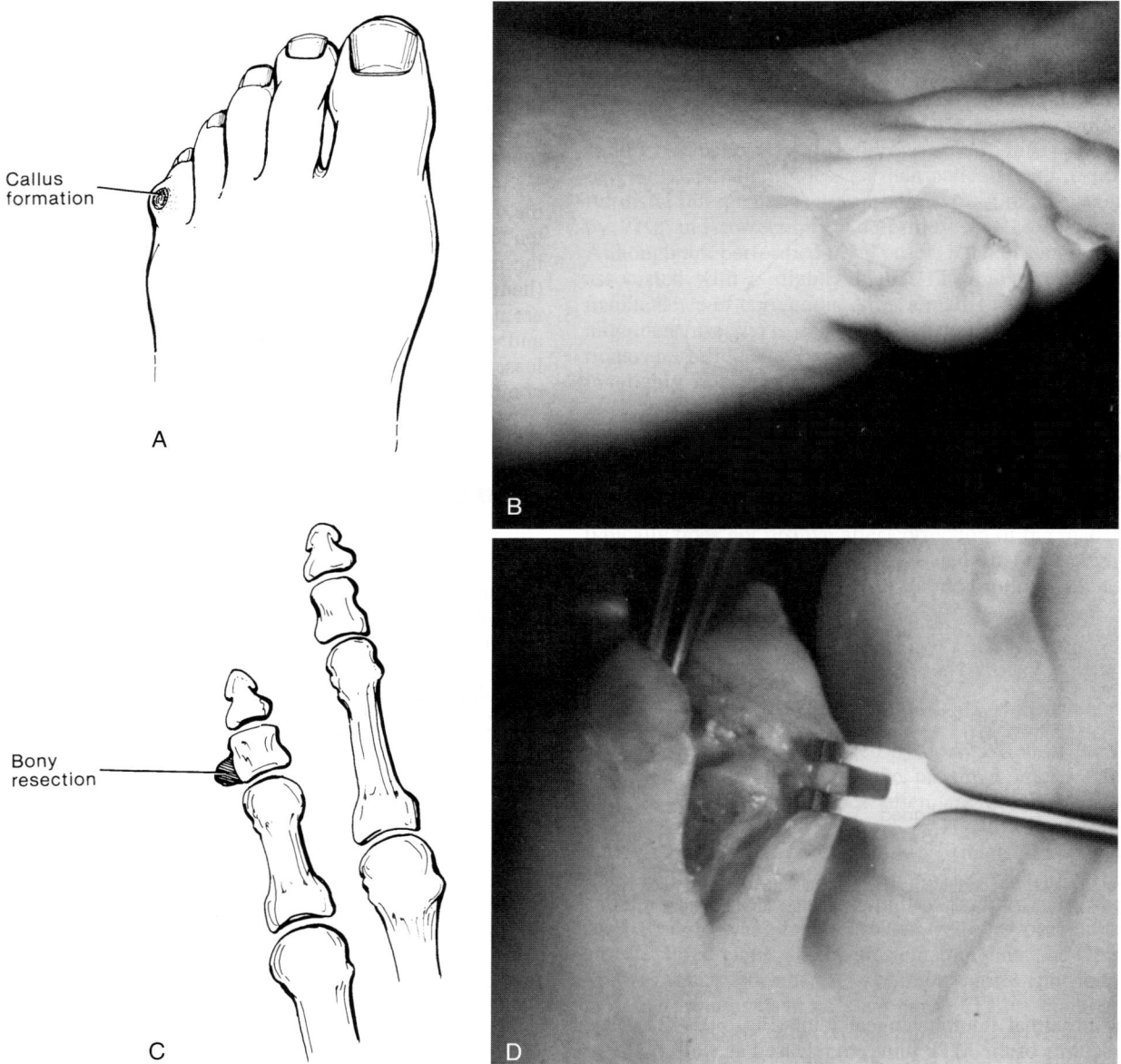

Figure 30J–123. *A* and *B*, Hard corn. *C* and *D*, Resection of lateral condyle to correct hard corn. Capsular repair helps prevent postoperative deformity. (*A* and *C*, from Mann RA, Coughlin MJ: Video Textbook of Foot and Ankle Surgery. St. Louis, Medical Video Production, 1991, p 50; *B* and *D*, © M. J. Coughlin. Used by permission.)

Treatment Options

Conservative Treatment

Exchanging a constricting shoe for a shoe with a roomy toe box is the most important aspect of conservative care. The bony prominence over the lateral aspect of the fifth toe may be padded, and the keratotic lesion may be shaved as well.[304] When conservative care does not relieve symptoms, the exostosis underlying a hard corn may be resected.[297, 304, 305, 311]

Technique of Hard Corn Repair

A dorsal longitudinal incision is centered over the interphalangeal joint of the fifth toe.[304, 311, 321] Usually a digital

anesthetic block is performed. The interphalangeal joint is exposed, and the capsule is peeled off the lateral condyle. If only the lateral condyle is prominent, it may be excised (Fig. 30J–123*B*).[305] When the base of the middle phalanx is prominent, it may be shaved with a rongeur. When a contracture of the interphalangeal joint is present, resection of the condyles of the proximal phalanx may achieve a more long-lasting repair.[304] A technique similar to that used for a fixed hammer toe deformity is employed (see previous description). An intramedullary Kirschner wire is used to stabilize the toe. Sutures and pins are removed 3 weeks after surgery, then the fifth toe is taped to the adjacent fourth toe for approximately 6 weeks. The patient initially ambulates in a postoperative shoe and later in a closed toe shoe.

Soft Corns

A soft corn is a hypertrophic keratotic lesion that occurs between the lesser toes either along the shaft or in the web space.[297, 304, 305] Soft corns develop because of pressure exerted between two prominent areas on adjacent toes (Fig. 30J–124A). Because there frequently is maceration between the lesser toes, the abnormality is termed a *soft corn* (Fig. 30J–124B). This lesion often is mistaken for a fungal infection because of this maceration.[305] Occasionally, a secondary infection may occur as well.

At times, the patient may complain of symptoms of recurrent infection, and in such cases a sinus tract is found extending into a mass of subcutaneous scar tissue. Occasionally, patients may have been treated for a long time

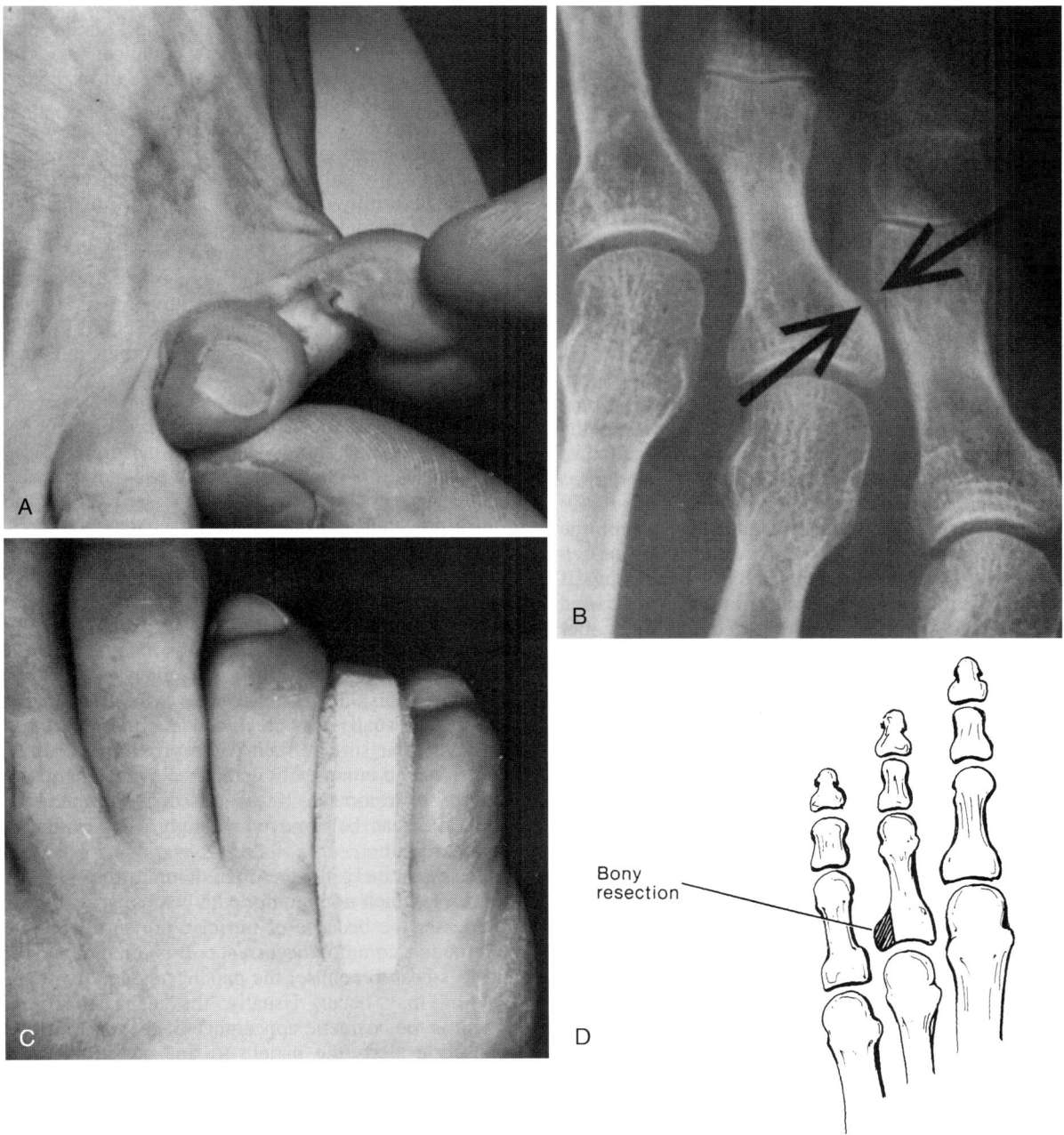

Figure 30J–124. *A*, Soft corn in web space. *B*, Radiograph shows area of bone impingement between distal aspect of proximal phalanx of fifth toe and proximal aspect of proximal phalanx of fourth toe. *C*, Padding may be placed in a symptomatic web space to relieve symptoms. *D*, Resection of condyle responsible for soft corn in web space. (*A–C* from Mann RA, Coughlin MJ: Video Textbook of Foot and Ankle Surgery. St. Louis, Medical Video Production, 1991, p 51.)

hallux valgus. The cause and anatomic variations that are present with a bunionette appear to be much more complex, however, than those originally described by Kelikian[364] and Davies.[350] An enlarged fifth metatarsal head may lead to a bunionette deformity (Fig. 30J–125A).[355, 357, 386, 387] Although

hypertrophy of the lateral condyle of the fifth metatarsal head may occur,[355, 387] Throckmorton and Bradlee[386] and later Fallat and Buckholz[357] reported that with pronation of the forefoot, the lateral plantar tubercle of the fifth metatarsal head rotates to a more lateral position, creating the

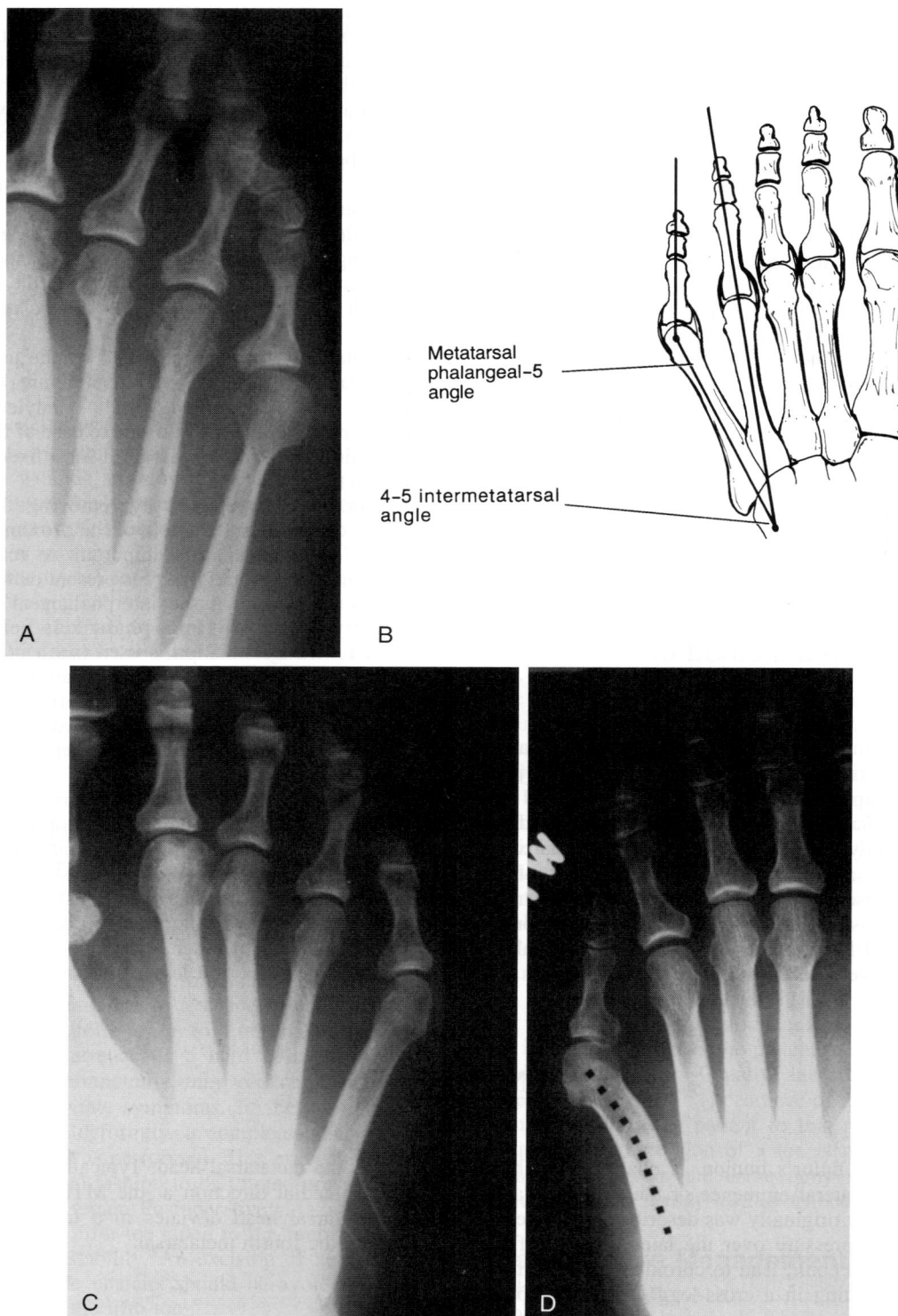

Figure 30J–125. *A,* Enlarged metatarsal head. *B,* The 4–5 intermetatarsal angle and metatarsophalangeal 5 angle. *C,* Increased 4–5 intermetatarsal angle. *D,* Lateral angulation of the distal fifth metatarsal. (*A, C,* and *D,* © M. J. Coughlin. Used by permission.)

radiographic impression of fifth metatarsal head enlargement. These investigators noted an average increase of the fourth-fifth (4–5) IM angle of 3 degrees with pes planus. Whether there is true hypertrophy of the fifth metatarsal head or a prominence of the fifth metatarsal head owing to pronation of the foot, the lateral condyle of the metatarsal head may become symptomatic without divergence of the fifth metatarsal.

The pertinent angular measurements that define a bunionette deformity are the 4–5 IM angle and the MTP-5 angle (Fig. 30J–125B). The MTP-5 angle is the magnitude of medial deviation of the fifth toe in relation to the fifth metatarsal shaft. The 4–5 IM angle calculates the divergence of the fourth and fifth metatarsals and is measured by the intersection of lines bisecting the base and neck of the fourth and fifth metatarsals.[381] A 4–5 angle of greater than 8 degrees is considered abnormal.[345, 356, 381, 387] A prominent fifth metatarsal head may develop owing to divergence of the fourth and fifth metatarsals (Fig. 30J–125C); however, an IM angle of more than 8 degrees may be asymptomatic and require no medical treatment.

Lateral bowing of the fifth metatarsal diaphysis can lead to the development of a bunionette deformity (Fig. 30J–125D).[355–357, 372, 389] Although the proximal fifth metatarsal appears to be in normal alignment, the diaphyseal region is characterized by a lateral curvature or bowing that results in prominence of the lateral metatarsal condyle. Nestor and colleagues,[376] in reporting on the anatomic variations in patients with symptomatic bunionettes, found that an increased 4–5 IM angle frequently was associated with a bunionette deformity, whereas fifth metatarsal bowing and an enlarged fifth metatarsal head were seen much less frequently. Coughlin[349] noted a type 1 deformity (an enlarged fifth metatarsal head) occurred in 27% of cases, a type 2 deformity (lateral bowing of the fifth metatarsal head) occurred in 23% of cases, and a type 3 deformity (enlarged 4–5 IM angle) occurred in 50% of cases in which a surgical repair was performed.

Biomechanics

In general, a bunionette deformity is a static deformity that is exacerbated by excess pressure of footwear against a prominent fifth metatarsal head. Anatomic variations, such as an increased 4–5 IM angle, fifth metatarsal bowing, or an enlarged fifth metatarsal head, may lead to symptoms in the athletic population. Repetitive activity, such as running or jogging, may lead to a thickened or inflamed bursa and may be associated with formation of a hyperkeratotic lesion overlying this deformity. A pes planus deformity may lead to a relative enlargement of the fifth metatarsal head and, with repetitive activity, may be associated with irritation and discomfort over the bunionette. Reduction of excessive pronation with an orthotic device may alleviate symptoms.

Clinical Evaluation

The major subjective complaints of an athlete are pain and irritation caused by friction between the underlying bony abnormality and restricting footwear. On clinical evaluation, an inflamed bursa,[360, 385, 386] a plantar keratosis,[359, 360, 374] a lateral keratosis,[353] or a combined plantar-lateral keratosis[353, 362] may be noted. Diebold and Bejjani[353] noted that two thirds of the patients in their series had significant pes planus. Diebold and Bejjani[353] noted that one third of the patients had a plantar lesion, and half had a lateral keratotic lesion.

A bunionette may develop as an isolated problem or may occur in combination with a hallux valgus deformity. An increased 1–2 IM angle combined with an increased 4–5 IM angle results in a wide or splay foot abnormality.[345, 350, 360, 363, 384]

Radiographic evaluation includes standing AP and lateral radiographs. Force plate studies or imprints that evaluate the pressure concentration on the plantar aspect of the foot are helpful in the analysis of a plantar keratosis.

Treatment Options

Conservative Treatment

The recognition by an athlete that the use of constricting footwear may be a significant cause of symptoms is important. Pain, swelling, and chronic irritation over the lateral bursa of the fifth metatarsal head may be reduced significantly by the use of properly fitted shoes.[350, 351, 364, 369, 372, 385] Padding of the prominent metatarsal head[369, 372] and shaving of the hypertrophic callus may afford significant relief of symptoms. An orthotic device may be used to control pronation and secondarily to reduce discomfort over the prominent fifth metatarsal head.

Operative Techniques

Numerous operative techniques have been proposed for surgical correction of a symptomatic bunionette deformity, including lateral condylectomy,[351, 355, 359, 365, 370, 372, 373, 385] metatarsal head resection,[354, 364, 366, 374] fifth ray resection,[346] distal metatarsal osteotomy,* diaphyseal osteotomy,[348, 349, 352, 358, 362, 380, 383, 387] and proximal fifth metatarsal osteotomy (Fig. 30J–126).[345, 356, 357, 362, 371, 378]

Lateral Condylectomy

When an isolated enlargement of the fifth metatarsal head or lateral condyle occurs without lateral deviation of the fifth metatarsal shaft from an increased 4–5 IM angle, a lateral condylectomy may be performed. Pes planus is not a contraindication to surgery if a symptomatic bunionette is the only deformity present.

A longitudinal skin incision is centered directly over the lateral condyle of the fifth metatarsal. The dorsal cutaneous nerve of the fifth toe is protected. An inverted L-type capsular incision (Fig. 30J–127) detaches the dorsal and proximal capsular attachments, allowing exposure of the

---

*See references 347, 360–363, 367, 368, 369, 375, 379, 384, and 390.

nence. The abductor digiti quinti is released, and the lateral eminence is resected with an osteotome or sagittal saw. An oblique osteotomy of the metaphyseal neck of the metatarsal is carried out using either a saw (Fig. 30J–131*A*) or a double action bone cutter.[368] This osteotomy is oriented in a distal lateral-to-proximal medial direction. The resected bone is displaced medially on the metatarsal and impacted on the proximal fragment (Fig. 30J–131*B* and *C*). The osteotomy is not fixed routinely.[368] The foot is wrapped in a soft gauze and tape dressing, and the patient ambulates in a postoperative shoe. Sutures are removed 3 weeks after surgery, and the toe is taped in the proper alignment for 4

more weeks. Kitaoka and Leventen[368] reported an average of 5 degrees of correction of the 4–5 IM angle and a diminished forefoot width of 4 mm with 87% patient satisfaction after this procedure. Sponsel,[384] who advocated an oblique distal osteotomy, noted an 11% delayed union rate, and Keating and coworkers[363] reported 75% of patients to have transfer lesions with a 12% recurrence rate. Pontious and colleagues[377] reported a much higher rate of success in oblique osteotomies that were internally fixed (Fig. 30J–132).

Technique of Distal Chevron Procedure. An alternative procedure is to resect the prominent lateral condyle in

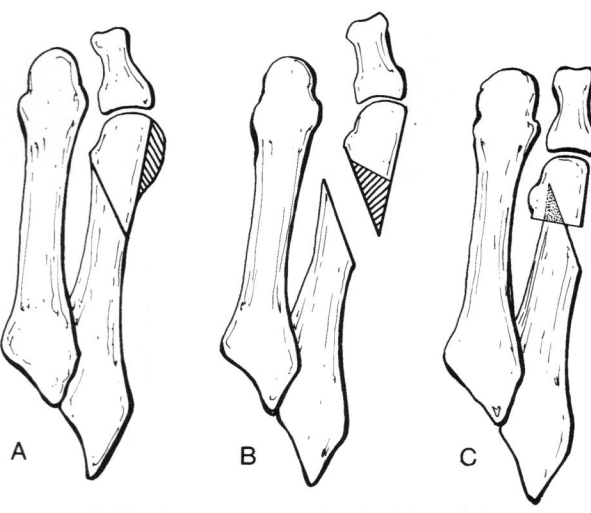

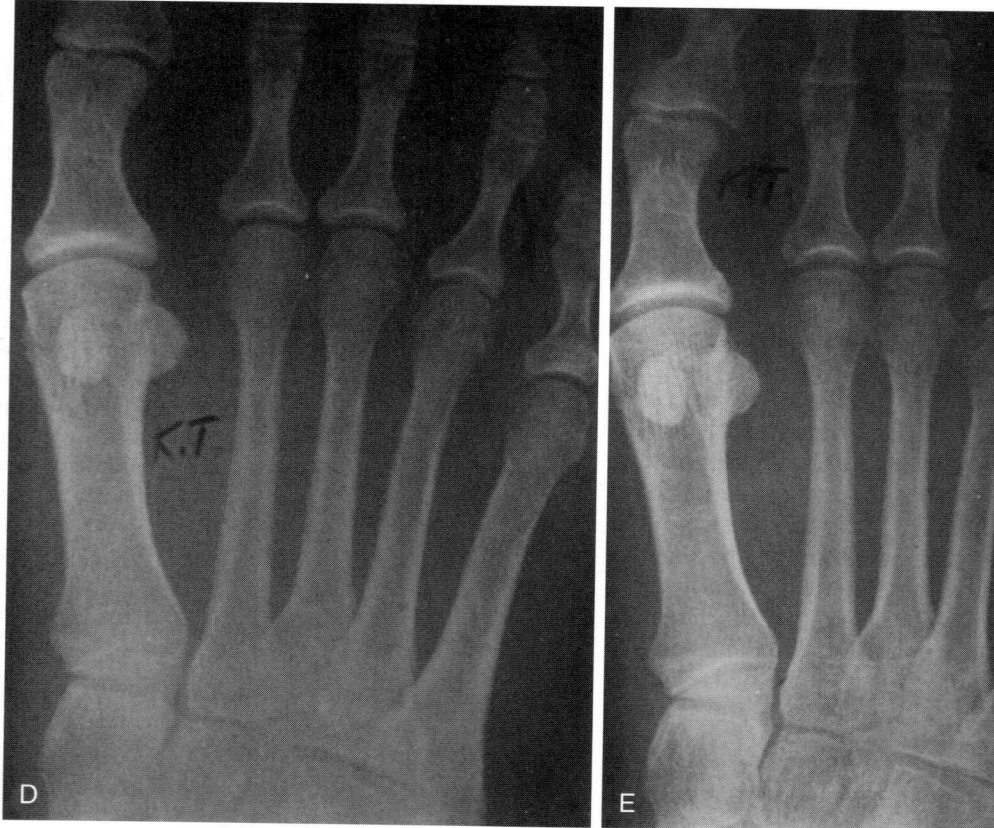

Figure 30J–131. *A,* Distal oblique osteotomy coupled with lateral eminence resection. *B,* Resection of fifth metatarsal metaphysis with distal oblique osteotomy. *C,* Impaction of osteotomy site. *D* and *E,* Preoperative and postoperative radiographs of distal oblique osteotomy. *Shaded areas* are resected. (*D* and *E,* © M. J. Coughlin. Used by permission.)

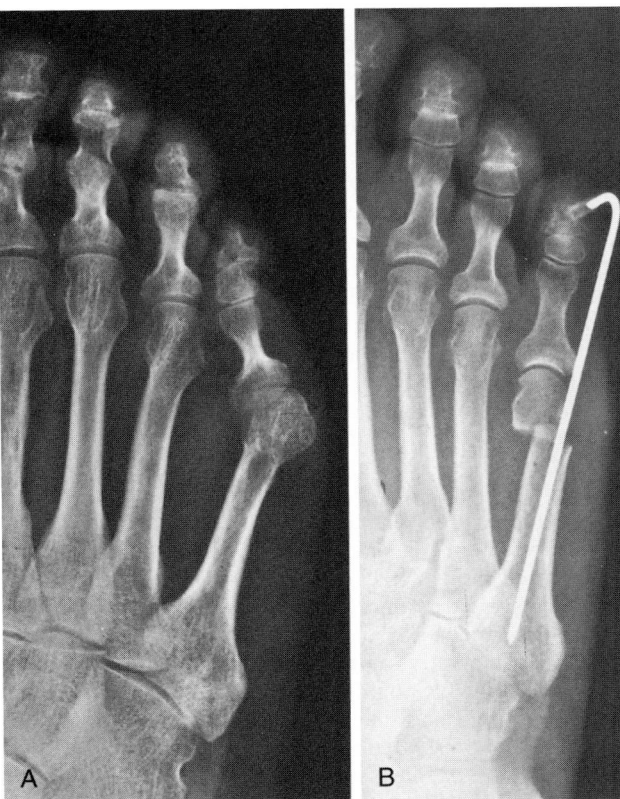

Figure 30J–132. *A,* Preoperative radiograph shows severe bunionette deformity. *B,* After distal oblique osteotomy with internal fixation. (Courtesy of H. Zollinger-Kies, Zurich, Switzerland.)

lent results with the chevron osteotomy. Kitaoka and associates[367] reported the 4–5 IM angle was reduced an average of 2.6 degrees, and the metatarsal-5 angle was reduced an average of 8 degrees with this procedure. Moran and Claridge[375] stressed that there was a low margin of error with this osteotomy and that there was a high risk of either recurrence or overcorrection and encouraged the use of Kirschner wire stabilization of the osteotomy site.

Diaphyseal Osteotomy

The indications for a diaphyseal fifth metatarsal osteotomy are a bunionette deformity associated with either an increased 4–5 IM angle or lateral bowing of the distal metatarsal. MTP joint realignment with a lateral eminence resection is performed simultaneously if necessary.

Technique of Midshaft Osteotomy. A diaphyseal metatarsal osteotomy has been used to correct a bunionette deformity.[348, 349] Voutey[387] carried out a transverse osteotomy in the diaphysis but described problems with rotation, angulation, and pseudarthrosis. Yancey[389] used a double transverse closing wedge osteotomy in the diaphyseal region to correct a bunionette deformity characterized by

combination with a distal chevron osteotomy. A midlateral longitudinal skin incision is made over the lateral eminence. An inverted L-type capsular incision releases the dorsal and proximal capsule and exposes the lateral eminence. Minimal soft tissue stripping should be performed to avoid vascular insult to the distal metatarsal fragment. Approximately 2 mm of the lateral eminence is removed with an osteotome or a sagittal saw. A drill hole in the midportion of the metatarsal is used to mark the apex of the osteotomy. A sagittal saw is used to create a horizontal chevron osteotomy. The osteotomy is based proximally with an angle of 60 degrees (Fig. 30J–133*A*). The osteotomy is oriented in a lateral-to-medial direction. The distal fragment is displaced approximately 2 to 3 mm in a medial direction and is impacted onto the proximal phalanx (Fig. 30J–133*B*). The fifth MTP medial capsular structures are not released because release might impair the circulation to the fifth metatarsal head. Although internal fixation is optional, it should be employed if there is any instability or tendency toward angulation at the osteotomy site. Kirschner wire fixation is used when necessary. A sagittal saw is used to remove any remaining prominent bone in the metaphyseal region of the fifth metatarsal. The lateral capsule is reefed to the abductor digiti quinti or the dorsal periosteum of the fifth metatarsal. Occasionally, drill holes in the metaphysis may be placed for use in repairing the lateral capsular structures. Throckmorton and Bradlee[386] and others[347, 367, 369] reported high levels of good and excel-

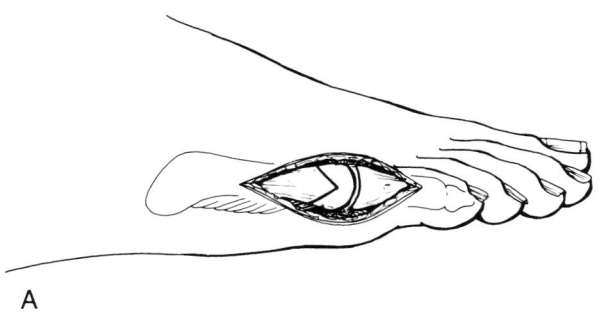

A

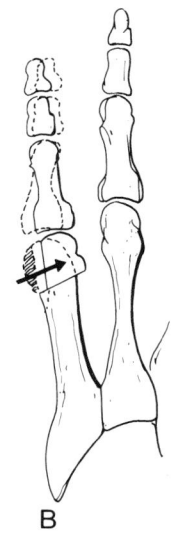

B

Figure 30J–133. *A,* Lateral view of a fifth metatarsal chevron osteotomy. *B,* Anteroposterior view after chevron osteotomy.

lateral angulation of the fifth metatarsal. Gerbert and colleagues[358] recommended use of a biplane osteotomy for a combined plantar-lateral keratotic lesion to displace the distal fragment in a medial direction. Mann[372] and Coughlin[348, 349] used an oblique diaphyseal fifth metatarsal osteotomy to treat diffuse keratotic lesions on either the plantar or plantar-lateral aspects of the fifth metatarsal. The oblique orientation of the metatarsal osteotomy permits a dorsal-medial translation of the metatarsal as the distal fragment is rotated. Internal fixation was recommended with either a small fragment screw or wire loop or a Kirschner wire. Mann[372] did not realign the fifth MTP joint with this procedure, and no results were reported, although one case of nonunion was noted.

Coughlin[348] modified Mann's oblique diaphyseal osteotomy by performing a fifth MTP joint realignment and lateral eminence resection. With this technique, a midlateral longitudinal incision is extended from the base of the fifth metatarsal to the middle of the proximal phalanx (Fig. 30J–134A). The dissection is carried down to the fifth metatarsal shaft, and the dorsal cutaneous nerve is protected. The abductor digiti quinti is retracted in a plantar direction exposing the diaphysis of the fifth metatarsal. An L-type capsular incision (see Fig. 30J–127) is used to expose the lateral eminence. The lateral eminence is excised using an oscillating saw or osteotome. The osteotomy is performed in a line parallel with the metatarsal shaft. The medial capsule of the fifth MTP joint is released (as described earlier) to allow realignment of the fifth MTP joint.

A diaphyseal osteotomy of the fifth metatarsal is performed with an oscillating saw. If a lateral keratosis is present, a direct horizontal osteotomy is made in a dorsal proximal-to-plantar distal plane (Fig. 30J–134B). Before final displacement of the osteotomy site, the fixation holes are drilled. A gliding hole is drilled in the dorsal distal fragment, and a tapped fixation hole is made in the proximal plantar fragment. The osteotomy is completed and displaced by rotating the distal fragment medially (Fig. 30J–134C). The osteotomy is fixed with either a small fragment compression screw or two minifragment compression screws. Distally, the fifth MTP joint capsule is repaired, and the fifth toe is brought into proper alignment (Fig. 30J–134D and E). Closure is begun by approximating the abductor digiti quinti and the MTP capsule. If necessary, the capsule is reattached through drill holes on the dorsal aspect of the metaphysis. The patient is allowed to ambulate in a wooden-soled shoe. Casting may be used for an unreliable patient or if the patient has some difficulty with ambulating. A compression gauze and tape dressing is used for 6 weeks.

If a combination plantar-lateral keratosis is present, the oblique osteotomy is oriented in a cephalad direction to create an elevating effect on the distal fragment, then the fragment is rotated (Fig. 30J–134F to H). The fifth MTP joint is realigned, and closure is performed in a similar fashion. Postoperative management is similar to that previously described. Coughlin[349] reported on 30 feet that had undergone a midshaft diaphyseal metatarsal osteotomy. All went on to successful union. The average 4–5 IM angle was reduced 10 degrees, and the MTP-5 angle was reduced 16 degrees. No transfer lesions developed, and a 93% patient satisfaction rate was reported. The average foot width was reduced 6 mm.

Midshaft osteotomies do not appear to have an increased nonunion rate. As Shereff and associates[382] noted, more

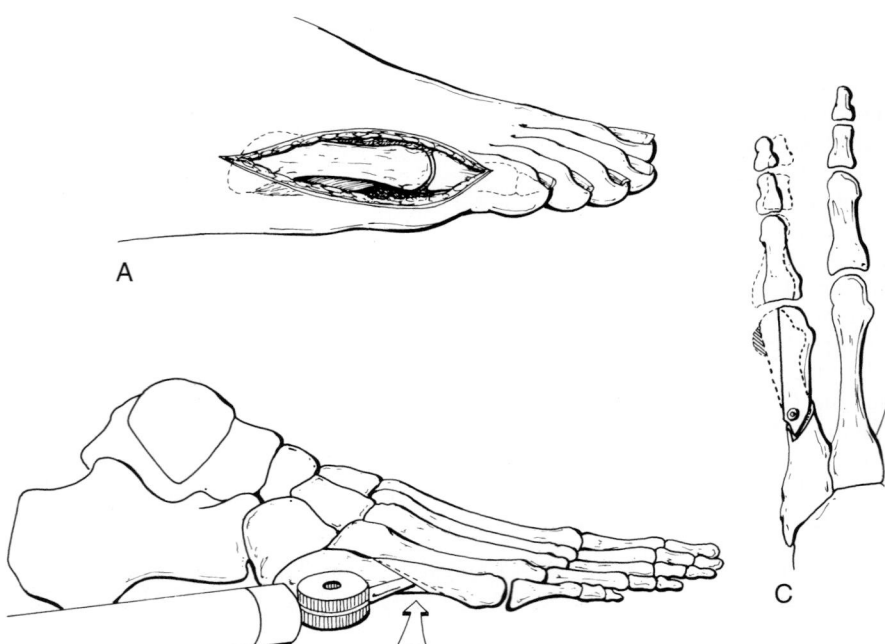

A

B

C

Figure 30J–134. *A,* Incision for a fifth metatarsal diaphyseal osteotomy. *B,* The horizontal osteotomy is performed from a proximal-dorsal to a plantar-distal site. *C,* The osteotomy is rotated.

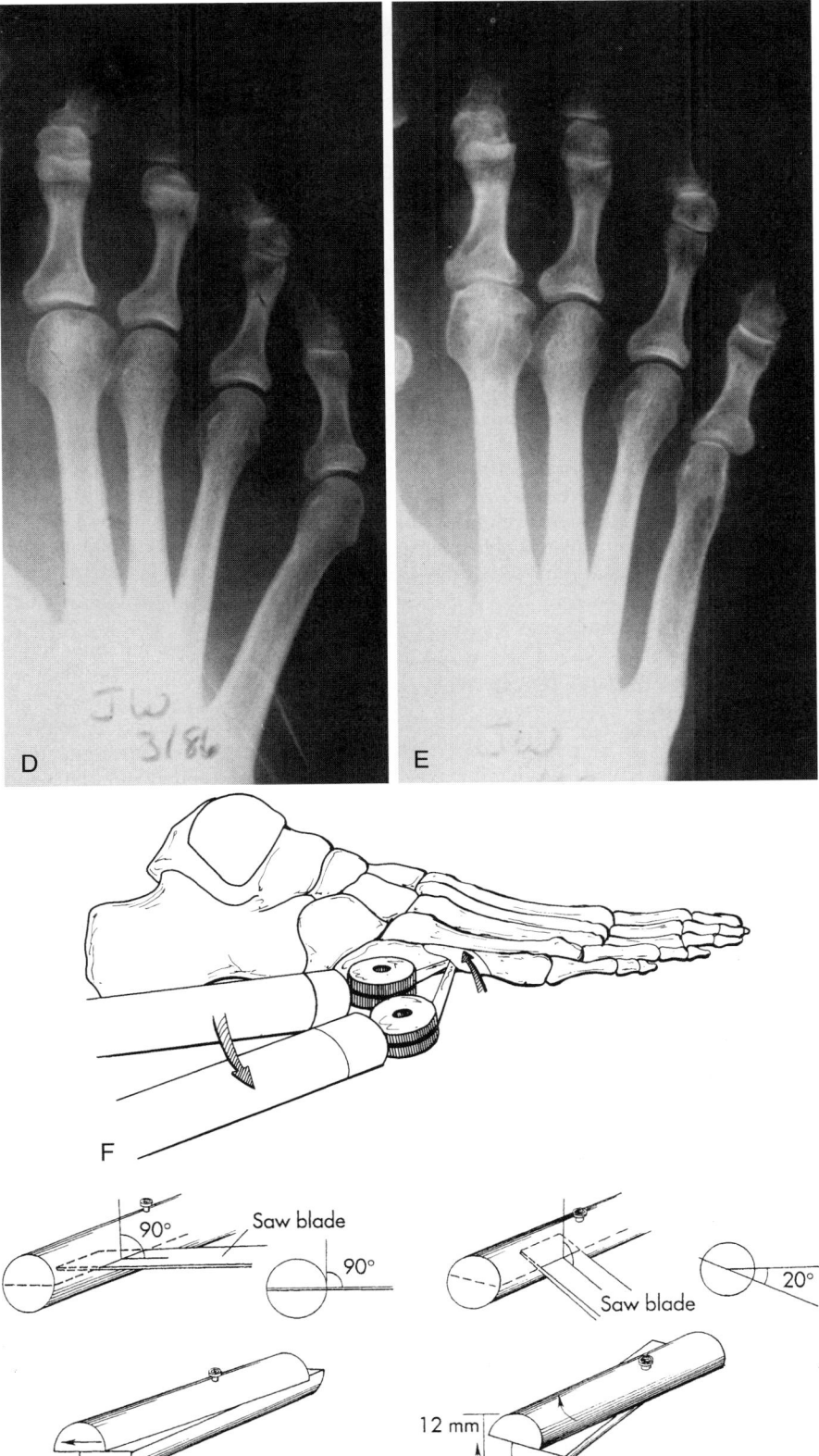

Figure 30J–134 *Continued. D*, Preoperative radiograph. *E*, Postoperative radiograph after oblique osteotomy. *F*, To achieve elevation of the fifth metatarsal head, the saw is oriented in a cephalad direction, and the osteotomy site is rotated. *G*, Schema illustrating effect of horizontal osteotomy. With the saw blade oriented in a lateral-to-medial direction, the osteotomy site is rotated and does not elevate the distal metatarsal. *H*, Schema illustrating effect of oblique osteotomy. With the saw blade oriented in a medial-to-lateral but also superior direction, as the osteotomy site is rotated, the distal fragment is elevated. (*D* and *E*, © M. J. Coughlin. Used by permission; *G* and *H*, adapted from Lutter L: Atlas of Adult Foot and Ankle Surgery. St. Louis, Mosby, 1997, pp 110–111.)

proximally positioned osteotomies may be at risk for delayed healing, however, as a result of interruption of the interosseous and extraosseous blood supply to the proximal fifth metatarsal (Fig. 30J–135).

Postoperative Management and Rehabilitation

Although recovery from bunionette surgery usually is relatively rapid, conservative methods often are used either to alleviate symptoms or to help postpone surgery until the off-season. After fifth MTP joint surgery or fifth metatarsal osteotomy, soft gauze and tape dressings are used to hold the fifth metatarsal and toe in proper alignment. The patient typically ambulates in a wooden-soled postoperative shoe. A below-knee cast may be used if a surgeon is concerned about fixation or about the reliability of the patient. Weight-bearing in a postoperative shoe usually is carried out by having the patient bear more weight on the inner aspect of the foot. By 3 weeks, a plantigrade stance and gait pattern can be used. Sutures are removed at the 3-week postoperative visit.

Criteria for Return to Sports Participation

Return to athletic activities can be expected earlier after a lateral condylectomy or MTP joint realignment than after a fifth metatarsal osteotomy. After a lateral condylectomy,

usually aggressive walking can be initiated at 4 weeks with running at 6 weeks after surgery. After a distal osteotomy or a diaphyseal osteotomy, internal fixation is removed at 6 weeks under local anesthesia. At 7 weeks, aggressive walking can be initiated, and if no complications are encountered, jogging and running can be started progressively at 10 weeks postoperatively. Roomy footwear with an adequate toe box is more comfortable during initiation of athletic activities.

Complications

Recurrence of deformity is the most common complication after lateral condylectomy. Fifth MTP joint realignment may be complicated by joint subluxation or dislocation. An adequate capsular joint repair may help to avoid this complication. Any dissection in this area may injure the lateral cutaneous nerve to the fifth toe (a branch of the sural nerve), leading to numbness or formation of neuroma.

A distal metatarsal osteotomy may be complicated by dorsal angulation with development of an IPK or transfer lesion beneath the fourth metatarsal head. Delayed union or nonunion may develop as well. The use of internal fixation may reduce the incidence of malunion and nonunion after floating fifth metatarsal osteotomies.

Although a diaphyseal oblique osteotomy may be complicated by malunion, delayed union, nonunion, or transfer metatarsalgia, the nature of the osteotomy coupled with rigid internal fixation has minimized these complications. Typically, this type of osteotomy is well healed by the sixth postoperative week.

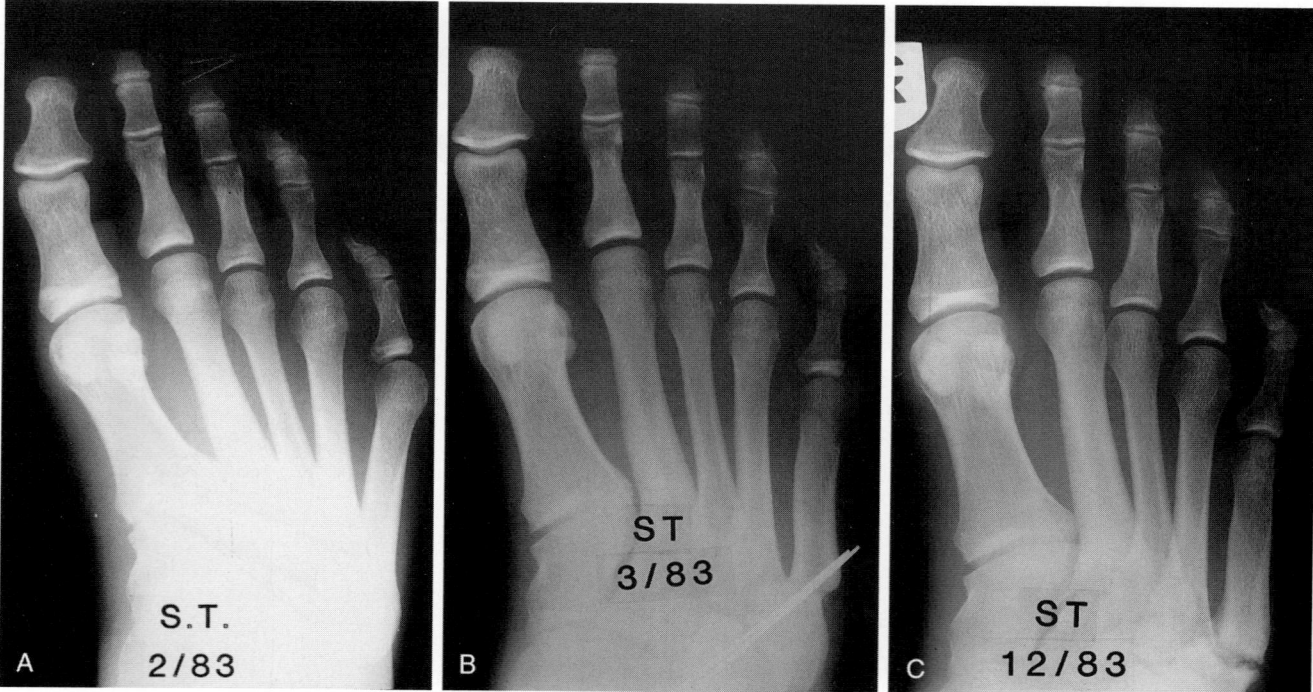

Figure 30J–135. *A,* Preoperative radiograph shows moderate bunionette deformity. *B,* After proximal fifth metatarsal osteotomy. *C,* Symptomatic nonunion after proximal osteotomy. This osteotomy took approximately 12 months to heal and prevented the patient from participating in high school athletics for that season. (From Mann RA, Coughlin MJ [eds]: Surgery of the Foot and Ankle, 6th ed. St. Louis, Mosby, 1993.)

Author's Preferred Method of Treatment

Conservative management of a symptomatic tailor's bunion should include the use of padding, shaving of keratotic lesions, and the use of roomy footwear. In many cases, an athlete can continue sports activities with the use of orthotic devices or pads. Development of chronic bursal thickening, blistering, and symptomatic keratoses may lead to operative treatment in certain patients. Because of the risk of transfer lesions and recurrence of deformity and of malunion, delayed union, or nonunion of osteotomy sites, surgical intervention should be delayed until a patient experiences significant difficulty in sports activities.

Surgical versatility in the treatment of a bunionette deformity is important. Attention to the underlying pathology helps to determine whether a condylectomy with a distal soft tissue repair, a distal metatarsal osteotomy, or a diaphyseal biplane osteotomy would offer the best treatment for the symptomatic bunionette deformity in the athlete. Analysis of the physical findings and examination of the plantar aspect of the foot for the presence of keratotic lesions help to differentiate the type of bunionette present and the appropriate treatment. Evaluation of radiographs is necessary to analyze the nature of the deformity.

Many different procedures have been advocated for treatment of a bunionette deformity. Lateral eminence resection, metatarsal head resection, and fifth ray resection as well as distal diaphyseal and proximal metatarsal osteotomies have been performed with and without MTP arthroplasties. The lack of adequate follow-up for most of these procedures and the anecdotal reports of success with different techniques raise significant questions about the long-term success rate. The presence of anatomic variations in patients with bunionette deformities complicates the decision-making process required in surgical intervention.

When an enlarged fifth metatarsal head or medial eminence is present (with or without a pronated foot or fifth ray), lateral condylectomy with MTP joint realignment or distal metatarsal osteotomy is the treatment of choice. The presence of a pure lateral keratotic lesion makes a chevron osteotomy preferable because of the stability of this osteotomy. Kirschner wire fixation often helps to stabilize the osteotomy site. When a plantar lateral keratotic lesion is present (with or without an increased 4–5 IM angle or lateral deviation), a distal oblique osteotomy as described by Kitaoka and Leventen[368] is preferable to the chevron procedure. A diaphyseal biplane osteotomy also may be used in this situation. When there is an abnormally wide 4–5 IM angle or when the less common lateral deviation of the distal fifth metatarsal is present, a diaphyseal biplane osteotomy affords an excellent means of correction.

Although there is some disagreement about the need for internal fixation after a fifth metatarsal osteotomy,[377] the development of delayed union, malunion, nonunion, or transfer lesions in patients in whom floating osteotomies have been performed indicates a need for internal fixation.

References

Hallux Valgus

1. Akin OA: The treatment of hallux valgus: A new operative procedure and its results. Med Sentinel 33:678–679, 1925.

2. Austin DW, Leventen EO: A new osteotomy for hallux valgus: A horizontally directed "V" displacement osteotomy of the metatarsal head for hallux valgus and primus varus. Clin Orthop 157:25–30, 1981.

3. Baxter DE: Treatment of bunion deformity in the athlete. Orthop Clin North Am 25:33–39, 1994.

4. Bonney G, Macnab I: Hallux valgus and hallux rigidus: A critical survey of operative results. J Bone Joint Surg Br 34:366–385, 1952.

5. Cedell CA, Astrom M: Proximal metatarsal osteotomy in hallux valgus. Acta Orthop Scand 53:1013–1018, 1982.

6. Cleveland M, Winnant EM: An end result study of the Keller operation. J Bone Joint Surg Am 32:163–175, 1950.

7. Colloff B, Weitz EM: Proximal phalangeal osteotomy in hallux valgus. Clin Orthop 54:105–113, 1967.

8. Corless JR: A modification of the Mitchell procedure. J Bone Joint Surg Br 58:138, 1976.

9. Coughlin MJ: Die operative Korrektur des Hallux valgus bei Jugendlichen mit proximaler Metatarsale-Osteotomie und distaler Weichteilrekonstruktion. Oper Orthop Traumatol 11:137–148, 1999.

10. Coughlin MJ: Hallux valgus. J Bone Joint Surg Am 78:932–966, 1996.

11. Coughlin MJ: Hallux valgus in the athlete. Sports Med Arthrosc Rev 2:326–340, 1994.

12. Coughlin MJ: Hallux valgus, causes, evaluation and treatment. Postgrad Med 75:174–187, 1975.

13. Coughlin MJ: Hallux valgus in men: Effect of the distal metatarsal articular angle on hallux valgus correction. Foot Ankle Int 18:463–470, 1997.

14. Coughlin MJ: Juvenile hallux valgus. In Coughlin MJ, Mann RA (eds): Surgery of the Foot and Ankle, 7th ed. St. Louis, Mosby–Year Book, 1999, pp 270–319.

15. Coughlin MJ: Juvenile hallux valgus: Etiology and treatment. Foot Ankle Int 16:682–697, 1995.

16. Coughlin MJ: Proximal first metatarsal osteotomy. In Johnson KA (ed): The Foot and Ankle, Master Techniques in Orthopaedic Surgery. New York, Raven Press, 1994, pp 85–105.

17. Coughlin M, Carlson RE: Treatment of hallux valgus with an increased distal metatarsal articular angle: Evaluation of double and triple first ray osteotomies. Foot Ankle Int 20:762–770, 1999.

18. Coughlin MJ, Mann RA: Arthrodesis of the first metatarsophalangeal joint as salvage for the failed Keller procedure. J Bone Joint Surg Am 69:68–75, 1987.

19. Coughlin MJ, Mann RA: The pathophysiology of the juvenile bunion. Instr Course Lect 36:122–136, 1987.

20. Coughlin M, Thompson F: The high price of high fashion footwear. Instr Course Lect 44:371–377, 1995.

21. Durman DC: Metatarsus primus varus and hallux valgus. Arch Surg 74:128–135, 1957.

22. DuVries HL: Static deformities. In DuVries HL (ed): Surgery of the Foot. St. Louis, CV Mosby, 1959, pp 381–388.

23. Funk FJ Jr, Wells RE: Bunionectomy—with distal osteotomy. Clin Orthop 85:71–74, 1972.

24. Goldberg I, Bahar A, Yosipovitch Z: Late results after correction of hallux valgus deformity by basilar phalangeal osteotomy. J Bone Joint Surg Am 69:64–67, 1987.

25. Goldner JL, Gaines RW: Adult and juvenile hallux valgus: Analysis and treatment. Orthop Clin North Am 7:863–887, 1976.

26. Hara B, Beck JC, Woo RA: First cuneiform closing abductory osteotomy for reduction of metatarsus primus adductus. J Foot Surg 31:434–439, 1992.

27. Hardy RH, Clapham JCR: Observations on hallux valgus. J Bone Joint Surg Br 33:376–391, 1951.

28. Hattrup SJ, Johnson KA: Chevron osteotomy: Analysis of factors in patients' dissatisfaction. Foot Ankle Int 5:327–332, 1985.

29. Hirvensalo E, Bostman O, Tormala P, et al: Chevron osteotomy fixed with absorbable polyglycolide pins. Foot Ankle Int 11:212–218, 1991.

30. Hohmann G: Fuss und Bein, 4th ed. Munich, JF Bergman, 1948, p 167.

31. Horne G, Tanzer T, Ford M: Chevron osteotomy for treatment of hallux valgus. Clin Orthop 183:32–36, 1984.

32. Hutton WC, Dhanendran M: The mechanics of normal and hallux valgus feet—a quantitative study. Clin Orthop 157:7–13, 1981.

33. Johnson KA, Cofield RH, Morrey BF: Chevron osteotomy for hallux valgus. Clin Orthop 142:44–47, 1979.

Abnormalities of the Toenail: Ingrown Toenails

160. Burzotta JL, Turri RM, Tsouris J: Phenol and alcohol chemical matrixectomy. Clin Podiatr Med Surg 6:453–468, 1989.
161. Cameron PF: Ingrowing toenails: An evaluation of two treatments. BMJ 283:821–822, 1981.
162. Ceh SE, Pettine KA: Treatment of ingrown toenail. J Musculoskel Med 7:62–82, 1990.
163. Clarke BG, Dillinger KA: Surgical treatment of ingrown toenail. Surgery 21:919–924, 1946.
164. Coughlin MJ: Toenail abnormalities. In Coughlin MJ, Mann RA (eds): Surgery of the Foot and Ankle, 7th ed. St. Louis, Mosby–Year Book, 1999, pp 1033–1070.
165. Dixon GL: Treatment of ingrown toenail. Foot Ankle Int 3:254–260, 1983.
166. Dockery GL: Nails: Fundamental conditions and procedures. In McGlamary ED (ed): Comprehensive Textbook of Foot Surgery. Baltimore, Williams & Wilkins, 1987, pp 3–37.
167. Dykyj D: Anatomy of the nail. Clin Podiatr Med Surg 6:215–228, 1989.
168. Gabriel SS, Dallos V, Stevenson DL: The ingrown toenail: A modified segmental matrix excision operation. Br J Surg 66:285–286, 1979.
169. Gallocher J: The phenol/alcohol method of nail matrix sterilization. N Z Med J 86:140–141, 1977.
170. Hashimoto K: Ultrastructure of the human toenail: Cell migration, keratinization, and formation of the intercellular cement. Arch Dermatol Forsch 240:1–22, 1971.
171. Heifetz CJ: Ingrown toenail. Am J Surg 38:298–315, 1937.
172. Johnson M: The human nail and its disorders. In Lorimer DL: Neale's Common Foot Disorders: Diagnosis and Management: A General Clinical Guide, 4th ed. Edinburgh, Churchill-Livingstone, 1993, pp 123–139.
173. Johnson M, Comaish J, Shuster S: Nail is produced by the normal nail bed: A controversy resolved. Br J Dermatol 125:27–29, 1991.
174. Keyes EL: The surgical treatment of ingrown toenails. JAMA 102:1458–1460, 1934.
175. Kuwada G: Long-term evaluation of partial and total surgical and phenol matrixectomies. J Am Podiatr Med Assoc 81:33–36, 1991.
176. Lewis BL: Microscopic studies of fetal and mature nail and surrounding soft tissue. Arch Dermatol 70:732–747, 1954.
177. Lloyd-Davies RW, Brill GC: The etiology and outpatient management of ingrowing toenail. Br J Surg 50:592–597, 1963.
178. Mann RA, Coughlin MJ: Toenail abnormalities. In Coughlin MJ (ed): The Video Textbook of Foot and Ankle Surgery. St. Louis, Medical Video Productions, 1991, pp 56–66.
179. Murray WR: Onychocryptosis. Clin Orthop 142:96–102, 1979.
180. Murray WR, Bedi BS: The surgical management of ingrowing toenail. Br J Surg 62:409–412, 1975.
181. Palmer BV, Jones A: Ingrowing toenails: The results of treatment. Br J Surg 66:575–576, 1979.
182. Pettine KA, Cofield RH, Johnson KA, Bussey RM: Ingrown toenail: Results of surgical treatment. Foot Ankle Int 9:130–134, 1988.
183. Ramsay G, Caldwell D: Phenol cauterization for ingrown toenails. Arch Emerg Med 3:243–246, 1986.
184. Robb JE, Murray WR: Phenol cauterization in the management of ingrowing toenails. Scott Med J 27:236–239, 1982.
185. Samman PD: The human toenail: Its genesis and blood supply. Br J Dermatol 71:296–302, 1959.
186. Thompson TC, Terwilliger C: The terminal Syme operation for ingrown toenail. Surg Clin North Am 31:575–584, 1951.
187. Townsend AC, Scott PJ: Ingrowing toenail and onychogryph. J Bone Joint Surg 48:354–358, 1966.
188. Wadhams P, McDonald J, Jenkin W: Epidermal inclusion cysts complication of nail surgery. J Am Podiatr Med Assoc 80:610, 1990.
189. Winograd AM: A modification in the technique for ingrown nail. JAMA 91:229–230, 1929.
190. Winograd AM: Results in operation for ingrown toenail. Illinois J 70:197–198, 1936.
191. Zadik FR: Obliteration of the nail bed of the great toe without shortening of the terminal phalanx. J Bone Joint Surg 328:66–67, 1950.
192. Zaias N: The Nail in Health and Disease. New York, SP Medical & Scientific Books, 1980, pp 1–43.

Abnormalities of the Toenail: Subungual Exostosis

193. Bendl BJ: Subungual exostosis. Cutis 26:260–262, 1980.
194. Breslow AM, Dorfman HD: Dupuytren's (subungual) exostosis. Am J Surg Pathol 12:368–378, 1988.
195. Cavolo DJ, D'Amelio JP, Hirsch AL, Patel T: Juvenile subungual osteochondroma: Case presentation. J Am Podiatr Med Assoc 71:81–83, 1981.
196. Chinn S, Jenkin W: Proximal nail groove pain associated with an exostosis. J Am Podiatr Med Assoc 76:506–508, 1986.
197. Cohen HJ, Frank SB, Minkin W: Subungual exostosis. Arch Dermatol 107:431–432, 1973.
198. Dal Cin P, Pauwels P, Poldermans LJ, et al: Clonal chromosome abnormalities in a so-called Dupuytren's subungual exostosis. Genes Chromosomes Cancer 24:162–164, 1999.
199. dePalma L, Gigane A, Specchia N: Subungual exostosis of the foot. Foot Ankle Int 17:758–763, 1996.
200. Dockery GL: Nails: Fundamental conditions and procedures. In McGlamry ED (ed): Comprehensive Textbook of Foot Surgery. Baltimore, Williams & Wilkins, 1987, pp 5–10.
201. Fickry T, Dkhissi M, Harfaoui A, et al: Les exostoses sous-ungueales etude retrospective d'une serie de 28 cas. Acta Orthop Belg 64:35–40, 1998.
202. Grisafi PJ, Lombardi CM, Sciarrino AL, et al: Three select subungual pathologies: Subungual exostosis, subungual osteochondroma, and subungual hematoma. Clin Podiatr Med Surg 6:355–364, 1989.
203. Ippolito E, Falez F, Tudisco C, et al: Subungual exostosis: Histological and clinical considerations on 30 cases. Ital J Orthop Traumatol 13:81–87, 1987.
204. Jahss MJ: Disorders of the Foot. Philadelphia, WB Saunders, 1982.
205. Johnston JA: Affections of the foot. In Mann RA (ed): Surgery of the Foot. St. Louis, CV Mosby, 1986, p 353.
206. Letts M, Davidson D, Nizalk E: Subungual exostosis: Diagnosis and treatment in children. J Trauma 44:346–349, 1998.
207. Norton LA: Nail disorders. J Am Acad Dermatol 2:457, 1980.
208. Oliviera ADS, Picoto A, Verde SF, Martins O: Subungual exostosis: Treatment as an office procedure. J Dermatol Surg Oncol 6:555–558, 1980.
209. Stephens H, Walling A: Subungual exostosis: A simple technique of excision. Foot Ankle Int 16:88–91, 1995.
210. Wang T, Wu Y, Su H: Subungual exostosis [letter to the editor]. J Dermatol 26:72–74, 1999.

Interdigital Neuroma

211. Amis J, Siverhus S, Liwnicz B: An anatomic basis for recurrence after Morton's neuroma excision. Foot Ankle Int 13:153–156, 1992.
212. Bassadonna P, Rucco V, Gasparini D, Onorato A: Plantar fat pad atrophy after corticosteroid injection for an interdigital neuroma. Am J Phys Med Rehabil 78:283–285, 1999.
213. Benedetti R, Baxter D, Davis P: Clinical results of simultaneous adjacent interdigital neurectomy in the foot. Foot Ankle Int 17:264–268, 1996.
214. Bennett G, Graham C, Mauldin D: Morton's interdigital neuroma: A comprehensive treatment protocol. Foot Ankle Int 16:760–763, 1995.
215. Beskin JL, Baxter DE: Recurrent pain following interdigital neurectomy—a plantar approach. Foot Ankle Int 9:34–39, 1988.
216. Betts LO: Morton's metatarsalgia: Neuritis of the fourth digital nerve. Med J Aust 1:514–515, 1940.
217. Bickel W, Dockerty M: Plantar neuromas, Morton's toe. SGO 85:111–116, 1947.
218. Bourke G, Owen J, Machet D: Histological comparison of the third interdigital nerve in patients with Morton's metatarsalgia and control patients. Aust N Z J Surg 64:421–424, 1994.
219. Bradley N, Miller W, Evans J: Plantar neuroma: Analysis of results following surgical excision in 145 patients. South Med J 69:853–854, 1976.
220. Coughlin MJ: The crossover second toe deformity. Foot Ankle Int 8:29–39, 1987.
221. Coughlin MJ: Lesser toe deformities. In Coughlin MJ, Mann RA (eds): Surgery of the Foot and Ankle, 7th ed. St. Louis, Mosby–Year Book, 1999, pp 320–391.
222. Coughlin MJ: Second metatarsophalangeal joint instability in the athlete. Foot Ankle Int 14:309–319, 1993.

223. Coughlin MJ: Soft tissue afflictions. In Chapman M (ed): Operative Orthopaedics. Philadelphia, JB Lippincott, 1988, pp 1819–1821.
224. Coughlin MJ: Subluxation and dislocation of the second metatarsophalangeal joint. Orthop Clin North Am 20:539–551, 1989.
225. Coughlin MJ: When to suspect crossover second toe deformity. J Musculoskel Med 4:39–48, 1987.
226. Coughlin MJ, Thompson FM: The high price of high-fashion footwear. Instr Course Lect 44:371–377, 1995.
227. Curtiss PH: Neurologic diseases of the foot. In Giannestras N (ed): Foot Disorders: Medical and Surgical Management, 2nd ed. Philadelphia, Lea & Febiger, 1973, pp 493–516.
228. Deese JM, Baxter DE: Compressive neuropathies of the lower extremity. J Musculoskel Med 68–91, 1988.
229. Dereymaeker G, Schroven I, Steenwreckx A, Stuer P: Results of excision of the interdigital nerve in the treatment of Morton's metatarsalgia. Acta Orthop Belg 62:22–25, 1996.
230. Friscia D, Strom D, Parr J, et al: Surgical treatment for primary interdigital neuroma. Orthopedics 14:669–672, 1991.
231. Gauthier G: Thomas Morton's disease: A nerve entrapment syndrome: A new surgical technique. Clin Orthop 142:90–92, 1979.
232. Graham CE, Graham DM: Morton's neuroma: A microscopic evaluation. Foot Ankle Int 5:150–155, 1984.
233. Graham CE, Johnson KA, Ilstrup DM: The intermetatarsal nerve: A microscopic evaluation. Foot Ankle Int 2:150–152, 1981.
234. Greenfield J, Rea J, Weld F: Morton's interdigital neuroma: Indications for treatment by local injections versus surgery. Clin Orthop 185:142–144, 1984.
235. Hauser ED: Interdigital neuroma of the foot. Surg Gynecol Obstet 133:265–267, 1971.
236. Hoadley AE: Six cases of metatarsalgia. Chicago Med Rec 5: 32, 1893.
237. Johnson JE, Johnson KA: Continued webspace pain following interdigital neuroma resection—results of reoperation. Proceedings of the American Orthopaedic Foot and Ankle Society. Foot Ankle Int 7:310–311, 1987.
238. Jones JR, Klenerman L: A study of the communicating branch between the medial and lateral plantar nerves. Foot Ankle Int 4: 313–315, 1984.
239. Karges DE: Plantar excision of primary interdigital neuromas. Foot Ankle Int 9:120–124, 1988.
240. Keh R, Ballew K, Higgins K, et al: Long-term follow-up of Morton's neuroma. J Foot Surg 31:93–95, 1992.
241. Klenerman L, MacClellan G, Guiloff R, Scadding J: Morton's metatarsalgia: A retrospective and prospective study (proceedings and reports of universities, colleges, councils, associations, and societies). J Bone Joint Surg Br 65:220–221, 1983.
242. Levitsky K, Alman B, Jevsevar D, Morehead J: Digital nerves of the foot: Anatomic variations and implications regarding the pathogenesis of interdigital neuroma. Foot Ankle Int 14:208–214, 1993.
243. Mann RA: Diseases of the nerves of the foot. In Mann RA (ed): Surgery of the Foot, 5th ed. St. Louis, CV Mosby, 1985, pp 199–208.
244. Mann RA, Reynolds JC: Interdigital neuroma: A critical clinical analysis. Foot Ankle Int 3:238–243, 1983.
245. Mendicino S, Rockett M: Morton's neuroma: Update on diagnosis and imaging. Clin Podiatr Surg Med 14:303–311, 1997.
246. McElvenny RT: The etiology and surgical treatment of intractable pain about the fourth metatarsophalangeal joint. J Bone Joint Surg 25:675–679, 1943.
247. McKeever DC: Surgical approach for neuroma of the plantar digital nerve. J Bone Joint Surg Am 34:490, 1952.
248. Morton TG: A peculiar painful affection of the fourth metatarsophalangeal articulation. Am J Med Sci 71:37–45, 1876.
249. Mulder JD: The causative mechanism in Morton's metatarsalgia. J Bone Joint Surg Br 33:94–95, 1951.
250. Murphy PE, Baxter DE: Nerve entrapment of the foot and ankle in runners. Clin Sports Med 4:753–763, 1985.
251. Rasmussen M, Kitaoka H, Patzer G: Nonoperative treatment of plantar interdigital neuroma with a single corticosteroid injection. Clin Orthop 326:188–193, 1996.
252. Reddy P, Zelicof S, Ruotolo C, Holder J: Interdigital neuroma: Local cutaneous changes after corticosteroid injection. Clin Orthop 317: 185–187, 1995.
253. Reed R, Bliss B: Morton's neuroma: Aggressive and productive intermetatarsal elastofibrosis. Arch Pathol 95:123–129, 1973.
254. Richardson E, Brotzman S, Graves S: The plantar incision for procedures involving the forefoot. J Bone Joint Surg Am 75:726–731, 1993.
255. Sarrafian SK: Nerves. In Sarrafian SK: Anatomy of the Foot and Ankle: Descriptive, Topographic, Functional. Philadelphia, JB Lippincott, 1983, pp 315–325.
256. Sartoris D, Brozinsky S, Resnick D: Magnetic resonance images. J Foot Surg 28:78–82, 1989.
257. Shapiro P, Shapiro S: Sonographic evaluation of interdigital neuromas. Foot Ankle Int 16:604–606, 1995.
258. Teasdall R, Saltzman C, Johnson K: A practical approach to Morton's neuroma. J Musculoskel Med 10:39–52, 1993.
259. Terk M, Kwong P, Suthar M, et al: Morton neuroma: Evaluation with MR imaging performed with contrast enhancement and fat suppression. Radiology 189:239–241, 1993.
260. Thompson F, Deland J: Occurrence of two interdigital neuromas in one foot. Foot Ankle Int 14:15–17, 1993.
261. Turan I, Lindgren U, Sahlstedt T: Computed tomography for diagnosis of Morton's neuroma. J Foot Surg 30:244–245, 1991.
262. Unger H, Mattoso P, Drusen M, Neumann C: Gadopentetate-enhanced magnetic resonance imaging with fat saturation in the evaluation of Morton's neuroma. J Foot Surg 31:244–246, 1992.
263. Wu K: Morton's interdigital neuroma: A clinical review of its etiology, treatment, and results. J Foot Ankle Surg 35:112–119, 1996.
264. Youngswick F: Intermetatarsal neuroma. Clin Podiatr Med Surg 11: 579–592, 1994.

Intractable Plantar Keratoses

265. Coughlin MJ: Crossover second toe deformity. Foot Ankle Int 8: 29–39, 1987.
266. Coughlin MJ: Lesser toe deformities. Orthopaedics 10:63–75, 1987.
267. Coughlin MJ: Second metatarsophalangeal joint instability in the athlete. Foot Ankle Int 14:309–319, 1993.
268. Coughlin MJ: Subluxation and dislocation of the second metatarsophalangeal joint. Orthop Clin North Am 20:539–551, 1989.
269. Coughlin MJ: When to suspect crossover second toe deformity. J Musculoskel Med 4:39–48, 1987.
270. Coughlin MJ, Mann RA: Lesser toe deformities. Instr Course Lect 36:137–160, 1987.
271. Coughlin MJ, Mann RA: Lesser toe deformities. In Coughlin MJ, Mann RA (eds): Surgery of the Foot and Ankle, 7th ed. St. Louis, Mosby–Year Book, 1999, pp 320–391.
272. Dreeben SM, Noble PC, Hammerman S, et al: Metatarsal osteotomy for primary metatarsalgia: Radiographic and pedobarographic study. Foot Ankle Int 9:214–218, 1989.
273. DuVries HL: Disorders of the skin. In DuVries HL (ed): Surgery of the Foot, 2nd ed. St. Louis, CV Mosby, 1965, pp 168–190, 456–462.
274. DuVries HL: New approach to the treatment of intractable verruca plantaris (plantar wart). JAMA 152:1202–1203, 1953.
275. Giannestras NJ: Shortening of the metatarsal shaft in the treatment of plantar keratosis. J Bone Joint Surg Am 49:61–71, 1958.
276. Hatcher RM, Goller WL, Weil LS: Intractable plantar keratoses: A review of surgical corrections. J Am Podiatr Assoc 68:377–386, 1978.
277. Helal B: Metatarsal osteotomy for metatarsalgia. J Bone Joint Surg Br 57:187–192, 1975.
278. Helal B, Greiss M: Telescoping osteotomy for pressure metatarsalgia. J Bone Joint Surg Br 66:213–217, 1984.
279. Holmes GB: Quantitative determination of intermetatarsal pressure. Foot Ankle Int 13:532–535, 1992.
280. Idusuyi CB, Kitaoka HB, Patzer GL: Oblique metatarsal osteotomy for intractable plantar keratosis: 10-year follow-up. Foot Ankle Int 19:351–355, 1998.
281. Jahss MH: The abnormal plantigrade foot. Orthop Rev 7:31–37, 1978.
282. Jacoby RP: V osteotomy for correction of intractable plantar keratosis. J Foot Surg 12:8–10, 1973.
283. Kitaoka HB, Patzer GL: Chevron osteotomy of lesser metatarsals for intractable plantar callosities. J Bone Joint Surg Br 80:516–518, 1998.
284. Mann RA: Intractable plantar keratosis. Instr Course Lect 33:287–309, 1984.
285. Mann RA: Keratotic disorders of the plantar skin. In Mann RA (ed):

Mann-DuVries Surgery of the Foot, 5th ed. St. Louis, CV Mosby, 1986, pp 180–198.

286. Mann RA, Coughlin MJ: Intractable plantar keratosis. In Coughlin MJ (ed): Video Textbook of Foot and Ankle Surgery. St. Louis, Medical Video Productions, 1991, pp 85–95.

287. Mann RA, Coughlin MJ: Keratotic disorders of the plantar skin. In Coughlin MJ, Mann RA (eds): Surgery of the Foot and Ankle, 7th ed. St. Louis, Mosby–Year Book, 1999, pp 392–435.

288. Mann RA, DuVries MD: Intractable plantar keratosis. Orthop Clin North Am 4:67–73, 1973.

289. Mann RA, Wapner K: Tibial sesamoid shaving for treatment of intractable plantar keratosis under the tibial sesamoid. Foot Ankle Int 13:196–198, 1992.

290. Pedowitz WJ: Distal oblique osteotomy for intractable plantar keratosis of the middle three metatarsals. Foot Ankle Int 9:7–9, 1988.

291. Pontious J, Lane GD, Moritz JC, Martin W: Lesser metatarsal V-osteotomy for chronic intractable plantar keratosis: Retrospective analysis of 40 procedures. J Podiatr Med Assoc 88:323–331, 1998.

292. Trnka J, Muhlbauer M, Zetti R, et al: Comparison of the results of the Weil and Helal osteotomies for the treatment of metatarsalgia secondary to dislocation of the lesser metatarsophalangeal joints. Foot Ankle Int 20:72–79, 1999.

293. Van Enoo RE, Cane EM: Tibial sesamoid planing for intractable plantar keratoses. Clin Podiatr Med Surg 8:41–47, 1991.

294. Winson IG, Rawlinson J, Broughton NS: Treatment of metatarsalgia by sliding distal metatarsal osteotomy. Foot Ankle Int 9:2–6, 1988.

Lesser Toe Deformities

295. Alvine FG, Garvin KL: Peg and dowel fusion of the proximal interphalangeal joint. Foot Ankle Int 1:90–94, 1980.

296. Barbari SG, Brevig K: Correction of clawtoes by Girdlestone-Taylor flexor-extensor transfer procedure. Foot Ankle Int 5:67–73, 1984.

297. Brahms MA: Common foot problems. J Bone Joint Surg Am 49:1653–1664, 1967.

298. Branch HE: Pathologic dislocation of the second toe. J Bone Joint Surg 19:978–984, 1937.

299. Cahill B, Connor D: A long-term follow-up on proximal phalangectomy for hammer toes. Clin Orthop 86:191–192, 1972.

300. Conklin M, Smith R: Treatment of the atypical lesser toe deformity with basal hemiphalangectomy. Foot Ankle Int 15:585–594, 1994.

301. Coughlin MJ: Crossover second toe deformity. Foot Ankle Int 8:29–39, 1987.

302. Coughlin MJ: The high cost of fashionable footwear. J Musculoskel Med 11:40–53, 1994.

303. Coughlin MJ: Lesser toe abnormalities. In Chapman M (ed): Operative Orthopaedics. Philadelphia, JB Lippincott, 1993, pp 2213–2224.

304. Coughlin MJ: Lesser toe deformities. Orthopaedics 10:63–75, 1987.

305. Coughlin MJ: Mallet toes, hammer toes, claw toes, and corns—causes and treatment of lesser toe deformities. Postgrad Med 75:191–198, 1984.

306. Coughlin MJ: Operative repair of the mallet toe deformity. Foot Ankle Int 16:109–116, 1995.

307. Coughlin MJ: Second metatarsophalangeal joint instability in the athlete. Foot Ankle Int 14:309–319, 1993.

308. Coughlin MJ: Subluxation and dislocation of the second metatarsophalangeal joint. Orthop Clin North Am 20:539–551, 1989.

309. Coughlin MJ: When to suspect crossover second toe deformity. J Musculoskel Med 4:39–48, 1987.

310. Coughlin MJ, Dorris J, Polk E: Operative repair of the fixed hammertoe deformity. Foot Ankle Int 21:94–104, 2000.

311. Coughlin MJ, Mann RA: Lesser toe deformities. In Coughlin MJ, Mann RA (eds): Surgery of the Foot, 7th ed. St. Louis, Mosby–Year Book, 1999, pp 320–391.

312. Coughlin MJ, Thompson FM: The high price of high-fashion footwear. Instr Course Lect 44:371–377, 1995.

313. Creer WS: Treatment of hammertoe. BMJ 1:527–528, 1935.

314. Daly P, Johnson K: Treatment of painful subluxation or dislocation at the second and third metatarsophalangeal joints by partial proximal phalanx excision and subtotal webbing. Clin Orthop 278:164–170, 1992.

315. DuVries HL: Dislocation of the toe. JAMA 160:728, 1956.

316. Ford LA, Collins KB, Christensen JC: Stabilization of the subluxed second metatarsophalangeal joint: Flexor tendon transfer versus primary repair of the plantar plate. J Foot Ankle Surg 37:217–222, 1998.

317. Girdlestone GR: Physiotherapy for hand and foot. J Chartered Soc Physiotherapy 32:167, 1947.

318. Glassman F, Wolin I, Sideman S: Phalangectomy for toe deformity. Surg Clin North Am 29:275–280, 1949.

319. Kuwada G: A retrospective analysis of modification of the flexor tendon transfer for correction of hammer toe. J Foot Ankle Surg 27:57–59, 1988.

320. Lehman D, Smith R: Treatment of symptomatic hammertoe with a proximal interphalangeal joint arthrodesis. Foot Ankle Int 16:535–541, 1995.

321. Mann RA, Coughlin MJ: Lesser toe deformities. Instr Course Lect 36:137–159, 1987.

322. Mann RA, Coughlin MJ: Lesser toe deformities. In Jahss MH (ed): Disorders of the Foot, 2nd ed. Philadelphia, WB Saunders, 1991, pp 1205–1228.

323. Mann RA, Coughlin MJ: Lesser toe deformities. In Coughlin MJ (ed): Video Textbook of Foot and Ankle Surgery. St. Louis, Medical Video Productions, 1991, pp 47–49.

324. Mann RA, Mizel MA: Monoarticular nontraumatic synovitis of the metatarsophalangeal joint: A new diagnosis. Foot Ankle Int 6:18–21, 1985.

325. McConnell BE: Correction of hammertoe deformity: A 10-year review of subperiosteal waist resection of the proximal phalanx. Orthop Rev 8:65–69, 1975.

326. McConnell BE: Hammertoe surgery: Waist resection of the proximal phalanx: A more simplified procedure. South Med J 68:595–598, 1975.

327. Ohm O, McDonnell M, Vetter W: Digital arthrodesis: An alternate method for correction of hammertoe deformity. J Foot Ankle Surg 29:207–211, 1990.

328. Parish TF: Dynamic correction of clawtoes. Orthop Clin North Am 4:97–102, 1973.

329. Pyper JB: The flexor-extensor transplant operation for claw toes. J Bone Joint Surg Br 40:528–533, 1958.

330. Sarrafian SK: Anatomy of the Foot and Ankle. Philadelphia, JB Lippincott, 1983.

331. Sarrafian SK, Topouzian L: Anatomy and physiology of the extensor apparatus of the toes. J Bone Joint Surg 51A:669–679, 1969.

332. Sarrafian SK: Correction of fixed hammertoe deformity with resection of the head of the proximal phalanx and extensor tendon tenodesis. Foot Ankle Int 16:449–451, 1995.

333. Scheck M: Etiology of acquired hammertoe deformity. Clin Orthop 123:63–69, 1979.

334. Schlefman B, Fenton C, McGlamry E: Peg in hole arthrodesis. J Am Podiatr Med Assoc 73:187–195, 1983.

335. Soule RA: Operation for the correction of hammertoe. N Y Med J 91:649–650, 1910.

336. Taylor RG: An operative procedure for the treatment of hammertoe and claw-toe. J Bone Joint Surg 22:608–609, 1940.

337. Taylor RG: The treatment of claw toes by multiple transfers of flexor into extensor tendons. J Bone Joint Surg Br 33:539–542, 1951.

338. Thompson F, Deland J: Flexor tendon transfer for metatarsophalangeal instability of the second toe. Foot Ankle Int 14:385–388, 1993.

339. Threthowen WH: Treatment of hammertoe. Lancet 1:1312–1313, 1925.

340. Trnka J, Muhlbauer M, Zetti R, et al: Comparison of the results of the Weil and Helal osteotomies for the treatment of metatarsalgia secondary to dislocation of the lesser metatarsophalangeal joints. Foot Ankle Int 20:72–79, 1999.

341. Young CS: An operation for the correction of hammertoe and clawtoe. J Bone Joint Surg 20:715–719, 1938.

342. Zeringue G, Harkless L: Evaluation and management of the web corn involving the fourth interdigital space. J Am Podiatr Med Assoc 76:210–213, 1986.

343. Zingas C, Katcherian D, Wu K: Kirschner wire breakage after surgery of the lesser toes. Foot Ankle Int 16:504–509, 1995.

Bunionettes

344. Adante J, Chin M, Makower B, et al: Surgical correction of tailor's bunion with resection of fifth metatarsal head and Silastic implant: An 8-year follow-up study. J Foot Surg 25:315–320, 1986.

345. Bishop J, Kahn A, Turba JE: Surgical correction of the splayfoot: The Giannestras procedure. Clin Orthop 146:234–238, 1980.

346. Brown JE: Functional and cosmetic correction of metatarsus latus (splay foot). Clin Orthop 14:166–170, 1959.
347. Campbell D: Chevron osteotomy for bunionette deformity. Foot Ankle Int 2:355–356, 1982.
348. Coughlin MJ: Etiology and treatment of the bunionette deformity. Instr Course Lect 39:37–48, 1990.
349. Coughlin M: Treatment of bunionette deformity with longitudinal diaphyseal osteotomy with distal soft tissue repair. Foot Ankle Int 11:195–203, 1991.
350. Davies H: Metatarsus quintus valgus. BMJ 664–665, 1949.
351. Dickson FD, Diveley RL: Functional Disorders of the Foot, 3rd ed. Philadelphia, JB Lippincott, 1953, p 230.
352. Diebold PF: Basal osteotomy of the fifth metatarsal for the bunionette. Foot Ankle Int 12:74–79, 1991.
353. Diebold PF, Bejjani FJ: Basal osteotomy of the fifth metatarsal with intermetatarsal pinning: A new approach to tailor's bunion. Foot Ankle Int 8:40–45, 1987.
354. Dorris M, Mandel L: Fifth metatarsal head resection for correction of tailor's bunions and sub-fifth metatarsal head keratoma: A retrospective analysis. J Foot Surg 30:269–275, 1991.
355. DuVries H: Surgery of the Foot, 2nd ed. St. Louis, CV Mosby, 1965, pp 456–462.
356. Estersohn H, Scherer P, Bogdan R: A preliminary report on opening wedge osteotomy of the fifth metatarsal. Arch Podiatr Med Foot Surg 1:317–327, 1974.
357. Fallat LM, Buckholz J: An analysis of the tailor's bunion by radiographic and anatomical display. J Am Podiatr Assoc 70:597–603, 1980.
358. Gerbert J, Sgarlato TE, Subotnik SI: Preliminary study of a closing wedge osteotomy of the fifth metatarsal for correction of a tailor's bunion deformity. J Am Podiatr Assoc 62:212–218, 1972.
359. Giannestras NJ: Other problems of the foot. In Giannestras NJ (ed): Foot Disorders: Medical and Surgical Management. Philadelphia, Lea & Febiger, 1973, pp 420–421.
360. Haber JH, Kraft J: Crescentic osteotomy for fifth metatarsal head lesions. J Foot Ankle Surg 19:66–67, 1980.
361. Hohmann F: Fuss und Bein. Munich, JG Bergman, 1951, pp 172–173.
362. Kaplan EG, Kaplan G, Jacobs AM: Management of fifth metatarsal head lesion by biplane osteotomy. J Foot Ankle Surg 15:1–8, 1976.
363. Keating SE, DeVincentis A, Goller WL: Oblique fifth metatarsal osteotomy: A followup study. J Foot Ankle Surg 21:104–107, 1982.
364. Kelikian H: Deformities of the lesser toe. In Kelikian H (ed): Hallux Valgus, Allied Deformities of the Forefoot and Metatarsalgia. Philadelphia, WB Saunders, 1965, pp 327–330.
365. Kitaoka H, Holiday A: Lateral condylar resection for bunionette. Clin Orthop 278:183–192, 1992.
366. Kitaoka H, Holiday A: Metatarsal head resection for bunionette, long-term follow-up. Foot Ankle Int 1:345–349, 1991.
367. Kitaoka H, Holiday A, Campbell D: Distal chevron metatarsal osteotomy for bunionette. Foot Ankle Int 12:80–85, 1991.

368. Kitaoka H, Leventen E: Medial displacement metatarsal osteotomy for treatment of the painful bunionette. Clin Orthop 243:172–179, 1988.
369. Leach RE, Igou R: Metatarsal osteotomy for bunionette deformity. Clin Orthop 100:171–175, 1974.
370. LeLievre J: Exostosis of the head of the fifth metatarsal bone, tailor's bunion. Le Concours Medical 78:4815–4816, 1956.
371. LeLievre J: Pathologie du Pied, 5th ed. Paris, Masson, 1971, pp 526–528.
372. Mann RA: Keratotic disorders of the plantar skin. In Mann RA (ed): Surgery of the Foot, 5th ed. St. Louis, CV Mosby, 1986, pp 194–198.
373. McGlamry ED: Metatarsal shortening: Osteoplasty of head and osteotomy of shaft. J Am Podiatr Assoc 59:394, 1969.
374. McKeever DC: Excision of the fifth metatarsal head. Clin Orthop 13:321–322, 1959.
375. Moran M, Claridge R: Chevron osteotomy for bunionette. Foot Ankle Int 16:684–688, 1994.
376. Nestor B, Kitaoka H, Bergmann A: Radiologic anatomy of the painful bunionette. Foot Ankle Int 11:6–11, 1990.
377. Pontious J, Brook J, Hillstrom H: Tailor's bunion: Is fixation necessary? J Am Podiatr Med Assoc 86:63–73, 1996.
378. Regnauld B: Technique Chirurgicales du Pied. Paris, Masson, 1974, p 23.
379. Sakoff M, Levy A, Hanft J: Metaphyseal osteotomy for the treatment of tailor's bunions. J Foot Ankle Surg 28:537–541, 1989.
380. Schabler J, Toney M, Hanft J, Kashuk K: Oblique metaphyseal osteotomy for the correction of tailor's bunion: A 3-year review. J Foot Surg 31:79–84, 1992.
381. Schoenhaus H, Rotman S, Meshon A: A review of normal metatarsal angles. J Am Podiatr Assoc 63:88–95, 1973.
382. Shereff M, Yang W, Kummer F, et al: Vascular anatomy of the fifth metatarsal. Foot Ankle Int 11:350–353, 1991.
383. Shrum D, Sprandel D, Marshall H: Triplanar closing base wedge osteotomy for tailor's bunion. J Am Podiatr Med Assoc 79:124–127, 1989.
384. Sponsel KH: Bunionette correction by metatarsal osteotomy. Orthop Clin North Am 7:808–819, 1976.
385. Stewart M: Miscellaneous affections of the foot. In Edmonson ES, Crenshaw AH (eds): Campbell's Operative Orthopaedics, 6th ed. St. Louis, CV Mosby, 1980, p 1733.
386. Throckmorton JK, Bradlee N: Transverse V sliding osteotomy: A new surgical procedure for the correction of tailor's bunion deformity. J Foot Surg 18:117–121, 1978.
387. Voutey H: Manueal de Chirurgie Orthopaedique et de Reeducational du Pied. Paris, Masson, 1978, pp 149–151.
388. Weisberg MH: Resection of the fifth metatarsal head in lateral segment problems. J Am Podiatr Assoc 57:374–376, 1967.
389. Yancey HA: Congenital lateral bowing of the fifth metatarsal. Clin Orthop 62:203–205, 1969.
390. Zvijac J, Janecki C, Freeling R: Distal oblique osteotomy for tailor's bunion. Foot Ankle Int 12:171–175, 1991.

Section K

Osteochondroses and Related Problems of the Foot and Ankle

S. Terry Canale, MD

The term *osteochondrosis* has been applied to more than 50 eponymic entities to describe a variety of conditions characterized by abnormal endochondral ossification of physeal growth.[1, 2, 5, 8] Osteochondrosis is defined as a disease of the growth or ossification centers in children that begins as a degeneration or necrosis followed by regeneration or recalcification. Osteochondritis dissecans is defined as an osteochondritis (inflammation of both bone and cartilage) that results in splitting of pieces of cartilage into the joint. Because normal endochondral ossification does not always present a uniform radiographic pattern, the differentiation of osteochondrosis from normal growth is often difficult.[1, 2, 5, 8] Diagnosis of an osteochondrosis includes abnormal radiographic findings in conjunction with local symptoms.

The etiology of osteochondritic changes has been described as traumatic, constitutional, idiopathic, and hereditary.[1, 2, 5, 6, 8, 10] Most authors now believe that these changes are caused by multifactorial elements. For example, excessive physical demands during athletic activity may incite osteochondral changes in growing bone made vulnerable by constitutional factors. Certainly, once the process has begun, repetitive trauma or pressure may prolong recovery and contribute to deformity. All osteochondroses heal, but treatment may be required to relieve pain or to prevent residual deformity, especially in those osteochondroses about the foot and ankle in the athlete.

Numerous classifications of the osteochondroses have been proposed on the basis of etiology, anatomic location, and type of growth center, but none has had much practical application. Siffert[10] proposed a clinically oriented classification that divides the osteochondroses into three fundamental groups—articular, nonarticular, and physeal (Table 30K–1). Osteochondroses involving the foot and ankle are generally articular or nonarticular. Articular osteochondroses, such as Freiberg's and Köhler's diseases, may result in degenerative arthritis, pain, and limitation of motion, and treatment should be aimed at minimizing the epiphyseal deformity and encouraging joint congruity. Nonarticular osteochondroses, such as Sever's disease of the os calcis, cause local pain with activity and local tenderness, usually occur in adolescents, and are self-limited conditions. Treatment of any osteochondritic condition must be individualized to allow the athlete a rapid, safe return to activity and to minimize sequelae of the condition.

A number of osteochondritic conditions in the foot and ankle have been described,[1–4, 7, 9] but many of these are rare and usually asymptomatic. The most common osteochondroses that may cause symptoms and require treatment affect the talus, calcaneus, navicular, cuneiforms, metatarsals, and sesamoids (Fig. 30K–1). Because an osteochondrosis or osteochondritis may have its onset in a child or adolescent but not become evident until adulthood, it is

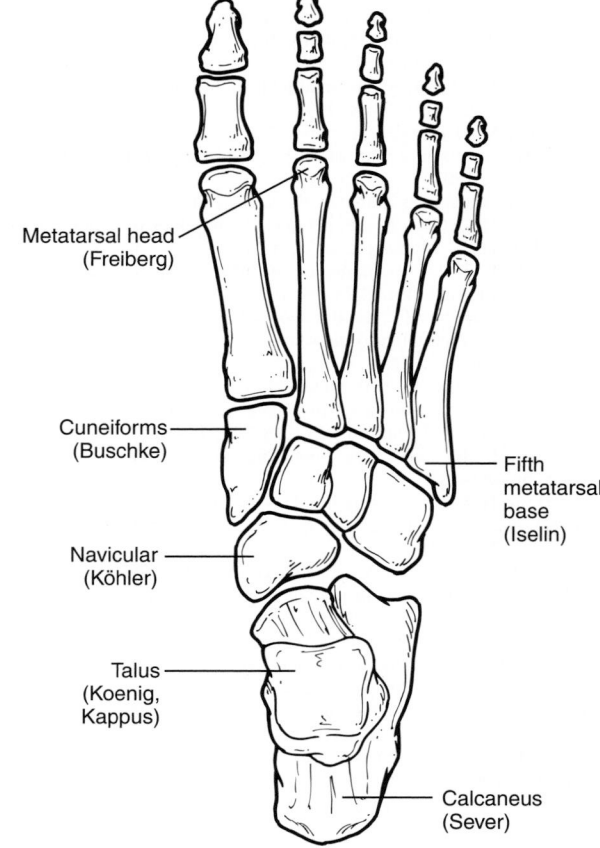

Figure 30K–1. Common sites of osteochondrosis in the foot. Specific form of disease is mentioned in parentheses.

difficult to divide these conditions into clear-cut adult and pediatric categories.

Osteochondritis Dissecans of the Talus

Etiology and Epidemiology

In 1888, Konig[34] first used the term *osteochondritis dissecans* to describe loose bodies in the knee joint, theorizing that they were caused by spontaneous necrosis of bone. In 1922, Kappis[31] noted the similarity of lesions of the ankle to those found in the knee and referred to osteochondritis dissecans of the ankle. In 1932, Rendu[45] reported an intra-articular fracture of the talus that appeared to be similar in nature to the lesion of osteochondritis dissecans. In 1953, Roden and colleagues[46] reported 55 osteochondritis dissecans–like lesions of the talus. They concluded that almost all of the lesions occurring laterally in the talus were secondary to trauma, rarely healed spontaneously, caused more symptoms than did lesions occurring in other locations in the ankle, and, because early arthritis developed, required early operation. Conversely, a large percentage of the medial lesions in their series were not secondary to trauma, had fewer symptoms, frequently healed sponta-

TABLE 30K–1
Classification of Osteochondroses

Articular osteochondroses
  Primary involvement of articular and epiphyseal cartilage and
    subjacent endochondral ossification (e.g., humeral condylosis,
    Freiberg's disease)
  Secondary involvement of articular and epiphyseal cartilage as a
    consequence of avascular necrosis of subjacent bone (e.g., Legg-
    Calvé-Perthes syndrome, Köhler's osteochondritis dissecans)
Nonarticular osteochondroses
  At tendon attachments (e.g., Osgood-Schlatter disease)
  At ligament attachments (e.g., vertebral ring, epicondyles)
  At impact sites (e.g., Sever's disease)
Physeal osteochondroses
  Long bones (e.g., tibia vara)
  Vertebrae (Scheuermann's disease)

From Siffert RS: Classification of osteochondroses. Clin Orthop 158:12, 1981.

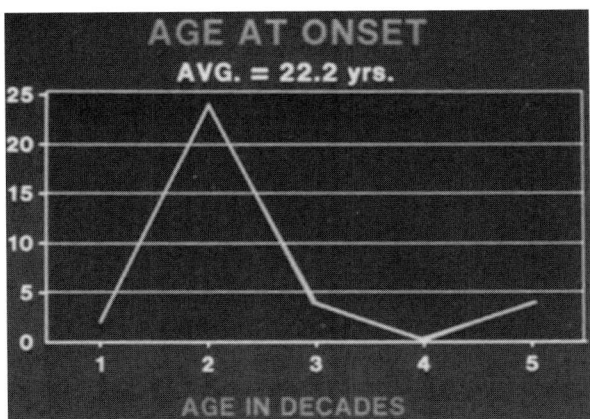

Figure 30K–2. Onset of symptoms in 31 patients with osteochondral lesions of the talus. The *vertical axis* indicates the number of patients.

neously, and, because little or no arthrosis developed, needed late excision only if a loose body was causing symptoms.

In 1959, Berndt and Harty[15] demonstrated that both the medial and lateral lesions of osteochondritis dissecans of the talus were in reality transchondral (osteochondral) fractures caused by trauma. In their classic work, 43% of the lesions were noted to be in the lateral portion, usually the middle third of the talus, whereas 57% were noted to be in the medial portion, usually the posterior third. In experiments with cadavers, the lateral lesion was produced by inversion and strong dorsiflexion; the medial lesion was caused by inversion, plantar flexion, and lateral rotation of the tibia on the talus.

Of the 31 lesions treated at the Campbell Clinic,[17, 18] 14 were medial, 15 were lateral, and 2 were central. Symptoms began in the second decade of life in 21 patients (Fig. 30K–2). Twenty-five of the lesions—9 medial, 15 lateral, and 1 central—were associated with a history of trauma. A history of pure inversion injury was associated with one medial and seven lateral lesions. Two lateral lesions were associated with a history of pure eversion and pure dorsiflexion injury. The 15 remaining lesions were associated with crushing trauma or poorly described twisting injuries. Of the lesions with no history of trauma, five were medial and one was central. According to the classification of Berndt and Harty, there were no stage I lesions, and only one lateral lesion was a stage II lesion. Of 24 stage III lesions, 13 were medial, 10 were lateral, and 1 was central. Of the six stage IV lesions, one was medial, four were lateral, and one was central.

Although osteochondritis dissecans of the talus is generally considered a condition of adulthood, Higuera and coworkers[30] reported 19 ankles with osteochondritis dissecans lesions in 18 young patients (average age, 13 years; range, 8 to 16 years). A history of trauma was confirmed in 10 of the 19 ankles. The lesion was painful in all ankles except for the right ankle of a patient with bilateral lesions. Inflammation in the region was found in 10, significant restriction of movement occurred in 7, and lesions of the external lateral ligament were found in 4. They obtained excellent or good results in 95% of patients, most of whom were treated conservatively.

In a meta-analysis of 32 articles in the literature that included 582 patients (average age, 27 years), Tol and associates[51] found that 44% of the talar dome lesions were lateral and 56% were medial. Lateral lesions were associated with previous ankle trauma in 94%, and medial lesions were associated with trauma in 62%; 67% of the patients were men and 33% were women.

Classification

Berndt and Harty[15] classified the lesion or fracture into four different stages (Fig. 30K–3): stage I, a small area of compression of subchondral bone; stage II, a partially detached osteochondral fragment; stage III, a completely detached osteochondral fragment remaining in the crater; and stage IV, a displaced osteochondral fragment.

Anderson and colleagues[11] added a stage IIb to the Berndt and Harty classification to include subchondral cyst formation. Loomer and coworkers,[38] using predominantly computed tomographic (CT) scans of osteochondral lesions, confirmed the frequency (77%) of "radiolucent lesions" or subchondral cysts and added stage V to the classification. Ferkel[23] described a classification based on CT findings (Fig. 30K–4), and Hepple and associates[28] proposed a new classification based on magnetic resonance imaging (MRI) features (Fig. 30K–5) because of a lack of correlation between the radiologic stages of Berndt and Harty and the stages they discovered using MRI. Of their 18 patients with osteochondral lesions, 12 had medial lesions, 5 had lateral lesions, and 1 had a posterior lesion.

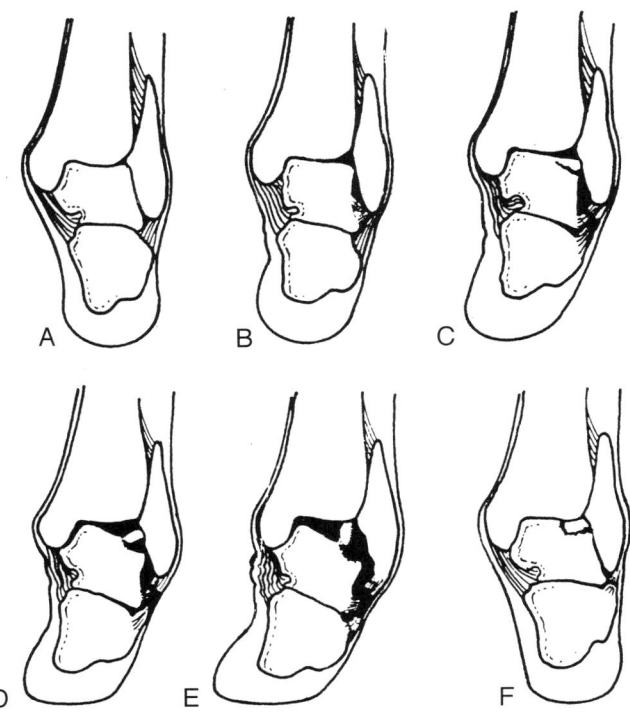

Figure 30K–3. Four stages of osteochondritis dissecans of the talus. *A,* Normal talus. *B,* Stage I. *C,* Stage II. *D,* Stage III. *E,* Stage IIIa. *F,* Stage IV. (Redrawn from Berndt AL, Harty M: Transchondral fracture of the talus. J Bone Joint Surg Am 41:988, 1959.)

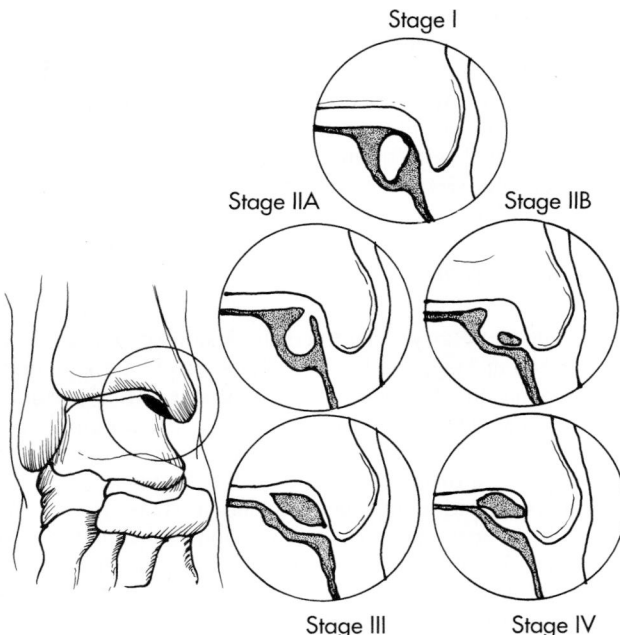

Figure 30K–4. Classification of osteochondritis dissecans of the talus based on computed tomographic scanning. Stage I, cystic lesion within talar dome, intact roof on all views. Stage IIA, cystic lesion with communication to talar dome surface. Stage IIB, open articular surface lesion with overlying nondisplaced fragment. Stage III, nondisplaced lesion with lucency. Stage IV, displaced fragment. (From Ferkel RD: Arthroscopy of the foot and ankle. In Coughlin MJ, Mann RA [eds]: Surgery of the Foot and Ankle, 7th ed. St Louis, Mosby, 1999, p 1272.)

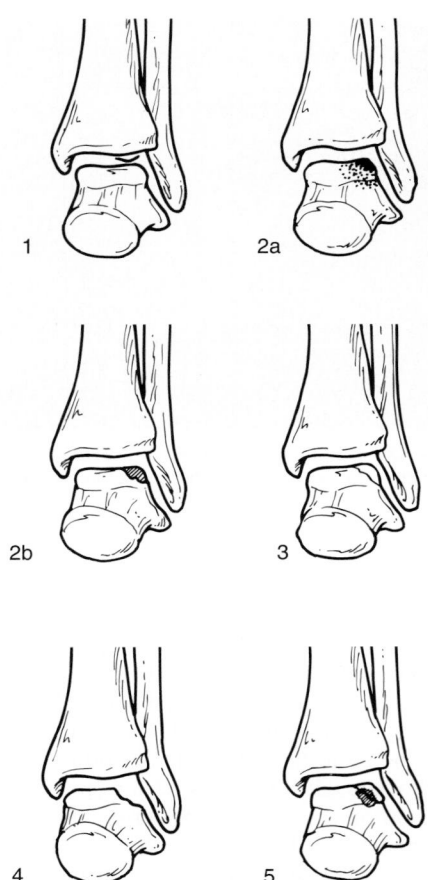

Figure 30K–5. Modified classification of osteochondritis dissecans of the talus based on magnetic resonance imaging appearance. Stage 1, articular cartilage damage only. Stage 2a, cartilage injury with underlying fracture and surrounding bone edema. Stage 2b, stage 2a without bone edema. Stage 3, detached but undisplaced fragment. Stage 4, detached and displaced fragment. Stage 5, subchondral cyst formation. (From Hepple S, Winson IG, Glew D: Osteochondral lesions of the talus: A revised classification. Foot Ankle Int 20:789–793, 1999.)

Taranow and colleagues[49] developed a classification based on preoperative MRI changes, with final staging of the articular cartilage determined during arthroscopy. Cartilage is classified as viable and intact (grade A) or breached and nonviable (grade B). The bone component is described as stage 1, a subchondral compression or bone bruise that appears as high signal on T_2-weighted images; stage 2, subchondral cysts that are not seen acutely but develop from stage 1 lesions; stage 3, partially separated or detached fragments in situ; and stage 4, displaced fragments. The condition of the cartilage and bone together was used to determine the type of surgical treatment.

Medial lesions are more cup shaped and deeper and look like osteochondritis dissecans; lateral lesions are more wafer shaped and shallow and resemble an osteochondral fracture (Fig. 30K–6). Medial lesions tend to stay within the crater and produce fewer symptoms than do lateral lesions, which tend to become detached.

Diagnosis

When an ankle sprain does not resolve, osteochondral fracture of the talus (osteochondritis dissecans) should be considered.[13, 19] Baker and associates[13] reported that 80% of patients with traumatic osteochondritis dissecans have a history of seemingly benign ankle sprain. If there is persistent effusion, delayed synovitis, or locking or giving way of the joint, radiographic examination should be performed 4 to 5 weeks after injury. Oblique and plantar flexed views

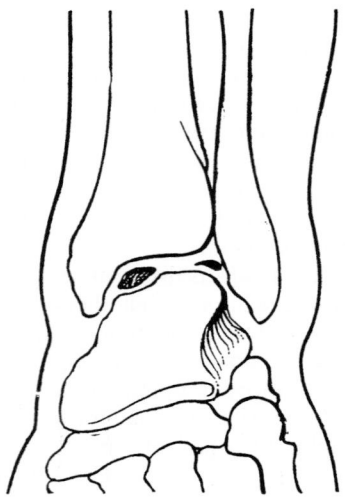

Figure 30K–6. Morphologic appearance of osteochondritis dissecans lesions in the talus. Lateral lesions are wafer shaped; medial lesions are deeper and cup shaped. (Redrawn from Canale ST, Belding RH: Osteochondral lesions of the talus. J Bone Joint Surg Am 62:97–102, 1980.)

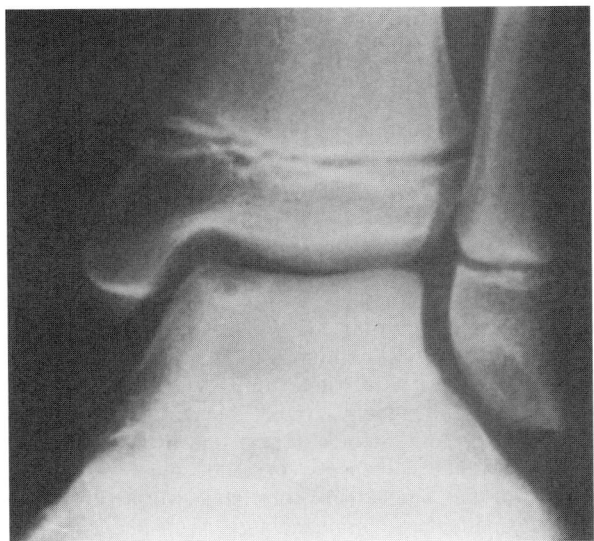

Figure 30K–7. Oblique plantar flexed view shows large extent of lesion.

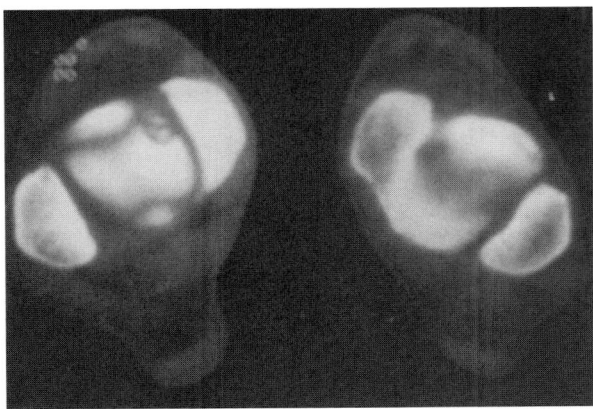

Figure 30K–9. Computed tomographic scan in axial plane defines ante-romedial lesion.

that avoid tibial overlap generally show the lesion more clearly than do plain films (Fig. 30K–7). If osteochondral fracture is suspected, bone scanning with use of a pinhole collimator should be done. Once the lesion is localized,

tomograms can determine its depth and size. Preoperative planning can be aided by CT scanning (Fig. 30K–8); axial cuts (Fig. 30K–9) determine the location of the lesion (anterior, medial, or posterior) and the necessity of osteotomy of the medial malleolus. If the fragment appears to be floating in the crater (Fig. 30K–10), it is usually inverted so that cartilage apposes the crater and cancellous bone apposes the ankle joint (Fig. 30K–11). Tomograms are helpful in localizing the floating lesion.

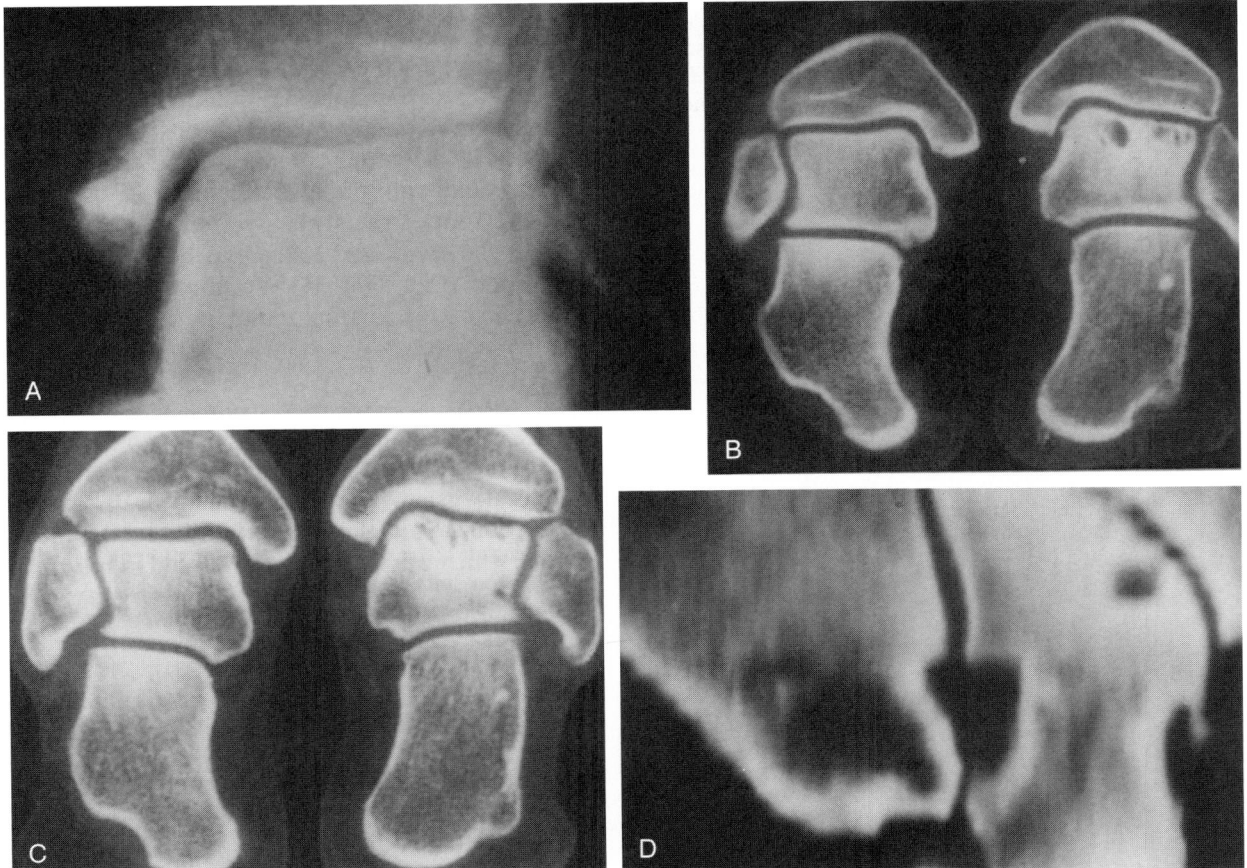

Figure 30K–8. *A,* Radiograph shows apparent osteochondritic medial lesion. *B* to *D,* Computed tomographic scan shows involvement of entire talus, possibly with avascular necrosis or osteonecrosis rather than osteochondritis dissecans.

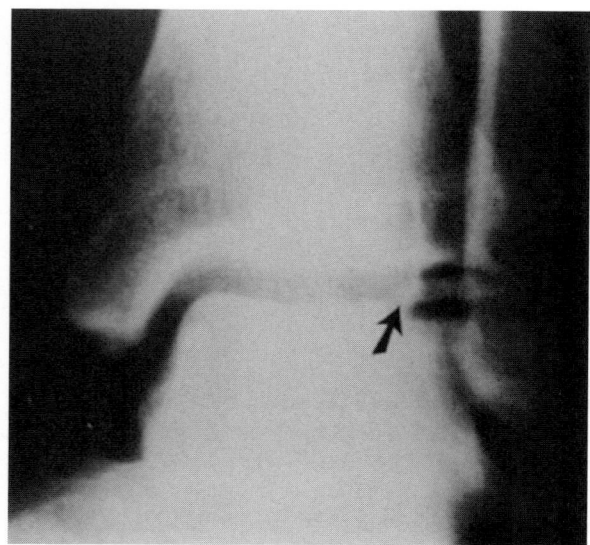

Figure 30K–10. Inverted fragment appears to be floating in crater. (*Arrow* points to articular cartilage surface of fragment.)

Several studies[11, 20, 21, 29, 36, 47] have confirmed the usefulness of MRI for both preoperative evaluation and follow-up examination (Fig. 30K–12). Anderson and colleagues[11] demonstrated that the low signal intensity in T_1-weighted images is useful for early and definitive diagnosis, even of stage I lesions. A high signal rim between the osteochondral fragment and the talar bed is considered indicative of instability of the fragment, with the presence of joint fluid or fibrous granulation tissue as a result of the mobility of these fragments. Lahm and colleagues[36] noted

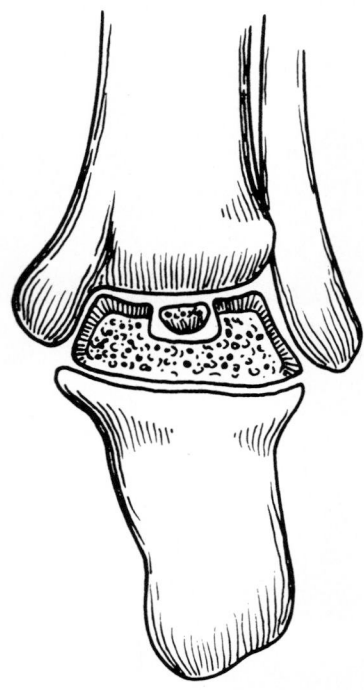

Figure 30K–11. Position of inverted fragment within the ankle joint; cartilage is apposed to crater, and cancellous bone is apposed to tibial articular cartilage.

that the diameter of the lesion measured on MRI was significantly larger than indicated on radiographs, an important factor in preoperative planning. They recommended MRI evaluation to detect changes that provide information about the detachment and viability of the fragment and help make the decision to preserve or to excise the fragment. Schneider and coworkers[47] also suggested that MRI allows more appropriate treatment because it delineates the lesion more accurately than either radiography or CT scanning does. DeSmet and associates[20] compared MRI and arthroscopic findings in 14 ankles with osteochondral lesions and concluded that the presence of a high signal rim in the T_2-weighted images indicated instability of the fragment. In a study of 22 ankles with osteochondral talar lesions, Higashiyama and colleagues[29] found that the low and high signal rims present before surgery disappeared in 100% and 77% of ankles, respectively. A decrease in or disappearance of the signal rim correlated well with clinical results; no patient in whom the signal rim persisted had a good result.

Treatment

In their meta-analysis of 32 articles in the literature concerning osteochondritis dissecans of the talus, Tol and associates[51] found that in 582 patients, the highest rate of success was obtained by excision, curettage, and drilling (85%), followed by excision and curettage (78%) and excision alone (38%). The average success rate of nonoperative treatment was 45%. Stage I and some stage II lesions, either medial or lateral, usually heal spontaneously or can be treated conservatively. Stage II and stage III medial lesions, which are usually not displaced in the crater, have fewer symptoms and result in traumatic arthritis less frequently than do stage III lateral lesions. Because of this stable, nondisplaced configuration, stage III medial lesions can often be treated conservatively, but stage III lateral lesions usually require excision in adults because they are less likely to heal, cause more symptoms, and more often result in traumatic arthritis.[37, 40, 48] In children with open physes, however, a trial period of conservative treatment is warranted to avoid producing a crater in the talus. Nonoperative treatment consists of the application of a short cast, a double upright patellar tendon weight-bearing brace, arch supports, or leather lace-up ankle corsets. If severe pain and limitation of activities persist after at least 6 months of conservative treatment, surgical treatment is indicated. Options for surgical treatment, open or arthroscopic, include excision, excision and curettage with or without drilling, cancellous bone grafting, internal fixation, and osteochondral transplantation.

The fragment can be excised by either arthrotomy or arthroscopy. A number of arthroscopic techniques have been described for treatment of osteochondritis dissecans of the ankle joint, but ankle arthroscopy is difficult and requires considerable expertise with arthroscopic instrumentation.[12, 14, 16, 22, 26, 32, 39, 42–44] A well-performed arthrotomy is preferable to a poorly done arthroscopic procedure. If excision of the entire fragment is not certain after arthroscopy, arthrotomy should be performed immediately.

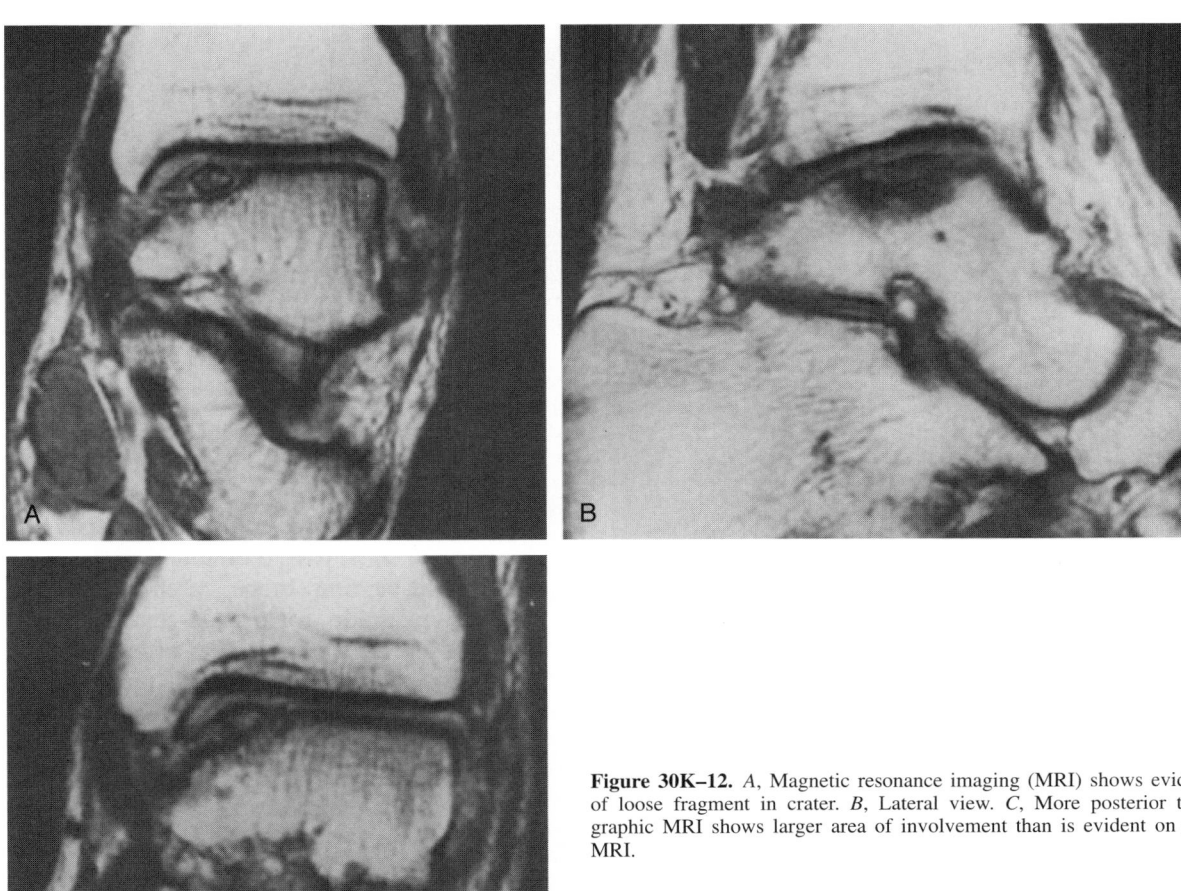

Figure 30K–12. *A,* Magnetic resonance imaging (MRI) shows evidence of loose fragment in crater. *B,* Lateral view. *C,* More posterior tomographic MRI shows larger area of involvement than is evident on plain MRI.

A small, 2-inch arthrotomy of the ankle has less morbidity than does arthrotomy of the knee joint and can often be performed as an outpatient procedure.

Because most of the lesions are small and because the distal tibia articulates with the sides of the crater, excision of the fragment has been reported to be successful in approximately 87% of patients with osteochondritis dissecans of the talus. On occasion, if the fragment is larger (>1.5 cm in diameter) and on the weight-bearing surface of the joint, open reduction and internal fixation may be indicated. The fragment should be attached and have viable subchondral cancellous bone on its undersurface (Fig. 30K–13) for the best chance of union. Conversely, a chronic, loose (unattached) body consisting only of cartilage is least likely to heal. If the fragment does not heal, a second operation is necessary to remove the fragment, and internal fixation may be necessary. This should be explained to the patient before surgery. Ogilvie-Harris and Sarrosa[41] described eight patients who required arthroscopic treatment of persistent ankle problems after open surgery for removal of an osteochondral fragment. The preferred approach is through an anterior arthrotomy.[52] The fragment is pinned retrograde.

Arthrotomy can be performed initially or in conjunction with arthroscopy. Lateral lesions are exposed more easily than are medial lesions because the lateral malleolus is more posterior than the medial malleolus. CT scanning is helpful in locating medial lesions; if the lesion is posterior, medial malleolar osteotomy may be necessary, but this should be avoided, if possible, when the distal tibial physis is open. Positioning the foot in plantar flexion allows inspection of more posterior lesions on the medial dome of the talus. Medial malleolar osteotomy has been used for this exposure, but osteotomy of the medial malleolus is fraught with complications such as malunion, nonunion, and necessity of later screw removal. Extensive plantar flexion of the toes should be avoided to prevent damage to the dorsal neurovascular structures and tendons, and the incision should be extended carefully to prevent rupture or cutting of the extensor tendons. Arthrotomy is most commonly performed through an anteromedial approach, but Thompson and Loomer[50] described a posteromedial approach to be used if the osteochondral fragment cannot be exposed through an anteromedial incision. In this technique, a flap is reflected posteriorly through the anteromedial incision, avoiding the neurovascular bundle and tendi-

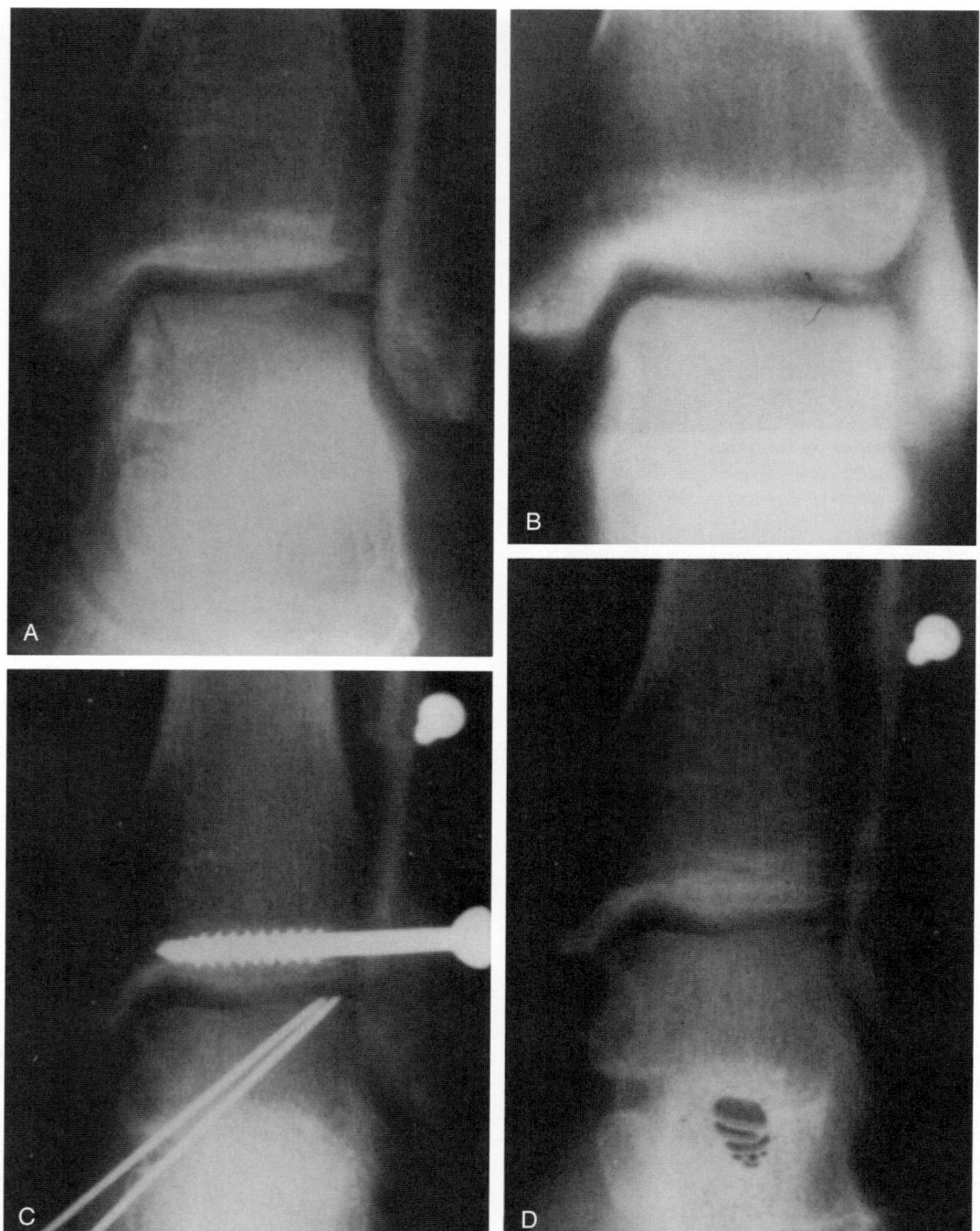

Figure 30K–13. *A* and *B,* Large stage III lateral lesion. *C,* After pinning; fibular osteotomy was performed for better exposure. *D,* Good healing at follow-up.

nous structures behind the posterior medial malleolus, and a capsular incision is made to expose the posterior aspect of the talus. Flick and Gould[24] described tibial "grooving," in which a small area is grooved out of the distal tibia with a gouge to expose the posteromedial lesion (Fig. 30K–14).

Although removal of weight-bearing cartilage to improve exposure appears to be indicated in no other joint of the body, it has been beneficial in several of my patients. Until the long-term effect is known, it should probably be avoided if at all possible.

Technique of Arthrotomy of the Ankle

If arthrotomy is done after arthroscopy, a second sterile drape is applied, gloves and gowns are changed, and arthrotomy is continued through either the anterolateral or anteromedial arthroscopy portal. Otherwise, a vertical incision approximately 1.5 inches long is made either anterolateral or anteromedial, with care taken to avoid the extensor tendons and neurovascular bundle. The foot is plantar flexed to expose the lesion, which is excised with a grasper

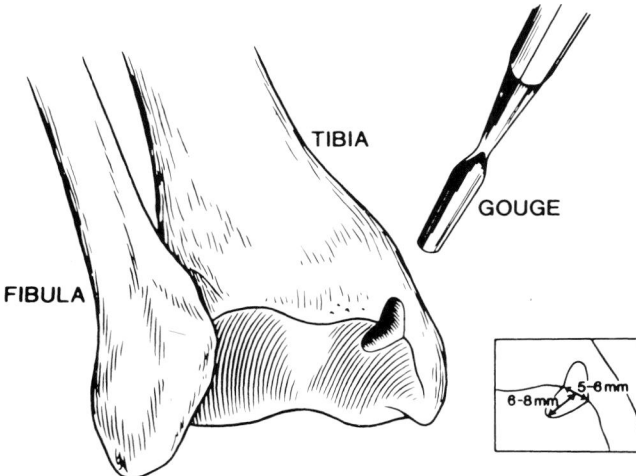

Figure 30K–14. Flick and Gould technique of "grooving" of distal tibia for exposure of posteromedial lesions without osteotomy of medial malleolus. (From Flick AB, Gould N: Osteochondritis dissecans of the talus [transchondral fractures of the talus]: Review of the literature and new surgical approach for medial dome lesions. Foot Ankle 5:165, 1985. ©American Orthopaedic Foot and Ankle Society, 1985.)

or curet. Curettage of the area is performed down to bleeding bone, and three or four holes are drilled with a small drill bit. This can be accomplished through a transmalleolar approach under direct vision if necessary. Medial malleolar osteotomy is rarely necessary and is required primarily for medial lesions. If it is needed, the medial malleolus is

predrilled with a 4.5 or 6.0 cannulated cancellous screw (Fig. 30K–15A), and the medial malleolus is then osteotomized obliquely through metaphyseal bone and retracted to expose the lesion (Fig. 30K–15B). After the lesion is resected and the crater drilled, the osteotomy site is secured with the cancellous bone screw (Fig. 30K–15C). The wounds are closed, and a sterile dressing and a short-leg patellar tendon–bearing cast are applied.

Return to Athletic Activity. After 2 weeks of non–weight-bearing in the cast, the cast and sutures are removed. A patellar tendon–bearing brace is fitted and worn for 10 weeks. Return to full activity is usually allowed at 4 to 6 weeks. Longer restriction of sports activities may be necessary if osteotomy of the medial malleolus is performed.

Technique of Thompson and Loomer

In the technique of Thompson and Loomer,[50] a 10-cm curved incision is made, convex posteriorly and centered posterior to the medial malleolus, and the medial capsule is exposed. A 2-cm longitudinal incision is made in the anteromedial capsule, extending from the tibia to the talus (Fig. 30K–16A). The foot is maximally plantar flexed, and the anterior half to two thirds of the superomedial rim of the talus is inspected. If inspection, curettage, and drilling of the defect cannot be completely accomplished from this approach, a curved incision is made directly over the tibialis posterior tendon. Anterior retraction is applied, and an incision is made in the deep surface of the flexor retinacu-

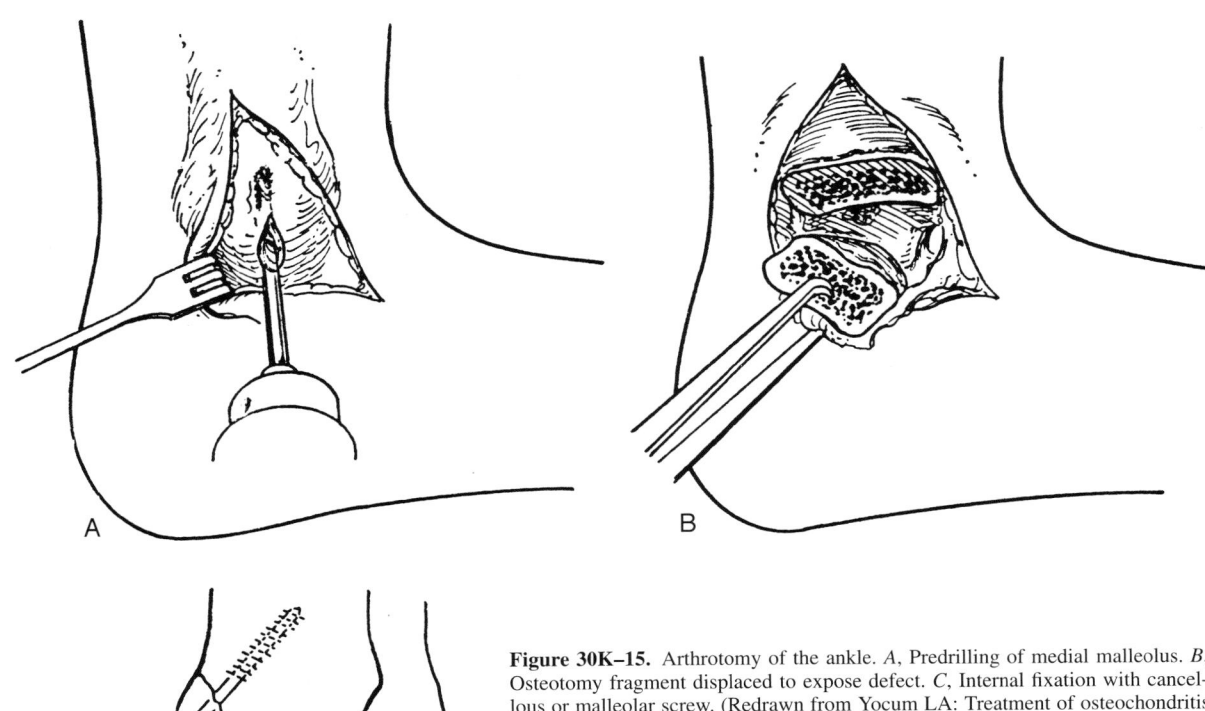

Figure 30K–15. Arthrotomy of the ankle. *A*, Predrilling of medial malleolus. *B*, Osteotomy fragment displaced to expose defect. *C*, Internal fixation with cancellous or malleolar screw. (Redrawn from Yocum LA: Treatment of osteochondritis dissecans of the talus. In Shields CL Jr [ed]: Manual of Sports Surgery. New York, Springer-Verlag, 1987.)

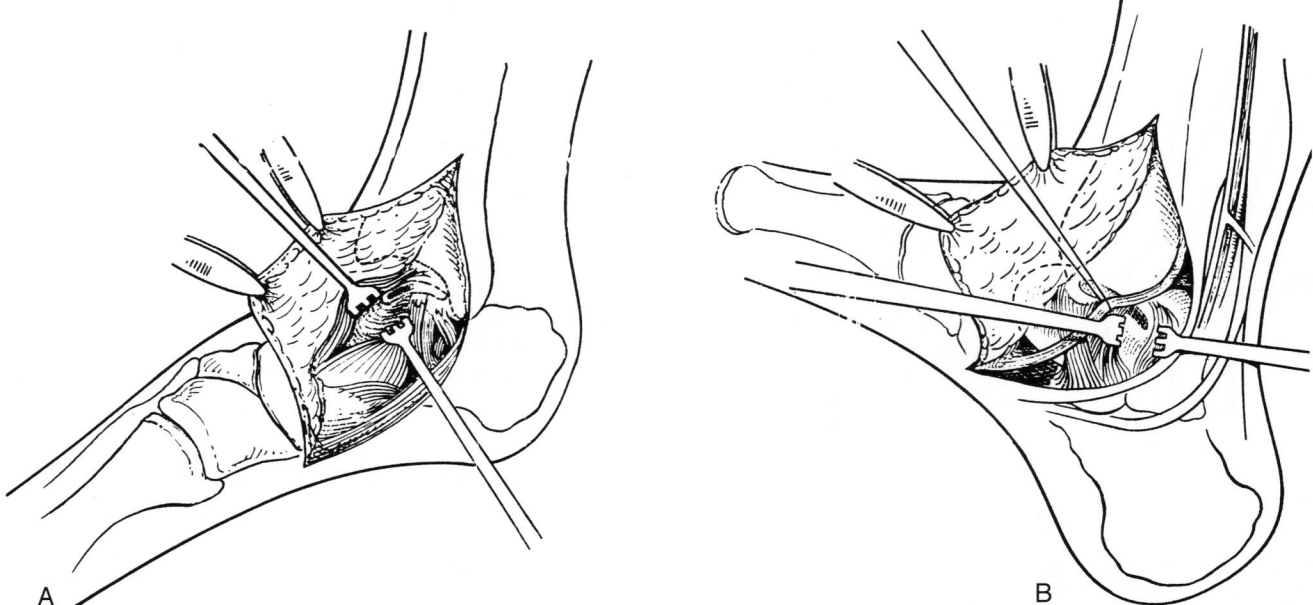

Figure 30K–16. *A*, Anteromedial exposure of talus with foot in maximal plantar flexion. *B*, Posteromedial exposure through same skin incision with foot in maximal dorsiflexion. (Redrawn from Thompson JP, Loomer RL: Osteochondral lesions of the talus in a sports medicine clinic. A new radiographic technique and surgical approach. Am J Sports Med 12:460–463, 1984.)

lum (Fig. 30K–16*B*). With gentle posterior traction, the remainder of the contents of the tarsal tunnel are retracted without exposure or examination. By maximal dorsiflexion of the foot, the posterior half of the superomedial border of the talus can be observed; the lesion is inspected and treated appropriately by excision and curettage.

Return to Athletic Activity. Range of motion exercises are begun immediately after surgery, and weight-bearing ambulation is allowed as soon as it can be tolerated. Return to full competition is usually possible at 12 to 16 weeks.

Technique of Open Reduction and Internal Fixation of the Fragment

The fragment and crater are exposed through an anterior incision. The fragment is elevated but, if possible, left attached. Its undersurface is inspected for cancellous bone. Both the fragment and the crater are freshened, and then the fragment is reduced into the crater. With small (2- to 3-mm) threaded Steinmann pins drilled from proximal to distal, the fragment is fixed in the crater. For ease of insertion, the pins can be placed through the malleoli. The pins are drilled out of the anterior talus, the drill is re-attached to the pins, and both are brought out of the talus so that the fragment remains reduced but the pins are not in the joint. The pins are cut off beneath the skin so that they can easily be removed at 6 to 12 weeks. The wound is closed, and a short-leg cast is applied.

The cast is changed and the sutures are removed at 2 weeks. At 12 weeks, the pins are removed, and a patellar tendon weight-bearing cast is applied, to be worn for 12 weeks.

Large lesions can be replaced, pinned, and grafted with techniques similar to those used for osteochondral lesions in the knee, but the fragment must have viable subchondral cancellous bone. Pinning and grafting are technically difficult, and nonunion may necessitate later removal of the pins and the fragment. Hangody and colleagues[27, 33] described the use of the mosaicplasty technique in 11 patients with talar defects larger than 10 mm. Osteochondral cylindrical grafts from the ipsilateral knee were placed into the talar defect by use of specially designed tube chisels. Early results were excellent.

Technique of Osteochondral Grafting

In the technique of Hangody and colleagues,[27] with the patient under general anesthesia, the affected lower extremity is prepared from the foot to well above the knee. The ankle is examined arthroscopically to delineate the chondral lesion further. If the lesion is more than 10 mm in diameter and is on the weight-bearing surface of the talus, the procedure should be performed open. Lateral lesions are approached through an anterior sagittal incision, and if necessary, a medial malleolar osteotomy is made for access to medial lesions. Once the lesion is exposed, curettage of all cartilage thought to be diseased is done to a sharply defined rim, and the subchondral base is abraded. Holes of 4.5 and 3.5 mm are drilled perpendicular to the surface of the talus to a depth of 15 mm.

Through a small incision, a graft is obtained arthroscopically from the medial or lateral femoral condyle of the ipsilateral knee (Fig. 30K–17). A specially designed tubular chisel is used to obtain osteochondral grafts 4.5 mm and 3.5 mm in diameter and 10 mm in length. After the grafts are removed from the tube, they are compressed and contoured, then carefully inserted into the recipient drill holes and press-fit by hand with special instruments. Range of

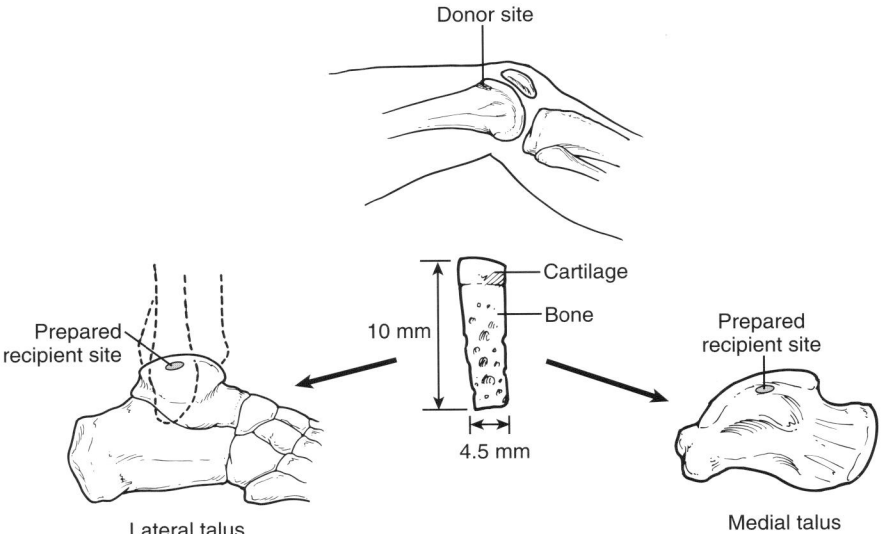

Figure 30K–17. Osteochondral grafting (mosaicplasty) using graft from ipsilateral knee to lateral and medial talar dome osteochondral defects. (From Hangody L, Kish G, Kárpáti Z, et al: Treatment of osteochondritis dissecans of the talus: Use of the mosaicplasty technique—a preliminary report. Foot Ankle Int 18:628–634, 1997.)

motion of the ankle is tested to ensure that the graft is well seated and secured. The incision and osteotomy are closed in the usual fashion. A drain is placed in the knee, and a compressive dressing is applied to the ankle.

Return to Athletic Activity. The patient is non–weight-bearing for 4 to 6 weeks.

Arthroscopic Treatment

These lesions can also be treated arthroscopically. Arthroscopic principles for the ankle are the same as those for the knee, but a small-joint system includes a 4-mm arthroscope with 30- and 70-degree angles; a smaller 2.7-mm arthroscope can also be used. Three anterior portals—lateral, central, and medial—are generally employed (Fig. 30K–18). Shaving the synovium anteriorly and use of some form of ankle distraction provide better visibility. Ankle distraction can be obtained with an external fixator by securing a skeletal traction pin through the distal tibia and a parallel skeletal traction pin through the os calcis. Application of longitudinal traction through the external fixator opens the joint sufficiently to expose all but the most posterior lesions. Guhl[26] successfully used skeletal traction for better exposure. A "uniplanar" distractor on the appropriate side is usually sufficient for medial or lateral lesions, and two distractors can be used for central or multiple lesions. The uniplanar distractor is similar to the femoral distractor used at the knee; 5/64-inch skeletal pins can be used. If skeletal traction is applied for ankle distraction, pins must avoid the tibial and fibular physes in the child. In athletes, drill holes in the distal tibia, os calcis, or talus may serve as stress risers, and return to strenuous activity should be delayed to avoid pathologic fracture. Neurologic complications have also been reported after overzealous distraction.

Return to Athletic Activity. A patellar tendon–bearing cast is used for several weeks postoperatively, and then a

patellar tendon–bearing brace is worn for 8 to 12 weeks to unload the ankle joint. Full return to competition is usually possible within 4 to 6 months.

Technique of Arthroscopy of the Ankle

Most osteochondral lesions are anterolateral or posteromedial. Anterolateral lesions can be viewed through an anteromedial portal, with instruments for drilling, excision, or pinning inserted through an anterolateral portal; portals are changed as necessary for optimal viewing and fixation.

Posteromedial lesions can be more difficult to view and treat. With noninvasive distraction and use of a small, 2.7-mm scope in the anterolateral portal, most posteromedial lesions can be treated through anteromedial and posterolateral portals. A small, curved curet or curved microfracture awl is used to make the perforations in the subchondral bone. Once the lesion is freed, it can be extracted with a grasper (Fig. 30K–19). If needed, a small trough can be made on the anteromedial tibia to improve access to posterior lesions. When the lesion is not accessible with this technique, image intensification can be used to guide placement of a Kirschner wire through the medial malleolus for drilling of the lesion (Fig. 30K–20). For pinning of larger lesions, an osteotomy of the malleolus may be necessary. Other instruments that are helpful include an open-end curet, a small (2.7-mm) full-radius resector, and a small (2.7-mm) bur. The arthroscopic portals are closed with nylon sutures, and a sterile compressive dressing is applied.

Return to Athletic Activity. The dressing is changed at 48 hours. Weight-bearing to tolerance is progressed during 7 to 10 days, after which crutches are discontinued. Active range of motion exercises are begun immediately, and a progressive strengthening program is implemented when soft tissue reaction subsides. If arthroscopic pinning has been done, non–weight-bearing is continued for 6 to 8

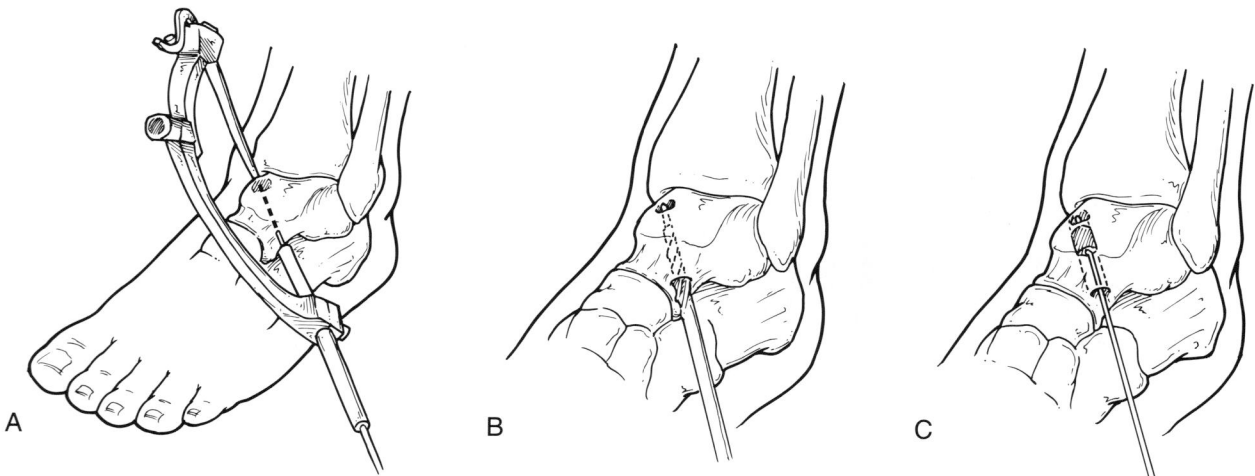

Figure 30K–22. Retrograde drilling of osteochondritis dissecans of the talus. *A,* Drill guide positioned over lesion and wire inserted through nonarticular junction of neck and body of talus. *B,* Cannulated drill placed over guidewire. *C,* Bone graft deposited beneath subchondral plate. (From Taranow WS, Bisignani GA, Towers JD, Conti SF: Retrograde drilling of osteochondral lesions of the medial talar dome. Foot Ankle Int 20:474–480, 1999.)

excision of the lesion. A history of pain relieved by aspirin is an important finding to distinguish pain caused by osteoid osteoma from that caused by other conditions. Plain radiographs and bone scans are helpful, but CT scanning and MRI are best for definitive diagnosis.

Tarsal Coalition or Osteochondral Fracture

Snyder and coworkers[84] and O'Neil and Micheli[79] reported a high incidence of tarsal coalition associated with ankle sprains in children and adolescents, including fibrous coalitions, cartilaginous coalitions, and bony coalitions (Fig. 30K–26). Osteochondral fracture may also mimic ankle sprain. Ankle sprain symptoms that do not resolve

after 4 to 5 weeks of conservative treatment should initiate appropriate imaging studies, including bone scan, CT, or tomography, and further evaluation to rule out tarsal coalition or osteochondral fracture of the talus.

Impingement Syndromes

Impingement syndromes were described as osteochondral ridges by O'Donoghue.[77] The anterior impingement syndrome occurs frequently in runners and jumpers, most commonly in the distal tibia, where it is always anterior and usually lateral.[64, 68, 80] Pain is usually the first symptom; it begins as a vague discomfort and becomes sharper and more localized to the front of the ankle. Ankle joint motion may also be limited (Fig. 30K–27). Symptomatic exostoses

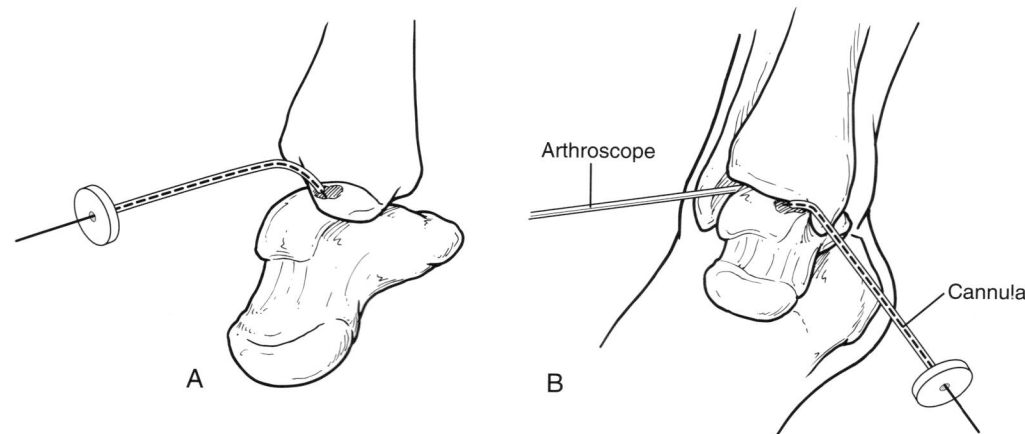

Figure 30K–23. Drilling of osteochondral lesion with use of meniscal repair instrumentation; no transmalleolar portal is required. *A,* For posteromedial lesions, arthroscope is placed in lateral portal, ankle is maximally plantar flexed, and curved cannula is inserted through anteromedial portal and is placed on the lesion. *B,* Trocar point needle is inserted through cannula, and osteochondral defect is drilled. Multiple holes can be drilled by moving malleable cannula to different locations on the lesion. (From Bryant DD, Siegel MG: Osteochondritis dissecans of the talus: A new technique for arthroscopic drilling. Arthroscopy 9:238–241, 1993.)

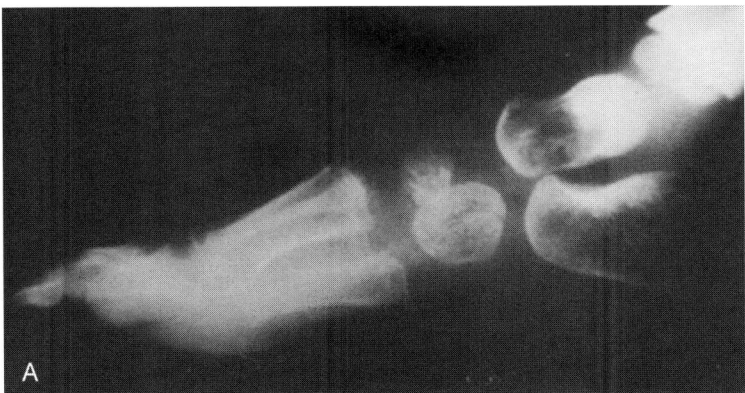

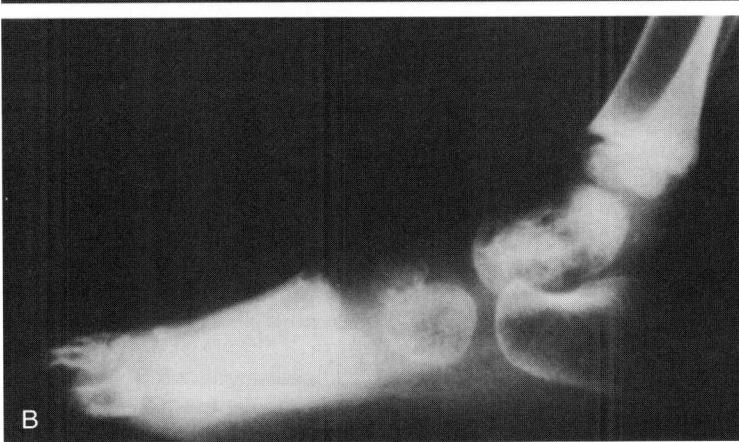

Figure 30K–24. Eosinophilic granuloma may cause symptoms of ankle sprain. *A*, Lesion in head and neck of talus. *B*, After excision and bone grafting.

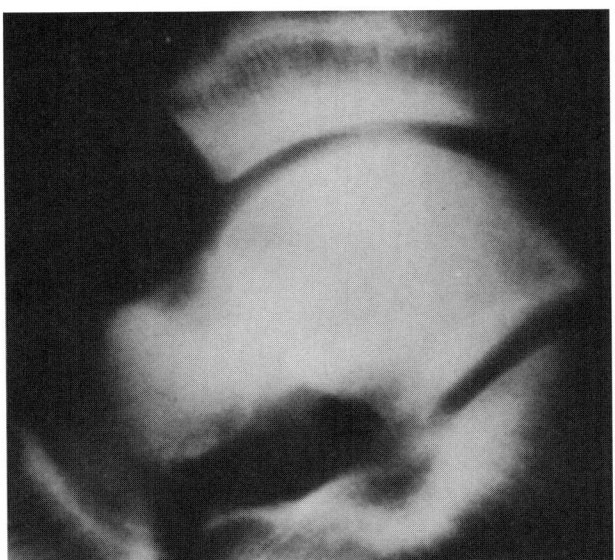

Figure 30K–25. Pigmented villonodular synovitis eroding into superior portion of talar neck caused symptoms of ankle sprain in young athlete.

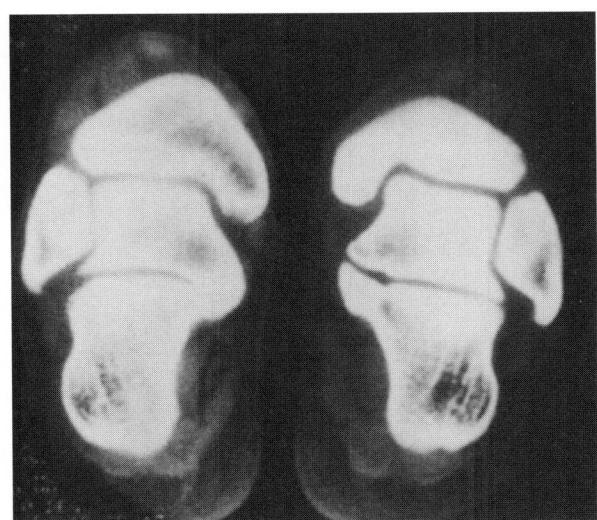

Figure 30K–26. Computed tomographic scanning shows medial facet tarsal coalition of talus and os calcis.

Normal

Bony Impingement

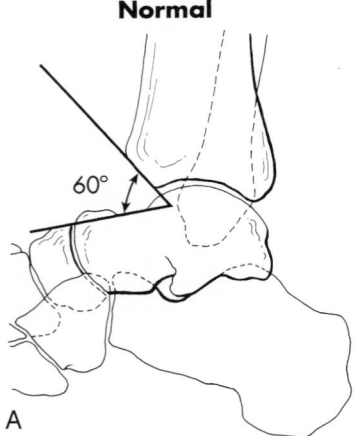

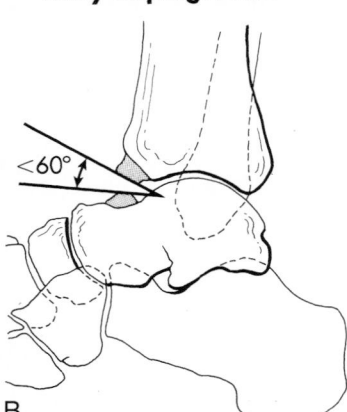

Figure 30K–27. Anterior impingement syndrome. *A*, Normal angle between distal tibia and talus is 60 degrees or more. *B*, Osteophytes on distal tibia and talar neck decrease angle to less than 60 degrees. (From Ferkel RD: Arthroscopy of the foot and ankle. In Coughlin MJ, Mann RA [eds]: Surgery of the Foot and Ankle, 7th ed. St Louis, Mosby, 1999, p 1277.)

are tender, and a large exostosis may be palpable. Routine lateral radiographs show the exostoses; non–weight-bearing lateral flexion and extension views also show the tibiotalar contact, and posterior joint space widening may be visible on weight-bearing lateral views.

Restriction of activities is usually sufficient treatment in younger patients, although older children may benefit from anti-inflammatory medication or cortisone injection. Arthroscopy or arthrotomy is occasionally required for excision of a bone spur or osteophyte in the distal tibia or talar neck, especially in older adolescents and adults (Fig. 30K–28). Scranton and McDermott[82] described a classification of anterior impingement based on preoperative radiographic appearance (Table 30K–2). Of 43 ankles treated with open or arthroscopic excision of the spurs, only 2 were grade I, 18 were grade II, 14 were grade III, and 9

were grade IV. Their criteria for surgery were radiographic evidence of an impinging anterior tibiotalar spur and no relief of symptoms after at least 3 months of conservative treatment. Conservative treatment consisted of rest, a ½-inch heel lift, nonsteroidal anti-inflammatory drugs, and at least one intra-articular injection of 1% lidocaine (Xylocaine) and 40 mg of methylprednisolone (Depo-Medrol). They found a predictable correlation between the grade of lesion and time to recovery, ranging from 5 weeks in patients with grade I lesions to 10 weeks in those with grade IV lesions. Recovery time was also shorter for the 22 ankles treated with arthroscopy (5 weeks) than for the 22 treated with arthrotomy (8 weeks). Arthroscopic débridement was recommended for grades I, II, and III lesions but not for grade IV lesions. Ogilvie-Harris and associates[78] also reported "significant" improvement in

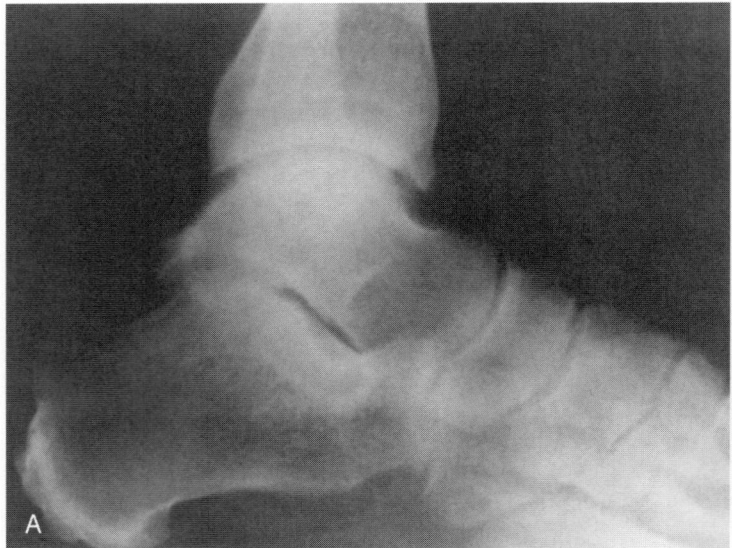

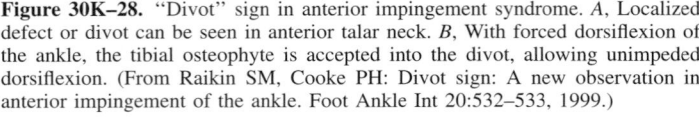

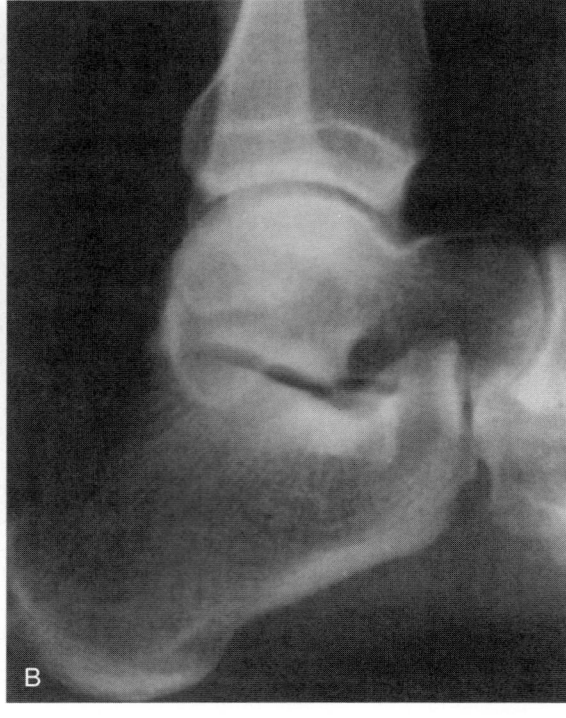

Figure 30K–28. "Divot" sign in anterior impingement syndrome. *A*, Localized defect or divot can be seen in anterior talar neck. *B*, With forced dorsiflexion of the ankle, the tibial osteophyte is accepted into the divot, allowing unimpeded dorsiflexion. (From Raikin SM, Cooke PH: Divot sign: A new observation in anterior impingement of the ankle. Foot Ankle Int 20:532–533, 1999.)

TABLE 30K–2
Classification of Anterior Impingement

Grade I	Synovial impingement: Radiographs show inflammatory reaction, up to 3-mm spur formation. Dorsiflexion stress view confirms impingement. Bright-light examination of lateral view confirms anterior soft tissue swelling.
Grade II	Osteochondral reaction exostosis: Radiographs show osseous spur formation larger than 3 mm. No talar spur present. Dorsiflexion view shows impingement. MRI confirms moderate osteoblastic and chondral hyperplastic reaction.
Grade III	Significant exostosis with or without fragmentation, with secondary spur formation on dorsum of talus, often with fragmentation of osteophytes.
Grade IV	Pantalocrural arthritic destruction: Radiographs suggest medial, lateral, or posterior degenerative arthritic changes.

From Scranton PE, McDermott JI: Anterior tibiotalar spurs: A comparison of open versus arthroscopic débridement. Foot Ankle 12:125–128, 1992.

pain, swelling, stiffness, limping, and activity level in 15 of 17 ankles with arthroscopic removal of bone spurs. Only one patient failed to return to sporting activities.

Raikin and Cooke[81] described the development of a localized "divot" in the anterior talar neck of high-level and professional soccer players (see Fig. 30K–28). They proposed that this divot, which accepts the growing tibial spur during ankle dorsiflexion, prevents the formation of an osteophyte on the anterior talar neck and allows unimpeded dorsiflexion. Pain seemed to be caused by the rubbing of the osteophyte against the raw bone at the base of the divot; arthroscopic resection of the tibial osteophyte was recommended for treatment.

A similar mechanism was proposed by Kim and associates[67] for the development of "tram track" lesions in six professional or collegiate soccer players. They suggested that repeated carving by a prominent osteophyte on the anterior tibial lip formed a longitudinal trough with variable width and a full-thickness cartilage defect well demarcated from the healthy margin of the articular cartilage of the talar dome. This lesion was found in 6 of 68 ankles treated arthroscopically for anterior impingement syndrome. None of the six patients was able to recall any significant traumatic events. The predominant symptom was pain in the anteromedial aspect of the ankle during running. At an average 27-month follow-up after arthroscopic excision of osteophytes and Kirschner wire drilling of the lesions, three patients had excellent results, two had good results, and one had a fair result. Five of the six returned to preoperative levels of competition.

Posterior impingement syndrome (talar compression syndrome or os trigonum syndrome) occurs often in ballet dancers and runners.[55, 56, 65] Pain and tenderness are localized at the posterolateral aspect of the ankle behind the peroneal tendons. This syndrome can also be effectively treated by restriction of activity and anti-inflammatory medication. Brodsky and Khalil[55] reported excision of the os trigonum for symptomatic posterior impingement syndrome in six professional ballet dancers. Marumoto and Ferkel[70] described arthroscopic excision of the os trigonum in 11 patients (Fig. 30K–29). As advantages of this technique, they cited decreased scarring, less surgical morbidity, and faster recovery than with open excision. All 11 patients reached maximal recovery levels within 3 months,

compared with recovery times of up to 12 months reported after open excision.[55, 63, 69]

Waller[89] described an anterolateral corner compression syndrome in which pain is localized to the anteroinferior border of the fibula and the anterolateral surface of the talus. The patient usually gives a history of inversion injuries to the foot. The heel is in valgus alignment, and the foot is pronated. Pain is relieved by tightening the posterior tibial tendon and releasing the peroneal tendons, which also makes the patient more susceptible to inversion injuries. Most authors believe that this condition is a chondromalacia of the lateral wall of the talus with associated synovial reaction.

Author's Preferred Method of Treatment

Restriction of activities is usually sufficient treatment in younger patients, although older children may benefit from anti-inflammatory medication or cortisone injection. The use of heel lifts can also help relieve pain. Arthroscopy or arthrotomy is occasionally required for excision of a bone spur or osteophyte in the distal tibia or talar neck, especially in older adolescents and adults (Fig. 30K–30). Arthroscopic excision of a painful os trigonum can be effective for dancers or other high-performance athletes.

Fractures of the Calcaneus and the Talus

Fractures of the anterior process of the calcaneus and posterior or lateral process of the talus can be mistaken for ankle sprains. Misdiagnosis of these injuries can lead to nonunion, which can cause ankle pain that limits athletic activity. Clark and associates[58] reviewed ankle radiographs of 1153 patients with acute ankle trauma to determine the presence of a fracture and the extent of ankle effusion. In 11 of 33 patients with ankle effusions but no detectable fracture on radiographs, tomography identified occult fractures: 4 osteochondral fractures of the talar dome and 1 fracture each of the neck of the talus, medial malleolus, anterior tibial rim, posterior tibial rim, tibial plafond, lateral malleolus, and anterior process of the calcaneus. They concluded that an ankle effusion of 13 mm or more had a positive predictive value of 82% for occult fracture and should prompt additional imaging.

Fractures of the Anterior Process of the Calcaneus. Fractures of the anterior process of the calcaneus are of two distinct types, avulsion and compression. Avulsion fractures usually occur with inversion ankle injuries, and compression fractures occur with forceful abduction of the forefoot with compression of the calcaneocuboid joint. Patients usually report a sudden twist of the ankle with immediate pain on the outer aspect of the midportion of the foot and discomfort with weight-bearing. Pain and tenderness are located in the region of the sinus tarsi, with maximal tenderness 2 cm anterior and 1 cm inferior to the anterior talofibular ligament, which helps to distinguish this lesion from a lateral ankle sprain. The avulsion fracture is best seen on a lateral oblique projection, and the compression fracture is best seen on the lateral view of the hindfoot.

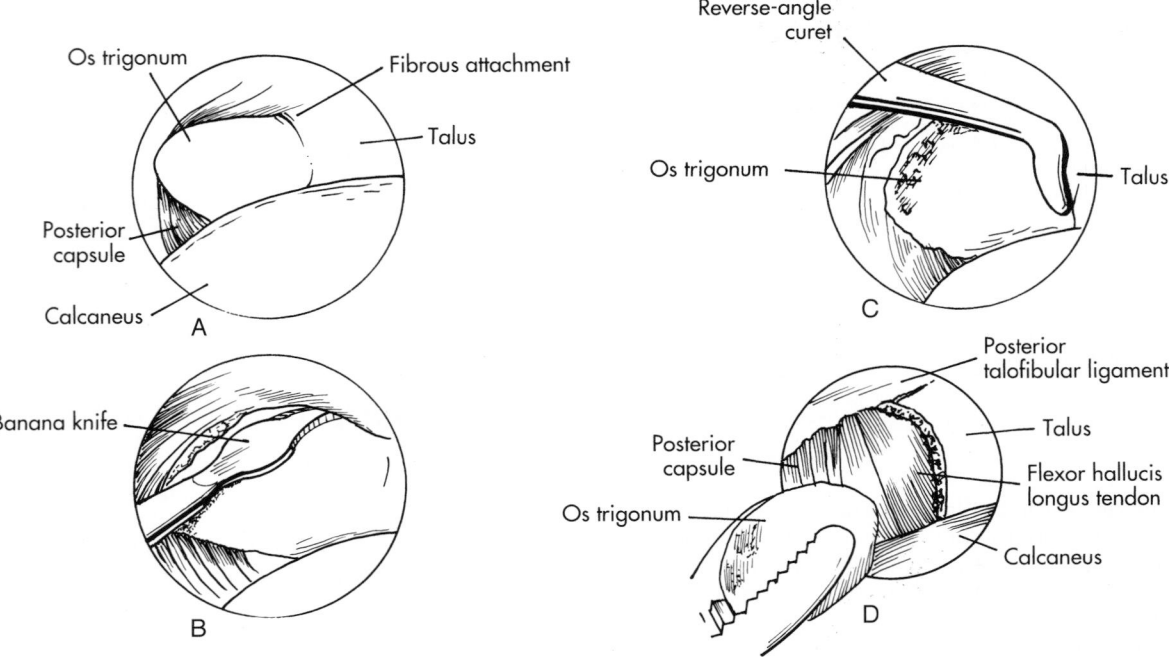

Figure 30K–29. Arthroscopic excision of os trigonum. *A*, Fibrous attachment of os trigonum can be identified through central portal. *B*, Banana knife through posterolateral portal is used to release soft tissues, taking extreme care to avoid cutting flexor hallucis longus tendon and neurovascular bundle medially. *C*, Reverse-angle curet is used to release soft tissue attachments to os trigonum. *D*, Once os trigonum is completely free, a grasper is used to remove it through the posterolateral portal. (From Ferkel RD: Arthroscopy of the foot and ankle. In Coughlin MJ, Mann RA [eds]: Surgery of the Foot and Ankle, 7th ed. St Louis, Mosby, 1999, p 1287.)

The more common avulsion fracture is generally treated with short-leg cast immobilization for 4 weeks. In the rare compression fracture, displaced articular fragments may require open reduction and internal fixation. Trnka and coworkers[86] described a patient in whom the fracture remained undiagnosed for 2 years and who had a Watson-Jones procedure done for ankle instability; after excision of the ununited fragment, she was asymptomatic at the site of the fracture, but progressive arthrosis caused pain with exercise and intensive walking.

Fractures of the Posterior Process of the Talus. There are two bone processes (posterior and lateral) of the

talus, both of which are subject to fracture either as an isolated event or in conjunction with other ankle or talar injuries.[59, 74–76, 87] The posterior process of the talus consists of two tubercles, medial and lateral, that are separated by the groove for the flexor hallucis longus tendon (Fig. 30K–31). The posterior fibers of the deltoid (talotibial) ligament insert into the medial tubercle, and the posterior talofibular ligament inserts into the lateral tubercle.

Fractures of the posterior process most commonly involve the lateral tubercle (Fig. 30K–32). In almost 50% of ankles, the os trigonum (fused or separate) is just posterior to the lateral tubercle of the posterior talar process and

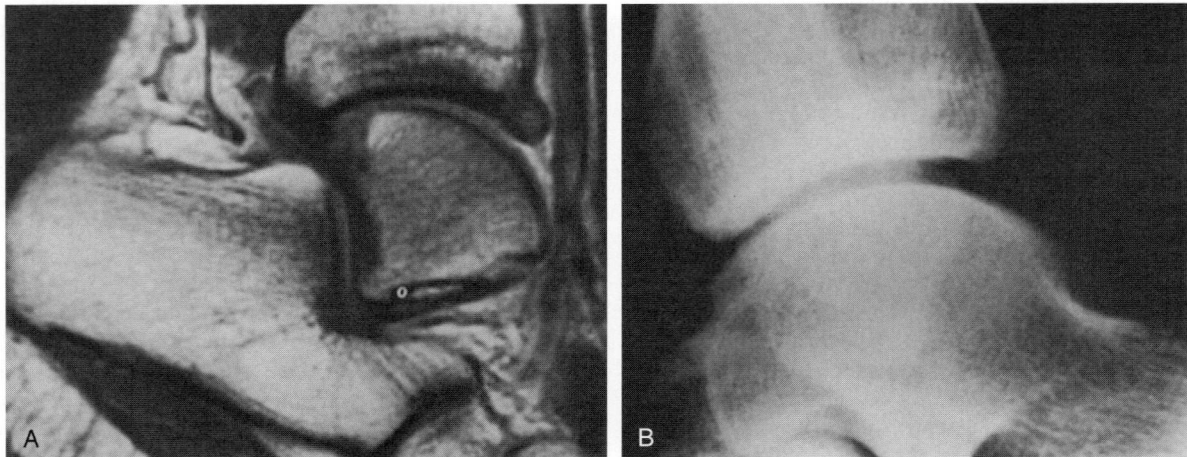

Figure 30K–30. *A*, MRI shows bone spur on anterolateral aspect of talar neck (impingement syndrome). *B*, After excision of bone spur.

may be mistaken for a fracture.[61, 65] Fracture of the lateral tubercle of the posterior process can be caused by avulsion or direct compression. Most often, the lateral tubercle is compressed between the calcaneus and the posterior lip of the tibia when the ankle is forced into extreme equinus. Repetitive moderate trauma can also produce this fracture, and several have been reported in athletes, particularly football and rugby players. Patients with fractures of the lateral tubercle of the posterior talar process usually have symptoms of "ankle sprains." Pain on palpation localized to the region of the lateral tubercle is the most common symptom. Edema is localized to either side of the tendo Achilles. Patients often relate a history of plantar flexion injury to the ankle with pain on ambulation that is made worse by plantar flexion of the foot. Differentiation of this fracture from a nonunited secondary ossification center is best made on the lateral radiograph. Most fractures of the lateral tubercle of the posterior talar process are nondisplaced or minimally displaced and can be treated in a short-leg cast or compression dressing and protected from full weight-bearing for 4 to 6 weeks. Nadim and colleagues[74] described open reduction and internal fixation of a displaced fracture, with healing of the fracture and no evidence of osteonecrosis of the fragment or talar body. They suggested that early diagnosis and operative treatment are essential to a good outcome of these injuries.

Nonunion of these fractures can cause persistent pain in the ankle, especially with extreme plantar flexion and with strenuous physical activity, and limitation of ankle and subtalar joint motion.[62] Veazey and coworkers[88] described nine patients with ununited fractures of the posterior process in whom the diagnosis was delayed 2 to 36 months (average, 9 months). After surgical excision of the ununited fragment, five patients had excellent results, one patient had a good result, one patient had a fair result, and two patients had poor results. The poor results were in a patient with an associated fracture of the anterior process of the calcaneus and in a patient with a painful sural neuroma. These authors recommended bone scanning as the most useful diagnostic imaging technique and excision of an ununited fragment through a lateral approach, with care taken to protect the sural nerve.

Fractures of the medial tubercle of the posterior process are much less frequent than those of the lateral tubercle.[85] Cedell[57] originally described the fracture in four athletes as occurring from a pronation-dorsiflexion force that caused avulsion of the insertion of the posterior talotibial ligament. Others have reported occurrence of the fracture in motor vehicle accidents[54, 59, 66] and in one soccer player who was kicked in the posteromedial aspect of the ankle.[90] Clinical findings of a nonunion usually include a tender, firm mass posterior to the medial malleolus, with no ankle instability or limitation of motion. Radiographs may show the mass, and CT scanning can confirm a nonunion.

Fractures of the entire posterior process (both lateral and medial tubercles) are rare.[59, 74–76] Nyska and coworkers[76] described four patients with fractures of the entire posterior talar process that were missed on initial examination. The mechanism of injury was inversion and plantar flexion of the foot. All four had poor results at 2- to 3-year follow-up. Because both the ankle and subtalar joints are involved in this fracture, malunion and early degenerative changes

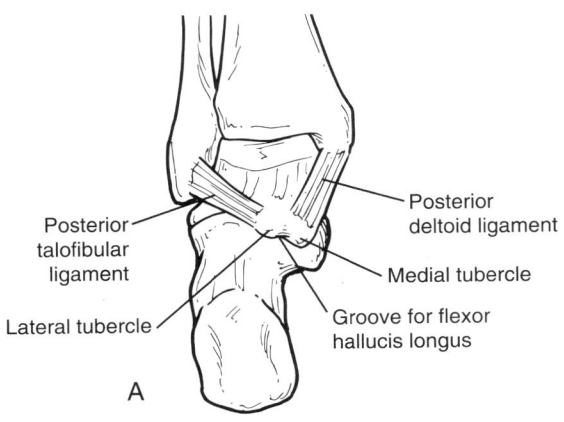

A

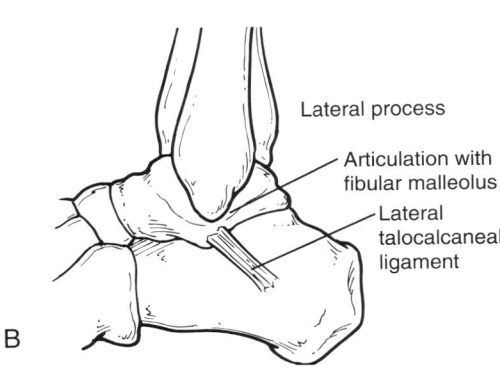

B

Figure 30K–31. *A,* Posterior process of the talus. *B,* Lateral process of the talus. (From Heckman JD: Fractures and dislocations of the foot. In Rockwood CA Jr, Green DP, Bucholz RW, Heckman JD [eds]: Rockwood and Green's Fractures in Adults, vol 2, 4th ed. Philadelphia, Lippincott-Raven, 1996, pp 2267–2405.)

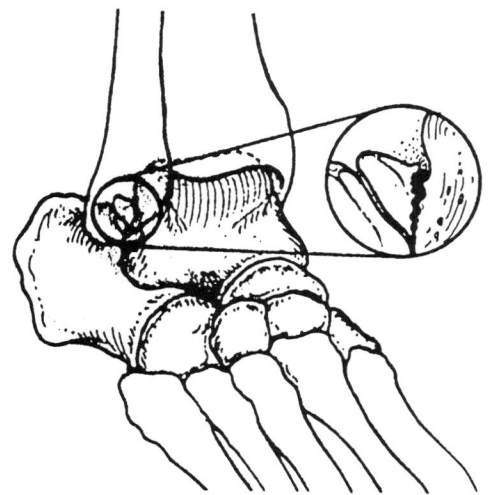

Figure 30K–32. Fracture of posterolateral talar tubercle. (Redrawn from Amis JA, Gangl PM: When inversion injury is more than a "sprained ankle." J Musculoskel Med Sep:68, 1987.)

postulated that delayed ossification might be the earliest event in the changes leading to irregular ossification and suggested that lateness of ossification of the navicular subjects it to more pressure than the bony structures can withstand. Abnormal ossification may be a response of the unprotected, growing nucleus to normal stresses of weight-bearing. If osseous vessels are compressed as they pass through the junction between cartilage and bone, ischemia results, leading to reactive hyperemia and pain.[103]

Cowell and Williams,[102] in a review of 21 patients with osteochondrosis of the tarsal navicular, found the diagnosis to be a clinical one requiring the presence of pain and tenderness in the area of the tarsal navicular associated with radiographic changes of sclerosis and diminished size of the tarsal navicular (Fig. 30K–38). They emphasized that the appearance of multiple ossification centers with no increase in density (sclerosis) should not be confused with Köhler's disease and that radiographic findings similar to Köhler's disease in an asymptomatic foot should be considered irregularities of ossification.

The most common symptoms are pain and limp. Tenderness in the area of the tarsal navicular is the most consistent physical finding, and the most common radiographic finding is a variable degree of sclerosis and flattening of the navicular (Alka-Seltzer-on-end appearance). Loss of the trabecular pattern and fragmentation are also common. The remaining bones of the foot are usually normal.

Köhler's disease is self-limited, and the final outcome is not affected by treatment. Cowell and Williams,[102] however, found that cast immobilization resulted in faster reso-

lution of symptoms (3.2 months) than did conservative treatment without casting (15.2 months). They recommended the use of a short-leg walking cast for 8 weeks. Borges and colleagues[101] examined 14 patients an average of 31.5 years after diagnosis of Köhler's disease and found that those treated without casting had symptoms for an average of 10 months, whereas those treated with casting were completely asymptomatic in an average of 3 months. Immobilization in a short-leg walking cast for 8 weeks or more was the most effective treatment. Orthoses have not been found to be effective.

Author's Preferred Method of Treatment

Initial treatment usually consists of rest and activity modification, followed by cast immobilization, usually for 6 to 8 weeks, if symptoms are not improved.

Return to Athletic Activity

Full competition can usually be resumed once symptoms have resolved, usually within 8 to 10 weeks if cast immobilization is used.

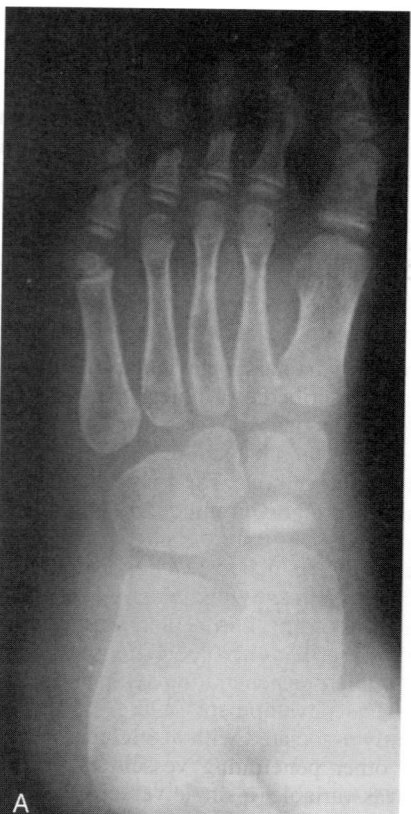
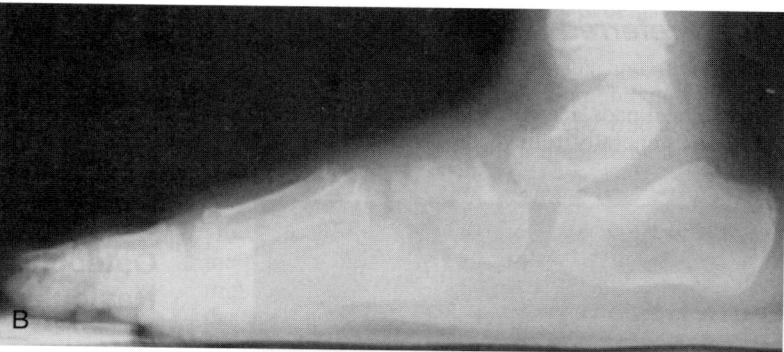

Figure 30K–38. Increased sclerosis and narrowing (Alka-Seltzer-on-end appearance) of the navicular (Köhler's disease) in a young athlete with complaints of pain in medial midfoot area.

Accessory Navicular

Pain over the medial inferior aspect of the navicular is called prehallux syndrome or accessory navicular (Fig. 30K–39A to D).[109] It is often associated with supple pes planus,[107, 108, 112, 115] tendinitis of the posterior tibialis tendon, and a bone prominence over the medial aspect of the navicular. An accessory navicular is present in approximately 14% of all feet,[115] although most of these are asymptomatic and eventually fuse with the navicular. Separation of the synchondrosis between the accessory navicular and the main body of the navicular may cause symptomatic fragmentation of the accessory navicular. If the accessory navicular persists into adolescence, it may become a painful ossicle. Although flatfeet are not associated with an increased incidence of accessory navicular, they are more often associated with symptomatic accessory navicular because of shoe pressure and mechanical stress on the tibialis posterior tendon.

Kiter and associates[111] compared MRI studies of 27 feet with accessory naviculars and 22 normal feet. They found two major anatomic differences: (1) the posterior tibial tendon inserted directly in the accessory navicular bone without any continuity with the sole of the foot or with a slip less than 1 mm thick in 20 of 27 feet with an accessory navicular, whereas this insertion anomaly was not present in any of the normal feet and the posterior tibial tendon had continuity with the sole of the foot and was at least 4 mm thick; (2) a mass with the consistency of fibrocartilage tissue was found between the tendon and bone in 20 of 27 feet with accessory navicular bones instead of the fatty tissue found in all 22 normal feet.

Most patients with an accessory navicular respond to conservative measures, such as an orthosis designed to relieve pressure over the prominent navicular tuberosity. A scaphoid pad is not recommended because it may cause increased pressure on the prominence, thus increasing symptoms. Removal of the accessory navicular may be

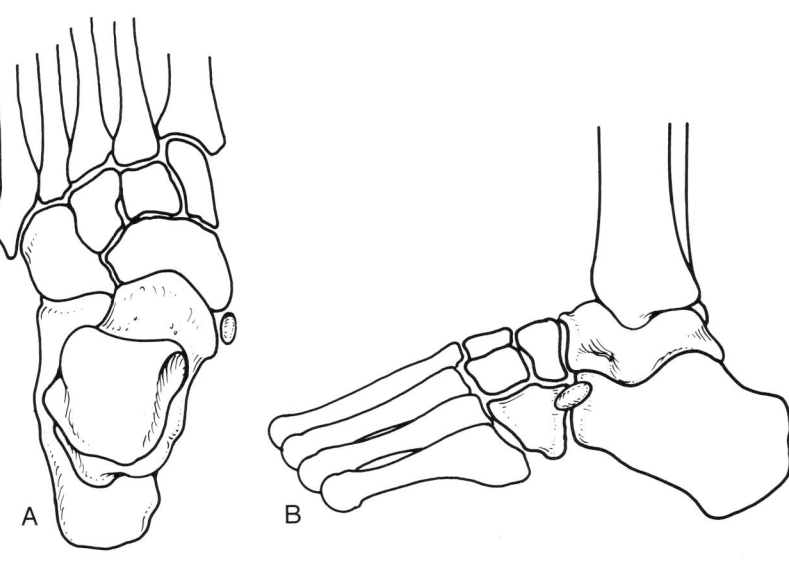

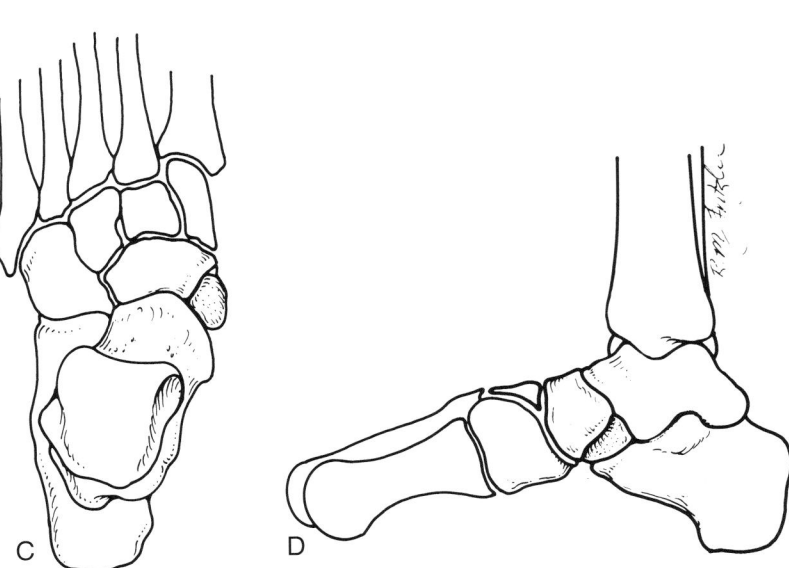

Figure 30K–39. Accessory navicular. *A* and *B*, type I. *C* and *D*, type II. (Redrawn from MacNicol MF, Voutsinas S: Surgical treatment of the symptomatic accessory navicular. J Bone Joint Surg Br 66:218–226, 1984.)

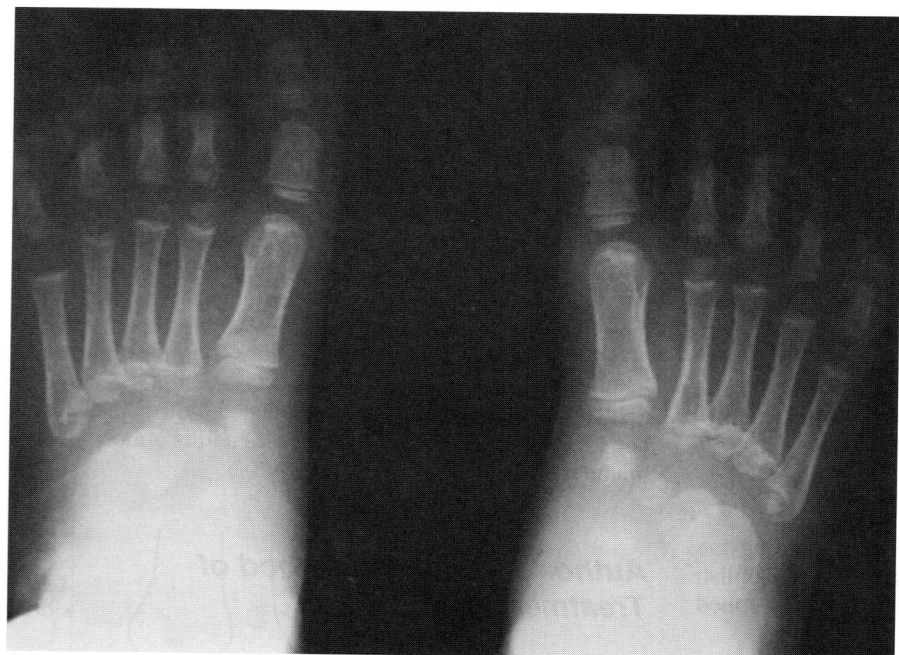

Figure 30K–42. Increased sclerosis and fragmentation of first cuneiform (Buschke's disease) in a child who complained of pain in the medial midfoot area.

first toe and longer second toe), and about 7% of patients have bilateral involvement.[127, 133]

Treatment includes metatarsal relief pads and cessation of all running and jumping activity. On occasion, a short-leg walking cast with a toe extension may be used for 6 to 12 weeks to resolve acute symptoms. Surgical treatment is indicated if conservative measures do not relieve the symptoms. The procedure chosen depends on the severity of the symptoms, the age of the patient, and the presence of loose bodies. For patients in adolescence and early adulthood, joint débridement and remodeling of the metatarsal head, as recommended by Freiberg,[126] are usually successful. For the rare severe deformity and loose bodies

in the joint (Fig. 30K–45), simple excision of the loose bodies is usually sufficient. The Smillie procedure,[130] in which the sclerotic bone is removed down to viable bone and the defect is packed with cancellous bone graft, may be required in a few patients with severe involvement. Metatarsal head replacement has been advocated for disabling involvement in the adult. Gauthier and Elbaz[126] recommended dorsal closing wedge osteotomy (Fig. 30K–46) for severe deformity in patients who bear excessive weight on the involved metatarsal head. Although this procedure has been infrequently reported in the English literature, Kinnard and Lirette[128] reported excellent results in 15 patients (average age, 29 years) after dorsiflexion osteotomy

TABLE 30K–3
Staging and Classification Systems for Freiberg's Disease

Katcherian	Smillie	Gauthier and Elbaz	Thompson and Hamilton	Description	Radiographs
Level A	Stage I	Stage 0 + 1	Type 1	Earliest form; fissure in epiphysis	Radiographs normal; bone scan may detect
Level B	Stage II	Stage 2	Type 2	Progression of subchondral fracture with bone resorption; collapse of dorsal central portion of MT head and alteration of articular surface	Radiographs may show slight widening of joint, sclerosis of epiphysis, collapse and flattening of articular surface
Level C	Stage III	Stage 2	Type 2	Further deformation and collapse of central portion of head	Progressive flattening of MT head with osteolysis and collapse; zone of rarefaction around sclerotic bone as healing and revascularization take place; premature physeal closure may be present
Level D	Stage IV	Stage 3	Type 3	Fracture and separation of central portion and peripheral projections of involved MT head resulting in loose bodies	Fragmentation of epiphysis, early joint narrowing, multiple loose bodies
Level E	Stage V	Stage 4	Type 3	Advanced arthrosis secondary to progressive flattening and deformity of MT head	Joint space narrowing, hypertrophy of MT head, irregularity of base of proximal phalanx with osteophyte formation

MT, metatarsal.
Modified from Katcherian DA: Treatment of Freiberg's disease. Orthop Clin North Am 25:69–81, 1994.

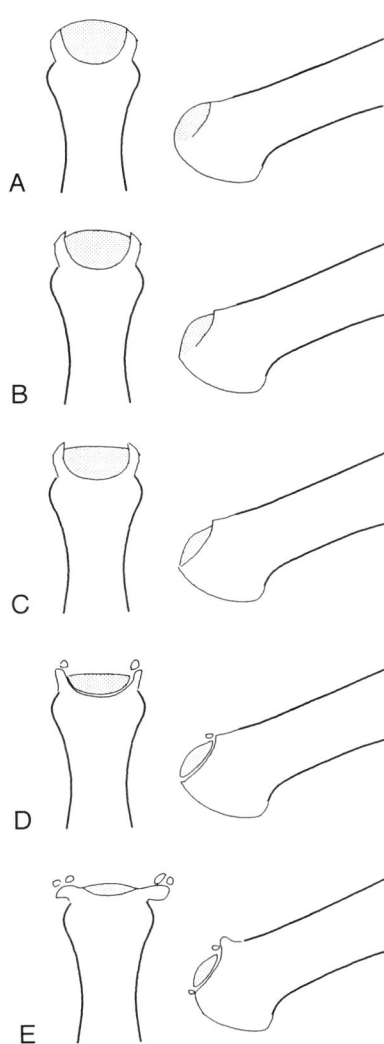

Figure 30K–43. Levels of progression of Freiberg's disease. *A,* Early fracture of subchondral epiphysis. *B,* Early collapse of dorsal central portion of metatarsal with flattening of articular surface. *C,* Further flattening of metatarsal head with continued collapse of central portion of articular surface with medial and lateral projections; plantar articular cartilage remains intact. *D,* Loose bodies form from fractures of lateral projections and separation of central articular fragment. *E,* End-stage degenerative arthrosis with marked flattening of metatarsal head and joint space narrowing. (From Katcherian DA: Treatment of Freiberg's disease. Orthop Clin North Am 25:69–81, 1994.)

fixed with transosseous sutures (Fig. 30K–47). They recommended this procedure as simple, reliable, nondestructive, and applicable to any stage of Freiberg's disease. Smith and coworkers[131] reported good results in 14 of 15 patients treated with metatarsal shortening osteotomy fixed with a small-fragment plate and screws. As advantages of this method, they cited the ease of the procedure and the avoidance of damage to the metatarsal head; however, it does not restore normal motion at the metatarsal joint, and a second procedure is required for plate removal. El-Tayeby[123] described an interpositional arthroplasty with use of the extensor digitorum longus tendon of the affected toe as a spacer. Of the 13 adolescents with this procedure, 10 had excellent results, 1 had a good result, and 2 had fair

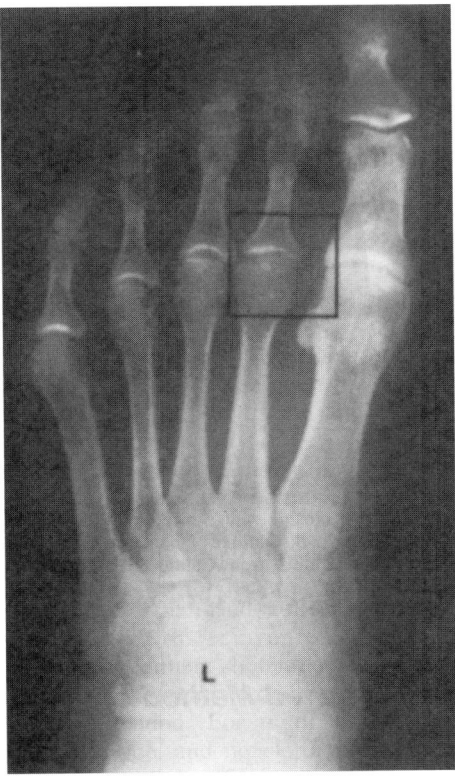

Figure 30K–44. Freiberg's infarction in an unusual area of the third metatarsal head in an adolescent athlete. (From Richardson EG: The foot in adolescents and adults. In Crenshaw AH [ed]: Campbell's Operative Orthopaedics, 7th ed. St Louis, Mosby, 1987.)

results. Although most patients had significant pain relief that allowed higher levels of activity, metatarsophalangeal range of motion did not improve, and eight patients had weak toe extension that gradually improved.

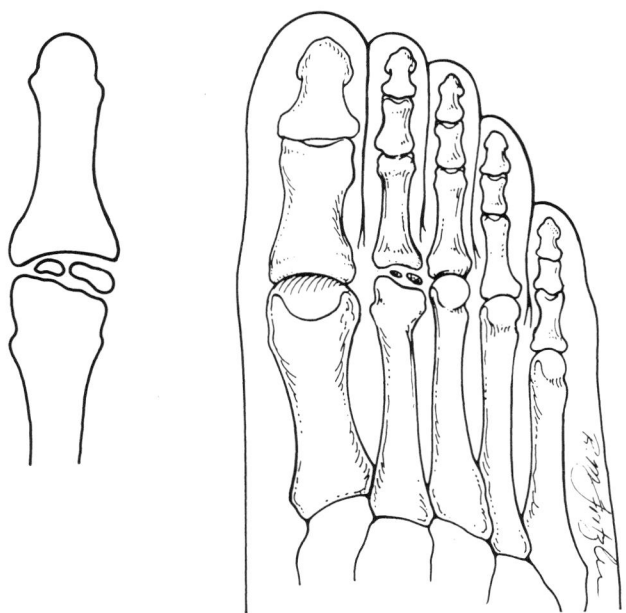

Figure 30K–45. Freiberg's infarction with loose bodies in joint.

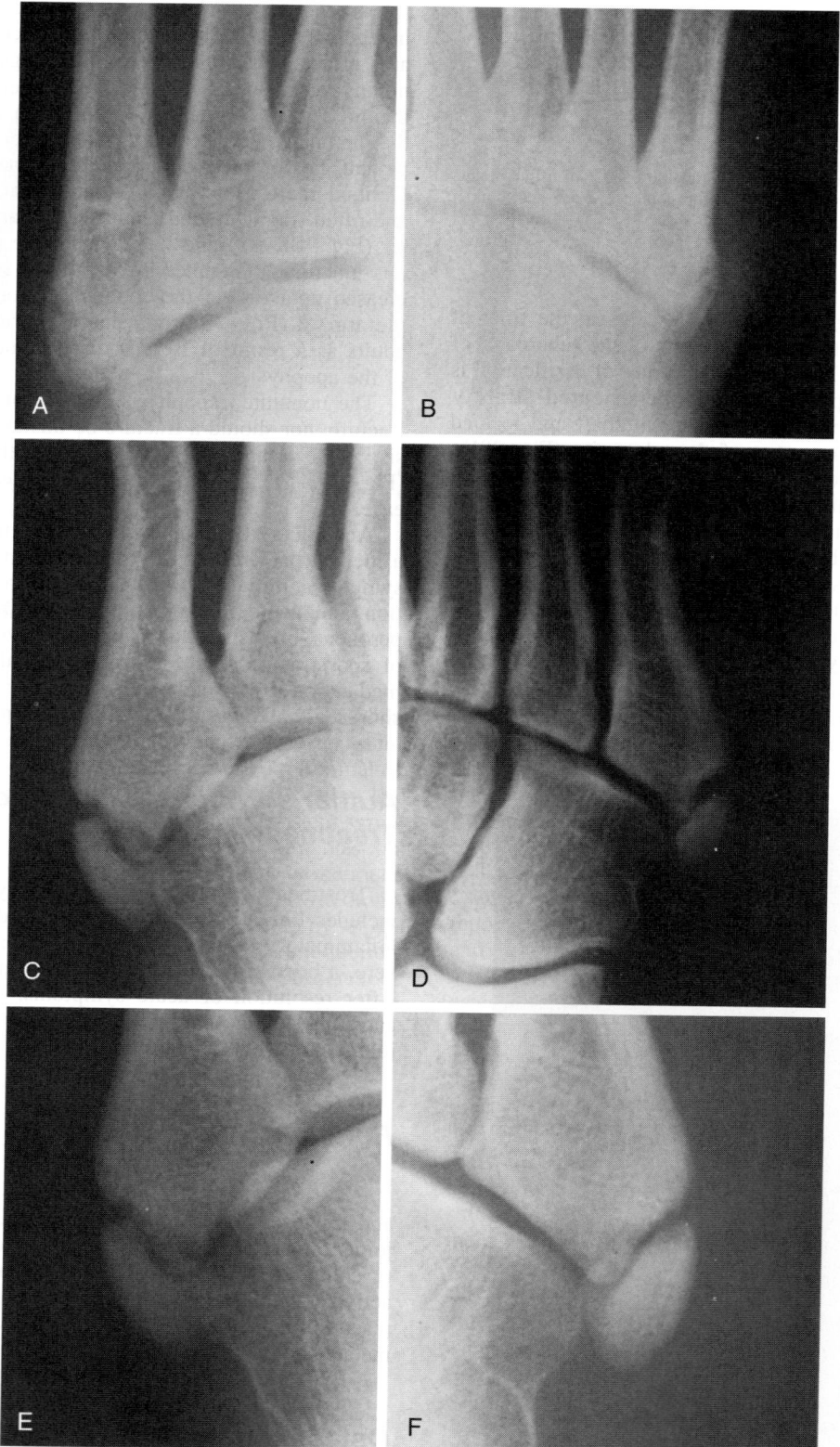

Figure 30K–50. *A* and *B*, Oblique radiographs of a 13-year-old basketball player with bilateral Iselin's disease. *C* and *D*, The same patient as a college freshman (18 years old) with nonunited secondary ossification centers that were asymptomatic. *E* and *F*, The patient as a college senior (21 years old); there is definite evidence of bilateral Iselin's disease and nonunion, but only the left foot is symptomatic.

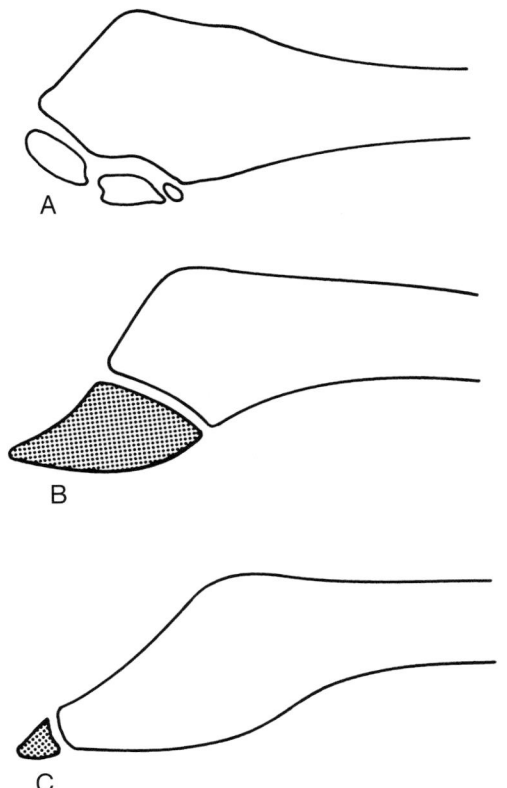

Figure 30K–51. Iselin's disease should not be confused with fracture (*A*), nonunion of the apophysis (*B*), or os vesalianum (*C*). (Redrawn from Sarrafian SK: Anatomy of the Foot and Ankle. Philadelphia, JB Lippincott, 1983.)

of the metatarsophalangeal joint and sesamoids may be difficult to determine, it is generally a stress fracture of the sesamoid and sesamoiditis.

Galen, in AD 180, named these small bones the sesamoids because of their resemblance to flat, oval sesame seeds.[160, 161] During the seventh or eighth week of embryonic life, both sesamoid bones of the hallux appear as islands of undifferentiated connective tissue between the first metatarsal heads. The fibular sesamoid is present slightly sooner than the tibial sesamoid. Ossification begins around year 8 to 9 in girls and in year 10 to 11 in boys. There may be two or more centers of ossification, with the tibial sesamoid being bipartite at skeletal maturity in approximately 10% to 25% of the population; the fibular sesamoid is rarely bipartite.[153, 159, 162] The sesamoids appear to have two anatomic functions (Fig. 30K–52). They act as a pulley system around which the medial and lateral heads of the flexor hallucis brevis musculotendinous units course before attaching to the base of the proximal phalanx.[153] In their location within the substance of the plantar plate, the sesamoids also serve as "shock absorbers" by disbursing impact forces on the metatarsal heads.[148]

Osteochondrosis of the sesamoids was first reported by Renander[158] in 1924. Treves,[164] in 1928, described a painful condition of the hallucal sesamoid in which radiographs showed a mottled appearance instead of the homogeneous appearance typical of normal cancellous bone. Although Finochetto[149] reported that sesamoiditis and osteochondritis were the same entity, Burman and Lapidus[145] and Ilfeld and Rosen[152] concluded that osteochondritis of the sesamoid is a separate clinical entity characterized by fragmentation, irregularity, and mottling of the symptomatic sesamoid. Whether there is a difference between osteochondrosis and osteochondritis of the sesamoid remains controversial. Histologic examination confirms the presence of bone necrosis and attempted bone repair in mottled and fragmented areas. An osteochondritis may develop in a sesamoid "at risk" from earlier osteochondrosis, and repetitive microtrauma may gradually result in mottling, fragmentation, and collapse.

Pain beneath the first metatarsal head may be difficult to treat. Richardson[160, 161] reported that the diagnosis of sesamoid injury constitutes a spectrum of abnormality rather than an isolated injury. Depending on the stage at which the patient is first seen, the diagnosis may range from bursitis over the tibial sesamoid[164] to the vague entity sesamoiditis, which encompasses both osteochondrosis and osteochondritis. In later stages, the diagnosis may include stress fracture,[151, 165, 166] traumatic or degenerative arthritis,[159] and chondromalacia[162] (Fig. 30K–53). Hematogenous

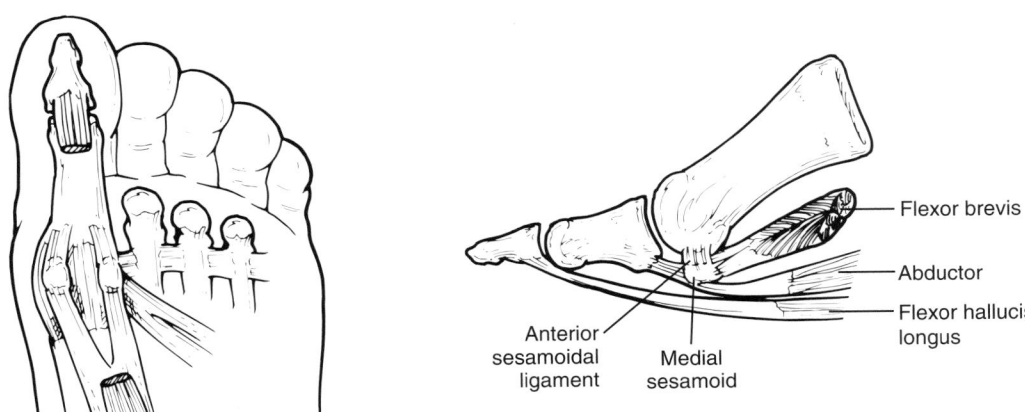

Figure 30K–52. Anatomy of the sesamoids. (From Leventen EO: Sesamoid disorders and treatment: An update. Clin Orthop 269:236–240, 1991.)

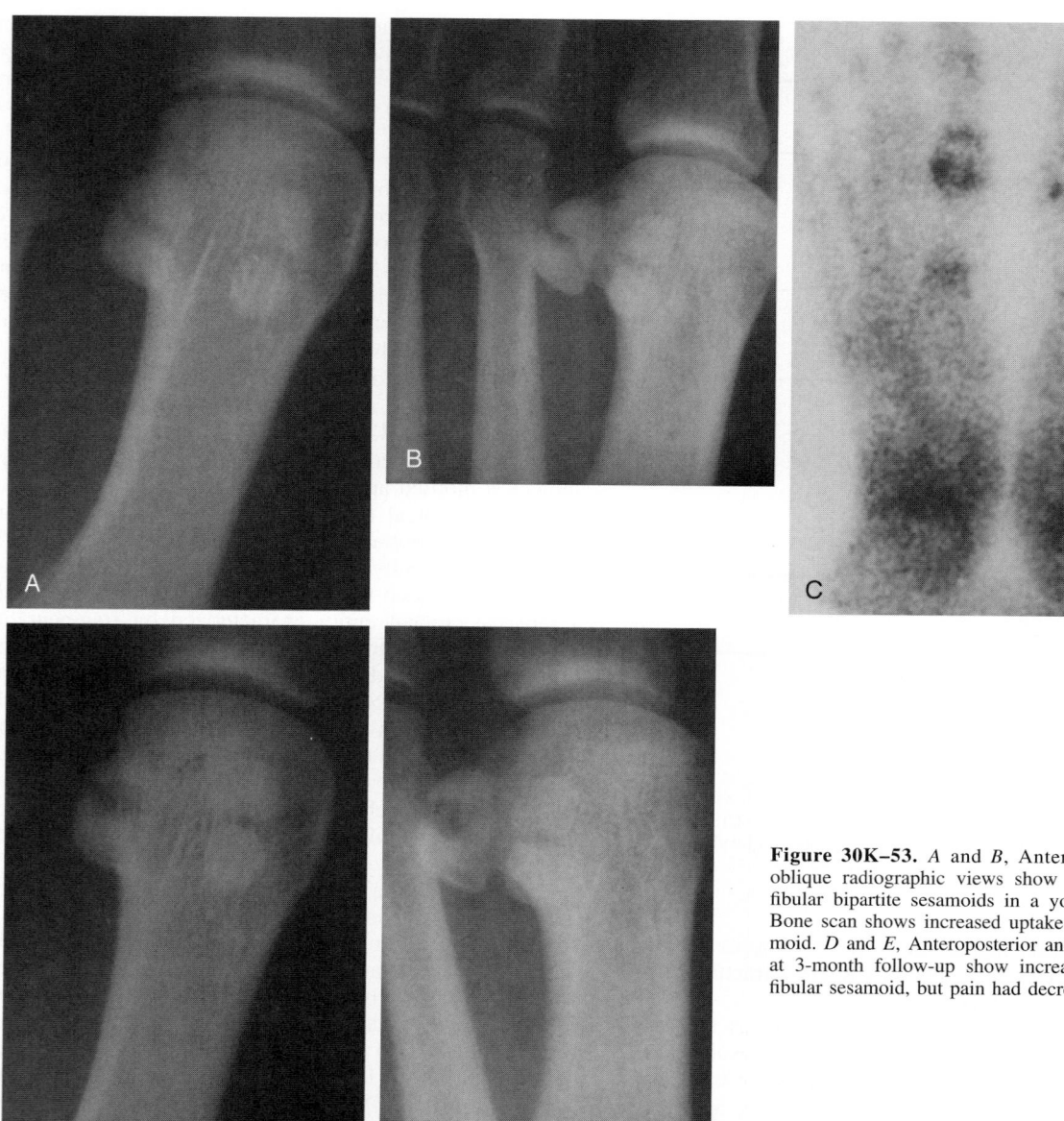

Figure 30K–53. *A* and *B*, Anteroposterior and oblique radiographic views show both tibial and fibular bipartite sesamoids in a young athlete. *C*, Bone scan shows increased uptake in fibular sesamoid. *D* and *E*, Anteroposterior and oblique views at 3-month follow-up show increased lucency in fibular sesamoid, but pain had decreased.

osteomyelitis of the sesamoid[150] should also be considered in the differential diagnosis, and sesamoid periostitis may occur in athletes with one of the rheumatoid variants, such as psoriasis, Reiter's syndrome, and ankylosing spondylitis.[159]

Routine radiographs are of little benefit. Oblique views should be made so that the tibial sesamoid is not overlapped by the first metatarsal. Radiographs of the opposite foot may be helpful in distinguishing a bipartite sesamoid from a fracture. If the symptomatic sesamoid shows more separation of the fragment or less distinct smooth edges at the adjacent bone margins than the asymptomatic side does, stress fracture or further disruption of a bipartite sesamoid should be suspected. The tibial sesamoid can be seen best

on films made with the foot and ankle in the lateral position, the metatarsophalangeal joints extended 50 to 60 degrees, and the x-ray beam angled 15 degrees cephalad and centered at the medial eminence of the first metatarsal. The single most important radiograph is the axial sesamoid view, which can be obtained in a variety of ways. The Muller technique (Fig. 30K–54) is preferred. Bone scanning is helpful to determine whether the problem is related to the sesamoid and to which sesamoid but does not distinguish sesamoiditis, osteochondrosis, osteochondritis, and stress fracture (see Fig. 30K–53). Bone scanning may reveal subclinical sesamoid injury or the "sesamoid at risk" (indicated by increased but still less uptake than that seen in the symptomatic sesamoid), and the athlete can be

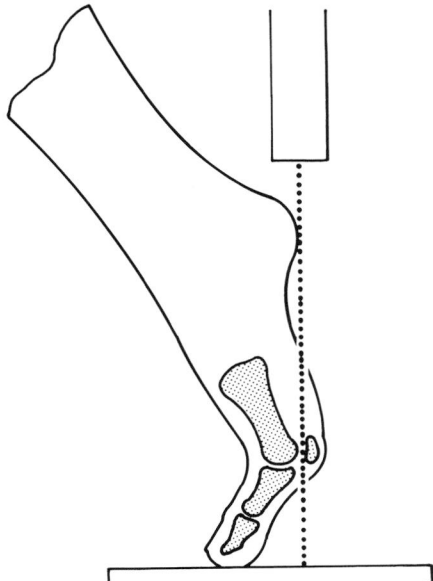

Figure 30K–54. The Muller radiographic technique for axial sesamoid view. (Redrawn from Richardson EG: Injuries to the hallucal sesamoids in the athlete. Foot Ankle Int 7:229, 1987. ©American Orthopaedic Foot and Ankle Society, 1987.)

warned of the possibility of osteochondrosis, osteochondritis, or stress fracture in the area.[146]

Osteochondritis or sesamoiditis should be suspected in the young athlete with local tenderness over a sesamoid and no evidence of swelling or redness about the joint, which would indicate infection or bursitis.[156, 157, 161, 163] Increased uptake at the tibial sesamoid on bone scanning or fragmentation and mottling of the sesamoid on radiographs further support the diagnosis. Treatment includes reduction of activity and the use of molded shoe inserts to which a metatarsal relief bar can be attached. The supports should be worn at all times for a minimum of 6 months, even if symptoms resolve quickly, and should be resumed if symptoms recur after 6 months. Axe and Ray[144] reported that orthotic treatment was effective in 8 of 10 athletes with sesamoid pain regardless of its cause. The advantage of orthotic treatment is that it allows the athlete to continue participation without loss of practice or competition time and delays the necessity of surgical treatment. If stress fracture of a bipartite or non-bipartite sesamoid occurs, cast treatment may be tried, but according to Richardson,[160, 161] it is usually not effective. Stress fractures may be difficult to diagnose in the absence of wide separation of the fragments and callus formation but should be suspected in the athlete with continued symptoms in spite of prolonged rest and conservative management. Because a flattened, fragmented, mottled, symptomatic sesamoid in an athlete probably indicates avascular necrosis, extended periods of conservative care are usually unwarranted and ineffective.[160, 161] If symptoms from displaced or nondisplaced fractures, sesamoiditis, osteochondrosis, or osteochondritis are not relieved by 3 to 6 months of conservative treatment, surgical excision of the sesamoid is generally recommended.[147, 154, 155, 160, 161] Fortunately, only the tibial sesamoid

is usually involved, and excision of both sesamoids is not required because this makes repair of the flexor hallucis brevis technically difficult. Loss of flexor hallucis brevis function after removal of both sesamoids usually results in an intrinsic-minus, cock-up deformity of the great toe, which is just as disabling to the athlete as the original condition.

The tibial sesamoid can be removed through a straight midline medial incision (Fig. 30K–55A) in the internervous plane between the medial plantar digital branch of the medial plantar nerve and the most medial branch of the superficial peroneal nerve dorsally.[160, 161] The retinacular hood overlying the medial capsule and the abductor hallucis tendon are incised in the same plane as the skin incision. An angled probe is inserted proximally, and the investing layer of deep fascia is gently lifted off the abductor hallucis to allow identification of the dorsal edge of the abductor hallucis tendon (Fig. 30K–55B). A longitudinal medial capsular incision is made along the dorsal border of the abductor hallucis tendon (Fig. 30K–55C), and the plantar aspect of the capsule is retracted plantarward and medially to expose the sesamoids. For removal of either sesamoid, the intersesamoid ligament is incised longitudinally (Fig. 30K–55D). By use of a small blade, the sesamoid is removed, staying close to its borders. If only one sesamoid is excised, repair of the plantar plate is not necessary; the capsule is closed (Fig. 30K–55E), and a bulky forefoot dressing is applied with a rigid dressing as a second layer. If both sesamoids are excised, the metatarsophalangeal joint is plantar flexed and the defect is repaired with a firm, absorbable suture; the joint is held in neutral flexion-extension with a smooth Kirschner wire inserted obliquely across the joint.

Author's Preferred Method of Treatment

Initial treatment includes nonsteroidal anti-inflammatory medication, activity modification, and full-length shoe orthoses with a metatarsal pad and a relief beneath the first metatarsal pad. If no relief is obtained, a period of cast immobilization is tried. Persistent symptoms are an indication for excision of the sesamoids.

Return to Athletic Activity

If one sesamoid has been excised, the cast is removed 5 to 7 days after surgery, and range of motion exercises are begun. At 10 to 14 days, the sutures are removed, and toe curls, toe stands, and manual passive flexion and extension exercises are begun. Full return to competitive athletics is not allowed for 6 weeks.

If both sesamoids have been excised, the Kirschner wire is removed 3 weeks after surgery, and non–weight-bearing is continued for another 3 weeks. Competitive athletics are not allowed for 12 weeks.

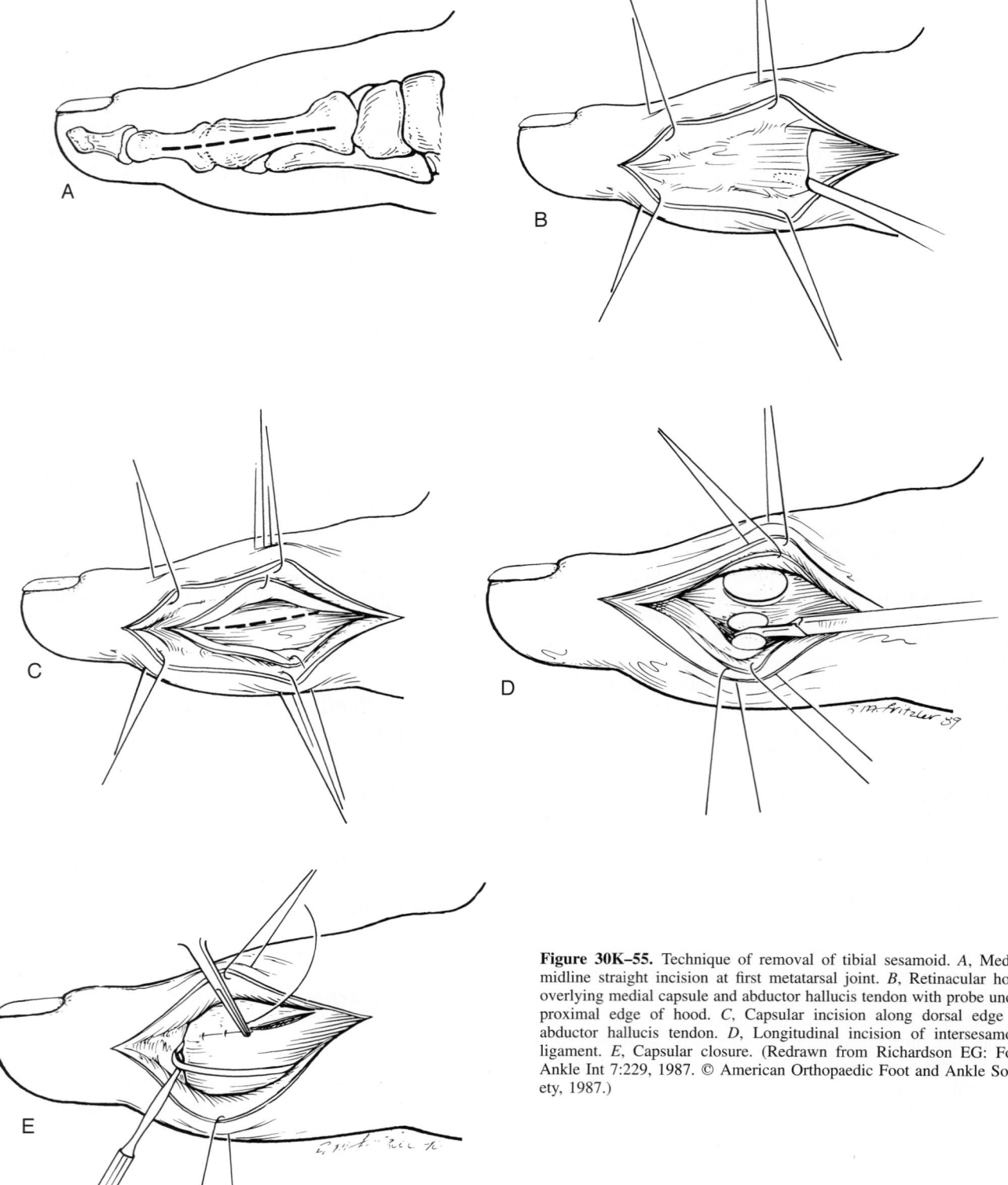

Figure 30K–55. Technique of removal of tibial sesamoid. *A*, Medial midline straight incision at first metatarsal joint. *B*, Retinacular hood overlying medial capsule and abductor hallucis tendon with probe under proximal edge of hood. *C*, Capsular incision along dorsal edge of abductor hallucis tendon. *D*, Longitudinal incision of intersesamoid ligament. *E*, Capsular closure. (Redrawn from Richardson EG: Foot Ankle Int 7:229, 1987. © American Orthopaedic Foot and Ankle Society, 1987.)

References

General

1. Breck L: An Atlas of the Osteochondroses. Springfield, Ill, Charles C Thomas, 1971.

2. Brower AC: The osteochondroses. Orthop Clin North Am 14:99–117, 1983.

3. Daniels TR: Osteochondroses of the foot. In Myerson MS (ed): Foot and Ankle Disorders, vol 2. Philadelphia, WB Saunders, 2000, pp 785–799.

4. Gregg JR, Das M: Foot and ankle problems in the preadolescent and adolescent athlete. Clin Sports Med 1:131–147, 1982.

5. Hoerr NL, Pyle SI, Francis CC: Radiographic Atlas of Skeletal Development of the Foot and Ankle. Philadelphia, JB Lippincott, 1983.

6. Perlman M, Leveille D, DeLeonibus J, et al: Inversion lateral ankle trauma: Differential diagnosis, review of the literature, and prospective study. J Foot Surg 26:95–135, 1987.

7. Roy DR: Accessory naviculars and the osteochondroses of the foot and ankle in the child and adolescent. Foot Ankle Clin 3:737–751, 1998.

8. Sarrafian SK: Anatomy of the Foot and Ankle. Philadelphia, JB Lippincott, 1983.

9. Sachenck RC Jr, Goodnight JM: Current concepts review: Osteochondritis dissecans. J Bone Joint Surg Am 78:439–456, 1996.

10. Siffert RS: Classification of osteochondroses. Clin Orthop 158:10–18, 1981.

Osteochondritis Dissecans of the Talus

11. Anderson IF, Crichton KJ, Grattan-Smith T, et al: Osteochondral fractures of the dome of the talus. J Bone Joint Surg Am 71:1143–1152, 1989.

12. Andrews JR, Previte WJ, Carson WG: Arthroscopy of the ankle: Technique and normal anatomy. Foot Ankle 6:29–33, 1985.

13. Baker CL, Andrews JR, Ryan JB: Arthroscopic treatment of transchondral talar dome fractures. Arthroscopy 2:82–87, 1986.

14. Baker CL, Morales RW: Arthroscopic treatment of transchondral talar dome fractures: A long-term follow-up study. Arthroscopy 15:197–202, 1999.

15. Berndt AL, Harty M: Transchondral fracture of the talus. J Bone Joint Surg Am 41:988–1029, 1959.

16. Bryant DD III, Siegel MG: Osteochondritis dissecans of the talus: A new technique for arthroscopic drilling. Arthroscopy 9:238–241, 1993.

17. Canale ST, Beaty JH: Osteochondral lesions of the talus. In Hamilton WC (ed): Traumatic Disorders of the Ankle. New York, Springer-Verlag, 1984, pp 227–254.

18. Canale ST, Belding RH: Osteochondral lesions of the talus. J Bone Joint Surg Am 62:97–102, 1980.

19. Davidson AM, Steel HD, MacKensie DA, Penny JA: A review of twenty-one cases of transchondral fractures of the talus. J Trauma 7:378–415, 1967.

20. DeSmet AA, Fisher DR, Burnstein MI, et al: Value of MR imaging in staging osteochondral lesions of the talus (osteochondritis dissecans). AJR Am J Roentgenol 154:555–558, 1990.

21. Dipaola JD, Nelson DW, Colville MR: Characterizing osteochondral lesions by magnetic resonance imaging. Arthroscopy 7:101–104, 1991.

22. Drez D, Guhl JF, Gollehan DL: Ankle arthroscopy—technique and indications. Foot Ankle 2:138–143, 1981.

23. Ferkel RD: Arthroscopy of the foot and ankle. In Coughlin MJ, Mann RA (eds): Surgery of the Foot and Ankle, 7th ed. St Louis, Mosby, 1999, pp 1257–1277.

24. Flick AB, Gould N: Osteochondritis dissecans of the talus (transchondral fractures of the talus): Review of the literature and new surgical approach for medial dome lesions. Foot Ankle 5:165–185, 1985.

25. Gepstein R, Conforty B, Weiss RE, Hallel T: Closed percutaneous drilling for osteochondral dissecans of the talus. Clin Orthop 213:197–200, 1986.

26. Guhl JF: New techniques for arthroscopic surgery of the ankle: Preliminary report. Orthopedics 9:261–269, 1986.

27. Hangody L, Kish G, Karpati Z, et al: Treatment of osteochondritis dissecans of the talus: Use of the mosaicplasty technique—a preliminary report. Foot Ankle Int 18:628–634, 1997.

28. Hepple S, Winson IG, Glew D: Osteochondral lesions of the talus: A revised classification. Foot Ankle Int 20:789–793, 1999.

29. Higashiyama I, Kumai T, Takakura Y, Tamail S: Follow-up study of MRI for osteochondral lesion of the talus. Foot Ankle Int 21:127–133, 2000.

30. Higuera J, Laguna R, Meral M, et al: Osteochondritis dissecans of the talus during childhood and adolescence. J Pediatr Orthop 18:328–332, 1998.

31. Kappis M: Weitere Beitrage zur traumatisch-mechanischen Entstehung der "spontanen" Knorpelablosungen (sogen. Osteochondritis dissecans). Dtsch Z Chir 171:13, 1922.

32. Kelbérine F, Frank A: Arthroscopic treatment of osteochondral lesions of the talar dome: A retrospective study of 48 cases. Arthroscopy 15:77–84, 1999.

33. Kish G, Módis L, Hangody L: Osteochondral mosaicplasty for the treatment of focal chondral and osteochondral lesions of the knee and talus in the athlete: Rationale, indications, techniques, and results. Clin Sports Med 18:45–68, 1999.

34. Konig F: Über freie Korper in den Gelenken. Dtsch Z Chir 27:90, 1888.

35. Kumai T, Takakura Y, Higashiyama I, Tamai S: Arthroscopic drilling for the treatment of osteochondral lesions of the talus. J Bone Joint Surg Am 81:1229–1235, 1999.

36. Lahm A, Erggelet C, Steinwachs M, Reichelt A: Arthroscopic management of osteochondral lesions of the talus: Results of drilling and usefulness of magnetic resonance imaging before and after treatment. Arthroscopy 16:299–304, 2000.

37. Lehman RC, Gregg JR: Osteochondritis dissecans of the midfoot. Foot Ankle 7:177–182, 1986.

38. Loomer R, Fisher C, Lloyd-Smith R, et al: Osteochondral lesions of the talus. Am J Sports Med 21:13–19, 1993.

39. Martin DF, Baker CL, Curl WW, et al: Operative ankle arthroscopy: Long-term followup. Am J Sports Med 17:16–23, 1989.

40. Mukherjee SK, Young AB: Dome fracture of the talus: Report of ten cases. J Bone Joint Surg Br 55:319–326, 1973.

41. Ogilvie-Harris DJ, Sarrosa EA: Arthroscopic treatment after previous failed open surgery for osteochondritis dissecans of the talus. Arthroscopy 15:809–812, 1999.

42. Ogilvie-Harris DJ, Sarrosa EA: Arthroscopic treatment of osteochondritis dissecans of the talus. Arthroscopy 15:805–808, 1999.

43. Parisien JS: Arthroscopic treatment of osteochondral lesions of the talus. Am J Sports Med 14:211–217, 1986.

44. Parisien JS: Diagnostic and surgical arthroscopy of the ankle: Technique and indications. Bull Hosp Joint Dis 45:38–47, 1985.

45. Rendu A: Fracture intra-articulaire parcellaire de la poulie astraglienne. Lyon Med 150:220, 1932.

46. Roden S, Tillegard P, Unander-Scharin L: Osteochondritis dissecans and similar lesions of the talus. Report of five cases with special reference to etiology and treatment. Acta Orthop Scand 23:51, 1953.

47. Schneider T, Fink B, Jerosch J, et al: The value of magnetic resonance imaging as postoperative control after arthroscopic treatment of osteochondritis dissecans. Arch Orthop Trauma Surg 117:235–239, 1998.

48. Shea MR, Manoli A: Osteochondral lesions of the talar dome. Foot Ankle 14:48–55, 1993.

49. Taranow WS, Bisignani GA, Towers JD, Conti SF: Retrograde drilling of osteochondral lesions of the medial talar dome. Foot Ankle Int 20:475–480, 1999.

50. Thompson JP, Loomer RL: Osteochondral lesions of the talus in a sports medicine clinic—a new radiographic technique and surgical approach. Am J Sports Med 12:460–463, 1984.

51. Tol JL, Struijs PAA, Bossuyt PMM, et al: Treatment strategies in osteochondral defects of the talar dome: A systematic review. Foot Ankle Int 21:119–126, 2000.

52. Yocum LA: Treatment of osteochondritis dissecans of the talus. In Shields CL Jr (ed): Manual of Sports Surgery. New York, Springer-Verlag, 1987, pp 183–199.

Lesions of the Talus That May Mimic Ankle Sprains

53. Amis JA, Gangl PM: When inversion injury is more than a "sprained ankle." J Musculoskel Med Sep:68–70, 1987.

54. Banks AS, Caldarella D: Fractures of the posteromedial process of the talus. J Am Podiatr Med Assoc 84:66–70, 1994.
55. Brodsky AE, Khalil MA: Talar compression syndrome. Am J Sports Med 14:472–476, 1986.
56. Bureau NJ, Cardinal E, Hobden R, Aubin B: Posterior ankle impingement syndrome: MR imaging findings in seven patients. Radiology 215:497–503, 2000.
57. Cedell CA: Rupture of the posterior talotibial ligament with the avulsion of a bone fragment from the talus. Acta Orthop Scand 45:454–461, 1974.
58. Clark TW, Janzen DL, Ho K, et al: Detection of radiographically occult ankle fractures following acute trauma: Positive predictive value of ankle effusion. AJR Am J Roentgenol 164:1185–1189, 1995.
59. Ebraheim NA, Padanilam TG, Wong FY: Posteromedial process fractures of the talus. Foot Ankle Int 11:734–739, 1995.
60. Ebraheim NA, Skie MC, Podeszwa DA, Jackson WT: Evaluation of process fractures of the talus using computed tomography. J Orthop Trauma 8:332–337, 1994.
61. Grogan DP, Walling AK, Ogden JA: Anatomy of the os trigonum. Unpublished data, 1989.
62. Haddad FS, Bartlett M, Singh D: Case report: The sequelae of posterior talar fractures. Injury 31:107–111, 2000.
63. Hamilton WG, Geppert MJ, Thompson FM: Pain in the posterior aspect of the ankle in dancers. Differential diagnosis and operative treatment. J Bone Joint Surg Am 78:1491–5000, 1996.
64. Hontas MJ, Haddad RJ, Schlesinger LC: Conditions of the talus in the runner. Am J Sports Med 14:486–490, 1986.
65. Johnson RP, Collier BD, Carrera GF: Os trigonum syndrome: Use of bone scan in the diagnosis. J Trauma 24:761–764, 1984.
66. Kanube K, Kubota H, Hasegawo A, Udagawa E: Fracture of the posterior medial tubercle of the talus treated by internal fixation: A report of two cases. Foot Ankle Int 16:164–166, 1995.
67. Kim S-H, Ha K-I, Ahn J-H: Tram track lesion of the talar dome. Arthroscopy 15:203–206, 1999.
68. Kleiger B: Anterior tibiotalar impingement syndromes in dancers. Foot Ankle 3:69–73, 1982.
69. Marotta JJ, Micheli LJ: Os trigonum impingement in dancers. Am J Sports Med 20:533–536, 1992.
70. Marumoto JM, Ferkel RD: Arthroscopic excision of the os trigonum: A new technique with preliminary clinical results. Foot Ankle Int 18:777–784, 1997.
71. McManama GB: Ankle injuries in the young athlete. Clin Sports Med 7:547–552, 1988.
72. Monroe MT, Manoli A II: Osteoid osteoma of the lateral talar process presenting as chronic sprained ankle. Foot Ankle Int 20:461–463, 1999.
73. Mosier–La Clair SM, Monroe MT, Manoli A: Medial impingement syndrome of the anterior tibiotalar fascicle of the deltoid ligament on the talus. Foot Ankle Int 21:385–391, 2000.
74. Nadim Y, Tosic A, Ebraheim N: Open reduction and internal fixation of fracture of the posterior process of the talus: A case report and review of the literature. Foot Ankle Int 20:50–52, 1999.
75. Nasser S, Manoli A II: Fracture of the entire posterior process of the talus: A case report. Foot Ankle 10:235–238, 1990.
76. Nyska M, Howard CB, Matan Y, et al: Fracture of the posterior body of the talus—the hidden fracture. Arch Orthop Trauma Surg 117:114–117, 1998.
77. O'Donoghue DH: Impingement exostosis of the talus and tibia. J Bone Joint Surg Am 39:835, 1957.
78. Ogilvie-Harris DJ, Mahomen N, Demaziere A: Anterior impingement of the ankle treated by arthroscopic removal of bony spurs. J Bone Joint Surg Br 75:437–450, 1993.
79. O'Neil DB, Micheli LJ: Tarsal coalition: A followup of adolescent athletes. Am J Sports Med 17:544–549, 1989.
80. Parkes JC II, Hamilton WG, Patterson AH, Rawles JG Jr: The anterior impingement syndrome of the ankle. J Trauma 20:895–898, 1980.
81. Raikin SM, Cooke PH: Divot sign: A new observation in anterior impingement of the ankle. Foot Ankle Int 20:532–533, 1999.
82. Scranton PE, McDermott JI: Anterior tibiotalar spurs: A comparison of open versus arthroscopic débridement. Foot Ankle 13:125–128, 1992.
83. Snow SW, Sobel M, DiCarlo EF, et al: Chronic ankle pain caused by osteoid osteoma of the neck of the talus. Foot Ankle Int 18:98–101, 1997.
84. Snyder RB, Lipscomb AB, Johnston RK: The relationship of tarsal coalitions to ankle sprains in athletes. Am J Sports Med 9:313–317, 1981.
85. Stefko RM, Lauerman WC, Heckman JD: Tarsal tunnel syndrome caused by an unrecognized fracture of the posterior process of the talus (Cedell fracture). J Bone Joint Surg Am 76:116–118, 1994.
86. Trnka HJ, Zettl R, Ritschl P: Fracture of the anterior superior process of the calcaneus: An often misdiagnosed fracture. Arch Orthop Trauma Surg 117:300–302, 1998.
87. Tucker DJ, Feder JM, Boylan JP: Fractures of the lateral process of the talus: Two case reports and a comprehensive literature review. Foot Ankle Int 19:641–646, 1998.
88. Veazey BL, Heckman JD, Galindo MJ, McGanity PLJ: Excision of ununited fractures of the posterior process of the talus: A treatment for chronic posterior ankle pain. Foot Ankle 13:453–457, 1992.
89. Waller JF Jr: Hindfoot and Midfoot Problems of the Runner. Symposium on the Foot and Leg in Running Sports. St Louis, CV Mosby, 1982.
90. Wolf RB, Heckman JD: Case report: Fracture of the posterior medial tubercle of the talus secondary to direct trauma. Foot Ankle Int 19:255–258, 1998.

Calcaneal Apophysitis

91. Ferguson AB, Gingrich RM: The normal and abnormal calcaneal apophysis and tarsal navicular. Clin Orthop 10:87–95, 1957.
92. Hughes E: Painful heels in children. Surg Gynecol Obstet 86:64–68, 1948.
93. Lokiec F, Wientroub S: Calcaneal osteochondritis: A new overuse injury. J Pediatr Orthop B 7:243–245, 1998.
94. Madden CC, Mellion MB: Sever's disease and other causes of heel pain in adolescents. Am Fam Physician 54:1995–2000, 1996.
95. Micheli LJ, Ireland ML: Prevention and management of calcaneal apophysitis in children: An overuse syndrome. J Pediatr Orthop 7:34–38, 1987.
96. Moreau G, Letts M: Unicameral bone cyst of the calcaneus in children. J Pediatr Orthop 14:101–104, 1994.
97. Peck DM: Apophyseal injuries in the young athlete. Am Fam Physician 51:1897–1898, 1995.
98. Shopfner CE, Coin CG: Effect of weight-bearing on the appearance and development of the secondary calcaneal epiphysis. Radiology 86:201–206, 1966.
99. Sever JW: Apophysitis of the os calcis. N Y Med J 95:1025–1029, 1912.
100. Winiker H, Scharli AF: Hematogenous calcaneal osteomyelitis in children. Eur J Pediatr Surg 1:216–220, 1991.

Osteochondrosis of the Tarsal Navicular

101. Borges JLP, Guille JT, Bowen JR: Köhler's bone disease of the tarsal navicular. J Pediatr Orthop 15:596–598, 1995.
102. Cowell HR, Williams FA: Köhler's disease of the tarsal navicular. Clin Orthop 158:53–59, 1981.
103. Ferguson AB, Gingrich RM: The normal and the abnormal calcaneal apophysis and tarsal navicular. Clin Orthop 10:87–94, 1957.
104. Karp MB: Köhler's disease of the tarsal scaphoid. J Bone Joint Surg 19:84–96, 1937.
105. Köhler A: A frequent disease of individual bones in children, apparently previously unknown. Munch Med Wochenschr 55:1923–1925, 1908.
106. Waugh W: The ossification and vascularization of the tarsal navicular and their relation to Köhler's disease. J Bone Joint Surg Br 40:765, 1958.

Accessory Navicular

107. Barry RJ, Scranton PE Jr: Flatfeet in children. Clin Orthop 181:68–75, 1983.
108. Bordelon RL: Hypermobile flatfoot in children. Clin Orthop 181:7–14, 1983.
109. Gregg JR, Das M: Foot and ankle problems in the preadolescent and adolescent athlete. Clin Sports Med 1:131–147, 1982.
110. Kidner FC: The prehallux (accessory scaphoid) in its relation to flatfoot. J Bone Joint Surg 11:831–837, 1929.
111. Kiter E, Erdag N, Karatosun V, Günal I: Tibialis posterior tendon

abnormalities in feet with accessory navicular bone and flatfoot. Acta Orthop Scand 70:618–621, 1999.

112. Leonard MH, Gonzales S, Breck LW, et al: Lateral transfer of the posterior tibial tendon in certain selected cases of pes planovalgus (Kidner operation). Clin Orthop 40:139–144, 1965.

113. MacNicol MF, Voustsinas S: Surgical treatment of the symptomatic accessory navicular. J Bone Joint Surg Br 66:218–226, 1984.

114. Malicky ES, Levine DS, Sangeorzan BJ: Modification of the Kidner procedure with fusion of the primary and accessory navicular bones. Foot Ankle Int 20:53–54, 1999.

115. Richardson EG: Pes planus. In Canale AH (ed): Campbell's Operative Orthopedics, 9th ed. St Louis, Mosby–Year Book, 1998, pp 1725–1732.

Osteochondrosis of the Cuneiform

116. Buchman J: Osteochondroses of the internal cuneiform. J Bone Joint Surg 15:225–232, 1933.

117. Haboush EJ: Bilateral disease of internal cuneiform bone with associated disease of the right scaphoid bone (Köhler's). JAMA 100:41–42, 1933.

118. Leeson MC, Weiner DS: Osteochondrosis of the tarsal cuneiforms. Clin Orthop 196:260–264, 1985.

119. Martin JV, Vicente-Herrera E, de Lamo JP, Fernandez CV: Case report: Osteochondritis of the medial cuneiform. J Pediatr Orthop B 8:69–71, 1999.

120. Meilstrup DB: Osteochondritis of the internal cuneiform, bilateral. AJR Am J Roentgenol 58:329–330, 1947.

121. Mubarak SJ: Osteochondrosis of the lateral cuneiform: Another cause of a limp in a child. J Bone Joint Surg Am 74:285–289, 1992.

122. Zimberg J, Levitt JCA, Brahim F: Osteochondrosis of the medial cuneiform: A case report. J Am Podiatr Assoc 75:538–539, 1985.

Freiberg's Disease

123. el-Tayeby HM: Freiberg's infarction: A new surgical procedure. J Foot Ankle Surg 37:23–27, 1998.

124. Falkenberg MP, Dickens DRV, Menelaus MB: Case report: Osteochondritis of the first metatarsal epiphysis. J Pediatr Orthop 10:797–799, 1990.

125. Freiberg AH: The so-called infarction of the second metatarsal bone. J Bone Joint Surg 8:257–261, 1926.

126. Gauthier G, Elbaz R: Freiberg's infarction: A subchondral bone fatigue fracture. A new surgical treatment. Clin Orthop 142:93–95, 1978.

127. Katcherian DA: Treatment of Freiberg's disease. Orthop Clin North Am 25:69–81, 1994.

128. Kinnard P, Lirette R: Freiberg's disease and dorsiflexion osteotomy. J Bone Joint Surg Br 73:864–865, 1991.

129. Kinoshita M, Okuda R, Morikawa J, et al: Osteochondral lesions of the proximal phalanx of the great toe: A report of two cases. Foot Ankle Int 19:252–254, 1998.

130. Smillie IS: Freiberg's infarction (Köhler's second disease). J Bone Joint Surg Br 39:580, 1957.

131. Smith T, Stanley T, Rowley D: Treatment of Freiberg's disease: A new operative technique. J Bone Joint Surg Br 73:129–130, 1991.

132. Sproul J, Klaaren H, Mannarino F: Surgical treatment of Freiberg's infarction in athletes. Am J Sports Med 21:381–384, 1993.

133. Stanley D, Betts R, Rowley D, et al: Assessment of etiologic factors in the development of Freiberg's disease. J Foot Surg 29:444–447, 1990.

134. Thompson FM, Hamilton WG: Problems of the second metatarsophalangeal joint. Orthopedics 10:83–89, 1987.

Iselin's Disease

135. Canale ST, Williams KD: Iselin's disease. J Pediatr Orthop 12:90–93, 1992.

136. Case JT: Borderlands of the Normal and Early Pathologic in Skeletal Roentgenology, 10th ed. New York, Grune & Stratton, 1956.

137. Dameron TB: Fractures and anatomical variations of the proximal portion of the fifth metatarsal. J Bone Joint Surg Am 57:788, 792, 1975.

138. Hoerr NL, Pyle SI, Francis CC: Radiographic Atlas of Skeletal Development of the Foot and Ankle. Springfield, Ill, Charles C Thomas, 1962.

139. Holland CT: The accessory bone of the foot, with notes on a few other conditions. In The Robert Jones Birthday Volume. Edinburgh, Oxford University Press, 1928, pp 157–182.

140. Iselin H: Wachtumsbeschwerden zur Zeit der Knochernen Entwicklung der Tuberositas metatarsi quint. Dtsch Z Chir 117:529–535, 1912.

141. Lehman RC, Gregg JR, Torg E: Iselin's disease. Am J Sports Med 14:494, 496, 1986.

142. Ralph BG, Barrett J, Kenyherca C, DiDomenico LA: Iselin's disease: A case presentation of nonunion and review of the differential diagnosis. J Foot Ankle Surg 38:409–416, 1999.

Osteochondrosis (Osteochondritis) of the Sesamoids

143. Anderson RB, McBryde AM Jr: Autogenous bone grafting of hallux sesamoid nonunions. Foot Ankle Int 18:293–296, 1997.

144. Axe MJ, Ray RL: Orthotic treatment of sesamoid pain. Am J Sports Med 16:411–416, 1989.

145. Burman MS, Lapidus PW: The functional disturbances caused by the inconsistent bones and sesamoids of the foot. Arch Surg 22:936–975, 1931.

146. Chisin R, Peyser A, Milgrom C: Bone scintigraphy in the assessment of the hallucal sesamoids. Foot Ankle Int 16:291–294, 1995.

147. Coughlin MJ: Sesamoid pain: Causes and surgical treatment. Instr Course Lect 39:23–35, 1990.

148. deBritto SR: The first metatarso-sesamoid joint. Int Orthop 6:61–67, 1982.

149. Finochetto R: Sesamoideos. Semana Médica 1:1451–1470, 1929.

150. Gordon SL, Evans C, Greer RB III: *Pseudomonas* osteomyelitis of the metatarsal sesamoid of the great toe. Clin Orthop 99:188–189, 1974.

151. Hulkko A, Orava S, Pellinen P, Puranen J: Stress fractures of the sesamoid bones of the first metatarsophalangeal joint in athletes. Arch Orthop Trauma Surg 104:113–115, 1985.

152. Ilfeld FW, Rosen V: Osteochondrosis of the first metatarsal sesamoid. Report of two cases. Clin Orthop 85:38–41, 1972.

153. Jahss MH: The sesamoids of the hallux. Clin Orthop 157:88–97, 1981.

154. Kaiman ME, Piconna R: Tibial sesamoidectomy: A review of the literature and retrospective study. J Foot Surg 22:286–289, 1983.

155. Leventen EO: Sesamoid disorders and treatment: An update. Clin Orthop 269:236–240, 1992.

156. McBryde AM Jr, Anderson RB: Sesamoid foot problems in the athlete. Clin Sports Med 7:51–60, 1988.

157. Quirk R: Common foot and ankle injuries in dance. Orthop Clin North Am 25:123–133, 1994.

158. Renander A: Two cases of typical osteochondropathy of the medial sesamoid bone of the first metatarsal. Acta Radiol 3:521–527, 1924.

159. Resnick D, Niwayama G, Feingold ML: The sesamoid bones of the hands and feet: Participators in arthritis. Radiology 123:57–62, 1977.

160. Richardson EG: Injuries to the hallucal sesamoids in the athlete. Foot Ankle 7:229–244, 1987.

161. Richardson EG: Hallucal sesamoid pain: Causes and surgical treatment. J Am Acad Orthop Surg 7:270–278, 1999.

162. Scranton PE, Rutkowski R: Anatomic variations in the first ray: Anatomic aspects related to bunion surgery and disorders of the sesamoid. Clin Orthop 151:244–246, 1980.

163. Taylor JAM, Sartoris DJ, Huang GS, Resnick DL: Painful conditions affecting the first metatarsal sesamoid bones. Radiographics 13:817–830, 1993.

164. Treves A: Un cas de sésamoidite interne du gros orteil. Rev Orthop 15:411–415, 1928.

165. Van Hal ME, Keene JS, Lange TA, Clancy WG Jr: Stress fractures of the great toe sesamoids. Am J Sports Med 10:122–128, 1982.

166. Zinman H, Keret D, Reis ND: Fracture of the medial sesamoid bone of the hallux. J Trauma 21:581–582, 1981.

INDEX

Note: Page numbers followed by the letter f refer to figures;
and those followed by the letter t refer to tables.

A

A band, in skeletal muscle, 3–4
AAS. *See* Anabolic-androgenic steroids.
ABCDE mnemonic, in on-field emergencies, 752–753
Abdomen
  examination of, in preparticipation evaluation, 743
  strengthening exercises for, 432f, 1547, 1548f
  stretching exercises for, 1547–1548, 1549f
Abdominal sports trauma, management of, 267–268, 267f, 759–760
Abdominal wall muscle, injuries to, vs. adductor injuries, 1495, 1516
Abduction maneuver, for reduction of anterior shoulder dislocation, 1037
Abductor digiti quinti, nerve to
  anatomy of, 2459, 2460f, 2461f, 2477f
  entrapment of, 2476–2478
    diagnosis of, 2477
    etiology of, 2477
    symptoms of, 2476–2477
    treatment of, 2477–2478
Abductor hallucis, 2486, 2486f
Abductor pollicis longus tendon
  peritendinitis of, 30
  tenosynovitis of, 1359, 1359f
Ability, vs. disability, 656
Abrasion, definition of, 57t
Abrasion arthroplasty, for knee osteoarthritis, 1881
Acceleration, in throwing, 1070, 1070f
  and elbow injuries, 1271, 1271f
  biomechanics of, 1237, 1254–1255, 1254f, 1256f
Acceleration-deceleration head injury, in children and adolescents, 775
Accessory motion, vs. physiologic motion, 323
Accessory navicular. *See* Navicular, accessory.
Accessory nerve
  anatomy of, 1158
  palsy of, 1158–1159
    clinical evaluation of, 1158, 1159f
    sports implicated in, 1159
    treatment of, 1158–1159
Accessory ossification center
  of acromion. *See* Os acromiale.
  of patella. *See* Patella, bipartite.
Accessory soleus muscle, 2195
Acclimatization
  thermal, and heat illness, 535
  to altitude, 552, 555
Acetabular labrum, tears of, 1457–1458, 1458f
  in children and adolescents, 1475, 1476f
Acetabular rim syndrome, 1475, 1476f
Acetabulum
  anatomy of, 1444
  fractures of, computed tomography of, 568, 568f
  physeal fractures of, 1465

Acetaminophen, for knee osteoarthritis, 1880
Acetazolamide, for acute mountain sickness, 553
Acetic acid, in iontophoresis, 350
Achilles tendon
  allograft from
    for combined anterior and posterior cruciate ligament reconstruction, 2117, 2117f
    for patellar tendon rupture, 1852
    for popliteofibular ligament reconstruction, 1990–1991, 1991f
    for popliteus reconstruction, 1925, 1927f, 1990–1991, 1991f
    for posterior cruciate ligament reconstruction, 2099
    for triceps tendon rupture, 1231, 1232f
  imaging of, normal, 2195, 2195f
  injuries to, 2429–2433
    anatomical considerations in, 2429–2430
    clinical evaluation of, 2430
    imaging of, 2195–2196, 2196f–2200f
    magnetic resonance imaging of, 586–587, 588f–589f
    postoperative management and rehabilitation of, 2432
    treatment of
      author's preferred method in, 2433
      nonoperative, 2430–2431
      operative, 2431–2432
  overuse injuries of, 29
  peritendinitis of, 30, 2195–2196, 2197f, 2429, 2430
  rupture of, 2433–2442
    clinical evaluation of, 2434–2435, 2435f
    corticosteroid injection and, 2431
    treatment of
      author's preferred method in, 2440–2442, 2441f
      controversies in, 2435–2436, 2435t, 2436t
      nonoperative, 2436
      operative, 2435t, 2436–2440, 2436t, 2437t, 2438f, 2439f
  tendinosis of, 2195, 2196f, 2429, 2430
    insertional, 2446, 2452–2453, 2454
  tightness of, and foot and ankle injuries, 2238
Achilles tendon protector, of sports shoe, 2280f, 2284
ACL. *See* Anterior cruciate ligament.
Acquired immunodeficiency syndrome. *See* Human immunodeficiency virus (HIV) infection.
Acromioclavicular joint
  anatomy of, 841, 841f, 912–913, 912f
  biomechanics of, 864, 912–913, 912f, 913f
  dislocation of, with coracoid process fracture, 996, 997, 998f, 999, 1001f
    treatment of, 1004, 1004f
  hypertrophy of, 888, 889f
  imaging of, 920

Acromioclavicular joint *(Continued)*
  injuries to
    acromioclavicular ligament repair for, 924, 924f
    classification of, 64, 64t, 914, 915f, 931
    complications of, 930
    coracoclavicular ligament repair for, 924–925, 925f
    coracoclavicular ligament transfer for, 925
    cross-arm adduction test for, 916, 917f
    diagnosis and physical examination of, 914, 916–920, 917f–920f
    distal clavicle resection for
      arthroscopic, 926–927, 927t
      with coracoclavicular ligament reconstruction, 925–926, 926f
    dynamic muscle transfer for, 924, 924f
    in children and adolescents, 931–932, 932f
    mechanisms of, 914, 915f
    O'Brien test for, 916–917, 917f
    postoperative care in, 929
    radiography in, 919–920, 921f, 922f
    treatment of, 920–929
      author's preferred method for, 927–929, 928f–929f
      in children and adolescents, 932
      nonoperative, 921–923, 922f–924f
      operative, 923–927
    type I, 917
    type II, 917, 918f
    type III, 917–918, 918f, 921–922
    type IV, 918, 919f
    type V, 918–919, 920f
    type VI, 919
  innervation of, 916, 916f
  intra-articular fractures of, 931
  motion of, 913–914, 914f
  reduction of, loss of, 930
  surgical anatomy of, 860–861, 861f
Acromioclavicular ligaments
  in acromioclavicular joint stability, 913, 913f
  repair of, 924, 924f
Acromion
  accessory ossification center of. *See* Os acromiale.
  anatomy of, 1096–1097
  downsloping of, 887, 887f
  enthesophyte of, 887, 888f
  fractures of, 931
    return to sports after, 993
    treatment of, 987–988, 992–993
  imaging of, 885–888, 885f–889f
  magnetic resonance imaging of, 886–888, 886f–889f
  ossification of, 981, 982f
  shape of
    and rotator cuff tear, 886f, 887, 1067, 1068f
    classification of, 60, 61f
  stress fractures of, 987–988
  surgical anatomy of, 859–860
Acromioplasty, anterior, for rotator cuff disorders, 1084

Osteoporosis
  age-related, 105
  corticosteroids and, 128
  laboratory studies in, 105
  postmenopausal, 105
  prevention of, 105
  risk factors for, 510t
  treatment of, 105
Osteotomy
  for knee osteoarthritis, 1883
  for slipped capital femoral epiphysis, 1467
  metatarsal. See Metatarsal osteotomy.
  tibial, high. See High tibial osteotomy.
Otoform-K, for hand splinting, 1426, 1426t
Outerbridge classification, of articular cartilage
    lesions, 60–61, 61t
Outsole, of sports shoe, 2280f, 2284–2285
  rubber and plastic technology for,
    2286–2287, 2287t
Oval ring concept, in wrist stability, 1339,
    1340f
Overhand loop knot, 241, 242
Overtubulation, 599–600
Overuse injuries. See also Stress fractures.
  in children and adolescents, 703–711, 1365,
    1365t
    nonosseous, 703–711
      diagnosis of, 704–705, 705t, 706f
      sites of, 703, 703f, 704f
      sources of, 704–705, 704f
      treatment of, 705–706, 706t
    of thoracolumbar spine, 1574
    of wrist, 1368–1369, 1369f, 1369t
    osseous, 706–711
      causes of, 707, 707t
      diagnosis of, 707–708, 708f–710f
      treatment of, 708, 711, 711f
  with cerebral palsy, 678
  in disabled athlete, 529
  in disabled child athlete, 663
  of distal clavicle, 930, 931f
  physeal, 725, 727f, 728
  to tendons, 28–29
Oxaprozin, properties of, 123t
Oxford technique, of resistance exercise,
    328–329
Oxygen, partial pressure of, at altitude, 552
Oxygen consumption (Vo₂)
  in dynamic exercise, 291
  in static exercise, 291–292
Oxygen uptake
  in children and adolescents, 617, 617f
  maximum
    at altitude, 552
    in children and adolescents, 616–617
    in female vs. male athletes, 506
    weight training in women and, 512

P

p, in research
  calculation of, 161
  examples of, 165t
Pacinian corpuscle, in proprioception, 398
Pad
  metatarsal, for intractable plantar keratosis,
    2543, 2543f
  of sports shoe, definition of, 2289
Paget-Schroetter syndrome, thoracic outlet
    syndrome and, 1163, 1164f
Pain
  after anterior cruciate ligament
    reconstruction, 2045

Pain (Continued)
  electrical stimulation for, 349–350
  gate theory of, 349
  in adductors, in myositis ossificans, 1496,
    1516
  in back. See Back pain.
  in foot, in child athlete with systemic illness,
    2390
  in groin, in adductor tendinitis, 1496,
    1515–1516
  in heel. See Heel pain.
  in knee
    anterior. See Patellofemoral pain.
    referred, 1962–1963, 1964f–1965f, 1967,
      2008f–2009f, 2009–2010
  in lateral retinaculum, 1794, 1795f
  in medial tuberosity, plantar fasciitis with.
    See Plantar fasciitis, with medial
      tuberosity pain.
  in shoulder instability, 1025
  patellofemoral. See Patellofemoral pain.
  postoperative, nonsteroidal anti-inflammatory
    drugs for, 124
  sympathetically maintained, 442, 442f
Pain dysfunction syndrome, 441, 441t. See also
    Complex regional pain syndrome.
Paired organ(s), sports-related loss of, 264–270
  legal considerations in, 269
  prevention of, 265–269
  risk of, 264
  sports participation recommendations related
    to, 269–270
Palmaris longus tendon, for ulnar collateral
    ligament reconstruction, 1243–1244, 1244f
Palpation, cardiac, in highly trained athletes,
    273, 273t
Palumbo Knee Sleeve, for patellofemoral pain,
    2132
Panacryl suture, tensile strength of, 171
Pancreas, injuries to, on-field management of,
    760
Panner's disease, 1260, 1262
  definition of, 1270
  vs. osteochondritis dissecans of capitellum,
    1284, 1285f
Paradoxical disrobing, in hypothermia, 546
Paraffin bath, for heat therapy, 357
Paralabral cyst, 893, 894f, 905–906
Parallel pitch lines, 2449, 2450f
Paralympics, 505, 683–684, 684f
Paraplegia, exercise physiology and, 526
Paraspinal muscle, posterior, exercise and
    stretching regimen for, 1548
Paratendinitis, definition of, 2410
Paratenon
  function of, 20, 21f
  structure of, 20, 21f
Paratenonitis
  definition of, 1843t
  with tendinosis, definition of, 1843t
Parathyroid hormone
  in bone, 104, 104t
  osteoblast receptor for, 100, 100t
Paravertebral sympathetic ganglion blockade, in
    complex regional pain syndrome, 448, 454
Parental pressure, on child athlete, 690
Paroxysmal supraventricular tachycardia,
    exercise and, 281–282
Pars interarticularis
  defect of, in pediatric spondylolisthesis,
    1570–1572, 1570f, 1571f
  stress reactions of, 1537–1538, 1537f,
    1558–1560
Passive motion, threshold to detection of, and
    proprioception, 331

Passive patellar tilt test, in patellofemoral joint
    disorders, 1720, 1721f
Passive stretch, for muscle strain, 16
Patella
  abnormalities of, 1816, 1817f
  absence of, 1816
  accessory ossification centers of. See Patella,
    bipartite.
  anatomy of, 1761–1762, 1761f, 1816, 1816f,
    2136, 2136f
  bony, 1711, 1772–1773, 1773f
  arthrofibrosis of, after high tibial osteotomy,
    1933–1934
  articular surface of, 1761, 1761f, 1816, 1816f
  biomechanics of, 1816–1817, 1817f–1818f
  bipartite, 1763, 1818–1823, 1819f–1822f
    classification of, 1763, 1763f, 1819, 1820f
    treatment of, 1820, 1821f
  blood supply to, 1761
  chondromalacia of, 1641–1643, 1643f, 1733f,
    1799–1808. See also Patellofemoral
      arthrosis.
  "Cyrano" long-nosed, 1773, 1773f
  dislocation of
    acute, 1697–1708
      anatomy and biomechanics of,
        1698–1700, 1699f–1700f, 1701t
      chondral or osteochondral injury in,
        1700, 1701f, 1702, 1702f, 1751,
        1751f
        imaging of, 1703–1704, 1752–1753,
          1752f
        treatment of, 1753
      clinical presentation in, 1698, 1698f
      epidemiology of, 1697–1698
      immobilization after, 1704–1705, 1735,
        1743
      in children and adolescents, 1749–1754
        clinical evaluation of, 1751–1752,
          1751f
        complications of, 1754
        imaging of, 1752–1753, 1752f–1753f
        pathophysiology of, 1753
        prognosis in, 1754
        treatment of, 1753–1754
      injuries associated with, 1700,
        1701f–1703f, 1702
      mechanism of injury of, 1698
      physical examination in, 1700, 1701f
      radiological findings in, 1702–1704,
        1703f–1704f
      rehabilitation after, 1707
      return to sports after, 1707
      treatment of, 1704–1707
        author's preferred method in,
          1707–1708, 1742–1743
        nonoperative, 1704–1705, 1707–1708,
          1735–1736, 1735f
        operative, 1705–1707, 1707f, 1708,
          1736–1738, 1737f
          indications for, 1705
          techniques for, 1706–1707, 1707f
        results of, 1708
    after extensor mechanism reconstruction,
      1741
    "miserable malalignment syndrome" in,
      test for, 1715–1716, 1716f
    predisposition to, 1697, 1714, 1755,
      1755f
    recurrent, 1710–1747
      age at initial injury and, 1697
      anatomy related to, 1710–1714,
        1710f–1714f
      clinical evaluation of, 1715–1735
      complications of, 1740–1742, 1741f

Spinocerebellar pathways, in proprioception, 397f, 398–399
Spinoglenoid ligament, 1154, 1154f
Spiral fracture
 of fingers, 1404–1408, 1405f–1407f
 of humeral shaft, 1181–1183, 1182f, 1185f
  clinical evaluation in, 1182–1183
  pathogenesis of, 1181, 1182f
  rehabilitation after, 1183
  return to sports after, 1183
  treatment of, 1183, 1184f–1185f
Spirometry, in exercise-induced asthma, 305, 308
Spit tobacco, 488–489, 489f
Spleen
 enlargement of, in mononucleosis, 255–256
 injuries to, on-field management of, 759–760
Splenius muscle, 1526
Splinting
 for boutonnière deformity, 1394–1395, 1395f
 for carpal tunnel syndrome, 1357
 for displaced humeral shaft fracture, 1196, 1198f
 for mallet finger, 1396–1398, 1397f–1398f
 for proximal interphalangeal joint fractures, 1390, 1390f
 for tendinitis of wrist, 1358
 for triquetrolunate instability, 1348, 1348f
 of forearm, for fractures, 1298, 1298f
 of hand, 1423–1428, 1425f–1426t, 1427f. *See also* Hand, splinting of.
 of wrist, protective, 1360, 1360f
Split peroneus brevis technique, for lateral ankle ligament reconstruction, 2340, 2341f
Spoiled gradient echo recall (SPGR) imaging, 592–593
Spondylolysis and spondylolisthesis, 1558–1560
 author's preferred method in treatment of, 1560
 bone scintigraphy in, 562, 564f
 in children and adolescents, 1570–1572, 1570f, 1571f
 radiographic evaluation of, 1537f, 1558, 1558f
 return to sports after, 1560
 treatment of, 1558–1560, 1559f
Spongiosum
 primary, 714
 secondary, 714
Sports
 classification of
  by contact, 747t
  by dynamic and static components, 291t, 295
  by strenuousness/intensity, 747t
  by type and intensity, 272, 272t
 contact. *See* Contact sports.
 disabled. *See* Disabled athlete(s).
 recreational, head injury from, 770
Sports drinks, 463
Sports feet, 665, 667f
Sports injuries
 bone scintigraphy in, 562, 563f–564f, 564
 cognitive appraisal of, 493, 495–496
 disruptive nature of, 501
 experience of, 497
  description of, 494–495
 imaging of, 557–593. *See also specific body part and specific imaging modality.*
 in children and adolescents
  from strength training, 732
  rates of, 828–829
  to shoulder, 1133–1137, 1133f–1138f
  with disabilities, 661–664

Sports injuries *(Continued)*
 in disabled child athlete, 661–664
 in older adult, 494
 neurodevelopment and, 640
 on-field management of, 749, 751–763
  ABCDE mnemonic in, 752–753
  airway in, 752
  AVPU mnemonic in, 753
  breathing in, 752
  cardiopulmonary resuscitation in, 753, 753t
  circulation in, 753
  disability in, 753
  exposure in, 753
  general assessment in, 752–753, 754f
  logroll in, 752, 752f
  needle cricothyroidotomy in, 752, 752f
  preparation for, 749, 751–752
 prevalence of, 493–494
 psychological issues in, 493–502, 692–693, 698. *See also* Sports psychology.
 rate of, 151, 151t–152t
 response to
  disruption/interference with life and, 496
  emotional nourishment and, 496
  four-stage model of, 693
  past coping and, 496–497
  research directions concerning, 501
  two-factor model of, 495–497
 stress and, 692–693
 treatment of
  corticosteroids in, 51–52
  nonsteroidal anti-inflammatory drugs in, 51
Sports medicine
 classification systems for, 58–65
  confusion among, 59
  descriptive, 63–65, 63t–65t, 64f
  involving anatomic changes from pathologic conditions, 60–61, 60f–61f, 61t
  involving grading and measurement, 59–60
  involving physical examination findings, 61–63, 62t
 terminology for, 56–58, 57t–58t
Sports medicine team, relationship of, to team physician, 764
Sports participation
 athlete's right to, 765–766
 by athlete with single paired organ, recommendations for, 269–270
 by children/adolescents
  detrimental effects of, 689–694
  motivation for, 688–689
  psychological aspects of, 687–698. *See also* Sports psychology.
  rewards of, 688–689
 by disabled children, guidelines for, 674–683, 676t
 clearance for, 744–747, 745t–748t
  in young athlete, 650
  team physician role in, 738
 evaluation for. *See* Preparticipation evaluation.
 neurodevelopmental disabilities and, 640
 neurodevelopmental readiness for, 628, 629f
  and training, 639–640
  during early adolescence, 637
  during late adolescence, 639
  during middle adolescence, 638
  during middle childhood, 632–633
  during preschool years, 630–631
  in early vs. late maturers, 636

Sports prostheses, 666f, 667f, 669f, 684
Sports psychologist
 as clinician, 498–499
 as consultant, 499–500
 as educator, 499
 as facilitator, 499
 training of, 500–501
Sports psychology. *See also* Sports injuries, response to.
 definition of, 498
 developmental considerations in, 688
 for children/adolescents, 687–698
  anxiety management in, 695–696
  attention control in, 696
  burnout in, 689, 698
  coach pressure and, 690–691
  competition and cooperation in, 691–692, 698
  counseling in, 698
  goal setting in, 697
  injury and, 692–693, 698
  management techniques in, 694–698
  mental practice/imagery in, 696–697
  motivation, activation, and psych-up in, 697
  parental pressure and, 690
  peer pressure and, 691
  performance anxiety in, 693–694
  reward and reinforcement in, 688–689, 697–698
  self-esteem and confidence building in, 697
  stress management in, 695–696
  toughness and aggression in, 698
  winning vs. losing in, 691–692
 relaxation techniques in, 695
Sports shoes. *See* Shoes.
Sprain, 57, 57t. *See also specific anatomic site.*
Spring ligament
 imaging of, 2206, 2209f
 tears of, 2206, 2209f
Spurling's maneuver, 798f
Square knot, 239–240, 239f
Squat test, for meniscal tears, 1673
Squatting
 in cruciate ligament rehabilitation, 337
 lower extremity muscle function during, 338–339, 339f
 patellar function during, 340
Squeeze test, in tibiofibular syndesmosis injury evaluation, 2328, 2328t, 2353
Stabilization. *See* Immobilization.
Stahl's classification, of Kienböck's disease, 1353, 1353f
Stair climbing ergometry, 363–366
 cadence in, 365
 clinical application of, 365–366
 duration of, 365–366
 in cruciate ligament rehabilitation, 337–338
 kinematics in, 363
 kinetics in, 364–365
 muscular activity in, 363–364
 setup in, 365, 365f
StairMaster, 363–366
Standard deviation, 161
State anxiety, competitive, 694
Static exercise
 cardiac effects of, 292, 295
 in sports classification, 291t
Static flexibility, 381
Static stretching, 323
Statics, in biomechanics, 136–139, 137f–139f
 forces and moments in, 136, 138, 138f
 free-body diagrams and, 136, 137f
 Newton's third law and, 138